KU-740-091

CLINICAL RESPIRATORY MEDICINE

second edition

Richard K. Albert
Professor of Medicine, University of Colorado
Chief, Medical Service
Denver Health Medical Center
Denver, Colorado
United States

Stephen G. Spiro
Professor of Respiratory Medicine
Consultant Physician, General and Thoracic Medicine
University College London Hospitals NHS Trust
The Middlesex Hospital
London
United Kingdom

James R. Jett
Professor of Medicine, Mayo Medical School
Consultant in Pulmonary Medicine and Medical Oncology
Mayo Clinic
Rochester, Minnesota
United States

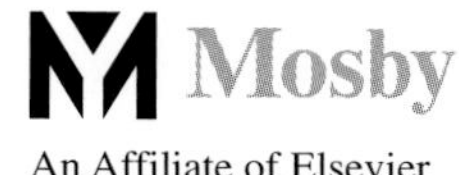

An Affiliate of Elsevier

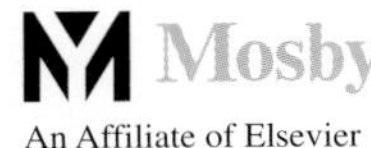

An Affiliate of Elsevier

170 S Independence Mall W 300E
Philadelphia, Pennsylvania 19106-3399

Clinical Respiratory Medicine, 2/e ISBN 0-323-02497-1
Copyright 2004, Mosby, Inc. All rights reserved.

No part of this publication may be reproduced, stored in a retrieval system, or transmitted in any form or by any means, electronic, mechanical, photocopying, recording, or otherwise, without prior permission of the publisher (Mosby Inc., 11830 Westline Industrial Drive, St. Louis, MO).

Notice

Medicine is an ever-changing field. Standard safety precautions must be followed, but as new research and clinical experience broaden our knowledge, changes in treatment and drug therapy may become necessary or appropriate. Readers are advised to check the most current product information provided by the manufacturer of each drug to be administered to verify the recommended dose, the method and duration of administration, and contraindications. It is the responsibility of the treating physician, relying on experience and knowledge of the patient, to determine dosages and the best treatment for each individual patient. Neither the Publisher nor the editor assumes any liability for any injury and/or damage to persons or property arising from this publication.

The Publisher

First Edition 1999.

Library of Congress Cataloging-in-Publication Data

Clinical respiratory medicine / [edited by] Richard K. Albert, Stephen G. Spiro, and James R. Jett.—2nd ed.
p.; cm.
Rev. ed. of: Comprehensive respiratory medicine, c1999.
Includes bibliographical references and index.
ISBN 0-323-02497-1
1. Respiratory organs—Diseases. I. Albert, Richard K. II. Spiro, Stephen G. III. Jett, James R. IV. Comprehensive respiratory medicine.
[DNLM: 1. Respiratory Tract Diseases. WF 140 C641 2004]
RC732.C565 2004
616.2—dc22 2003066605

Acquisitions Editor: Todd Hummel
Development Editor: Joanne Husovski
Senior Project Manager: Natalie Ware

Printed in China.
Last digit is the print number: 9 8 7 6 5 4 3 2 1

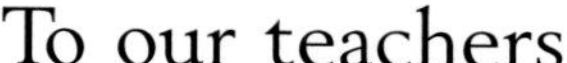
To our teachers

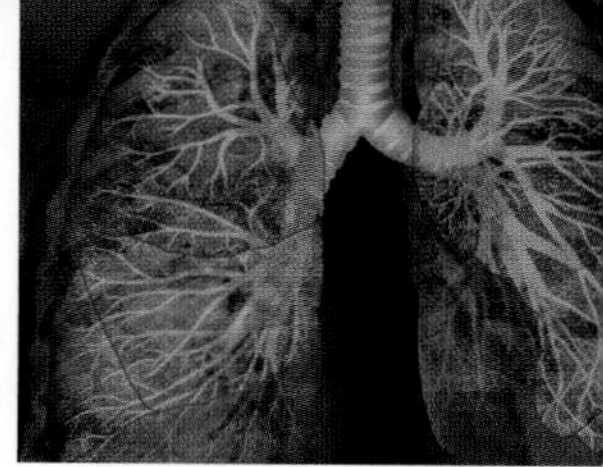

Contributors

Carlo Agostini, MD
Senior Investigator, also Deputy
Clinical Immunology Branch
Department of Clinical and Experimental Medicine
Padua University School of Medicine
Padova, Italy
Noninfectious Conditions

Richard K. Albert, MD
Professor of Medicine
University of Colorado
Chief, Medical Service
Denver Health Medical Center
Denver, Colorado
Chest Pain; Obesity

Mark S. Allen, MD
Professor of Surgery
Mayo Medical School
Chair, Division of General Thoracic Surgery
Mayo Foundation
Rochester, Minnesota
Diagnostic Thoracic Surgical Procedures

Selim M. Arcasoy, MD
Associate Professor of Clinical Medicine
Medical Director Lung Transplantation Program
Pulmonary, Allergy, and Critical Care Division
Department of Medicine
New York Presbyterian Hospital
Columbia University College of Physicians and Surgeons
New York, New York
Disorders of the Mediastinum

Charles W. Atwood, Jr, MD
Fellow, Pulmonary and Critical Care Medicine
University of Pittsburgh School of Medicine,
University of Pittsburgh Medical Center, and VA Pittsburgh Healthcare System
Pittsburgh, Pennsylvania
Obstructive Sleep Apnea; Central Sleep Apnea and Other Forms of Sleep-Disordered Breathing

Marie Christine Aubry, MD
Assistant Professor of Pathology
Mayo Medical School
Consultant in Pathology
Mayo Clinic
Rochester, Minnesota
Malignant Pleural Mesothelioma

Ronald Balkissoon, MD
Associate Professor of Medicine
Division of Pulmonary Sciences and Critical Care Medicine
National Jewish Medical and Research Center
University of Colorado School of Medicine
Denver, Colorado
Chronic Obstructive Pulmonary Disease: Management of Chronic Disease

Alexander A. Bankier, MD
Associate Professor of Radiology
University of Vienna
Vienna, Austria
Pulmonary Embolism

Alan F. Barker, MD
Professor of Medicine
Pulmonary and Critical Care Medicine
Oregon Health and Science University
Portland, Oregon
Bronchiectasis

Peter J. Barnes, MD
Professor of Thoracic Medicine
Department of Thoracic Medicine
National Heart and Lung Institute
Imperial College
London, United Kingdom
Beta-Agonists, Anticholinergics, and Other Nonsteroid Drugs

John B. Bass, Jr, MD
Chairman, Department of Internal Medicine
University of South Alabama College of Medicine
Mobile, Alabama
Tuberculosis and Disease Caused by Atypical Mycobacteria

Surinder S. Birring, BSc, MRCP
Specialist Registrar in Respiratory Medicine
Institute for Lung Health
Glenfield Hospital
Leicester, United Kingdom
Cough

Andrew Bradbeer, MB, BS
Senior Registrar
Royal Brompton Hospital
London, United Kingdom
Connective Tissue Disorders

Luca Brazzi, MD
Assistant Professor in Anesthesia and Intensive Care
Istituto di Anestesia e Rianimazione
Ospedale Maggiore di Milano IRCCS
Milan, Italy
Acute Respiratory Distress Syndrome

John R. Britton, MD
Professor of Respiratory Medicine
University of Nottingham
City Hospital
Nottingham, United Kingdom
Idiopathic Pulmonary Fibrosis and Other Idiopathic Interstitial Pneumonias

William A. Broughton, MD
Professor of Medicine
University of South Alabama College of Medicine
USA Knollwood Hospital Sleep Disorders Center
Mobile, Alabama
Tuberculosis and Disease Caused by Atypical Mycobacteria

Roy G. Brower, MD
Professor of Medicine
Medical Director, Medical Intensive Care Unit
Johns Hopkins University School of Medicine
Baltimore, Maryland
Pulmonary Circulation

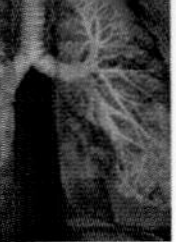

Otto Burghuber, MD
Professor of Medicine
Chief, Department of Medicine
Krankenhaus Korneuburg
Korneuburg, Austria
Pulmonary Embolism

Philippe Camus, MD
Faculté de Médecine
Université de Bourgogne
Centre Hospitalier Universitaire de Dijon
Dijon, France
Inflammatory Bowel Disease

Stephen D. Cassivi, MD
Assistant Professor of Surgery
Mayo Clinic College of Medicine
Staff Surgeon, Division of General Thoracic Surgery
Mayo Clinic
Rochester, Minnesota
Chest Tube Insertion and Management; Diagnostic Thoracic Surgical Procedures

Moira Chan-Yeung, MD
Professor of Medicine
Department of Medicine
University of British Columbia
Vancouver General Hospital
Vancouver, Canada
Occupational Asthma

Thomas Colby, MD
Consultant in Surgical Pathology
Department of Pathology
Mayo Clinic
Scottsdale, Arizona
Inflammatory Bowel Disease

Chris J. Corrigan, MD
Reader and Consultant Physician
Guy's, King's, and St. Thomas' School of Medicine
King's College, University of London
London, United Kingdom
Extrinsic Allergic Alveolitis

Ulrich Costabel, MD
Professor of Medicine
University of Essen
Chief, Department of Pneumologie and Allergologie
Rurhlandklinik
Essen, Germany
Idiopathic Pulmonary Fibrosis and Other Idiopathic Interstitial Pneumonias

Stephen W. Crawford, MD
Staff Physician
Pulmonary Medicine
Naval Medical Center San Diego
San Diego, California
Hematopoietic Stem Cell Transplantation

Bruce H. Culver, MD
Associate Professor of Medicine
Division of Pulmonary and Critical Care
University of Washington School of Medicine
Seattle, Washington
Respiratory Mechanics; Gas Exchange in the Lung; Pulmonary Circulation; Acid-Base Balance and Control of Ventilation; Pulmonary Function and Exercise Testing

Claude Deschamps, MD
Professor of Surgery
Mayo Clinic College of Medicine
Consultant, Division of General Thoracic Surgery
Mayo Foundation
Rochester, Minnesota
Chest Tube Insertion and Management

Roland M. du Bois, MD, FRCP
Professor of Respiratory Medicine
Imperial College of Science, Technology, and Medicine
Interstitial Lung Disease Unit
Royal Brompton Hospital
London, United Kingdom
Connective Tissue Disorders

Jim Egan, MD
Consultant Respiratory Physician
The Mater Misericordiae Hospital and St. Vincents University Hospital
University College Dublin
Dublin, Ireland
Pneumonia in the Non-HIV Immunocompromised Host

Timothy W. Evans, MD
Consultant in Intensive Care and Respiratory Medicine
Royal Brompton Hospital
London, United Kingdom
Pulmonary Hypertension

Stanley B. Fiel, MD
Regional Chairman
Department of Medicine
Atlantic Health Systems
The deNeufville Professor and Chair
Department of Medicine
Morristown Memorial Hospital
Morristown, New Jersey
Cystic Fibrosis

Jean-William Fitting, MD
Associate Professor of Respiratory Medicine
Service de Pneumologie, Centre Hospitalier Universitaire Vaudois
Lausanne, Switzerland
Acute and Chronic Neuromuscular Disorders

Luciano Gattinoni, MD
Consultant Physician
Istituto di Anestesia e Rianimazione
Milan, Italy
Acute Respiratory Distress Syndrome

E. Brigitte Gottschall, MD, MSPH
Assistant Professor
Division of Environmental and Occupational Health Sciences
National Jewish Medical and Research Center
Department of Medicine
University of Colorado Health Sciences Center
Denver, Colorado
Asbestosis; Toxic Inhalational Lung Injury

David M. Hansell, MD
Professor of Thoracic Imaging
Royal Brompton Hospital
London, United Kingdom
Imaging

Christian J. Herold, MD
Professor of Radiology and Radiologic Sciences
Director, Diagnostic Imaging
Department of Radiology
University of Vienna
Vienna, Austria
Pulmonary Embolism

Pieter S. Hiemstra, MD
Associate Professor
Department of Pulmonology
Leiden University Medical Center
Leiden, The Netherlands
Asthma: Cell Biology

Nicholas S. Hill, MD
Professor of Medicine
Tufts University School of Medicine
Boston, Massachusetts
Noninvasive Mechanical Ventilation

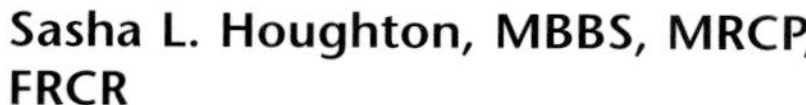

Sasha L. Houghton, MBBS, MRCP, FRCR
Specialist Registrar
Department of Radiology
University College London Hospitals
London, United Kingdom
Other Biopsy Procedures

Gérard J. Huchon, MD
Head of Service de Pneumologie et Réanimation
Hôpital de l'Hôtel-Dieu
Professor of Respiratory Medicine
Université René Descartes
Paris, France
Bacterial Pneumonia; Non-bacterial Pneumonia

James R. Jett, MD
Professor of Medicine
Vice-Chairman, Division of Medicine
Head, Section of Respiratory Therapy
Mayo Clinic
Rochester, Minnesota
Lung Tumors; Malignant Pleural Mesothelioma

Andrew T. Jones, MD
Consultant in Intensive Care and Respiratory Medicine
Guy's and St. Thomas' NHS Trust
St. Thomas' Hospital
London, United Kingdom
Pulmonary Hypertension

Rudolf A. Jorres, PhD
Senior Scientist, Research Laboratory
Center for Pneumology and Thoracic Surgery
Hospital Grosshansdorf
Grosshansdorf, Germany
Air Pollution

Sanjay Kalra, MD
Consultant, Division of Pulmonary and Critical Care Medicine
Assistant Professor of Medicine
Mayo Clinic and Mayo Medical School
Rochester, Minnesota
Eosinophilic Lung Disease and Bronchiolitis Obliterans Organizing Pneumonia

Huib A. M. Kerstjens, MD, PhD
Professor of Pulmonology
Department of Pulmonary Diseases
University Hospital Groningen
Groningen, The Netherlands
Asthma: Epidemiology and Risk Factors

John W. Kreit, MD
Associate Professor of Medicine
Division of Pulmonary, Allergy, and Critical Care Medicine
University of Pittsburgh School of Medicine
Pittsburgh, Pennsylvania
Hemoptysis

Michael J. Krowka, MD
Professor of Medicine
Division of Pulmonary and Critical Care Medicine
Division of Gastroenterology and Hepatology
Mayo Clinic
Rochester, Minnesota
Hepatic and Biliary Diseases

Stephen E. Lapinsky, MD
Education Director
Division of Respirology
Mount Sinai Hospital
Associate Professor of Medicine
University of Toronto
Toronto, Canada
Pregnancy

Sylvie Leroy, MD
Chef de Clinique
Centre Hospitalier Universitaire de Lille
Clinique des Maladies Respiratoires
Hôpital A. Calmette
Lille, France
Silicosis and Coal Workers' Pneumoconiosis

Marc C. I. Lipman, MD, FRCP
Consultant Physician
Royal Free Hospital
London, United Kingdom
Pulmonary Infections

Robert Loddenkemper, MD
Professor of Medicine
Zentralklinik Emil von Behring/Humboldt University
Berlin, Germany
Pleural Effusion

William MacNee, MD
Professor of Respiratory and Environmental Medicine
University of Edinburgh
Consultant Physician
Clinical Director Respiratory Medicine
Lothian University NHS Trust
Edinburgh, United Kingdom
Chronic Obstructive Pulmonary Disease: Epidemiology, Physiology, and Clinical Evaluation

Helgo Magnussen, MD
Medical Director
Hospital Grosshansdorf
Grosshansdorf, Germany
Air Pollution

Barry Make, MD
Director, COPD Program and Pulmonary Rehabilitation
National Jewish Medical and Research Center
Professor of Medicine
Division of Pulmonary Sciences and Critical Care Medicine
University of Colorado School of Medicine
Denver, Colorado
Chronic Obstructive Pulmonary Disease: Management of Chronic Disease

Jean-Luc Malo, MD
Professor of Respiratory Medicine
Hôpital du Sacré-Coeur de Montréal
Montréal, Québec, Canada
Occupational Asthma

R. N. Maskell, MD
Consultant Physician
Southmead Hospital
Bristol, United Kingdom
Bacterial Pneumonia

David E. Midthun, MD
Associate Professor of Medicine
Mayo Clinic School of Medicine
Consultant, Pulmonary and Critical Care Medicine
Mayo Clinic
Rochester, Minnesota
Lung Tumors

Rob F. Miller, MD
Clinical Senior Lecturer/Consultant Physician
Royal Free and University College Medical School
London, United Kingdom
Pulmonary Infections

Peter R. Mills, MD
Pulmonary Fellow
St. Bartholomew's and Royal London School of Medicine and Dentistry
London Chest Hospital
London, United Kingdom
Management of Exacerbations in Chronic Obstructive Pulmonary Disease

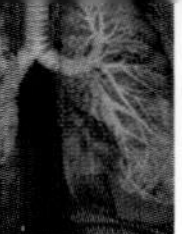

Erich Minar, MD
Associate Professor of Medicine
Department of Medicine II
Division of Angiology
University of Vienna—AKH
Vienna, Austria
Pulmonary Embolism

David Mitchell, MD
Consultant Physician and Honorary Senior Lecturer in Medicine
Chest and Allergy Clinic
St. Mary's Hospital and Imperial College School of Medicine
London, United Kingdom
Rhinitis and Sinusitis

David R. Moller, MD
Associate Professor of Medicine
The Johns Hopkins University School of Medicine
Baltimore, Maryland
Sarcoidosis

Rodrigo E. Morales, MD
Clinical Instructor
University of South Alabama College of Medicine
Department of Internal Medicine
Division of Pulmonary Diseases, Critical Care, and Sleep Medicine
Mobile, Alabama
Tuberculosis and Disease Caused by Atypical Mycobacteria

Jeffrey L. Myers, MD
Consultant, Division of Anatomic Pathology
Professor of Pathology
Mayo Clinic and Mayo Medical School
Rochester, Minnesota
Eosinophilic Lung Disease and Bronchiolitis Obliterans Organizing Pneumonia; Other Diffuse Lung Diseases

Lee S. Newman, MD, MA
Professor of Medicine
Head, Division of Environmental and Occupational Health Sciences
National Jewish Medical and Research Center
Professor of Medicine, Division of Pulmonary Science and Critical Care Medicine
Professor of Preventive Medicine and Biometrics
University of Colorado Health Science Center
Denver, Colorado
Asbestosis; Toxic Inhalational Lung Injury

Anthony J. Newman-Taylor, MSc, FRCP
Professor of Occupational and Environmental Medicine
National Heart and Lung Institute
Imperial College
London, United Kingdom
Extrinsic Allergic Alveolitis

Paul M. O'Byrne, MD
EJ Moran Campbell Professor
Chairman, Department of Medicine
McMaster University
Hamilton, Ontario, Canada
Corticosteroids

Eric J. Olson, MD
Consultant, Division of Pulmonary and Critical Care Medicine
Assistant Professor of Medicine
Mayo Clinic and Mayo Medical School
Rochester, Minnesota
Other Diffuse Lung Diseases

Simon P. G. Padley, MD
Consultant Radiologist
Department of Radiology
Chelsea and Westminster Hospital
London, United Kingdom
Imaging

Martyn R. Partridge, MD, FRCP
Professor of Respiratory Medicine
Imperial College London
Charing Cross Hospital Campus
London, United Kingdom
Asthma: Clinical Features, Diagnosis, and Treatment

Ian D. Pavord, MD
Consultant Physician and Honorary Reader in Respiratory Medicine
Glenfield Hospital
Leicester, United Kingdom
Cough

Paolo Pelosi, MD
Assistant Professor in Anesthesia and Intensive Care
University of Milan
Clinical Assistant
Istituto di Anestesia e Rianimazione
Milan, Italy
Acute Respiratory Distress Syndrome

Anthony C. Pickering, MD
Consultant Physician
North West Lung Centre
Wythenshawe Hospital
Manchester, United Kingdom
Berylliosis, Byssinosis, and Occupational Chronic Obstructive Pulmonary Disease

David J. Pierson, MD
Professor of Medicine
Division of Pulmonary and Critical Care Medicine
Department of Medicine
University of Washington
Medical Director of Respiratory Care
Harborview Medical Center
Seattle, Washington
Invasive Mechanical Ventilation

Venerino Poletti, MD
Department of Pulmonary Medicine
Ospedale Maggiore
Bologna, Italy
Noninfectious Conditions

Michael I. Polkey, MRCP, PhD
Consultant Physician and Reader in Respiratory Medicine
Royal Brompton Hospital/National Heart and Lung Institute
London, United Kingdom
Overview of Respiratory Muscle Function

Dirkje S. Postma, MD
Professor of Pulmonology
Department of Pulmonology
University Hospital Groningen
Groningen, The Netherlands
Asthma: Epidemiology and Risk Factors

Udaya B. S. Prakash, MD
Scripps Professor of Medicine
Mayo Medical School
Mayo Graduate School of Medicine
Consultant, Pulmonary, Critical Care, and Internal Medicine
Director of Bronchoscopy
Mayo Medical Center
Rochester, Minnesota
Bronchoscopy

Antoine Rabbat, MD
Praticien Hospitalier
Assistance Publique Hôpitaux de Paris
Pneumologie and Réanimation
Hôtel-Dieu
Paris, France
Bacterial Pneumonia; Non-bacterial Pneumonia

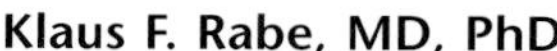

Klaus F. Rabe, MD, PhD
Head, Pulmonology Department
Leiden University Medical Center
Leiden, The Netherlands
Asthma: Cell Biology

Melissa L. Rosado de Christenson, MD, FACR
Adjunct Professor of Radiology
Department of Radiology and Nuclear Medicine
Uniformed Services University of the Health Sciences
Bethesda, Maryland
Disorders of the Mediastinum

Robin M. Rudd, MD
Consultant Physician
London Chest Hospital
London, United Kingdom
Disability Evaluation

Jay H. Ryu, MD
Consultant, Division of Pulmonary and Critical Care Medicine
Professor of Medicine
Mayo Clinic and Mayo Medical School
Rochester, Minnesota
Eosinophilic Lung Disease and Bronchiolitis Obliterans Organizing Pneumonia; Other Diffuse Lung Diseases

Glenis Scadding, MD, FRCP
Consultant Physician in Rhinology, Allergy, and Immunology
Rhinology Department
Royal, National Throat, Nose, and Ear Hospital
London, United Kingdom
Rhinitis and Sinusitis

Daniel V. Schidlow, MD
Professor and Chair, Department of Pediatrics
Senior Associate Dean, Pediatric Clinical Campus
Drexel University College of Medicine
Chief Medical and Academic Officer
St. Christopher's Hospital for Children
Philadelphia, Pennsylvania
Cystic Fibrosis

Marvin I. Schwarz, MD
The James C. Campbell Professor of Pulmonary Medicine
Head of the Division of Pulmonary Sciences and Critical Care Medicine
University of Colorado Health Sciences Center
Denver, Colorado
Pulmonary Vasculitis and Hemorrhage

Gianpietro Semenzato, MD
Professor of Medicine
Department of Clinical and Experimental Medicine
Padua University School of Medicine
Padova, Italy
Noninfectious Conditions

Jonathan E. Sevransky, MD
Assistant Professor of Medicine
Medical Director, JHMBC ICU
Division of Pulmonary and Critical Care Medicine
Johns Hopkins Asthma and Allergy Center
Baltimore, Maryland
Pulmonary Circulation

Penny J. Shaw, MD
Consultant Radiologist
University College Hospital
London, United Kingdom
Other Biopsy Procedures

David W. Shimabukuro, MDCM
Assistant Professor
UCSF Department of Anesthesia and Perioperative Care
University of California, San Francisco
San Francisco, California
Airway Management

Anita K. Simonds, MD
Consultant in Respiratory Medicine
Royal Brompton Hospital
London, United Kingdom
Scoliosis and Kyphoscoliosis

S. David Singh, MD
Senior Lecturer
Respiratory Medicine and Clinical Pharmacology
North West Lung Research Centre
South Manchester University Hospitals Trust
Manchester, United Kingdom
Dyspnea

Arthur S. Slutsky, MD
Professor of Medicine, Surgery, and Biomedical Engineering
Director, Interdepartmental Division of Critical Care
University of Toronto
Vice President (Research), St. Michael Hospital
Toronto, Ontario, Canada
Pregnancy

Gregory I. Snell, MD
Head, Lung Transplant Service (Medical)
Department of Allergy, Immunology, and Respiratory Medicine
Alfred Hospital and Monash University
Melbourne, Victoria, Australia
Lung Transplantation

Stephen G. Spiro, MD
Professor of Respiratory Medicine
Consultant Physician General and Thoracic Medicine
University College London Hospitals NHS Trust
The Middlesex Hospital
London, United Kingdom
Thoracentesis and Closed Pleural Biopsy

Robert G. Stirling, MB, BS
Consultant Physician
Department of Allergy, Immunology, and Respiratory Medicine
Alfred Hospital
Prahran, Victoria, Australia
Connective Tissue Disorders

Diane C. Strollo, MD
Clinical Associate Professor of Radiology
Deparment of Radiology
University of Pittsburgh Medical Health System
Pittsburgh, Pennsylvania
Disorders of the Mediastinum

Patrick J. Strollo, Jr, MD
Associate Professor of Medicine
Division of Pulmonary, Allergy, and Critical Care Medicine
Medical Director, Sleep Disorders Laboratory
University of Pittsburgh Medical Center
Pittsburgh, Pennsylvania
Obstructive Sleep Apnea; Central Sleep Apnea and Other Forms of Sleep-Disordered Breathing

Edward W. Swenson, MD
Professor of Medicine, Emeritus
Benicia, California
Preoperative Pulmonary Evaluation

Erik R. Swenson, MD
Professor of Medicine
University of Washington
VA Puget Sound Health Care System
Seattle, Washington
Preoperative Pulmonary Evaluation

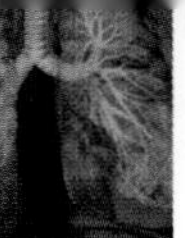

Nick H. T. Ten Hacken, MD
Consultant in Respiratory Medicine
University Hospital
Groningen, The Netherlands
Asthma: Epidemiology and Risk Factors

Galen B. Toews, MD
Professor of Internal Medicine
Chief, Division of Pulmonary and Critical Care Medicine
Department of Internal Medicine
University of Michigan Health System
Ann Arbor, Michigan
Host Defenses

Antoni Torres, MD
Director of Institut Clinic de Pneumologia I Cirurgia Toracica
Associate Professor of Medicine
Hospital Clinic de Barcelona
Barcelona, Spain
Hospital-Acquired Pneumonia

Franco Valenza, MD
Assistant Professor in Anesthesia and Intensive Care
Istituto di Anestesia e Rianimazione
Ospedale Maggiore di Milano IRCCS
Milan, Italy
Acute Respiratory Distress Syndrome

Sandra van Wetering, PhD
Research Fellow
Department of Pulmonology
Leiden University Medical Center
Leiden, The Netherlands
Asthma: Cell Biology

Roland G. J. R. A. Vanderschueren, MD, PhD, FACCP
Director
Department of Pulmonary Diseases
St. Antonius Ziekenhuis
Niuwegen, The Netherlands
Pneumothorax

Benoit Wallaert, MD
Professor of Medicine
Clinique des Maladies Respiratoires
Hôpital A. Calmette
CHRU
Lille, France
Silicosis and Coal Workers' Pneumoconiosis

Herbert H. Watzke, MD
Assistant Professor of Medicine
University of Vienna
Vienna, Austria
Pulmonary Embolism

Jadwiga A. Wedzicha, MD
Professor of Respiratory Medicine
Academic Unit of Respiratory Medicine
St. Bartholomew's and Royal London School of Medicine and Dentistry
London, United Kingdom
Management of Exacerbations in Chronic Obstructive Pulmonary Disease

Athol Wells, MD
Consultant Physician
Royal Brompton Hospital
London, United Kingdom
Approach to Diagnosis of Diffuse Lung Disease

Dorothy A. White, MD
Assistant Professor of Medicine
Memorial Sloan-Kettering Cancer Center
New York, New York
Drugs and the Lungs

Jeanine P. Wiener-Kronish, MD
Professor of Anesthesia and Medicine
Vice-Chairman, Department of Anesthesia and Perioperative Care
Investigator, Cardiovascular Research Institute
University of California San Francisco
San Francisco, California
Airway Management

Trevor J. Williams, MD
Clinical Director
Department of Allergy, Immunology, and Respiratory Medicine
Alfred Hospital
Monash University Clinical School
Melbourne, Australia
Lung Transplantation

Ashley A. Woodcock, MD, FRCP
Consultant in Respiratory Medicine
Department of Respiratory Medicine
North West Lung Research Centre
South Manchester University Hospitals Trust
Manchester, United Kingdom
Dyspnea

Mark A. Woodhead, MD
Honorary Lecturer
University of Manchester
Consultant Physician
Manchester Royal Infirmary
Manchester, United Kingdom
An Approach to the Diagnosis of Pulmonary Infection

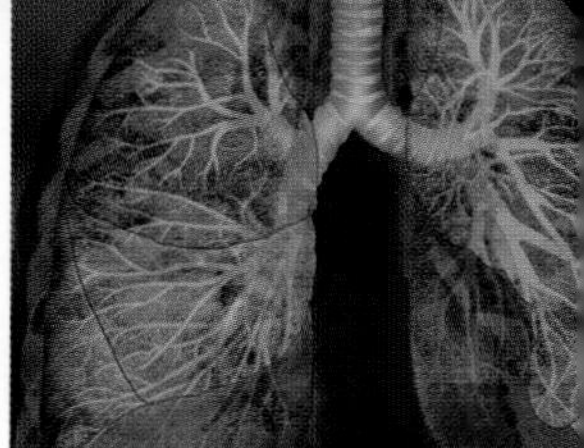

Preface

The first edition of this book was published in 1999 with the intent of (1) bringing the ideas of the world community of respiratory medicine together into a single publication, (2) utilizing the extraordinary advances in computer graphics and publishing to emphasize a visual, as opposed to a textual, presentation of material, and (3) combining detailed presentations of lung structure and physiology with clinical material. We were gratified by the resulting product, the praise given the book by its reviewers, the comments we received from numerous readers, and its acceptance by our colleagues around the world. This second edition maintains this same focus. The book is written by 113 authors (many are new contributors) from 11 different countries. We again have emphasized a visual presentation, and every chapter has been scrutinized for the opportunity to use figures and graphics over text. Each figure in the first edition was reviewed to determine whether it added to the presentation or could be improved.

The Structure and Function section has been completely reorganized for this edition. The Physiology section has been completely revised, dividing it into six new chapters with expanded discussions of most areas, a new chapter on the respiratory muscles, and the inclusion of a discussion of exercise physiology. The chapter on Host Defense has been expanded to include considerable new information about signaling, trafficking, cell-cell interactions, and apoptosis.

The editors have reviewed each chapter in the first edition in detail, deleting some of the material because we felt the topics were more appropriate for general physicians than respiratory medicine specialists. The Infectious Disease section has been completely reorganized to match how clinicians approach patients with these diseases, and to include recommendations from up-to-date guidelines. New chapters on bronchiectasis and on the cell biology of asthma have been added. The discussion of interstitial lung diseases has incorporated new diagnostic categories, and the chapter on sarcoidosis has been expanded to include new information on genetics and the use of alternative immunosuppressive treatments. New authors have provided updated discussions on silicosis and lung transplantation.

Because of the ease of web-based literature searches, we have elected to reduce the number of references provided to a few "Selected Readings."

The second edition remains directed at students and house officers, trainees in respiratory medicine, physicians practicing general or family medicine, and all respiratory medicine clinicians. The discussion of critical care topics is not intended to be comprehensive but rather is limited to those specific areas in which respiratory medicine practitioners should have special expertise.

The administrative difficulties associated with bringing a book to publication are extraordinary. Accordingly, the editors would like to acknowledge the contributions of our Development Editor, Joanne Husovski. Without her efforts, work on this second edition would not have been as successful. How she cajoled, organized, and kept the project on schedule while maintaining her outward calm and delightful demeanor remains a mystery. It was our very great pleasure to have her guidance.

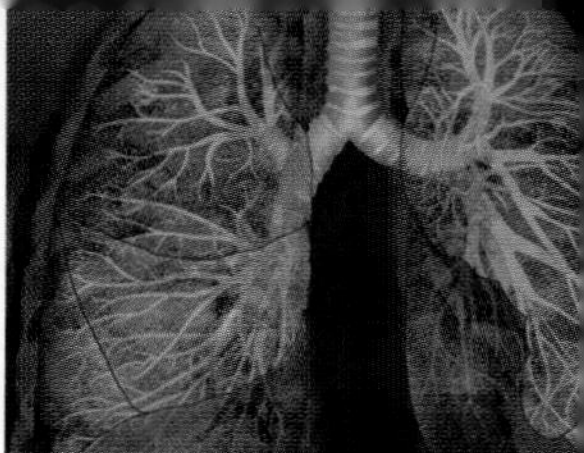

Contents

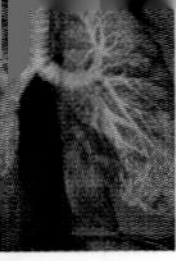

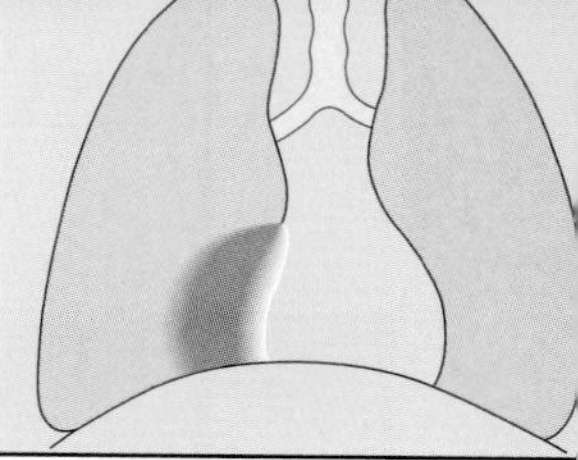

CHAPTER 1

Imaging

David M. Hansell and Simon P.G. Padley

IMAGING TECHNIQUES

Clinicians have two main imaging techniques at their disposal for the investigation of patients with chest disease: the chest radiograph, which produces a projectional image, and computed tomography (CT), which provides a cross-sectional view. Other techniques, such as magnetic resonance imaging (MRI), radionuclide scanning, and ultrasonography, can provide valuable additional information but rarely are performed in patients who have not undergone chest radiography or CT. Because imaging is an integral part of the practice of respiratory medicine, an understanding of the strengths and weaknesses of these various techniques is vital. The advent of high-resolution CT (HRCT) and spiral CT has lent further precision to the investigation of patients with suspected chest disease, but the use of such sophisticated tests should not be indiscriminate; the accurately interpreted chest radiograph remains the mainstay of thoracic imaging.

Plain Chest Radiography

TECHNICAL CONSIDERATIONS

The views of the chest most frequently performed are the erect posteroanterior (PA) and the lateral projections, taken with the patient holding the breath at total lung capacity. On a frontal PA chest radiograph, just under half the lung is free from overlying structures such as the ribs and diaphragm. Many technical factors, notably the kilovoltage and film-screen combination, determine how well the lungs are shown. Because of the characteristics of radiographic film, perfect exposures of the least dense and densest parts of the chest cannot be obtained in a single radiograph. Methods for overcoming this handicap of radiographic film include the use of high-kilovoltage techniques, asymmetrical film-screen combinations, and sophisticated devices that control regional x-ray exposure.

Because the coefficients of x-ray absorption of bone and soft tissue approach one another at high kilovoltage, the skeletal structures do not obscure the lungs on high-kilovoltage radiographs to the extent seen on low-kilovoltage radiographs. High-kilovoltage radiographs therefore show much more of the lungs. Improved penetration of the mediastinum also allows some of the central airways to be seen. Although high-kilovoltage radiographs are preferable for routine examinations of the lungs and mediastinum, low-kilovoltage radiographs provide good detail of unobscured lung because of the improved contrast between lung vessels and the surrounding lung (Fig. 1.1). Furthermore, dense lesions (e.g., calcified pleural plaques) are particularly well demonstrated on low-kilovoltage films.

One of the most important major advances in plain-film radiography was the introduction of more sensitive phosphorescent screens. Screens luminesce when an x-ray beam falls on them, are housed in a film cassette, and are in contact with the radiographic film, which records the image. The improved light emission from the latest rare-earth phosphors compared with older calcium screens results in shorter exposure times and therefore sharper images. A significant advance in film-screen combinations for chest imaging was the development of an asymmetrical combination of a thin front screen and high-contrast film emulsion on one side of the film base and a thicker back screen and a low-contrast film emulsion on the other side. Because of this design, the wide spectrum of transmission of x-rays through the thorax can be accommodated. Such a film-screen combination shows significantly more detail in the mediastinum and lung obscured by the diaphragm and heart.

To overcome the considerable differences in density between the mediastinum and the lungs, attempts have been made to produce a more uniformly exposed chest radiograph (Fig. 1.2). Newer devices modulate the exposure for each part of the chest by means of an electronic feedback system. One of the mostly widely used is the advanced multiple beam equalization radiography (AMBER) system. The AMBER unit uses a horizontal scanning slit-beam that is divided into segments, each being modulated by an electronic feedback loop from corresponding detectors on the far side of the patient. Such a system is particularly good at demonstrating lung pathology that is obscured by the heart and diaphragm.

The frontal and lateral projections are sufficient for most purposes in chest radiography. Other radiographic views are less frequently required, but they should not be overlooked because they may offer a quick and inexpensive solution to a particular problem. The lateral decubitus view is not, as its name implies, a lateral view. It is a frontal view taken with a horizontal beam with the patient lying on his or her side. The main purpose of this view is to demonstrate the movement of fluid in the pleural space (Fig. 1.3). A modification of the lateral decubitus view is the "lateral shoot-through" sometimes used in bed-bound patients, in which a lateral radiograph of the supine patient is taken to show an anterior pneumothorax behind the sternum (not always visible on a frontal chest radiograph; Fig. 1.4). If a pleural effusion is not loculated, it gravitates to some extent to the dependent part of the pleural cavity. If the patient lies on his or her side, the fluid layers between the chest wall and the lung edge. This view may also be useful for demonstrating a small pneumothorax, because the visceral pleural edge of the lung falls away from the chest walls in the nondependent hemithorax.

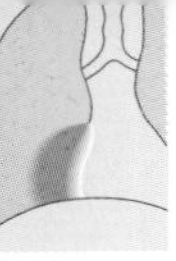

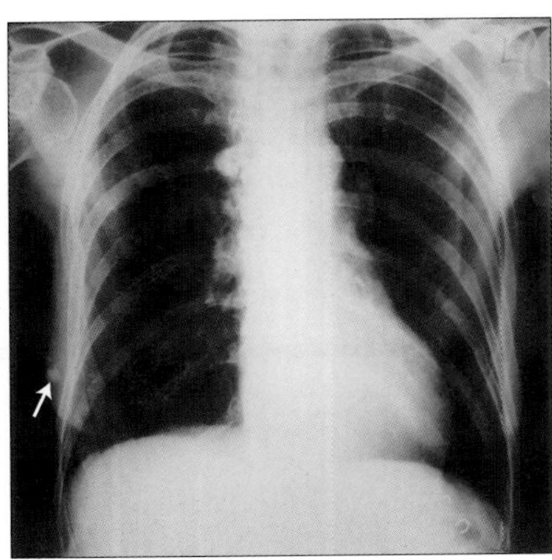

A

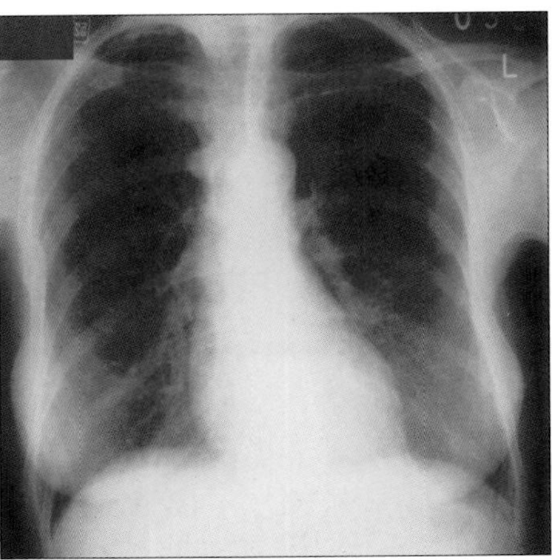

B

Figure 1.1 The effects of low and high kilovoltage on the chest radiograph. A, Low-kilovoltage chest radiograph showing good detail of the bones. Note the calcified fibroadenoma within the right breast *(arrow)*. **B,** A high-kilovoltage radiograph of the same patient shows better soft-tissue detail within the mediastinum but less definition of bony structures. Note the loss of visualization of the calcified fibroadenoma in the right breast.

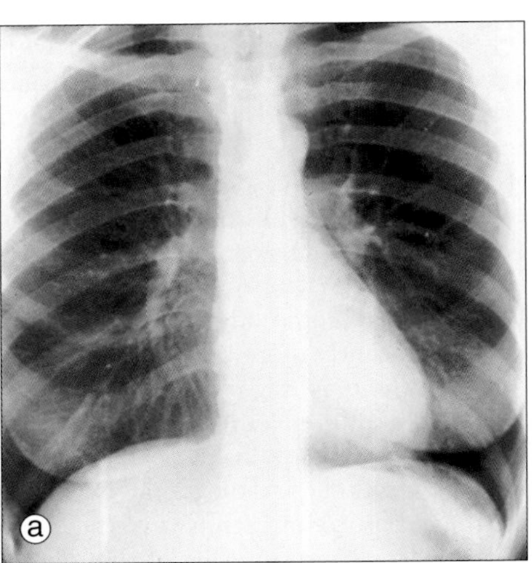

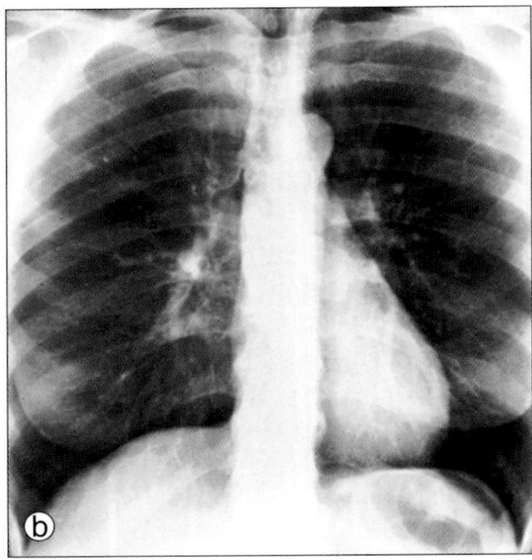

Figure 1.2 Comparison of conventional and advanced multiple beam equalization radiographs. A, Conventional high-kilovoltage chest radiograph. **B,** Advanced multiple beam equalization radiograph (scanning equalization radiograph) of the same patient, revealing increased lung detail behind the heart and right hemidiaphragm.

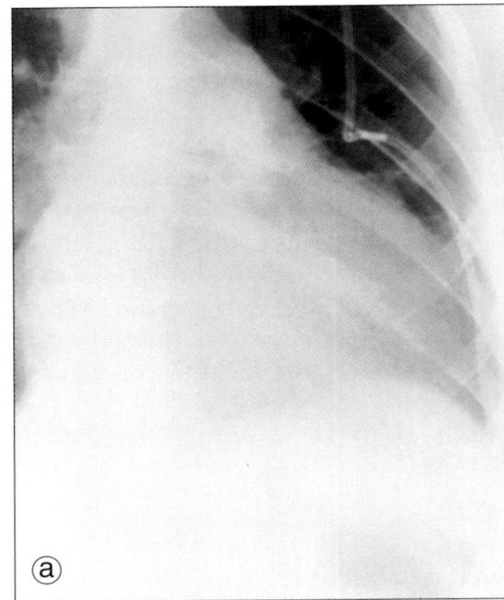

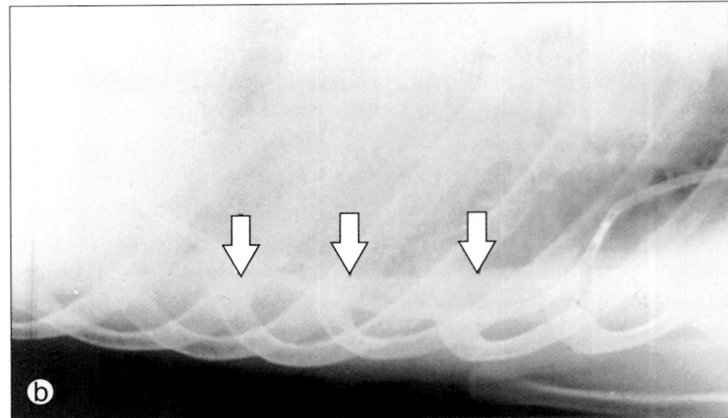

Figure 1.3 Demonstration of small effusions. A, Posteroanterior (PA) chest radiograph of a patient who has a ventriculoperitoneal shunt. More soft tissue than usual is present between the gastric air bubble and the base of the lung because of a subpulmonic effusion. **B,** Decubitus film shows redistribution of fluid to the dependent part of the chest *(arrows)*.

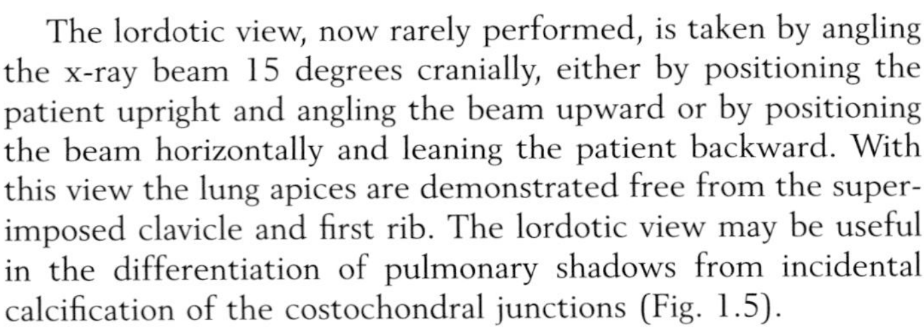

The lordotic view, now rarely performed, is taken by angling the x-ray beam 15 degrees cranially, either by positioning the patient upright and angling the beam upward or by positioning the beam horizontally and leaning the patient backward. With this view the lung apices are demonstrated free from the superimposed clavicle and first rib. The lordotic view may be useful in the differentiation of pulmonary shadows from incidental calcification of the costochondral junctions (Fig. 1.5).

PORTABLE CHEST RADIOGRAPHY

Portable or mobile chest radiography has the obvious advantage that the examination can be carried out without moving the patient from the ward. However, the portable radiograph has many disadvantages. The shorter-focus film distance results in undesirable magnification, and high-kilovoltage techniques cannot be used because portable machines are unable to deliver high kilovoltage. Furthermore, the maximum current is limited so that

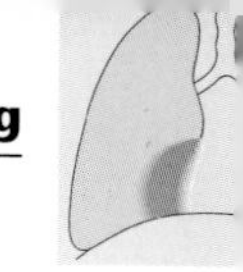

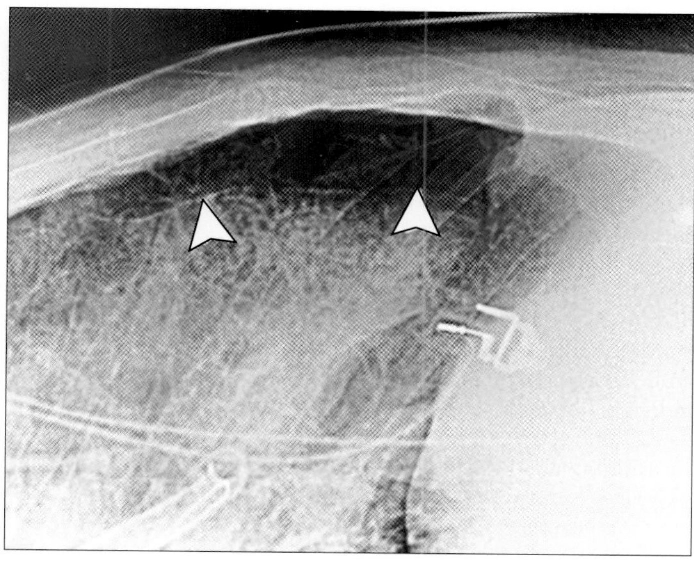

Figure 1.4 Lateral shoot-through digital radiograph of a patient in the intensive care unit. The anterior pneumothorax (note the visceral pleural edge—*arrowheads*) was not obvious on the anteroposterior portable radiograph.

long exposure times are needed, which potentially increases blurring of the image. Portable lateral radiographs are even less likely to be successful because of the extremely long exposure times required.

The positioning of patients for portable radiography is difficult, and the resulting radiographs are often suboptimal. Even with the patient in the so-called "erect" position (i.e., sitting up), the chest is rarely as vertical as it is in a standing patient. Because many patients are unable to move to the radiography department for a formal radiograph, any method for improving the quality of a portable chest radiograph, such as digital radiography, is a significant advance.

DIGITAL CHEST RADIOGRAPHY

Digital technology is integral to techniques such as CT and MRI. Conventional film radiography as a means of image capture, storage, and display represents something of a compromise, and it has become apparent that digital image acquisition, transmission, display, and storage can be advantageously applied to chest radiography.

Digital chest radiographs are produced by three methods. In the first, optical drum scanners or laser scanners are used to digitize conventional film radiographs. Although few indications call for this approach, much useful information has been derived from observer performance studies of digitized conventional film to establish the parameters for clinically acceptable digital radiographs.

The second technique is the use of a dedicated digital chest unit to digitally acquire the image (as opposed to digitization of a conventional radiograph). The prototypical device was described more than 10 years ago and used a scanning slit beam and 1024 solid-state detectors. The number of detectors limited the spatial resolution of this system and it has not been further developed.

The third method involves use of conventional radiographic equipment but with a reusable photostimulatable plate (selenium or phosphor derivatives) instead of conventional film. Phosphor-plate computed, or digital, radiography is used in many hospitals, often as a substitute for portable film radiography. The phosphor plate, which is housed in a "filmless" cassette, stores some of the energy of the incident x-ray as a latent image. When the plate is scanned with a laser beam, the stored energy is emitted as light that is detected by a photomultiplier and converted into a digital signal. The digital information is then manipulated, displayed, and stored in whatever format is

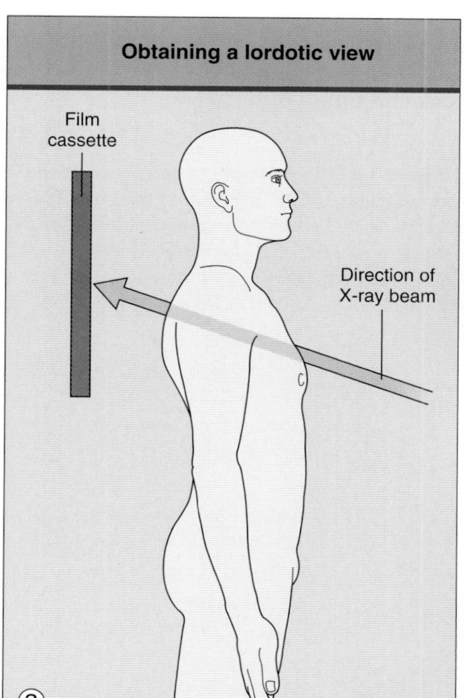

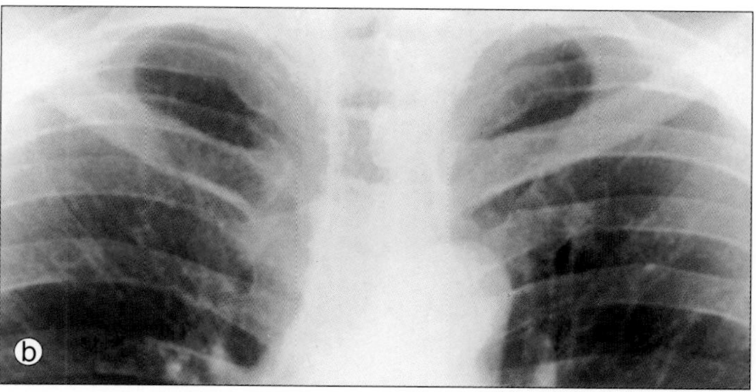

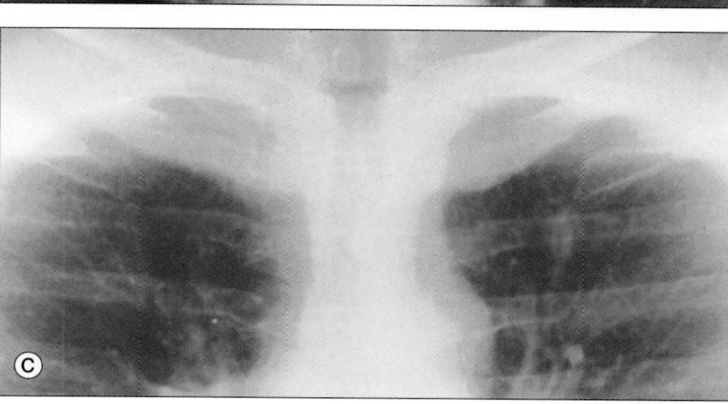

Figure 1.5 The value of lordotic views. A, Method of obtaining a lordotic view of the lung apices. The x-ray beam is angled upward. **B,** Selective view of the upper zones of a patient with hemoptysis, with a suggestion of a small opacity projected over the anterior end of the left first rib. **C,** A lordotic view confirms that the small opacity is intrapulmonary (rather than calcified costochondral cartilage).

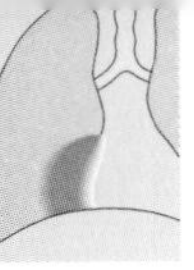

desired. The phosphor plate can be reused once the latent image has been erased by exposure to light. Most currently available computed radiography systems produce a digital radiograph with a picture element (pixel) size of 0.2 mm. The fundamental requirement to segment the image into a finite number of pixels has resulted in much work to determine the relationship between pixel size, which affects spatial resolution, and the detectability of focal abnormalities. Although it might seem desirable to aim for an image composed of pixels of the smallest possible size, an inverse relationship occurs between pixel size and the cost and speed of data handling. Thus, pixel size is ultimately a compromise between image quality and ease of data processing and storage.

An unequivocal advantage of digital computed radiography over conventional film radiography is the linear photoluminescence-dose response, which is much lower with conventional film. This extremely wide latitude coupled with the facility for image processing produces diagnostic images over a wide range of exposures.

Observer performance studies have shown that computed radiography can equal conventional film radiography for virtually any task. However, postprocessing of the digital image has to be used to match the digital radiograph to the specific task. Enhancement of the image for one purpose often degrades it for another. Reports conflict as to whether digital chest radiographs can be satisfactorily interpreted on television monitors, as opposed to laser-printed film, but it is increasingly apparent that high-resolution monitors are adequate for making primary diagnoses from digital chest radiographs.

Computed Tomography

Film radiography and CT are based on the same basic principle—the absorption of x-rays by tissues that contain constituents of different atomic numbers. Through use of multiple projections and computed calculations of radiographic density, slight differences in x-ray absorption result in the display of a cross-sectional image. The components of a CT scanner, contained within the gantry, include an x-ray tube that rotates around the patient and an array of x-ray detectors. The patient lies on the examination couch, which moves through the aperture of the CT gantry. The data acquired are then processed by the CT computer, resulting in the final images that are displayed on the CT monitor and traditionally printed onto film.

Spiral (also known as volume or helical) scanning entails continuous scanning and table movement into the CT gantry. With this method a continuous data set or "spiral" of information may be acquired in a single holding of the patient's breath (Fig. 1.6). The information is reconstructed into axial sections, perpendicular to the long axis of the patient, that are identical to conventional CT sections. The main advantage of spiral CT is that truly contiguous scanning is possible with no gap between the individual axial images.

An alternative technology that dispenses with the mechanical rotating anode is electron beam ultrafast CT scanning. The patient is surrounded by a tungsten target ring, and a focused electron beam sweeps around the tungsten ring at high speed to produce an x-ray beam. Such machines can acquire an image in 100 msec or less, and therefore real-time studies are possible, with images acquired at 17 frames per second at a given level. Rapid-acquisition studies allow the evaluation of normal and abnormal dynamic structural changes (e.g., lung density during the respiratory cycle or the excursion of the tracheal wall during forced respiratory maneuvers).

The speed advantages of ultrafast CT have been significantly eroded by a number of developments in conventional CT systems. The speed with which a mechanical CT scanner acquires a data set depends on the time it takes to rotate the anode around the patient and the speed with which the patient is fed through the aperture of the scanner. Reductions in rotation time and increases in patient feed speed have resulted in shorter and shorter examination times. The most significant development in CT hardware to facilitate these changes has been the widespread and rapid introduction of CT scanners that acquire 4, 8, or 16 slices per gantry rotation. These different systems are most simply described as 4-, 8-, or 16-channel scanners, with the number relating to the number of rows of detectors that are irradiated at one time.

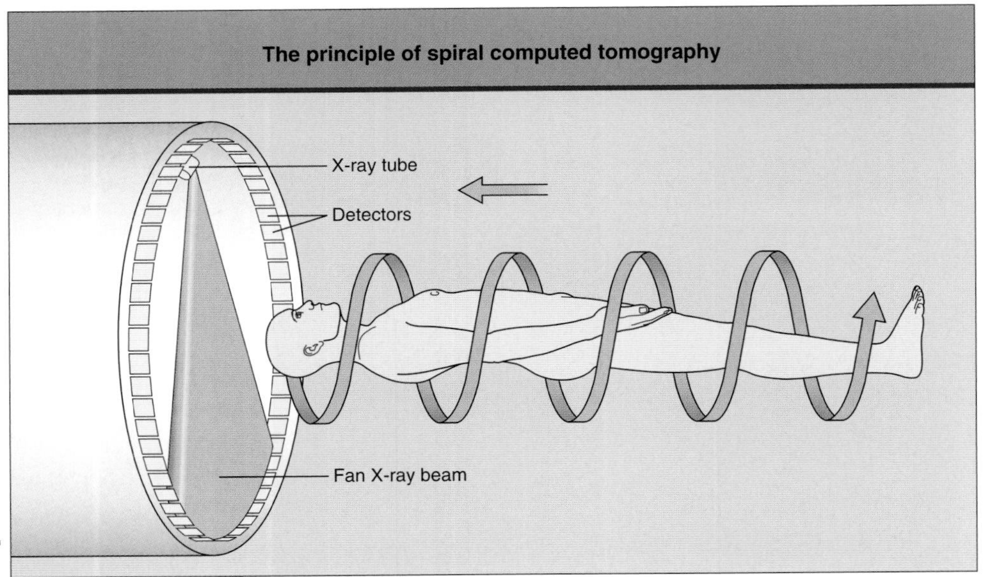

Figure 1.6 The principle of spiral computed tomography (CT). The patient moves into the scanner with the x-ray tube continuously rotating and the detectors acquiring information. The rapidity of data acquisition allows a complete examination of the thorax to be performed in a single holding of the patient's breath.

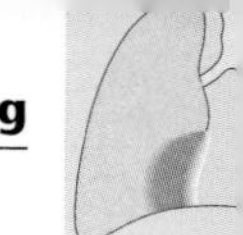

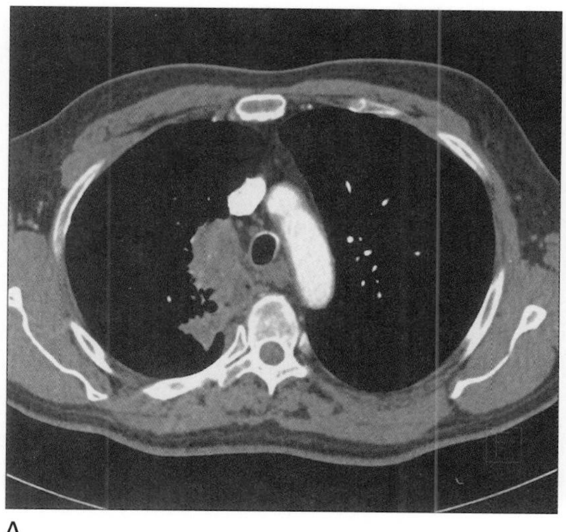

A

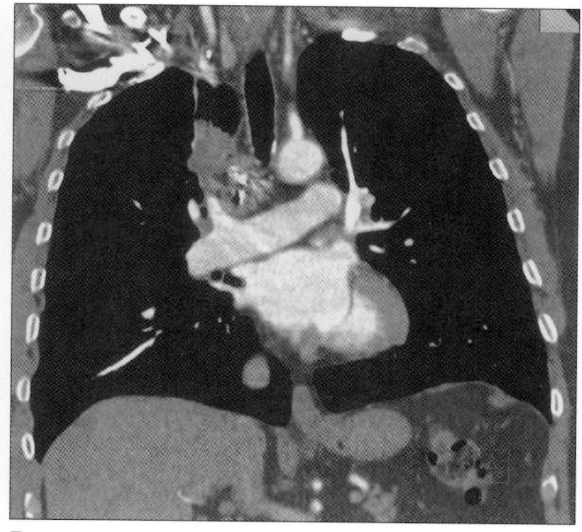

B

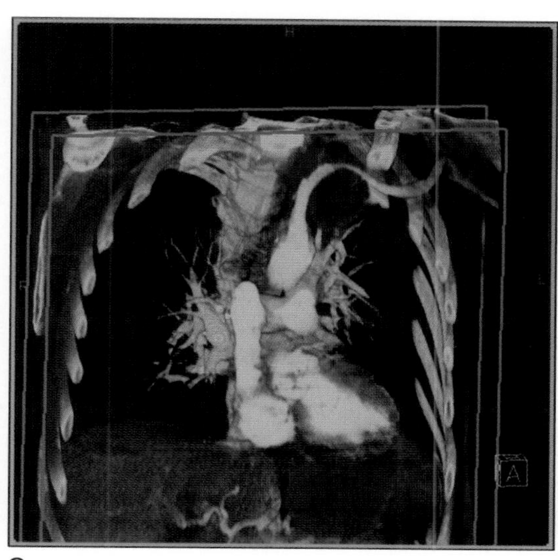

C

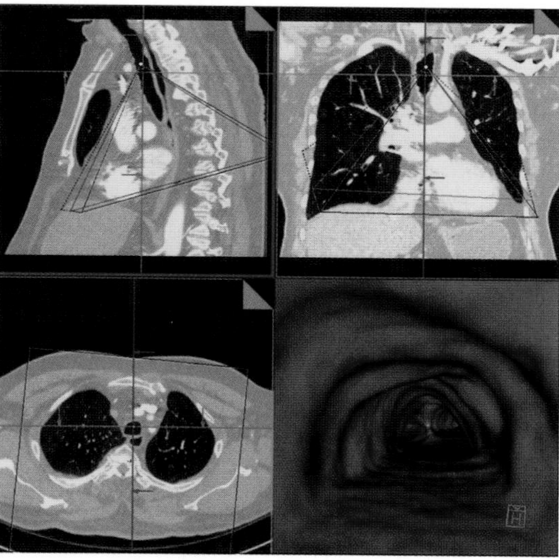

D

Figure 1.7 Data set from a 16-channel computed tomography (CT) system. A, This axial image demonstrates a bronchogenic carcinoma lying in a right paratracheal position. **B,** A reformat from the same data demonstrates the same abnormality in the coronal plane without loss of image resolution. **C,** A coronal volume rendered image of a different patient demonstrating a left superior sulcus tumor encasing the left subclavian artery (*arrows*). **D,** Virtual bronchoscopic image from a normal patient, demonstrating the orientation of the endoluminal view in sagittal, coronal, and axial planes.

Temporal resolution has been further reduced by data reconstruction algorithms that allow CT images to be generated from a partial rotation of the gantry. Temporal resolution of as little as 125 msec is now possible and enables modern multichannel CT scanners to acquire cardiac gated images that effectively freeze cardiac motion, which allows analysis of coronary artery calcification and narrowing.

Traditionally, the signal from the x-ray detectors is reconstructed by a computer, displayed on the computer console, and laser-printed onto film. However a 16-channel CT system can now scan the thorax and abdomen at 0.75 mm of collimation in under 20 seconds. These images may be reconstructed with a small overlap, resulting in a stack of images that may contain 500 individual slices. This many images would occupy many sheets of film, rendering traditional printing impractical. Radiologists, therefore, are now routinely analyzing the data sets on workstations. Because multichannel scanners now generate a volume of data rather than a series of axial images, the data set may be reconstructed in any plane without loss of detail. Additional reconstructive techniques allow interactive volume rendering and virtual bronchoscopy to be performed rapidly (Fig. 1.7).

TECHNICAL CONSIDERATIONS

The CT image is composed of a matrix of picture elements (pixels). A fixed number of pixels make up the matrix, so the size of each pixel varies according to the diameter of the circle to be scanned. A typical matrix in a modern CT system is 512 × 512 pixels. The smaller the circle size, the smaller the area represented by a pixel and the higher the spatial resolution of the image. In practical terms, the size of the field of view is adjusted to the size of the area of interest, usually the chest diameter.

Often a marked difference exists in the appearances of images produced on different CT scanners. This is largely the result of differences in software—the algorithms for reconstruction that are used to smooth the image, to a greater or lesser extent, by averaging the densities of neighboring pixels. The lung is a high-contrast environment, so less smoothing is needed than in other parts of the body. Higher spatial-resolution algorithms (which make image "noise"—a granular appearance—more conspicuous) are generally more desirable for scanning of the lungs.

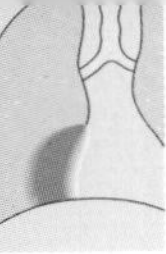

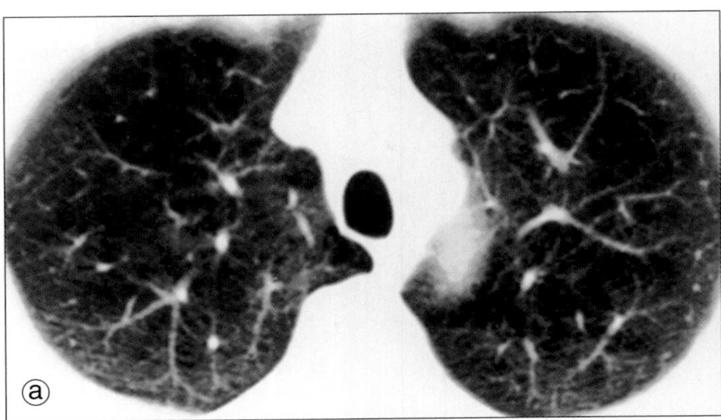

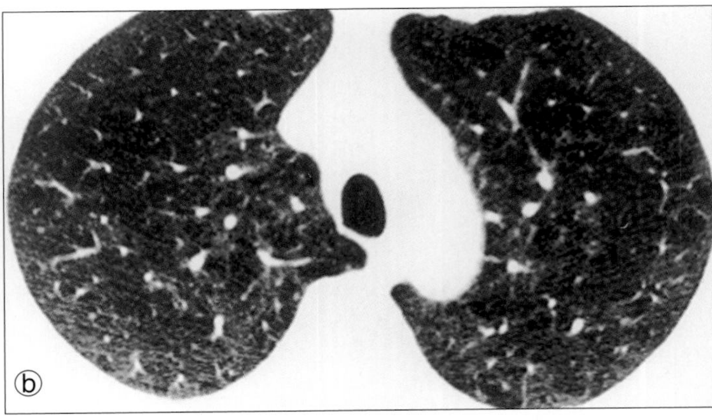

Figure 1.8 The partial volume effect on computed tomography (CT). A, This 10-mm CT section shows a poorly defined opacity adjacent to the left superior mediastinum, apparently within the lung. **B,** The 1.5-mm section through the same region reveals that the appearance in **A** results from a partial volume effect, that is, the aortic arch is partially included in the 10-mm thick sections.

Section Thickness

Although a CT section is viewed as a two-dimensional image, it has a third dimension: the depth. The depth, or section thickness, is determined by the width of the slit through which the x-ray beam passes (beam collimation) or, in the case of multichannel systems, by the width of the detector elements. Because a section has a predetermined thickness, each pixel has a volume. This three-dimensional element is referred to as a *voxel*. The computer calculates the average radiographic density of tissue within each voxel, and the final CT image consists of a representation of the numerous voxels (not individually visible without magnification) in the section. The single attenuation value of a voxel represents the average of the attenuation values of all the various structures within the voxel. The thicker the section, the greater the chance that different structures will be included within the voxel and so the greater the averaging that occurs. This is known as the partial volume effect; the easiest way to reduce this effect is to use thinner sections (Fig. 1.8).

When the whole chest is examined, contiguous 5-mm–thick sections are usually reconstructed for analysis. If the study is undertaken on a multichannel system, the data set may be reconstructed at thinner intervals predetermined by the thickness of the detector rows, and these thinner sections may be used for reporting or for multiplanar reconstructions. Thinner sections are also used to study fine detail and complex areas of anatomy, such as the aortopulmonary window and subcarinal regions. Another case in which narrow sections may be useful for the display of differential densities (which would otherwise be lost because of the partial volume effect) is the small foci of fat or calcium that are sometimes seen within a hamartoma.

Although little difference exists in the patient's total dose of radiation between conventional single-channel CT and 4-, 8-, or 16-channel systems, there is a striking difference in the patient's radiation dose between contiguous sections and interspaced fine sections. The effective dose to the patient with interspaced fine sections (e.g., 1 or 2 mm) every 10 mm, such as used for HRCT of the lung parenchyma, is considerably less than the dose imposed by single or multichannel spiral CT of the entire chest volume.

Window Settings

The average density of each voxel is measured in Hounsfield units (H); the units have been arbitrarily chosen so that 0 represents the density of water and −1000 represents the density of air. The span of Hounsfield units in the thorax is wider than in any other part of the body, ranging from aerated lung (approximately −800 H) to ribs (700 H). Two variables allow the operator to select the range of densities to be viewed—window width and window center (or level).

The window width determines the number of Hounsfield units to be displayed. Any densities greater than the upper limit of the window width are displayed as white, and any below the limit of the window are displayed as black. Between these two limits, the densities are displayed in shades of gray. The median density of the window chosen is the center or level, and this center can be moved higher or lower at will, thus moving the window up or down through the range. The narrower the window width, the greater the contrast discrimination within the window. No single window setting can be used to show the wide range of densities encountered in the chest on a single image. For this reason, at least two sets of images are required to demonstrate the lung parenchyma and soft tissues of the mediastinum, respectively (Fig. 1.9). Standard window widths and centers for thoracic CT vary among departments, but generally for the soft tissues of the mediastinum a window width of 400 to 600 H and a center of 30 H are appropriate. For the lungs, a wide window of 1500 H and a center of approximately −500 H are usually satisfactory. For bones, the best settings are the widest possible window setting and a center of 30 H.

Window settings have a profound influence on the size and conspicuity of normal and abnormal structures. Nonetheless, it is impossible to prescribe precise window settings because of the element of observer preference and the differences among machines. The most accurate representation of an object appears to be achieved if the value of the window level is halfway between the density of the structure to be measured and the density of the surrounding tissue. For example, the diameter of a pulmonary nodule as measured using soft-tissue settings appropriate for the mediastinum will be grossly underestimated. When inappropriate window settings are used, smaller struc-

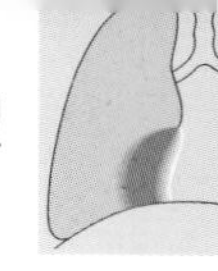

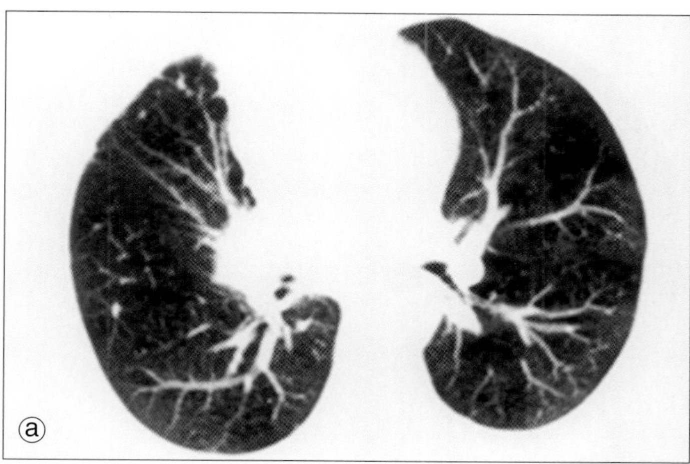

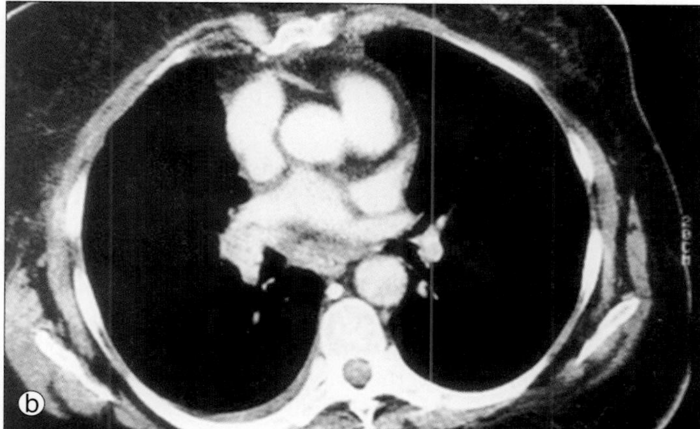

Figure 1.9 The effect of window settings on computed tomography (CT) scans. A 6-mm thick CT section displayed on different window settings. **A,** On lung windows (center 600 H, width 1000 H), nodules in the right lung and pulmonary vessels are clearly visible. Note the lack of mediastinal detail. **B,** On soft-tissue windows (center 35 H, width 400 H), the contrast-enhanced chambers of the heart and a small right pleural effusion are visible.

tures (e.g., the peripheral pulmonary vessels) are affected proportionately much more than larger structures.

Intravenous Contrast Enhancement

Intravenous contrast enhancement is performed only in specific circumstances because of the high contrast on CT between vessels and surrounding air in the lung and between vessels and surrounding fat within the mediastinum. Intravenous contrast enhancement may, for example, aid in distinguishing between hilar vessels and a soft-tissue mass. The exact timing of the injection of contrast media depends most on the amount of time the CT scanner requires to scan the thorax. With multichannel CT scanners, the circulation time of the patient becomes an important factor.

Contrast medium rapidly diffuses out of the vascular space into the extravascular space, so that opacification of the vasculature after a bolus injection via a power injector quickly declines and structures such as lymph nodes steadily increase in density over time. Such dynamics result in a point at which a solid structure may have exactly the same density as an adjacent vessel. The timing and duration of the contrast-medium infusion must therefore be taken into account when a contrast-enhanced CT scan is interpreted. Rapid scanning protocols with automated injectors tend to improve contrast enhancement of vascular structures at the expense of enhancement of solid lesions because of the rapidity of scanning. With spiral CT it is possible to achieve good opacification of all the thoracic vascular structures using small volumes of contrast media. Optimal contrast enhancement is a prerequisite for the diagnosis of pulmonary embolism (PE) or aortic and great vessel abnormalities. For the achievement of optimal contrast enhancement, many CT systems now include an automated triggering system. When the pulmonary arteries are examined, a low-dose repeating scan monitors the density in the pulmonary outflow tract once every second. When a predetermined density threshold is reached as a result of the arrival of intravenous contrast, the preplanned examination is triggered. The couch rapidly moves the patient from the monitoring position to the start position, the patient is instructed by a prerecorded message from a loudspeaker to hold the breath, and the data acquisition commences.

During examination of inflammatory lesions such as the reaction around an empyema, it may be necessary to delay scanning by 30 seconds to allow the contrast medium to diffuse into the extravascular space. When the liver and adrenals in a patient with suspected lung cancer are examined, the optimal phase of contrast enhancement to maximize the conspicuity of hepatic metastases is during the portal venous phase of contrast enhancement, which occurs 60 to 80 seconds after injection of contrast medium.

High-resolution Computed Tomography

TECHNICAL CONSIDERATIONS

In the past 10 years the development of HRCT has had great impact on the approach to the imaging of diffuse interstitial lung disease and bronchiectasis. Images of the lung produced by HRCT correlate closely with the macroscopic appearances of pathologic specimens, so in the context of diffuse lung disease, HRCT represents a substantial improvement over chest radiography. Three factors significantly improve the spatial resolution of CT and result in the designation "high-resolution": narrow beam collimation, a high spatial reconstruction algorithm, and a small field of view.

Narrow collimation of the x-ray beam reduces volume averaging within the section and so increases spatial resolution compared with standard 10-mm collimation. For routine HRCT scanning, 1.5-mm beam collimation is generally regarded as optimal. Narrow collimation has a marked effect on the appearance of the lungs, notably the vessels and bronchi; the branching vascular pattern seen particularly in the midzones on standard 10-mm sections has a more nodular appearance with narrow sections, because shorter segments of the obliquely running vessels are included in the section (Fig. 1.10).

In HRCT of the lung, a high–spatial-frequency algorithm is used to take advantage of the inherently high-contrast environment of the lung. The high–spatial-frequency algorithm (also known as the "edge-enhancing," "sharp," or formerly "bone" algorithm) reduces image smoothing and makes structures visibly sharper, but at the same time makes image noise more obvious.

Several artifacts are consistently identified on HRCT images, but they do not usually degrade the diagnostic content of the

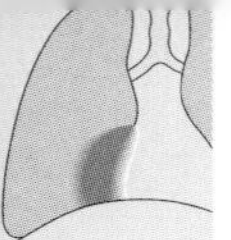

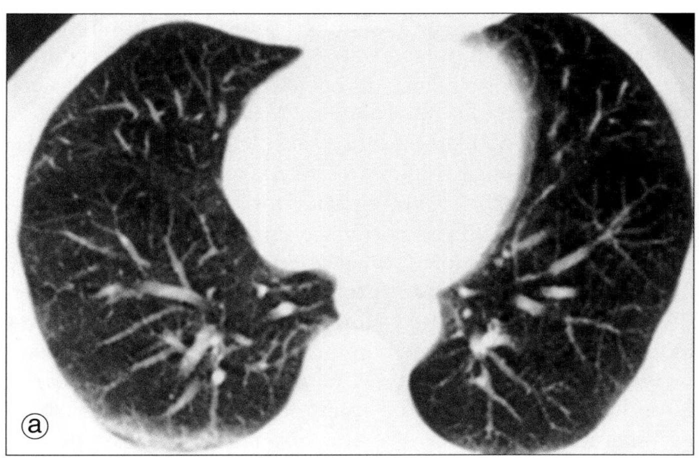

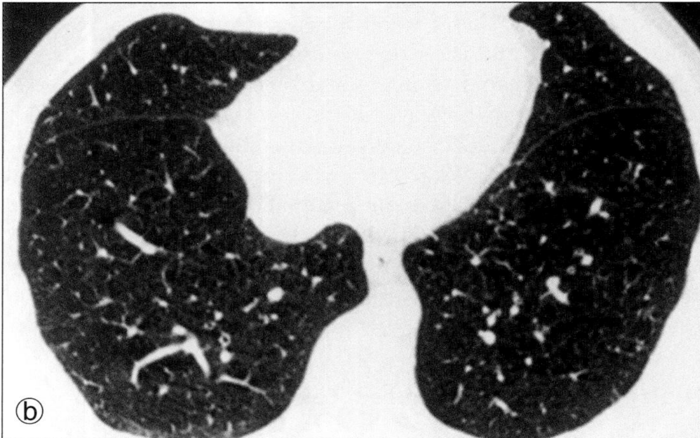

Figure 1.10 The effect of computed tomography (CT) section thickness on resolution. A, This 10-mm CT section through the lower lobes shows normal lung parenchyma and vessels. **B,** In the 1.5-mm high-resolution CT at the same level as **A,** the vessels are sharper and appear as more nodular opacities (less of their length is included in the plane of section). Note the increased clarity of the oblique fissures and bronchi.

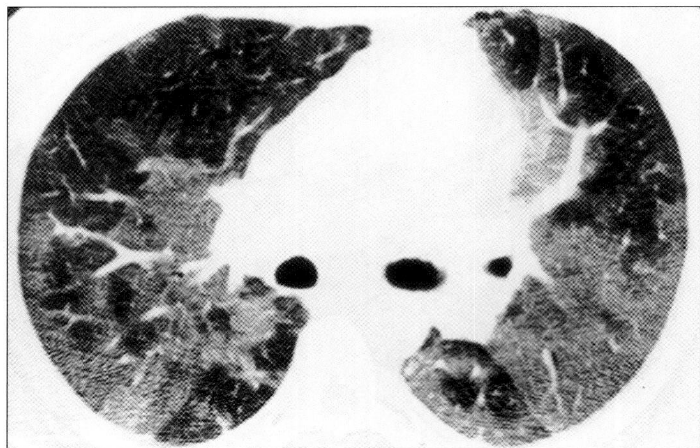

Figure 1.11 High-resolution computed tomography (HRCT) image demonstrating artifact caused by aliasing and quantum mottle. Detail is obscured in the posterior parts of the lungs. The patchy parenchymal opacification results from desquamative interstitial pneumonitis.

images. Nevertheless, it is useful to be able to recognize the more common ones. Probably the most frequently encountered artifact is a streaking caused by patient motion. Cardiac motion sometimes causes movement of the adjacent lung and therefore degradation of image quality. Some CT scanners are able to eliminate this artifact by triggering the acquisition of the slice from the electrocardiogram (ECG) trace and so collect the data during diastole when cardiac motion is minimized. To optimize this technique the scanner must have a short rotation time and also be capable of acquiring a CT image from data from a partial rotation. This reduces the data acquisition time window to as little as 360 msec.

The size of the patient has a direct effect on the quality of the lung image—the larger the patient, the more conspicuous the noise (which appears as granular streaks) because of increased x-ray absorption by the patient. This artifact is particularly evident in the posterior lung adjacent to the vertebral column. The phenomenon of aliasing results in a fine, streaklike pattern radiating from sharp, high-contrast interfaces. The severity of the aliasing artifact is related to the geometry of the CT scanner. Unlike quantum mottle, aliasing is independent of the radiation dose. These artifacts are exaggerated by the non-smoothing, high–spatial-resolution reconstruction algorithm but do not mimic normal anatomic structures and are rarely severe enough to obscure important detail in the lung parenchyma (Fig. 1.11).

The degree to which HRCT samples the lung depends primarily on the spacing between the thin sections. An HRCT examination also may vary in terms of the number of sections, the position of the patient, the phase in which respiration is suspended, the window settings at which the images are displayed, and the manipulation of the image by postprocessing. No single protocol can be recommended to cover every eventuality. However, the simplest protocol entails 1.5-mm collimation sections at 20-mm intervals from apex to lung bases. Any given scanning protocol may need to be modified—a patient referred with unexplained hemoptysis ideally is scanned with contiguous standard sections through the major airways (to show a small endobronchial abnormality) and interspaced narrow sections through the remainder of the lungs (to identify bronchiectasis).

When early interstitial disease is suspected (e.g., in asbestos-exposed individuals who have an apparently normal chest radiograph), HRCT scans are often performed with the patient in the prone position to prevent any confusion with the increased opacification seen in the dependent posterior-basal segments of many normal individuals scanned in the usual supine position. The increased density seen in the posterior dependent lung in the supine position disappears in normal individuals when the scan is repeated at the same level with the patient in the prone position. No advantage is gained by scanning a patient in the prone position if no obvious diffuse lung disease is found on a contemporary chest radiograph.

A limited number of scans taken at end expiration can reveal evidence of air trapping caused by small-airway disease, which may not be detectable on routine inspiratory scans. Areas of air trapping range from a single secondary pulmonary lobule to a cluster of lobules that give a patchwork appearance of areas of low attenuation adjacent to higher-attenuation, normal lung parenchyma (Fig. 1.12).

Alterations in window settings sometimes make detection of parenchymal abnormalities on HRCT images impossible when

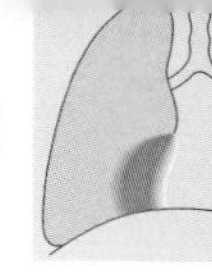

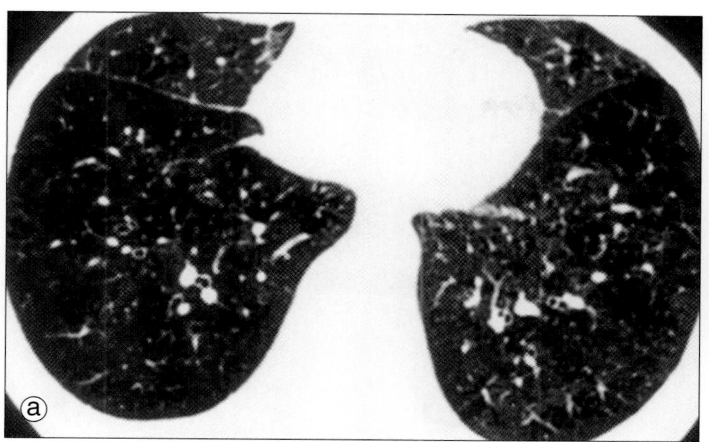

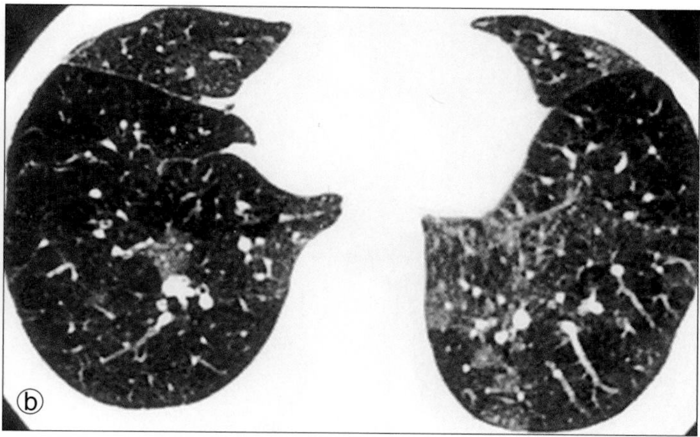

Figure 1.12 High-resolution computed tomography (HRCT) scan through the lower lobes of a patient who has severe dyspnea and rheumatoid arthritis. A, Minor inhomogeneity of the density of the lung parenchyma and some dilatation of the bronchus. **B,** HRCT scan taken at end expiration emphasizes the density differences. Appearances are consistent with obliterative bronchiolitis.

there is a subtle increase or decrease in attenuation of the lung parenchyma. Uniformity of window settings from patient to patient aids in consistent interpretation of lung images. In general, a window level of −500 to −800 H and a width of between 900 and 1500 H are usually satisfactory. Modification of the window settings for particular tasks is often desirable; for example, in looking for pleuroparenchymal abnormalities in asbestos-exposed individuals, a wider window of up to 2000 H may be useful. Conversely, a narrower window of approximately 600 H may emphasize the subtle density differences that characterize emphysema and small-airway disease.

A relatively high radiation dose to the patient is inherent in all CT scanning. The radiation burden to the patient is considerably less with HRCT than with conventional CT. It has been estimated that the mean radiation dose delivered to the skin with HRCT using 1.5-mm sections at 20-mm intervals is 6% that of conventional 10-mm contiguous-scanning protocols. A method of further reducing the radiation burden to the patient is to decrease the milliamperage; it is possible to reduce the milliamperage by up to tenfold and still obtain comparably diagnostic images. Although future refinements in CT technology may reduce the radiation burden to patients, CT still subjects patients to a relatively high radiation dose, and therefore must not be performed indiscriminately.

CLINICAL APPLICATIONS

Increasingly, HRCT is used to confirm or refute the impression of an abnormality seen on a chest radiograph. It may also be used to achieve a histospecific diagnosis in some patients who have obvious but nonspecific radiographic abnormalities.

It is probably impossible to determine the frequency with which HRCT reveals significant parenchymal abnormalities when the chest radiograph appears normal. Studies of individual diseases show that HRCT demonstrates abnormalities despite normal chest radiographs in 29% of patients with systemic sclerosis and in up to 30% of patients with asbestosis. For patients with hypersensitivity pneumonitis, the percentage may be even higher. Based on the average sensitivity results of several studies, HRCT appears to have a sensitivity of approximately 94% compared with 80% for chest radiography; this increased sensitivity does not seem to be achieved at the expense of decreased specificity.

In patients with clinical, radiographic, and lung-function evidence of diffuse lung disease, much evidence now indicates that results of HRCT are predictive of the correct histologic diagnosis more often and with a greater degree of confidence than chest radiography allows. In the original study that compared the diagnostic accuracy of chest radiography with CT in the prediction of specific histologic diagnoses in patients with diffuse lung disease, Mathieson and colleagues showed that three observers could make a confident diagnosis in 23% of cases on the basis of chest radiographs and in 49% of cases using CT; the correct diagnoses were made in 77% and 93% of these readings, respectively (Fig. 1.13).

Another study showed that for three observers the high-confidence diagnoses made on the basis of chest radiography findings alone were correct in 29%, 34%, and 19% of cases, whereas in HRCT the results were 57%, 55%, and 47%, respectively. Moreover, the intraobserver agreement for the proposed diagnosis was improved with HRCT compared with chest radiography. These studies show that HRCT is clearly useful in the assessment of patients suspected of having diffuse lung disease but for whom the clinical features and chest radiograph do not allow a confident diagnosis to be made. Even without clinical information, a number of diffuse lung diseases can, in the hands of experienced chest radiologists, have a diagnostic appearance on HRCT; these include fibrosing alveolitis, sarcoidosis, Langerhans-cell histiocytosis, lymphangioleiomyomatosis, pneumoconiosis, and hypersensitivity pneumonitis (Fig. 1.14). The ability of HRCT to allow observers to provide correct histospecific diagnoses appears to be maintained in advanced end-stage disease.

However, HRCT is sometimes used indiscriminately for patients in whom the high certainty of diagnosis from clinical and radiographic findings does not justify the extra cost and radiation burden. No evidence shows that an HRCT examination adds anything of diagnostic value for a patient who has progressive shortness of breath, finger clubbing, crackles at the lung bases, and the typical radiographic pattern and lung-function profile of fibrosing alveolitis. Nevertheless, the ability of HRCT

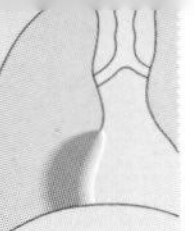

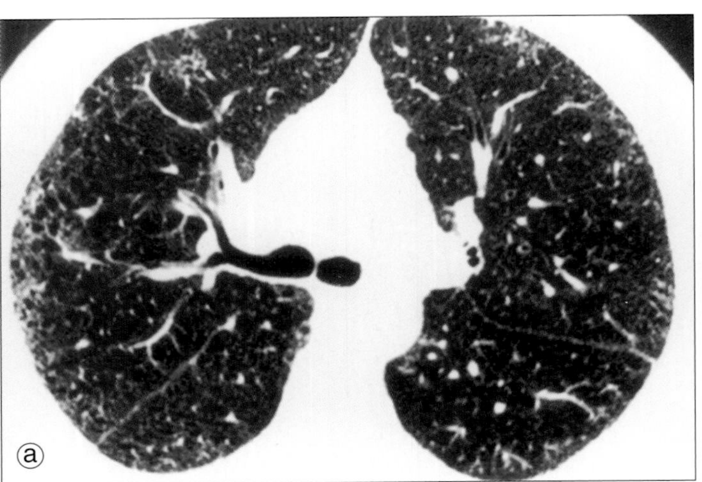

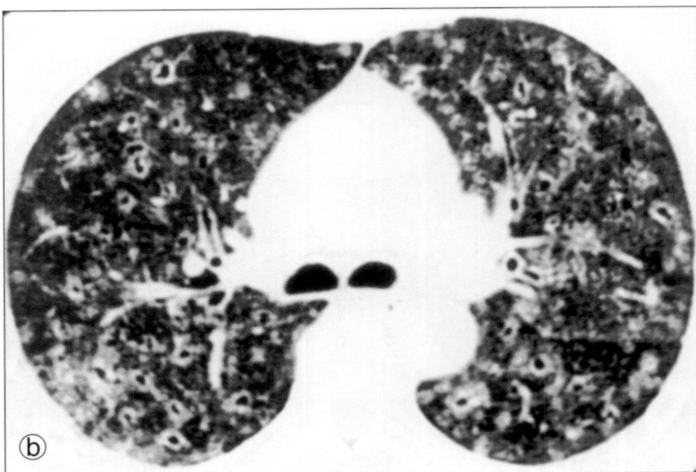

Figure 1.13 High-resolution computed tomography (HRCT) patterns. A, Subpleural reticular pattern typical of established fibrosing alveolitis. **B,** Numerous cavitating nodules, several of which have odd shapes; sections through the lung bases were normal. This HRCT pattern and distribution are virtually pathognomonic of Langerhans-cell histiocytosis.

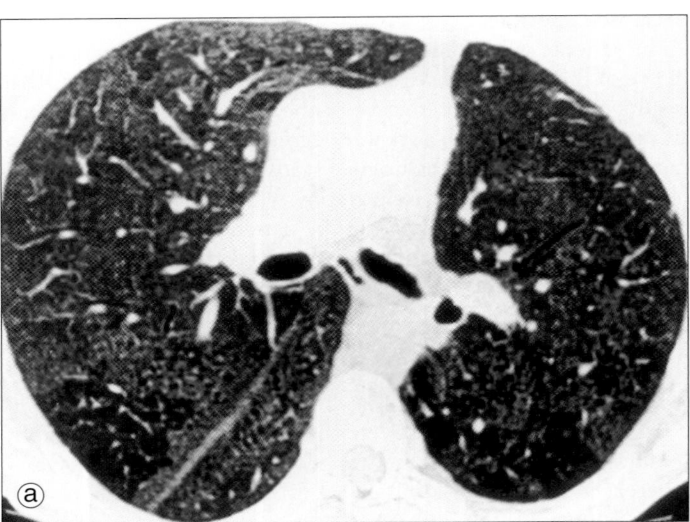

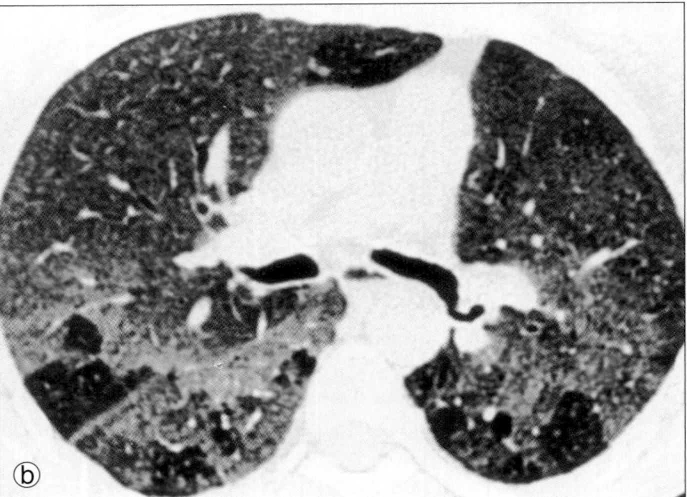

Figure 1.14 High-resolution computed tomography (HRCT) of a patient with subacute hypersensitivity pneumonitis. A, Widespread nodular and ground-glass patterns. **B,** Note the areas of decreased attenuation posteriorly, made more obvious on this scan obtained in expiration.

Table 1.1
Causes of ground-glass opacification

Pneumocystis jiroveci or cytomegalovirus pneumonia
Acute respiratory distress syndrome/acute interstitial pneumonia
Hypersensitivity pneumonitis – subacute
Desquamative interstitial pneumonitis
Pulmonary edema
Idiopathic pulmonary hemorrhage
Bronchioloalveolar cell carcinoma
Alveolar proteinosis
Lymphocytic interstitial pneumonia
Respiratory bronchiolitis – interstitial lung disease

to characterize disease, and often to deliver a definite and correct diagnosis in patients with nonspecific radiographic shadowing, is frequently helpful.

Much interest has been shown in defining the role of HRCT in the staging of disease activity, particularly for fibrosing alveolitis, in which cellular histology indicates disease activity and is used to predict both responses to treatment and prognosis. There is now evidence that a predominance of ground-glass opacification in fibrosing alveolitis is predictive of a good response to treatment and increased actuarial survival compared with patients with a more reticular pattern, which denotes established fibrosis. Similar observations about the potential reversibility of disease can be made through the use of HRCT on patients with sarcoidosis, in whom a ground-glass or a nodular pattern predominates. In other conditions the identification of ground-glass opacification on HRCT, although nonspecific, almost invariably indicates a potentially reversible disease—for example, extrinsic allergic alveolitis, diffuse pulmonary hemorrhage, and *Pneumocystis jiroveci* pneumonia (Table 1.1). An important exception is bronchoalveolar cell carcinoma, in which there may be areas of ground-glass opacification that merge into areas of frank consolidation or a more nodular pattern. Another caveat is associated with the situation in which fine, intralobular fibrosis is seen on HRCT as widespread ground-glass opacification; in this rare occurrence evidence of traction bronchiectasis is usually present within the areas of ground-glass opacification.

The ability of CT to show differences among various patterns of disease has clarified the reasons for the sometimes complex mixed obstructive and restrictive functional deficits found in some diffuse lung diseases. A good example is hypersensitivity pneumonitis, in which both interstitial and small-airway disease coexist; patterns caused by these different pathologic processes can be readily seen on HRCT scans. The extent of the various HRCT patterns correlates with the expected functional indices of restriction and obstruction. Other conditions in which CT is able to tease out the morphologic abnormalities responsible for complex functional deficits include fibrosing alveolitis with coexisting emphysema and sarcoidosis, in which interstitial fibrosis may exist in combination with small-airway obstruction by peribronchiolar granulomata.

In patients in whom lung biopsy is deemed necessary, HRCT may be invaluable for determination of which type of biopsy procedure is likely to be successful in obtaining diagnostic material. The broad distinction between peripheral disease and central and bronchocentric disease is easily made on HRCT examination. Disease with a subpleural distribution, such as fibrosing alveolitis, is most unlikely to be sampled by transbronchial biopsy, whereas diseases in which a bronchocentric distribution is revealed on HRCT, such as sarcoidosis and lymphangitis carcinomatosa, are consistently accessible to transbronchial biopsy. In patients in whom an open or thoracoscopic lung biopsy is contemplated, HRCT assists in determining the optimal biopsy site. Pathologic examination of a lung biopsy specimen can still justifiably be regarded as the final arbiter for the presence or absence of subtle interstitial lung disease. Because HRCT images provide an in vivo "big picture," many lung pathologists now combine the imaging and pathologic information before assigning a final diagnosis, and in many centers the benefits of a team approach to the diagnosis of diffuse lung disease are recognized. The indications for HRCT that have been developed over the past 10 years are summarized in Table 1.2.

Magnetic Resonance Imaging and Magnetic Resonance Angiography

Plain radiographs, CT, ultrasound, contrast angiography, and isotope scanning form the mainstay of the imaging of thoracic diseases. Although MRI complements these techniques, it generally remains a problem-solving tool rather than a technique of first choice.

Table 1.2
Indications for high-resolution computed tomography of the lungs

Indications
Narrow the differential diagnosis or make a histospecific diagnosis in patients with obvious but nonspecific radiographic abnormalities
Detect diffuse lung disease in patients with normal or equivocal radiographic abnormalities
Elucidate unexpected pulmonary function test results
Investigate patients presenting with hemoptysis
Evaluate disease reversibility, particularly in patients who have fibrosing alveolitis
Guide the type and site of lung biopsy

MRI entails placing the subject in a very strong magnetic field (typically 0.2 to 1.5 tesla) and then irradiating the area under examination with pulses of radio waves. Anatomic MRI is dependent on the presence of water within tissue to produce the signal required for interpretation. Protons within this water exist within different local atomic environments, and consequently they have different properties. These differences can be exploited by sequence manipulation to generate differences in contrast between tissues in the final MRI scan. The frequency of the radio frequency pulse transmitted into the patient is carefully selected so that it causes hydrogen protons within water to be disturbed from the orientation they have assumed as a result of being placed inside the powerful magnetic field within the bore of the magnet. After the transient disturbance caused by the radio frequency pulse, these protons, which behave like small bar magnets, relax back into their original resting positions. As they do this they release energy in the form of another pulse of radio waves, which are detected by the receiver coils that are located in the wall of the bore of the magnet, or more commonly in a variety of receiver coils placed more directly around the area under investigation. The coils (frequently designated according to the body part being examined, e.g., knee coil, head coil, neck coil, body coil) are placed appropriately at the start of the examination. In the case of thoracic imaging the body coil usually is composed of a pair of coil mats placed in front of and behind the patient.

Historically the main strengths of MRI are the high intrinsic soft-tissue contrast generated, the lack of artifact from bone, the lack of ionizing radiation, and the ability to produce images in any chosen plane. The major weaknesses of MRI in the thorax have, until recently, been its susceptibility to image degradation resulting from respiratory and cardiac motion and the relatively long times required to perform an examination. In general the quality of MRI scans is related to the field strength of the scanner and the peak power and speed of the amplifiers that generate the interrogating radio frequency pulses.

For thoracic imaging, ECG triggering facilities, whereby the acquisition of imaging data can be coordinated with the cardiac cycle to reduce flow artifact, are essential. Various methods of compensation for respiratory motion have been developed. Some use external devices such as respiratory bellows, which detect movement of the chest wall, with data collection occurring when motion is at its least. Other methods are essentially software developments, which compensate for respiratory disruption of magnetic spins. Most of these techniques have been superseded on modern scanners by the ability to acquire images of the thorax while the patient applies breath-holding techniques.

MEDIASTINAL AND CHEST WALL IMAGING

The most common indication for MRI in respiratory disease is for imaging of neoplastic disease, most commonly bronchogenic carcinoma. In addition to the primary disease, secondary complications such as cerebral conditions, spinal metastases, and retroperitoneal fibrosis all lend themselves to MRI. MRI also allows assessment of invasion of mediastinal structures such as the major airways, heart and great vessels, chest wall, and diaphragm and allows differentiation among forms of soft tissue, fluid, hemorrhage, local hematoma, and aneurysms (Figs. 1.15 and 1.16). With modern multichannel CT,

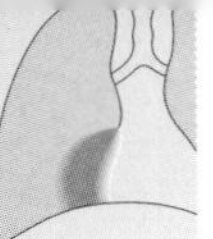

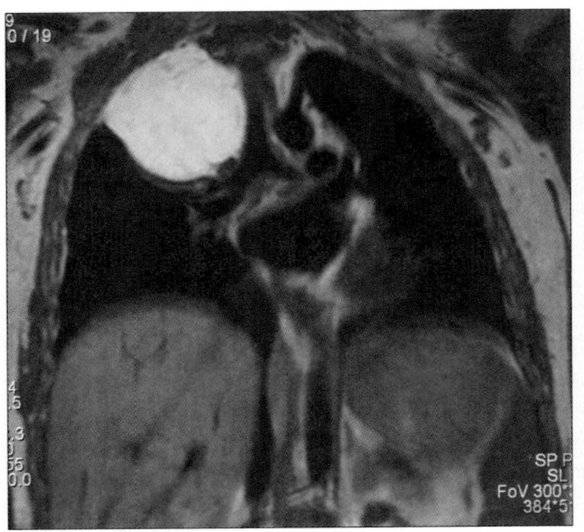

A

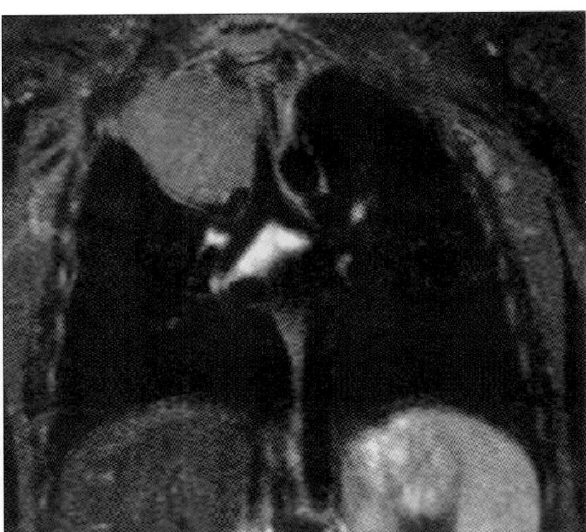

B

Figure 1.15 Right upper zone mass in an 11-year-old boy. **A,** A coronal T1-weighted sequence demonstrates a high–signal-intensity apical mass. **B,** With the addition of fat saturation and subsequent reduction in the signal returned from fat, the signal intensity in the mass falls significantly. This confirms the fatty nature of the mass, which is a large pleural lipoma.

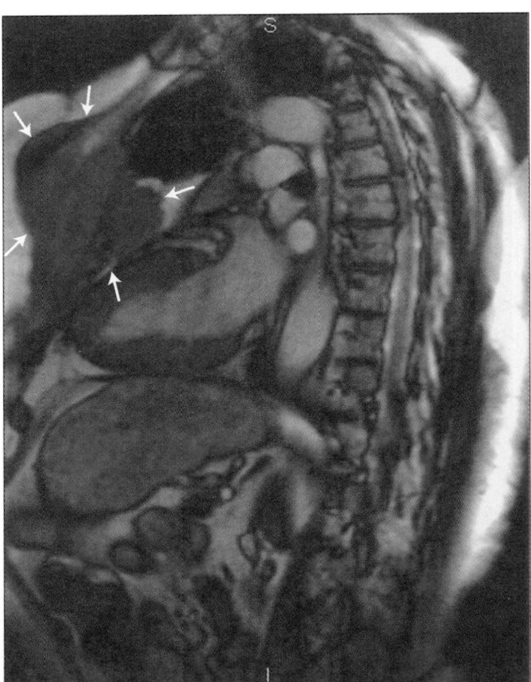

Figure 1.16 Chest wall invasion demonstrated with magnetic resonance imaging (MRI). Oblique sagittal T2-weighted image through the long axis of the left ventricle demonstrates an adjacent chest wall mass *(arrows)* extending through the interior chest wall into the overlying breast tissue. This was the result of recurrent breast carcinoma.

MRI has relatively little advantage over CT in assessment of chest wall invasion except in the case of superior sulcus tumors. MRI may be superior to CT for the assessment of diaphragmatic and mediastinal invasion (Fig. 1.17). However, in general, the clinical benefits of using MRI instead of CT are questionable, and commensurate improvements in outcome to compensate for the more lengthy and expensive procedure have not been shown.

LUNG PARENCHYMAL IMAGING

The lungs present an enormous challenge to MRI examiners for a number of reasons. First, they are constantly moving because of respiratory and cardiac motion. Second, because they have a low water content relative to other biological tissues, they have a low proton density and return relatively little signal. Third, because of the multiple interfaces between air and soft tissue, innumerable small disturbances exist in the magnetic field. This loss of homogeneity at air-tissue interfaces results in a phenomenon known as magnetic susceptibility artifact, which further reduces signal and increases noise. Therefore, with standard spin-echo sequences, normal lung exhibits little signal and is often obliterated by artifacts. Various attempts to tackle these problems by designing particular pulse sequences have met with little success during the past 10 to 15 years. Paradoxically the lack of signal from the lung may in some situations be an advantage, because abnormalities that contain relatively greater amounts of tissue water may become more obvious.

VENTILATION STUDIES

Another area of intense interest has been the use of polarized gases (helium 3 and xenon 129) to show pulmonary ventilation. With this technique a process of heating and irradiating with polarized light produces polarized gases. The gases (which have a short half-life) are inhaled and imaged by means of optimized sequences. The use of dual-frequency probes allows gas and proton images to be acquired and registered, enabling function and anatomy to be correlated.

MAGNETIC RESONANCE ANGIOGRAPHY

Magnetic resonance can also be used to demonstrate vascular anatomy by generation of contrast between flowing blood and stationary tissue, which may be achieved with or without intravenous magnetic resonance contrast agents. Generally the use of contrast media increases the signal returned from blood, increases the signal-to-noise ratio, and allows acquisition times to be shorter. Magnetic resonance angiography (MRA) can be used for observation of venous or arterial flow, together or separately (see Fig. 1.17).

The contrast agents used in magnetic resonance generally and MRA in particular are almost exclusively based on gadolinium chelates. Most are extracellular-space agents and cause shortening of the T1 relaxation time, thereby increasing the signal from the enhanced tissue on T1-weighted sequences. The distribution of these agents is very similar to the iodinated contrast agents used routinely in CT.

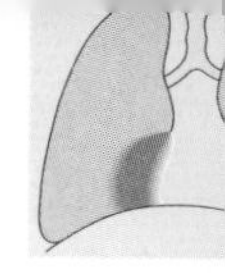

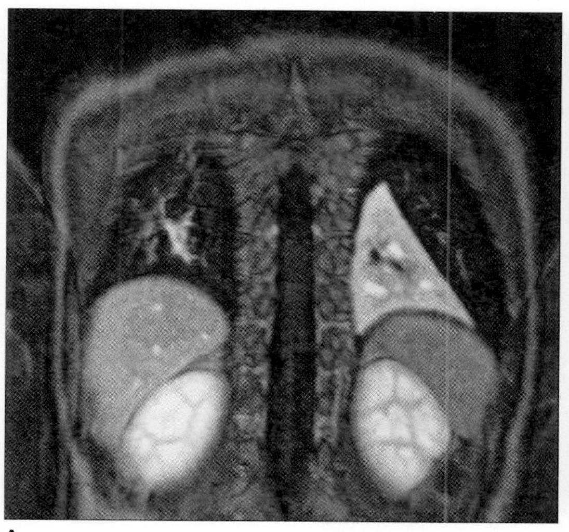

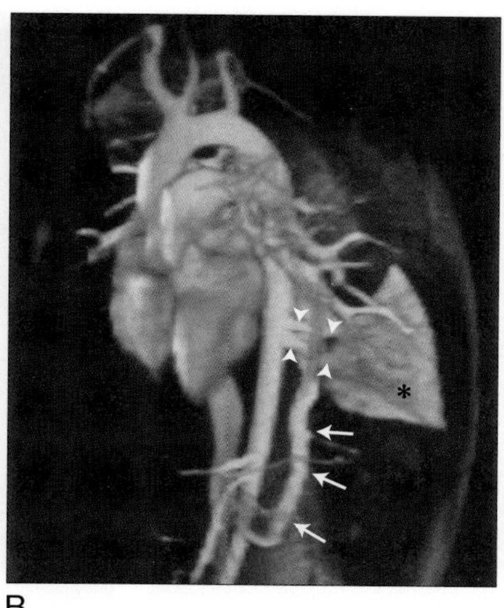

A B

Figure 1.17 Extralobar pulmonary sequestration. A, A coronal contrast-enhanced image with the patient's breath held demonstrates the avidly enhancing pulmonary sequestration at the left lung base. Note the clear plane between the triangular sequestrated segment and the diaphragm and underlying spleen. **B,** Volume rendered angiographic image demonstrating the same triangular sequestrated segment *(asterisk)* with two supplying branches from the aorta *(arrowheads)* and complex venous drainage. The largest vein drains subdiaphragmatically *(arrows)* into the left renal vein.

PULMONARY EMBOLI AND INFARCTION

At present, magnetic resonance is not routinely used in patients with suspected PE and infarction, but it has been the subject of much research. A number of published series have demonstrated that pulmonary MRA with the patient's breath held can now show fifth-order pulmonary vessels and allow diagnosis of emboli to segmental level. The presence of smaller pulmonary emboli can be inferred by lack of segmental and subsegmental perfusion. Three-dimensional MRA data sets can be acquired and displayed on work stations as moving projections, which can reveal areas of deficient perfusion.

VASCULAR MALFORMATIONS AND CONGENITAL ANOMALIES

Evidence is increasing that magnetic resonance can clearly define a number of vascular and developmental anomalies of the lungs by combining anatomic and flow imaging. These include the scimitar syndrome, hypogenetic lung syndrome, pulmonary artery agenesis, bronchopulmonary sequestration, and vascular malformations (see Fig. 1.17).

CARDIOVASCULAR IMAGING

Magnetic resonance is now regarded as the definitive technique for imaging the aorta for dissection and in the treatment of aneurysms and coarctation. Magnetic resonance is widely used for the assessment of congenital heart disease. It can also be used to assess cardiac anatomy and function, and software has been developed to allow rapid and accurate assessment of wall motion, ejection fraction, stress testing for reversible ischemia, hibernating myocardium, and valvular disease. The ultimate challenge, namely, the accurate imaging of the coronary arteries, is under intense investigation but is not yet practiced routinely. Nevertheless, MRI is now able to provide comprehensive noninvasive cardiac assessment that is likely to challenge more-established techniques such as nuclear medicine and echocardiography.

PET Scanning and PET Computed Tomography

Positron emission tomography (PET) has now been in clinical use for the past decade, and great interest has developed regarding the potential application of the technology. Availability remains significantly limited despite the apparent benefits of this technique, largely because of the cost and complexity of producing the short-lived isotopes and the expense of the PET imaging equipment itself. Nevertheless, in the United States PET now has approval for reimbursement from Medicare and Medicaid for certain conditions.

Most studies of PET relevant to chest pathology use a short–half-life radionuclide, flourine 18, which is incorporated into a molecule that mimics glucose metabolism, flourodeoxyglucose. This tracer is called 18F-flourodeoxyglucose, or 18F-FDG. Because cancer cells have altered glucose metabolism and consume glucose at far greater rates than normal cells, tracer activity is greatly increased in many cancers. This increased concentration of tracer activity can then be detected and directly or indirectly coregistered against conventional anatomic imaging studies. Although it is possible to perform PET scans using gamma camera coincidence imaging (GCI), this technology is inferior to full detector ring dedicated PET. Moreover, most of the research evidence produced has been based on this more-sophisticated full ring detector technology.

Lung cancer staging is one of the very few areas in which meaningful randomized trials of PET have been completed. These trials have demonstrated that PET studies will bring about a change in management in a significant number of patients, compared with a management plan derived from conventional staging.

Positron emission testing can be directly combined with a conventional CT study in the most current systems. These allow a multichannel CT examination to be conducted on the same gantry used for the full detector ring PET study, with the two data sets immediately coregistered to provide CT/PET fusion images (Fig. 1.18).

In the future, PET is likely to become a routine imaging tool in all cancer centers for early diagnosis, staging, and restaging of an increasing variety of cancers, and these applications are likely to use 85% to 90% of the work capacity of any given PET unit.

Pulmonary Angiography

Pulmonary angiography is used to investigate the pulmonary circulation when other, less-invasive methods have failed to provide the requisite information. The most frequent indication is for

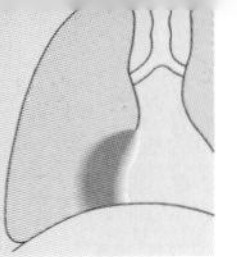

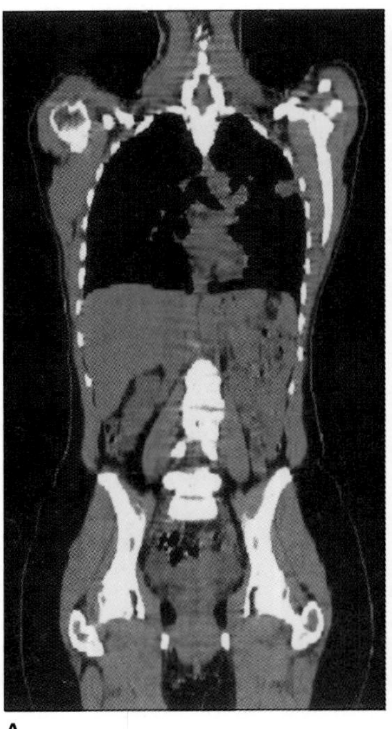

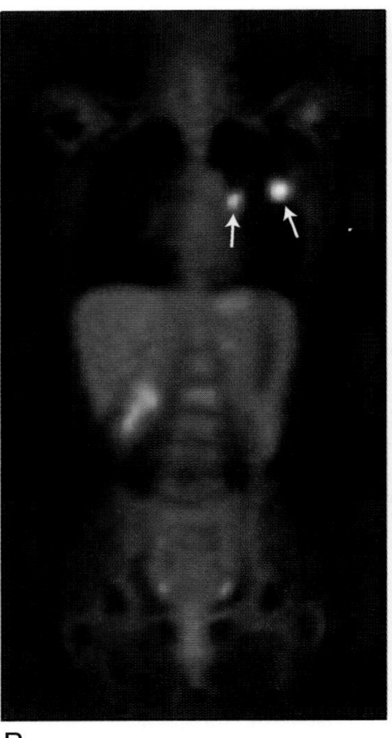

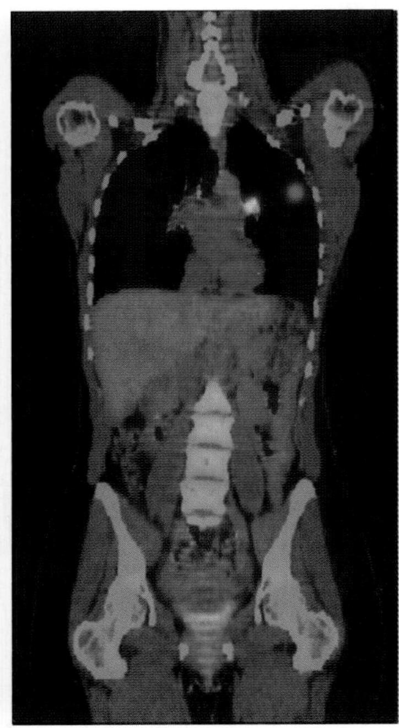

Figure 1.18 Combined computed tomography (CT) and positron emission tomography (PET) scans of a patient with a peripheral bronchiogenic carcinoma in the left lung and involved left hilar nodes. A, Coronal whole-body CT image demonstrating the peripheral lung nodule. **B,** Coronal whole-body PET image demonstrating intense signal activity within the nodule and within the left hilar node. **C,** CT/PET fusion image demonstrating both sets of data on a single image.

suspected PE, usually after a nondiagnostic ventilation-perfusion (V/Q) scan. Ideally the angiogram is undertaken within 24 hours of acute presentation of a patient with suspected embolism. However, a delay of 48 to 72 hours should not preclude the use of pulmonary angiography, although the diagnostic yield progressively declines because of fragmentation of thrombi over time, especially if anticoagulation has been instituted.

Pulmonary angiography is a technique that tends to be underused for a variety of reasons. Apart from the expense and relatively invasive nature of angiography, it is perceived to have a high complication rate (although this is not supported by the published evidence). The mean imbalance between the number of times V/Q scan and angiography are performed is striking, and it has been estimated that only one angiogram is requested for every 100 V/Q scans. This is a ratio that flatters the diagnostic abilities of V/Q scanning, which in most series yields an equivocal result in 30% to 60% of patients. The frequently quoted complications of angiography, namely respiratory compromise, arrhythmia, renal failure, and transient hypersensitivity reactions, are based on historical data that suggested a mortality rate of up to 0.5%, a major nonfatal complication rate of 1%, and a minor complication rate of 5%. More recent evaluation suggests that pulmonary angiography is much safer. This improvement is attributed predominantly to the change from ionic contrast media to low, osmolar nonionic agents. In addition, the use of more flexible, small-gauge pigtail catheters has reduced the incidence of myocardial injury.

The technique of pulmonary angiography involves fluoroscopically directed insertion of a guide wire, followed by a modified pigtail catheter into the right and left main pulmonary arteries in turn, with injection of a nonionic contrast agent at an appropriate flow rate. At least two views per side are required, with additional oblique or magnification views as necessary. Catheter access is usually via the femoral vein, with the internal jugular and subclavian veins as possible alternatives. Despite

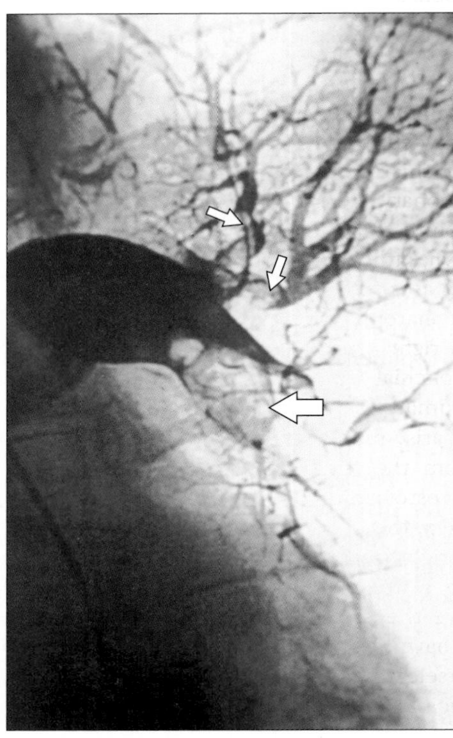

Figure 1.19 Digital subtraction pulmonary angiogram. A large thrombus causes a filling defect within the contrast in the artery of the left lower lobe *(large arrow)*. Smaller thrombi are present within the proximal branches to the upper lobe *(small arrows)*.

the desirable high resolution of conventional film-screen angiography, most departments now undertake angiography with digital subtraction vascular equipment (Fig. 1.19). Problems with misregistration artifacts, inherent in digital subtraction systems and caused by respiratory or cardiac cycle-phase differences between the mask image and the contrast image, can usually be overcome by the acquisition of a series of mask views before contrast medium is injected. Crossing of the tricuspid valve may induce an arrhythmia that is usually transient. Therefore, ECG monitoring is mandatory, and the use of prophylactic, antiarrhythmic agents or temporary pacing-wire insertion is common practice in some centers.

When a pulmonary embolus is present, it most frequently is situated in the posterior segments of the lower lobe. Thrombi beyond the segmental vessel level are detected less reliably than more central thrombi. However, the significance of thrombi confined to subsegmental vessels is unclear. The typical angiographic findings of PE are vascular cutoff or, when vascular occlusion is not complete, an intraluminal filling defect with the passage of contrast medium around and beyond the clot. Indirect signs of embolism include areas of relatively delayed or reduced perfusion, late filling of the venous circulation, and vessel tortuosity. When the angiogram is undertaken to investigate suspected chronic thromboembolic disease, the vascular changes include local stenosis or thin webs, luminal ectasia, and irregularities in the normal tapering pattern.

The high threshold for proceeding to pulmonary angiography when the diagnosis of PE remains in doubt has been central to the developing role of contrast-enhanced spiral CT scanning in the diagnosis of PE.

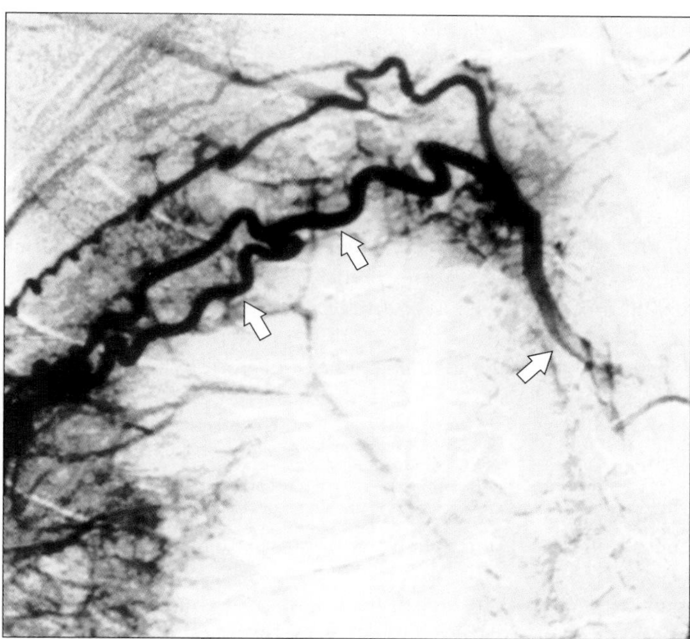

Figure 1.20 Bronchial arteriogram in a patient with hemoptysis. Marked hypertrophy of the intercostal and bronchial arteries is present *(arrows)*. These changes were caused by chronic thromboembolic disease.

Bronchial Artery Embolization

Bronchial artery embolization is usually performed to stop massive hemoptysis in patients who are not suitable candidates for surgical management. The most common causes of bronchial artery hypertrophy and consequent hemorrhage are suppurative lung diseases (particularly bronchiectasis) and fibrocavitary disease that involves mycetomas. Less-common causes of hemorrhage from the bronchial circulation include bronchial carcinoma, chronic pulmonary abscess, and congenital cyanotic heart disease. No absolute contraindications to bronchial artery embolization are known, although the patient should be hemodynamically stable and able to cooperate.

The most common anatomic arrangement on bronchial arteriography is one main right bronchial artery that arises from a common intercostobronchial trunk, which comes off the thoracic aorta at approximately the level of T5, and two left bronchial arteries that arise more inferiorly. However, bronchial arteries may arise from the thyrocervical trunk, the internal mammary artery, the costocervical trunk, the subclavian artery, a lower intercostal artery, the inferior phrenic artery, or even the abdominal aorta. The right intercostal bronchial trunk takes off from the aorta at an acute upward angle, whereas the left bronchial arteries leave the aorta more or less at right angles, and special catheters have been designed to facilitate selective catheterization. Superselective catheterization of the bronchial circulation allows precise delivery of embolic material and so prevents spillover into the aorta or inadvertent embolization of the spinal artery.

Fiberoptic bronchoscopy is often advocated before bronchial artery embolization to establish the site of hemorrhage. However, a large hemoptysis almost invariably results in vigorous coughing, and so blood is spread throughout the bronchial tree, which makes localization impossible. Few criteria exist to determine which angiographically demonstrated bronchial arteries should be embolized. Guidelines are particularly relevant when several bronchial arteries have been identified and the site of hemorrhage is not obvious based on prior thoracic imaging. Embolization is directed at the vessels considered most likely to be the source of hemorrhage (Fig. 1.20). Bronchial arteries of diameter >3 mm are considered pathologically enlarged. In patients with diffuse, suppurative lung disease, most commonly cystic fibrosis, attempts are made to embolize all significantly enlarged bronchial arteries bilaterally. If no abnormal bronchial arteries are identified, a systematic search is made for aberrant bronchial arteries. When a patient continues to have hemoptysis after embolization of all suspicious systemic arteries, it may be necessary to investigate the pulmonary circulation for a source of hemorrhage.

A variety of embolic materials has been used for the embolization of bronchial arteries, ranging from particles of polyvinyl foam to small pieces of Gelfoam. Although coils lodged proximally in the bronchial artery have been used, they prevent subsequent catheterization.

After bronchial artery embolization, many patients experience transient fever and chest pain; after 2 days some patients cough up a small amount of blood, which possibly arises from limited infarction of the bronchial mucosa. Serious complications after bronchial artery embolization are rare, the most serious being transverse myelitis, probably caused by contrast toxicity rather than inadvertent embolization. Inadvertent spillover of embolization material into the thoracic aorta may cause distant ischemia in the legs or abdominal organs.

The aim of bronchial artery embolization is the immediate control of life-threatening hemoptysis, which is achieved in more than 75% of patients. Failures usually result from nonidentification of significant bronchial arteries and an inability to maintain the catheter position and proceed to embolization. Up to 20% of patients rebleed within 6 months of an initially successful bronchial artery embolization. The reasons cited for recurrent hemorrhage are recanalization of previously embolized vessels, incomplete initial embolization, and hypertrophy of

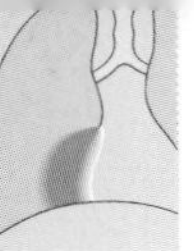

small bronchial arteries not initially embolized. However, bronchial artery embolization usually can be satisfactorily repeated in patients who rebleed.

Superior Vena Cava Stents

Superior vena cava obstruction (SVCO) is characterized by facial and upper limb swelling, headache, and shortness of breath and is usually caused by advanced mediastinal malignancy. Conventional palliative treatment relies on radiotherapy, chemotherapy, and sometimes surgery. Radiotherapy usually produces an initial improvement, although subsequent recurrence of symptoms is frequent. Balloon angioplasty of both benign and malignant causes of SVCO has been reported, but, as might be expected, symptoms are liable to recur soon after angioplasty alone.

The percutaneous placement of metallic stents for the treatment of SVCO has several attractions. With increasing experience, clinicians report reliable and successful palliation of SVCO with the use of stents of various designs. A superior venacavogram is necessary to identify the length of the stenosis and its site in relation to the confluence of the brachiocephalic veins and the right atrium. Identification of an intraluminal thrombus or tumor is an absolute contraindication to the procedure. After balloon dilatation of the superior vena cava stricture, the stent is positioned across the stricture and a postplacement venacavogram is performed to confirm free flow of blood into the right atrium (Fig. 1.21). After angioplasty and stent placement, relief of SVCO symptoms is usually rapid and dramatic. Recurrence of symptoms may be caused by venous thrombosis or tumor progression distal to the stent. Although rupture of the superior vena cava at the time of angioplasty is a risk, this complication seems to be extremely rare, possibly because of the tamponade provided by surrounding tumor or postirradiation fibrosis.

The role of intravascular stents in nonmalignant SVCO has not yet been defined. Patients with SVCO caused by benign fibrosing mediastinitis have been treated successfully, although occlusion of the stent by the progression of the mediastinal fibrosis or by endothelial proliferation may occur.

NORMAL RADIOGRAPHIC ANATOMY

Mediastinum and Hilar Structures

The mediastinum is delineated by the lungs on both sides, the thoracic inlet above, the diaphragm below, and the vertebral column posteriorly. Because the various structures that make up the mediastinum are superimposed on one another, they cannot be separately identified on a two-dimensional chest radiograph; for this reason the normal anatomy of the individual components of the mediastinum is considered in more detail in the section on CT of the mediastinum. Nevertheless, because a chest radiograph is usually the first imaging investigation, the clinician must be able to identify the normal appearance of the mediastinum and the considerable possible variations that result from the patient's body habitus and age.

The mediastinum is conventionally divided into superior, anterior, middle, and posterior compartments (Fig. 1.22). Some texts add a superior compartment. The practical purpose of these arbitrary divisions is related to the fact that specific mediastinal pathologies show a definite predilection for individual compartments (e.g., a superior mediastinal mass is most frequently caused by intrathoracic extension of the thyroid gland; a middle mediastinal mass usually results from enlarged lymph nodes). However, localization of a mass within one of these compartments does not normally allow a specific diagnosis to be made, nor do the arbitrary boundaries preclude disease from involving more than one compartment.

Only the outline of the mediastinum and the air-containing trachea and bronchi (and sometimes the esophagus) are clearly seen on a normal PA chest radiograph. On a chest radiograph, the right brachiocephalic vein and superior vena cava form the right superior mediastinal border. This border is usually vertical

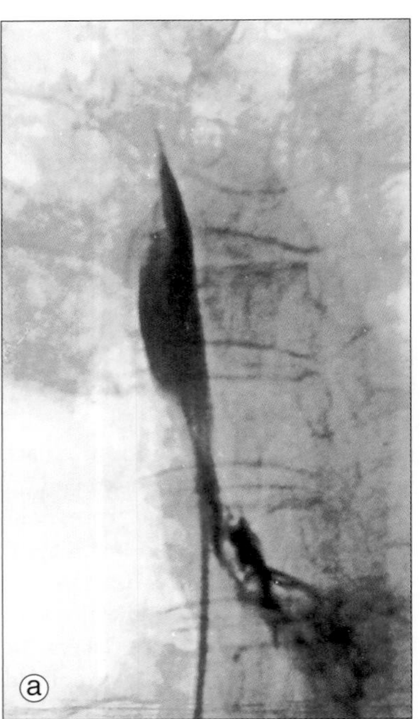

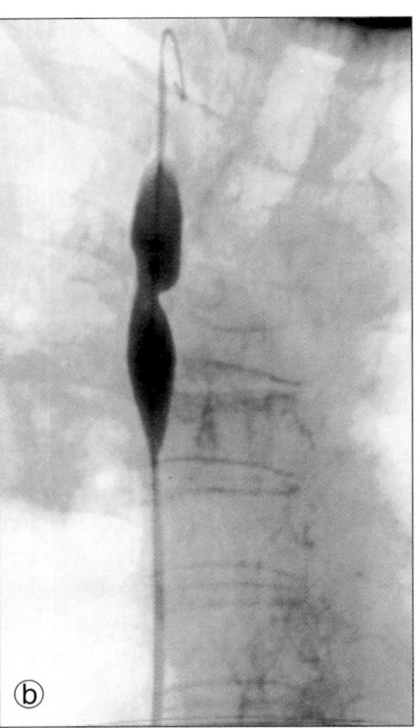

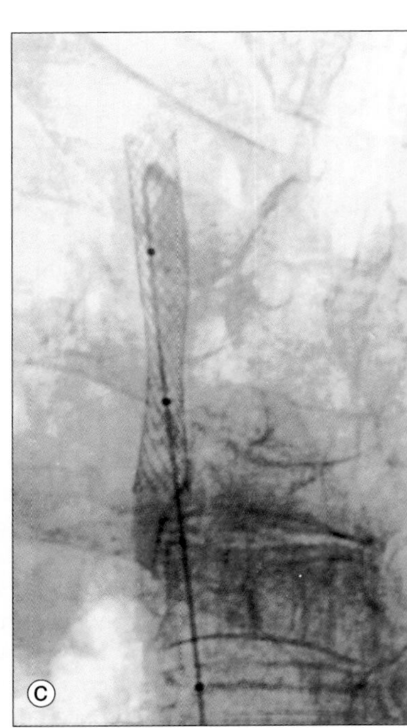

Figure 1.21 Stenting of superior vena cava obstruction (SVCO). The patient had a SVCO caused by mediastinal malignancy. **A,** Superior venacavogram showing a tight stricture in the mid-superior vena cava. **B,** Balloon dilatation of the stricture. **C,** Placement of a meshed-wire stent in the patent superior vena cava.

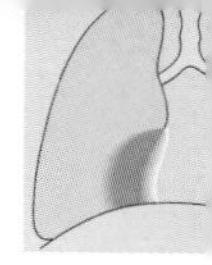

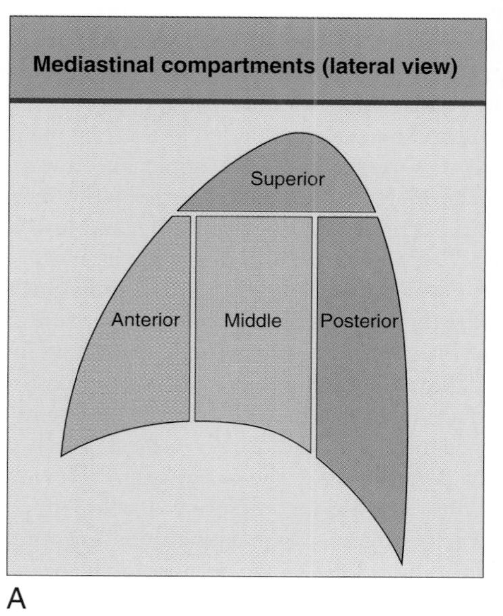

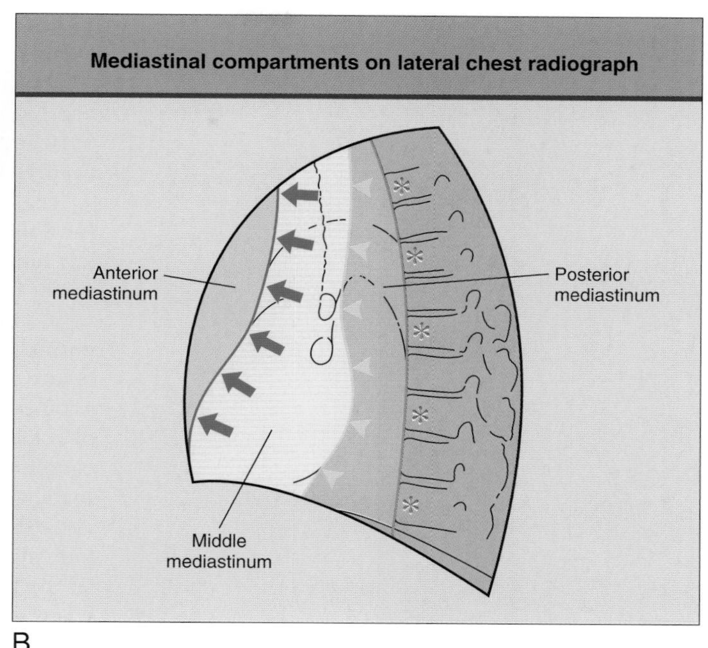

Figure 1.22 The mediastinal compartmental divisions. A, Arbitrary division of the mediastinum into superior, anterior, middle, and posterior compartments. **B,** An alternative scheme omits the superior mediastinal compartment. The area posterior to the sternum and anterior to the heart and great vessels *(arrows)* defines the anterior mediastinum in both cases. Likewise, a line placed along the posterior aspect of the trachea and heart *(arrowheads)* defines the middle from the posterior mediastinum, which is defined posteriorly by the vertebrae *(asterisks)*.

and straight (in contrast to the situation in which right paratracheal lymphadenopathy exists, where the right superior mediastinal border tends to be undulate), and it becomes less distinct as it reaches the thoracic inlet. The right side of the superior mediastinum can appear considerably widened in patients who have an abundance of mediastinal fat (Fig. 1.23); these individuals often have prominent cardiophrenic fat pads. The mediastinal border to the left of the trachea above the aortic arch is the result of summation of the left carotid and left subclavian arteries, together with the left brachiocephalic and jugular veins. The left cardiac border comprises the left atrial appendage, which merges inferiorly with the left ventricle. The silhouette of the heart should always be sharply outlined. Any blurring of the border results from loss of immediately adjacent aerated lung, usually because of collapse or consolidation.

The densities of the heart shadow to the left and to the right of the vertebral column should be identical; any difference indicates pathology (e.g., an area of consolidation or a mass in a lower lobe). On a well-penetrated film, a density with a convex lateral border is frequently seen through the right heart border. This apparent mass is caused by the confluence of the right pulmonary veins as they enter the left atrium and is of no clinical significance.

The trachea and main bronchi should be visible through the upper and middle mediastinum. The trachea is rarely straight and often lies to the right of the midline at its midpoint. In older individuals, the trachea may be markedly displaced by a dilated aortic arch below. In approximately 60% of normal subjects the right wall of the trachea (the right paratracheal stripe) can be identified as a line of uniform thickness (<4 mm in width); when visible, it excludes the presence of any adjacent space-occupying lesion, usually lymphadenopathy. The angle between the main bronchi, which forms the carina, is usually somewhat less than 80 degrees. Splaying of the carina is a relatively crude sign of subcarinal disease, either in the form of a massive subcarinal lymphadenopathy or a markedly enlarged left atrium. A more-sensitive sign of subcarinal disease is obscuration of the upper part of the azygoesophageal line, which is usually visible in its entirety on a well-penetrated chest radiograph (Fig. 1.24). The origins of the lobar bronchi, when they are projected over the mediastinal shadow, can usually be identified, but segmental bronchi within the lungs generally are not seen on plain radiography.

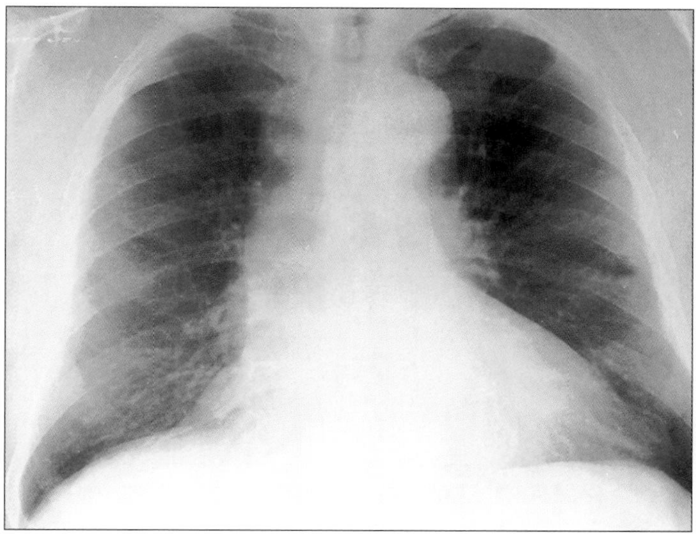

Figure 1.23 Widening of the superior mediastinum caused by abundance of mediastinal fat. In addition, bilateral cardiophrenic fat pads are present.

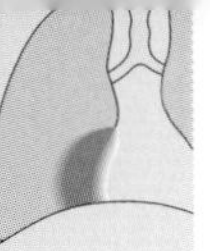

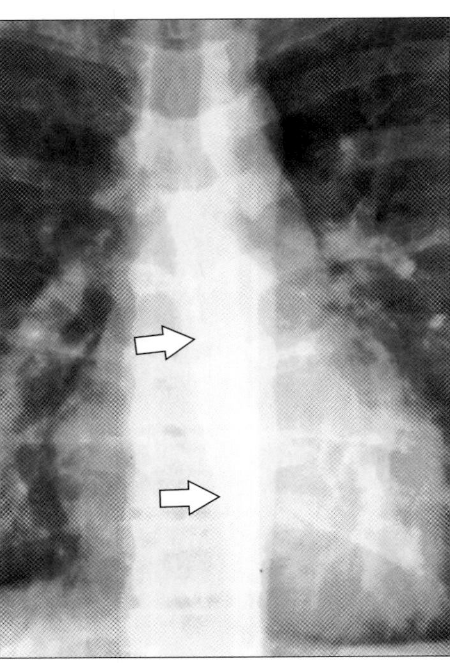

Figure 1.24 Amber chest radiograph. The normal azygoesophageal line is demonstrated *(arrows)*.

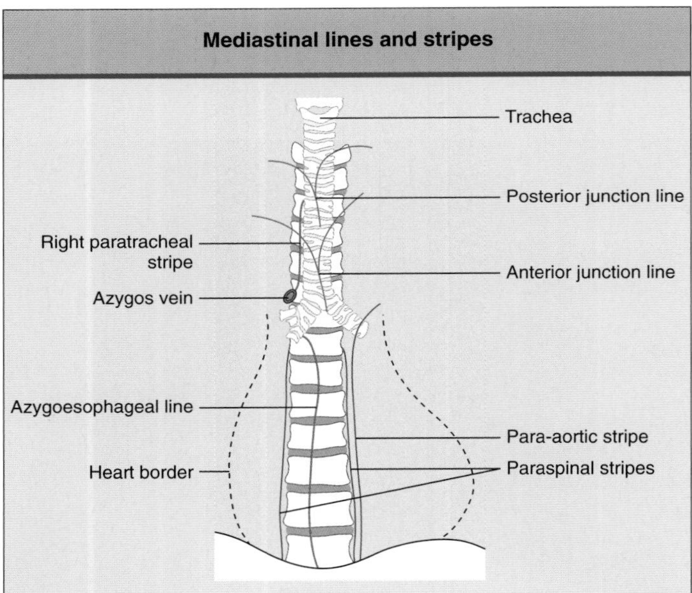

Figure 1.25 Some of the mediastinal lines and stripes frequently seen on a frontal chest radiograph.

The normal hilar shadows on a chest radiograph represent the summation of the pulmonary arteries and veins, with little contribution from the overlying bronchial walls or lymph nodes of normal size. The hila are approximately the same size, and the left hilum normally lies between 0.5 cm and 1.5 cm above the level of the right hilum. The size and shape of the hila show remarkable variations among normal individuals, making subtle abnormalities difficult to identify.

Pulmonary Fissures, Vessels, and Bronchi

The two lungs are separated by the four layers of pleura behind and in front of the mediastinum. The resultant posterior and anterior junction lines are often visible on frontal chest radiographs as nearly vertical stripes, with the posterior junction line lying higher than the anterior (Fig. 1.25). Because these junction lines are not invariably seen (their visibility is largely dependent on whether the pleural reflections are tangential to the x-ray beam), their presence or absence is not usually of significance.

The lobes of lung are surrounded by visceral pleura; the major (or oblique) fissure separates the upper and lower lobes of the left lung. The major fissure and the minor (horizontal or transverse) fissure separate the upper, middle, and lower lobes of the right lung. The minor fissure is visible in more than half of normal PA chest radiographs. In normal individuals, the minor fissure is slightly bowed upward and runs horizontally; any deviation from this configuration is usually caused by loss of volume of a lobe. The major fissures are not visible on a frontal radiograph and are inconsistently identifiable on lateral radiographs. Inability to detect a fissure usually indicates that the fissure is not exactly in the line of the x-ray beam. However, in a few individuals, fissures are incompletely developed, a point familiar to thoracic surgeons who sometimes encounter difficulty when performing a lobectomy because of incomplete cleavage between lobes. Accessory fissures are occasionally seen (e.g., in the left lung a minor fissure can be present that separates the lingula from the remainder of the upper lobe).

All of the branching structures seen within normal lungs on a chest radiograph are pulmonary arteries or veins. The pulmonary veins may sometimes be differentiated from the pulmonary arteries; the superior pulmonary veins have a distinctly vertical course. However, it is often impossible to differentiate arteries from veins in the lung periphery. On a chest radiograph taken with the patient in the erect position, a gradual increase in the diameter of the vessels is seen, at equidistant points from the hilum, traveling from lung apex to base; this gravity-dependent effect disappears if the patient is supine or in cardiac failure.

The lobes of the lung are divided into segments, each of which is supplied by its own segmental pulmonary artery and accompanying bronchus. The walls of the segmental bronchi are rarely seen on the chest radiograph, except when the patient is lying parallel with the x-ray beam (in which case they are seen end-on as ring shadows that measure up to 8 mm in diameter). The most frequently identified segmental airways are the anterior segmental bronchi of the upper lobes.

Diaphragm and Thoracic Cage

The interface between aerated lung and the hemidiaphragms is sharp, and the highest point of each dome is normally medial to the midclavicular line. The right dome of the diaphragm is higher than the left by up to 2 cm in the erect position, unless the left dome is elevated by air in the stomach. Laterally, the hemidiaphragm forms an acute angle with the chest wall. Filling in or blunting of these costophrenic angles usually represents pleural disease—either pleural thickening or an effusion. In the elderly, localized humps on the dome of the diaphragm, particularly posteriorly (thus most obvious on a lateral radiograph) are common and indicate minor weaknesses or defects of the diaphragm. Interposition of the colon in front of the right lobe of the liver is a frequently seen normal variant (so-called Chilaiditi syndrome).

Apparent pleural thickening along the lateral chest wall in the midzones is a frequent observation in obese individuals; this thickening is caused by the bulging inward of subpleural fat. Deformities of the thoracic cage may cause distortion of the normal mediastinum and so simulate disease. One of the most common deformities is pectus excavatum, which, by compressing the heart between the depressed sternum and vertebral column, causes displacement of the apparently enlarged heart to the left and blurring of the right heart border (Fig. 1.26). A similar appearance may arise from an unusually straight thoracic spine, referred to as *straight back syndrome* (Fig. 1.27).

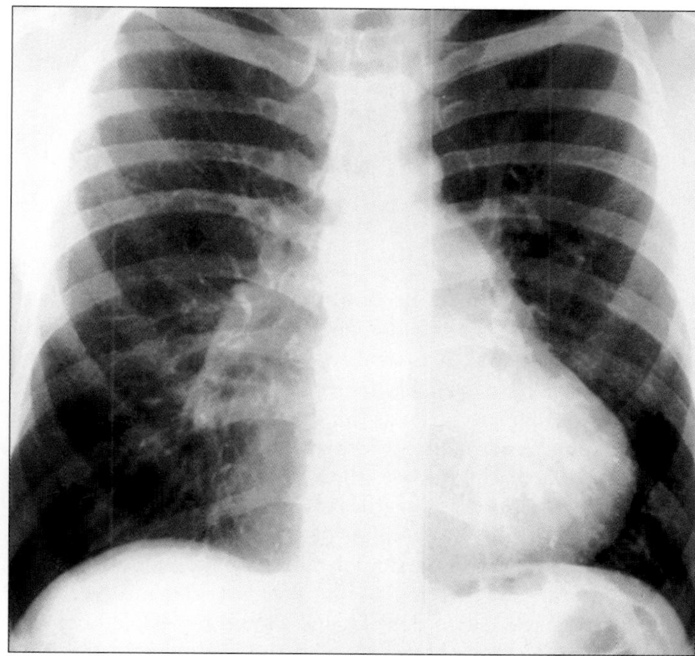

Figure 1.26 Frontal chest radiograph of a patient who has marked pectus excavatum. The blurring of the right heart border and apparent increase in heart size are a direct consequence of a depressed sternum. Note the '7' configuration of the ribs.

Anatomy on the Lateral Chest Radiograph

Consistent viewing of lateral chest radiographs in the same orientation, whether a right or left lateral projection, improves the ability to detect deviations from normal. In the lateral view, the trachea is angled slightly posteriorly as it runs toward the carina, and its posterior wall is always visible as a fine stripe (Fig. 1.28). The posterior walls of the right main bronchus and the right intermediate bronchus are outlined by air and are also seen as a continuous stripe on the lateral radiograph. The overlying scapulae are invariably seen running almost vertically in the upper part of the lateral radiograph (and may be misinterpreted as intrathoracic structures). Additional confusing shadows are formed by the soft tissues of the outstretched arms, which project over the upper mediastinum. The carina is not visible as such on the lateral radiograph, and the two transradiancies projected over the lower trachea represent the right main bronchus (superiorly) and the left main bronchus (inferiorly).

Overlying structures on a lateral radiograph obscure most of the lung. In normal individuals, the unobscured lung in the retrosternal and retrocardiac regions should be of the same transradiancy. Furthermore, as the gaze travels down the spine, a gradual increase in transradiancy should be apparent. The loss of this phenomenon suggests the presence of disease in the posterior-basal segments of the lower lobes (e.g., fibrosing alveolitis; Fig. 1.29).

The two major fissures are seen as diagonal lines, of a hair's breadth, that run from the upper dorsal spine to the anterior surface of the diaphragm. Care must be taken not to confuse the obliquely running rib edges with fissures. The minor fissure extends horizontally from the mid-right major fissure. Often, the confident differentiation of the right from the left major fissure is not possible. Similarly, although the two hemidiaphragms may be identified individually (especially if the gastric bubble is visible under the left dome of the diaphragm), differentiation between the right and the left hemidiaphragms is often impossible. A useful sign is the relative heights of the two

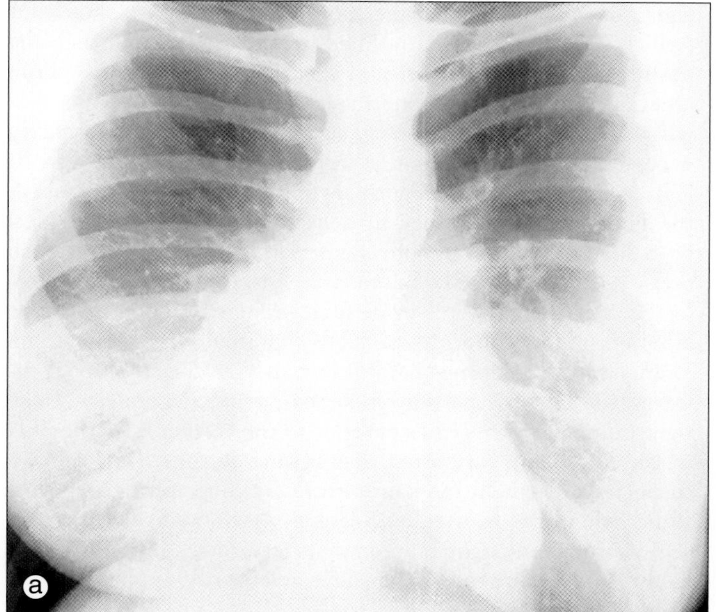

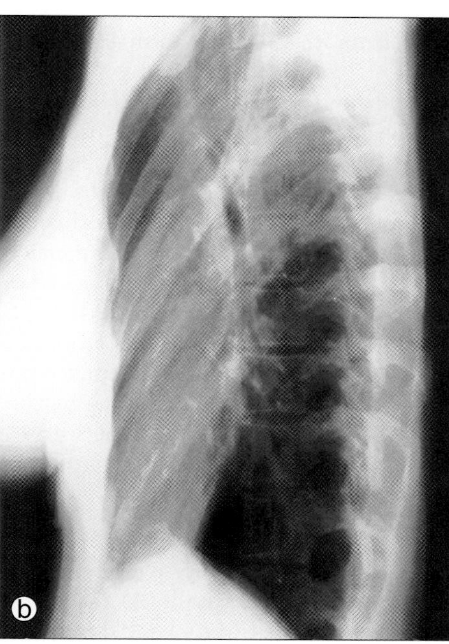

Figure 1.27 The effect of a straight spine. A, Loss of the right heart border. **B,** The loss is caused by complete lack of the normal spinal kyphosis, which results in a reduction of the anteroposterior diameter of the chest.

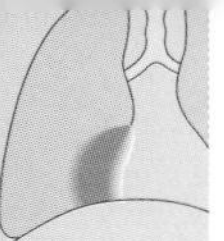

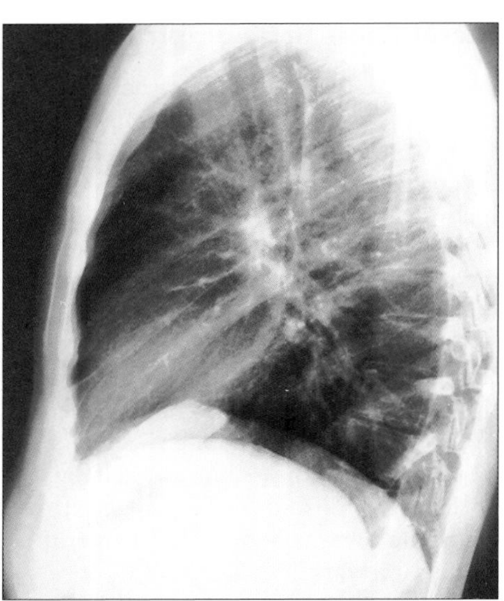

Figure 1.28 The lateral radiograph in a normal subject.

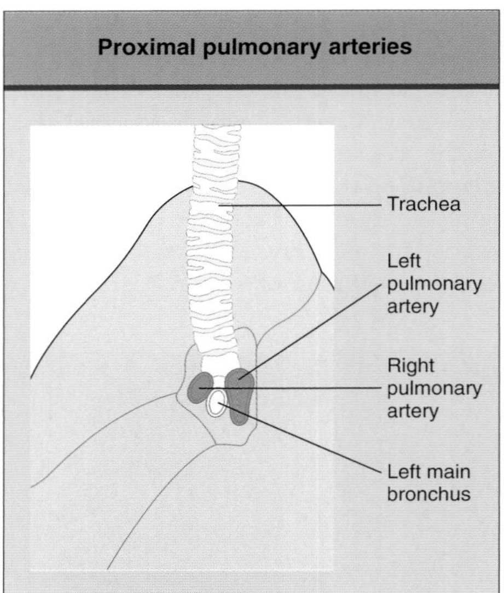

Figure 1.30 The position of proximal pulmonary arteries as shown on a lateral chest radiograph.

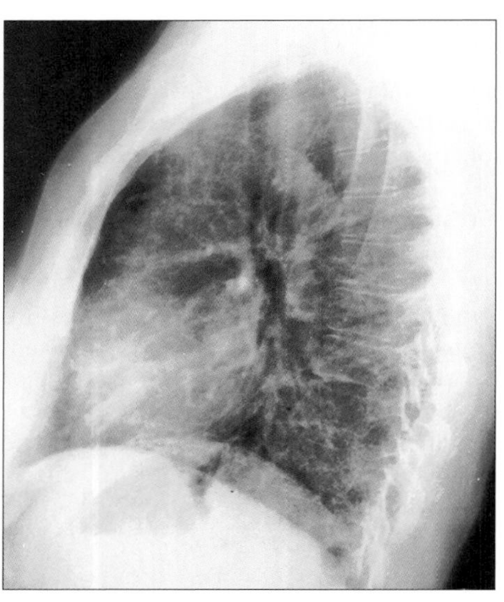

Figure 1.29 Loss of the normal increase in transradiancy toward the lower part of the dorsal spine in a patient with fibrosing alveolitis.

domes; the dome farthest from the film is normally higher because of magnification.

The summation of both hila on the lateral radiograph generates a complex shadow. However, one general point is useful in the interpretation of radiographs of this difficult area: the right pulmonary artery lies anterior to the trachea and right main bronchus, whereas the left pulmonary artery arches over the left main bronchus so that a large part of it lies posterior to the major bronchi (Fig. 1.30).

A bandlike opacity is often seen along the lower third of the anterior chest wall behind the sternum. It represents a normal density and occurs because less-aerated lung is in contact with the chest wall as a result of the occupation of the space by the heart. This opacity should not be confused with pleural disease.

POINTS IN THE INTERPRETATION OF A CHEST RADIOGRAPH

Even when an obvious radiographic abnormality is present, the chest radiograph must be reviewed systematically. As the interpreter gains increasing experience, identification of deviations from normal appearances becomes rapid, which leads quickly to a directed search for related abnormalities. Before a chest radiograph is interpreted, it is vital to establish whether any previous radiographs are available for comparison; the sequence and pattern of change are often as important as the identification of a radiographic abnormality. Information gained from earlier radiographs, particularly if they show that no serial change has occurred, often prevents needless further investigation.

A check that the radiograph is of satisfactory quality includes an estimation of the adequacy of radiographic exposure, depth of inspiration, and position of the patient. The intervertebral disc spaces of the entire dorsal spine should be visible on a correctly exposed chest radiograph, and the midpoint of the right hemidiaphragm lies at the level of the anterior end of the sixth rib if the (normal) subject has taken a satisfactory breath. The medial ends of the clavicles should be equidistant from the spinous processes of the cervical vertebral bodies.

The order in which the various parts of a chest radiograph are examined is unimportant. A suggested sequence is to first check the position of the trachea, then the mediastinal contour (which should be sharply outlined in its entirety), and then the position, outline, and density of the hilar shadows. The certain identification of a hilar abnormality often requires comparison with a previous radiograph; any suspicion of a hilar abnormality necessitates the retrieval of any previous chest radiographs. At least as important as an abnormal contour in detecting a mass at the hilum is a discrepancy in density between the two sides; both hilar shadows, at equivalent points, should be of equal density, and a mass at the hilum (or an intrapulmonary mass projected over the hilum) is evident as an increased density of the affected hilum. For a questionably abnormal hilum, the lateral radiograph is sometimes helpful in clarifying the situation, providing the normal anatomy is kept in mind (i.e., most of the right pulmonary artery lies anterior to the trachea, and the bulk of the left pulmonary artery lies behind the trachea). Thus, a suspected right hilar mass on a frontal radiograph that appears to be behind the trachea on a lateral view is unlikely to represent a prominent right pulmonary artery and is therefore most likely to be an abnormal mass (the converse rule applies to a suspicious left hilum).

Table 1.3
Causes of consolidation

Common	Rare
Infection	Allergic lung diseases
Infarction	Connective tissue diseases
Cardiogenic pulmonary edema	Drug reactions
Noncardiogenic pulmonary edema	Hemorrhage
Adult respiratory distress syndrome	Lymphoma
Neurogenic edema	Radiation
Drug-induced edema	Amyloid
Miscellaneous	Eosinophilic lung disease
	Sarcoid
	Alveolar proteinosis

The lungs may then be examined in terms of their size, the relative transradiancy of each zone, and the position of the horizontal fissure. Pulmonary vessels are seen as far out as the outer third of the lung, and the number of vessels should be roughly symmetrical on the two sides. Next, the position and clarity of the hemidiaphragms should be noted, followed by an assessment of the ribs and soft tissues of the chest wall. Before a chest radiograph is regarded as normal, areas that are poorly demonstrated or sometimes misinterpreted should be reviewed; these include the central mediastinum (where even a large mass may be invisible on the PA view); the lungs behind the diaphragm and heart; the lung apices (often obscured by the overlying clavicles and ribs); and the lung and pleura just inside the chest wall.

Radiographic Signs

CONSOLIDATION

Consolidation, or air-space shadowing, is caused by opacification of the air-containing spaces of the lung. The causes of consolidation are numerous (Table 1.3) and include almost any pathologic process that results in the filling of the normal alveolar spaces and small airways. The responsible material is almost invariably of fluid density, and usually the volume of the displacing fluid equals the volume of air displaced. This normally results in no net change in size of the lobar anatomy. Typically the radiologic appearances do not reveal what has caused the air-space filling, especially in the absence of a clinical history. The possible exception to this generalization is air-space shadowing resulting from cardiogenic alveolar edema, when associated signs of congestive cardiac failure are found. When analyzing an area of pulmonary opacification, the presence of a number of radiologic characteristics allows the confident characterization of air-space shadowing.

Typically, the shadowing is ill-defined, except where it directly abuts a pleural surface (including the interlobar fissures), in which case it is sharply demarcated (Fig. 1.31). Although consolidation respects lobar boundaries, there are no such barriers that prevent spread into adjacent lung segments, which are frequently contiguously involved. Thus, an area of consolidation within a single lobe often enlarges in an irregular manner, and a discrete, well-defined opacity (so-called "round pneumonia") is the exception and not the rule (Fig. 1.32).

The vascular markings within an area of consolidation usually become obscured, as the contrast between the air-containing

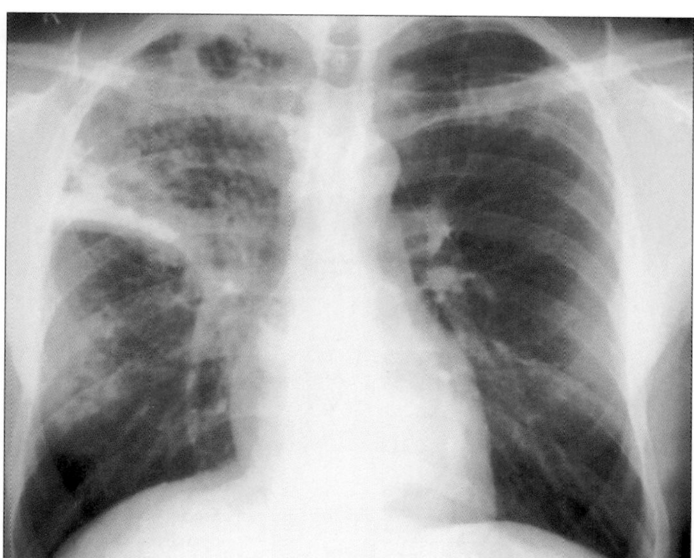

Figure 1.31 Patchy consolidation caused by tuberculosis. Where this abuts the horizontal fissure, the inferior surface of the consolidation is sharply defined.

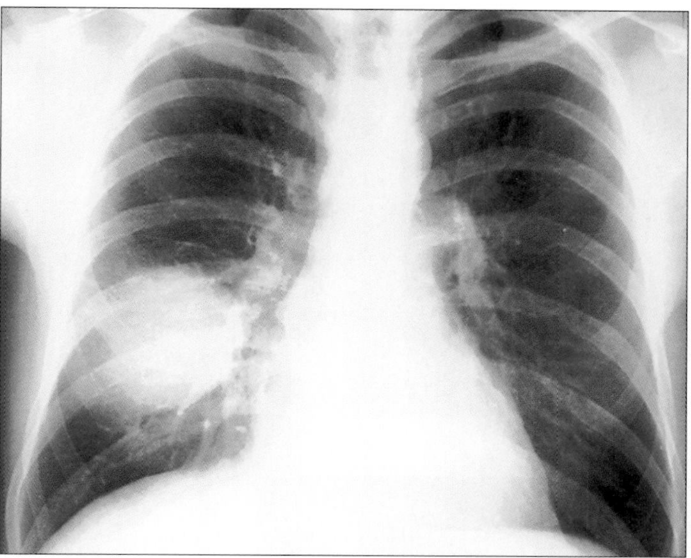

Figure 1.32 Well-defined, rounded opacity in the right midzone, which fades out peripherally. Round pneumonia caused by pneumococcal infection.

lung and the soft-tissue–density vascular markings is lost. The bronchi, however, which are usually too thin walled to be differentiated from the surrounding lung parenchyma, become apparent in negative contrast to the air-space opacification and thereby produce the true hallmark of consolidation, the air bronchogram (Fig. 1.33). A relatively uncommon but very suggestive radiologic sign of consolidation is the acinar shadow, which results when an individual secondary pulmonary lobule becomes opacified but remains surrounded by normally aerated lung. The resultant soft-tissue–density nodule is usually on the periphery of a more confluent area of consolidation and normally measures 0.5 to 1 cm in diameter. These acinar opacities are most commonly seen in association with mycobacterial and varicella-zoster pneumonias but can occur with consolidation resulting

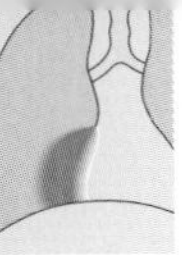

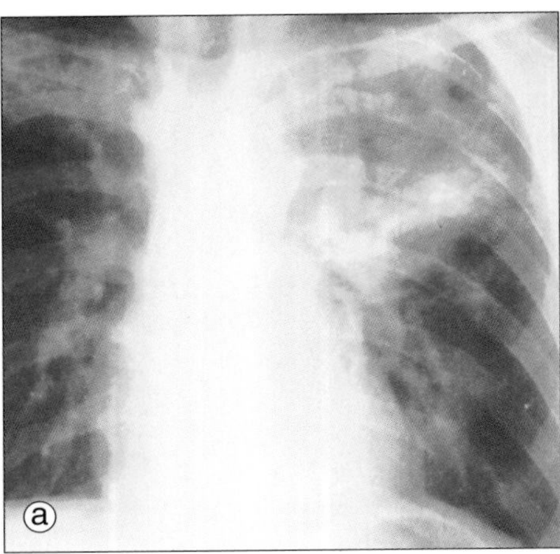

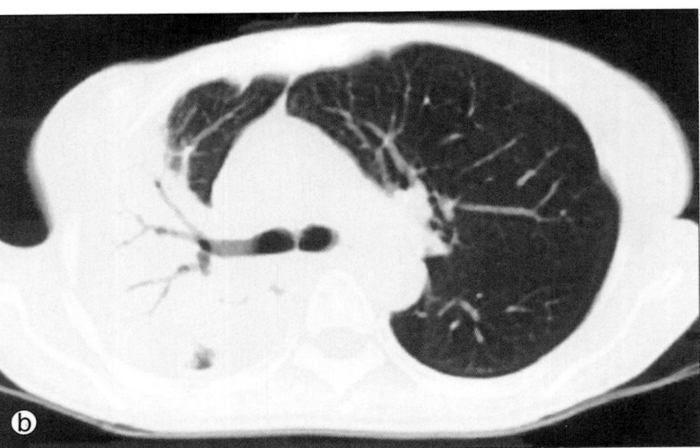

Figure 1.33 Air bronchogram in consolidation. A, Left, upper-zone tuberculosis demonstrating an air bronchogram. **B,** Computed tomography (CT) scan through the carina demonstrates an extensive air bronchogram in a different patient who has lobar pneumonia.

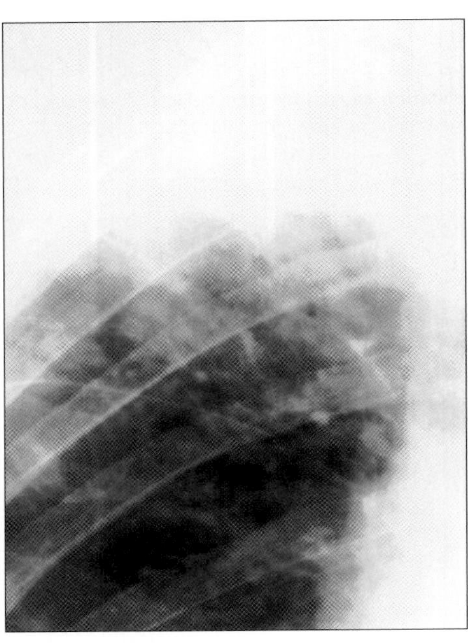

Figure 1.34 Acinar opacities seen at the periphery of confluent right upper lobar consolidation in a patient who has tuberculosis. Note the elevation of the horizontal fissure.

from any other cause (Fig. 1.34). Occasionally, an acinus is left normally aerated but surrounded by opacified air spaces; this radiologic sign has been termed the *air alveologram*. When consolidation is not fully developed and has caused only partial filling of the air spaces, the resultant radiographic appearance is ground-glass opacification (Fig. 1.35). Again, there is a wide range of possible causes, and in addition to causes of consolidation this pattern may result from interstitial lung infiltration.

When an area of consolidation undergoes necrosis because of either infection or infarction, liquefaction may result, and if either a gas-forming organism is present or communication with the bronchial tree occurs, an air-fluid level may develop in addition to cavity formation (Fig. 1.36). Consolidation frequently produces a silhouette sign, as described by Felson and Felson. Although this radiographic sign may be seen in association with a wide number of intrapulmonary pathologic processes, it is best demonstrated with the many forms of consolidation because of the relatively transitory nature of the shadowing. The original description stated that when an intrathoracic lesion touches a border of the heart, aorta, or diaphragm, it obliterates that

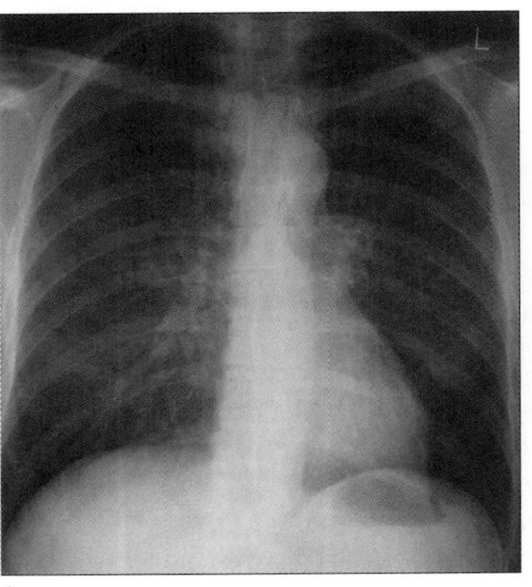

A

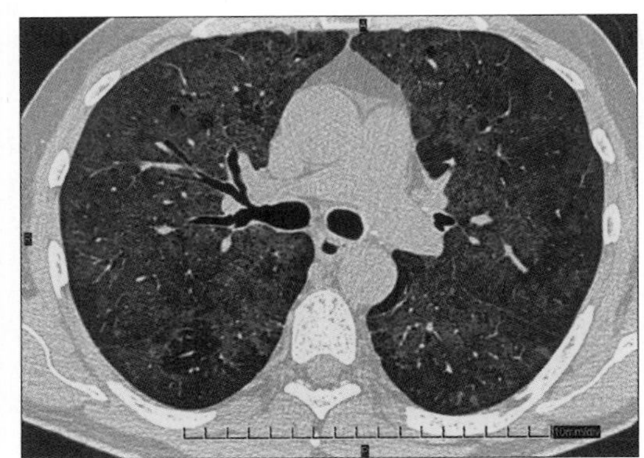

B

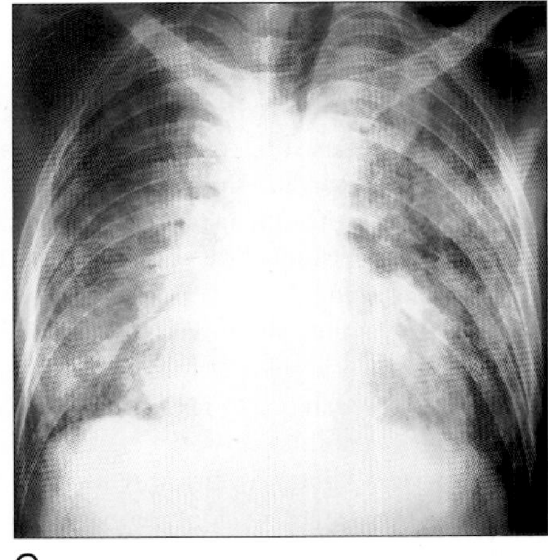

C

Figure 1.35 Ground-glass opacification in the midzone and lower zone. A, Chest radiograph of a 35-year-old, human immunodeficiency virus (HIV)–positive man with *Pneumocystis jiroveci* pneumonia. Note perihilar, poorly defined increased (ground-glass) density. **B,** High-resolution computed tomography (HRCT) image of the same patient, demonstrating variation of lung attenuation with markedly black airways highlighted by the ground-glass patchy infiltrate. **C,** Diffuse and severe ground-glass and air-space infiltrate in a different patient with *P. jiroveci* pneumonia.

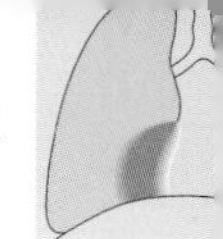

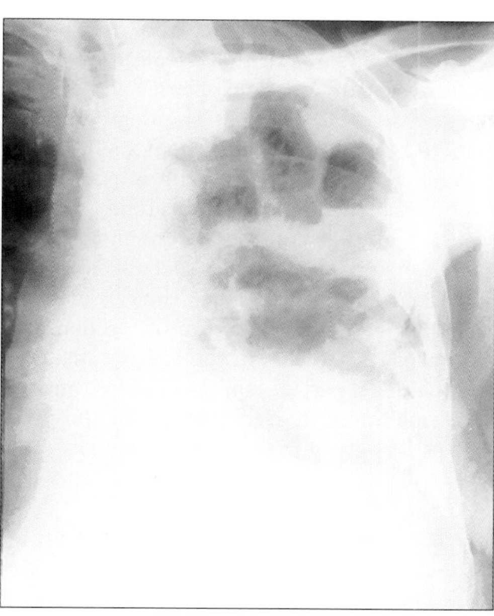

Figure 1.36 Multiple cavities, some containing air-fluid levels within the left lung. The patient has necrotizing pneumonia.

border on the radiograph. Furthermore, a small area of consolidation may obliterate a normal air–soft-tissue interface as effectively as a large area. This is demonstrated well by the obliteration of the right heart border by subtle middle-lobar consolidation that might otherwise be overlooked.

Understanding the significance of the silhouette sign allows the observer to localize an area of consolidation or other pulmonary opacity. Only if an area of consolidation lies in direct contact with a normal structure is the silhouette of that structure lost. If an area of consolidation and a normal structure–lung interface merely lie along the same x-ray path, then they are superimposed on the radiograph but do not demonstrate the silhouette sign. Thus, lingular consolidation is likely to obscure the heart border, but left lower lobar consolidation usually does not (Figs. 1.37 and 1.38). There are several potential causes for a falsely positive silhouette sign. Some relatively common anatomic variants that result in a reduced AP diameter of the thorax, such as pectus excavatum or straight back syndrome, cause loss of the right heart border as the depressed sternum distorts the normal anatomy (see Fig. 1.26). Occasionally a sco-

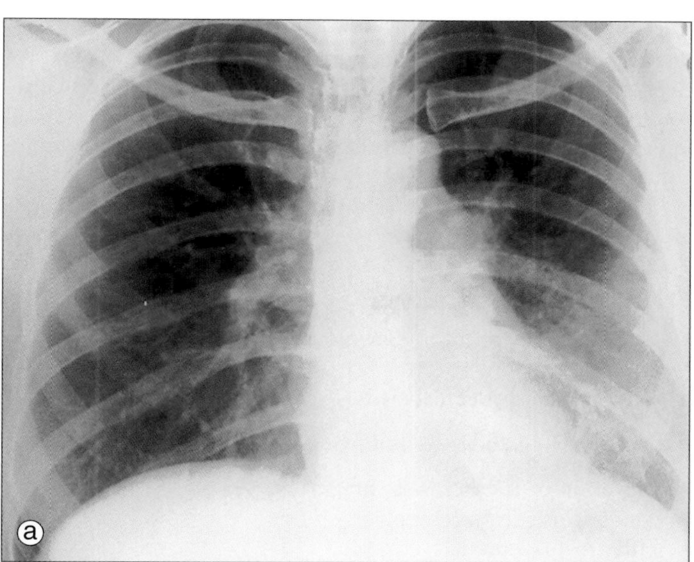

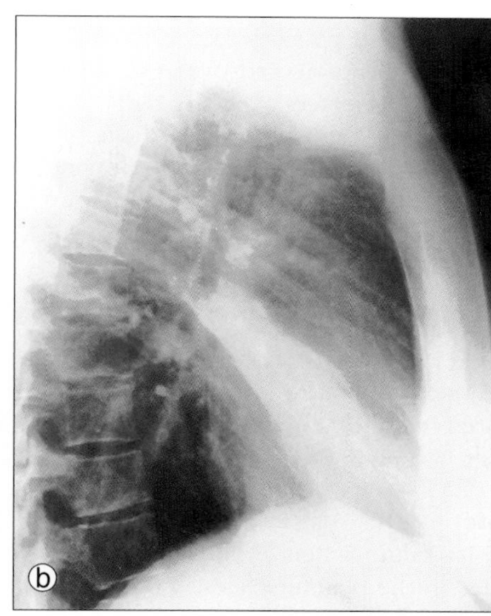

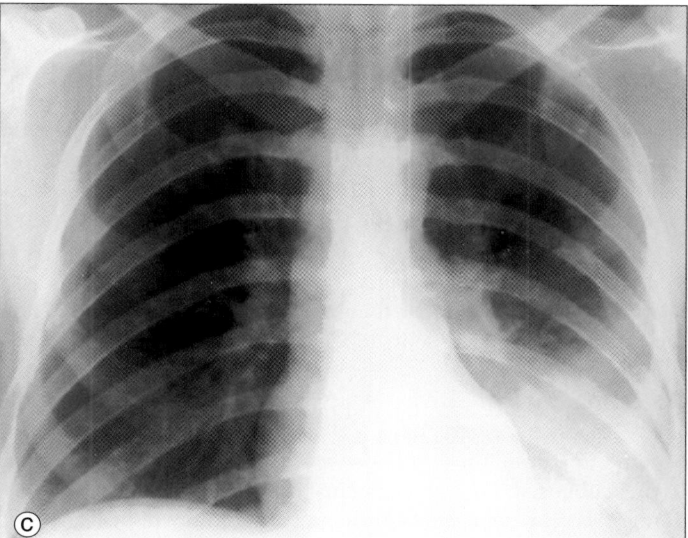

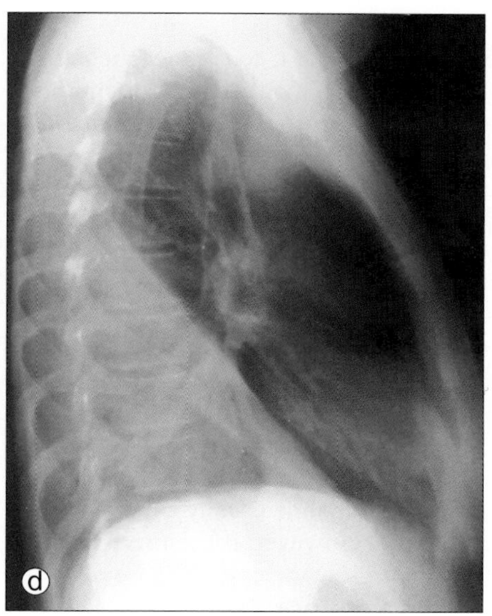

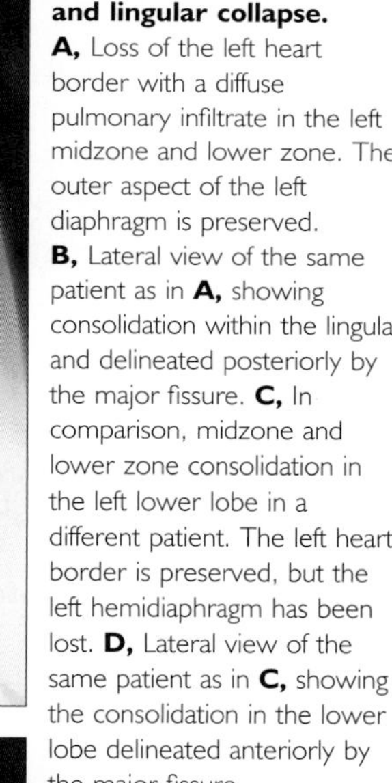

Figure 1.37 Lower lobar and lingular collapse. **A,** Loss of the left heart border with a diffuse pulmonary infiltrate in the left midzone and lower zone. The outer aspect of the left diaphragm is preserved. **B,** Lateral view of the same patient as in **A,** showing consolidation within the lingula and delineated posteriorly by the major fissure. **C,** In comparison, midzone and lower zone consolidation in the left lower lobe in a different patient. The left heart border is preserved, but the left hemidiaphragm has been lost. **D,** Lateral view of the same patient as in **C,** showing the consolidation in the lower lobe delineated anteriorly by the major fissure.

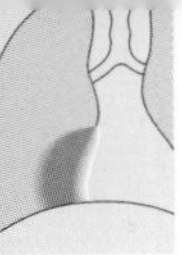

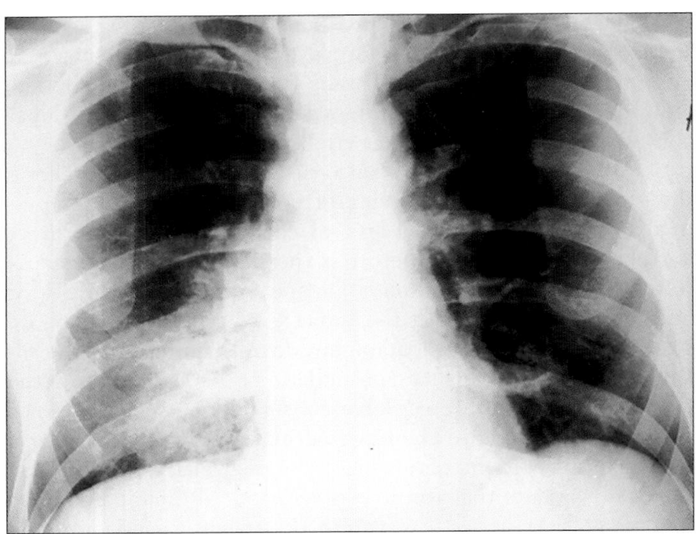

Figure 1.38 Right lower lobar consolidation. The right heart border is clearly defined. Because the consolidation is not complete the hemidiaphragm has not been effaced.

liosis, usually concave to the left and possibly relatively trivial, causes the right heart border to be projected over the spine. Only when the heart border is projected over the right lung can the silhouette sign be elicited. Underexposed radiographs may appear to demonstrate the silhouette sign, so it is imperative that the technical quality of the radiograph is taken into account.

COLLAPSE

When partial or complete volume loss occurs in a lung or lobe, this is referred to as *collapse* or *atelectasis*. The terms are essentially interchangeable, and they imply a diminished volume of air in the lung with associated reduction in lung volume. Several different mechanisms result in lung or lobar collapse.

Relaxation or Passive Collapse

The lung retracts toward its hilum when air or an abnormal amount of fluid accumulates in the pleural space.

Cicatrization Collapse

The normal expansion of the lung, and for it to contact the parietal pleura, depends on a balance between outward forces in the chest wall and opposite elastic forces in the lung. If the lung is abnormally stiff, this balance is disturbed, lung compliance is decreased, and the volume of the affected lung is reduced. Perhaps the best example of this phenomenon is volume loss associated with pulmonary fibrosis.

Adhesive Collapse

In the normal lung the forces that govern surface tension become more pronounced as the surface area of the air space is reduced. Hence, the collapse of smaller airways and alveoli tends to occur at lower lung volumes, a tendency that is offset by surfactant, which reduces the surface tension of the fluid that lines the alveoli. In the normal lung this reduction is usually sufficient to overcome the tendency to collapse. However, if the mechanism is disturbed, as in respiratory distress syndrome, collapse of the alveoli occurs, and typically the larger airways remain patent.

Reabsorption Collapse

In acute bronchial obstruction, gases in the alveoli are steadily taken up by the blood in the pulmonary capillaries and are not replenished, which causes alveolar collapse. The degree of collapse may be counteracted by collateral air drift if the obstruction is distal to the main bronchus, and also by infection and accumulation of secretions. If the obstruction becomes chronic, subsequent reabsorption of intra-alveolar secretions and exudate may result in complete collapse—the usual mechanism of collapse seen in carcinoma of the bronchus. When the cause of collapse is a proximal obstructing mass, the S sign of Golden may be apparent. This sign takes its name from the S shape made by the relevant fissure as the distal part of a lobe collapses, but the proximal part of a lobe maintains its bulk because of the presence of a tumor.

Radiographic Signs of Lobar Collapse

The radiographic appearance in pulmonary collapse depends on a number of factors, including the mechanism of collapse, the extent of collapse, the presence or absence of consolidation in the affected lung, and the pre-existing state of the pleura. This last factor includes the presence of underlying pleural tethering or thickening and the presence of pleural fluid. Pre-existing lung disease, such as fibrosis and pleural adhesions, may alter the expected displacement of anatomic landmarks in lung collapse. An air bronchogram is rare in reabsorption collapse but is usual in passive and adhesive collapse and may be seen in cicatrization collapse if fibrosis is particularly dense.

Signs of collapse may be direct or indirect. Indirect signs are the result of compensatory changes that occur as a consequence of the volume loss. Direct signs of collapse include the following:

- Displacement of interlobar fissures
- Loss of aeration
- Vascular and bronchial signs

Indirect signs include the following:

- Elevation of the hemidiaphragm
- Mediastinal displacement
- Hilar displacement
- Compensatory hyperinflation
- Crowding of the ribs

There tends to be a reciprocal relationship among the individual compensatory signs of collapse, so that if there is a mediastinal shift to the side of collapse, significant diaphragmatic elevation is unlikely to be present. In lower lobar collapse, for example, if hemidiaphragmatic elevation is marked, hilar depression is less marked.

Displacement of Interlobar Fissures

Displacement of interlobar fissures is the most reliable sign, and the degree of displacement depends on the extent of collapse.

Loss of Aeration

The increased density of a collapsed area of lung may not become apparent until collapse is almost complete. However, if the collapsed lung is adjacent to the mediastinum or diaphragm, the presence of the silhouette sign may indicate loss of aeration.

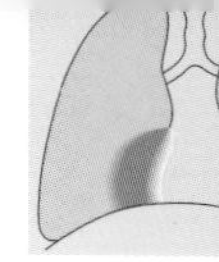

Vascular and Bronchial Signs

If a lobe is partially collapsed, crowding of its vessels may be visible; also, if an air bronchogram is visible, the bronchi may appear crowded together.

Elevation of the Hemidiaphragm

Elevation of the hemidiaphragm may be seen in lower lobar collapse but is uncommon in collapse of the other lobes.

Mediastinal Displacement

In upper lobar collapse the trachea is often displaced toward the affected side; in lower lobar collapse the heart may be displaced to the same side.

Hilar Displacement

The hilum may be elevated in upper lobar collapse and depressed in lower lobar collapse.

Compensatory Hyperinflation

The remaining normal lung may become hyperinflated and therefore may appear more transradiant, with the vessels more widely spaced than in the corresponding area of the contralateral lung. With considerable collapse of a lung, compensatory hyperinflation of the contralateral lung may occur, with herniation of lung across the midline.

Crowding of the Ribs

On the side of the collapse the intercostal spaces are often narrowed, with crowding together of the ribs, which reflects the diminished overall volume of the affected hemithorax.

Complete Lung Collapse

When complete collapse of an entire lung occurs (in the absence of an accompanying pneumothorax, large pleural effusion, or extensive consolidation), complete opacification of that hemithorax is seen, with displacement of the mediastinum to the affected side and elevation of the hemidiaphragm. Compensatory hyperinflation of the contralateral lung occurs, often with herniation across the midline. Herniation occurs most often in the retrosternal space, anterior to the ascending aorta, but may occur posterior to the heart (Fig. 1.39).

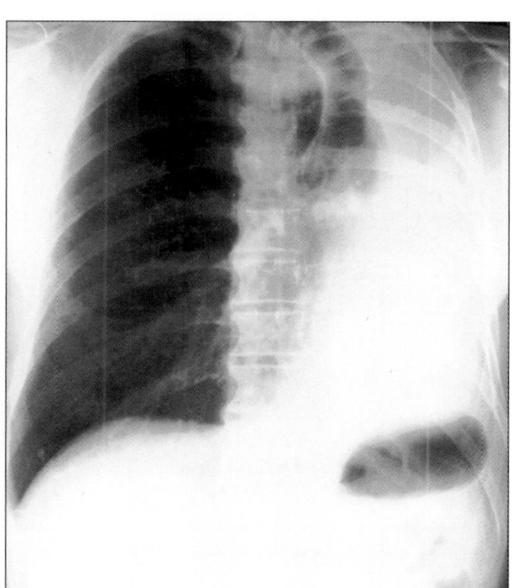

Figure 1.39 Collapse of the left lung. There is a proximal obstructing tumor within the left main bronchus, with complete collapse of the left lung and a mediastinal shift to the left.

Individual or Combined Lobar Collapse

The descriptions that follow apply to collapse of individual lobes, uncomplicated by pre-existing pulmonary or pleural disease. The alterations to the positions of the fissures, mediastinal structures, and diaphragms are shown in Figure 1.40.

Right Upper Lobar Collapse

As the right upper lobe collapses (Fig. 1.41), the horizontal fissure rotates around the hilum and the lateral end moves upward and medially toward the superior mediastinum. The anterior end moves upward, toward the apex. The upper half of the oblique fissure moves anteriorly. The two fissures become concave superiorly. In severe collapse the lobe may be flattened against the superior mediastinum and may obscure the upper pole of the hilum. The hilum is elevated, and its lower pole may be prominent. Deviation of the trachea to the right is usual, and compensatory hyperinflation of the right middle and lower lobes may be apparent.

Middle Lobar Collapse

In right middle lobar collapse (Fig. 1.42), the horizontal fissure and lower half of the oblique fissure move toward each other, a feature best seen on the lateral projection. Because the horizontal fissure tends to be more mobile, it usually shows the greater displacement. On the frontal radiograph, middle lobar collapse may be subtle because the horizontal fissure may not be visible, and increased opacity does not become apparent until collapse is almost complete. Critical analysis of the radiograph sometimes reveals obscuration of the right heart border as the only clue. The lordotic AP projection is rarely required but may be used to bring the displaced fissure into the line of the x-ray beam, and occasionally may elegantly demonstrate middle lobar collapse. Because the volume of this lobe is relatively small, indirect signs of volume loss are rarely obvious.

Left Lower Lobar Collapse

In left lower lobar collapse (Fig. 1.43), the normal oblique fissures extend from the level of the fourth thoracic vertebra posteriorly to the diaphragm, close to the sternum anteriorly. The position of these fissures on the lateral projection is the best index of lower lobar volumes. When a lower lobe collapses, the oblique fissure moves posteriorly but maintains its normal slope. In addition to posterior movement, the collapsing lower lobe causes medial displacement of the oblique fissure, which may become visible in places on the frontal projection.

Right Lower Lobar Collapse

Right lower lobar collapse (Fig. 1.44) causes partial depression of the horizontal fissure, which may be apparent on the frontal projection. Increased opacity of a collapsed lower lobe also is usually visible on the frontal projection. A completely collapsed lower lobe may be so small that it flattens and merges with the mediastinum to produce a thin, wedge-shaped shadow. In left lower lobar collapse the heart may obscure this opacity, and a penetrated view may be required to demonstrate it. Mediastinal structures and parts of the diaphragm adjacent to the nonaerated lobe are obscured. When significant lower lobar collapse occurs, especially when the collapsed lobe is so small as to be invisible as a separate opacity, confirmatory evidence is usually apparent from close inspection of the relevant hilum. The hilum

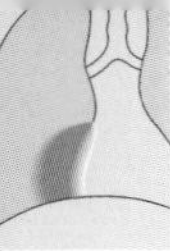

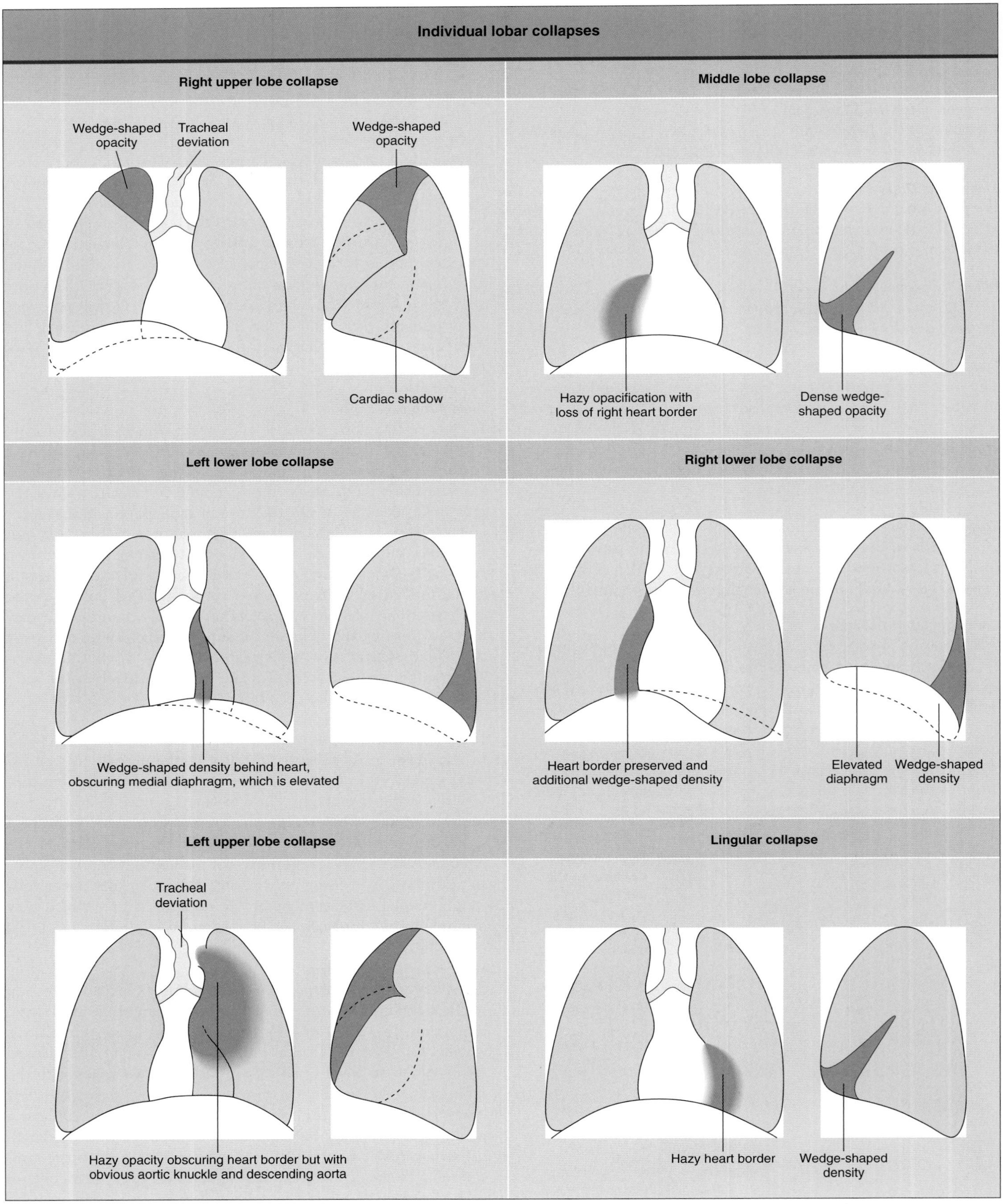

Individual lobar collapses

Right upper lobe collapse

Wedge-shaped opacity
Tracheal deviation
Wedge-shaped opacity
Cardiac shadow

Middle lobe collapse

Hazy opacification with loss of right heart border
Dense wedge-shaped opacity

Left lower lobe collapse

Wedge-shaped density behind heart, obscuring medial diaphragm, which is elevated

Right lower lobe collapse

Heart border preserved and additional wedge-shaped density
Elevated diaphragm
Wedge-shaped density

Left upper lobe collapse

Tracheal deviation
Hazy opacity obscuring heart border but with obvious aortic knuckle and descending aorta

Lingular collapse

Hazy heart border
Wedge-shaped density

Figure 1.40 Individual lobar collapses. Compare these representations with the radiographic examples in Figures 1.37 through 1.41.

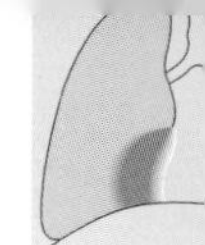

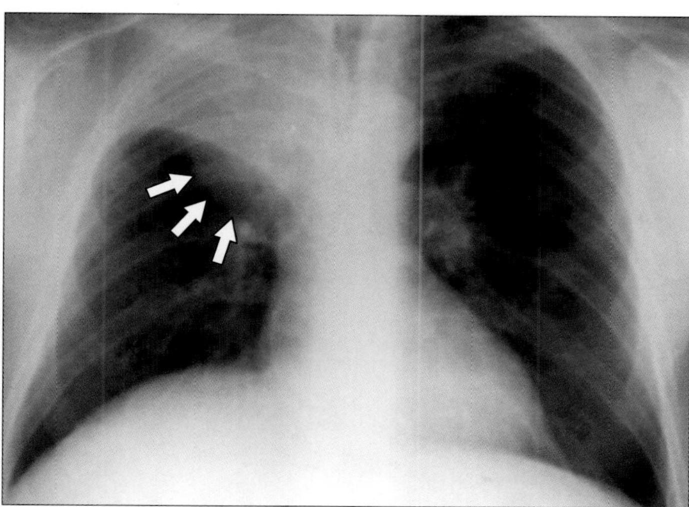

Figure 1.41 Right upper lobar collapse caused by a right hilar tumor. The horizontal fissure takes on an 'S' configuration, known as the S sign of Golden *(arrows)*.

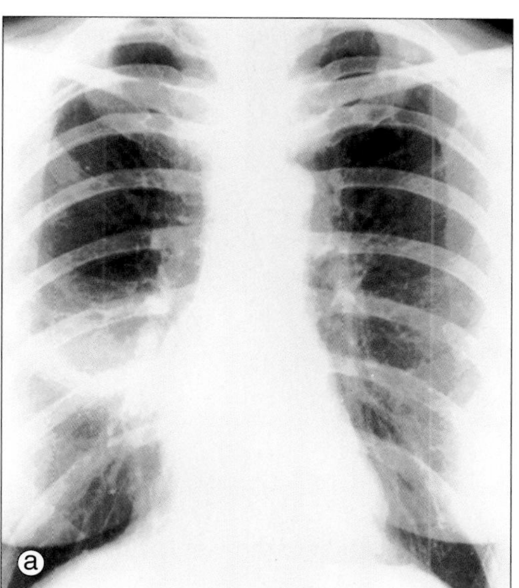

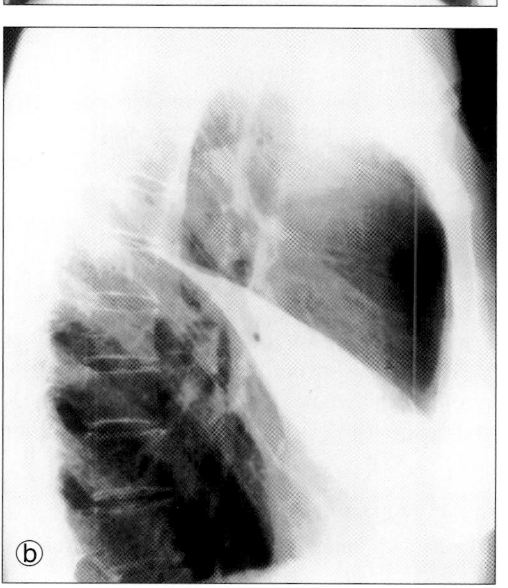

Figure 1.42 Middle lobar collapse. Loss of the right heart border is seen on the frontal radiograph. **B,** A well-defined wedge-shaped opacity on the lateral radiograph is delineated by the horizontal and oblique fissures.

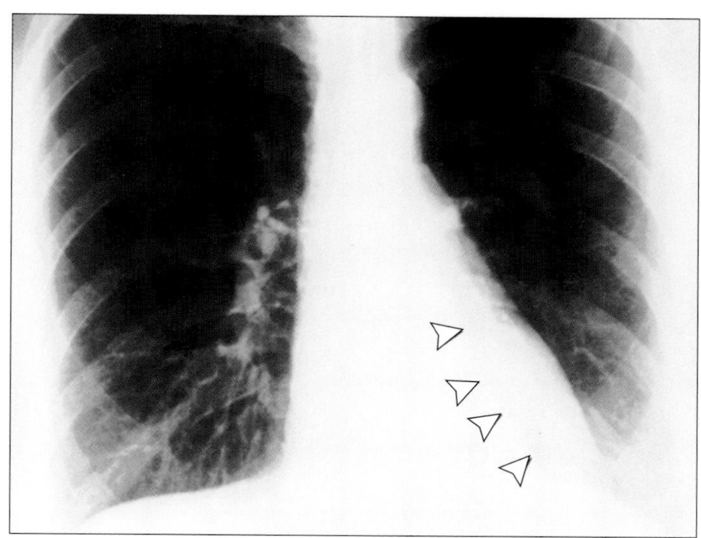

Figure 1.43 Left lower lobar collapse in a patient who has asthma and mucus plugging. The left hemithorax is of reduced volume, and loss of the normal silhouette of the left lower lobar pulmonary artery exists. The left lower lobe has contracted behind the cardiac silhouette *(arrowheads)*.

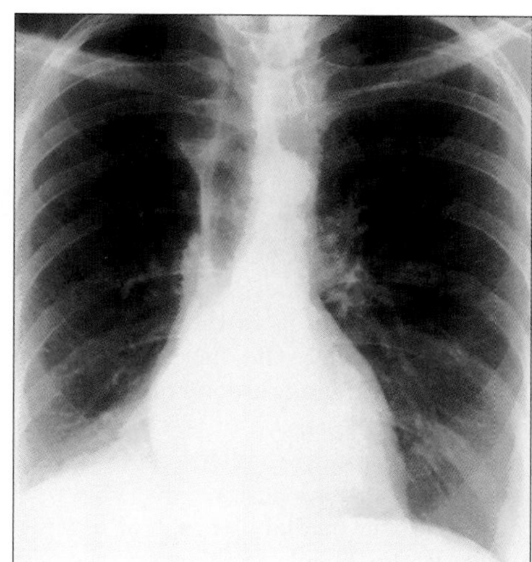

Figure 1.44 Right lower lobar collapse in the same patient as shown in Figure 1.43, but on a different occasion. The right heart border has been preserved, but the volume of the right hemithorax has been reduced and the trachea has shifted to the right side.

is usually depressed and rotated medially, with loss of the normal hilar vascular structures, which is made even more obvious if a previous film is available for comparison. In addition, indirect signs of collapse, such as upper lobar hyperinflation, are present. Diaphragmatic elevation is unusual.

Lingula Collapse

The lingula is often involved in collapse of the left upper lobe, but occasionally it may collapse individually. When this occurs, the radiographic features are similar to those seen with middle lobar collapse. However, the absence of a horizontal fissure on the left makes anterior displacement of the lower half of the oblique fissure and increased opacity anterior to it important signs. On the frontal projection, the left heart border becomes obscured.

Left Upper Lobar Collapse

The pattern of upper lobar collapse is different in the two lungs. Left upper lobar collapse (Fig. 1.45) is apparent on the lateral

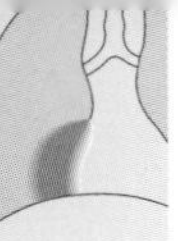

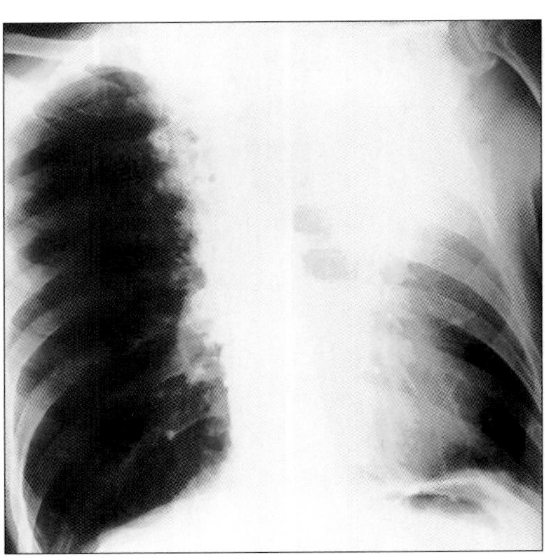

Figure 1.45 Left upper lobar collapse with shift of the mediastinum to the left and loss of definition of the mediastinal structures. The opacification fades out more inferiorly.

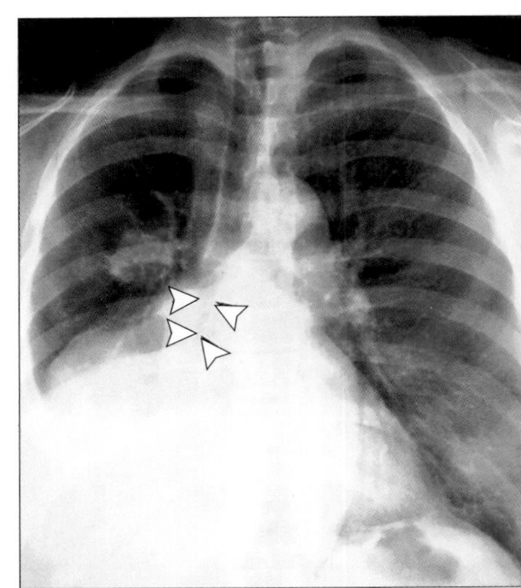

Figure 1.46 Right middle and lower lobar collapse caused by an obstructing lesion in the bronchus intermedius. A bronchial cut-off sign is visible *(arrowheads)*. A separate pulmonary mass is present in the right upper lobe.

projection as anterior displacement of the entire oblique fissure, which becomes oriented almost parallel to the anterior chest wall. With increasing collapse the upper lobe retracts posteriorly and loses contact with the anterior chest wall. With complete collapse the left upper lobe may lose contact with the chest wall and diaphragm and retract medially against the mediastinum. On a lateral film, therefore, left upper lobar collapse appears as an elongated opacity that extends from the apex and reaches, or almost reaches, the diaphragm; it is anterior to the hilum and is bounded by the displaced oblique fissure posteriorly and by the hyperinflated lower lobe.

A collapsed left upper lobe does not produce a sharp outline on the frontal view. An ill-defined, hazy opacity is present in the upper, middle, and sometimes lower zones, the opacity being densest near the hilum. Pulmonary vessels in the hyperinflated lower lobe are usually visible through the haze. The aortic knuckle is usually obscured, unless the upper lobe has collapsed anterior to it, in which case hyperexpansion of the lower lobar apical segment may occur and separate the collapsed upper lobe from the mediastinal silhouette and aortic knuckle. This produces an unusual but characteristic medial crescent of lucency termed the *Luftsichel sign.* If the lingula is involved, the left heart border is obscured. The hilum is often elevated, and the trachea deviated to the left.

Combined Lobar Collapses

Right Lower and Middle Lobar Collapse

Because the right lower and middle lobes originate from the bronchus intermedius, an extensive lesion at that site may cause combined collapse. The appearances are similar to right lower lobar collapse (Fig. 1.46), except that the horizontal fissure is not apparent and the opacification reaches the lateral chest wall on the frontal radiograph and similarly extends to the anterior chest wall on the lateral view.

Right Upper and Middle Lobar Collapse

Combined collapse of the right upper and middle lobes is unusual because of the distance between the origins of their bronchi; it can generally be taken to imply the presence of more than one lesion. This combination produces appearances (Fig. 1.47) that are almost identical to those of left upper lobar collapse. On occasion, isolated right upper lobar collapse also pro-

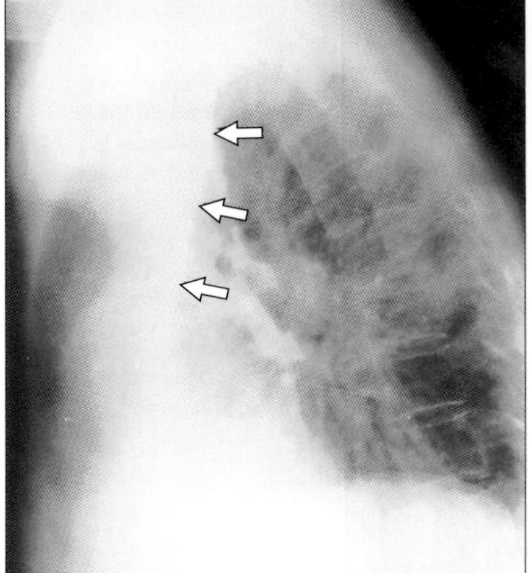

Figure 1.47 Right middle and upper lobar collapse. Lateral radiographic changes are similar to those seen on the opposite side with a left upper lobar collapse. The major fissure shifts anteriorly *(arrows)* and extends from the lung apex to the anterior costophrenic recess.

duces appearances that are identical to those of left upper lobar collapse.

Rounded Atelectasis

Rounded atelectasis is an unusual form of pulmonary collapse that may be misdiagnosed as a pulmonary tumor. The plain film shows an opacity that may be several centimeters in diameter, frequently with ill-defined edges. Rounded atelectasis is always pleura based and associated with pleural thickening. Vascular shadows may radiate from part of the opacity, said to resemble a comet's tail (Fig. 1.48). The appearance is caused by the folding in on itself of peripheral lung tissue. Rounded atelectasis is usually related to previous asbestos exposure but may also occur secondary to any exudative pleural effusion. It is not of any other pathologic significance, although when present it often raises the question of a malignancy. The CT appearance is usually sufficiently diagnostic to allow differentiation from other pulmonary masses (Fig. 1.49).

UNILATERAL INCREASED TRANSRADIANCY

The most common causes of increased unilateral transradiancy are technical factors, such as patient rotation, poor beam cen-

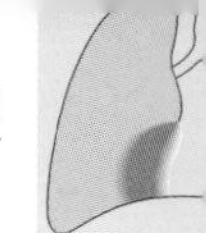

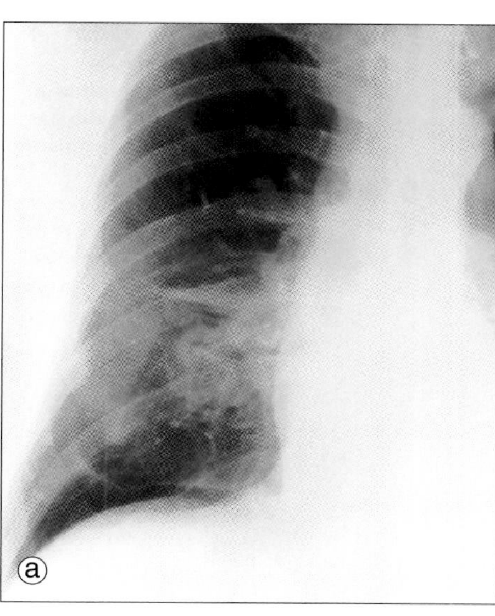

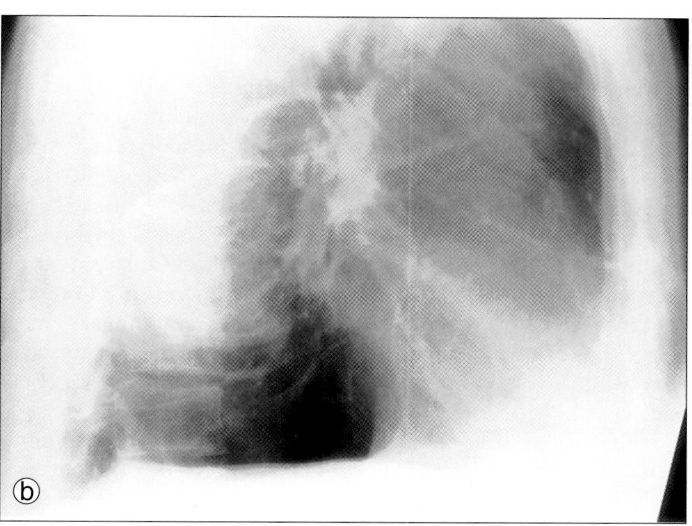

Figure 1.48 Rounded atelectasis. A, A poorly defined opacity is visible on the frontal radiograph. **B,** The lateral film reveals that the cause is a radiating parenchymal band that extends from the posterior chest wall.

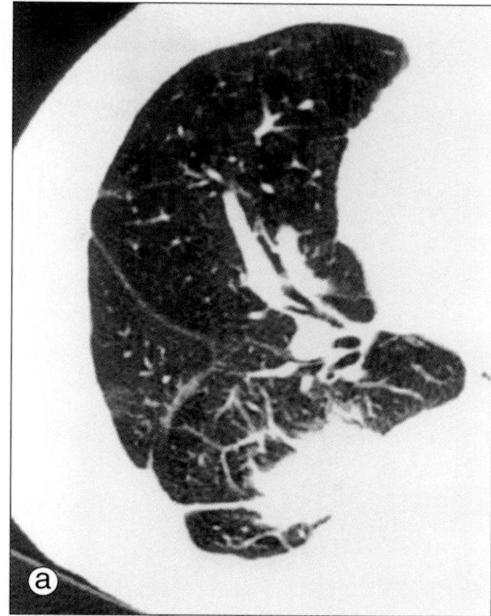

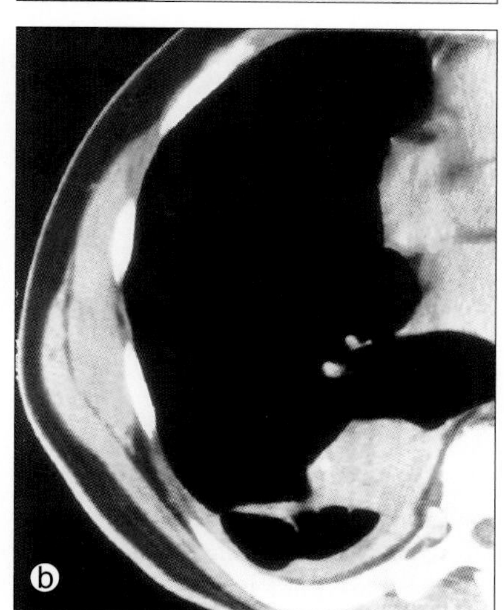

Figure 1.49 Rounded atelectasis. A, Computed tomography (CT) scan reveals the characteristic pleurally based mass with radiating bronchovascular strands. **B,** Mediastinal window settings demonstrate a fleck of calcification, in keeping with previous asbestos exposure.

tering, and an offset grid. Usually, hypertransradiancy caused by technical factors can be identified by comparison of the soft tissues around the shoulder girdle, and particularly over the axillae. Nevertheless, there are a number of pathologic causes of unilateral increased transradiancy.

Chest Wall

A hemithorax may have increased transradiancy (i.e., may appear blacker) if the x-rays are less attenuated because of a reduction in the amount of overlying soft tissue. The most common cause for this is a mastectomy. Rarely, the same phenomenon may be seen in patients with congenital unilateral absence of pectoral muscles, known as Poland's syndrome (Fig. 1.50). This may be accompanied by associated skeletal abnormalities in the ipsilateral ribs but may be recognized by loss of the normal axillary skin fold.

Reduced Vascularity

Interruption or significant reduction in the blood supply to one lung, either congenital or acquired, results in increased transradiancy in that lung (Fig. 1.51).

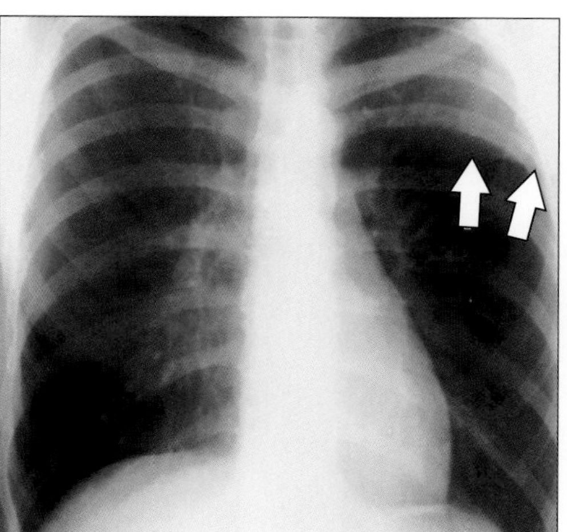

Figure 1.50 Poland's syndrome. Incidental finding on a chest radiograph of congenital absence of the left pectoralis major muscle. Note the alteration in the left axillary skin fold compared with the right *(arrows)*.

Lung Hyperexpansion

If a lung is overexpanded because of either air trapping secondary to the presence of a foreign body or asymmetrical emphysema, then that hemithorax may demonstrate increased transradiancy. When the whole lung is affected, the hemithorax

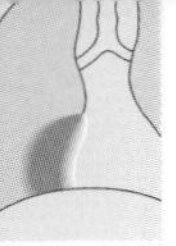

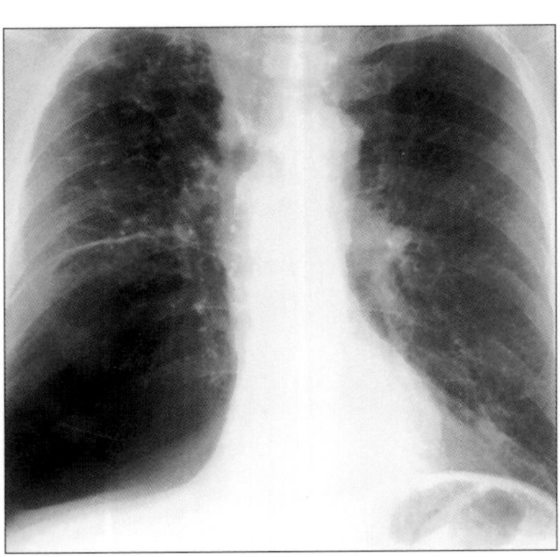

Figure 1.51 Increased transradiancy in the right lower zone. A large emphysematous bulla occupies the lower half of the right lung, and the apical changes are in keeping with previous tuberculosis.

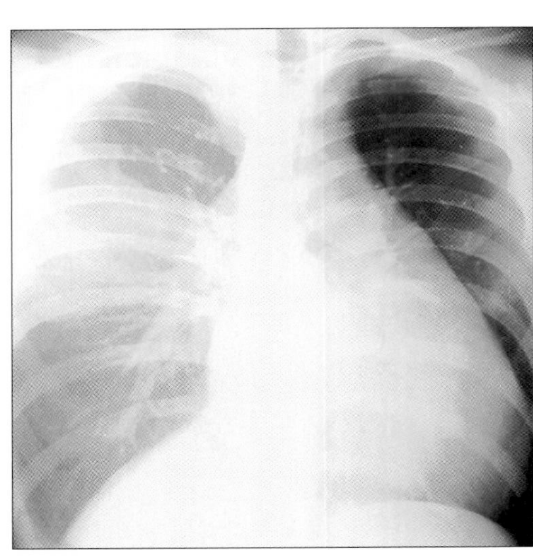

Figure 1.52 Supine radiograph of a patient who has a large right pleural effusion. The generalized increase in radiopacity of the right side is caused by posterior layering of a pleural effusion.

is usually relatively larger than the opposite side. However, the same phenomenon may occur with compensatory emphysema, because of collapse or removal of an ipsilateral lobe. In this case the transradiant hemithorax may be of normal volume, and the presence of the increased transradiancy should prompt a search for other evidence of collapse or prior surgery.

A relatively increased transradiancy of one hemithorax with no obvious cause suggests the possibility of a generalized increase in radiopacity of the opposite side—for example, the posterior layering of a pleural effusion in a supine patient (Fig. 1.52).

The Pulmonary Mass

The finding of a solitary pulmonary nodule on the chest radiograph requires careful analysis, because the diagnostic possibilities are numerous. Once a pulmonary mass has been identified, the observer must decide first if the lesion is genuine and second whether the lesion is truly intrapulmonary. The possibility of a cutaneous lesion should not be forgotten, especially if only a part of the nodule is well defined. If doubt remains, repeat radiographs are obtained, with a lateral view and, if relevant, nipple markers. What appears at first glance to be a solitary pulmonary mass may on closer inspection actually be the most obvious of a number of pulmonary nodules. The radiology of multiple pulmonary nodules is discussed later.

When a pulmonary mass is clearly defined around its entire circumference and is projected over the lung on frontal and lateral projections, the mass is truly intrapulmonary (Fig. 1.53). However, if a surface is in contact with another soft-tissue structure, the possibility that an extrapulmonary mass is projecting into the lung must be considered. Analysis of the breadth of the base of the lesion, the angle made with the adjacent structure, and the presence of bone destruction often allows the observer to differentiate between an extrapulmonary mass that extends into the adjacent lung and an intrapulmonary mass that has grown to contact the mediastinum, diaphragm, or chest wall.

The analysis of a solitary pulmonary mass relies on a number of radiologic and clinical factors. The latter include patient age, geographic and ethnic origins, smoking history, and medical history. The likelihood that a pulmonary nodule represents a malignancy in a young nonsmoker who comes from an area in which histoplasmosis is endemic is clearly different from that in an elderly patient with a lifelong history of smoking.

Radiographic features of a pulmonary nodule that should be analyzed include size, density, margins, vascular markings, and growth rate.

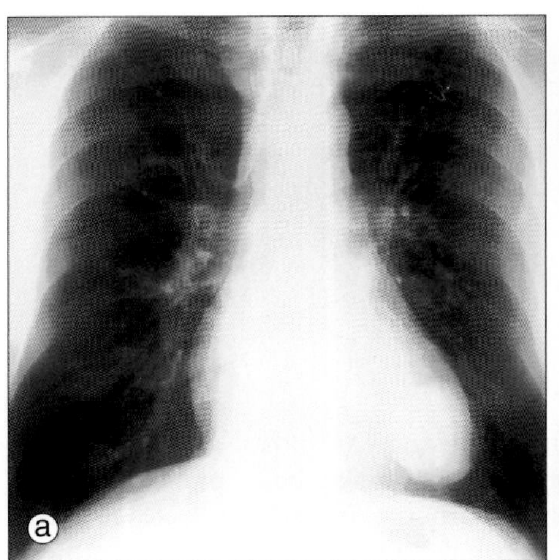

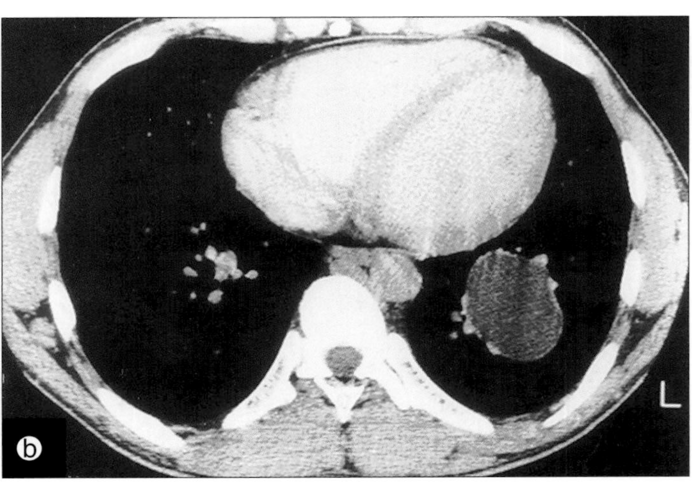

Figure 1.53 A rounded pulmonary mass. **A,** Posteroanterior (PA) radiograph of a patient who has a well-defined pulmonary mass. The entire circumference is shown on the film, which indicates no surface of contact with the mediastinal structures. **B,** Computed tomography (CT) of this mass demonstrates it is of fluid density—a hydatid cyst.

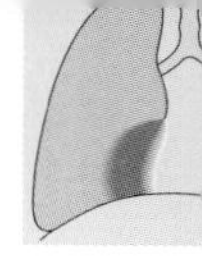

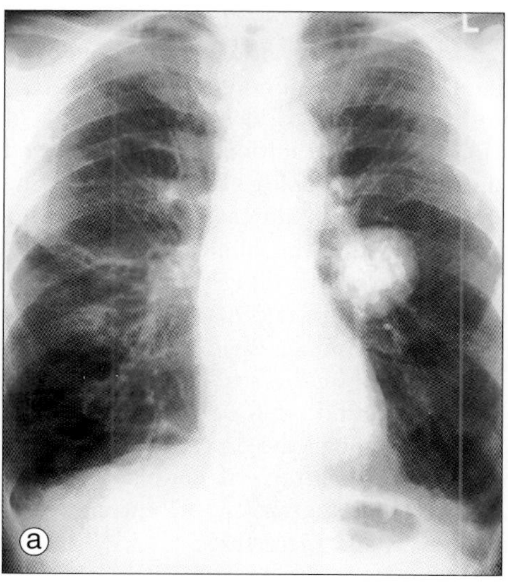

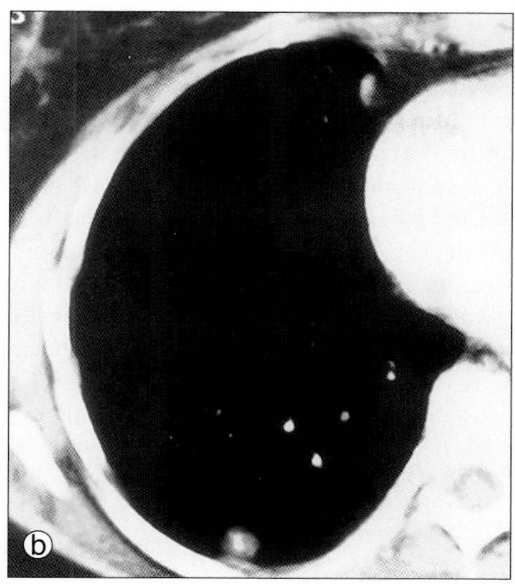

Figure 1.54 Examples of pulmonary calcification. **A,** Posteroanterior (PA) chest radiograph of a mass that projects over the left hilum. The mass is smoothly marginated and contains central popcorn calcification; it is unusually large but otherwise a typical pulmonary hamartoma. **B,** Computed tomography (CT) scan through a small, peripherally based lung nodule. A well-defined fleck of central calcification is visible. These are the typical appearances of subacute histoplasmosis.

SIZE

Generally, the likelihood of malignancy is greater with increasing size, although the opposite argument is not reliable.

DENSITY

Most pulmonary masses are of soft-tissue density. However, careful inspection must be made for the presence of calcification, because certain patterns of calcification are typical of benign lesions that may be safely observed rather than resected. A completely or centrally calcified nodule is diagnostic of a tuberculoma or histoplasmoma. Often, CT is required to confirm this pattern of calcification. Likewise, concentric rings of calcification are typical of healed histoplasmosis infection. Popcorn calcification within the matrix of a pulmonary nodule is highly suggestive of a hamartoma (Fig. 1.54). Other forms of calcification do not reliably indicate whether a nodule is benign or malignant, and dystrophic calcification within a pulmonary malignancy is relatively common.

MARGINS

Perfectly smooth, round lesions are likely to be benign (see Fig. 1.53). However, this rule is not completely reliable, because some primary lung malignancies and secondary deposits, particularly from soft-tissue sarcomas, may be perfectly spherical. In contrast, lobulated or spiculated masses are much more likely to represent malignancy.

VASCULAR MARKINGS

A rare, benign, but important cause of a pulmonary nodule is an arteriovenous malformation. The diagnosis may be suggested on the plain radiograph if a prominent feeding artery or draining vein is identified.

GROWTH RATE

Review of the previous radiographs, when available, may establish whether a lesion is static or increasing in size. Usual practice is to express the growth of a pulmonary tumor in terms of the time it takes to double in volume, which equates to an increase in diameter of 25%, assuming that the tumor is roughly spherical, as is usually the case. Tumors with a doubling time of less than 30 days or greater than 2 years are very unlikely to result from malignancy. However, often no previous films are available, and thus the use of growth rate as a diagnostic aid is limited.

When a solitary lung mass is evident on the chest radiograph, and no features suggest whether it is of benign cause or a malignant lesion, the lesion is assumed to be a primary lung carcinoma until proved otherwise. In the assessment of a potential lung primary tumor, certain guidelines may be helpful.

Approximately half of primary lung carcinomas arise centrally in a proximal or segmental bronchus and as a result take the form of a hilar mass.

Because carcinoma of the bronchus arises in the bronchial mucosa, the tumor is likely to grow into the bronchial lumen and around the bronchus. As the bronchial lumen narrows, the distal lung may become consolidated and lose volume. Depending on the site of the tumor, a malignant solitary lung mass may be associated with lobar or segmental collapse (Fig. 1.55) or even collapse of an entire lung (see Fig. 1.39).

Peripheral tumors usually appear as solitary nodules or masses, but no features on plain films reliably differentiate a

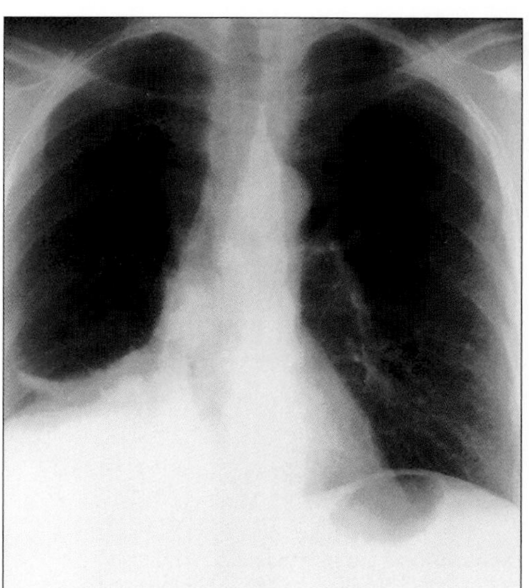

Figure 1.55 Right lower and partial middle lobar collapse secondary to a proximal bronchogenic carcinoma.

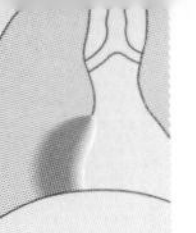

benign from a malignant pulmonary nodule. As described previously, malignant tumors are often larger, poorly defined, spiculated, or lobulated. Satellite opacities around a mass are more commonly seen with benign lesions, notably granulomatous diseases (see Fig. 1.34). At least 5% of bronchial carcinomas cavitate because of central necrosis or abscess formation; the resultant cavity is typically thick walled with an irregular inner margin (Fig. 1.56). Peripheral tumors may invade the ribs or spine directly. Bone destruction must be specifically sought and, when present, almost invariably indicates malignancy (Fig. 1.57).

Multiple Pulmonary Nodules

The differential diagnosis of multiple pulmonary nodules is extensive (Table 1.4), but analysis of the chest radiograph and review of the clinical status of the patient rapidly narrow the

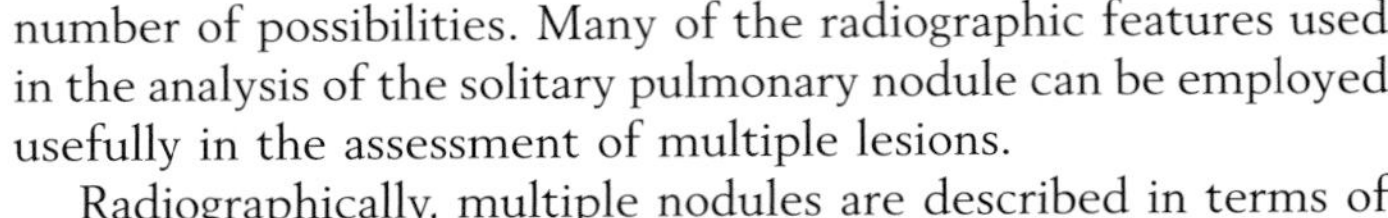

number of possibilities. Many of the radiographic features used in the analysis of the solitary pulmonary nodule can be employed usefully in the assessment of multiple lesions.

Radiographically, multiple nodules are described in terms of size, number, distribution, density, definition, cavitation, speed of growth (if serial films are available), and accompanying pleural, mediastinal, or skeletal abnormalities. Additional important clinical clues may come from the clinical status of the patient. Evidence of infection, systemic illness, and prior malignancy is specifically sought (Figs. 1.58, 1.59, and 1.60). Miliary nodules are a particular form of nodular shadowing. The term *miliary* derives from the likening of the size and shape of the nodules to millet seeds, being round, well defined, and 2 to 3 mm in diameter (Fig. 1.61). Although the description is usually associated with tuberculosis, this pattern of nodular infiltrate may also result from *Histoplasmosis* infection, organic and inorganic dust diseases, sarcoidosis, and metastases.

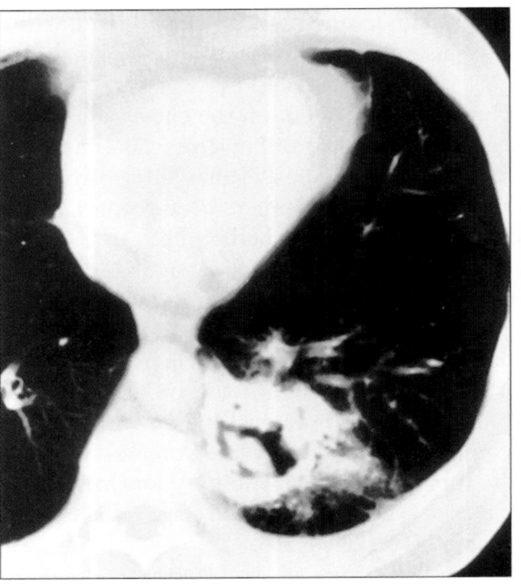

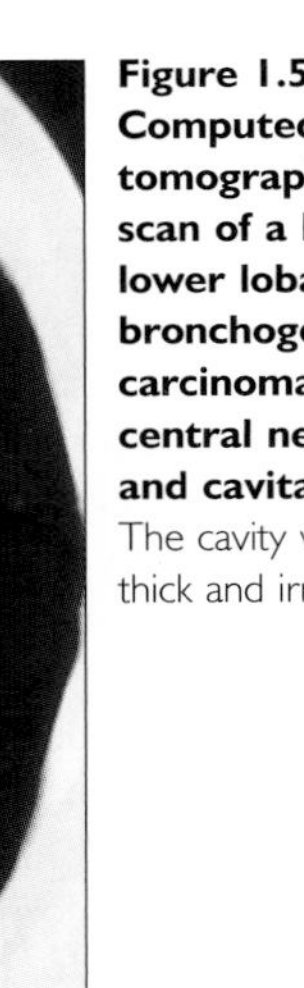

Figure 1.56 Computed tomography (CT) scan of a left lower lobar bronchogenic carcinoma with central necrosis and cavitation. The cavity wall is thick and irregular.

Table 1.4
Causes of acquired pulmonary nodules

Acquired	
Neoplastic	Inflammatory
Benign	Infectious
Hamartomas	Granulomatous infections
Papillomatosis	Multiple embolic abscesses
Bronchogenic cysts	Round pneumonias
Malignant	Viral infections – chickenpox and measles
Metastases	Parasites – hydatid and paragonimiasis
Lymphoma	Noninfectious
Multifocal tumor	Caplan's syndrome and rheumatoid nodules
Kaposi's sarcoma	Wegener's granulomatosis
Bronchoalveolar cell carcinoma	Sarcoidosis
	Others
	Progressive massive fibrosis
	Amyloid
	Infarcts
	Bronchial impaction

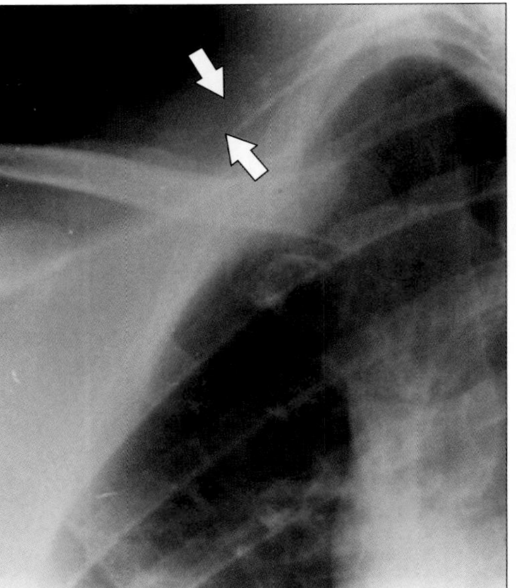

Figure 1.57 Oblique view of the right apex demonstrating bone destruction within the first rib *(arrows)*. The patient has peripheral bronchogenic carcinoma.

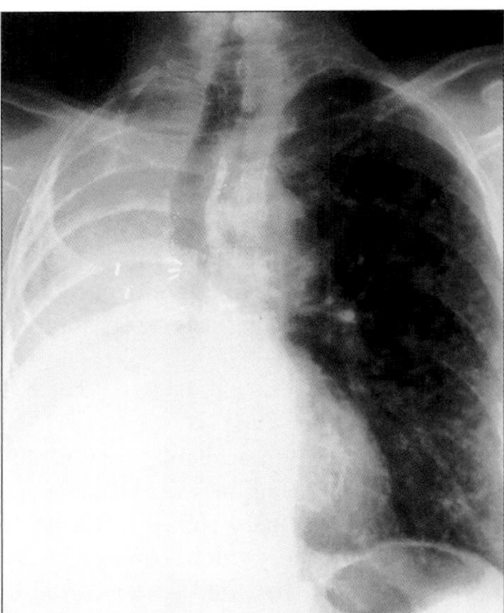

Figure 1.58 Chest radiograph of a patient who had a previous right pneumonectomy for adenocarcinoma. Multiple pulmonary nodules are now within the lung because of secondary deposits.

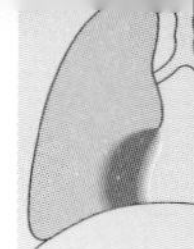

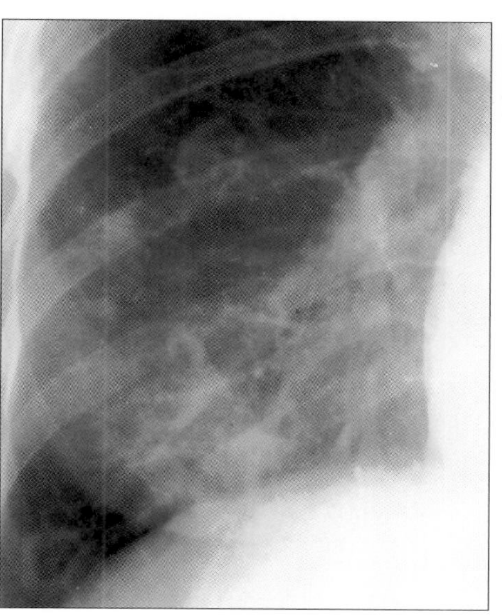

Figure 1.59 Magnified view of the right lower zone. The multiple pulmonary nodules are cavitating in this case of multiple staphylococcal abscesses in an intravenous drug abuser.

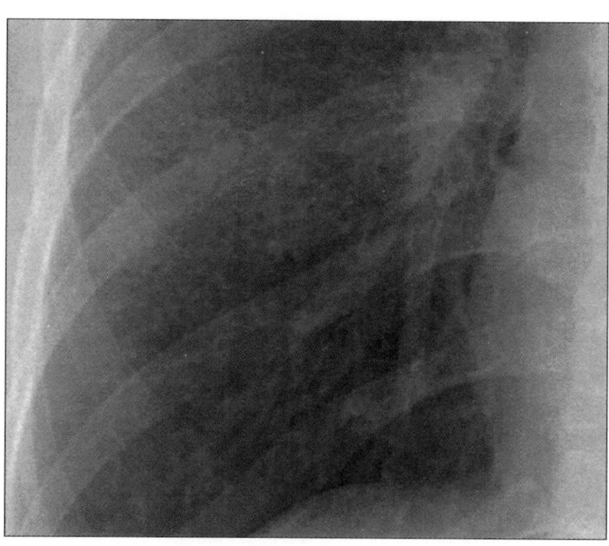

Figure 1.61 Miliary tuberculosis. Close-up of the right lower zone demonstrating innumerable 2- to 3-mm soft-tissue nodules.

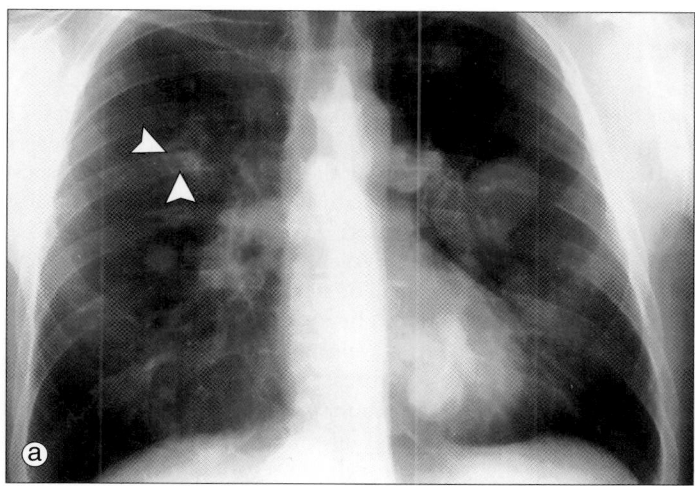

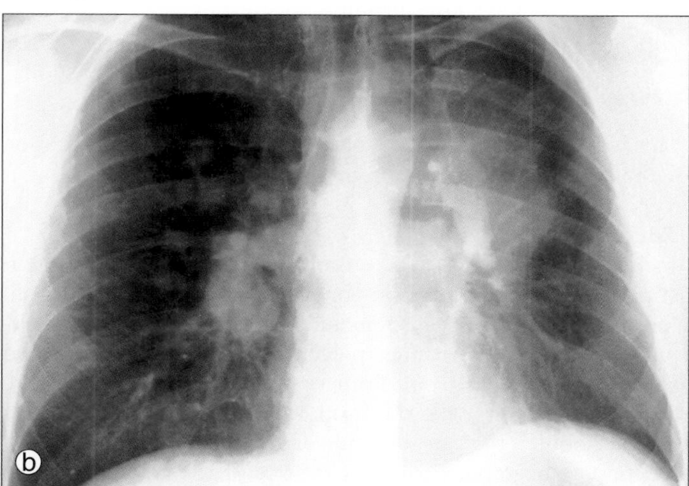

Figure 1.60 Multiple pulmonary nodules. A, The multiple pulmonary nodules are smoothly defined and vary in size; some are cavitating *(arrowheads)*. **B,** Subsequent chest radiograph obtained shortly afterward. The left perihilar nodules are no longer visible because they lie within the now collapsed left upper lobe. The patient has multiple metastases from soft-tissue sarcoma.

Diffuse Shadowing

Many diseases cause diffuse lung shadowing on chest radiography. Careful analysis is required to correctly determine the nature of the abnormality and narrow the differential diagnosis. Appearances on the chest radiograph can be misleading, and the pattern of disease demonstrated at pathologic or HRCT examination may differ considerably from the pattern of abnormality suggested by the chest radiograph. The summation of multiple, small, linear opacities on the chest radiograph may produce the appearance of multiple small nodules. Likewise, the superimposition of multiple small nodules may produce a granular or ground-glass pattern. A variety of descriptive terms is used in the analysis of a chest radiograph in this context, and frequently appearances are classified as being either interstitial or air space. However, a number of processes is capable of producing both patterns, so the differential diagnosis may be erroneously narrowed at an early stage of analysis. Therefore, it is preferable to analyze the pattern in purely descriptive terms, such as reticular or nodular shadowing, to avoid this pitfall.

RETICULAR SHADOWING

Reticular or linear shadowing (Fig. 1.62) is made up of multiple, short, irregular linear densities, usually randomly oriented and often overlapping to produce a netlike pattern. When profuse they may summate to form ring shadows or sometimes a nodular pattern. Occasionally the linear shadows may be oriented at right angles to the pleural surface, so-called "Kerley's B lines" (Fig. 1.63), a phenomenon that indicates thickening of the interlobular septa. When the linear opacities are extremely profuse or coarse, the impression of a ring or honeycomb pattern is given.

NODULAR OPACITIES

Nodules may be well or poorly defined and of varying densities, ranging from soft-tissue density to calcific (Fig. 1.64). They may be discrete or coalescent, with areas of confluence producing consolidation. When the nodules are greater than a few mil-

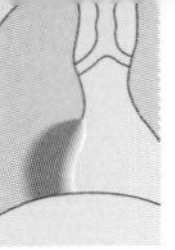

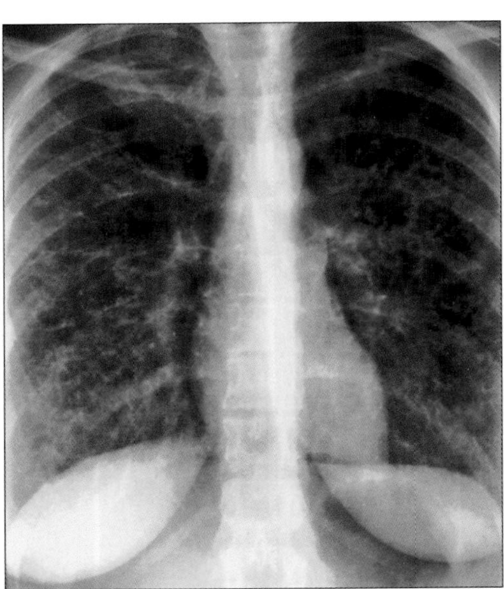

Figure 1.62 Extensive reticular infiltrate in a patient who has normal-volume lungs. The patient has Langerhans-cell histiocytosis.

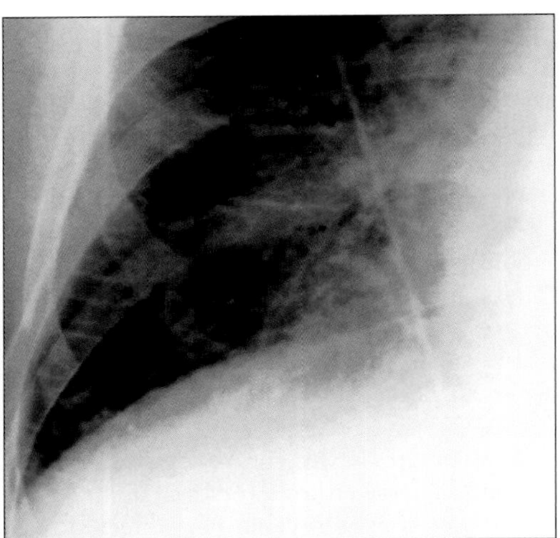

Figure 1.63 Kerley's B lines in a patient with heart failure. Note that the reticular opacities are oriented at right angles to the pleural surface.

limeters in diameter the differential diagnosis changes. Larger discrete nodules are discussed in a previous section.

RETICULONODULAR SHADOWING

Often the examiner is unable to confidently assign a pattern of diffuse shadowing to one of the two previously described categories because they overlap. The reticulonodular pattern is probably the most common form of diffuse lung shadowing.

GROUND-GLASS SHADOWING

The term *ground-glass shadowing* (see Fig. 1.35) refers to a generalized increase in density of the lung, which may be diffuse or patchy but is most commonly bilateral and midzonal and lower zonal or perihilar. The underlying vascular branching pattern is not totally obscured, as it is in consolidation, but the vessels become less distinct; likewise, the hila and diaphragms may appear less sharply. This subtle abnormality is considerably easier to appreciate when a previous normal film is available for comparison.

In addition to determination of the radiographic pattern of diffuse abnormality, a number of other features must be sought,

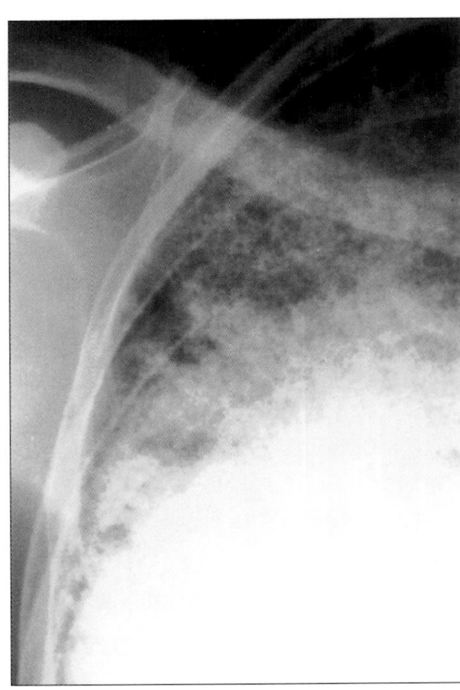

Figure 1.64 Very profuse nodular shadowing, coalescent in the midzone and lower zone. The individual nodules are of high density. The patient has alveolar microlithiasis.

including whether the distribution of disease is central or peripheral, whether it occurs in the upper, middle, or lower zone, and whether distortion of the lung architecture is associated. Additional important features include signs of cardiac failure or fluid overload, such as increased heart size, equalization of upper and lower lobar vein size, and pleural effusions. Hilar or mediastinal enlargement caused by lymph nodes or vascular enlargement should also be specifically sought. The bones and soft tissues of the chest wall may provide important clues, such as evidence of previous breast surgery or an erosive arthritis. The accuracy of radiographic analysis is reduced in the absence of appropriate clinical information. For example, ascertaining whether the patient is well, acutely or chronically unwell, of normal immune status, or immunocompromised can dramatically narrow a wide radiologic differential diagnosis.

Airway Disease

Plain tomography has been replaced by CT as the investigation of choice for the examination of airway abnormalities.

TRACHEAL NARROWING

Tracheal narrowing may be caused by an extrinsic mass mediastinal fibrosis or an intrinsic abnormality of the tracheal wall. Chronic inflammatory causes include fibrosing mediastinitis, sarcoidosis, chronic relapsing polychondritis (Fig. 1.65), and Wegener's granulomatosis. Primary tumors of the trachea are rare. Benign tumors take the form of small, well-defined, intraluminal nodules that are difficult or impossible to visualize on the chest radiograph. Malignant tumors of the trachea tend to occur close to the carina (Fig. 1.66), although they may be quite extensive and cause a long stricture (Fig. 1.67). Tracheal-wall thickening and tracheal luminal narrowing can be detected on the plain chest radiograph, especially when specifically sought. The right lateral wall of the trachea (the right paratracheal stripe) above the level of the azygos vein is typically a 2-mm

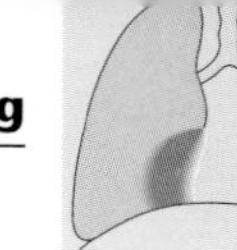

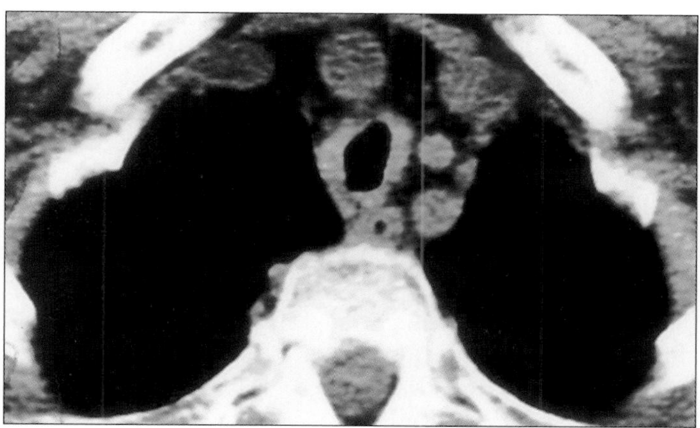

Figure 1.65 Circumferential tracheal-wall thickening with tracheal narrowing. This is a case of relapsing polychondritis.

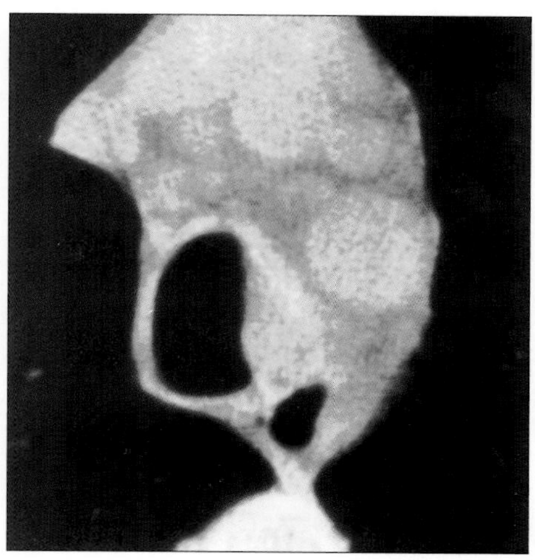

Figure 1.66 Focal carcinoma within the tracheal wall.

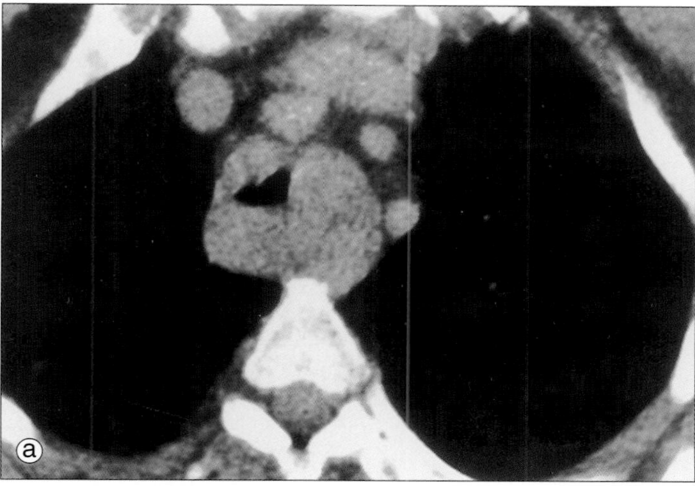

Figure 1.67 Adenoid cystic carcinoma. Extensive tracheal tumor. **A,** Circumferential soft-tissue tumor of the trachea at the level of the great vessels. **B,** Coronal reformation showing extensive tracheal-wall thickening measuring, on the left, almost 2 cm *(arrow)*.

thick, soft-tissue stripe, and tracheal-wall thickening can easily be seen if this portion of the airway is involved (Fig. 1.68).

TRACHEAL WIDENING

The normal dimensions of the trachea have been assessed by means of a variety of techniques, most recently CT. The trachea becomes slightly larger with increasing age. On CT scanning, the maximal coronal diameter of the trachea is 23 mm in men and 20 mm in women. Dilatation of the trachea is rare and may result from a generalized defect of connective tissue (Fig. 1.69). On the plain radiograph, shift of the right paratracheal stripe to the right is often the only sign of tracheal widening, and because the trachea is frequently not central, it is only if the left wall of the trachea is also identified that tracheal widening can be recognized.

BRONCHIECTASIS

The chest radiograph is relatively insensitive for the detection of bronchiectasis, and in most series a significant portion of plain radiographs of patients with bronchiectasis are judged to be normal (Fig. 1.70). HRCT, the use of which is discussed subsequently, is now the investigation of choice for bronchiectasis. Abnormalities present on the chest radiograph are as follows.

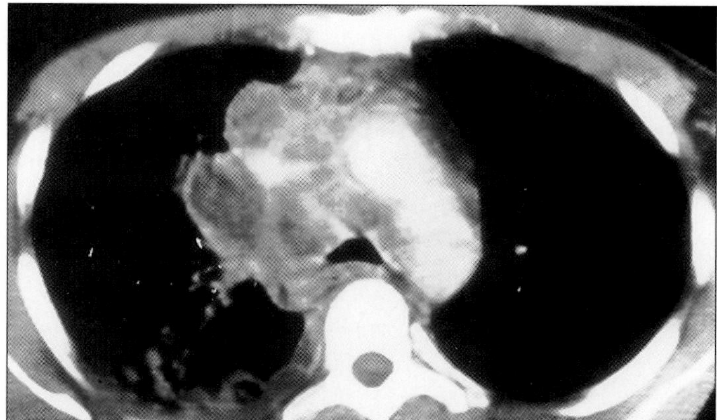

Figure 1.68 Computed tomography (CT) scan demonstrating an extensive, necrotic, metastatic, mediastinal, lymph-node enlargement, which is causing tracheal narrowing.

Bronchial-wall thickening is evident as parallel, linear opacities radiating from the hilum, with lack of the normal convergence more peripherally. Ring shadows occur when the dilated airway is seen end on; they may be thick or thin walled and may contain secretions that produce an air-fluid level. Bronchiectatic

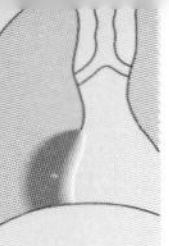

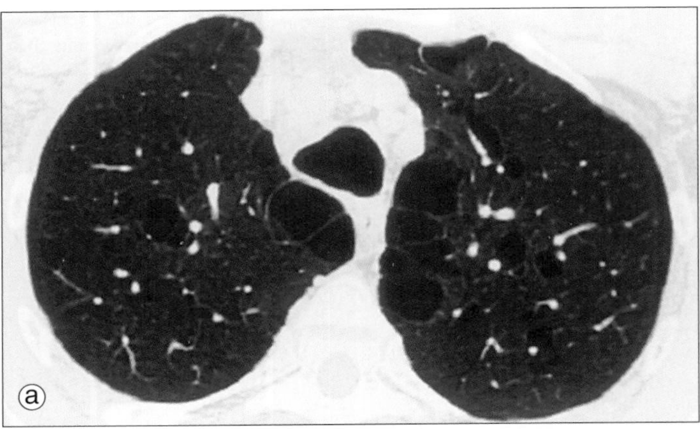

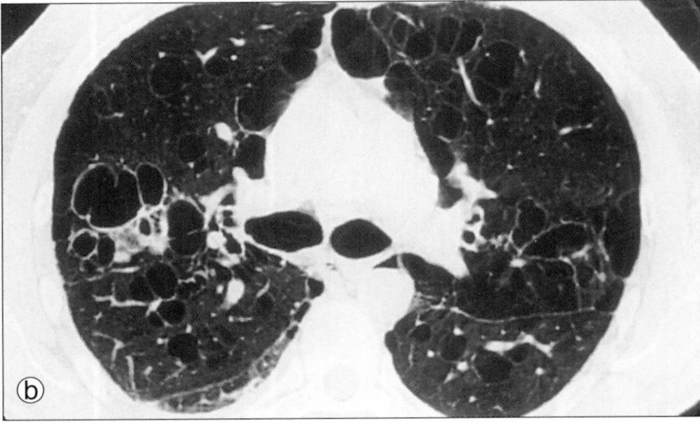

Figure 1.69 Tracheobronchomegaly. Computed tomography (CT) scans showing diffuse moderate dilatation of the trachea and main bronchi in association with cystic bronchiectasis. **A,** At the level of the trachea. **B,** At the level of the carina.

airways that become plugged with secretions may produce tubular, soft-tissue–density opacities radiating from the hilum, more commonly in the lower lobes.

Distortion of the lobar anatomy with volume loss and crowding together of bronchovascular structures may be associated. However, patients with cystic fibrosis, also characterized by bronchiectasis, may have significant air trapping, which results in overexpansion. Even severe bronchiectasis may be invisible within a completely collapsed lobe.

Cylindrical (or tubular) bronchiectasis produces a dilated bronchus with parallel walls; in varicose bronchiectasis the walls are irregular; and in saccular (or cystic) bronchiectasis the airways terminate as round cysts. More than one pattern is usually seen in a patient. Bronchiectasis usually involves the peripheral bronchi more severely than the central bronchi. Although it has long been held that in allergic bronchopulmonary aspergillosis this pattern may be reversed, overall the distribution and morphology demonstrated by CT give no more than clues to the underlying cause.

Mediastinal Abnormalities

The normal radiographic anatomy of the mediastinum is discussed in a previous section of this chapter. When a mediastinal abnormality is present on the PA radiograph, a lateral view should be obtained to aid in anatomic localization. The imaging of mediastinal masses depends heavily on CT scanning, which is discussed elsewhere. However, a familiarity with normal anatomy is required for the detection of mediastinal masses that at first appear to be subtle distortions of the normal mediastinal contours. A considerable volume of mediastinal tumor or lymph-node enlargement may be present in the face of an apparently normal chest radiograph.

The most common cause of mediastinal enlargement visible on the chest radiograph in children is the normal thymus, which may enlarge and contract in certain disease states but normally remains relatively prominent, especially on CT scans, until puberty (Fig. 1.71). Lymphadenopathy, tumor, hiatal hernia, and vascular abnormalities account for most mediastinal masses seen in adults.

MEDIASTINAL LYMPHADENOPATHY

Lymph nodes are present in all compartments of the mediastinum but are visible on the chest radiograph only when they are calcified or enlarged. Causes of mediastinal nodal enlargement are discussed elsewhere. The chest radiograph is a relatively insensitive indicator of lymphadenopathy. Enlargement of right paratracheal nodes is identified more easily than those of left paratracheal nodes, aortic-pulmonary nodes, and subcarinal

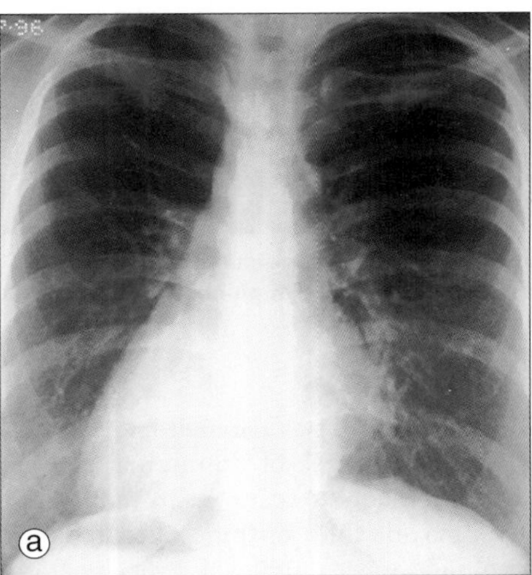

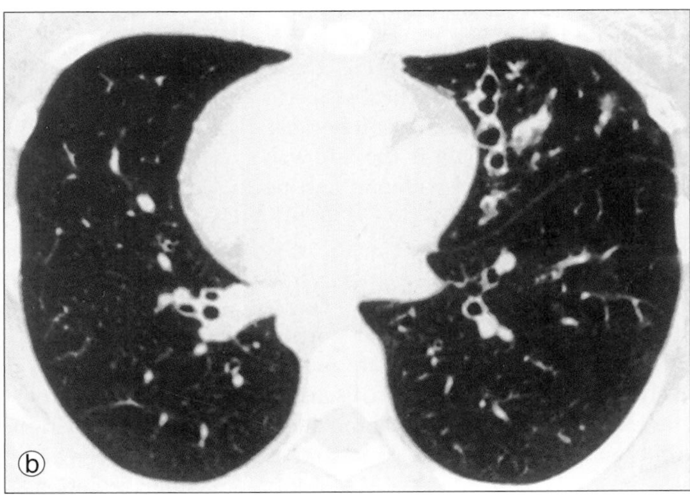

Figure 1.70 Bronchiectasis. A, The chest radiograph of a patient who has primary ciliary dyskinesia. Dextrocardia is present. Some questionable bronchial-wall thickening adjacent to the left heart border is obscured. **B,** The changes of bronchiectasis are much more convincingly demonstrated on high-resolution computed tomography (HRCT).

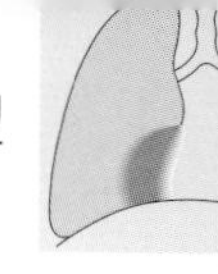

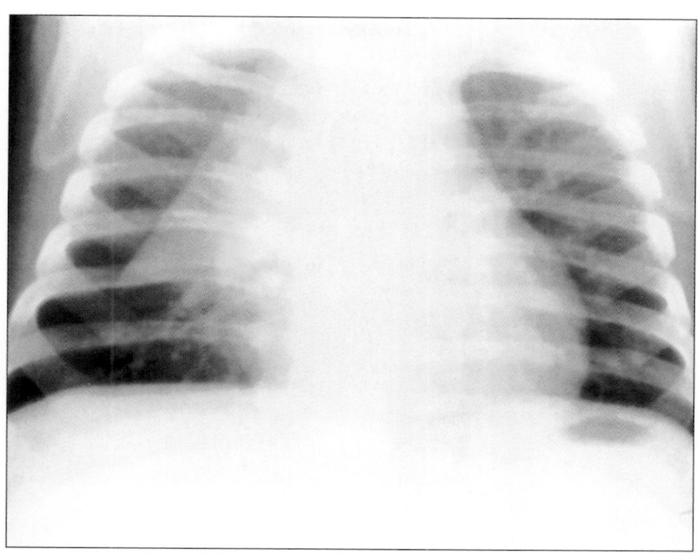

Figure 1.71 A prominent, but normal, thymic silhouette in an infant. Note the characteristic sail shape of the thymus as it projects over the right lung, and the typically slightly lobulated contour as it conforms to the overlying ribs.

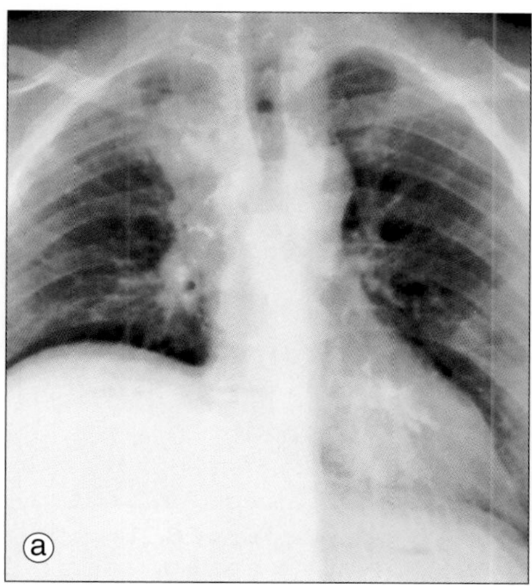

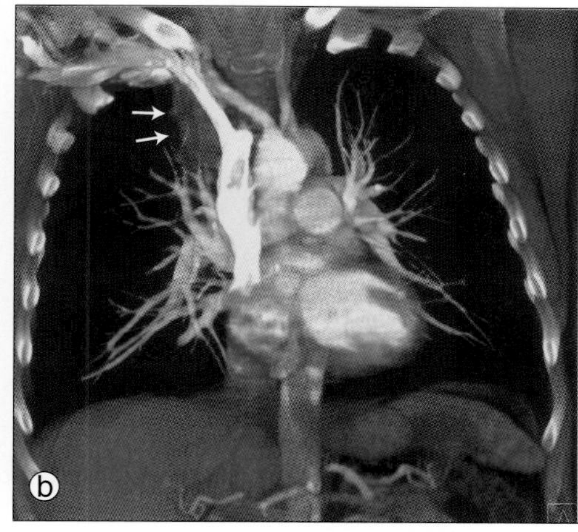

Figure 1.72 Right paratracheal lymph-node enlargement caused by bronchogenic carcinoma. A, A right phrenic nerve palsy results in elevation of the right hemidiaphragm. **B,** Coronal volume rendered slab image from a multidetector CT from a different patient. Again, right paratracheal lymph node enlargement is present (*arrows*), with the enlarged nodes abutting but not distorting the right brachiocephalic vein and superior vena cava.

lymph nodes (Fig. 1.72). Barium swallow is a simple method of identifying some cases of subcarinal lymphadenopathy, but CT is the most comprehensive and accurate method of assessing mediastinal nodes.

ABNORMALITIES OF THE THORACIC AORTA

The thoracic aorta arises in the middle mediastinum and then arches through the anterior, middle, and posterior mediastinal compartments. The greater vessels arise from the aortic arch in the superior mediastinum (Fig. 1.73). Dilatation or tortuosity of the aortic arch or its branches may cause widening of the mediastinal shadow. So-called "unfolding of the aorta" is a common finding in the chest radiograph of elderly patients or those with hypertension. Aneurysm of the aorta most often results from atherosclerosis (Fig. 1.74). Cystic medial necrosis (Marfan's syndrome), infection (mycotic aneurysm), syphilitic aortitis, and a history of trauma are less-common causes. Most aortic aneurysms are asymptomatic and appear as a mediastinal opacity on the radiograph, sometimes with curvilinear calcification visible in the wall. Aneurysms of the ascending aorta are best appreciated on the lateral radiograph as a filling in of the retrosternal window. Aneurysms of the arch and descending aorta are frequently evident on the frontal radiograph, but a lateral view is often required for more accurate localization, and cross-sectional imaging is often required to confirm that the mediastinal abnormality in question is of vascular origin.

In the acutely injured patient, traumatic aortic rupture may be suspected from chest radiographic findings, and confirmation of injury usually requires angiography (Fig. 1.75). However, when the chest radiograph is equivocal and the degree of trauma is less than that usually associated with aortic injury, a spiral CT scan may be performed in the stable patient to exclude a mediastinal hematoma. If any doubt remains, the patient should proceed to angiography. If the aortic injury remains undetected and the patient survives, an aneurysm secondary to the trauma may develop subsequently. This is almost always confined to the junction of arch and descending aorta. Aortic abnormalities may produce pressure changes in adjacent skeletal structures.

Aneurysm of the ascending aorta may erode the posterior surface of the sternum, and descending aortic aneurysms may

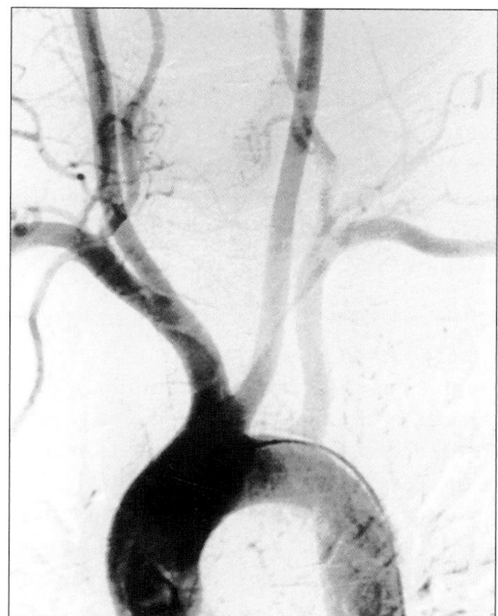

Figure 1.73 Digital subtraction arch aortogram. This patient has two vessels arising from the arch, a common variant of the normal three vessels. The image was obtained with the patient in a 30-degree left anterior oblique position.

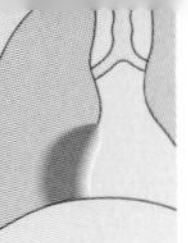

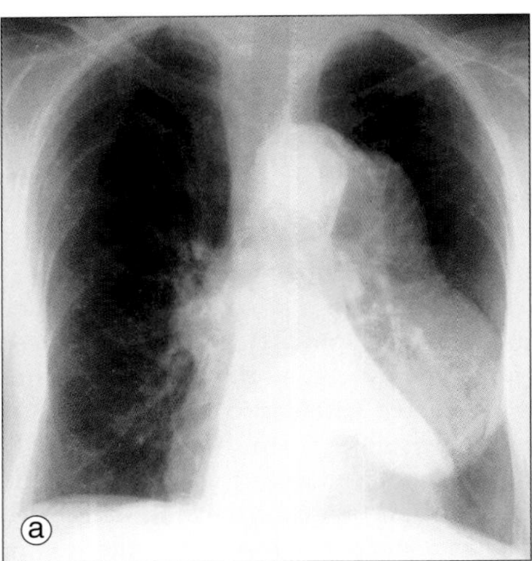

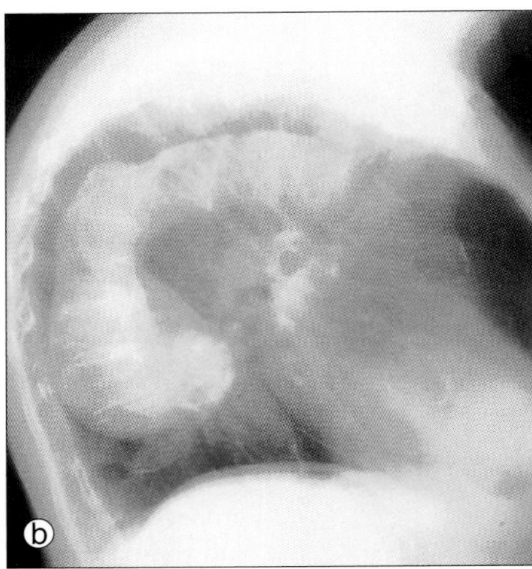

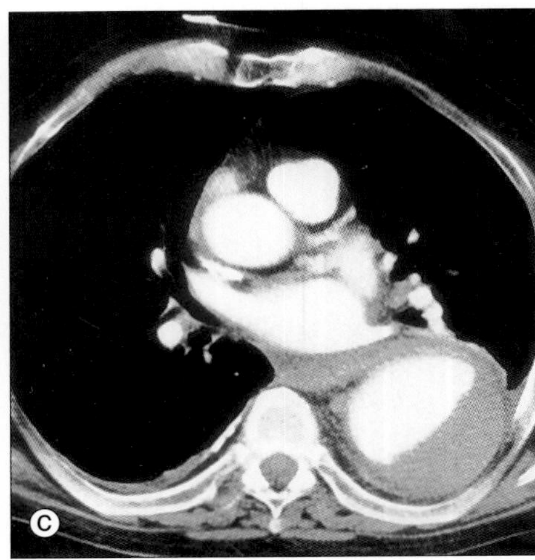

Figure 1.74 Thoracic aortic aneurysm. A, Marked dilatation and tortuosity of the descending thoracic aorta is present. Note how the left heart border is still evident, indicating the abnormality is likely to lie in the posterior thorax. **B,** Lateral view in the same patient demonstrates that the aneurysm involves the posterior arch and descending thoracic aorta. Note calcification within the ascending aorta. **C,** Computed tomography (CT) demonstrating extensive mural thrombus.

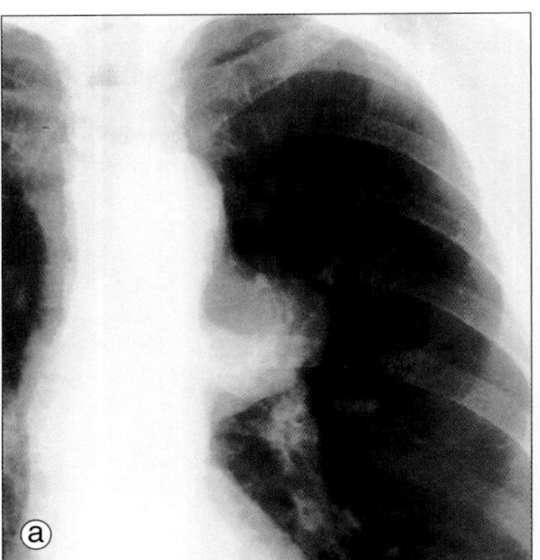

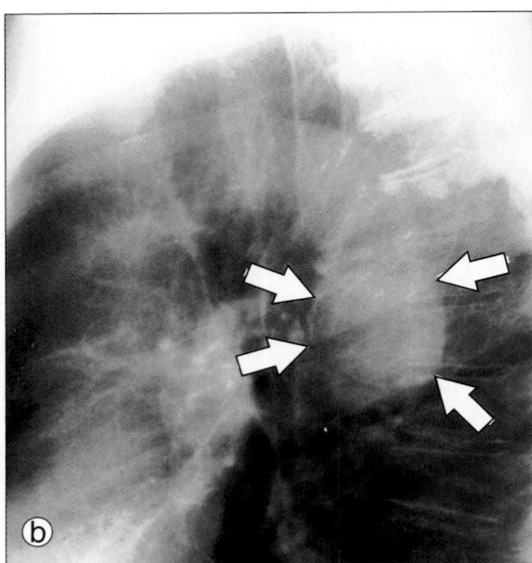

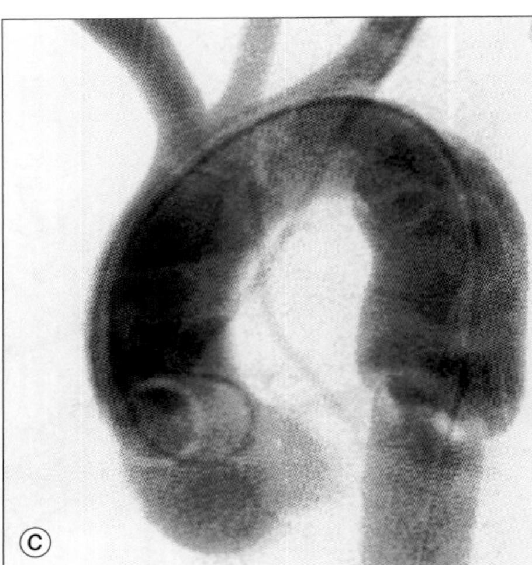

Figure 1.75 Traumatic aortic aneurysm. A, On the posteroanterior (PA) radiograph, a soft-tissue density mass projects over the left hilum. Note how the left lower lobar artery is still visible through this mass, which indicates that it is separate from the hilum *(arrows)*. The medial surface blends smoothly with the mediastinal structures, indicating it is likely to be extrapulmonary. **B,** The lateral view confirms an aneurysm secondary to previous trauma at the typical site, the junction of the posterior arch and descending thoracic aorta *(arrows)*. **C,** The arch aortogram confirms the diagnosis of an acute aortic injury at the typical site.

cause scalloping of the spine. Tortuosity of the innominate artery is a common cause of widening of the superior mediastinum in the elderly. Right-sided aortic arch (Fig. 1.76) and pseudocoarctation of the aorta are two anomalies that may alter the appearance of the mediastinum and suggest a mass.

ABNORMALITIES OF THE ESOPHAGUS

Abnormalities of the esophagus are relatively common. They include infection, inflammation, trauma, perforation, and benign and malignant neoplastic processes. Esophageal abnormalities may be associated with diseases that also involve the lungs. For example, in systemic sclerosis, esophageal motility disorders that result in significant dilatation and reflux may be encountered in conjunction with pulmonary fibrosis and the results of recurrent aspiration (Fig. 1.77).

DILATATION OF CENTRAL VEINS

The superior vena cava and azygos veins may dilate because of increased pressure, increased flow, obstruction, or congenital abnormality. Increased flow in the superior vena cava is seen in supracardiac, total, anomalous pulmonary venous drainage (Fig. 1.78) and in the azygos vein in the congenital absence of the inferior vena cava. Rarely, aneurysmal dilatation of the superior mediastinal veins produces an abnormal mediastinal silhouette. Likewise, obstruction of the superior vena cava may cause dilatation of the great veins in the superior mediastinum, which results in widening of the mediastinal contour. However, the clinical features are likely to be obvious by the time radiographic abnormalities become significant.

OTHER MEDIASTINAL ABNORMALITIES

Pneumomediastinum or mediastinal emphysema is the presence of air between the tissue planes of the mediastinum. This may

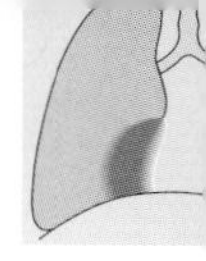

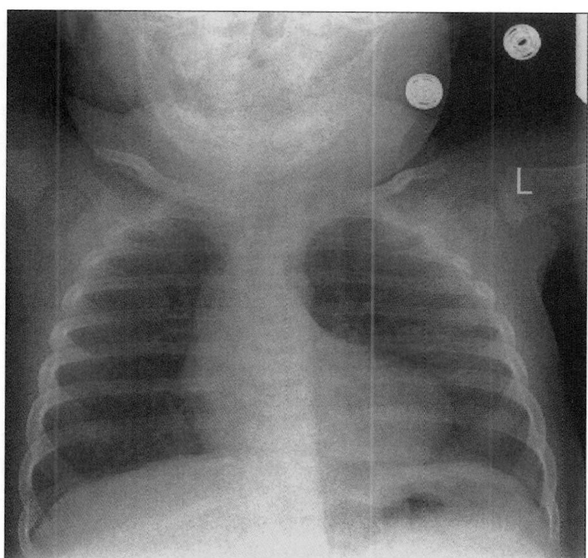

Figure 1.76 Tetralogy of Fallot. There is a right-sided aortic arch in addition to elevation of the ventricular apex because of developing ventricular hypertrophy. Note the relatively oligemic lungs.

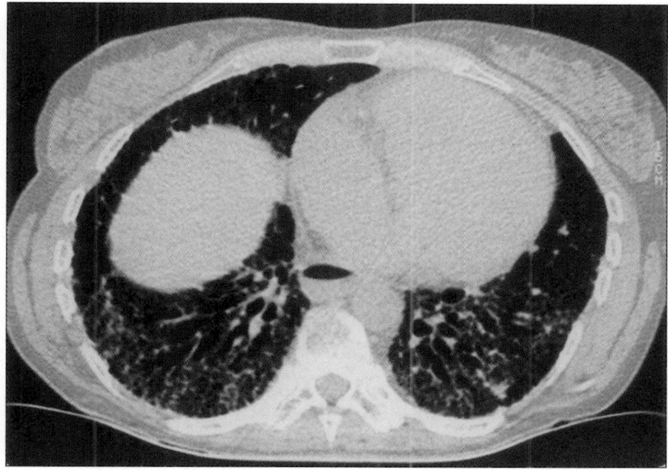

Figure 1.77 Systemic sclerosis with esophageal involvement. There is a coarse bibasal reticular infiltrate with marked traction bronchiectasis. In addition, the esophagus is moderately dilated and contains an air-fluid level.

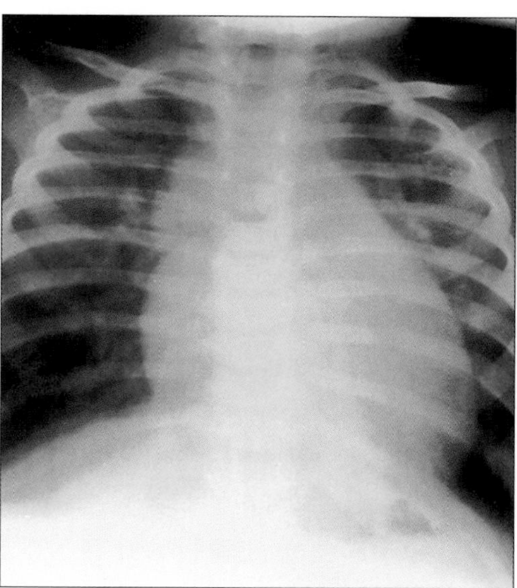

Figure 1.78 Total anomalous pulmonary venous drainage. Widening of the superior mediastinum caused by dilatation of the superior vena cava.

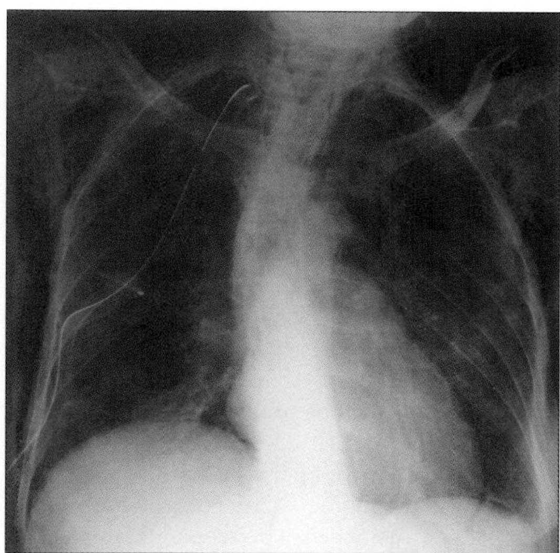

Figure 1.79 Pneumomediastinum. Air separates the tissue planes within the mediastinum and extends into the soft tissues of the neck and chest. A right-sided intercostal drain is in situ.

occur secondary to interstitial pulmonary emphysema (most often caused by mechanical ventilation); perforation of the esophagus, trachea, or a bronchus; or a penetrating chest injury. Chest radiography may show vertical, translucent streaks in the mediastinum, which represent air separating the soft-tissue planes (Fig. 1.79). The air may extend up into the neck and over the chest wall (causing subcutaneous emphysema) and also over the diaphragm. The mediastinal pleura may be displaced laterally and then be visible as a thin stripe alongside the mediastinum.

Acute mediastinitis is usually caused by perforation of the esophagus, pharynx, or trachea, and a chest radiograph usually shows widening of the mediastinum. A pneumomediastinum is often apparent, and fluid levels may be visible in the mediastinum. Chronic or fibrosing mediastinitis usually manifests as SVCO. Mediastinal hemorrhage may occur as a result of venous or arterial bleeding. The mediastinum appears widened, and blood may be seen to track over the lung apices. Identification of a life-threatening cause such as aortic rupture is obviously imperative.

Hilar Abnormalities

Having identified a hilar abnormality, the observer must differentiate between a vascular and a nonvascular cause. Vascular prominence is often bilateral and accompanied by enlargement of the main pulmonary artery (Fig. 1.80). Although the hila are large, they are of relatively normal density, and usually the pulmonary artery branches can be traced continuously from the adjacent lung to their point of convergence with the interlobar arteries—the "hilar convergence" sign. In comparison, enlargement caused by lymph nodes or hilar tumors usually produces a lobulated hilar contour, with discernible lateral or inferior borders. Frequently, the normal hilar point is obliterated and, on the left, the aortopulmonary angle is filled in (Fig. 1.81).

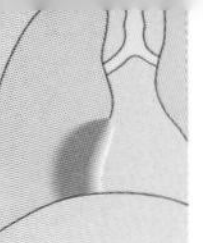

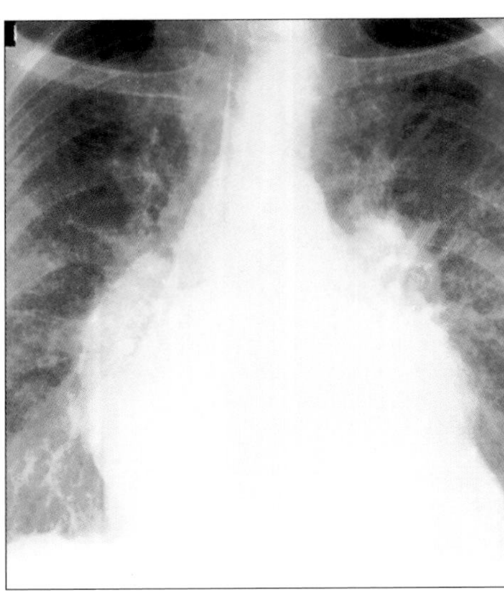

Figure 1.80 Atrioseptal defect results in marked dilatation of the proximal pulmonary arteries. The cardiac silhouette is enlarged.

Occasionally a pulmonary lesion is superimposed directly on the hilum on the frontal radiograph, which produces a spuriously large or dense hilum. The true position of the abnormality is revealed on the lateral radiograph (see Fig. 1.75). A further pitfall is encountered when the vessels to the lingula or, more commonly, the right middle lobe are superimposed on the lower part of the hilar shadow, particularly when the film is taken anteroposteriorly, in a lordotic projection, or with a poor inspiratory effort. A lateral radiograph usually confirms the vascular nature of the shadowing.

Pleural Disease

PLEURAL FLUID

The most dependent recess of the pleural space is the posterior costophrenic angle, which is where a small effusion tends to collect. As little as 100 to 200 mL of fluid accumulated in this recess can be seen above the dome of the diaphragm on the frontal view. Even smaller effusions may be seen on a lateral radiograph, and it is possible to identify effusions of only a few milliliters through use of decubitus views with a horizontal beam, ultrasound, or CT. Eventually, the costophrenic angle on the frontal view fills in, and with increasing fluid a homogeneous opacity spreads upward, obscuring the lung base (Fig. 1.82). The fluid usually demonstrates a concave upper edge, higher laterally than medially, and obscures the diaphragm. Fluid may track into the fissures. A massive effusion may cause complete opacification of a hemithorax with passive atelectasis. The space-occupying effect of the effusion may push the mediastinum toward the opposite side, especially when the lung does not collapse significantly (Fig. 1.83).

Lamellar effusions are shallow collections between the lung surface and the visceral pleura, sometimes with sparing of the costophrenic angle. Subpulmonary effusions accumulate between the diaphragm and under surface of a lung, mimicking elevation of the hemidiaphragm (see Fig. 1.3). Usually the contour to the top of such an effusion differs from the normal diaphragmatic contour, the apparent apex being more lateral than usual. Also, some blunting of the costophrenic angle or tracking of fluid into fissures may be visible. On the left side, increased distance between the gastric air bubble and lung base may be apparent. A subpulmonary effusion may be confirmed by ultrasound. However, because the fluid is free to shift within the pleural cavity with changes in patient position, a decubitus film may be needed for confirmation.

Encapsulated or encysted fluid may be difficult to differentiate from an extrapleural opacity, parenchymal lung disease, or mediastinal mass. However, an encysted effusion is often associated with free pleural fluid or other pleural shadowing and may extend into a fissure (see Fig. 1.82). Loculated effusions tend to have comparatively little depth but considerable width, rather like a biconvex lens. The appearance of these effusions, therefore, depends on whether they are viewed face on, in profile, or obliquely. Extrapleural opacities tend to have a much sharper outline, with tapered, sometimes concave edges where they meet the chest wall. Peripheral, pleurally based lung lesions may show an air bronchogram that differentiates them from true pleural disease. The differentiation between pleural thickening or mass and loculated pleural fluid may be difficult on plain films; CT and ultrasound are particularly useful in this context.

Fluid may become loculated in the interlobar fissures and is most frequently seen in heart failure. Fluid that collects in the horizontal fissure produces a lenticular, oval, or round shadow,

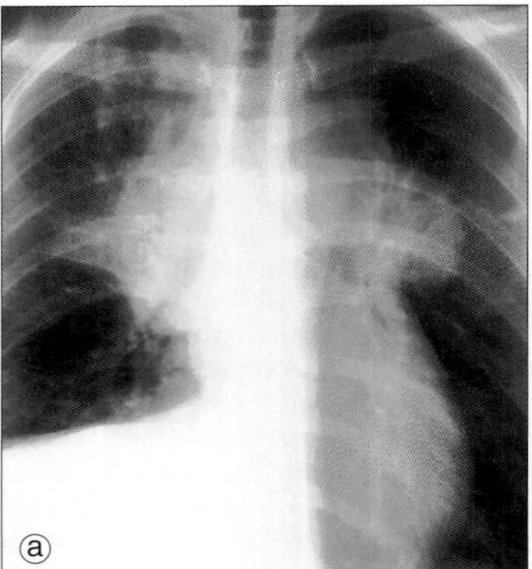

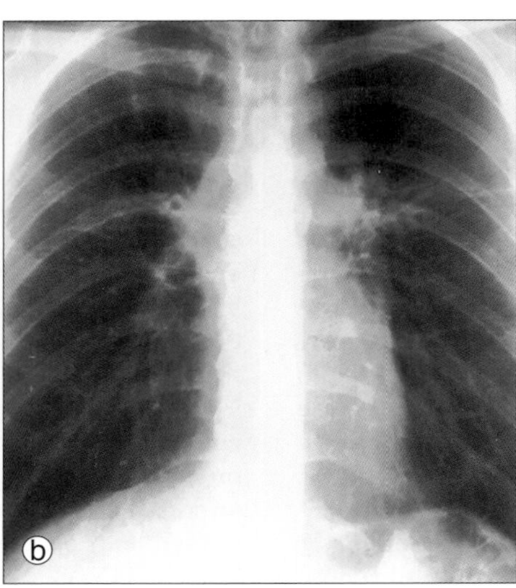

Figure 1.81 Non-Hodgkin's lymphoma. A, Bilateral hilar lymph-node enlargement, with obliteration of the normal aortopulmonary angle and subcarinal nodes. A right-sided pleural effusion is present. **B,** The same patient showing residual abnormality after chemotherapy.

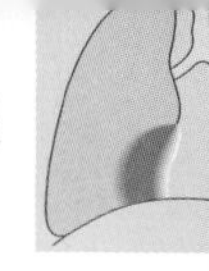

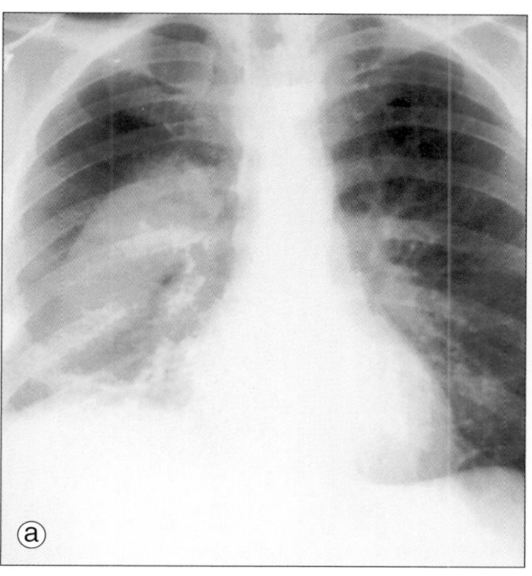

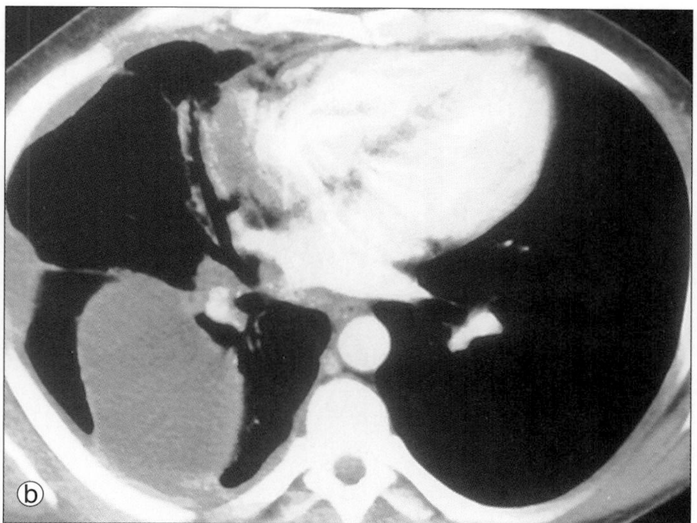

Figure 1.82 Small, right pleural effusion. A, The lentiform opacity in the right midzone is caused by a loculated interlobar effusion. **B,** Computed tomography (CT) scan on mediastinal settings demonstrating the position of the loculated fluid within the oblique fissure.

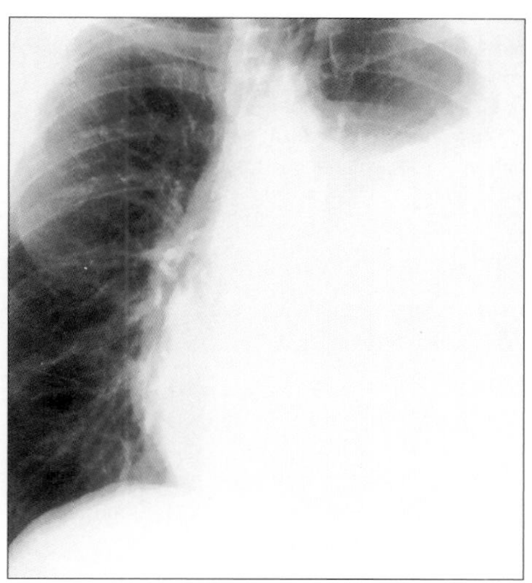

Figure 1.83 Large, left pleural effusion. There has been a previous mastectomy on the right and the pleural effusion is malignant. The mediastinal shift to the right results from the space-occupying effects of the fluid.

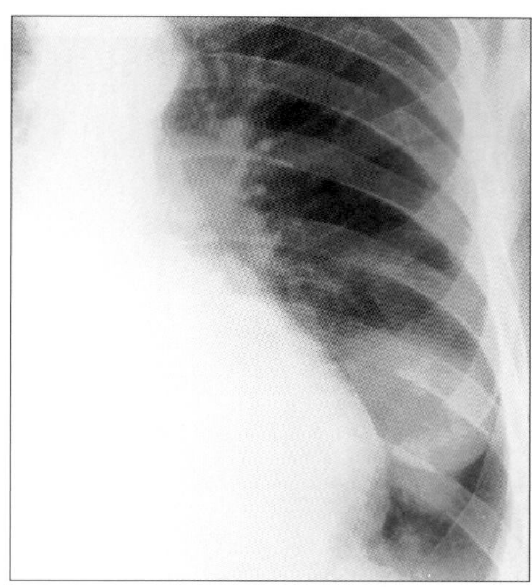

Figure 1.84 Small, left basal pleural effusion. The opacity in the left midzone is caused by fluid loculated in the oblique fissure.

with well-demarcated edges. Loculated fluid in an oblique fissure may be poorly defined on a frontal radiograph, but a lateral film is usually diagnostic because the fissure is seen tangentially, and the typical lenticular configuration of the effusion is demonstrated. Loculated interlobar effusions can appear rounded on two views and may disappear rapidly; therefore, they are sometimes known as *pulmonary pseudotumors* (Fig. 1.84). With subsequent episodes of heart failure they may return at the same site.

Diagnosis of an empyema usually requires thoracentesis. Nevertheless, radiographically the diagnosis may be suspected on examination of a plain film because of the spontaneous appearance of an air-fluid level in a pleural effusion, because this usually equates with loculation and communication with the tracheobronchial tree or the presence of a gas-forming organism. Loculation is best demonstrated with ultrasound.

PNEUMOTHORAX

A small pneumothorax is easily overlooked and, in an erect patient, usually collects at the apex. The lung retracts toward the hilum, and on a frontal chest film the sharp white line of the visceral pleura is visible, separated from the chest wall by the radiolucent pleural space, which is devoid of lung markings. This pleural region should not be confused with a skin fold (Fig. 1.85). The lung usually remains aerated, although perfusion is reduced in proportion to ventilation, and therefore the radiodensity of the partially collapsed lung remains relatively normal. A closed pneumothorax is easier to see on an expiratory film, although expiratory radiographs are not routinely required for the detection of clinically significant pneumothoraces. A lateral decubitus film with the affected side uppermost is occasionally helpful, as the pleural air can be seen along the lateral chest wall. This view is particularly useful in infants, because the air tends to collect anteriorly and medially and therefore small pneumothoraces are difficult to see on supine AP films.

A large pneumothorax may lead to complete relaxation and retraction of the lung, with some mediastinal shift toward the normal side (Fig. 1.86). Because tension pneumothorax is a medical emergency, it is often treated before a chest radiograph is obtained. However, if a radiograph is taken in this situation it shows marked displacement of the mediastinum (Fig. 1.87). Radiographically, the lung may be squashed against the mediastinum or may herniate across the midline, and the ipsilateral hemidiaphragm may be depressed.

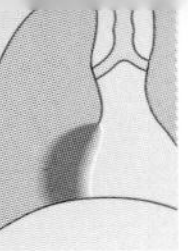

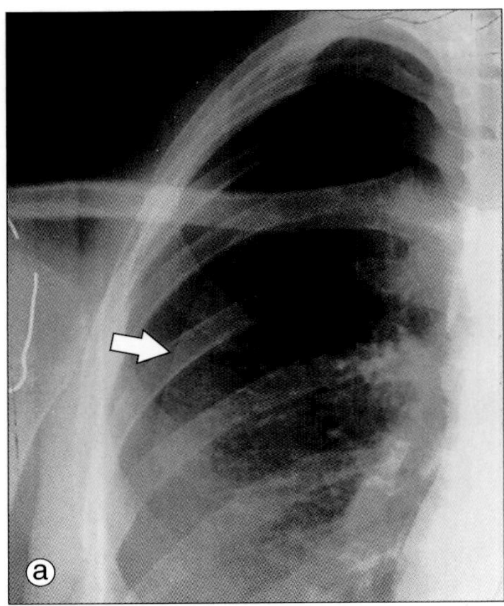

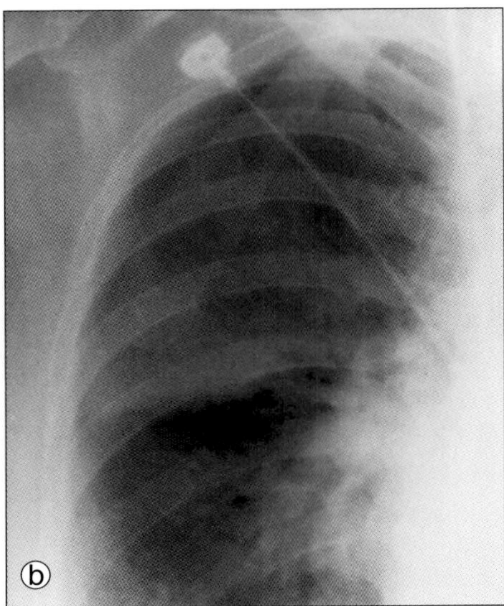

Figure 1.85 Shallow right pneumothorax. A, A discrete pleural white line is seen. Peripheral to this, there are no lung markings. **B,** In this skin fold, although a change in density parallels the chest wall, no discrete pleural line is present, and lung markings are seen to extend beyond the apparent lung edge. This appearance is caused by a superficial fold of skin produced by the x-ray cassette.

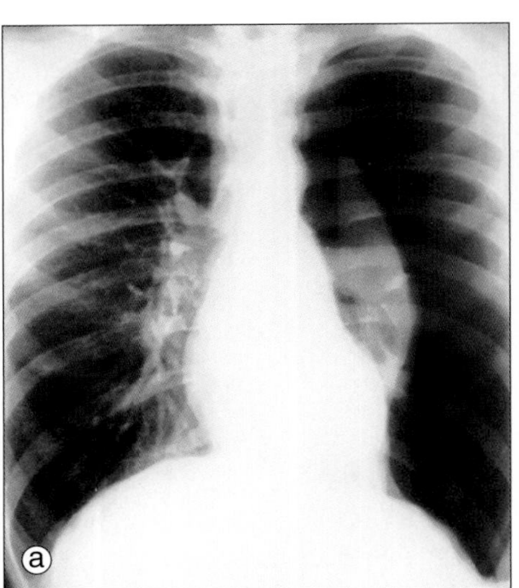

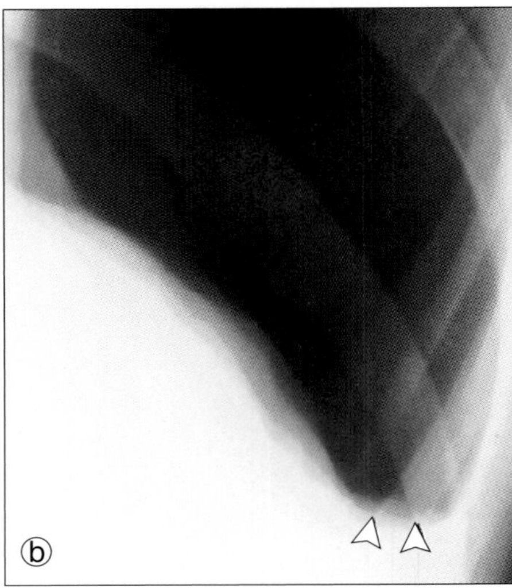

Figure 1.86 Left-sided pneumothorax. A, Complete collapse of the left lung, which is retracted to the left hilum. **B,** Magnified view of the left lower zone demonstrates the short air-fluid level commonly seen in a costophrenic angle when a pneumothorax is present *(arrowheads)*.

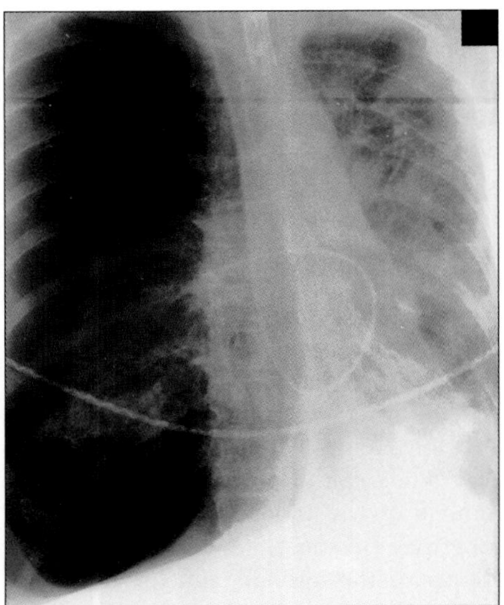

Figure 1.87 Tension pneumothorax after insertion of a Swan-Ganz catheter. Note the shift of the mediastinum toward the left and reversal of the normal contour of the right hemidiaphragm.

Complications of Pneumothorax

Pleural adhesions may limit the distribution of a pneumothorax and result in a loculated or encysted pneumothorax. The usual appearance is an ovoid air collection adjacent to the chest wall, which may be radiographically indistinguishable from a thin-walled, subpleural pulmonary cyst or bulla. Pleural adhesions are occasionally seen as line shadows that stretch between the two pleural layers; they prevent relaxation of the underlying lung. Rupture of an adhesion may produce a hemopneumothorax. Collapse or consolidation of a lobe or lung in association with a pneumothorax is important because it may delay re-expansion of the lung.

Because the normal pleural space contains a small volume of fluid, blunting of the costophrenic angle by a short fluid level is commonly seen with a pneumothorax (see Fig. 1.86). In a small pneumothorax, this fluid level may be the most obvious radiologic sign. A larger fluid level usually signifies a complication and represents exudate, pus, or blood, depending on the cause of the pneumothorax (Fig. 1.88).

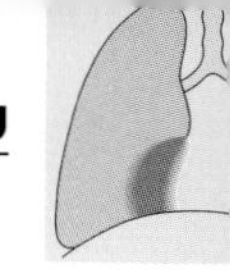

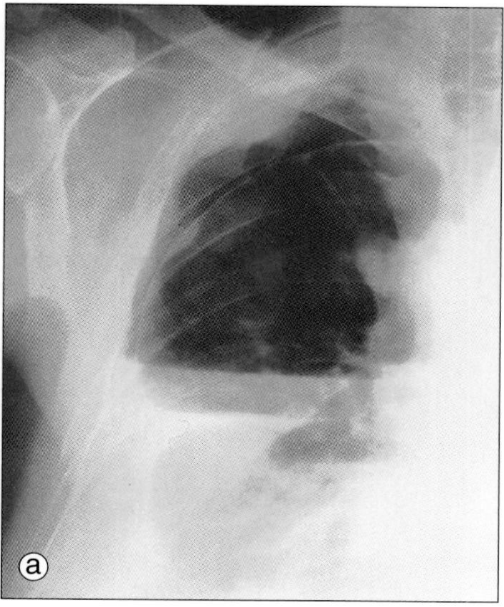

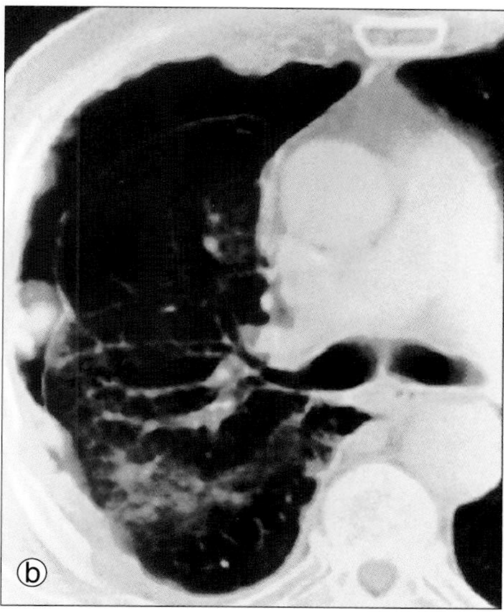

Figure 1.88 Hydropneumothorax in a patient with a mesothelioma. A, Note the normal thickness of the visceral pleura, but the lobulated soft-tissue shadowing caused by tumor within the parietal pleura. **B,** Computed tomography (CT) scan in the same patient that demonstrates the lobulated pleural tumor.

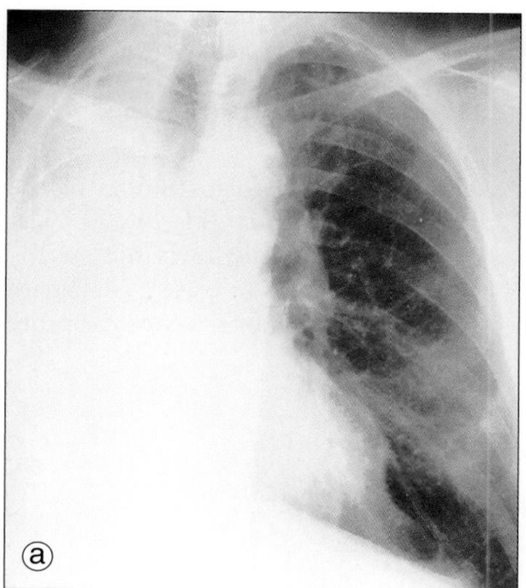

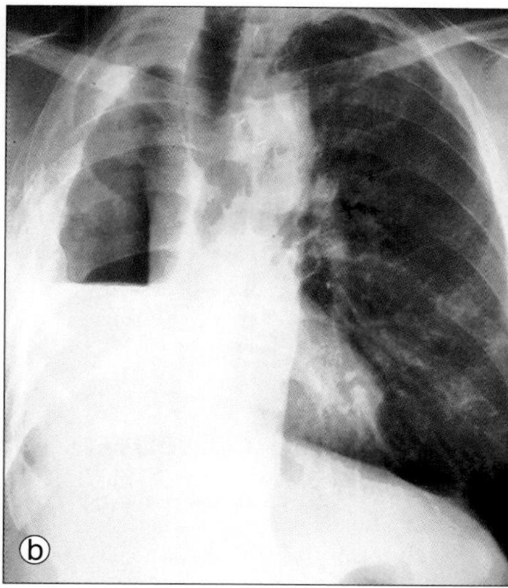

Figure 1.89 Pneumonectomy—appearances and complications. A, Chest radiograph showing the normal appearances after a right pneumonectomy.
B, Spontaneous development of an air-fluid level caused by a bronchopleural fistula from local recurrence.

The usual radiographic appearance of a hydropneumothorax is that of a pneumothorax that contains a horizontal fluid level that separates opaque fluid below from lucent air above. A hydropneumothorax or pyopneumothorax may arise as a result of a bronchopleural fistula (an abnormal communication between the bronchial tree and the pleural space). This may be a complication of surgery, but may occur as a complication of a subpleural lung tumor (Fig. 1.89).

PLEURAL THICKENING

Blunting of a costophrenic angle is a common observation and usually is caused by localized pleural thickening secondary to previous pleuritis. In the asymptomatic patient and in the absence of other radiologic abnormalities, this blunting is of no significance other than that it may simulate a pleural effusion. When relevant, the possibility of pleural fluid may have to be excluded by other techniques. Localized pleural thickening that extends into the inferior end of an oblique fissure may produce so-called "tenting" of the diaphragm and is of similar significance, although a similar appearance may result from scarring caused by pulmonary infection or infarction.

Bilateral apical pleural thickening is common and usually symmetrical, occurs more frequently in elderly patients, and does not necessarily indicate previous tuberculosis. The cause is uncertain, but in some individuals the caps represent extrapleural fat that has descended because of scarring and consequent retraction of the upper lobes. In contrast, asymmetrical or unilateral apical pleural thickening may be highly significant, especially if associated with pain. Asymmetrical apical pleural shadowing may represent a Pancoast tumor, and evidence of bone destruction should be specifically sought (Fig. 1.90).

More extensive unilateral pleural thickening is usually the result of a previous thoracotomy or an exudative pleural effusion. A simple transudate usually resolves completely, but empyema and hemothorax are likely to resolve with pleural fibrosis. The thickened pleura may calcify (Fig. 1.91), and the entire lung may become surrounded by fibrotic pleura, which may be as much as a few centimeters thick (Fig. 1.92). Bilateral (parietal) pleural plaques are a common manifestation of asbestos exposure, and occasionally, more-diffuse, visceral pleural thickening is seen.

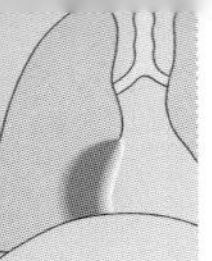

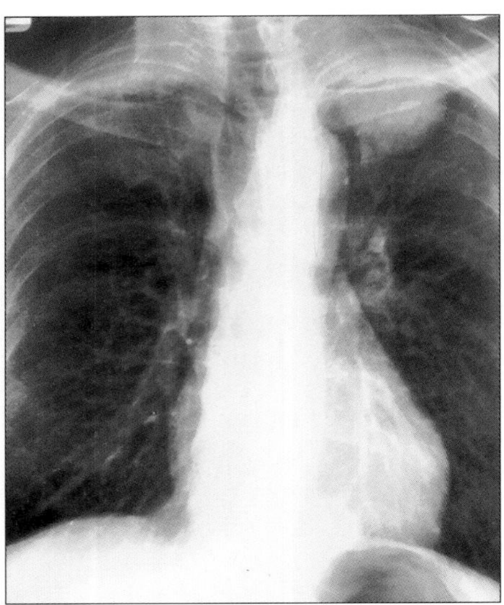

Figure 1.90 Apical abnormalities. Benign apical pleural thickening is visible on the right; on the left there is also a Pancoast tumor.

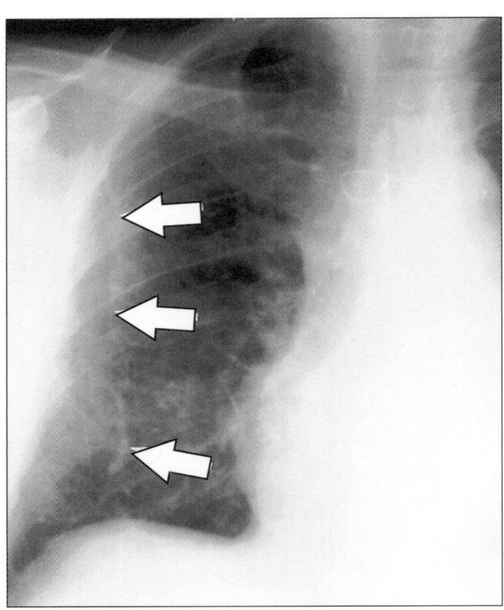

Figure 1.91 Previous thoracotomy (note sternotomy sutures) for mitral valve replacement. Pleural calcification is seen on the right side *(arrows)*.

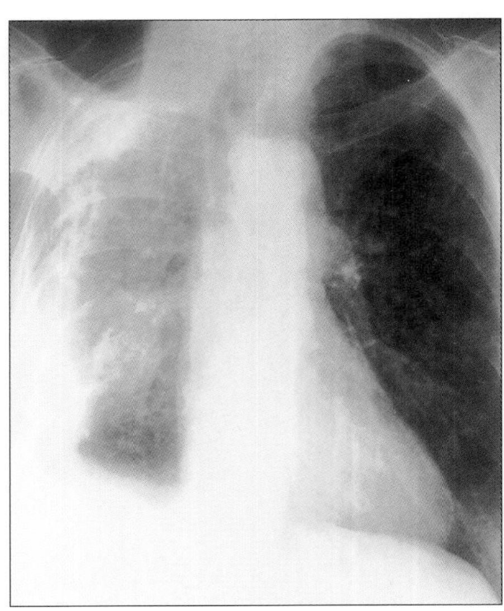

Figure 1.92 Previous tuberculosis. Extensive right-sided pleural thickening and calcification, with reduction in volume of the right hemithorax.

PLEURAL CALCIFICATION

In general, pleural calcification has the same causes as pleural thickening. Unilateral pleural calcification is, therefore, likely to be the result of previous empyema or hemothorax, and bilateral calcification occurs after asbestos exposure (Fig. 1.93). Pleural calcification may be discovered in a patient who is not aware of previous chest disease.

The calcification associated with previous pleurisy, empyema, or hemothorax occurs in the visceral pleura (Fig. 1.94); associated pleural thickening is almost always present and separates the calcium from the ribs. The calcium may be in a continuous sheet or in discrete plaques, which usually produce dense, coarse, irregular shadows, often sharply demarcated laterally. When a plaque is viewed face on, it may be less well defined and may mimic a pulmonary infiltrate.

PLEURAL MASSES

Primary tumors of the pleura are rare. Benign tumors of the pleura include pleural fibroma and lipoma (Fig. 1.95). The most common malignant disease of the pleura is metastatic, usually adenocarcinoma from the bronchus or breast. Malignant mesothelioma is usually associated with prior asbestos exposure (Fig. 1.96).

COMPUTED TOMOGRAPHY

Anatomy of the Mediastinum

The soft-tissue contrast provided by CT, along with its cross-sectional nature, make the diagnostic information it reveals far superior to that provided by two-dimensional radiography.

Figure 1.93 Extensive bilateral pleural thickening secondary to asbestos exposure.

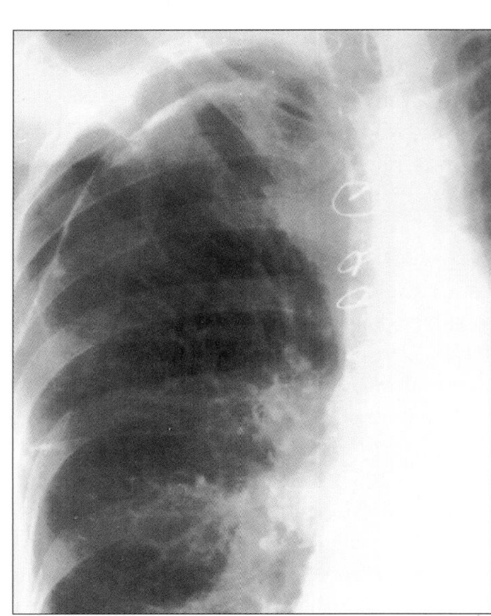

Figure 1.94 Previous sternotomy resulting in pleural thickening and calcification. A small pneumothorax is visible. Note how the pleural thickening is associated with the visceral pleura.

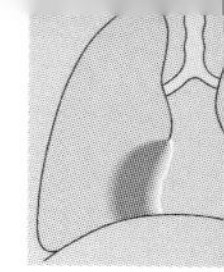

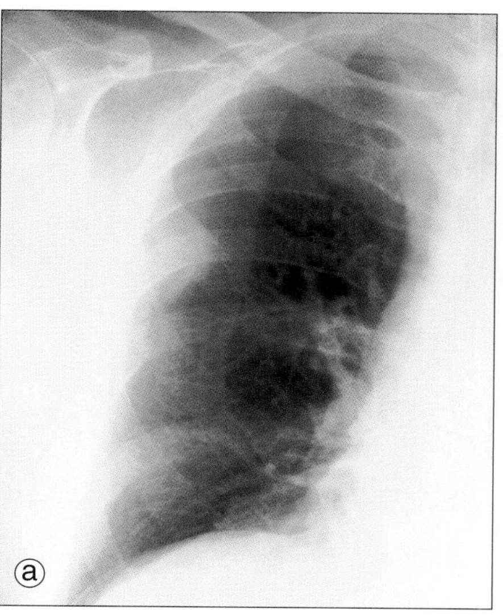

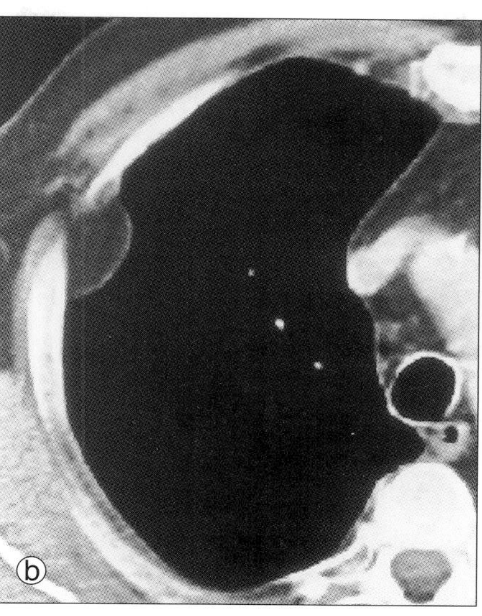

Figure 1.95 The appearances of a pleural lipoma. A, Localized view of the right lung from a posteroanterior (PA) chest radiograph. There is a pleurally based opacity in the right midzone, well-defined medially but fading out laterally. **B,** Computed tomography (CT) scan of the same right lung. The opacity is caused by a pleural lipoma. Note the identical CT attenuation of this mass compared with the subcutaneous fat.

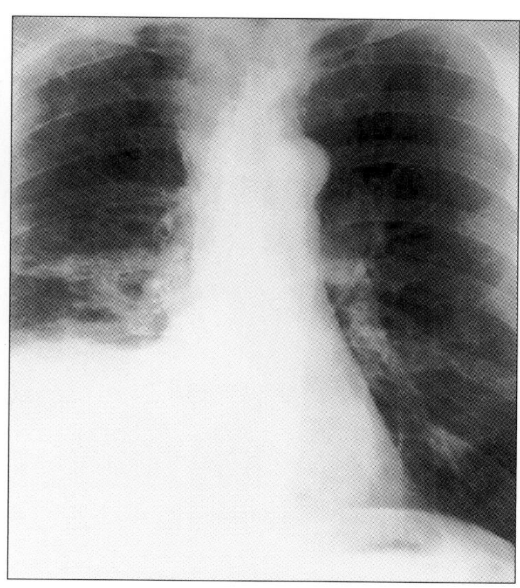

Figure 1.96 Malignant mesothelioma. A lobulated pleural thickening extends from the right apex down to the right diaphragm, which appears elevated. The overall volume of the right hemithorax is reduced.

Modern CT scanners can acquire a volume of information that includes the whole of the mediastinum within the time taken by a single held breath. This three-dimensional data set can then be displayed as continuous or overlapping axial slices, free from breathing-related movement artifacts. Usually a collimation and slice width of between 5 and 10 mm is used, and it is usual but not always essential to give intravenous contrast medium. The normal mediastinal anatomy is demonstrated in Figures 1.97 through 1.101.

GREAT VESSELS

The great vessels form the most familiar anatomic landmarks within the mediastinum. Knowledge of the relationship of these vessels to other mediastinal components allows accurate description of the location of pathology and has important implications for planning the approach to either open operation or mediastinoscopy. The most common branching pattern of the aortic arch is for three arteries to arise from the upper arch—the right innominate, left common carotid, and left subclavian arteries (see Fig. 1.97). However, many variations on this basic anatomy exist (see Fig. 1.73). The transverse portion of the aortic arch is the most readily recognizable vascular structure within the mediastinum (see Fig. 1.98). The great veins lie anterior to the arterial structures. The left brachiocephalic vein is situated above and anterior to the aortic arch and aortic branches, although its position is variable. The right brachiocephalic vein descends more directly in the anterior right mediastinum to merge with its counterpart and form the superior vena cava. As CT contrast medium is administered into one arm, one brachiocephalic vein is heavily opacified while the other remains of soft-tissue density.

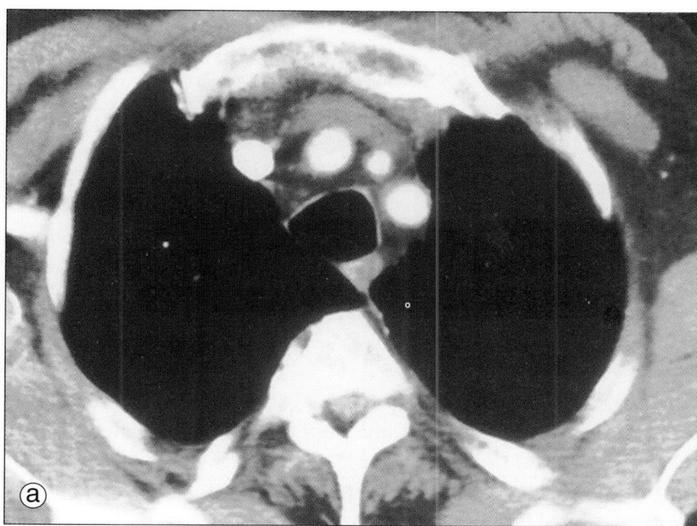

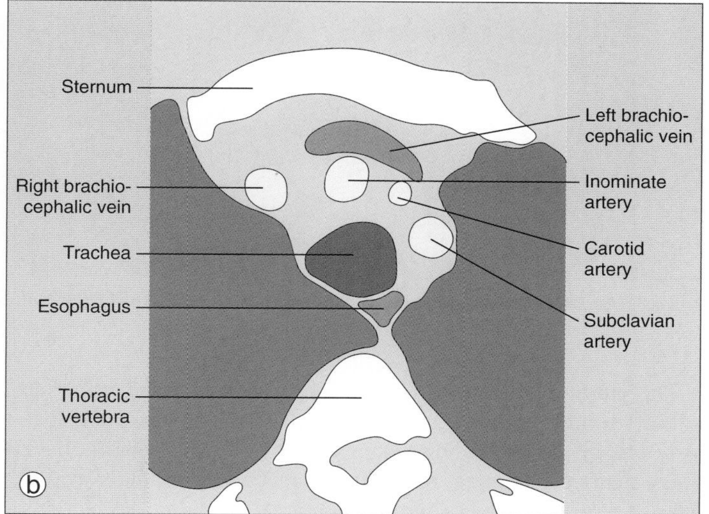

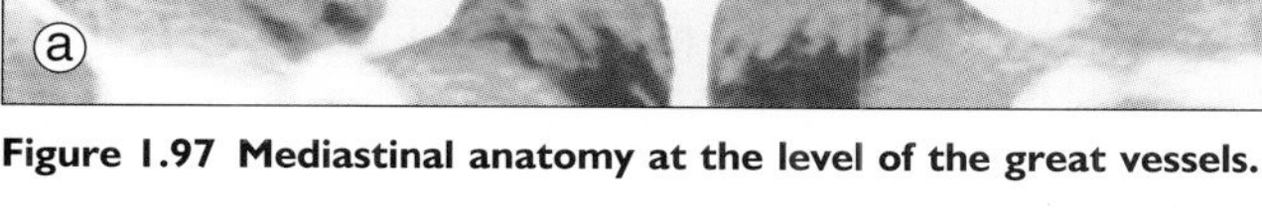

Figure 1.97 Mediastinal anatomy at the level of the great vessels.

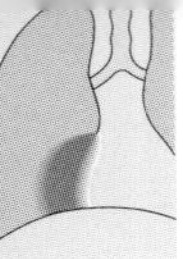

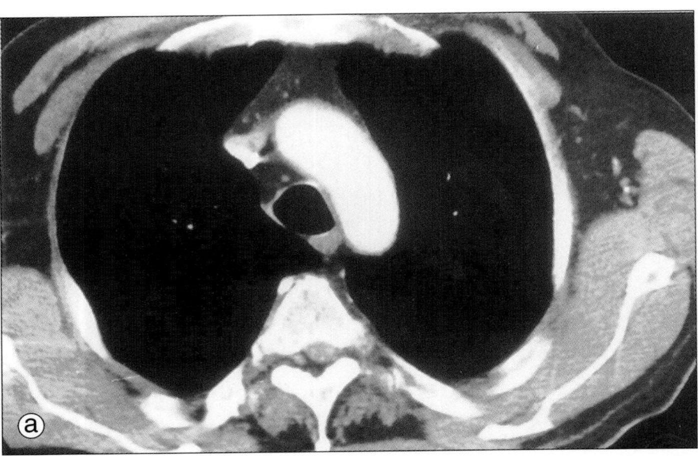

Figure 1.98 Mediastinal anatomy at the level of the aortic arch.

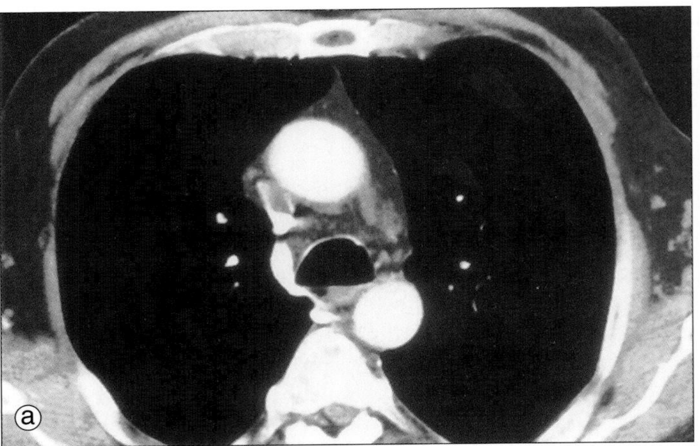

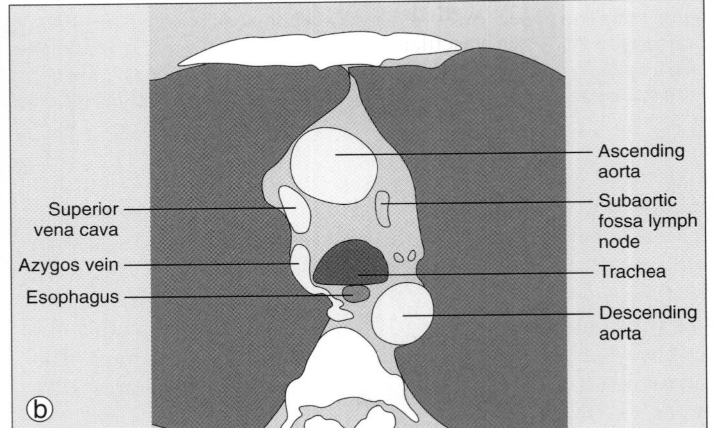

Figure 1.99 Mediastinal anatomy at the level of the subaortic fossa.

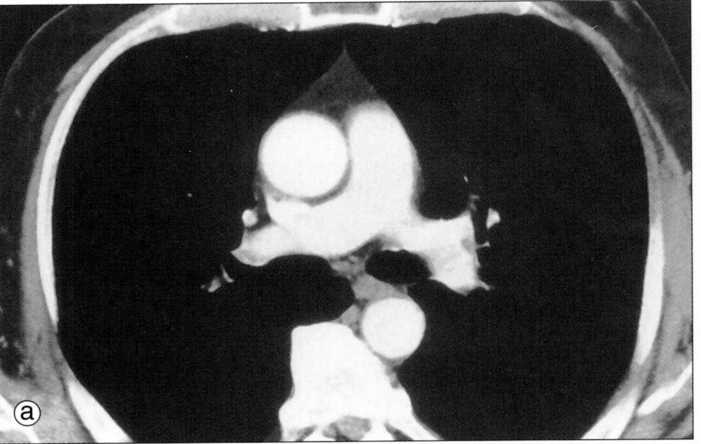

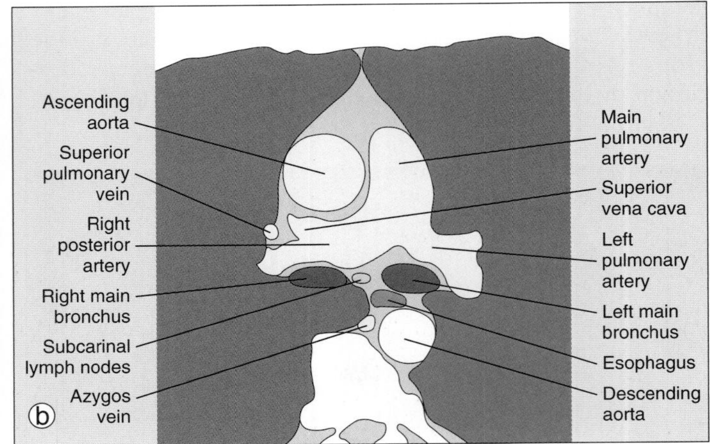

Figure 1.100 Mediastinal anatomy through the division of the main pulmonary artery.

The pulmonary outflow tract ascends, usually outlined by fat within the pericardium, to divide at a point adjacent and just posterior to the ascending aorta. Usually the main pulmonary artery diameter is equal to or less than the ascending aorta as measured on CT. When the pulmonary artery diameter exceeds the aortic diameter, underlying pulmonary hypertension is likely. The right pulmonary artery swings dorsally and to the right, behind the ascending aorta and superior vena cava and anterior to the right main bronchus (see Fig. 1.100). After giving a branch to the upper lobe, it descends posterolaterally to the bronchus intermedius. The left pulmonary artery follows a shorter course and arches up and over the left main bronchus.

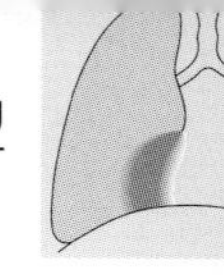

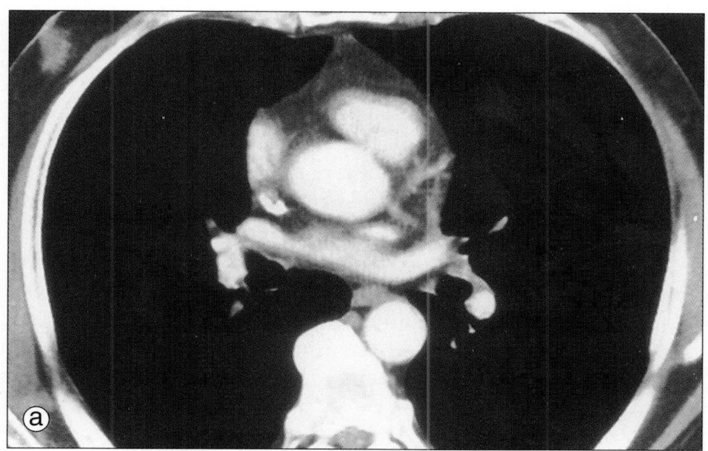

Figure 1.101 Mediastinal anatomy through the aortic root.

Hilar anatomy is well demonstrated on contrast-enhanced CT, especially when vascular structures are traced sequentially over contiguous images. Knowledge of normal anatomy enables differentiation of vascular structures from normal or enlarged mediastinal lymph nodes, even on unenhanced scans; however, if there is any cause for doubt, intravenous contrast always clarifies the situation (Fig. 1.102).

AIRWAYS

The trachea descends through the thoracic inlet, where reduction in caliber may occur, and usually appears rounded on scans obtained in full inspiration. If scans are obtained during expiration, the membranous posterior wall of the trachea is seen to bow forward into the tracheal lumen. The wall of the trachea is only 2 mm thick, and any intramural thickening is well demonstrated on CT. Modern scanners also allow reformatting of the data in sagittal or coronal planes, thus providing more elegant demonstration of tracheal abnormalities. The anatomy of the bronchial tree can be traced from the tracheal carina out into the lungs, at least to the segmental level, with excellent correlation between CT and bronchoscopic findings. Furthermore, the three-dimensional data set acquired on modern spiral scanners can be manipulated to provide a computer simulation of the bronchoscopic appearances (see Fig. 1.7D).

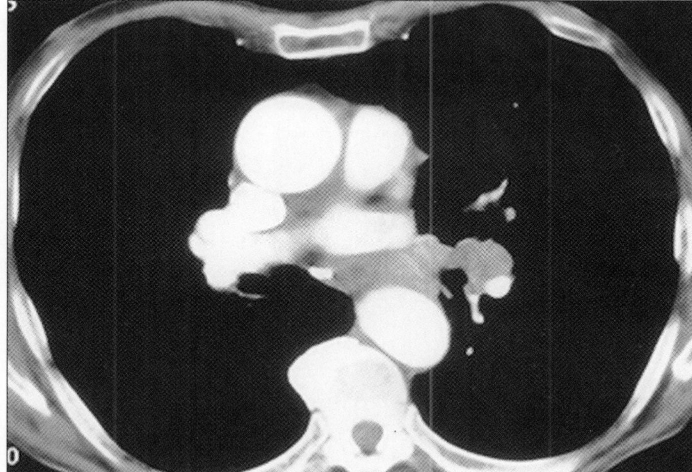

Figure 1.102 Contrast-enhanced computed tomography (CT) scan. Left hilar lymph-node enlargement with extension of abnormal tissue anterior to the descending aorta.

THYMUS

In the normal state the thymus is not visible on the chest radiograph of the adult patient, but the thymic remnant is frequently evident on CT. The thymus reduces in size after puberty. It lies in the anterior mediastinum, just in front of the root of the aorta, and is bi-lobed; the left lobe usually is the larger. Generally, the thymus is assessed by examining the contours of the gland (which should be concave) and the thickness of the individual lobes. In children the thymus is of soft-tissue density on CT scanning, but after puberty it starts to involute and the gland undergoes atrophy and fatty replacement. Traces of thymic tissue within the anterior mediastinal fat are frequently identifiable on CT in young adults.

THYROID

Usually the thyroid is confined to the neck, but frequently mediastinal extension occurs with thyroid enlargement (see discussion later in this chapter). Typically, the thyroid lies on either side of the extrathoracic trachea and is bounded laterally by the carotid artery and internal jugular vein. On contrast enhancement, normal thyroid tissue enhances avidly and is usually of relatively high attenuation on unenhanced scans because of its relatively high iodine content.

ESOPHAGUS

Often the esophagus is completely collapsed on CT scanning, and therefore inconspicuous, but it can be identified easily if it contains air or contrast medium. Initially the esophagus lies directly posterior to the trachea, and below the bifurcation it usually deviates slightly to the left and lies adjacent to the aorta. The esophageal wall is usually only 2 to 3 mm in thickness.

LYMPH NODES

Numerous lymph nodes are present within the mediastinum, usually less than 1 cm along the long axis and discrete; they may not be visible on CT scanning. Previous granulomatous disease may result in extensive mediastinal lymph-node calcification,

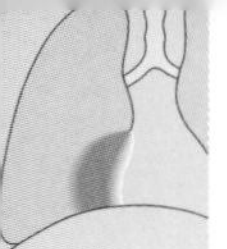

which reveals the true extent of normal mediastinal lymph-node distribution (Fig. 1.103). An extensive chain of lymph nodes also accompanies the internal mammary vessels bilaterally. Additional nodes are present in the intercostal chain adjacent to the heads of the ribs in a posterior, paraspinal position and alongside the esophagus and descending thoracic aorta. These merge with the retrocrural lymph-node chain, and the para-aortic nodes on the abdomen.

PERICARDIUM

The pericardial membrane is composed of visceral and parietal layers and surrounds the heart. The visceral layer is separated from the myocardium by a variable amount of epicardial fat. The parietal layer is variably fused with the mediastinal pleura. Where they are separate, mediastinal fat may accumulate (such as in the epiphrenic fat pad). Fluid within the pericardial sac may be evident on the chest radiograph, CT scan, or ultrasonogram.

Computed Tomographic Evaluation of Mediastinal Masses

In most patients with a mediastinal mass the local compressive or invasive effects of the mediastinal mass cause symptoms, but in a surprising number of patients the mass is discovered on a chest radiograph taken for an unrelated cause. Generally, the PA and lateral chest radiographs enable localization of the mass to one of the compartments of the mediastinum, which refines the differential diagnosis. However, current practice is for patients with a mediastinal mass to undergo a contrast-enhanced CT scan, or sometimes MRI.

The differential diagnosis of a mediastinal mass is wide. Masses can arise from any of the normal structures in the mediastinum, as well as from metastatic disease from a distant primary site. In addition, mediastinal abscesses may also manifest as a mass. The diagnosis is considerably narrowed by CT, which enables the organ of origin of the mass to be assessed, defines the attenuation and enhancement characteristics, and reveals evidence of invasion of adjacent structures. Mediastinal masses are usually classified according to the anatomic portion of the mediastinum from which they appear to arise (Fig. 1.104).

SUPERIOR MEDIASTINAL MASSES

Thyroid

An enlarged thyroid may extend inferiorly into the superior mediastinum and may be large enough to reach into the middle mediastinum. However, this rarely presents a diagnostic problem because the mass is obviously continuous with the cervical thyroid tissue and enhances avidly after intravenous administration of contrast medium. Frequently, the enlarged gland contains low-density cysts and areas of calcification, particularly within cyst walls. Large thyroid masses may cause tracheal deviation or narrowing and may enlarge acutely if hemorrhage into the gland occurs (Fig. 1.105). Although the thyroid originates anterior to the trachea, there may be exten-

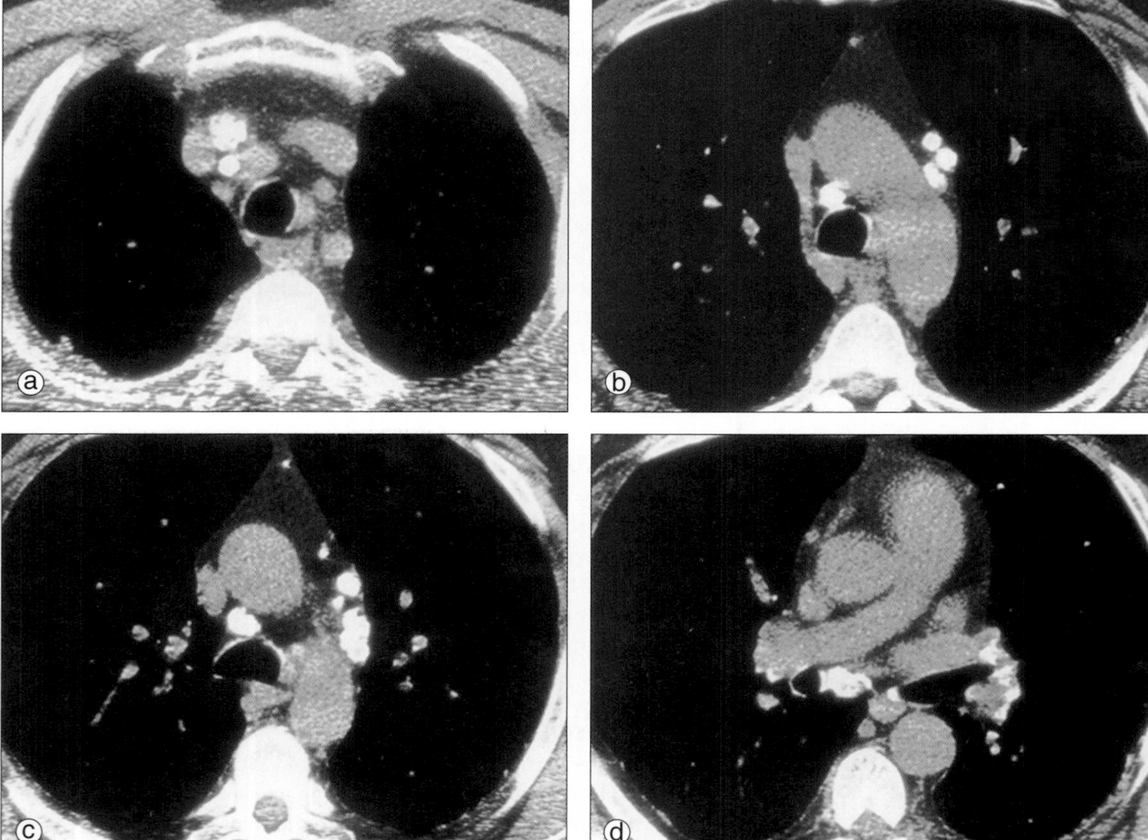

Figure 1.103 Calcified mediastinal lymph nodes secondary to previous granulomatous disease on an unenhanced computed tomography (CT) scan through the thorax. Compare with Figures 1-97 through 1–101.

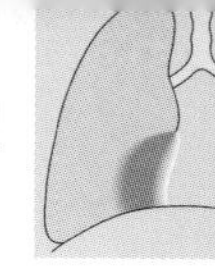

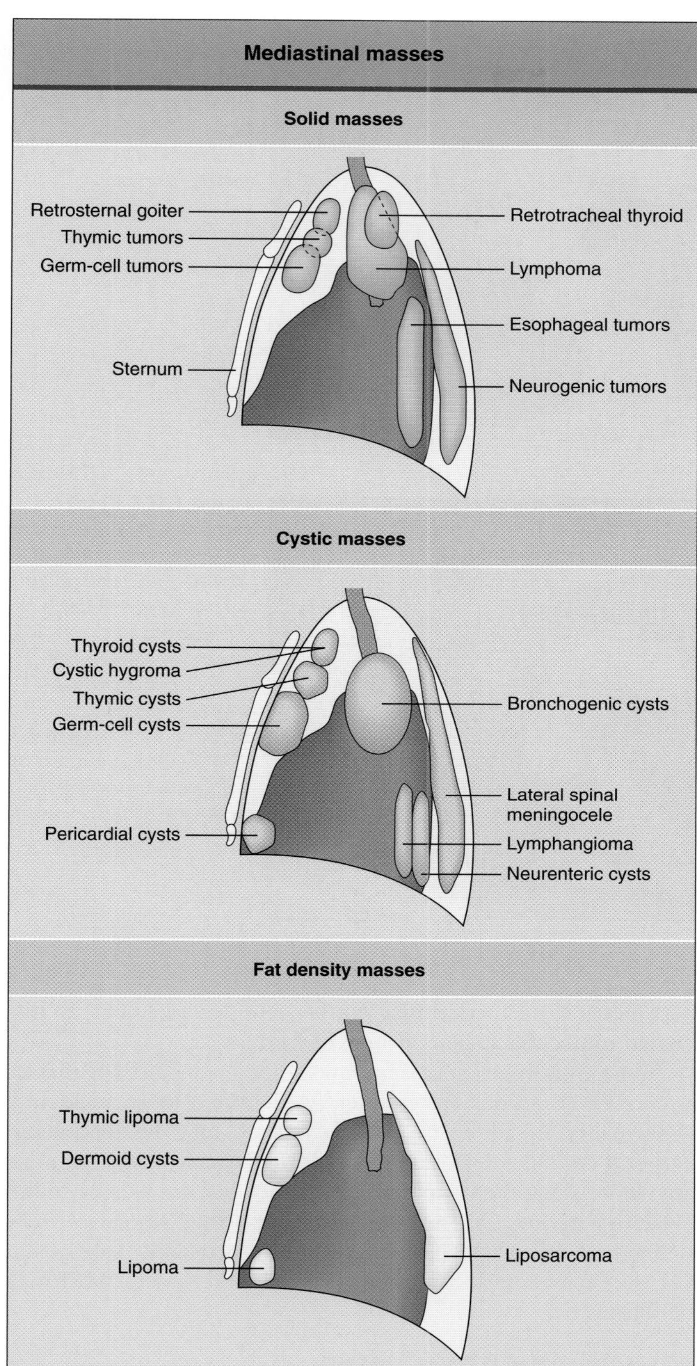

Figure 1.104 Distribution and classification of mediastinal masses depending on density derived from computed tomography (CT).

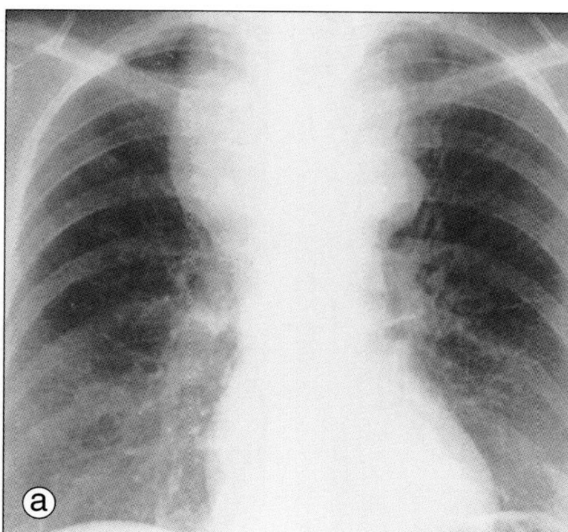

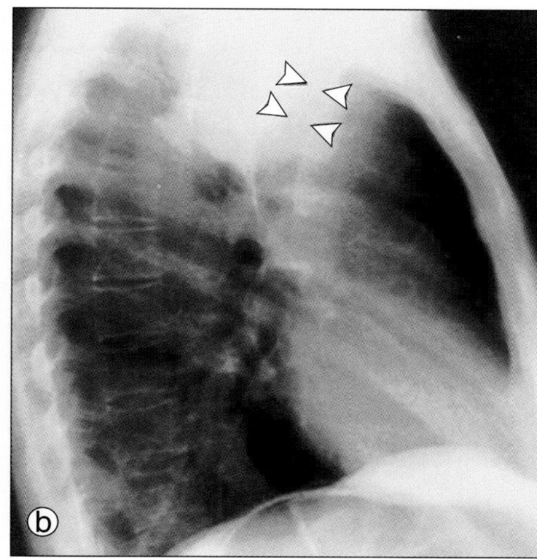

Figure 1.105 Retrosternal thyroid mass. A, Posteroanterior (PA) chest radiograph with a large superior mediastinal mass mainly to the right of the trachea. **B**, The lateral view demonstrates an extension behind the trachea, which is narrowed in its anteroposterior dimension *(arrowheads)*. The thyroid frequently extends into a retrotracheal position in the upper mediastinum.

sion to the right and even posterior to the trachea within the upper mediastinum.

Lymphatic Malformations

Lymphatic malformations are rare and may occur in the superior mediastinum. The most common of these is the cystic hygroma, which usually occurs in infants as a cervical mass with an extensive intrathoracic component. Although considered benign, these lesions are difficult to completely resect because of their tendency to spread around normal structures.

ANTERIOR MEDIASTINAL MASSES

The majority of anterior mediastinal masses arise from the thymus, the thyroid (see earlier discussion), germ-cell tumors, and enlarged lymph nodes.

Thymus

The normal thymus involutes after puberty but may show reactive enlargement in certain disease states or after chemotherapy. However, intrinsic neoplasia of the thymus is a relatively common cause of an anterior mediastinal mass in adult life. Causes of thymic neoplasia include thymoma, thymic carcinoma, thymic cysts (Fig. 1.106), thymic lipoma, thymic carcinoid, and thymic lymphoma. With CT, fat or fluid elements may be identified within a thymic mass, and invasion of adjacent structures can be shown. With the exception of thymolipoma and thymic cysts, histology is usually required for definitive diagnosis.

Teratomas and Germ-cell Tumors

Teratomas and germ-cell tumors originate from primitive stem cell rests. These neoplasms can be separated into benign and malignant forms; the former consists of benign cystic teratomas (synonymous with dermoid cysts). Benign cystic teratomas (Fig. 1.107) may contain differentiated elements and therefore on CT may display a variety of densities, ranging from that of fat to that of calcified tissue and even that of teeth. The malignant teratomas constitute a variety of tumors that usually arise in the

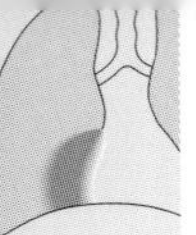

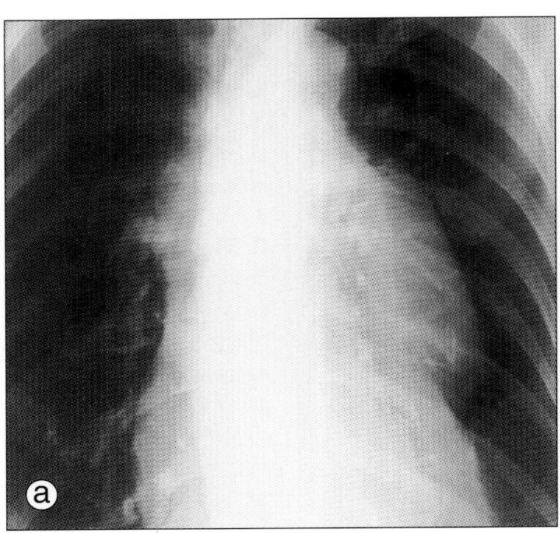

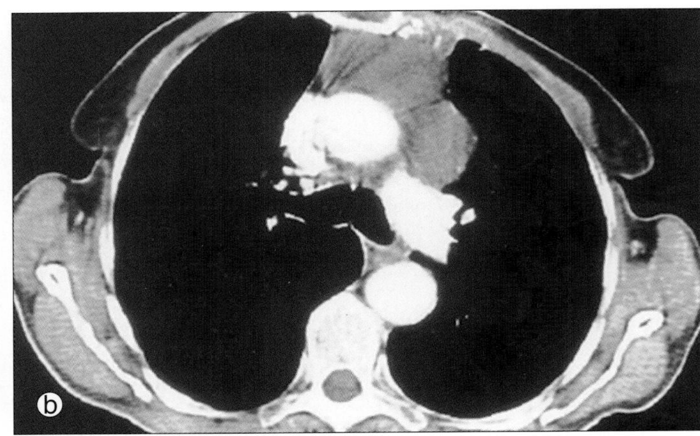

Figure 1.106 Thymic cyst. A, Anteroposterior chest radiograph with mediastinal widening. **B,** Contrast-enhanced computed tomography (CT) confirms an anterior mediastinal abnormality of fluid density.

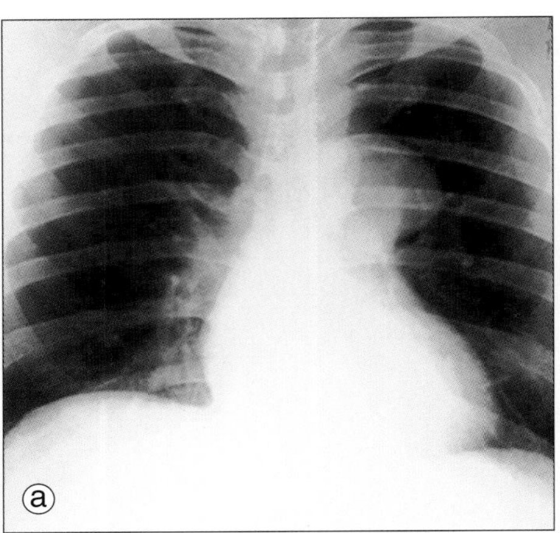

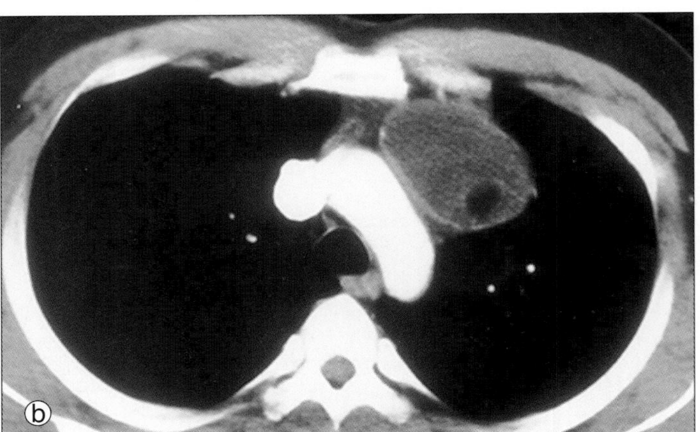

Figure 1.107 Cystic teratoma. A, Posteroanterior (PA) erect chest radiograph showing a mass arising from the mediastinum. Note how the posterior aortic arch and descending aorta are still visualized, which indicates an anterior position. **B,** Computed tomography (CT) scan shows fluid and fat elements within an anterior mediastinal mass.

testes, namely seminomas, teratocarcinomas, embryonal carcinomas, yolk sac tumors, and choriocarcinomas. Some mediastinal germ-cell tumors may be secondary to a primary tumor arising within the gonads. Malignant germ-cell tumors are usually found in young men, secrete tumor markers, and are chemosensitive.

Lymph Node Enlargement

Lymph-node enlargement is a common cause of an anterior mediastinal mass, although many processes that involve lymph nodes cause generalized mediastinal nodal enlargement. These processes may be infective (such as tuberculosis or histoplasmosis), neoplastic, reactive, or of unknown cause (such as sarcoidosis).

Lymphoma

Hodgkin's disease and, to a lesser extent, non-Hodgkin's lymphoma and lymphatic leukemia frequently involve the mediastinum, especially the paratracheal, tracheobronchial, and anterior mediastinal nodes. Typically the lymph-node enlargement is asymmetrical.

MIDDLE MEDIASTINAL MASSES

Middle mediastinal masses are most frequently malignant, usually from metastatic nodal enlargement. However, the presence of enlarged nodes is not an accurate predictor of malignancy, because reactive enlargement is also common. The classification of mediastinal lymph-node enlargement is discussed under the staging of lung cancer.

Some important developmental middle mediastinal masses occur. These lesions are frequently identified as an incidental abnormality in adult life, although they may be discovered earlier if complications supervene. Bronchogenic cysts may arise anywhere along the course of the trachea but are usually found close to a carina. On the chest radiograph they appear as well-defined, round masses that may, on rare occasions, calcify. On CT they may appear as either cystic or solid masses. MRI may be diagnostic.

POSTERIOR MEDIASTINAL MASSES

The posterior mediastinum contains neural elements, which give rise to a range of benign and malignant neural tumors. These may grow to considerable size before presentation, and modeling abnormalities may occur in the adjacent ribs and spine, which provide clues to the chronicity of the tumors. On CT scanning, they are typically paraspinal and of soft-tissue density, with patchy calcification. Also, CT may show the typical dumbbell extension of a neurofibroma from an extraspinal position through an intervertebral foramina. In the assessment of neurogenic tumors, MRI has distinct advantages over CT because of its ability to definitively confirm or exclude tumor extension into the spinal canal (Fig. 1.108).

The esophagus lies in the posterior mediastinum. Esophageal carcinoma usually is associated with dysphagia or weight loss

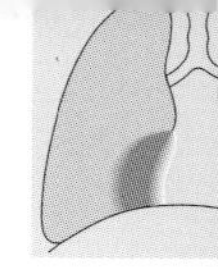

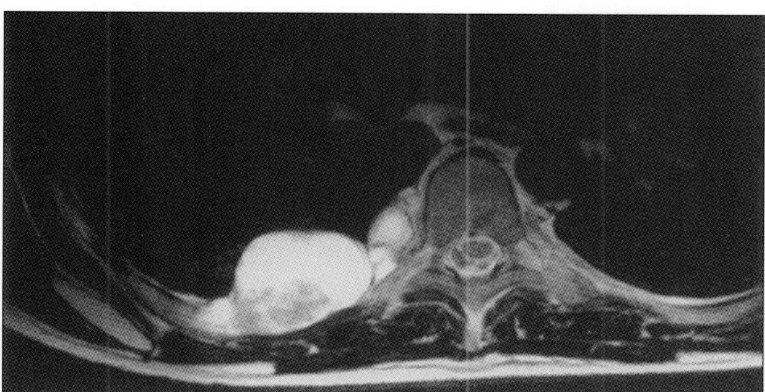

Figure 1.108 Paraganglionoma in an adult. A right paraspinal high T2-weighted signal lobulated mass is present. There is no extension into the soft tissues of the chest wall or through the neural foramina into the spinal canal.

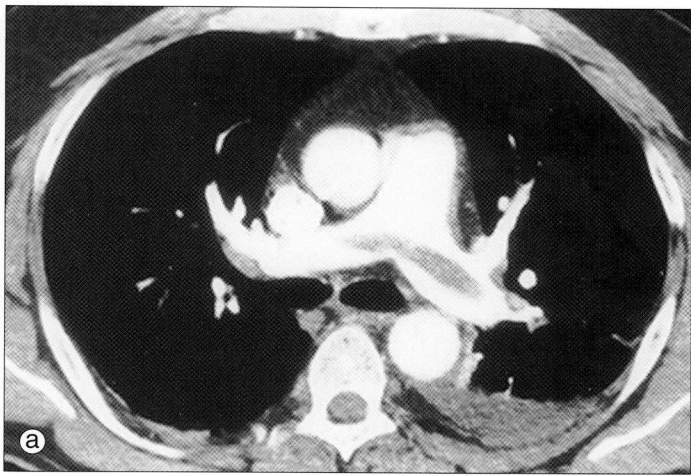

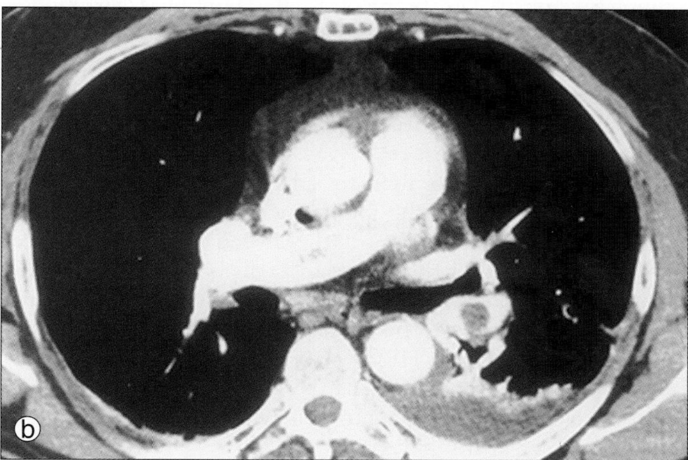

Figure 1.109 Spiral computed tomography (CT) for pulmonary embolism (PE). A, Contrast-enhanced CT scan through the division of the main pulmonary artery showing a saddle thrombus. **B,** Sections slightly more inferiorly showing further thrombus extending down into the left main pulmonary artery.

without the presence of an apparent mass on the chest radiograph. Usually, CT is reserved for the staging of esophageal malignancy, in addition to the assessment of local tumor bulk. Benign esophageal lesions may reach a considerable size before symptoms occur, and as a result such large masses may be apparent on the plain radiograph. Such tumors include fibroma, leiomyoma, and lipomas.

Neuroenteric cysts are rare congenital masses that occur in the posterior mediastinum, usually inseparable from the esophagus, and sometimes within the esophageal wall. If a vertebral or neural canal abnormality is present, these masses are known as *neuroenteric cysts*, but if not, they are termed *esophageal duplication cysts*. Posterior mediastinal masses may arise directly from the spinal column and may represent primary or secondary tumors, infective processes, or the results of trauma or degeneration.

Spiral Computed Tomography for Pulmonary Embolism

The potential for CT diagnosis of PE, first reported in 1980, was realized well before sophisticated scanners became available. With recent advances in CT hardware and software came the ability to acquire, within the duration of a single holding of the breath, a volume of data large enough to include the entire thorax. This rapid acquisition allows excellent contrast opacification of the pulmonary arterial tree for the duration of the scan, thereby revealing any thrombus within the central pulmonary vessels (Fig. 1.109). Subsequently, a series of studies evaluated helical and electron beam CT in the diagnosis of acute pulmonary embolus, with excellent reported sensitivity and specificity for the detection of clots down to the segmental level. Most of these studies also identified an important additional advantage of CT: the ability to provide an alternative diagnosis that explains the symptoms of chest pain or dyspnea in those patients who do not have PE.

When CT is compared with pulmonary angiography for the detection of subsegmental clot, the sensitivity and specificity of CT are not as good. Isolated, subsegmental thrombi may be relatively common. Indeed, in one series 30% of the patients had emboli confined to the subsegmental vessels, and many of the emboli would have been missed on CT. In comparison, the Prospective Investigation of Pulmonary Embolism Diagnosis (PIOPED) study suggested a prevalence of only 6% for isolated subsegmental emboli. The clinical significance of isolated subsegmental emboli remains uncertain.

The argument that CT plays a major role in the diagnostic algorithm for PE has been proposed recently. Although some authorities have suggested that V/Q scanning may be omitted as part of the diagnostic workup, others have supported a continuing role for V/Q scanning in patients with normal chest radiographs. The rationale is that the V/Q scan, with its lower cost and radiation dose, is likely to be conclusive in patients who have otherwise normal lungs.

Cost is always an issue in the acceptability of any new test. A cost-effectiveness analysis of 15 combinations of five commonly used tests in PE, including angiography, CT, and V/Q scanning, revealed that all the best outcomes included helical CT, when both effectiveness (mortality) and marginal cost effectiveness (cost per life saved) were assessed. Even when the assumed sensitivity fell below 85%, CT maintained its economic advantage.

Despite the rapid developments in this area (including a potential role for MRI), it seems likely that for some time to come spiral CT scanning will have an important role in the diagnosis of PE, especially in view of the widespread high threshold for performing pulmonary angiography.

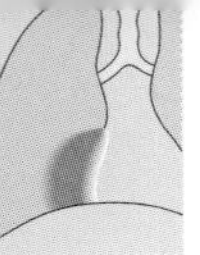

INTERPRETATION OF HIGH-RESOLUTION COMPUTED TOMOGRAPHY OF THE LUNGS

Appearance of Normal Lung Anatomy

Accurate interpretation of HRCT of the lung requires an understanding of the normal appearances of the bronchi, the blood vessels, and the secondary pulmonary lobule. The close correspondence between the appearances of gross pathologic specimens and HRCT features enables the use of anatomic terms to describe the patterns of lung disease depicted by HRCT.

Throughout the lung, the bronchi and pulmonary arteries run together and taper slightly as they travel radially; this is easiest to appreciate in the bronchovascular bundles that run within and parallel to the plane of the HRCT section. At any given point, the diameter of the bronchus is the same as its accompanying pulmonary artery. The bronchovascular bundle is surrounded by connective tissue from the hilum to the bronchioles in the lung periphery. The concept that connected components make up the lung interstitium is useful for the understanding of HRCT findings in interstitial lung disease; the peripheral interstitium around the surface of the lung beneath the visceral pleura extends into the lung to surround the secondary pulmonary lobules. Within the lobules, a finer network of septal, connective-tissue fibers support the alveoli. The "axial" fibers form a sheath around the bronchovascular bundles. Thus, the connective tissue stroma of these three separate components is in continuity and so forms a fibrous skeleton for the lungs.

In normal individuals, HRCT shows a clear and definite interface between the bronchovascular bundle and surrounding lung. Any thickening of the connective tissue interstitium results in apparent bronchial-wall thickening and blurring of this interface. The size of the smallest subsegmental bronchi visible on HRCT is determined by the thickness of the bronchial wall rather than by the bronchial diameter. In general, bronchi with a diameter less than 3 mm and walls less than 300 mm thick are not consistently identifiable on HRCT. Airways reach this critical size approximately 2 to 3 cm from the pleural surface. The secondary pulmonary lobule is the smallest anatomic unit of the lung that is surrounded by a connective-tissue septum (Fig. 1.110). Within the septa lie lymphatic vessels and venules. The lobule contains 5 to 12 acini, each of which measures approximately 6 to 10 mm in diameter. Each lobule is approximately 2 cm in diameter and polyhedral, and often these lobules resemble truncated cones. In the lung periphery, the bases of the cone-shaped lobules lie on a visceral pleural surface. In the central parts of the lung, the interlobular septa—and therefore the lobules—are less well developed. The centrilobular bronchiole and accompanying pulmonary artery enter through the apex of the lobule.

The interlobular septa measure approximately 100 μm in thickness. The lower limit of resolution of HRCT is approximately 200 μm, so normal septa are infrequently identified on HRCT. The few interlobular septa that are visible in normal individuals are seen as straight lines 1 to 2 cm in length that terminate at a visceral pleural surface. Sometimes several septa that join end to end are seen as a nonbranching, linear structure, which can measure up to 4 cm in length; these are most frequent at the lung bases, just above the diaphragmatic surface.

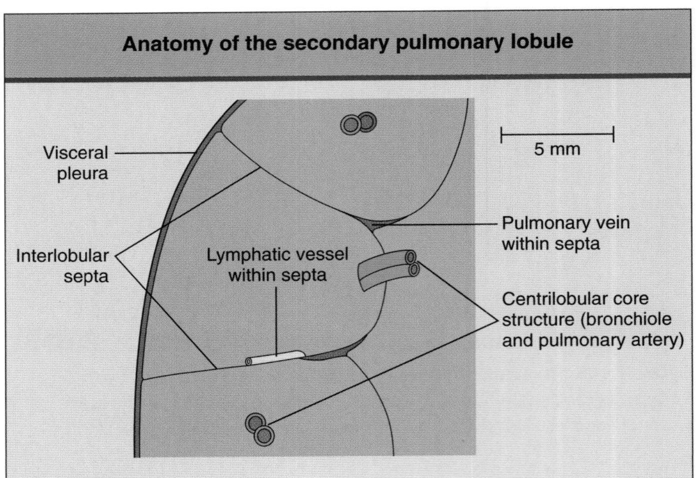

Figure 1.110 Anatomy of the secondary pulmonary lobule.

The secondary pulmonary lobule is supplied by a centrilobular artery and bronchiole that are approximately 1 mm in diameter as they enter the lobule. In the normal state, the core structures, effectively the 500-μm–diameter centrilobular artery, are visible as dots 1 cm deep to the pleural surface. On standard window settings the lung parenchyma is of almost homogeneous low density, marginally greater than that of air.

Patterns of Parenchymal Disease

Vague terms traditionally used in the lexicon of plain chest radiography can be replaced by precise descriptions derived from an understanding of HRCT anatomy. Abnormal patterns on HRCT that represent pulmonary disease can usually be categorized into one of four patterns: reticular and linear opacities, nodular opacities, increased lung density, and cystic air spaces with areas of decreased lung density.

Although these HRCT patterns generally have a corresponding pattern on chest radiography, they are seen with much greater clarity on the cross-sectional images of HRCT, and the precise distribution of disease can be more readily appreciated. Conformity in the terminology used to describe the HRCT abnormalities of diffuse, infiltrative lung diseases is increasing.

RETICULAR PATTERN

A reticular pattern on HRCT always indicates significant pathology. A reticular pattern caused by thickening of interlobular septa is a cardinal sign of many interstitial lung diseases. Numerous interlobular septa that join up to form an obvious network indicate an extensive interstitial abnormality caused by infiltration with fibrosis, abnormal cells, or fluid (e.g., fibrosing alveolitis, lymphangitis carcinomatosa, and pulmonary edema, respectively). Interlobular septal thickening that results from fibrosing alveolitis is often associated with intralobular, interstitial thickening (beyond the resolution of HRCT) and a coarse reticular pattern that contains cystic air spaces and produces the honeycomb pattern of destroyed lung. Thickening of the interlobular septa may be smooth or irregular, but this distinction is not always obvious. Irregular septal thickening is a feature of lymphangitic spread of tumor, whereas pulmonary edema and alveolar proteinosis cause smooth thickening. Sarcoidosis is typ-

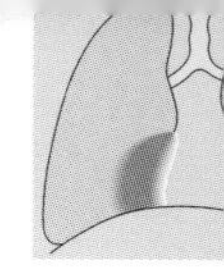

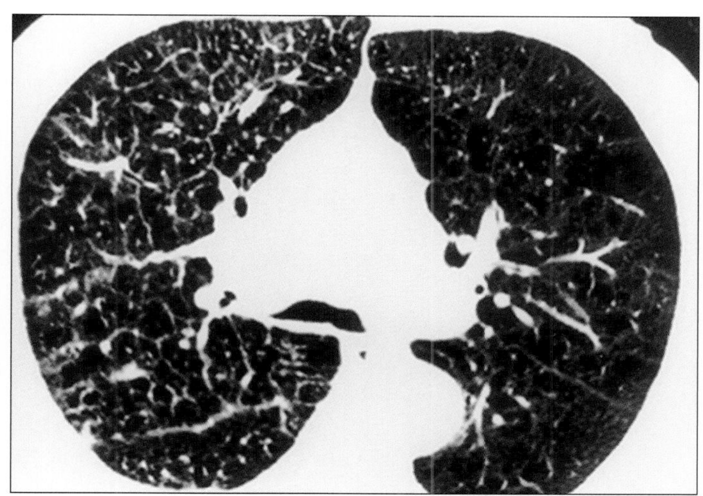

Figure 1.111 High-resolution computed tomography (HRCT) showing generalized, irregular thickening of the interlobular septa in both lungs. The patient has lymphangitis carcinomatosa.

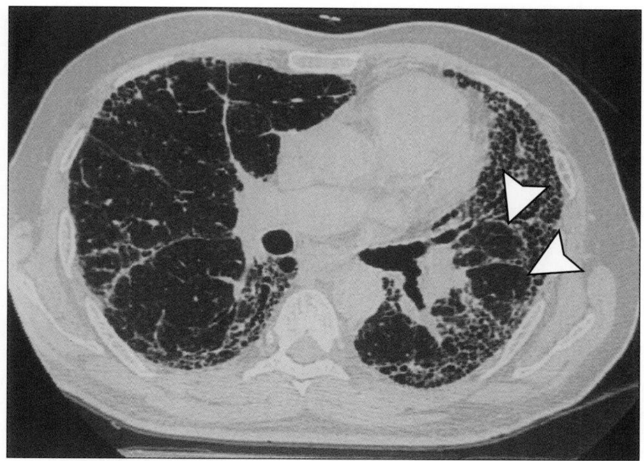

Figure 1.112 High-resolution computed tomography (HRCT) of end-stage pulmonary fibrosis. Small cystic spaces are visible throughout much of the left lung base. Less marked changes are present on the right. Traction bronchiectasis is evident within the affected lung *(arrows)*.

ified by some nodular septal thickening, although widespread septal thickening is not characteristic of this condition.

Because the various parts of the lung interstitium are in continuous, widespread interstitial disease that causes interlobular septal thickening also results in bronchovascular interstitial thickening (e.g., by lymphangitis carcinomatosa). The bronchovascular thickening seen on HRCT is equivalent to the peribronchial "cuffing" seen around end-on bronchi on chest radiography. The HRCT finding of peribronchovascular thickening in isolation must be interpreted with caution, because it may be seen in reversible pure airway disease (e.g., asthma). Thickening of the subsegmental and segmental bronchovascular bundles (e.g., as caused by lymphangitis carcinomatosa) sometimes gives the interface between the thickened bronchial wall and surrounding lung a feathery appearance (Fig. 1.111).

The coarseness of the network that makes up the reticular pattern on HRCT is determined by the level at which the interstitial thickening is most severe. Thickening of the intralobular septa results in a very fine reticular pattern on HRCT, visible on only an optimal HRCT scan. Some of the very delicate linear structures that make up such a fine reticular pattern are so small as to be below the resolution limits of HRCT, even with the narrowest collimation. The result is an amorphous increase in lung density (ground-glass opacification, described later) caused by volume averaging within the section.

Extensive pulmonary fibrosis causes complete destruction of the architecture of the secondary pulmonary lobules, which results in a coarse reticular pattern made up of irregular, linear opacities. The reticular pattern of end-stage fibrotic or honeycomb lung mirrors the appearance on chest radiography and is characterized by cystic spaces that measure a few millimeters to several centimeters across and are surrounded by discernible walls (Fig. 1.112). Paradoxically, thickened interlobular septa are not an obvious feature of advanced fibrosing alveolitis, probably because of the severe disturbance of the normal lung architecture. The distortion that accompanies interstitial fibrosis may result in irregular dilatation of the segmental and subsegmental bronchi, a phenomenon termed *traction bronchiectasis* (Fig. 1.113).

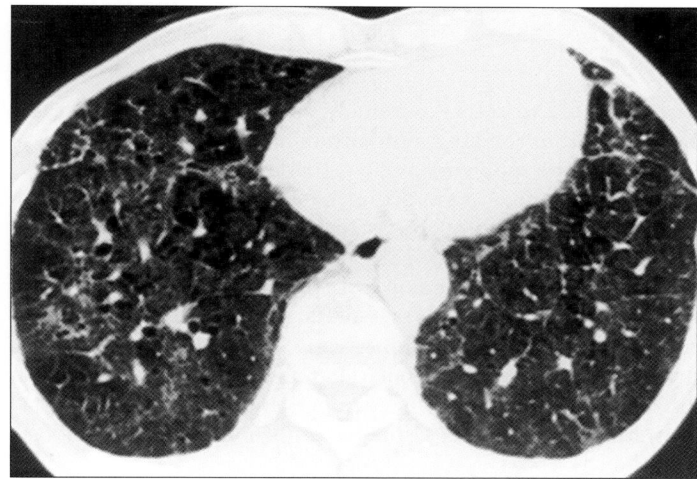

Figure 1.113 Widespread reticular pattern with architectural distortion. The patient has pulmonary fibrosis caused by chronic hypersensitivity pneumonitis. In the right lower lobe the airways are dilated ("traction bronchiectasis").

NODULAR PATTERN

A nodular pattern on HRCT is composed of innumerable, small, discrete opacities that range in diameter from 1 mm to 10 mm. The nodular pattern is a feature of both interstitial and air-space diseases. The location of nodules in relation to the lobules and bronchovascular bundles, as well as their density, clarity of outline, and uniformity of size, may indicate whether the nodules lie predominantly within the interstitium or air spaces. Because most diffuse lung pathologies have both interstitial and air-space components, this distinction does not always aid in the diagnosis. Whether pulmonary nodules can be detected on CT depends on their size, profusion, density, and on the scanning technique. Narrow-collimation HRCT is clearly superior to conventional CT for the detection of micronodular disease, because there is less partial-volume effect, which can average out the attenuation of tiny nodules. A further refinement is the use of maximum-intensity projection images obtained

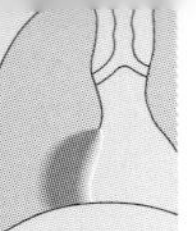

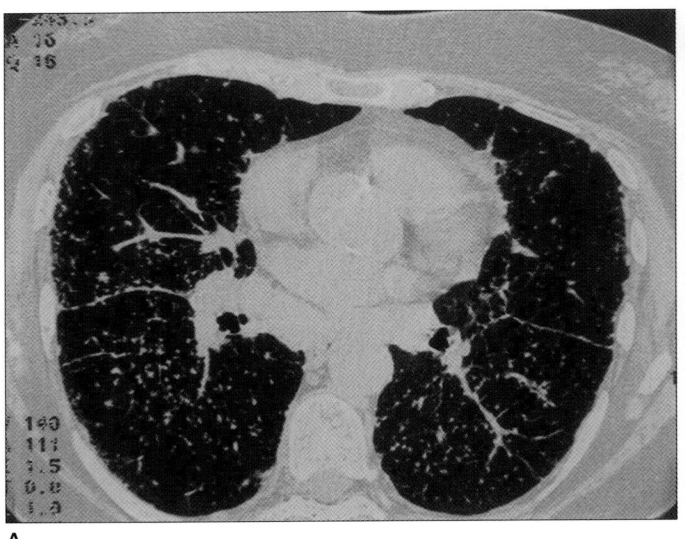

Figure 1.114 High-resolution computed tomography (HRCT) of sarcoidosis. A, Thickening and beading of the bronchovascular bundles, particularly in the left lower lobe, typical of sarcoidosis. Note the marked beading of the right oblique fissure resulting from subpleural nodularity, which can also be detected adjacent to the right anterolateral chest wall. **B,** Silicosis. Compare with **A.** In silicosis the nodules tend to be more posterior and are not subpleural or bronchovascular in distribution and are frequently less irregular in outline.

with spiral CT to detect extremely subtle micronodular disease. Nodules within the lung interstitium are seen in the interlobular septa, in the subpleural regions (particularly in relation to the fissures), and in a peribronchovascular distribution. Nodular thickening of the bronchovascular interstitium results in an irregular interface between the margins of the bronchovascular bundles and the surrounding lung parenchyma. These features are most pronounced in cases of sarcoidosis, in which coalescent, perilymphatic granulomas cause a beaded appearance of the thickened bronchovascular bundles. The bronchovascular distribution of nodules, in conjunction with a perihilar concentration of disease, is virtually pathognomonic of sarcoidosis (Fig. 1.114).

The nodular pattern seen in coal-worker's pneumoconiosis and silicosis is generally more uniform in distribution; centrilobular nodules may be distributed more in the upper zone and subpleurally, but overall they tend to be more evenly spread throughout the lung parenchyma than those seen in sarcoidosis.

When the air spaces are filled or partially filled with exudate, individual acini may become visible as poorly defined nodules approximately 8 mm in diameter. Acinar nodules may merge with areas of ground-glass opacification and are sometimes seen around the periphery of areas of dense parenchymal consolidation (Fig. 1.115). Such nodules are usually centrilobular, although this may be difficult to appreciate if the nodules are very profuse. Conditions in which this nonspecific pattern is seen include organizing pneumonia, hypersensitivity pneumonitis (Fig. 1.116), endobronchial spread of tuberculosis, idiopathic pulmonary hemorrhage, and some cases of bronchoalveolar cell carcinoma.

INCREASED LUNG DENSITY

An amorphous increase in lung density on HRCT is often described as having the appearance of ground-glass opacification (Fig. 1.117). Unlike the equivalent abnormality on chest radiography, in which the pulmonary vessels are often indistinct, a

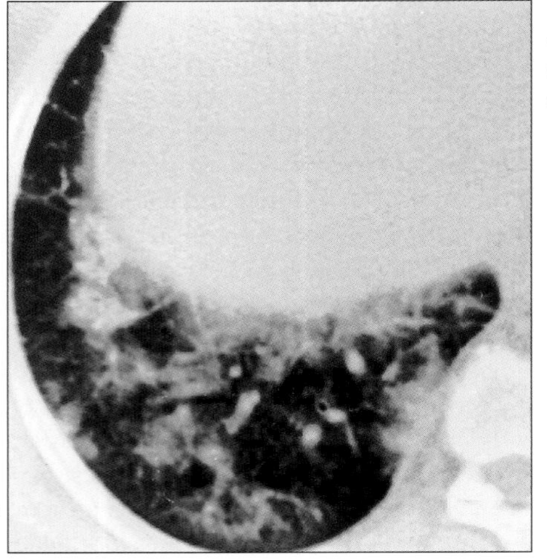

Figure 1.115 Poorly defined acinar nodules and patchy consolidation. The patient has cardiogenic pulmonary edema.

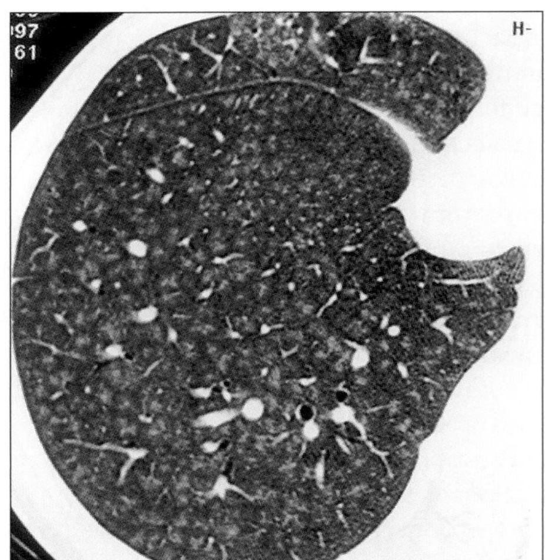

Figure 1.116 High-resolution computed tomography (HRCT) showing poorly defined nodular opacities merging with ground-glass opacification. The patient has subacute hypersensitivity pneumonitis.

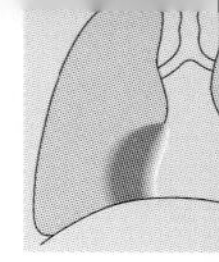

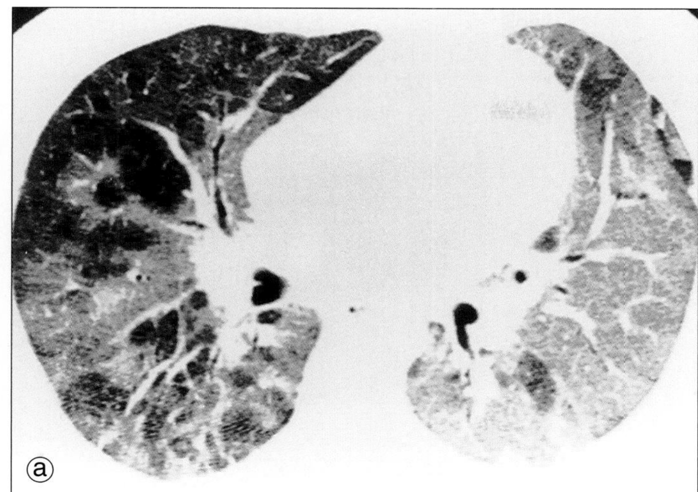

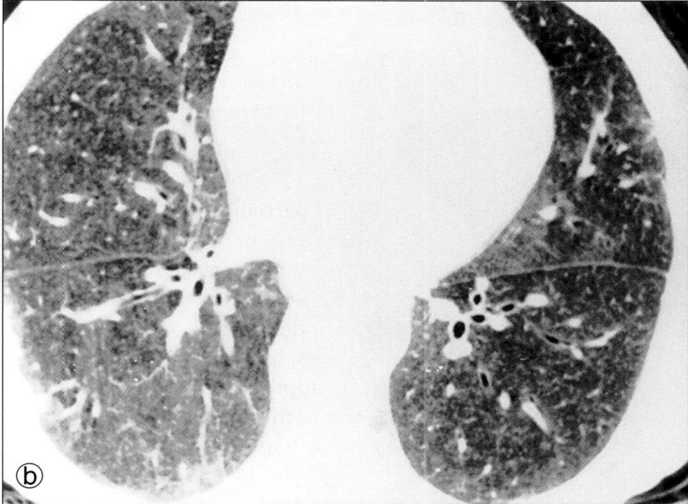

Figure 1.117 Ground-glass appearance on high-resolution computed tomography (HRCT). A, Extensive ground-glass opacification in a patient who has desquamative interstitial pneumonitis. Note that the vessels are visible within the areas of ground-glass opacification. **B,** Generalized ground-glass opacification in a patient who has lymphocytic pneumonitis (note the marked contrast between the density of air within the bronchi and the density of the lung parenchyma).

ground-glass pattern on HRCT does not obscure the pulmonary vasculature. In cases in which the presence of a ground-glass pattern is equivocal, HRCT is often useful to compare the density of the lung parenchyma with air in the bronchi; in the normal state, the difference in density is marginal. Although this HRCT abnormality is usually easily recognizable, particularly when it is interspersed with areas of normal lung parenchyma, subtle degrees of increased parenchymal opacification may not be obvious. It is important to recognize that a normal increase in parenchymal density, indistinguishable from a generalized opacification caused by infiltrative lung disease, resulting in a ground-glass pattern is seen in patients who hold their breath at end of expiration (Fig. 1.118).

On a pathologic level, the changes responsible for ground-glass opacification are complex and include partial filling of the air spaces and thickening of the interstitium or a combination of the two. Conditions that are characterized by these pathologic changes and result in the nonspecific pattern of ground-glass opacification include fibrosing alveolitis in the active cellular phase, *Pneumocystis jiroveci* pneumonia, subacute hypersensitivity pneumonitis, sarcoidosis, drug-induced lung damage, diffuse pulmonary hemorrhage, and acute lung injury. The amorphous ground-glass density seen on HRCT in these conditions usually represents a potentially reversible process. However, mild thickening of the intralobular interstitium by irreversible fibrosis may rarely produce a ground-glass appearance in fibrosing alveolitis. Furthermore, ground-glass opacification may be seen in areas of bronchoalveolar cell carcinoma, usually in conjunction with patches of denser, consolidated lung (Fig. 1.119).

A pitfall in identifying a ground-glass pattern on HRCT occurs when regional differences in pulmonary perfusion are present; regional alterations in pulmonary blood flow, caused by thromboembolism, for example, may result in striking differences in lung density (Fig. 1.120). The density difference between the underperfused lung and the normal lung may give the appearance of a ground-glass density in normal (but relatively overperfused) lung parenchyma. These areas of different densities have often been termed *mosaic oligemia*. A similar appearance is seen in patients who have patchy air trapping caused by small-airway disease, for example, an obliterative bronchiolitis; the relatively transradiant areas of underventilated and therefore underperfused lung make the normal lung parenchyma appear more than usually dense and thus simulate a ground-glass infiltrate. This potential pitfall can often be recognized for what it is by the relative paucity of vessels in the underventilated parts of the lungs caused by hypoxic vasoconstriction. The vessels in the relatively normal lung of higher density are engorged because of shunting of blood to these regions (see Fig. 1.120).

CYSTIC AIR SPACES

The term *cystic air space* describes a clearly defined, air-containing space that has a definable wall 1 to 3 mm thick. Many conditions are characterized by a profusion of cystic air spaces, which may not be recognizable as such on chest radiography (Fig. 1.121), whereas the size and distribution of these cysts on HRCT may suggest the diagnosis.

The destruction of alveolar walls that characterizes emphysema produces areas of low attenuation on HRCT, which often merge imperceptibly with normal lung (Fig. 1.122). In patients who have predominantly centrilobular emphysema, circular areas of lung destruction may resemble cysts; however, the centrilobular core is usually visible as a dotlike structure in the center of the apparent cyst. Although bullae of varying sizes are clearly seen on HRCT in patients with emphysema, usually a background permeative, destructive parenchyma prevents confusion with other conditions in which cystic air spaces are a prominent feature.

Cystic air spaces as the dominant abnormality are seen in only a few conditions, which include lymphangioleiomyomatosis, Langerhans-cell histiocytosis, end-stage fibrosing alveolitis, and postinfective pneumatoceles. In lymphangioleiomyomatosis, the cysts are usually uniformly scattered throughout the lungs, with normal lung parenchyma intervening; the individual cysts are rarely larger than 4 cm in diameter (Fig. 1.123). As the disease progresses, the larger cystic air spaces coalesce, the circumferential, well-defined walls of the cysts become disrupted, and the HRCT pattern of advanced lymphangioleiomyomatosis, and indeed of Langerhans-cell histiocytosis may be practically indis-

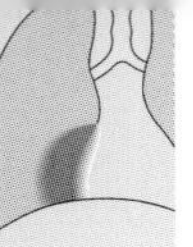

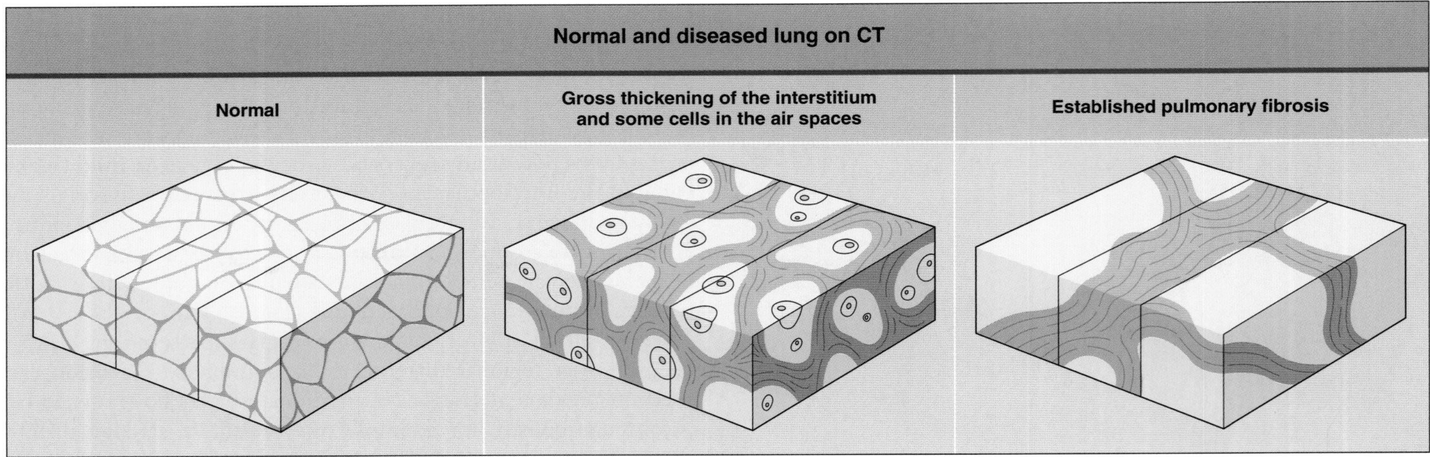

Figure 1.118 Normal and diseased lung voxels. A, In the normal state, most of the volume of these voxels is made up of air. **B,** Gross thickening of the interstitium and some cells within the air spaces causes displacement of air and therefore an increase in density within the voxels. This produces ground-glass opacification on a high-resolution computed tomography (HRCT) image. **C,** In established pulmonary fibrosis, the strands of fibrotic lung occupy much of the volume of individual voxels, which is reflected in their density; pulmonary fibrosis therefore has a reticular pattern on HRCT.

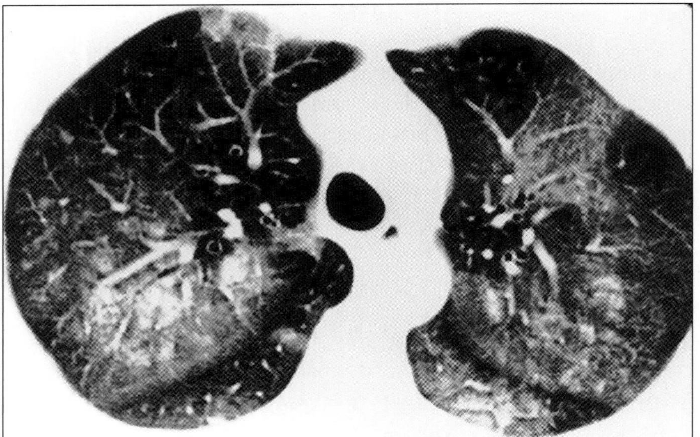

Figure 1.119 Patchy areas of ground-glass opacification in a patient who has biopsy-proved bronchoalveolar cell carcinoma.

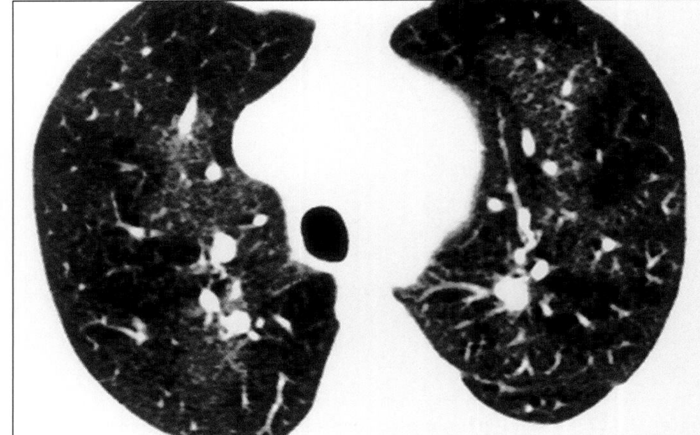

Figure 1.120 Uneven density of the lung parenchyma caused by perfusion inhomogeneity. The patient has chronic thromboembolism (note the dilatation of the segmental pulmonary arteries). The denser (relatively overperfused) lung has a ground-glass appearance.

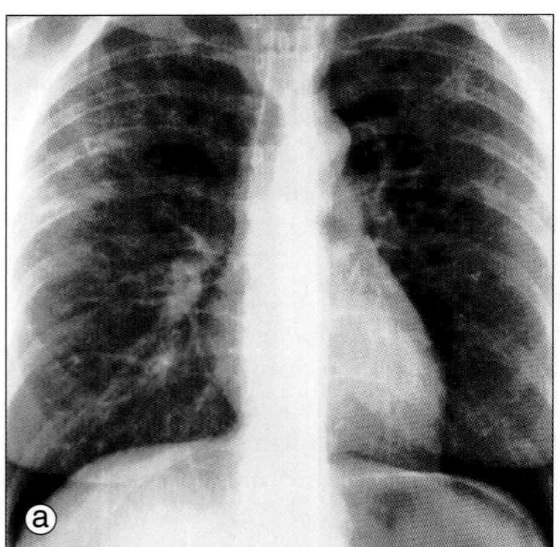

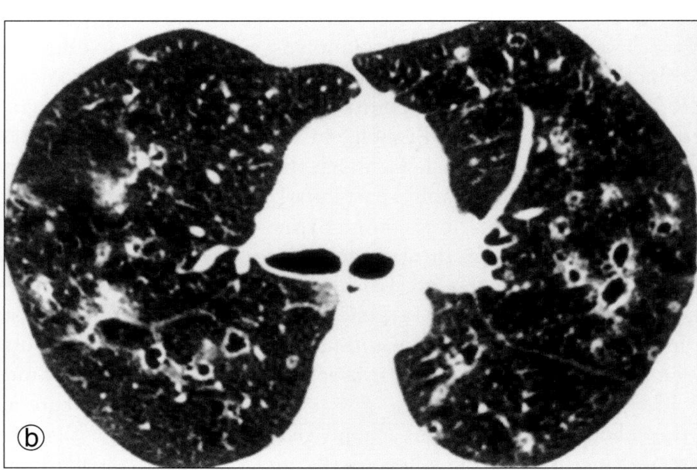

Figure 1.121 Cystic air spaces. A, Nonspecific shadowing on a chest radiograph, with the suggestion of a cavitating nodule in the right upper zone. **B,** High-resolution computed tomography (HRCT) through the upper lobes reveals multiple, oddly shaped, cavitating lesions, typical of Langerhans-cell histiocytosis.

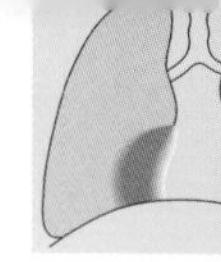

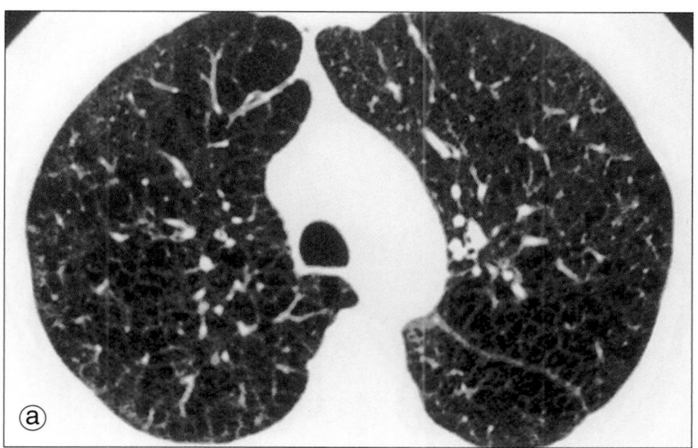

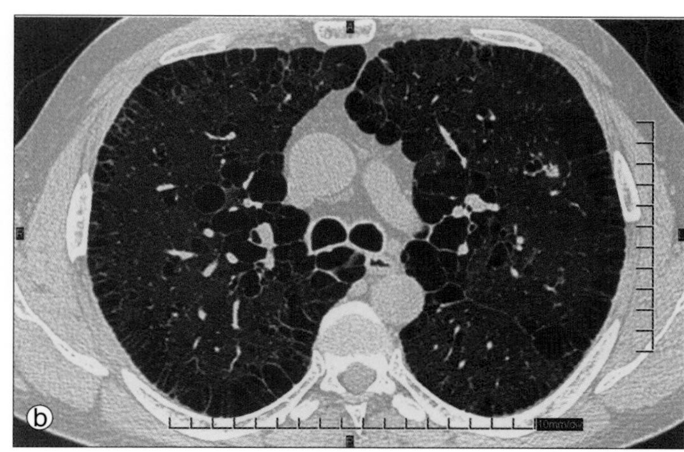

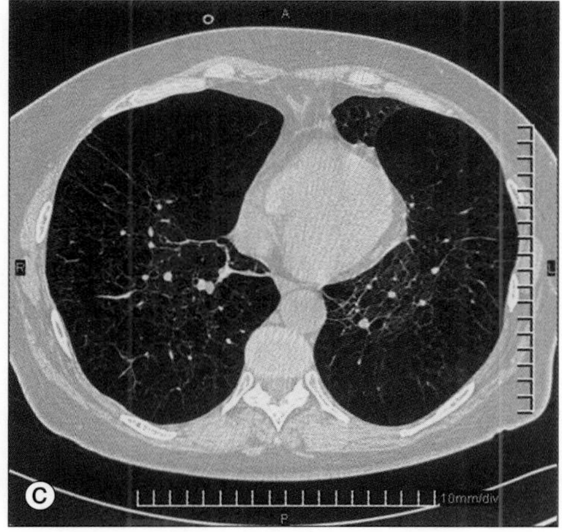

Figure 1.122 High-resolution computed tomography (HRCT) of centrilobular emphysema. **A,** Centrilobular emphysema. Note the permeative destruction of the lung parenchyma with scattered centrilobular lucent areas. **B,** Paraseptal emphysema. Note, however, that the disease is concentrated in the subpleural lung. **C,** Panacinar emphysema. Large swathes of completely destroyed lung are evident, with almost no vascular or soft tissue structures demonstrated within.

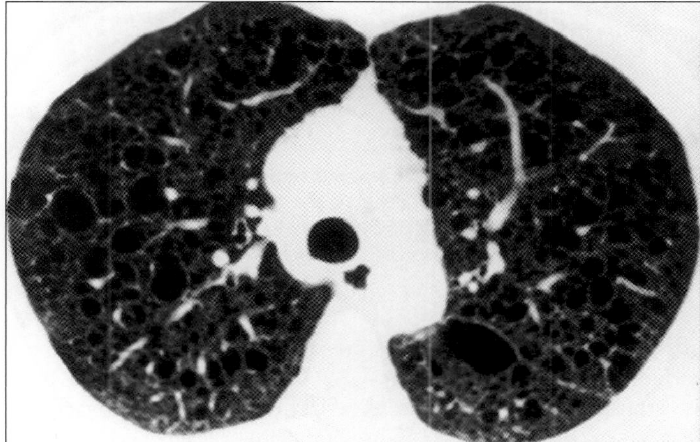

Figure 1.123 High-resolution computed tomography (HRCT) of advanced lymphangioleiomyomatosis. Note the coalescence of cystic air spaces, which resembles severe centrilobular emphysema.

tinguishable from severe centrilobular emphysema. Distinction of the delicate, lacelike reticular pattern of lymphangioleiomyomatosis on HRCT from that of end-stage fibrosing alveolitis is usually possible because the cystic air spaces in a fibrotic honeycomb lung are smaller and have thicker walls. Furthermore, the tendency for fibrosing alveolitis to have a peripheral distribution, even in its end stage, is usually still obvious in the upper zones.

Similar, confluent cystic air spaces that give a delicate pattern on HRCT are seen in patients with advanced Langerhans-cell histiocytosis. However, earlier in the disease, a nodular component is present, and some of the nodules cavitate. The combination of cavitating nodules, some of which have curious shapes (e.g., cloverleaf), and cystic air spaces with a predominantly upper zone distribution is virtually pathognomonic for the diagnosis (see Fig. 1.121). Serial HRCT scans show the natural history of nodules, which cavitate, become cystic air spaces, and, in the end stages, coalesce. In a few cases the cavitating nodules and cystic air spaces may resolve, with the lung parenchyma reverting to a normal appearance. Some of the cavitating nodules in Langerhans-cell histiocytosis superficially resemble bronchiectatic airways, but there is a lack of continuity between these lesions on adjacent sections, and the segmental bronchi, where they can be identified, do not have any of the HRCT features of bronchiectasis.

Diseases of the Airways

The imaging test of choice for the detection of bronchiectasis is now HRCT. The diagnosis of bronchiectasis on chest radiography can rarely be made with certainty unless the disease is severe. The opportunity for prospective studies to compare the

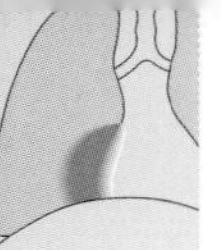

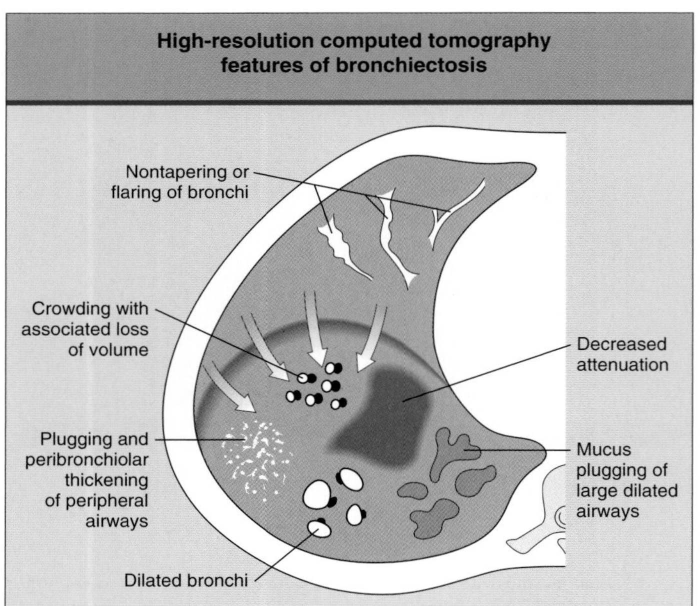

Figure 1.124 High-resolution computed tomography (HRCT) features of bronchiectasis. Nontapering or flaring of bronchi lying within the plane of section. Signet ring sign of dilated bronchi runs perpendicular to the plane of CT section. Mucous plugging of large, dilated airways and plugging and peribronchiolar thickening of small peripheral airways are present. Crowding has occurred with associated loss of volume (see position of oblique fissure). Areas of decreased attenuation are present, which reflects associated small-airway disease.

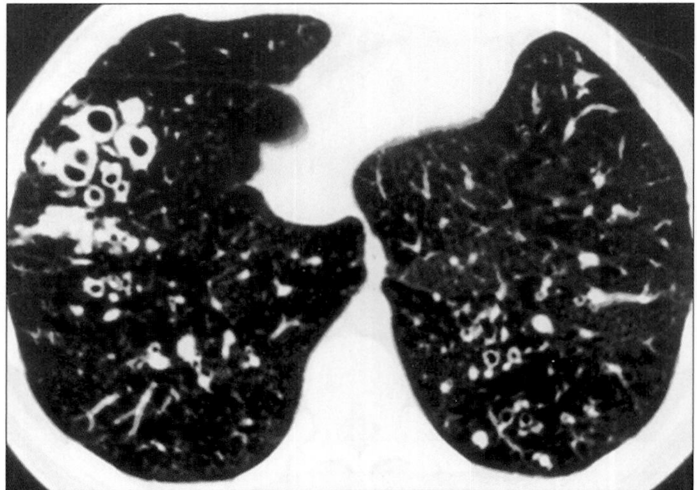

Figure 1.125 Severe bronchiectasis in the right lower lobe with plugging of the dilated bronchi. Mild, cylindrical bronchiectasis in the left lower lobe showing the signet ring sign.

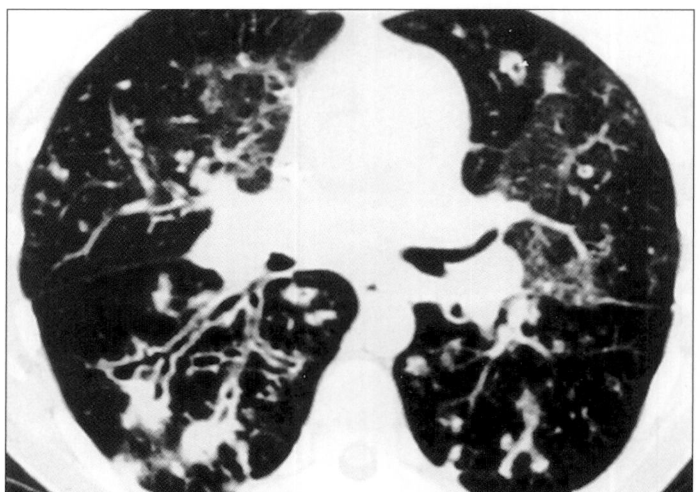

Figure 1.126 High-resolution computed tomography (HRCT) of a patient with cystic fibrosis. Nontapering and flaring of the bronchiectatic airways is visible in the apical segment of the right lower lobe. In addition, mosaic perfusion is present, reflecting associated small-airway disease.

accuracy of HRCT with that of what used to be the gold standard, bronchography, has passed. Most of the evidence that suggests HRCT is at least as good as bronchography is based on small, retrospective studies with different bronchographic and CT techniques. However, now that bronchography is rarely performed, no other imaging technique begins to compare in sensitivity and specificity with an optimal HRCT examination.

Bronchiectasis is defined as damage to the bronchial wall that results in irreversible dilatation of the bronchi, whatever the cause. Therefore, the main feature of bronchiectasis on HRCT is dilatation of the bronchi with or without bronchial-wall thickening. Criteria for the HRCT identification of abnormally dilated bronchi depend on the orientation of the bronchi in relation to the plane of the HRCT section (Fig. 1.124).

Vertically orientated bronchi are seen in the transverse section, so reference can be made to the accompanying pulmonary artery that in normal individuals is of approximately the same caliber; any dilatation of the bronchus results in the so-called "signet ring sign" (Fig. 1.125). Although this is generally a reliable sign of abnormal bronchial dilatation, care must be taken when comparing the diameter of the bronchi with adjacent pulmonary arteries just below the division of the lower lobar bronchus. At this level, pairs of segmental and sometimes subsegmental bronchi converge, and the resulting fusion of the two bronchi may give the spurious impression of an abnormally dilated bronchus. Bronchi that have a more horizontal course on CT, particularly the anterior segmental bronchi of the upper lobes and the segmental bronchi of the lingula and right middle lobe, are demonstrated along their length, and abnormal dilatation is seen as nontapering parallel walls or even flaring of the bronchi as they course distally (Fig. 1.126). In more severe cases of bronchiectasis, the bronchi are obviously dilated and have a varicose or cystic appearance.

Bronchial-wall thickening is a frequent, but not invariable, feature of bronchiectasis. The definition of what constitutes abnormal bronchial-wall thickening remains a point of contention, particularly because mild degrees of wall thickening are seen in normal subjects, asymptomatic smokers, asthmatic individuals, and patients affected by an acute, lower–respiratory tract, viral infection. In brief, no robust and reproducible criterion for the identification of abnormal bronchial-wall thickening exists, so bronchial-wall thickening remains a subjective sign with an attendant high variation in observer interpretation. However, it is the presence of peribronchial thickening that renders the smaller peripheral airways visible on HRCT. Although there is no exact level beyond which visualization of the bronchi can be regarded as abnormal on HRCT, normal

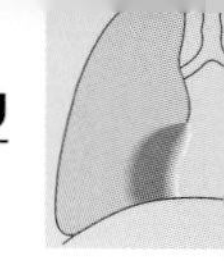

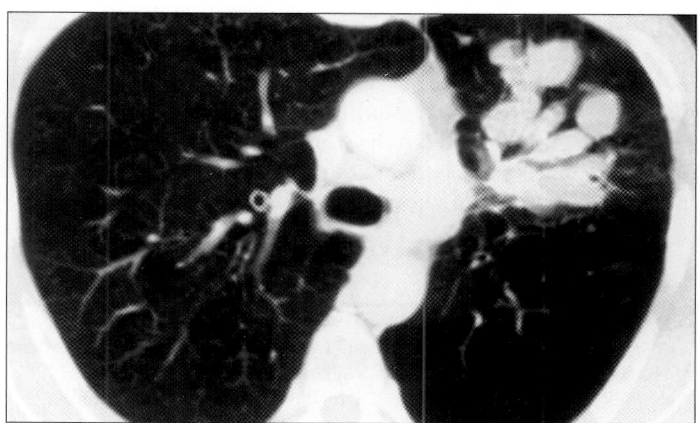

Figure 1.127 Severe bronchiectasis in the left upper lobe. The bronchi are completely filled with fluid, which results in multiple round and elliptical opacities. The patient has allergic bronchopulmonary aspergillosis.

bronchi should not be visible within 2 to 3 cm of the pleural surface. The appearance of large elliptical and circular opacities, which represent secretion-filled, dilated bronchi, is a sign of gross bronchiectasis and is almost invariably seen in the presence of other obviously dilated bronchi, some of which may contain air-fluid levels (Fig. 1.127). When mucous plugging of the smaller airways occurs, minute branching structures or dots in the lung periphery may be identifiable. In some cases, plugging of the numerous centrilobular bronchioles gives a curious nodular appearance to the lungs (Fig. 1.128).

Supplementary HRCT signs of bronchiectasis include crowding of the affected bronchi, with obvious volume loss of the lobe as shown by the position of the major fissures. In many lobes affected by bronchiectasis, areas of decreased attenuation of the lung parenchyma adjacent to the abnormal airways can be identified; this pattern of mosaic attenuation is thought to reflect accompanying small-airway disease, and the extent of the pattern correlates well with functional evidence of airflow obstruction, particularly indices of small-airway dysfunction.

A positive diagnosis of bronchiectasis on HRCT is straightforward in patients with moderate and severe disease. However, in some situations subtle signs of bronchiectasis may be obscured by technical artifacts. Conversely, the HRCT appearances of bronchiectasis may be mimicked by other lung pathologies. Some of the causes of false-negative and false-positive diagnoses of bronchiectasis are listed in Table 1.5.

Interest in the ability of HRCT to reveal small-airway disease is increasing. In the exudative form of bronchiolar disease (typified by Japanese panbronchiolitis), HRCT directly shows the plugged small airways as small irregular branching opacities. The HRCT signs of constrictive obliterative bronchiolitis (e.g., in patients with rheumatoid arthritis or post-viral obliterative bronchiolitis) are indirect; areas of decreased attenuation occur, within which the vessels are of reduced caliber (but not distorted, in contrast to what is seen with emphysema). The areas of decreased attenuation may merge with those of more normal lung or may have sharply demarcated, "geographic" boundaries (mosaic attenuation pattern). The density differences that characterize constrictive obliterative bronchiolitis may be extremely subtle, but because they represent areas of reduced ventilation, and therefore air trapping, they may be dramatically emphasized

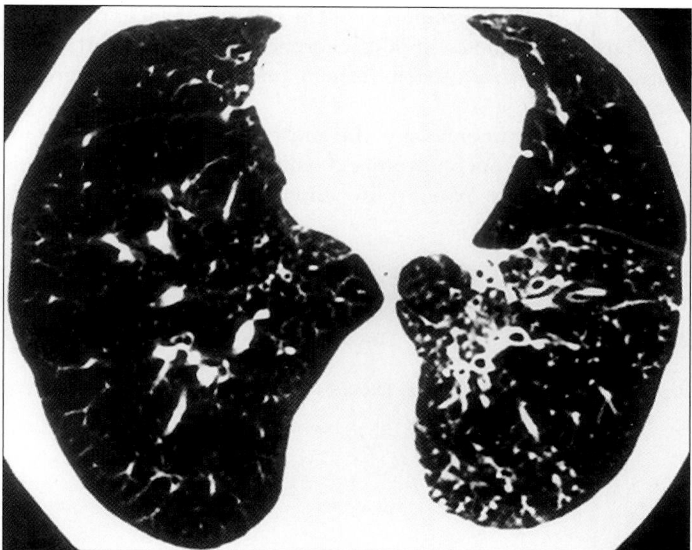

Figure 1.128 Numerous small irregular opacities in the left lower lobe representing plugged bronchioles. This is a case of panbronchiolitis.

Table 1.5
Causes of false-positive and false-negative diagnoses of bronchiectasis on high-resolution computed tomography

False negatives	False positives
Inappropriately thick computed tomography section	Cardiac pulsation causing 'double vessels'
Movement artifact obscures lung detail	Confluence of subsegmental bronchi may give spurious impression of bronchiectasis, at a single level (particularly in the lower lobes)
Focal, inconspicuous, thin-walled bronchiectasis	Cavitating nodules mimicking bronchiectasis (e.g. Langerhans cell histiocytosis)
Bronchiectatic airways masked by surrounding fibrosis	Reversible dilatation of bronchi with acute pneumonic consolidation

on scans performed at end expiration. The majority of patients affected by small-airway disease has some bronchiectatic changes on HRCT, which tend to be more severe in those who have immunologically mediated obliterative bronchiolitis (e.g., after lung transplantation).

High-resolution Computed Tomography and Pulmonary Infections in Immunocompromised Patients

Pulmonary opportunistic infections are a common complication in immunocompromised patients. The pulmonary complications associated with human immunodeficiency virus (HIV) and acquired immunodeficiency syndrome (AIDS) are covered in Chapters 30 and 31. Chest disease in the non-HIV population frequently results in radiographic appearances that are nonspecific. High morbidity and mortality rates are associated with chest infection in these patients. For the diagnostic yield of radiography and HRCT to be maximized, the underlying cause of immunodeficiency, type of immunosuppressive therapy, white blood cell count, and overall medical status of the patient must be known. The introduction of HRCT now makes it possible to offer earlier and more specific diagnostic information. Further-

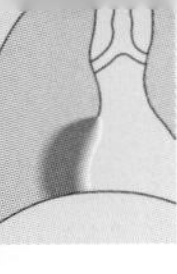

more, HRCT allows prediction of the relative chances of obtaining a positive diagnosis from transbronchial versus percutaneous biopsy, particularly when other techniques have proved nondiagnostic.

Bacterial pneumonias are the most frequent pulmonary infection in immunocompromised patients. Usually, HRCT is reserved for those patients in whom the chest radiograph is equivocal for the presence of abnormality or in whom infective complications require further assessment. Invasive aspergillosis may occur in patients after solid organ or bone marrow transplantation. Diagnosis may be difficult, and an early CT examination has been suggested to be useful in the investigation of the immunocompromised patient who has clinical evidence of chest infection but a normal chest radiograph.

SUGGESTED READING

Armstrong P, et al: Imaging Diseases of the Chest. London, Mosby, 2000.

Fraser RS, et al: Diagnosis of Diseases of the Chest. Philadelphia, WB Saunders, 1999.

Naidich D, et al: Computed Tomography and Magnetic Resonance of the Thorax. Philadelphia, Lippincott Williams and Wilkins, 1998.

Webb WR, et al: High Resolution CT of the Lung. Philadelphia, Lippincott Williams and Wilkins, 2001.

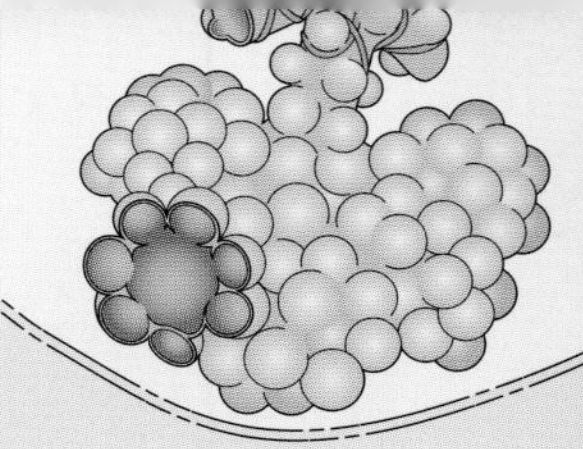

CHAPTER 2

Respiratory Mechanics

Bruce H. Culver

This chapter describes the physical properties of the lungs and chest wall involved in the cyclic processes of ventilation supporting the metabolic needs of the body. The respiratory muscles are introduced, but their function is more fully described in Chapter 6. Clinical measurements of some of these mechanical properties are an important part of pulmonary function testing at rest and with exercise, as discussed in Chapter 7.

STRUCTURE OF THE THORAX AND LUNGS

Thorax

The bony thorax protects the lungs, heart, and great vessels, but it also allows the lungs to change volume from a minimum of 1.5 to 2 L to a maximum of 6 to 8 L. This large expansion is made possible by the articulation of the ribs with the spine and the sternum, the arrangement of the muscles, and the motion of the diaphragm. The ribs articulate with the transverse processes of the thoracic vertebrae and have flexible cartilaginous connections with the sternum. The ribs angle down, both from back to front and from midline to side, so that as they elevate, both the anteroposterior and the transverse dimensions of the thorax increase (Fig. 2.1). The external intercostal muscles, which angle down from posterior to anterior (Fig. 2.2), are well situated to elevate the ribs. With deep inspiratory efforts, the first and second ribs are elevated and stabilized by the accessory muscles of respiration in the neck. If the upper extremities are fixed, the pectoral muscles can also act to raise the ribs (e.g., holding on to a chair back or leaning against a wall when out of breath). Expiration is normally passive because of the elastic recoil of the lung, but it can be assisted by the internal intercostal muscle. Forced expiration (or coughing) requires the abdominal muscles to force the diaphragm upward.

The diaphragm is dome shaped in its relaxed position and can be pulled flatter by muscle contraction. The diaphragm is most often described as fixed at the periphery so that its action pulls down the center of the dome, lengthening the lungs. However, if it is fixed centrally by the pressure of the abdominal contents, the peripheral attachments will lift the ribs, which swing outward when elevated, increasing the transverse diameter of the chest. In addition, the increase in abdominal pressure associated with descent of the diaphragm acts on the lower ribs in the “zone of apposition” to impart an outward force. The actual action of the diaphragm is a combination of these mechanisms, in a proportion that varies with position and abdominal wall tension.

The intercostal muscles are innervated from the thoracic spine at their own level, and the abdominal muscles are innervated from the lower thoracic and lumbar levels, but the diaphragm is served by the phrenic nerves, which originate at the cervical level (C3–C5). Thus, the diaphragm remains functional in patients who have spinal injuries below the midcervical level. The long course of each phrenic nerve along the mediastinum, however, makes it vulnerable to both transient and permanent interruptions by disease, injury, or surgery. Occasionally, local irritation of a phrenic nerve leads to intractable singultus (i.e., hiccups). The respiratory muscles are more fully discussed in Chapter 6.

Pleural Space

The lungs are covered by a thin visceral pleura, which is invaginated into the lobar fissures. The inner aspect of each hemithorax (and top of the diaphragm) is lined with the parietal pleura, which also covers the mediastinum and joins the visceral pleura on each side at the lung hilum. The pleural space extends deeply into the posterior and lateral costophrenic recesses and consists of a potential space, normally containing only a few milliliters of fluid to serve a lubricating function.

The inspiratory forces of the chest wall and diaphragm are transmitted to the lung by the creation of a more negative pressure in this potential space. In pathologic states, pleural effusions may form and make the lung volume smaller by occupying part of the intrathoracic space. Penetration of the chest wall or rupture of the lung surface can allow air to enter the pleural space and create a pneumothorax.

Airways

The upper respiratory passages (nasal cavities and pharynx) conduct, warm, and moisten air as it moves into the lungs. The respiratory system develops as an offshoot from the digestive system and, like the digestive system, has an absorptive function. The entire system is continuously exposed to particulate and infective agents and, accordingly, is protected by a well-developed lymphoid barrier and, more superficially, a mucous barrier. The upper respiratory passages contain the olfactory areas and also conduct and help shape the sounds that produce speech.

The larynx opens off the lowest part of the pharynx. During swallowing, the larynx is closed off from both the pharynx above and the esophagus posteriorly by the epiglottis. The trachea begins at the lower border of the cricoid cartilage of the larynx, at the level of the sixth cervical vertebra. The lumen of the trachea is held open by incomplete, C-shaped cartilaginous rings. The posterior membranous portion contains smooth muscle. When the intrathoracic pressure exceeds the intraluminal pressure, the membranous portion becomes invaginated, the ends of the rings may overlap, and the lumen is greatly nar-

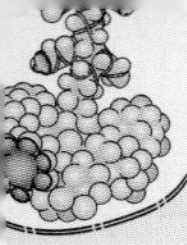

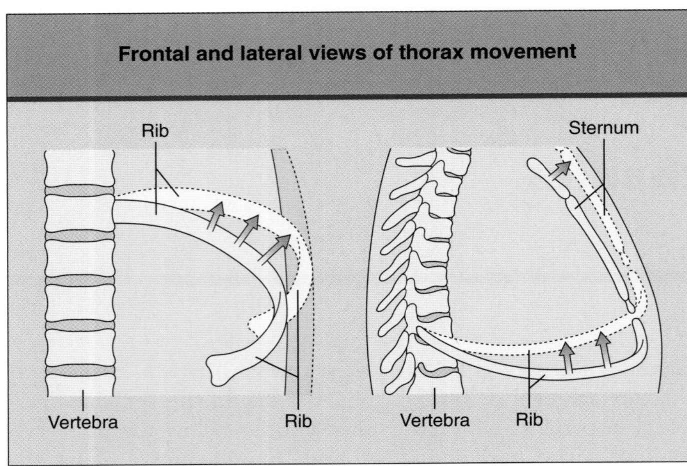

Figure 2.1 Frontal and lateral views of thorax movement. With rib elevation, both the transverse and the anteroposterior dimensions increase.

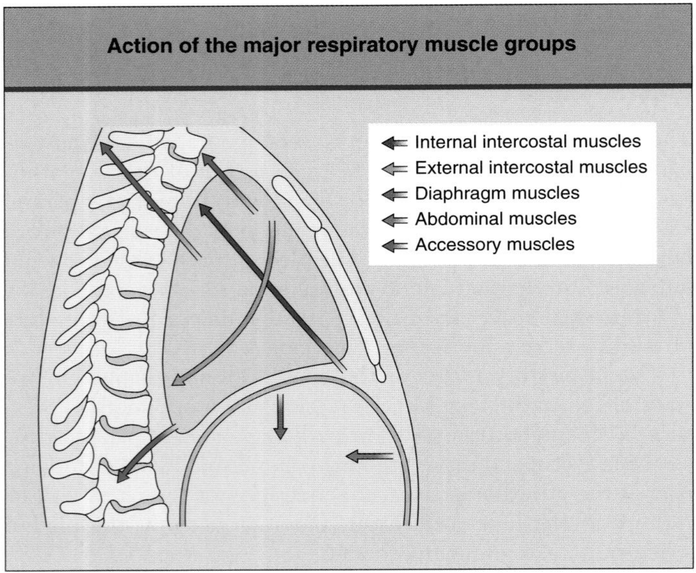

Figure 2.2 Action of the major respiratory muscle groups (intercostals, accessories, diaphragm, and abdominal).

rowed. Smooth muscle contraction narrows the lumen but increases its rigidity. With deep inspiration, the trachea enlarges and lengthens. The trachea bifurcates into the main bronchi, which in turn become lobar, segmental, and subsegmental bronchi and end in bronchioles, which lack cartilage and are about 1 mm in diameter. Beyond these are the respiratory bronchioles, alveolar ducts, sacs, and alveoli that make up the respiratory zone in which gas exchange and other functions take place.

The intraparenchymal bronchi are invested with overlapping helical bands of smooth muscle, wound in clockwise and counterclockwise fashion. The amount of smooth muscle increases proportionately in the smaller bronchioles to occupy about 20% of the wall thickness. Elastic fibers are a well-developed component at every level of the respiratory system. They stretch when the lungs are expanded in inspiration, and their recoil helps return the lungs to their end-exhalation volume. Elastic

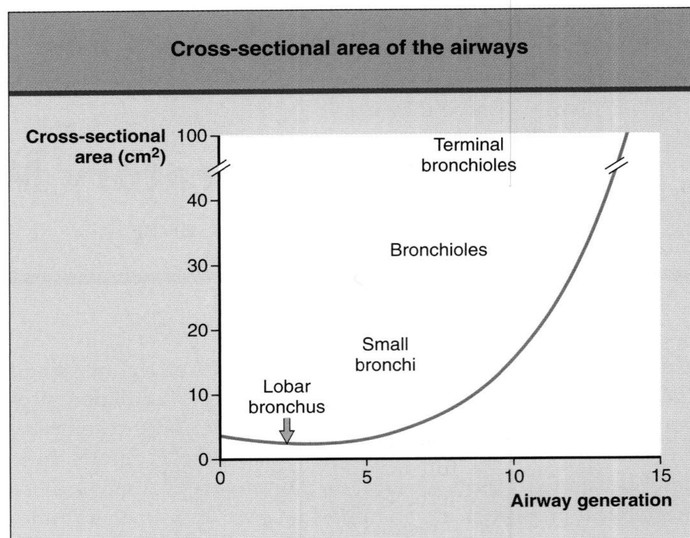

Figure 2.3 Total cross-sectional area of the airways. The aggregate luminal area increases greatly, from about 2.5 cm^2 in the trachea and major airways to more than 100 cm^2 at the level of the terminal bronchioles. Modified with permission from Culver BH [ed]: The Respiratory System. Seattle, ASUW Publications, 1997. Weibel ER: Morphometry of the Human Lung. Berlin and New York, Springer-Verlag, 1963.

fibers are a rich component of the connective tissue in the smaller bronchi and bronchioles. The smooth muscle stops at the portals of the respiratory zone, but elastic and collagen fibers contribute to the alveolar wall and form an irregular, wide-meshed net of delicate, interlacing fibers.

The number of airway generations required to reach the respiratory zone varies with pathway length, so that areas near the hilum may be reached in 15 generations, while those in the periphery may require 25. Although the sizes of individual airways become smaller, the number of airways approximately doubles with each new generation, so that the total cross-sectional area of the combined air path increases. This is especially so in the smaller bronchi and bronchioles, where the "daughters" of each division are only slightly smaller than the "parent." The rapidly increasing total cross-sectional area of small airways, shown diagrammatically in Figure 2.3, means that their contribution to airflow resistance in the lungs is small. Thus, diseases that affect these peripheral airways may be functionally "silent" until an advanced state.

Interdependence in the Lung

Because the lung parenchyma is made up of interconnected alveolar walls, interstitial tissues, and fibers, any local distortion in a given region is opposed by the surrounding tissue. That is, if a small zone of alveoli within a lobe begins to collapse, the surrounding tissue is stretched and thus tends to pull the zone back open. This property is termed *structural interdependence*. It, along with surfactant and the presence of collateral air pathways, helps prevent alveolar collapse, even when small bronchioles become plugged. When collapsed areas of lung cannot expand despite distention of the surrounding alveoli, lung injury may develop as a result of extremely large forces that are generated at the interface. Because the bronchi and blood vessels travel

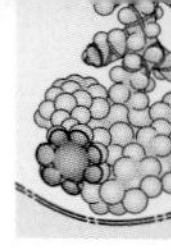

through, and have attachments to, the lung parenchyma, they too are affected by the surrounding tissue. As the lung expands, the caliber of these channels also increases, and at low lung volume, airway closure may occur.

RESPIRATORY MECHANICS

The properties of the lung and chest that affect and effect the movement of air in and out of the lungs are central to understanding both normal and abnormal lung function.

Lung Volumes

The total gas-containing capacity of the lungs can be divided into a series of volumes, as shown in Figure 2.4 which, in combination, give lung capacities. The largest amount of air that can be held in the lungs at full inspiration is the total lung capacity (TLC). After a complete forced exhalation, the lungs are not empty but contain a residual volume (RV). The difference between TLC and RV—that is, the greatest volume of air that can be inhaled or exhaled—is the vital capacity (VC). The VC can be affected by factors that limit either lung expansion or lung emptying.

A normal breath has a tidal volume (V_T) that is only a small portion of the VC (about 10%), and even during strenuous exercise, V_T increases to only 50% to 60% of VC. Increases in V_T occur by using parts of the inspiratory reserve and expiratory reserve volumes, as shown in Figure 2.4. At the end of a relaxed tidal exhalation, the lungs return to a resting volume, which is normally about 50% of TLC. The volume contained in the lungs at this end-tidal position is the functional residual capacity (FRC), and the volume that can be inhaled from this point is the inspiratory capacity (IC).

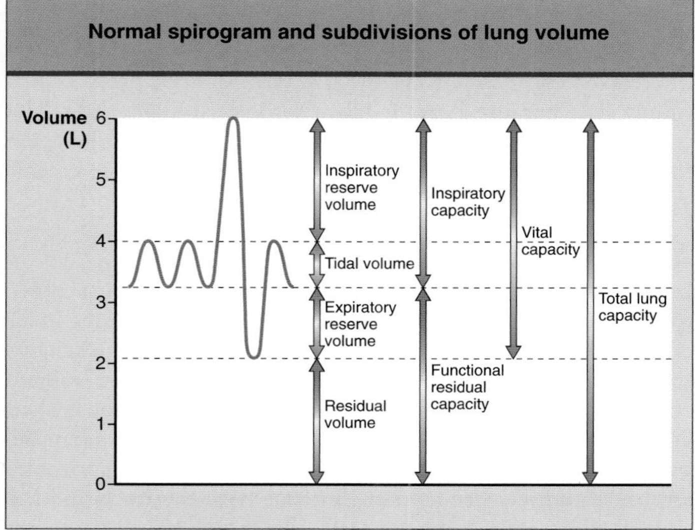

Figure 2.4 The normal spirogram and subdivisions of lung volume. By convention, *volume* is used to describe the smallest subdivisions that do not overlap (residual volume, expiratory reserve volume, tidal volume, and inspiratory reserve volume), and *capacity* is used to describe combinations of these volumes (functional residual capacity, inspiratory capacity, vital capacity, and total lung capacity). From Pulmonary terms and symbols: A report of the ACCP-ATS Joint Committee on Pulmonary Nomenclature: Chest 67:583-593, 1975.

Lung–Chest Wall System

Understanding the process of normal breathing, special maneuvers such as coughing, and the effects of positive-pressure ventilators requires knowledge of the mechanical properties of the thorax. Three primary forces are involved:

1. Elastic recoil properties of the lung
2. Elastic recoil properties of the chest wall
3. Muscular efforts of the chest wall, diaphragm, and abdomen

In combination, these result in changes in lung (and thorax) volume, alveolar pressure, and intrapleural pressure.

VOLUMES OF ELASTIC STRUCTURES

The recoil tendency of a spring can be expressed in terms of its unstressed or resting length and its length-tension relationship. Similarly, for expandable volumetric structures, the relevant properties are the unstressed volume and the relationship between the volume and the transmural pressure required to achieve that volume (Fig. 2.5). By convention, transmural pressures are expressed as the difference between the pressure inside (P_{IN}) and the pressure outside (P_{OUT}) the structure ($P_{IN} - P_{OUT}$). It is convenient to think of this as the distending pressure required to achieve a certain volume. In addition, this distending pressure represents the recoil pressure, or the tendency of the structure to return to its unstressed volume (where transmural pressure is zero). A positive recoil pressure indicates a tendency to become smaller. A structure distorted to a volume below its unstressed volume has a negative recoil pressure, which indicates its tendency to become larger.

ELASTIC PROPERTIES OF THE LUNG

The lungs are elastic structures with a tendency to recoil to a small unstressed volume (usually slightly less than RV). To maintain any lung volume larger than this unstressed volume requires a force that distends the lungs; this force is the difference between the alveolar pressure (P_A) and the pressure surrounding the lungs, the intrapleural pressure (P_{PL}). The elastic properties of the lungs and their tendency to recoil are represented by a plot of the relationship between lung volume and transmural pressure (Fig. 2.6). Such graphs apply to an excised lung inflated by a pump, an in vivo lung inflated by a ventilator, or the more physiologic normal lung inflated by expanding the chest (to create a more negative pleural pressure). In each case, the curve of volume versus the transpulmonary pressure difference ($P_A - P_{PL}$) is the same.

The slope of this pressure-volume curve represents the compliance of the lungs (C_L), as represented by equation 2.1.

$$\text{EQUATION 2.1: } C_L = \Delta V/\Delta P$$

The C_L decreases as the lungs near the limit of their distensibility at TLC. Usually, C_L is measured just above FRC in the tidal breathing range. Because it is normally expressed in absolute volume units (e.g., L/cmH_2O), C_L is strongly dependent on lung size. For example, for the same pressure change, a single lung has only 50% of the volume change of two lungs. A small child's normal C_L is considerably lower than an adult's. For this reason, C_L is often divided by lung volume to give the volume-independent specific compliance.

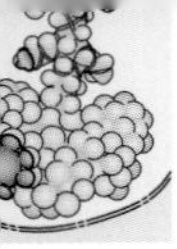

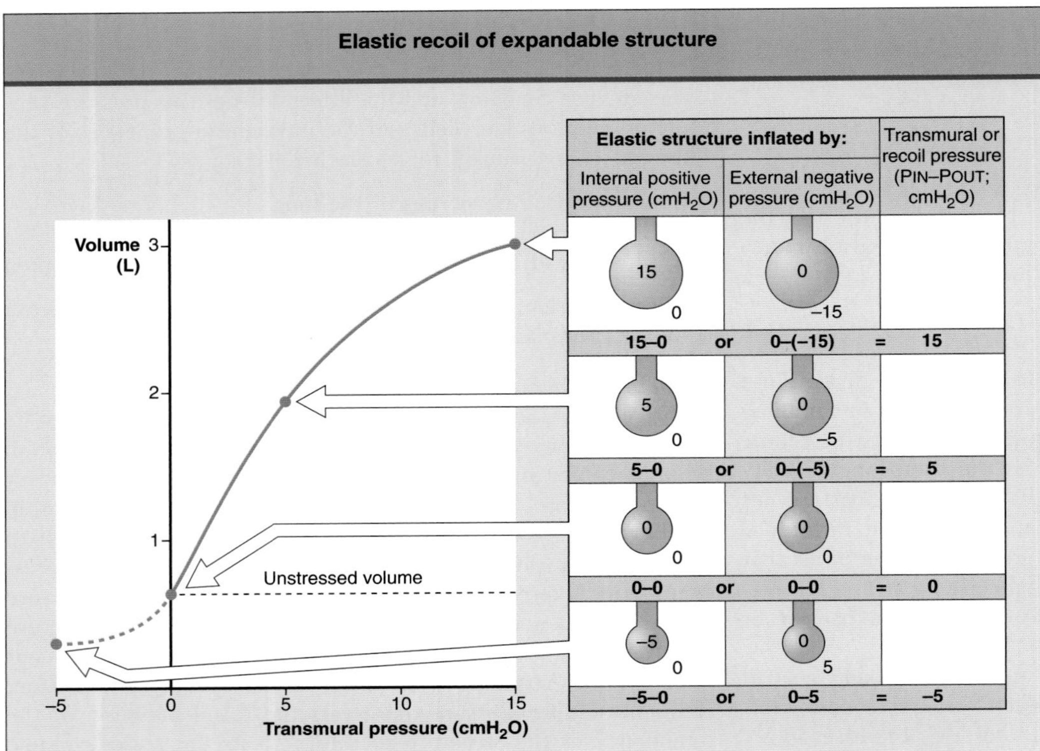

Figure 2.5 Elastic recoil of an expandable structure. The transmural pressure ($P_{IN} - P_{OUT}$) associated with each volume indicates the tendency to return to the unstressed volume. Positive pressure and negative pressure inflation are equivalent.

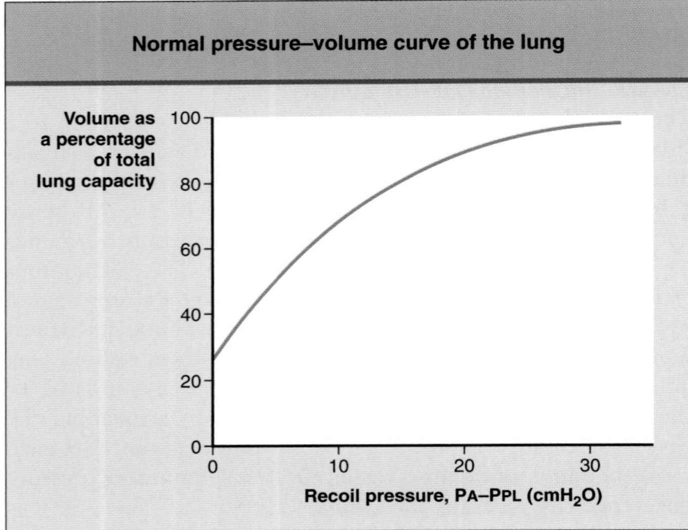

Figure 2.6 Normal pressure-volume curve of the lung. The elastic recoil pressure of the lung as obtained during a very slow expiration from total lung capacity (the curve on inspiration is somewhat different). Modified with permission from Culver BH [ed]: The Respiratory System. Seattle, ASUW Publications, 1997.

Table 2.1
Recoil pressures

Transmural pressure	Pressure inside – pressure outside
Lungs	Alveolar pressure (P_A) – pleural pressure (P_{PL})
Chest wall	P_{PL} – atmospheric pressure (P_{ATM}), or simply P_{PL}
Respiratory system	($P_A - P_{PL}$) + ($P_{PL} - P_{ATM}$) = $P_A - P_{ATM}$

ELASTIC PROPERTIES OF THE CHEST WALL

The chest wall has elastic properties that can be expressed in the same way as those of the lung (Fig. 2.7). The chest wall differs from many common elastic structures, in that its unstressed volume (where recoil pressure is zero) is normally quite high. When expanded above its unstressed volume, it recoils inward, but if the chest wall is "distorted" to a smaller volume, its tendency is to recoil outward. Recoil pressure for the relaxed chest wall is $P_{PL} - P_{ATM}$ (atmospheric pressure), or simply P_{PL}, because P_{ATM} is taken to be zero (Table 2.1). The compliance of the chest wall is similar to that of the lungs in the midvolume range, but note that at TLC the chest remains as distensible as it is at FRC.

LUNG AND CHEST WALL: THE RESPIRATORY SYSTEM

In the intact thorax, the lungs and chest wall must move together. The muscular effort required to inspire a volume of air or the pressure that must be developed by a ventilator to achieve the same volume change is determined by the pressure-volume curve of the combined respiratory system, shown by the dashed line in Figure 2.7. The lungs and chest wall normally contain the same volume of air, so that only points at the same horizontal level in Figure 2.7 can coexist. Because both the lungs and the chest wall are expanded together, the distending pressure for the respiratory system is the sum of the distending pressures required by the lungs and the chest wall. The transmural pressure for the respiratory system is $P_A - P_{ATM}$ (Table 2.1). Figure 2.7 shows that a greater pressure change is required to add volume to the respiratory system than to either of its components alone, and thus the compliance of the respiratory system

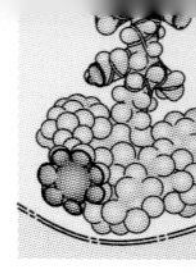

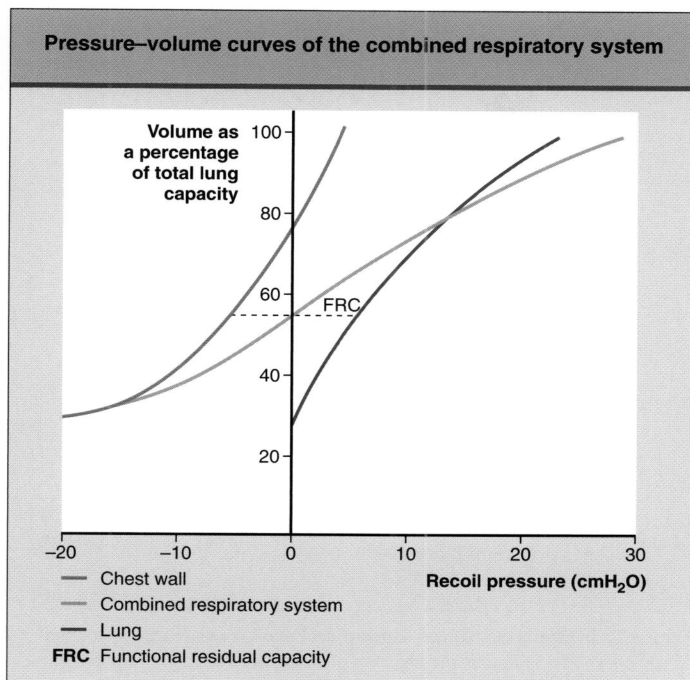

Figure 2.7 Pressure-volume curves of the combined thoracic system. The relaxed chest wall has a relatively high unstressed volume. The recoil of the combined respiratory system is the sum of the recoil of the chest wall plus lung. Modified with permission from Culver BH [ed]: The Respiratory System. Seattle, ASUW Publications, 1997. based on Rahn H, Otis AB, Chadwich LE, Fenn WO: The pressure-volume diagram of the thorax and lung. Am J Physiol 146:161-178, 1946.

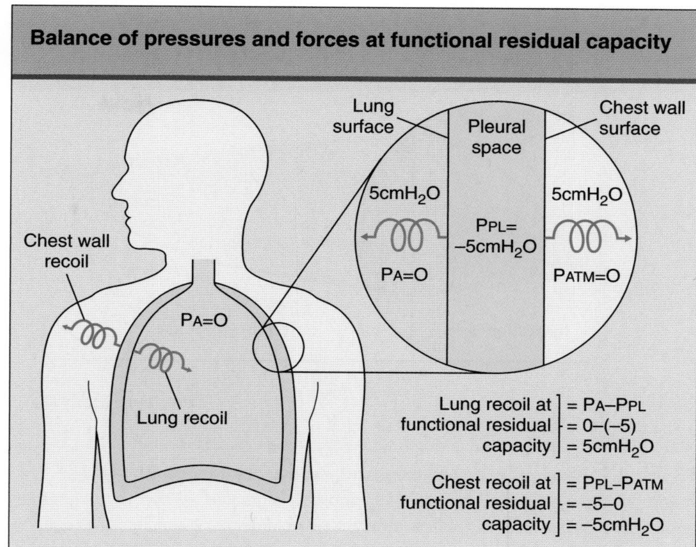

Figure 2.8 Balance of pressures and forces at functional residual capacity. The opposing recoils of lung and chest wall create a negative intrapleural pressure. Modified with permission from Culver BH [ed]: The Respiratory System. Seattle, ASUW Publications, 1997.

is lower than that of either lungs or chest wall at the same volume. At first, this may seem paradoxical, because the chest wall's tendency to expand might be thought to help lung expansion; however, as the system volume is increased, the outward recoil of the chest wall decreases, and this force must be replaced by additional work.

The third mechanical factor, muscle force, is not considered in Figure 2.7. Thus, the pressure difference across the lung, which has no muscle, can always be taken from its curve, but the pressure across the chest wall (and diaphragm) may reflect muscle tension and is described by this curve only during complete relaxation. Similarly, the curve for the respiratory system shows the pressure that would be measured by a manometer held tightly in the mouth after a subject has inhaled or exhaled to a particular volume, and then relaxed all muscle effort.

At the resting end-tidal position of the respiratory system (FRC), no active muscular forces are applied and PA = PATM (distending pressure = 0). The lung is distended above its low unstressed volume, and the chest wall is held below its relatively high unstressed volume. The relaxed FRC is the volume at which the opposing tendencies of the lungs to recoil inward and the chest wall to recoil outward are evenly balanced. Any change in the unstressed volume or the compliance of the lungs or chest wall results in a new FRC. For example, obesity reduces the unstressed volume of the chest wall and thus reduces the FRC (and expiratory reserve volume; see Chapter 69). Emphysema increases both compliance and unstressed volume of the lung, which results in a higher FRC and a "shift to the left" of the respiratory system pressure-volume curve.

The opposing forces of lung and chest wall create a subatmospheric (negative) pressure in the intrapleural space at the FRC (Fig. 2.8). Because the lungs and chest wall are not directly linked, it is actually the intrapleural pressure that opposes lung recoil and chest wall recoil. Thus, at a relaxed FRC, it must have the same magnitude as each of these recoil forces. The average pleural pressure is normally about –5 cmH_2O at FRC.

Events of the Respiratory Cycle

Inspiration is an active process. Contraction of the inspiratory muscles (primarily the intercostals and the diaphragm) tends to expand the thorax, which creates a more negative intrapleural pressure, which in turn causes the alveolar pressure to become negative with respect to the atmosphere and draws air into the lungs. This process continues until the lung volume increases to a point where its recoil pressure is increased to balance the combined muscular and elastic forces of the chest wall. At this point, alveolar pressure becomes zero, and the inspiratory flow stops because a pressure gradient no longer exists along the airways.

During normal breathing, expiration is a passive process. The inspiratory muscles relax, and the balance of forces shifts so that lung recoil predominates. The alveolar pressure becomes positive, and the air moves from the alveoli through the airways to the outside atmosphere until FRC conditions are reached, when the forces are balanced again and the alveolar pressure is zero. Note that with a typical small VT, the chest wall remains below its unstressed volume, with a small outward recoil force, and pleural pressure can be negative throughout the cycle. During active expiration, this process can be assisted by contraction of the expiratory muscles (intercostal and abdominal wall muscles), which makes pleural pressure positive.

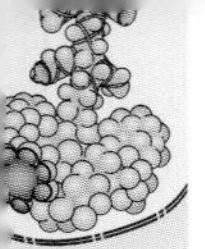

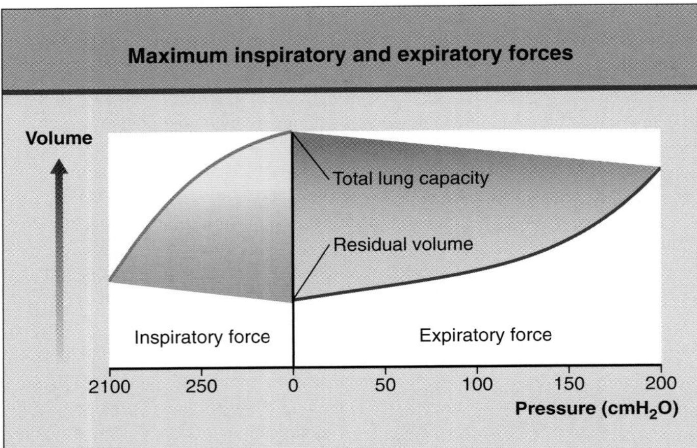

Figure 2.9 Maximum inspiratory and expiratory forces. The normal maximum force generated by inspiratory muscles is greatest at low lung volume, and the expiratory force is greatest at high lung volume. Lung volume decreases with pressure due to gas compression. Modified with permission from Culver BH [ed]: The Respiratory System. Seattle, ASUW Publications, 1997.

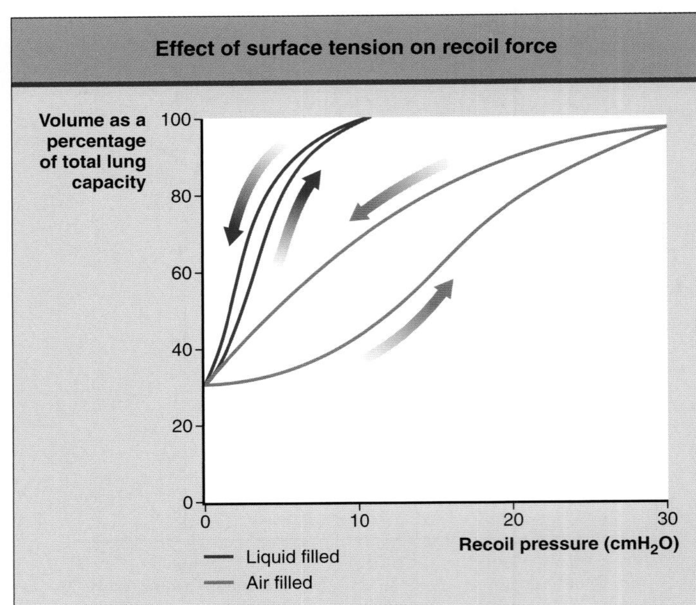

Figure 2.10 Effect of surface tension on recoil force. Pressure-volume curves obtained on inflation and deflation of a normal air-filled lung and the same lung when filled with saline. The horizontal difference between the curves reflects the effect of surface tension, which is greater on inspiration than on expiration and is abolished when the lung is filled with liquid. Modified with permission from Culver BH [ed]: The Respiratory System. Seattle, ASUW Publications, 1997. Data from Bachofen H, Hildebrandt J, Bachofen M: Pressure-volume curves of air- and liquid-filled excised lungs—surface tension in situ. J Appl Physiol 29:422-431, 1970.

Respiratory Muscle Effort

The maximum inspiratory and expiratory pressures measure the maximal efforts of the respiratory muscles (Fig. 2.9). That is, if one tried to inhale against a closed pressure manometer, the negative pressure that could be generated at the mouth would be about 100 cmH_2O at a low lung volume. At TLC, no negative pressure can be generated, and thus no more air can be drawn into the chest. Maximum expiratory pressures are somewhat greater, 150 to 200 cmH_2O at a high lung volume, and they fall to zero at RV.

Surface Tension

At the surface of a liquid, the intramolecular forces are not balanced by the more widely spaced molecules of the gas phase, which creates a surface tension. The surface tension of the air-liquid interface that lines the alveoli contributes an important part of the elastic properties of the lung shown by the pressure-volume curve. If a lung is filled with liquid, surface forces are abolished, and the resultant pressure-volume curve (Fig. 2.10) reflects only the tissue properties of the lung. This liquid-filled curve is shifted to the left, indicating that the lung can be distended with much less pressure. The air-filled lung, in addition to requiring greater pressures, demonstrates marked hysteresis; that is, the pressure-volume curve during inflation is different from that during deflation.

The air-filled deflation curve approaches the liquid-filled curve at a low lung volume, indicating that the pressure from surface tension becomes small at this volume. Given no other parameters, however, the prediction would be that pressure from surface forces should *increase* as alveoli become smaller. Laplace's law relates the pressure within a sphere to wall tension (T) and radius (r): $P = 2T/r$; for a cylinder, $P = T/r$. If the surface tension remains constant as the radius decreases (smaller alveoli or airway), the pressure from the surface tension should rise. This situation is avoided in the lung by the presence of a unique surface-lining material, surfactant, which not only reduces surface tension but also does so in a volume-dependent manner. As lung volume and surface area decrease, the lining layer compresses, and surface tension decreases until it is nearly abolished at RV. This property has important consequences in the lung including:

- The work needed to expand the lungs is greatly reduced.
- The stability of alveoli and terminal airways is maintained. (If pressure increased within an alveolus as it became smaller, the alveolus would tend to empty into interconnected, larger alveoli with lower pressure.)
- Inwardly directed forces of surface tension in the "corners" of alveoli act to draw fluid from the capillaries and interstitium into the alveoli, so lowering surface tension helps prevent alveolar edema (discussed in Chapter 4).

Pulmonary surfactant is produced in alveolar type II cells in the form of lamellar bodies. It appears in the liquid alveolar lining as tubular myelin, then spreads as a monolayer at the air-liquid interface. The major component, and the component primarily responsible for the surface tension–lowering effects, is dipalmitoyl phosphatidylcholine (DPPC). DPPC has a non-polar end made up of two saturated fatty acid chains and a polar end that tends to have a positive charge. At the air-liquid interface, the molecules orient with the hydrophilic polar end in the liquid and the fatty acid chains projecting into the air (Fig. 2.11). Both ends have a similar cross-sectional area, allowing them to pack closely together. The molecules may also adsorb directly to the epithelial surface, which tends

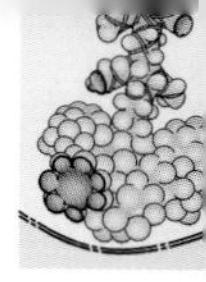

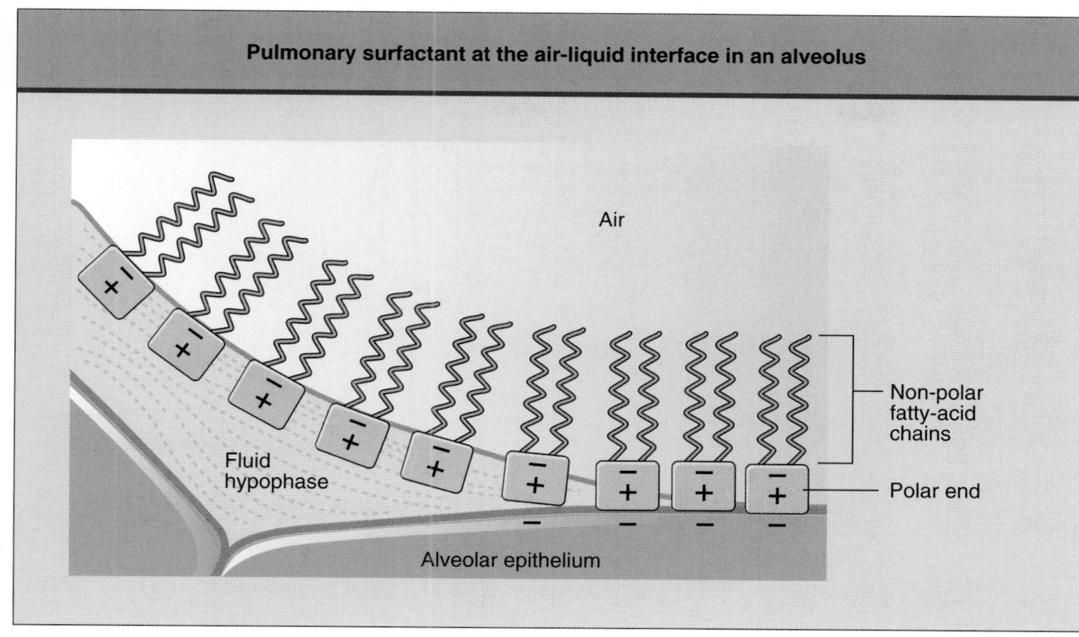

Figure 2.11 Pulmonary surfactant at the air-liquid interface in an alveolus. The nonpolar fatty acid chains project into the alveolar gas phase. The hydrophilic polar end lies within the surface of the liquid phase, or it may be able to bond directly to the epithelium. The close arrangement of the molecules facilitates their surface tension–lowering properties. The fluid hypophase tends to fill alveolar corners and surface irregularities.

to have a negative charge, in areas where a liquid subphase is absent.

Flow Resistance

Airflow between the atmosphere and alveolar gas is dependent on the driving pressure (i.e., alveolar – atmospheric) and the airway resistance, as shown in equation 2.2.

EQUATION 2.2: $\text{Flow} = \dot{V} = \Delta P/R = (P_A - P_{ATM})/R_{AW}$

The normal airway resistance (R_{AW}) during quiet breathing (or a panting maneuver, as it is usually measured clinically) is less than 2 cmH_2O/L per second. Airflow resistance is affected by:

- Viscosity of air
- Length of airways (R_{AW} is directly proportional to length)
- Caliber of airways (R_{AW} is proportional to l/r^4)

Thus, a doubling of length doubles resistance, but a halving of caliber causes a 16-fold increase in resistance. Airway caliber is affected by:

- Position of the airway in the bronchial tree
- Lung volume
- Bronchial muscle tone
- Mucus secretion
- Pressure across the airway wall

All these factors are similar during both inspiration and expiration, except the last. During inspiration, the intrathoracic pressure that surrounds airways is more negative than the intra-airway pressure, so airways tend to be distended (Fig. 2.12). With active expiratory efforts, the pleural pressure becomes positive; concurrently, the intraluminal pressure decreases progressively in airways mouthward of the alveoli. This reflects both frictional losses and a decrease in lateral pressure through the Bernoulli effect as the decreasing cross-sectional area of the composite airway requires a marked increase in the velocity of air movement (convective acceleration). Because their cartilaginous structure is incomplete, airways are compressed under such forces. This leads to flow limitation; that is, a greater effort does not yield higher airflow during forced expiration.

Maximum airflow rates are evaluated by having the subject take a full inspiration to TLC and then blow the air out as forcefully and completely (to RV) as possible. Using a spirometer, this forced vital capacity (FVC) is recorded as an expiratory spirogram (volume versus time), or, if the flow rate is also measured, the same information can be recorded as a maximum expiratory flow versus volume curve (Fig. 2.13). A remarkable feature of this maneuver is that the maximum flow rate for any volume, except the highest lung volumes near the beginning of the exhalation, is achieved with submaximal effort and cannot be exceeded with further effort. The mechanism of flow limitation is related to the rate of propagation of a pressure wave through a compliant tube, but the result can be understood with a simpler conceptual model of dynamic compression. Because this compression begins when intra-airway pressure falls below pleural pressure, the effective driving pressure becomes $P_A - P_{PL}$ ($30 - 20 = 10$ cmH_2O in Figure 2.13, forced expiration). This is the same as the elastic recoil pressure of the lung and is a function of lung volume, not effort. For example, in Figure 2.13, if a greater expiratory effort is made and the pleural pressure is raised to 40 cmH_2O at the same lung volume, the alveolar pressure becomes 50 cmH_2O and the effective driving pressure is 10 cmH_2O (50 – 40), so the resultant flow rate remains unchanged.

This mechanism may have its major physiologic significance in normal individuals during a cough. Although overall airflow rate (L/second) out of the lungs is not increased by the high pleural pressure generated, the airflow velocity (m/second)

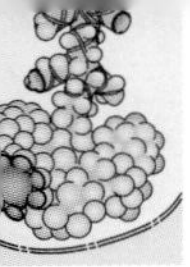

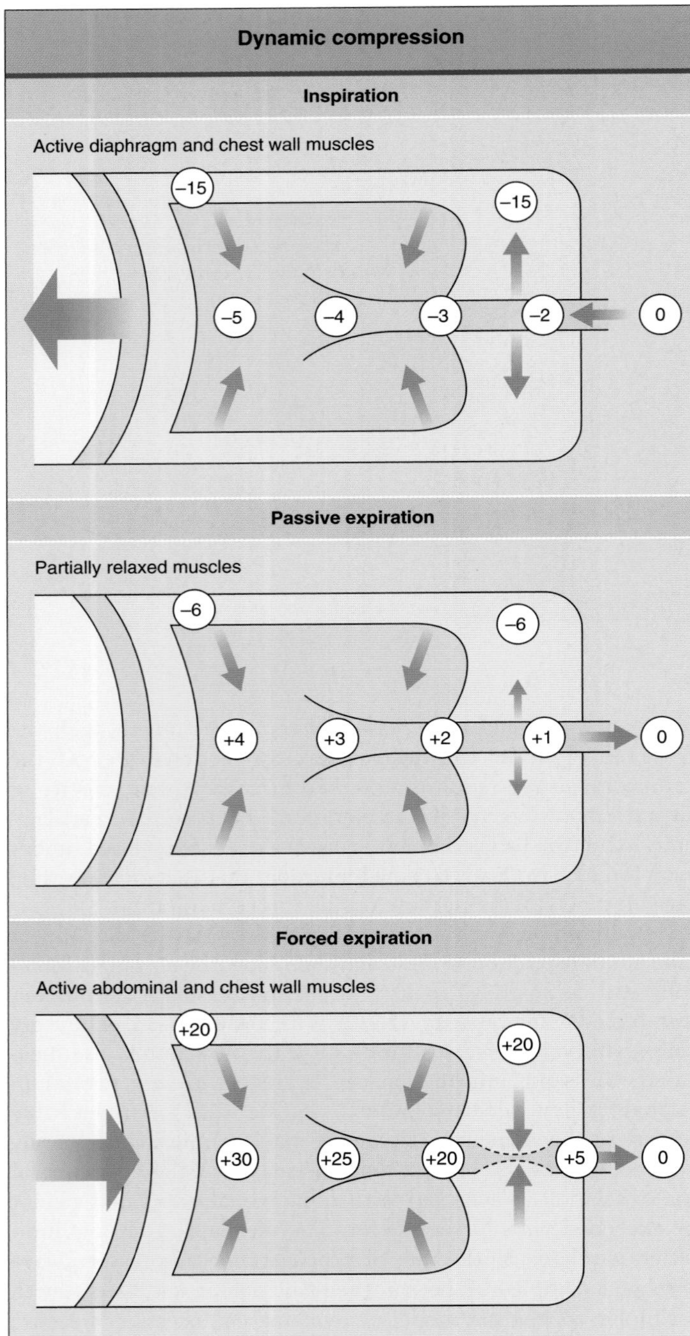

Figure 2.12 Dynamic compression. Comparison of intrathoracic and intraluminal pressures during inspiration, passive expiration, and forced expiration. In each case, the lung volume is the same, with a recoil pressure of 10 cmH_2O. During inspiration, the intrathoracic airways tend to be distended, which lowers airway resistance. In passive expiration, although intrapleural pressure may remain slightly negative, a positive alveolar pressure is generated by lung elastic recoil. Central airways are less distended during passive expiration than during inspiration. In forced expiration, high intrapleural pressure plus lung recoil creates a large, positive alveolar pressure to drive flow, but it also compresses central airways. Flow is limited once dynamic compression begins downstream from the point where intraluminal pressure falls below pleural pressure (the equal pressure point). Further effort increases alveolar driving pressure but also increases compression. Airway resistance becomes high and varies with the degree of effort.

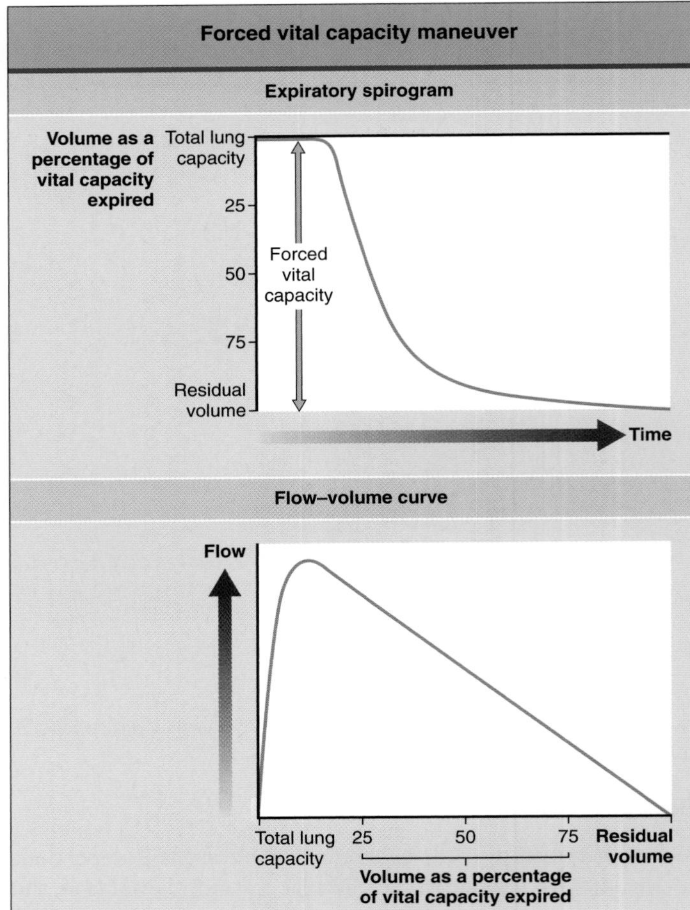

Figure 2.13 Forced vital capacity maneuver. This common breathing test can be displayed as an expiratory spirogram or as a flow-volume curve. Volume axes show percentage of vital capacity expired. Modified with permission from Culver BH [ed]: The Respiratory System. Seattle, ASUW Publications, 1997.

through the narrowed major airways is greatly increased, which aids the removal of secretions and foreign material.

Work of Breathing

The muscle effort required to raise lung volume above the FRC during inspiration is a form of work. Part of this is the elastic work used to stretch the tissues and the surface lining of the lung, and another part is the frictional work required to overcome airflow resistance in the airways. The elastic work stored in stretched fibers on inspiration provides the energy needed to push air out on the subsequent passive exhalation. With active expiratory efforts, additional muscle work is done on expiration as well.

The elastic and frictional components of respiratory work are affected differently by lung volume. At low lung volumes, airways are narrower, and resistance (and thus frictional work) increases rapidly (resistance is proportional to $1/r^4$). At higher lung volumes, the muscles must do more elastic work to keep the lungs stretched. The relaxed FRC is the volume at which the static recoil forces of the lung and chest wall are balanced. Figure 2.15 shows that FRC is also the volume at which the

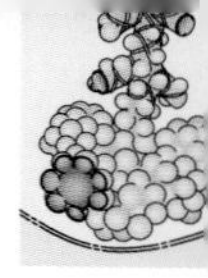

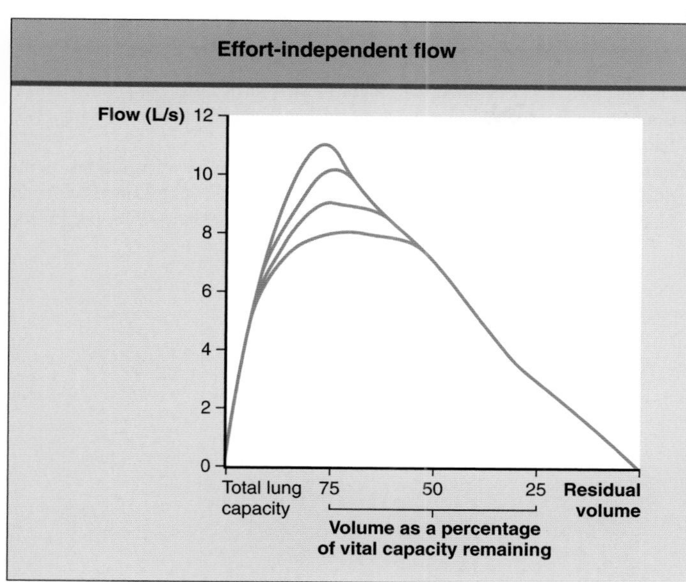

Figure 2.14 Effort-independent flow. The top curve represents maximum expiratory effort, and the lower curves show the flow that results from progressively less effort. At lower lung volumes, the maximum flow rate is relatively independent of effort. Modified with permission from Bates DV, Macklem PT, Christie RV: Respiratory Function in Disease, 2nd ed. Philadelphia, WB Saunders, 1971, pp 10-95

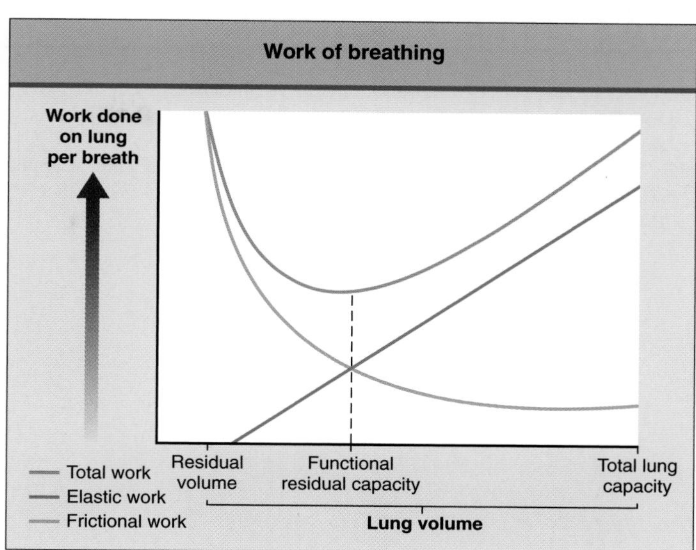

Figure 2.15 Work of breathing. The combined work of lung and chest wall expansion (elastic) and airflow resistance (frictional) is normally lowest near functional residual capacity. Modified with permission from Culver BH [ed]: The Respiratory System. Seattle, ASUW Publications, 1997.

work of breathing is least. If either the elastic or the frictional contributions to the work of breathing change, FRC may change rapidly, or chronically.

The narrowed airways in obstructive disease increase frictional work, and the volume at which the work of breathing is least increases. The accompanying shift of the tidal breathing range to a higher volume may occur quite suddenly in an asthma attack, or it may develop slowly with chronic obstructive disease. When airflow rates increase, frictional work becomes relatively more important, so that patients who have obstructive disease may shift to a higher end-expiratory volume during exercise or voluntary hyperventilation.

Restrictive disease processes reduce C_L, Accordingly, the force required by the muscles to stretch the lung increases. The elastic work required to breathe at any lung volume is higher, and this shifts the volume for least work lower. Increased C_L, as with emphysema, has the opposite effect. Figure 2.7 shows that the static forces predict the same changes in FRC (greater lung recoil results in lower FRC volume, and vice versa).

Normally, the energy consumed by breathing is very small. In metabolic terms, it requires less than 1 mL/minute of oxygen consumption for each liter per minute of ventilation, or only 1% to 2% of a person's total body oxygen consumption at rest. With severe airway obstruction, the energy cost of breathing becomes much higher (as much as 30% during an acute exacerbation).

Distribution of Ventilation

The incoming air of each tidal breath is not distributed evenly to all alveoli in the lung. Pleural pressure is not the same throughout the chest, but has a vertical gradient of several centimeters of water because of the effects of gravity, the configuration of the chest and diaphragm, the presence of the heart and mediastinal structures, and the need for the lung to fit within the thorax irrespective of the shape of either the lung or the thorax. At FRC in upright humans, $-5\ cmH_2O$ is an average value at chest midlevel, but near the apices, the pressure outside the lung might be $-8\ cmH_2O$, and near the bases only $-2\ cmH_2O$. Because alveoli throughout the lung appear to have similar maximum volume and pressure-volume relationships, and because alveolar pressure is the same everywhere, those alveoli near the top of the lung are held at a larger volume (distending pressure of $8\ cmH_2O$) than those near the bottom (distending pressure of $2\ cmH_2O$). This places the lower alveoli on a steeper (more compliant) portion of their pressure-volume curve. In addition, the proximity of the basal alveoli to the motion of the diaphragm exposes them to a greater increase in distending pressure with inspiration. These two factors combine to give the lower portion of the normal lung a relatively greater proportion of the tidal ventilation than the apices.

A second consequence of the higher (i.e., less negative) pleural pressure in the basal portions of the lung is that the distending pressure of the small airways is also less. At RV, airways close, and the dependent portions of the lung reach this closing volume first, while higher portions of the lung are still partially distended. Thus, a patient who breathes at very low lung volumes, near RV (e.g., obese patients), may have basal airway closure and consequently little ventilation to the lung bases.

In summary, respiratory units in the basal portion of the lung contain less gas but receive more ventilation as long as they remain open. However, they are more susceptible to airway closure and loss of ventilation at low lung volumes.

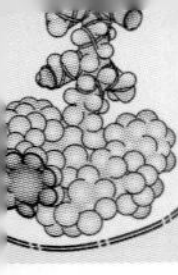

SUGGESTED READINGS

Gibson GJ: Lung volumes and elasticity. In Hughes JMB, Pride NB (eds): Lung Function Tests: Physiologic Principles and Clinical Applications. London, WB Saunders, 1999, pp 45-56.

Hills BA: Surface-active phospholipids: a Pandora's box of clinical applications. Part I: The lung and air spaces. Intern Med J 32: 170-178, 2002.

Pride NB: Airflow resistance. In Hughes JMB, Pride NB (eds): Lung Function Tests: Physiologic Principles and Clinical Applications. London, WB Saunders, 1999, pp 27-44.

Schurch S, Bachofen H, Possmeyer F: Alveolar lining layer: functions, composition, structures. In Hlastala MP, Robertson HT (eds): Lung Biology in Health and Disease, vol 121. New York, Marcel Dekker, 1998, pp 35-98.

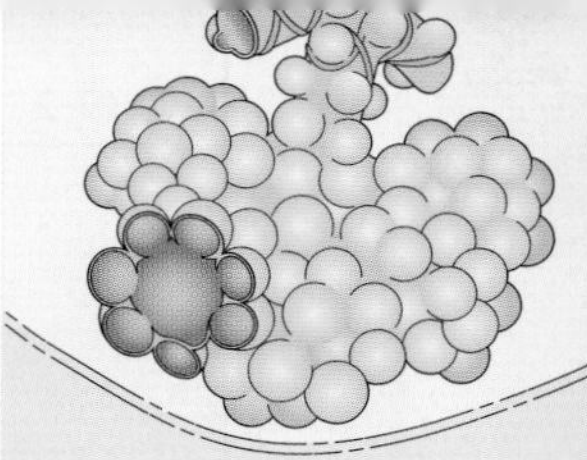

CHAPTER 3 Gas Exchange in the Lung

Bruce H. Culver

The primary function of the lung is to provide adequate oxygenation of the blood and to remove carbon dioxide, as first described by Lavoisier in 1777:

> Eminently respirable air that enters the lung, leaves it in the form of chalky aeriform acids [carbon dioxide] . . . in almost equal volume. . . . Respiration acts only on the portion of pure air that is eminently respirable [which he later named *oxygine*] . . . the excess [nitrogen], is a purely passive medium which enters and leaves the lung . . . without change or alteration. The respirable portion of air has the property to combine with blood and its combination results in its red color.
>
> (Quoted in West JB [ed]: Pulmonary Gas Exchange, vol 1. New York, Academic Press, 1980)

This gas exchange process can be considered in three parts:

1. Ventilation of the lungs, which determines the alveolar levels of oxygen and carbon dioxide
2. Storage and transport of these gases in the blood
3. Process of equilibration between alveolar gas and arterial blood

The terminology and abbreviations particular to gas exchange are introduced in Table 3.1.

FUNCTIONAL ANATOMY OF GAS EXCHANGE

The lung can be functionally divided into a conducting zone of air passages and a respiratory zone that consists of the last few branches of airways and alveoli, where gas exchange with blood takes place. In the conducting zone, from the upper respiratory tract to the terminal bronchioles, essentially no exchange of respiratory gases with the atmosphere occurs. These airways warm and humidify the incoming air and can remove some gaseous and particulate pollutants.

The terminal bronchioles are succeeded by two to five generations of respiratory bronchioles (Fig. 3.1), which have increasing numbers of alveoli in their walls. The next branches are alveolar ducts, which are completely alveolated, with no ciliated epithelium remaining, and terminate in alveolar sacs and individual alveoli. Helical bands of smooth muscle extend to the alveolar ducts and may aid in controlling the distribution of ventilation. The entire respiratory unit served by one terminal bronchiole is an acinus. Several adjacent acini make up a pulmonary lobule, which has incomplete connective tissue septae that separate it from adjacent lobules. The collateral communication of both airflow and blood flow is better within a lobule than between lobules, although canals of Lambert apparently connect bronchioles of adjacent lobules.

Alveoli are irregular polyhedrons approximately 250 μm in diameter. They increase in number in early childhood to the average adult total of 300 million (varying with body size). The total alveolar surface area is 85% to 90% covered with capillaries, which provides an impressive surface area of 70 m^2 for gas exchange. Adjacent alveoli are connected by pores of Kohn that provide routes for collateral airflow, fluid movement, phagocyte mobility, and bacterial spread.

Most of the alveolar surface is covered by epithelial cells that have very attenuated cytoplasm sitting directly on a basement membrane. The capillary endothelial cells are also very thin (except where their nuclei bulge) and also sit directly on a basement membrane. Over much of the area where gas exchange takes place, these basement membranes are fused into one membrane, with no intervening interstitial space (Fig. 3.2). Thus, the diffusion distance from alveolar gas to plasma may be less than 0.5 μm. The distance to a red cell or even within a red cell (about 8 μm) may be much greater than that across the alveolar and capillary membrane itself.

Despite the anatomic complexity of the lung, its gas exchange function can be well described by simple models that consist of a conducting zone (branched tube) and a respiratory zone (usually depicted as one or more giant alveoli) with blood flow.

AMBIENT GAS PARTIAL PRESSURES (TENSIONS)

Atmospheric or barometric pressure (P_B) is the total pressure exerted by the kinetic energy of all the molecules in the atmospheric mixture. It varies with altitude, but at sea level, it raises a column of mercury in an evacuated tube to a height of 760 mm (equivalent to 29.9 inches of mercury, or 100 kPa) and varies slightly from day to day.

In discussing lung mechanics, the pressure in the chest or lungs is measured relative to atmospheric pressure (P_{ATM}), which is set at zero. This is termed *gauge pressure* and is commonly used, for example, to measure blood pressure or tire pressure. However, gas pressures in the atmosphere, alveoli, and blood are reported in absolute pressure terms, expressed as millimeters of mercury (mmHg) or torr. An alveolar pressure of

---

Units in this chapter are expressed in mmHg, torr, or cmH_2O. For SI units, the conversion factors are:

$$1\ cmH_2O = 0.1\ kPa$$
$$1\ mmHg = 1\ torr = 0.132\ kPa$$
$$1\ kPa = 7.6\ mmHg \text{ or torr } = 10\ cmH_2O$$

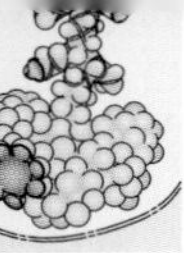

Table 3.1
Gas exchange terminology and abbreviations

Symbol	Definition	Units
P	Pressure or partial pressure; e.g., PO_2 = partial pressure of oxygen	mmHg (millimeters of mercury) or torr (1 torr = 1 mmHg under standard gravitational conditions, i.e., sea level)
		kPa (kiloPascal; 1 kPa = 7.6 mmHg or torr)
		cmH_2O (centimeters of water; 1 mmHg = 1.3 cmH_2O)
F	Fraction of a given gas present in a mixture (F x 100 = percentage concentration)	–
V	Volume of gas	L (liters) or mL (milliliters)
$\dot{V}$	Flow (volume per time)	mL/min (milliliters per minute; e.g., oxygen consumption, $\dot{V}O_2$)
		L/min (e.g., ventilation, $\dot{V}$E)
		L/s (e.g., airflow rates)

The symbols and modifiers used in this chapter are based on those recommended in the *American Medical Association Manual of Style* and the ATS-ACCP Joint Committee on Nomenclature. Main symbols indicating the type of measurement are in capital letters followed by one or more modifiers to indicate location or the gas measured. By convention, locations related to ventilation are given in small capital letters (e.g., I, inspired; E, expired, A, alveolar), and vascular locations are given in lower-case letters (e.g., a, arterial; v, venous; c, capillary).

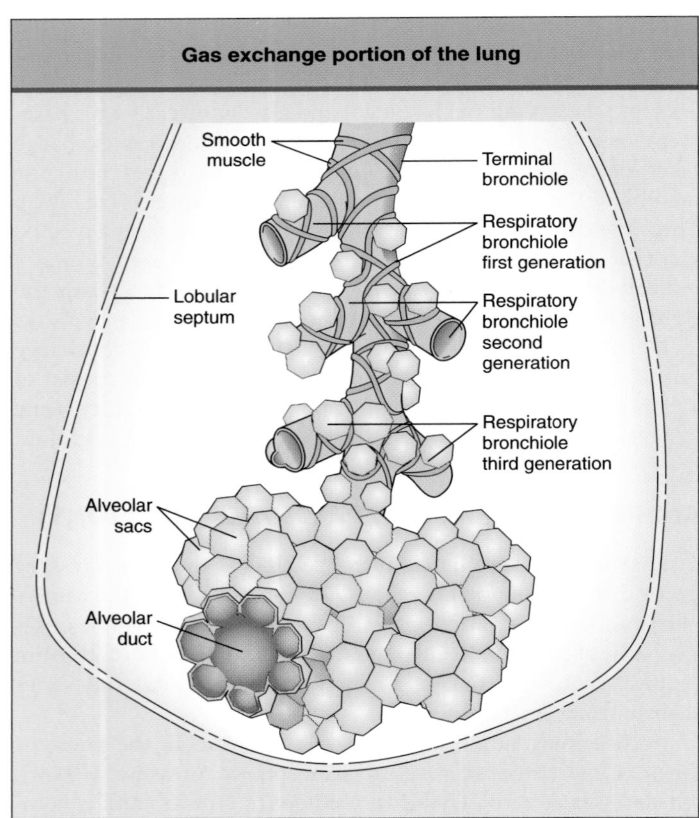

Figure 3.1 Gas exchange portion of the lung.

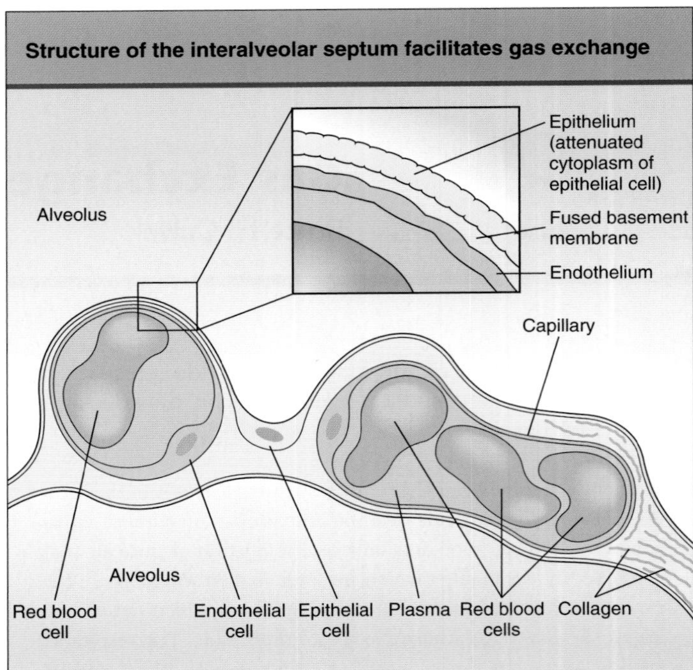

Figure 3.2 Structure of the interalveolar septum facilitates gas exchange. Capillaries tend to lie asymmetrically within the septum, with most of the interstitial space, structural elements, and cell nuclei on the "thick side." The "thin side" presents a very short path for gas diffusion. Based on information from Siegwart B, Gehr P, Gil J, Weibel E: Morphometric estimation of pulmonary diffusing capacity. IV. The normal dog lung. Respir Physiol 13:141-159, 1971.

13 cmH_2O, or 10 mmHg (gauge), is equivalent to 770 mmHg in absolute pressure.

Atmospheric air is a mixture that consists of oxygen (20.95%), nitrogen (78.09%), argon (0.93%), and carbon dioxide (0.03%), with water vapor that varies from 0% to 2% and dilutes the other gases accordingly. For practical purposes, air is considered to be 21% oxygen and 79% nitrogen; carbon dioxide and other trace gases are ignored. Water vapor requires special consideration (discussed later).

Concept of Partial Pressure

In a mixture of gases, the pressure exerted by the kinetic energy of each separate gas is referred to as its *partial pressure*. If the mixture is enclosed in a sealed container, it develops a pressure on the walls of the container by the mechanism of collisions between the gas molecules and the container walls. The force or pressure developed by all the molecules of the mixture as they bounce off the container walls is the total pressure developed by the gas. The partial pressure of any component is the pressure developed by the molecules of that component acting alone. Because the random motion that causes collisions is the same motion that allows diffusion to take place, the partial pressure of a gas is a measure of its tendency to diffuse through either gas or fluid media.

The total pressure of a mixture of gases is equal to the sum of the partial pressures of each gas in the mixture (Dalton's law). Because the alveoli and airways are open to the atmosphere, the sum of the partial pressures in the lung must add up to the barometric pressure (equation 3.1).

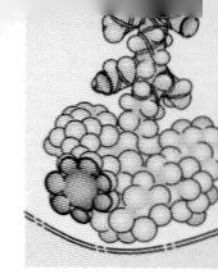

EQUATION 3.1: DALTON'S LAW

$$P_{ATM} = P_{CO_2} + P_{O_2} + P_{N_2} + P_{H_2O}$$

The small variations in alveolar pressure during the respiratory cycle are ignored.

In the gas phase, partial pressure is proportional to concentration. By convention, gas fractions are measured after water vapor has been removed ("dry" gas). Thus, the partial pressure of a gas is found by multiplying the concentration or fraction of the gas by the total pressure of dry gases (i.e., no water vapor).

The concept of partial pressure also applies to gases in a liquid, including plasma or blood. When a gas-free liquid is in contact with air, gas molecules move into the liquid by diffusion until the partial pressures in the liquid and air are the same. The relationship between the partial pressure of a gas in a liquid and the content of that gas depends on solubility and any chemical binding that takes place. For example, nitrogen and oxygen are both poorly soluble, but large amounts of oxygen are bound to hemoglobin (Hb).

Water Vapor

Water vapor requires special consideration, because water is present as both a gas and a liquid in the body. When a gas mixture is in contact with liquid and is saturated with the vapor of that liquid, the partial pressure of that vapor is a function of temperature (Table 3.2).

Atmospheric gas is cooler than body temperature, and although it contains some water, it is rarely 100% saturated. Inspired gas that enters the upper portion of the respiratory system is rapidly warmed to body temperature and becomes fully saturated with water vapor. The small volume change associated with warming and added water vapor can be calculated from gas laws, if necessary (Table 3.3). At 37°C, water vapor has a partial pressure of 47 mmHg. This pressure does not vary with changes in barometric pressure or changes in the other components in the gas mixture. Thus, if P_B is 760 mmHg and P_{H_2O} is 47 mmHg, the difference, 713 mmHg, is the partial pressure of the remaining dry, inspired gases. Of this total, 21% is oxygen and 79% is nitrogen, so $P_{IO_2} = 0.21 \times 713 = 150$ mmHg, and $P_{IN_2} = 0.79 \times 713 = 563$ mmHg.

Air has the same relative concentration of gases, even when P_B is lowered. For example, at the top of Mt. Everest (altitude about 29,000 feet), $P_B = 253$ mmHg, and the atmospheric $P_{O_2} = 0.21 \times 253 = 53$ mmHg.

Table 3.2
Water vapor pressure

Temperature (°C)	Water Vapor Pressure	
	mmHg	kPa
0	4.6	0.6
20	17.5	2.3
37	47.0	6.2
100	760.0	100

The partial pressure due to water vapor at full saturation varies with temperature.

Table 3.3
Gas conditions and corrections

The volume occupied by an amount of gas is directly proportional to its absolute temperature (°Kelvin), is inversely proportional to its total pressure, and is further affected by the volume of water vapor present.

Exhaled gas collected in a spirometer or bag is saturated at ambient temperature and pressure (ATPS).

Lung and ventilatory volumes are conventionally converted into body temperature and pressure, saturated (BTPS) conditions, a volume expansion of 9%–10%.

Gas transfer quantities ($\dot{V}O_2$, $\dot{V}CO_2$, and diffusing capacity) are conventionally expressed at standard temperature (273°K), pressure (760 mmHg), and dry (STPD) conditions.

While necessary for quantitative calculations, these conversions can be largely ignored for conceptual understanding.

For quantitative calculations, gas volumes must be corrected for changes in temperature and added water vapor.

VENTILATION

The total ventilation per minute ($\dot{V}_E$ = volume exhaled per minute) can be determined by collecting exhaled gas for a measured time. The volume of gas exhaled during one normal respiratory cycle is V_T. The total ventilation is equal to V_T multiplied by the breathing frequency, f ($\dot{V}_E = V_T \times f$).

Alveolar Ventilation and Dead Space

Gas exchange occurs in alveoli when freshly inspired air comes in contact with capillary blood. However, not all of each inspired breath reaches the alveoli to participate in gas exchange. Inspired air must first pass through the conducting airways, from the nose to the distal bronchioles, which contain no alveoli and do not participate in gas exchange. At the end of inspiration, the volume of air that remains in the conducting airways, and therefore does not participate in gas exchange, is the anatomic dead space. The effect of the conducting airways on ventilation and gas exchange can be considered in two ways. After inspiration, atmospheric air (plus a little water vapor) remains in these airways and leaves as the first gas out on the subsequent exhalation. After expiration, alveolar gas (with carbon dioxide added and oxygen partially removed) fills the anatomic dead space and re-enters the alveoli with the next breath. Thus, a tidal breath may inspire 500 mL of air and result in a 500 mL expansion of the alveolar volume followed by the expiration of 500 mL, but the volume of fresh air delivered to the alveoli and the volume of alveolar air exhaled to the atmosphere are each less than 500 mL by an amount equal to the volume of the anatomic dead space.

In addition to the conducting airways, any alveoli that are ventilated with air but not perfused with blood cannot participate in gas exchange. The volume of ventilation that goes to these alveoli is also wasted and is called alveolar dead space. Ventilation to areas of lung that have reduced, but not absent, perfusion can be treated as if a portion were going to alveoli with normal perfusion and a portion to alveoli with no perfusion. This latter portion is also part of the alveolar dead space (Fig. 3.3). The sum of anatomic and alveolar dead space makes up the physiologic dead space.

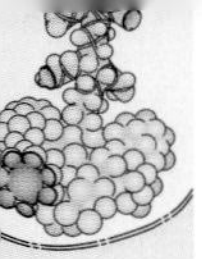

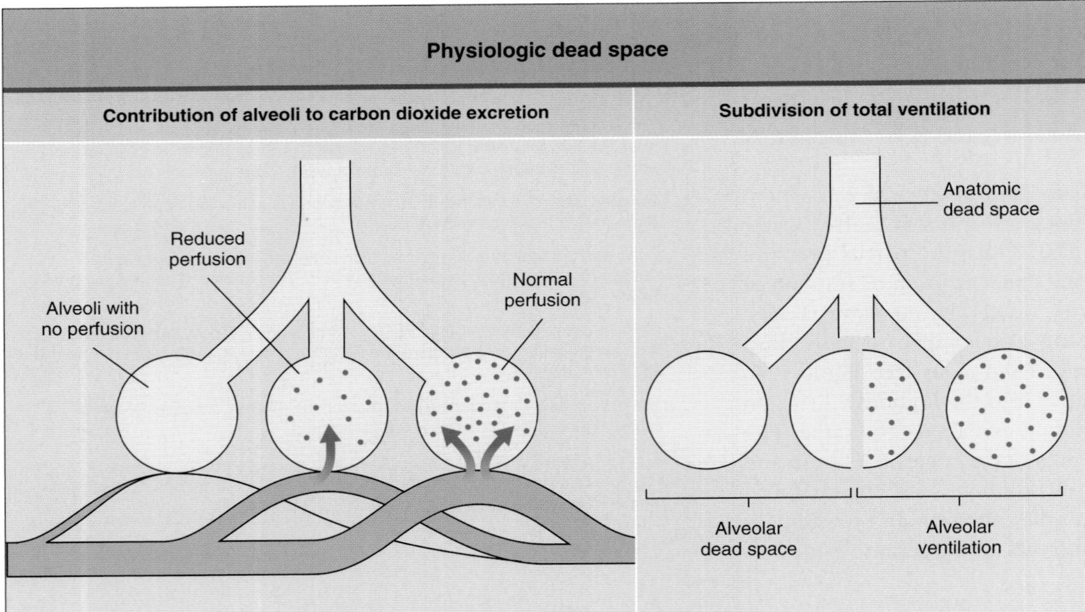

Figure 3.3 Physiologic dead space. Alveoli with no perfusion, reduced perfusion, and normal perfusion, and their contribution to carbon dioxide excretion. Total ventilation is subdivided into anatomic dead space, alveolar dead space with no perfusion, and alveolar ventilation with ideal perfusion. Modified from Culver BH [ed]: The Respiratory System. Seattle, ASUW Publications, 1997.

The volume of the anatomic dead space ($V_{D_{an}}$) in a normal adult male is 150 to 180 mL (approximately equal to the lean body weight in pounds). In a young, normal individual, the volume of the physiologic dead space (V_D) is only slightly greater than this, or about 25% to 35% of an average V_T (referred to as the V_D/V_T ratio). The anatomic dead space is not fixed; it increases at higher lung volumes because the intrapulmonary airways increase in size, along with the surrounding lung tissue, via interdependence. Thus, breathing with a large V_T and the accompanying larger end-inspiratory lung volume is associated with a modest decrease in V_D/V_T ratio. With exercise, V_T may increase to 2.5 to 3 L and V_D/V_T normally falls to 15% or less, but an important additional factor is the increase in pulmonary blood flow, which tends to eliminate any poorly perfused alveolar dead space. At the other extreme, it would seem that as V_T becomes small, approaching the anatomic dead space, alveolar ventilation should fall to zero and gas exchange become impossible. However, with high-frequency ventilation, it has been demonstrated that gas exchange can be maintained even with V_T equal to or less than the measured anatomic dead space. Some fresh gas reaches alveoli because some path lengths are shorter than others and because airway gas exchanges with alveolar gas by diffusion and by physical mixing induced by the heartbeat.

The physiologic dead space and wasted ventilation may be considerably increased with diseases of the air spaces and vasculature, primarily because of an increase in the alveolar component. (Importantly, increases in the physiologic dead space are almost always abnormal, i.e., pathologic.) The fraction of ventilation "wasted" by going to physiologic dead space can be calculated from arterial and expired gas values. Dead space has the effect of diluting the carbon dioxide content of expired gas below the alveolar level, and the equation derived in Table 3.4 is simply a calculation of this dilution. Because the body needs to eliminate a certain volume of carbon dioxide per minute, the effect of a low P_ECO_2 is to require more total ventilation to maintain homeostasis.

Table 3.4
Physiologic dead space calculations

The physiologic dead space, made up of ventilation to anatomic dead space plus that to unperfused alveoli and a portion of that to poorly perfused alveoli, is not an anatomically identifiable volume, but an 'as if' volume may be obtained by calculation from a collection of exhaled gas over 1–3 minutes.

Using a 'conservation of mass' concept, the total expired volume of gas per minute is considered to have two sources:

- ideal alveoli with equal alveolar and arterial partial pressures of carbon dioxide ($P_ACO_2 = P_aCO_2$); and
- unperfused areas (conducting airways or alveolar dead space) with P_ACO_2 = inspired $PCO_2 = 0$.

The total expired volume of carbon dioxide comes entirely from the effective (nondead space) alveolar ventilation ($V_E - V_D$).

$$(\dot{V}CO_2 = \dot{V}_E \times F_LCO_2 = (\dot{V}_E - \dot{V}_D) \times F_ACO_2$$

Algebraic manipulation yields:

$$(\dot{V}_D = F_ACO_2 = \dot{V}_E \times F_ACO_2 - \dot{V}_E \times F_ECO_2$$

$$\dot{V}_D\dot{V}_E = (F_ACO_2 - F_ECO_2)/F_ACO_2$$

Multiplying top and bottom by ($P_{ATM} - 47$) converts fractions to partial pressure:

$$\dot{V}_D/\dot{V}_E = (P_ACO_2 - P_ECO_2)/P_ACO_2$$

P_ACO_2 cannot be readily measured, but in these assumed ideal alveoli $P_ACO_2 = P_aCO_2$, so the measured arterial blood gas value can be substituted to create the final equation below. P_ECO_2 is obtained from a collection of expired gas.

By convention, the results are reported as the $\dot{V}_D/\dot{V}_T$ or wasted fraction of each tidal breath, but actually they are measured as the average wasted ventilation over 1–3 minutes.

$$\dot{V}_D/\dot{V}_T = \dot{V}_D/\dot{V}_E = (P_aCO_2 - P_ECO_2)/P_aCO_2$$

Multiplying this fraction by the tidal volume or minute ventilation gives the volume of physiologic dead space or wasted ventilation. [in carrying out this measurement, it must be remembered that the volume of air in mouthpiece, connections, and valve (mechanical dead space) also contribute air free of carbon dioxide to the expired collection.]

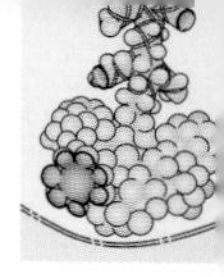

The volume of air that participates in gas exchange because it is in contact with perfused alveoli is termed the *alveolar ventilation* ($\dot{V}A = \dot{V}E - \dot{V}D$). The volume per minute of alveolar ventilation is critical, because it determines the amount of air presented to alveoli into which carbon dioxide can be excreted and from which oxygen can be removed. Note that *alveolar ventilation* as defined here and as widely used in respiratory physiology is a conceptual term and might better be called *gas exchange ventilation*. It is not the same as the volume of gas that enters or leaves alveoli each minute.

Carbon Dioxide Elimination

Because the body's carbon dioxide production ($\dot{V}CO_2$) is eliminated only by ventilation, it must equal the volume of carbon dioxide exhaled per minute minus the volume of carbon dioxide inhaled, which is negligible and can be disregarded. All the carbon dioxide expired must come from alveolar ventilation and is equal to the volume of this ventilation times the concentration of carbon dioxide in the effective gas-exchanging space ($FACO_2$) (equation 3.2).

EQUATION 3.2: CARBON DIOXIDE PRODUCTION

$$\dot{V}CO_2 = \dot{V}A \times FACO_2$$

Rearranging this equation demonstrates that for a given level of metabolic carbon dioxide production, a reciprocal relationship exists between alveolar ventilation and the level of alveolar carbon dioxide (equation 3.3).

EQUATION 3.3: RELATIONSHIP OF ALVEOLAR VENTILATION AND CO_2 PRODUCTION

$$FACO_2 = \dot{V}CO_2/\dot{V}A$$

Multiplying both sides of equation 3.3 by the total pressure of dry gases in the alveoli ($PB - 47$) converts the fraction into the partial pressure units in which carbon dioxide is commonly measured and yields the useful relationship in equation 3.4, which states that alveolar PCO_2 is directly related to the production of carbon dioxide and inversely related to alveolar ventilation ($\dot{V}A$).

EQUATION 3.4: CO_2 EQUILIBRIUM

$$PACO_2 = (\dot{V}CO_2/\dot{V}A) \times (PB - 47)$$

The body maintains a normal alveolar (and arterial) PCO_2 of 40 mmHg by adjusting ventilation appropriately for the $\dot{V}CO_2$ dictated by metabolic demand.

Hyperventilation is defined as ventilation in excess of metabolic needs. Therefore, a $PACO_2$ below normal indicates alveolar hyperventilation. Conversely, a $PACO_2$ greater than normal indicates alveolar hypoventilation.

Any depression in central nervous system function can change $\dot{V}E$ and therefore $\dot{V}A$; for example, many drugs such as narcotics and sedatives can reduce $\dot{V}E$. Any increase in VD will reduce $\dot{V}A$ unless $\dot{V}E$ increases proportionally. Many disease processes increase physiologic dead space, which is a contributory cause of ventilatory failure when the patient can no longer increase total ventilation.

The alveolar PCO_2 level reflects a balance among the carbon dioxide that enters the alveoli, that which escapes from the blood to the alveoli, and that which leaves with exhaled gas. In a steady state, production and excretion must be the same. Under resting conditions, $\dot{V}CO_2$ is relatively constant, at approximately 200 mL/minute for an individual of normal size. If a person hyperventilates, initially carbon dioxide is exhaled at a greater rate than it is produced; $PACO_2$ falls (and with it, arterial PCO_2). As $PACO_2$ falls, the carbon dioxide exhaled per minute decreases, because less is loaded into exhaled air, until carbon dioxide elimination is again equal to carbon dioxide production and a new steady state is established. In hypoventilation, the rate of carbon dioxide exhalation initially falls, so $PACO_2$ and $PaCO_2$ rise until a new steady state is reached at which excretion again equals production, with less ventilation but with each liter of gas leaving the alveoli carrying more carbon dioxide. This mechanism allows patients who have severe lung disease and high work of breathing to excrete their carbon dioxide production at less energy cost.

Alveolar Oxygen

The level of alveolar oxygen also reflects a balance of two processes:

1. Oxygen delivery to the alveoli by ventilation
2. Oxygen removal from the alveoli by capillary blood

Oxygen delivery to alveoli is determined by their ventilation ($\dot{V}A$) and the fraction of inspired oxygen (FIO_2), but oxygen is also carried away in exhaled air. The gas that leaves alveoli has the alveolar oxygen concentration (FAO_2). So the net oxygen taken up from alveoli is expressed as $\dot{V}A \times (FIO_2 - FAO_2)$, which can be written as a conservation of mass equation that states that the oxygen consumed to meet metabolic demand ($\dot{V}O_2$) equals that removed from the alveolar ventilation (none is removed from dead space ventilation).

EQUATION 3.5: OXYGEN DELIVERY—CONSERVATION OF MASS

$$\dot{V}O_2 = \dot{V}A(FIO_2 - FAO_2)$$

Rearranging this equation demonstrates that for a given level of metabolic oxygen consumption, a reciprocal relationship exists between alveolar ventilation and the fraction of oxygen removed from the incoming air. That is, when alveolar ventilation is decreased, more oxygen must be extracted from each unit of that incoming ventilation, which results in a lower residual level of alveolar oxygen (equation 3.6).

EQUATION 3.6: OXYGEN DELIVERY—RECIPROCAL RELATIONSHIP BETWEEN ALVEOLAR VENTILATION AND FRACTION OF OXYGEN REMOVED

$$FIO_2 - FAO_2 = \dot{V}O_2/\dot{V}A$$

Conversion of equation 3.6 into partial pressure by multiplying both sides by $PB - 47$ gives equation 3.7.

EQUATION 3.7: OXYGEN DELIVERY—CONVERSION INTO PARTIAL PRESSURE

$$PIO_2 - PAO_2 = (\dot{V}O_2/\dot{V}A) \times (PB - 47)$$

Equation 3.7 shows that PAO_2 is determined by PIO_2, $\dot{V}A$, and $\dot{V}O_2$. If PIO_2 and $\dot{V}O_2$ are constant and $\dot{V}A$ increases, PAO_2 must also increase, and if $\dot{V}A$ decreases, PAO_2 must also decrease. Oxygen removal from inspired air is governed by tissue oxygen consumption and varies with activity, but under resting conditions it is approximately 250 mL/minute for a person of average size. In a steady state, PAO_2 does not change, so the removal of oxygen from inspired air matches the transfer of oxygen to the blood. In hyperventilation, initially alveolar oxygen is added at a greater rate than it is consumed, and PAO_2 rises. As PAO_2 rises, the amount of oxygen exhaled increases and that unloaded to the alveoli decreases, until a new steady state is established at a higher PAO_2. In hypoventilation, the rate of oxygen delivery to the alveoli initially falls, and PAO_2 falls until a new steady state is reached with less ventilation, but each liter of gas that leaves the alveoli has given up more oxygen.

ESTIMATING THE ALVEOLAR PARTIAL PRESSURE OF OXYGEN

Abnormalities in oxygenation often cause a wide disparity between the level of alveolar oxygen and that measured in the arterial blood. To fully understand the clinical arterial blood gas values, it is necessary to estimate quantitatively the PAO_2, but this cannot be readily obtained from equation 3.7 because neither $\dot{V}O_2$ nor $\dot{V}A$ is easily measured. However, because carbon dioxide production is the metabolic product of oxygen consumption, the quantities $\dot{V}CO_2$ and $\dot{V}O_2$ are tightly linked, and their ratio, $\dot{V}CO_2/\dot{V}O_2$, is the respiratory exchange ratio (R). If these values are identical (R = 1), the solutions to equations 3.4 and 3.7 are identical and show that the fall in PO_2 from inspired to alveolar air is exactly the same as the rise in PCO_2 from zero to the alveolar level. With a more typical R of 0.8, the consumption of five molecules of oxygen results in the production of four molecules of carbon dioxide, and it follows that in the lung, the addition of carbon dioxide to a level of 40 mmHg in alveolar air would be associated with a PAO_2 that showed a 50 mmHg reduction from the inspired air (equation 3.8).

EQUATION 3.8: OXYGEN DELIVERY—ESTIMATED

$$PAO_2 = PIO_2 - (PACO_2/R)$$

Because the measured $PaCO_2$ is very close to $PACO_2$, this simplified version of the alveolar gas equation can be rewritten as equation 3.9.

EQUATION 3.9: ALVEOLAR GAS EQUATION—SIMPLIFIED

$$PAO_2 = PIO_2 - (PaCO_2/R)$$

For typical normal values, R = 0.8, $PIO_2 = 0.21(760 - 47)$, and $PaCO_2 = 40$ (equation 3.10).

EQUATION 3.10: ALVEOLAR GAS—NORMAL VALUES

$$PAO_2 = 150 - (40/0.8) = 100\,mmHg$$

The alveolar gas equation is often misinterpreted as indicating that inspired oxygen is displaced by carbon dioxide in the alveoli, but this is incorrect. The removal of oxygen and the addition of carbon dioxide proceed as independent processes in the lung, but because the normal respiratory quotient (see later) in the tissues is typically 0.8 to 1, loss of oxygen from the inspired air to the blood is approximately equal to the gain in carbon dioxide.

Appropriate interpretation of arterial blood gas values always requires thinking through the alveolar gas equation. This helps, for example, to establish whether a low PaO_2 is explained by hypoventilation or whether the PaO_2 is appropriate for the FIO_2. Table 3.5 gives examples of the use of the alveolar gas equation.

Metabolism and the Respiratory Exchange Ratio

Energy necessary for life processes is produced by the oxidation of carbohydrates, proteins, and fats, which produces principally carbon dioxide and water as breakdown products. The respiratory quotient (RQ) is the ratio of metabolic carbon dioxide production to oxygen consumption of the tissues ($\dot{V}CO_2/\dot{V}O_2$). When carbohydrate is metabolized, RQ = 1; when fat is metabolized, RQ = 0.7; and when protein is metabolized, RQ averages 0.8. Thus, the RQ for the entire body varies with the percentages of carbohydrate, fat, and protein being oxidized at any given time. The respiratory exchange ratio (R) relates to the volume of carbon dioxide eliminated and the net volume of oxygen taken up in the lungs. In a steady state or over a long period, R must equal RQ, but R may vary transiently with factors other than metabolism. For example, if an individual suddenly increases ventilation, R rises because carbon dioxide is "blown off" from blood and tissue stores (but little oxygen can be added). During exercise, R may reach 1.4 because of hyperventilation and continued excretion of carbon dioxide while an oxygen debt is contracted.

TRANSPORT OF GASES IN THE BLOOD

Oxygen Transport

Respiratory gases are carried in blood in physical solutions by binding proteins and (for carbon dioxide) through chemical conversion. The small quantities carried in physical solution are cal-

Table 3.5
Applying of the alveolar gas equation

	Normal Ventilation	Hyper-ventilation	Hypo-ventilation
$PIO_2 = (0.21 \times 713)$ (mmHg)	150	150	150
$PaCO_2$ (mmHg)	40	20	64
R	0.8	0.8	0.8
$PAO_2 = PIO_2 - (PaCO_2/R)$ (mmHg)	150–50 = 100	150–25 = 125	150–80 = 70

The amount of ventilation relative to metabolic need markedly affects the PAO_2 available to equilibrate with capillary blood; this can be estimated using the alveolar gas equation. The PAO_2 calculated, which ranges from 70 to 125 mmHg in these examples, is a somewhat theoretical value for average alveoli; some areas of the lung may have higher or lower values.

culated in Table 3.6. For oxygen, with only 3 mL of oxygen per liter in physical solution at a normal arterial PO_2, it would be impossible to pump enough blood to meet tissue demand without the large additional transport provided by hemoglobin.

HEMOGLOBIN

Hemoglobin is a complex protein consisting of four polypeptide chains (two α-chains and two β-chains), with four heme groups to bind oxygen. One mole of Hb can carry four moles of oxygen, so the theoretical maximum oxygen carrying capacity is calculated as 1.39 mL/g of Hb (but the actual maximum appears to be slightly less, as some sites are not available). Normal blood has an Hb concentration of 15 g/100 mL blood and can potentially carry about 20 mL oxygen per 100 mL of blood as oxyhemoglobin.

The Hb sites fill with oxygen in relation to its partial pressure in solution; the percentage of saturation of Hb indicates the portion of the total oxygen-binding sites actually occupied. The relationship between PO_2 and Hb oxygen content or percentage saturation is nonlinear (Fig. 3.4). The curve is S-shaped, which has particular physiologic advantages. In the normal arterial range, the curve is fairly flat, so that moderate decreases in arterial PO_2 cause only small decrements in arterial oxygen saturation (SaO_2) and content. A normal saturation of 97.5% occurs at a PO_2 of 100 mmHg. A decrease in PO_2 to 60 mmHg still allows the Hb to be 90% saturated. The curve is fairly steep in the normal range of systemic venous PO_2 (PvO_2), which allows further unloading of oxygen to active tissues, with only a small reduction in the partial pressure that drives oxygen diffusion to the cells. The oxygen unloaded under normal resting conditions leaves a PvO_2 of 40 mmHg and a saturation of 75%.

Factors that Affect the Affinity of Hemoglobin for Oxygen

The relative affinity of Hb for oxygen is described by the parameter P_{50} (the PO_2 at 50% saturation). Decreased P_{50} or a curve shift to the left means increased affinity or more oxygen bound for any PO_2; increased P_{50} or a curve shift to the right means decreased affinity (Fig. 3.5). Physiologic factors that affect the affinity of Hb for oxygen include pH, PCO_2, and temperature.

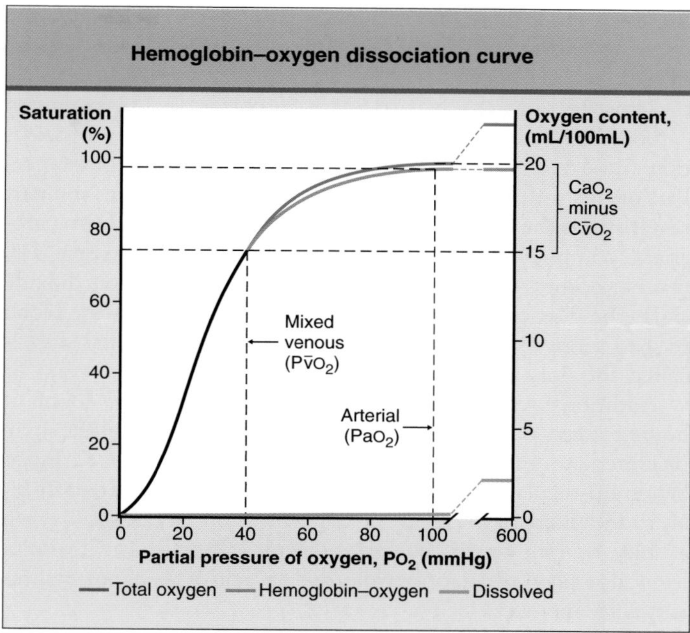

Figure 3.4 Hemoglobin-oxygen (Hb-O_2) dissociation curve shows the percentage saturation of hemoglobin at each PO_2. When the hemoglobin concentration is known, the content of oxygen can be calculated. The total content includes the small additional content of oxygen in solution, which becomes significant at high levels of PO_2. The saturation scale on the left applies only to the Hb-O_2 line. The scale on the right shows content values for a normal hemoglobin level of 15 g/100 mL blood. Modified from Hlastala MP: Blood gas transport. In Culver BH [ed]: The Respiratory System. Seattle, ASUW Publications, 1997, pp 43-52.

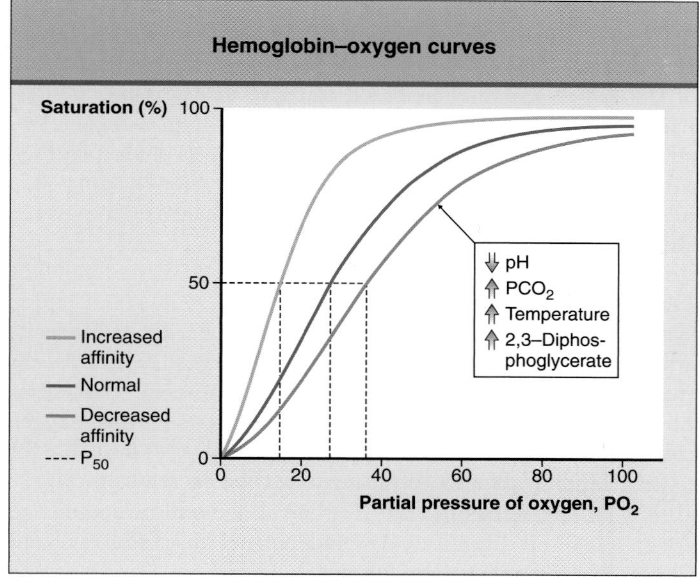

Figure 3.5 Normal, increased affinity (left shift), and decreased affinity (right shift) hemoglobin-oxygen curves. Note that decreased affinity means a higher PO_2 at a given saturation (e.g., 50%) or a lower saturation at a given PO_2 (e.g., 40). Modified from Hlastala MP: Blood gas transport. In Culver BH [ed]: The Respiratory System. Seattle, ASUW Publications, 1997, pp 43-52.

Table 3.6
Gases in physical solution

The content of a gas (oxygen, carbon dioxide, or nitrogen) carried in physical solution in the blood is proportional to its partial pressure and solubility (Henry's law), where C is the concentration (mL/100mL blood), P is the partial pressure (mmHg), and α is the solubility (mL/100 mL blood per mmHg].

Henry's Law

$C = \alpha P$

The solubility of gases in liquid decreases as temperature increases. For blood at 37°C, the solubility of oxygen (αO_2) is 0.003 mL/100mL blood per mmHg, and αCO_2 is 0.072 mL/100mL blood per mmHg.

The amount of oxygen stored in blood in physical solution at a normal arterial PO_2 of 13.3 kPa (100 mmHg) is given by the following equation:

$CO_2 = \alpha O_2 \times PO_2 = 0.003 \times 100 = 0.3$ mL/100 mL blood

The amount of carbon dioxide stored in blood in physical solution at a normal arterial PCO_2 of 5.3 kPa (40 mmHg) is given by the following equation:

$CCO_2 = \alpha CO_2 \times PCO_2 = 0.072 \times 100 = 2.9$ mL/100mL blood

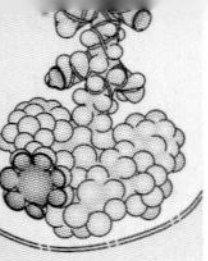

Increases in all these, as seen in an exercising muscle, shift the curve to the right, which decreases affinity and helps unload oxygen at the tissues.

The effect of PCO_2 is particularly important as the loading of carbon dioxide in tissues produces a right shift of the dissociation curve and enhances the simultaneous unloading of oxygen. Part of this shift is caused by the associated pH change, and part results from the binding of carbon dioxide with Hb to form carbamino compounds, which have a lower affinity for oxygen. The reverse occurs in the lungs as the unloading of carbon dioxide shifts the dissociation curve to the left, which enables the blood to load more oxygen at a given PaO_2. This bidirectional shift is called the Bohr effect.

Additional regulation of Hb-O_2 affinity over a time frame of hours to days occurs via 2,3-diphosphoglycerate (2,3-DPG), an intermediate metabolite in the red cell metabolic pathway. When up-regulated by a stimulus such as chronic hypoxia (e.g., altitude), increased 2,3-DPG concentration decreases oxygen affinity by binding to the Hb molecule. Changes in 2,3-DPG level also play an adaptive role during acid-base abnormalities and with anemia.

Affinity for oxygen can also be affected by variation in the Hb polypeptides. At 37°C and pH 7.4, normal adult Hb A has a P_{50} of 27 mmHg, and human fetal Hb has a P_{50} of 20 mmHg. Several abnormal hemoglobin types have been identified that have either high or low oxygen affinity.

The physiologic advantage of a curve shift for oxygen delivery depends on the conditions of loading and unloading. An increased affinity means that the blood that leaves the alveoli, equilibrated with the alveolar PO_2, has a slightly higher oxygen content, but when it is required to give up 5 mL/100 mL or more of its content to metabolically active tissue, the PO_2 at the delivery point has to fall to a lower than normal value (see Fig. 3.5). A decreased affinity means that the blood leaving the alveoli has a slightly lower content, but not very much lower because of the nearly flat top of the Hb-O_2 curve. This blood can give up the same amount (5 mL/100 mL) to the tissues and still maintain a higher PO_2 at the delivery point. Thus, at near-normal levels of alveolar PO_2, a right shift is usually advantageous, but when loading at a markedly reduced PO_2 (e.g., via placental exchange or at extreme altitude), a left shift is more helpful.

CARBON MONOXIDE

Carbon monoxide is a particularly dangerous gas because its affinity for Hb is 200 to 250 times that of oxygen, which means that it can fully saturate Hb at a very low ambient concentration. The presence of carbon monoxide decreases the oxygen carrying capacity by functionally removing Hb sites available for oxygen binding. It also causes an effective increase in oxygen affinity of the remaining Hb. Carbon monoxide poisoning can create a marked disparity between a normal measured PaO_2 and a severely reduced oxygen content.

ARTERIAL BLOOD OXYGEN CONTENT

The equilibration of blood with alveolar gas in the pulmonary capillaries determines the partial pressure of oxygen in plasma, and it would do so even if Hb were totally absent. The PO_2 in the plasma is in equilibrium with the Hb in the red cells, which yields an oxygen saturation determined by the shape and position of the Hb-O_2 curve. The arterial oxygen content (CaO_2) is determined by this saturation and by the concentration of Hb present, plus a small contribution of dissolved oxygen. With a normal Hb concentration of 15 g/100 mL, the normal arterial oxygen content is about 20.5 mL/100 mL (Table 3.7). Blood with a decreased Hb concentration (anemia) holds less oxygen, and that with an increased Hb concentration (polycythemia) holds an increased amount of oxygen.

VENOUS BLOOD OXYGEN CONTENT

A portion of the oxygen carried in arterial blood is given up to the tissues to meet metabolic needs, which leaves a lower oxygen content in the venous blood that returns to the right heart and lungs. This mixed venous oxygen content ($C\bar{v}O_2$) depends on arterial oxygen content and the balance between tissue oxygen consumption ($\dot{V}O_2$) and blood flow ($\dot{Q}$). It is described by the Fick equation (equation 3.11), which states that the volume of oxygen consumed per minute is equal to the cardiac output times the content of oxygen removed from each unit volume of blood (Table 3.8).

EQUATION 3.11: VENOUS OXYGEN CONTENT—FICK EQUATION

$$\dot{V}O_2 = \dot{Q} \times (CaO_2 - C\bar{v}O_2)$$

An increased oxygen demand in the face of a constant blood flow requires an increased arterial-venous (a-$\bar{v}$) oxygen content difference. Alternatively, an increased blood flow in the face of a constant metabolic demand yields a decreased (a-$\bar{v}$) oxygen difference.

The mixed venous partial pressure of oxygen ($P\bar{v}O_2$) is determined by the venous oxygen content and the oxygen dissociation curve. The venous oxygen content and PO_2 vary in the blood that returns from different capillary beds, depending on the matching of blood flow to metabolic demand. For example, blood that leaves exercising muscle may have a very low venous oxygen content, whereas the kidneys have high blood flow and relatively little oxygen extraction. After these flows combine in the right heart, the mixed venous (designated by the symbol $\bar{v}$) content reflects total body oxygen extraction.

Carbon Dioxide Transport

As the blood passes through the lung, carbon dioxide equilibrates with the alveolar gas so that arterial PCO_2 is very close to

Table 3.7
Normal arterial oxygen content

Parameter	Value
Arterial partial pressure of O_2	90–100 mmHg
Arterial saturation of O_2	97%
Hemoglobin (Hb) content	15 g/100 mL
O_2 carrying capacity of Hb	1.39 mL/g Hb
Arterial O_2 content	O_2 bound to Hb plus dissolved O_2 = (15 x 1.39 x 0.97) + (0.003 x 100) = 20.2 + 0.3 mL/100 mL = 20.5 mL/100 mL

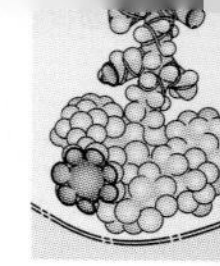

Table 3.8
The Fick equation, $\dot{V}O_2 = \dot{Q} \times (CaO_2 - C\bar{v}O_2)$

Parameter	Symbol	Typical normal values at rest
Oxygen consumption	$\dot{V}O_2$	250mL/min
Cardiac output	$\dot{Q}$	5L/minute
Difference between alveolar and mixed venous oxygen content	$CaO_2 - C\bar{v}O_2$	50mL/L blood (or 5mL/100mL blood)
Arterial oxygen content	CaO_2	200mL/L blood (or 20mL/100mL blood)
Mixed venous oxygen content	$C\bar{v}O_2$	150mL/L blood (or 15mL/100L blood)
Mixed venous partial pressure of oxygen	$P\bar{v}O_2$	~40mmHg

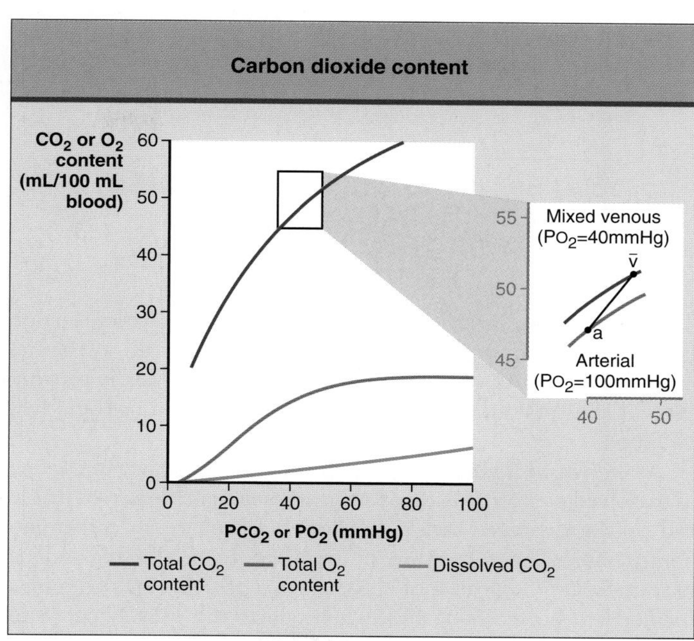

Figure 3.6 The curve of carbon dioxide content versus PCO_2 is steeper than the hemoglobin-oxygen curve, shown for comparison. It includes carbon dioxide bound to hemoglobin plus bicarbonate (the largest fraction) and dissolved carbon dioxide. Inset: Increasing the PO_2 decreases the carbon dioxide content for any PCO_2 (Haldane effect). As the blood shifts between the oxygenated and the deoxygenated curves, the functional steepness (i.e., $\Delta CCO_2/\Delta PCO_2$) between the arterial point and mixed venous point is increased. Modified from Hlastala MP: Blood gas transport. In Culver BH [ed]: The Respiratory System. Seattle, ASUW Publications, 1997, pp 43-52.

alveolar PCO_2. The alveolar PCO_2, and hence arterial PCO_2, is determined by the balance between alveolar ventilation and carbon dioxide production. Under normal conditions, arterial PCO_2 is regulated near 40 mmHg, with an arterial carbon dioxide content related to partial pressure in a nonlinear fashion, normally 47 mL/100 mL.

The venous carbon dioxide is determined by the arterial carbon dioxide content and the relationship between blood flow and carbon dioxide production, again described by the Fick principle. With a typical RQ of 0.8, a resting oxygen consumption of 250 mL/minute is associated with a carbon dioxide production of 200 mL/minute and, at a cardiac output of 5 L/minute, requires the loading of an additional 4 mL/100 mL of carbon dioxide into the systemic venous blood. This increase to a venous carbon dioxide content of 51 mL/100 mL occurs with only a modest rise in mixed venous partial pressure to a $P\bar{v}CO_2$ of 46 mmHg.

CARBON DIOXIDE DISSOCIATION CURVE

The overall relationship between carbon dioxide content (CCO_2) and PCO_2 is curvilinear, as indicated in Figure 3.6, but the curve is essentially linear over the limited range between arterial and venous PCO_2 (40 to 46 mmHg). Although the quantity of carbon dioxide exchanged is similar to that of oxygen (as governed by the RQ), this narrow range of arterial-to-venous PCO_2 is made possible by the steepness of the carbon dioxide dissociation curve. Oxygenation of Hb decreases its ability to carry carbon dioxide, which facilitates the unloading of carbon dioxide at the lung, whereas the opposite effect occurs at tissues. This shift between the dissociation curves of venous and oxygenated blood increases the "physiologic" slope of the carbon dioxide curve (as shown in the inset in Fig. 3.6). The ability to load or unload carbon dioxide with minimal change in PCO_2 helps minimize the change in pH between arterial and venous blood.

CARBON DIOXIDE STORAGE IN BLOOD

Carbon dioxide is stored in physical solution and in chemical combination with Hb, but in addition, a major portion of carbon dioxide is stored in the blood as bicarbonate (HCO_3^-). The blood stores of carbon dioxide are greater than those of oxygen, and because bicarbonate is also present in the extravascular interstitial fluid, the body stores of carbon dioxide are much greater than those of oxygen. Thus, with a change in ventilation or if breathing ceases (apnea or asphyxia), the carbon dioxide level changes much more slowly than the level of oxygen does.

Because the solubility of carbon dioxide is more than 20 times that of oxygen, a greater content of carbon dioxide is carried in physical solution at physiologic partial pressures (see Table 3.6). This is normally 2.9 mL/100 mL, representing about 6% of the total amount of carbon dioxide carried in arterial blood.

Carbon dioxide binds with Hb to form carbamino compounds and also, to a small extent, binds with other proteins. At a normal arterial PCO_2, carbamino binding of carbon dioxide amounts to about 2.1 mL/100 mL blood, or 4% of the total carbon dioxide content. Formation of carbamino compounds tends to weaken the Hb-O_2 affinity (the Bohr effect). Conversely, as Hb binds oxygen, carbamino-compound formation decreases (the Haldane effect). These interactions assist in the appropriate loading and unloading of oxygen and carbon dioxide in the lungs and tissues. Even though carbamino binding makes up only a small part of the blood carbon dioxide storage, it undergoes a relatively large change between venous and arterial blood, so that it accounts for more than 25% of the carbon dioxide loaded in tissue and unloaded at the lung.

By far the major storage of carbon dioxide in blood is in the form of bicarbonate ion. In blood, carbon dioxide combines with water to form carbonic acid, which then dissociates to form

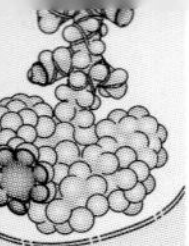

hydrogen ion and bicarbonate ion. The first reaction is slow unless it is catalyzed by carbonic anhydrase (CA), present in the red cell and other tissues (equation 3.12).

EQUATION 3.12: CARBON DIOXIDE STORAGE IN BLOOD

$$CO_2 + H_2O \Leftrightarrow H_2CO_3 \Leftrightarrow H^+ + HCO_3^-$$

The whole-blood bicarbonate concentration of carbon dioxide is equivalent to approximately 42 mL/100 mL at a normal arterial PCO_2, with most of that in the plasma. This is roughly 90% of the total amount of carbon dioxide stored in the arterial blood.

As shown in Figure 3.7, carbon dioxide is carried in plasma as dissolved carbon dioxide or as bicarbonate and is carried inside red cells as dissolved carbon dioxide, bicarbonate, or carbamino compounds. The formation of bicarbonate in the red cell is extremely rapid because of the presence of CA. Hydrogen ions formed are buffered by Hb, which shifts the Hb-O_2 curve to the right and thus enhances oxygen release. As a result of the high concentration of bicarbonate formed, some bicarbonate diffuses out into the plasma and, to maintain charge neutrality, chloride diffuses into the cell. The uncatalyzed formation of bicarbonate extracellularly is extremely slow. Thus, even though the majority of blood carbon dioxide content is carried in plasma HCO_3^-, the red cell plays an important role in facilitating its interconversion to and from diffusible gas and in buffering the associated hydrogen ions.

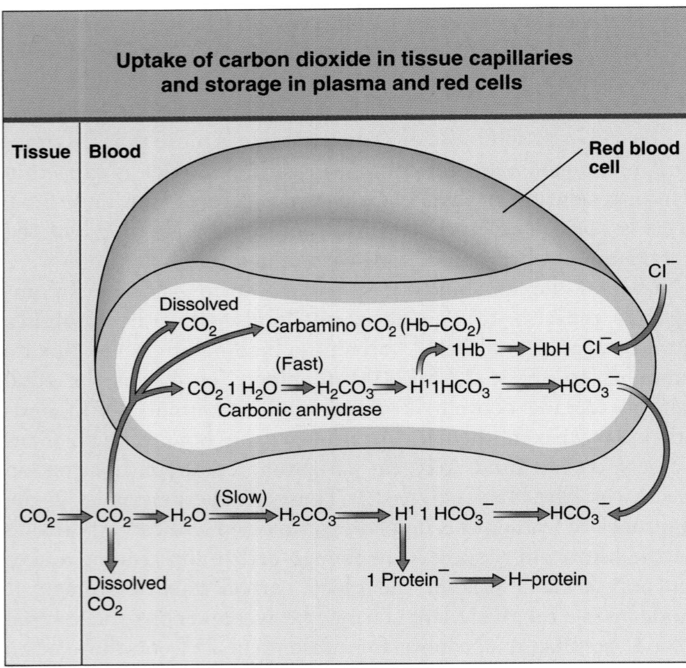

Figure 3.7 Uptake of carbon dioxide in tissue capillaries and storage in plasma and red cells. In the pulmonary capillaries, all the reactions and diffusions are reversed. Modified from Hlastala MP: Blood gas transport. In Culver BH [ed]: The Respiratory System. Seattle, ASUW Publications, 1997, pp 43-52.

ALVEOLAR-ARTERIAL OXYGEN EQUILIBRATION

In the discussion of alveolar ventilation, the factors that determine the average alveolar PO_2 of the lung were shown to be the inspired PO_2 and the relationship of alveolar ventilation to oxygen consumption. In an ideal cardiorespiratory system, the arterial blood would be perfectly equilibrated with the alveolar PO_2, but even normal individuals fall somewhat short of this; thus, an alveolar-arterial difference in PO_2 [$P(A - a)O_2$] occurs. With lung disease or circulatory abnormalities, $P(A - a)O_2$ may become quite wide. The three factors involved in alveolar-arterial equilibration are diffusion, shunt, and ventilation-perfusion matching.

Diffusion

Oxygen moves from alveolar gas to arterial blood by a passive process of diffusion from higher to lower partial pressure. The flux of a gas across a membrane is equal to a coefficient called the diffusion capacity (DL) times the partial pressure gradient, which in the case of the lung is between alveolar gas and capillary blood. In the gas phase, diffusion is proportional to the inverse of the square root of the molecular weight (i.e., smaller molecules move faster). In a liquid, diffusion is proportional to solubility divided by the square root of the molecular weight. In the lung, diffusion is also dependent on the nature and length of the diffusion pathway and the total surface area available for diffusion, which reflects the effective alveolar capillary bed. The total diffusion capacity of the lung is made up of two components:

1. Diffusion through the alveolar membrane itself
2. Effective resistance of the red cell plus the process of chemical combination with Hb

The average red blood cell spends about 0.75 second in the alveolar capillaries (the capillary transit time). With a normal diffusion capacity, enough oxygen crosses the membrane to bring the red cell Hb to equilibrium with the alveolar PO_2 in 0.25 second or less. A diffusion abnormality slows the rate at which oxygen crosses, but usually a sufficient time reserve is available for the red cell to be fully oxygenated by the time it leaves the capillary (Fig. 3.8). Only when the diffusion capacity is severely limited (<25% of normal) or the transit time is markedly shortened is it possible for the blood that leaves the alveolar capillaries to have a lower PO_2 than that of the alveolar gas. Thus, a diffusion abnormality, although present in many diseases, is rarely the physiologic cause of a low PaO_2 at rest. If a diffusion limitation for oxygen exists when breathing air, it may be virtually eliminated by breathing oxygen, because the very high driving pressure of oxygen in alveolar gas increases the rate of equilibration. Thus, on 100% oxygen ($PAO_2 \approx 670$ mmHg) it can be arbitrarily stated that diffusion limitation makes no contribution to any $P(A - a)O_2$.

Although it may not indicate the physiologic reason for hypoxemia, it is often useful to measure the diffusion capacity of the lung to help establish the condition of the alveolar-capillary membrane (i.e., the alveolar surface area and capillary volume). Because it is technically difficult to estimate the back pressure of capillary PO_2 (it is changing, of course, from $P\bar{v}O_2$ to PaO_2), the clinical measurement of diffusion capacity is established with carbon monoxide. The test is described in Chapter 7.

Carbon dioxide also moves from blood to alveolus by diffusion. Although it is a larger molecule, diffusion in a liquid is

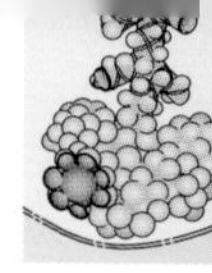

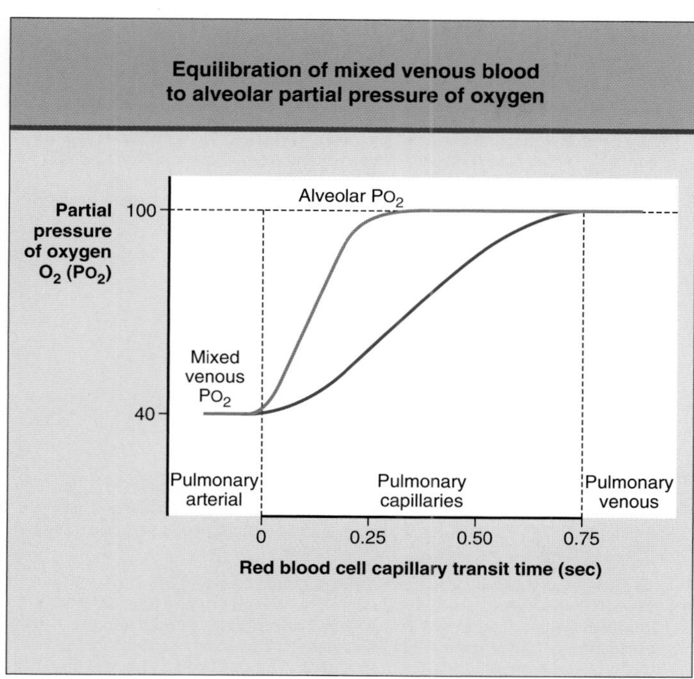

Figure 3.8 Mixed venous blood equilibrates to the alveolar PO_2 level by diffusion during transit through the pulmonary capillaries. Even when the diffusion rate is abnormally slow (blue line), the blood may be fully oxygenated within the normal transit time.

proportional to solubility, so carbon dioxide diffuses through the alveolar wall more readily than oxygen by a factor of 20. However, the transfer of carbon dioxide out of the blood also depends on chemical reaction rates (remember that much carbon dioxide is carried as HCO_3^-, which must be converted, via CA, into carbon dioxide). As a result of this, plus the much lower initial driving pressure difference for carbon dioxide unloading, the equilibration rates between blood and alveolus are similar for carbon dioxide and oxygen.

Alveolar-Arterial Oxygen Difference

Because the lung is not a single unit but consists of approximately 300 million alveoli, one might expect differences from one region to another. All alveoli do not receive the same amount of ventilation ($\dot{V}A$) or perfusion ($\dot{Q}$), nor is the matching of ventilation to blood flow ($\dot{V}A/\dot{Q}$) the same for each alveolus. Because of this, gas partial pressures vary from one alveolus to the next. A diffusion limitation, if it exists, would create a difference between the alveolar gas partial pressure and that in the capillary leaving it, which would lead directly to a measured alveolar-arterial oxygen difference. In considering ventilation-perfusion abnormalities and shunt, it is assumed that each capillary is in complete equilibrium with the alveolus that it passes, but the subsequent mixture of blood from different areas of the lung results in an arterial PO_2 less than the value calculated for alveolar PO_2, that is, a positive $PAO_2 - PaO_2$, or a $P(A - a)O_2$ difference.

Shunt

Shunt refers to blood that passes from the systemic venous to arterial system (i.e., right to left) without going through gas exchange areas of the lung. Some normal shunting of blood always occurs as a result of the bronchial arterial blood that drains to the pulmonary veins after having perfused and given up oxygen to the bronchial tissues, and a small amount of coronary venous blood, which drains directly into the cavity of the left ventricle through the thebesian veins. An abnormal shunt may occur through congenital defects in the heart or blood vessels or, more commonly, through areas of atelectasis or consolidation in the lung. For example, if one lung collapses but continues to receive half the cardiac output, deoxygenated blood mixes with oxygenated blood (Fig. 3.9) to cause a marked reduction in the oxygenation of the arterial blood. Note that because of the shape of the Hb-O_2 dissociation curve, the final PO_2 is much closer to that of the shunted blood than to that leaving well-ventilated units.

If a patient who has a 50% shunt breathes 100% oxygen, the alveolar gas equation shows that the PAO_2 in well-ventilated units increases to about 670 mmHg, but this causes only a small increase in the oxygen content of the blood that leaves them. The shunt blood continues to have a mixed venous content, which will be slightly higher if oxygen extraction $[C(a - \bar{v})O_2]$ remains constant. The mixed arterial blood remains somewhat hypoxemic, with a very large $P(A - a)O_2$ difference.

The effect of shunting can also be visualized graphically from the Hb-O_2 dissociation curve (Fig. 3.10). Because Hb is fully saturated above a PaO_2 of 150 mmHg, the additional content results from dissolved oxygen and is linearly related to PO_2. Thus, a fixed relationship exists in this range between an increasing shunt fraction (movement of Ca toward $C\bar{v}$ on the vertical axis) and a decreasing PaO_2. For a normal $C(a - \bar{v})O_2$ value of 5 mL/100 mL, this calculates to a fall in PO_2 of about 20 mmHg below the alveolar value for each 1% shunt. This rule of thumb is useful to esti-

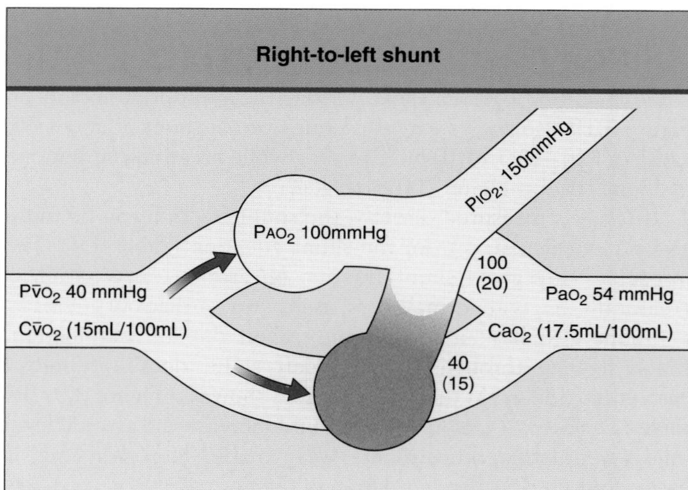

Figure 3.9 Shunt is blood flow not exposed to alveolar gas. To find the PO_2 of the mixed arterial blood (PaO_2), the relative blood flow (50 : 50 in this example) and oxygen *content* (shown in parentheses) contributed by each side must be considered; that is, CaO_2 = (shunt fraction × mixed venous content) + (nonshunt fraction × ventilated capillary content). After determining the content (or percentage saturation) of the mixture, the resultant PaO_2 can be found from the hemoglobin-oxygen dissociation curve. (In this example, $CaO_2 - C\bar{v}O_2$ has narrowed to 2.5 mL/100 mL, which implies an increase in cardiac output. If this does not occur, then $C\bar{v}O_2$ must drop below 15, and the final PaO_2 will be lower than shown.) Culver BH [ed]: The Respiratory System. Seattle, ASUW Publications, 1997.

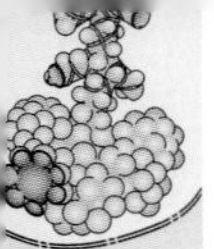

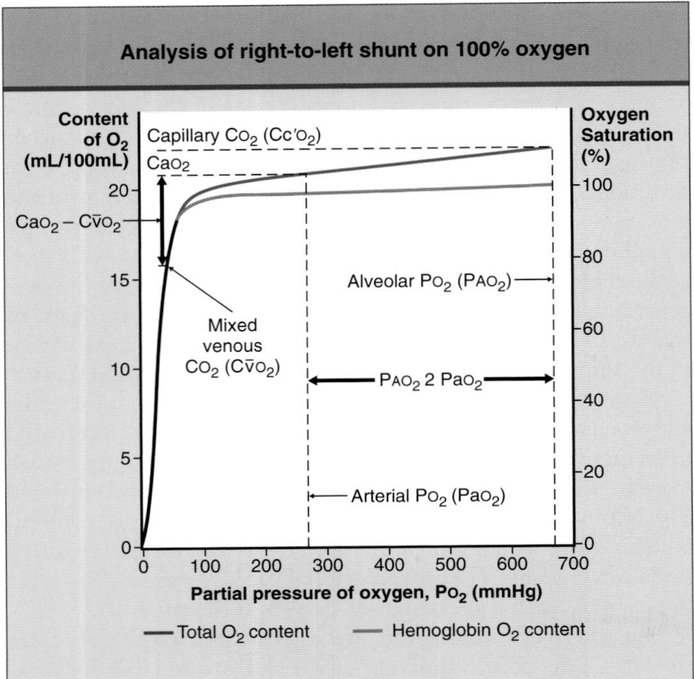

Figure 3.10 Analysis of right-to-left shunt in a patient who is breathing 100% oxygen. In this example, the shunt fraction is 20% of cardiac output, so the arterial oxygen content (CaO_2) represents the mixture of one part venous blood and four parts fully oxygenated blood from alveolar capillaries. On 100% oxygen, the PO_2 of well-ventilated alveoli is about 670 mmHg; the content in capillary blood leaving them is shown as $Cc'O_2$. A normal $CaO_2 - C\bar{v}O_2$ difference gives the mixed venous content shown. With a 20% shunt, the arterial blood content (CaO_2) is one fifth the distance from $Cc'O_2$ to $C\bar{v}O_2$ on the vertical axis. Projecting horizontally gives the PaO_2 associated with this content. Modified from Culver BH [ed]: The Respiratory System. Seattle, ASUW Publications, 1997.

mate the shunt fraction from arterial blood gas values obtained while breathing 100% oxygen. Plotting the appropriate points on Figure 3.10 also shows why the same normal shunt of about 5% causes a $P(A-a)O_2$ of 10 to 15 mmHg while breathing air but one of about 100 mmHg on 100% oxygen.

If $C\bar{v}O_2$ is measured directly, the shunt fraction can be more accurately calculated from the shunt equation (Table 3.9). The impact of any given shunt fraction on arterial oxygenation is greater if $C\bar{v}O_2$ is abnormally low, as in a low cardiac output state.

Shunt also has an impact on carbon dioxide elimination. Blood flowing through a right-to-left shunt does not unload carbon dioxide, so in the 50% example shown in Figure 3.9, the mixed venous PCO_2 of about 46 would increase the arterial level unless ventilatory adjustments were made. However, this is easily corrected. If the ventilation in the normal alveoli increases enough for their PCO_2 to decrease to 34, the final arterial mixture would have a PCO_2 of 40. (Unlike oxygen, the relationship of carbon dioxide content and partial pressure is nearly linear in this range.) To some extent, this adjustment may occur automatically as ventilation that is unable to reach closed or filled alveoli is diverted to the open units. Any tendency for arterial PCO_2 to rise would stimulate respiratory centers to increase ventilation further. This problem manifests clinically in patients who are unable to increase their minute ventilations because of disease or because of dependence on mechanical ventilators.

Table 3.9
Shunt calculation

The oxygen transported in arterial blood is considered to come from two sources – shunt flow ($\dot{Q}S$) with mixed venous oxygen content ($C\bar{v}O_2$) and nonshunt flow (total flow minus shunt flow, or $\dot{Q}T - \dot{Q}S$), with an oxygen content in equilibrium with well-ventilated alveoli ($Cc'O_2$ for capillary oxygen content), hence:

$$\dot{Q}TCaO_2 = \dot{Q}SCvO_2 + (\dot{Q}T - \dot{Q}S)Cc'O_2$$

Algebraic manipulations yield:

$$\dot{Q}TCaO_2 = QSCvO_2 + QTCc'O_2 - QSCc'O_2$$
$$\dot{Q}SCc'O_2 - \dot{Q}SCvO_2 = \dot{Q}TCc'O_2 - \dot{Q}TCaO_2$$
$$\dot{Q}S(Cc'O_2 - CvO_2) = \dot{Q}T(Cc'O_2 - CaO_2)$$
$$\dot{Q}S/\dot{Q}T = (Cc'O_2 - CaO_2)/(Cc'O_2 - CvO_2)$$

CaO_2 and $C\bar{v}O_2$ are measured from appropriate blood samples; $Cc'O_2$ is obtained by assuming that $Pc'O_2 = PAO_2$ calculated from the alveolar gas equation ($PIO_2 - PCO_2/R$) or, if the subject is breathing 100% oxygen, only ($PIO_2 - PCO_2$).

To truly calculate shunt fraction the subject must be breathing 100% oxygen. If the measurements are made breathing air or any fraction of inspired oxygen other than 1.0, the 'shunt' calculated is termed venous admixture (or 'physiologic shunt') because it includes any contribution of low V/Q areas as well as diffusion limitation. The calculation answers the question: if the observed reduction in PaO_2 were entirely caused by shunt, how large would that shunt have to be? Thus, for example, a calculation of 10% venous admixture in a patient breathing air might be caused by a 10% true shunt, or to a larger volume of blood flowing through low $\dot{V}/Q$ areas, or to some combination of true shunt, low, and high V/Q areas.

Ventilation-Perfusion Abnormalities

The average $\dot{V}A/\dot{Q}$ ratio is about 4 L/min:5 L/min, which is 0.8, but this average derives from alveoli with $\dot{V}A/\dot{Q}$ ranging from near zero (unventilated) to nearly infinity (unperfused). In the normal lung, the regional distribution of blood flow is influenced by the vascular branching pattern, gravity, and other factors resulting in more perfusion being directed to the dorsal, caudal lung regions and less to the cephalad regions. A number of mechanical factors cause ventilation to be greater in the dorsal, caudal regions as well. However, the difference in perfusion from the bottom to top of the lung is greater than the difference in ventilation. Accordingly, the ratio of ventilation to perfusion is low at the bottom of the lung and high at the top of the lung. Because the matching of ventilation and perfusion varies, the PAO_2 and $PACO_2$ are different in different areas of the lung. In lung diseases, the scatter of $\dot{V}A/\dot{Q}$ around the mean may be much greater than normal.

For alveolar gas in individual alveoli, groups of alveoli, or regions of lung, the partial pressures of oxygen and carbon dioxide are determined by the balance of influx and efflux of each gas, respectively. Thus, with a decrease in ventilation (or an increase in perfusion), the $\dot{V}A/\dot{Q}$ ratio of an alveolus is decreased, which causes PAO_2 to fall. That is, when ventilation is low relative to the amount blood flow that carries oxygen away, more oxygen molecules must be removed from each unit of incoming air, the local PAO_2 falls, and as it does, less oxygen is loaded onto the perfusing blood until a new local steady state is reached.

The normal balance of ventilation and oxygen uptake causes the PO_2 to fall from 150 mmHg in inspired air to 100 mmHg in ideally ventilated and perfused alveoli. As the $\dot{V}A/\dot{Q}$ ratio falls toward zero (near shunt), PAO_2 falls toward the mixed venous value (about 40 mmHg), and $PACO_2$ rises toward its mixed venous value (about 46 mmHg). Accordingly, with $\dot{V}A/\dot{Q}$ ratios below normal, any PAO_2 from 100 down to 40 mmHg is possible ($PACO_2$ values are in the range of 40 to 46 mmHg). The range of possible values can be displayed on a PO_2-PCO_2 graph (Fig. 3.11). The specific $\dot{V}A/\dot{Q}$ ratio in a given lung unit and the rise in oxygen content in the capillaries leaving that unit determine the extraction of oxygen from inspired air, which in turn determines the magnitude of the drop in PO_2 from inspired air to alveolar air. When blood perfuses alveoli with lower levels of PAO_2, the PAO_2 in the draining capillary is reduced (as the gas tensions equilibrate). When the blood containing these lowered PAO_2 values mixes with blood coming from normal alveoli, the resulting mixture of contents causes arterial hypoxemia (Fig. 3.12).

Figure 3.13 shows that, unlike a shunt, if the inspired PO_2 is raised even moderately, PAO_2 in these poorly ventilated alveoli rises sufficiently so that hypoxemia is eliminated, although $P(A-a)O_2$ is still large. If a patient with a low ratio of $\dot{V}A/\dot{Q}$ is placed on 100% oxygen, the inert gas nitrogen is washed out of the alveoli and blood. (Even if alveoli are very poorly ventilated, the nitrogen is washed out by the blood perfusing them and is subsequently eliminated via more functional units.) Once this occurs, oxygen, carbon dioxide, and water are the only gases left in the lung, and their partial pressures must add up to PB (if not, more gas is drawn in from the airways, or the alveolus shrinks). If the uptake of oxygen by blood is faster than the inflow of oxygen through a severely obstructed bronchiole ($\dot{V}A/\dot{Q} < 0.1$), the alveoli shrink and eventually collapse in a process known as *absorption atelectasis*, after which they behave as a shunt—one reason to avoid the use of 100% oxygen. Because

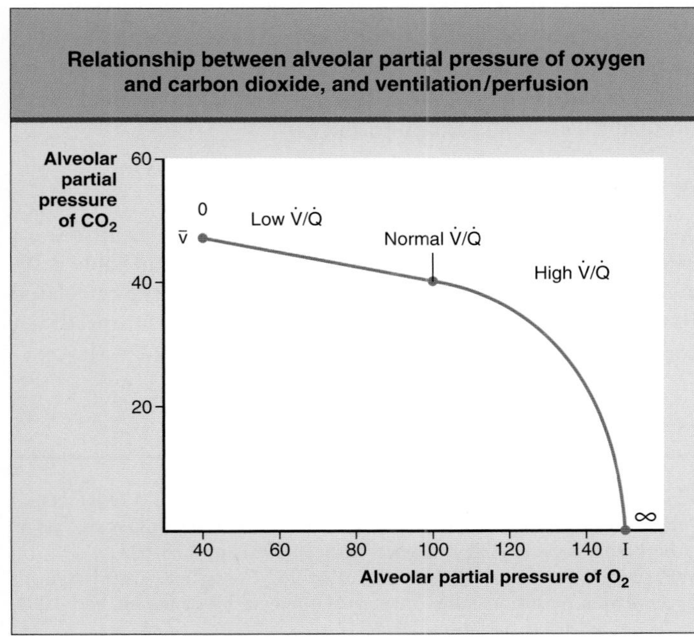

Figure 3.11 Spectrum of alveolar PO_2 and PCO_2 values possible as the ventilation-perfusion ratio ($\dot{V}/\dot{Q}$) ranges from zero to infinity. The values follow a line from the mixed venous point ($\bar{v}$) to that representing inspired gas (I).

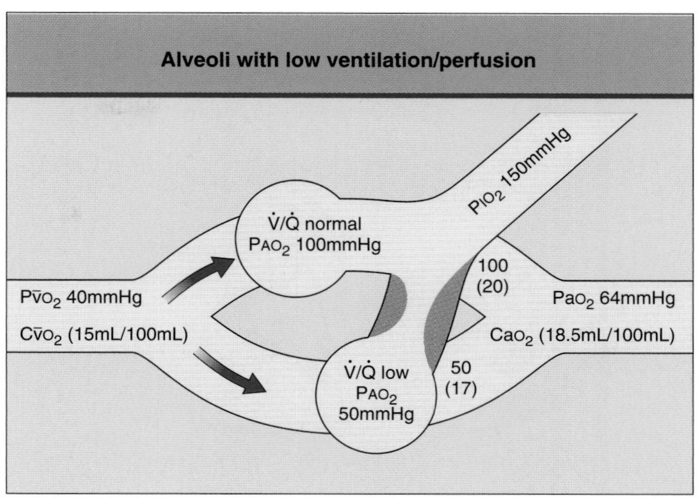

Figure 3.12 In alveoli with a low ventilation-perfusion ratio ($\dot{V}/\dot{Q}$), the alveolar PO_2 (PAO_2) is low, as more oxygen is removed from the incoming air. In this example, the $\dot{V}/\dot{Q}$ ratio has arbitrarily been chosen to result in a PAO_2 of 50 mmHg, and blood flow is equally divided. The mixture of contents (shown in parentheses) yields a PAO_2 well below normal.

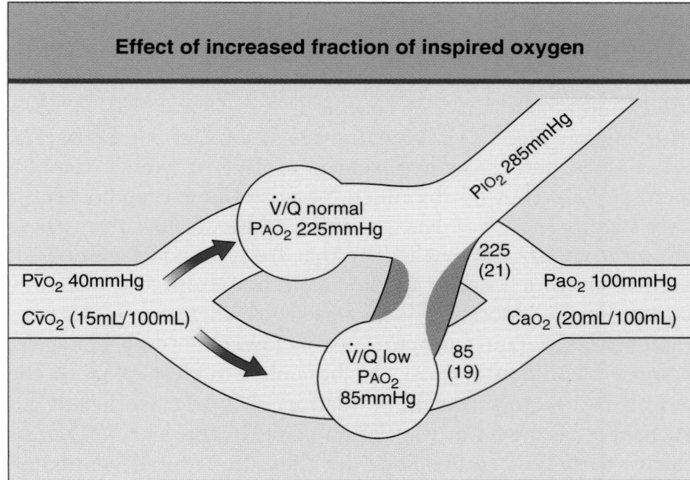

Figure 3.13 Effect of increased fraction of inspired oxygen (FIO_2) when low ventilation-perfusion ($\dot{V}/\dot{Q}$) alveoli are present. Ventilation and perfusion are identical to the example in Figure 3.12, but the FIO_2 has been increased to 0.4, which results in a normal arterial PO_2. Unlike the case with shunt, the added oxygen increases the PO_2 in both low and normal $\dot{V}/\dot{Q}$ areas. The drop in PO_2 from inspired to alveolar air on the obstructed side (285 – 85 = 200 mmHg) is now twice as large as it was on room air, because it takes twice as much oxygen to raise the blood content from 15 to 19 versus 15 to 17 mL/100 mL; this is also seen to a smaller extent on the normal side.

PAH_2O is fixed at 47 mmHg and $PACO_2$ cannot exceed $P\bar{v}CO_2$, the PaO_2 of any open alveolus is more than 650 mmHg no matter how low its $\dot{V}A/\dot{Q}$ ratio falls. Thus, on 100% oxygen, the effect of abnormal $\dot{V}A/\dot{Q}$ ratios on the equilibration of mixed arterial blood with alveolar PO_2 is completely eliminated; that is, $\dot{V}A/\dot{Q}$ mismatching no longer contributes to the observed $P(A-a)O_2$ difference.

If an alveolus is unperfused (e.g., vessels blocked by an embolus), no oxygen can be removed from it or carbon dioxide

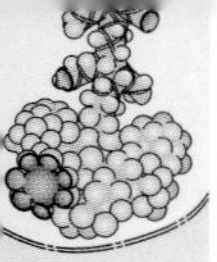

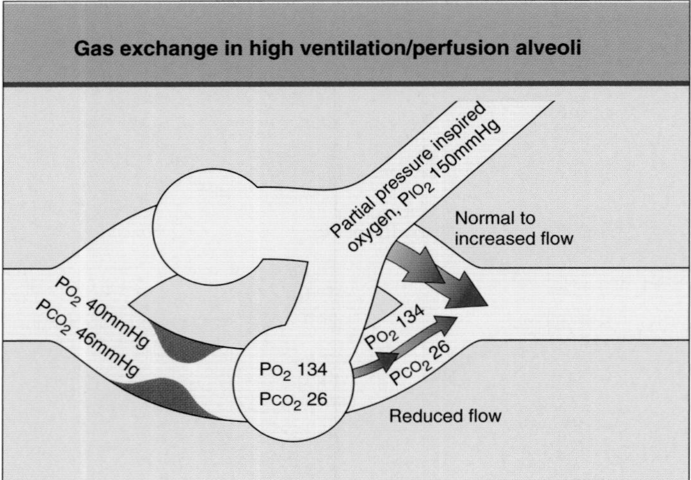

Figure 3.14 Gas exchange in high ventilation-perfusion ($\dot{V}/\dot{Q}$) alveoli. In this example, blood flow is reduced to about one fourth normal. (The missing blood flow must be shifted elsewhere, which affects the ratio of "normal" alveoli.) In the high $\dot{V}/\dot{Q}$ alveoli, P_{O_2} is increased and arterial P_{CO_2} decreased. (The specific values are for illustration only; as a result of the interaction of $\dot{V}/\dot{Q}$ and blood gas contents, these values are most easily obtained from tables or nomograms.)

Table 3.10 Physiologic mechanisms of hypoxemia
Decreased alveolar partial pressure of oxygen (P_{AO_2}); normal alveolar minus arterial difference ($P_{AO_2} - Pa_{O_2}$)
Decreased P_{IO_2}:
Lower atmospheric pressure (PATM) with normal fraction of inspired oxygen (F_{IO_2})(e.g., high altitude)
Lower F_{IO_2} with normal PATM (e.g., iatrogenic)
Alveolar hypoventilation:
$P_{AO_2} = P_{IO_2} - Pa_{CO_2}/R$ (e.g., depressed respiratory drive)
Increased $P_{AO_2} - Pa_{O_2}$
Diffusion limitation — blood leaving an alveolus fails to reach equilibration with alveolar gas; rarely significant as a cause of clinical hypoxemia
Ventilation-perfusion ($\dot{V}/\dot{Q}$) mismatching — specifically, the low $\dot{V}_A/\dot{Q}$ areas cause hypoxemia by contributing blood with reduced content to the arterial mixture
Shunt — the extreme of low $\dot{V}/\dot{Q}$; shunt flow of deoxygenated blood has no contact with alveolar gas
On 100% oxygen ($F_{IO_2} = 1.0$) only the shunt mechanism contributes to the $P_{AO_2} - Pa_{O_2}$ difference. Breathing air or on any $F_{IO_2} < 1.0$, both shunt and low $\dot{V}/\dot{Q}$ areas (plus any diffusion limitation) contribute to the $P_{AO_2} - Pa_{O_2}$ difference. This combined effect is termed *venous admixture* and has also been called *physiologic shunt*.

added to it. With less severe underperfusion (or overventilation), the $\dot{V}_A/\dot{Q}$ ratio rises toward infinity, and the alveolar gas values approach that of inspired gas ($P_{O_2} = 150$, $P_{CO_2} = 0$ mmHg; see Fig. 3.11). Note that a high $\dot{V}_A/\dot{Q}$ abnormality (Fig. 3.14) does not cause hypoxemia; in fact, it would tend to increase Pa_{O_2} (but not by much, because the oxygen content is only slightly increased and the reduced blood flow from these alveoli is greatly outweighed by that from an equal number of normal alveoli). Carbon dioxide excretion from the high $\dot{V}/\dot{Q}$ portion of the blood flow is increased, which gives a lower end-capillary Pc_{CO_2} (and a proportionately lower content), but again, because blood flow is small, this has only a modest effect on the overall Pa_{CO_2}. In terms of ventilation, this is an inefficient gas exchange, because the ventilation going to the high $\dot{V}/\dot{Q}$ units carries away less carbon dioxide; thus, the overall ventilation must increase to maintain homeostasis. These alveoli then contribute to physiologic dead space or "wasted ventilation."

Disease processes may cause both low and high $\dot{V}_A/\dot{Q}$ areas simultaneously, possibly with a normal overall mean $\dot{V}_A/\dot{Q}$. However, the shape of the Hb-O_2 curve shows that little oxygen content is added as the P_{O_2} increases above 100. Thus, the blood from these high $\dot{V}/\dot{Q}$ units is unable to compensate for the drop in oxygen content contributed by the low $\dot{V}/\dot{Q}$ areas. In addition, by definition, less blood comes from high $\dot{V}/\dot{Q}$ units than from an equal volume of low $\dot{V}/\dot{Q}$ units. Thus, even a process that results in both high and low $\dot{V}/\dot{Q}$ areas results in arterial hypoxemia.

Abnormal $\dot{V}_A/\dot{Q}$ relationships also interfere with the elimination of carbon dioxide, but an elevation of Pa_{CO_2} is not commonly seen in such patients because the normal response to a rising Pa_{CO_2} is to increase overall ventilation. This increases the carbon dioxide excretion in both high and low $\dot{V}/\dot{Q}$ areas, which brings Pa_{CO_2} back to normal. The increase in ventilation also increases P_{AO_2} somewhat, which improves the oxygen content of blood that leaves low $\dot{V}/\dot{Q}$ alveoli but does little for that of high $\dot{V}/\dot{Q}$ areas. The net result of this ventilatory response is to normalize Pa_{CO_2} and improve, but not fully correct, Pa_{O_2}.

Arterial Hypoxemia

Arterial hypoxemia (i.e., a low Pa_{O_2}) can result from one or more of five physiologic mechanisms, summarized in Table 3.10. Two of these lower P_{AO_2} but do not contribute to the calculated $P(A - a)O_2$ difference. The remaining three mechanisms all act to lower Pa_{O_2} below P_{AO_2} and therefore widen $P(A - a)O_2$.

SUGGESTED READINGS

Anthonisen NR, Fleetham JA: Ventilation: total, alveolar and dead space. In Fahri LE, Tenney SM (eds): Handbook of Physiology, vol 4, The Respiratory System, sec 3, Gas Exchange. Bethesda, American Physiological Society, 1987, pp 113-130.

Baumann R, Bartels H, Bauer C: Blood oxygen transport. In Fahri LE, Tenney SM (eds): Handbook of Physiology, vol 4, The Respiratory System, sec 3, Gas Exchange. Bethesda, American Physiological Society, 1987, pp 147-172.

Klocke RA: Carbon dioxide transport. In Fahri LE, Tenney SM (eds): Handbook of Physiology, vol 4, The Respiratory System, sec 3, Gas Exchange. Bethesda, American Physiological Society, 1987, pp 173-197.

Wagner PD, Laravuso RB, Uhl RR, West JB: Continuous distribution of ventilation-perfusion ratios in normal subjects breathing air and 100% O_2. J Clin Invest 54:54-68, 1974.

CHAPTER 4

Pulmonary Circulation

Bruce H. Culver, Jonathan Sevransky, and Roy Brower

The lungs are served by two circulations—the pulmonary circulation, which accommodates the entire cardiac output from the right heart through a low-pressure circulation, and the bronchial circulation, which arises from branches off the aorta with systemic pressures and usually carries less than 1% of the cardiac output.

CIRCULATORY STRUCTURE

Pulmonary Circulation

The pulmonary arteries lie near and branch with the airways in the bronchovascular bundle. They are much thinner than systemic arteries and have, proportionately, more elastic tissue in their walls. The walls of the arterioles (diameter <100 μm) are so thin, relative to their systemic counterparts, that fluid and gas can move across them. Within the gas-exchanging zone, the arterioles give rise to a network of pulmonary capillaries in the alveolar walls that is continuous throughout the lungs. They are so numerous that, when distended, blood flows almost as an unbroken sheet between the air spaces (Fig. 4.1). "Sheet flow" reduces vascular resistance and optimizes gas exchange. When the transmural pressure difference between the inside and outside of the vessels is low, some of the capillary segments are closed, but they are easily opened and recruited into the pulmonary vascular bed as needed and may be further distended when increased flow leads to an increased transmural pressure. A red cell that follows a capillary path from the pulmonary artery to a vein may cross several alveoli, with the average transit time through the vessels engaged in gas exchange calculated to be about 0.75 second. The capillaries unite to form larger alveolar microvessels, which become venules and then veins that run between the lobules toward the hila, where upper and lower pulmonary veins from each lung empty into the left atrium.

Bronchial Circulation

The bronchial arteries arise directly from the aorta or from intercostal arteries to supply the walls of the trachea and bronchi and also to nourish the major pulmonary vessels, nerves, interstitium, and pleura. Extensive small-vessel anastomoses occur between these (systemic) vessels and both the pre- and post-capillary pulmonary vasculatures. The bronchial veins from the larger airways and hilar region drain via the systemic veins (particularly the azygos system) into the right atrium. However, bronchial flow to the intrapulmonary structures connects to the pulmonary circulation and drains via the pulmonary veins into the left atrium. This small contribution of desaturated blood contributes to the normal (2% to 5%) anatomic shunt, which may become increased when the bronchial circulation hypertrophies to supply inflammatory and neoplastic lesions. The bronchial circulation has a role in the regulation of temperature and humidity in the airways and supplies the fluid for secretion through the airway mucosa.

Lymphatic Circulation

Pulmonary lymphatics are not found in alveolar walls but originate in interstitial spaces at the level of the respiratory bronchioles and at the pleural surface, then follow the bronchovascular bundles to the hila. The lymph flows through the right lymphatic duct and the thoracic duct into the right and left brachiocephalic veins. The total flow from the lungs is quite low under normal conditions (<0.5 mL/minute in experimental animals) but can increase many fold with pulmonary edema. The lymphatics have valves to prevent backflow and can generate sufficient pressures to maintain flow when systemic venous pressure is as high as 20 cmH_2O.

CIRCULATORY PHYSIOLOGY

The pulmonary circulation conducts the entire cardiac output with a remarkably low driving pressure between the pulmonary artery (mean Ppa = 15 to 20 mmHg) and the left atrium (Pla = 7 to 12 mmHg). Like the airways, the branching pattern of vessels leads to an increase in total cross-sectional area as the alveolar vessels are approached, but (unlike the airways) this increase is not associated with a decrease in resistance. Total cross-sectional area increases at a branching point if the number of daughter branches (n) is greater than the ratio of the parent-to-daughter radii squared, $(a/b)^2$, but resistance decreases only if n is greater than $(a/b)^4$. The latter case occurs in the peripheral airways but not in the vessels, so although small peripheral airways contribute little to normal airflow resistance, pulmonary microvessels make up a substantial portion of vascular resistance. Efforts to partition the pressure drop longitudinally suggest that about 20% to 30% is in the arterial portion (including arterioles), 40% to 60% in the microvascular portion, and the remainder in the veins. With increases in flow, recruitment occurs mainly at the microvascular level, so their relative contribution to resistance becomes less.

Pulmonary vascular resistance, R, is calculated as transvascular driving pressure, ΔP (mean upstream Ppa minus mean downstream Pla), divided by the flow, $R = \Delta P/Q$. The calculated resistance must be interpreted in the context of flow because the relationship of driving pressure to flow is usually not linear and does not pass through zero. As shown in Figure 4.2, pulmonary vascular resistance decreases as flow and pressure increase with the attendant recruitment and distention of vessels.

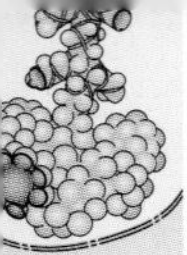

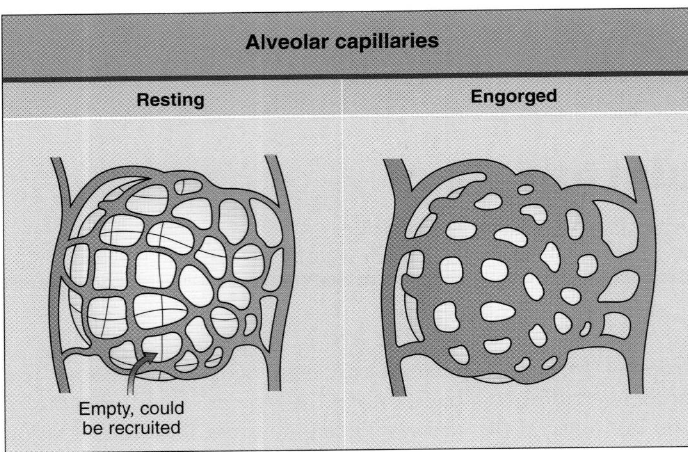

Figure 4.1 Alveolar capillaries. The normal cardiac output requires only a portion of the sheet of capillaries; any remaining vessels can be recruited when cardiac output rises during exercise. Modified with permission from Butler J: The circulation of the lung. In Culver BH [ed]: The Respiratory System. Seattle, ASUW Publications, 1997, pp 111-122.

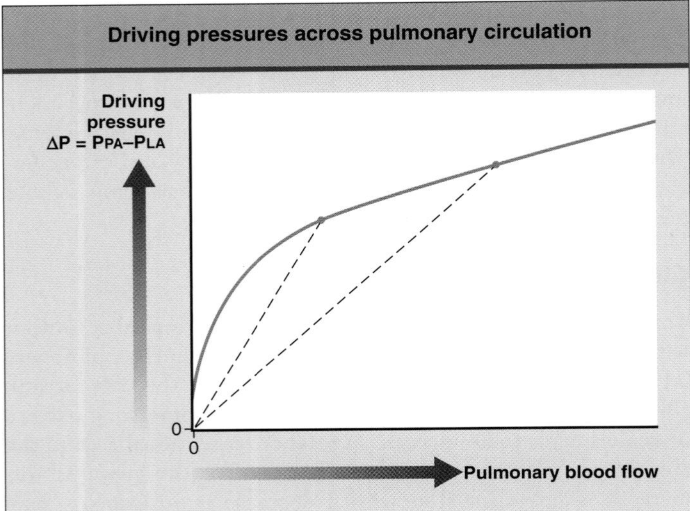

Figure 4.2 Driving pressure across the pulmonary circulation (mean pulmonary artery pressure [Ppa] minus mean left atrial pressure [Pla]) increases nonlinearly with cardiac output. Resistance, represented by the slope from the origin to any point on the line, decreases with increased pulmonary blood flow, which reflects recruitment and distention of vessels.

The resistance to flow through a vessel increases with its length, with the viscosity of the fluid, and, most importantly, with the inverse of the radius to the fourth power. In addition to muscle activity in the wall, the caliber of a distensible vessel depends passively on the transmural pressure difference between intravascular and extravascular pressure. This is particularly important in the lungs, where the vessels are embedded in expandable parenchyma. It is convenient to consider separately the effect of lung expansion on the extra-alveolar arterial and venous vessels, which differs from the effect on the microvessels of the alveolar zone. With lung volume increase, extra-alveolar vessels are distended as the pressure is lowered in the expanding perivascular space around them (Fig. 4.3), and they are elongated as the lung expands.

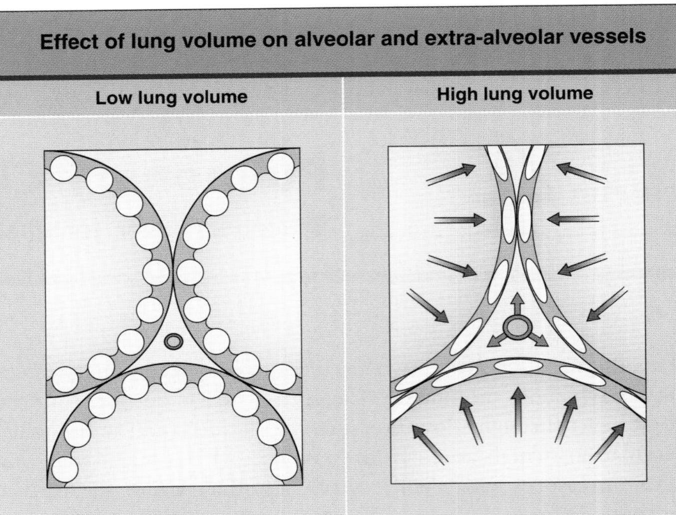

Figure 4.3 Lung volume affects alveolar and extra-alveolar vessels differently. At high lung volume, alveolar microvessels are stretched and compressed as vascular pressures fall relative to alveolar pressure. Extra-alveolar vessels, however, tend to be expanded as the pressure surrounding them decreases. Modified with permission from Butler J: The circulation of the lung. In Culver BH [ed]: The Respiratory System. Seattle, ASUW Publications, 1997, pp 111-122.

By contrast, the alveolar microvessels in the alveolar walls are elongated but partially collapsed by lung inflation because the alveolar pressure that surrounds them tends to increase relative to the intravascular pressure. This is easy to recognize with positive pressure ventilation, but it also occurs with spontaneous inspiration, because intravascular pressures fall relative to atmospheric and alveolar pressure. The sheets of capillaries in the alveolar walls are protected from the full compressive force of the alveolar pressure by the surface tension of the fluid that lines curved portions of the alveolar surface. Microvessels in the corners, where alveolar walls meet, are more fully protected from compression by the sharper curvature of the surface film and perhaps by local distending forces, analogous to the extra-alveolar vessels (Fig. 4.4). The pulmonary vascular resistance is the sum of that through alveolar and extra-alveolar vessels and thus has a complex relationship with lung volume. It is lowest at about the normal lung volume (functional residual capacity) but increases at higher and lower volumes.

BLOOD FLOW DISTRIBUTION

Anatomy and gravity influence the distribution of blood flow within the lung. If the upright lung is viewed as a stacked series of slices, a vertical gradient occurs in which the average flow of the slice rises progressively down the lung, largely influenced by gravity. However, within each slice, a marked variability of blood flow is found among regions, with high-flow areas distributed dorsally. The tendency of blood flow to be higher in dorsal and basal regions is largely preserved even when the gravitational direction is opposite, which indicates that anatomic branching patterns are a major determinant of flow distribution.

The gravitational effect has been conceptualized by dividing the lung into four zones, one above another, based on the rela-

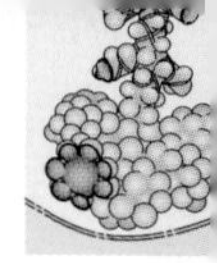

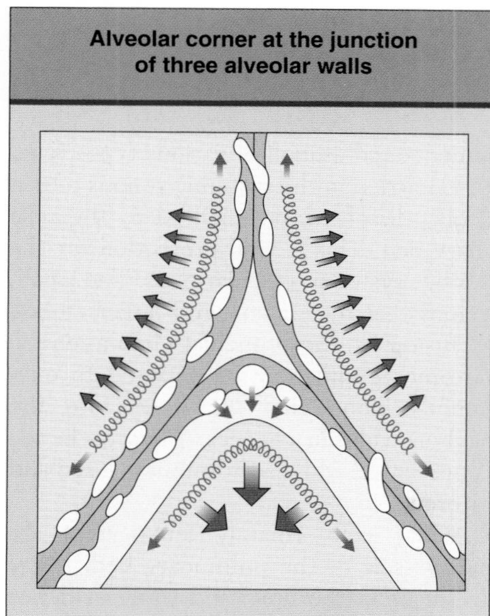

Figure 4.4 Alveolar "corner" at the junction of three alveolar walls. Surface tension (depicted by springs) holds vessels open, particularly in corners, and promotes fluid transudation by lowering the pressure around vessels. Modified with permission from Butler J: The circulation of the lung. In Culver BH [ed]: The Respiratory System. Seattle, ASUW Publications, 1997, pp 111-122.

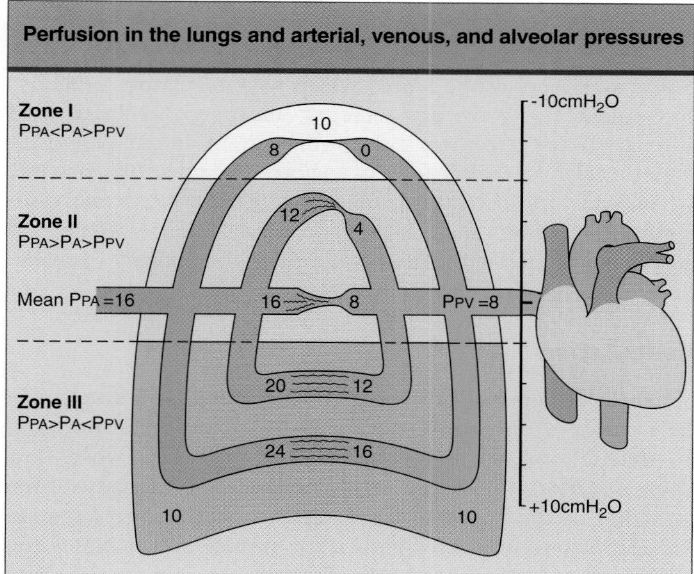

Figure 4.5 Perfusion in the lungs is influenced by the relationship of arterial and venous pressures to alveolar pressure. In this example, the alveolar pressure is 10 cmH_2O, as might be found in a patient who receives positive pressure ventilation. Modified with permission from Culver BH: Hemodynamic monitoring: physiologic problems in interpretation. In Fallat RJ, Luce JM [eds]: Cardiopulmonary Critical Care. Edinburgh, Churchill Livingstone, 1988.

tionship of vascular and alveolar pressures (Fig. 4.5). Intravascular pressures are higher at the bottom of the lung than at the top by an amount equal to a vertical hydrostatic column as high as the lung. Near the lung apex, zone I, the pressure in the alveoli (PA) exceeds that in both the pulmonary arteries (Ppa) and pulmonary vein (Ppv) and collapses the alveolar vessels, except those in the alveolar corners, which remain patent and allow flow to continue. Below this, in zone II, Ppa exceeds PA, but PA is greater than Ppv, so flow depends on the pressure difference between Ppa and PA. The vessels remain open but are critically narrowed at the downstream end, where venous pressure is lower than alveolar pressure. This creates independence of flow from the downstream venous pressure, analogous to a waterfall in which a stream that flows over a precipice is unaffected by a rising level in the pool below until it rises above the level of the lip. In the mid to lower portion of the lung, zone III, both Ppa and Ppv exceed PA, the vessels are distended, and blood flow is the highest. Zone IV is restricted to a small area in the most dependent region where flow diminishes. It has been postulated that this reduction is the result of increased vascular resistance generated by low lung volumes in this area. It has been observed, however, that flow reduction in the most dorsal lung regions occurs regardless of whether they are dependent or nondependent. Accordingly, other explanations are needed.

Although the vertical zone concept contributes to the average increase in flow down the lung, it does not explain the observed variability in flow within an isogravitational slice, which implies that other anatomic or vasoregulatory factors are important at this level. Rather than defined levels, these conditions may be more dispersed within the lung, based on local microvascular pressure.

REGULATION OF PULMONARY BLOOD FLOW

Besides their responses to passive mechanisms (anatomy, gravity, lung volume, alveolar pressure), the pulmonary vessels show vasomotor activity as a result of both neural and non-neural factors. Motor efferents from three autonomic networks are in anatomic proximity to the vasculature—sympathetic, parasympathetic, and nonadrenergic noncholinergic fibers. The sympathetic efferents probably have little effect, whereas parasympathetic stimulation dilates constricted vessels. Although acetylcholine is a potent pulmonary vasodilator, there is little cholinergic innervation of the pulmonary resistance vessels. The nonadrenergic noncholinergic system is inhibitory, constantly releasing small vasodilatory peptides at the ganglia and postganglionic ends of its unique network. This, vasodilator function is augmented with exercise.

Pulmonary arteries demonstrate intrinsically low tone as they remain relaxed when isolated from the lung. This represents a balance of endothelium-derived vasoconstrictor and vasodilator substances. Although their relative roles are yet to be clarified, many vasoactive peptides are found in the lung. Those having vasoconstrictor activity on the pulmonary circulation include angiotensin II, arginine vasopressin, endothelin 1, peptide tyrosine Y, and substance P. Vasodilatory peptides include adrenomedullin, atrial naturetic peptide, calcitonin gene-related peptide, endothelin 3, somatostatin, and vasoactive intestinal peptide.

Nitric oxide is produced in endothelial cells in the pulmonary circulation and elsewhere and is now recognized as an important mediator of vasodilatation. The oxidation of a nitrogen from L-arginine is catalyzed by nitric oxide synthase, present in both a constitutive form and a form that is inducible by products of inflammation. Nitric oxide activates guanylate cyclase, which increases cyclic guanosine monophosphate within vascular smooth muscle cells. This, in turn, reduces intracellular Ca^{++} by several mechanisms, leading to vascular relaxation. Nitric oxide is also abundantly produced in the nasal sinuses, providing an intriguing mechanism whereby inhaled nitric

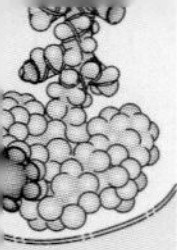

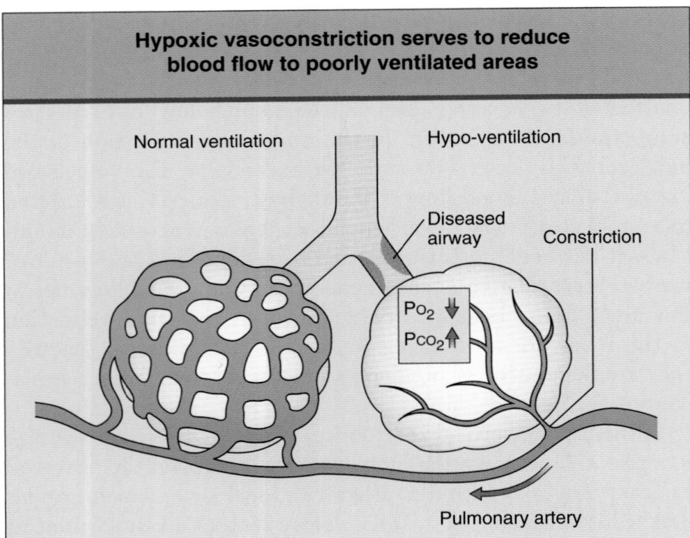

Figure 4.6 Hypoxic vasoconstriction reduces blood flow to poorly ventilated areas. This improves $\dot{V}/\dot{Q}$ matching and oxygenation but, if generalized, contributes to pulmonary hypertension. Modified with permission from Butler J: The circulation of the lung. In Culver BH [ed]: The Respiratory System. Seattle, ASUW Publications, 1997, pp 111-122.

oxide could enhance blood flow to the best-ventilated areas of lung.

Although the role of nasal nitric oxide in ventilation-perfusion matching is still speculative, the role of alveolar hypoxia in vasoregulation has been recognized for more than 50 years, but the mechanisms involved are still uncertain. The arterioles constrict when the Po_2 in the alveoli they serve falls, and additional vasoconstriction results if alveolar Pco_2 rises (Fig. 4.6). This hypoxic vasoconstriction appears to be a response to a low Po_2 in the air spaces rather than in the intraluminal blood, which is normally desaturated in these pre-alveolar vessels. The site and mechanism of this local signal pathway are unclear, but the microvascular endothelium seems to be necessary to signal the constriction of the more proximal arteriolar smooth muscle. When ventilation is decreased by an obstructed airway or other injury, local hypoxic pulmonary vasoregulation decreases blood flow to the affected region, which tends to restore the local ventilation-perfusion ($\dot{V}/\dot{Q}$) ratio toward normal and thereby improve the Po_2 of the blood that leaves that area. The diverted blood flow can be directed to better-ventilated regions, which further contributes to an improvement in overall matching.

Considerable individual variability is found in the hypoxic vasoconstrictor response, and it may be diminished by vasodilating drugs. Diversion of blood flow is most effective in the atelectatic lung, in which hypoxic vasoconstriction is unopposed by the radial traction of surrounding expanded lung tissue. A reciprocal reflex in the airways also contributes to better matching, as small airways constrict when intraluminal Pco_2 falls and dilate when it rises. Hypoxic vasoconstriction is a helpful, adaptive response to local or regional lung abnormalities, but when alveolar hypoxia is generalized (e.g., hypoventilation or altitude), the increased resistance can lead to pulmonary hypertension.

NONRESPIRATORY FUNCTIONS OF THE PULMONARY CIRCULATION

Filtering

Aggregates of blood elements and emboli of various types (e.g., fat, air, particulate matter) carried in the systemic venous return are continually filtered out, dissolved, or engulfed by the cells of the pulmonary capillary bed. This is vital protection for the cerebral, coronary, and other systemic vascular beds. The small, potentially ischemic regions that may occur with larger emboli may receive limited perfusion by the bronchial circulation via bronchopulmonary anastomoses and may be exposed to oxygenated pulmonary venous blood that backflows into the occluded region during lung volume changes. Thus, ischemic damage to the alveoli is prevented while a thrombus is lysed and the pulmonary flow restored.

Large numbers of white cells (mainly leukocytes) are sequestered in the small vessels of the pulmonary bed. Many reticuloendothelial cells occur in the lung, and some evidence suggests that the vascular endothelial cell itself can be phagocytic when stimulated.

Modification of Mediators

Some mediators in the blood, which have regulatory functions throughout the body, are secreted, taken up, or inactivated through specific receptors and enzyme systems in the pulmonary endothelial cells. Best known is angiotensin-converting enzyme, which converts inactive angiotensin 1 into the systemic vasoconstrictor angiotensin 2. Histamine, bradykinin, serotonin, and acetylcholine are largely inactivated by the pulmonary endothelium in one passage through the lungs.

Coagulation

When local injury is present, pulmonary endothelial cells can be a source of thromboplastin and tissue plasminogen activator. In spite of vascular stasis and closure of vessels when flow decreases, clots do not form in pulmonary vessels because of the structure of the endothelial surface and because the secretion of anticlotting substances bathes the surface and prevents the adherence of platelets and cells. Embolic thrombi are dissolved remarkably quickly by local thrombolytic secretions.

FLUID EXCHANGE IN THE PULMONARY CIRCULATION

The fluid flux across the pulmonary vascular endothelium is influenced by the same pressure relationship as in the systemic capillaries, summarized in the modified Starling equation (Table 4.1). The hydrostatic pressure in the pulmonary microvessels (Pmv) exceeds the interstitial hydrostatic pressure (Ppmv) outside the microvessels. This effect favors filtration. The interstitial tissue fluid protein osmotic pressure is probably about two thirds that in the vessel; thus, the net osmotic force is absorptive and inward. The components of this equation make it convenient to categorize abnormal fluid flux into the lung into two broad types: hydrostatic edema, when the primary abnormality is an increase in Pmv minus Ppmv, and permeability edema, when endothelial injury increases fluid conductivity across the membrane (incorporated into the permeability factor) and

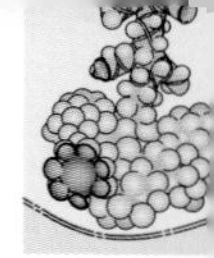

Table 4.1
The Starling equation

$F = Kf[(Pmv - Ppmv) - \sigma(\pi v - \pi t)]$

Symbol	Description
F	Net fluid flux out of vessels
Kf	Permeability factor
σ	Reflection coefficient to oncotic agents
Pmv	Pressure in microvessels
Ppmv	Perimicrovascular pressure
pv	Osmotic pressure in vessels
pt	Osmotic pressure of tissues

decreases the osmotic reflection coefficient and osmotic gradient. The terms *cardiogenic* and *noncardiogenic* are also commonly used for these two mechanisms of edema formation.

Fluid flux is sensitive to small intravascular or perivascular pressure changes. Intravascular pressure rises may originate downstream (left heart failure) or may follow overall vascular volume increments (overhydration) or displacement of blood from the systemic to the pulmonary vessels. Fluid is exchanged across the capillary walls, but the interstitial space around alveolar microvessels is tightly restricted by the collagen network between the alveolar walls. The two alveolar epithelial layers and the contained capillary bed form an inexpansible sandwich, so leakage is limited. The extra-alveolar arterioles and venules, which are not so confined and are also very thin walled, may be an additional important site of fluid leakage.

Surface tension in the fluid film that lines the alveoli opposes alveolar pressure and tends to lower the interstitial pressure around pulmonary microvessels, particularly in corner areas (see Fig. 4.4). An increase in surface tension may contribute to edema when surfactant is lost in an injured lung. Interstitial pressure around the extra-alveolar vessels is close to intrathoracic (pleural) pressure and falls as the lungs are distended, which favors relatively more leakage from them at high rather than low lung volumes (see Fig. 4.3).

Interstitial Edema

Normally, a net outflow of fluid from the upstream capillaries is reabsorbed into the downstream capillaries, where the intravascular pressure is lower.

Several factors tend to keep the lung from becoming edematous. Fluid leakage causes local perivascular pressures to rise, particularly in the "sandwich" between the alveolar walls, which reduces the outward fluid flux. It may also compress the vessels, which reduces the total surface available for leakage. Because the fluid that leaks through intact endothelium is largely protein free, it dilutes and washes out the interstitial protein. This reduces the perivascular osmotic pressure of tissues and thus increases the inward osmotic pressure difference and reduces the local fluid leak. If excess leakage does occur, the fluid moves from the alveolar walls, where it could interfere with gas exchange, into the low-pressure interstitial zones around the bronchovascular bundles, where it forms relatively innocuous venous, arterial, and peribronchial cuffs. This fluid may be absorbed in part by the rich bronchial vascular network and by the many lymphatics in the adventitia of the airways and vessels. Edema fluid may also reach the pleural space, where it is absorbed by the pleural lymphatic and blood vessels. Finally, experimental data suggest that all the blood perfusing the capillaries in alveolar walls must first pass through capillaries located in alveolar corners, and that the negative interstitial pressure surrounding these corner capillaries (and, accordingly, the transmural pressure) is critically dependent on alveolar surface tension. When surface tension is eliminated by alveolar flooding, interstitial pressure around these vessels increases, thus serving to compress the corner vessels and diminish flow through the capillaries in the alveolar wall of these flooded alveoli. This mechanism provides for much more precise control of perfusion, virtually on an alveolus-to-alveolus basis, compared with the effects of alveolar hypoxia, which are directed to much more proximal vessels.

When the capillary endothelium is injured, locally or through the effect of circulating mediators, the vascular permeability to fluids and solutes is increased so that even a modest outward pressure gradient causes a large fluid leak. The ability to retain large molecules is lost, protein-rich plasma leaks out, and the osmotic pressure in tissues approaches that in vessels, so that the osmotic force opposing intravascular hydrostatic pressure is lost. This high-permeability or "leaky capillary" edema can be a fulminant process and lead to severe abnormalities of gas exchange.

Alveolar Edema

The epithelial cells that line the air spaces have tight junctions along their apical surface, so this membrane is normally much less permeable than the endothelial membrane, protecting alveolar spaces as interstitial edema increases. After total lung water has increased by about 50%, the edema fluid appears in the alveoli. A structural failure, at the epithelial cell junctions or elsewhere, is suspected, as there is no protein gradient between interstitial and alveolar edema fluid. Fluid is initially seen only in the corners of the alveoli, where the pressure below the curved fluid film is lowest. As more fluid accumulates, the alveoli rapidly become completely filled, again because of surface tension effects. As alveoli fill, the radius of the curvature of the meniscus of the fluid becomes shorter, and the effect of surface tension becomes greater (Laplace's law), which pulls fluid in more strongly (Fig. 4.7). Thus, the sequence of edema development progresses from the perimicrovascular interstitium to peribronchovascular "sump" to patchy alveolar flooding.

Fluid and ions normally exchange across the bronchial and alveolar epithelial surfaces to regulate the character of the mucous blanket and maintain the subphase film beneath the surfactant that lines the alveoli. Alveolar edema can be cleared by an active process of sodium reabsorption with water following osmotic transport. The type II epithelial cells take in sodium through channels on their apical surface and move it by active Na^+,K^+-ATPase pumping on the basolateral surfaces into the interstitium. The type I cells appear to have similar, though less prominent, apparatus and, because they make up 95% of the surface, might have a significant role. This has not been demonstrated, however, as type I cell culture models are lacking. Fluid removal may also occur in distal airways where epithelial and

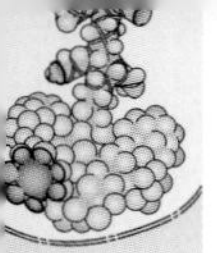

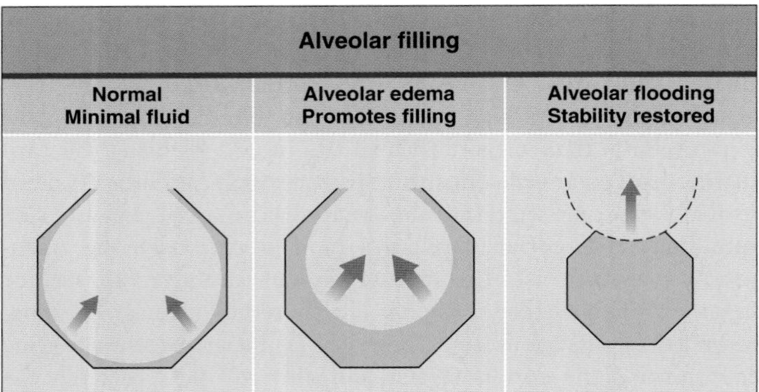

Figure 4.7 Alveoli tend to fill with fluid in an "all-or-none" fashion. In the normal alveolus, a small amount of fluid rounds off the corners. Alveolar edema decreases the radius, which increases the inward force of surface tension and pulls in more fluid. When the alveolus is filled, the radius of the surface increases, so stability is regained. Modified with permission from Butler J: The circulation of the lung. In Culver BH [ed]: The Respiratory System. Seattle, ASUW Publications, 1997, pp 111-122.

Clara cells actively transport sodium. These active mechanisms are also crucial in the initial clearance of fetal lung fluid at birth. In experimental models, fluid clearance from air spaces is enhanced by β_2-agonists and blocked by the antagonist propranolol.

High-Altitude Pulmonary Edema

Some individuals traveling or climbing to high altitude develop pulmonary edema that may be severe and life threatening. The mechanisms are becoming better understood and seem to involve both hydrostatic and permeability factors. The underlying abnormality in individuals who are susceptible to high-altitude pulmonary edema (HAPE), and who are subject to repeated episodes with repeated exposures, is an exaggerated elevation of pulmonary artery pressure in response to hypoxia that is further increased by exertion. Susceptible individuals have slight elevations of Ppa at rest or during routine activities when breathing air at sea level and have a greater increase in response to exercise than control subjects do. In response to a hypoxic challenge, HAPE-susceptible subjects have a rise in Ppa that is three- to fourfold higher than that of controls. At altitude, typically greater than 3000 m, Ppa in these individuals would be expected to rise rapidly in response to alveolar hypoxia and to increase further with the exertion that is common to mountaineering activities. Symptomatic edema develops over 24 hours to a few days but rarely occurs after 5 days at altitude. The few hemodynamic measurements made under these circumstances have shown marked elevation of Ppa systolic pressure, as high as 80 to 100 mmHg, but usually normal pulmonary arterial occlusion pressure. Thus, although high hydrostatic forces are involved, this is not a typical cardiogenic mechanism with elevation of left atrial pressure reflected into the pulmonary microvasculature. The site of hypoxic vasoconstriction is in small pulmonary arteries and arterioles, although there is some venoconstriction that could contribute to a pressure increase at the capillary level. It has been hypothesized that a heterogeneous distribution of the increased pulmonary vascular resistance might divert relatively high blood flow to low-resistance arterioles, increasing local microvascular pressure sufficient to cause the patchy edema pattern typically seen in radiographs of those with HAPE. Interestingly, bronchoalveolar lavage fluid obtained from climbers on Mt. Whitney and elsewhere with symptomatic HAPE has shown high levels of protein, which is consistent with increased vascular permeability, and red cells, suggesting further loss of barrier function. Because granulocytes and inflammatory markers are seen in modest quantities and more likely later in the course, this is believed to be a noninflammatory permeability change. This may be explained by the stretching of pores under hydrostatic forces or, in more severe cases, by overt capillary stress failure with endothelial, epithelial, and basement membrane disruption, as described in rabbit lungs subjected to high intravascular pressure. Although the cellular mechanisms responsible for the exaggerated pulmonary vascular response are yet to be elucidated, there is now a plausible sequence of events leading to pulmonary edema in HAPE-susceptible individuals.

RESPIRATORY-CIRCULATORY INTERACTIONS

Spontaneous Breathing

The phasic changes of intrathoracic pressure and lung volume of the respiratory cycle alter the preload and afterload of the right and left heart, which interact to vary cardiac output and blood pressure with the respiratory cycle. The changes are modest during normal tidal breathing but can be more notable in pathologic states. During inhalation, the decrease in intrathoracic pressure enhances systemic venous return to the chest. The right atrium and ventricle fill, and right heart output to the pulmonary vessels increases as the alveoli fill with air. Lung expansion dilates the extra-alveolar pulmonary arterial vessels, which reduces their resistance and helps to accommodate the increased flow. Ppa stays almost constant relative to PA. The increase in right ventricular volume tends to stiffen or compress the left ventricle within the common pericardium, but the surge of pulmonary flow reaches the left heart after two to three beats, so that systemic output and blood pressure begin to rise in late inspiration or early expiration. This preload effect is normally dominant, but the inspiratory drop in intrathoracic pressure can also add effective afterload to the left ventricle. When the pressure outside the heart is lower, the myocardium must generate a greater transmural pressure difference to maintain the same stroke volume. Accordingly, systemic blood pressure falls a few millimeters of mercury coincident with inspiration and rises a few millimeters of mercury during exhalation. Depending on the respiratory rate, this direct pressure effect may be enhanced or countered by the arrival at the left ventricle of the inspiratory surge of pulmonary flow.

When intrathoracic pressure swings are exaggerated, as occurs during an asthma attack or an exacerbation of chronic obstructive pulmonary disease, the inspiratory drop in blood pressure can be 20 to 30 mmHg, creating the clinical finding of pulsus paradoxus. Interestingly, such markedly negative inspiratory pressures do not generate a proportionate increase in systemic venous return because of a flow-limiting, or waterfall, mechanism in the central veins. When the intraluminal pressure falls in these veins, the vessels collapse at the point where they are first exposed to atmospheric pressure, in the neck, axilla, and abdomen, and their flow becomes independent of the increasingly negative downstream right atrial pressure.

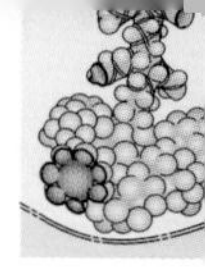

When the pericardial space is limited (e.g., pericardial effusion, constrictive pericarditis, enlarged heart), the interaction between the two ventricles is more prominent. Inspiratory filling of the right heart limits the diastolic expansion of the left heart. This ventricular interaction contributes to an inspiratory decrease in systemic outflow and blood pressure and allows them to increase when the right heart is less full during expiration.

Positive Pressure Ventilation

When patients are mechanically ventilated with positive inspiratory pressure, the same mechanisms seen in spontaneous breathing are involved, but the pressure effects shift the phase of the tidal cycle. For example, the pressure outside the left ventricle rises during inspiration, so the same contraction yields a higher blood pressure early in the inspiratory phase. This may be augmented by blood pushed out of the capillaries by the positive alveolar pressure (see Fig. 4.3). During late inspiration or early expiration, the blood pressure decreases as the effect of an inspiratory decrease in venous return to the right heart reaches the left side. If the expiratory phase is long enough, the blood pressure will begin to rise, reflecting enhanced venous return to the right heart earlier in expiration.

In addition to the cyclic changes, there are overall effects on cardiac output when spontaneous breathing is replaced by positive pressure ventilation, particularly when positive end-expiratory pressure (PEEP) is added. The mean airway pressure and mean intrathoracic pressure are both higher, and the latter is reflected in the pressure outside the right heart. This, in turn, causes the right atrial pressure to be higher, which may decrease the pressure difference, driving venous flow from the systemic capacitance vessels (alternatively, the increase in lung volume may partially compress the inferior vena cava as it runs through the lung just above the diaphragm, thereby increasing resistance to venous return). A resultant decrease in cardiac output is typically seen, accompanied by a decrease in right atrial transmural pressure and a decrease in right ventricular end-diastolic volume, particularly if intravascular volume is low. This may be opposed by a rise in abdominal pressure as thoracic volume increases and by increased venous tone to help restore the driving pressure for venous return.

When an increase in end-expiratory lung volume is recruited by PEEP, the chest wall must also be passively expanded, and its pressure-volume relationship (see Fig. 2.7) would predict at least a modest increase in pleural pressure. However, direct measurements with suitable flat devices show that when the lungs are distended with PEEP, the pressure in the cardiac fossa may rise more than that measured by an esophageal balloon, and the pressure in the pericardium may be still higher. Bedside measurements of a decreased cardiac output accompanied by a higher pulmonary arterial occlusion pressure may suggest a decrease in cardiac function or contractility, but when accurate measurements of juxtacardiac pressure or left ventricular end-diastolic volume are made, the ventricle is seen to be operating at a lower preload on the same function curve. The same phenomenon may be seen when patients with severe airflow obstruction develop dynamic hyperinflation with an associated increase in cardiac fossa pressure.

High levels of PEEP and of end-inspiratory alveolar pressure compress alveolar septal capillaries, outweighing any distention of extra-alveolar vessels with the lung volume increase, and thus increase pulmonary vascular resistance and right ventricular afterload. If this effect becomes dominant, a decrease in cardiac output may be associated with an increase in right ventricular end-diastolic volume.

The increase in juxtacardiac pressure with PEEP decreases the stroke work the left ventricle must do to maintain any given systemic blood pressure, thus effectively decreasing left ventricular afterload. In most circumstances, the preload effect previously described dominates, but a failing ventricle is quite sensitive to afterload, and this effect becomes more important in patients with severe heart disease.

HEMODYNAMIC MONITORING IN CRITICAL ILLNESS

Many critically ill patients require frequent or continuous assessments to identify potentially life-threatening conditions and to guide the use of life-sustaining treatments. Hemodynamic monitoring devices aid clinicians in assessing circulatory function, arterial blood oxygenation, and oxygen delivery to systemic tissues. Devices used frequently in intensive care units include central venous catheters, pulmonary artery catheters, pulse oximeters, and systemic arterial catheters. The rationale for the use of each of these monitoring devices is reviewed in this section. Fine points and caveats for data interpretation are discussed.

Central Venous Catheters

A catheter placed in the superior vena cava allows measurement of central venous pressure (CVP), which is usually similar to right ventricular end-diastolic pressure. It may, accordingly, reflect right ventricular preload and therefore be used to estimate right ventricular end-diastolic volume (preload). Because both right and left ventricular end-diastolic volumes are primary determinant of stroke volume and cardiac output, CVP is sometimes useful in the assessment of patients with circulatory dysfunction. For example, a low CVP in a patient with hypotension suggests that vascular volume is inadequate and that administration of intravenous fluids or blood products may be appropriate. A high CVP in a patient with diffuse pulmonary infiltrates and hypoxemia may suggest volume overload or congestive heart failure and the need for diuretics and fluid restriction. Central venous catheters are also frequently necessary for the intravenous administration of vasoactive drugs and caustic infusates.

The reader is referred elsewhere for detailed instructions on the placement of central venous catheters. New evidence suggests that complications of placement can be minimized by using maximal barrier precautions and chlorhexidine antisepsis and avoiding the femoral site. The most common sites of insertion of central venous catheters are the internal jugular vein and the subclavian vein. Under some circumstances, the external jugular, brachial, cephalic, and femoral sites are used.

SITES OF CENTRAL VENOUS CATHETERIZATION

The decision of which vessel to cannulate should take into consideration the patient's clinical status, risk of infectious and mechanical complications, anatomy, and operator experience.

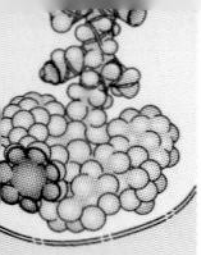

Table 4.2
Advantages and disadvantages of major routes of access for central line insertion

Site	Advantages	Disadvantages
Internal jugular	↓ Risk of pneumothorax	Landmarks may be obscured with intubated patient or patients who have a tracheostomy
	Easily compressible	More difficult in hypovolemic patient
	Higher rate success with inexperienced operators	?↑ Risk of infection
Subclavian	Consistent landmarks	Noncompressible site
	Patient comfort	May be higher risk of complications with inexperienced operators
	Most reliable access in hypovolemic patient	↑ Risk of pneumothorax
Femoral	Easily accessed during cardiopulmonary resuscitation	Difficult access in hypovolemic patient
	Compressible site	?↑ Risk of infection
	No need for Trendelenburg	?↑ Risk of thromboembolism
		May be less effective for monitoring central venous pressure in some patients

The subclavian vein may be the preferred approach in a patient who is hypovolemic and has normal coagulation parameters. It is also the preferred site to minimize infectious complications. During cardiopulmonary resuscitation, the femoral site might be preferred while the airway is being secured. In patients with uncorrected coagulopathies, the cephalic, brachial, and femoral sites may be preferred because they can be more easily compressed to reduce bleeding. If possible, the subclavian vein should be avoided in patients with hyperinflated lungs or bullae, which predispose to pneumothorax. In patients with ascites or elevated pleural pressures, a femoral CVP may not accurately reflect right atrial pressure. The risks and benefits of the different approaches to central venous access are compared in Table 4.2.

COMPLICATIONS OF CENTRAL VENOUS CATHETERIZATION

All catheters represent potential sources of infection. To prevent catheter-related bloodstream infections, sterile procedure and maintenance techniques should be strictly followed. The femoral site is more prone to infectious complications and venous thrombosis compared with the subclavian site. Other complications of central catheters are often related to the site of insertion. The most frequent mechanical complications from internal jugular cannulation are carotid artery puncture, hematoma, and pneumothorax. With subclavian vein catheterization, patients are at risk for pneumothorax, subclavian artery puncture, hemothorax, and hematoma. Risks of femoral vein catheterization include femoral artery puncture, which may cause a retroperitoneal hematoma; an increased incidence of catheter-related bacteremia; and venous thrombosis. All central venous catheters can cause venous thrombosis, but the clinical significance of these clots is not clear. Mechanical complications of central venous catheterization are included in Table 4.2.

The risk of complications, both mechanical and infectious, is directly proportional to the number of attempts at catheterization. In some studies, the incidence of complications was substantially higher when the procedures were performed by less experienced operators. As a general rule, operators who are unsuccessful at gaining access at a single site with two to three passes should attempt to obtain access from another site or seek assistance from a more experienced operator. Recent studies suggest that the use of real-time sonographic devices may minimize complications, especially for inexperienced operators, but the value of such devices for experienced operators is unclear. When attempts to obtain access via the subclavian or internal jugular route are unsuccessful, a chest radiograph should be obtained to rule out pneumothorax before attempting insertion on the contralateral site.

LIMITATIONS OF CENTRAL VENOUS PRESSURE MONITORING

In many clinical situations, CVP does not accurately reflect left ventricular end-diastolic pressure and therefore cannot be used to estimate left ventricular preload. For example, a patient with pulmonary hypertension might have elevated CVP but normal or low left ventricular end-diastolic pressure and volume. In patients with acute left ventricular myocardial infarction, CVP may be modestly elevated, while left atrial and left ventricular end-diastolic pressures are severely increased, with radiographic and clinical evidence of pulmonary edema. In patients with ascites or elevated pleural pressures, the pressures measured in the femoral vein may not accurately reflect right atrial pressure. Moreover, changes in CVP frequently do not predict the changes in left heart pressures.

In more than 25% of patients with mitral valve disease, right atrial pressure is discordant with left atrial. In some of these patients, fluid loading causes right and left atrial pressures to diverge, and responses of right atrial pressure and left ventricular end-diastolic volume to pressor agents are inconsistent. Thus, in many critically ill patients, CVP may provide misleading information about left heart pressure and preload or response to therapy. Additional methods for evaluating cardiac filling pressures and function are frequently required.

Pulmonary Artery Catheters

In 1970, Swan and colleagues reported the development of a balloon-tipped flow-directed catheter to measure pulmonary artery pressure and estimate left ventricular end-diastolic pressure (Fig. 4.8). The catheter was introduced through a central vein, such as the subclavian or internal jugular, and advanced through the chambers of the right heart into a medium-sized pulmonary artery. When positioned in a pulmonary artery and inflated, the small balloon at the catheter tip caused cessation of blood flow distal to the catheter, resulting in a stagnant column of blood from the pulmonary capillary bed to a confluence of medium-sized veins where flow was continuing. Thus, the pressure measured at the catheter tip immediately distal to the balloon—pulmonary arterial occlusion pressure (Ppao)—reflected a pressure close to the left atrium and therefore could, under most circumstances, be used to estimate left ventricular end-diastolic pressure. Use of Ppao avoids some of the previously described limitations of CVP for assessing vascular filling and ventricular preload.

Several years after the introduction of the balloon-tipped flow-directed catheter, techniques were developed by which cardiac output could also be measured via a pulmonary artery catheter (PAC) using a modification of the catheter developed

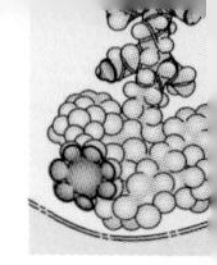

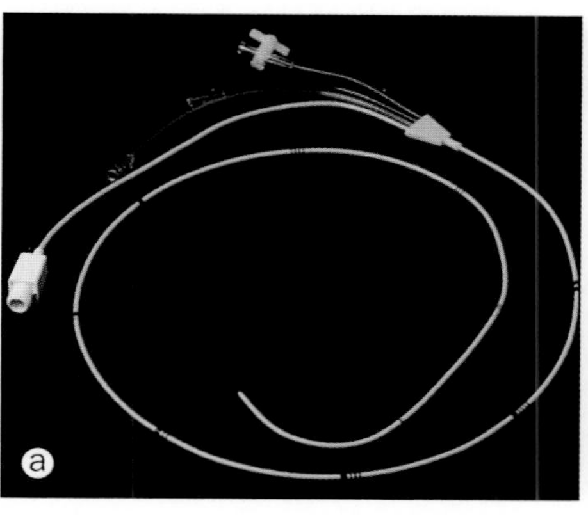

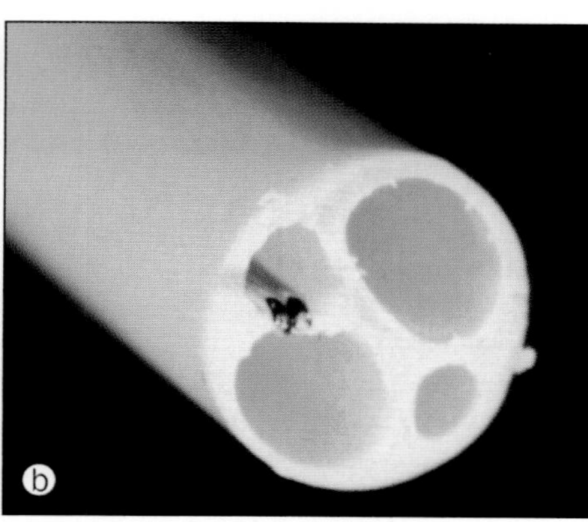

Figure 4.8 Pulmonary artery catheter. A, Red—channel for balloon inflation; blue—channel to proximal port (for right atrial pressure and injectate); yellow—channel to distal port (for measurement of pulmonary artery pressure and pulmonary capillary wedge pressure); bright yellow—thermistor connection. **B,** Cross section of pulmonary artery catheter. Clockwise from left: thermistor wire, distal port channel, balloon channel, proximal port channel.

by Swan. Cooled fluid is injected through a separate channel of the catheter, exiting the channel through a side hole in the right heart. Blood temperature is monitored with a thermistor at the catheter tip. When the change in blood temperature is graphed against time, analysis of the area and shape of the curve allows a calculation of flow (cardiac output) between the sites of cool fluid injection and the thermistor at the distal catheter tip. With concomitant measurements of blood pressure, right and left atrial pressures, and arterial and mixed venous blood gases, the PAC allows the determination of systemic and pulmonary vascular resistance, systemic oxygen delivery, and oxygen extraction by systemic tissue. Since its development and introduction to clinical practice, the PAC has become an important part of the hemodynamic monitoring armamentarium of many intensivists.

INTERPRETATION OF DATA

Several assumptions are required to use Ppao to estimate left ventricular end-diastolic volume (Fig. 4.9). These assumptions pertain to two key questions: (1) How well does Ppao represent left ventricular end-diastolic pressure (see Fig. 4.9, assumptions a, b, c and d)? (2) How well does left ventricular end-diastolic pressure represent left ventricular end-diastolic volume (see Fig. 4.9, assumptions e and f)? Intensivists must consider these assumptions to avoid errors when reading Pcw tracings and interpreting their significance.

Some mechanically ventilated patients require high levels of PEEP or continuous positive airway pressure (CPAP) to improve oxygenation. This raises juxtacardiac pressure and tends to cause a misleading elevation in Ppao (see Fig. 4.9, assumption f). To correct for this effect, some workers have advocated measuring Ppao approximately 1 second after briefly disconnecting the ventilator from the endotracheal tube. However, this could cause hypoxemia from abrupt decreased alveolar derecruitment or could contribute to lung injury from repeated closing and reopening of small airways. Another approach is to assume that approximately 25% of the PEEP or CPAP is transmitted to the juxtacardiac pressure space and subtract this amount from the measured Ppao (after correcting for the difference in units, as PEEP and CPAP are reported in cmH_2O and Ppao is measured in mmHg). As a rule of thumb, this adjustment can be made by subtracting 25% of the PEEP or CPAP value from Pcw.

It is important to read the Ppao at end-expiration. This is the point in the respiratory cycle when the juxtacardiac pressure is closest to atmospheric pressure (regardless of the level of PEEP

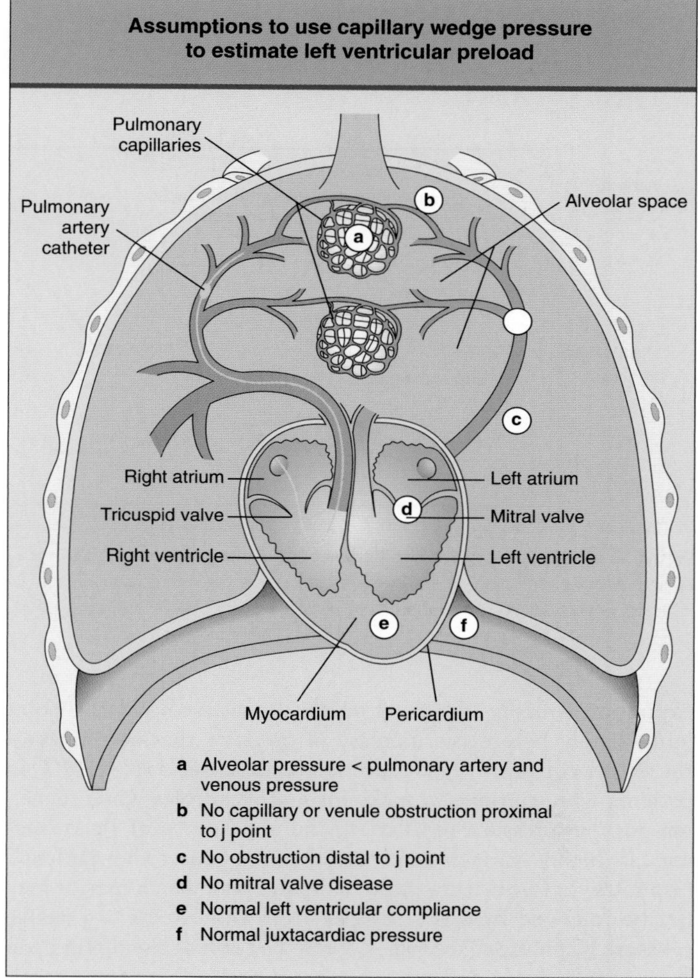

Figure 4.9 Assumptions required to use capillary wedge pressure to estimate left ventricular preload.

or CPAP; see Fig. 4.9, assumption f). Identifying the point of end-expiration on the Ppao tracing is straightforward in patients breathing spontaneously, without positive pressure ventilatory assistance: the Ppao should be read immediately before the dip in pressure that signifies the beginning of inspiration (Fig. 4.10*A*). In patients receiving positive pressure ventilation and who are making no inspiratory efforts of their own, end-

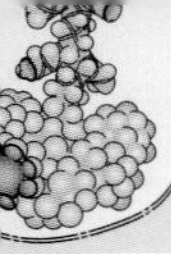

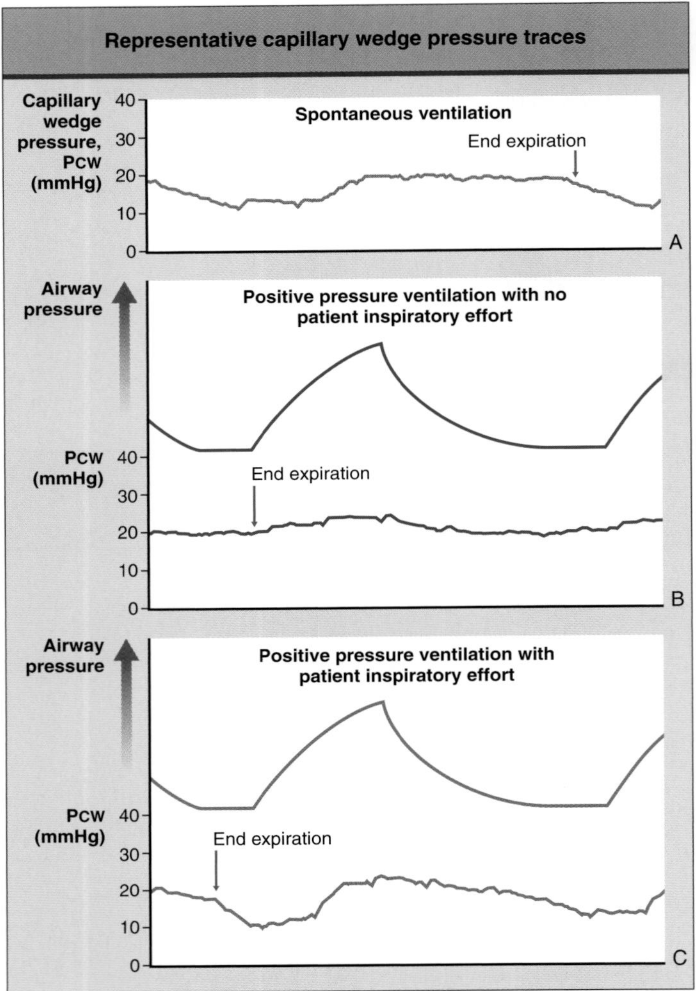

Figure 4.10 Representative capillary wedge pressure traces. Shown are **A,** spontaneous ventilation, **B,** positive pressure ventilation with no patient inspiratory effort, and **C,** positive pressure ventilation with patient inspiratory effort.

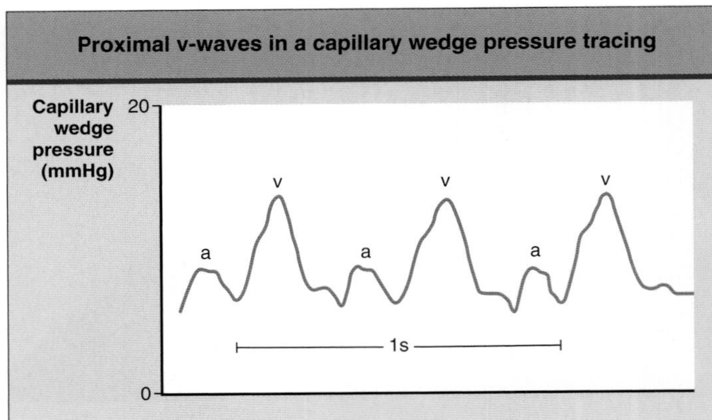

Figure 4.11 Proximal v waves in a capillary wedge pressure tracing.

expiration is easily identified on the Ppao tracing as the point immediately before the increase in pressure that accompanies the effects of positive pressure inspiration (see Fig. 4.10*B*). In patients who continue to make inspiratory efforts while receiving positive pressure ventilation, the appearance of Ppao tracings is highly variable and often ambiguous. The patient's inspiratory effort usually causes a dip in Ppao, which may or may not be followed by a rise in Ppao from the effects of positive pressure inspiration (see Fig. 4.10C). The size of the dip in Ppao in early inspiration and the subsequent rise in Ppao from ventilator pressure depend on the magnitude of the patient's effort in relation to the ventilator flow rate. In patients with vigorous inspiratory efforts, Ppao tracings resemble those of patients breathing spontaneously without positive pressure assistance: the rise in Ppao due to ventilator assistance may not occur at all. Regardless of the magnitudes of these dips and rises in Ppao, it is critical to read Ppao at end-expiration. Reading Ppao at the wrong point in the cycle can lead to wrong treatment decisions.

The effect of left ventricular end-diastolic compliance must also be considered when interpreting a Ppao value (see Fig. 4.9, assumption e). In a patient with normal left ventricular end-diastolic compliance, a Ppao of 12 mmHg may reflect ample diastolic filling. In contrast, in a patient with reduced diastolic compliance, as in hypertrophic cardiomyopathy, a Ppao of 12 mmHg may reflect inadequate end-diastolic volume.

When there is increased atrial filling during ventricular systole, as in mitral regurgitation, the Ppao tracing may show enlarged v waves (Fig. 4.11). These may also appear in other conditions, such as mitral stenosis and hypervolemia. If the mean Ppao is read in the presence of large v waves, left ventricular end-diastolic pressure and diastolic filling may be overestimated. To avoid this error, the Ppao tracing should be read immediately before the start of the v wave, as close as possible to end-expiration. This usually appears around the time of the T wave during simultaneous electrocardiogram recordings.

ROLE OF THE PULMONARY ARTERY CATHETER

Experienced physicians frequently have difficulty using common clinical and laboratory data to assess circulation in critically ill patients. This is especially true in patients requiring mechanical ventilation. Noninvasive techniques such as echocardiography are often not helpful in distinguishing among the different forms of shock.

In a study of patients in whom PACs were placed, attending intensivists and critical care fellows were correct in slightly more than 50% of their estimations of cardiac index, Ppao, and mean pulmonary artery pressure based on their clinical assessments. Changes in therapy were made in almost half of patients based on information subsequently obtained from PACs.

In general, PACs should be considered when two conditions occur together:

1. Usual clinical observations and laboratory data are ambiguous with respect to the assessment of circulation, particularly in the presence of hypotension. For example, a patient may have hypotension and low urine output, suggesting low cardiac output from inadequate vascular volume. However, the same patient may also have clinical or radiographic findings consistent with pulmonary edema and diffuse pulmonary infiltrates, suggesting volume overload or cardiac dysfunction.
2. Consequences of the wrong treatment decision may worsen the physiologic abnormalities. If the patient just described

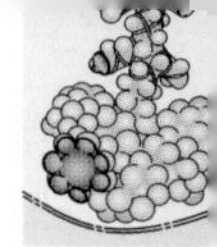

Table 4.3
Hemodynamic equations and normal values

Parameter	Formula	Normal values
Mean arterial pressure (MAP)	[(Diastolic pressure x 2) + systolic pressure]/3	10.6–13.3 kPa (80–100 mmHg)
Cardiac index (CI)	Cardiac output/body surface area	2.5–4.0 L/min per m^2
Stroke index (SI)	CI/heart rate	30–65 mL/beat per m^2
Systemic vascular resistance	[(MAP – Right atrial pressure) x 80]/Cardiac output	1200–1600 dyn . sec . cm^{25}
Pulmonary vascular resistance	{[Mean pulmonary arterial pressure (MPAP) – pulmonary capillary wedge pressure (Pcw)] x 80}/cardiac output	200–400 dyn . sec . cm^{25}
Left ventricular stroke work index	(MAP – Pcw) x SI x 0.0136	45–60 g/beat per m^2
Right ventricular stroke work index	(MPAP – central venous pressure) x SI x 0.0136	5–10 g/beat per m^2
Oxygen delivery	CI x 10 x Cao_2	500–750 mL/min per m^2
Arterial oxygen content (Cao_2)	1.34 x Hemoglobin x Sao_2 + [0.0031 x arterial partial pressure of oxygen (Pao_2)]	16–20 mL/dL
Mixed venous oxygen content (Cvo_2)	1.34 x Hemoglobin x Svo_2 + (0.0031 x Pao_2)	13–15 mL/dL
Difference between Cao_2 and Cvo_2	$Cao_2 - Cvo_2$	3.5–5.0 mL/dL
Oxygen consumption	($Cao_2 - Cvo_2$) x CI x 10	100–175 mL/min per m^2

were truly hypovolemic but a diuretic were prescribed, shock would worsen. If the patient were in congestive heart failure but intravenous fluids and blood products were given, pulmonary edema would worsen. It is necessary to carefully adjust preload and afterload to maximize cardiac output.

Under most other circumstances, it may be prudent to attempt a trial of therapy based on clinical impressions before PAC placement. For example, in a young hypotensive patient with apparent sepsis, warm extremities, and marginal urine output, intravenous fluids followed by vasopressors may be prescribed. If improvement is not apparent or if the patient deteriorates over the next several hours, perhaps with worsening azotemia and hypotension, the decision to place a PAC can be reconsidered. In the absence of pulmonary edema, hypotension and low urine output should always be treated rapidly with additional volume.

Appropriate use of the PAC can also provide valuable information on physiologic parameters pertaining to circulation, oxygenation, and organ perfusion. Hemodynamic parameters that are directly or indirectly obtained with PACs are summarized in Table 4.3. A common problem in critically ill patients is hypotension. PAC data allow the distinction between hypotension from low cardiac output versus that caused by low systemic vascular resistance. When hypotension is caused by low cardiac output, Ppao values indicate whether low cardiac output is the result of inadequate preload or poor cardiac performance. Typical hemodynamic profiles in various shock conditions are shown in Table 4.4. The PAC is frequently useful for guiding therapy with intravenous fluids and blood products, vasopressors, and inotropic drugs in patients with circulatory failure. The PAC can also be diagnostic of cardiac tamponade.

Table 4.4
Typical hemodynamic parameters of shock

Cardiac index	Pulmonary capillary wedge pressure	Central venous pressure	Systemic vascular resistance	Diagnosis
↑	↓⇔	↓	↓	Distributive shock (e.g., septic shock, anaphylactic shock)
				Cardiogenic shock
↓	↑	↑	↑	Left ventricular myocardial infarction
↓	↓⇔	↑	↑	Right ventricular myocardial infarction
↓	↓	↓	↑	Hypovolemic shock (e.g., massive gastrointestinal hemorrhage)
				Extracardiac obstructive
↓	↑	↑	↑	Tension pneumothorax
↓	↓	↑⇔	↑	Massive pulmonary embolism
↓	↑	↑	↑	Pericardial tamponade

COMPLICATIONS OF PULMONARY ARTERY CATHETERIZATION

As with any invasive procedure, PAC insertion can cause complications. These can be grouped into several categories. First, there are mechanical complications of vascular access, as outlined in Table 4.2. Second, there are mechanical complications of PAC placement, as outlined in Table 4.5. The third group of complications includes infections involving the insertion site, the catheter itself, and the tricuspid and pulmonic valves. Finally, there are complications caused by the incorrect interpretation and use of PAC data.

Arterial Pressure Monitoring

Arterial pressure must be assessed frequently to identify life-threatening changes in circulatory status and to monitor the effectiveness of life-sustaining treatments, such as blood products and vasopressors. Traditional blood pressure assessment by sphygmomanometry is impractical in critically ill patients

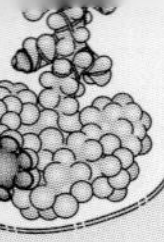

Table 4.5 Complications of pulmonary artery catheterization		
Complication	**Risk factor for complication**	**Measures to avoid complication**
Arrhythmia	Catheter coiled in right ventricle Balloon not inflated while advancing	Familiarity with usual distance to wedged position Check balloon
Complete heart block	Left bundle branch block	Have transvenous or external pacer available
Balloon rupture	Overinflation	Check balloon prior to insertion Use only 1.5 mL air to inflate balloon
Pulmonary artery rupture	Inflation of balloon too distal Use of more than 1.5 mL air for inflation Catheter use during coronary artery bypass surgery during cold cardioplegia	Do not overwedge Use only 1.5 mL air to inflate balloon Remove pulmonary artery catheter to right atrium during coronary artery bypass surgery
Pulmonary infarction	Catheter tip too distal Prolonged balloon inflation	Check chest radiograph Always deflate balloon
Catheter-associated thrombosis and embolism	Prolonged catheterization	Remove catheter as soon as feasible
Infection	Prolonged catheterization	Remove catheter as soon as feasible Maximal barrier precautions during insertion
Valvular or papillary muscle damage	Knotting of catheter around papillary muscle Withdrawal of catheter with balloon inflated	Familiarity with usual distance to wedge position Deflate balloon prior to catheter withdrawal
Cardiac rupture	Myocardial infarction Stiff catheter Small ventricular chamber	Keep catheter tip out of right ventricle Remove catheter to right atrium during coronary artery bypass surgery

because of the time required for each measurement. Invasive blood pressure monitoring allows continuous measurement through an indwelling vascular catheter. Automated noninvasive techniques allow frequent blood pressure measurements with an inflatable pneumatic cuff wrapped around the upper or lower extremity.

INVASIVE ARTERIAL PRESSURE MONITORING

Measurement of arterial blood pressure by an indwelling vascular catheter is more accurate than other methods of measurement. Moreover, a graphic display of arterial pressure can be viewed in "real time" to provide diagnostic and therapeutic information that is not available with other techniques (Fig. 4.12). Invasive pressure monitoring is of greatest value in conditions in which large changes in arterial pressure occur quickly, such as shock, or when intravenous vasodilators are used for hypertensive emergencies. Another advantage of invasive arterial pressure monitoring is that arterial blood gases can be drawn frequently through the catheter. This is especially important in patients with severe acid-base disorders or acute respiratory failure requiring mechanical ventilation.

AUTOMATED NONINVASIVE BLOOD PRESSURE MONITORING

This technique provides intermittent measurements of arterial blood pressure. An inflatable pneumatic cuff is wrapped around the upper arm and inflated to a pressure that exceeds arterial systolic pressure. The cuff pressure is then slowly deflated while pressure in the cuff is continuously monitored by the automated system. When cuff pressure decreases below arterial systolic pressure, oscillations in cuff pressure are created by the pulsations of arterial blood. Analysis of the pressures at which these oscillations begin, become maximal, and cease provides estimations of systolic, mean, and diastolic pressures.

Automated noninvasive blood pressure measurements can be obtained at frequent intervals, such as every 5 minutes.

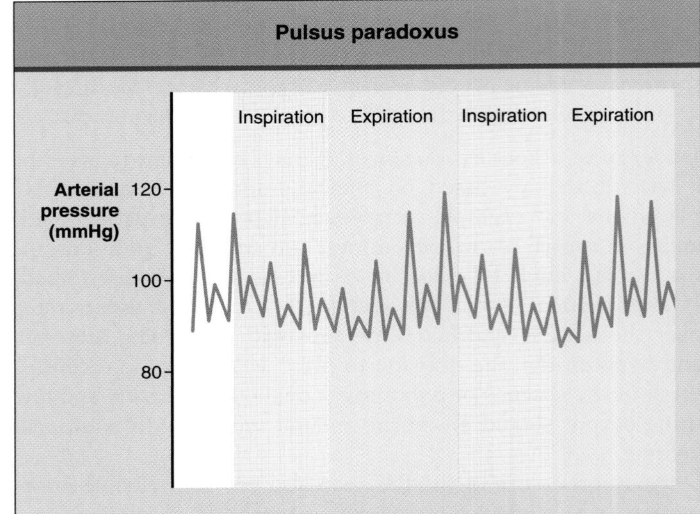

Figure 4.12 Arterial pressure tracing showing pulsus paradoxus. Systolic pressure falls by greater than 1.3 kPa (>10 mmHg) during inspiration.

However, these pressure measurements are not as accurate as those obtained by an indwelling vascular catheter, especially when there is systemic vasodilatation, as in septic shock. Moreover, intermittent measurements of arterial pressure with noninvasive techniques do not provide graphic displays (see Fig. 4.12).

Pulse Oximetry

Pulse oximetry provides a virtually continuous assessment and digital display of oxyhemoglobin saturation, which is one of the key determinants of oxygen delivery to systemic tissues. Light-emitting diodes are applied comfortably to the skin or

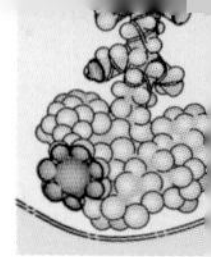

Table 4.6
Factors that affect accuracy of pulse oximetry

Poor circulation (low cardiac output, vasoconstriction)
Low true oxygen saturation (<90%)
Ambient light
Effects of nail polish, skin pigmentation
Carboxyhemoglobin and methemoglobin
Motion artifact

fingernail. Light absorbance by oxyhemoglobin and reduced hemoglobin during arterial pulsations is compared with light absorbance between pulsations. This allows adjustments for absorbance by tissue, skin pigmentation, and capillary and venous blood. Because pulse oximeters are relatively inexpensive, noninvasive, and easily applied and usually provide useful data, they are widely employed in the care of critically ill patients.

Several limitations of pulse oximetry are listed in Table 4.6. Pulse oximetry provides fairly accurate estimations of oxygen saturation when true oxygen saturation exceeds 90%. Some studies suggest 90% confidence limits of approximately ± 4% for pulse oximetry values greater than 90%. However, the confidence limits increase substantially when pulse oximetry values fall below 90%. Thus, pulse oximetry values greater than 92% can usually be interpreted as "safe." Values below 92% should trigger additional investigations to confirm the accuracy of the pulse oximetry value.

CONTROVERSIES IN HEMODYNAMIC MONITORING

Health care workers are frequently tempted to adopt new methods of hemodynamic monitoring. The rationale for rapid and more accurate assessment of the circulatory status is compelling, and the aura of new technology is seductive. However, many new "advances" in monitoring entail risks to patients, and complications may outweigh any beneficial effects.

Although PACs have been used in critically ill patients for more than 25 years, it is not yet clear that patient outcomes improve with this monitoring technique; nor is it clear in which patients such monitoring is likely to be beneficial. Although some studies suggest that physicians' clinical assessments of circulatory status are frequently inaccurate, and that information from PACs allows a beneficial redirection of treatment, other studies suggest that the use of PACs is associated with worse outcomes. Complications from PACs (see Table 4.5) may substantially reduce a patient's chance of recovery.

In a recent retrospective analysis of outcomes among critically ill patients, survival was significantly worse in patients in whom PACs were used on the first day in the intensive care unit than in those in whom PACs were not used. This study was notable in that the patient groups were carefully matched to avoid the confounding effects of uncontrolled variables such as age and severity of illness. This study strongly suggests that health care workers should reconsider the use of PACs. However, although this study demonstrated a clear association between PAC use and increased mortality, it did not prove a causal relationship. Although the risks of PAC insertion and use may outweigh the beneficial effects, other factors could have influenced the results of this study. For example, it is likely that some clinical information that triggered PAC insertion was not available to the investigators. If so, then the two groups would not have been matched for risk of death, tilting the table in favor of patients who did not receive PACs. Another explanation is that physicians with less critical care experience may be more likely to rely on information from PACs. PAC data may improve the outcomes in patients under the care of less experienced physicians. However, the same patients might fare better if cared for by more experienced physicians who are less reliant on technology.

Measurements from both pulmonary artery and central venous catheters have been used to optimize oxygen delivery in select patient subgroups. However, the use of PACs to reach supranormal physiologic goals has not led to improved outcomes in either critically ill patients in the medical intensive care unit or high-risk surgical patients. One study suggested that patients with severe sepsis and renal failure may benefit from early goal-directed therapy based on central venous oxygen saturation on presentation to the emergency room.

Another controversial issue in hemodynamic monitoring is the optimal period to leave a vascular catheter in place before removing it. The risk of catheter-related infection increases substantially with the length of time a catheter remains in place, and each infection contributes substantially to intensive care unit length of stay, hospital cost, and mortality. Some policies require the removal of catheters after 3 days, replacing them in new sites if necessary. However, each new catheter placement involves risks, and the costs of catheter replacement are not trivial. In a recent study, the incidence of bloodstream infections and mechanical complications was compared in groups of patients randomized to receive catheter replacements either every 3 days or when clinically indicated. As expected, frequent catheter reinsertion was associated with more mechanical complications such as pneumothorax. However, the incidence of bloodstream infection was not higher in patients whose catheters were changed only when clinical signs suggested infection. This study strongly suggests that the risks of new catheter placement outweigh the benefits of reduced infectious complications. However, the risks associated with catheter placement vary with the experience of the operator, and the likelihood of infectious complications may also vary with insertion and maintenance techniques. It is possible that different results would occur under different conditions.

SUGGESTED READINGS

Bartch P, Swenson ER, Maggiorini M: Update: high altitude pulmonary edema. Adv Exp Med Biol 502:89-106, 2001.

Bhattacharya J: Physiological basis of pulmonary edema. In Matthay M, Ingbar D (eds): Pulmonary Edema. Vol 116 of Lenfant C (ed): Lung Biology in Health and Disease. New York, Marcel Dekker, 1998.

Butler J (ed): The Bronchial Circulation. Vol 57 of Lenfant C (ed): Lung Biology in Health and Disease. New York, Marcel Dekker, 1992.

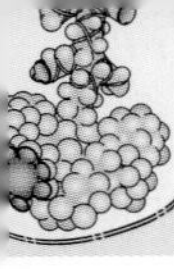

Cobb DK, High KP, Sawyer RG, et al: A controlled trial of scheduled replacement central venous and pulmonary-artery catheters. N Engl J Med 327:1062-1068, 1992.

Cohn JN, Tristani FE, Khatri IM: Studies in clinical shock and hypotension. J Clin Invest 48:2008-2018, 1969.

Connors AF, McCaffree DR, Gray BA: Evaluation of right-heart catheterization in the critically ill patient without acute myocardial infarction. N Engl J Med 308:263-267, 1983.

Connors AF, Speroff T, Dawson NV, et al: The effectiveness of right heart catheterization in the initial care of critically ill patients. JAMA 276:889-897, 1996.

Glenny RW: State of the art: blood flow distribution in the lung. Chest 114:8S-16S, 1998.

Joynt GM, Buckley TA, Oh TE, et al: Comparison of intrathoracic and intra-abdominal measurements of central venous pressure. Lancet 347:1155-1157, 1996.

Mansfield PF, Hohn DC, Fornage BD, et al: Complications and failures of subclavian-vein catheterization. N Engl J Med 331:1735-1738, 1994.

Matthay M, Folkesson HG, Clerici C: Lung epithelial fluid transport and the resolution of pulmonary edema. Physiol Rev 82:569-600, 2002.

O'Grady NP, Alexander M, Dellinger EP, et al: Guidelines for the prevention of intravascular catheter-related infections Infect Control Hosp Epidemiol 2002, pp. 759-769.

Raad I: Intravascular-catheter-related infections. Lancet 351:893-898, 1998.

Rivers E, Nguyen B, Havstad S, et al: Early goal-directed therapy in the treatment of severe sepsis and septic shock. N Engl J Med 345:1368-1377, 2001.

Swan HJC, Ganz W, Forrester J, et al: Catheterization of the heart in man with use of a flow-directed balloon-tipped catheter. N Engl J Med 283:447-451, 1970.

Tyberg JV, Grant DA, Kingma I, et al: Effects of positive intrathoracic pressure on pulmonary and systemic hemodynamics. Respir Physiol 119:163-171, 2000.

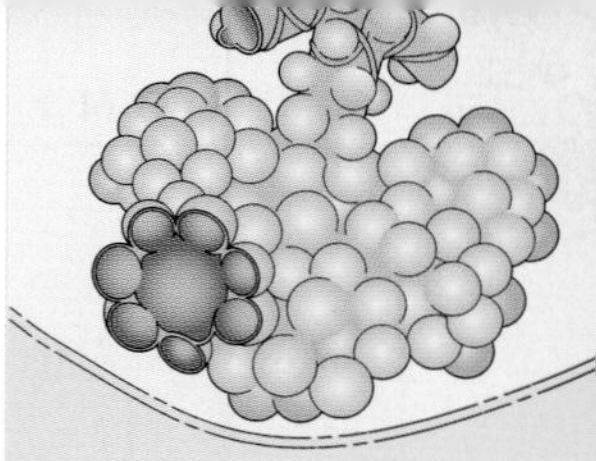

CHAPTER 5

Acid-Base Balance and Control of Ventilation

Bruce H. Culver

ACID-BASE BALANCE

The respiratory system is closely interrelated to the acid-base status of the body because the carbon dioxide produced by tissue metabolism dissolves in water in the tissues or blood and becomes hydrated to form carbonic acid. In red blood cells, as well as some other cells of the body, the hydration reaction is greatly accelerated by carbonic anhydrase (CA) (equation 5.1).

EQUATION 5.1: CARBONIC ACID SYSTEM

$$CO_2 + H_2O \overset{CA}{\leftrightarrow} H_2CO_3 \leftrightarrow H^+ + HCO_3^-$$

Normal values for the components of the carbonic acid system are given in Table 5.1, and the quantitative relationship among them is expressed by the Henderson-Hasselbalch equation.

It is convenient to consider acids produced by the body to be of two types—carbonic acid from the preceding reaction, and noncarbonic or metabolic acids such as phosphoric, sulfuric, and a variety of organic acids. Carbonic acid can be effectively removed or regulated through the lung as carbon dioxide, whereas the metabolic acids must be either excreted, primarily through the kidney, or metabolized. Changes in the carbonic acid component, which present as changes in $PaCO_2$, are termed respiratory acid-base abnormalities, and changes in the handling of metabolic acid or alkali result in metabolic acid-base derangements. Based on measurements of arterial pH, PCO_2, and $[HCO_3^-]$, it is possible to quantify the clinical acid-base status of a patient in terms of a respiratory component, indicated by $PaCO_2$, and a metabolic component, reflected by changes in $[HCO_3^-]$.

From inspection of the reaction (see equation 5.1), it is apparent that an increase in PCO_2, and thus in $[CO_2]$, drives the reaction to the right, which increases $[H^+]$ and leads to a respiratory acidosis, whereas a decrease in PCO_2 has the opposite effect, leading to a respiratory alkalosis. Similarly, the addition of H^+ from a metabolic source drives the reaction to the left, consuming HCO_3^- and creating additional carbon dioxide, which can be removed via ventilation. The magnitude of metabolic acidosis is reflected by the decrement in $[HCO_3^-]$. With an excess of a metabolic base, H^+ ions are removed from the right side of the equation, and the resultant shift of equilibrium causes $[HCO_3^-]$ to rise in relationship to the magnitude of the metabolic alkalosis. Understanding these relationships quantitatively requires a more detailed analysis and is further complicated in the body by the concurrent activity of other buffer systems.

Note that the concentration of hydrogen ions $[H^+]$ in body fluids is about a million times less than the concentration of other ions. Small changes in absolute $[H^+]$ can produce significant physiologic alterations, yet the body tolerates a wide range of relative activity. The range of viable arterial pH, from about 7.7 to 6.8, represents an eightfold change in $[H^+]$, from 20 to 160 nmol/L (and gastric $[H^+]$ is a million times higher).

Handling of Metabolic Acids

Metabolic (noncarbonic) acid or alkali is buffered by carbonic acid plus its salt, primarily sodium bicarbonate in extracellular fluid (ECF), as in equation 5.2.

EQUATION 5.2: METABOLIC ACID

$$\begin{array}{c} HCl + NaHCO_3 \\ \Updownarrow \\ H^+ + HCO_3^- \leftrightarrow H_2CO_3 \leftrightarrow CO_2 + H_2O \\ + \\ NaCl \end{array}$$

Some true chemical buffering occurs because the resultant carbonic acid is a weaker acid than the HCl added, but the major buffering in the body is physiologic, as virtually all the carbonic acid formed is excreted by the lungs under conditions of constant $PaCO_2$.

The effects of adding metabolic acid to water, to a bicarbonate solution, and to physiologic ECF are shown in Table 5.2. Quantitatively, if 12 mmol HCl are added to 1 L of water, it dissociates, and the resultant $[H^+]$ is 12 mmol/L, a pH of 1.9. However, if 12 mmol HCl are added to 1 L of a solution that contains 24 mmol $NaHCO_3^-$, the added H^+ ions combine with HCO_3^-, ultimately to form carbon dioxide. If the solution is equilibrated to a constant PCO_2 of 40 mmHg, all the carbon dioxide formed is removed, and the reaction continues until the 12 mmol of H^+ added has reacted with 12 mmol of HCO_3^-, which reduces its concentration from 24 to 12 mmol/L. Solving the Henderson-Hasselbalch equation (see Table 5.1) for PCO_2 = 40 mmHg and $[HCO_3^-]$ = 12 mmol/L yields a pH of 7.1 and an $[H^+]$ of 80 nmol/L. Thus, in this example, 12 million nanomoles of H^+ are added as HCl, but $[H^+]$ increases by only 40 nmol/L. Virtually all the carbonic acid formed is eliminated as carbon dioxide, as long as PCO_2 is kept constant, and the change in $[HCO_3^-]$ is equal to the amount of acid added.

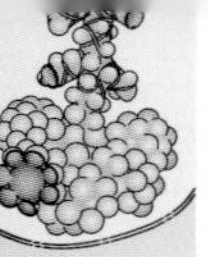

Table 5.1
Carbonic acid system

$CO_2 + H_2O \rightleftharpoons H_2CO_3 \rightleftharpoons H^1 + HCO_3^-$

Component	Value
$[HCO_3^-]$	~ 24mmol/L, as sodium bicarbonate
$[H^+]$	~ 40 3 10^{-9} mol/L at a normal arterial pH = 7.40 By convention $[H^+]$ is expressed as its negative logarithm: pH = –log $[H^+]$
$[CO_2]$	~ 1.2mmol/L at a normal arterial P_{CO_2} $[CO_2]$ includes the CO_2 in physical solution in plasma plus the very small amount of undissociated carbonic acid (H_2CO_3)

The Henderson–Hasselbalch equation for the carbonic acid system is:

pH = 6.1 1 log ($[HCO_3^-]$/0.03P_{CO_2})

If any two of the components are measured, the third can be calculated

Table 5.2
Handling of metabolic acid

	Effect of Adding 12 mmol/L of a Metabolic Acid to		
	Water	Bicarbonate Solution	Extracellular Fluid
Initial $[HCO_3^-]$ (mmol/L)	0	24	24
Final $[HCO_3^-]$ (mmol/L)	0	12	14
Final $[H^+]$	12 mmol/L	80 nmol/L	68 nmol/L
Final pH	1.9	7.1	7.2

In the body, however, the ECF contains additional buffers, and to the extent that these take up some of the added H^+, the change in HCO_3^- is less than the added metabolic acid. To mitigate a pH change from either carbonic or metabolic aberrations, H^+ can be taken up by, or donated from, hemoglobin (Hb), plasma proteins, and inorganic chemical buffers. If the same experiment is carried out with 12 mmol of HCl added to 1 L of ECF, again equilibrated to a P_{CO_2} of 40 mmHg, the result is a decrease in $[HCO_3^-]$ to 14, with a pH of 7.2 and an $[H^+]$ of 68 nmol/L. The pH change is less, as more total buffering has occurred, but the decrement in $[HCO_3^-]$ is only 10, which indicates that 2 mmol of H^+ have been buffered by the noncarbonic buffers. Empirical evidence such as this shows that the buffering capacity of the noncarbonic system in normal ECF is about 1 mmol/L per 0.1 change in pH. That is, with an increase in $[H^+]$ sufficient to lower the pH by 0.1 unit, the buffers take up 1 mmol/L of H^+, or release the same amount for a change in the opposite direction.

Handling of Respiratory Acid

The effect of adding carbonic acid to a bicarbonate solution is shown in Table 5.3. In this example, when P_{CO_2} is increased from 40 to 80 mmHg, the increase in $[CO_2]$ drives the reaction to the right, and because the P_{CO_2} is doubled, the final product of reactants on the right must also be doubled. This occurs when 40 nmol of H^+ have been formed, increasing $[H^+]$ to 80 nmol/L (pH falls from 7.4 to 7.1). Each new H^+ formed is associated with one new HCO_3^-, and thus $[HCO_3^-]$ also increases by

Table 5.3
Handling of respiratory acid

		P_{CO_2} (mmHg)	pH	$[H^+]$ (nmol/L)	$[HCO_3^-]$ (mmol/L)
	$CO_2 + H_2O \rightleftharpoons H_2CO_3 \rightleftharpoons H^1 + HCO_3^-$				
Effect of doubling P_{CO_2} in a bicarbonate solution	Initial	40	7.40	40	24
	Final	80	7.10	80	24.000040
	KHb + $CO_2 + H_2O \rightleftharpoons H_2CO_3 \rightleftharpoons H^1 + HCO_3^-$ ⇅ HHb + K^1 HCO_3^-				
Effect of doubling P_{CO_2} in physiologic extracellular fluid	Initial	40	7.40	40	24
	Final	80	7.15	71	26.5

40 nmol/L, but this is negligible compared with the 24 mmol/L of HCO_3^- originally present. Thus, $[HCO_3^-]$ does not change measurably when carbon dioxide is added to an HCO_3^- solution with no other buffers present.

In the ECF of the body, however, the presence of noncarbonic buffers alters this relationship as well. Quantitatively, the most important of these is Hb, which is used, with its potassium salt, to represent all the noncarbonic buffers in the example shown (see Table 5.3). Again, the P_{CO_2} is increased from 40 to 80 mmHg, this time in the presence of Hb equivalent to the amount distributed in normal ECF. In the simple bicarbonate solution, the reaction reaches equilibrium after only 40 nmol/L of H^+ have been formed, but in ECF, some of the newly formed H^+ can be taken up by Hb, so the reaction continues to the right and HCO_3^- ions accumulate. The plasma $[HCO_3^-]$ rises by an amount that reflects the number of H^+ ions buffered by Hb. As the pH decreases by 2.5 units to 7.15, the Hb and other noncarbonic buffers accept about 2.5 mmol of H^+, and the $[HCO_3^-]$ increases by 2.5 mmol/L. Again, the participation of noncarbonic buffers allows a smaller pH change than that observed in the bicarbonate solution.

A decrease in P_{CO_2} and the associated increase in pH of a respiratory alkalosis results in a fall in plasma $[HCO_3^-]$. When P_{CO_2} goes up or down, the buffering effect of noncarbonic buffers can be measured as the change in $[HCO_3^-]$ for a given change in pH and expressed as a buffer value, $b = -\Delta[HCO_3^-]/\Delta pH$, with the negative sign indicating that the $[HCO_3^-]$ change is opposite to the change in pH. The units of this ratio (mmol/L per pH) are more simply referred to as slykes (sl).

The greater the concentration of Hb and other noncarbonic buffers present, the greater the buffering of H^+ for a given change of pH. For blood with 15 g/100 mL Hb, b = 30 sl. In the body, however, the blood and its plasma are in equilibrium for these ions with the extravascular interstitial fluid (but not readily with the intracellular fluid). Interstitial fluid contains no Hb and very little protein, so it contributes little to noncarbonic buffering, but as H^+ ions are buffered in the blood and HCO_3^- levels are altered, these ions come into diffusional equilibrium with the interstitial fluid over 10 to 30 minutes. In effect, the buffering capacity of the blood is diluted by the interstitial fluid, and because blood volume is about one third the total ECF

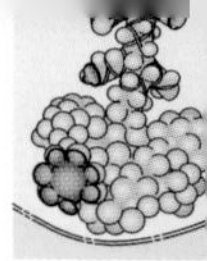

volume, the buffering capacity of ECF is about one third that of blood. For total ECF, $b \cong \frac{1}{3} \times 30 \cong 10$ sl.

Primary Acid-Base Disorders

Before acid-base abnormalities can be understood, the presence and extent of the four primary disorders must be recognized.

- Respiratory acidosis results from a high PCO_2, which reflects hypoventilation and is present, by definition, whenever PCO_2 is greater than 43. It is associated with a small increase in HCO_3^-, predictable as $\Delta[HCO_3^-] \cong -10 \times \Delta pH$, or 1 mEq/L per 0.1 pH unit fall.
- Respiratory alkalosis results from a low PCO_2, which reflects hyperventilation and is present, by definition, whenever PCO_2 is less than 37. It is associated with a small decrease in HCO_3^-, predictable as $\Delta[HCO_3^-] \cong -10 \times \Delta pH$, or 1 mEq/L per 0.1 pH unit rise.
- Metabolic acidosis is recognized by a decrement in HCO_3^- greater than that expected for the pH effect alone and can be quantitated as a decrease in base excess (defined later and in Table 5.4).
- Metabolic alkalosis is recognized by a rise in HCO_3^- greater than that expected for the pH effect alone and can be quantitated as an increase in base excess.

Note that the terms *acidosis* and *alkalosis* are applied to the pathophysiologic processes that tend to cause an excess or deficit of H^+. It is possible—indeed, common—to have processes of both acidosis and alkalosis present simultaneously (e.g., respiratory acidosis plus metabolic alkalosis) with a pH that is low, high, or normal, depending on their relative magnitude. *Acidemia* and *alkalemia* are more precise terms when referring to blood pH.

As a first approximation, metabolic abnormalities are recognized by a deviation of $[HCO_3^-]$ from the normal value of 24, but it must be remembered that because of the action of the noncarbonic buffers, even a pure respiratory abnormality is associated with changes in $[HCO_3^-]$ of $\pm$ 3 mmol/L over the pH range 7.1 to 7.7. The base excess (BE) or base deficit (usually expressed as a negative BE) of the ECF is a better quantification of any metabolic component present. At a pH of 7.4, the noncarbonic buffers hold only their normal complement of H^+ ions and thus do not contribute to buffering. The BE calculates any deviation of $[HCO_3^-]$ from 24 that would exist at a pH of 7.4 and thus is equal in magnitude to the amount of excess metabolic acid or base added to the system, just as in a simple HCO_3^- solution. Many laboratories report this value along with blood gas measurements, but it can be estimated with a simple mental calculation (see Table 5.4) or obtained from a graphic display, as described later.

Table 5.4
Base excess calculation

Base excess (BE) is defined as the difference between the patient's $[HCO_3^-]$ after correction to pH 7.40 by change of PCO_2 and the normal $[HCO_3^-]$ at pH 7.40 of 24.0 mmol/L.

Because the blood gas sample is usually not measured at a pH of 7.4, it is necessary to calculate an adjustment to this pH, which must be done by manipulation of PCO_2 so that the metabolic component of interest is not altered. As PCO_2 is hypothetically moved up or down to adjust the pH, the hypothetic $[HCO_3^-]$ changes from its measured value as determined by the noncarbonic buffer slope:

$\Delta[HCO_3^-] \approx -10 \times \Delta pH$, or −1 mmol/L per 0.1 pH unit rise.

Example 1

Consider the situation in Table 5.2 where 12 mmol/L of excess acid was added to a patient's extracellular fluid and ventilation was maintained normal. The resultant blood gas measurements include pH, 7.2; PCO_2, 40 mmHg; $[HCO_3^-]$, 14 mmol/L.

The pH must be adjusted up 0.2 units to 7.4, which requires a decrease in PCO_2.

At pH = 7.4, the hypothetic $[HCO_3^-]$ is adjusted by $\Delta[HCO_3^-] \approx -10 \times 0.2 = -2$

The hypothetic $[HCO_3^-]$ equals the measured value of 14–2 = 12

BE = $[HCO_3^-]$ at 7.4 − 24 = 12 − 24 = −12 mmol/L

The negative base excess of 12 mmol/L is equal to the excess acid load added.

Example 2

Consider a patient with the measured values: pH, 7.1; PCO_2, 95 mmHg; and $[HCO_3^-]$, 29 mmol/L.

The pH is adjusted up 0.3 units to 7.4.

$\Delta[HCO_3^-]$	$\approx -10 \times 0.3$	= −3
Hypothetic $[HCO_3^-]$	= 29–3	= 26
BE	= 26–24	= 2 mmol/L

While at first this patient may appear to have a significant metabolic alkalosis, which suggests partial compensation for the respiratory acidosis and therefore some chronicity, BE is small and within the normal limit of ±2, so this suggests acute hypoventilation.

Note that as the pH is hypothetically corrected to 7.4, PCO_2 or $[HCO_3^-]$ may move in an abnormal direction. It is convenient to remember that, consistent with the hydration reaction for CO_2, the $[HCO_3^-]$ adjustment is always in the same direction as the PCO_2 change.

In the examples above, the measured HCO_3^- is hypothetically adjusted to a pH of 7.4 and compared with the normal value of 24 mmol/L. Alternatively, the same relationship can be used to adjust the normal HCO_3^- to the normal value expected at the measured pH and subtract the measured HCO_3^-. In Example 2, a 'normal' HCO_3^- is calculated at pH 7.1 to be 27 mmol/L and the BE to be 29 − 27 = 2 mmol/L. This is what happens visually on the Davenport diagram when the vertical distance of a point above or below the 10 sl line is assessed.

Compensation for Acid-Base Disorders

If the underlying pathology prevents the body from correcting a primary acid-base disorder (e.g., by restoring hypoventilation to normal), mechanisms come into play to minimize the deviation of pH from normal. The immediate effects of buffering are aided by a second type of homeostatic mechanism, termed *physiologic compensation*. The Henderson-Hasselbalch equation shows that pH is a function of the ratio of $[HCO_3^-]$ to PCO_2, so pH is improved if this ratio is restored toward normal. If, for example, the primary disorder is a metabolic acidosis, $[HCO_3^-]$ is low and the physiologic compensation is to lower PCO_2 by increasing ventilation. This restores the $[HCO_3^-]/PCO_2$ ratio closer to normal, even though the absolute values of both $[HCO_3^-]$ and PCO_2 are now abnormal. This response, and the opposite one in the case of a metabolic alkalosis, demonstrates ventilatory compensation for a primary metabolic acid-base disorder.

If the primary derangement is ventilatory in origin (e.g., respiratory acidosis with a high PCO_2), the body responds by increasing $[HCO_3^-]$ and restoring the $[HCO_3^-]/PCO_2$ ratio and pH toward normal. This metabolic compensation for primary respiratory disorders involves both renal retention or excretion

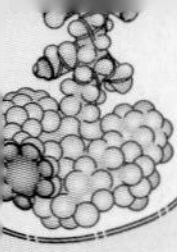

Table 5.5 HCO$_3^-$ change with respiratory acidosis and alkalosis
Respiratory Acidosis
Acute: the increase in HCO$_3^-$ = 0.1 × the increase in PaCO_2
Chronic: the increase in HCO$_3^-$ = 0.3 × the increase in PaCO_2.
Respiratory Alkalosis
Acute: the fall in HCO$_3^-$ = 0.2 × the decrease in PaCO_2
Chronic: the fall in HCO$_3^-$ = 0.4 × the decrease in PaCO_2.

of HCO_3^- and physicochemical binding, which occurs in bone and intracellular proteins. The time course of these mechanisms of metabolic compensation is about 3 days, as opposed to the ventilatory compensations, which are immediate. Thus, respiratory acid-base disturbances can be divided into those that are uncompensated and therefore likely to be of short duration (i.e., acute) and those that are compensated (chronic) processes. This is not possible for metabolic acid-base disturbances, as their normal ventilatory compensation develops concurrently.

Davenport Diagram

In general, compensations for primary acid-base alterations do not completely restore pH to 7.4. The primary acid-base disorders and their mechanisms and limits of compensation can be displayed in one of several graphic formats. Renal adaptation to respiratory alkalosis results in decreases in serum HCO_3^-. Decreases in serum HCO_3^- are mediated by down-regulation of HCO_3^- reabsorption in the proximal tubule. This occurs rapidly, so the distinction between acute and chronic respiratory alkalosis is approximately 24 hours.

A number of formulas have been developed to depict this compensatory relationship (Table 5.5).

The Davenport diagram is a commonly used visual display of acid-base relationships (Fig. 5.1) and is a graphic representation of the Henderson-Hasselbalch equation in which any point shows a potentially coexisting combination of the three variables.

Respiratory disorders are shown by moving from the normal central point to higher or lower values of PCO_2. The sloping line that passes through the center shows the 10 sl buffer value of the noncarbonic buffers and thus indicates the expected values for pH and [HCO_3^-] as PCO_2 rises or falls in a pure respiratory acidosis or alkalosis. Vertical displacements above or below this line indicate that a metabolic disorder (either primary or compensatory) has caused an excess or deficit of base in the ECF. If no compensation occurred for a primary metabolic disorder, the values would follow the line that represents PCO_2 = 40. The Davenport diagram is a convenient way to visualize the paths of primary disorders and their compensation. Figure 5.2 shows, for example, the development of an acute respiratory acidosis with subsequent metabolic compensation. Figure 5.3 shows the range

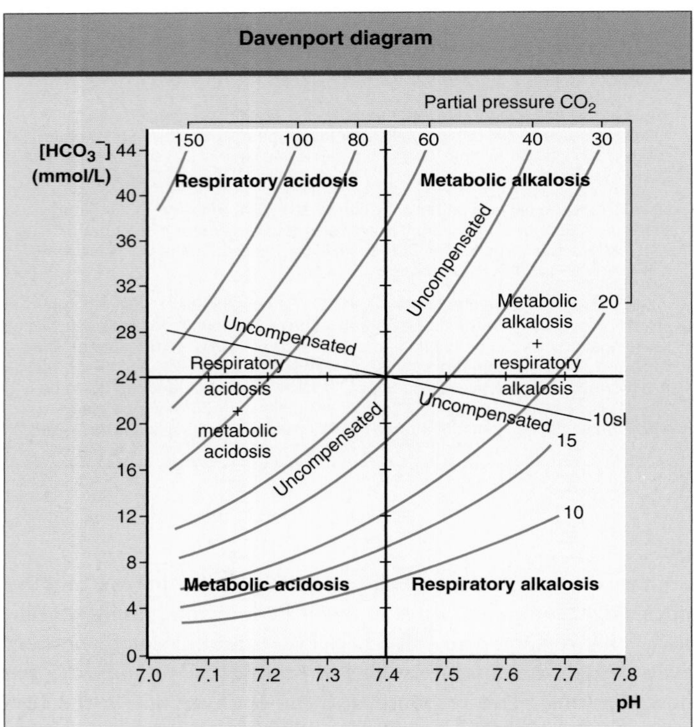

Figure 5.1 Davenport diagram. This graphic display plots plasma HCO_3^- against plasma pH, with lines of equal carbon dioxide partial pressure (PCO_2) curving across the graph (intermediate values of PCO_2 can be interpolated along vertical lines).

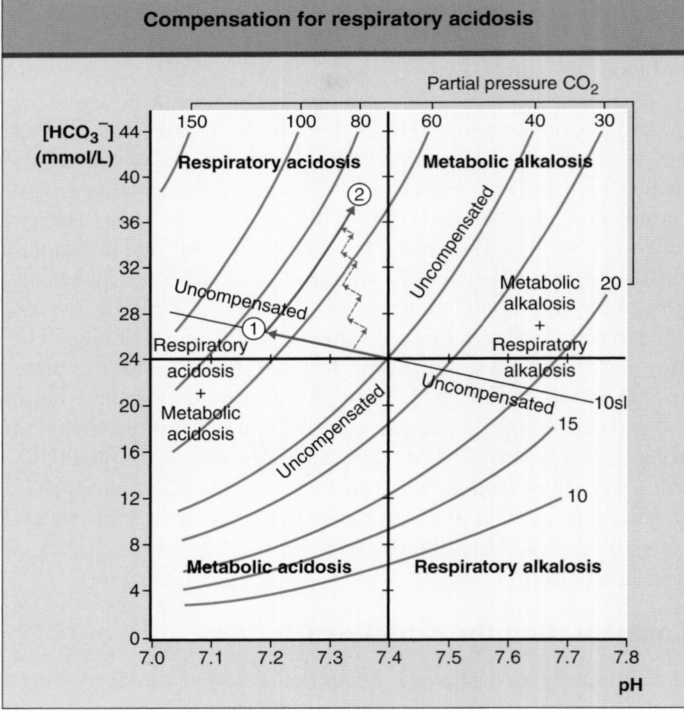

Figure 5.2 Compensation for a respiratory acidosis. Rapid development of hypoventilation, in which carbon dioxide partial pressure rises from 40 to 70 mmHg, would follow the 10 sl line of acute respiratory acidosis to point 1. If this level of hypoventilation were maintained for days, metabolic compensation would increase HCO_3^- and improve the pH toward point 2. More likely, a progressive decline in ventilation over days might follow the stuttering, dotted path to the same end point.

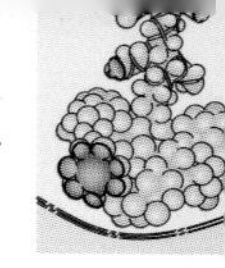

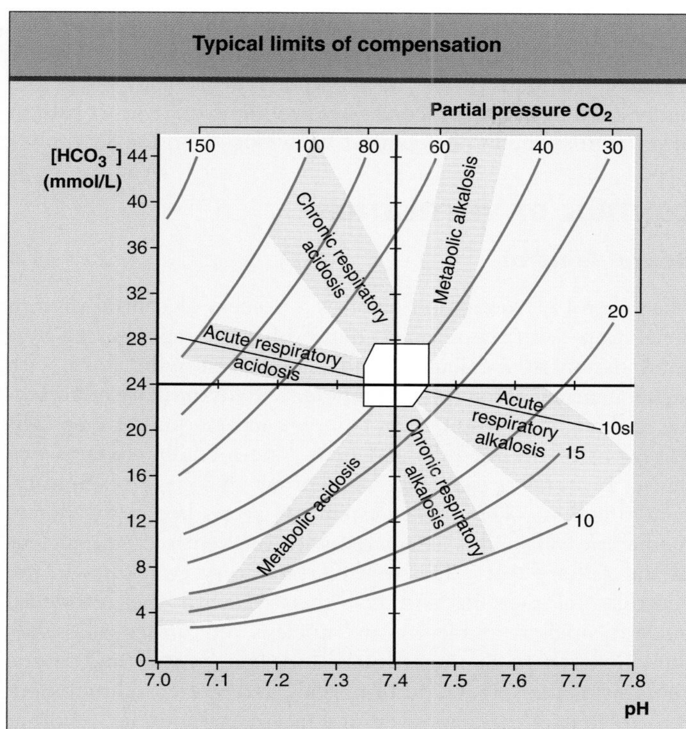

Figure 5.3 Typical limits of compensation are conveniently displayed on the Davenport diagram. Modified with permission from Hornbein TF: Acid-base balance. In Culver BH [ed]: The Respiratory System. Seattle, ASUW Publications, 6:15, 2002. Data from Goldberg M, Greene SB, Moss ML, et al: Computer based instruction and diagnosis of acid-base disorders. JAMA 223:269-275, 1973.

of values seen in common acid-base disorders and illustrates the usual limits of compensation.

Clinical Acid-Base Disorders

RESPIRATORY ACIDOSIS

Hypoventilation is defined as alveolar ventilation inadequate for metabolic demand and is indicated by an elevation of arterial PCO_2 above the normal 40 ± 3 mmHg (at sea level; it is lower at altitude). It results from an inadequate drive to breathe, from mechanical impairments of the chest wall or lung parenchyma, or (most commonly) from severe airflow limitation (e.g., asthma or chronic obstructive pulmonary disease [COPD]).

An elevated $PaCO_2$ defines the presence of respiratory acidosis regardless of the arterial pH.

Acute Respiratory Acidosis

Acute respiratory acidosis is identified by high $PaCO_2$, fall in pH, and increase in [HCO_3^-] that approximates 1 mmol/L for each 0.1 decrement in pH (i.e., BE ≈ 0). On the Davenport diagram, the values follow the 10 sl line to the left (see Fig. 5.1).

Chronic Respiratory Acidosis

Chronic respiratory acidosis is identified by a high $PaCO_2$, a variable decrement in pH, and an increase in [HCO_3^-] that exceeds 1 mmol/L for each 0.1 decrement in pH (i.e., BE > 2). On the Davenport diagram, the values are in the left upper quadrant above the 10 sl line (see Fig. 5.1). Metabolic compensation probably begins within hours by the redistribution of HCO_3^- within bone and intracellular stores. Over the course of several days, renal retention of HCO_3^- in response to excess H^+ can produce nearly complete compensation for moderate elevations of $PaCO_2$ (the change in [HCO_3^-] representing approximately 75% of the change in $PaCO_2$) and brings the pH very near to 7.4 (see Figs. 5.2 and 5.3). At higher levels of $PaCO_2$, renal tubular reabsorption of HCO_3^- is not sufficient to restore the normal [HCO_3^-]/PCO_2 ratio, and the pH remains increasingly acid. Patients with fully compensated respiratory acidosis may be quite stable despite considerable elevations of $PaCO_2$. Accordingly, the decrement in pH is a better indication of clinical risk.

RESPIRATORY ALKALOSIS

Hyperventilation is defined as alveolar ventilation in excess of metabolic demand and is indicated by a fall in arterial PCO_2 below the normal 40 ± 3 mmHg. It results from an excessive drive to breathe, which may result from pain or anxiety, but is also stimulated by hypoxemia and the derangements of many pulmonary diseases, including mild to moderate asthma, pulmonary emboli, pulmonary hypertension, and interstitial pulmonary fibrosis; by systemic illnesses, including head injury, shock, and bacteremia; and by ingestion of aspirin. Respiratory alkalosis is easily induced by excessive mechanical ventilation.

A low $PaCO_2$ defines the presence of respiratory alkalosis regardless of the arterial pH.

Acute Respiratory Alkalosis

Acute respiratory alkalosis is identified by a low $PaCO_2$, a rise in pH, and a decrease in [HCO_3^-] that approximates 1 mmol/L per 0.1 increment in pH (i.e., BE ≈ 0). On the Davenport diagram, the values follow the 10 sl line to the right (see Fig. 5.1). The empirical data plotted in Figure 5.3 show that patients who have more severe degrees of acute hyperventilation may have somewhat lower [HCO_3^-] values than expected for the immediate effects of noncarbonic buffers.

Chronic Respiratory Alkalosis

Chronic respiratory alkalosis is identified by a low $PaCO_2$, a variable but small increase in pH, and a decrease in [HCO_3^-] that exceeds 1 mmol/L per 0.1 increment in pH (i.e., BE < −2). On the Davenport diagram, the values are in the right lower quadrant below the 10 sl line (see Fig. 5.1). The mechanisms of metabolic compensation described earlier, but in the reverse direction, can produce almost complete compensation to a pH near 7.4 (see Fig. 5.3) when hyperventilation is sustained, as, for example, in those living at high altitudes or in patients with restrictive lung disease.

Metabolic Disorders

METABOLIC ACIDOSIS

Metabolic acidosis is defined by a decrement in [HCO_3^-] greater than that expected for the pH effect alone and is quantified by calculation of a base deficit or negative BE. A negative BE defines the presence of a component of metabolic acidosis regardless of the arterial pH.

Two general types of metabolic acidosis occur—those that result from excess acid accumulation with the subsequent loss of HCO_3^- via ventilation, as described earlier, and those that result from a primary loss of HCO_3^- from the body. Examples of excess acid include:

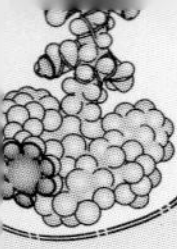

- Production of lactic acid when tissue oxygen demand outstrips supply, as in exercising muscle, low cardiac output states, or conditions of low arterial oxygen content
- Ketoacidosis associated with insulin deficiency
- Inadequate excretion of acid in acute or chronic renal failure

Bicarbonate loss may occur from defects in renal tubular function and from intestinal secretions in diarrhea. Although the base deficit quantifies the net acidosis from any of these causes, it does not differentiate between the two types, which is done by calculating the unmeasured anions, or "anion gap." Ionic balance must be maintained in the ECF, so the sum of the positive ions (mainly Na^+ and K^+) must equal the sum of the negative ions (Cl^-, HCO_3^-, and unmeasured anions). The difference, $(Na^+ + K^+) - (Cl^- + HCO_3^-)$, gives the anion gap (although K^+ is often ignored in the clinical calculation) and is normally less than 8 to 12. The anion gap remains normal with primary HCO_3^- losses, as these are typically balanced by retention of Cl^-, but is increased by the accumulation of the unmeasured anions left behind when excess acid (other than HCl) is buffered by the bicarbonate system.

METABOLIC ALKALOSIS

Metabolic alkalosis is defined by an increase in $[HCO_3^-]$ greater than expected for the pH effect alone and is quantified by calculation of a positive BE. A positive BE defines the presence of a metabolic alkalosis, regardless of the arterial pH.

Metabolic alkalosis is most commonly caused by loss of acid via gastric secretions (vomiting or gastric suction) or by retention of HCO_3^- with diuretic therapy. Both are associated with chloride depletion, with a decrease in serum chloride concentration roughly equivalent to the increase in plasma $[HCO_3^-]$.

RESPIRATORY COMPENSATION

Respiratory compensation for primary metabolic disorders is rapid but does not result in complete compensation (see Fig. 5.3). Respiratory drive is stimulated by low pH, so hyperventilation in response to an acid stimulus can result in more than a doubling of alveolar ventilation (driving Pa_{CO_2} to <20 mmHg). Metabolic alkalosis generally results in moderate degrees of hypoventilation, with Pa_{CO_2} rarely exceeding 60 mmHg unless pulmonary abnormalities are present as well. The hypoxemia associated with hypoventilation when breathing air provides a ventilatory drive to limit a further rise in P_{CO_2}. Figure 5.3 shows that the maximum extent of ventilatory compensation observed with a chronic metabolic acidosis or alkalosis results in a pH that is about halfway between that which would have existed in the absence of any ventilatory compensation (at Pa_{CO_2} = 40 mmHg) and complete compensation (pH = 7.4). Metabolic acid-base derangements of shorter duration show less complete compensation, presumably related to the rate of readjustment of brain ECF acid-base balance.

Combined Disorders

Not all acid-base disorders fit neatly into the primary and compensatory patterns described. Combined primary disorders may occur, such as an acute cessation of ventilation (asphyxia) that causes both respiratory and metabolic (lactic) acidoses. More complex disorders may also be seen. For example, the superimposition of a short-term increase in ventilation or of diuretic therapy on a chronic, well-compensated respiratory acidosis may result in an alkalotic pH. The blood pH, P_{CO_2}, and HCO_3^- are sufficient to identify the net components present, but a full understanding of the processes involved in an individual patient often requires additional clinical knowledge or prior data.

CONTROL OF VENTILATION

Neural Control

The control of ventilation involves a process of central rhythm generation, with the rate and depth of breathing adjusted by a combination of mechanical and chemical stimuli, along with higher central nervous system inputs. The rhythmicity of breathing is thought to result from complex interactions among cells in regions of the medulla and pons. The medulla contains two dense, bilateral aggregations of neurons that have respiratory-related activity. The dorsal respiratory group lies in the dorsomedial medulla and is associated with the ventrolateral nucleus of the solitary tract. The ventral respiratory group lies in the ventrolateral medulla and is associated with the retrofacial nucleus, nucleus ambiguus, and nucleus retroambigualis. Outputs from these neurons descend via the ventral and lateral columns of the spinal cord to phrenic and intercostal motoneurons to control the diaphragm and intercostal muscles. Another important respiratory area is located in the dorsolateral pons, associated with the nucleus parabrachialis medialis, and is commonly called the pneumotaxic center. This region may play a role in switching between the inspiratory and expiratory phases.

Although the average ventilation level is normally set predominantly by chemical stimuli, mechaniconeural receptors may also modify the ventilatory pattern. Although these receptors can be demonstrated in animals, their roles in humans are less clear. They include the following:

- Slowly adapting pulmonary stretch receptors located in the airways with vagal afferents that are stimulated by increases in lung volume. For example, when functional residual capacity is raised or when lung volume is held at its end-inspiratory level, a reduction in respiratory frequency results primarily from prolongation of the expiratory period (inflation reflex of Hering-Breuer). A reduction in activity of these receptors with lung deflation stimulates inspiratory onset (deflation reflex) and may contribute to the tachypnea that accompanies atelectasis.
- Rapidly adapting pulmonary stretch receptors concentrated near the carina and central bronchi, also with vagal afferents, are stimulated both mechanically and chemically to generate the cough reflex.
- C-fiber endings attached to unmyelinated afferent fibers are found close to the pulmonary capillaries, where they have been called type J (juxtapulmonary capillary) receptors, and are also present in the bronchi in proximity to the bronchial circulation. Both types of C-fiber endings are stimulated by endogenously produced substances, including histamine, some prostaglandins, bradykinin, and serotonin, and may have a role in conditions such as asthma, pulmonary venous congestion, and pulmonary embolism. C-fiber endings also are mechanically sensitive and can be activated by lung hyperinflation.

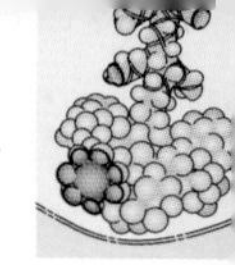

- Musculoskeletal afferents stimulated by the stretching of skeletal muscle increase ventilation and may contribute to the initial hyperpnea of exercise.

Chemical Stimuli

The influence of ventilation on the levels of carbon dioxide and oxygen in the blood is described in Chapter 3. In turn, these levels are sensed and modulate neural inputs to the respiratory centers to complete a feedback loop. Receptors responsive to changes in levels of oxygen, carbon dioxide, and pH are located peripherally in the aortic and carotid bodies and centrally on the brain side of the blood-brain barrier.

PERIPHERAL CHEMORECEPTORS

The carotid bodies lie close to the carotid bifurcation on either side of the neck, and the aortic bodies lie near the aortic arch. Each of these receives an extremely high blood flow relative to their size, which results in tissue blood-gas partial pressures very close to the arterial level. Arterial oxygen partial pressure, rather than oxygen content, is the principal chemical stimulus to these peripheral receptors. Experiments in which blood oxygen content is lowered by anemia or carbon monoxide administration show little or no change in peripheral chemosensor output when Pa_{O_2} is not reduced simultaneously. Receptor neural output is minimal above a Pa_{O_2} of 200 mmHg, increases gradually with lower levels, and increases much more rapidly below a Pa_{O_2} of 60 mmHg.

The peripheral chemoreceptors are also sensitive to arterial pH. A decrease in pH (acidemia) increases the firing rate and stimulates ventilation, whereas an increase in pH has the opposite effect. Pa_{CO_2} stimulates the peripheral receptors, in addition to its pH effect. These two chemical stimuli, hypoxia and acidity, interact and are more than additive in their combined influence on chemoreceptor discharge and ventilation.

CENTRAL CHEMORECEPTORS

Chemosensitive areas have been demonstrated near the ventrolateral surface of the medulla in the cat and rat. The stimulus to this receptor appears to be primarily the pH or hydrogen ion content of brain ECF, and again, acidosis increases the ventilatory signal. The stimulus is similar with pH reduction of either respiratory or metabolic origin, but because the blood-brain barrier is much more permeable to carbon dioxide than to HCO_3^-, the effect of respiratory acid-base disturbances is much more immediate.

INTERACTION OF CHEMICAL STIMULI

The acute ventilatory increase in response to hypoxia appears to be mediated entirely by the peripheral receptors, whereas hypoxia, if anything, depresses central output. The response is initially attenuated by the effect of hypocapnic alkalosis on both peripheral and central chemoreceptors, but if hypoxia persists, such as at altitude, and metabolic compensation occurs, the ventilation can increase further.

The ventilatory response to an acute rise in Pa_{CO_2} results primarily (about 80%) from the central chemoreceptors, with the remainder attributable to peripheral chemoreceptors. For the same arterial pH change, the ventilatory response to respiratory acidosis is greater than that seen with metabolic acidosis. This results from a difference in central chemoreceptor activity because of the effect of the blood-brain barrier. Carbon dioxide, like other gases, readily crosses the blood-brain barrier, so that brain ECF P_{CO_2} is similar to that in blood, but most ions, including H^+ and HCO_3^-, cross the blood-brain barrier much more slowly. Respiratory acidosis stimulates both peripheral and central chemoreceptors as the carbon dioxide crosses the blood-brain barrier to acidify brain ECF. The resultant ventilatory response reflects the sum of the signals from both receptors. With metabolic acidosis, the peripheral chemoreceptor response is similar to that with carbon dioxide, but because the hydrogen ion does not readily reach the central chemosensor, central stimulation does not occur. Instead, the hypocapnia that results from peripheral chemoreceptor stimulation creates a central nervous system alkalosis, and the resultant ventilatory response reflects the net effect of an increased peripheral drive partially offset by a decreased central drive.

Although the blood-brain barrier is poorly permeable to H^+ and HCO_3^-, redistribution of these ions does occur over several hours. The blood-brain barrier and choroid plexus may regulate ECF composition of the brain, much as the kidney does for the rest of the body. However, equilibrium across the blood-brain barrier may develop over hours, whereas renal adjustments may require days.

Measurement of Ventilatory Drive

The classic methods of measuring ventilatory drive alter the stimulus (P_{CO_2} or P_{O_2}) and measure the response in ventilation per minute. A major drawback to these methods is that they depend on normal lungs and chest wall. Because ventilation is the index of response, any mechanical impairment of the breathing apparatus (restrictive or obstructive disease) tends to reduce the measurement. An attempt to make more meaningful measurements in patients who have lung disease led to the development of the mouth occlusion pressure technique, in which the inspiratory pressure developed against a shutter transiently closed during the first 100 msec of a tidal breath ($P_{0.1}$) is taken as an index of respiratory center output. This technique tends to parallel phrenic nerve traffic, but its accuracy may be reduced in severe COPD, where the time constant for transmission of an inspiratory pressure change to the mouth may be prolonged.

VENTILATORY PATTERN

The total ventilation per minute is the product of the tidal volume and the respiratory frequency. ($\dot{V}_E = V_T \times f$). The ventilatory pattern can be further described by measurement of the time during inspiration in relationship to the total tidal cycle (T_I/T_{TOT}), and the average inspiratory flow rate is given by V_T/T_I. Ventilation is typically measured using a mouthpiece and nose clips, but these tend to alter the pattern. To avoid this, research studies may use calibrated magnetometers or inductance belts.

RESTING PARTIAL PRESSURE OF ARTERIAL CARBON DIOXIDE

Human alveolar ventilation is normally regulated to maintain Pa_{CO_2} between 37 and 43 mmHg at sea level. In the absence of serious mechanical impediments to ventilation, a Pa_{CO_2} above this range may be interpreted as reflecting low respiratory drive, whereas a low Pa_{CO_2} in a spontaneously breathing individual reflects increased drive.

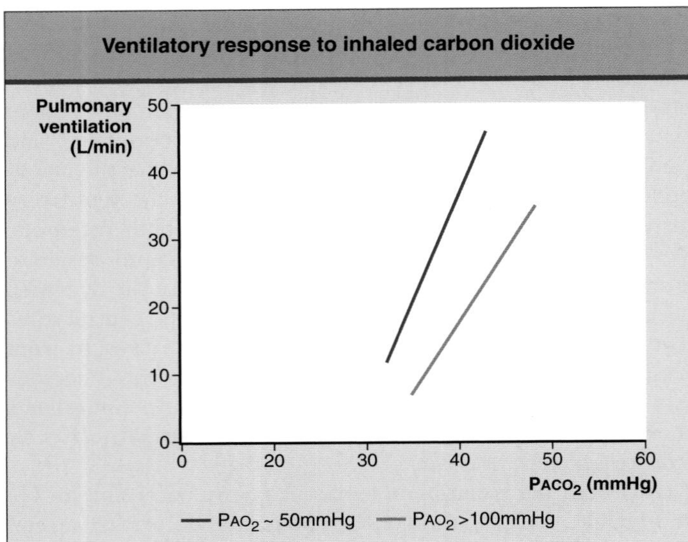

Figure 5.4 Ventilatory response to inhaled carbon dioxide at two different levels of alveolar partial pressure of oxygen (PAO_2). Minute ventilation increases as $PACO_2$ (and with it, $PaCO_2$) is elevated. The slope showing ventilatory sensitivity to $PACO_2$ increases with the added stimulus of low PaO_2.

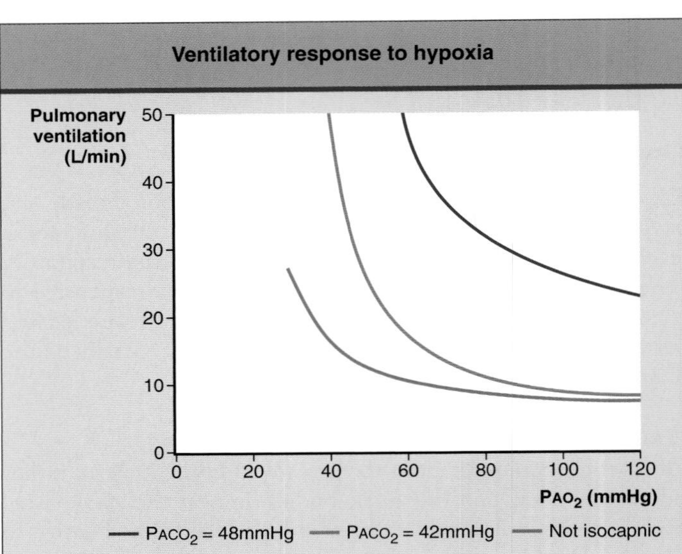

Figure 5.5 Ventilatory response to hypoxia. Minute ventilation increases in a nonlinear fashion as PAO_2 is decreased (with constant $PACO_2$). The response is greater with the added stimulus of higher PCO_2. The lowest line shows a diminished response when PCO_2 is permitted to fall (not isocapnic) as hyperventilation is stimulated by hypoxia. Modified from Hlastala MP, Berger AJ: Physiology of Respiration. New York, Oxford University Press, 1996, pp 176-195.

CARBON DIOXIDE RESPONSE CURVES

Carbon dioxide is introduced into the inspired gas to raise $PaCO_2$ or, alternatively, endogenous carbon dioxide is built up by rebreathing from a closed system while the increase in ventilation is monitored. Both are done with a high inspired oxygen level to eliminate the influence of fluctuations in PaO_2. In the physiologic range of $PaCO_2$, a straight line is obtained in a plot of minute ventilation versus $PaCO_2$ (Fig. 5.4). The slope of this line, a measurement of the sensitivity of the respiratory system to $PaCO_2$, is normally 2 to 5 L/minute per mmHg $PaCO_2$. A decrease in this slope in the absence of ventilatory impairment is an indication of a decreased respiratory drive.

HYPOXIA RESPONSE CURVES

Changes in ventilation in response to decreasing arterial oxygen partial pressures tend to follow a hyperbolic curve (Fig. 5.5). The response is quite modest at PaO_2 levels in the high-normal range, but VE increases sharply as PaO_2 falls below 60 mmHg. If $PaCO_2$ is allowed to decrease as ventilation increases, the response is attenuated by the offsetting pH effect, so carbon dioxide may be progressively added to maintain isocapneic conditions. The alinearity makes it difficult to express drive numerically, but a left shift or flattening of the curve is interpreted as decreased hypoxic drive. When the results of such a test are plotted as ventilation versus arterial oxygen saturation, the inverse relationship is typically linear. This is a coincidental outcome of the two curvilinear relationships, as the signal for ventilation is PaO_2, not SaO_2. The range of hypoxic sensitivity among normal individuals is wide.

Because the hypoxic drive is rather modest for PaO_2 greater than 60 mmHg, it is generally held that the carbon dioxide response is mainly responsible for maintaining the level of ventilation in normal humans at sea level. The range of measured drives among normal individuals is wide, largely determined genetically, and hypoxic and hypercapnic drives do not correlate well with each other. The ventilatory sensitivities to carbon dioxide and to hypoxia tend to decrease with age and are depressed by anesthetics, sedatives, and narcotics. The impact of a low ventilatory drive is most likely to become manifest when the system is stressed by high ventilatory demand or by the increased work of airflow obstruction.

VENTILATORY LOADING

Respiratory drive may be further examined by studying the response of subjects to an imposed external load, such as an added inspiratory resistance or a threshold of negative pressure. With an added load, normal subjects typically show a decreased ventilatory response to hypercapnia or hypoxia but an increase in neural drive, as reflected by phrenic activity or mouth occlusion pressure. Similarly, with advanced COPD, ventilatory responses to chemical stimuli are reduced, but $P_{0.1}$ values tend to be high. A potential contributor to hypercapnia in COPD and asthma is a failure to perceive or respond to the added load.

SUGGESTED READINGS

Berger AJ, Hornbein TF: Control of breathing. In Patton HD, et al (eds): Textbook of Physiology, vol 2, 21st ed. Philadelphia, WB Saunders, 1989, ch 54.

Calverley PMA: Control of breathing. In Hughes JMB, Pride N (eds): Lung Function Tests: Physiologic Principles and Clinical Application. London, WB Saunders, 1999, pp 107-120.

Hlastala MP, Berger AJ: Physiology of Respiration, 2nd ed. New York, Oxford University Press, 2001.

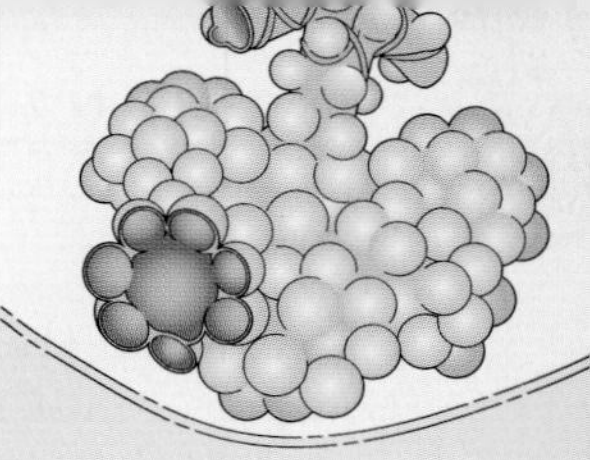

CHAPTER 6

Overview of Respiratory Muscle Function

Michael I. Polkey

Even in the presence of normal lung parenchyma, maintenance of blood gas homeostasis can be achieved only if there is movement of air into and out of the thorax, an activity that requires respiratory muscle activity. This chapter describes the function of the respiratory muscles and a clinical approach to the evaluation of patients with possible respiratory muscle dysfunction.

Anatomy

In humans the most important inspiratory muscle is the diaphragm, which accounts for approximately 70% of minute ventilation in normal individuals. The diaphragm has two components: the costal and crural diaphragms. Although these components are known to have different mechanical actions in vitro, they always act in tandem in vivo. The costal diaphragm arises from the seventh through the twelfth ribs and inserts into a central, noncontractile tendon. The crural diaphragm, in contrast, arises from the first three lumbar vertebrae and is therefore fixed. The nerve supply to the diaphragm arises from the third, fourth, and fifth cervical roots and unites to form the phrenic nerves, which traverse the neck and descend in the mediastinum to the diaphragm. Because of their long course the phrenic nerves are susceptible to damage from a variety of conditions and medical procedures.

Some extradiaphragmatic muscles also have inspiratory activity, in particular the scalene and the sternomastoid muscles. Expiration is normally a passive process, but expiratory muscles can, in the absence of flow limitation, serve to increase minute ventilation and have important functions in relation to cough (and therefore sputum clearance). The most important respiratory muscles are the abdominals (transversus abdominis, rectus abdominis, and external oblique). Intercostal muscles have both inspiratory and expiratory functions.

Physiology

Structurally, all the respiratory muscles are skeletal in nature (rather than cardiac) and are subject to the same pathophysiologic processes as other skeletal muscles. The diaphragm is composed, in healthy humans, of 50% type I fatigue-resistant fibers, 25% type IIa fibers, and 25% type IIb fibers. Contraction of muscle fibers is triggered by the arrival of a nerve impulse at the motor end plate. Acetylcholine is released and depolarizes the muscle cell membrane. This depolarization is directed inward, causing intracellular calcium release. The calcium is taken up by troponin, which then permits cyclic attachment and detachment of cross-bridges between actin and myosin. The consequent contraction of the muscle fiber creates either tension if the muscle length is constant or shortening if it is free to move. Alterations at the cellular level have been observed and at least partially explain the clinical observation that diaphragmatic fatigue is rare in patients with chronic obstructive pulmonary disease (COPD). In particular, as airway obstruction increases there develops a predominance of type I fatigue-resistant fibers as well as an increase in mitochondria; moreover, available evidence suggests that the mitochondria work with enhanced efficiency. Animal models of emphysema have suggested that the muscle might reach a new optimal length by a process of sarcomere loss; however, available data suggest that the human diaphragm in COPD develops sarcomere shortening rather than loss. Whether there is a shorter optimal diaphragmatic length in patients with COPD remains a matter of controversy.

Diaphragmatic contraction results in a caudal movement of the central tendon, which causes pressure to increase below the diaphragm (in the abdomen) and to become more subatmospheric above the diaphragm (in the chest). The rise in intra-abdominal pressure caused by diaphragmatic contraction manifests as an outward movement of the anterior abdominal wall, visible on inspection. The pressure is also transmitted through the zone of apposition to the lower rib cage wall, which also moves outward in inspiration. Unopposed diaphragmatic contraction causes inward movement of the upper thoracic cage (as in high quadriplegia), but normally this movement is counterbalanced by co-contraction of the extradiaphragmatic inspiratory muscles.

The endurance properties of the respiratory muscles may be as important clinically as their strength. At present no routinely applicable clinical test that can measure respiratory muscle endurance exists, but laboratory studies have shown that maximal voluntary ventilation can be sustained only for 10 to 15 seconds, after which exponential decay occurs. After approximately 60 seconds a plateau that can be sustained indefinitely is reached. The plateau is approximately 55% of maximum breathing capacity.

Factors Influencing Respiratory Muscle Function

PHYSIOLOGIC FACTORS

Stimulus Frequency

For the isometric muscle a single impulse gives rise to a "twitch." If multiple impulses are given in succession the twitches summate to cause a tetanic contraction. The plot of tension generated against stimulus frequency is termed the *force-frequency*

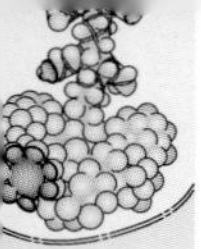

curve (Fig. 6.1). The usual rate of motor unit discharge in humans is 5 to 15 Hz, which is on the steep portion of the force-frequency curve; therefore, small changes in the nerve discharge rate in the physiologic range cause large changes in force output. The forces generated during a maximum voluntary effort (such as the static mouth pressure maneuver discussed in a later section) are considered to represent brief high frequencies (e.g., greater than 50-Hz maneuvers), but these discharge frequencies cannot be sustained for more than a brief time.

Length

Like other skeletal muscles, the respiratory muscles exhibit a length-tension relationship; specifically there is an optimal length (L_O) at which a given stimulus produces maximal force. If the muscle length is shorter or longer than this, tension is reduced. For the diaphragm in vivo, L_O lies below residual volume (RV). Therefore, at all lung volumes higher than this, respiratory muscle strength is reduced (Fig. 6.2). This has clinical implications in diseases such as COPD, in which the inspiratory muscles are chronically shortened.

Fatigue

Fatigue is a reduction in force-generating capacity of the muscle that results from activity under load and that is reversible by rest. The simplest measure of force-generating capacity is a brief maximal voluntary maneuver, but this is a high-frequency maneuver and therefore not typical of muscle contraction in vivo. Moreover, a force decrement obtained this way could occur at any point from the diaphragmatic motor area in the cortex to the interior of the diaphragmatic muscle cell. The form of fatigue currently thought to have the most clinical relevance, therefore, is a force decrement elicited by physiologic stimulation frequencies (termed *low-frequency fatigue*); this type of fatigue is also recognized to be of long duration (sometimes greater than 24 hours). Low-frequency fatigue is characterized by a reduction in force (or pressure) elicited when a muscle is stimulated at low (e.g., 10 Hz) but not high (e.g., 50 to 100 Hz) frequencies (see Fig. 6.1). In a peripheral muscle (e.g., the quadriceps), trains of electrical stimuli may be applied at different frequencies to a portion of the muscle, allowing in construction of a force-frequency curve. However, tetanic stimulation is both technically difficult to achieve for the phrenic nerve in vivo and extremely painful. As a consequence many investigators prefer to work with an unpotentiated single stimulus. With this approach a long-lasting reduction in twitch transdiaphragmatic pressure can be observed in laboratory volunteers; the reduction is considered evidence of diaphragmatic fatigue (Fig. 6.3). It has not been possible, however, to demonstrate diaphragmatic fatigue in clinical situations in which it might be expected to occur—such as in patients with COPD or those who require mechanical ventilation. Voluntary maneuvers (e.g., the static mouth pressure, discussed later in this chapter) are assumed to be of high frequency and therefore are not suitable for the assessment of low-frequency respiratory muscle fatigue.

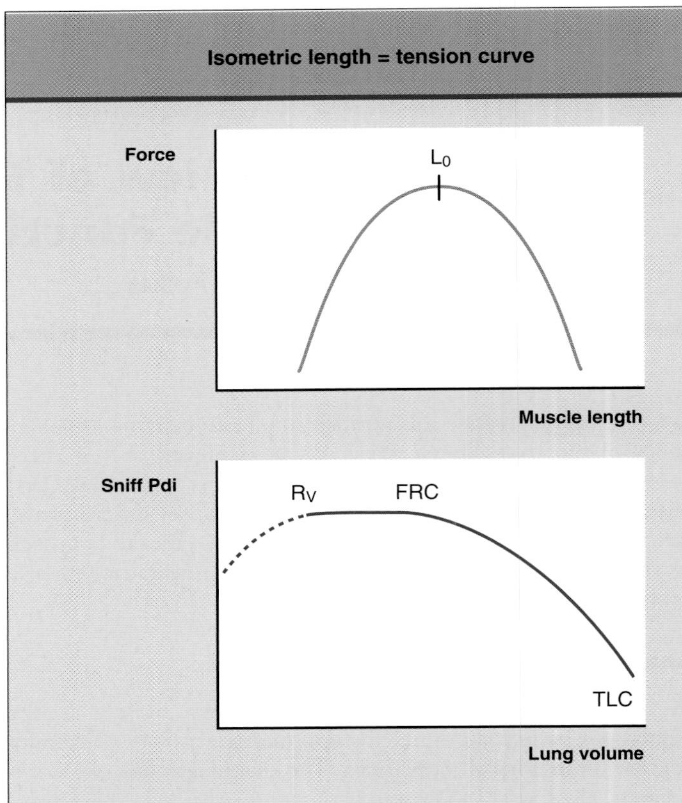

Figure 6.2 Schematic representation of the isometric length-tension curve in humans. The upper panel shows the properties of respiratory muscle in vitro, and the lower panel shows the in vivo properties of human respiratory muscle, measured as maximal sniff transdiaphragmatic pressure. (Adapted from Wanke T, Schenz G, Zwick H, et al: Dependence of maximal sniff generated mouth and transdiaphragmatic pressures on lung volume. Thorax 45:352-355, 1990.)

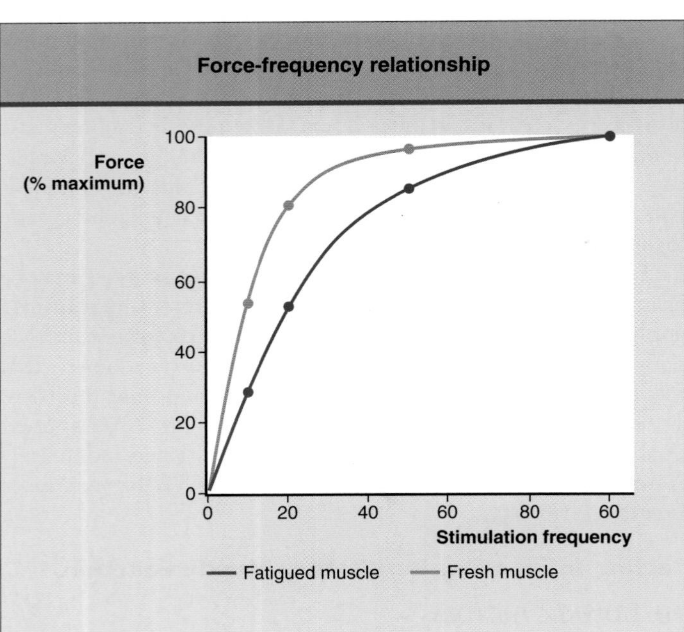

Figure 6.1 Force-frequency relationship of in vivo human respiratory muscles. The force-frequency curve of the fresh muscle is shown in red, and the relationship after a fatiguing task is shown in blue; a disproportionate force loss at low stimulation frequencies is observed. (Redrawn from Moxham J, Wiles CM, Newham D, Edwards RHT: Ciba Found Symp 82:197-212, 1981.)

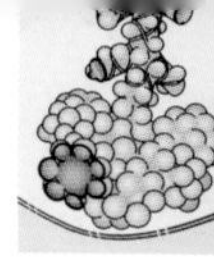

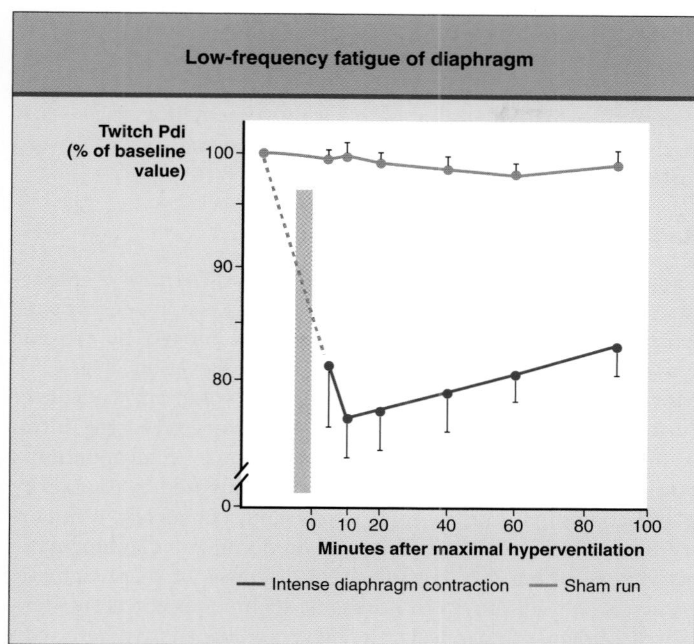

Figure 6.3 Demonstration of low-frequency fatigue of the diaphragm in normal subjects. The mean twitch tension (twitch transdiaphragmatic pressure; Tw Pdi) is shown before and at intervals up to 90 minutes after intense diaphragmatic contraction (in this case, a 2-minute period of maximal normocapnic hyperventilation) in nine healthy adults *(blue symbols)*. Data in the same subjects after a sham ("normal breathing") run is shown in red. A significant decline in Tw Pdi is observed that has only partially recovered at 90 minutes, which confirms the presence of low-frequency diaphragmatic fatigue. (Data from Hamnegård C-H, Wragg SD, Kyroussis D, et al: Diaphragm fatigue following maximal ventilation in man. Eur Respir J 9:241-247, 1996.)

PATHOLOGIC CONDITIONS

A variety of pathologic conditions may cause clinically relevant diaphragmatic dysfunction; a classification of causes is suggested in Table 6.1. Any individual clinician's exposure depends on the nature of the practice, but in my experience, in a significant proportion of patients with isolated diaphragmatic paralysis the cause of the dysfunction is not confirmed or the patient receives a clinical diagnosis of neuralgic amyotrophy.

Table 6.1
Causes of respiratory muscle weakness by aetiology and site

Acute	
Nerve	Guillain Barré Organophosphate poisoning Poliomyelitis
Neuromuscular junction	Botulism Envenomation/shellfish poisoning Drugs with neuromuscular blocking effects (as main or side effect)
Muscle	Biochemical disturbance; e.g., hypokalaemia Periodic paralysis
Chronic	
Nerve	Motor neuron disease Neuralgic amytrophy (idiopathic and familial) Critical illness polyneuropathy Chronic inflammatory demylinating polyneuropathy Trauma (iatrogenic; e.g., motor vehicle accident) Hereditary sensorimotor neuropathy Toxins (e.g., lead) Drugs (e.g., vincristine) Porphyria, diabetes mellitus Lymphomatous/malignant infiltration Vasculitis
Neuromuscular junction	Myasthenia gravis Lambert Eaton syndrome
Muscle	Muscular dystrophies Myopathies Acid maltase deficiency Hypothyroidism

RECOGNIZING RESPIRATORY MUSCLE WEAKNESS

Pursuit of the diagnosis of respiratory muscle weakness can be straightforward once the diagnosis is considered. Four clinical pictures are particularly characteristic of respiratory muscle weakness (Table 6.2). When confirmation or refutation of respiratory muscle weakness is sought, a stepwise approach is suggested (Fig. 6.4). It should be remembered that although there are various reasons why a particular test may yield a low value, a high value reliably excludes respiratory muscle weakness.

Table 6.2
Clinical syndromes characteristic of respiratory muscle weakness

1.	Patient with breathlessness unexplained by chest x-ray findings or obstructive lung disease
2.	Patient with restrictive ventilatory defect on lung function testing with a low TL_{CO} but normal or supernormal K_{CO}
3.	Patient with chronic respiratory failure unexplained by obstructive lung disease or known cause (e.g., scoliosis)
4.	Patient intubated for acute respiratory failure but found to require low pressures and low supplemental oxygen needs

Clinical Consultation

The patient may give a history that suggests the cause of respiratory muscle weakness (e.g., recent surgical procedures or symptoms of generalized neurologic disease). Symptoms that suggest isolated bilateral diaphragmatic paralysis include orthopnea and dyspnea on bending forward. However, these symptoms may be associated with other pulmonary conditions. A specific symptom of bilateral diaphragmatic paralysis is breathlessness on standing in water once the level rises higher than the costal margin. The mechanism for this is a reduction in vital capacity (VC) due to a reduced total lung capacity. Pain at the shoulder tip (or tips) or radiating down the arms suggests neuralgic amyotrophy as the cause.

Examination may confirm evidence (e.g., surgical scars in the neck) of iatrogenic injury. Evidence of neuromuscular disease

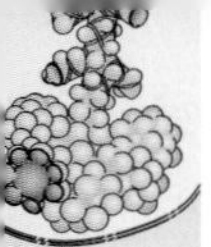

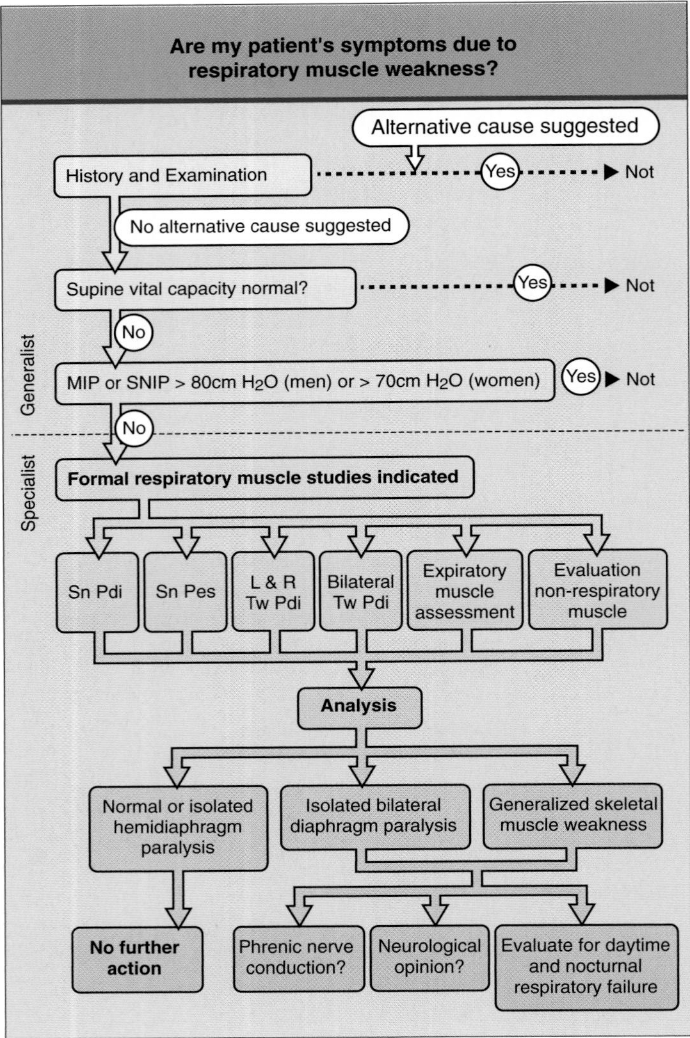

Figure 6.4 Suggested protocol for the investigation of respiratory muscle function. L, left; MIP, maximal inspiratory pressure; R, right; SNIP, sniff nasal inspiratory pressure; Sn Pdi, sniff diaphragmatic pressure; Sn Pes, sniff esophageal pressure; Tw Pdi, twitch transdiaphragmatic pressure.

should be sought; signs of denervation (wasting and fasciculation) are particularly helpful. Patients with isolated diaphragmatic paralysis and intact upper abdominal muscles exhibit the symptom of paradoxical abdominal movement (Fig. 6.5)—that is, during inspiration the anterior abdominal wall moves inward instead of outward.

Radiology

Radiology is of little or no value in the assessment of diaphragmatic function. On plain chest x-ray films, poor concordance exists between diaphragmatic function as judged by phrenic nerve stimulation and hemidiaphragmatic elevation (Fig. 6.6). Movement of the diaphragm during a voluntary maneuver (usually a sniff) can be detected by fluoroscopic screening, ultrasound, and magnetic resonance imaging. However, an apparently normal diaphragmatic movement can be simulated by expiratory phase abdominal muscle contraction, and, conversely, a minority of patients (6%) sniff without predominant diaphragmatic activity, resulting in a false-positive diagnosis of diaphragmatic paralysis. In addition, even if imaging techniques correctly identify diaphragmatic paralysis, they give no quantitative data with regard to severity. The finding of basal atelectasis on computed tomography is common in patients with respiratory muscle weakness, and so this diagnosis should be considered when these appearances are found without a clear cause.

Tests of Respiratory Muscle Strength

VITAL CAPACITY

Whenever respiratory muscle weakness is suspected, spirometry should be performed with the patient standing and lying. A reduced VC is observed in patients with respiratory muscle weakness but is clearly a nonspecific finding. Additional disadvantages are that reductions in VC are not linearly related to respiratory muscle strength and that patients with neuromuscular disease may have difficulty forming a seal around the mouthpiece and therefore generate a falsely low VC. Classically in patients with isolated diaphragmatic weakness, a fall in VC of greater than 20% is observed when the patient moves from the erect to the supine position, but this may not be observed in those patients with small VCs because of advanced respira-

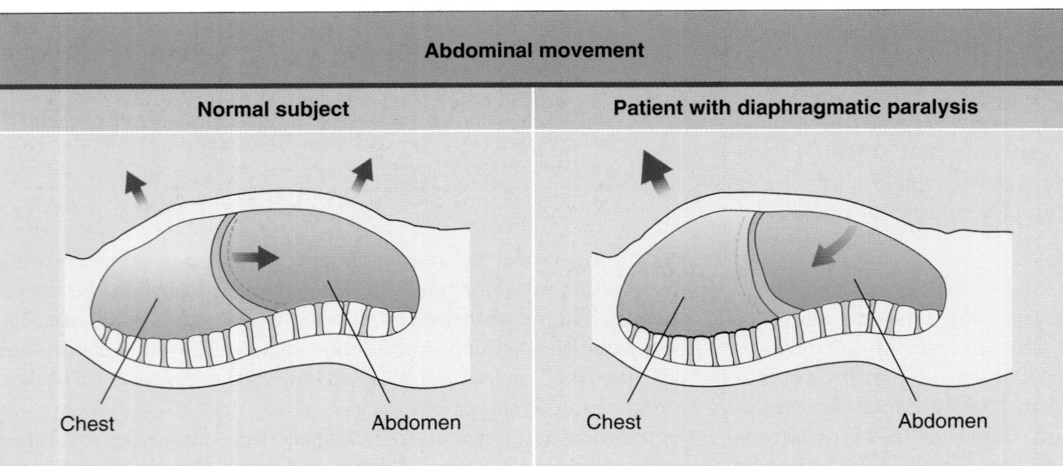

Figure 6.5 Schematic demonstration of normal abdominal and rib cage movement *(left panel)* and the paradoxical abdominal motion of isolated diaphragmatic paralysis *(right panel)*. The diaphragm at resting end-expiration is shown as a solid line and after inspiration as a dashed line. In the normal subject *(left)*, the diaphragm moves caudally, and in the patient with diaphragmatic paralysis *(right)*, the diaphragm moves in a cephalad direction.

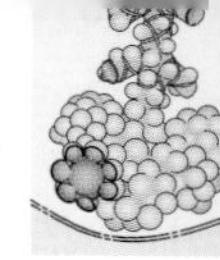

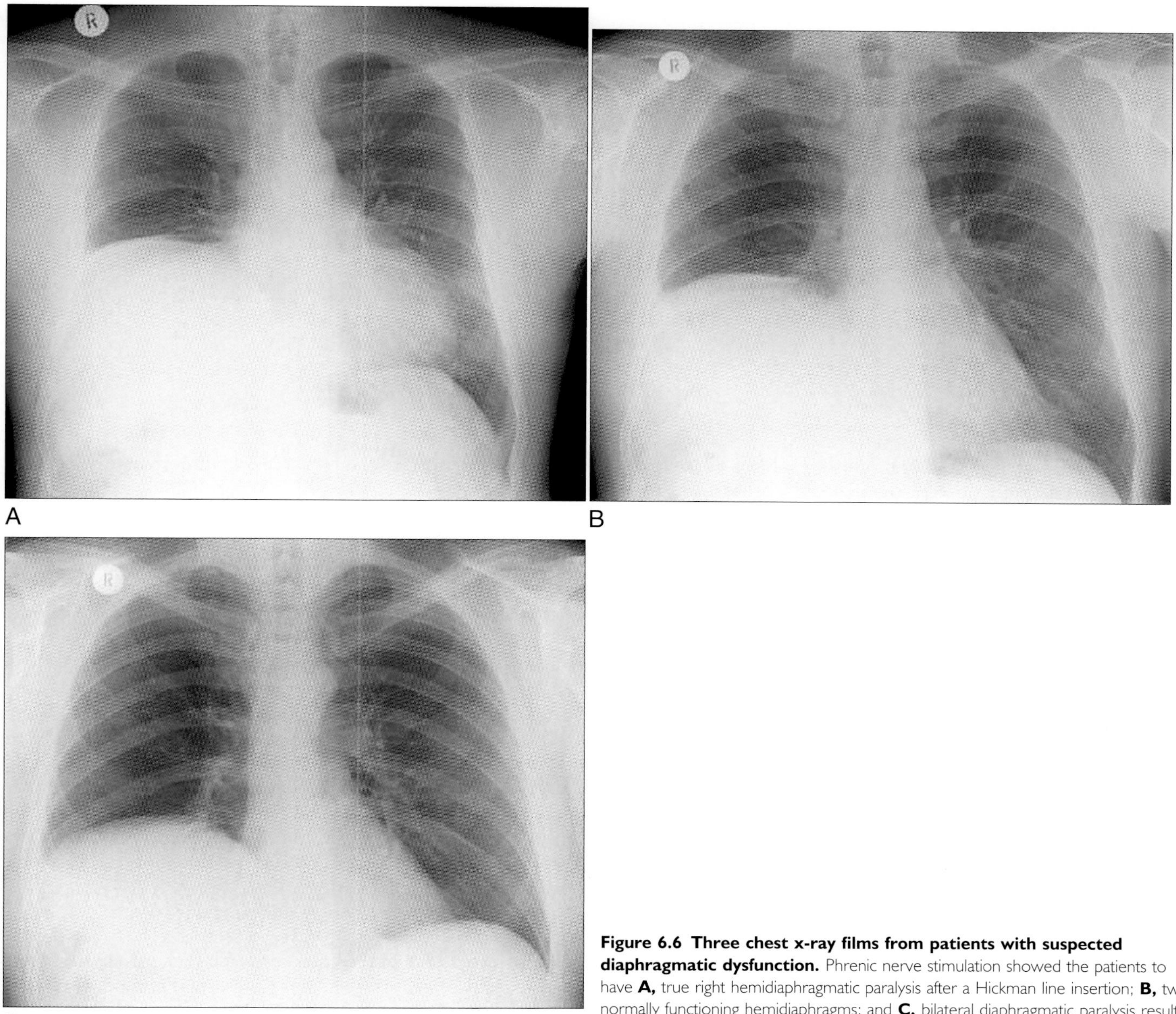

Figure 6.6 Three chest x-ray films from patients with suspected diaphragmatic dysfunction. Phrenic nerve stimulation showed the patients to have **A,** true right hemidiaphragmatic paralysis after a Hickman line insertion; **B,** two normally functioning hemidiaphragms; and **C,** bilateral diaphragmatic paralysis resulting from diabetes mellitus.

tory muscle weakness. Nevertheless, a normal (i.e., within 1.6 standard residuals) supine VC excludes clinically significant respiratory muscle weakness.

Standard pulmonary function testing may suggest an extrathoracic restrictive defect (low total lung capacity, low single-breath carbon monoxide diffusion (TL_{CO}), or normal or supranormal transfer coefficient (K_{CO}), but these abnormalities are also present in skeletal chest wall disorders and obesity. Fluttering on the flow volume loop is a recognized feature of diseases that have vocal cord involvement (e.g., amyotrophic lateral sclerosis).

STATIC INSPIRATORY AND EXPIRATORY MOUTH PRESSURES

The maximum pressure generated during a static inspiratory or expiratory effort against a closed airway is a direct reflection of respiratory muscle strength. Values for this test have been obtained in large series in normal subjects, but normal values fall within a wide range. In addition, obtaining an accurate result depends on the ability to seal the lips around the mouthpiece, which poses a problem in patients with neuromuscular disease. A final problem is that a significant learning effect seems to exist. Nevertheless, unequivocally normal static pressures can exclude clinically significant respiratory muscle weakness.

SNIFF NASAL INSPIRATORY PRESSURE

A recently developed test, measurement of the sniff nasal inspiratory pressure is an alternative noninvasive method for the evaluation of inspiratory muscle function and may have particular application in patients unable to complete a static mouth pressure maneuver. Pressure is measured by means of a bung placed

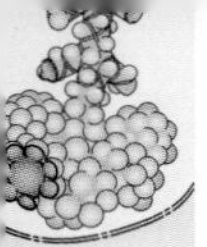

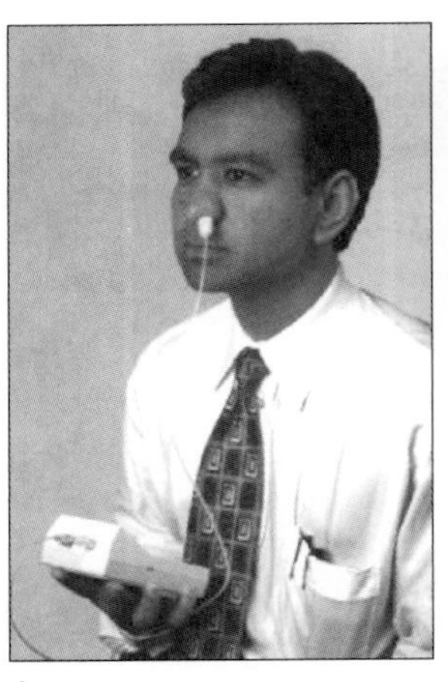

A

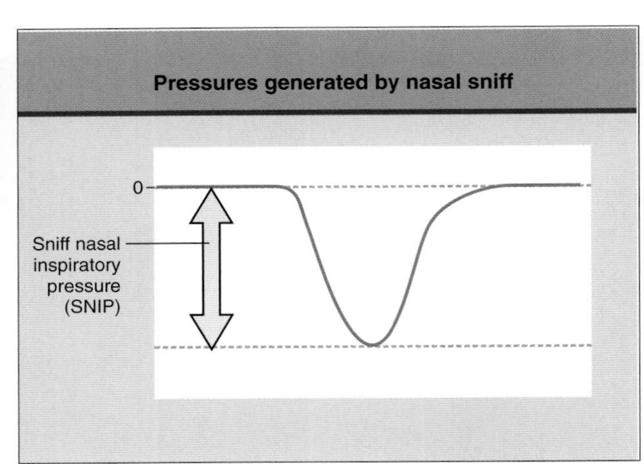

B

Figure 6.7 The sniff maneuver, which makes use of a nasal bung and an adapted pressure meter. **A,** Measurement setup. **B,** The trace produced. The meter returns a numerical value that is the amplitude of the pressure swing between atmospheric (0) pressure and the nadir.

in the occluded nostril (Fig. 6.7) while the subject performs a maximal voluntary sniff through the unoccluded nostril.

FORMAL RESPIRATORY MUSCLE TESTING

In many cases the forgoing tests exclude respiratory muscle weakness as the cause of the patient's symptoms. However, in a few cases additional tests are required to resolve matters, and these are normally conducted in specialist laboratories. A recent joint task force of the American Thoracic Society and the European Respiratory Society has provided a detailed guide to this type of testing.

Measurement of Intrathoracic Pressure

Contraction of the inspiratory muscles leads to tension generation followed by muscle shortening and then a fall in intrathoracic pressure. Although measurement of pressure at the mouth or nose is adequate for the exclusion of respiratory muscle weakness in many patients, incomplete transmission of pressure between the thorax and the upper airway may occur, particularly in patients with coexistent obstructive lung disease and during short maneuvers such as the sniff or phrenic nerve stimulation test (see "Phrenic Nerve Stimulation" later in this chapter). Therefore, very accurate assessment of respiratory muscle strength requires passage of esophageal (to measure pleural pressure) and gastric catheters. Once in place the catheters also have the advantage of permitting measurement of dynamic lung compliance as well as estimation of intrinsic positive end-expiratory pressure. Transdiaphragmatic pressure is the arithmetic difference between intra-abdominal and intrathoracic pressures (Fig. 6.8).

Experience indicates that such catheters can be passed even in patients with advanced medical conditions and diseases, like amyotrophic lateral sclerosis in which bulbar dysfunction is present. A variety of catheter systems are available, including air-filled, water-filled, and solid-state types; all are adequate for the clinical evaluation of respiratory muscle strength.

Maximal Voluntary Sniff

Although it is possible to measure esophageal and transdiaphragmatic pressure during a maximal voluntary maneuver, there are two fundamental objections to this approach. First, a wide range of normal values may be obtained (in one study as low as 18 cm H_2O), so the test is poorly discriminatory. Second, variation in the type of maneuver performed (e.g., purely inspiratory or combined inspiratory-expiratory) can substantially influence the transdiaphragmatic pressure obtained. Therefore, it is best to examine pressure generation during a maximal voluntary sniff; this maneuver is predominantly diaphragmatic, at least when performed by subjects without experience with the procedure.

Figure 6.8 shows a typical sniff recording in a healthy subject and one in a patient with bilateral diaphragmatic paralysis. The normal lower limit for sniff diaphragmatic pressure is 70 cm H_2O in women and 80 cm H_2O in men. Typical values in bilateral diaphragmatic paralysis are much lower than this (e.g., 20 cm H_2O), but patients with hemidiaphragmatic paralysis may approach the normal range, and these patients can be identified with confidence only by the use of phrenic nerve stimulation. The sniff esophageal pressure is a useful indicator of global inspiratory muscle function.

Phrenic Nerve Stimulation

Stimulation of each phrenic nerve in isolation or together offers a unique way of assessing the most important component of the respiratory muscle pump. The indications for phrenic nerve stimulation are as follows:

- Measurement of phrenic nerve conduction time to elucidate cause or prognosis
- Investigation of hemidiaphragmatic function
- Accurate measurement of respiratory muscle function when previous tests have been inconclusive or when accurate sequential monitoring is required to guide therapy

The classic technique for phrenic nerve stimulation is electrical stimulation of the phrenic nerve. This technique is still useful for measurement of phrenic nerve conduction time (Fig. 6.9). The disadvantages of electrical stimulation are that it may be painful and that difficulty exists in determining whether an absent response indicates diaphragmatic paralysis or failure to locate the nerve. As a consequence of these factors the lower limit of normal values for the transdiaphragmatic pressure elicited by the bilateral twitch transdiaphragmatic pressure (Tw Pdi) is also low, and so this test is relatively nondiscriminatory except in cases of severe diaphragmatic weakness.

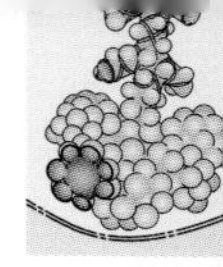

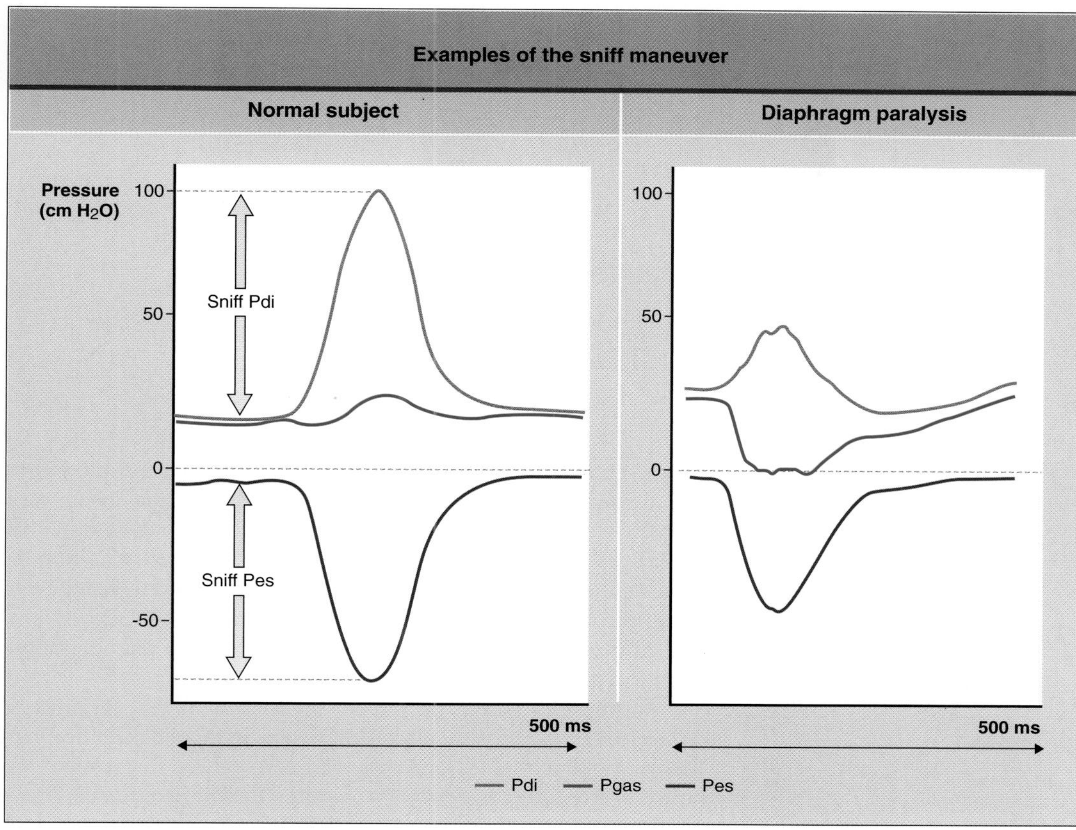

Figure 6.8 Examples of the sniff maneuver. Left panel shows a recording from a healthy subject. Note that the esophageal (pleural) pressure change is subatmospheric, whereas the intra-abdominal pressure becomes more positive. Measurement conventions for the sniff esophageal (Sn Pes) and sniff transdiaphragmatic pressures (Sn Pdi) are illustrated. The right panel shows an example from a patient with bilateral diaphragmatic paralysis. Note that there is now a negative pressure change in the abdominal compartment, because the diaphragm fails to prevent pressure transmission from the thorax.

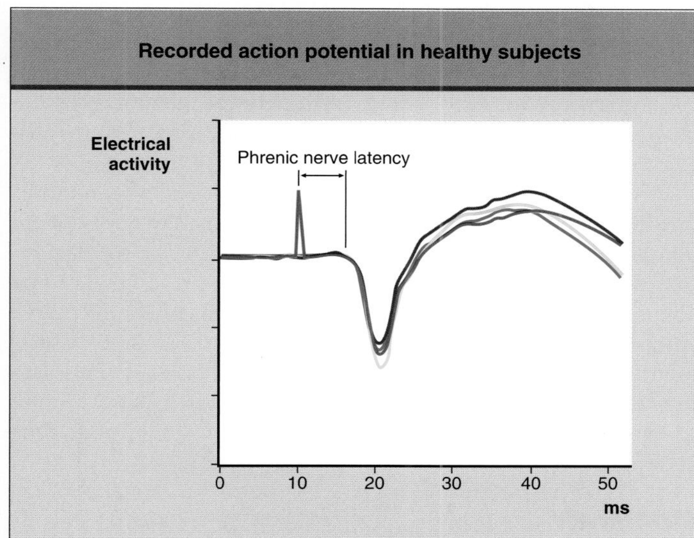

Figure 6.9 Example of an action potential recorded from surface electrodes in a healthy subject after electrical phrenic nerve stimulation.

A newly developed alternative is magnetic nerve stimulation. With this technique a brief pulsed magnetic field is created by the discharge of a large quantity of electrical energy (approximately 5000 V) through a stimulator coil. The shape of the field is determined by the shape of a coil; for example, the commonly used 90-mm circular coil produces a "volcano-shaped" field (Fig. 6.10).

Unlike electrical energy, the field passes through biologic material to a depth of up to 10 cm, depending on coil configuration. With the exception of patients with cardiac pacemakers, in whom stimulator use is contraindicated, magnetic stimulation is much better tolerated than electrical stimulation. Measurement of twitch Pdi in response to cervical magnetic stimulation is the simplest nonvolitional method of measuring diaphragmatic strength, and unilateral magnetic stimulation of the phrenic nerve may be used to assess hemidiaphragmatic function (Fig. 6.11).

Clinical Use of Respiratory Muscle Strength Data

The diagnosis of respiratory muscle weakness is useful for avoiding unnecessary diagnostic investigations directed at elucidating the cause of a patient's breathlessness or other symptoms. It may also be useful for anticipating the need for mechanical ventilation. For acute respiratory muscle weakness (the most common problem in the developed world being the Guillain-Barré syndrome), it is usual to measure the VC. Values less than 15 ml/kg indicate the need for urgent mechanical ventilation, although this threshold must be revised upward in the case of coexistent pulmonary or other disease, such as obesity, that places a load on the respiratory system. For diseases with a slower course, such as amyotrophic lateral sclerosis, more detailed tests are appropriate, and the "field" test with the best predictive power with regard to daytime hypercapnia is measurement of the sniff nasal inspiratory pressure. The finding of a low sniff nasal inspiratory pressure in a normocapnic patient

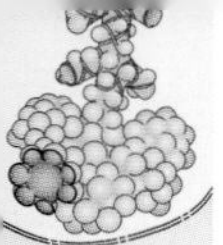

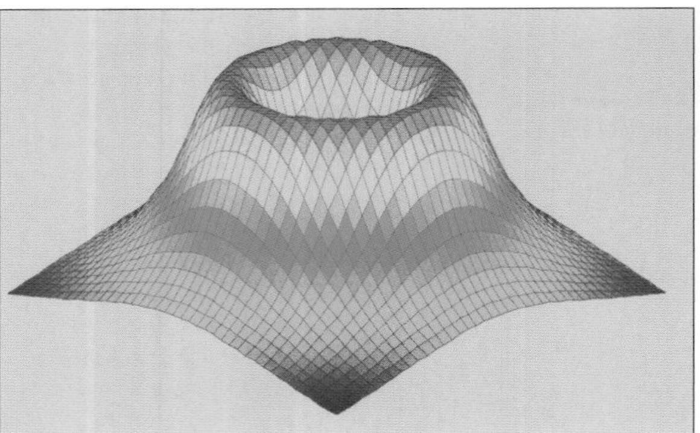

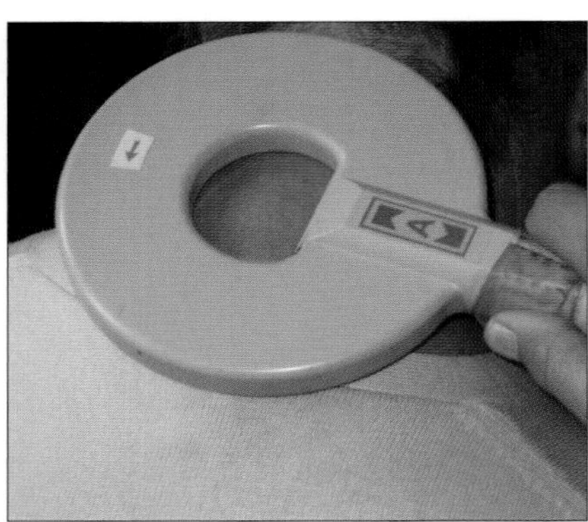

Figure 6.10 Cervical magnetic stimulation. The left panel shows the field created by discharge of a 90-mm circular coil. The right panel shows the coil in position over the cervical nerve roots for percutaneous stimulation of the phrenic nerves.

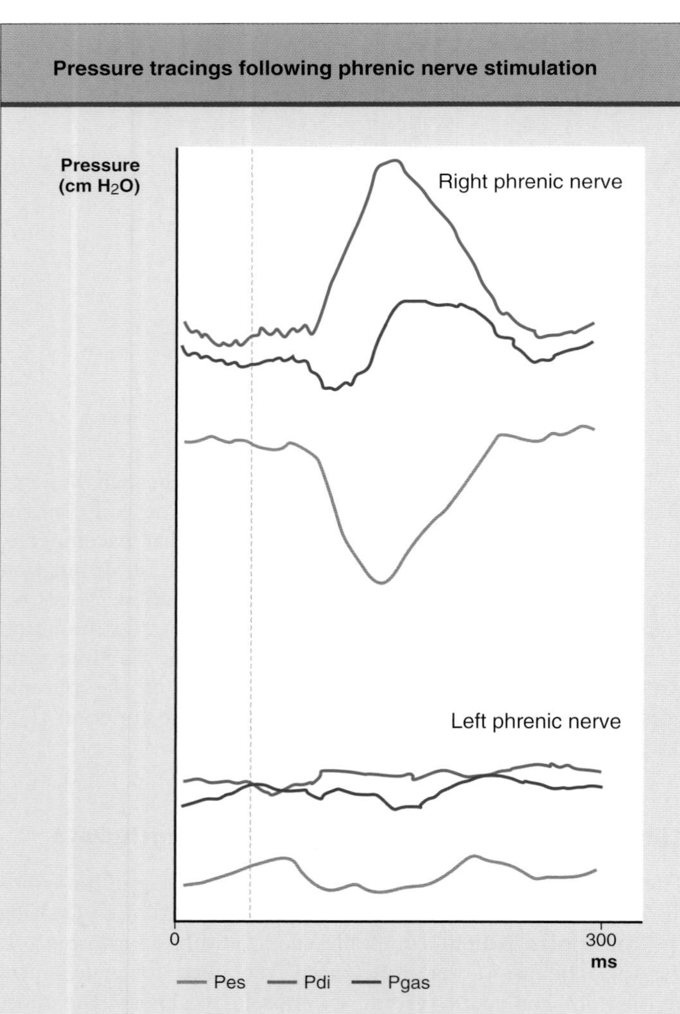

Figure 6.11 Examples of pressure tracings produced after left and right phrenic nerve stimulation in a patient with left phrenic nerve injury. The time of stimulation is shown by the dashed line.

with motor neuron disease should prompt discussion about the patient's preferences with regard to noninvasive ventilation.

Special Situations

Some situations arise in which clinical measurement of respiratory muscle strength is difficult. One such situation is in children, in whom it may be difficult to obtain a true maximum from voluntary maneuvers. In practice the sniff nasal inspiratory pressure measurement has well defined normal values down to age 5 years. Magnetic stimulation is feasible in children, infants, and neonates in whom assessment of diaphragmatic function is required; in these situations the major clinical concern is how much discomfort is justified when attempting to pass measurement catheters.

Another situation in which measurement of respiratory muscle strength is difficult is the patient with advanced emphysema. Such patients may generate low values for respiratory muscle strength for two reasons other than impaired diaphragmatic contractility. The first is that where functional residual capacity is increased, as is usual because of expiratory flow limitation, then inspiratory (but not expiratory) muscle strength is reduced by virtue of the force-length relationship discussed previously. Second, tests measuring the pressure generated in the upper airway, especially measurement of the sniff nasal inspiratory pressure, may be poorly reflective of pleural pressure change because of impaired pressure transmission through diseased airways.

A more common problem is the adult patient who requires invasive mechanical ventilation. Such patients may have critical illness polyneuropathy and therefore be at high risk for respiratory muscle pump dysfunction, yet they also are unlikely to be able to make a maximal voluntary contraction. A phrenic nerve stimulation technique is therefore essential for accurate assessment of the respiratory muscle pump. To obtain accurate data in this situation, the investigator must pay particular attention to ensuring that the airway is occluded and to monitoring lung volume.

SUMMARY

When the cause of breathlessness or respiratory failure is unknown, then respiratory muscle weakness deserves consideration, particularly when predisposing factors are present. Very often, simple tests can confirm or refute the possibility. When necessary, specialized tests can be diagnostic and may also give clues regarding the cause of the condition. Identification of respiratory muscle weakness may save the patient other unnecessary investigations. The condition can be palliated using noninvasive positive pressure ventilation.

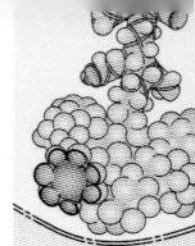

SUGGESTED READINGS

American Thoracic Society, European Respiratory Society: ATS/ERS statement on respiratory muscle testing. Am J Respir Crit Care Med 166:518-624, 2002.

Hamnegård C-H, Wragg SD, Kyroussis D, et al: Diaphragm fatigue following maximal ventilation in man. Eur Respir J 9:241-247, 1996.

Hamnegård C-H, Wragg SD, Mills GH, et al: Clinical assessment of diaphragm strength by cervical magnetic stimulation of the phrenic nerves. Thorax 51:1239-1242, 1996.

Lyall RA, Donaldson N, Polkey MI, et al: Respiratory muscle strength and ventilatory failure in amyotrophic lateral sclerosis. Brain 124:2000-2013, 2001.

Moxham J, Wiles CM, Newham D, Edwards RHT: Contractile function and fatigue of the respiratory muscles in man. Ciba Found Symp 82:197-212, 1981.

Polkey MI, Green M, Moxham J: Measurement of respiratory muscle strength. Thorax 50:1131-1135, 1995.

Polkey MI, Moxham J: Clinical aspects of respiratory muscle dysfunction in the critically ill. Chest 119:926-939, 2001.

Rafferty GF, Leech S, Knight L, et al: Sniff nasal inspiratory pressure in children. Pediatr Pulmonol 29:468-475, 2000.

Wanke T, Schenz G, Zwick H, et al: Dependence of maximal sniff generated mouth and transdiaphragmatic pressures on lung volume. Thorax 45:352-355, 1990.

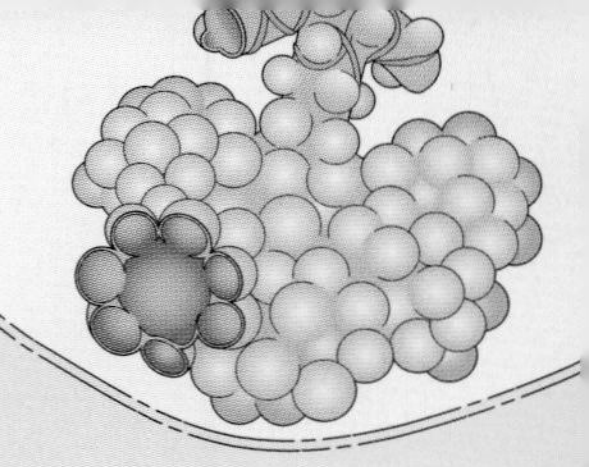

CHAPTER 7

Pulmonary Function and Exercise Testing

Bruce H. Culver

PULMONARY FUNCTION TESTING

Pulmonary function testing encompasses a range of measurements, from those that can be readily obtained at the bedside or in the home to complex physiologic assessments made in a referral laboratory.

Spirometry performed in the office is useful to screen for abnormalities of airflow or lung volume, to test bronchodilator responsiveness, and to periodically assess patients who have asthma or chronic obstructive pulmonary disease (COPD). Screening spirometry is now recommended for middle-aged smokers and former smokers to identify airflow obstruction at an earlier stage, before presentation with dyspnea. Testing in the pulmonary function laboratory allows further classification and quantification of lung disease by adding data from the evaluation of lung volumes and gas exchange through the measurement of diffusing capacity and arterial blood gases and the testing of gas distribution. Special testing is available for prethoracotomy evaluation, measurement of upper airway obstruction, and bronchoprovocation challenge testing and to assess exercise response.

Spirometry

Assessments of vital capacity (VC) and airflow are based on the forced expiratory volume maneuver, in which the subject inhales maximally to total lung capacity (TLC), then exhales forcefully and completely to residual volume (RV). The expiratory flow rate at any point during this maneuver is determined by the driving pressure for airflow and the airway resistance. During a forceful exhalation, the intrathoracic pressure that surrounds the central airways exceeds the intraluminal pressure, causing dynamic compression of the airway (see Chapter 2, Fig. 2.13). As a result, the effective driving pressure becomes the difference between alveolar pressure and the pleural pressure that compresses airways. This pressure difference is equivalent to the elastic recoil pressure of the lung tissue. Thus, even during a forceful effort, the intrinsic elastic properties of the lung are a major determinant of airflow. Airway resistance upstream from the point of compression is determined primarily by airway caliber, which varies directly with lung volume. Throughout exhalation from TLC, both recoil pressure and airway caliber progressively decrease, so that airflow rates, after an early peak, also progressively decrease.

To obtain a satisfactory spirogram, the preceding inspiration must be maximal, and the forced expiratory volume maneuver must be continued to cessation of flow or, when emptying is slowed, for at least 6 to 10 seconds. The resultant information is commonly displayed in one of two formats. The traditional spirogram (Fig. 7.1) plots volume versus time, with flow rate indicated by the steepness of the plot. The orientation of the axes varies with equipment, with time moving either left or right and exhaled volume either up or down. In the flow-volume display (Fig. 7.2), the flow rate is measured and plotted on the vertical axis, with volume on the horizontal axis. Time is not shown on this plot but may be indicated by tick marks. With this display, the reproducibility of successive efforts and some patterns of abnormality may be more easily seen. It is important to recognize that both the traditional spirogram and the expiratory flow-volume display are obtained from the same maneuver but emphasize different aspects of the same information.

EXPIRATORY FLOW MEASUREMENTS

Basic measurements from the forced expiratory volume maneuver include the forced vital capacity (FVC), the forced expiratory volume in 1 second (FEV_1), and the ratio of FEV_1 to FVC. The FVC or total volume exhaled is equivalent in normal individuals to a VC measured after a complete but *not forceful* exhalation. Patients who have advanced obstructive airway disease often manifest exaggerated dynamic compression (i.e., more severe narrowing of airways with forceful efforts), so that the FVC is smaller than the slow VC. A reduction in VC reflects a reduction in TLC, an increase in RV, or a combination of both. The FEV_1 is readily obtained from the traditional spirogram by observing the volume exhaled in the first second of effort. This measurement cannot be seen on the flow-volume display but can be calculated by the microprocessors in most modern equipment that uses this display. The FEV_1/FVC ratio is easily obtained from simple equipment and provides the best index of airflow limitation. When the slow VC is also available, and if it is larger than the FVC, it should be substituted for the FVC, as this may increase the ratio's sensitivity for detecting airway obstruction. This ratio is commonly expressed as a percentage and referred to as the percent FEV_1; however, this terminology may cause confusion, because the FEV_1 itself is expressed as a percentage of its predicted value.

An additional flow measurement commonly reported from the spirogram is the average forced expiratory flow rate between 25% and 75% of the exhaled VC (FEF_{25-75}), formerly referred to as the maximum midexpiratory flow rate. This measurement shows wider variability than does FEV_1 or the FEV_1/FVC ratio, both within and between individuals. When this variability is appropriately accounted for, the FEF_{25-75} is no

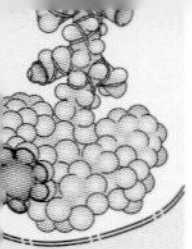

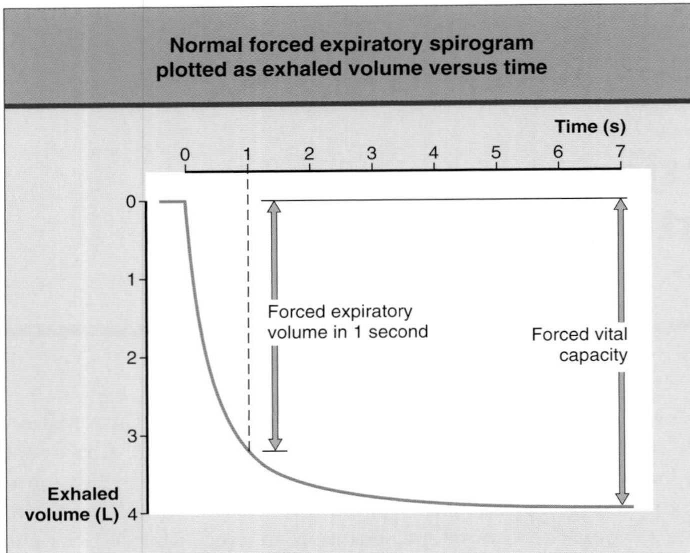

Figure 7.1 Normal forced expiratory spirogram plotted as exhaled volume versus time. The forced expiratory volume at 1 second (FEV_1) and forced vital capacity (FVC) are indicated by arrows. In this example, FEV_1 is 3.35 L, FVC is 4 L, and the FEV_1/FVC ratio is 84%. (Modified with permission from Culver BH: Pulmonary function testing. In Kelly WN [ed]: Textbook of Internal Medicine. Philadelphia, JB Lippincott, 1988.)

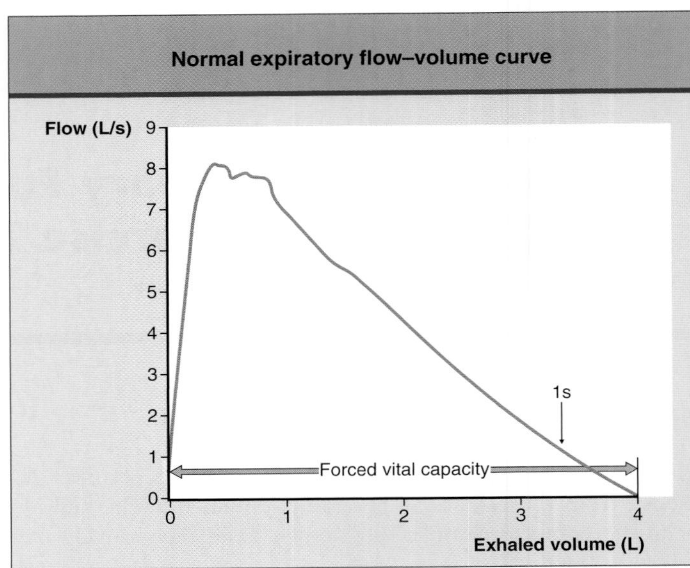

Figure 7.2 Normal expiratory flow-volume curve. The same forced expiratory volume maneuver shown in Figure 7.1 is plotted here as a flow-volume curve. The airflow rate reaches a peak early in the exhalation, then decreases progressively until airflow ceases at residual volume.

more sensitive than the FEV_1/FVC ratio for the detection of airflow limitation.

Numerous other flow measurements can be obtained from the forced expiratory volume maneuver, but they are highly interdependent with those already mentioned and add little new information. The $FEV_{0.5}$ may be used to assess the initiation of effort but adds little diagnostic information. The FEV_3 and particularly the FEV_3/FVC ratio have been shown to be slightly more sensitive than the FEV_1/FVC ratio for the detection of early airflow obstruction. This is because the measurement is extended later in the spirogram and is thus influenced more by flow at low lung volumes, where early airway disease is first manifest.

The peak expiratory flow rate achieved during the FVC maneuver cannot be accurately calculated from a spirogram display but is readily seen on the flow-volume display and can be calculated by microprocessors. It can show considerable effort-to-effort variability, even when FEV_1 and FVC measurements are nearly identical. A peak flow measurement can also be obtained by simple hand-held devices, which are useful for interval follow-up and for home management of patients who have reactive airway disease, but they are less accurate and less sensitive than spirometry for screening. Whereas spirographic flow measurements are obtained over a time interval or volume interval, measurements from the flow-volume display or current microprocessors can be reported at specific lung volumes. Maximum flow rates at 50% and 75% of exhaled volume are commonly reported, but nomenclature varies, and the latter is often designated as the flow rate at 25% of remaining VC.

The maximum voluntary ventilation (MVV) can be measured on some office spirometers, but this test is primarily a laboratory measurement. The subject is instructed to breathe deeply and rapidly, typically 60 to 70 breaths per minute, and the total volume of ventilation over a 12- to 15-second period is extrapolated to liters per minute. Historically, this was the initial dynamic test for obstructive disease, but it has now been supplanted by the forced expiratory maneuver for the diagnosis of airflow limitation. It is used as a global assessment of ventilatory capacity in the evaluation of dyspnea, the interpretation of exercise limitation, disability assessment, and some preoperative testing, and to evaluate neuromuscular disease of the chest wall and diaphragm.

PREDICTION EQUATIONS AND LIMITS OF NORMALITY

Numerous prediction equations have been derived from spirometric surveys of normal populations. Currently accepted studies exclude all smokers as well as individuals who have any thoracic or cardiopulmonary disease. Most studies have found that spirometric parameters can be predicted on the basis of gender, age, and height and that the addition of other body size measurements does not improve the accuracy of the equations.

The prediction equations give the midpoint of the normal range, which, unfortunately, is wide for most spirometric measurements. The lower limit of normal (LLN) must be established from the variability among individuals who have the same prediction parameters. For each test, the LLN is best determined by subtracting a fixed quantity, the confidence interval, from the predicted value. For most spirometric measurements, this quantity is different for males and females but does not vary with height, age, or magnitude of the predicted value.

Use of a percentage of the predicted value as a lower limit is convenient but less accurate, because it causes the normal range to vary with the magnitude of the predicted value. A lower limit value equal to 80% of the predicted value has been widely used in spirometric interpretation. Although this is a reasonable approximation for FEV_1 and FVC in young individuals, it is overly sensitive for older or smaller individuals. An 80% lower limit is quite inappropriate for FEF_{25-75}, where the normal range

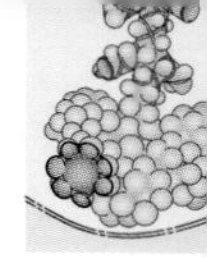

may extend to 50% to 60% of the predicted value. The predicted value for the FEV_1/FVC ratio varies little with body size but does decline progressively with age (e.g., from 87% to 77% in females, 84% to 74% in males). The LLN is approximately 8 to 10 percentage points below the predicted percentage. Because the ratio is typically expressed as a percentage, reporting this value as a percent of the predicted value is confusing and should be avoided.

The lower limit values are chosen to exclude 5% of a normal population; that is, 5% will be mislabeled as having disease. In screening a generally healthy population for a rare disease, a borderline low result is more likely to represent this mislabeling than true identification of disease. However, because spirometry is often used to test symptomatic individuals for a common disease, the probability that a borderline result reflects a true abnormality is much higher.

INTERPRETATION OF SPIROMETRIC ABNORMALITIES

Obstructive

A decrease in airflow is the hallmark of the obstructive diseases; this physiologic diagnosis rests primarily on the demonstration of an FEV_1/FVC ratio below the LLN. Typically, FVC is normal early in the course of disease but is reduced in more severe disease as the RV is increased because of trapped air. The severity of obstructive impairment is quantified by the decrement in FEV_1. When the FEV_1/FVC ratio is low, even individuals with an FEV_1 equal to 80% to 100% of the predicted value (and with a high-normal FVC) are considered to have mild airflow obstruction and have been shown to have increased morbidity over time.

Restrictive

A restrictive defect is defined by a reduction in TLC (which cannot be measured by simple spirometry), but restriction in lung volume can be inferred from spirometry when a matched decrement occurs in FVC and FEV_1 so that the FEV_1/FVC ratio is normal or high. A decrement in FVC because of the increased RV of obstruction should not be classified as a restrictive defect, because lung volumes are large. When FVC and the FEV_1/FVC ratio are both decreased, restriction can be determined only by an assessment of TLC.

Reversibility

The usefulness of spirometry in the office or clinic is often enhanced by the assessment of bronchodilator response. Spirometry is repeated after the administration of an inhaled bronchodilator, waiting 15 minutes after a β-agonist or 30 minutes after ipratropium bromide. An increase of 12% to 15% in the FEV_1 represents a significant response in an individual who has near-normal spirometry. With more severe obstructive disease, the magnitude of improvement should also be at least 200 mL to differentiate the pharmacologic response from test-to-test variability. Often FVC improves in parallel with FEV_1. An improvement in FVC by more than 15% in the absence of a change in FEV_1 may reflect either an improvement in flow rates after the first second or simply a longer duration of effort.

Although the FEV_1/FVC ratio is the most useful test for the diagnosis of airflow limitation, it may remain the same or even decrease following the use of a bronchodilator, depending on the relative change in its two components, and thus is not a useful index of reversibility. Because of its large intraindividual variability, FEF_{25-75} must show an increase of 30% to 40% to represent a significant bronchodilator effect. Occasionally, this parameter changes little or even decreases despite a clear improvement in FEV_1 or (particularly) FVC. This is because the bronchodilator has allowed exhalation to continue to a lower RV, so that the 25% to 75% increment is now measured at a lower lung volume, with consequent lower flow rates.

Lung Volumes

Spirometry can measure only those subdivisions of lung volume that lie within the VC range (see Chapter 2, Fig. 2.4). Measurement of TLC or of the volume of gas in the chest at functional residual capacity (FRC) requires a method of measuring the gas that remains in the lungs at RV. Typically, the gas volume contained in the lungs at FRC is measured, with TLC and RV determined by adding or subtracting the appropriate increments from an accompanying spirogram.

METHODS OF MEASUREMENT

The most common methods of measuring lung volumes are helium dilution, nitrogen washout, and body plethysmography. TLC can also be determined quite accurately from planimetry of posteroanterior and lateral chest radiographs or from computed tomography scans, using one of several geometric models.

Helium Dilution

A spirometer is filled with a known volume and concentration of an inert gas, typically 10% helium (Fig. 7.3). While the patient is breathing through a mouthpiece with the nose occluded, a valve is turned at end-exhalation (i.e., at FRC) to connect him or her to this closed system. As normal tidal breathing continues over the course of a few minutes, the gas in the patient's lung equilibrates with gas in the spirometer, and the helium concentration, which is continuously monitored, falls to a new, lower, steady-state level. Carbon dioxide is removed from the closed system by soda lime absorption, and a low flow of oxygen is added to compensate for the patient's ongoing oxygen consumption by keeping the mixing chamber or spirometer volume constant. The ratio of the initial to the final concentration of helium allows calculation of the unknown volume (the FRC) present in the system. A continuous tracing of the spirogram, including a maximum inspiratory and expiratory effort, allows calculation of the subdivisions of lung volume and correction for any offset from the relaxed FRC at the moment the valve was opened to start the test.

Nitrogen Washout

Nitrogen washout is also based on the principle of conservation of mass of an inert gas, in this case, the nitrogen normally contained in the lungs. The patient breathes through a mouthpiece and, at the end of a relaxed tidal exhalation, is connected to an inspiratory source of 100% oxygen (Fig. 7.4). The patient's exhaled gas is directed by one-way valves into a collection bag previously flushed with oxygen so that it contains no nitrogen. The resident nitrogen is washed out of the lungs progressively and monitored with continuous analysis. When the exhaled nitrogen concentration falls to less than 2%, the test is termi-

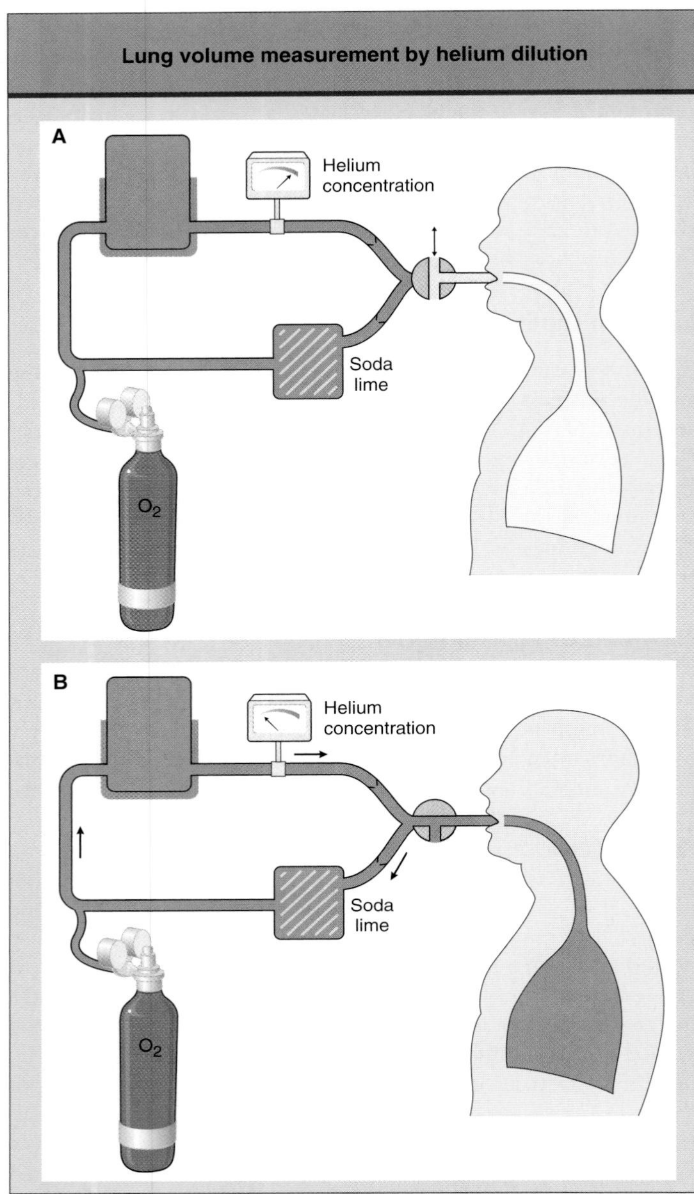

Figure 7.3 Lung volume measurement by helium dilution. A, The spirometer and circuit are prepared with a known gas volume and concentration of helium. **B,** The subject breathes through the circuit, as carbon dioxide is absorbed and oxygen consumption is replaced, until a new lower helium concentration is established. The unknown lung volume added to the circuit when the valve was turned is calculated from the dilution of the initial helium concentration: $[He]_{initial} \times Vol_I = [He]_{final} \times (Vol_I + FRC)$.

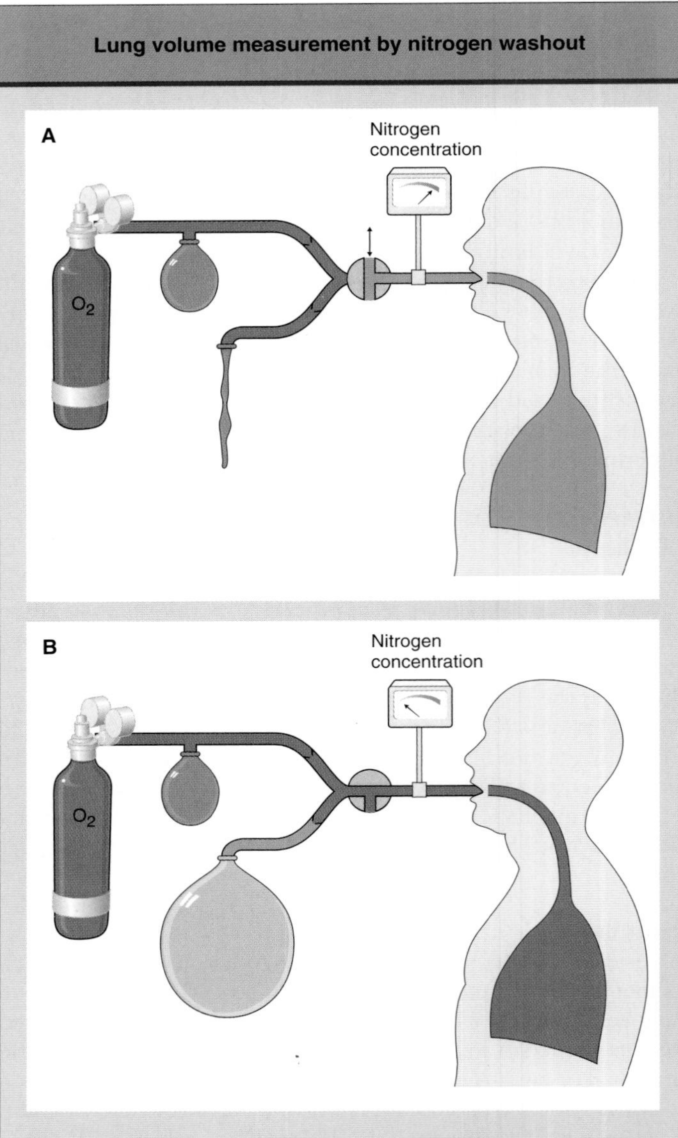

Figure 7.4 Lung volume measurement by nitrogen washout. A, Before the test, as the subject breathes air, the lungs are filled with 80% nitrogen and the collection system is flushed free of nitrogen. **B,** The subject inhales 100% oxygen and exhales into the collection bag until the exhaled N_2 concentration approaches zero. The total volume of the bag and its final N_2 concentration are measured, and the unknown initial lung volume (including valve and mouthpiece dead space) is calculated: $[N_2]_{bag} \times Vol_{bag} = 0.80 \times FRC$.

nated and the volume of nitrogen collected is measured. The FRC can be calculated on the basis that this nitrogen volume represents 80% of the lung gas contained at the beginning of the test. Instead of the collection bag, current microprocessors use a calculation based on an instantaneous, breath-by-breath measurement of exhaled volume times nitrogen concentration. Washout can be completed in 3 to 4 minutes in normal subjects but may require more than 15 minutes in patients with severe obstructive airway disease so that the gas volume in slowly mixing spaces can be measured.

Body Plethysmography

The volume of all the gas within the thorax, whether in communication with airways or not, can be measured by this technique, based on the physical principles of gas compression described by Boyle's law. The subject sits within a fully enclosed rigid box and breathes through a mouthpiece connected through a shutter to the internal volume of the box (Fig. 7.5). Sensitive manometers monitor the pressure at the airway and inside the chamber. The apparatus is calibrated with the subject in place, so that the volume addition required within the chamber to raise the chamber pressure by 1 cmH_2O is known. At the end of a tidal exhalation, the airway shutter is closed and the subject is

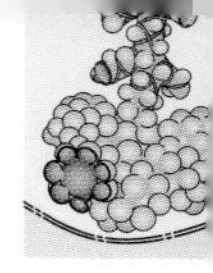

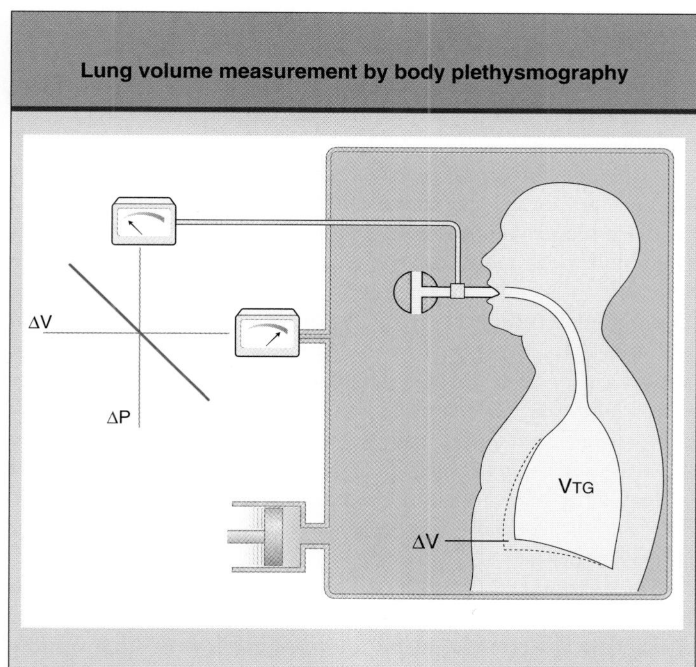

Figure 7.5 Lung volume measurement by body plethysmography. As the subject makes panting efforts against a closed airway shutter valve, the product of pressure and thoracic gas volume (V_{TG}) stays constant (Boyle's law). Thus, $P_B \times V_{TG} = (P_B - \Delta P) \times (V_{TG} + \Delta V)$. Solving for V_{TG} yields: $V_{TG} = P_B (\Delta V/\Delta P) - \Delta V$. Because ΔV is very small relative to V_{TG}, it is ignored, so $V_{TG} = P_B (\Delta V/\Delta P)$. ΔP is obtained directly from the airway pressure transducer, and ΔV is obtained from the pressure change in the plethysmograph, after calibration by cycling a known volume with a piston pump. V_{TG} is obtained from the slope of this relationship plotted during the panting maneuver.

asked to make panting efforts with the glottis open. An effort to expand the chest decompresses intrathoracic gas and reciprocally compresses that in the chamber, and the opposite occurs during an expiratory effort.

Under conditions of constant temperature, well maintained by the high blood flow through the lungs, the product of airway pressure and lung gas volume is a constant. The slope of the relationship between the change in airway pressure and the change in thoracic volume, which can be calculated continuously or plotted on an oscilloscope, is inversely related to the intrathoracic volume. Because this technique is sensitive to gas volume that is *not* in free communication with the airways, such as that in bullae or even a pneumothorax, the measurement is often called the thoracic gas volume and may commonly exceed the FRC measured by gas dilution techniques. Advantages of this method, besides its inclusion of "trapped" gas, are that several measurements can be repeated rapidly, and airway resistance can be measured with the same apparatus when panting is continued with the shutter open.

INTERPRETATION OF LUNG VOLUME ABNORMALITIES

Inspiration is limited at TLC when the maximum inspiratory force that can be applied by the chest muscles and diaphragm is opposed equally by the increasing recoil force of the lungs as they are distended to higher volumes. Usually, TLC is limited primarily by the elastic properties of the lungs, as variations in muscle strength have only a small effect on total chest expansion until weakness becomes quite marked. Parenchymal restrictive diseases reduce lung compliance, so greater distending pressure is required to achieve any volume change and, eventually, lower TLC. The displacement of intrathoracic gas volume by effusions, edema, intravascular volume, and inflammatory cells also contributes to a reduction in measured lung gas volumes. Except for pleural effusions, these quantities are relatively small and are outweighed by the frequently associated changes in lung elastic properties.

The minimum lung volume, or RV, is determined by a combination of two factors. The first is the amount of squeeze the chest wall and abdominal muscles can provide, and this is the dominant factor determining the RV in youth. The second factor is airway closure. With progressive age and the normal loss of tissue elastic recoil forces, the lung volume at which small airways close and trap remaining gas behind them increases, and this becomes the dominant factor in determining RV.

Restrictive Disease

Restrictive lung diseases are defined as those that cause a significant decrease in TLC. In most parenchymal infiltrative processes, this is accompanied by parallel decrements in FRC, RV, and VC, although a reduction in only RV may be seen in early stages of disease as increased tissue recoil delays airway closure. Obesity shows a different pattern, in that the primary effect is on the relaxed end-expiratory volume or FRC. The large abdomen and heavy chest wall reduce the outward recoil of the thoracic cage, which opposes the inward recoil of the lung parenchyma and maintains normal FRC. However, RV is determined by airway closure and is little affected, and the TLC achievable using maximum inspiratory force is only minimally reduced until obesity becomes extreme. Thus, the typical spirogram in obesity shows an FRC that approaches RV (i.e., the expiratory reserve volume is markedly reduced), but with a relatively large inspiratory capacity and a near-normal TLC and VC.

Obstructive Disease

Obstructive diseases cause airway closure that stops exhalation at a higher lung volume because of the combined effects of airway inflammation and loss of tissue recoil on luminal caliber. This results in a progressive increase in RV (Fig. 7.6), as increasing amounts of gas are trapped behind closed airways. These patients breathe at an increased FRC because of the combined effects of a decrease in lung recoil force from emphysema and the need to increase luminal caliber to minimize the resistive work of airflow. The TLC is normal to high, which again reflects the loss of lung recoil forces. Because RV increases to a greater extent than does TLC, the VC decreases with severe airway obstruction.

Diffusion Capacity

The diffusion capacity (D_L), also called transfer factor, measures the capacity to transfer gas from alveolar spaces into the alveolar capillary blood. This process occurs by passive diffusion and is a function of the pressure difference that drives gas, the surface area over which exchange takes place, and the resistance to gas movement through the membrane and into chemical com-

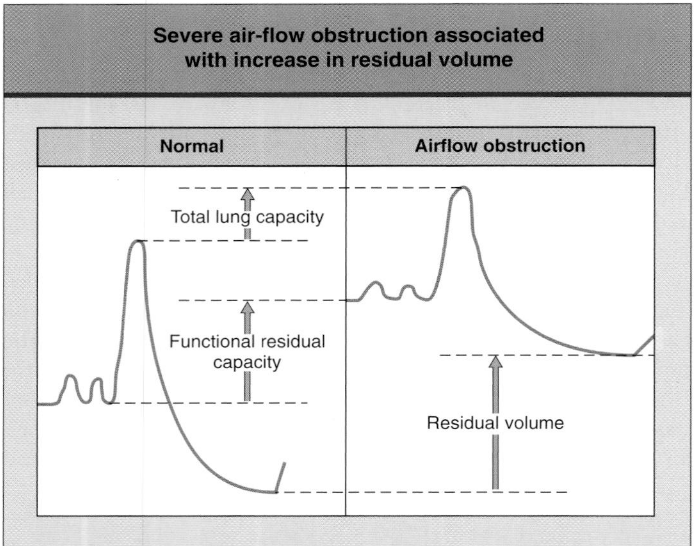

Figure 7.6 Severe airflow obstruction is associated with an increase in residual volume. Prolonged expiratory airflow may continue until the subsequent inhalation, and alveolar gas is trapped behind narrowed and closed airways. The functional residual capacity at which tidal breathing occurs is also increased, and total lung capacity may be high as well. (Modified with permission from Culver BH: Pulmonary function testing. In Kelly WN [ed]: Textbook of Internal Medicine. Philadelphia, JB Lippincott, 1988.)

bination with the blood. The units are milliliters per minute per millimeter mercury of driving pressure (mL/minute per mmHg). (In SI units, 1 mole/minute per kPa = 2.896 mL/minute per mmHg.) Carbon monoxide is used for the clinical test of diffusing capacity (DLCO) because its extreme avidity for hemoglobin allows the backpressure to diffusion to be considered negligible.

In the widely used single-breath method, the subject exhales to RV, then takes a VC inhalation of the test gas, which contains a low level of carbon monoxide (0.3%) and an inert gas (e.g., 10% helium). After holding at full inspiration for 8 to 10 seconds, the subject exhales quickly. The initial portion of the expirate, which includes anatomic dead space, is discarded, and a sample of the subsequent alveolar gas is collected or measured. The reduction in helium concentration in the alveolar sample allows calculation of the alveolar volume at TLC into which carbon monoxide was distributed and of the initial carbon monoxide concentration after its dilution by the resident RV. The final concentration of carbon monoxide measured in the exhaled alveolar sample allows calculation of the volume of carbon monoxide transferred out of alveoli and a calculation, for which an exponential decline is assumed, of the mean carbon monoxide driving pressure during the breath-holding period. An effective residence time is calculated from the breath-holding period plus a portion of the time of inspiration and sample collection.

A significant problem with the diffusing capacity measurement is that numerous variations in the handling of small correction factors (for gas conditions, apparatus dead space, timing measurement, and so on) can cumulatively cause the calculated value to vary substantially. Although reproducibility within a laboratory can be acceptable, the accuracy of comparisons between laboratories or to published normal standards is much less consistent, as reflected by published predicted values that vary by 20% or more. It is essential that each laboratory choose prediction equations that are appropriate to the nuances of its equipment and technique.

Although diffusion is often thought of as a function of alveolar membrane thickness, the dominant factor is usually the capillary blood volume, which influences both the surface area available for exchange and the volume of blood and hemoglobin available to accept carbon monoxide. The influence of hemoglobin concentration [Hb] can be accounted for by theoretical or empirical correction factors. The rate of blood flow is not important, because carbon monoxide is taken up even by stagnant blood (or extravasated blood, in the case of pulmonary hemorrhage), but the recruitment of capillaries during high-flow conditions such as exercise or with congenital left-to-right shunt increases the measured diffusing capacity. The LLN needs to be determined according to the same principles described earlier for spirometry.

Many laboratories also report the diffusing capacity as a ratio to the alveolar volume (DL/VA). This is also called the transfer coefficient (KCO). The implication is that loss of lung volume because of mechanical abnormalities is accompanied by a parallel loss of diffusion capacity. This, however, is not the case with a voluntary limitation of inspiration, in which capillaries remain perfused and DL/VA rises, or with pneumonectomy, in which capillaries are recruited in the remaining lung and DL/VA is again high. Diffusing capacity is commonly reduced in parenchymal inflammatory diseases, primarily because of the loss of available capillaries. The most common pattern in diseases such as sarcoidosis and interstitial fibrosis is for DL to be reduced and DL/VA to be slightly low or "normal," as volume is also lost. Both DL and DL/VA are low with the loss of capillary surface area and blood volume in emphysema and in diseases that are primarily vascular, such as vasculitis, recurrent emboli, and pulmonary hypertension. Clinical interpretation of diffusion abnormality should be based primarily on the DL, with small published correction factors available for [Hb] and lung volume, rather than the DL/VA ratio.

Tests of Gas Distribution

Abnormalities of spirometry and airflow rate reflect overall narrowing of airways, but most lung diseases affect airways irregularly, which leads to abnormalities of gas distribution that may be more sensitive indicators of early airway disease.

CLOSING VOLUME

As lung volume decreases, the smaller, intraparenchymal airways decrease in caliber until they close at low lung volume, and ventilation to or from alveoli beyond these points of closure ceases. Because there is a vertical gradient in the pleural pressure that surrounds the lungs (when subjects are supine, standing, sitting, or in either lateral decubitus position), the lung is less distended in dependent regions than it is higher in the thorax. In late exhalation, dependent airways close (and these areas reach their regional RV), while air continues to flow from the upper portions of the lung until they too close, and overall RV is reached. The beginning of this wave of ascending airway closure can be detected by physiologic tests and is termed *closing volume.*

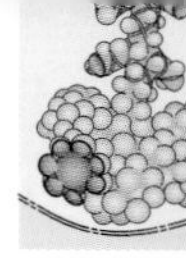

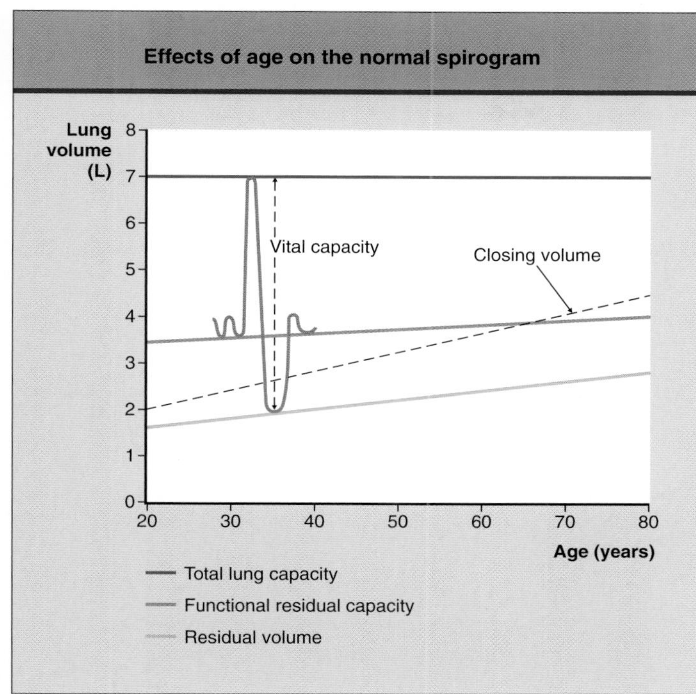

Figure 7.7 Effects of age on the normal spirogram. Residual volume progressively increases, with an associated small reduction in vital capacity. The functional residual capacity (FRC) increases slightly, but the closing volume, at which dependent airways cease to ventilate, increases more steeply and exceeds the normal FRC in older ages. (Modified with permission from Culver and Butler.) Culver BH, Butler J: Alterations in pulmonary function. In Andres R, Bierman E, Hazzard W [eds]: Principles of Geriatric Medicine. New York, McGraw-Hill, 1985.

Closing volume is usually expressed as a percentage of VC. That is, a closing volume of 20% means that airway closure can be detected during a slow exhalation when 20% of the VC remains before reaching RV (Fig. 7.7). Alternatively, when RV is measured, this can be added to closing volume, and the sum, termed the *closing capacity*, is expressed as a percentage of TLC.

Both these measures have been used as tests of early airway dysfunction in the natural history of COPD. Abnormalities can be detected in a high percentage of smokers, but the diagnostic usefulness is limited because this includes many who do not go on to develop progressive airflow limitation. On an individual patient basis, the closing volume is most helpful in its relationship to the lung volume at which tidal breathing occurs. When airway closure occurs at a volume below FRC, the airways are open throughout the lungs during tidal breathing, but when airway closure occurs above FRC, the affected alveoli are underventilated. Because the dependent regions are well perfused, this creates a region with a low ventilation-to-perfusion ratio, which contributes to hypoxemia. This occurs when the closing volume is increased by normal aging, COPD, and the effect of peribronchial edema in left ventricular failure. Similar consequences follow when FRC is reduced by recumbent posture or by obesity.

Arterial Blood Gas Measurement

Measurement of pH, PCO_2, and PO_2 in arterial blood is commonly included in the complete pulmonary function assessment of patients suspected of having lung disease. Both pH and PCO_2 are directly measured, and the accompanying bicarbonate concentration is calculated from the Henderson-Hasselbalch equation. (The value of this "calculated" data must not be discounted; it is every bit as accurate as the pH and PCO_2 measurements from which it is derived.)

An increase in arterial PCO_2 means that alveolar ventilation is low relative to carbon dioxide production because total ventilation is low, the effective alveolar ventilation is reduced by excessive wasted ventilation, or the carbon dioxide production level has increased without a concomitant increase in ventilation. The matching of ventilation to the needed carbon dioxide elimination is a function of both mechanical capabilities and ventilatory drive. Most patients who suffer hypercapnia have severe mechanical impairments, but those who also have relatively low drive are more likely to retain carbon dioxide. Patients who have an FEV_1 greater than 1 L rarely retain carbon dioxide unless lack of drive is a major factor. Despite the airflow obstruction present during an acute asthma attack, multiple stimuli tend to increase drive and ventilation. However, when obstruction becomes extreme, again with an FEV_1 around 1 L or below for an adult, the development of acute hypercapnia is likely. Most parenchymal restrictive diseases tend to be associated with mild hyperventilation, presumably from mechanical stimuli to the respiratory centers, until the functional abnormalities become very severe.

The normal PCO_2 remains in a narrow range (around 40 mmHg at sea level) throughout life, but the normal PO_2 diminishes progressively with age, and the decline is more marked when measured in the supine position. In both cases, this reflects the progressive increase in closing volume with age (see Fig. 7.7). Abnormal reductions in PO_2 are caused by hypoventilation, as reflected by an increase in PCO_2, or by the combined effects of pulmonary blood flow to poorly ventilated areas (low $\dot{V}/\dot{Q}$ ratio) and right-to-left shunting. Diffusion abnormalities, unless extremely severe, rarely contribute to a low PO_2 among patients at rest. The low PO_2 commonly seen in patients who have diffusion abnormalities reflects the concomitant presence of $\dot{V}/\dot{Q}$ abnormalities associated with their disease. Diffusion limitation may make a small contribution to the reduction in PO_2 observed during exercise, but again, the major component is a worsened effect of the ventilation-perfusion abnormalities.

Special Testing

UPPER AIRWAY OBSTRUCTION

Obstruction in the central airways (e.g., tracheal tumor or stenosis) affects the expiratory flow-volume relationship in a different way than does the more common peripheral airway obstruction of COPD. The latter has its predominant effect late in expiration, with slowing of terminal flow rates, so that peak flow tends to be relatively maintained while the remaining flow-volume curve becomes progressively convex toward the horizontal axis (Fig. 7.8). Central obstructions have their primary effect early, which results in a truncated, flat-topped flow-volume curve (Fig. 7.9), reflecting a steady effort against a constant resistance. In the latter portion of expiration, the decreasing lung volume and airway caliber shift the site of major resistance to the more peripheral airways, so that the latter portion of the flow-volume curve is normal.

When a central obstruction is in the extrathoracic airway and has some variability (e.g., vocal cord paralysis), its effect

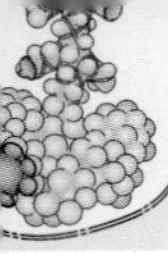

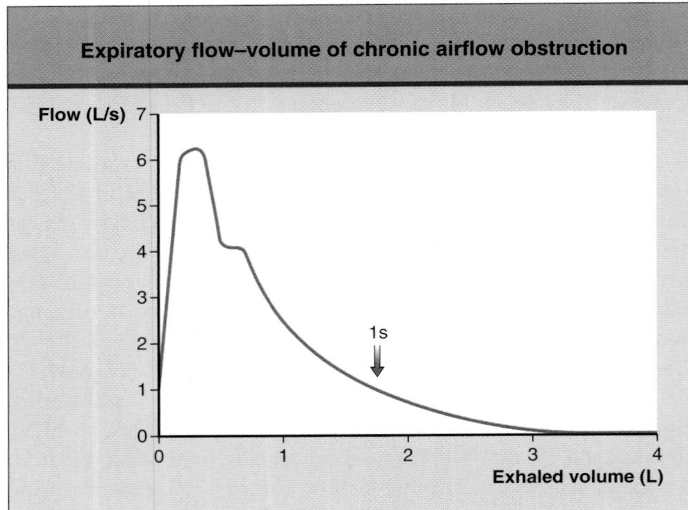

Figure 7.8 Expiratory flow-volume curve of chronic airflow obstruction. Airflow rates are markedly reduced at mid to lower lung volumes, with a curve that is convex to the horizontal axis. In this example, just under 50% of the vital capacity has been exhaled in 1 second. (Modified with permission from Culver BH: Pulmonary function testing. In Kelly WN [ed]: Textbook of Internal Medicine. Philadelphia, JB Lippincott, 1988.)

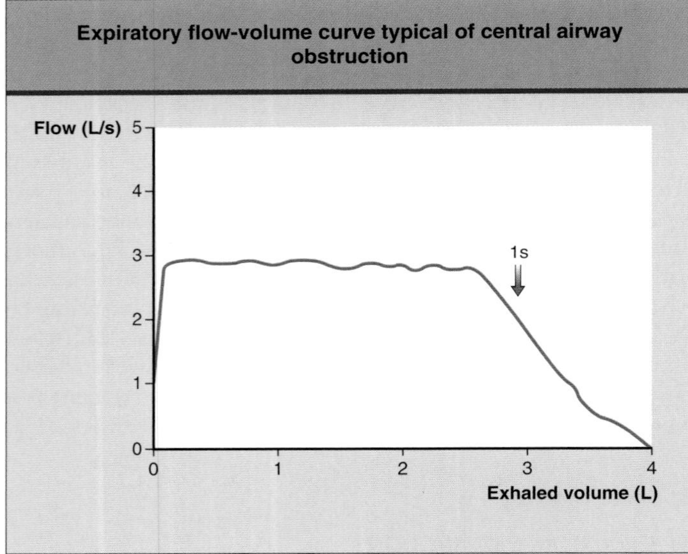

Figure 7.9 Expiratory flow-volume curve shows the pattern typical of central airway obstruction. Peak flow is markedly truncated, but the flow rates at low lung volume are unaffected. Despite the dramatic effect on the flow-volume curve, the FEV_1/FVC ratio is only modestly affected—71% in this example. (Modified with permission from Culver BH: Pulmonary function testing. In Kelly WN [ed]: Textbook of Internal Medicine. Philadelphia, JB Lippincott, 1988.)

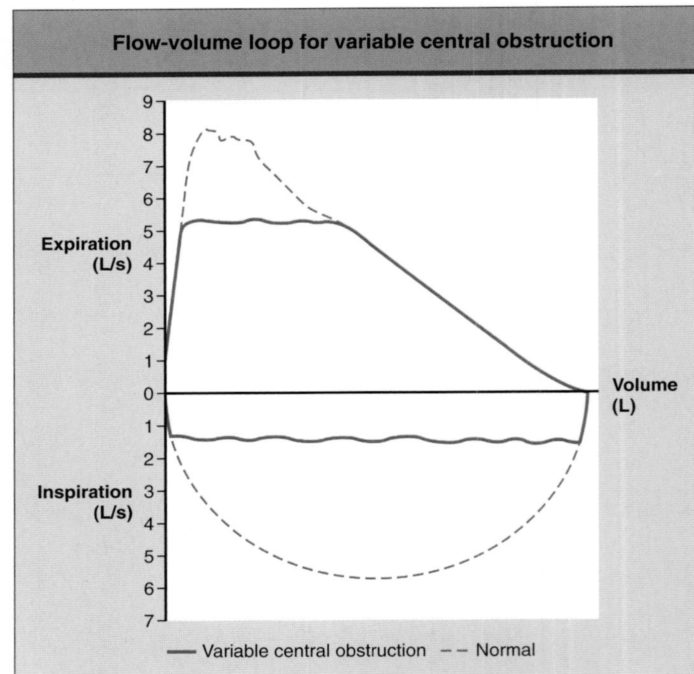

Figure 7.10 Flow-volume loop showing both forced expiratory and inspiratory airflows. The expiratory peak flow is somewhat truncated, consistent with a mild central obstruction during exhalation, whereas inspiratory flow is markedly reduced compared with the normal curve. This pattern is typical of a flexible, extrathoracic obstruction such as that caused by paralyzed vocal cords. (Modified with permission from Culver BH: Pulmonary function testing. In Kelly WN [ed]: Textbook of Internal Medicine. Philadelphia, JB Lippincott, 1988.)

is much greater during inspiratory flow than expiratory flow. The negative intraluminal pressure generated during inspiration narrows the airway, which exacerbates the obstruction, whereas during expiration, the positive airway pressure below the site of obstruction tends to distend the airway, which reduces the abnormality. These lesions are assessed by recording on the flow-volume display the maximum-effort inspiratory flow pattern, as well as that during expiration, to complete a flow-volume "loop." The normal inspiratory flow pattern has a hemicircular shape with peak inspiratory flow at midvolume that consistently exceeds midvolume expiratory flow (Fig. 7.10).

BRONCHOPROVOCATION TESTING

Patients who have suspected reactive airway disease frequently have normal spirometry readings when they are asymptomatic. When the diagnosis is unclear, provocation testing may be used in an attempt to explain symptoms or predict future risks. A common clinical provocation of asthma is the airway mucosal cooling and drying effect of exercise hyperpnea, or cold-air inhalation. Provocation testing with exercise can use free running, treadmill running, or bicycle pedaling, with the yields of abnormal tests being in that order. To provide a sufficient ventilatory stimulus, the exercise level is increased over 2 to 3 minutes to reach 70% to 90% of maximal capability, as estimated from heart rate, after which it is sustained for an additional 4 to 6 minutes. Spirometry is done before exercise and repeated after exercise, with the most marked decrease in flow rates noted at 5 to 10 minutes after exercise. A reduction in FEV_1 of 10% is considered significant, as normal subjects typically show a small increase shortly after exercise. Cold-air challenge, in which spirometry is done before and after isocapneic hyperventilation of air that has been dehumidified and cooled to 4°C, is less widely available as a provocation.

Methacholine responsiveness is a nonspecific indicator of airway reactivity. Patients are tested starting with a single inhalation at a very low concentration, and the doses are progressively

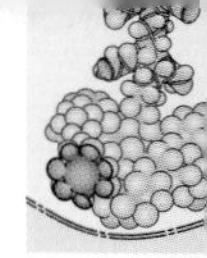

increased until either a predetermined maximum dose has been achieved or the FEV_1 has decreased by 20%. Normal individuals do not respond to the maximum dose, whereas patients with asthma usually respond to very low to intermediate doses. A negative response at the maximum dose in a patient suspected of having asthma makes that diagnosis very unlikely, but positive responses are less specific. Subjects who have a family history of asthma or hay fever symptoms may show intermediate responses, as may patients with COPD or cystic fibrosis and some normal subjects in the recovery period after viral respiratory infections.

In selected circumstances, provocation testing may be carried out with specific suspected allergens or occupational exposures. Dose preparation needs to be done carefully to avoid an excessive and dangerous response. Studies may be designed to mimic the circumstances of the patient's clinical or occupational exposure. Testing may need to be continued for several hours to seek a late-phase reaction.

RESPIRATORY AND CARDIAC RESPONSES TO EXERCISE

Cardiopulmonary exercise testing is carried out to assess a patient's exercise capacity objectively, to observe the response of the components of the oxygen delivery system to this stress, and to determine, if possible, the factor or factors that limit exercise capacity or cause exertional dyspnea. Testing procedures can range from simple measurements, such as the distance walked in 6 minutes, to a complex array of continuously monitored parameters during an incremental work protocol programmed on a calibrated ergometer or treadmill.

Normal Exercise

The work of exercise requires additional oxygen delivery to and uptake by muscles, which in turn produces more carbon dioxide. These processes require higher levels of alveolar ventilation, cardiac output, and muscle blood flow, and additional oxygen extraction from the blood. When the capacity of aerobic glycolysis approaches its limit, additional adenosine triphosphate can be generated, albeit much less efficiently, through anaerobic pathways that result in lactate production and metabolic acidosis. As these additional H^+ ions are buffered, HCO_3^- is consumed and additional carbon dioxide is produced, so that the rate of carbon dioxide output relative to oxygen uptake, the respiratory exchange ratio (R), rises. In addition, stimulation by the metabolic acidosis drives up ventilation even more near maximal exercise, and the resultant washout of carbon dioxide from the blood contributes to a further increase in R.

VENTILATORY RESPONSE

The ventilatory response to exercise is characterized by an increase in minute ventilation ($\dot{V}_E$) caused by increases in both frequency (f) and tidal volume (V_T) ($\dot{V}_E = f \times V_T$). At maximal exercise, the respiratory rate is about 40 to 50 breaths per minute, and V_T approaches about 60% of VC as end-expiratory lung volume decreases below resting FRC and end-inspiratory lung volume increases to about 80% of TLC. The effective, gas-exchanging alveolar ventilation increases further as the increased pulmonary blood flow recruits vessels, which allows less wasted ventilation in poorly perfused regions. The ratio of the volume of physiologic dead space (V_D) to V_T typically falls from about 30% to 15% to 20% with exercise, reflecting both this recruitment and the increase in tidal volume relative to anatomic dead space. Ventilation is not limiting in normal subjects, as the minute ventilation at maximal exercise is only about two thirds of the MVV measured during pulmonary testing or estimated from FEV_1. Newer techniques, plotting the tidal flow-volume loop at increasing levels of exercise within the maximum flow-volume envelope available to the patient, give additional insight into mechanisms of ventilatory response and limitation. Young normals show a comfortable reserve, but the increased ventilatory demand of highly fit athletes causes both inspiratory and expiratory flows to approach their limits. Older normals, particularly those fit enough to reach a high $\dot{V}O_2max$, show expiratory flow limitation in the latter half of the tidal volume, while both inspiratory flow and end-inspiratory lung volume may exceed 90% of their limiting values, indicating little ventilatory reserve.

CARDIAC RESPONSE

The cardiac response to exercise is dominated by a progressive increase in heart rate, as stroke volume increases modestly to a maximum value relatively early in exercise. Heart rate can increase three- to fourfold to a maximum approximated as $210 - (\text{age} \times 0.65)$. The lower resting heart rate of a well-conditioned individual, which reflects a larger stroke volume, allows a greater relative increase over resting output. Oxygen delivery to active tissues is further increased by a progressively greater extraction, from a resting value of 25% of arterial content to about 80%. The venous PO_2 levels that leave maximally exercising muscle may be less than 10 mmHg, with tissue mitochondrial levels probably less than 1 mmHg. Effective redistribution of blood flow to exercising muscle is an important, but not readily measurable, aspect of the cardiovascular response. The need for heat dissipation through increased skin blood flow compromises maximal oxygen uptake when exercise is prolonged or in a hot environment. Exercise capacity in normal subjects is limited by the maximum blood flow that can be delivered to the active muscle and, ultimately, by cellular hypoxia and acidosis. The resultant drive to ventilation may cause the sensation of dyspnea, which makes it appear that respiratory function is limiting.

BLOOD GAS RESPONSE

The blood gas response to exercise in a normal subject typically shows mild hyperventilation, with a late increase caused by acidosis, and well-maintained oxygenation. The alveolar-arterial PO_2 difference typically widens from less than 10 at rest to 20 to 25 at maximal exercise, due to a greater degree of $\dot{V}/\dot{Q}$ mismatch and the very low mixed venous oxygen, which increases the effect of any venous admixture. Despite the widened $P(A - a)O_2$, the concurrent increase in PAO_2, reflecting a greater increase in ventilation than in oxygen consumption, allows arterial PO_2 to remain normally high. (This increase in end-exercise PAO_2 will be underestimated by the alveolar gas equation [see Chapter 3, equation 3.9] unless it is recognized that R increases from 0.8 at rest to >1 at maximal exercise.) Small decrements in PO_2 have been noted at very high levels of exercise in athletic subjects, apparently due to a variable com-

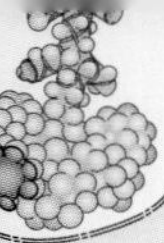

Table 7.1
Cardiopulmonary exercise testing

Parameter		Discussion
Oxygen consumption, $\dot{V}O_2max$ (L/min or mL/min) or $\dot{V}O_2/kg$ (mL/kg/min)		Reference data show an increase with body size and decline with age, but vary quite markedly from sedentary to regularly exercising "normal subjects"
		The expected capacity of obese subjects is better predicted from height than weight
Heart rate (beats/min)		Compare maximum value with 220 – age or 210 – (.65 x age); with variability of 10-15 beats around the predicted value
		Lower values may reflect chronotropic insufficiency (sometimes drug related), incomplete effort, or noncardiac limitation
		Electrocardiogram is also analyzed for arrhythmias and ischemic change
Oxygen pulse, $\dot{V}O_2$/beat (mL)		Reflects the product of stroke volume times arterial – venous O_2 content difference
		Its progressive increase during exercise results mainly from increasing extraction, but as maximum extraction is similar among individuals the maximum O_2 pulse is a surrogate for stroke volume
Blood pressure (mmHg)		Systolic pressure normally increases with exercise
		A failure to increase, or especially a decrease, reflects failure of the right ventricle (pulmonary hypertension) or LV (ischemia, aortic stenosis) to meet the output demand and is an indication to stop the test
Ventilation, $\dot{V}Emax$ (L/min)		Compare with measured maximum voluntary ventilation or with 40 x FEV_1
		Ventilatory limitation is suggested if exercise VE approaches these benchmarks
		The pattern of increase of respiratory rate and tidal volume is quite variable
Ventilatory equivalent, $\dot{V}E/\dot{V}O_2$ (L/L)		Normally about 25–30 at mid-exercise, increasing near maximum
		High values suggest either hyperventilation or excessive wasted ventilation
Anaerobic threshold, AT (mL/min or percentage of VO_2max)		Inferred from an increase in the slope of $\dot{V}CO_2$ vs $\dot{V}O_2$, $\dot{V}E$ vs $\dot{V}O_2$ or from an increase in $R > 1$
		Failure to demonstrate an AT may reflect submaximal effort
		An early AT suggests cardiac disease or poor conditioning
Wasted ventilation, $\dot{V}DS/\dot{V}T$ (%)		Calculated from $PaCO_2$ or less accurately from end-tidal PCO_2
		A failure to decrease normally with exercise shows lack of recruitability and suggests pulmonary vascular disease with a reduction in available capillary bed
Arterial blood gases:	$PaCO_2$	Low values throughout exercise suggest anxiety or excessive drive to ventilate
		A rising value above 40mmHg at end exercise is good evidence for ventilatory limitation
	PaO_2	A significant decrease with exercise usually reflects low $\dot{V}/\dot{Q}$ areas contributing increasingly desaturated blood as extraction increases and mixed venous content falls
		Flow may be redistributed to low $\dot{V}/\dot{Q}$ areas during exercise as hypoxic vasoconstriction is opposed by higher pulmonary artery pressure
		With pulmonary hypertension, shunt may develop via the foramen ovale
		Diffusion limitation probably plays a minor role, if any

bination of an excessive increase in $P(A - a)O_2$, an inadequate hyperventilatory response, and the development of diffusion limitation.

Early in exercise, arterial PCO_2 is slightly lower than normal, which reflects an increased drive that may originate from muscle receptors. As anaerobic metabolism develops, metabolic acidosis initially becomes apparent as the $PaCO_2$ drops without a corresponding increase in pH. As heart rate and cardiac output limitations are reached, more lactate is released. The capacity of a subject to continue past this point is largely a function of training and determination, perhaps enhanced by an inherently low ventilatory drive. It is not unusual for a well-motivated subject to exercise to a pH of 7.15.

Exercise Testing

Clinical cardiopulmonary exercise testing is most commonly carried out using a progressive work protocol, performed on either a treadmill with increasing speeds and slopes or a stationary bicycle pedaled at a constant rate with a variable resistance to apply an increasing load. Load is increased in a continuous ramp or at intervals ranging from 20 to 180 seconds. In simple screening tests, the electrocardiogram is monitored for heart rate, rhythm, and ischemia, and oxygenation is monitored by pulse oximetry. In more complete testing, the subject breathes through a mouthpiece for measurement of respiratory rate and VT, and minute ventilation and gases are analyzed either by interval collections or by continuous monitoring with integration over time. For blood gas information beyond oximetry, arterial blood gases can be sampled at the end of exercise, or a radial artery catheter is placed for sequential measurement.

The standard measurement of exercise capacity is the oxygen uptake per minute, $\dot{V}O_2$, and the maximum value that can be achieved during a progressive work test. The value depends to some extent on the volume of muscle that is active, so that bicycle tests yield maximums that are about 10% lower than those of treadmill tests, in which more upper body activity is

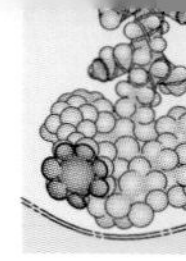

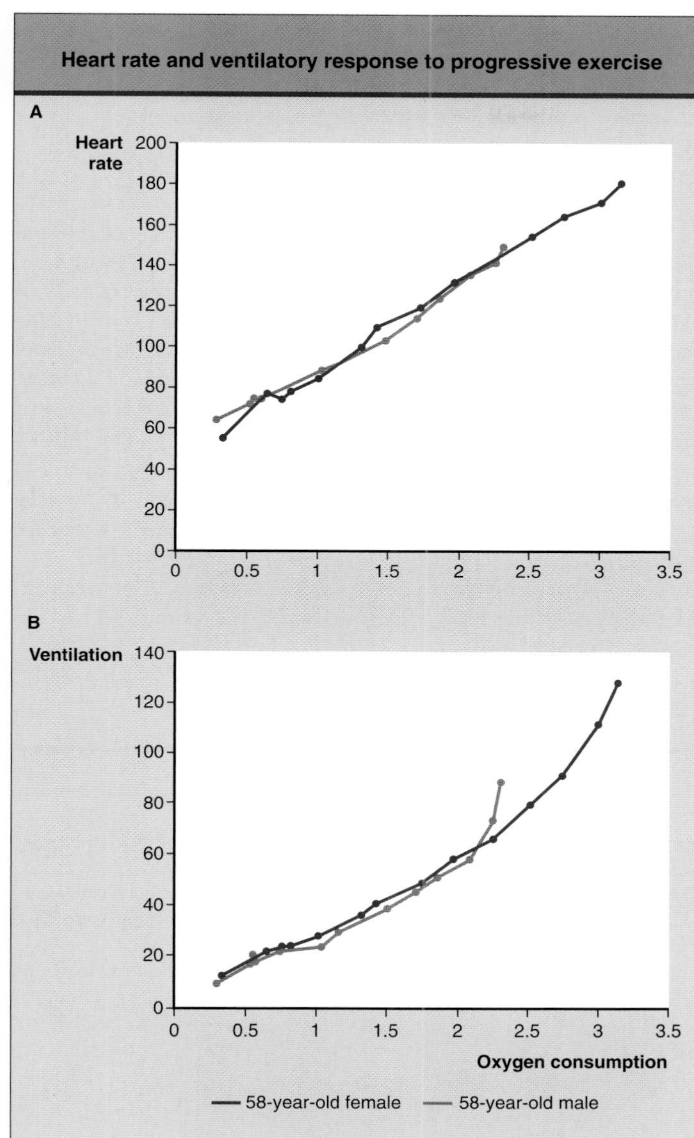

Figure 7.11 Heart rate and ventilatory response to progressive exercise. A, Heart rate is plotted for a 58-year-old man and a 38-year-old woman during a bicycle ergometer exercise test with a continuously increasing work rate to a symptom-limited maximum. Heart rate increases similarly and nearly linearly with oxygen consumption for both subjects, but the younger individual achieves an expected higher maximum. A higher stroke volume is suggested for the athletically fit woman by a lower resting heart rate and a greater calculated value for oxygen consumed per heartbeat (O_2 pulse of 18 vs. 15 mL) at maximal exercise. **B,** Both individuals have a similar ventilatory response at submaximal exercise, reflecting a normal ventilatory equivalent of about 25 L per liter of $\dot{V}O_2$. Ventilation increases disproportionately near maximal exercise but is not limiting for either subject, as each stopped well below his or her measured maximum voluntary ventilation.

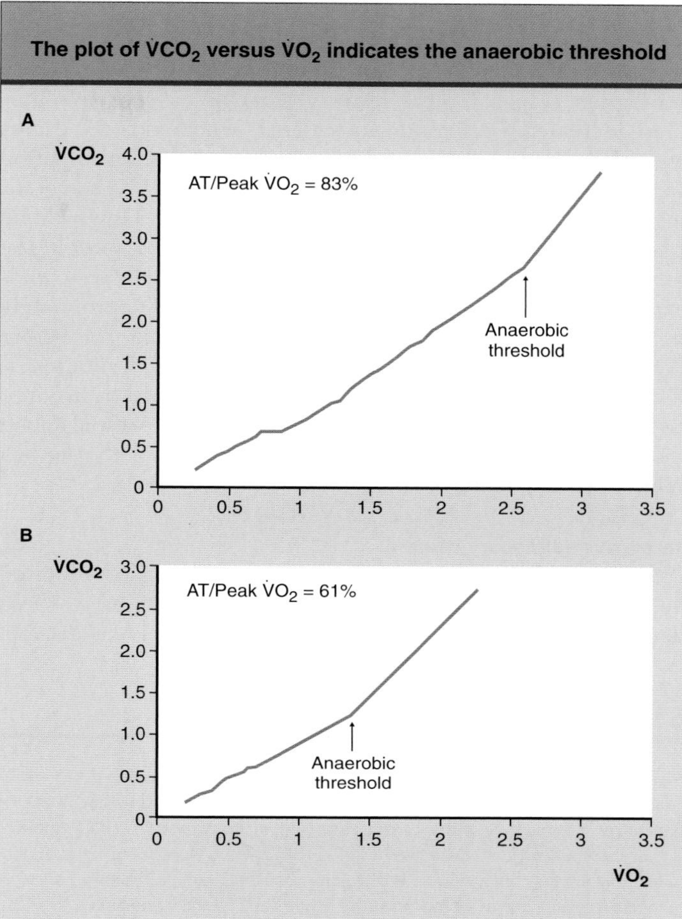

Figure 7.12 The plot of $\dot{V}CO_2$ versus $\dot{V}O_2$ indicates the anaerobic threshold. The inflection point on this plot reflects a relative increase in carbon dioxide elimination, associated with developing metabolic acidosis. Both subjects are in the normal range, but values closer to $\dot{V}O_2$max are associated with a higher level of training and fitness.

required. Because the relationships between heart rate and both cardiac output and oxygen consumption are quite linear, some information can be projected from submaximal responses, but the maximum $\dot{V}O_2$ and limits to exercise are best determined by continuing the test until the patient can no longer maintain the pace or is limited by symptoms.

The elements typically reported in the interpretation of exercise testing are given in Table 7.1. Data from exercise tests on two normal individuals, a 58-year-old man and a fit 38-year-old woman, are shown in Figures 7.11 and 7.12.

PATTERNS OF ABNORMAL EXERCISE PERFORMANCE

Cardiac Disease

Patients who have valvular cardiac impairment can reach a normal maximum heart rate, but they do so at low levels of work. A high heart rate relative to the low $\dot{V}O_2$max means the calculated oxygen pulse is low, which suggests a small forward stroke volume. The minute ventilation is also somewhat higher than expected, particularly toward the end of exercise, consistent with the early onset of an anaerobic threshold because of poor oxygen delivery. Patients who have ischemic heart disease or cardiomyopathy similarly have a low $\dot{V}O_2$ and oxygen pulse, but they often fail to reach their predicted heart rate. With the heart rate further slowed by pharmacologic treatment, these patients may show a normal or even high oxygen pulse. Patients with heart failure have been noted to breathe at low lung volume and may demonstrate expiratory flow limitation but have an adequate end-inspiratory reserve and do not approach their MVV unless there is concomitant respiratory disease.

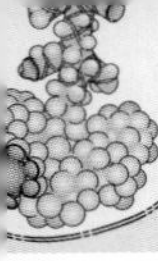

Obstructive Pulmonary Disease

Patients with severe airflow obstruction commonly have their exercise performance limited by ventilatory mechanics. Minute ventilation is high for the level of work or oxygen consumption (increased ventilatory equivalent), which reflects excess wasted ventilation. At maximal exercise, the minute ventilation approaches or even exceeds the maximum level expected for the degree of obstruction (MVV or 40 × FEV_1). Flow-volume analysis shows expiratory flow limitation throughout most of the tidal breath and dynamic hyperinflation with a shift up in end-expiratory lung volume. The heart rate increases appropriately for the work level, but maximal exercise is reached well before the predicted maximum for age. If ventilatory limitation is severe, the anaerobic threshold may not be reached or may not be demonstrated as an increase in ventilation. Arterial blood gases may show a normal or elevated P_{CO_2}, but rarely the low value expected at maximal exercise.

Restrictive Pulmonary Disease

Patients who have severe restrictive disease may also be limited by ventilatory mechanics and have similar responses to those described previously. With restrictive parenchymal lung disease, $\dot{V}_{Emax}$ may reach or exceed the MVV or FEV_1 × 40, and the ventilatory response is more likely to be characterized by a rapid rate with low V_T. Many restrictive disorders also involve a component of pulmonary vascular disease, as described next.

Pulmonary Vascular Disease

Patients who have loss of pulmonary vasculature are less able to recruit additional vascular capacity to handle the increased blood flow of exercise. Pulmonary artery pressure increases more than normal, and if pulmonary hypertension is severe, the capacity of the right heart to maintain cardiac output may be the limiting factor. Heart rate is higher than normal for the work level but may not reach the predicted maximum for age. Likewise, minute ventilation is higher than predicted at all levels, but $\dot{V}_{Emax}$ is still well below that predicted by MVV. The V_D/V_T ratio remains higher than expected with progressive exercise, which reflects the lack of significant recruitment of vessels. Exercise blood gases usually show hypocapnia and progressive hypoxemia, as the significant elevation in pulmonary artery pressure may overcome the hypoxic vasoconstriction in poorly ventilated areas of the lung, which increases the venous admixture to the arterial blood.

SUGGESTED READINGS

American Thoracic Society: Guidelines for methacholine and exercise challenge testing—1999. Am J Respir Crit Care Med 161:309-329, 2000.

American Thoracic Society: Standardization of spirometry—1994 update. Am J Respir Crit Care Med 136:1107-1136, 1995. (New documents updating spirometry, lung volumes, diffusing capacity, and pulmonary function interpretation are in preparation by a joint ATS/ERS committee.)

American Thoracic Society/American College of Chest Physicians: ATS/ACCP statement on cardiopulmonary exercise testing. Am J Respir Crit Care Med 167:211-277, 2003.

Crapo RO, Jensen RL, Wanger JS: Single-breath carbon monoxide diffusing capacity. Clin Chest Med 22:637-649, 2001.

Ferguson GT, Enright PL, Buist AS, Higgins MW: Office spirometry for lung health assessment in adults. Chest 117:1146-1161, 2000.

Hankinson JL, Odencratz JR, Fedan KB: Spirometric reference values from a sample of the general US population. Am J Respir Crit Care Med 159:179-187, 1999.

Hughes JMB, Pride NB: Lung Function Tests: Physiologic Principles and Clinical Applications. London, WB Saunders, 1999.

CHAPTER 8 Host Defenses

Galen B. Toews

The exchange of gases to support tissue metabolism is the primary function of the lung. This function requires that each day the lung come in contact with approximately 10,000 L of inhaled ambient air. The inhalation of airborne particulate matter and microbes is an unavoidable consequence of respiration. Elaborate host defenses have evolved to eliminate deposited microorganisms before their multiplication and invasion have deleterious effects on the host. The processes involved in microbial elimination are also able to injure the delicate respiratory apparatus; therefore, these responses must be tightly regulated locally to balance efficient gas exchange and host defense. Pulmonary host defenses are distributed throughout the respiratory tract. The coordinated interactions of cells or cells and soluble factors are involved in most components of pulmonary host defenses. Pulmonary host defenses can be divided into the following four components:

1. Structural defenses
2. Innate immunity
3. Inflammatory responses
4. Specific immune responses

STRUCTURAL DEFENSES

Nasopharyngeal Airways

The nose almost completely traps all particles greater than 10 mm in diameter and is a relatively effective filter for particles greater than 5 mm in diameter. The nasopharynx also absorbs both soluble and reactive gases. Sulfur dioxide, a very soluble gas, is almost completely absorbed by the nose under normal breathing conditions. Rapid changes in direction of airflow in the posterior nasopharynx favor inertial deposition of large particles. Impacted particles are removed from the nasopharyngeal airways by sneezing, coughing, or swallowing.

Ciliated mucosa is present on the nasal septum and turbinates. Mucociliary action sweeps mucus toward the posterior pharynx, where secretions are swallowed or cleared from the throat.

Conducting Airways

MUCOCILIARY ESCALATOR

Airway epithelial cells form a continuous lining of the airways (Fig. 8.1). Particles greater than 2 mm in diameter enter the conducting airway and become trapped in mucus. Mucociliary clearance and cough are the principal means of clearing particulate matter and microbes from the conducting airway. The removal of an inhaled microbe that encounters the mucous blanket covering the larger airways depends on the coordinated beating of cilia. Cough alone cannot remove mucus efficiently.

The respiratory secretions in the conducting airway contain two distinct layers (Fig. 8.2). An upper viscous layer is formed by mucins, a group of highly glycosylated proteins synthesized by epithelial cells. Mucin-synthesizing cells include goblet cells in the surface epithelium and mucous cells in the submucosal glands. A watery sublayer underlies the upper viscous layer. The underlying watery layer provides a minimally resistant material that allows the underlying cilia to beat. The tip of the beating cilia just catches the lower edge of the thicker gel phase, which propels the mucus forward. Mucins give the upper viscous layer the stickiness it requires to trap particulate matter and also present potential carbohydrate receptors for more specific interactions. *Haemophilus influenzae*, *Streptococcus pneumoniae*, and *Staphylococcus aureus* bind avidly to mucins. Bacterial binding probably enhances bacterial clearance in the presence of a normal mucociliary escalator. Conversely, it provides a foothold that allows bacterial growth and colonization in the absence of normal, efficient mucociliary clearance.

Mucus is propelled through the respiratory tract by pseudostratified, ciliated epithelium. Each ciliated cell possesses approximately 200 cilia, with a ciliary beat frequency of 12 to 14 beats per second. Microbes can be cleared from the trachea with a half-time of 30 minutes and from distal airways with a half-time of hours.

The products of immune effector cells play an important role in altering and regulating mucociliary clearance. Oxidants, which include hydrogen peroxide and superoxide, impair ciliary function, and proteases, such as elastase, damage cilia and decrease mucociliary activity. Platelet-activating factor impairs ciliary motility and decreases mucociliary clearance. Factors released from inflammatory cells can increase ciliary activity. Interferon (IFN)-γ, tumor necrosis factor (TNF)–α, and interleukin (IL)-1 increase ciliary beating by a mechanism that is dependent on nitric oxide. Neural and hormonal mediators upregulate ciliary beat frequency.

AIRWAY SECRETIONS

Airway epithelial cells secrete a variety of nonmucin constituents that are important in host defense. These include iron-binding proteins, antioxidants, and antiproteases.

Most microbes require iron for their survival. The iron is normally sequestered in cells or firmly complexed to transport proteins. Microbes compete for iron with their own transport proteins, known as siderophores. Lactoferrin, which is released by serous cells, avidly binds iron. This property is used both to inhibit the iron-dependent growth of bacteria at mucosal surfaces and to protect tissues from injury induced by hydroxyl radicals.

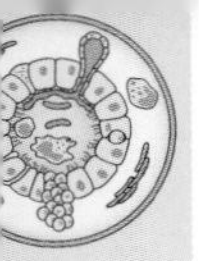

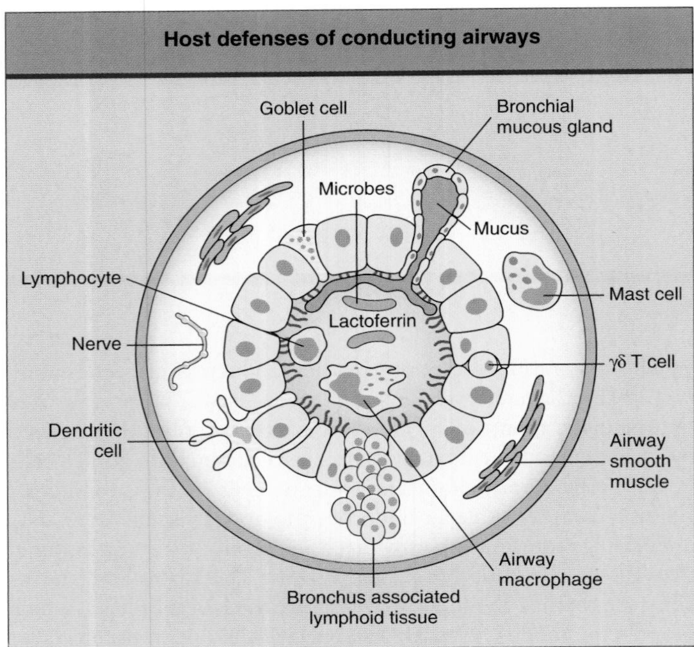

Figure 8.1 Host defenses of conducting airways. The conducting airways of the lung are complex structures composed of approximately 50 different cell types. Ciliated pseudostratified columnar epithelium lines the conducting airways and moves mucus generated by goblet cells and bronchial glands toward the mouth, where it is expectorated or swallowed. Airway macrophages move across the epithelium and recognize, ingest, and kill deposited airborne bacteria. The initiation of specific immune responses requires dendritic cells (DCs), which are present beneath and between airway epithelial cells. Lymphocytes are present within the airway, throughout the submucosa and lamina propria, and within lymphoid nodules and bronchus-associated lymphoid tissue. Lymphocytes are present between epithelial cells of the bronchial mucosa and intraepithelial lymphocytes bear γδ–T-cell receptors.

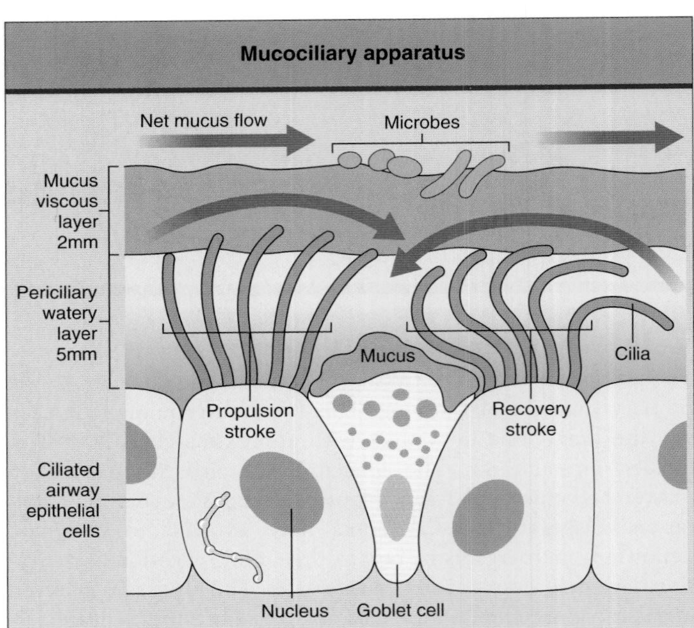

Figure 8.2 Mucociliary apparatus. The mucous blanket that coats the airways consists of two parts: an upper viscous layer and a watery sublayer. The viscous upper layer is moved in a cephalad direction by the force of the effective stroke of cilia, which just penetrate the lower edge of the gel phase. The recovery stroke of cilia takes place in a thin, watery layer in which cilia beat in an energy-conserving fashion.

Lysozyme is an enzyme that is secreted in large quantities in human airways (10 to 20 mg/day), where it helps to defend against bacterial and fungal infection by catalyzing the hydrolysis of bonds between constituents of the cell walls of most bacteria. Lysozyme lyses *S. pneumoniae,* is toxic to *Cryptococcus neoformans* and *Coccidioides immitis,* and can reduce the tissue-damaging effects of inflammation by inhibiting chemotaxis and the production of toxic oxygen radicals by stimulated neutrophils.

Leukocytes and bacteria are the major sources of proteases in human airway secretions. Neutrophil elastase can degrade a wide range of extracellular matrix components, including elastin, laminin, fibronectin, and collagen. *Pseudomonas aeruginosa, S. aureus, H. influenzae,* and *S. pneumoniae* all produce bacterial proteases, which degrade elastin, immunoglobulins (Ig), lysozyme basement membrane, and complement components. Conducting airways must be protected from degradation. To counteract the potentially damaging effects of these proteases, the airway secretions contain both serum-derived proteases (alpha$_1$-antitrypsin, alpha$_2$-antichymotrypsin, and alpha$_2$-macroglobulin) and airway epithelial cell–derived proteases (the secretory leukoprotease inhibitor, elafin, which is derived entirely from the pulmonary epithelium). Elafin is produced by Clara cell lines and may also contribute to the antiprotease defenses of the airway.

INNATE IMMUNITY

The immune system is divided into innate and adaptive components. All multicellular organisms have innate immune defenses. The essential difference between the two systems is the means by which they recognize microbes. Innate immune recognition is mediated by germ line–encoded receptors. Each receptor has evolved to recognize specific infectious microorganisms by natural selection.

Innate Immune Recognition

Recognition of microbes is problematic because microbes mutate frequently and are heterogeneous. The innate immune response has evolved to allow recognition of a few highly conserved structures present in large groups of microorganisms. The receptors recognize molecular patterns rather than particular structures and therefore have been termed *pathogen recognition receptors* (PRRs). The innate immune system uses several hundred receptors to accomplish this task. The patterns recognized by PRRs are termed *pathogen-associated molecular patterns,* or PAMPs. Characteristic PAMPs include lipopolysaccharides (LPSs) and teichoic acids, shared by gram-negative and gram-positive bacteria, respectively; mannans (conserved components of yeast cell walls); and unmethylated CpG motifs, characteristic of bacterial, but not mammalian, DNA. Although PAMPs are chemically distinct, they share common features. PAMPs are produced only by microbes; are essential for survival of the microbe or for microbial pathogenicity; and are invariant structures shared by classes of pathogens.

Cells that bear innate immune or germ line–encoded PRRs include macrophages, dendritic cells (DCs), mast cells,

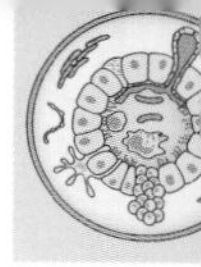

neutrophils, eosinophils, and natural killer (NK) cells. The principal functions of pattern recognition receptors include opsonization, activation of complement and coagulation cascades, phagocytosis, induction of inflammatory cytokines, and induction of apoptosis. Pattern recognition receptors trigger these effector cells to perform their effector functions immediately.

PATTERN RECOGNITION RECEPTORS

PRRs can be divided along functional lines into three classes: secreted, endocytic, and signaling receptors. Mannan-binding lectin (MBL), serum amyloid protein (SAP), and C-reactive protein (CRP) are secreted pattern recognition molecules produced by the liver during the acute phase response to infection. CRP and SAP are members of the pentraxin family; both function as opsonins following binding to phosphorylcholine on bacterial surfaces. CRP and SAP also bind to C1q and activate the classic complement pathway. MBL is a member of the collectin family, which also includes pulmonary surfactant proteins A (SP-A) and D (SP-D). Collectins typically form oligomeric receptors. MBL binds to mannose residues, which are abundant on the surface of many microbes. MBL also associates with and activates MBL-associated serum proteinases (MASPs), which initiate the lectin pathway of complement by cleaving C2 and C4 proteins.

PRRs also mediate phagocytosis of microorganisms. Macrophage mannose receptor (MMR) is a member of the C-type lectin family. MMR interacts with a variety of gram-positive and gram-negative bacteria and fungal pathogens and mediates phagocytosis and delivery of microbial pathogens into the lysosomal compartment, where they are degraded by lysosomal enzymes. DEC205, a receptor expressed on DCs, is closely related to MMR. The function and ligand specificity of DEC205 are unknown. Macrophage scavenger receptor (MSR) is another phagocytic PRR. MSR belongs to the scavenger receptor type A (SR-A) family and has a broad specificity to a variety of ligands, including double-stranded RNA, LPS, and lipoteichoic acid. MSR protects against endotoxic shock by scavenging LPS. MSR-deficient mice have an increased susceptibility to *Listeria monocytogenes,* herpes simplex virus, and malarial infections. MSR plays a role in lipid homeostasis by binding and endocytosing acetylated low-density lipoproteins. MARCO, another SR-A family member, binds to bacterial cell walls and LPS and mediates phagocytosis of bacterial pathogens.

Toll-like Receptors

Signaling PRRs recognize pathogen-associated molecular patterns and activate signal transduction pathways that induce expression of a variety of inflammatory cytokines and costimulatory molecules. Toll-like receptors (TLRs) are signaling PRRs.

Ten TLRs have been described in humans and mice. TLRs are type I transmembrane proteins that are evolutionarily conserved between insects and humans. TLRs differ from one another in ligand specificities, expression patterns, and possibly the target genes they can induce. A few thousand TLR molecules per cell are expressed on monocytes, and a few hundred TLR molecules are expressed on immature DCs. TLR expression is observed in a variety of cells, including vascular endothelial cells, adipocytes, cardiac myocytes, and epithelial cells. Each of these cells, therefore, can be considered to be components of the innate immune system.

Identification of TLR4 as the receptor for gram-negative bacterial LPS and TLR2 as the receptor for gram-positive peptidoglycan and lipopeptides led to an initial model in which each of the TLRs was expected to recognize a broad class of microbes. The discovery of additional ligands for TLR2 and TLR4 has changed the model to explain microbial recognition. Innate immune cells likely use several different TLRs to detect different features of an organism simultaneously; this permits information about the nature of the microbe to be transmitted into the cell. The innate immune system uses this information to generate a response that is tailored to the nature of the microbial threat.

TLR4, however, is not the sole receptor involved in recognition of LPS. LPS initially interacts with a serum protein, LPS-binding protein (LBP), which transfers LPS to CD14, a receptor on macrophages. MD-2, a cell surface protein, is required for TLR4-mediated recognition of LPS. The LPS-recognition complex likely consists of three molecular components: CD14, TLR4, and MD-2. The binding of LPS to CD14 presumably leads to the association of CD14 with the TLR4–MD-2 complex. Assembly of this complex may induce the dimerization of TLR4. TLR4 activation results in the recruitment of the adaptor protein MyD88, which eventually leads to NF-κB activation. NF-κB moves into the nucleus and induces transcriptional activation of a wide variety of inflammatory–immune-response genes. In addition to LPS, TLR4 has been implicated in the recognition of lipoteichoic acid, the heat-shock protein hsp60, and the fusion protein of the respiratory syncytial virus.

TLR2 recognizes more ligands than any other PRR. Ligands for TLR2 include peptidoglycan, bacterial lipoproteins, certain LPS molecules that differ in structure from the LPS of gram-negative bacteria, zymosan (a component of yeast cell walls), and a lipid from *Trypanosoma cruzi*. TLR2 does not recognize these PAMPs independently but functions by forming heterodimers with either TLR1 or TLR6. Both TLR2 and TLR6 are required for recognition of MALP-2, a mycoplasma-derived diacylated lipoprotein. Heterodimerization of TLR2 with either TLR6 or TLR1 is required for the induction of signaling.

TLR5 recognizes flagellin, the principal structural component of bacterial flagella. A significant feature of flagellin as a TLR ligand is that it is a pure protein stimulus without lipid or carbohydrate moieties. TLR9 recognizes unmethylated CpG motifs present in bacterial DNA. The logic of this recognition is that most of the mammalian genome is methylated, whereas bacteria lack CpG methylation enzymes. TLR9 likely recognizes its ligand intracellularly, perhaps in endosomes or lysosomes, presumably after bacterial lysis.

Activation of TLRs induces transcriptional activation of a wide variety of inflammatory and immune-response genes. Molecules induced by TLR activation include inflammatory mediators such as TNF-α, IL-1, IL-6, IFN-α, IFN-β, and chemokines; costimulatory molecules of T-cell activation, CD80 and CD86; and signals that regulate the differentiation of lymphocytes including IL-4, IL-5, IL-10, IL-12, transforming growth factor (TGF)-β, and IFN-γ. Activation of TLRs also results in upregulation of microbicidal killing mechanisms. TLR signaling induces inducible nitric oxide synthase (iNOS) mRNA

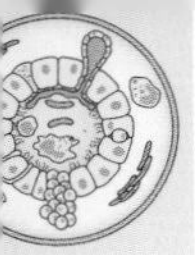

and the production of nitric oxide (NO). Although TLR2 stimulation activates the production of NO, inhibition of NO does not block TLR2-stimulated killing of intracellular microbes, which suggests that TLR2 activates other potent microbicidal mechanisms as well.

Alveolar Macrophages

Resident pulmonary macrophages constitute the first line of defense against microbes that reach the alveolar surface. Resident pulmonary macrophages can be found within the interstitium, lining the alveoli, and within the airways, both in the lumen and within the epithelial lining. These macrophages have two origins—pulmonary and alveolar. Pulmonary macrophages differentiate from monocytes that enter the lung from the circulation. Alveolar macrophages are also derived from proliferating macrophage precursors within the interstitium of the lung, and their microbicidal function is dependent on four critical attributes (Fig. 8.3)—signal recognition, migration in response to stimuli, microbe ingestion, and secretion of mediators. Macrophages recognize signals in their microenvironment via surface receptors (PRRs). Macrophages also express two distinct receptors for the third component of complement (the major soluble protein effector of innate immunity). Complement receptor 1 (CR1) preferentially binds C3b but also binds C3bi and C4b. Complement receptor 3 (CR3, CD11b/18, MAC-1, Mo-1), a member of the β_2 integrin family, is a receptor for C3bi but also recognizes LPS and fibrinogen. *Histoplasma capsulatum* binds directly to CR3. Direct binding of microbes to CR3 is an important recognition mechanism of microbes before the onset of specific immunity. Patients who have a genetic deficiency in the CD18 complex have recurrent life-threatening infections, which documents the critical role of CR3 in host defenses against infectious agents.

Phagocytosis occurs after recognition of the microbe. Particle engulfment requires receptor-ligand interactions, which guide pseudopod extensions of macrophages from points of initial local contact to circumferential envelopment (zipper hypothesis). Phagocytosis therefore requires engagement of specific receptors and the generation of transmembrane signals.

Following phagocytosis, the microbe is initially contained within a phagosome that subsequently fuses with one or more lysosomes. Resident alveolar macrophages are not fully activated for microbicidal killing. Activation stimuli for resident alveolar macrophages come from the following four sources:

1. The microorganism itself
2. Responding macrophages
3. Secreted products of other innate immune cells
4. Plasma proteins

LPS, a cell wall component of bacteria, is a potent macrophage-activating signal (Fig. 8.4). Interaction of the macrophage with LPS can occur either during engulfment of the microorganism or after LPS has been released by intracellular killing and/or digestion. Macrophage-activating stimuli are produced by macrophages themselves. The release of IFN-α and/or IFN-β, induced by LPS, provides the priming signal to augment macrophage microbicidal activity. Similarly, granulocyte-macrophage colony-stimulating factor (GM-CSF) can be a potent stimulator of macrophage activation. Cells of types other than macrophages provide important activating stimuli. Interactions with microbes lead to the nonimmune production of IFN-γ by NK cells.

Oxidative and nonoxidative processes are used by alveolar macrophages to kill ingested microbes. Resident macrophages have considerably less antimicrobial activity than monocytes. A decrease in the magnitude of the respiratory burst and the loss of granule peroxidase account for the decline. Because resident alveolar macrophages contain minimal myeloperoxidase (MPO), their MPO-H_2O_2-halide system is defective.

Figure 8.3 Alveolar macrophage functions. Macrophage functions are dependent on the ability of macrophages to recognize signals, migrate in response to stimuli, ingest microbes, and secrete mediators.

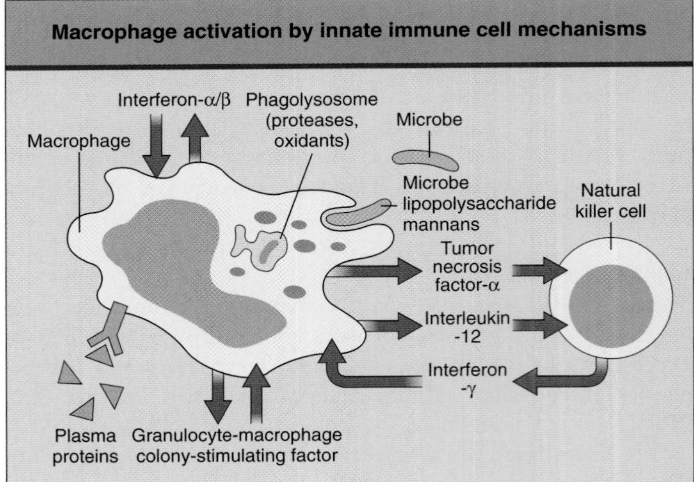

Figure 8.4 Macrophage activation by innate immune cell mechanisms. Resident macrophages that ingest microbes or interact with microbial products via cell-surface receptors produce a number of activating cytokines (interferon [IFN]-α, IFN-β, granulocyte-macrophage colony-stimulating factor [GM-CSF], tumor necrosis factor [TNF]-α, interleukin [IL]-12). Some cytokines function in an autocrine or paracrine fashion to activate macrophages. TNF-α and IL-12 induce natural killer (NK) cells to produce IFN-γ, a potent activator of macrophage microbicidal activity.

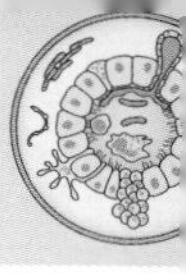

Microbes can also be killed by macrophage-dependent nonoxidative mechanisms. Defensins are a multiple-member family of cytotoxic peptides that kill many gram-positive organisms (*S. aureus*) and gram-negative species (*Escherichia coli, Klebsiella pneumoniae, P. aeruginosa*). Defensins also kill fungi and inactivate certain viruses.

Natural Killer Cells

The lung contains NK cells. Macrophage–NK cell interactions are probably critical to the activation of macrophages during innate immune responses. The interaction of macrophages with microbes produces IL-12, which, together with TNF-α, induces IFN-γ production by NK cells. Early IFN-γ activates macrophages and enhances their microbicidal activity.

Complement

Complement is the major soluble protein effector of innate immunity and is activated when either the alternative pathway interacts with carbohydrate-rich particles that lack sialic acid or the classic pathway is triggered by the binding of collectin to certain carbohydrates. Normal alveolar lavage fluids contain a functional alternative complement pathway. Complement activation generates C3b, an opsonin that promotes receptor-mediated phagocytosis of microbes by macrophages. Complement activation also produces C5a, which is an important chemoattractant for polymorphonuclear neutrophil leukocytes (PMNs). Activation of the entire complement pathway results in the assembly of the C5b-C9 complex on microbial membrane surfaces. Assembly of this membrane attack complex on the surface of a microbe results in lysis and killing of the microbe.

Surfactant

Alveolar epithelial cells secrete proteins that play important roles in innate immune responses. SP-A and SP-D are members of a group of molecules called *collectins*. Although SP-A may not function as a true opsonin, it facilitates alveolar macrophages and type II alveolar epithelial cell uptake of microbes trapped in lipid–SP-A complexes. In vitro exposure of alveolar macrophages to SP-A results in enhanced phagocytosis of *S. aureus* and *P. aeruginosa*. Also, SP-A directly binds to and opsonizes *H. influenzae* type A, promotes chemotaxis of alveolar macrophages, increases secretion of GM-CSF and IL-3, and modifies macrophage production of oxidants. Type II alveolar epithelial cells and nonciliated bronchiolar Clara cells produce SP-D, which mediates agglutination of gram-negative bacteria. Surfactant also has a role in extracellular killing of microbes through its detergent effect.

INFLAMMATORY RESPONSES

The clearance of most bacteria requires a dual phagocytic system that involves both resident alveolar macrophages and recruited polymorphonuclear leukocytes. In the setting of a low bacterial burden or exposure to minimally virulent organisms, alveolar macrophages can effectively phagocytose and kill invading organisms. However, when the bacterial burden is large, the bacteria are more virulent, or encapsulated gram-negative organisms such as *P. aeruginosa* or *K. pneumoniae* gain access to the lower air spaces, the recruitment of neutrophils is essential for effective containment and clearance of bacteria.

Recruitment of PMNs into the alveoli is initiated by the generation of chemotaxins within the alveolar space (Fig. 8.5). Complement activation occurs early via the alternative complement pathway, which can be activated by a wide variety of substances, including complex polysaccharides, LPSs (bacterial endotoxins), and surface components of certain bacteria and fungi.

Alternative complement pathway activation leads to cleavage of C5. The cleavage fragments of the C5 molecule are important chemotaxins during the early phases of pulmonary host defenses against bacterial microbes. C5-deficient mice have reduced PMN recruitment to the lung after intratracheal inoculation of *S. pneumoniae*, *P. aeruginosa*, and *H. influenzae* compared with congenic C5-sufficient mice.

Complement fragments have chemotaxic activity for both polymorphonuclear leukocytes and macrophages. Thus, complement fragments lack the specificity to account for the dominant recruitment of PMN noted in the acute inflammatory response to bacteria. A supergene family of chemotaxic cytokines, chemokines, possesses relatively high degrees of specificity for PMN and mononuclear cells. Accordingly, they provide a potential mechanism for the selective recruitment of peripheral-blood leukocytes to specific sites of inflammation.

Four closely related families of chemotaxic cytokines, referred to as CXC, CC, C, and CXXXC chemokines, have been characterized. The CXC chemokine family, which includes IL-8, MIP-2, GRO, ENA-78, and NAP-2, has stimulatory and chemotactic activity predominantly for PMN. The CC family, which includes MCP-1, MCP-2, MCP-3, RANTES, MIP-1α, and MIP-1β, has chemotaxic and/or activating effects on macrophages, lymphocytes, eosinophils, basophils, and mast cells. Lymphotactin is the only identified C chemokine, and fractalkine is the only identified CXXXC chemokine.

Macrophages are crucial to the initiation of chemokine-induced inflammatory responses. Bacterial products stimulate alveolar macrophage production of CXC chemokines. Additionally, bacterial products stimulate the production of TNF-α and IL-1, both of which induce gene expression and secretion of CXC chemokines from endothelial cells, pulmonary epithelial cells, and fibroblasts. Thus, the alveolar capillary membrane is viewed as a dynamic assembly of immune and nonimmune cells that, in aggregate, generate the quantities of both CXC and CC chemokines required to recruit specific inflammatory cells.

CXC chemokines are important in pulmonary host defenses in both patients and animal models. Respiratory secretions from patients with acute pulmonary bacterial infections contain increased amounts of IL-8. Both TNF-α and MIP-2 are rapidly induced in murine lungs following pulmonary infections with *K. pneumoniae*. Treatment of infected mice with anti–MIP-2 antibodies results in decreased clearance of *K. pneumoniae*.

When contact is established between a neutrophil and a microbe, the particle is ingested by phagocytosis. Whereas the acidic environment within phagocytic vacuoles can limit the growth of some bacteria, effective killing requires products of molecular oxygen, granule constituents, or both. Hydrogen peroxide is produced by PMNs, as well as highly reactive unstable intermediates such as superoxide ion radicals, hydroxyl radicals, and singlet oxygen molecules. Although it is not entirely clear

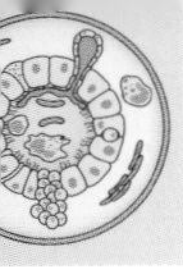

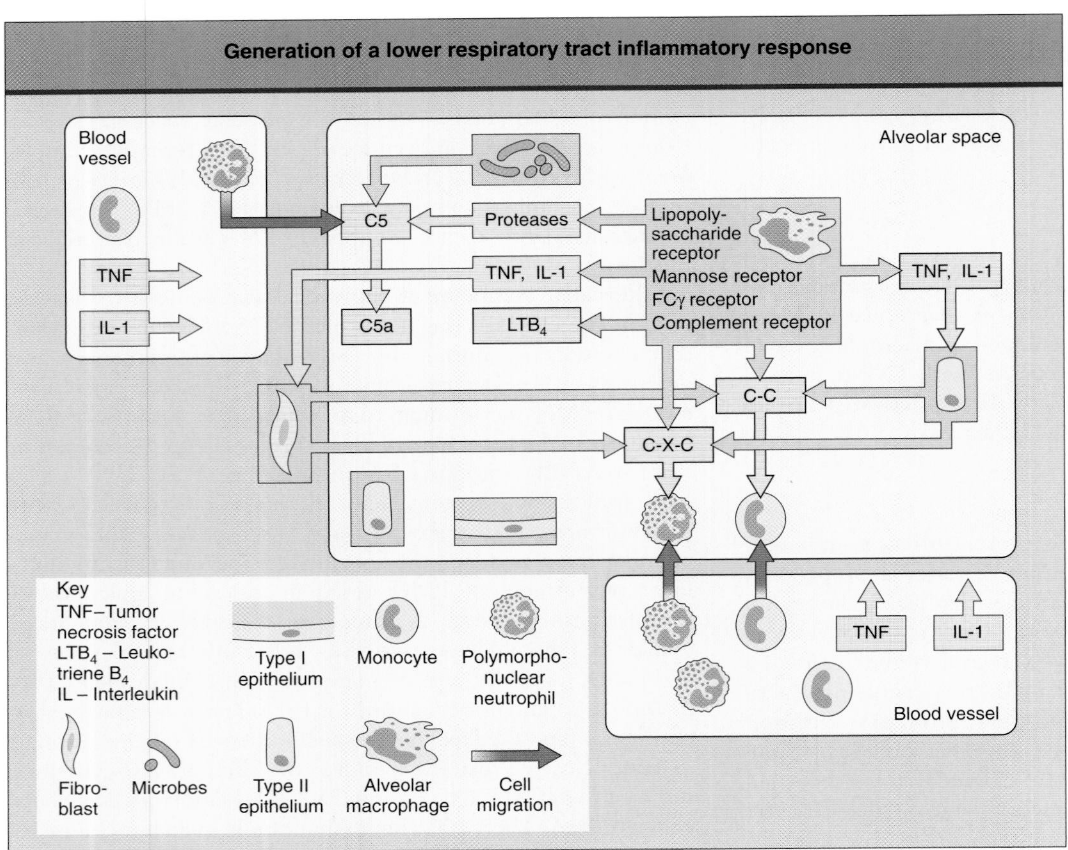

Figure 8.5 Generation of a lower respiratory tract inflammatory response. Bacteria or bacterial products that enter the alveolus are recognized by alveolar macrophages. Complement activation occurs early and generates C5a. Microbial products stimulate alveolar macrophage production of tumor necrosis factor (TNF)-α, interleukin (IL)-1, IL-8, and leukotrienes. TNF-α and IL-1β induce chemokine gene expression and chemokine production by epithelial cells and fibroblasts present in the lower respiratory tract. The entire alveolar capillary wall is engaged in the tightly regulated recruitment of inflammatory cells.

how products of the MPO–hydrogen peroxide–halide system alter the viability of bacteria and fungi, it is well established that this system participates in oxygen-dependent killing by neutrophils.

Phagocytes are also able to kill some microorganisms effectively by oxygen- and MPO-independent systems. A variety of microbicidal products are stored in cytoplasmic granules. Lactoferrin limits proliferation of bacteria by virtue of its ability to chelate iron, an essential growth factor for many microbial species. Lysozyme, found in both specific and azurophil granules of human neutrophils, efficiently hydrolyzes certain bacterial cell walls. Elastase, cathepsin G, and other cationic proteins found in neutrophil azurophil granules are capable of killing bacteria. Finally, human neutrophils contain defensins, which kill fungal organisms and a wide variety of gram-positive and gram-negative bacteria.

SPECIFIC IMMUNE RESPONSES

Specific immune responses consist functionally of two major effector systems, antibody- and cell-mediated immunities, which are generated by B and T lymphocytes, respectively. Using products of the *RAG1* and *RAG2* genes, B and T lymphocytes rearrange their Ig and T-cell receptor (TCR) genes to create approximately 10^{11} different clones of B and T lymphocytes that express distinct antigen receptors. The receptors on B lymphocytes recognize native antigens, which may be simple chemical groups, carbohydrates, or proteins. T-lymphocyte receptors recognize only peptides that are derived from protein antigens. These peptide antigens are bound to cell-surface proteins that make up what is termed the *major histocompatibility complex* (MHC) classes I and II. Clones of lymphocytes that have receptors of adequate affinity are triggered by antigen-presenting cells (APCs) to proliferate and develop into effector cells. After elimination of an infection, antigen-specific clones remain expanded as "memory" lymphocytes that provide a more rapid response to a second exposure to the antigen.

Selection of Antigens for Specific Immune Responses

T-helper lymphocytes (THs) orchestrate specific immune responses by promoting intracellular killing of microbes by macrophages, antibody production by B lymphocytes, and clonal expansion of cytotoxic T lymphocytes. The interaction between antigenic peptides presented in association with MHC class II membrane proteins on the surface of APCs and the TCRs of T cells triggers cellular activation (Fig. 8.6). The peptides are generated from exogenous antigens (bacteria, mycobacteria, fungi) that have been ingested through phagocytosis or pinocytosis. Proteins are proteolytically digested into polypeptide fragments 10 to 20 amino acids in length. Polypeptides that contain immunodominant epitopes are bound to the antigen-binding groove of the MHC glycoprotein complex and are delivered to the surface of the APC. The MHC-antigen-TCR interaction provides specificity for T-lymphocyte activation. A second costimulatory signal is required to activate T lymphocytes to produce cytokines. The costimulatory signal is delivered by CD28, a membrane protein of TH cells that, together with TCRs, costimulates the transcription of the gene encoding IL-2 and

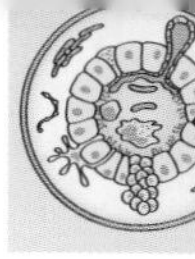

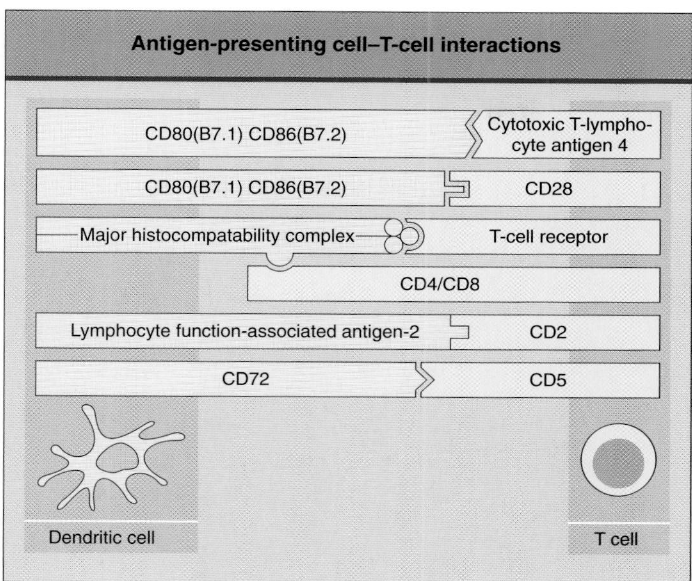

Figure 8.6 Interactions between antigen-presenting cells (APCs) and T cells. A wide variety of cell surface molecules on dendritic cells (DCs) interact with cell surface molecules on T cells. These include antigen-presenting and antigen-recognition structures such as major histocompatibility complex II, the T-cell receptor (TCR), and CD4/CD8. Costimulatory molecules such as B7 and CD28 are required for T lymphocytes to be activated. Interactions between antigen-presenting cells and T cells take place within an "immunologic synapse" formed by close cell contact between APCs and T cells.

stabilizes IL-2 messenger RNA (mRNA). The second signal is provided by the expression of the CD28 ligands, B7.1 (CD80), and B7.2 (CD86), on APCs. Cell-cell contact and transmembrane signaling are also promoted by the interaction of lymphocyte function–associated antigen (LFA) molecules on T lymphocytes with intercellular adhesion molecules (ICAMs) on APCs. As CD2 interacts with LFA-3 and CD4 interacts with MHC class II molecules, the processes that select proteins for endocytosis by APCs augment the expression of B7.1 or B7.2 or of adherence molecules and also determine which antigens activate TH cells.

Dendritic Cell Maturation and Differentiation

APCs provide an essential link between innate and adaptive immunities (Fig. 8.7). DCs are the most potent APC for T cells. DCs are localized at epithelial borders throughout the mammalian host, where they recognize pathogens and microenvironmental tissue damage and signal the presence of "danger" to cells of adaptive immunity; DCs capture antigens, migrate to draining lymphoid organs, and, after a process of maturation, select antigen-specific lymphocytes to which they present processed antigen, thereby initiating adaptive immune responses. DCs at different maturational stages may differ in phenotype, function, and localization. At least three stages of maturation have been delineated, including precursor DCs found in blood and lymphatics, tissue-residing immature DCs, and mature DCs present within secondary lymphoid organs.

DC progenitors represent a small fraction of $CD34^+$ hematopoietic progenitor cells in bone marrow or peripheral blood. GM-CSF and TNF-α stimulate growth and differentiation of DC progenitors into DC precursors. This process is modulated by multiple cytokines including c-KIT ligand, Flt-3 ligand, IL-3, TGF-β, IL-4, and IL-13. Myeloid DCs are closely related to monocytes. Monocytes generate myeloid DC when cultured with GM-CSF and IL-4. Conversely, immature myeloid DCs differentiate to macrophage phenotypes when cultured with M-CSF. Whether a monocyte becomes a DC or a macrophage may in part be influenced in vivo by the endothelium. Monocytes that transmigrate the endothelium in the abluminal-to-luminal direction (during entry to lymphatics) become DCs; those that remain in the tissues become macrophages.

Dendritic Cell Migration

Chemokines and chemokine receptors play a major role in directing the right cells to the right places. Immature DCs as well as monocytes express various receptors for inflammatory chemokines such as CCR1 (receptor for RANTES); CCR2 (receptor shared by MCP-1 through MCP-4); CCR3 (receptor for eotaxin); CCR5 (receptor for MIP-1α, MIP-1β, and RANTES); and CCR6 (receptor for MIP-3α). As a result of these receptor-ligand interactions, monocytes and immature DCs are rapidly recruited to organs undergoing inflammatory responses. After arrival at sites of inflammation, DCs capture antigens. Proteins internalized by macropinocytosis are degraded, and the resultant peptides, associated with newly synthesized MHC class II molecules, form complexes that are expressed at the plasma membrane. Larger particulates, such as microbes, are internalized by phagocytosis. Microbial glycoconjugates are taken up through specialized receptors.

Dendritic Cell Maturation

DC maturation occurs at the site of inflammation. Maturation of pulmonary DCs might occur through two different pathways following antigen exposure (see Fig. 8.7). First, microbial products such as LPS might bind to TLRs on epithelial cells, macrophages, and DCs. TLR ligand interactions on epithelial cells and macrophages would then lead to the release of cytokines. TLRs would also induce cytokine expression and expression of CD80 and CD86 molecules on the surface of APCs. Because PAMPs occur only on pathogens, TLRs induce CD80 and CD86 molecules only in the presence of infection. T cells require at least two signals to become activated; one is a complex of a peptide and an MHC molecule, and the other is a costimulatory signal mediated by molecules such as CD80 and CD86 on the surface of APCs. Accordingly, a T cell receives both of the signals required for activation only if its receptor binds to the peptide that was derived from the pathogen that induced the expression of CD80 or CD86 molecule through its PAMP. This mechanism ensures that, normally, only pathogen-specific T cells are activated. Recognition of an antigen in the absence of CD80 or CD86 molecules leads to permanent inactivation or apoptosis of T cells. Innate immune recognition thus controls all major aspects of the adaptive immune response through the recognition of infectious microbes and the induction of signals required for the triggering of specific immunity.

The maturation process also leads to migration to secondary lymphoid organs. Maturing DCs downregulate CCR1, CCR5, and CCR6. Conversely, receptors for constitutive chemokines, CCR4, CCR7, and CXCR4 are upregulated in maturing DCs.

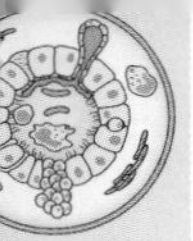

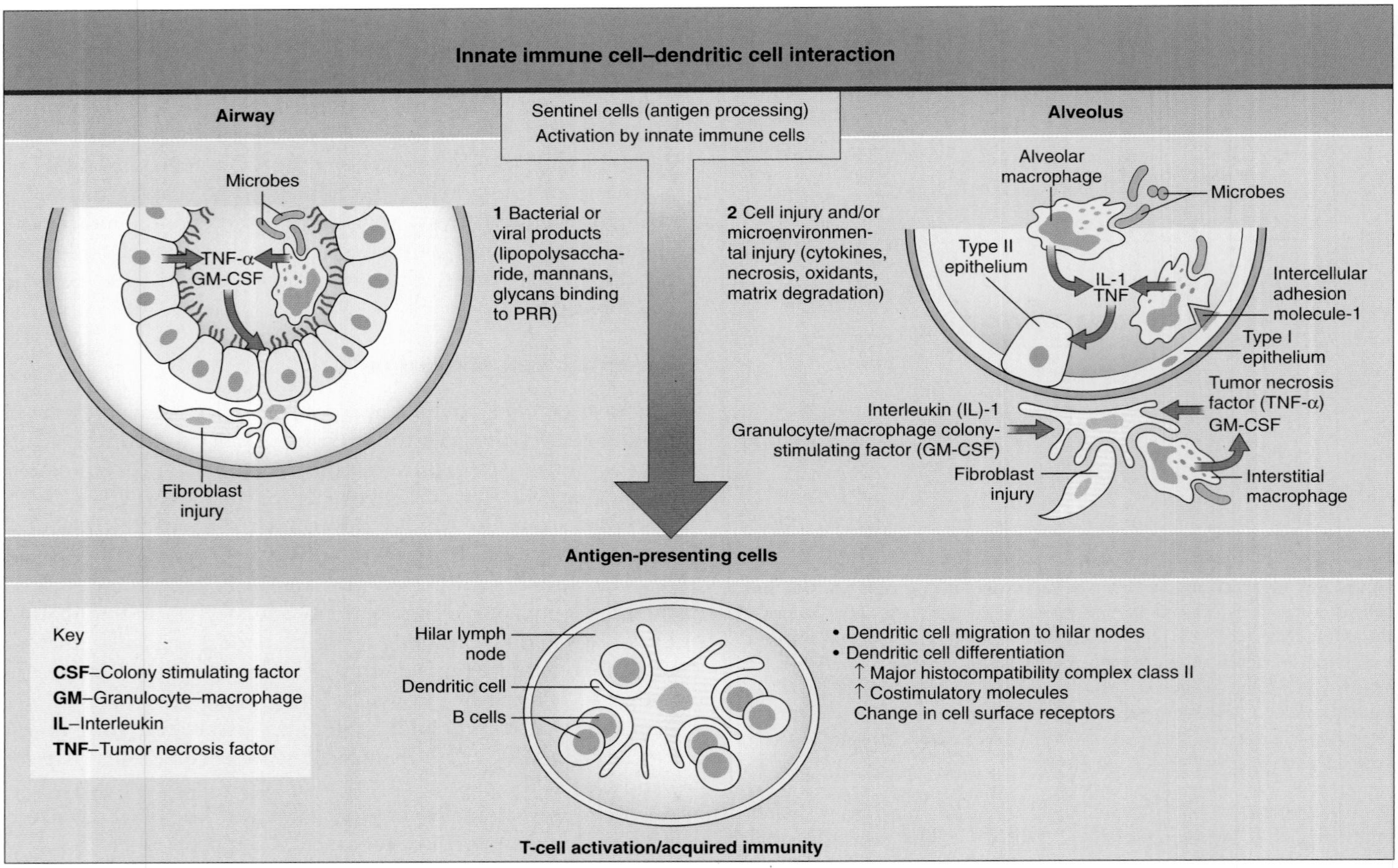

Innate immune cell–dendritic cell interaction

Airway

Sentinel cells (antigen processing)
Activation by innate immune cells

Alveolus

Microbes

TNF-α

GM-CSF

Fibroblast injury

1 Bacterial or viral products (lipopolysaccharide, mannans, glycans binding to PRR)

2 Cell injury and/or microenvironmental injury (cytokines, necrosis, oxidants, matrix degradation)

Alveolar macrophage

Microbes

Type II epithelium

IL-1

TNF

Intercellular adhesion molecule-1

Type I epithelium

Tumor necrosis factor (TNF-α)

GM-CSF

Interleukin (IL)-1

Granulocyte/macrophage colony-stimulating factor (GM-CSF)

Fibroblast injury

Interstitial macrophage

Antigen-presenting cells

Key

CSF–Colony stimulating factor

GM–Granulocyte–macrophage

IL–Interleukin

TNF–Tumor necrosis factor

Hilar lymph node

Dendritic cell

B cells

- Dendritic cell migration to hilar nodes
- Dendritic cell differentiation
  - ↑ Major histocompatibility complex class II
  - ↑ Costimulatory molecules
  - Change in cell surface receptors

T-cell activation/acquired immunity

Figure 8.7 Innate immune cell–dendritic cell (DC) interaction. Generation of pulmonary immune responses requires maturation and/or activation of pulmonary DCs. Precursor DCs are located in the periphery of the lung, in contact with either airway epithelial cells or alveolar epithelial cells. These "sentinel" cells are efficient antigen-processing cells but are inefficient antigen-presenting cells (APCs). DCs become activated as a result of interaction with microbial products or products of cell or microenvironmental tissue injury. DC activation and maturation lead to DC migration to hilar nodes and the differentiation of DCs into potent APCs. Pulmonary epithelial cells and pulmonary macrophages are essential regulatory links in the generation of microbe-specific T-cell immunity.

CCR7 is likely of particular importance to the movement of mature DCs into lymphatics, because the ligand secondary lymphoid tissue chemokine (SLC) is produced by lymphatic endothelial cells. DCs enter lymphatics and drain to lymph nodes, where the final positioning within the T-cell area may be controlled by other CCR7 ligands, including ELC, produced by resident mature DCs and MIP-3β.

Macrophage Antigen Presentation

Alveolar macrophages are ineffective APCs for naive T lymphocytes or resting memory cells but can restimulate recently activated T lymphocytes. Alveolar macrophages fail to effectively activate CD4 T lymphocytes because they bind resting T lymphocytes poorly and do not express B7 costimulatory cell surface molecules.

Resident alveolar macrophages actively suppress T lymphocyte activation and proliferation induced by antigens. Depletion of alveolar macrophages in vivo dramatically enhances the capacity of experimental animals to mount an immune response. The potential value of such a steady-state downregulatory control mechanism in the lung is self-evident, as the lung is frequently exposed to antigens. Immune responses must be restricted and downregulated within the pulmonary parenchyma, because immune reactions inevitably result in significant damage to gas-exchange surfaces. Conversely, unchecked microbial growth can also result in significant damage to gas-exchange surfaces. Accordingly, alveolar macrophage suppressive activity can be reversed. Both GM-CSF and TNF-α significantly reduce alveolar macrophage suppressive activity and increase DC maturation. Thus, microbial stimuli (e.g., LPS) lessen the downregulatory tone of alveolar macrophages by inducing GM-CSF production by macrophages and/or alveolar and airway epithelial cells and TNF production by macrophages, and simultaneously enhance the immunostimulatory activity of DCs. In aggregate, these LPS-induced changes in APCs allow local T-cell activation in the face of microbial challenges.

Selection of the Type of Immune Response

The elimination of different microbes requires different types of responses. Type 1 responses are mediated primarily by activated macrophages and involve the phagocytosis and intracellular killing of microorganisms. Type 2 responses are mediated by noncytotoxic antibodies, mast cells, and eosinophils. Type 1 immune responses are mediated by TH1 cells, which secrete IL-2, IFN-γ, TNF-α, and GM-CSF. Type 2 responses are mediated by TH2 cells, which produce IL-4, IL-5, IL-6, and IL-10.

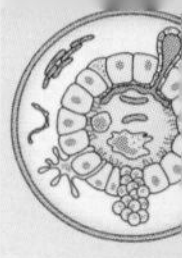

TH1 AND TH2 CELLS

Both TH1 and TH2 cells develop in response to signals derived from the innate immune system (Fig. 8.8). Activation of tissue macrophages through cell surface carbohydrate pattern receptors or by CD14 to which LPS has been bound causes secretion of IL-12 and TNF-α. The differentiation of naive TH cells to the TH1 phenotype is induced by IL-12 through its ability to maximize IFN-γ and curtail IL-4 production by T cells. Also, LPS causes macrophages to produce IFN-γ–inducing factor, which has similar effects. Both IL-2 and TNF-α synergize with IL-2 from T cells or with IL-15 from activated macrophages to induce production of IFN-γ by NK cells. In turn, IFN-γ augments IL-12 secretion and activity through its capacity to activate both IL-12 production by macrophages and the expression of IL-12 receptors on T and NK cells. Thus, IFN-γ and IL-12 comprise an autocrine positive feedback system that amplifies the levels of IFN-γ for macrophage activation and IL-12 for the proliferation and activation of NK and TH1 cells.

The development of TH2 cells requires IL-4 during the priming of naive T cells. Basophils and mast cells produce IL-4 after exposure to certain antigens. A subpopulation of T cells that express NK 1.1 markers and are CD4$^+$ rapidly produce large amounts of IL-4.

Cytokines produced by the developing TH1 and/or TH2 cells contribute to the control of polarized responses. The development of TH2 cells is suppressed by IFN-γ produced by TH1 cells. Both IL-10 and IL-4 produced by TH2 cells suppress the development of TH1 cells. Chronic exposure to antigen is required to produce highly segregated TH1 or TH2 responses.

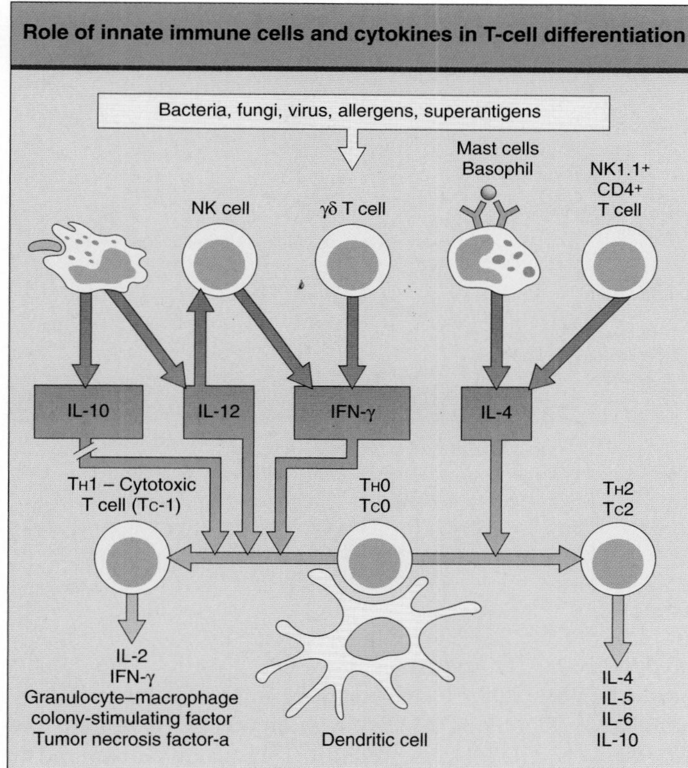

Figure 8.8 Role of innate cells and cytokines in T-cell differentiation. Innate immune cells are a major source of cytokines that control the development of T-helper (TH) 1 and TH2 cells. After ingestion of microbes, macrophages produce interleukin (IL)-12, which powerfully induces the development of TH1 cells from naive CD4 cells after their interaction with antigen-bearing dendritic cells (DCs). IL-12 also induces interferon (IFN)-γ secretion by natural killer (NK) cells. γδ-T lymphocytes also secrete IFN-γ after interactions with microbes. IFN-γ enhances IL-12 production and suppresses the development of TH2 cells. IL-4 is required for the development of the TH2 cells. Following interaction of naive CD4 cells with antigen-bearing DCs, basophils, mast cells, γδ-T lymphocytes, and NK1.1$^+$, CD4$^+$ T lymphocytes found in lymphoid tissues produce IL-4. IL-10 and IL-4 suppress the development of TH1 cells.

Regulatory T Cells

T-cell activation is initiated by the interaction of APCs with naive T cells. T-cell activation is also regulated by regulatory T cells. The best characterized subsets of T regulatory cells are CD4$^+$/CD25$^+$ cells. These cells constitute 5% to 10% of peripheral CD4$^+$ T cells in naive mice. Regulatory T lymphocytes are the main sources of soluble mediators that downregulate immune responses. Cytokines produced by these cells are believed to have key roles in the induction of anergy or active suppression. Regulatory T cells include TH2 lymphocytes that produce IL-4 or IL-10, TH3 lymphocytes that produce high levels of TGF-β alone or in conjunction with very low levels of IL-4, IL-10, or IFN-γ, and TR1 cells that produce high levels of IL-10 in conjunction with low levels of TGF-β.

LOWER RESPIRATORY TRACT IMMUNE RESPONSES MEDIATED BY T CELLS

Immunity mediated by T cells appears to be especially important for host defense against fungi, mycobacteria, and viruses. The kinetics of immune responses mediated by T lymphocytes in the lower respiratory tract has been defined almost exclusively from serial studies of murine models of these infections (Fig. 8.9).

CRYPTOCOCCUS NEOFORMANS

Host defenses against C. *neoformans* are dependent on CD4 and CD8 T cells. Mice depleted of CD4 T cells have earlier dissemination of C. *neoformans* from the lung, and their burden of C. *neoformans* is greater in extrapulmonary organs. Survival of mice depleted of CD4 cells is reduced. Mice depleted of CD8 lymphocytes have both reduced survival and impaired pulmonary clearance. Cellular recruitment of macrophages to the lung is significantly reduced in both CD4 and CD8 T cell–deficient mice. Depletion of both CD4 and CD8 T cells ablates inflammation and completely abrogates pulmonary clearance.

Effective clearance of C. *neoformans* requires the generation of a robust T1 response. Induction of TNF-α appears to be a critical early step in the afferent phase of T1 cell-mediated immunity against C. *neoformans.* A single dose of anti–TNF-α antibodies at the onset of a C. *neoformans* infection results in ineffective pulmonary clearance and dissemination of C. *neoformans* to the brain. Delaying the induction of TNF-α alters the usual, protective T1 response induced by C. *neoformans* to a nonprotective T1 response. These phenomena suggest that TNF-α–induced activation of DCs is required for effective production of IL-12.

Chemokine signaling also plays a role in T1 and T2 immune response polarization within the lung after C. *neoformans* infections. In mice lacking CCR2, the primary receptor for MCP-1,

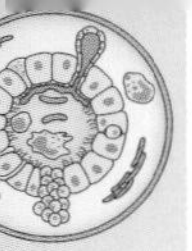

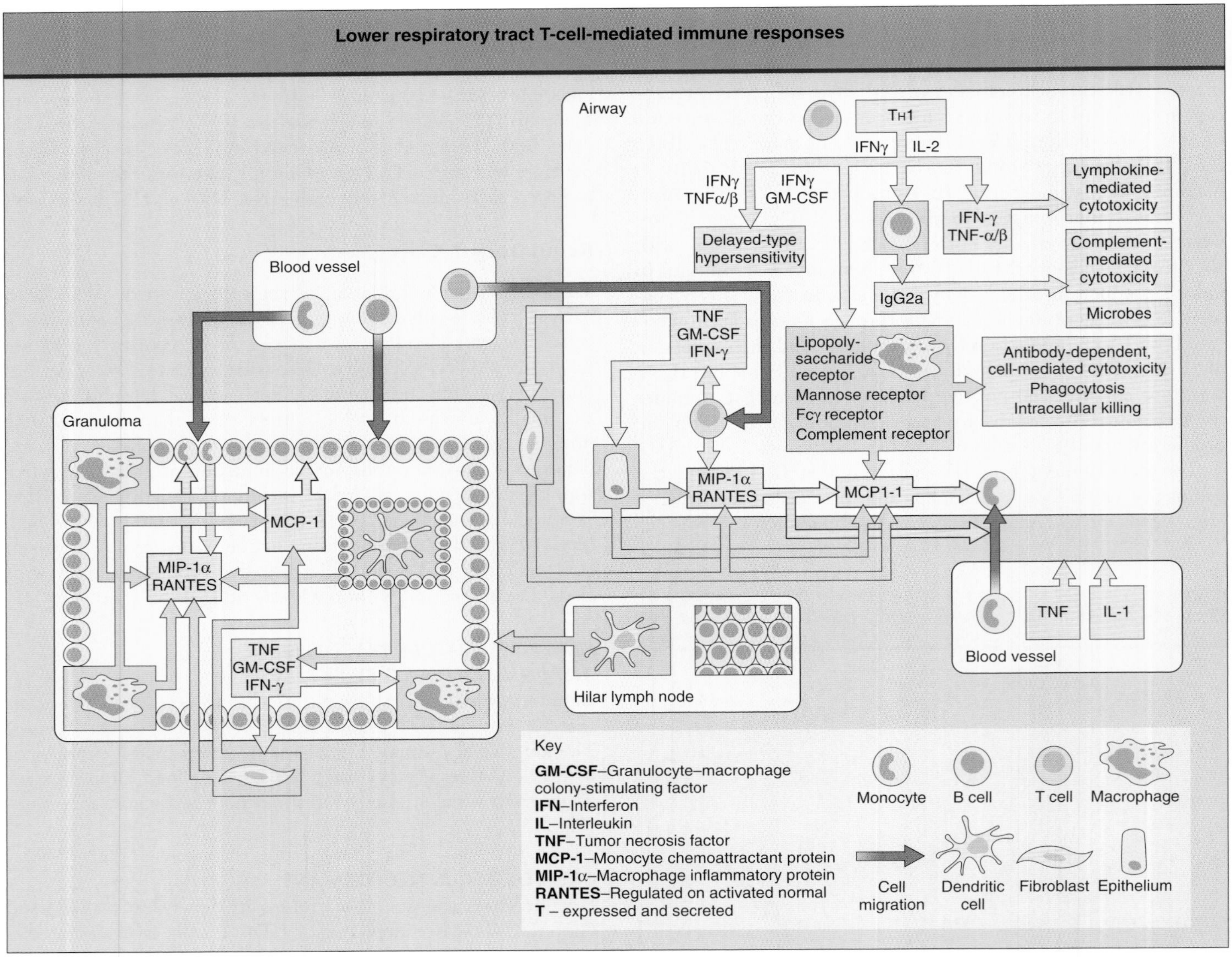

Figure 8.9 Lower respiratory tract T-cell–mediated immune responses. T-cell activation occurs in draining hilar lymph nodes. Activated T lymphocytes recirculate from hilar nodes to sites of microbial multiplication in the lower respiratory tract via a series of highly regulated events involving adherence molecule expression by both lymphocytes and endothelial cells and cell recruitment events in response to cytokines. TH1 lymphocytes are stimulated by resident antigen-presenting cells (APCs) to produce high levels of tumor necrosis factor (TNF), granulocyte-macrophage colony-stimulating factor (GM-CSF), and interferon (IFN)-γ. C-C chemokines (MCP-1, MIP-1α) produced in response to microbial products and TNF secretion recruit mononuclear phagocytes, which are crucial to granuloma formation and to the clearance of certain pathogens.

intratracheal inoculation with C. *neoformans* results in delays in macrophage and CD8 T-cell recruitment and cryptococcal clearance. CCR2-deficient mice exhibit significant dissemination of C. *neoformans* to the spleen and brain 6 weeks after infection. In contrast to the T1 response generated by CCR2-expressing mice, CCR2-deficient mice produce a strong T2 response to pulmonary C. *neoformans*. $CCR2^{-/-}$ mice generate an immune response that is characterized by chronic pulmonary eosinophilia, crystal deposition in the lungs, pulmonary leukocyte production of IL-4 and IL-5 but not IFN-γ, and increased serum IgE. A lack of CCR2 results in a switch to a T2-type immune response.

CCR2-deficient mice show evidence of defective macrophage and $CD8^+$ T-cell recruitment to the lung. CD8 depletion during C. *neoformans* infections results in the production of predominantly T2 cytokines by CD4 T cells. Thus, IFN-γ production by $CD8^+$ T cells might be important for the development of T1-type CD4 T-cell immunity to C. *neoformans*. Alternatively, CD8 T-cell–produced IFN-γ may be required to prime macrophages and/or DCs for IL-12 production. Lack of recruitment of the appropriate DCs to the lung might also explain the CCR2-induced defect.

Participation of CD8 T cells in microbial activity against C. *neoformans* could involve one or more of the following three mechanisms:

1. $CD8^+$ T cells could act directly on the microbe to inhibit or kill it.
2. Cytotoxic CD8 T lymphocytes could lyse infected target cells.

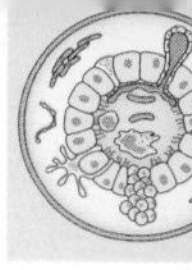

3. CD8^{+} T cells could enhance the antimicrobial activity of immune cells, particularly monocytes and macrophages, by producing cytokines.

Development of delayed hypersensitivity to live or heat-killed *C. neoformans* organisms depends on CD8^{+} T cells. In the absence of CD8^{+} T cells, CD4^{+} T lymphocytes produce predominantly TH2 cytokines (IL-4, IL-5, IL-10) in vitro.

The molecular signals required for the recruitment of mononuclear phagocytes to the lung after *C. neoformans* infection have been defined. The recruitment of monocytes is dependent on both MIP-1 and MIP-1α. Specific T lymphocytes generate GM-CSF, IFN-γ, and TNF-α, all of which activate monocytes, endothelial cells, fibroblasts, and epithelial cells to produce MCP-1. Additionally, activated T lymphocytes produce MIP-1α and RANTES. Studies carried out using neutralizing anti–MCP-1 or anti–MIP-1α–specific antiserum document the importance of these two molecules in mononuclear cell recruitment. The functional network of multiple chemokines is required for effective clearance of *C. neoformans*. MCP-1 plays an important role in the initial recruitment of cells (CD4^{+} and CD8^{+} T lymphocytes and a small number of monocytes) that produce MIP-1α. In turn, MIP-1α mediates the bulk of monocyte recruitment into the lungs.

Fungi (e.g., *Blastomyces dermatitidis, Candida albicans, C. neoformans, H. capsulatum*) continue to grow within resident pulmonary macrophages. Macrophage-activating cytokines are required to increase the antimicrobial activity of pulmonary macrophages to allow these phagocytes to kill intracellular microbes. Macrophages treated with the T-cell cytokines IFN-γ or GM-CSF exhibit significant fungicidal activity. Of these, GM-CSF but not IFN-γ increases complement-dependent phagocytosis with cryptococci. Depletion of CD4^{+} T cells in vivo inhibits multinucleated giant-cell formation, which is one mechanism for containing *C. neoformans* in the lung.

Mycobacterium tuberculosis

Antigen specific CD4 T lymphocytes isolated from mice infected with *M. tuberculosis* produce IL-2, IFN-γ, and small amounts of IL-4. A combination of TH1, TH2, and/or TH0 cells is involved in pulmonary host responses to *M. tuberculosis*. Class I restricted CD8 lymphocytes also participate in the immune response to mycobacteria; CD8 lymphocytes are present in the outer mantle of many granulomatous lesions.

γδ-T lymphocytes are also involved in immune responses to mycobacteria. Mice immunized with *M. tuberculosis* have γδ-T lymphocytes that respond vigorously to *M. tuberculosis* antigens. It is interesting to note that an extraordinarily high percentage of murine γδ–T-cell hybridomas thus far generated react with purified protein derivative. γδ-T lymphocytes can be expanded by in vitro stimulation of peripheral blood cells from patients affected by *M. tuberculosis*. Mycobacteria-stimulated γδ-T lymphocytes have various functions that are relevant to defense against intracellular microbes, which include secretion of TNF-α and IFN-γ and the ability to lyse target cells infected by mycobacteria.

The recruitment of monocytes and lymphocyte populations to the site of infection is required for granuloma formation. Infection of murine macrophages in vitro with several strains of *M. tuberculosis* induces rapid expression of genes that encode for murine chemokines, MIP-1α, MIP-2, IP-10, and MCP-1. Induction of these chemokine mRNAs was also found in the lungs of mice after aerosol infection. Purified protein derivative, *M. tuberculosis* culture filtrates, and whole bacilli also stimulate TNF-α production from human monocytes and alveolar macrophages in vitro. An important immunoprotective role is played by TNF-α in tuberculosis infection in mice via mechanisms that appear to be related to nitric oxide production and granuloma formation. Anti–TNF-α antibody inhibits granuloma formation after bacille Calmette-Guérin (BCG) challenge and results in a progressive, lethal BCG infection. Thus, proinflammatory cytokines and chemokines secreted during mycobacterial infections play an important role in mobilizing and activating cellular immune responses and contribute to granuloma formation.

Following phagocytosis of *M. tuberculosis* by mononuclear phagocytes, the bacteria reside in a membrane-bound phagosome. Survival of *M. tuberculosis* within mononuclear phagocytes is partially related to the absence of phagosome-lysosome fusion. The ability of *M. tuberculosis* to reside within endosomes allows macrophages to eventually present *M. tuberculosis* antigens, but it also enables the acquisition of nutrients by *M. tuberculosis*.

A central role is played by IFN-γ in activating antimicrobial activity in mycobacterium-containing macrophages. Studies of mice that have IFN-γ deletions (IFN-$\gamma^{-/-}$) and IFN-γ receptor deletions (IFN-γ-$R^{-/-}$) demonstrate the crucial role of IFN-γ. *M. tuberculosis*–infected IFN-$\gamma^{-/-}$ mice develop granulomas with caseous necrosis, widespread tissue destruction, and widespread dissemination of infection. Both IFN-$\gamma^{-/-}$ and IFN-γ-$R^{-/-}$ animals fail to produce nitric oxide, which is essential for antimicrobial killing in mice. Both IFN-γ and TNF-α are synergistic in activating the tuberculostatic capacities of murine phagocytes. Both TNF-α and GM-CSF can also cooperate to induce significant intracellular destruction of mycobacteria. Mechanisms for growth inhibition of mycobacteria in murine macrophages have been shown to involve nitric oxide. The mechanisms for killing or growth inhibition of *M. tuberculosis* in human mononuclear phagocytes remain elusive.

Viruses

Antigen-specific, CD8-cytotoxic T lymphocytes are crucial to the defense of the lung against viral infection. Specific cytotoxic CD8 T cells appear in the parenchyma of the lung within 1 week after pulmonary viral infection. Induction of this CD8 T-cell response is believed to involve replication of viral particles in the cytosol of infected epithelial cells, presentation of viral antigens on the surface of infected cells in conjunction with MHC class I molecules, and the eventual generation of mature CD8 cytotoxic cells. Viral infections are eradicated by CD8 T lymphocytes that recognize MHC class I–associated viral antigens on the surface of infected cells and destroy these infected cells.

LOWER RESPIRATORY TRACT IMMUNE RESPONSES MEDIATED BY B CELLS

Production of Ig is the hallmark of an immune response mediated by B lymphocytes. Instillation of antigen into the lower respiratory tract induces pulmonary antibody responses. A dose

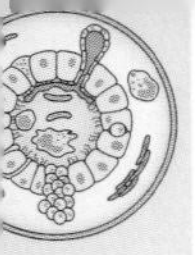

of antigen sufficient to overwhelm nonspecific clearance mechanisms and induce pulmonary inflammation is required for the induction of an antibody response. In such circumstances, the antigen is translocated from the lung to the draining lymph nodes, which are the primary site for the induction of antibody responses to intralobar antigen. Antibody-forming cells (AFCs) are generated in hilar nodes and released into efferent lymphatics and blood, through which they reach the lung parenchyma; pulmonary inflammation promotes the recruitment of AFCs to the lungs.

Localized antigen exposure also leads to recruitment and/or production of memory cells within the lobe in which antigen is deposited. Memory cells have several important functions:

- They allow a subsequently challenged lung to mount antibody responses to far lower doses of antigen than are initially required to induce these responses
- They induce AFC responses of far greater magnitude than occur after primary immunization
- Memory B cells within the lung interstitium retain the ability to produce antibody after localized rechallenge for years

B-Cell Activation, Differentiation, and Immunoglobulin Isotype Switching

B cells are activated by specific antigens through surface immunoglobulins that act as the antigen receptor. Most antigens require T-cell help from antigen-specific T cells to generate an antibody response. This dependence results from the need for direct interaction of T cells and B cells for lymphocyte differentiation into immunoglobulin-secreting B cells and subsequently into memory B cells or plasma cells. This first step in B-cell activation that is antigen specific takes place when B cells bind native antigens and receive accessory signals that are provided by T cells activated by DCs. Antigen-specific B cells are activated by cross-linking of surface Ig by native antigen, and T cells are activated by processed antigens presented on MHC class II by DCs. Costimulation of T cells is mediated by CD40/CD40L and B7/CD28 interactions between DCs and T cells. Cognate-specific interactions between peptide bound to MHC class II molecules on B cells and antigen-specific TCRs on CD4 T cells must also occur. This interaction triggers the T cell to make membrane and secreted molecules that drive B-cell proliferation and differentiation (Fig. 8.10).

During an antibody-mediated immune response, individual B cells switch Ig isotype expression. Cells that produce IgM switch to the production of IgE or one of the IgG or IgA subclasses. Isotype switching is regulated by T lymphocytes; T cells affect isotype switching in B cells both through cell-surface interactions between CD40L on T cells and CD40 on B cells and by the secretion of cytokines. Cytokine production is why TH2 responses are associated with strong antibody production; TH2 cells provide B-cell help much more efficiently because they produce cytokines that preferentially induce switching to certain isotypes and because they secrete a variety of B-cell stimulatory cytokines. With appropriate stimulation, activated B cells undergo 6 to 10 cycles of cell division and can produce up to 1000 plasma cells. Plasma cells are efficient producers of protective antibody, secreting as many as 30,000 molecules of Ig per minute. B-cell activation and differentiation also lead to the production of memory B cells.

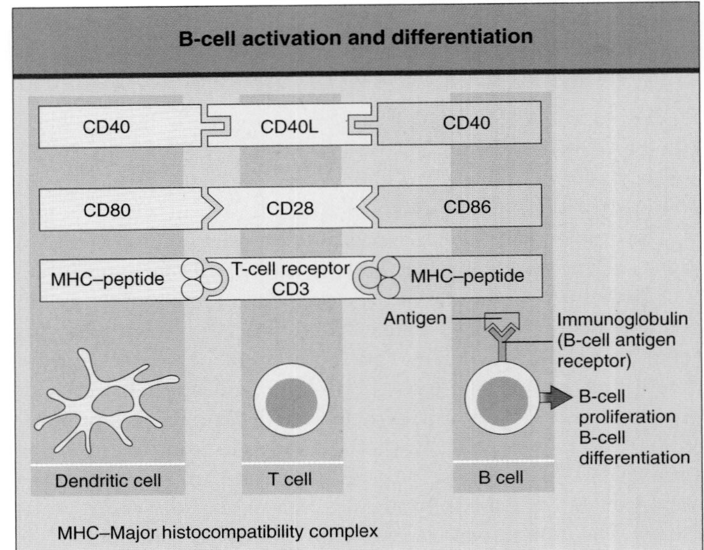

Figure 8.10 B-cell activation and differentiation. B-cell activation and differentiation involve cell-cell interactions among dendritic cells (DCs), T-helper cells, and B cells. Antigen-specific B cells are activated by cross-linking of the B-cell antigen receptor by native antigen; T cells are activated by processed antigens presented on major histocompatibility complex (MHC) class II by DCs. Costimulation of T cells by CD40/CD40L and CD80/CD28 interactions is required to activate T-helper (TH) cells. Interactions between antigen expressed by MHC class II on B cells and the T-cell receptor are essential for B-lymphocytic differentiation. Costimulation by CD40/CD40L and CD80/CD28 interactions is crucial in the B cell–T cell interaction as well. CD40/CD40L interactions occur only if the T cell recognizes the antigen presented by the B cell and expresses CD40L. These interactions are required for B-cell proliferation, differentiation, and maturation and immunoglobulin (Ig) isotype switching.

Respiratory immunoglobulins

Immunoglobulins are a major protein constituent of normal respiratory secretions. Approximately 20% of the total protein present in bronchoalveolar lavage fluids consists of IgG, IgM, and IgA. Relative concentrations of IgA progressively decrease, whereas IgG concentration aggressively increases as sample collection moves from the oral cavity to the alveolus.

Humans produce more IgA than any other Ig class. Secretory IgA found in external secretions consists of two molecules of IgA polymerized together by a joining **J** chain and by a secretory component, a glycoprotein produced by epithelial cells. Secretory IgA is derived from mucosal B cells; the secretory component is required for the transport of IgA through epithelial cells and bronchial glands. The primary site for induction of IgA responses within the lung is bronchus-associated lymphoid tissues.

The role of IgA in pulmonary defenses is enigmatic. Most IgA antibodies have antiviral specificities. Specific IgA antibodies are present in patients infected with influenza A. Because IgA has four binding sites, it is an effective agglutinating antibody. Accordingly, IgA may inhibit bacterial adherence to the respiratory epithelium. Specific IgA antibodies against *Bordetella pertussis* toxin have been isolated from respiratory secretions.

Human alveolar macrophages bear Fc receptors that bind IgA1 and IgA2. The latter is important for mucosal immunity because it is resistant to bacterial proteases specific to the hinge

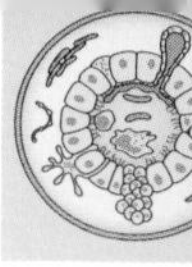

region of IgA1. Bacterial proteases for IgA are produced by *S. pneumoniae* and *H. influenzae*.

The major circulating plasma Ig class is IgG, which is also the major class of Ig found in the lower respiratory tract, and can be divided into four subclasses, each with a unique heavy-chain structure. The major role of respiratory tract IgG is to function as an opsonin and to interact with soluble factors such as the complement system. Opsonization facilitates phagocytosis by interactions with Fc receptors on inflammatory cells such as neutrophils, monocytes, macrophages, and NK cells.

The Fc domain of IgG is recognized by three Fcγ receptors (FcγRs). All classes of FcγR have at least two mRNA transcripts. All transcripts have closely related extracellular and transmembrane regions, but they differ in their cytoplasmic domains. All FcγRs function as signal-transducing molecules.

Role of Antibody in Lower Respiratory Tract Defense

Models of bacterial clearance in experimental animal models have defined mechanisms of accumulation of AFCs in the lung, the production of immunoglobulins, and the role of immunoglobulins. Systemic immunization enhances pulmonary clearance of *H. influenzae* and *P. aeruginosa*. After immunization, specific antibodies directed against the microbe appear in both serum and bronchoalveolar lavage fluid. Two major sources for respiratory tract immunoglobulins are the following:

1. Passive transudation from the vascular compartment into the alveolar space
2. Intrapulmonary antibody synthesis

The rate of transudation is dependent on plasma Ig concentration and resistance to diffusion. Transudation rates increase during states of increased permeability, such as inflammation. Because antibody specificities of serum and alveolar antibodies are identical, it seems likely that alveolar antibodies are derived in large part from serum in these models.

Serum IgG can clearly gain access to the alveolar space during inflammation, when large changes in alveolar permeability occur. Intravenous injection of a murine IgG monoclonal antibody specific for a cell surface–exposed epitope of nontypeable *H. influenzae* results in enhanced pulmonary clearance. Accordingly, direct airway immunization should not be required for the production of protective antibodies in the lung.

CONCLUSION

The lung contains a remarkably complex system of host defenses. This provides the means to differentiate innocuous from potentially harmful substances rapidly. This also enables the generation of highly specific and highly protective responses to the myriad pathogenic microorganisms that inhabit the environment. Memory lymphocytes enable acquired immunologic defenses to construct, by selective processes, responses that are appropriate for contemporary infectious agents. Important information regarding the regulation of inflammatory and immune responses has been generated from animal models of infectious diseases. It is hoped that application of this knowledge will continue to provide paradigms for therapies to stimulate deficient responses and suppress harmful responses to microbial pathogens that enter the lung.

SUGGESTED READINGS

Aderem A, Ulevitch RJ: Toll-like receptors in the induction of the innate immune response. Nature 406:782-787, 2000.

Bungel P-R, Nadel JA: Mucus and mucin-secreting cells. In Barnes P, Drazen J, Rennard S, Thomson N (eds): Asthma and COPD: Basic Mechanisms and Clinical Management. San Diego, Academic Press, 2002, pp 155-165.

Fearon DL, Lockley RM: The instructive role of the innate immunity in the acquired immune response. Science 272:50-54, 1996.

Huffnagle GB, Toews GB: Mechanisms of macrophage recruitment into infected lung. In Lipscomb MF, Russel SW (eds): Lung Macrophages and Dendritic Cells in Health. New York, Marcel Dekker, 1997, pp 373-407.

Kunkel SL, Chensue SW, Colletti L, et al: Cytokine networks and leukocyte recruitment. In Nelson S, Martin TR (eds): Cytokines in Lung Disease: Infection and Inflammation. New York, Marcel Dekker, 2000, pp 19-36.

Maloy KJ, Powric F: Regulatory T cells in the control of immune pathology. Nat Immunol 2:816-822, 2001.

Medzhitov R, Janeway C Jr: Innate immunity. N Engl J Med 343:338-344, 2000.

Moore BB, Toews GB: Humoral immunity in the lung. In Neidermann MS, Sarosi GA, Glassroth J (eds): Respiratory Infection Textbook. Philadelphia, Lippincott Williams and Wilkins, 2001, pp 27-44.

Moser M, Murphy KM: Dendritic cell regulation of Th1-Th2 development. Nat Immunol 1(3):199-205, 2000.

Reis e Sousa C, Sher A, Kaye P: The role of dendritic cells in the induction and regulation of immunity to microbial infection. Curr Opin Immunol 11:392-399, 1999.

Schlesinger LS: The role of mononuclear phagocytes in tuberculosis. In Lipscomb MF, Russel SW (eds): Lung Macrophages and Dendritic Cells in Health. New York, Marcel Dekker, 1997, pp 437-480.

Toews GB: Macrophages. In Barnes' P, Drazen J, Rennard S, Thompson N (eds): Asthma and COPD. San Diego, Academic Press, 2002, pp 99-109.

Traynor TR, Kuziel WA, Toews GB, Huffnagle GB: CCR2 expression determines T1 vs T2 polarization during pulmonary *Cryptococcus neoformans* infection. J Immunol 164:2021-2027, 2000.

Underhill DM, Ozinsky A: Toll-like receptors: Key mediators of microbe detection. Curr Opin Immunol 14:103-110, 2002.

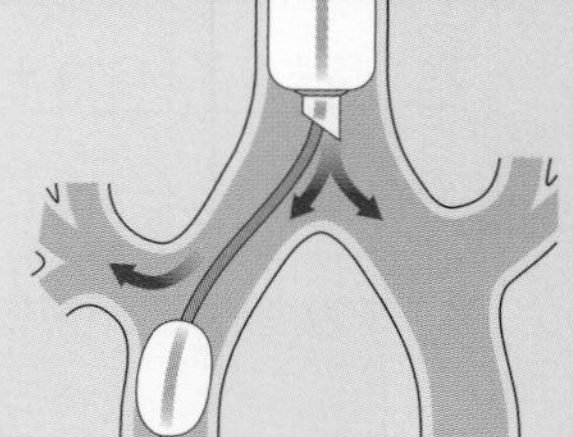

CHAPTER 9

Bronchoscopy

Udaya B. S. Prakash

The first bronchoscopy was performed in 1897 by Killian, who used a laryngoscope to examine the trachea and main bronchi. Subsequently the rigid bronchoscope was developed, and for the next 65 years it was the only instrument used to evaluate the airways (Fig. 9.1). The next major milestone was when Ikeda developed and introduced the flexible fiberoptic bronchoscope into clinical use in the early 1970s (Fig. 9.2). Both the rigid and the flexible bronchoscopes have undergone many modifications, and currently both are employed in the management of respiratory disorders. Bronchoscopy is now the most commonly used invasive procedure in pulmonology. In the United States alone, more than 500,000 bronchoscopies are performed each year.

BRONCHOSCOPES

The Rigid Bronchoscope

The rigid bronchoscope, also known as the "open-tube" or "ventilating" bronchoscope, is used in laser bronchoscopy, dilatation of tracheobronchial stenoses, airway placement of silicone stents, extraction of airway foreign bodies, and management of massive hemoptysis. Rigid bronchoscopy can be safely performed with the patient under intravenous sedation or general anesthesia. A major advantage of the rigid bronchoscope is its ability to accomplish quick and effective resolution of obstruction of larger airways caused by neoplasms, airway stenoses, foreign bodies, and other processes. The rigid bronchoscope itself can be used as a coring or dilating instrument to remove large obstructing masses. The rigid bronchoscope can also be used as a conduit for the passage of the flexible bronchoscope to reach distal airways to apply palliative therapy. This technique combines the safety of the rigid bronchoscope and the maneuverability of the flexible bronchoscope. The acquisition of skill in rigid bronchoscopy requires special training and extensive practice.

The Flexible Bronchoscope

The flexible fiberoptic bronchoscope is used in over 95% of all bronchoscopic procedures. The versatility and the relative ease of use permit the operator to reach the distal airways and lung parenchyma to obtain samples not easily attainable by the rigid bronchoscope (see Fig. 9.2). Almost all flexible bronchoscopies can be safely performed with administration of topical anesthesia, in an outpatient setting, or at the patient's bedside. The instrument can be inserted nasally, orally, or via tracheotomy stoma. Many ancillary instruments are available for diagnostic and therapeutic applications.

Flexible bronchoscopes with larger channels permit insertion of larger biopsy forceps, balloon catheters, laser fibers, and other instruments, thereby enhancing the diagnostic and therapeutic results. An ultrathin flexible bronchoscope is used for the examination of infants and neonates. A disposable suction apparatus at the proximal end of the newer bronchoscopes has minimized the risk of cross-contamination. The videoflexible bronchoscope has a charge-couple device at its distal tip to capture digital images, which are visualized on a monitor. This system is excellent for teaching purposes. However, the ability to visualize the airways directly through the bronchoscope is lost. The digital images can be stored in a variety of digital formats. The disadvantages include the added expense of video equipment, computer terminal, and larger working and storage space.

INDICATIONS AND CONTRAINDICATIONS FOR BRONCHOSCOPY

Indications

The indications for diagnostic and therapeutic bronchoscopy are numerous and are listed in Tables 9.1 and 9.2. The most common diagnostic indications for bronchoscopy include lung mass, nodule, suspicion of cancer, and lung infiltrates. Some of these indications are discussed at length in the following sections. In many patients, diagnostic and therapeutic bronchoscopy may be required simultaneously.

Contraindications

Bronchoscopy has very few absolute contraindications. Bronchoscopic visualization of the airways and bronchoalveolar lavage (BAL) can be performed without correction of coagulation abnormalities. Hypoxemia or pulmonary dysfunction alone does not pose contraindications, as long as supplemental oxygen is provided during the procedure.

Absolute contraindications to bronchoscopy include an unstable cardiovascular status, life-threatening cardiac arrhythmias, severe refractory hypoxemia, an uncooperative patient, and an inadequately trained bronchoscopist and bronchoscopic team. Contraindications to rigid bronchoscopy, in addition to those just listed, include an unstable neck, a severely ankylosed cervical spine, and severely restricted motion of the temporomandibular joints.

Complications

Bronchoscopy and bronchoscopic procedures are among the safest diagnostic pulmonary procedures and carry low morbidity and mortality. Complications from the flexible and rigid

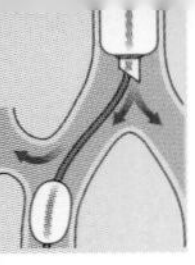

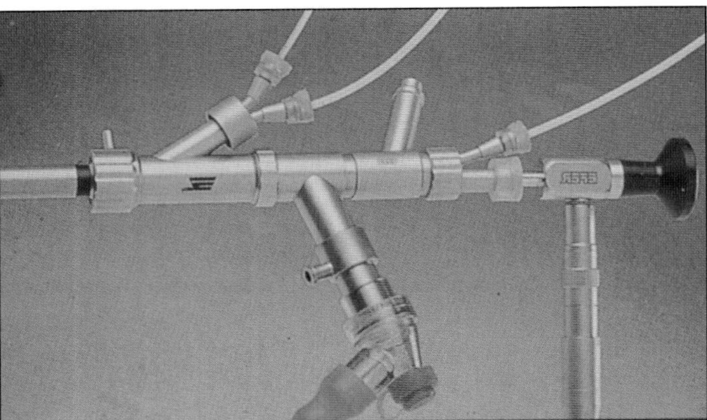

Figure 9.1 Modern rigid bronchoscope demonstrates numerous attachments and portals at its proximal end. These modifications permit adequate ventilation of the patient and use of various ancillary instruments. (Courtesy of Professor Jean-Francois Dumon.)

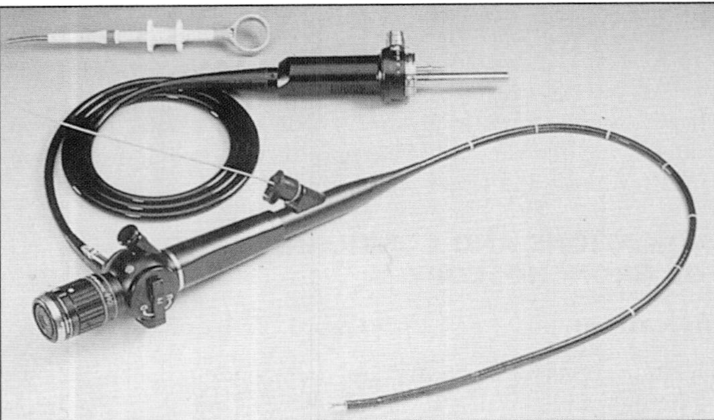

Figure 9.2 Flexible bronchoscope with biopsy forceps introduced through its working channel. The flexibility of the distal tip permits easy maneuverability in all lobar and segmental bronchi. (Courtesy of Olympus Corporation.)

Table 9.1
Indications for diagnostic bronchoscopy

Cough	Tracheobronchial strictures and stenoses
Hemoptysis	Chemical and thermal burns of tracheobronchial tree
Wheeze and stridor	Thoracic trauma
Abnormal chest radiograph	Vocal cord paralysis and hoarseness
Diagnostic bronchoalveolar lavage:	Diaphragmatic paralysis
Pulmonary infections	Pleural effusion
Diffuse lung disease	Persistent pneumothorax
Intrathoracic lymphadenopathy or mass	Miscellaneous
Bronchogenic carcinoma	Suspected tracheoesophageal or bronchoesophageal fistula
Positive or suspicious sputum cytology	Bronchopleural fistula
Staging of bronchogenic carcinoma	Bronchography
Follow-up of bronchogenic carcinoma	Assessment of endotracheal tube placement
Metastatic carcinoma	Assessment of potential endotracheal-tube-related injury
Esophageal and mediastinal tumors	Postoperative assessment of tracheal, tracheobronchial, or bronchial anastomosis
Foreign body in the tracheobronchial tree	

Table 9.2
Indications for therapeutic bronchoscopy

Retained secretions, mucous plugs, clots, and necrotic debris	Lung abscess
Foreign body in the tracheobronchial tree	Mediastinal cysts
Neoplasms of the tracheobronchial tree	Bronchogenic cysts
Bronchoscopic removal	Pneumothorax
Laser therapy	Bronchopleural fistula
Brachytherapy	Miscellaneous
Placement of tracheobronchial stent	Intralesional injection
Strictures and stenoses	Endotracheal tube placement
Bronchoscopic dilatation	Cystic fibrosis
Laser therapy	Asthma
Balloon dilatation	Thoracic trauma
Stent placement	Therapeutic lavage (pulmonary alveolar proteinosis)

Table 9.3
Factors associated with increased risk of complications during bronchoscopy

Lack of patient cooperation	Severe asthma
Lack of skilled personnel	Severe coagulopathy
Lack of appropriate facilities	Significant tracheal obstruction
Unstable angina	Mechanical ventilation
Uncontrolled arrhythmias	High positive end-expiratory pressure
Refractory hypoxia	Bronchoscopic lung biopsy
Severe hypercapnia	Prolonged bronchoscopic procedure
Severe bullous emphysema	

Adapted with permission from Semin Resp Med 18:583–589, 1997. (Prakash)

bronchoscopes are similar. The factors that increase the risk of complications are listed in Table 9.3. Premedications, sedatives, topical anesthetics, and vagus-mediated mechanisms can cause respiratory depression, hypoventilation, hypotension, and syncope. Topical anesthetics can also cause laryngospasm, bronchospasm, seizures, or cardiorespiratory arrest. Nearly one third of patients develop fever after bronchoscopy and BAL. The transient fever is most likely related to the procedure-induced release of proinflammatory cytokines.

Methemoglobinemia is an uncommon but important complication of bronchoscopy. It results from the oxidation of ferrous iron to ferric iron within the hemoglobin molecule. Topical anesthetics like benzocaine and prilocaine are well known to cause methemoglobinemia. In bronchoscopy, methemoglobinemia has resulted most often from the use of benzocaine. Lidocaine has also caused this complication. Infants and the elderly are more likely to develop toxic methemoglobinemia from benzocaine. Methemoglobinemia may also result from enhanced absorption of local anesthetic from the nasopharynx or trachea as a result of candidiasis. Higher levels of methemoglobin (greater than 30% to 40%) can be life threatening. Treatment of significant methemoglobinemia requires administration of intravenous methylene blue, 1 to 2 mg/kg, over a 10-minute period.

Rigid bronchoscopy has the potential to damage the teeth, dentures, and oropharyngeal structures. Bronchoscopic proce-

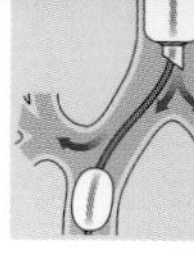

dures such as brushing, biopsy, and lavage are occasionally complicated by bronchospasm, laryngospasm, hypoxemia, cardiac arrhythmias, fever, pneumonia, pneumothorax, and hemorrhage.

The major complication of bronchoscopic lung biopsy is pneumothorax, which occurs in less than 1% of cases when fluoroscopic guidance is used. The risk of pneumothorax is higher without fluoroscopic guidance. Routine hospitalization is not required after bronchoscopic lung biopsy. Bronchoscopic lung biopsy can be performed in patients on mechanical ventilators, but the pneumothorax rate can be as high as 14%.

Significant hemorrhage (>25 mL) following bronchoscopic lung biopsy occurs in less than 5% of cases. The hemorrhage is almost always controllable by bronchoscopic techniques. Formation of excess granulation at the site of stent insertion is a complication of metallic stents. Silicone stents are more likely to migrate.

Bronchoscopy-induced infection or infection transmitted through a bronchoscope from an infected patient to an uninfected patient is uncommon. However, several publications have reported bronchoscopic transmission of bacterial and mycobacterial infections from infected patients to uninfected patients, sometimes with fatal outcomes. Bronchoscopic procedures have led to pseudo-outbreaks of *Pseudomonas aeruginosa* and *Serratia marcescens* infections. The pseudoinfection indicates isolation of an infectious agent from the bronchoscopic specimens obtained from an uninfected patient. Here, the pseudoinfection is the result of an inadequately cleaned and sterilized bronchoscope used in the uninfected patient after it was used to examine an infected patient. Improper bronchoscope cleaning and disinfecting procedures have been responsible for several outbreaks of pseudoinfections.

TECHNIQUE

Preparation of the Patient

Discussions with the patient regarding the indication for bronchoscopy, goals, risks, and potential complications are an integral aspect of bronchoscopy practice. The pre-bronchoscopy evaluations should include an accurate and pertinent medical history with attention to the presence of potential risk factors, a cardiopulmonary examination, and a chest radiograph (Table 9.4). Other imaging procedures and special tests should be individualized. An otherwise healthy patient should not require a complete blood count, a clotting screen, chemistry profile, and urinalysis. Measurements of prothrombin time, activated partial thromboplastin time, bleeding time, and platelet count are required in individuals on anticoagulant therapy and those with active bleeding, known or clinically suspected bleeding disorders, liver disease, renal dysfunction, malabsorption, malnutrition, or other coagulopathies.

Bronchoscopy for visualization of the airways, bronchial washings, diagnostic BAL, and therapeutic bronchoscopy for removal of secretions and mucous plugs can be performed safely in patients with severe coagulation problems. Biopsies and resection of airway lesions should be attempted only after coagulation abnormalities have been corrected. Although platelet dysfunction is common in renal insufficiency, the increased risk of bleeding is difficult to predict. Generally, a blood urea nitrogen level of greater than 30 mg/dL or a serum creatinine level of greater than 3 mg/dL is considered a relative contraindication

Table 9.4
Prebronchoscopy checklist

1.	Is there an appropriate indication for bronchoscopy?
2.	Has there been a previous bronchoscopy?
3.	If the answer to the above question is yes, were there any problems or complications?
4.	Does the patient [and close relative(s) if patient is unable to communicate] fully understand the goals, risks, and complications of bronchoscopy?
5.	Does the patient's past medical history (allergy to medications or topical anesthesia) and present clinical condition pose special problems or predispose to complications?
6.	Are all the appropriate tests completed and the results available?
7.	Are the premedications appropriate and the dosages correct?
8.	Does the patient require special consideration before bronchoscopy (e.g., corticosteroids for asthma, insulin for diabetes mellitus, or prophylaxis against endocarditis) or during bronchoscopy (e.g., supplemental oxygen, extra sedation)?
9.	Is the plan for postbronchoscopy care appropriate?
10.	Are all the appropriate instruments and personnel available to assist during the procedure and to handle the potential complications?

Adapted from Prakash UBS, Cortese DA, Stubbs, SE: Technical solutions to common problems in bronchoscopy. In Prakash UBS (ed): Bronchoscopy. New York, Raven, 1994. Copyright Mayo Foundation.

to bronchoscopic lung biopsy. Patients with platelet counts less than 50,000/dL should receive 6 to 10 units of platelets before undergoing bronchoscopic lung biopsy.

Routine arterial blood gas analysis and pulmonary function tests are unnecessary, because even the severe impairment of pulmonary function in patients with diffuse pulmonary infiltrates is only a relative contraindication to bronchoscopy. Noninvasive techniques such as sphygmomanometry, electrocardiographic monitoring, and pulse oximetry provide adequate information regarding the patient's cardiopulmonary status during the procedure. If a patient is scheduled to undergo both bronchoscopy and pulmonary function testing within a period of 72 hours, it is recommended that pulmonary function tests be performed first, because bronchoscopy can cause bronchial mucosal edema and lead to falsely abnormal pulmonary functions. Patients should forego oral fluid or food intake for at least 6 hours before the procedure.

Premedication, Sedation, and Anesthesia

Premedication consisting of an antisialagogue and an anxiolytic drug may be administered 30 to 40 minutes before the procedure. Many bronchoscopists use an anticholinergic drug such as atropine or glycopyrrolate (0.3 to 0.5 mg intramuscularly for either agent). If adequate sedation is used, the routine use of premedications is not necessary. Midazolam is currently the drug of choice for sedation in almost all flexible bronchoscopies. The dosages of preoperative and intraoperative sedatives should be titrated to achieve antegrade amnesia, relaxation, and cooperation. The usual dose of midazolam for conscious sedation is 0.07 mg/kg, but the choice and dosage of sedatives should be tailored for each patient, with attention given to the potential for complications with oversedation. Propofol, administered intravenously, is an excellent sedative. It is used more commonly for lengthy procedures and rigid bronchoscopy.

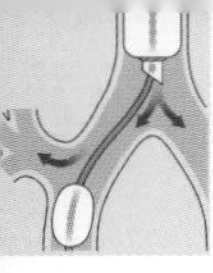

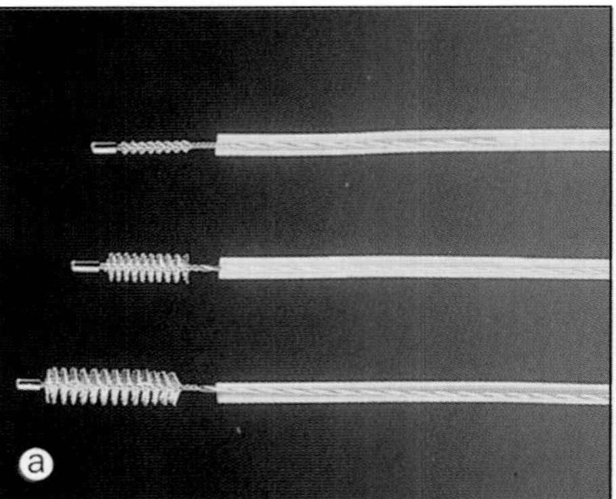

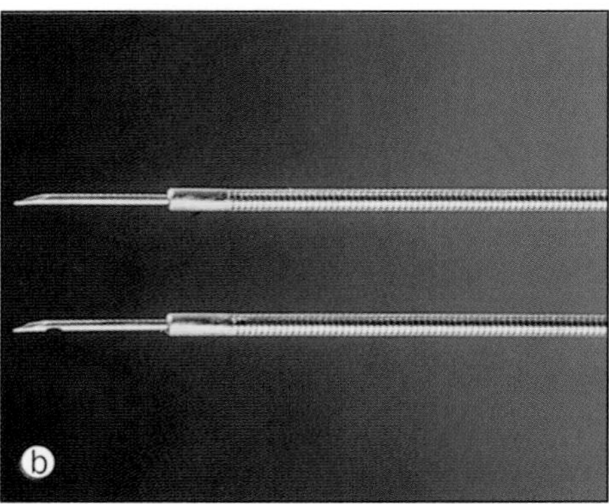

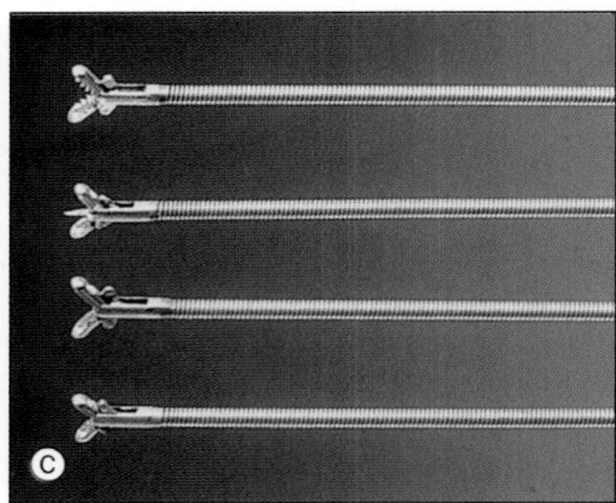

Figure 9.3 Bronchoscopy brushes **(A)**, needles **(B)**, and biopsy forceps **(C)** are available in various sizes and types. (Courtesy of Olympus Corporation.)

Almost all flexible bronchoscopic procedures can be performed with administration of topical anesthesia; lidocaine is the drug of choice. Lidocaine is used to anesthetize the upper airways and is administered with a hand-held atomizer. Lidocaine is also instilled through the channel of the flexible bronchoscope during the procedure. Even though research studies have recommended a maximum lidocaine dose of up to 600 mg, the clinically recommended dose is less than 300 mg or less than 4.5 mg/kg per procedure. General anesthesia may be required for rigid bronchoscopy, complicated and lengthy flexible bronchoscopic procedures, and most pediatric bronchoscopies and when the patient is intensely anxious.

Hypoxemia is common during bronchoscopy, even in those without preexisting hypoxemia. Routine administration of oxygen during bronchoscopy is now a common practice. Patients with preexisting hypoxemia require higher fractions of supplemental oxygen. Pulse oximetry should be used to assess oxygenation. Other prebronchoscopic precautions, such as prophylactic administration of antibiotics to prevent bacterial endocarditis, should be individualized.

Technique

Flexible bronchoscopy can be performed with the patient seated or supine, in a bed, in the intensive care unit, or in the outpatient setting. Ideally, outpatient examinations are performed in an operating room or a dedicated room. Fluoroscopy for bronchoscopic lung biopsy, procedures performed with the patient under general anesthesia, therapeutic bronchoscopies in critical care units, and urgent bronchoscopies require special preparation and locations. Equipment and drugs should be readily available to deal with emergencies.

The flexible bronchoscope is commonly inserted either nasally or orally with or without an endotracheal tube. It can also be inserted through a tracheostomy stoma or a rigid bronchoscope. Every bronchoscopist should be able to perform bronchoscopy by the nasal or oral route. The oral route, which involves use of an endotracheal tube, permits the bronchoscopist to easily remove and reinsert the instrument at will to clean the lens and remove mucous plugs from the channel. The bronchoscope can be withdrawn and reinserted quickly if bleeding and clots become obstacles. If the oral route is used, a "bite block" is placed between the incisors to prevent the patient from biting and damaging the flexible bronchoscope. If the nasal route is used, the nasal passage itself serves as a stent for the passage of the instrument, allowing excellent examination of the upper airways. The nasal route is also suitable for a brief examination when manipulation of the airway is not contemplated, such as for postoperative scrutiny after a bronchoplasty procedure, placement of brachytherapy catheters, and assessment of results of treatment for major airway obstruction.

Nasal prongs or a mask can provide supplemental oxygen for the nasal approach. If an orotracheal tube is used, an adapter attached to the oxygen supply provides supplemental oxygen.

A normal flexible bronchoscopic examination includes a thorough evaluation of the supraglottic airways as well as the laryngeal structures and function during phonation. The examination proceeds with the evaluation of the trachea and its movements during phases of respiration and coughing. Then, each side is examined so that all segmental bronchi and their branches have been visually inspected for abnormalities of the mucosa, luminal narrowing, and bronchial obstruction. After complete examination of trachea and both bronchial trees, brushings and biopsies are obtained from the luminal or parenchymal abnormalities. Appropriate procedures and instruments (brushes, needles, or forceps) are selected for obtaining tissue samples.

Endobronchial lesions are sampled with cytology brushes, catheters, needles, and biopsy forceps. Each of these instruments is available in different sizes from various manufacturers (Fig. 9.3). Frequent performance of these procedures is essential for the acquisition and maintenance of proficiency. Visible endobronchial lesions that appear suspicious should be subjected to biopsy unless contraindicated by an underlying coagulopathy. Proper handling and processing of the bronchoscopically obtained specimens are important. Communication among the bronchoscopist, pathologist, microbiologist, and the patient's physician is crucial if the results of the bronchoscopy are to be maximized.

Bronchoscopic lung biopsy is obtained via the flexible bronchoscope (Fig. 9.4). Fluoroscopic guidance helps the bronchoscopist to select the maximally abnormal areas for biopsies. It also permits accurate placement of the forceps in the periphery of the lung for lung biopsy near the pleura and for biopsy of lung nodules (Fig. 9.5). The use of fluoroscopy obviates routine chest radiography after bronchoscopic lung biopsy. One study observed that the incidence of pneumothorax was 1.8% when fluoroscopy was used and significantly increased to 2.9% when it was not used. Four to five biopsies are required in most patients, although a smaller number may be adequate in sar-

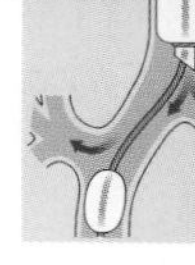

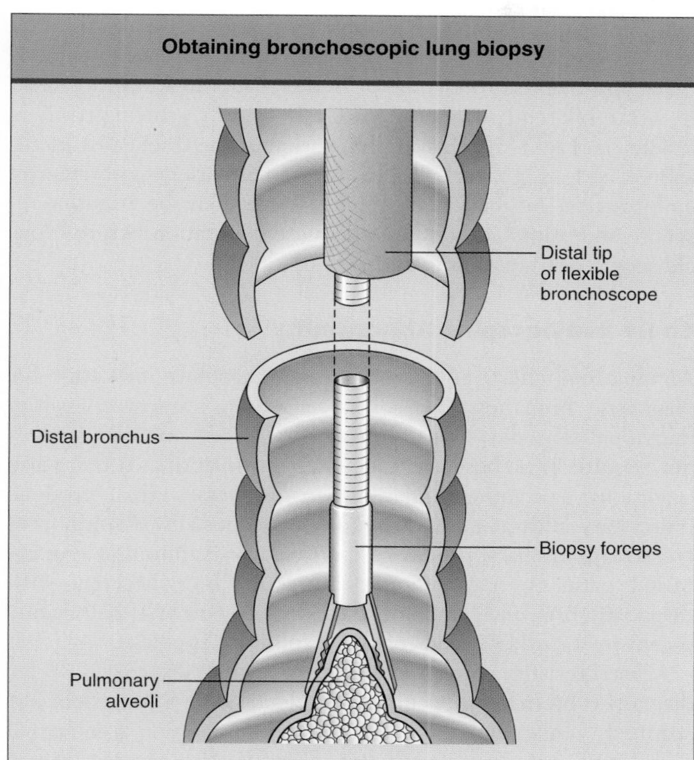

Figure 9.4 The mechanism by which bronchoscopic lung biopsy is obtained. The biopsy forceps pinches off the lung tissue located between two branches of terminal bronchi.

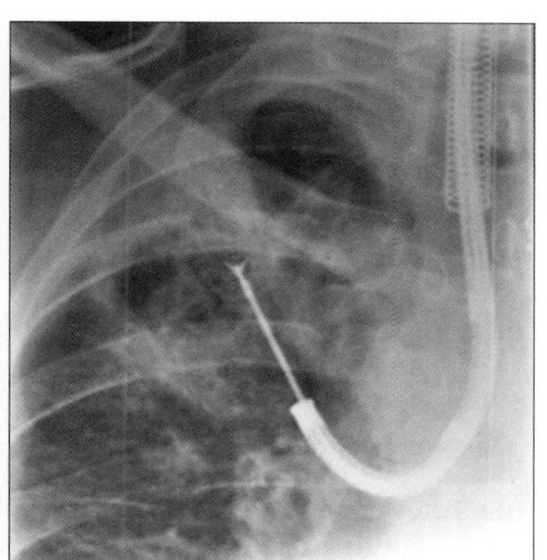

Figure 9.5 Bronchoscopic lung biopsy under fluoroscopic guidance assures that the tissue sample obtained is truly representative of the disease process depicted on chest radiograph or computed tomographic (CT) scan. Fluoroscopic technique significantly reduces the risk of pneumothorax.

coidosis (<4), and a larger number may be necessary in lung transplant patients (up to 8). Routine hospitalization is not necessary after bronchoscopic lung biopsy.

Rigid bronchoscopy, laser therapy, dilatation of airway strictures, stent placement, brachytherapy, electrocoagulation, needle aspiration, ultrasound, and other procedures require specialized training and equipment. These procedures are discussed later in this chapter.

Postbronchoscopy Care

Most adult patients tolerate bronchoscopy well and are able to care for themselves within a short period after bronchoscopy,

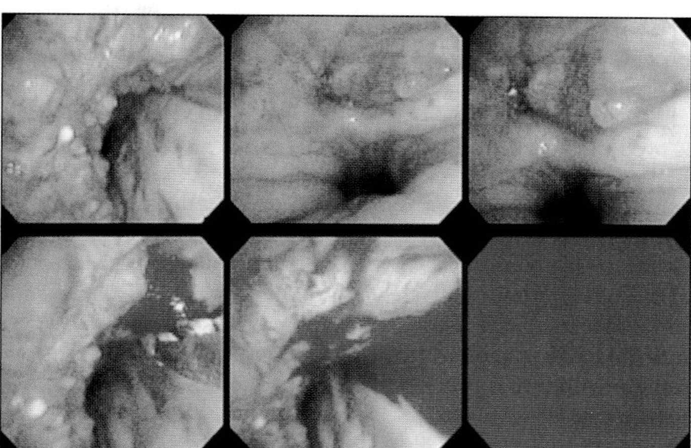

Figure 9.6 Postbiopsy bleeding. Depicted in a consecutive series of bronchoscopic images obtained before and soon after biopsy of mucosal lesion in a patient with small-cell carcinoma.

provided no general anesthesia has been used. A brief period of observation in a suite adjoining the bronchoscopy suite should suffice. The bronchoscopist should watch for pneumothorax and bleeding (Fig. 9.6). The patient should be advised not to drink or eat until normal sensation returns to the oropharynx. Driving soon after bronchoscopy should be avoided if sedatives have been used.

SYMPTOMS AND SIGNS REQUIRING BRONCHOSCOPY

Cough

Chronic cough is among the most common indications for bronchoscopy. However, bronchoscopy has a diagnostic yield in the range of 4% in patients with chronic cough and normal chest radiograph. In carefully selected patients, a diagnostic rate of 28% has been reported. The main reason for bronchoscopy is to exclude a tracheobronchial cause for a chronic cough. Lesions of the trachea and main bronchi may cause cough, with an initially normal chest radiograph. Bronchoscopy can be most helpful in such patients. Chronic cough associated with hemoptysis, localized wheeze, or an abnormal chest radiograph is a more compelling indication for bronchoscopy. In patients with chronic cough (>3 months), diagnostic bronchoscopy may be considered if methacholine challenge, otorhinolaryngologic examination, and barium swallow (and/or esophageal pH study) are nondiagnostic.

Hemoptysis

Hemoptysis can arise from various vascular sources including bronchial arteries, pulmonary arteries, pulmonary veins, pulmonary capillaries, and neovascularization following trauma or radiation therapy. Important causes of massive hemoptysis include tuberculous cavities, neoplasms of the tracheobronchial tree, pulmonary mycetomas, bronchiectasis, pulmonary alveolar hemorrhage syndromes, and cystic fibrosis.

Chronic or intermittent streaky hemoptysis is common in patients with chronic bronchitis and may not require bronchoscopy. Any significant or new hemoptysis requires

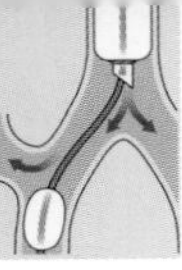

bronchoscopic evaluation. Bronchoscopy is more likely to provide helpful information if the chest x-ray film is abnormal. If bronchoscopy reveals blood in the airways, it should be traced as far distally as possible to assure that an endobronchial lesion is not missed (Fig. 9.7). Ultrathin flexible bronchoscopes permit the examination of the distal bronchial tree. Bronchoscopy should be performed as soon as possible after the patient is found to have hemoptysis because bronchoscopy performed during active hemoptysis is more likely to yield a diagnosis than a procedure performed after hemoptysis has ceased. Obvious vascular abnormalities such as prominent submucosal capillaries, bronchial inflammation, and subtle mucosal abnormalities are valuable findings. Bronchoscopic specimens should be collected for appropriate studies depending on the clinical situation.

Wheeze and Stridor

Generalized wheeze is not an indication for bronchoscopy. If clinical examination identifies a localized or unilateral wheeze, and if there is no known reason for it, a diagnostic bronchoscopy should be considered (Fig. 9.8). Localized wheezing may indicate an obstructing lesion. Stridor usually denotes urgency, and emergency laryngoscopy and bronchoscopy may be required. If the stridor is caused by a foreign body or a significant lesion in the large airway, a combined diagnostic and therapeutic bronchoscopy may be necessary. Acute stridor is more common in children than in adults. The most common causes in children include epiglottitis, croup, laryngomalacia, laryngeal papillomata, and tracheal foreign body. Acute stridor in adults is caused by acute bilateral vocal cord paralysis, rapidly growing tracheal lesions, and acute extrinsic compression of the trachea by mediastinal and esophageal lesions. In some patients, emergency endotracheal intubation or tracheostomy may be required to secure an optimal airway and adequate ventilation before bronchoscopic examination is undertaken.

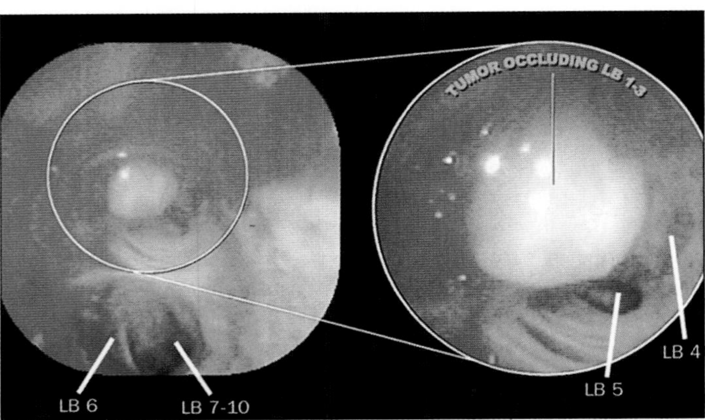

Figure 9.7 Subacute hemoptysis. A patient with subacute hemoptysis of 3 months' duration had bronchoscopy, which showed mucosal inflammation. A later examination revealed the source: metastatic cancer in the left upper lobe.

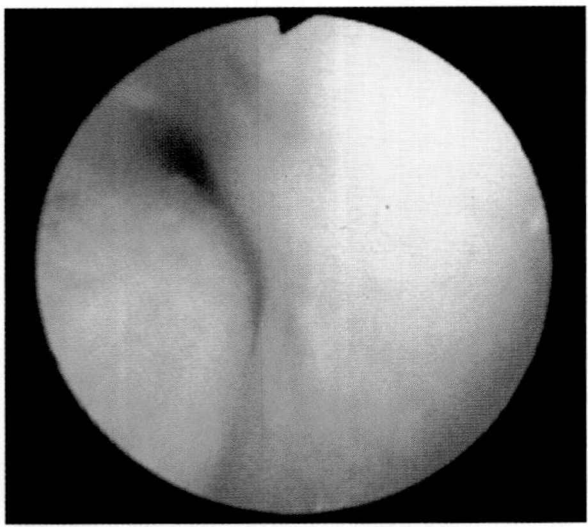

Figure 9.8 Tracheal buckling. Bronchoscopic examination revealed localized upper tracheal buckling on hyperflexion of the neck. Symptoms cleared after three tracheal rings were resected. Pathologic analysis showed localized tracheomalacia.

Chest Radiographic Abnormality

An abnormal chest radiograph is not an absolute indication for diagnostic bronchoscopy. For instance, an otherwise healthy individual who develops community-acquired pneumonia does not require bronchoscopy. Likewise, the majority of the acute infectious and other inflammatory processes that produce pulmonary infiltrates do not require bronchoscopy. Rapidly progressive pulmonary processes, particularly in immunocompromised patients, may require emergency bronchoscopy with diagnostic BAL and lung biopsy to identify potential pathogenic organisms or other causes of the respiratory problem.

Characteristic chest radiologic abnormalities that call for diagnostic bronchoscopy include atelectasis of a lung, lobe, or segment; enlarging or suspicious pulmonary parenchymal nodules; cavitated pulmonary lesions; mediastinal masses; diffuse parenchymal processes without an established diagnosis; rapidly progressive pulmonary infiltrates in immunosuppressed patients; and sudden disruption of tracheobronchial air bronchogram. Hilar, mediastinal, or subcarinal lymphadenopathy is another indication for diagnostic bronchoscopy with needle aspiration.

Pulmonary Infections

Bronchoscopy is useful in the diagnosis of all types of pulmonary infections. The main purpose is the collection of respiratory samples for special stains and cultures. The samples include bronchial washings, BAL, protected-catheter brushings, and bronchoscopic lung biopsy (Table 9.5). Bronchoscopy with BAL is commonly used to identify infectious organisms in mechanically ventilated patients with pneumonia and in immunocompromised patients with pulmonary infiltrates.

BACTERIAL INFECTIONS

Bacterial infections of the lower respiratory tract can be diagnosed by BAL or protected-catheter brush. Presently, the routine use of protected-catheter brush has been replaced by BAL. Specimens obtained by protected-catheter brush indicate active infection when bacterial count is greater than 10^3 cfu/mL. In patients with ventilator-associated pneumonia, identification of less than 10^3 cfu/mL indicates that pneumonia is unlikely. When more than 10^3 cfu/mL organisms are identified, more than 75% of patients are likely to have pneumonia. If a BAL specimen demonstrates a bacterial count that exceeds 10^4 cfu/mL, it is considered positive for bacterial infection of the lower respiratory tract.

MYCOBACTERIAL INFECTIONS

Bronchoscopy is helpful in the diagnosis of tuberculosis. The diagnostic rates range from 58% to 96%, with an average rate of

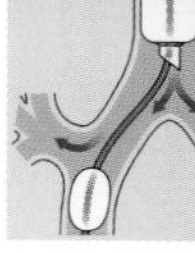

Table 9.5
Bronchoscopic techniques and applications in respiratory infections

Bronchoscopic technique	Clinical application
Bronchoscopy (visualization)	1. Assessment of mucosal, intraluminal, and extraluminal pathology 2. Evaluation of endobronchial tuberculosis, mycoses, viral vesicles (in AIDS) 3. Invasive tracheobronchial aspergillosis, candidiasis, and others 4. Follow-up of endobronchial disease (tuberculosis, etc.)
Bronchial washings	Culture of mycobacteria, fungi, and viruses, and Pneumocystis smears
Bronchoalveolar lavage	Culture of all organisms, especially for identification of mycobacteria, fungi, cytomegalovirus, and other viruses, and Pneumocystis smears
Protected specimen brushing	Culture of aerobic and anaerobic bacteria
Nonprotected bronchial brushing	Stains and culture for mycobacteria, fungi, *Pneumocystis carinii*, and viruses
Endobronchial biopsy	1. Mucosal lesions caused by mycobacteria, fungi, protozoa, etc. 2. Removal of obstructing lesions responsible for infection (tumor, foreign body, etc.) 3. Drainage of lung abscess, piecemeal removal of mycetomas (aspergillomas and other fungus balls)
Bronchoscopic needle aspiration	1. Stains and culture of extrabronchial lymph nodes for identification of mycobacteria and fungi 2. Drainage of bronchogenic cyst and instillation of sclerosing agent
Bronchoscopic lung biopsy	Stains and culture of all organisms, especially for identification of *Pneumocystis carinii*, mycobacteria, and fungi; also detection of parasitic lung infections
Rigid or flexible bronchoscope	Insertion of tracheobronchial prosthesis (stent) to overcome airway obstruction caused by intrinsic stenosis (post-tuberculous or fungal), extrinsic compression caused by mediastinal fibrosis due to histoplasmosis

72%. Bronchoscopy is the only procedure to provide the diagnosis in up to 45% of patients with active tuberculosis. In contrast, routine culture of bronchoscopic specimens has a diagnostic yield of 6%. If bronchoscopic specimens are routinely cultured for mycobacteria, in only 5% of patients with tuberculosis is bronchoscopy likely to be the only procedure to yield the diagnosis. In patients with miliary tuberculosis, in whom sputum smears are frequently negative, bronchoscopic brushings, washings, and bronchoscopic lung biopsy are diagnostic in up to 80% of patients, and bronchoscopy is the only procedure to provide the diagnosis in up to 10%. In all patients suspected of having tuberculosis, sputum and gastric washings should be tested and bronchoscopy performed only if these studies are negative.

In endobronchial tuberculosis, the bronchoscopic examination may reveal mucosal and submucosal granulomas, mucosal ulcerations, endobronchial polyps, bronchial stenosis, and bronchial erosion by a mediastinal lymph node that may mimic a neoplasm (Fig. 9.9).

MYCOTIC INFECTIONS

Bronchoscopy plays an important role in the diagnosis of pulmonary mycoses. If bronchoscopy leads to identification of organisms that cause histoplasmosis, coccidioidomycosis, blastomycosis, cryptococcosis, nocardiosis, and mucormycosis, then it is indicative of respiratory infection. In contrast, growth of

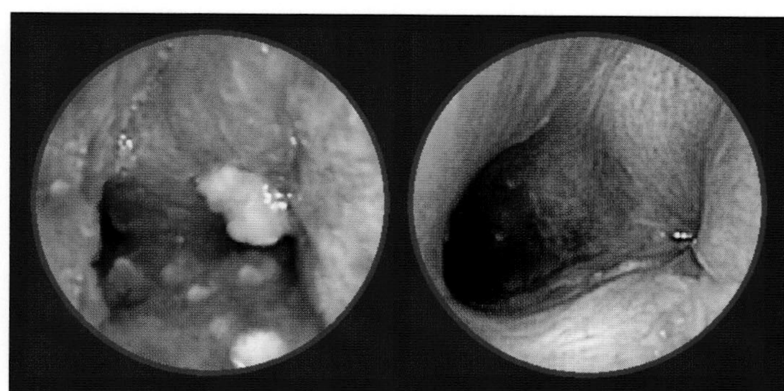

Figure 9.9 Endobronchial tuberculosis involving distal trachea and main bronchi. Figure on left was obtained before chemotherapy, and the post-therapy appearance is shown on the right. Endobronchial tuberculosis is commonly mistaken for bronchogenic carcinoma.

Aspergillus and *Candida* species from bronchoscopic washings does not establish the diagnosis of respiratory mycosis, because these organisms frequently colonize the respiratory tract. Therefore, the presence of hyphae in bronchoscopic specimens should be correlated with clinical findings. Negative results do not exclude the diagnosis, and further procedures or empirical therapy may be necessary. In patients with hemoptysis caused by an aspergilloma, bronchoscopy helps in identifying the site of bleeding so that appropriate therapy can be planned.

Histoplasmosis of the respiratory system can involve the lung parenchyma as well as the airways. Bronchoscopy is useful in documenting the diagnosis in patients with cavitated lesions, localized infiltrates, and miliary disease caused by histoplasmosis. In up to 10% of patients with histoplasmosis, bronchoscopy is the only technique to provide the diagnosis. However, bronchoscopy is not very useful in patients with pulmonary nodules caused by histoplasmosis.

Histoplasmosis occasionally leads to complications such as mucosal granulomas, increased mucosal vascularity, bronchial stenosis from extrinsic compression caused by mediastinal fibrosis, and broncholithiasis. Bronchoscopy is helpful in the diagnosis and treatment of some of these complications.

In patients with acquired immunodeficiency syndrome (AIDS), endobronchial obstructing lesions secondary to aspergillosis and *Pneumocystis jiroveci* have been described. In patients with severe neutropenia, tracheobronchial invasive aspergillosis leads to airway obstruction and respiratory distress.

Actinomycosis of the lungs rarely requires bronchoscopy for the diagnosis. However, it is not uncommon for this organism to be isolated from secretions obtained from the location of obstructive airway lesions. When detected in bronchoscopically obtained specimens in patients with endobronchial neoplasms, foreign bodies, and strictures, it usually represents a saprophytic growth.

IMMUNOCOMPROMISED PATIENTS

Bronchoscopy is the most commonly used invasive diagnostic procedure in immunocompromised patients with pulmonary infiltrates. Overall sensitivity of bronchoscopic procedures in the identification of infections in these patients is 90%. If the results of bronchoscopy are negative for an infectious cause of respiratory illness, the probability that infection is not present may be as high as 94% (negative predictive value). BAL is the most

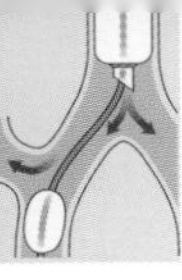

helpful and most frequently used technique in this group of patients.

HUMAN IMMUNODEFICIENCY VIRUS INFECTION

In patients with AIDS, clinical suspicion of *P. jiroveci* pneumonia is a common indication for bronchoscopy. BAL and bronchoscopic lung biopsy have about equal sensitivity (over 90%) when used alone for diagnosing *P. jiroveci* pneumonia, and bronchoscopic lung biopsy has sensitivity of 94%. Combinations of BAL and lung biopsy increase the diagnostic yield to almost 100%. Empirical therapy for more than 24 hours significantly impairs the diagnostic yield of BAL in detecting the respiratory pathogens in patients with HIV infection. Therefore, bronchoscopy with BAL should be carried out before commencement of therapy, or as soon as possible after empiric treatment is begun.

Bronchoscopy with BAL and lung biopsy is also helpful in identifying respiratory infections caused by cytomegalovirus, *Mycobacterium avium-intracellulare*, *Cryptococcus neoformans*, *M. tuberculosis*, *Coccidioides immitis*, *Histoplasma capsulatum*, and *Blastomyces dermatitidis*. Lung biopsy specimens should be submitted for cultures.

LUNG ABSCESS

The indications for bronchoscopy in lung abscess include collection of culture specimens, exclusion of an endobronchial obstruction (neoplasm or foreign body) responsible for the abscess, and, in some patients, bronchoscopic drainage of the abscess. Patients who undergo bronchoscopic attempts to empty the abscess may slowly expectorate the contents over a period of hours or days. However, bronchoscopic drainage is not uniformly successful unless the abscess cavity can be reached directly with the bronchoscope (Fig. 9.10).

Diffuse Lung Disease

Bronchoscopy is frequently used in the diagnosis of diffuse lung diseases, and the bronchoscopic procedures employed are BAL (Fig. 9.11) and bronchoscopic lung biopsy (see Figs. 9.4 and 9.5).

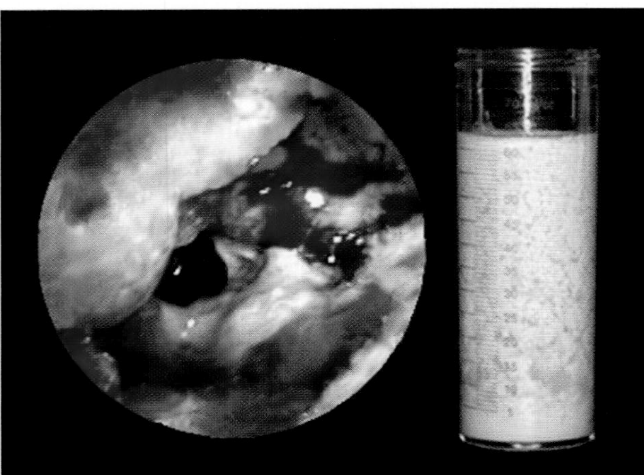

Figure 9.10 Bronchoscopic appearance of a large cavity in the right upper lobe *(left)*. This patient had received radiotherapy for lung cancer. Pus suctioned from the cavity is shown on the right.

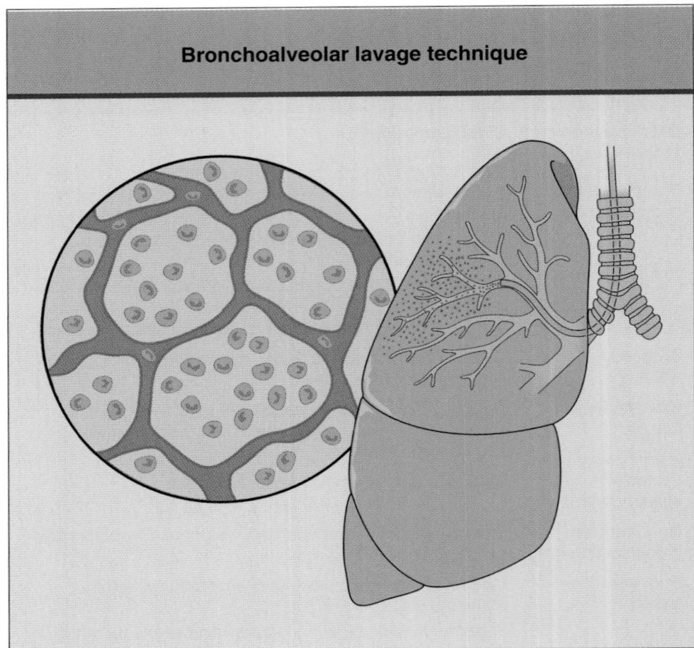

Figure 9.11 Bronchoalveolar lavage (BAL) is performed by wedging the tip of the flexible bronchoscope in the segmental bronchus leading to the parenchymal abnormalities detected by imaging techniques. Normal saline, 100 to 150 mL, in aliquots of 10 to 50 mL, is instilled through the bronchoscope channel and suctioned back into a container for analysis.

BAL has been employed to diagnose various interstitial lung diseases, pulmonary malignancies, and pulmonary infections. BAL has been used to analyze cellular constituents at the alveolar level and thus follow the status of the alveolitis and its response to therapy. In current clinical practice, however, BAL has a limited role in the diagnosis and treatment of idiopathic pulmonary fibrosis and lung disease associated with collagen diseases.

BAL alone is diagnostic of several pulmonary disorders when the results of the lavage correlates with clinical and imaging studies (Table 9.6 and Fig. 9.12). The CD4/CD8 ratio may distinguish sarcoidosis from hypersensitivity pneumonitis; in the former, CD4/CD8 may be as high as 10:1 to 20:1, and in the latter, the ratio is decreased or reversed. Similar reversal of CD4/CD8 ratio is seen in patients with AIDS and lymphocytic

Table 9.6
Bronchoalveolar lavage in respiratory diseases

BAL is diagnostic	BAL is supportive
• Langerhans-cell granuloma	• Alveolar hemorrhage
• Fat embolism syndrome	• Radiation-induced organizing pneumonitis
• Lipoid (mineral oil) pneumonia	• Amiodarone
• Alveolar proteinosis	• Methotrexate
• Eosinophilic pneumonia	• Sarcoidosis
• Lymphangitic cancer	• Rheumatoid lung
• Pulmonary endometriosis	• Scleroderma
• PCP, TBC, legionella, etc	• Silicosis
	• BOOP

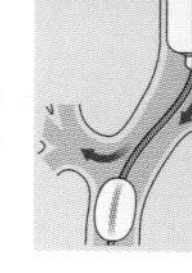

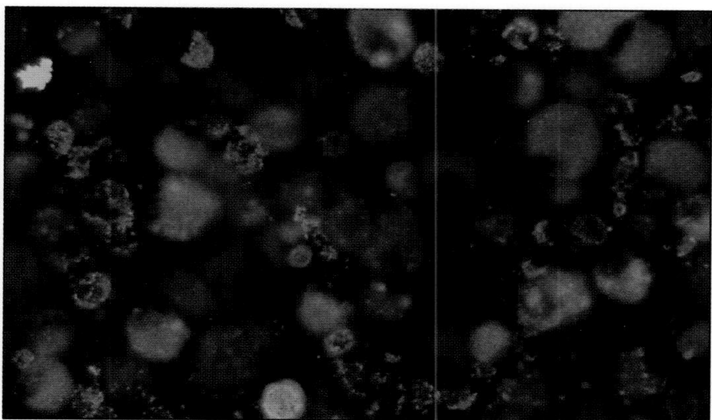

Figure 9.12 Bronchoalveolar lavage sample treated with special stain shows numerous CD1a (OKT6) cells (orange-colored cells) in a patient with pulmonary Langerhans cell histiocytosis of the lung.

interstitial pneumonitis. BAL has a diagnostic rate of greater than 75% in lymphangitic pulmonary metastasis. In alveolar proteinosis, the lavage effluent appears somewhat turbid (sandy) and layered, with proteinaceous material settling to the bottom of the container. This typical feature alone is diagnostic of the disorder when imaging and clinical data suggest the diagnosis. In alveolar hemorrhage syndrome, the later aliquots of lavage effluent become bloodier, and increased number of hemosiderin-laden macrophages (>20%) in the BAL effluent indicate pulmonary alveolar hemorrhage. The lavage effluent can be subjected to special stains such as lipid stains (Congo red or Sudan black), iron stains, and immunochemical techniques. Lipid stain helps in documenting fat embolism by demonstrating greater than 5% lipid-laden macrophages in 60% of patients with acute chest syndrome caused by sickle cell disease. Lipid stain also helps identify lipoid pneumonia caused by respiratory aspiration of gastric contents.

Bronchoscopic lung biopsy averts open lung biopsy in a significant number of patients. Bronchoscopic lung biopsy should be considered when a diffuse or localized interstitial, alveolar, miliary, or fine nodular pattern of disease is present and when the diagnosis cannot be established by BAL, high-resolution computed tomography (HRCT) of the chest, or other less invasive techniques. Bronchoscopic lung biopsy is very useful in certain diffuse pulmonary disorders (Table 9.7). A stronger indication for biopsy is the case in which histologic diagnosis is imperative. The diagnosis of idiopathic pulmonary fibrosis by bronchoscopic lung biopsy alone is controversial, because a histologic diagnosis consistent with idiopathic pulmonary fibrosis is

Table 9.7
Pulmonary diseases in which bronchoscopic lung biopsy provides high diagnostic yield

Sarcoidosis	*Pneumocystis jiroveci* infection
Hypersensitivity pneumonitis	Mycobacterioses
Eosinophilic granuloma (histiocytosis-X)	Mycoses
Alveolar proteinosis	Cytomegalovirus infection
Lymphangitic metastasis	Pneumoconioses
Diffuse pulmonary lymphoma	Rejection process in lung transplant recipients
Diffuse alveolar cell carcinoma	

present in many pulmonary diseases. The usefulness of bronchoscopic lung biopsy in immunocompromised patients, including those with *P. jiroveci* pneumonia, and fungal lung infections is discussed above.

Presently, HRCT of the chest permits diagnosis of typical features of usual interstitial pneumonia, pulmonary lymphangioleiomyomatosis, lymphangitic pulmonary metastases, and pulmonary Langerhans cell histiocytosis. In these disorders, BAL and lung biopsy may not be necessary unless discrepancies exist between clinical features and HRCT images.

Intrathoracic Lymphadenopathy and Mass

Bronchoscopy is indicated in patients with radiologic diagnosis of intrathoracic lymphadenopathy or mass. Bronchoscopy will confirm the mucosal involvement of the airway mucosa or the extrinsic compression of the airways. A bronchoscopic diagnosis of malignancy in the lymph nodes may preclude mediastinoscopy and/or thoracotomy.

The flexible bronchoscope is used to obtain needle aspiration biopsy specimens of paratracheal, hilar, subcarinal, or mediastinal lymph nodes. Multiple needle aspirations can be safely obtained from the same site. A 21-gauge needle provides aspirates for cytologic analysis, and a 19-gauge needle can be used to obtain a core of tissue for histologic preparation. The overall yield in malignant disease is about 75%. The diagnostic sensitivity is 80% to 89%, especially if a 19-gauge needle is used. The diagnostic accuracy of a cytologic examination with positive results is very high, but false-positive results occur if cancer cells are aspirated from an endobronchial neoplasm. The predictive value of a negative result on cytologic examination is low (<25%). Immediate on-site analysis of specimens increases the diagnostic yield. Bronchoscopic needle aspiration may be useful in establishing a benign diagnosis. In patients with suspected sarcoidosis, the technique reveals noncaseous granulomas in about 65% of patients. When bronchoscopic needle aspiration is combined with mucosal biopsy, the diagnosis of sarcoidosis has been reported to increase to more than 70%. The bronchoscopic needle aspiration is safe. Negligible bleeding is seen at the site of needle puncture. Hemomediastinum, pneumothorax, pneumomediastinum, and bacteremia have occurred sporadically.

Bronchogenic Carcinoma

Bronchoscopy is probably the most important procedure in the diagnosis of bronchogenic carcinoma (Fig. 9.13). It is also helpful in the staging, early detection, and follow-up of patients treated for lung cancer. In patients with suspected lung cancer, bronchoscopic brushings, needle aspirations, and biopsies from the abnormal tracheobronchial mucosa or mass lesions in the lung parenchyma establish the diagnosis. Additionally, bronchial washings add to the diagnostic yield. Diligent examination of the tracheobronchial mucosa is imperative before biopsy specimens are obtained. If obvious changes are not present, subtle abnormalities should be sought. Multiple biopsies and brushings may be needed in some patients, and various types of brushes and biopsy forceps are available for this purpose (see Fig. 9.3).

Bronchoscopy plays a major role in the staging of primary lung cancer. Simple visualization of the extent of tracheobronchial involvement by the tumor helps determine if the lesion is

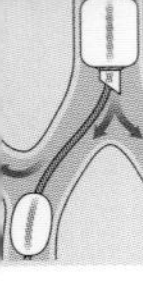

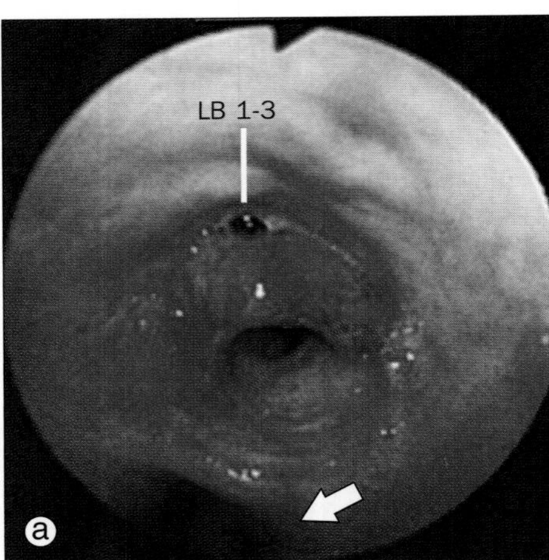

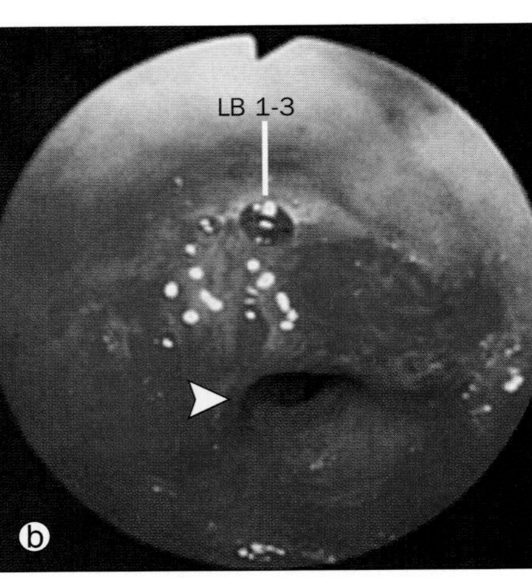

Figure 9.13 Squamous cell carcinoma of left upper lobe **(A)**; a close-up **(B)**. Partial obstruction to the bronchus leading to anterior and apical-posterior segments can be seen. Bronchus seen at the 7 o'clock position (arrow) in **A** leads to left lower lobe, and the lower bronchus in **B** is the bronchus to lingular segments (arrow).

surgically resectable. For instance, the involvement of the main carina may place a patient in category T4 or stage IIIB. Similarly the bronchoscopic identification of vocal cord paralysis denotes a worse prognosis. If the bronchoscopic biopsy reveals small-cell lung cancer, surgical therapy is excluded. A bronchoscopic biopsy may indicate a metastatic cancer in the bronchus or lung, and this information may drastically alter the therapeutic approach. The staging of lung cancer by bronchoscopic needle aspiration of mediastinal lymph nodes is discussed in a previous section.

Early detection, localization, and aggressive treatment of bronchogenic or preinvasive stages of lung cancer result in 5-year survival rates of 70% to 80%. Once a radiologically occult cancer is suspected, based on positive results of the cytologic examination, cancer of oropharynx and larynx should be excluded. In the majority of patients with positive sputum cytology and a normal chest radiograph (so-called "occult cancer"), localization of lung cancer can be accomplished by bronchoscopic visualization and biopsy of the airway mucosa. Over 50% of radiologically occult cancers demonstrate mucosal abnormalities at the first bronchoscopic inspection.

In some patients with occult lung cancer, localization is difficult because the tumor may not produce bronchoscopically visible mucosal abnormalities. Such patients require repeated bronchoscopic examinations over several months before localization is established. Autofluorescence bronchoscopy is an option in such patients.

Autofluorescence bronchoscopy is a technique to detect early malignant changes in the airway epithelium. The technique is based on the premise that during bronchoscopy, the light reflected from the abnormal respiratory mucosa is different from the light reflected by the normal mucosa. In patients suspected of having bronchogenic cancer or diagnosed with an occult lung cancer, a standard "white-light" bronchoscopy is performed. If it shows no mucosal changes, the procedure is immediately repeated using a bronchoscopic light source with a different wavelength. If mucosal abnormalities are present, the mucosa will appear different in color from normal mucosa. Specimens are obtained from the abnormal mucosa for histologic analysis. A multicenter study of 700 biopsy specimens from 173 high-risk subjects concluded that the relative sensitivity of standard bronchoscopy and autofluorescence bronchoscopy combined was 6.3 times that of standard bronchoscopy alone for detecting dysplasia and carcinoma in situ and 2.7 times that of standard bronchoscopy alone for detecting moderate or severe (i.e., high-grade) dysplasia, carcinoma in situ, and invasive carcinoma. However, another study found no difference in the diagnostic efficacy of combined standard bronchoscopy and autofluorescence bronchoscopy in smokers. Angiogenic squamous cell dysplasia is a morphologic entity commonly found in preneoplastic tissue. One study has noted that autofluorescence technique detected 75% of angiogenic squamous dysplasias, in contrast to standard bronchoscopy, which detected only 15% of such lesions.

Follow-up bronchoscopy may be required in some patients who have undergone cancer treatments. The indication for bronchoscopy is dependent on clinical findings. Surgical treatment involving complicated procedures, such as tracheoplasty and reanastomosis, often requires intraoperative or immediately postoperative bronchoscopy to assess the results of the surgical procedure.

Metastatic Cancer in the Thorax

Intrathoracic metastases from nonpulmonary malignancies have varying respiratory manifestations. Four clinical presentations that often require bronchoscopy include extrinsic compression of the tracheobronchial tree, endobronchial metastasis, pulmonary parenchymal nodule, and interstitial infiltration secondary to lymphangitic spread. The bronchoscopic diagnostic approaches are similar to those in primary lung cancer. Endobronchial metastasis is more likely from Hodgkin's lymphoma, hypernephroma, and cancer of the breast or colon. The role of BAL in the diagnosis of lymphangitic metastasis is discussed in a previous section.

Cancers of the esophagus and mediastinum may produce extrinsic compression or may extend directly into the tracheobronchial tree. Another complication of these tumors is the occasional occurrence of tracheoesophageal or tracheomediastinal fistula. Because of these possibilities, it is advisable to perform bronchoscopy before extensive surgical resections are undertaken. Routine cytologic analysis of bronchoscopic aspirates in patients with cancer limited to the esophagus may yield false-positive results, because the esophageal secretions aspirated into the airways may contain exfoliated cancer cells from esophageal cancer.

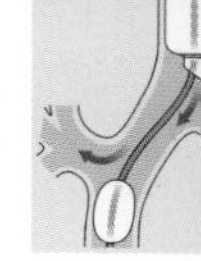

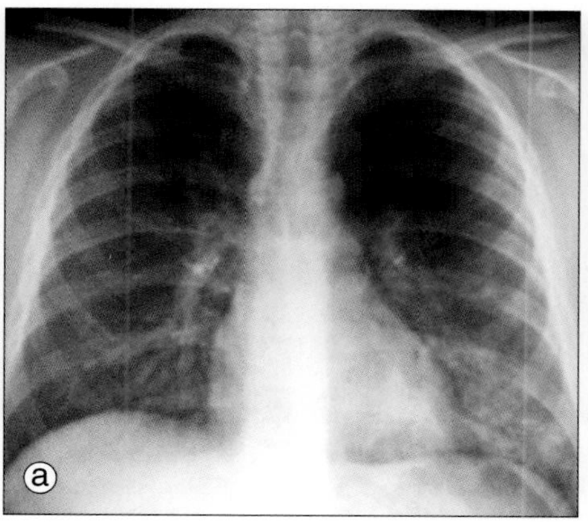

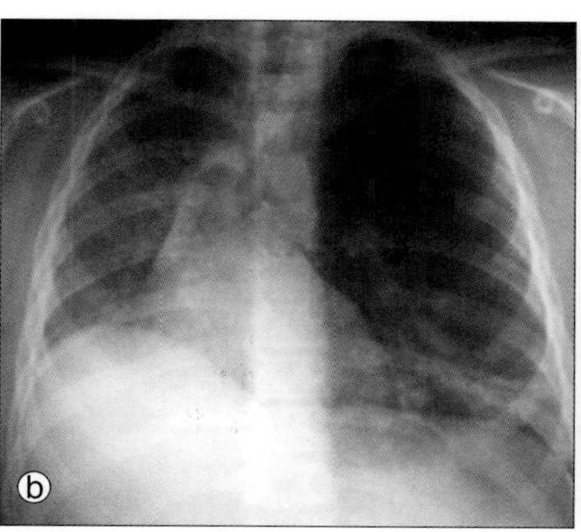

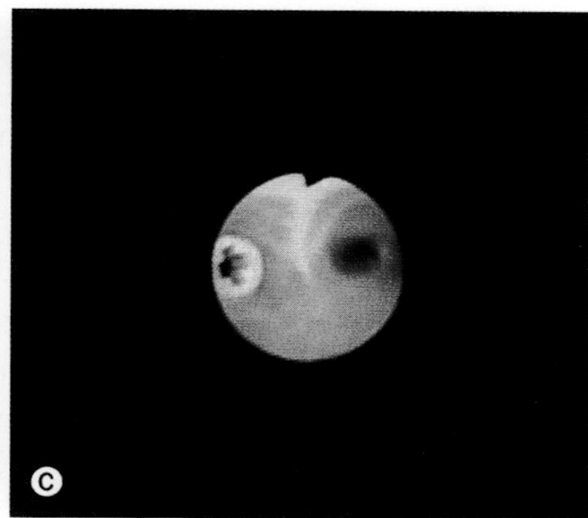

Figure 9.14 Chest radiographs of an 8-year-old boy who had cough and wheeze of 7 weeks' duration. A, Image obtained during full inspiration shows good expansion of both lungs. **B,** Image obtained after full expiration reveals hyperinflation of left lung caused by "check-valve"obstruction of the left main-stem bronchus by a previously aspirated piece of a toy **(C)**.

Tracheobronchial Foreign Body

Foreign body aspiration is always suspected in children with acute or subacute pulmonary symptoms. It is, however, rarely considered in adults with subacute or chronic respiratory symptoms without a clear history of aspiration. The singular diagnostic factor leading to consideration of foreign body aspiration is a high clinical index of suspicion. The diagnosis can be verified by visualizing the foreign body by chest x-ray or via bronchoscopy. A nonradiopaque foreign body may be easily missed on a chest x-ray film but may be suggested by associated atelectasis or infiltration in the postobstructive region or by air trapping and hyperinflation on postexhalation chest film (Fig. 9.14). Common foreign bodies include vegetable matter, seeds, straight pins, and safety pins. The treatment of tracheobronchial foreign bodies is discussed under therapeutic bronchoscopy.

Tracheobronchial Strictures and Stenoses

Tracheobronchial strictures and stenoses are caused by benign and malignant diseases. In the majority of patients with significant stenoses, clinical information should point toward the diagnosis, although an incorrect diagnosis of asthma is not uncommon. The cause of luminal narrowing can be intraluminal, extraluminal or within the wall of the airways. Benign strictures result from diverse processes including injury from tracheal intubation, crush injury of the neck, infections such as histoplasmosis and tuberculosis, mediastinal granulomatosis, Wegener's granulomatosis, and relapsing polychondritis (Fig. 9.15). The role of bronchoscopy in airway malignancy is discussed in a previous section. In benign strictures, bronchoscopy may show atrophic mucosa, mucosal edema, or granularity. In all newly suspected benign airway strictures with abnormal mucosa, multiple biopsies should be obtained to exclude malignancy. The presence of granulomas in biopsy specimens may indicate an infectious process or sarcoidosis. Often, the cause of benign strictures cannot be established.

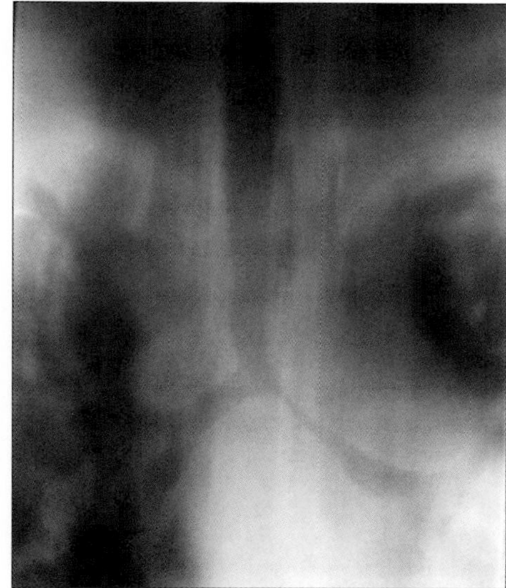

Figure 9.15 Tomographic representation of distal tracheal narrowing, significant stenosis of left main-stem bronchus, and moderate stenosis of right main-stem bronchus in a patient with relapsing polychondritis. This patient required bronchoscopic dilatation and silicone stent placement.

Chemical and Thermal Burns

The inhalation of certain chemicals, gases, and superheated air can produce acute, subacute, and chronic airway and pulmonary parenchymal complications. These include acute severe edema and erythema of the tracheobronchial mucosa and mucosal sloughing. Smoke inhalation may result in diffuse soot deposition in the tracheobronchial tree. Unconsciousness in these victims poses the threat of aspiration of orogastric contents into the airways. Diagnostic bronchoscopy to assess the extent of mucosal damage should also be used to exclude and treat aspirated gastric contents and foreign bodies. Bronchoscopy in the subacute stage may reveal necrosis of the tracheobronchial mucosa and hemorrhagic tracheobronchitis and, in the chronic phase, scarring and stenoses of tracheobronchial tree, bronchiectasis, formation of granulation tissue, and bronchiolitis obliterans on lung biopsy.

Thoracic Trauma

Diagnostic bronchoscopy is often indicated for victims of major thoracic trauma. The main indication in patients with recent chest trauma is the exclusion of serious airway injury, such as fracture of the tracheobronchial tree. Bronchoscopy helps in the management of other trauma-related problems such as atelectasis of the lung, lobe, or segment. Bronchoscopy may also reveal aspirated material or thick secretions and mucous plugging, which can be removed at the time of diagnostic bronchoscopy. Unsuspected foreign bodies of the airways are occasionally encountered in victims of trauma. Bronchoscopy for evaluation of hemoptysis following chest trauma may reveal oozing of blood from lung periphery as a result of pulmonary contusion and tissue laceration.

Paralysis of Vocal Cords and Diaphragm

The anatomic course of the left recurrent laryngeal nerve takes it around the left hilar structures. Pathologic lesions of the left hilar structures can compress or destroy the nerve and cause paralysis of the left vocal cord. Paralysis of the right vocal cord by an intrathoracic process is less common. Diagnostic bronchoscopy may be indicated if symptoms of vocal cord paralysis are associated with left hilar mass.

Neoplastic involvement of hilar or mediastinal lymph nodes or lymph nodes in the path of the phrenic nerves should be considered when evaluating diaphragmatic paralysis. Tumors that cause diaphragmatic paralysis are usually large and visible on the chest radiograph. Chest computed tomography (CT) may aid in the detection of subtle hilar lymphadenopathy. Bronchoscopy with needle aspiration and/or biopsy of the perihilar lymph nodes is a diagnostic option.

Pleural Effusion and Persistent Pneumothorax

Pleural effusion has been used as an indication for diagnostic bronchoscopy even though the diagnostic yield is low. An occult endobronchial obstructing lesion may contribute to the persistence of pneumothorax or continued air leak following placement of a chest tube. Bronchoscopy is performed occasionally to exclude an inapparent bronchial lesion.

Other Conditions

In patients with bronchiectasis, bronchoscopy has been used to obtain culture specimens. In cases of suspected bronchiectasis, bronchography has often been used to confirm the diagnosis and to assist in planning medical or surgical management. A water-soluble contrast material can be instilled via flexible bronchoscope to perform bronchography to detect bronchiectasis. The HRCT has essentially replaced bronchography to diagnose bronchiectasis.

Bronchoscopy is extremely useful in certain airway disorders. In patients with broncholithiasis, relapsing polychondritis, tracheobronchomalacia, airway-esophageal fistula, tracheopathia osteoplastica, and amyloidosis, bronchoscopy is frequently the only technique to evaluate the dynamics of airway motion and establish the diagnosis (Fig. 9.16).

THERAPEUTIC BRONCHOSCOPY

Therapeutic aspects of bronchoscopy are as important as the diagnostic indications. Often, simultaneous diagnostic and therapeutic bronchoscopies are indicated. Lobar or segmental atelectasis caused by retained secretions or mucous plugs is the most common indication for therapeutic bronchoscopy. Among patients in critical care units, up to 75% of bronchoscopies are performed for therapeutic purposes. The other indications for therapeutic bronchoscopy are listed in Table 9.2.

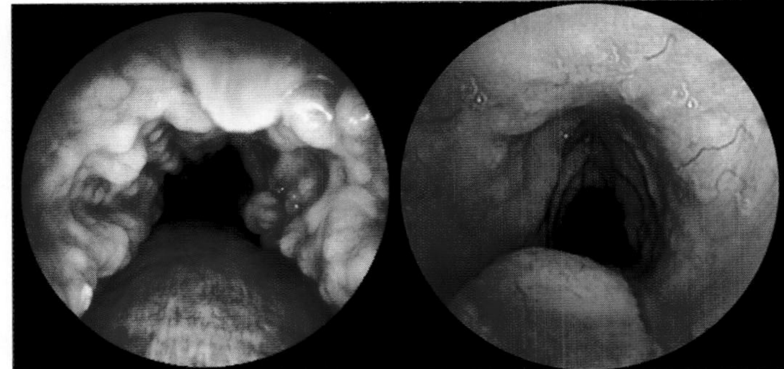

Figure 9.16 Bronchoscopic appearance of the trachea in tracheopathia osteoplastica *(left)* and tracheobronchial amyloidosis *(right)*. The former disorder typically spares the posterior membranous part of the airways. Amyloidosis of the airways produces a "golden-yellow, oily" appearance of the mucosal lesions. Although the bronchoscopic appearance itself is diagnostic of tracheopathia, a biopsy is necessary to document amyloidosis. Image on left from Prakash UBS (ed): Bronchoscopy. New York, Raven, 1994.

Retained Secretions, Mucous Plugs, and Clots

Retention of secretions and mucous plugs is a common clinical problem in patients with impaired cough and clearance mechanisms due to altered level of consciousness, poor pulmonary function or weakness, recurrent aspiration, ventilator dependence, or post-thoracotomy state. Inspissated mucus and resultant mucous plug may cause segmental or lobar atelectasis. Blood clots formed from pulmonary lesions, after trauma, or after thoracic surgery pose special problems because such clots are usually tenacious and more difficult to remove than the mucous plugs. Therapeutic bronchoscopy is also indicated in patients who develop a pseudomembrane in the tracheobronchial tree following photodynamic therapy of airway neoplasms and necrotic debris following chemical or thermal burns of the tracheobronchial mucosa.

Immediate therapeutic bronchoscopy is indicated if atelectasis is responsible for respiratory distress. In less urgent cases, nonbronchoscopic means should be first attempted. It should be noted that not all patients with segmental or even lobar atelectasis show uniform benefit from therapeutic bronchoscopy. In such cases, the etiology of hypoxemia may not be related to atelectasis.

A flexible bronchoscope with a large channel can help to quickly aspirate the thick and tenacious mucous and blood clots from the airways. A soft orotracheal tube permits administration of supplemental oxygen during the procedure. It also enables the operator to remove the bronchoscope from the airways for the cleaning of the instrument channel. The patient's coughing during the bronchoscopic suction also helps move the mucous secretions and plugs proximally. Very thick and tenacious secretions and mucous plugs may require removal by biopsy forceps. Forceps may be required to remove necrotic mucosa, pseudomembrane, and necrotic debris resulting from various airway diseases.

In hypoxemic patients who require vigorous suctioning, the oxygenation should be monitored by pulse oximetry so that the preexisting hypoxemia does not worsen. Large-channel flexible bronchoscopes are more likely to aggravate this problem because of their ability to suck large volumes of gas. Supplemental oxygenation permits safe performance of the procedure.

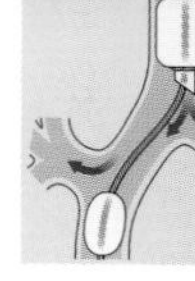

Table 9.8 Bronchoscopic control of hemoptysis
Repeated suctioning (to keep open the airways)
Iced saline irrigation
Vasoactive drugs (epinephrine, vasopressin analogs)
Bronchoscopic tamponade
Balloon tamponade
Tamponade with gauze or Gelfoam
Thrombin/fibrinogen instillation
Laser coagulation
Argon plasma coagulator
Electrocautery
Cryotherapy*
Bronchoscopic brachytherapy**
Isolation of bronchial tree (double-lumen ET tube, etc)

* Not suitable for massive hemoptysis
** Not suitable for massive hemoptysis or acute control hemoptysis

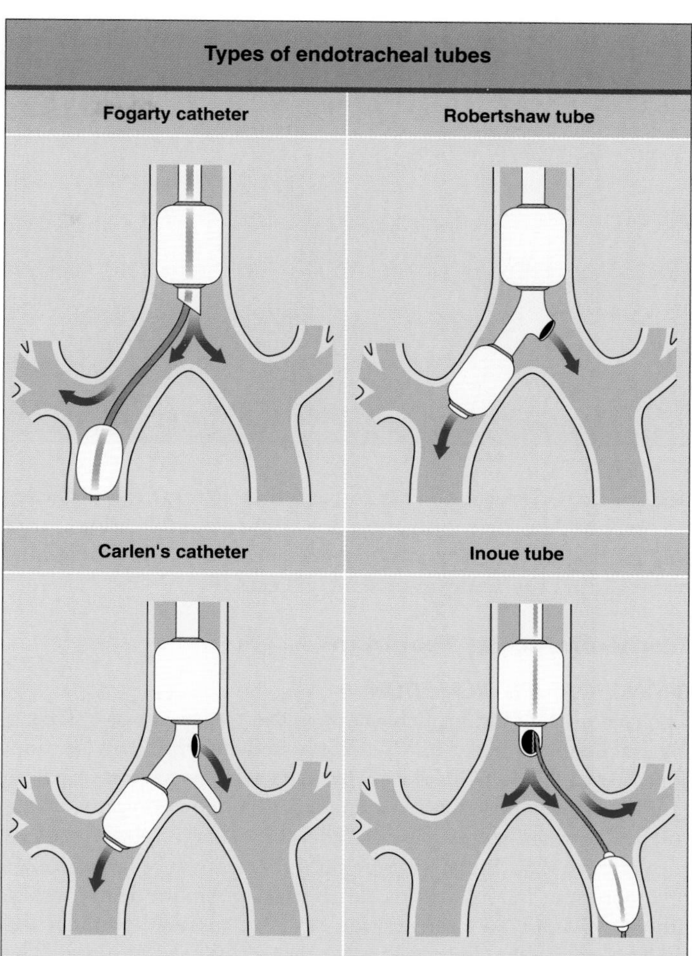

Figure 9.17 Types of endotracheal tubes available to simultaneously control massive hemoptysis and provide adequate ventilation. When a Fogarty catheter is used through an endotracheal tube (size >8), or if an Inoue tube is used, a standard flexible bronchoscope can be passed easily. Only an ultrathin flexible bronchoscope can pass through either a Carlen tube or a Robertshaw tube.

In patients with refractory atelectasis, bronchoscopic bronchial balloon occlusion with application of positive pressure ventilation delivered through the balloon catheter lumen has resulted in the re-expansion of atelectatic segments.

Bronchial tamponade via the bronchoscope is aimed at isolating a pulmonary segment or subsegment distal to the location of the tamponade. The bronchial tamponade technique has been used for the bronchoscopic treatment of bronchial or pulmonary hemorrhage, refractory pneumothorax, persistent air leaks following thoracotomy, and bronchopleural fistula. The therapeutic results from these maneuvers are not uniformly successful.

Hemoptysis

Hemoptysis is a commonly encountered symptom. However, massive bleeding is seen in less than 5% of patients with hemoptysis. Asphyxiation rather than exsanguination causes death following massive hemoptysis. To prevent this and to treat continued bleeding, hemodynamic status and oxygenation are stabilized. Then, bronchoscopy is performed to localize the site of bleeding and treat it bronchoscopically, if feasible (Table 9.8). A bronchoscope with a large working channel passed through an orotracheal tube is recommended. Uncontrollable or excessive bleeding may require the use of the rigid bronchoscope. If bleeding originates in a distal segment, the bronchoscope tip should tamponade the bronchus. Iced saline irrigation, using 10 to 20 mL at a time, usually slows and stops the bleeding that may result from bronchoscopic lung biopsy. Bronchoscopic instillation of 1:10,000 epinephrine, bronchoscopic balloon tamponade, and fibrin glue tamponade are some of the methods used. Fibrin glue technique is usually unsuccessful in massive hemoptysis because the blood flushes away the fibrin glue.

It is important to enable adequate ventilation and oxygenation by suctioning the aspirated blood and blood clots from the uninvolved airways. If the bleeding is from a visible tumor or an area where tamponade technique is not feasible, bronchoscopic coagulation of the lesion may be necessary. Smaller lesions can be coagulated with the laser; lower energy (approximately 15 W) is suitable for coagulation. Bronchoscopic electrocautery, argon plasma coagulation, and cryotherapy are alternatives to laser application.

If the aforementioned measures fail, tamponade with a rigid bronchoscope may be required to prevent asphyxiation. If rigid bronchoscopy is not available or possible, a double-lumen orotracheal tube can be used to isolate the lungs (Fig. 9.17). If the double-lumen tubes are used, it should be recognized that examination of airways is possible only with a smaller-caliber flexible bronchoscope because of the smaller inner diameter of the double-lumen tubes.

Tracheobronchial Foreign Body

Rigid bronchoscopy has been the instrument of choice in tracheobronchial foreign body extraction, particularly in children. However, most of the airway foreign bodies in adults can be extracted with a flexible bronchoscope (Fig. 9.18). Small-caliber flexible bronchoscopes and special extraction instruments have been used effectively to remove foreign bodies from pediatric airways (see Fig. 9.14). Flexible bronchoscopy is particularly

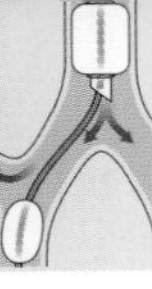

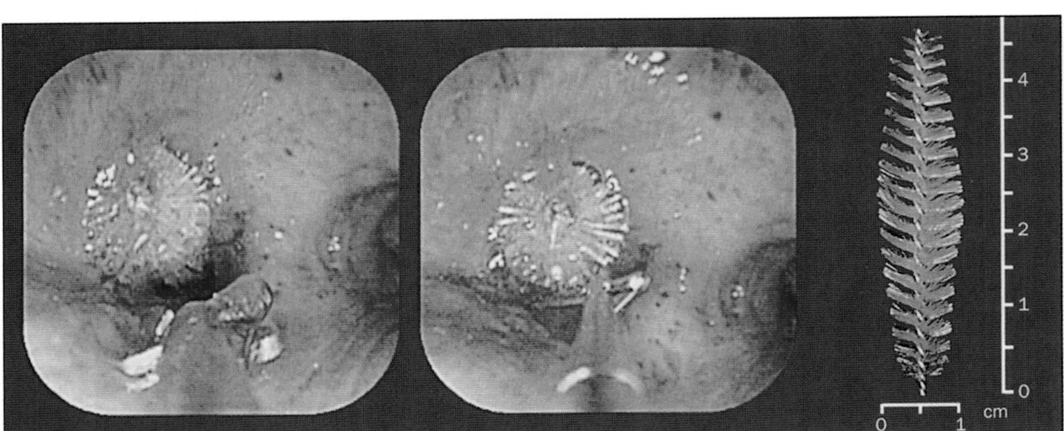

Figure 9.18 A foreign body (a fractured tracheostomy cleaning brush) lodged in the right bronchus intermedius. This was extracted using a flexible bronchoscope and long-toothed ureteral stone forceps passed through the biopsy channel of the flexible bronchoscope.

helpful if the foreign body is impacted in airways too distal for access with the rigid bronchoscope. Acute complications from foreign body extraction are uncommon. Mucosal bleeding may occur during the removal of sharp objects.

Tracheobronchial Neoplasms

BRONCHOSCOPIC RESECTION

The role of the rigid bronchoscope in the treatment of obstructing tracheobronchial tumors is discussed in a previous section. This treatment is palliative in patients who require immediate relief of airway obstruction secondary to large neoplasms in the trachea or main-stem bronchi. The use of large biopsy forceps through the rigid bronchoscope permits removal of large masses of obstructing neoplastic tissue. If this technique leads to significant bleeding, a large suction catheter inserted through the rigid bronchoscope helps keep the airways cleared of blood. The flexible bronchoscope is ill suited for this purpose because of the small working channel and its inability to permit removal of large pieces of tumor and large volumes of blood. However, the flexible bronchoscope can be used effectively to coagulate and remove airway neoplasms using laser therapy, electrocautery, argon plasma coagulation, and other palliative therapies. Various types of bronchoscopic therapies employed in the treatment of airway stenoses, both benign and malignant, are listed in Table 9.9.

LASER BRONCHOSCOPY

Laser therapy provides immediate relief of occlusion in over 90% of patients with large airway tumors. The laser energy causes cell death by intense heat, coagulation, and evaporation of tissue. Assorted types of lasers are available for the treatment of tracheobronchial neoplasms through both the flexible and rigid bronchoscopes, with the neodymium:yttrium-aluminum-garnet (Nd:YAG) laser being the most popular. The rigid bronchoscope is better suited for laser bronchoscopy. Usually, laser therapies are palliative and are indicated for the relief of the obstruction caused by tumors of trachea and major bronchi. Laser therapy, however, has been used to cure both benign and malignant airway tumors. Special training in the use of the laser is required.

Precautions during laser therapy include the use of low FIO_2, noncombustible anesthetic gases, and protection of eyes of the bronchoscopy team. Complications include hemorrhage, pneumothorax, air embolism, and death. Peripheral bronchial tumors rarely require laser therapy unless relief of postobstructive pneumonia is clinically indicated.

Table 9.9
Bronchoscopic therapies

Therapy	Type of lesion	Type of bronchoscope	Rapidity of positive result	Repeatability of therapy
Mechanical débridement	Endoluminal or submucosal	Rigid or flexible (rigid preferable)	++++	+++
Laser	Endoluminal	Rigid or flexible (rigid preferable)	++++	++++
Argon plasma	Endoluminal	Rigid or flexible	++++	++++
Brachytherapy	Endoluminal or submucosal	Flexible	+	+
Cryotherapy	Endoluminal	Rigid or flexible	++	+++
Balloon dilatation	Endoluminal or submucosal with extraluminal compression	Rigid or flexible (rigid preferable)	++++	++++
Photodynamic therapy	Endoluminal	Flexible	++	+++
Electrocautery	Endoluminal	Rigid or flexible	+++	++++
Stent	Endoluminal with extraluminal compression	Rigid or flexible (Dumon stent requires rigid bronchoscope; Wall stents and Gianturco stents require fluoroscopy)	++++	+++

++++, most rapid or repeatable.

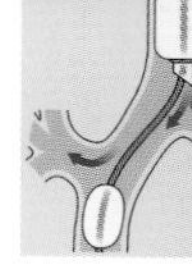

ARGON PLASMA COAGULATOR

Argon is an inert gas in its natural state. When argon is ionized by electricity, the electrically conducting argon plasma medium is formed. The argon plasma coagulator uses the argon plasma medium to deliver high-frequency current and high temperatures via a rigid or flexible bronchoscope probe to coagulate, devitalize, and destroy malignant tissue in the airways. As target surface becomes less electrically conductive, argon plasma seeks adjacent tissue with less electrical resistance. Once the malignant tissue is thus treated, the devitalized tissue is mechanically removed with grasping forceps. The technique is easier to perform than laser application, and the unit is less expensive than the laser units. Therapeutic results in airway malignancies and bleeding are similar to those with laser therapy.

Precautions are similar to those for laser bronchoscopy. Additionally, the patient should be protected from electrical shock by grounding the patient so that the electrical circuit is complete. Complications of argon plasma therapy include perforation of the airways and damage to the inner lining of flexible bronchoscope.

BRONCHOSCOPIC ELECTROCAUTERY

Bronchoscopic electrocautery uses the standard electrocautery technique through the bronchoscope to apply electrical current to coagulate and desiccate the obstructing tissue in the airways. The therapeutic results are similar to those from laser and argon plasma therapy. Special equipment is required for use with the flexible bronchoscope. The technique is easier to perform than laser application, and the unit is less expensive than the laser and argon plasma units. Precautions and complications are similar to those associated with use of the laser and the argon plasma coagulator.

BRONCHOSCOPIC CRYOTHERAPY

Bronchoscopic cryotherapy, used to treat both benign and malignant airway lesions, makes use of extreme hypothermia to destroy malignant cells and scar tissue. The technique requires either a flexible or rigid bronchoscopic cryoprobe, through which liquid nitrogen or nitrous oxide is circulated. This causes the probe tip to develop a very cold temperature. When the cold probe comes into contact with the tumor or stenotic tissue for several minutes, it freezes the tissue. The treated tissue undergoes cold necrosis over the next 48 to 72 hours. The necrotic tumor is sometimes expectorated. Objective improvement occurs in 50% to 70% of patients. The disadvantage of cryotherapy is that it requires prolonged, often repeated bronchoscopies. Therefore, it is not suited for acute airway obstructions that require emergent therapy. Cryotherapy has been used to extract thick mucous plugs and foreign bodies from the airways. Cryotherapy equipment is less expensive than laser and argon plasma equipment.

BRACHYTHERAPY

Brachytherapy is the delivery of ionizing radiation therapy from a source of ionizing radiation placed within or very near the tissue being treated. The bronchoscope is used to place the brachytherapy catheter in the affected airway to palliate tracheobronchial malignancies in patients who cannot receive external beam radiation or other types of treatment. Brachytherapy is usually preceded by airway débridement by rigid bronchoscopy, laser therapy, or other methods. The most commonly used isotope is iridium 192, but others include cesium 137, cobalt 60, gold 198, and iodine 125. Both low- and high-dose brachytherapy techniques are available. The high-dose treatment can be completed rapidly. Low-dose brachytherapy is slightly prolonged (24 to 48 hours) and requires hospitalization. Reduction in hemoptysis in 60% of patients and increase in airway diameter in 85% of patients have been described. However, some studies have reported increased risk of significant, occasionally massive hemoptysis following high-dose brachytherapy. Other complications include severe radiation bronchitis, airway necrosis, airway-mediastinal fistula, and esophagitis.

PHOTOTHERAPY

Phototherapy of tracheobronchial cancers is a therapeutic alternative in patients deemed unsuitable for surgical treatment. Fluorescent compounds, such as hematoporphyrin derivative (HpD) and dihematoporphyrin ether (DHE), function as cancer "tags." When administered, these chemicals are retained in malignant tissue at higher concentrations than in normal tissue. Several hours after intravenous administration of HpD or DHE, a special light with the appropriate wavelength is shone on the bronchial mucosa using the bronchoscope. The resultant photodynamic chemical reactions lead to the intracellular production of toxic radicals including singlet oxygen, hydroxyl ion, and hydrogen peroxide. These events result in death of malignant cells. Phototherapy has demonstrated at least a 50% complete response in tumors that measure less than 3 cm^2 in largest surface area.

Complications from photodynamic therapy are infrequent and include a burn on the face and/or hands that resembles sunburn, hemoptysis, and expectoration of gray necrotic material. Therapeutic bronchoscopy may be needed to extract the necrotic pseudomembrane.

Airway Stenosis

Symptomatic benign strictures and stenoses of the tracheobronchial tree often require surgical treatment. Bronchoscopic dilatation using the rigid bronchoscope, balloons, laser, electrocautery, and placement of airway stent may obviate the need for surgery. These treatments are best suited for short strictures or strictures caused by membranous or weblike lesions. Thick transmural strictures and long strictures are least likely to respond to laser ablation.

BRONCHOSCOPIC DILATATION

Bronchoscopic dilatation is applicable in patients whose airway strictures cannot be treated surgically. Both benign and malignant airway lesions can be treated by bronchoscopic techniques. In benign strictures, the passage of rigid bronchoscopes of gradually increasing diameters may dilate the trachea and main-stem bronchi. Balloon dilatation through either the flexible or rigid bronchoscope can be accomplished if the stenosis is limited to a short segment of the airway (Fig. 9.19). Repeated dilatations may be required to treat recurrent stenosis. Dilatation is unlikely to relieve the airway stenosis caused by extrinsic lesions. In most patients who require stent placement, preliminary dilatation is necessary.

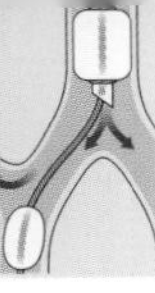

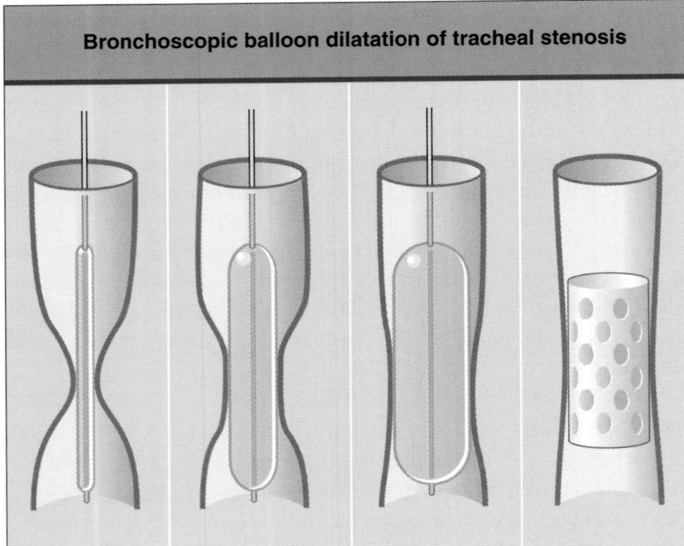

Figure 9.19 Bronchoscopic balloon dilatation of tracheal stenosis, diagrammatic depiction. This can be accomplished with a flexible or rigid bronchoscope, using graduated dilating balloons. After optimal dilation, a silicone stent (placed with a rigid bronchoscope) relieves airway obstruction.

AIRWAY STENTS

Airway prosthesis or stents relieve airway obstruction caused by malignant or benign disease. The advantage is that stents can be used in airway stenoses caused by intramural, transmural, and extramural processes. Airway dilatation and debulking are often necessary before stent insertion. Stents work best in the trachea and main-stem bronchi (Figs. 9.20 and 9.21). They are not well suited for lobar and distal bronchial stenoses. In any case, stent placement is seldom indicated for distal airway lesions. The types of stents include products of expandable metal wire, molded silicone, and combinations of both.

Rigid bronchoscopy is essential for the insertion, manipulation, and removal of most silicone stents. Flexible, self-expanding metal stents can be inserted by flexible bronchoscopy with or without fluoroscopic guidance (see Fig. 9.21). Special training in the technique is necessary. Complications from tracheobronchial stents include migration of the stent; increased mucous secretions with somewhat decreased clearing by cough; and growth of granulation tissue. Migration is more likely with silicone stents, and metallic stents are more likely to cause granulation tissue.

Bronchopleural Fistula and Pneumothorax

Bronchopleural fistulas and persistent pneumothoraces are challenging problems in the ventilated patient. The closure of the bronchopleural fistula by the bronchoscopic application of various sealing agents (fibrin glue, stent, bone, ethanol, and so on) has been tried with limited success.

Bronchogenic Cysts and Mediastinal Cysts

Bronchogenic cysts and mediastinal cysts occasionally become filled with liquid and compress the tracheobronchial lumen. Bronchoscopic drainage of these cysts has been performed to relieve the airway compression. The bronchoscope also has been used to drain lung abscesses (see Fig. 9.10), fluid-filled cysts, pericardial effusion, and other lesions in the mediastinum and the lung.

Endotracheal Tube Placement

Patients with endotracheal tubes often require bronchoscopy for the replacement of the tube. The flexible bronchoscope is helpful in intubating patients with cervical spine trauma or massive facial injuries and for replacing or changing such tubes. The flexible bronchoscope has been used to assess the pathogenic factors leading to laryngotracheal injury due to tracheal intubation in critically ill patients and to replace endotracheal tubes in patients on mechanical ventilation who require change of tube.

Therapeutic Lavage

Alveolar proteinosis is a condition in which a diffuse intraalveolar deposition of lipoproteinaceous material leads to progressive respiratory distress. The treatment for this rare disorder has been the insertion of the double-lumen endotracheal tube, followed by instillation of several liters of normal saline to wash out the intraalveolar material. This requires general anesthesia and special equipment and personnel. Several reports have described the use of a flexible bronchoscope to therapeutically wash individual segments. Such procedures are time consuming and may also require deep sedation or general anesthesia.

Broncholithiasis

Broncholiths are calcified peribronchial lymph nodes that encroach upon adjacent airways and cause clinical and

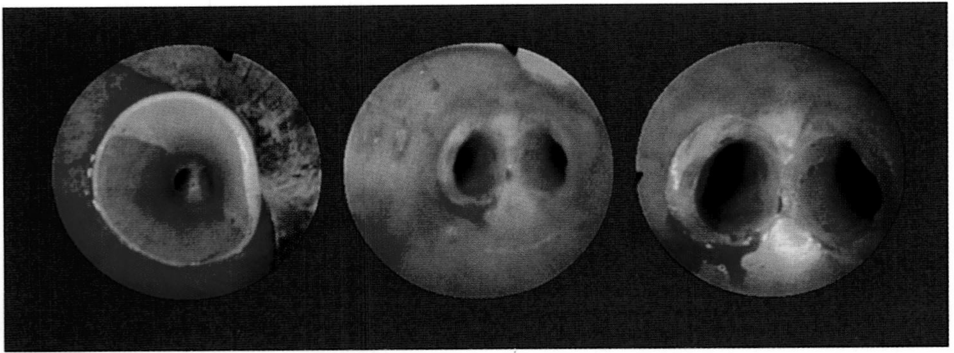

Figure 9.20 Rigid bronchoscopic placement of a silicone ⅄ stent over the main carina. This was to provide ventilation of both main-stem bronchi in a patient with squamous cell carcinoma involving the main carina and proximal main-stem bronchi.

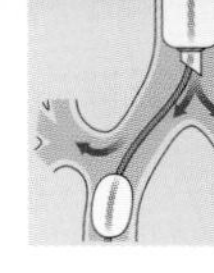

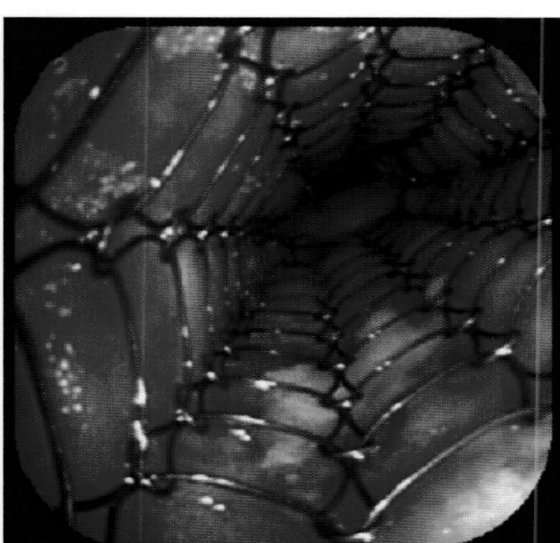

Figure 9.21 Expandable metallic stent placed in the right main-stem bronchus with flexible bronchoscopic guidance. These stents can be placed under fluoroscopic guidance, without bronchoscopy. However, manipulation and removal requires bronchoscopy, often with a rigid bronchoscope.

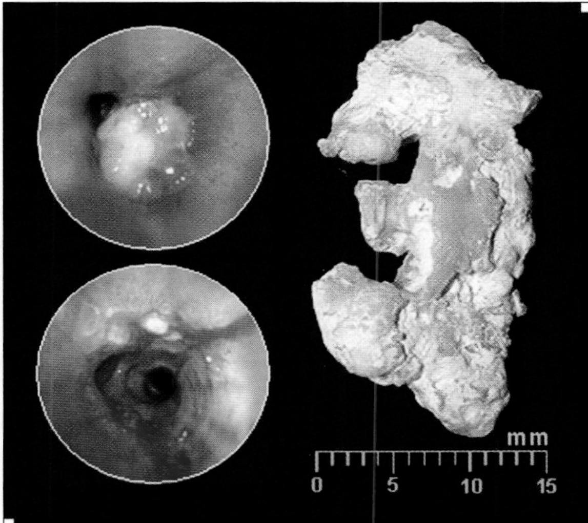

Figure 9.22 Broncholith and associated granulation tissue in the left main-stem bronchus *(upper left)*, and the left main-stem bronchus immediately after rigid bronchoscopic removal of the broncholith *(lower left)*. The extracted broncholith is shown on the right.

roentgenographic abnormalities. Most broncholiths are sequelae of fungal or mycobacterial granulomatous lymphadenitis. Symptoms develop when the calcified lymph node impinges on or erodes into the airway lumen. Broncholiths cause chronic cough, hemoptysis, stone expectoration (lithoptysis), recurrent pneumonia, and fistulas between the bronchi and adjacent mediastinal structures. Bronchoscopy is perhaps the most important test in the management of broncholithiasis. When the broncholith is free within the airway lumen, bronchoscopic extraction is successful in almost all patients (Fig. 9.22).

MISCELLANEOUS

Lung Transplant

Lung transplant recipients are prone to develop airway complications as well as pulmonary complications. Interventional bronchoscopy is required in greater than 25% of lung transplant recipients, and many patients require repeated bronchoscopies for the assessment and management of complications. The post-transplant complications include anastomotic stenosis and dehiscence, airway malacia, granuloma formation, difficulty in clearing mucus, tracheobronchial aspergillosis, transplant rejection, progressive bronchiolitis, and opportunistic infections of the lungs. Bronchoscopic therapeutic procedures include airway dilatation, stent placement, and laser or forceps excision of stenosis. Many transplant centers perform “surveillance” bronchoscopy, a routinely scheduled (sometimes monthly) bronchoscopic lung biopsy to detect rejection.

Bronchoscopic Lung Volume Reduction

Advanced emphysema leads to severe respiratory insufficiency through different mechanisms. The hyperinflation of lungs produces dyspnea by severely limiting the excursion of chest cage during breathing. Surgical resection of 20% to 30% of both lungs has been shown to improve respiratory mechanics and diminish symptoms. Because surgical lung volume reduction is associated with significant morbidity and mortality, bronchoscopic lung volume reduction is being tested in selected patients. Preliminary reports in small numbers of patients have described bronchoscopic occlusion of segmental bronchi by balloons, fibrin glue, metallic coils, and one-way silicone-metal stents. The bronchoscopic “resizing” of the overexpanded lung has the potential to become a common procedure. However, the long-term results of bronchoscopic lung volume reduction in larger numbers of patients remain to be seen. It is also unclear whether this type of therapy needs to be repeated if and when the lung volumes increase. Currently, the procedure is in experimental stages.

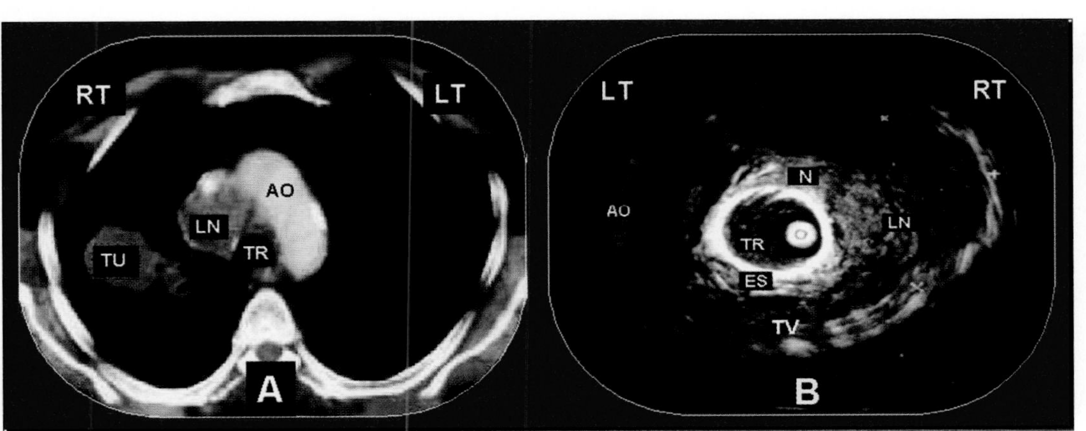

Figure 9.23 Bronchoscopic ultrasound. A, Computed tomography (CT) shows the tumor in the right upper lobe (TU) and enlarged right paratracheal lymph node; the trachea (TR) and aortic arch (AO) are also identified. **B,** Bronchoscopic ultrasound images at the level of the AO shows the enlarged right paratracheal lymph nodes (LN), which can be clearly separated from the tracheal wall. A smaller lymph node is visible anterior to the trachea (N), and the esophagus is visible posterior to the trachea (ES). The thoracic vertebral column (TV) also can be seen. (Courtesy of Heinrich Becker, MD.)

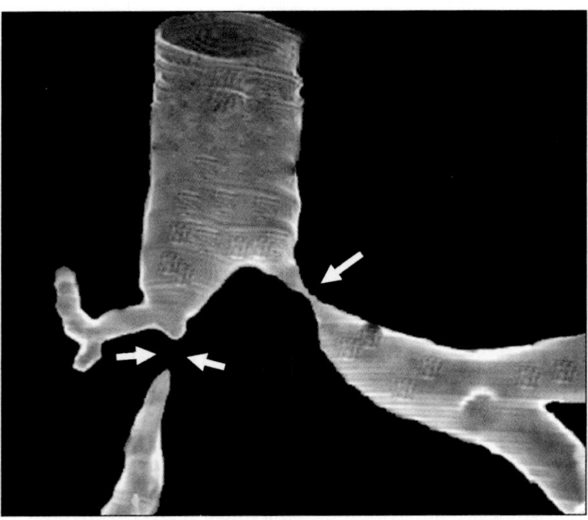

Figure 9.24 Virtual bronchoscopy. Computed tomographic (CT) images are manipulated to create a three-dimensional image of the major airways. In this figure, severe narrowing of the left main-stem bronchus *(longer arrow)* and complete occlusion of the bronchus intermedius *(shorter arrows)* were thought to be the result of mediastinal fibrosis.

Bronchoscopic Ultrasonography

This technique requires an echographic camera, a bronchoscopic ultrasonic probe, and a video monitor to obtain the echographic images. Ultrasound-guided detection of paratracheal, hilar, or mediastinal lymphadenopathy may help in the staging of lung cancer (Fig. 9.23). Currently, the clinical role of this technique is limited. Development of technology for simultaneous ultrasound visualization and needle aspiration of abnormal lesions may make it clinically useful.

Virtual Bronchoscopy

Virtual bronchoscopy demonstrates three-dimensional images of airway anatomy and intraluminal and extraluminal abnormalities without the performance of bronchoscopy. The virtual reality images are derived from data obtained with chest CT. Virtual bronchoscopy can be used to identify endobronchial tumor, airway distortion, stenosis, and ectasia (Fig. 9.24). It also permits identification and mapping of extrabronchial anatomy—specifically, the relationship of the tracheobronchial tree to the surrounding structures, including blood vessels and lymph nodes. Virtual bronchoscopy has been used for grading and follow-up of airway strictures, presurgical assessment of airway dynamics, bronchoscopy training, and endobronchial therapy. Even though virtual bronchoscopy reveals the endoluminal and extraluminal lesions, real bronchoscopic procedures are required to obtain tissue diagnosis. Currently, virtual bronchoscopy has a limited clinical role.

BRONCHOSCOPY TRAINING

The development of newer techniques in bronchoscopy has led to increased requests from novice and expert bronchoscopists for guidelines in various procedures. In 2002 and 2003 the major professional societies published guidelines regarding the number of procedures required to attain and maintain proficiency in the many procedures described in this chapter. The initial enthusiasm for certain procedures like laser therapy has waned because of the high cost of equipment, the limited number of patients who require this therapy, and the difficulty in obtaining optimal training. The competing procedures, namely HRCT of the chest, transesophageal ultrasound-guided needle aspiration of mediastinal lymph nodes, and video-assisted thoracoscopy, have led to decreased numbers of bronchoscopic procedures in certain respiratory disorders.

SUGGESTED READINGS

Bolliger C, Mathur P (eds): Interventional Bronchoscopy. Prog Respir Res; Basel, Karger, 2000.

Bolliger CT, Mathur PN, Beamis JF, et al: European Respiratory Society/American Thoracic Society. ERS/ATS statement on interventional pulmonology. Eur Respir J 19:356-373, 2002.

Colt HG, Prakash UBS, Offord KP: Bronchoscopy in North America: Survey by the American Association for Bronchology, 1999. J Bronchol 7:8-25, 2000.

Ernst A, Silvestri GA, Johnstone D, ACCP Interventional/Diagnostic Procedures Network Steering Committee: Interventional pulmonary procedures. Guidelines from the American College of Chest Physicians. Chest 123:1693-1717, 2003.

Goldberg M, Patchefsky AS (eds): Uncommon tumors of the tracheobronchial tree: Diagnosis and Management. Chest Surg Clin North Am 13:1-174, 2003.

Mehta AC (ed): Flexible bronchoscopy update. Clin Chest Med 22:224-383, 2001.

Prakash UBS (ed): Bronchoscopy. New York, Raven, 1994.

Prakash UBS, Offord KP, Stubbs SE: Bronchoscopy in North America: the ACCP survey. Chest 100:168-175, 1991.

Wang KP, Mehta AC, Turner JF, Jr. (eds): Flexible Bronchoscopy. Malden, Massachusetts, Blackwell Scientific, 2004.

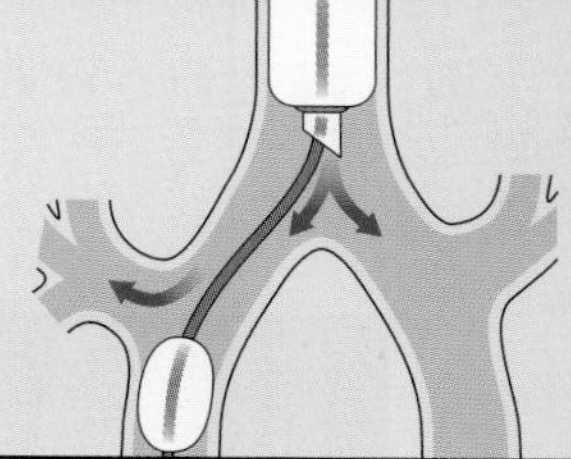

CHAPTER 10

Thoracentesis and Closed Pleural Biopsy

Stephen G. Spiro

Pleural effusions are most commonly caused by malignancy and infection—in particular parapneumonic and tuberculous—and may need to be investigated by means of closed pleural biopsy if an initial aspirated sample is negative for malignant cytology or an obvious infection. Most malignant causes are diagnosed on the cytologic examination of a 20-mL aliquot of the effusion, which can be aspirated by inserting a needle through the chest wall under local anesthesia. In cases of tuberculosis, the fluid rarely yields acid-fast bacilli when direct smears are examined, but it is predominantly lymphocytic and usually has a reduced glucose content. Pyogenic infection or parapneumonic effusions may be milky and have a purulent appearance, may show a lesser shade of turbidity, or even may be clear but contain neutrophils. Empyemas tend to appear creamy and sometimes have a fecal smell. The rare chylous effusion is paler and more milky in appearance.

INDICATIONS AND CONTRAINDICATIONS

If the initial pleural aspiration is not diagnostic, it should be repeated, and a closed pleural biopsy performed at the same time. The biopsy is especially useful in cases of suspected tuberculosis, as the pleural histology may yield granulomata in up to 50% of cases. Pleural biopsy adds 2% to 10% to the yield of cytology for malignancy and is particularly important in the diagnosis of mesothelioma.

TECHNIQUE

A variety of needles are available. The Cope needle was introduced in 1958, but the Abrams needle remains the most popular. The Raja needle is a modification of the Abrams needle and was introduced in 1993. Tru-Cut biopsy needles are used under ultrasound control by radiologists to produce a core of tissue from obviously thickened pleural tissues for histologic examination. Finally, biopsy specimens can be taken from the parietal pleura using forceps during the course of a thoracoscopy, usually as a video-assisted thoracoscopic procedure.

Positioning the Patient

The patient should sit upright, leaning forward with arms folded across the chest, and leaning onto a pillow that rests on the bed-table. Position the patient's head also leaning forward onto the pillow for several minutes to allow comfortable breathing. The folding of the patient's arms lifts the scapula upward and outward and prevents them from impeding the procedure.

Anesthesia

After cleaning the skin, introduce 1% plain lidocaine (lignocaine) into the posterior axillary line with as small a needle as possible. Once the skin is anesthetized, a longer No. 1 needle is advanced. Push out lidocaine continuously and aim to advance beneath the rib until the pleura is penetrated and fluid can be drawn back into the attached syringe (Fig. 10.1). At this stage, use a second syringe that contains 1% lidocaine to widen the area of anesthesia, keeping the skin entry site as the apex of an imagined pyramid of anesthesia. Always withdraw the needle back to just under the skin before advancing it at a new angle. The best practice is to use a new syringe of lidocaine once the pleural cavity has been entered, as malignant pleural effusions can seed along the needle track from the pleura. A total of 10 mL of 1% lidocaine should be sufficient to anesthetize the chest wall of most subjects.

Incision

Next, make a stab incision with a No. 11 scalpel blade along the intended biopsy track. This easily can be widened and extended down to the pleural surface by blunt dissection with a pair of straight Spencer-Wells forceps (Fig. 10.2).

USE OF THE ABRAMS NEEDLE

The Abrams needle contains an inner stylus, which is removed and not used. The inner of the two remaining cylinders has a cutting edge that, when pulled back, opens a triangular aperture on the outer sheath of the needle and allows fluid to enter the inner cannula (Fig. 10.3). To open or close the window in the outer sheath, the ferrule is rotated clockwise or counterclockwise, respectively (Fig. 10.4). The ferrule lies in line with the closed aperture when turned clockwise as far as it can go. The hub of the needle is attached to a three-way tap with a hose to drain fluid for collection and to a large syringe with a Luer lock fitting.

The knob on the ferrule of the inner sheath must be in line with the needle aperture. With the aperture closed, use a rotating action to push the needle gently through the chest wall into the pleural cavity (Fig. 10.5). Blunt dissection (see "Incision," earlier in this chapter) enables the needle to pass easily and prevents it from bursting into the pleural cavity, thus avoiding the risk of trauma. The needle point is blunt, which also limits potential damage, for example, a pneumothorax.

Once the pleural cavity has been entered, open the needle and withdraw fluid (Fig. 10.6). Collect samples of 20 mL and

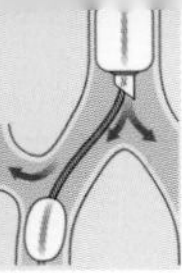

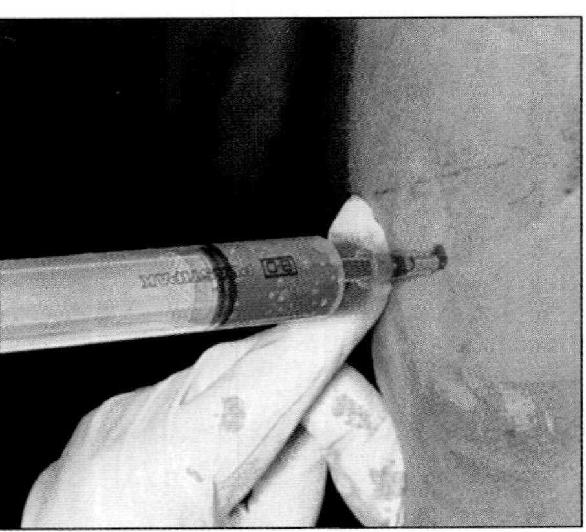

Figure 10.1 Infiltration of chest wall with local anesthetic. The needle penetrates the pleura, and fluid is aspirated back into the syringe.

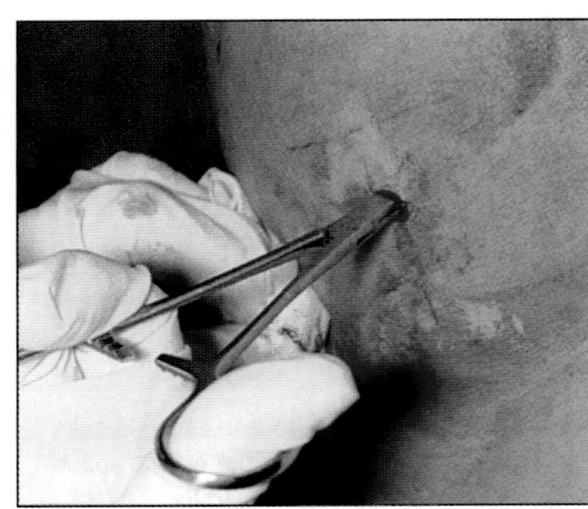

Figure 10.2 A blunt dissection down to and into the pleural cavity. The forceps are opened gently and pushed forward to tease apart the muscle fibers.

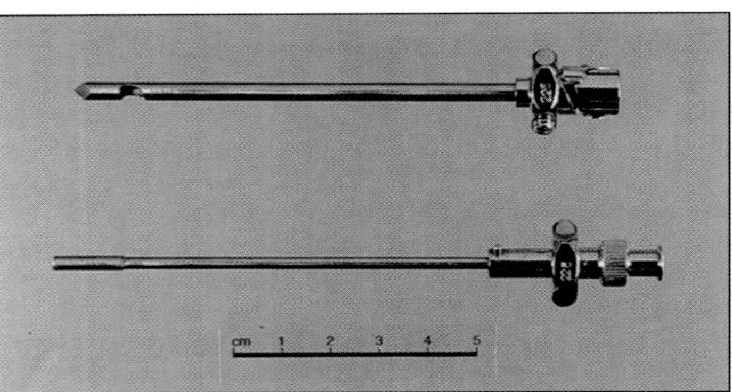

Figure 10.3 The inner and outer sheaths of an Abrams' needle showing the aperture in the outer sheath. The tip of the inner sheath cuts the biopsy.

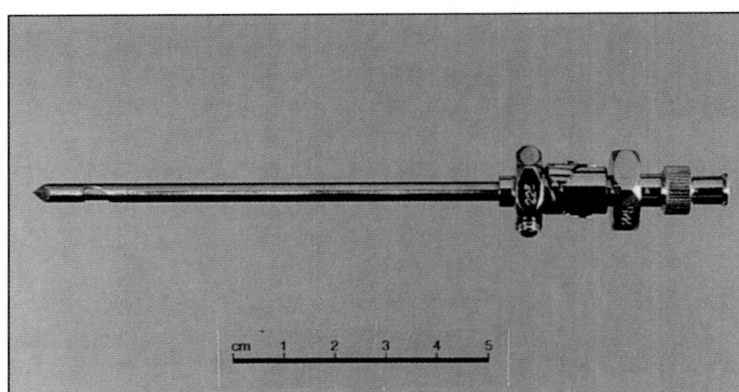

Figure 10.4 Needle assembled showing the ferrule that is rotated to cut the specimen.

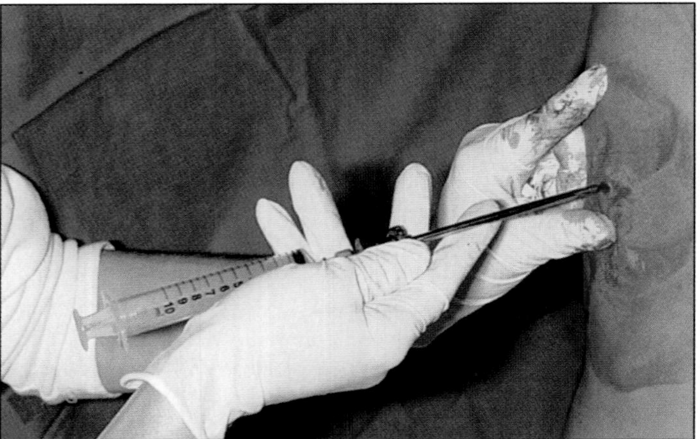

Figure 10.5 Gentle insertion of the closed needle into the pleural cavity. The needle, with aperture closed, should enter the pleural space with only gentle, rotating pressure by the hand of the operator.

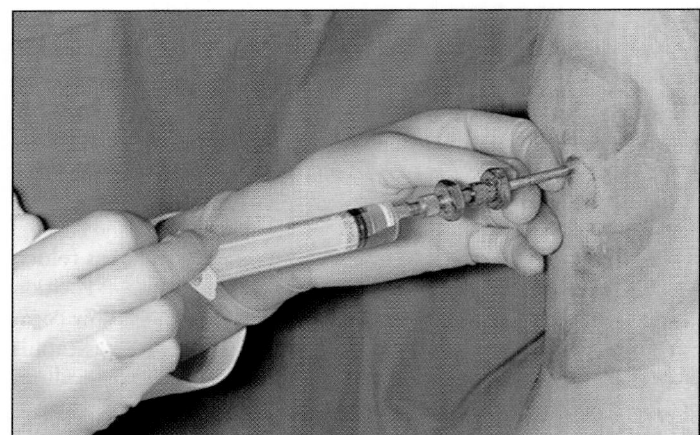

Figure 10.6 Fluid is withdrawn into the syringe with the needle aperture open. A three-way tap system can be added if fluid is to be collected for laboratory testing.

eject them into specimen containers using a three-way tap. After collecting the pleural fluid samples, attach the needle directly to a 20-mL syringe and then tilt it so that the aperture is felt snagging the pleural surface. When lateral pressure is exerted as the needle is slowly pulled back, the pleura is pushed into the aperture (Fig. 10.7). While tension is maintained, twist the ferrule closed (Fig. 10.8) and pull the needle out of the chest cavity sharply. Then, open the needle over either saline or formal saline (saline plus formaldehyde) and squirt the biopsy sample into a container or tease it off with a needle. Perform several biopsies at various clock positions, apart from the positions between 10 PM and 2 AM (to avoid damaging an intercostal nerve or vessel lying in the bed of the rib above). One biopsy sample should be placed into saline for culture for *Mycobacterium tuberculosis* and the others into formal saline.

The Abrams system is relatively easy to use and is recommended as the most effective method of obtaining pleural fluid

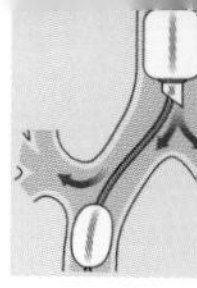

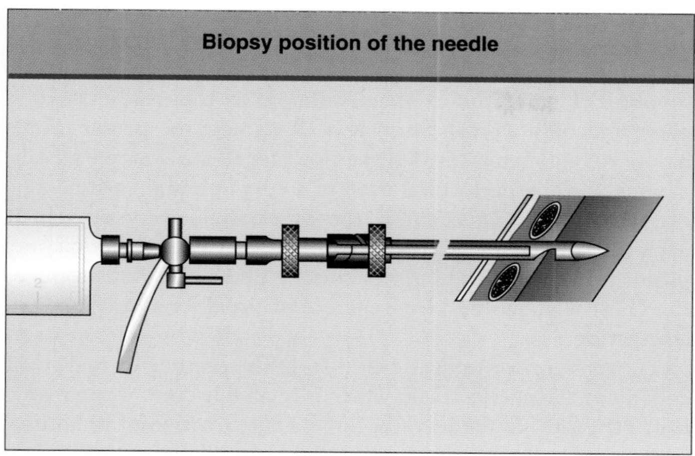

Figure 10.7 Biopsy position of the needle.

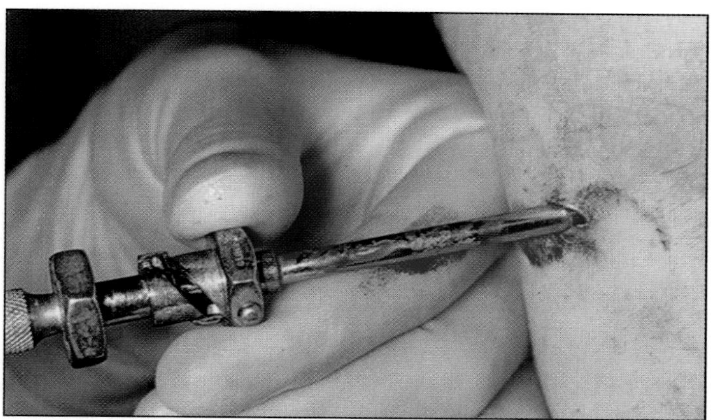

Figure 10.8 Taking a pleural biopsy by rotating the ferrule to close the aperture. Pull the whole apparatus sharply out of the chest.

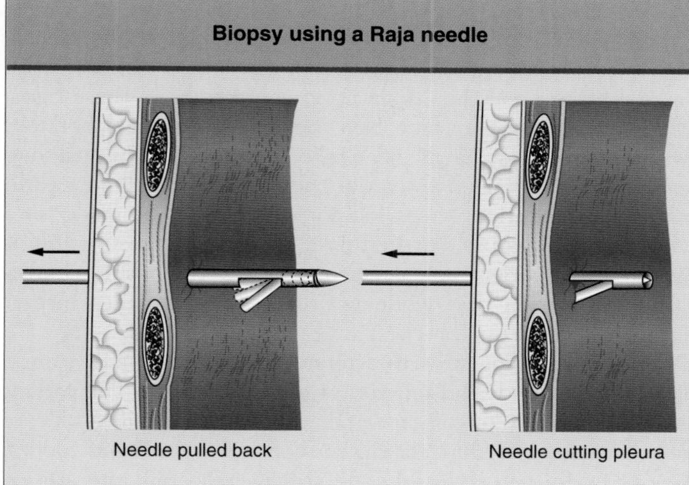

Figure 10.9 Method of biopsy using a Raja needle. The flap impinges on the pleura as the needle is pulled back and cuts off a piece of pleura on closure.

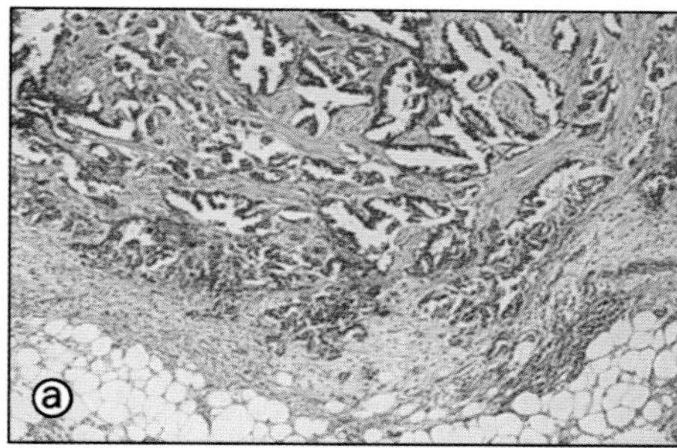

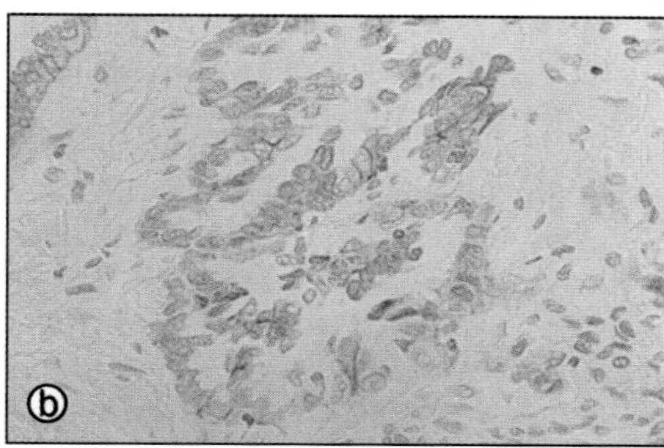

Figure 10.10 Pleural biopsy. Adenocarcinoma **(A)** and AUA1 immunostaining positive for adenocarcinoma **(B)**.

drawn via the needle and three-way tap, as well as for biopsy specimens.

THE RAJA NEEDLE

The Raja needle is a modification of the Abrams system; it has a biopsy flap that opens once the pleural cavity is entered and the inner sheath is pulled back. The flap fixes onto the parietal pleural surface and, when closed, cuts off a piece of pleura (Fig. 10.9). Comparisons with the more readily available Abrams needle have suggested a higher diagnostic yield.

SPECIMEN HANDLING

Always take important biopsy specimens directly to the laboratories. To prevent contamination of the fluid by additional bleeding, remove it for investigation before taking a biopsy. Send the fluid for routine bacterial culture, direct smear and culture for tuberculosis, cytology, and protein and glucose estimation (together with a serum glucose sample). Measurement of pleural fluid amylase and rheumatoid factor should be requested if necessary.

Between four and six biopsies are usually taken and sent in formal saline for histologic examination and in normal saline for culture.

Pleural biopsy is very successful in the identification of tuberculosis, but less so for malignancy (Fig. 10.10). Needle biopsies increase the yield for finding tuberculosis, especially if the biopsy sample is also sent for culture. In malignancy, needle biopsy has a 50% sensitivity compared with pleural fluid cytology but adds a little to the overall yield. Needle biopsy is, however, very useful for mesothelioma, which cannot easily be distinguished from adenocarcinoma in pleural fluid cytology.

CHOICE OF TECHNIQUE

Few studies have compared the different methods for closed pleural biopsy. The Abrams needle remains the most popular, and if an average of five biopsy specimens are taken, the yield (usually tumor or tuberculosis) is 60%. A comparison of the Raja and Abrams needles gives a diagnosis in about 80% and 50% of biopsies, respectively. Comparing the Abrams needle with the

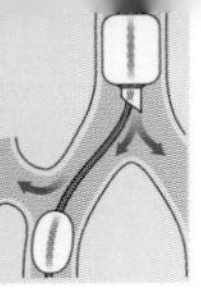

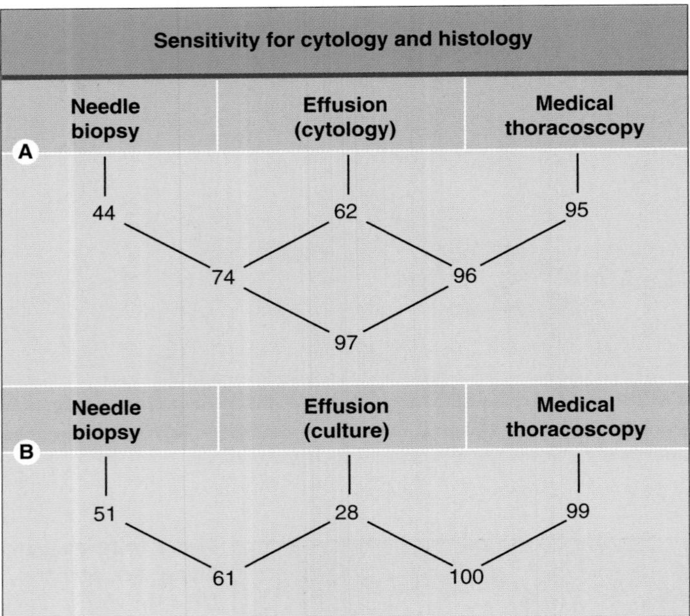

Figure 10.11 Sensitivity (%) for cytology and histology. A, Sensitivity for cytology and histology combined for the different biopsy techniques in 208 malignant pleural effusions. **B,** Sensitivity for cytology and histology in the diagnosis of 100 tuberculous pleural effusions using the different diagnostic techniques. (From Loddenkemper R: Thoracoscopy—state of the art. Eur Respir J 11:213-221, 1998.)

Tru-Cut biopsy needle demonstrates similar results, and use of fiberoptic thoracoscopes for biopsies in general is superior to using the Abrams needle. Rigid thoracoscopy may be even better. A comparison of cytology, closed pleural biopsy, and thoracoscopy for both malignant disease and tuberculosis shows that although the highest diagnostic yield is obtained with thoracoscopy, needle biopsy adds considerably to the number of cases diagnosed on examination of the pleural effusion, making thoracoscopy unnecessary in 74% of malignant and 61% of cases of tuberculosis (Fig. 10.11).

COMPLICATIONS

Very few complications of closed needle biopsy have been reported. Pneumothorax is uncommon, as the needle point is blunt and only a small amount of fluid need be present for a biopsy to be taken. Provided the two pleural surfaces part easily, a biopsy can be performed even in a "dry" pleural cavity.

Hemorrhage can occur if the intercostal artery or vein is damaged by taking a biopsy at the 12-o'clock position and pushing up against the inferior surface of a rib. A hematoma of the chest wall can develop rapidly but usually requires no specific action.

Longer-term complications include the seeding of malignant cells along the needle track, which is relatively common in malignant effusions. Should this occur, a single fraction of radiotherapy controls the developing nodule in most cases.

PITFALLS

In the case of a large pleural effusion, enough fluid should be aspirated both for testing and to make the patient more comfortable. It is becoming common to insert intercostal tubes into large effusions and then drain them completely. In these cases, pleural fluid samples may have been sent to the laboratory without any biopsy having been taken. Although additional fluid can easily be obtained from the chest tube if the fluid examinations are negative, a new incision will have to be made for a closed pleural biopsy. Furthermore, once an intercostal drain is inserted, the patient may need to remain in the hospital in discomfort for some days while awaiting results, and then further interventions across the chest wall may be required.

A preferred course is to aspirate about 1 L of fluid from a large effusion and send samples to the laboratories. The patient may then be able to go home and await results. If all results are negative, the procedure should be repeated and a closed pleural biopsy performed. If results are still negative and there is no systemic or other obvious cause for the effusion, a thoracoscopy should be performed with biopsies taken from the parietal pleura under direct vision. Even this may not provide a diagnosis but, in experienced hands, thoracoscopy adds about 10% to 30% to the overall yield of closed biopsy and cytology diagnoses.

SUGGESTED READINGS

Loddenkemper R, Boutin C. Thoracoscopy: Diagnostic and therapeutic indications. Eur Respir J 6:1544-1555, 1993.

McLeod DT, Ternouth I, Nkanza N: Comparison of the Tru-Cut biopsy needle with the Abrams punch for pleural biopsy. Thorax 44:794-796, 1989.

Mungall IPF, Cowen PN, Cooke NT, et al: Multiple pleural biopsy with the Abrams needle. Thorax 35:600-602, 1980.

Ogirala RG, Agarwal V, Vizioli LD, et al: Comparison of the Raja and the Abrams pleural biopsy needles in patients with pleural effusions. Am Rev Respir Dis 47:1291-1294, 1993.

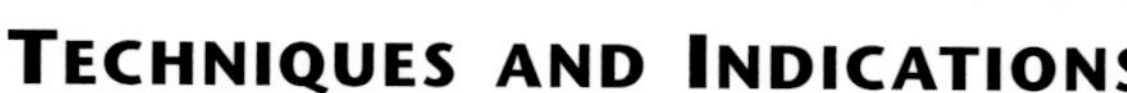

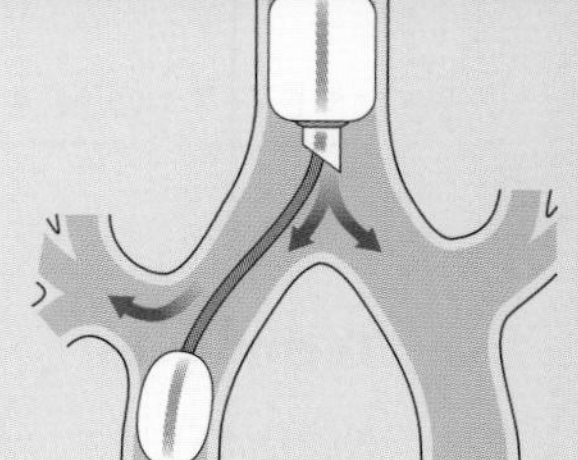

CHAPTER 11 Other Biopsy Procedures

Sacha L. Houghton and Penny J. Shaw

BIOPSY OF INTRAPULMONARY LESIONS

This section describes the equipment and techniques available to obtain diagnostic tissue from predominantly solid lesions within the lung parenchyma. The common lesions and sites biopsied are summarized in Figure 11.1, and the most frequent method of biopsy by site is summarized in Figure 11.2. Adequate tissue samples are obtained by needle, and the technique and its indications are different from those required to diagnose more diffuse intrapulmonary disease. The latter, which includes conditions such as idiopathic pulmonary fibrosis, requires an open lung biopsy via a minithoracotomy or video-assisted thoracoscopy.

Imaging plays an important role in confirming and identifying the site of the lesion, its size, and the quality of the surrounding lung tissue. It is also used to assess the extent of the pathology and the presence of other diseases. The radiologist determines whether the lesion is suitable for transthoracic biopsy and identifies the optimum site for biopsy and under which imaging modality it should be performed. The choice of needle takes into account the patient's safety, whether histology or cytology is required, and personal preference.

Indications and Contraindications

Transthoracic needle biopsy is an established and accepted technique for the diagnosis of malignant masses or nodules, with a sensitivity of 90% to 97%. The technique was previously limited by the low specificity for benign disease, but this has improved with needle placement under computed tomographic (CT) guidance and the use of coaxial transthoracic needle biopsy with an automated cutting needle. The main indication is in cancer patients to establish cell type in inoperable advanced disease with negative sputum cytology and bronchoscopy. It is also widely used when there are solitary or multiple masses with a known extrathoracic malignancy to confirm metastatic disease. During staging of a thoracic malignancy, a contralateral pulmonary nodule or mediastinal, hepatic, or adrenal mass may be discovered. For assessment of operability, it is then of paramount importance to biopsy such lesions. It is also an established technique for confirming a Pancoast tumor. However, biopsy of a solitary mass or nodule is more controversial. If there is a high clinical and radiologic index of suspicion that the lesion is malignant, and the patient is otherwise operable, the patient may go straight to surgery. However, if a solitary mass is thought clinically and radiologically to be benign, a biopsy (preferably a core biopsy) is the next useful step. Fine-needle aspiration (FNA) or biopsy for microorganisms is increasingly being used in the diagnosis of regions of consolidation or masses, especially in immunocompromised patients. Hilar and mediastinal lesions may also be biopsied percutaneously, which may be of particular value as an alternative to transbronchial biopsy, mediastinoscopy, or transesophageal biopsy.

The contraindications are largely relative and are summarized in Table 11.1. Biopsy of a lesion in patients with very poor lung function is possible, provided the lesion lies peripherally and a "safe" route that does not traverse the lung parenchyma is identified (usually with CT). When performing the biopsy, care should be taken to avoid a pneumothorax, which could be life threatening. A coagulation screen is performed if risk factors are present, for example, if the patient has hepatic metastases, has a history of alcohol ingestion, or is taking warfarin or aspirin. A prothrombin time less than 15 to 16 seconds and an international normalized ratio less than 1.4 are acceptable. Some hydatid lesions have been biopsied, but there is still an increased and probably unacceptable risk of an anaphylactic reaction in this group of patients.

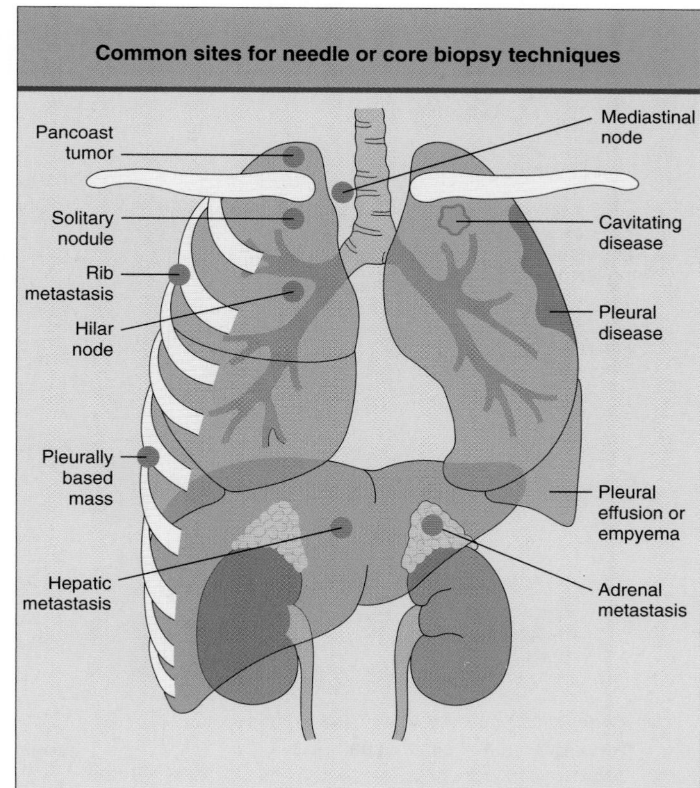

Figure 11.1 Common sites for needle or core biopsy techniques.

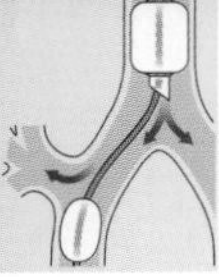

Techniques

NEEDLES

Many different needles are available but are generally either fine needles for aspiration for cytology or cutting needles that produce a core of tissue for histology. Fine needles include the Westcott, Chiba, and Franseen needles and those that have a corkscrew appearance, such as the Rotex needle (Fig. 11.3). They are usually 20- to 23-gauge and provide a specimen for cytology or culture. More flexible, 22-gauge needles can be difficult to position. The Westcott has an added advantage in that small fragments of tissue are frequently obtained in addition to the aspirate, in the small "notch" or slotted opening just proximal to the needle tip. This provides cores for histology in approximately 50% of biopsies.

Aspirates should be obtained only if there is local cytologic expertise available. Ideally, the cytologist attends the biopsy to ensure that an adequate specimen is obtained. Larger cutting needles (18- or 20-gauge) provide a core for histology and have greater rigidity, allowing greater control in placement. Commonly used cutting needles have a spring-loaded mechanism that fires the inner notched stylet and outer cutting cannula when a button is pushed; examples include the Bard Biopty biopsy system (Fig. 11.4) and the Bauer Temno biopsy device (Fig. 11.5). The "gun" or handle of the Bard system is reusable, and the needle is disposable.

Various sizes are available (14-, 18-, or 20-gauge needles), and a core of tissue is consistently produced. The "throw" of the gun is usually 11 or 23 mm, so lesions ideally need to be at least this size. The 23-mm throw produces better cores.

Table 11.1
Contraindications to needle biopsy

Type of contraindication	Comment
Relative	Uncooperative patient: uncontrollable cough inability to lie prone or supine
	Poor lung function/chronic obstructive pulmonary disease (forced expiratory volume in 1 second <1L or multiple bullae)
	Pneumonectomy
	Bleeding disorder
	Pulmonary hypertension
	Very small nodules, less than 5mm diameter
	Hydatid disease (because of the risk of anaphylactic reaction)
Absolute	Arteriovenous malformation with high pulmonary artery pressure

Historically, it has been suggested that cutting needles are associated with a higher complication rate than fine needles. A recent review of UK lung biopsy practice analyzed data from 5444 biopsies and found no difference between the two methods, a conclusion supported by other studies. The pneumothorax rate is related to the number of pleural passes made, which can be reduced by using a coaxial system that has an 18- or 19-gauge, thin-walled introducer needle through which a fine needle can be passed (Fig. 11.6), or by performing a fine-needle core biopsy. Fluid introduced into the pleural space can also be used to provide a safer route in some patients. The choice of

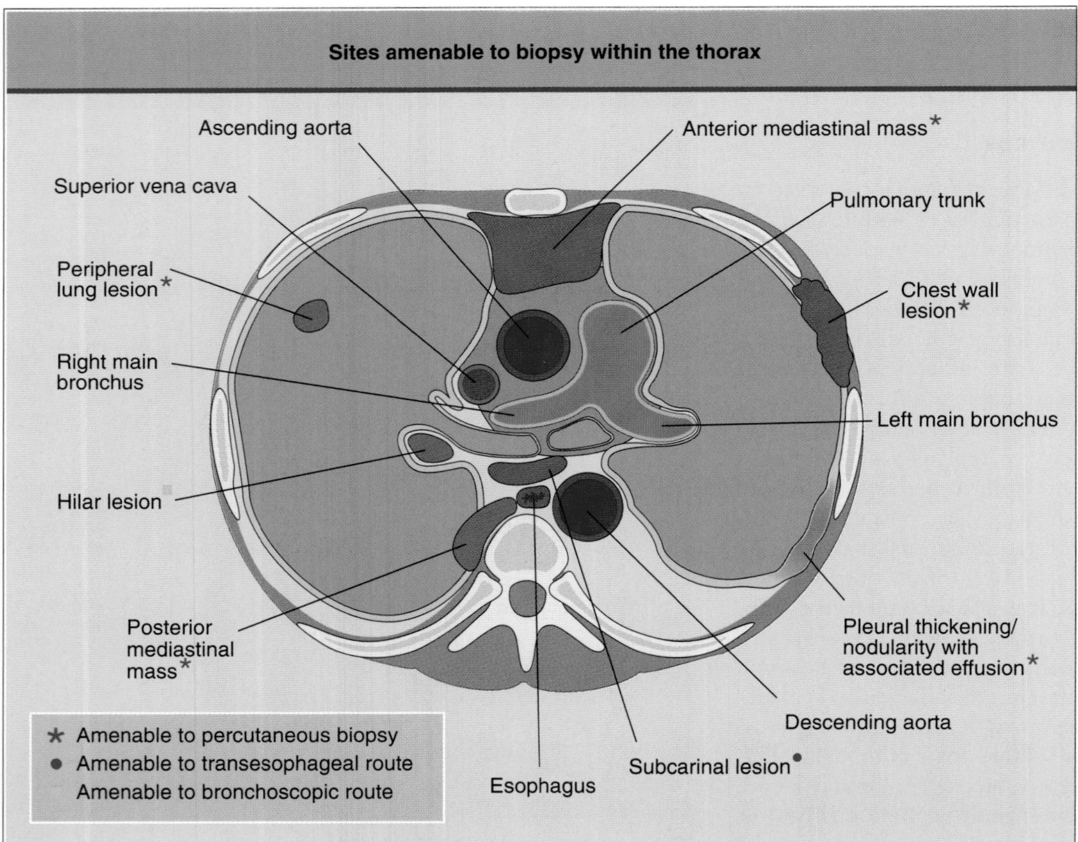

Figure 11.2 Common methods for biopsy according to site.

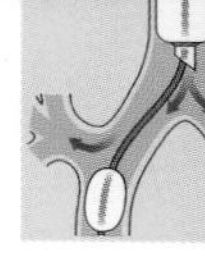

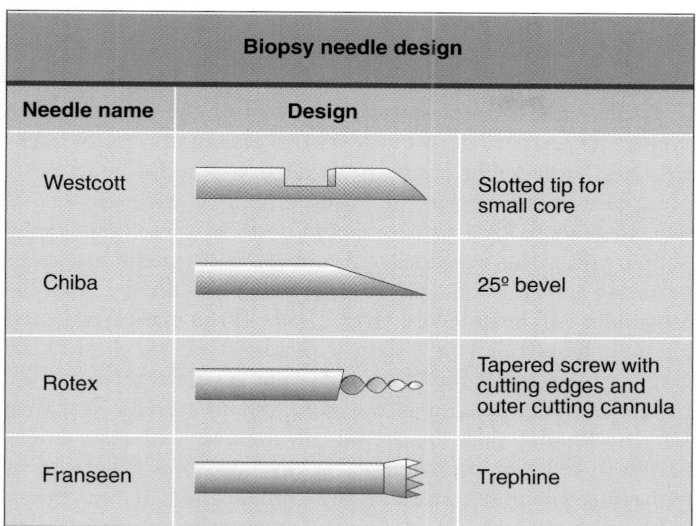

Figure 11.3 Needle tip design.

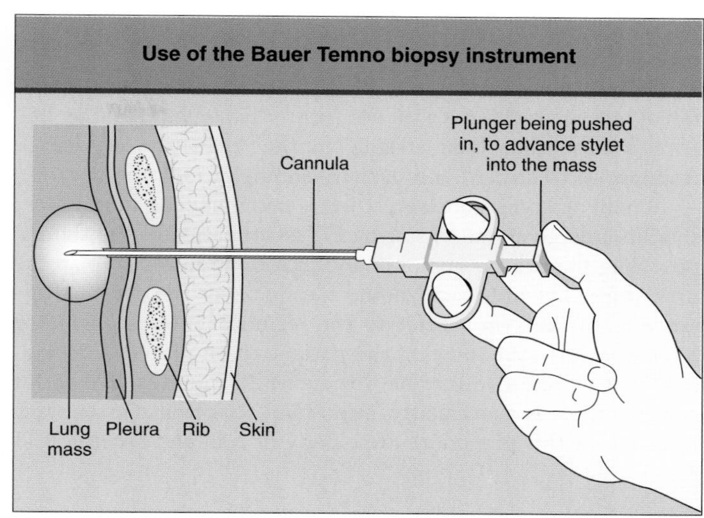

Figure 11.5 Use of the Bauer Temno biopsy instrument. The stylet is positioned within the lesion to be biopsied by pushing the plunger. The advantages are that the instrument requires one hand only, is lightweight, is easy to use under computed tomographic (CT) guidance, and produces a 2-cm core.

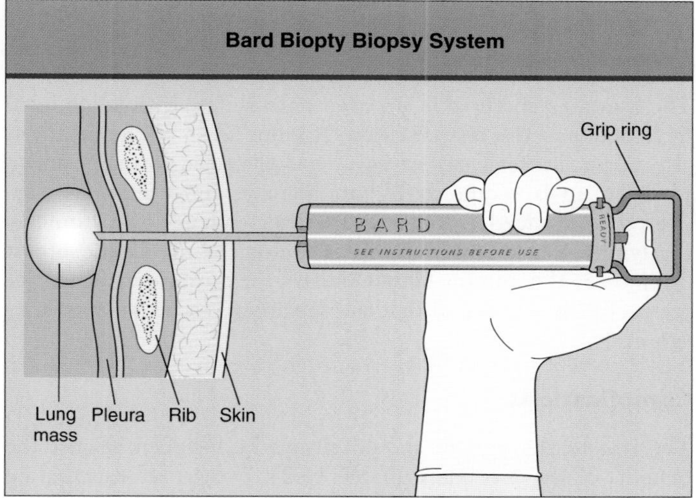

Figure 11.4 The Bard Biopty System. The needle is introduced into the patient so that the tip reaches the area in which biopsy will be performed.

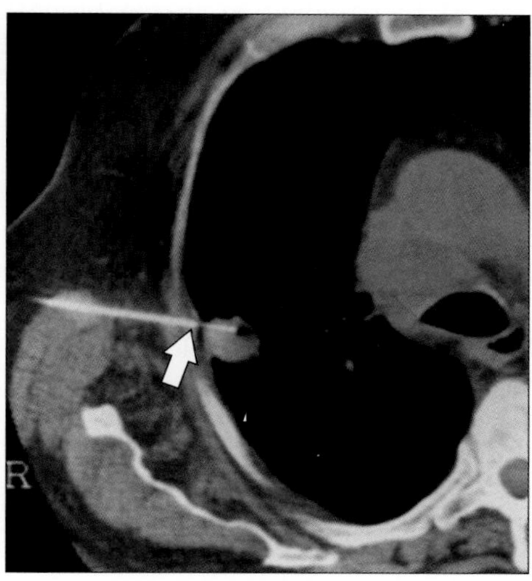

Figure 11.6 Coaxial systems. The arrow marks the distal end of the 18-gauge introducer needle, through which a 20-gauge needle has been passed into the nodule.

needle must primarily take into account the safety of the patient, but the approach and choice of the radiologist are also considerations.

IMAGE GUIDANCE

Fluoroscopy has been superseded by CT as the imaging modality for percutaneous biopsy, allowing precise positioning of the needle within the lesion and avoidance of vascular structures. Ultrasound guidance, used when the lesion is large and pleurally based, has the added advantage of not involving radiation.

Positron-emission tomography (PET) is rapidly becoming an established technique in the evaluation and staging of oncology patients. In lung cancer, it provides information regarding the pulmonary nodule or mass, mediastinal disease, and extrathoracic metastases. The positron emitting agent most frequently used is 18F-fluoro-2-deoxyglucose (FDG). The imaging technique is based on the higher rate of glucose metabolism within neoplastic cells as compared with surrounding normal tissue. FDG accumulates at these regions of increased glycolysis, which are imaged by the PET camera. In recent years the development of PET cameras combined with CT (PET-CT) has allowed more precise anatomic localization of these FDG-avid foci.

Whole-body imaging is usually performed, and the scanning process takes around 60 to 80 minutes. The use of PET in oncology patients both upstages and downstages disease in conjunction with other imaging techniques. It provides valuable information regarding disease activity for the planning of biopsy procedures.

Potential pitfalls in its sensitivity relate to the fact that a sufficient amount of metabolically active tissue is required for a PET diagnosis, making the imaging of lesions smaller than 1 cm unreliable. False-negative results may occur with tumors with relatively low metabolic activity, such as carcinoid tumors. False-positive results are produced by inflammatory conditions such as bacterial pneumonia, abscess, tuberculosis, and active sarcoidosis. These false positives are due to increased granulocyte activity.

Despite these limitations, PET complements other conventional imaging techniques. In the future this technique may find applications other than staging, in the evaluation of disease response to treatment and in the planning of radiotherapy.

A patient being considered for a percutaneous lung biopsy should undergo an initial staging CT examination of the thorax, providing the precise anatomic localization required to plan the procedure. The approach should ideally cover the shortest distance from the skin surface to the region of interest, avoiding fissures, while still allowing the patient to be placed in a position that will be comfortable for about 20 minutes. The latter consideration is particularly important, as often the patients referred for this procedure are elderly or frail and breathless at rest.

PROCEDURE

The patient should be fasted, and informed consent should be taken by the person performing the biopsy. The patient should be informed that after the procedure he or she may have a pneumothorax (possibly requiring a chest drain) or hemoptysis and, as occurs rarely, may need to be admitted to the hospital overnight. The radiologist should explain that more than one pass is usually needed. Sedation may be necessary in fragile or high-risk patients, and intravenous access should be obtained prior to the procedure. An electrocardiograph and pulse oximeter are necessary if sedation is used. With the patient comfortably positioned on the CT table, a short scan covering only the region of interest is performed in inspiration. This acquisition only takes a few seconds on a modern spiral CT scanner.

The exact site of the lesion is determined by correlating the images obtained with the position of the CT table. A mark can then be made on the patient's skin at this precise point, directing the entry point of the needle. The procedure is undertaken under full sterile conditions. Lidocaine (lignocaine) 1% (10 mL) or 2% (5 mL) should be administered, taking care that the lung parenchyma and visceral pleura are not punctured but that the pleura is anesthetized. The patient should be warned that it is not always possible to anesthetize the pleura fully because of the risk of pneumothorax from the anesthetic needle.

A slight "give" occurs when the biopsy needle enters the pleural space. The needle is advanced either in suspended respiration or in small rapid movements during the same phase of gentle respiration to reduce the trauma to the lung parenchyma. Accurate placement of the needle tip is essential and may take time with small nodules. The progression of the needle toward the lesion, and the final position of the tip, are intermittently checked by repeating the initial scan as required. If the lesion is cavitating or has central necrosis, then the specimen must be taken from the periphery. The number of passes will vary, but on average one to three will be required (fewer if the patient is at high risk). The aim is to obtain a diagnosis, but the safety of the patient is paramount. Once the needle is in position, the central stylet is removed and a finger is placed over the hub to prevent air embolism. A syringe is attached, suction applied, and gentle to-and-fro movements are made to obtain an aspirate, aiming the needle in slightly different directions. Pressure is released before the needle is withdrawn, or the specimen will be pulled back into the syringe. Saline (2 to 5 mL) can be injected into and then aspirated from a localized infiltrate to attempt to identify microorganisms. The specimen is dealt with immediately.

If the patient has dyspnea at the end of the procedure, an immediate scan will detect even a small pneumothorax. Sequential chest radiographs are then obtained at 1 and 4 hours post-procedure to ensure that the pneumothorax is not increasing in size. In general, each patient should undergo chest radiography 1 hour after the procedure. About 88% of pneumothoraces requiring intervention will be detected immediately, and the remainder will be detected after 1 hour. If the mass is large and pleurally based, and if the patient remains well, no chest radiograph is required. If the chest x-ray film is satisfactory or if the patient is well with a small but static pneumothorax (less than 30%) at 4 hours, then the patient can go home with instructions to return if he or she becomes symptomatic, as a delayed or expanding pneumothorax is a rare complication. If the patient is symptomatic or has a progressive pneumothorax, observation in the hospital is necessary, and the clinician must decide whether to aspirate or drain the pneumothorax. Hemoptysis is a worrying complication but rarely requires treatment.

Specimen Handling

The aspirated material is smeared onto slides, with some fixed in alcohol and the rest air-dried. A saline wash of the needle is also taken. Larger cores of tissue are placed in formalin unless fresh tissue is required (if lymphoma or infections are suspected). Advanced cytologic procedures such as flow cytometry for lymphoma, estrogen receptor status for metastatic breast carcinoma, and immunocytochemistry for prostate malignancies are useful. It is essential that the specimen reach the laboratory promptly.

Complications

The risk to the patient should always be weighed against the benefits of the procedure (Table 11.2). Deaths after aspiration are rare (1 in 5000 to 10,000 biopsies) and result from cardiac arrest, air embolism, tension pneumothorax, or hemorrhage.

Table 11.2
Complications of needle biopsy

Type	Complication
Early complications	Pneumothorax, 5–50%
	Hemoptysis, 5–10%
	Hemorrhage, 10–40%
	Air embolism, rare
Late complications	Tumor seeding, extremely rare
	Empyema
	Bronchopleural fistula
Increased risk of pneumothorax	If the patient has: • chronic obstructive pulmonary disease/bullae • uncontrollable coughing during the procedure • a difficult small central lesion Or if: • multiple pleural passes are made • fissure is crossed • procedure is prolonged

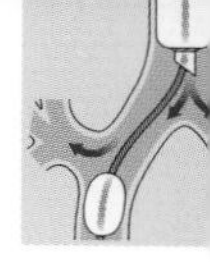

The pneumothorax rate with fine-needle aspirate and cutting needle biopsy is surprisingly similar and lies in the range of 3% to 42%. Patients may experience sharp chest pain as it occurs. Most pneumothoraces are small; however, some require treatment with a chest drain. The frequency of this complication lies in the range of 0% to 17%. Lying the patient with the puncture site dependent can reduce the rate of pneumothorax. Drainage through a one-way valve (Heimlich valve) is useful in emergency situations and also in patients who are recovering, as it allows the patient to remain ambulatory. Aspiration with an 18-gauge catheter attached to a three-way tap also reduces the need for chest tube placement in many patients.

Tension pneumothorax occurs within minutes and is a medical emergency. They are rare but occur in patients with emphysema.

Hemoptysis occurs in around 4%-5% of biopsies. It is more common in patients with pulmonary hypertension and is often preceded by a cough. Hemoptysis usually resolves rapidly and rarely requires treatment, but if it is massive it may be life threatening. Air embolism is rare, but should be considered if the patient breathes deeply and collapses. Coughing at the time of needle insertion suggests this possibility. Needles should always be removed during uncontrollable coughing to reduce the risk of this complication and also the chance of hemorrhage. Treatment includes administration of 100% oxygen, placement of the patient head down in a left lateral decubitus position, and transfer to a hyperbaric unit if available.

Pitfalls and Controversies

The yield in malignant disease is high (sensitivity of 90% to 95%) whether a fine-needle aspirate or cutting needle is used and even if the nodules are small. If no specific diagnosis is made, the biopsy should be repeated. This will enable an additional 5% to 10% of patients with undiagnosed but potentially curable malignancy to be identified.

The technique of fine-needle aspiration has been limited by a low rate of diagnosis of benign disease (sensitivity 20% to 50%), which has been improved (over 70%) by obtaining core biopsies for histology using coaxial systems and cutting needles.

Diagnostic difficulties occur in lesions with a high level of fibrosis, for example, metastatic breast carcinoma and Hodgkin's disease. Excessive mucous production as in bronchoalveolar carcinoma can also interfere with the diagnosis.

Small-needle core biopsies have an improved yield in benign disease, for example, cryptogenic organizing pneumonia, Wegener's granulomatosis, and some infections.

Biopsy of a solitary mass with suspected malignancy in a patient who is potentially operable remains controversial. The argument against performance of a biopsy is that the patient still requires surgery, and, therefore, the management is not altered by the procedure. The advantages are that the patient is better informed and the operation is better planned and faster as frozen sections are avoided.

MEDIASTINAL BIOPSIES

Mediastinal biopsies can be performed via mediastinoscopy; percutaneously if the mediastinal mass abuts the chest wall anteriorly or posteriorly, or with a transesophageal approach for central subcarinal or aortopulmonary nodes.

Techniques

PERCUTANEOUS ROUTE

Aspiration and cutting needles have been used, but core biopsies are usually necessary for primary mediastinal tumors, lymphomas, thymomas, and benign diseases. A safe route that avoids the lung parenchyma must be found (Fig. 11.7). This may involve a transpleural approach through an existing effusion or pneumothorax, or the patient can be positioned in the lateral decubitus position. This causes a slight shift of the mediastinum, and can help avoid the transpulmonary route. An approach through an effusion can be created by injecting saline into the pleural space. These alternative approaches reduce the incidence of complications. Biopsy is preferably carried out under CT guidance, which allows the vascular structures to be more easily identified and avoided.

TRANSESOPHAGEAL ENDOSCOPIC ULTRASOUND

Transesophageal endoscopic ultrasound-guided fine-needle aspiration (EUS-FNA) is a relatively new technique that may be used to sample central mediastinal lymph nodes, for example, nodes in the aortopulmonary, subcarinal, and paraesophageal regions (stations 5, 7, and 8, respectively). Sensitivities of 88% to 96%, specificities of 100%, and accuracies of 94% to 97% have been reported for diagnosis of malignancies by this technique.

Another attraction of EUS is its cost effectiveness. EUS-FNA precludes mediastinoscopy, a more costly procedure, in some patients. The main role of EUS-FNA in the mediastinum is in lung-cancer staging, esophageal cancer, and in the diagnosis of benign causes of lymphadenopathy such as sarcoidosis and tuberculosis. EUS has the capability of sampling nodes as small as 3 mm. Any contraindication to endoscopy is a contraindication to EUS.

The patient should be fasted, and informed consent should be obtained by the operator before the procedure. With the patient under conscious sedation, the endoscope is passed into the esophagus. Initial scanning is performed via a radial endoscopic ultrasound probe, positioned in the tip of the endoscope. This probe provides a 360-degree overview of the mediastinum, in a plane perpendicular to the long axis of the endoscope (Fig. 11.8A). Once an area of interest is identified, the radial probe is withdrawn and replaced with a linear array echoendoscope. This allows full visualization in a plane parallel to the scope and, therefore, a full view of the biopsy path. EUS-FNA is then performed, usually with a 22-gauge needle. The needle is placed into the node (Fig. 11.8B) and moved rapidly back and forth while a withdrawn syringe provides continuous suction. The suction is then released before the needle is withdrawn to prevent contamination of the sample by luminal contents. Structures within 5 cm of the esophageal lumen may be sampled, and, in addition, the left adrenal gland and the left lobe of the liver may be sampled via a transgastric approach. EUS aspiration of pleural fluid may be performed, providing further cytologic samples. Typically the procedure lasts approximately 30 minutes. The patient may be discharged home after a short recovery period.

EUS-FNA of mediastinal nodes is a very safe technique, with no reported complications in recent series from the United

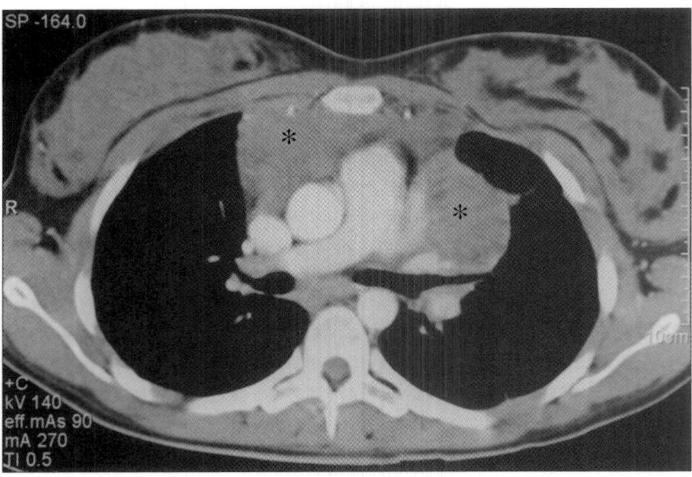

A

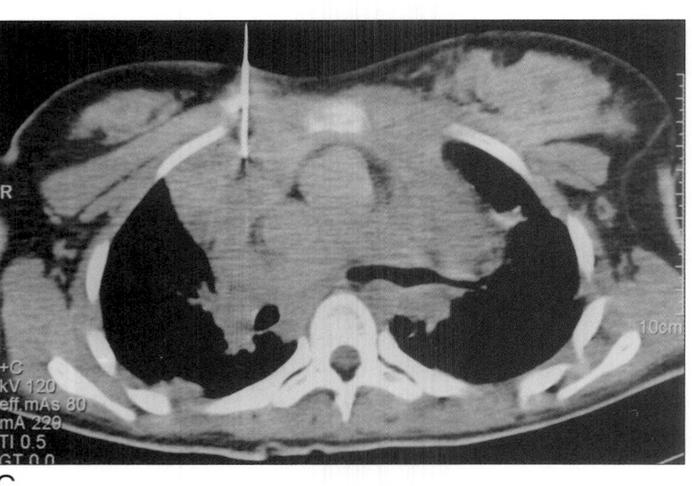

C

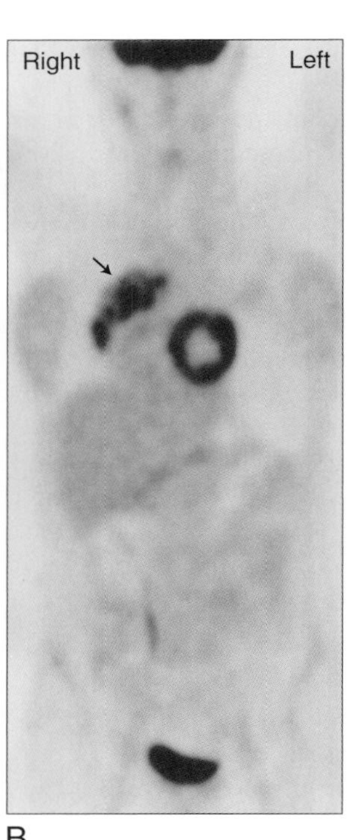

B

Figure 11.7 Mediastinal biopsy. A, Young patient with extensive mediastinal adenopathy following treatment for Hodgkin's disease. Note the right- and left-sided adenopathy *(stars)*. **B,** The PET scan guided the mediastinal biopsy, PET activity was present in the right side of the mediastinal mass *(arrow)*. **C,** Actual biopsy under CT guidance. Recurrent Hodgkin's lymphoma was confirmed.

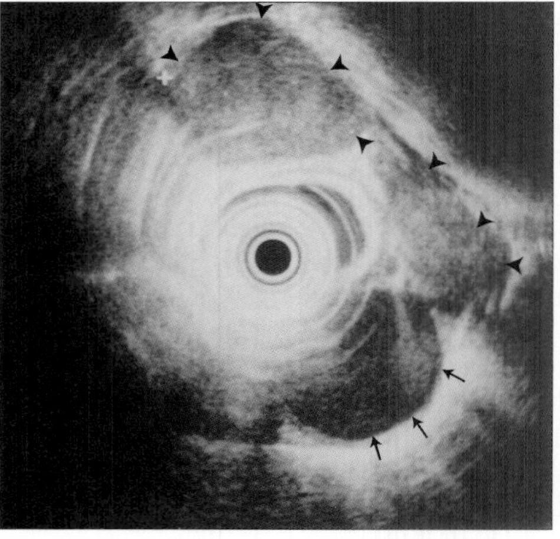

A

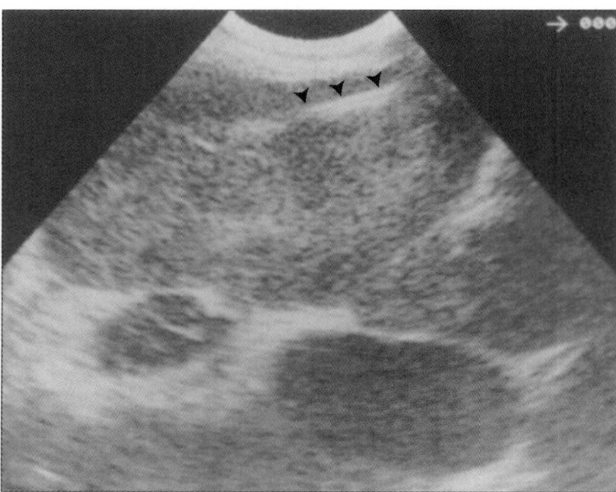

B

Figure 11.8 Endoscopic ultrasound of the mediastinum. A, A 360-degree view of mediastinal lymphadenopathy obtained with a radial probe. The descending aorta is shown by *arrows*. Nodal masses are delineated by *arrowheads*. **B,** The linear probe provides clear visualization of the needle within the lymph node being sampled *(arrowheads)*. A non–small-cell carcinoma was confirmed on cytologic examination. (Courtesy of Dr. Z. Amin, University College London Hospitals.)

States and Europe. Some patients may experience transient chest discomfort.

Granulomatous disease and lymphoma are difficult diagnoses to make based on an FNA sample from any source. In the future, development of a core biopsy needle used via the endoscopic route will resolve this shortcoming. The false-negative rate for EUS is around 13% because of micrometastatic nodal disease or selective involvement of different nodes in the same group. After a negative EUS-FNA, a patient may require more invasive staging techniques if there is a high suspicion of malignant mediastinal involvement.

MEDIASTINAL COLLECTIONS

Aspiration or catheter drainage of mediastinal abscesses secondary to esophageal perforation may be a useful alternative to surgery. It is valuable with advanced collections and in patients unfit for surgery, and it may be lifesaving.

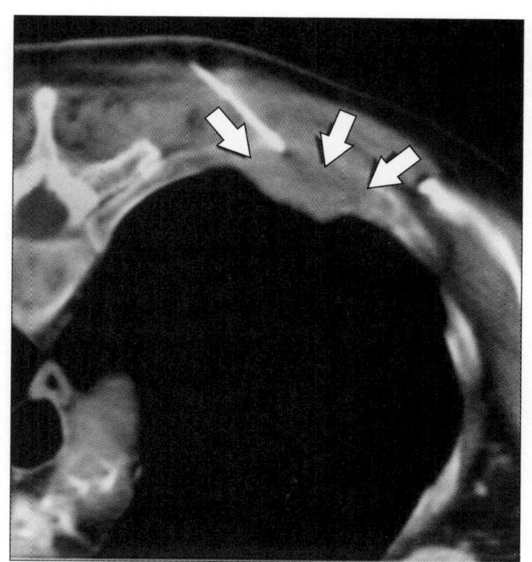

Figure 11.10 Biopsy of a rib metastasis. Non–small-cell carcinoma was confirmed on this "safe" biopsy, performed under computed tomographic (CT) guidance.

PLEURAL AND CHEST WALL BIOPSIES

Pleural and chest wall biopsies are performed under ultrasound (Fig. 11.9) or CT guidance (Fig. 11.10). Core biopsies are essential for peripheral masses to differentiate mesothelioma from metastatic adenocarcinoma. Usually at least three cores are desirable. If the pleura is not very thickened, multiple passes may be necessary. The optimum route is one that runs along the main axis of the pathology, allowing more of the lesion to be sampled but with less risk of a pneumothorax (Fig. 11.11). Radiologists favor the 18-gauge Bard Biopty biopsy system or Temno cutting needles over the Abrams needle. Specimens should be sent for microbiologic as well as histologic examination, including tests for acid-fast bacilli. Fresh specimens may be useful if a lymphoma is suspected.

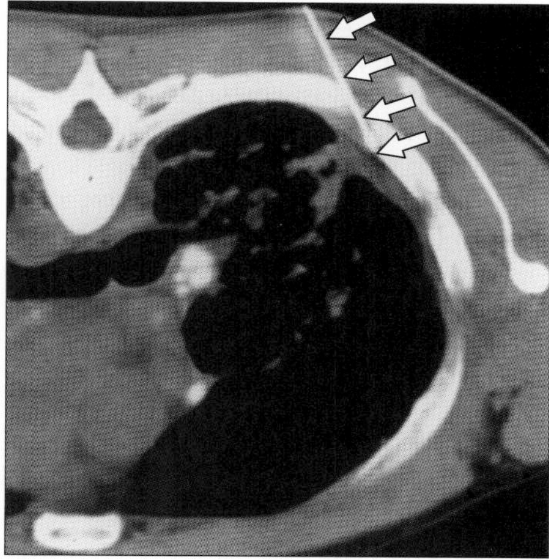

Figure 11.11 Oblique route of biopsy under computed tomographic (CT) guidance. Granulomatous disease was confirmed with a Biopty gun biopsy without complications.

EXTRATHORACIC BIOPSY

Lesions may be identified in the liver, adrenal glands, or ribs during the staging of patients with bronchogenic carcinoma. If appearances suggest metastases, it is essential to perform a biopsy to confirm inoperability. Biopsies of hepatic lesions are preferably performed under ultrasound guidance, where they are easily imaged and biopsy is rapid. Biopsies of adrenal lesions are usually performed under CT guidance (Fig. 11.12). It may be necessary even then to traverse the hepatic or pulmonary parenchyma to enter the adrenal mass. If the mass is on the side opposite the primary carcinoma, the pulmonary parenchymal route should be avoided, as a pneumothorax could delay surgery. A coaxial system is useful, as several aspirates or cores can be obtained with a single pass of the introducer needle.

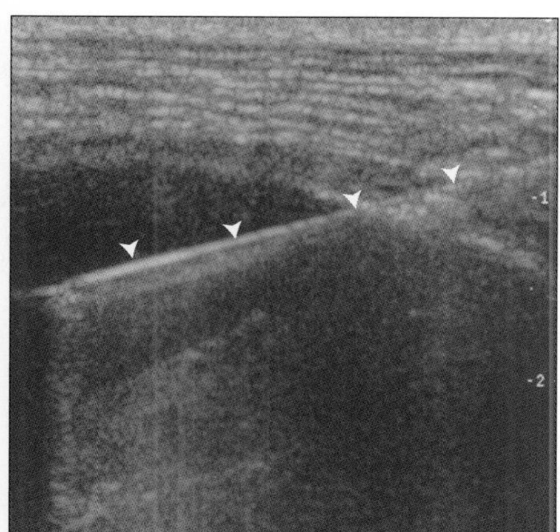

Figure 11.9 Ultrasound-guided pleural biopsy. The needle *(arrowheads)* passes through the chest wall across the pleura in the presence of a large pleural effusion.

PLEURAL DRAINAGE

The most common indications are a malignant effusion or an empyema. Of patients with a community-acquired pneumonia, 40% develop a parapneumonic effusion. The majority of such cases resolve spontaneously, but the effusion can progress to form an empyema. Early and rapid drainage of an empyema is essential to prevent fibrin deposition, which leads to pleural fibrosis and possibly a restrictive defect. An esophageal rupture or endobronchial lesion should always be considered in a patient with an empyema without an obvious predisposing cause.

Indications and Contraindications

A pleural effusion can be tapped for diagnostic purposes, and a pleural biopsy may be usefully performed at the same time. A

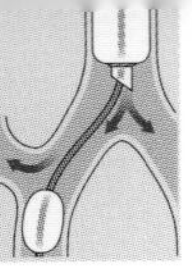

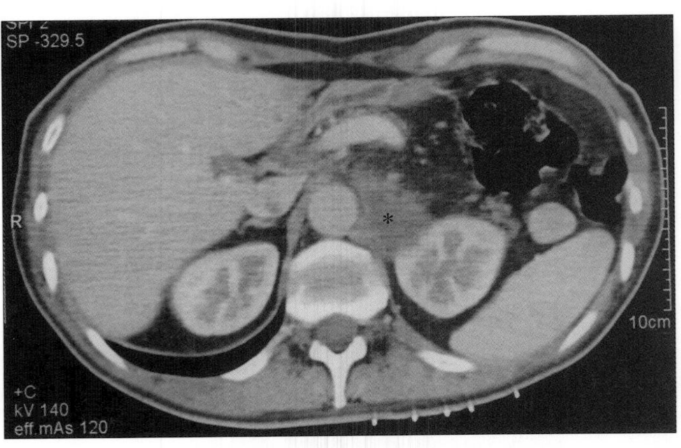

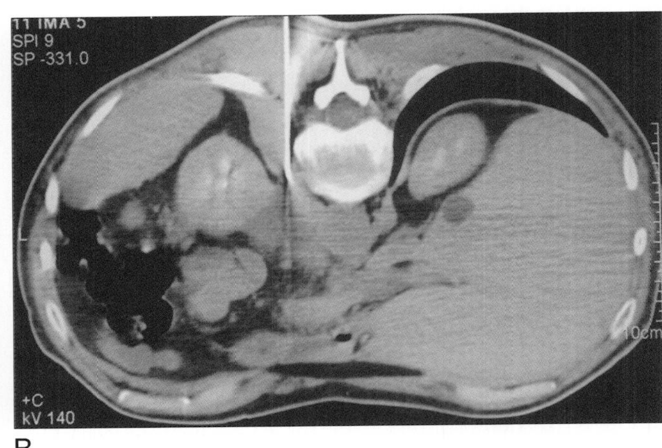

A B

Figure 11.12 Biopsy of an adrenal metastasis under computed tomographic (CT) guidance. A, Irregular left adrenal mass *(star)* anterior to the left kidney. **B,** Needle tip in adrenal mass with the patient prone. Inoperability due to this extrathoracic metastasis was confirmed.

pleural effusion can be drained for therapeutic purposes if it is large and the patient is symptomatic (usually with a malignant effusion); if it is infected or is an empyema (if the glucose is low, or the pH is less than 7.2); or if a hemothorax is present (usually after trauma). A bleeding disorder is a relative contraindication, predisposing to hematoma formation.

Technique

IMAGE GUIDANCE

Ultrasound is the easiest and quickest way to confirm the presence of pleural fluid and also indicates its volume. Echogenic fluid is almost diagnostic of an empyema. Ultrasound also demonstrates the presence of septae and multiple locules, which may hinder drainage and necessitate the use of multiple drainage tubes or intrapleural streptokinase.

CT has an advantage in evaluating any underlying lung or mediastinal pathology. In empyemas, the pleura is characteristically smooth and diffusely thickened and is enhanced after intravenous contrast injection.

PROCEDURE

A large effusion can be drained without image guidance, but smaller or multiloculated effusions are better drained under ultrasound or CT guidance. The patient sits down and leans forward, "hugging" a pillow against the chest to bring the arms forward and clear the scapulae from the back. A small stool under the feet makes the patient feel more comfortable, and the optimum skin position is marked. A sterile technique with local anesthetic is again used. The size of the catheter used varies among small, pigtail catheters or larger catheters for empyemas.

The depth of the effusion can be judged by both ultrasound and using the local anesthetic needle. The catheter can be positioned by means of a cannula and guidewire technique or via a single-step procedure. The latter is more commonly used. The catheter contains an introducing central stylet. Both catheter and stylet are simultaneously advanced into the pleural space. Once it has been entered, the catheter is advanced into the effusion while the central stylet is simultaneously withdrawn. The catheter is connected rapidly to a drainage bag with a three-way tap. Samples for cytologic, microbiologic, and chemical analysis can be taken. If drainage is for a short time (24 to 48 hours), a bag will normally suffice. If drainage is required for a longer duration (normal with empyemas) or if the effusion is large—presumably because of active fluid production—the catheter is connected to an underwater drainage system.

If aspiration is undertaken, no more than 1.5 L of fluid should be removed at one time because of the risk of pulmonary edema. Larger catheters can be used, but smaller catheters are usually adequate and more comfortable for the patient. The catheters should be securely fastened to the skin, and regular saline irrigation should be performed to maintain patency (20 mL of saline every 4 to 6 hours). Fibrinolytics (e.g., streptokinase) given early for treatment of empyemas may increase drainage with faster radiographic improvement.

Pleural fluid is sent for cytologic, microbiologic, and chemical analysis.

Complications

Complications are few, provided no bleeding disorder is present. Pneumothorax occurs in less than 5% of cases. Puncture of other viscera can be avoided by inserting the catheter under ultrasound guidance and using blunt dissection through the chest wall to avoid traumatizing the catheter. Pain may occur at the site of insertion, but this is eased by inserting the catheter laterally for patient comfort. Reactions to streptokinase are much fewer when the purified form is used, but previously have included anaphylaxis and bleeding, both intrapleurally and systemically, with larger doses.

Pitfalls and Controversies

Both chest physicians and radiologists insert catheters for pleural drainage. For multiloculated, multiple, or small collections, the procedure is performed under image guidance by a radiologist. The routine use of intrapleural streptokinase still has not been widely adopted because of the expense and the complications associated with the use of the less purified form, the occasional occurrence of large hemorrhages, and the use of larger doses. Its efficacy in the overall management of empyemas remains uncertain (see Chapter 23).

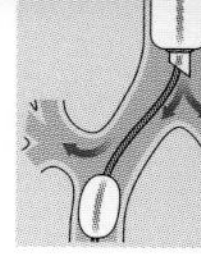

SUGGESTED READINGS

Arakawa H, Nakajima Y, Kurihara Y, et al: CT-guided transthoracic needle biopsy: A comparison between automated biopsy gun and fine needle aspiration. Clin Radiol 51:503-506, 1996.

Davies RJ, Traill ZC, Gleeson FV: Randomised controlled trial of intrapleural streptokinase in community acquired pleural infection. Thorax 52:416-421, 1997.

Fickling W, Wallace MB: Endoscopic ultrasound and lung cancer. American Society for Gastrointestinal Endoscopy. 56(Suppl. 4):518-521, 2002.

Lacasse Y, Wong E, Guyatt G, Cook D: Transthoracic needle aspiration biopsy for the diagnosis of localised pulmonary lesions: A meta-analysis. Thorax 54:884-893, 1999.

Lucidarme O, Howarth N, Finet J-F, Grenier PA: Intrapulmonary lesions: Percutaneous automated biopsy with a detachable, 18-gauge, co-axial cutting needle. Radiology 207:759-765, 1998.

Perlmutt LM, Braun SD, Newman GE, et al: Timing of chest film follow-up after transthoracic needle aspiration. AJR Am J Roentgenol 146:1049-1050, 1986.

Proptas Z, Westcott JL: Transthoracic needle biopsy of mediastinal lymph nodes for staging lung and other cancers. Radiology 199:489-496, 1996.

Richardson CM, Pointon KS, Manhire AR, Macfarlane JT. Percutaneous lung biopsies: A survey of UK practice based on 5444 biopsies. BJR 75:731-735, 2002.

Vansteenkiste JF: Imaging in lung cancer: Positron emission tomography scan. Eur Respir J 19(suppl 35):49s-60s, 2002.

Westcott JL, Rao N, Colley DP: Transthoracic needle biopsy of small pulmonary nodules. Radiology 202:97-103, 1997.

Westcott JL: Percutaneous transthoracic needle biopsy. Radiology 169:593-601, 1988.

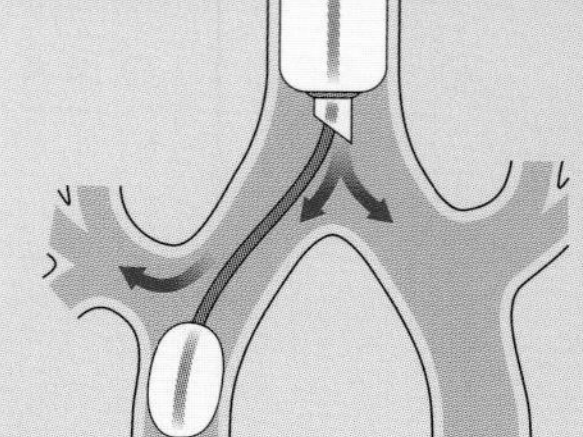

CHAPTER 12 Chest Tube Insertion and Management

Stephen D. Cassivi and Claude Deschamps

The pleural cavity can require drainage when, in pathologic states, it contains air (pneumothorax), blood (hemothorax), serum (pleural effusion), lymph (chylothorax), pus (empyema), or a combination of these. In the presence of these abnormal collections, the pleural cavity pressure may become positive, which allows the lung to collapse partially or fully, leading to hypoxemia. The most common procedure used to drain air or fluid collections is the insertion of a tube thoracostomy (chest tube). Optimally, this provides for drainage of air or fluid, allows the lung to re-expand, and re-establishes a negative intrapleural pressure. Correct use of a chest tube requires the skill to insert it safely and position it well, with minimal discomfort to the patient, as well as the judgment to know when it is indicated and how to manage it properly after insertion. This implies a sound knowledge of the principles of surgical drains and a working knowledge of the underwater seal drainage system being used.

INDICATIONS AND CONTRAINDICATIONS

Situations of acute or severe respiratory compromise are considered absolute indications for chest tube placement and include tension pneumothorax, large symptomatic pneumothorax, hemothorax, empyema, and surgical violation of the pleural space (Table 12.1). In other situations, appropriate judgment and experience are required to determine whether a chest tube is needed. Alternatives to chest tube placement, such as observation, thoracentesis, or formal operative drainage, must be considered and individualized, depending on the situation. Special caution is necessary when there is a possibility of coagulopathy, intrapleural adhesions, or abnormal intrathoracic anatomy. The only contraindications to chest tube placement are a fused pleural space or inadequate experience to perform the procedure safely and effectively. Both these circumstances should prompt a thoracic surgical consultation.

TECHNIQUE

The technique of chest tube insertion has been described in many publications. A focused, yet comprehensive history and physical examination should precede any surgical procedure, even when it is done at the bedside. Chest radiographs and computed tomograms, if available, should be thoroughly reviewed beforehand and should be readily available during the procedure. When possible, a full discussion with the patient, including the indications, risks, and postprocedure care, is required before insertion of a pleural drain.

Tube Selection

Currently, the most common tube used for chest drainage is a Silastic tube with multiple side holes. It usually has a linear radiopaque stripe running through the most proximal hole (allowing its location to be identified on chest radiographs) and markings to indicate distance in centimeters from the most proximal hole (Fig. 12.1). These tubes range in size up to 40 French. It should be noted that some tube insertion kits come with a central trocar within the chest tube. Routine use of this trocar is unnecessary, can be dangerous, and is discouraged.

The size of the drain depends on the indication for insertion and the size of the patient. In general, larger drains are more uncomfortable and more difficult to insert using local anesthesia. Conversely, smaller tubes are usually better tolerated but are more likely to clog with thick fluid or particulate matter, such as that encountered in a hemothorax or empyema. Smaller chest drains are also more prone to drainage problems due to kinking of the tubing. Most collections can be adequately drained using a 28 or 32 French chest tube. Usually, a simple pneumothorax requires only a 24 French chest tube.

Recently, in some North American institutions, a 19 French fluted, Silastic Blake drain has been used for standard postoperative drainage. It is smaller, less rigid, easily inserted, and better tolerated than the more conventional chest tube. It seems to be just as effective in uncomplicated postoperative situations but has the distinct disadvantage of being 10 times as expensive as its conventional counterpart.

Drain Insertion Site and Patient Positioning

Generally, the optimal site for placement of a chest tube is through the fourth or fifth interspace in the anterior to midaxillary line, just beyond the lateral edge of the pectoral muscle and breast tissue (Fig. 12.2). This insertion site has the advantage of relatively easy access, and it avoids the discomfort of a more posteriorly placed tube in patients who are often lying supine in a hospital bed. It is also usually high enough to avoid subdiaphragmatic placement yet low enough to adequately drain fluid. It should be noted that in patients who are lying supine in bed with free-flowing pleural fluid collections, the interspace level of placement is much less important than the posterior positioning of the tube within the pleural space. Placement of a chest tube in the second or third interspace anteriorly is to be avoided in most cases. It does not provide any advantage over the lateral position and is significantly more painful and disfiguring for the patient.

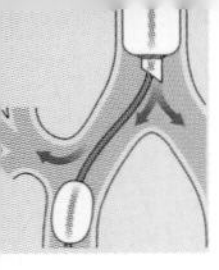

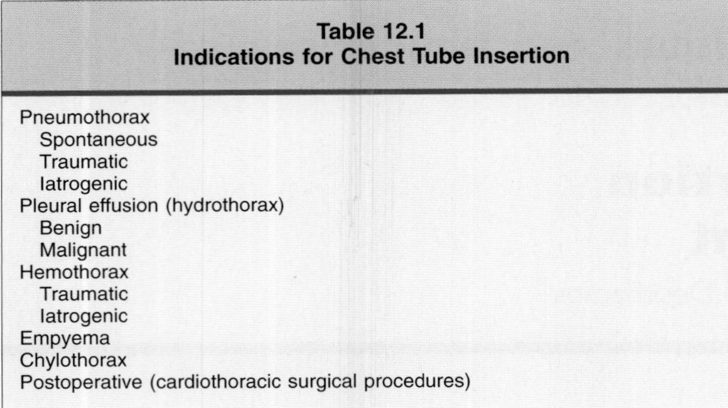

Table 12.1
Indications for Chest Tube Insertion

Pneumothorax
- Spontaneous
- Traumatic
- Iatrogenic

Pleural effusion (hydrothorax)
- Benign
- Malignant

Hemothorax
- Traumatic
- Iatrogenic

Empyema
Chylothorax
Postoperative (cardiothoracic surgical procedures)

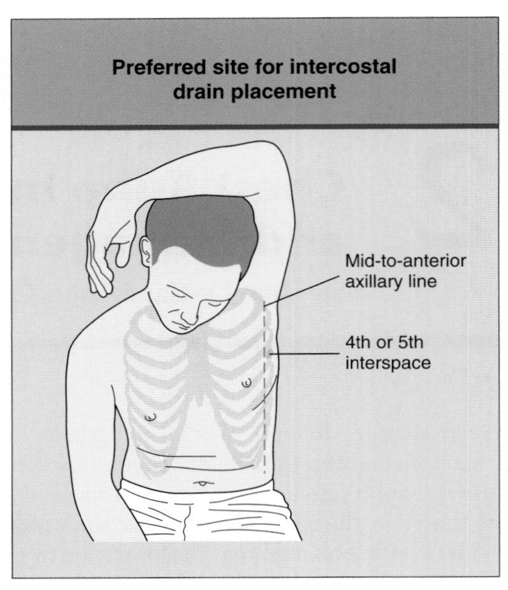

Figure 12.2 Preferred site for intercostal drain placement—mid-to-anterior axillary line, fourth or fifth interspace.

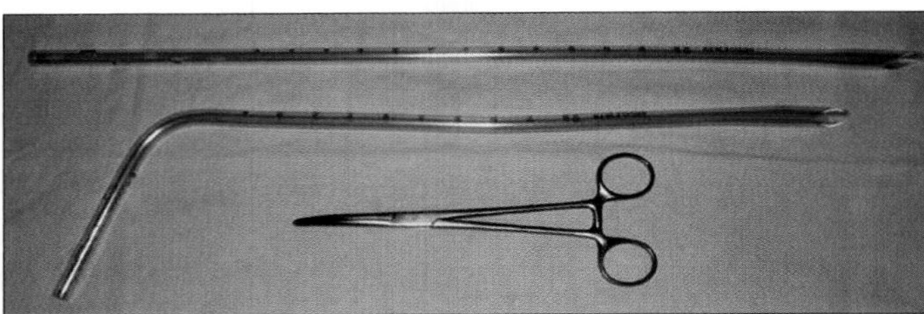

Figure 12.1 Silastic chest tubes. Multiholed straight and angled Silastic chest tubes and a Kelly clamp.

For elective chest drain insertion, the patient should be kept in a relatively comfortable position that facilitates tube placement in the location described previously. Usually, this can be achieved by placing the patient in the supine or semi-Fowler position (thorax and head elevated 30 to 45 degrees), with the involved side elevated approximately 30 to 45 degrees on wedges or pillows. To improve access to the lateral chest wall, the patient's arm on the involved side is brought above the head (Fig. 12.3). As with most thoracic procedures, the operator should stand at the patient's back.

Preparation, Anesthesia, and Incision

Before positioning the patient, all necessary equipment should be made available (Table 12.2). The chest wall is cleaned with antiseptic solution and draped in such a way as to provide an operative field of approximately 20 × 20 cm. The skin is infiltrated with 1% lidocaine at the chosen site of insertion using a 21-gauge needle. Further generous infiltration of the subcutaneous tissues can be done with a large-bore (18-gauge) needle. Aspirating before injecting with this needle prevents inadvertent vascular injection and indicates the direction and depth of the parietal pleura. The parietal pleura is extremely sensitive and therefore must be thoroughly anesthetized.

A 2-cm transverse incision is made using the scalpel. The incision is usually made one interspace below the interspace planned for insertion to allow "tunneling" over the superior border of the lower rib. At this stage, an O silk stitch can be placed at the

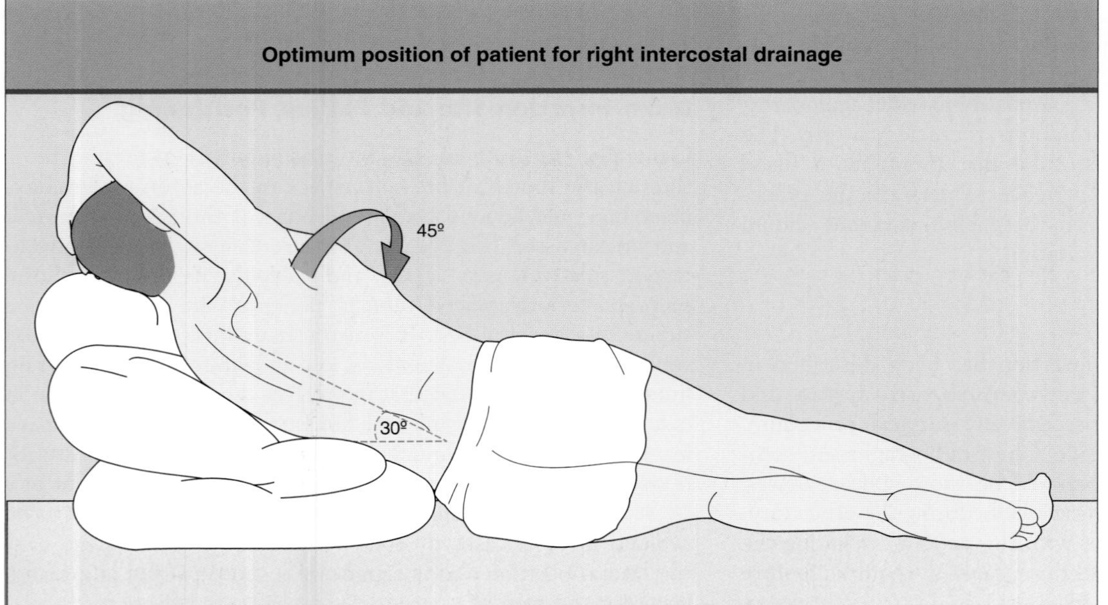

Figure 12.3 Patient positioned for right intercostal drainage. The head and trunk are elevated on pillows to a 30-degree angle, and the body is rotated by 45 degrees.

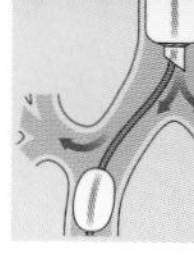

Table 12.2
Equipment required for chest tube insertion

Sterile gloves and gown
Antiseptic solution with swab applicators
Sterile drapes or towels
20-mL syringe
21-gauge needle
18-gauge needle
1% lidocaine
Scalpel with blade
Needle driver
O silk stitch (cutting needle)
Kelly clamp
Chest tube
Underwater seal chest drainage system
Gauze and dressing material

posterior margin of the incision and tied down, leaving the two ends even and uncut. This will be used later to secure the chest tube. Placing the stitch at this point, before initial dissection and entry into the pleural space, with its requisite drainage of fluid or air, is much easier. It allows a more efficient securing of the chest tube once it has been positioned in the pleural cavity. In an obese patient, it may be necessary to increase the size of the initial skin incision to permit adequate palpation of the ribs and interspaces.

Drain Insertion

Following the incision and placement of the securing stitch, a curved Kelly clamp is used to dissect a track for the chest tube within the subcutaneous and intercostal tissues. "Tunneling" of this track over the superior border of the lower rib prevents damage to the intercostal neurovascular bundle that resides along the inferior border of each rib. It also reduces the likelihood of air leakage at the time of chest tube removal and thereafter while the incision site heals.

Dissection using the Kelly clamp is done with incremental spreading and advancement of the clamp to create a track for the chest tube. It is important to dissect along only one track; this will avoid difficulties in finding the dissected path at the moment of tube insertion. This is especially relevant in obese patients. The pleura can be very taut or thick and sometimes presents a significant resistance to entry. Extreme care must be taken when entering the pleural cavity with the Kelly clamp to control its forward progress and prevent inadvertent entry into underlying structures. Entry into the pleural cavity is signaled by egress of air or fluid and a sudden decrease in resistance to the clamp's moving forward. For the patient, breaching of the parietal pleura is usually the most uncomfortable part of the procedure, and it is often useful to use more local anesthetic in the area before piercing the pleural cavity.

Once the parietal pleura has been breached, the clamp is withdrawn in the open position. The next step is to insert the index finger into the pleural cavity to ensure pleural entry (and exclude subdiaphragmatic placement) and assess for the presence of pleural adhesions and pleural lesions or nodularity (Fig. 12.4). The chest tube can then be guided into place using the Kelly clamp (Fig. 12.5). This is an important part of the procedure, but it is often rushed because of patient discomfort or

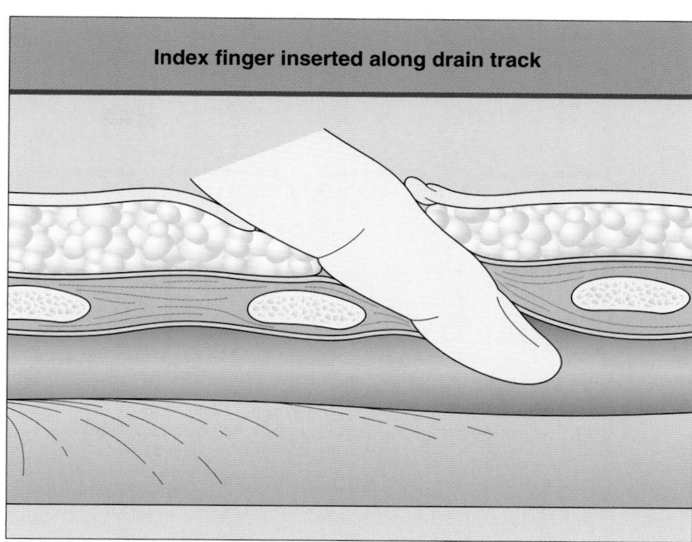

Figure 12.4 An index finger is inserted along the drain track to exclude adhesions and confirm entry into the chest cavity. Note that the track has been created in the interspace over the upper surface of the rib.

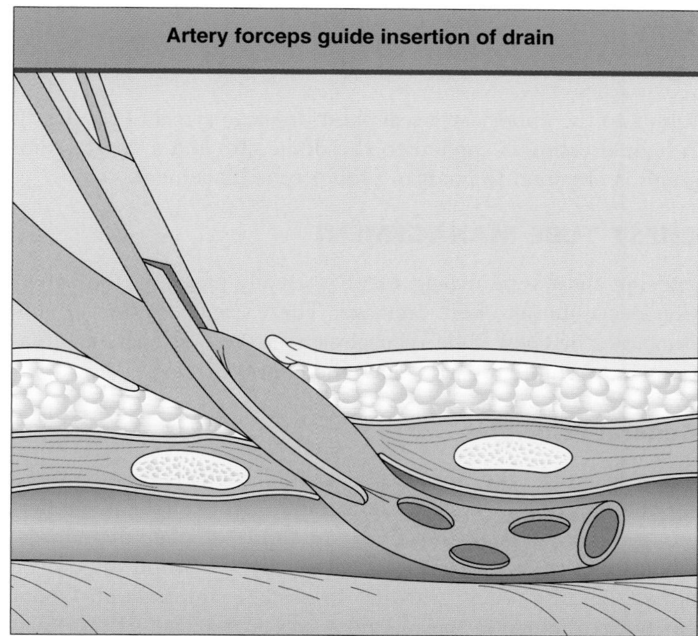

Figure 12.5 Use of a Kelly clamp to guide drain insertion.

ongoing fluid or air leakage. Proper functioning of the tube requires that care be taken at this point to deliberately direct the tube in the desired position. In the most common scenario—that is, a patient who will be mostly supine—the tube should be guided posteriorly and then directed cephalad. A tube positioned in this fashion will drain both air and fluid satisfactorily in the vast majority of cases. To ensure a posterior placement of the drain, once the tube is in the pleural cavity, its tip must be deliberately directed posteriorly before it is advanced. Failure to do this often leads to a poorly functioning tube positioned anteriorly or within the major fissure.

Once the chest tube is positioned correctly, it can be secured in place with the previously placed suture and connected by

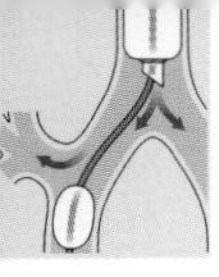

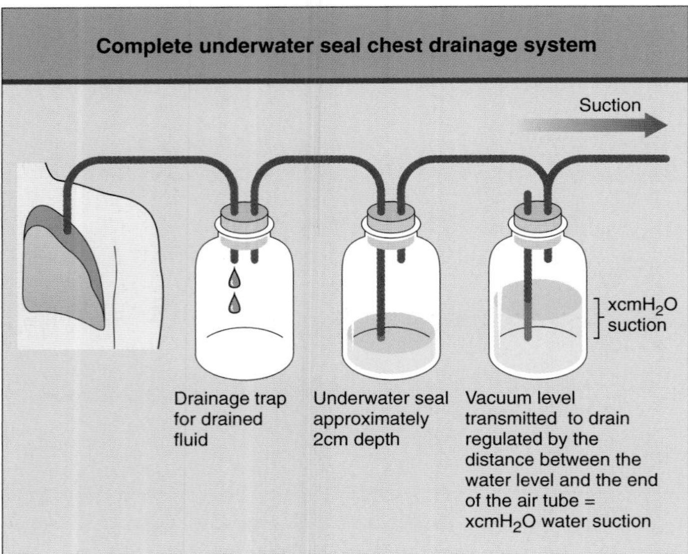

Figure 12.6 Complete underwater seal chest drainage system. In the most basic form, both the trap and vacuum regulation chambers are omitted. The latter is clearly irrelevant if suction is not applied. Commercial drain assemblies can incorporate all three chambers in one casing and may include a manometer to measure the intrapleural pressure.

tubing to the underwater seal chest drainage system (Fig. 12.6). A light dressing is applied to the drain site, and a chest radiograph is obtained to confirm proper tube placement.

CHEST TUBE MANAGEMENT

Specific chest tube management is usually based on the condition necessitating chest drainage. There are, however, general principles of chest tube management as well as specific situations that require a particular remedy or response.

General Principles

Once inserted, the chest tube should be closely monitored for the nature (air, fluid, or both) and quantity (slight, moderate, or large air leak or volume of fluid) of pleural drainage. Changes in these parameters, especially if abrupt, should be noted because they provide important information about current pathology in the pleural space or drainage system malfunction. The amount of fluid drained per 8-hour period should be recorded.

Suction is usually applied to the underwater seal device initially after tube placement to promote drainage and a negative intrapleural pressure. The amount of suction applied is usually −20 cm of water. It should be emphasized that suction is provided via the underwater seal device and never directly to the chest tube; the former is controlled, whereas the latter may lead to pulmonary or vascular injury. Suction can usually be discontinued and the patient left on "water seal" early in the course of chest tube management if drainage is adequate and the pleural process is resolving. There are certain circumstances in which chest tube suction should be avoided. This is the case if a chest tube is placed following a pneumonectomy or in patients with emphysema and a prominent air leak, such as those undergoing lung volume reduction surgery.

There are a number of observable clues to the functional status of the chest tube and the current status of the pleural space. Oscillation or "tidaling" of the fluid level in the water seal or in the tubing leading to the water seal device demonstrates, when it is synchronous with the patient's respiratory cycle, that the chest drain is patent and communicating with the pleural space. It also indicates that the lung has not completely re-expanded to fill the entire pleural space. Allowing fluid to pool in dependent portions of the tubing connecting the chest drain to the underwater seal device should be avoided. This condition creates an increased resistance to proper drainage of air and will delay resolution of the intrapleural process. This can be avoided by educating the nursing staff to this potential problem and having them intermittently drain the dependent loop of tubing.

Air Leak

When bubbling is observed in the underwater seal device, especially if this is a new or unexpected finding or if it is continuous (not in cycle with respiration), a thorough survey of the drainage apparatus must be undertaken. An air leak anywhere in the tubing, from the insertion site at the skin to the underwater seal device, as well as any connectors in between, can cause bubbling to appear in the water seal chamber. This can be assessed by placing a clamp as near to the insertion site as possible. Bubbling will continue if there is a leak in the tubing. The location of the tubing breach can be found by sequentially moving the clamp toward the underwater seal device and checking at each application for continued bubbling. Air leaks often occur at the connection joint of the chest drain to the underwater seal device's tubing. Once the leak has been located, the damaged tubing or connector should be replaced. The practice of taping the tubing connection joints is unlikely to prevent or treat occult air leaks but may be useful in reducing the incidence of inadvertent disconnection of the tubing. A disconnection can still occur, however, and it may not be easily noticeable underneath a layer of tape. At our hospital, we now "band" each connection point with a circumferential ratcheted plastic appliance.

Clamping

In general, chest tube clamping should be avoided. There are a few instances when clamping is necessary or can be a useful adjunct in tube management. Chest drains should be clamped proximally (nearer to the patient) when changing the tubing or underwater seal device. "Diagnostic" clamping may also be necessary to troubleshoot when a leak in the tubing system is suspected. Chest tube clamping at the time of drain insertion to prevent re-expansion pulmonary edema is described later in this chapter.

Before removing a chest tube that has a persistent low-grade leak or a wide oscillation of fluid in the tubing, it may be useful to simulate chest tube removal by clamping it for a short period (1 to 2 hours). A chest radiograph is then obtained. If the lung remains expanded and there is no evidence of increasing subcutaneous emphysema in spite of the tube being clamped, the chest tube can be removed. If, however, the radiograph shows a pneumothorax or increasing subcutaneous emphysema, or if the patient becomes symptomatic with shortness of breath or pain, the clamp should be promptly removed. Patients who have their chest tubes clamped for this reason must be closely monitored for symptoms and clinical signs of worsening dyspnea or reaccumulation of the pneumothorax. Routine tube clamping before chest tube removal is unnecessary.

Removal

Chest tubes are removed when the indication for their placement has resolved; that is, air leaks have stopped, fluid loss has diminished to a minimal rate (usually <300 mL/24 hours), and chest radiographs show the lung to be well expanded. Patients still requiring positive-pressure ventilation with high peak airway pressures are at high risk for new or recurrent air leaks due to barotrauma. In this situation, a chest tube, which otherwise would be removed because it has accomplished the intended drainage, should be left in place until the patient has been extubated or the risks of barotrauma have been minimized.

There are many techniques for chest tube removal. After cutting the drain stitch holding the tube in place at the skin, the patient is asked to take as deep a breath as possible and hold it. Once the patient reaches maximal inspiration, the drain is gently but swiftly removed. An airtight dressing is then applied to the drain exit site. This method has proved to be the most reliable way of avoiding ingress of air into the pleural cavity. At maximal inspiration, the patient has completed the portion of the respiratory cycle with the most negative intrapleural pressure. If the patient experiences any discomfort during removal of the chest drain, he or she will only be able to exhale, causing increased positive intrapleural pressure and favoring the egress of any pleural air.

Some clinicians emphasize the need to place a purse-string or mattress stitch at the time of tube insertion so that this can be tied down after drain removal to ensure wound closure. We do not believe that this is absolutely necessary and do not routinely use this technique; however, it might be useful when the chest tube has been in place for several weeks. Although the stitch assists in closing the drain site, it is associated with increased pain after removal and requires an early return visit to remove the stitch 5 to 7 days later.

SPECIAL CONSIDERATIONS

Insertion Difficulties

NEGATIVE ASPIRATION

The best opportunity to drain a pleural space is at the time of initial tube insertion. As mentioned earlier, needle aspiration at the time of local anesthetic administration allows for confirmation of the presence of air or fluid. If, during needle aspiration, no air or fluid is encountered, further attempts should be made through higher and lower interspaces. If neither air nor fluid (as appropriate) is found, the procedure should be postponed and the situation re-evaluated. Additional imaging, including image guidance techniques, or a more experienced physician or surgeon may be required. Failure to follow these precautions may convert a minor difficulty into an emergency, with inadvertent insertion of a drain into the lung or other viscera.

INTRAPLEURAL ADHESIONS

Patients with previous ipsilateral cardiothoracic procedures or a history of a prior pleural process are at increased risk for significant pleural adhesions. These factors should always be taken into consideration when deciding whether to place a chest tube. Intrapleural adhesions are detected by palpation. If the adhesions are thin and flimsy, they can often be swept away sufficiently to allow the drain to be inserted safely. If the adhesions are stout, they should be left in place, because attempts to take them down by finger sweeping may cause tearing and bleeding of the lung. Often, the chest tube can still be inserted and advanced gently to find its own way around various areas of adhesion. If, however, a complete pleural symphysis is encountered, the procedure should be aborted and its indications reconsidered.

SUBDIAPHRAGMATIC PLACEMENT

A chest tube may be incorrectly placed under the diaphragm if the insertion site is too low on the chest or the diaphragm is higher than expected. This error usually occurs when the operator incorrectly interprets a lower chest opacification as fluid, rather than considering the possibility of a raised hemidiaphragm. This mistake can usually be identified when the operator performs finger palpation after breaching the "pleura." If no intra-abdominal injuries have occurred, the insertion site can simply be closed and a higher insertion performed. Careful monitoring for abdominal injuries is continued after the procedure is properly completed.

As mentioned previously, this error can be avoided if one remembers that patients will generally be supine during the course of their chest drainage. Therefore, in free-flowing pleural fluid collections, the positioning of the tube in the pleural space posteriorly is much more important than a low-lying insertion site, which increases the risk of subdiaphragmatic placement.

IMPALED STRUCTURE

An impaled structure requires urgent surgical referral. As with many complications, the optimal management is to take every precaution to prevent its occurrence. As mentioned previously, the use of trocars to assist with chest tube placement may predispose to this type of injury. Using the technique of blunt finger palpation to guide the drain insertion avoids this serious injury in most cases.

Difficult Management Issues

SUBCUTANEOUS EMPHYSEMA

Subcutaneous emphysema is a result of leaking air that is under sufficient pressure to track into the subcutaneous tissues. As with any gas or fluid, air under pressure seeks the exit path of least resistance. If a chest drain is occluded either by clamping or clogging of the tubing with fibrinous material or clot, continued air leak from the pulmonary parenchyma will seek a different path of exit from the pleural space. This can also occur if there is a volume of "stagnant" fluid in a dependent loop of the connecting tubing, as described earlier. The increased intrapleural pressure promotes lung collapse and subsequent tracking of air via breaches in the parietal pleura into the subcutaneous tissues.

When subcutaneous emphysema is present, a thorough evaluation of the tubing and collection system must be carried out. A chest radiograph is important to assess the lung. Any obstruc-

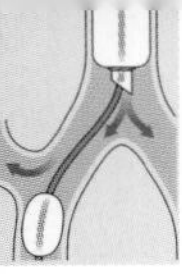

tion within the tubing must be cleared to favor egress of air via the drain over any other pathway. An initial maneuver to consider is to restart suction on the drain via the underwater seal device. If the tubing is patent, restarting the suction may be sufficient. Evaluation of the pleural space with computed tomography may help determine the area requiring further drainage. Occasionally, the parenchymal air leak is of such magnitude that a second chest tube is required. On rare occasions, surgical repair of the air leak might be necessary.

Subcutaneous emphysema can be quite disfiguring and therefore extremely distressing to patients and their families. It is often necessary to reassure them that although it is dramatic, this is rarely a dangerous situation. However, they should be advised that it usually takes more time to resolve than it took to appear, but ultimately, it will resolve.

PROLONGED AIR LEAK

A prolonged air leak is usually defined as one that persists for more than 1 week. This can be secondary to a number of causes. If the air leak is not amenable to surgical repair and is expected to eventually heal spontaneously, a prolonged hospital stay may be avoided with the use of a Heimlich valve (Fig. 12.7). This is a passive drainage system that employs a one-way flutter valve, allowing air and fluid to be expelled from the chest cavity while preventing air from entering the pleural space. The patient can be discharged with instructions to return on a weekly basis for a chest radiograph to evaluate the resolution of the air leak.

Special attention must be paid to ensure that the Heimlich valve is attached in the proper direction. Otherwise, air can be trapped in the pleural space, collapsing the lung and creating the potential for a tension pneumothorax.

DRAIN OBSTRUCTION

Occasionally, a chest drain may become occluded with fibrinous debris or frank clot. If the intrapleural process initially warranting the chest tube has not resolved, the chest tube occlusion must be cleared. This can often be achieved by “milking” or stripping the tubing. It should be remembered that such stripping of the tubing can create transient negative intrapleural pressures in excess of 400 cmH_2O. This maneuver is of questionable benefit and therefore should not be undertaken without the knowledge and consent of the primary surgeon or physician responsible for the chest tube. Another way to clear intraluminal blockage from the chest tube is to pass a Fogarty embolectomy catheter retrogradely up the tube and draw it back with the balloon inflated, thereby pulling out the debris. This should be done under meticulously sterile technique. If, after trying these techniques, the drain remains occluded, a new drain might have to be inserted and the occluded drain removed.

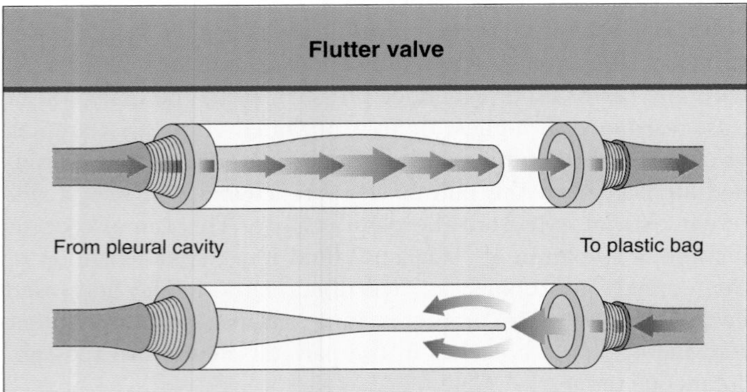

Figure 12.7 Heimlich valve. Air expelled from the pleural cavity opens the flutter valve (upper); when pleural pressure falls below atmospheric pressure, the flutter valve is compressed and sealed to prevent the inflow of air (lower).

FAILURE OF THE LUNG TO RE-EXPAND

Following insertion of a chest tube, a frontal chest radiograph should be obtained to assess positioning of the tube and clearance of the intrapleural process that required drain placement. If the lung has not fully re-expanded, an explanation must be sought from among the following scenarios.

In the case of a large air leak or initially following lung resection, the lung may not have had enough time to fully re-expand, and no immediate action is necessary. Otherwise, proper intrapleural placement must be confirmed. This may not be entirely possible with the two-dimensional radiograph, but it should be able to identify whether all the chest tube holes are within the pleural space. If this is not the case, the tube may be drawing outside air into the pleural space, preventing full re-expansion of the lung. A new sterile tube will have to be inserted in this case. If the radiograph suggests that all drain holes are appropriately within the pleural space but the lung is not fully expanded, this may be due to an extrapleural insertion of the tube. Observing a complete lack of any drainage (air or fluid) or oscillation in the tubing can identify this situation. A lateral chest radiograph can help to confirm this; however, a computed tomography scan is more sensitive.

In cases of hemothoraces, chronic pleural effusions, or empyemas, the underlying lung may not be able to fully re-expand owing to a fibrinous peel overlying the visceral pleura. Drainage of the fluid collection may be complete, yet it leaves an unresolved intrapleural space. If this space does not resolve after a few days of suction applied via the chest drain, a surgical decortication may be necessary. Alternatively, a bronchoscopy may be indicated to exclude an endobronchial blockage preventing re-expansion of the underlying lung parenchyma.

RE-EXPANSION PULMONARY EDEMA

When draining a large intrapleural fluid collection that is compressing underlying lung, consideration should be given to the extremely rare but potentially lethal phenomenon of re-expansion pulmonary edema. This process is due to rapid re-expansion of the previously compressed lung at the time of fluid drainage, leading to a rapid increase in blood flow and pulmonary capillary pressure. Fluid shift across the capillary and alveolar membranes causes excess extravascular fluid.

The first sign of this process is usually noted at chest tube insertion, when fluid drainage is rapid and the patient begins to cough uncontrollably. This usually occurs when between 800 and 1500 mL of fluid is acutely drained. When this is observed, the chest tube should be clamped immediately. This usually controls the patient’s urge to cough and prevents further progression of the underlying pathologic process. A controlled drainage is then performed by intermittently unclamping the tube until resolution of the effusion is observed.

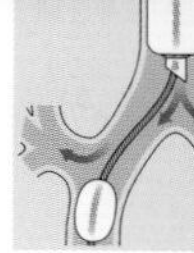

SUGGESTED READINGS

Cerfolio RJ, Bass CS, Pask AH, Katholi CR: Predictors and treatment of persistent air leaks. Ann Thorac Surg 73:1727-1730, 2002.

Duncan C, Erickson R: Pressures associated with chest tube stripping. Heart Lung 11:166-171, 1982.

Gayer G, Rozenman J, Hoffmann C, et al: CT diagnosis of malpositioned chest tubes. Br J Radiol 73:786-790, 2000.

Gift AG, Bolgiano CS, Cunningham J: Sensation during chest tube removal. Heart Lung 20:131-137, 1991.

Gordon PA, Norton JM, Guerra JM, Perdue ST: Positioning of chest tubes: effects on pressure and drainage. Am J Crit Care 6:33-38, 1997.

Grégoire J, Deslauriers J: Closed drainage and suction systems. In Pearson FG, Cooper JD, Deslauriers J, et al (eds): Thoracic Surgery, vol 1, 2nd ed. New York, Churchill Livingstone, 2002, pp 1281-1300.

Harriss DR, Graham TR: Management of intercostal drains. Br J Hosp Med 45:383-386, 1991.

Miller KS, Sahn SA: Chest tubes: indications, techniques, management and complications. Chest 91:258-264, 1987.

Obney JA, Barnes MJ, Lisagor PG, Cohen DJ: A method for mediastinal drainage after cardiac procedures using small Silastic drains. Ann Thorac Surg 70:1109-1110, 2000.

Sewell RW, Fewel JG, Grover FL, Arom KV: Experimental evaluation of reexpansion pulmonary oedema. Ann Thorac Surg 26:126-132, 1978.

Teplitz L: Update: are milking and stripping chest tubes necessary? Focus Crit Care 18:506-511, 1991.

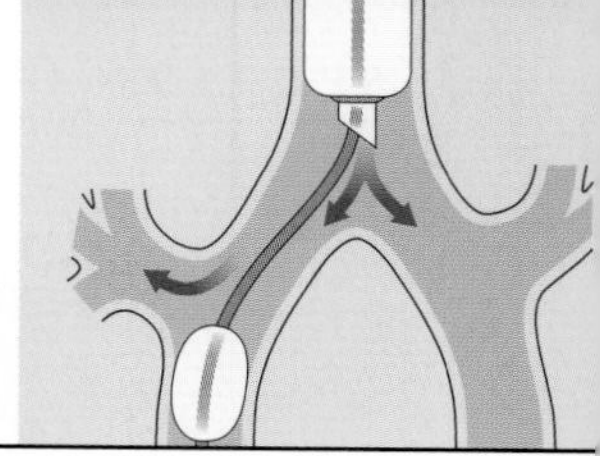

CHAPTER 13

Diagnostic Thoracic Surgical Procedures

Stephen D. Cassivi and Mark S. Allen

Despite the ever-increasing sensitivity of noninvasive diagnostic methods, especially in the field of diagnostic imaging, there remains an important role for diagnostic thoracic surgical procedures. Various thoracic surgical procedures add critical information in the diagnostic workup of patients with diverse thoracic diseases. To provide definitive tissue diagnosis and to assess stage and resectability of chest tumors, the general thoracic surgeon is vital in the diagnostic evaluation of patients.

Thoracic surgical procedures commonly employed for diagnosis include, in order of invasiveness, bronchoscopic, cervical, scalene and supraclavicular lymph node, pleural, mediastinal, and pulmonary biopsy procedures that involve endoscopic, thoracoscopic, or open surgical approaches. There is a spectrum of invasiveness to these procedures, with exploratory thoracotomy representing the most invasive of these diagnostic techniques. The choice of procedure is guided by the particular clinical question to be answered as well as specific patient characteristics and, at times, the individual surgeon's preference and experience. Overall, these procedures provide a high diagnostic yield with low morbidity and mortality rates. Complications, although rare, do occasionally occur, and it is therefore incumbent on referring physicians to possess a clear understanding of the nature of these procedures, their level of invasiveness, and their relative risk-to-benefit ratios.

PREOPERATIVE CONSIDERATIONS

Except for flexible bronchoscopy, which can be performed using topical anesthesia with minimal sedation, most diagnostic surgical interventions require general anesthesia. Determination of the appropriateness of the intervention should be a first consideration, because some degree of operative risk is always present. A general contraindication to these procedures would be excessive operative risk from comorbid conditions. The referring physician and ultimately the operating surgeon must assess the patient's overall medical status and ability to withstand the proposed procedure. Furthermore, a diagnostic surgical intervention, no matter how minimally invasive, is unnecessary and unwarranted if the findings of the procedure will not influence the treatment plan for the individual patient.

CLINICAL APPLICATION OF DIAGNOSTIC THORACIC SURGICAL PROCEDURES

The diagnostic thoracic surgical procedures discussed in this chapter have varied applications with relative advantages and disadvantages (Table 13.1). They are most commonly used in three broad areas:

1. Assessment of bronchogenic carcinoma
2. Diagnosis of interstitial lung disease
3. Sampling of indeterminate pleural, pulmonary, and mediastinal lesions

Bronchoscopy

FLEXIBLE BRONCHOSCOPY

As a diagnostic tool, flexible bronchoscopy offers a relatively noninvasive way to visualize and obtain tissue samples from the airways. This flexible characteristic allows access to subsegmental branches of the tracheobronchial tree. Although flexible bronchoscopy can be done via the endotracheal tube in an anesthetized and intubated patient, this procedure is commonly performed using topical anesthetic and conscious sedation.

Flexible bronchoscopy not only allows visualization of the tracheobronchial tree, but also provides access for obtaining tissue samples such as washings, brushings, and bronchoalveolar lavage for cytologic and microbiologic analyses. Endobronchial and transbronchial biopsies can also be obtained. Transbronchial needle (Wang) biopsies can be performed to assess mediastinal lymphadenopathy via the flexible bronchoscope. (See Chapter 9, Bronchoscopy.)

RIGID BRONCHOSCOPY

Rigid bronchoscopy is employed, for the most part, for therapeutic interventions of the airway (laser débridement, tumor debulking, placement of airway stents, foreign body retrieval), because most of the diagnostic uses have been supplanted by flexible bronchoscopy (Fig. 13.1). The rigid bronchoscope continues to be an important diagnostic tool in special circumstances such as those requiring a better tactile sense when assessing for possible extrinsic tumor invasion of the airway, or when larger biopsies are sought. It is also indispensable when airway control is in question because of hemoptysis or tumor invasion. (See Chapter 9, Bronchoscopy.)

Rigid bronchoscopy usually requires general anesthesia with a muscle relaxant and specific ventilatory strategies. The options most commonly employed include jet ventilation and continuous or intermittent insufflation. In patients in whom airway control is an overwhelming concern because of an obstructing airway lesion, muscle relaxants are avoided to maintain spontaneous breathing.

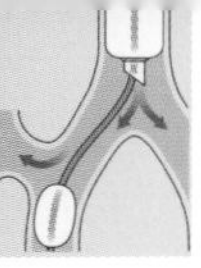

Table 13.1
Features of surgical investigative procedures

Procedure	Application	Advantages	Disadvantages
Rigid bronchoscopy	Diagnosis of carcinoma Clear airway obstruction	Removal of secretions/blood Large biopsy specimen may reveal submucosal tumor Opportunity to debulk inoperable tumors or excise benign lesions Assessment of carinal fixation	Poor view of secondary bronchial divisions
Cervical and scalene lymph node biopsy	Diagnosis of enlarged nodes	Safer technique than fine-needle aspiration (FNA) for deeper nodes Large tissue sample	Operative procedure Occasional technical difficulty
Mediastinoscopy	Diagnosis of middle mediastinal pathology (node/mass)	Direct access to mediastinal abnormality Much larger tissue sample than FNA	Operative field restricted to paratracheal and subcarinal areas
Mediastinotomy	Diagnosis of anterior mediastinal pathology (node/mass)	Reaches areas of anterior mediastinum not accessible to mediastinoscopy Useful for subaortic node sampling May be safer to use than mediastinoscopy in patients who have superior vena cava obstruction Much larger tissue sample than in FNA	Operative field restricted to upper anterior mediastinum More complex operative procedure
Thoracoscopy	Pleural biopsy Biopsy of visceral pleura deposits	Can be effected through single puncture Visually directed biopsy	Limited to small biopsies Dependent on pleural cavity being free of adhesions
Video-assisted thoracic surgery	Any ipsilateral biopsy or sampling procedure	Complementary to mediastinoscopy and mediastinotomy Excellent view and full operative intervention possible (e.g. wedge excision of pulmonary nodule or dissection of mediastinal mass)	Dependent on pleural cavity being free of adhesions Significant surgical expertise required

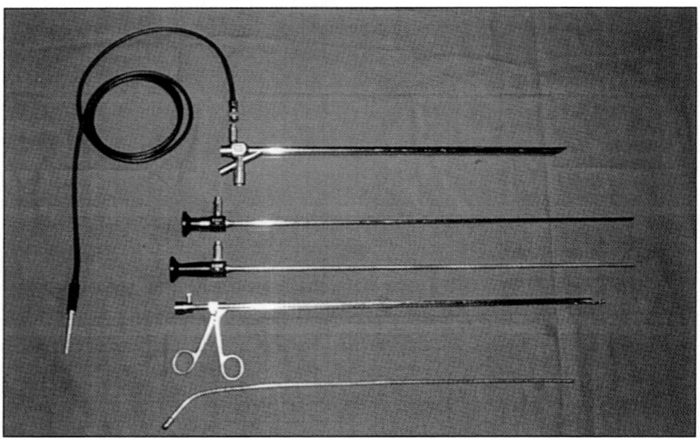

Figure 13.1 Rigid bronchoscopy equipment. Bronchoscope with light cable *(top)*, straight and right-angle surgical telescopes, biopsy forceps, and suction cannula *(bottom)*.

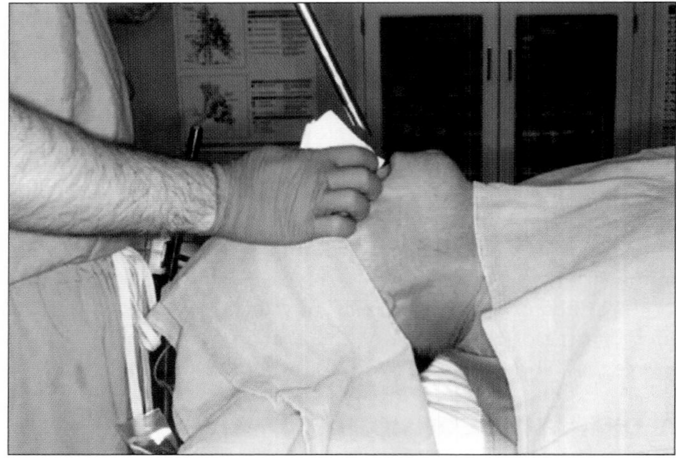

Figure 13.2 Positioning and insertion of rigid bronchoscope. The patient is positioned supinely with the neck extended. The rigid bronchoscope is inserted with the bevel down.

Technique

In general, the size of the rigid bronchoscope used for adult men is 8 or 9mm (outer diameter) and for adult women is 7 or 8 mm. Smaller sizes are available for children or smaller adults.

Following induction of anesthesia, the patient is positioned supinely with the neck extended into the "sniffing" position. Right-handed surgeons use the left thumb to further protect the patient's upper teeth and lips from injury and to serve as the fulcrum in positioning and supporting the bronchoscope throughout the procedure. Protection is also supplemented by using a rubber tooth guard or saline-soaked gauze sponge. The patient's eyes are also shielded from inadvertent injury with padded covers for the duration of the procedure.

The bronchoscope is inserted through the right side of the patient's mouth with the bevel down (Fig. 13.2). It is advanced toward the base of the tongue in the posterior oropharynx. The tip of the epiglottis is identified by carefully elevating the tongue as the scope is brought into a more horizontal position. The scope is then advanced a short distance past the tip of the epiglottis. The protruding superior lip of the bronchoscope is used to gently lift the tip of the epiglottis, allowing visualization of the vocal cords and laryngeal inlet. The surgeon rotates the bronchoscope 90 degrees along its long axis, placing the bevel in the anteroposterior plane to allow easy passage through the vocal cords. The bronchoscope can then be carefully advanced into the trachea under direct vision. To facilitate passage of the bron-

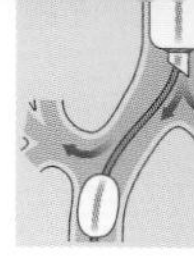

choscope into the left or right main-stem bronchus, the patient's head is turned to the contralateral side. Visualization of the segmental and subsegmental airways can be facilitated by insertion of a flexible bronchoscope via the lumen on the rigid bronchoscope.

Cervical, Scalene, and Supraclavicular Lymph Node Biopsy

Both bronchogenic and esophageal carcinoma may involve the lymph nodes in the cervical, scalene, and supraclavicular areas. Open biopsy of nonpalpable scalene lymph nodes is no longer a routine preoperative staging procedure since the advent of cervical mediastinoscopy. Clinically positive or palpable nodes in this area are now accessed most commonly by fine-needle aspiration. Some experts have advocated a role for ipsilateral scalene lymph node biopsy in patients with positive N2 disease found at mediastinoscopy in order to rule out unresectable N3 disease.

TECHNIQUE

A 3- to 4-cm-long skin crease incision is made at the level just above the insertion of the sternocleidomastoid muscle into the medial clavicle. Dissection can either proceed between the clavicular and sternal heads of this muscle, or both can be retracted medially. The scalene fat pad lies on the anterior scalene muscle and lateral to the internal jugular vein. The scalene fat pad receives its blood supply usually from the transverse cervical artery, entering the fat pad inferiorly. This should be identified, ligated, and divided. Injury to the phrenic nerve is possible owing to its location along the anterior surface of the anterior scalene muscle, deep to the fat pad. Other rare yet significant complications associated with this procedure include pneumothorax and thoracic duct injury with subsequent chylous fistula.

Cervical Mediastinoscopy

Cervical mediastinoscopy, currently a mainstay of lung cancer staging, was popularized in Europe by Carlens and in North America by Pearson in the 1960s. It is used not only for lung cancer staging but also to assess any lymphadenopathy in the pretracheal, paratracheal, and subcarinal areas. Lymph nodes that are accessible by the standard cervical approach are the upper and lower paratracheal and subcarinal levels (stations 2, 4, and 7, respectively, in the American Joint Committee on Cancer [AJCC] nomenclature) (see Chapter 41, Lung Cancer). The so-called "extended" cervical mediastinoscopy, introduced by Ginsberg, allows access to the aortopulmonary window and para-aortic lymph nodes (stations 5 and 6, respectively, in the AJCC nomenclature). Repeat mediastinoscopy, although technically possible, carries a higher risk of complications because of the loss of normal tissue planes to guide the usual dissection. Cervical mediastinoscopy can usually be performed as an outpatient procedure.

In spite of improvements in imaging of the mediastinum with modern computed tomography (CT) scanners and the recent advent of positron emission tomography (PET) scans, cervical mediastinoscopy remains the gold standard for staging the mediastinum in lung cancer. Of special note is that PET scans can have false-positive results in the mediastinal nodes. It is therefore imperative that a tissue diagnosis be obtained to document mediastinal metastases before surgical resection is denied. Cervical mediastinoscopy has a diagnostic accuracy of over 90%.

TECHNIQUE

With the patient intubated and under general anesthesia, a bolster is placed under his or her shoulders to provide adequate neck extension for the procedure. A 3-cm transverse incision is made approximately 1 cm above the sternal notch. The pretracheal fascia is exposed by splitting the strap muscles in the midline, with right-angle retractors used to retract the thyroid gland superiorly if necessary. The pretracheal fascia is incised transversely and bluntly dissected off the anterior surface of the trachea with the index finger. This allows direct palpation of the vascular structures, including the aortic arch and innominate vessels as well as any prominent lymphadenopathy. The mediastinoscope is introduced beneath the pretracheal fascia (Fig. 13.3). Further blunt dissection can be done under direct vision using the tip of the mediastinoscopy sucker. Systematic dissection and biopsy of the different lymph node levels is then possible.

A spinal needle attached to a syringe can be used to aspirate and thus differentiate between solid masses that can undergo biopsy and vascular structures that should be avoided. Most small bleeding can be controlled by judicious use of electrocautery or temporary packing. Because of the risk of significant hemorrhage from injury to the many nearby vascular structures, the operating staff should always be prepared for possible conversion to sternotomy or thoracotomy for definitive control of bleeding. Special care should also be taken when performing biopsies on lymph nodes in the left paratracheal area, as the left recurrent laryngeal nerve courses nearby and can be injured by aggressive biopsy procedures or injudicious use of electrocautery.

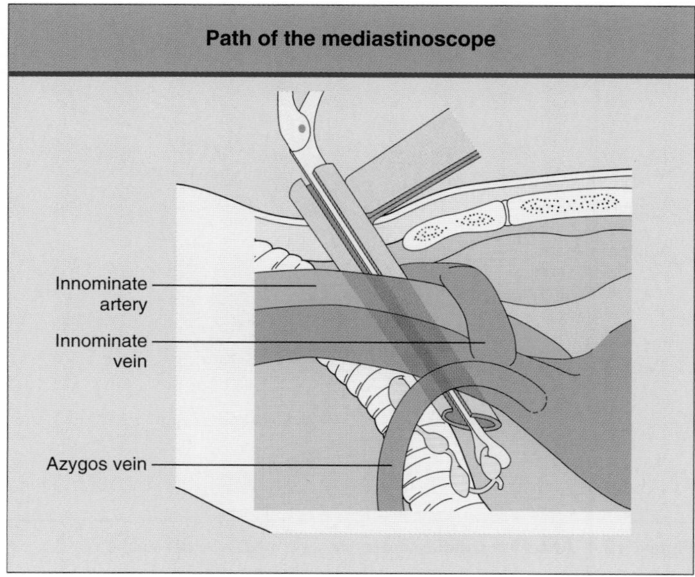

Figure 13.3 Path of the cervical mediastinoscope.

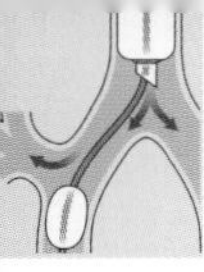

Anterior Mediastinotomy

Anterior mediastinotomy, also known as the "Chamberlain procedure," is a technique that provides access to the anterior mediastinum. It is typically used to sample lymph nodes in the aortopulmonary window and para-aortic lymph nodes (stations 5 and 6, respectively, in the AJCC nomenclature). These nodal stations can also be accessed by extended cervical mediastinoscopy or thoracoscopy. Although anterior mediastinotomy is to some extent more invasive than cervical mediastinoscopy, patients are usually able to leave the hospital on the day of surgery.

TECHNIQUE

A 4-cm transverse incision is usually made in the second interspace, just lateral to the lateral sternal border. The pectoral muscle can commonly be split along the line of its fibers without cutting through muscle. The intercostal muscle is then incised along the upper edge of the second costal cartilage. The internal mammary vessels, located medially, can usually be avoided and preserved. The mediastinal pleura is bluntly pushed laterally to avoid entry into the pleural space. The mediastinoscope is introduced to permit optimal visualization and obtain appropriate biopsy specimens (Fig. 13.4).

Anterior mediastinotomy

Station L6 nodes
Left phrenic nerve
Internal mammary artery
Internal mammary vein
Aortic arch
Aorto-pulmonary window
Station L5 nodes
Vagus nerve

Figure 13.4 Anterior mediastinotomy. The medial portion of the rib is removed here for pictorial purposes only. It is not generally removed in this operation.

Occasionally the mediastinal pleura is breached. A chest tube is generally not required if the visceral pleura has not been damaged. At the end of the procedure, a small catheter can be inserted into the pleural space via the mediastinotomy. The tube is pulled out once the overlying muscular tissues have been almost closed, with the anesthesiologist providing sustained positive pressure ventilation to evacuate any residual intrapleural air.

Thoracoscopy

Minimally invasive access to the lung, pleural space, and mediastinum can be obtained by thoracoscopy (Table 13.2). Also referred to as *video-assisted thoracic surgery* (VATS), this can be useful in the diagnosis of pleural pathology such as diffuse or focal thickening due to mesothelioma, pleural metastases, asbestos-related plaques, or benign inflammatory pleuritis. Thoracoscopy can also assist in the diagnosis and treatment of pleural fluid collections. In the staging of lung and esophageal cancer, thoracoscopy can provide access in a minimally invasive way to the paratracheal, prevascular, aortopulmonary window, para-aortic, subcarinal, paraesophageal, and inferior pulmonary ligament lymph node groups (stations 2 to 9, respectively, in the AJCC nomenclature). Tumor invasion of local structures and overall resectability can also be assessed. Thoracoscopy is also used to obtain biopsies of lung tissue to assess discrete nodules or diffuse lung disease.

Thoracoscopy is most effectively performed with single lung ventilation of the contralateral side using a double-lumen endotracheal tube or a bronchial blocker. This allows collapse of the lung on the operated side, permitting adequate visualization and maneuverability within the pleural space. Dense pleural adhesions are therefore a contraindication for effective thoracoscopy, as is the inability to tolerate single lung ventilation.

It should be noted that although thoracoscopy is a form of minimally invasive surgery, it remains a high-risk procedure when performed in high-risk patients. Of particular note are patients with interstitial lung disease requiring lung biopsy to tailor treatment options. These patients usually suffer from severe respiratory compromise before thoracoscopy. They are sometimes already on mechanical ventilation, and a significant proportion of these patients have elevated pulmonary arterial pressures. In the experience published from the Mayo Clinic, patients with interstitial lung disease undergoing thoracoscopic lung biopsy had an operative mortality of just under 6%.

TECHNIQUE

Thoracoscopy is performed using single lung ventilation of the contralateral side. The patient is positioned laterally similar to

Table 13.2 Video-assisted thoracic surgery techniques for diagnostic intervention
Pleural biopsy
Mediastinal biopsy
Indeterminate pulmonary nodule
Interstitial lung disease
Assessment of operability in bronchogenic carcinoma patients

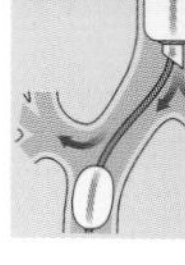

the positioning used for a posterolateral thoracotomy. When thoracoscopy is performed for drainage and evaluation of a pleural effusion, a single 2-cm port is usually sufficient. It is placed in the sixth or seventh interspace in the anterior axillary line. Through this port, the camera and a thin suction tip or biopsy forceps can be introduced and maneuvered. For most other applications, one or two additional ports are required and are commonly positioned separately along the fifth interspace, in the line of a potential posterolateral thoracotomy (Fig. 13.5). In this way, conversion to thoracotomy requires simply the extension of the incision between these two port sites. In the Mayo Clinic experience, one third of cases were converted to open thoracotomy, with the greatest number being for a nodule found to be malignant and requiring a formal resection (completion lobectomy).

Whereas biopsy for diagnosis of interstitial lung disease requires only defining several areas of representative pathology, wedge resection of an indeterminate pulmonary nodule first necessitates precise localization of the lesion. This is usually done using the surgeon's finger introduced through one of the thoracoscopy incisions (Fig. 13.6). It is clearly easier to locate larger and peripherally located lesions. Smaller or deeper lesions may not be accessible and may require conversion to open thoracotomy.

Once the area to be biopsied has been located, an endoscopic stapling device can be inserted through a thoracoport and used to perform a wedge resection (Fig. 13.7). After the specimen has been resected, it should be removed from the pleural cavity within an endoscopic specimen retrieval bag to avoid port site contamination. A more economical alternative is to use a surgical glove introduced through one of the port sites and held open with two Kelly clamps.

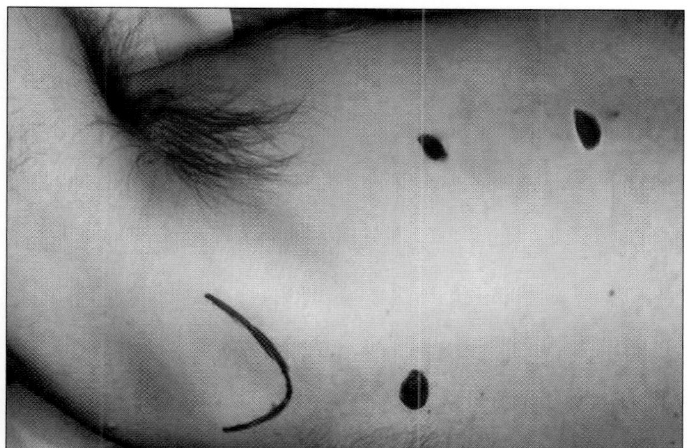

Figure 13.5 Location of thoracoscopic port sites. One port is placed at about the seventh interspace in the anterior axillary line. Further ports may be required and are usually placed along the line of a potential posterolateral thoracotomy incision at the level of the fifth interspace.

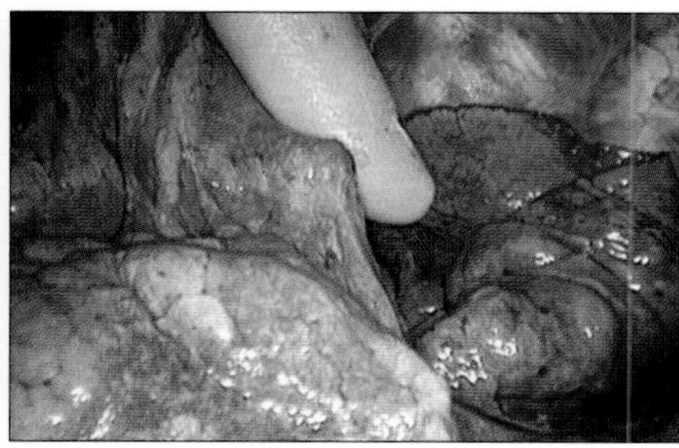

Figure 13.6 Palpation of intrapulmonary nodule during thoracoscopy.

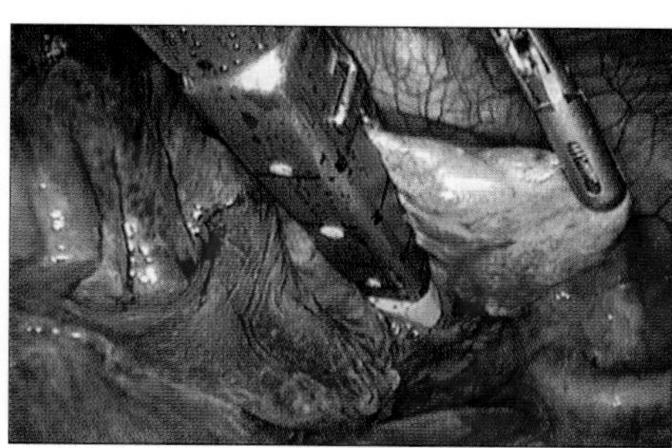

Figure 13.7 Use of endoscopic stapler during thoracoscopic lung biopsy.

The biopsy specimen should be processed initially on a sterile back table in the operating room. In the case of diffuse lung infiltrates, the staple line can be excised and used for microbiologic culture testing, while the remainder of the specimen is sent to pathology for histologic evaluation. When an indeterminate lung nodule is excised, a small portion should be kept for microbiologic cultures in the event that the evaluation of the rest of the nodule suggests a nonmalignant diagnosis.

After all biopsies have been performed, the pleural cavity should be reassessed for any bleeding or other injury. Special attention should be paid to the staple lines and port sites. Once hemostasis is ascertained, a single 28 French chest tube is introduced via the initial thoracoport in the seventh interspace anteriorly. It is guided posteriorly, and care is taken to avoid placement within the fissure. Barring a significant air leak, this tube can usually be removed within 12 to 24 hours and the patient discharged from hospital on the day after surgery.

Open Thoracotomy

Open thoracotomy is at the far end of the spectrum of morbidity for diagnostic thoracic surgical procedures. It is therefore usually the least preferred option. There are, however, several situations in which this procedure is indicated and is the best diagnostic modality available. These include patients who, because of a fused pleural space or the inability to withstand single lung ventilation, cannot safely undergo thoracoscopy.

Frequently patients referred for open lung biopsy are critically ill and have significant pulmonary compromise, often requiring mechanical ventilatory assistance. Although open lung biopsy is generally a very accurate diagnostic tool, most studies do not show a survival benefit in critically ill patients with diffuse lung disease even when a biopsy directs a change in therapy. Special care should be taken to assess the risk of such a procedure and its likely diagnostic yield in specific situations.

TECHNIQUE

Usually the patient undergoing thoracotomy is placed in the lateral position, with both arms flexed forward at the shoulder. The incision is made transversely approximately one to two finger-breadths beneath the scapular tip. This provides access to the fourth, fifth, or sixth interspace. Alternatively, the patient is positioned supinely, and an anterolateral thoracotomy is performed just beneath the mammary fold in the fourth or fifth interspace. As with the thoracoscopic approach, pulmonary

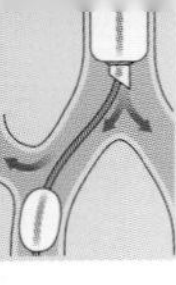

resection is performed with the assistance of surgical stapling devices. At the end of the procedure, before the wound is closed, a single 28 French chest tube is inserted via a separate incision beneath the main thoracotomy incision. It is guided into the pleural space and positioned posteriorly using a different interspace than the thoracotomy. It will remain until drainage of air or fluid ceases.

CONCLUSION

A spectrum of surgical procedures is available to assist in diagnosis of thoracic diseases. The choice of the optimal diagnostic approach is based on individual patient characteristics, the specific diagnostic dilemma, and the surgeon's preferences and experience. It is essential to have a thorough understanding of the particular clinical situation, the advantages and disadvantages of the procedural alternatives, and the therapeutic implications of each possible diagnostic finding. This allows the clinician asked to perform the procedure to provide the most useful diagnostic answer with the least risk to the patient. Only then does the clinician avoid being more than a mere technician.

SUGGESTED READINGS

Allen MS, Deschamps C, Jones DM, et al: Video-assisted thoracic surgical procedures: the Mayo experience. Mayo Clin Proc 71:351-359, 1996.

Ginsberg RJ, Rice TW, Goldberg M, et al: Extended cervical mediastinoscopy—a single staging procedure for bronchogenic carcinoma of the left upper lobe. J Thorac Cardiovasc Surg 94:673-678, 1987.

Hammoud ZT, Anderson RC, Meyers BF, et al: The current role of mediastinoscopy in the evaluation of thoracic disease. J Thorac Cardiovasc Surg 118:894-899, 1999.

Lee JD, Ginsberg RJ: Lung cancer staging: the value of ipsilateral scalene lymph node biopsy performed at mediastinoscopy. Ann Thorac Surg 62:338-341, 1996.

Olak J: Parasternal mediastinotomy (Chamberlain procedure). Chest Surg Clin N Am 6:31-40, 1996.

Rogers ML, Duffy JP: Surgical aspects of chronic post-thoracotomy pain. Eur J Cardiothorac Surg 18:711-716, 2000.

Temes RT, Joste NE, Qualls CR, et al: Lung biopsy: is it necessary? J Thorac Cardiovasc Surg 118:1097-1100, 1999.

Toloza EM, Harpole L, Detterbeck F, McCrory D. Invasive staging of non-small cell lung cancer: a review of the current evidence. Chest 123:S157-S166, 2003.

Wain JC: Rigid bronchoscopy: the value of a venerable procedure. Chest Surg Clin N Am 11:691-699, 2001.

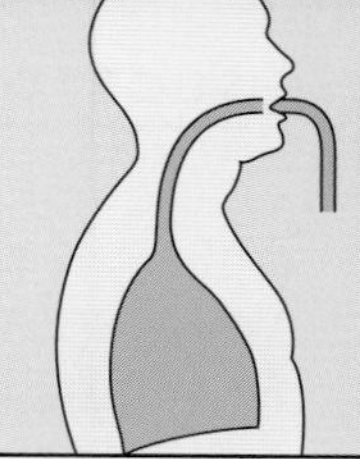

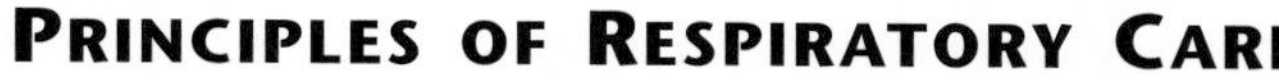

CHAPTER 14

Invasive Mechanical Ventilation

David J. Pierson

Although mechanical ventilation is a key component of intensive care, unfamiliar jargon and technical detail render it confusing and difficult for many clinicians. The rapidity and complexity of change in this area of respiratory medicine in recent years add to the problem.

Table 14.1 lists a number of factors that are central to a rational approach to mechanical ventilation in acute illness. It is also important that the fundamental goals and objectives of mechanical ventilation (Table 14.2) be understood, both in general and relative to the individual patient.

INDICATIONS AND CONTRAINDICATIONS

In the absence of a contraindication, mechanical ventilation is indicated whenever any of the circumstances listed under "Clinical Objectives" in Table 14.2 exists to a degree that threatens the life of the patient. Apart from apnea, few individual symptoms, signs, or laboratory findings by themselves mandate the initiation of ventilatory support. Rather, this therapy becomes necessary in the right clinical setting in combination with consideration of the severity and rapidity of the development or worsening of physiologic derangements.

A summary of the main categories of indications for invasive ventilatory support is given in Table 14.3.

Apnea and Impending Respiratory Arrest

Respiratory arrest is an indication the validity of which is so great that a controlled study of alternative therapies could not be done ethically. "Impending" respiratory arrest, however, is difficult to define prospectively, and attempts to study it as an indication for intubation and mechanical ventilation have so far proved unsuccessful. Intubation and mechanical ventilation are commonly instituted because the clinician judges the patient to be in severe respiratory distress, to be "tiring" or "about to arrest," but interobserver variation and the extent to which these subjective impressions predict an unfavorable outcome if intubation is not performed have never been investigated.

Acute Exacerbation of Chronic Obstructive Pulmonary Disease

The substantial number of studies of noninvasive positive pressure ventilation (NPPV) in acute exacerbations of chronic obstructive pulmonary disease (COPD) has not directly addressed the validity of the criteria used for intubation. The writing committee for the Global Initiative for Obstructive Lung Disease (GOLD), using what it considers to be the "best available evidence," recommends that invasive mechanical ventilation be used for patients with acute exacerbations of COPD who have cardiovascular instability, somnolence or other altered mental state, are uncooperative, have a high risk of aspiration, copious or very viscous respiratory tract secretions, any craniofacial condition (e.g., recent trauma or surgery) potentially rendering NPPV difficult, or extreme obesity. Very severe or progressive respiratory acidosis is also accepted as an indication, but agreement is lacking as to whether a pH of 7.25, a $PaCO_2$ of 60 mmHg, or some other arbitrary threshold should be used.

Acute Severe Asthma

Retrospective studies have shown that relatively few patients with acute severe asthma require invasive mechanical ventilation, but no clinical trials to define the specific indications have been reported. These indications may be similar to those for acute COPD exacerbations, although the potential for more rapid physiologic improvement in asthma and the fact that patients with asthma are typically younger and healthier than those with severe COPD raise doubts about this assumption.

Neuromuscular Disease

In acute respiratory insufficiency complicating neuromuscular disorders such as Guillain-Barré syndrome and myasthenia gravis, there is agreement among experienced clinicians that invasive mechanical ventilation should be initiated *before* the patient develops respiratory acidosis. Although the vital capacity and the maximum inspiratory pressure generated against an occluded airway have been used to assess the need for intubation in such patients, the thresholds shown in Table 14.3 have not been established through prospective studies.

Acute Hypoxemic Respiratory Failure

Severe hypoxemia by itself is seldom an indication for invasive mechanical ventilation. For example, isolated hypoxemia in patients with diffuse pneumonia or pulmonary edema can often be managed with high-flow oxygen by mask, with or without continuous positive airway pressure (CPAP). Typically, patients with severe hypoxemia in the setting of severe acute illness have other indications for ventilatory support, such as excessive work of breathing or a diminished ventilatory drive. There is no evidence to indicate what threshold of PaO_2/FIO_2 or other measure of oxygenation failure should be used as an independent indication for intubation and mechanical ventilation or, in fact, whether such a threshold exists.

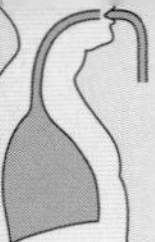

Table 14.1
Important factors in invasive mechanical ventilation

Clinical Setting
Postoperative or other "routine" mechanical ventilation in patients who have normal lungs Obstructive lung disease (chronic obstructive pulmonary disease, asthma) Acute lung injury, acute respiratory distress syndrome Asymmetric or unilateral pulmonary disease Neuromuscular disease Acute brain injury Flail chest
Patient's Underlying Pulmonary Status
No known pulmonary disease Obstructive lung disease (chronic obstructive pulmonary disease, asthma) Restrictive pulmonary disease Chronic ventilatory failure (underlying carbon dioxide retention)
Volume- versus Pressure-Targeted Ventilation
Volume-targeted: delivered tidal volume fixed, peak airway pressure variable Pressure-targeted: peak airway pressure fixed, delivered tidal volume variable
Full versus Partial Ventilatory Support
Full ventilatory support: ventilator does all the required work of breathing Partial ventilatory support: patient must provide at least a portion of required work of breathing

Table 14.2
Goals and objectives of mechanical ventilation

Goals
To replace in whole or in part the gas exchanging functions of the lungs and ventilatory pump in patients whose ability to maintain these functions is temporarily or permanently impaired To provide these functions with as little disruption of homeostasis and with as few complications as possible
Physiologic Objectives
To improve alveolar ventilation, as indicated by arterial pressure of carbon dioxide ($Paco_2$) and pH To improve arterial oxygenation, as indicated by Pao_2, saturation, and/or oxygen content To increase end-inspiratory lung inflation To increase end-expiratory lung volume (functional residual capacity) To reduce the work of breathing (i.e., to unload the ventilatory muscles)
Clinical Objectives
To reverse acute respiratory acidosis – relief of immediately life-threatening acidemia, rather than necessarily to make $Paco_2$ and/or pH normal To reverse hypoxemia – increase Pao_2 [generally such that arterial saturation is 90% or more, e.g., to ≥ 8 kPa (≥ 60 mmHg)] to reverse or prevent clinically important tissue hypoxia To relieve respiratory distress – improve patient comfort while the primary disease process resolves or improves To prevent or reverse atelectasis – avoid or correct adverse consequences of incomplete lung inflation To reverse ventilatory muscle fatigue – unload the ventilatory muscles and allow them to rest while the causes of increased workload are reversed or improved To permit sedation and/or neuromuscular blockade – render the patient unable to breathe spontaneously, as during surgery or certain intensive care unit procedures To decrease systemic or myocardial oxygen consumption in certain settings (e.g., severe, acute respiratory distress syndrome, cardiogenic shock), when spontaneous breathing or other muscular activity impairs systemic or cardiac oxygenation To reduce intracranial pressure - reduce intracranial blood volume through controlled hyperventilation in acute intracranial hypertension To stabilize the chest wall, as in chest wall resection or massive flail chest
From Slutsky AS: American College of Chest Physicians Consensus Conference on Mechanical Ventilation. Chest 104:1833–1859, 1993.

Table 14.3
Indications for invasive mechanical ventilation

Apnea or impending respiratory arrest Acute exacerbation of COPD* with dyspnea, tachypnea, and acute respiratory acidosis (hypercapnia and decreased arterial pH), plus at least one of the following: • Acute cardiovascular instability • Altered mental status or persistent uncooperativeness • Inability to protect the lower airway • Copious or unusually viscous secretions • Abnormalities of the face or upper airway that would prevent effective NPPV • Progressive respiratory acidosis or other deterioration despite intensive initial therapy, including NPPV
Acute ventilatory insufficiency in neuromuscular diseases, in the presence of any of the following: • Acute respiratory acidosis (hypercapnia and decreased arterial pH) • Progressive decline in vital capacity to less than 10-15 mL/kg • Progressive decline in maximum inspiratory pressure to less than 20-30 cm H_2O
Acute hypoxemic respiratory failure with tachypnea, respiratory distress, and persistent hypoxemia despite administration of high FIO_2 via high-flow system, or in the presence of any of the following: • Acute cardiovascular instability • Altered mental status or persistent uncooperativeness • Inability to protect the lower airway
Presence of the need for endotracheal intubation to maintain or protect the airway or to manage secretions, in the following settings: • Endotracheal tube 7.0 mm internal diameter or less with minute ventilation > 10 L/min • Endotracheal tube 8.0 mm internal diameter or less with minute ventilation > 15 L/min
In the absence of the above conditions, emergent intubation and IPPV are not necessarily indicated in the following circumstances before other therapies have been tried: • Dyspnea; acute respiratory distress • Acute exacerbation of COPD • Acute severe asthma • Acute hypoxemic respiratory failure in immunocompromised patients • Hypoxemia as an isolated finding • Traumatic brain injury • Flail test
*Also applies to acute severe asthma if respiratory acidosis or airflow obstruction has worsened despite aggressive management. COPD, chronic obstructive pulmonary disease; FIO_2, inspired oxygen fraction; IPPV, invasive pesitive pressure ventilation; NPPV, noninvasive positive-pressure ventilation.

Several studies of NPPV in various forms of acute hypoxemic respiratory failure have yielded inconclusive results, although preliminary data suggest that it may be possible to avoid intubation in some immunocompromised patients with the use of this modality. The initial improvements in gas exchange achieved by CPAP mask in some studies have not been associated with better outcomes or a reduction in the need for intubation. Cardiovascular instability, altered mental status, and the inability to adequately protect the lower airway are clear indications for intubation in acute hypoxemic respiratory failure; in the absence of these findings, it may be reasonable to attempt NPPV or at least a CPAP mask in an otherwise healthy patient, particularly if there is reason to believe that the patient's condition will improve rapidly.

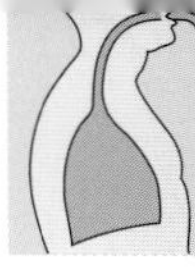

Heart Failure and Cardiogenic Shock

Available evidence on the management of cardiac pulmonary edema indicates that CPAP or NPPV may improve gas exchange—possibly with a reduced need for intubation—but that rates of clinical recovery and other outcomes are no different from those achieved without these interventions. Cardiogenic shock, however, may represent a separate indication for invasive mechanical ventilation to decrease the oxygen cost of breathing at a time of severely impaired cardiac function and potentially to functionally decrease left ventricular afterload by increasing intrathoracic and juxtacardiac pressures (see Chapter 4). Although this has not been subjected to a prospective clinical trial, retrospective studies of patients managed with intra-aortic balloon pumps have found higher rates of weaning from the pump and improved hospital mortality in patients who were intubated and ventilated.

Acute Brain Injury

Short-term hyperventilation can rapidly decrease intracranial pressure in patients with traumatic brain injury by constricting cerebral blood vessels and decreasing both cerebral blood flow and cerebral blood volume. Available evidence indicates, however, that routine hyperventilation in such patients does not improve survival or neurologic outcome and may, in fact, worsen the latter. Although brief periods of hyperventilation are used acutely to reduce sudden increases in intracranial pressure while more definitive measures are undertaken, the presence of acute brain injury is not by itself an indication for hyperventilation.

Flail Chest

When several ribs are each fractured in two or more places, the chest wall may become unstable, and paradoxical inward motion may be observed during spontaneous inhalation. At one time, this clinical finding was considered an indication for intubation and "internal pneumatic stabilization" until the fractures healed. Data from clinical series and experiments on animal models indicate, however, that both physiology and clinical outcome are determined more by the underlying lung injury than by the flail chest. Particularly in view of the potential complications, flail chest injury is not an indication for invasive mechanical ventilation in patients who do not have any of the other indications discussed here or listed in Table 14.3.

Contraindications to invasive mechanical ventilation are summarized in Table 14.4.

Table 14.4
Contraindications to invasive mechanical ventilation

No indication for ventilatory support exists (see Table 14.3)
Noninvasive ventilation is indicated in preference to invasive mechanical ventilation
Intubation and mechanical ventilation are contrary to the patient's expressed wishes
Life-support interventions, including mechanical ventilation, constitute medically futile therapy

TECHNIQUES

Types and Modes of Mechanical Ventilation

A confusing array of methods to mechanically ventilate a patient's lungs is available to clinicians, and these are distinguished by numerous variables. Phase variables are used to initiate one of the three phases (trigger, limit, and cycle) of the ventilatory cycle. The trigger variable, causing inspiration to begin, can be a preset pressure variation (pressure triggering), a preset volume (volume triggering), a designated flow change (flow triggering), or an elapsed time (time triggering). The limit variable is the pressure, volume, or flow target that cannot be exceeded during inspiration. Inspiration may thus be limited when a preset peak airway pressure is reached (pressure limiting), when a preset volume is delivered (volume limiting), or when a preset peak flow is attained (flow limiting). Cycling refers to the factors that terminate inspiration. A breath may be pressure, volume, or time cycled, terminating when a preset pressure, volume, or time interval, respectively, has been reached.

Three different types of breaths can be provided during mechanical ventilation, depending on whether the ventilator or the patient does the work and whether the ventilator or the patient initiates the breath: mandatory, assisted, and spontaneous breaths (Fig. 14.1). Mandatory breaths are machine cycled and are triggered, limited, and cycled by the ventilator. The patient is entirely passive, and the ventilator performs the work of breathing. Assisted breaths are like mandatory breaths, in that they are limited and cycled by the ventilator, but they are triggered by the patient. Breathing work is thus provided partly by the ventilator and partly by the patient. Spontaneous breaths are triggered, limited, and cycled by the patient, who performs all the work of breathing.

The relationship between the various types of breaths and the inspiratory-phase variables is called a mode of ventilation. Table 14.5 lists and describes the modes currently available for positive-pressure ventilatory support.

The distinction between volume-targeted and pressure-targeted ventilation is clinically important. Volume-targeted modes deliver a fixed tidal volume (VT) with each breath. This

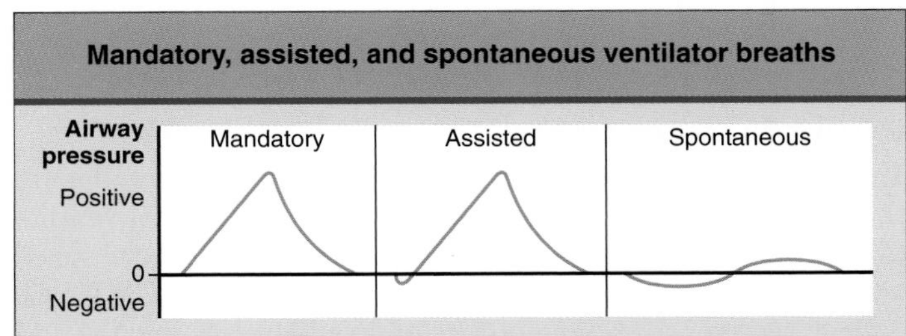

Figure 14.1 Mandatory, assisted, and spontaneous ventilator breaths. Pressures generated at the proximal airway during mandatory, assisted, and spontaneous breaths in a patient who receives mechanical ventilation. In a mandatory breath, all pressure change is positive, and all work is done by the ventilator. An assisted breath involves work by both ventilator and patient—it is delivered by the ventilator under positive pressure but is initiated (triggered) by the patient's muscular effort, which produces an initially negative pressure deflection. A spontaneous breath reflects only the patient's work, and airway pressure becomes positive only during exhalation as the tidal breath is expelled.

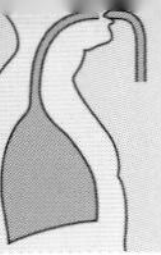

Table 14.5
Types and modes of positive-pressure ventilation

Type	Mode	Description
Conventional positive pressure ventilation: tidal volume (VT) preset (volume or time cycled)	Assisted mechanical ventilation or assist/control	All breaths machine delivered at preset VT Patient can increase rate (and thus minute ventilation) by triggering additional machine breaths if desired
	Controlled mechanical ventilation (CMV)	All breaths machine delivered at preset VT Fixed rate (and minute ventilation) cannot be increased by patient effort
	Intermittent mandatory ventilation (IMV)	Fixed rate of machine-delivered, set VT breaths Patient can also breathe spontaneously between machine-delivered breaths if desired
	Synchronized intermittent mandatory ventilation	As in IMV, except that machine-delivered breaths are initiated only after the patient exhales, which prevents 'stacking' on spontaneous breaths
Conventional positive pressure ventilation: peak pressure preset (flow or time cycled)	Pressure support ventilation	Patient breathes spontaneously and determines rate VT is determined by inflation pressure used and patient's lung–thorax compliance Minute ventilation varies, depending on inflation pressure used
	Pressure control ventilation	Inflation pressure, inspiratory time, and rate are fixed, with VT (and thus minute ventilation) determined by patient's lung–thorax compliance
	Airway pressure release ventilation	Patient breathes spontaneously at high level of continuous positive airway pressure (CPAP), which is intermittently dropped to a lower level to allow brief passive exhalation to a lower lung volume Minute ventilation determined by patient's spontaneous rate and inspiratory effort plus CPAP levels used and frequency of pressure release
High-frequency ventilation	High-frequency positive pressure ventilation	Preset (usually small) VT, as with assisted mechanical ventilation, CMV, or IMV, at cycling frequencies of 60–110 breaths/minute
	High-frequency jet ventilation	Bursts of high-pressure (jet) gas flow directly into patient's trachea at rates of 60–150 bursts/minute Delivered VT augmented by entrainment from a second, humidified gas source VT and minute ventilation are unknown
	High-frequency oscillatory ventilation	Oscillation of gas in the respiratory tract at 600–1200 cycles/minute (10–20 Hz) with both inspiration and expiration active

Adapted from Pierson DJ: Respiratory therapy techniques. In Kelly WN (ed): Textbook of Internal Medicine, 3rd ed. Philadelphia, Lippincott-Raven, 1999, pp 2127–2133

means that airway pressure during a given breath can vary, depending on the resistance to airflow during inspiration and on the patient's lung and chest wall compliance. As shown in Figure 14.2, the pressure profile of a volume-targeted breath has several components. Once the breath has been delivered, an end-inspiratory hold maneuver can be performed to measure the static or plateau pressure (Pplat). The latter is a reflection of respiratory system distention and is used to calculate the static compliance of the respiratory system ($\Delta V/\Delta P$). During inspiration, airway pressure reflects the resistance to flow as well as the compliance of the system. Thus, an increase in inspiratory flow, bronchospasm, or airway secretions increases PImax but does not affect Pplat.

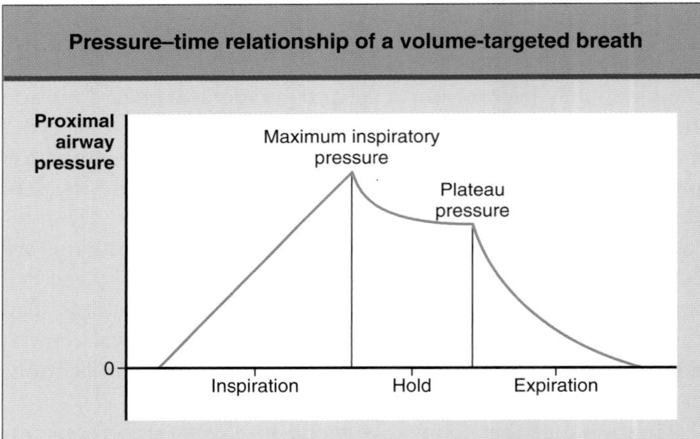

Figure 14.2 Pressure-time relationship of a volume-targeted breath. A single positive pressure breath, starting from zero end-expiratory pressure. An end-inspiratory hold maneuver is performed to determine static or plateau pressure (Pplat). Maximum inspiratory pressure (PImax) reflects airway resistance during inspiration and is higher than Pplat in this volume-targeted breath. Increased inspiratory flow or a narrowing of the airway increases PImax but does not affect Pplat.

VOLUME-TARGETED MODES

The most commonly used volume-targeted ventilator modes are shown in Figure 14.3. These are controlled mechanical ventilation (CMV), assist/control (A/C) ventilation, and synchronized intermittent mandatory ventilation (SIMV). With CMV, the patient receives a preset number of fixed-volume breaths and cannot increase minute ventilation by triggering more machine breaths or by breathing spontaneously between them. The difference between A/C ventilation and CMV is that, with the former, the patient may trigger additional fixed-volume machine breaths if desired. With intermittent mandatory ventilation (IMV), a fixed number of preset-volume breaths are delivered by the ventilator, but the patient (if capable) can also breathe spontaneously from the ventilator circuit. Conceptually, IMV is somewhat like being on both CMV and a T-piece at the same time. The theoretical risk of "stacking" a mandatory breath on top of a large spontaneous breath, which would produce barotrauma, means that most ventilators deliver IMV in such a way that mandatory breaths can be delivered only after expiration is sensed, called SIMV.

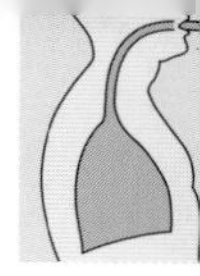

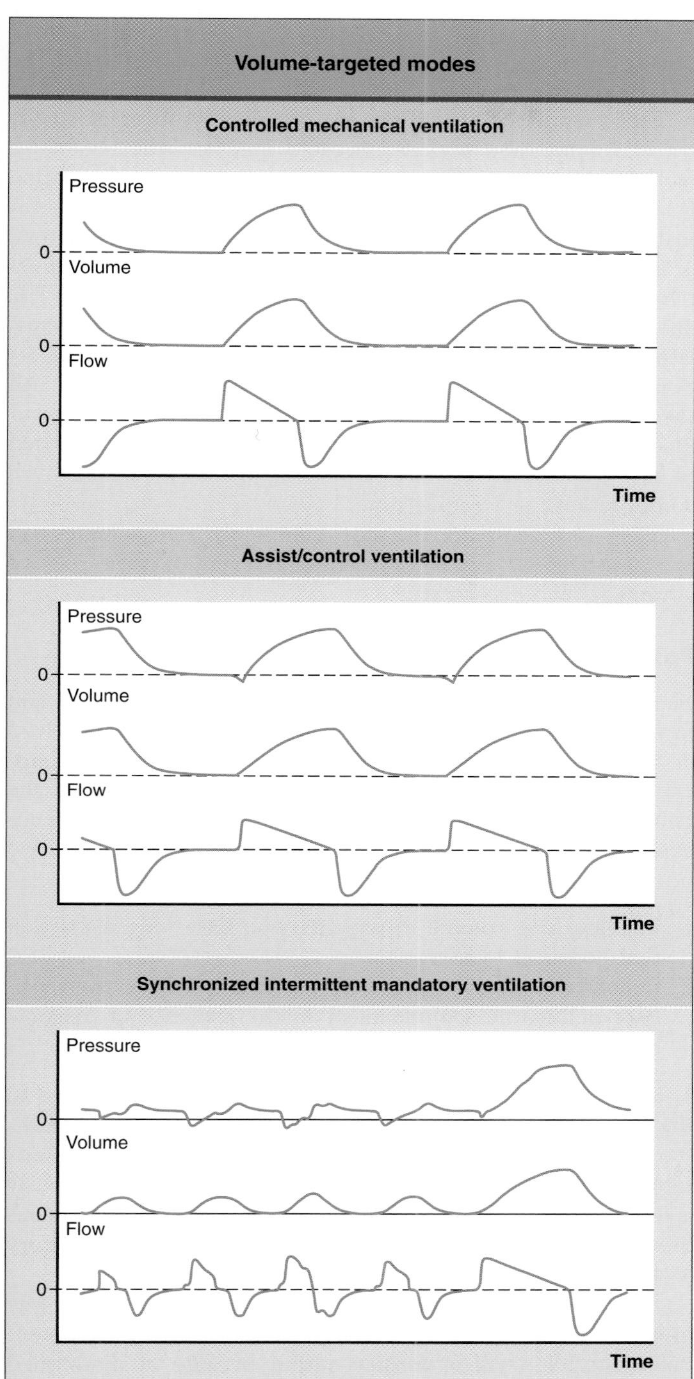

Figure 14.3 Volume-targeted modes. Changes in pressure at the airway opening, lung volume, and flow during controlled mechanical ventilation (CMV), assist/control (A/C) ventilation, and synchronized intermittent mandatory ventilation (SIMV). With CMV, all breaths are machine-triggered mandatory breaths, and the patient is passive throughout the cycle. Essentially, A/C ventilation is the same as CMV, except that the patient may, if desired, trigger the set-volume machine breaths at a more rapid rate. With SIMV, a set number of machine-triggered, mandatory breaths is delivered, as with CMV. However, in SIMV, the patient can also breathe spontaneously between mandatory breaths if desired. When the mandatory rate in SIMV is sufficient to provide all the ventilation the patient needs, this mode is effectively the same as CMV.

Full ventilatory support is provided by CMV, which means that all work performed on the respiratory system during ventilation is provided by the ventilator. In A/C ventilation, full ventilatory support is provided when the patient is not triggering, but partial ventilatory support is provided when the patient breathes at a rate greater than the fixed backup rate. In SIMV, full ventilatory support is provided when the patient is not attempting to breathe above the mandatory rate, and partial ventilatory support is provided when any spontaneous ventilation is present.

PRESSURE-TARGETED MODES

A number of modes are available that preset the maximum inflation pressure rather than a fixed VT. Most widely used among these are pressure support ventilation (PSV) and pressure control ventilation (PCV), illustrated in Figure 14.4.

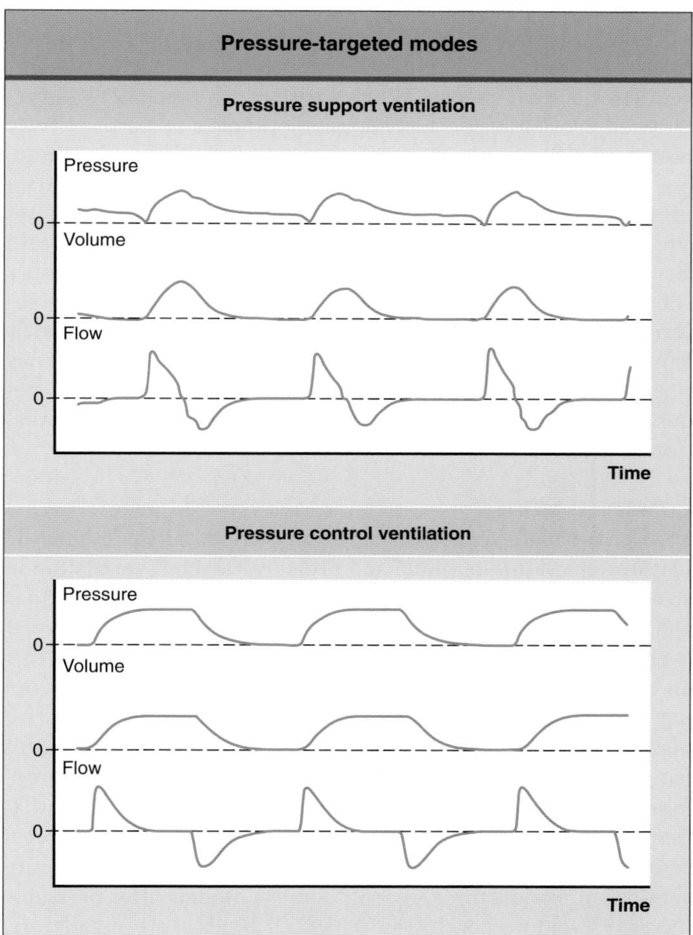

Figure 14.4 Pressure-targeted modes. Changes in pressure at the airway opening, lung volume, and flow during pressure support ventilation (PSV) and pressure control ventilation (PCV). The former is essentially spontaneous breathing with a preset positive pressure that boosts each inspiration. Patients on PSV receive no ventilation if apnea occurs. In that the rate is fixed and the patient cannot trigger additional breaths or breathe spontaneously between mandatory breaths, PCV is analogous to controlled mechanical ventilation (CMV; see Fig. 14.3); it differs from CMV in that maximum inspiratory pressure rather than tidal volume is fixed, and both tidal volume and minute ventilation can vary if the patient's lung-thorax compliance or airway resistance changes.

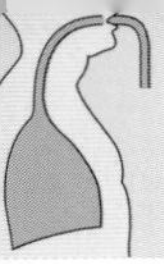

With PSV, the patient breathes spontaneously and is assisted with every breath to reach a preset inspiratory pressure target. This is conceptually the same as intermittent positive pressure breathing, although the technical aspects of its delivery are different. Pressure support can be combined with SIMV, so that when the patient takes a spontaneous breath over and above the set frequency of mandatory volume-targeted breaths, inspiration is assisted to the set pressure support level.

Similar to CMV, with PCV, the rate is fixed and cannot be increased by patient effort, but a difference is that the peak inflation pressure rather than the VT is set (see Fig. 14.4). Technically, the term for this mode is *pressure-controlled continuous mandatory ventilation*. On some ventilators, it is also possible to deliver pressure-controlled A/C ventilation and SIMV. Pressure-controlled inverse-ratio ventilation is not a separate mode; rather, it is PCV with the inspiratory phase longer than expiration. This variant of PCV has been used in patients who have severe hypoxemic respiratory failure in an attempt to improve oxygenation, but its popularity has waned because of the high incidence of hemodynamic compromise and barotrauma.

A key distinction between volume- and pressure-targeted modes is what happens when the mechanics of the patient-ventilator system change. When a patient who receives volume-targeted ventilation develops a pneumothorax or partial airway obstruction by inspissated secretions, the same VT is delivered, but at higher peak and static airway pressures. However, with pressure-targeted ventilation, maximal airway pressure is preset and cannot increase under these circumstances. Instead, with airway obstruction or a decrease in compliance, the pressure stays the same, and the delivered VT decreases. Thus, complications may be manifested differently in the different modes. When managing a patient whose pulmonary process may improve rapidly, as in acute asthma or pulmonary edema, frequent ventilator adjustments are needed when pressure ventilation is used.

COMBINED MODES

Most critical care ventilators of recent manufacture combine the features of volume-targeted and pressure-targeted ventilation in an attempt to avoid the high peak airway pressures of the former and the varying VTs that may occur with the latter. Of interest is the fact that peak airway pressure has no deleterious effect on the lung if the setting resulting in the elevated pressure does not simultaneously increase Pplat. Nonetheless, in a competitive market, manufacturers have attempted to make unique combinations, and several apparently new modes have appeared. Essentially, these combinations consist of either volume ventilation, with high inspiratory flow and a limitation on peak pressure, or pressure ventilation regulated to provide a preset minute ventilation. For example, recent Siemens models offer pressure-regulated volume control, in which all breaths are mandatory, the rate is fixed, and the inspiratory pressure is varied to maintain a preset VT. These same ventilators also offer volume support, a combined mode that consists of PSV with a preset target VT or minute volume, which the ventilator achieves by adding mandatory breaths; the inspiratory pressures of these breaths are varied as necessary to achieve the set volume goal. Auto-mode, a third variation provided on recent Siemens critical care ventilators, essentially combines pressure-regulated volume control and volume support. Auto-mode combines dual-control breath-to-breath time-cycled breaths with dual-control breath-to-breath flow-cycled breaths, with patient effort or the lack thereof determining how individual breaths are cycled.

Each manufacturer features its own slightly different blending of volume- and pressure-targeted modes. Other examples include auto-flow (Drager), adaptive pressure regulation (Hamilton), and volume-assured pressure support (Bird). Automatic tube compensation, a feature of recent Drager ventilators, is not a mode per se but rather an attempt to overcome the resistive work of breathing added by the endotracheal tube. The operator enters the endotracheal tube diameter, and the ventilator applies positive pressure to overcome the desired proportion of calculated tube resistance via closed-loop control. All these so-called combined modes are intended to give the manufacturers a market advantage, but none has been demonstrated to have a detectable effect on clinical outcomes such as survival, complications, or weaning time.

Table 14.6 compares the most commonly used volume- and pressure-targeted ventilator modes in terms of their relative advantages and disadvantages.

Positive End-Expiratory Pressure

Manipulation of inspiration by means of the phase variables and modes just discussed is one of the two main processes involved in mechanical ventilation. The other is manipulation of end-expiratory pressure, which may be kept equal to that of the atmosphere or deliberately raised to produce positive end-expiratory pressure (PEEP). The application of PEEP has two primary purposes:

1. Increase lung volume in patients who have lung restriction that produces hypoxemia.
2. Reduce the effort required for patients to trigger the ventilator or breathe spontaneously in the presence of dynamic hyperinflation and auto-PEEP (see later).

When PEEP is applied to the breathing circuit connected to the closed respiratory system of an intubated patient, all breaths start and end at a pressure above ambient. Continuous pressurization of the system from which a patient breathes spontaneously is referred to as CPAP, a term applicable only during spontaneous breathing. Whenever positive pressure above the end-expiratory level is applied during inspiration, the term PEEP is used.

Because end-expiratory, end-inspiratory, and mean airway pressures are all increased in the presence of PEEP, the potential exists for a fall in cardiac output because of diminished venous return to the right side of the heart. Regional or generalized lung overdistention can also stretch pulmonary vessels, which can either expand or narrow their caliber (depending on whether the vessels are alveolar or extra-alveolar in location) and can increase or decrease pulmonary vascular resistance. Resistance generally decreases, but this could be due to either vascular narrowing or the reduction in cardiac output that frequently occurs concurrently. In the presence of a reduced cardiac output secondary to either or both of these mechanisms, any gain in arterial oxygenation may be offset, and tissue oxygen delivery may actually fall. In addition, the application of PEEP may increase end-inspiratory lung volume to the point where individual lung units become overdistended and rupture alveolar membranes, leading to clinical barotrauma.

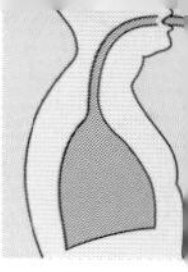

Table 14.6
Advantages and disadvantages of the different commonly used ventilator modes

Mode	Advantages	Disadvantages	Appropriate Clinical Circumstances	Inappropriate Clinical Circumstances
Assisted mechanical ventilation (AMV) or assist/control ventilation	Can respond to increased need for ventilation by increasing machine rate Decreased oxygen consumption in patients who have high work of breathing compared with low-rate intermittent mandatory ventilation (IMV) or spontaneous breathing	Higher mean intrathoracic pressure than with modes that provide partial ventilatory support Respiratory alkalosis in dyspneic or agitated patients if inspiratory flows and/or sedation is insufficient	Any patient who requires mechanical ventilation Increased work of spontaneous breathing, as in high minute ventilation or small endotracheal tube Depressed or fluctuating ventilatory drive	Respiratory alkalosis unresponsive to ventilator adjustment and/or sedation Use with Siemens Servo 900C ventilator in dyspneic patient who has normal or low minute ventilation (insufficient flow during inspiration)
Controlled mechanical ventilation (CMV)	Decreased oxygen consumption in patients who have high spontaneous work of breathing Rests ventilatory muscles Least complicated and least expensive mode for long-term ventilation	Cannot respond to increased need for ventilation by either machine-delivered or spontaneous breaths Patient distress if alert and dyspneic Usually requires heavy sedation with or without paralysis	Paralysis or neurologic injury rendering patient incapable of any spontaneous ventilation Deliberate hyperventilation to reduce intracranial pressure	Any patient who is capable of triggering a ventilator breath
Intermittent mandatory ventilation (IMV); synchronized IMV	May reduce patient–ventilator asynchrony Lower mean intrathoracic pressure than with AMV if used for partial ventilatory support Can provide periodic deep breaths to prevent atelectasis in intubated patients who have very low spontaneous tidal volumes (VTs)	Cannot respond to increased patient demand with increased ventilator minute volume Increased work of breathing for patient as compared with AMV when used for partial ventilatory support Tends to increase total time on ventilator when used for gradual weaning	Any patient who requires invasive mechanical ventilation, provided inappropriate circumstances (next column) are not present Use for partial ventilatory support in patients who have hypovolemia and hypotension on AMV As an alternative volume-targeted mode when patients do not tolerate AMV	Use as partial ventilatory support in patients who have depressed or fluctuating ventilatory drive, ventilatory muscle paralysis or weakness, or in the presence of a small-diameter endotracheal tube
Pressure support ventilation	Increased peak inspiratory flow as compared with volume modes Lower mean intrathoracic pressure than with AMV or IMV Less distressing than volume-preset modes for some patients Can provide smooth transition to spontaneous ventilation during weaning	VT and minute ventilation are not assured Hypoventilation or apnea if patient's ventilatory drive fluctuates Requires closer monitoring of gas exchange and mechanics in critically ill patients than does AMV or IMV Repeated triggering of apnea alarm in patients who have Cheyne-Stokes respiration	As a stand-alone mode for patients who have intact ventilatory drive and who require modest inflation pressures As a transitional mode during recovery from severe acute respiratory distress syndrome (ARDS) or other acute respiratory failure During weaning in any patient in whom decreasing the level of ventilatory support is appropriate	Absent or fluctuating ventilatory drive Rapidly changing lung or chest wall mechanics (e.g., bronchospasm, pulmonary edema) because of need for repeated pressure adjustments
Pressure control ventilation	Increased peak inspiratory flow as compared with volume modes Improved distribution of ventilation in some patients who have severe oxygenation failure, and may result in improved oxygenation and/or decreased alveolar pressure in comparison with AMV or IMV	VT and minute ventilation are not assured Requires closer monitoring of gas exchange and mechanics than does AMV or IMV Need to switch to another mode for weaning	Critically ill patients who have ARDS or other severe acute respiratory failure when appropriately skilled personnel are continuously available	Use for routine ventilatory support Use in any patient when personnel experienced with its use are not available on a continuous basis

POSITIVE END-EXPIRATORY PRESSURE TRIAL

Whenever feasible, a systematic, incremental PEEP trial should be performed in a controlled manner (Table 14.7). Ideally, only one variable—the amount of PEEP—is altered during the trial, with VT, fraction of inspired oxygen (FIO_2), position, and other factors that might affect oxygenation left unchanged. Both favorable and adverse PEEP effects are assessed at each level as PEEP is increased. Because the condition of the patient may change over time, the intervals at each level must be kept short.

As PEEP is increased, the occurrence of cardiac impairment becomes more likely. Direct measurement of cardiac output during the trial is recommended if any of the following circumstances exist:

- Levels of PEEP used are likely to impair cardiac function (e.g., $\geq 15\,cmH_2O$).
- Unexplained tachycardia or other manifestations of possible hypovolemia are present.
- The patient has underlying cardiac disease.

Changes in cardiac output and lung compliance are likely to occur rapidly following an increase in PEEP and should be sought within the first 3 to 5 minutes at each level.

As PEEP is increased, PaO_2 is measured sequentially as the primary index of a favorable response. If a substantial increase in PaO_2 occurs with no evidence of either cardiac impairment or alveolar overdistention (as assessed using static compliance),

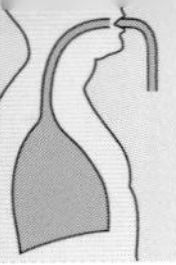

Table 14.7
Protocol for systematic positive end-expiratory pressure trial

Protocol	Comments
1. Obtain baseline respiratory and hemodynamic data before initiating positive end-expiratory pressure (PEEP) and at each level employed in trial	Respiratory data (all patients) – fraction of inspired oxygen (FIO_2), PEEP level, corrected tidal volume, respiratory rate (mandatory, total), peak inspiratory pressure, end-inspiratory plateau pressure, partial pressure of arterial blood gases (PaO_2, $PaCO_2$), and pH Additional respiratory data (in extremely ill or unstable patients, or for more aggressive management approach) – mixed venous PO_2 and saturation, arterial and mixed venous O_2 contents Hemodynamic data (all patients) – heart rate, blood pressure, continuous electrocardiographic monitoring Cardiac output measurement – recommended for use of PEEP >15 cmH_2O, suspected hypovolemia (unexplained tachycardia), or coexistent cardiac disease
2. Change only one variable at a time (i.e., PEEP level)	Keep tidal volume, FIO_2, and other ventilator settings the same at each level Avoid transfusion, position changes, changes in pressor infusions during trial if possible
3. Keep time intervals between PEEP increments short (e.g., 15–20 minutes)	To minimize confounding data from changes in patient's underlying condition
4. Apply PEEP in sequential increments (e.g., 5 cmH_2O)	Smaller increments may prolong trial Larger increments increase likelihood of adverse effects
5. Monitor for immediate adverse effects at each new PEEP level (e.g., after 3–5 minutes)	Hypotension or >20% fall in cardiac output Fall in respiratory system compliance Cardiac arrhythmias or increased intracranial pressure, where appropriate
6. Assess arterial oxygenation and other respiratory data collection as in step 1 above once patient has stabilized at each new PEEP level (e.g., 15 minutes)	–
7. Evaluate overall cardiorespiratory response at each PEEP level used	Favorable – improved oxygenation, improved compliance Unfavorable – hypotension, decreased cardiac output, decreased compliance, decreased oxygenation
8. Assess results in light of overall goals for PEEP therapy	If O_2 delivery has improved without adverse effects, leave patient on current PEEP level, reduce FIO_2 if possible, and re-evaluate frequently as indicated If oxygenation is still inadequate or FIO_2 is still unacceptably high, and no adverse effects have occurred, increase PEEP sequentially, applying steps 4–7 above If O_2 delivery has decreased or compliance has fallen significantly at new PEEP level, return patient to previous PEEP level and re-evaluate if: Deterioration results from decreased PO_2; reassess indications for PEEP Deterioration results from decreased cardiac output; consider volume loading or administration of pressor drugs Compliance has fallen but O_2 delivery has not decreased; consider reducing tidal volume to reduce risk of alveolar rupture and ventilator-induced lung injury

that PEEP level can be maintained and the FIO_2 titrated downward to maintain the target PaO_2. Improvements in PaO_2 tend to occur more slowly than do changes in cardiac function or compliance as PEEP is increased, and arterial blood gas specimens should be drawn 10 to 20 minutes after each change. Suggested guidelines are given in Table 14.8.

WEANING POSITIVE END-EXPIRATORY PRESSURE

Previously, empirical recommendations for applying and discontinuing PEEP were used. More recently, advances in the understanding of ventilator-induced lung injury, along with results from major clinical trials, have led to a new overall approach to the ventilator management of acute lung injury and the acute respiratory distress syndrome (ARDS). The lung-protective ventilation protocol summarized in Figure 14.5 and the FIO_2-PEEP "ladder" shown in Table 14.9 provide guidance for both PEEP trials and PEEP weaning as presented here.

Ventilator Management Based on Clinical Setting

Guidelines for ventilator management according to clinical setting are given in Table 14.8.

ROUTINE VENTILATORY SUPPORT

Most patients who require a period of invasive mechanical ventilation have relatively normal underlying lung function. What may be referred to as "routine" ventilatory support is encountered most frequently in the postoperative period or in the setting of short-term loss of spontaneous ventilation, such as with a drug overdose. In such settings, a volume-targeted mode is simplest and most reliable and usually requires fewer adjustments than does pressure-targeted ventilation. Some clinicians prefer to add 5 cmH_2O of PEEP routinely to counteract the modest drop in functional residual capacity (FRC) that has been shown to occur with endotracheal intubation. This is probably unnecessary in most patients, and most important, the

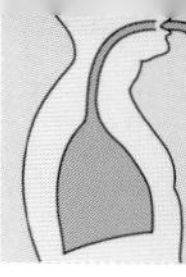

Table 14.8
Guidelines for ventilator settings according to diagnosis and clinical circumstances

Clinical Setting (Examples)	Clinical Objectives	Mode	Tidal Volume	Target pH/Partial Pressure of Carbon Dioxide ($Paco_2$)	Target Pao_2/ Oxygen Saturation by Pulse Oximetry (Spo_2)	Positive End-Expiratory Pressure (PEEP)	Comments
Routine (postoperative ventilation, drug overdose)	Prevent atelectasis, maintain normal acid–base balance, avoid hypoxemia, avoid O_2 toxicity	Volume	10–12 mL/kg	Normal	Normal	0–5 cmH_2O	These settings are appropriate for the majority of patients who require mechanical ventilation
Obstructive lung disease (chronic obstructive pulmonary disease, asthma)	Unload ventilatory muscles, prevent further hyperinflation, maintain acid–base balance appropriate for patient, facilitate weaning	Either volume or pressure	5–8 mL/kg	Permissive hypercapnia and acidemia (avoid acute alkalosis)	Normal	0–5 cmH_2O; more if auto-PEEP present (see Table 14.13)	Noninvasive ventilation is preferable if not contraindicated (see Chapter 12)
Acute lung injury and acute respiratory distress syndrome (ARDS)	Support oxygenation (Fio_2 versus PEEP); preserve circulatory function; avoid ventilator-induced lung injury and clinical barotrauma	Either volume or pressure	≤ 6 mL/kg (predicted body weight) to achieve goals for tidal volume and end-inspiratory plateau pressure	Permissive hypercapnia and acidemia (if not contraindicated)	Pao_2 55-70 mm Hg; Spo_2 88–94%	Sufficient to maintain target oxygenation without impairing cardiac function (see Fig. 14.6)	This 'lung-protective' ventilatory strategy requires appropriate sedation (see Table 14.9)
Focal or unilateral pulmonary disease (lobar pneumonia or atelectasis)	Avoid worsening hypoxemia, avoid clinical barotrauma, avoid circulatory compromise	Volume	10–12 mL/kg	Normal	Normal; may not be achievable in presence of large shunt effect	Avoid or use cautiously (see Table 14.7)	PEEP may worsen hypoxemia by overdistending uninvolved areas of lung and increasing shunt effect
Acute neuromuscular disease without acute lung injury (Guillain-Barré syndrome, cervical spinal cord injury)	Avoid atelectasis, minimize dyspnea	Volume	12–16 mL/kg	Normal or mild acute respiratory alkalosis	Normal (avoid even mild hypoxemia)	0–5 cmH_2O unless required for oxygenation	Such patients usually prefer high inspiratory flows and large tidal volumes, and often maintain a respiratory alkalosis
Acute brain injury (head trauma)	Avoid compromising cerebral perfusion pressure, decrease intracranial pressure	Volume	10–12 mL/kg	Normal or acute respiratory alkalosis [$Paco_2$ 3.3–4.0 kPa (25–30 mmHg)]	Normal	Avoid	Value of acute respiratory alkalosis disputed except for emergent, short-term reduction of very high intracranial pressure
Flail chest	Maintain adequate lung inflation and gas exchange	Volume	10–12 mL/kg unless acute lung injury also present	Normal	Normal	5 cmH_2O or as needed for support of oxygenation	Ventilatory support usually unnecessary unless acute lung injury also present

PEEP-induced increase in FRC is just as likely to come at the expense of overexpanding open alveoli rather than opening parts of the lung located below their closing volume.

Healthy individuals normally breathe with a VT of 5 to 7 mL/kg. However, diffuse microatelectasis and an increased difference in alveolar and arterial PO_2 ($PAO_2 - PaO_2$) soon develop because of decreased surfactant function if these individuals do not more fully expand their lungs several times per hour by sighing. The same problem exists with intubated patients who have normal lungs and who are ventilated with "normal" VTs in the absence of sigh breaths. The need for sighs, which in the presence of pulmonary disease might overdistend and rupture alveoli, can be obviated if a larger VT (10 to 12 mL/kg) is used.

The cycling rate and hence minute ventilation are adjusted to provide normal arterial pH and PCO_2 values (e.g., 7.40 ± 0.05 units and 5.3 ± 0.6 kPa [40 ± 5 mmHg], respectively). Enough supplemental oxygen is used to prevent hypoxemia, although maintaining PaO_2 greater than 13.3 kPa (>100 mmHg) is unnecessary.

OBSTRUCTIVE LUNG DISEASE

Patients with severe COPD or asthma are at increased risk for circulatory impairment and barotrauma when subjected to invasive mechanical ventilation, and a number of modifications of the routine approach are required.

Patients with COPD have hyperinflation as part of their stable disease (i.e., increased FRC), and the degree of hyperinflation increases during acute exacerbations. Patients with asthma generally do not have chronic hyperinflation (unless they are suboptimally treated), but they develop hyperinflation during acute exacerbations. The three main goals of invasive mechanical ventilation in patients who have acutely exacerbated COPD or acute severe asthma are to:

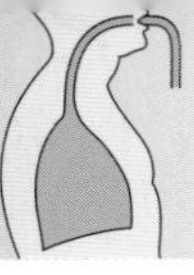

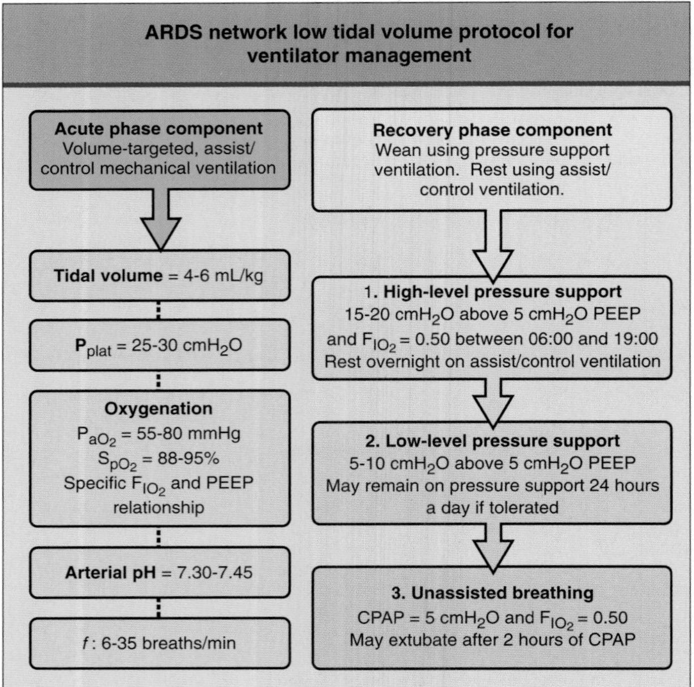

Figure 14.5 Acute Respiratory Distress Syndrome Network low tidal volume protocol for ventilator management. The protocol has two main components. The acute phase component (left) uses volume-targeted assist/control ventilation with five interdependent algorithm parts. The recovery phase component (right) uses graded pressure support ventilation to facilitate the patient's transition to unassisted breathing. CPAP, continuous positive airway pressure; f, respiratory rate; FIO_2, fraction of inspired oxygen; PaO_2, arterial partial pressure of oxygen; PEEP, positive end-expiratory pressure; Pplat, end-inspiratory plateau pressure; SpO_2, arterial oxygen saturation measured by pulse oximetry. (From Kallet RH, Corral W, Silverman HJ, Luce JM: Implementation of a low tidal volume ventilation protocol for patients with acute lung injury or acute respiratory distress syndrome. Respir Care 46:1024-1037, 2001.)

1. Rest the ventilatory muscles (thereby decreasing the work of breathing and the carbon dioxide production resulting from this increased work).
2. Avoid further dynamic hyperinflation.
3. Avoid overventilation and acute alkalemia.

Resting the ventilatory muscles can be achieved by providing full ventilatory support using volume-targeted ventilation (either A/C ventilation or SIMV), so that the patient makes no respiratory effort; by providing partial ventilatory support using PSV; or by providing PEEP to reduce the inspiratory work of breathing.

This is one of the two clinical settings in which permissive hypercapnia is appropriate, the other being acute lung injury (discussed later). When the degree of airflow limitation is severe, it may not be possible to provide a sufficient minute ventilation (i.e., respiratory rate × VT) to reduce the $PaCO_2$ enough to produce a normal pH without worsening the hyperinflation. In obstructive lung disease, PEEP serves a different function than in acute lung injury. Its purpose here is not to increase lung volume (which is already excessive) but to decrease the muscular effort required to trigger the ventilator or breathe spontaneously in the presence of dynamic hyperinflation and auto-PEEP.

Table 14.9
"PEEP-F_{IO_2} titration ladder" for determining ventilator settings during lung-protective ventilation

F_{IO_2}	PEEP (cm H_2O)
0.30	5
0.40	5
0.40	8
0.50	8
0.50	10
0.60	10
0.60	12
0.70	12
0.70	14
0.80	14
0.90	14
0.90	16
0.90	18
1.00	18
1.00	20+

ACUTE LUNG INJURY

The goals of mechanical ventilation in acute lung injury and ARDS are to:

- Support oxygenation.
- Limit or reduce circulatory compromise.
- Limit or reduce ventilator-induced lung injury.

The first of these goals is accomplished through manipulations of FIO_2 and PEEP, the aim of which is to balance the risks of pulmonary oxygen toxicity with those of raised intrathoracic pressures and lung volumes. Attempts to avoid ventilator-induced lung injury include a lung-protective ventilation strategy that involves low VT, limited alveolar pressure, and permissive hypercapnia (see Chapter 65).

Either volume- or pressure-targeted ventilation may be used to manage ARDS. Currently, best evidence indicates that a lung-protective ventilation strategy that keeps VT to a maximum of 6 mL/kg predicted body weight and avoids Pplat above 30 cmH_2O (as outlined in Fig. 14.5) minimizes ventilator-induced lung injury and reduces mortality. Because of the increasing prevalence of obesity throughout the world and the risk of unintended lung overdistention in overweight patients if admission weight rather than predicted body weight is used to determine VT, the following formulas are used to determine initial settings:

Males: Predicted body weight (kg) =
50 + 2.3 [(height in cm − 152) ÷ 2.54] =
50 + 2.3 (height in inches − 60)

Females: Predicted body weight (kg) =
45.5 + 2.3 [(height in cm − 152) ÷ 2.54] =
45.5 + 2.3 (height in inches − 60)

The rate must be adjusted so that auto-PEEP does not develop, a limitation that results in hypercapnia in a minority of patients. Most patients tolerate arterial pH values in the range of 7.2 to 7.3 without difficulty, and bicarbonate infusion is not used by most authorities unless the value falls well below this range.

In managing patients who have severe ARDS, the clinician may need to accept permissive hypoxemia as well as permissive hypercapnia. Although the goal is to maintain PaO_2 in the normal range, this may not be attainable in some patients without the use of potentially injurious levels of PEEP. When this occurs, most clinicians attempt a trial of prone positioning; this maneuver increases oxygenation to a clinically meaningful degree in two thirds to three fourths of the patients in whom it is tried. A PaO_2 of 6.6 to 8.0 kPa (50 to 60 mmHg) (oxygen saturation as measured by pulse oximetry [SpO_2] 80% to 90%) is usually well tolerated if hemoglobin concentration and cardiac function are adequate. Because both hypercapnia and hypoxemia can distress patients, appropriate sedation is required when pursuing the lung-protective ventilatory strategy in ARDS (see Fig. 14.5). The PEEP-FIO_2 "ladder" (see Table 14.9) titrates these two ventilator settings according to the original ARDS Network protocol, on which the scheme in Figure 14.5 is based. A second study comparing this "ladder" for setting PEEP and FIO_2 to a similar titration using higher PEEP levels and correspondingly lower FIO_2s found no difference in patient outcome.

UNILATERAL OR ASYMMETRICAL LUNG DISEASE

Patients who have lobar pneumonia, lobar or whole-lung atelectasis, and other markedly asymmetrical pulmonary involvement present a special problem, particularly in the presence of severe hypoxemia. Such patients illustrate why PEEP should not automatically be applied as treatment for hypoxemic respiratory failure. Respiratory system compliance is much higher in relatively normal areas of lung than in areas of consolidation or collapse. As a result, application of PEEP may have more deleterious effects on cardiac output, resulting in a fall in the mixed venous oxygen. When this occurs, the effect of any degree of shunt or ventilation-perfusion heterogeneity becomes magnified. Accordingly, applying PEEP can worsen rather than improve arterial oxygenation. Some patients who have hypoxemic respiratory failure and apparently asymmetrical lung involvement respond favorably to PEEP, however, which emphasizes the need to perform PEEP trials.

NEUROMUSCULAR DISEASE

Patients who have acute neuromuscular disease or cervical spinal cord injury and whose lung function is relatively normal may benefit from ventilator management at higher than usual V_Ts and flows. Such patients may experience dyspnea at V_Ts of 10 to 12 mL/kg, which improves when larger volumes (12 to 16 mL/kg) are used. Similarly, these patients typically prefer faster inspiratory flows (e.g., 80 to 100 L/minute). Such settings often result in a mild to moderate respiratory alkalosis, which is usually well tolerated and is soon accompanied by a compensatory metabolic acidosis. Alternatively, low levels of PEEP may accomplish the same relief of dyspnea as the attendant hyperventilation.

Many patients who have traumatic quadriplegia or other acute neuromuscular disorders experience recurrent atelectasis, which can cause more severe hypoxemia than is usually seen with lobar collapse in other clinical settings. Ventilation with larger than usual V_Ts, with or without the addition of low-level PEEP, is important in such patients to prevent recurrence. Frequent changes in posture may also be beneficial.

ACUTE BRAIN INJURY

Patients who have closed head injury or other acute brain insult may lose the normal autoregulation of cerebral perfusion pressure. In such patients, anything that decreases mean arterial pressure or raises central venous pressure must be avoided. Thus, PEEP is used cautiously, if at all, in patients who have acute brain injury, because the raised intrathoracic pressure is transmitted via the vertebral veins to the central nervous system. Maneuvers that induce coughing and may raise intracranial pressure, such as tracheal suctioning, are avoided whenever possible in these patients.

For many years, deliberate hyperventilation to arterial PCO_2 levels of 3.3 to 4.0 kPa (25 to 30 mmHg) was an integral part of ventilator management in patients who had acute brain injury. Results of recent studies call this practice into question, however, and hyperventilation is no longer used in many institutions, except as a temporary emergency measure while other treatments for intracranial hypertension are initiated.

FLAIL CHEST

Several studies demonstrate that the clinical course and outcome of flail chest injury are determined mainly by the underlying pulmonary injury rather than the flail segment per se. Patients who sustain multiple rib fractures without associated lung contusion or pneumonia generally recover uneventfully. Flail chest in the setting of acute lung injury typically follows the course of that illness, with little separate contribution from the chest wall instability.

Thus, mechanical ventilation in patients who have a flail chest injury is essentially intended to manage the underlying pulmonary condition. Attention must be given to pain control, however, particularly when only partial ventilatory support is used, because this forces the patient to use the intercostal muscles associated with the flail. Many clinicians prefer to use full ventilatory support until the patient is ready for weaning. Intercostal nerve blocks or the administration of epidural narcotics can greatly aid in pain control and ventilator weaning in such patients.

Weaning and Extubation

Clinicians have multiple options when reducing or discontinuing ventilatory support (Fig. 14.6), which has resulted in considerable controversy regarding the best approach.

BASIC APPROACH TO WEANING

In the recent past, there was a fundamental change in the approach to discontinuing invasive mechanical ventilation—from "predicting" to "checking." For the last 30 years, clinicians have used a variety of measures of ventilatory mechanics to identify the point at which a patient was ready to switch from full ventilatory support to fully spontaneous breathing. These predictive measures, or "weaning parameters," included spontaneous respiratory rate, often divided by the patient's average spontaneous V_T during a brief disconnection from the ventilator (f/V_T, or the "rapid shallow breathing index"); inspiratory

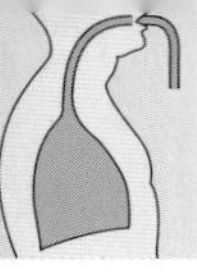

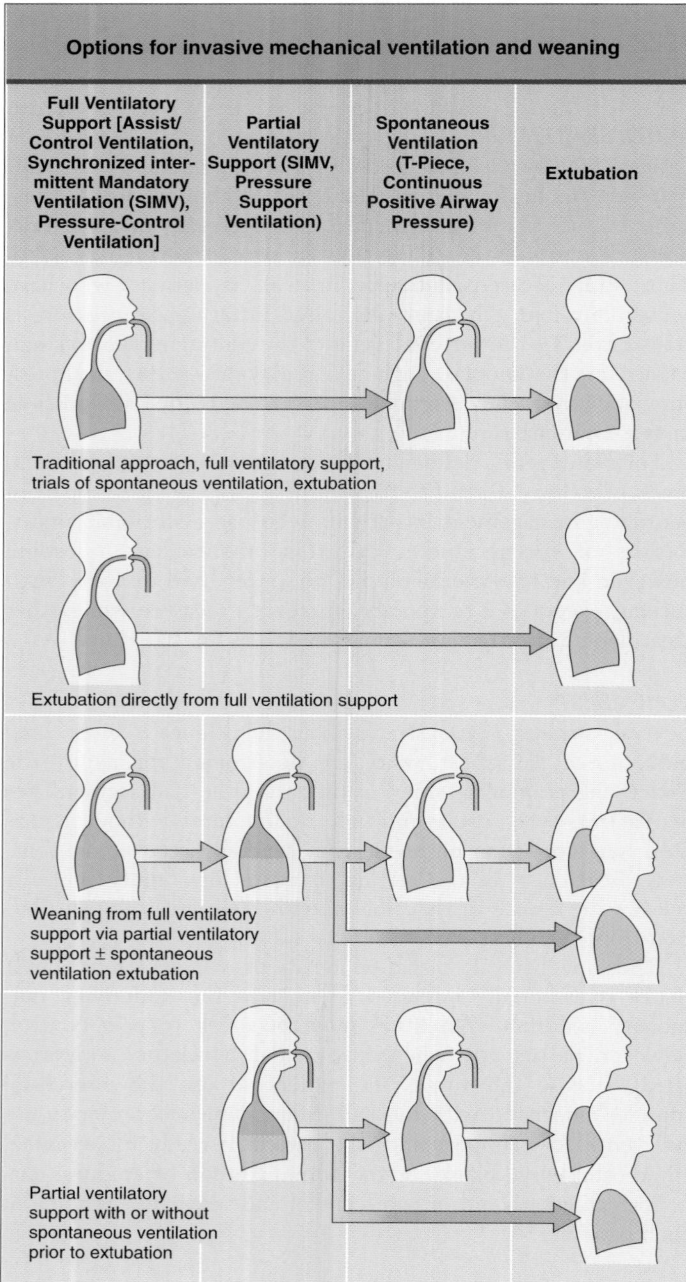

Figure 14.6 Options for invasive mechanical ventilation and weaning. Ventilator modes can be combined in a number of ways when discontinuing ventilatory support before extubation. The traditional approach uses full ventilatory support, one or more trials of spontaneous ventilation, and extubation if tolerated by the patient both clinically and by gas exchange criteria. Extubation directly from full ventilatory support is commonly carried out in the operating room or postanesthetic recovery room after anesthesia, but it is not recommended in managing patients who have acute respiratory failure. Other options are to wean from full ventilatory support using an intermediate stage of partial ventilatory support, with or without a trial of spontaneous ventilation before extubation, or management from the beginning using partial ventilatory support, with or without a trial of spontaneous ventilation before extubation. (Continuous positive airway pressure is either through the ventilator circuit or by means of a valve attached to a T-piece circuit.)

vital capacity; minute ventilation; and the maximum inspiratory pressure the patient could generate during end-expiratory airway occlusion. Most often, patients remained fully supported until threshold criteria were reached in one or more of these weaning parameters; then a trial of spontaneous breathing or progressively reduced inspiratory support was undertaken.

A systematic review of existing evidence for the efficacy of these weaning predictors, singly and in combination, was undertaken in conjunction with the development of practice guidelines by the American College of Chest Physicians, the American Association for Respiratory Care, and the American College of Critical Care Medicine (see Suggested Reading). Two important findings of this process were that no existing measurement, index, or combination of measurements could predict the ability to discontinue ventilatory support with sufficient accuracy, and that many patients considered to be "unweanable" or in need of a prolonged weaning regimen could, in fact, breathe without assistance if simply taken off ventilatory support. This led to the recommendation that, rather than attempting to predict when patients were ready for weaning, clinicians should simply "check," both early and repeatedly, to determine whether they were, in fact, ready. Table 14.10 summarizes the principles of weaning as recommended by the new guidelines.

Table 14.10
Principles of weaning from mechanical ventilation

- Assess every patient who requires ventilatory support for 24 hours or more for possible weaning and extubation
- Perform a spontaneous breathing trial (SBT) as soon as patient meets all five of the following criteria:
  1. Evidence of some reversal of the underlying cause of acute respiratory failure
  2. Adequate arterial oxygenation (e.g., arterial PO_2 at least 60 mmHg on 40% oxygen with positive end-expiratory pressure $\leq$5 cmH_2O)
  3. Acceptable acid-base balance (e.g., arterial pH $\geq$ 7.25)
  4. Hemodynamic stability (absence of active myocardial ischemia, and blood pressure supportable without significant vasopressor support)
  5. Sufficient ventilatory drive and neuromuscular function to initiate a spontaneous inspiratory effort
- Provide no more than minimal support during the SBT (i.e., T-piece, continuous positive airway pressure, and/or pressure support $\leq$ 5 cmH_2O).
- Strongly consider discontinuing ventilatory support if patient can sustain spontaneous ventilation for 30-120 minutes with reasonable comfort and acceptable arterial blood gas values
- Consider extubation separately from weaning, taking into consideration the abilities to maintain an adequate airway and clear respiratory tract secretions
- Investigate potential reasons for ventilator dependency if patient fails SBT
- Repeat SBT daily
- Between SBTs, provide a stable, nonfatiguing, comfortable form of ventilatory support

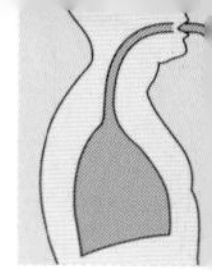

ASSESSMENT FOR READINESS TO WEAN

According to the new evidence-based guidelines, patients should be checked for readiness to wean when the following are present:

- Evidence of some reversal of the underlying cause for acute respiratory failure.
- Adequate arterial oxygenation (e.g., arterial P_{O_2} at least 60 mmHg on 40% oxygen with PEEP ≤5 cmH_2O).
- Acceptable acid-base balance (e.g., arterial pH 7.25 or higher).
- Hemodynamic stability (absence of active myocardial ischemia, and blood pressure supportable without significant vasopressor support).
- Sufficient ventilatory drive and neuromuscular function to initiate a spontaneous inspiratory effort.

SPONTANEOUS BREATHING TRIAL

Patients meeting the aforementioned criteria should have a spontaneous breathing trial (see Table 14.10). Although the time-honored T-piece method remains the favorite of many clinicians, this requires disconnecting the patient from the ventilator and interposing a different breathing circuit. A simpler alternative is to leave the patient connected to the ventilator circuit and switch to the CPAP mode, so that no mandatory or assisted breaths are provided. Low-level CPAP (e.g., 5 cmH_2O) can be provided during the trial at the discretion of the clinician, although adding more than 5 cmH_2O of inspiratory pressure support tends to defeat the purpose of the spontaneous breathing trial and should be avoided. Increasing the F_{IO_2} by 0.10 during the trial is recommended to avoid hypoxemia, as lung volumes and ventilation-perfusion matching may change during spontaneous breathing.

Patients should be observed closely during the trial for evidence of increasing respiratory distress (e.g., a progressively increasing respiratory rate over several minutes to ≥35 breaths/minute) or increasing tachycardia or systemic arterial hypertension, indicating that ventilatory support should be reinstituted. If spontaneous breathing is clinically tolerated for 30 minutes, an arterial blood specimen should be obtained for analysis to confirm that arterial oxygenation and acid-base status have not deteriorated unacceptably. The trial may be extended for up to 120 minutes if it is not initially clear whether it will be successful. However, there is little to gain by lengthening the period of spontaneous breathing beyond this point. Prompt extubation should be considered for patients who tolerate the trial clinically and maintain acceptable arterial blood gas values, provided no separate indication for an endotracheal tube is present (see later).

FAILURE OF SPONTANEOUS BREATHING TRIAL

An unsuccessful spontaneous breathing trial in a patient who fulfills the criteria for initiating it should be regarded as a diagnostic and therapeutic problem requiring deliberate attention. Figure 14.7 presents an algorithm for sorting out the reason or reasons for a failed trial. According to best available evidence, patients should undergo a spontaneous breathing trial once each day. Between trials, a level of support should be provided (e.g., A/C ventilation, or pressure support sufficient to prevent tachypnea and maintain patient comfort) that allows the patient to rest without developing ventilatory muscle fatigue.

For difficult cases, such as prolonged mechanical ventilation in acute respiratory failure or in patients with a serious underlying illness in other organ systems, it is helpful to approach weaning in a systematic fashion, considering possible impediments to success in the order of their likelihood, as summarized in Figure 14.7. In most cases of initial weaning failure, the reason becomes apparent on proceeding through the algorithm in a stepwise fashion. Perhaps the most common reason for inability to wean from mechanical ventilation among patients who have been critically ill for 1 week or more is that the primary illness has not improved sufficiently.

When patients are unable to be weaned because of a high minute ventilation requirement, as is commonly seen in ARDS, the clinician may be helped by an analysis of the physiologic mechanism responsible. Only three basic mechanisms can account for a higher than normal minute ventilation: hyperventilation (i.e., respiratory alkalosis), increased carbon dioxide production, and increased dead space ventilation (V_{DS}/V_T). Hyperventilation is readily identified by the presence of hypocapnia. Carbon dioxide production and V_{DS}/V_T can be assessed either by collecting expired gas in a bag or by using a metabolic cart (as used for determining nutritional requirements), in conjunction with an arterial blood sample. Making these simple measurements can help identify the reason for a high minute ventilation:

- If increased carbon dioxide production is the cause, the clinical problem is a systemic rather than a pulmonary one—perhaps the patient is receiving excessive nutritional support.
- If increased V_{DS}/V_T is responsible, the increased ventilation requirement results from the shunt seen in ARDS or pneumonia, dynamic hyperinflation, or pulmonary thromboembolism.

WEANING TECHNIQUE

The main techniques currently in use for gradual weaning from ventilatory support are the T-piece method and PSV. The T-piece method consists of repetitive periods of spontaneous ventilation (as described in Fig. 14.6) to the patient's tolerance, interspersed with periods of rest with full ventilatory support. When PSV is used in weaning, the patient is switched from full ventilatory support to PSV at an inspiratory pressure sufficient to provide the same V_T as before; inspiratory pressure is then gradually reduced, using the patient's respiratory rate (usually maintained below 30 breaths/minute) as a guide to the adequacy of support. Weaning with SIMV, which consists of gradually reducing the mandatory rate and thus progressively decreasing the ventilator's contribution to the required minute ventilation, using the total respiratory rate (mandatory plus spontaneous breaths) and other clinical signs as indicators of progress, is no longer recommended because multicenter clinical trials have shown it to prolong the process when compared with T-piece trials and PSV.

EXTUBATION

Discontinuation of ventilatory support and extubation are not the same thing. In most instances, both can be carried out

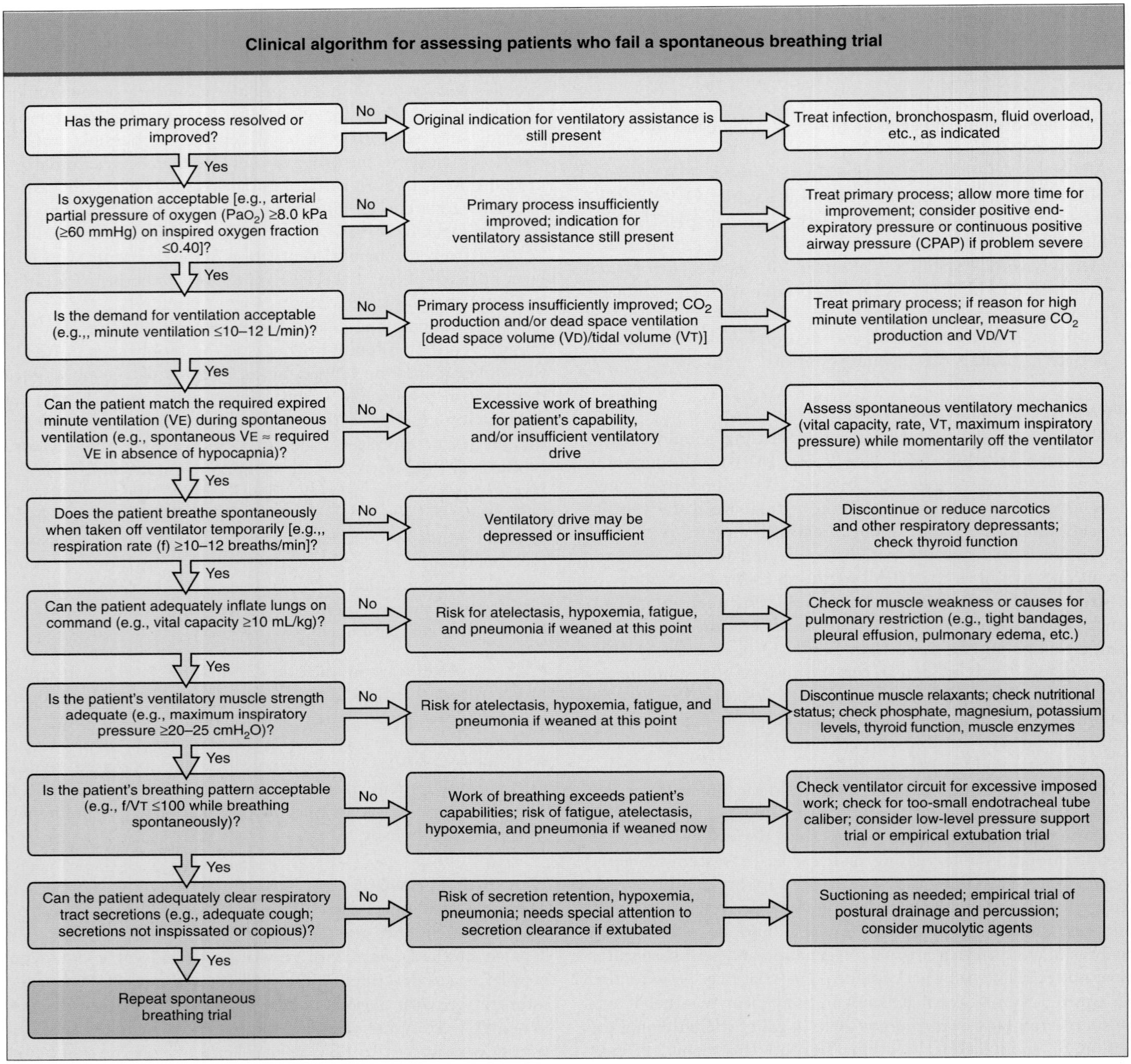

Clinical algorithm for assessing patients who fail a spontaneous breathing trial

Question (Yes → next question)	No	Action
Has the primary process resolved or improved?	Original indication for ventilatory assistance is still present	Treat infection, bronchospasm, fluid overload, etc., as indicated
Is oxygenation acceptable [e.g., arterial partial pressure of oxygen (PaO_2) ≥8.0 kPa (≥60 mmHg) on inspired oxygen fraction ≤0.40]?	Primary process insufficiently improved; indication for ventilatory assistance still present	Treat primary process; allow more time for improvement; consider positive end-expiratory pressure or continuous positive airway pressure (CPAP) if problem severe
Is the demand for ventilation acceptable (e.g.,, minute ventilation ≤10–12 L/min)?	Primary process insufficiently improved; CO_2 production and/or dead space ventilation [dead space volume (V_D)/tidal volume (V_T)]	Treat primary process; if reason for high minute ventilation unclear, measure CO_2 production and V_D/V_T
Can the patient match the required expired minute ventilation (V_E) during spontaneous ventilation (e.g., spontaneous $V_E \approx$ required V_E in absence of hypocapnia)?	Excessive work of breathing for patient's capability, and/or insufficient ventilatory drive	Assess spontaneous ventilatory mechanics (vital capacity, rate, V_T, maximum inspiratory pressure) while momentarily off the ventilator
Does the patient breathe spontaneously when taken off ventilator temporarily [e.g.,, respiration rate (f) ≥10–12 breaths/min]?	Ventilatory drive may be depressed or insufficient	Discontinue or reduce narcotics and other respiratory depressants; check thyroid function
Can the patient adequately inflate lungs on command (e.g., vital capacity ≥10 mL/kg)?	Risk for atelectasis, hypoxemia, fatigue, and pneumonia if weaned at this point	Check for muscle weakness or causes for pulmonary restriction (e.g., tight bandages, pleural effusion, pulmonary edema, etc.)
Is the patient's ventilatory muscle strength adequate (e.g., maximum inspiratory pressure ≥20–25 cmH_2O)?	Risk for atelectasis, hypoxemia, fatigue, and pneumonia if weaned at this point	Discontinue muscle relaxants; check nutritional status; check phosphate, magnesium, potassium levels, thyroid function, muscle enzymes
Is the patient's breathing pattern acceptable (e.g., $f/V_T \leq 100$ while breathing spontaneously)?	Work of breathing exceeds patient's capabilities; risk of fatigue, atelectasis, hypoxemia, and pneumonia if weaned now	Check ventilator circuit for excessive imposed work; check for too-small endotracheal tube caliber; consider low-level pressure support trial or empirical extubation trial
Can the patient adequately clear respiratory tract secretions (e.g., adequate cough; secretions not inspissated or copious)?	Risk of secretion retention, hypoxemia, pneumonia; needs special attention to secretion clearance if extubated	Suctioning as needed; empirical trial of postural drainage and percussion; consider mucolytic agents

Yes → Repeat spontaneous breathing trial

Figure 14.7 Clinical algorithm for weaning patients from mechanical ventilation. This step-by-step approach is especially helpful in patients who have failed previous weaning attempts or are otherwise difficult to wean. 10 cmH_2O = 1 kPa.

together—as after general anesthesia. However, failure to recognize the important exceptions can lead to serious problems. In addition to the need for mechanical ventilation, indications for translaryngeal intubation include upper airway problems, inability to protect the lower airways from aspiration of oropharyngeal or gastric contents, and inability to clear secretions without suctioning or other measures.

A convenient predictor of the need for upper airway protection is the cuff-leak test. If the patient can breathe around the endotracheal tube when the cuff is momentarily deflated, or if air can be heard passing into the mouth with a manual inflation pressure of no more than 20 cmH_2O, it is unlikely that the patient requires reintubation because of upper airway obstruction. The cuff-leak test is very sensitive but not very specific, in that a substantial number of patients can be extubated successfully in the absence of a demonstrable air leak.

Unfortunately, no specific tests or measurements are currently available to assess patients' ability to protect their airway from aspiration and their ability to clear secretions. A trial of extubation is often the best way to determine whether the

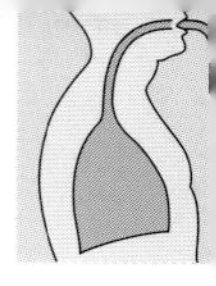

patient needs continued airway protection (with a tracheostomy, for example).

COMPLICATIONS

Although frequently lifesaving, invasive mechanical ventilation is also associated with numerous complications, some of which can be life threatening in themselves (Table 14.11). The expression "associated with" is important conceptually, because many adverse effects that occur while a patient is being mechanically ventilated cannot be shown conclusively to arise directly from the ventilator or its operation. Nosocomial pneumonia in the ventilated patient, for example, is more likely a consequence of critical illness and the breakdown of normal host defenses than of the ventilator per se. Because they are related temporally and clinically to intubation and mechanical ventilation, however, it is logical to consider all such complications together here.

Table 14.11
Complications of invasive mechanical ventilation

Adverse Physiologic Effects
Impaired cardiac function
Increased intracranial pressure
Gastric distention
Respiratory alkalosis
Renal and hepatic dysfunction
Dynamic Hyperinflation and Auto–Positive End-Expiratory Pressure
Clinical Barotrauma (Ventilator-Related Extra-Alveolar Air)
Pulmonary interstitial emphysema
Systemic air embolism
Pneumomediastinum
Pneumothorax
Pneumoretroperitoneum or pneumoperitoneum
Complications of Intubation, Tracheostomy, and Artificial Airways
During intubation or performance of tracheotomy
Difficult intubation; loss of airway
Tissue injury; hemorrhage
While tube is in place
Increased airway secretions
Loss of endogenous humidification system
Impaired mucociliary clearance
Mucosal injury
Alteration of mouth flora/lower airway colonization
Increased work of breathing
Loss of ability to speak
During extubation or decannulation
After extubation or decannulation
Immediate (laryngeal edema, vocal cord dysfunction)
Early (aspiration, pneumonia)
Late (tracheal stenosis)
Consequences of Ventilator Malfunction
Ventilator-Associated Pneumonia
Agitation and Respiratory Distress
Worsening Oxygenation
Ventilator-related problems
Progression of underlying disease
Onset of new medical problem
Effects of interventions/procedures
Medications
Technologic/Communication Problems

Physiologic Effects of Positive Pressure Ventilation

Initiating positive pressure mechanical ventilation in any patient alters pulmonary mechanics and respiratory function. Several of these changes are more "effects" than "complications," in that they are direct, predictable results of changes in lung volume and intrathoracic pressure. In several instances, although these effects have been well known for years, the precise mechanisms remain uncertain.

IMPAIRED CARDIAC FUNCTION

The effects of positive pressure ventilation on cardiac function are more common with the application of PEEP but may also occur when mechanical ventilation is used without PEEP, especially in volume-depleted patients and those who have preexisting cardiac disease.

Two mechanisms for decreased cardiac function have been postulated:

1. Reduced right ventricular preload as a result of raised mean intrathoracic pressure (which is an absolute effect of positive pressure ventilation).
2. Increased right ventricular afterload because of increased lung volume (which need not occur if gas trapping does not occur and if tidal residual volumes are physiologic).

Which one is more important remains unclear.

Compared with spontaneous breathing, positive pressure ventilation increases both peak and mean intrathoracic pressure and thus increases the pressure gradient that must be overcome by venous blood as it returns to the right atrium. Mean intrathoracic pressure is further increased by the application of PEEP, and in the presence of relative hypovolemia, even small amounts of PEEP can compromise cardiac function. Patients who have preexisting right ventricular dysfunction are at increased risk for cardiac impairment with the addition of PEEP. Some investigators have suggested that the reduction in venous return may be the result of an increase in inferior vena caval resistance because of the increase in lung volume compressing the inferior vena cava as it enters the thorax and becomes surrounded by lung parenchyma. Increases in lung volume cause an increase in pulmonary vascular resistance, but the change in volume must be very large. Over the physiologic range of lung volume, changes in resistance are trivial. If this occurs, however, it increases right ventricular afterload, which may compromise the forward output of that chamber. The increase in right ventricular volume associated with raised pulmonary vascular resistance may in turn impair left ventricular function, because both ventricles share the interventricular septum, pericardial sac, and certain circumferential muscle fibers.

Positive pressure ventilation does not always impair cardiac function, and in certain circumstances, it may even improve it. Although the work of spontaneous breathing normally accounts for a small proportion of overall oxygen consumption, this may increase drastically during acute respiratory failure. When cardiac function is severely impaired, as in cardiogenic shock, the heart may not be able to meet the demands imposed on it

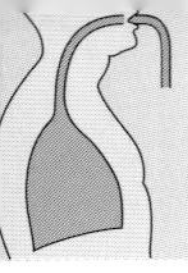

by this excessive work of breathing. In addition, the increase in juxtacardiac pressure that occurs as a result of the increase in intrathoracic pressure induced by positive pressure causes a functional reduction in left ventricular afterload.

INCREASED INTRACRANIAL PRESSURE

Positive pressure ventilation can increase jugular venous pressure, which in turn can impede venous return from the brain and raise intracranial pressure (ICP).

Normally, over a wide range of cerebral perfusion pressure (mean arterial pressure minus ICP), cerebral blood flow is kept constant through autoregulation, and changes in ICP or cardiac output have little effect. When ICP is elevated, however, as after head injury, autoregulation is lost, the relationship of cerebral blood flow to cerebral perfusion pressure becomes linear, and either an increase in ICP or a drop in cardiac output can reduce cerebral blood flow. Fortunately, conditions that require high levels of PEEP to support oxygenation, such as ARDS, also markedly reduce lung compliance, so that less pressure is transmitted to the jugular venous system.

GASTRIC DISTENTION

Gastric and intestinal distention with air may occur when manual ventilation with bag and mask raises mouth pressure above lower esophageal sphincter pressure. During mechanical ventilation via a cuffed endotracheal tube, it is not uncommon for patients who have low respiratory system compliance to develop gastric distention, presumably because tracheal pressure exceeds both cuff pressure and lower esophageal sphincter pressure in the presence of a closed or occluded mouth. Distention can be massive (meteorism), and gastric rupture has been reported. Placement of a small-bore nasogastric tube usually prevents or alleviates this problem.

RESPIRATORY ALKALOSIS

Respiratory alkalosis is among the most common adverse occurrences during mechanical ventilation. Severe alkalemia may precipitate cardiac arrhythmias or seizures. Unintentional respiratory alkalosis (pH > 7.55) developed in 11% of ventilated patients in one series and was associated with an increased overall mortality rate. Dyspnea, agitation, and pain are the most common causes in patients who do not suffer severe central nervous system dysfunction or chronic liver disease. Appropriate ventilator adjustment, occasionally combined with sedation as required, controls the alkalosis in most instances.

RENAL AND HEPATIC EFFECTS

Fluid retention and edema are common in patients who receive mechanical ventilation. Reductions in renal blood flow and impairment in renal function, especially with the use of PEEP, have been documented by a number of investigators, who postulate mechanisms such as elevation of serum antidiuretic hormone, excessive aldosterone effect, and (more recently) reduced levels of atrial natriuretic peptides.

Liver dysfunction is also fairly common in ventilated patients, which has led some investigators to conclude that positive pressure ventilation causes hepatic impairment. A fall in portal blood flow has been documented with PEEP therapy, but the clinical importance of this is unclear. As with a number of other adverse effects discussed here, it may be difficult to separate the effects of mechanical ventilation on renal and hepatic function from manifestations of the patient's underlying disease process.

Dynamic Hyperinflation and Auto–Positive End-Expiratory Pressure

PATHOGENESIS

As mentioned earlier, COPD and asthma are characterized physiologically by hyperinflation and expiratory airflow limitation. When airway obstruction is severe, there may be insufficient time to exhale a given tidal breath completely before the next inspiration. This means that the next breath begins at a higher lung volume. Over the course of several such breaths, the patient becomes progressively hyperinflated and reaches a new FRC that is considerably higher than when the sequence began. Patients who have severe COPD may experience this phenomenon spontaneously during panic attacks or at times of increased dyspnea, but it can be especially serious during positive pressure ventilation.

CLINICAL MANIFESTATIONS

As a result of the elastic recoil of the lung when distended above FRC (and of the chest wall at even larger lung volumes), dynamic hyperinflation is associated with positive end-expiratory alveolar pressure, or auto-PEEP (also called intrinsic PEEP, dynamic PEEP, or endogenous PEEP). The physiologic effect of auto-PEEP is the same as that of PEEP applied at the airway by adjusting the ventilator (i.e., extrinsic PEEP)—reductions in cardiac preload because of diminished venous return to the chest. The reduced cardiac output can lead to hypotension and, if severe, to pulseless electrical activity and cardiac arrest. Dynamic hyperinflation can also lead to local alveolar overdistention and rupture, followed by pneumothorax and other forms of extra-alveolar air (clinical barotrauma, discussed later).

Auto-PEEP is common in ventilated patients who have underlying COPD. Several other clinical circumstances suggest an increased likelihood of dynamic hyperinflation and auto-PEEP (Table 14.12). Of special importance is the situation in which the patient appears to exert unusual effort to trigger the ventilator or when airflow from the ventilator is not initiated with every inspiratory effort. Figure 14.8 illustrates why the latter occurs.

DETECTION AND MEASUREMENT

Unlike externally applied PEEP, which is indicated on the ventilator's pressure manometer, auto-PEEP cannot be detected unless an end-exhalation occlusion maneuver is performed to allow pressures in the patient's alveoli to equilibrate with the exhalation valve of the ventilator circuit at end-expiration (Table 14.13). When patients breathe spontaneously or attempt to trigger the ventilator, the end-expiratory occlusion technique cannot be used, and a different method such as stepwise addition of external PEEP must be used (see Table 14.13).

PREVENTION AND MANAGEMENT

The key to preventing dynamic hyperinflation, and to reducing its severity when present, is to increase expiratory time. Dynamic hyperinflation occurs because insufficient time is available to complete lung emptying after each positive pressure breath. Therefore, prevention and management hinge on mea-

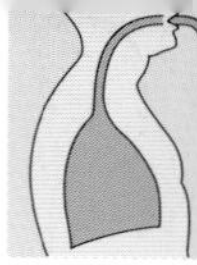

Table 14.12
When to suspect the presence of auto–positive end-expiratory pressure

- Known obstructive lung disease in any ventilated patient
- Development of otherwise unexplained tachycardia, hypotension, or pulseless electrical activity, especially immediately following initiation of positive pressure ventilation
- Patient appears to work very hard to trigger ventilator (in any mode)
- Patient's inspiratory efforts do not trigger airflow from ventilator every time
- If monitoring with graphics display, expiratory airflow continues to onset of next inspiration

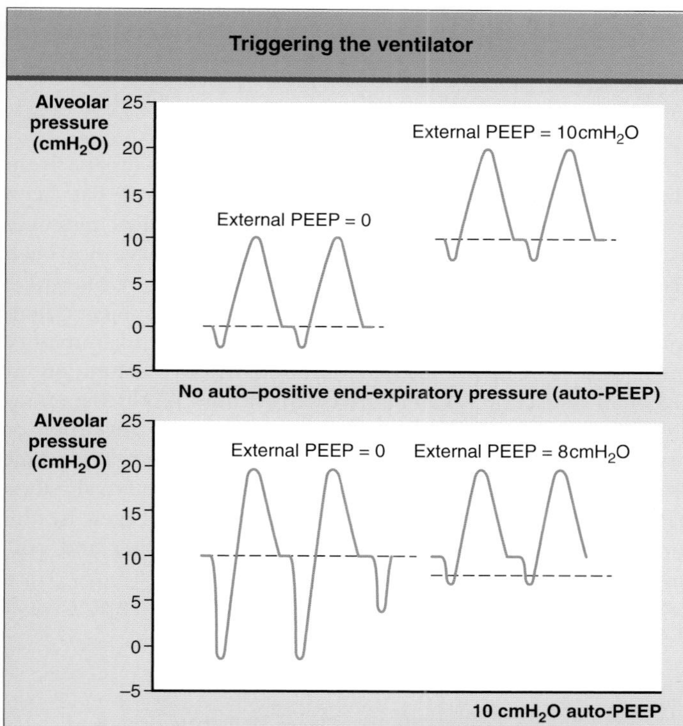

Figure 14.8 Patient's ability to trigger the ventilator. Impact of dynamic hyperinflation and auto–positive end-expiratory pressure (auto-PEEP), and the effect of adding external PEEP. In the absence of auto-PEEP, the addition of external PEEP does not affect the relative ease of initiating breaths from the ventilator. In the presence of $10\,cmH_2O$ of auto-PEEP but in the absence of external PEEP, to initiate inspiratory flow from the ventilator, the patient must generate enough ventilatory muscle contraction to overcome the $10\,cmH_2O$ of auto-PEEP and reduce tracheal pressure below zero. On occasion, insufficient force is generated to trigger the ventilator. When $8\,cmH_2O$ of external PEEP is added, the patient can trigger the ventilator more easily, because much less ventilatory muscle contraction is needed to bring tracheal pressure down to the external PEEP level. $10\,cmH_2O = 1$ kPa.

Table 14.13
Techniques for detecting and quantitating auto–positive end-expiratory pressure

Technique	Method
End-expiratory occlusion technique: manual expiratory circuit occlusion (measurement not possible if patient actively attempts to breathe)	Following inspiration, turn ventilator rate control to zero so that the next inspiration does not occur At the moment when the next inspiration should occur, occlude the expiratory line for 1–3 sec, and read total positive end-expiratory pressure (PEEP) from ventilator's pressure manometer Return ventilator rate control to previous setting
Use of ventilator's expiratory hold function (measurement not possible if patient actively attempts to breathe)	Following inspiration, depress expiratory hold button Keep button depressed throughout exhalation Read total PEEP level on ventilator's pressure manometer 1–3 sec after end-expiratory occlusion begins
Use of Braschi valve (measurement not possible if patient actively attempts to breathe)	Place Braschi valve in inspiratory circuit between ventilator and patient eye Remove valve cap during exhalation, so that next inspiration is vented to room Read total PEEP on ventilator's pressure manometer 1–3 sec after onset of ventilator's inspiratory cycle
Measurement of esophageal (pleural) pressure	Read pressure from esophageal balloon at end-expiration
Stepwise addition of external PEEP	Add 2–3 cmH_2O increments of external PEEP while monitoring peak and static inspiratory pressures If peak and static pressures do not change, external PEEP remains below auto-PEEP level If peak and/or static inspiratory pressure increase on addition of external PEEP, auto-PEEP level has been exceeded

Table 14.14
Prevention and management of auto–positive end-expiratory pressure

Goal	Method
Aggressively treat airflow obstruction	Inhaled bronchodilators Systemic corticosteroids Aggressive clearance of secretions
Maximize expiratory time	Decrease overall minute ventilation (especially if pH > 7.40) Increase inspiratory flow rate to 90–100 L/min Exchange large-bore disposable ventilator circuit for nondisposable, low compressible-volume circuit to reduce the tidal volume required of the ventilator
Decrease patient's inspiratory work of breathing when auto–positive end-expiratory pressure (auto-PEEP) is present	If patient makes spontaneous inspiratory efforts, add external PEEP to 80% of measured or estimated auto-PEEP level

sures to reduce airway obstruction and to decrease the time spent on inspiration during each minute. Table 14.14 lists practical steps that can be taken to prevent auto-PEEP in ventilated patients and to minimize it when present.

If the patient makes active inspiratory efforts, as shown in Figure 14.8, the addition of external PEEP decreases the muscular effort needed to trigger breaths from the ventilator, and thus decreases the work of breathing and increases patient comfort. The added external PEEP can be selected empirically (measurement of auto-PEEP is inaccurate in spontaneously breathing patients), or it can be set at about 80% of the measured or estimated auto-PEEP level; the latter is an average of various actual auto-PEEP levels in different lung regions, some of which are lower than the measured auto-PEEP. The level of auto-PEEP is checked frequently as the patient's condition changes, with adjustments in external PEEP made accordingly.

Barotrauma

Pneumothorax, pneumomediastinum, subcutaneous emphysema, and other forms of extra-alveolar air detected during mechanical ventilation are collectively termed *barotrauma*. Although this term implies that excessive pressure is the cause, it is more likely that alveolar disruption results from overdistention (i.e., excessive peak inflating volume) rather than high pressure per se. Extra-alveolar air that first becomes evident during ventilatory support may also be unrelated to the ventilator. Figure 14.9 shows how spontaneous alveolar rupture or other disruption of alveolar integrity can be followed by several kinds of clinical manifestations, depending on how much air enters the pulmonary interstitium and where the path of least resistance takes it.

Pneumomediastinum, pneumoperitoneum, and subcutaneous emphysema are rarely of physiologic significance and do not require specific treatment. However, pneumothorax is different, in that the air collects in a space (the pleural cavity) from which it cannot naturally escape as pressure increases. Pneumothorax in a patient who receives positive pressure ventilation can quickly progress to tension pneumothorax, which may rapidly cause cardiovascular collapse and death; for this reason, it must always be relieved promptly if ventilatory support cannot be immediately discontinued.

Table 14.15 outlines the steps for minimizing the risk of alveolar rupture and barotrauma during mechanical ventilation. These steps are especially important in high-risk patients, such as those who have obstructive or unevenly distributed lung disease, pulmonary infection, and late-phase ARDS (beyond 1 to 2 weeks).

Table 14.15
Prevention of barotrauma

Use small tidal volumes in patients who have obstructive lung disease or other cause for pulmonary hyperinflation
Decrease tidal volume as positive end-expiratory pressure (PEEP) is increased
Use PEEP cautiously in patients at increased risk: Unilateral, patchy, or cavitary lung disease Nosocomial pneumonia or sepsis syndrome Acute respiratory distress syndrome late in clinical course (e.g., after 1–2 weeks) Chronic obstructive pulmonary disease or asthma
Monitor respiratory system compliance during PEEP trials as a predictor of increased risk for alveolar rupture
Avoid or promptly correct right main-stem bronchus intubation
Avoid end-inspiratory pause
Keep short-inspiration:long-expiration ratio low
Monitor patient for auto-PEEP; follow steps in Table 14.13 to reduce it if present

Ventilator-induced parenchymal lung injury (apart from clinically apparent barotrauma, as discussed here) has been shown to affect both lung dysfunction and clinical outcome in acute lung injury. Although the mechanisms have not been clarified, current data suggest that it results from repetitive opening and closing of collapsed air spaces, which subjects them to high local pressures, leading to the activation of inflammatory mediators (so-called biotrauma). Similarly, overdistention of alveoli or lung regions can injure them without producing extra-alveolar air. Current evidence indicates that the prevention or reduction of ventilator-induced lung injury is an important reason for improved outcomes and increased survival when patients with acute lung injury or ARDS are managed by the lung-protective ventilatory strategy discussed earlier and outlined in Figure 14.5.

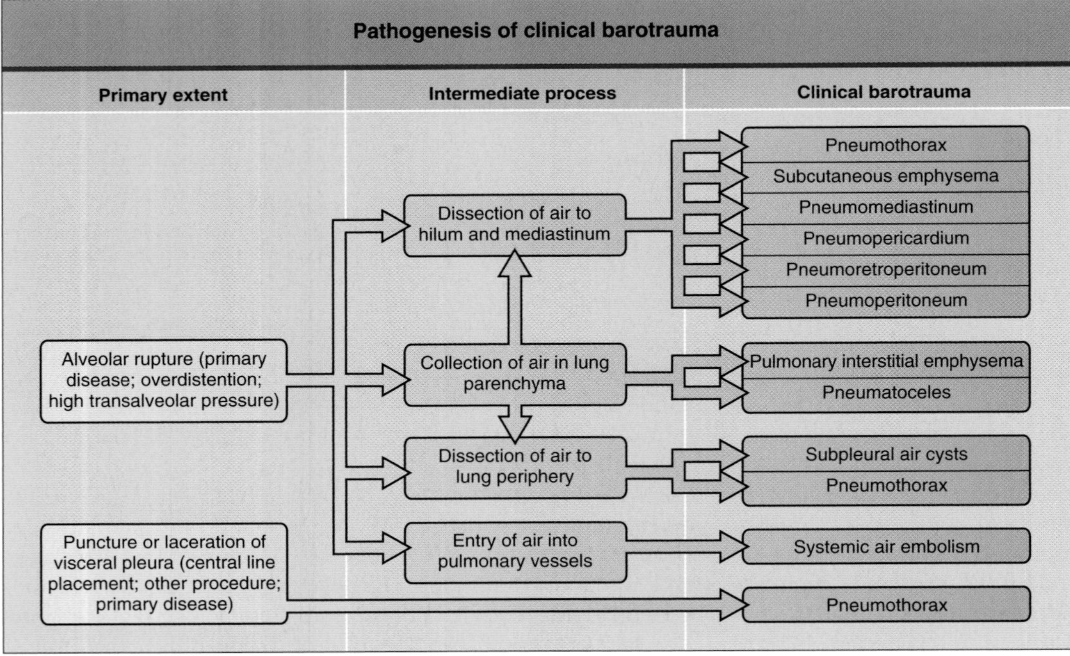

Figure 14.9 Pathogenesis of clinical barotrauma. The clinical manifestations of extra-alveolar air during mechanical ventilation can arise either from "spontaneous" alveolar rupture or from direct disruption of the integrity of the alveolus.

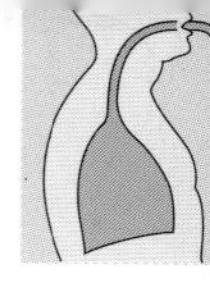

Other Complications

Several important complications associated with invasive mechanical ventilation are not discussed in this chapter. Complications associated with intubation, tracheotomy, and artificial airways are discussed in Chapter 16, and ventilator-associated pneumonia is covered in Chapter 26. A discussion of troubleshooting and other technical aspects of ventilators and their operation is beyond the scope of this chapter. However, three important topics that are not generally included in reviews of ventilator complications are briefly discussed here.

"FIGHTING THE VENTILATOR"

When agitation and respiratory distress develop in a patient on a mechanical ventilator who previously appeared comfortable, this is an important clinical circumstance for which the clinician needs an organized approach. The patient should not automatically be sedated but must instead be evaluated for several potentially life-threatening developments that can present in this fashion.

The ventilator is first disconnected from the patient, and the patient is ventilated manually using 100% oxygen and a self-inflating bag. If this procedure relieves the patient's distress, the problem lies proximal to the endotracheal tube, and the ventilator and its circuitry must be inspected or replaced. If agitation and respiratory distress persist, the airways are suctioned and a brief physical examination is performed, noting recent trends in vital signs and any other new developments in the hours preceding the onset of distress. If the likely cause is not apparent, a more detailed examination is required, which must include a new set of measurements of arterial blood gases and a bedside chest radiograph. On rare occasions, if the patient appears to be in extremis and tension pneumothorax cannot be excluded at the bedside, empirical measures to drain the chest may be warranted.

DETERIORATING OXYGENATION

Deteriorating arterial oxygenation during mechanical ventilation, a common reason for "fighting the ventilator," should initiate a systematic search for specific mechanisms and therapy rather than simply an increase in inspired oxygen fraction or level of PEEP. Possible causes for worsening oxygenation fall into several categories.

The problem could be with the ventilator and its circuitry. The patient's primary disease process (e.g., pneumonia, ARDS) could be worsening, or a new medical problem may have appeared. Examples of the latter include pneumothorax, acute lobar atelectasis, pulmonary edema from fluid overload, nosocomial pneumonia or sepsis, aspiration of gastric contents, retained secretions, and bronchospasm. A fall in cardiac output can also cause worsening oxygenation in a patient who has significant pulmonary venous admixture.

Interventions and procedures can also lead to a decline in oxygenation. Examples include the effects of airway suctioning, chest physical therapy, or even changes in body position, especially in patients affected by heterogeneously distributed pulmonary involvement. Bronchoscopy, thoracentesis, and hemodialysis can also lead to a decline in oxygenation. Finally, a number of drugs administered to patients undergoing mechanical ventilation can interfere with arterial oxygenation. Among these are vasodilators (which can decrease hypoxic vasoconstriction), β-blockers (which can depress cardiac output and induce bronchospasm), and bronchodilators (which can transiently alter ventilation-perfusion ratios).

SUBOPTIMAL VENTILATOR MANAGEMENT

Some adverse effects of mechanical ventilation are iatrogenic. With the increasing complexity of ventilators and their modes, it becomes more likely that the physician, nurse, or respiratory therapist who adjusts the ventilator may not fully understand the consequences of a given adjustment. Table 14.16 lists several such iatrogenic problems, the clinical circumstances in which they typically occur, and steps to prevent or correct them.

PITFALLS AND CONTROVERSIES

Few aspects of invasive mechanical ventilation rest on the firm foundation of scientific data. Because it is carried out in critically ill patients, in whom controlled trials are exceedingly difficult to conduct, mechanical ventilation remains empirical in many areas, driven by the biases of the individual clinician. In the literature, at conferences, and at the bedside, ongoing debate occurs about the best modes, the best monitors, and the best end points for the management of mechanical ventilation. In relatively few instances do good data support a "best" anything in this field.

Of the numerous areas of unresolved controversy, oxygen toxicity, the use of neuromuscular blocking agents, and the exercise or rest of ventilatory muscles are briefly discussed here.

Oxygen Toxicity

After the desire to avoid high peak airway pressures, the drive to prevent pulmonary oxygen toxicity is the dominant force in ventilator management in critically ill patients. In experimental animals and normal human volunteers, signs of oxygen toxicity appear within hours of exposure to high FIO_2, and 100% oxygen can be fatal in a day or two. The bountiful data that document these statements have led many intensivists to assume that serious or even fatal oxygen toxicity is a threat to the ventilated patient if the FIO_2 cannot be decreased to 0.50 or sometimes considerably less within one to several days.

Yet there is a discrepancy between the results of laboratory studies and observations in the intensive care unit. Although it is difficult to separate the signs of potential oxygen toxicity from those of ARDS or other primary processes that cause respiratory failure, it is not clear that any instance of oxygen toxicity has occurred in a critically ill patient, despite the administration of 70% or even 100% oxygen, when necessary, for many days. Evidence from animal experiments supports the notion that critical illness, and especially severe hypoxemia, prevents or ameliorates the toxic effects of oxygen on the lung.

Whether high FIO_2 is injurious to the lungs or not, the measures used to avoid oxygen toxicity have adverse effects that are unquestioned, frequent, and potentially life threatening.

How one balances the somewhat nebulous threat of oxygen toxicity against the likelihood of adverse effects from high levels of PEEP remains an individual decision. However, several guidelines seem prudent regardless of the philosophic approach used. A PEEP trial should be used to determine the best level for the patient, with adjustments guided by the patient's course. No

Table 14.16
Suboptimal ventilator management that adversely affects patients

Problem	Clinical Setting	Prevention or Correction
Unintended hyperventilation (acute respiratory alkalosis)	'Normalizing' arterial partial pressure of carbon dioxide ($PaCO_2$) in patient with 'acute-on-chronic' carbon dioxide retention	Recognize underlying metabolic alkalosis (high serum bicarbonate) Use arterial pH, not $PaCO_2$, as guide for ventilator adjustments
	Too-rapid ventilator cycling in assist-control mode	Adjust triggering sensitivity to minimum level that prevents spontaneous cycling (e.g., 1–1.5 cmH_2O) Make sure inspiratory flow is sufficient for patient's needs Sedate patient if needed
Unintended hypoventilation (acute respiratory acidosis)	Unstable or fluctuating ventilatory drive in patient on low synchronized intermittent mandatory ventilation (SIMV) rate (potential for variable patient contribution to required minute ventilation)	Increase SIMV rate to meet patient's total minute ventilation requirement Switch to A/C ventilation mode
	Backup rate set too far below patient's triggering rate in A/C ventilation	Increase backup rate to 2–3 breaths/min less than patient's stable triggering rate
Excessive patient work of breathing	Low SIMV rate with small-diameter endotracheal tube or weak and/or fatigued patient	Increase SIMV rate to provide all or most of patient's required minute ventilation Switch to A/C mode Add inspiratory pressure support sufficient to overcome tube resistance
	T-piece trial with small-diameter endotracheal tube A/C mode with excessive triggering effort	Add inspiratory pressure support sufficient to overcome tube resistance at patient's required minute ventilation Adjust trigger/assist sensitivity to 1–1.5 cmH_2O
Inappropriate use of neuromuscular blocking agents	Patient who previously was tolerant now "fighting the ventilator"	Disconnect patient from circuit and ventilate manually to make sure ventilator is functioning normally (volume; pressure; flow pattern) Rapidly assess airway patency, symmetry of chest expansion, vital signs, and other monitoring data Perform more complete patient assessment and adjust ventilator settings as clinically indicated
	Unintended hyperventilation (acute respiratory alkalosis)	Recognize underlying metabolic alkalosis (high serum bicarbonate) Use arterial pH, not $PaCO_2$, as guide for ventilator adjustments Sedate patient with appropriate agent (e.g., benzodiazepine) if above does not apply and assessment of patient and ventilator reveals no acute problem
	Neuromuscular blocking agent used without concomitant sedation	Administer sufficient sedative to calm patient and produce amnesia
Technology gap in patient management	Physician ordering ventilator mode or settings fails to appreciate technical or clinical problem with therapy as ordered	Discussion among physician, nurse, and respiratory therapist before therapy is carried out, initiated by any party (especially important with new or unfamiliar ventilator modes)
	Nurse or respiratory therapist unfamiliar or uncomfortable with ventilator, mode, or settings as ordered	–
Bedside communication failure	Those caring for patient at bedside (nurse, respiratory therapist) do not understand patient's problem or rationale for ordered therapy	Explanation by physician caring for patient about diagnosis, pathophysiology, and/or therapeutic rationale
	Failure on part of nurse or respiratory therapist to communicate concerns about above problem	Discussion with attending physician, initiated by concerned nurse or respiratory therapist

more oxygen should be used than is necessary to saturate the hemoglobin, and in severe ARDS, arterial saturation levels of 80% to 90% (PO_2 6.6 to 8.0 kPa [50 to 60 mmHg]) should be accepted. Consideration must be given to erythrocyte transfusion in the presence of anemia to increase arterial oxygen content. The FIO_2 must be adjusted downward as rapidly as possible as the patient improves.

Sedation and Paralysis

Use of neuromuscular blocking agents during mechanical ventilation has become more widespread in recent years. In some instances, this is because the modes of ventilation used, such as pressure control with inverse ratio ventilation, are uncomfortable for patients and result in "fighting the ventilator" if they are awake and alert. In others, it is part of an attempt to reduce peripheral oxygen utilization in the aggressive management of ARDS or sepsis. Sedation and muscle relaxation are necessary for operative surgery, certain diagnostic procedures such as angiography and computed tomographic scanning in uncooperative patients, and various invasive procedures performed in the intensive care unit. Some suggest using respiratory pressure-volume curves to guide the selection of PEEP level and VT, and this maneuver also requires paralysis. In general, however, neuromuscular blocking agents are overused.

Rendering a patient incapable of movement is a hazardous undertaking, associated with increased risks for venous thrombosis, nosocomial pneumonia, and skin breakdown, and it has extremely deleterious effects on the diaphragm.

Exercise or Rest for Ventilatory Muscles?

Controversy has existed for more than 30 years as to whether the ventilatory muscles of a patient who receives invasive mechanical ventilation need to be rested or exercised. Advocates of resting the muscles point out that failure of the ventilatory pump is the proximate cause of most cases of acute hypercapnic respiratory failure, especially in patients who have underly-

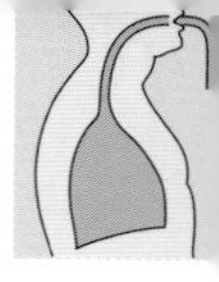

ing obstructive lung disease. Separating "failure" from the normal reduction in inspiratory respiratory muscle strength as total lung capacity is approached is impossible, however. To permit the fatigued ventilatory muscles to recover through rest seems intuitive. However, the opposite camp maintains a "use it or lose it" stance, pointing to evidence of rapid loss of skeletal muscle mass and functional capability when patients are immobilized. Advocates of exercising the ventilatory muscles often use partial ventilatory support throughout the period of mechanical ventilation, which makes the muscles do at least some of the work of breathing.

Studies that support both positions have been published, and the controversy is unresolved. However, because the work of breathing in relation to a patient's capabilities is a major determinant of dyspnea, it is important to address the issue in the context of patient comfort. Although the rationale behind partial ventilatory support for a patient who has ongoing respiratory failure and who is not ready to be weaned is understandable, any benefit derived from making that patient struggle to breathe seems questionable. When partial ventilatory support is used at any stage of management, whether via SIMV or PSV, enough support should be provided to keep the total respiratory rate below about 30 breaths per minute. Patients who breathe more rapidly are typically restless, tachycardic, and diaphoretic and are surely not deriving any benefit from exercising their ventilatory muscles.

Weaning from ventilatory support necessarily involves loading the patient's ventilatory muscles and hence stressing them. When weaning is not being actively attempted, however, patient comfort should be given a high priority. During weaning, particularly in difficult-to-wean patients who are undergoing a gradual weaning regimen, it may be important to provide sufficient support to rest the ventilatory muscles after each episode of spontaneous breathing in which fatigue is induced.

SUGGESTED READING

Acute Respiratory Distress Syndrome Network: Ventilation with lower tidal volumes as compared with traditional tidal volumes for acute lung injury and the acute respiratory distress syndrome. N Engl J Med 342:1301-1308, 2000.

Gladwin MT, Pierson DJ: Mechanical ventilation of the patient with severe chronic obstructive pulmonary disease. Intensive Care Med 24:898-910, 1998.

Hess DR, Kacmarek RM: Essentials of Mechanical Ventilation, 2nd ed. New York, McGraw-Hill, 2002.

Invasive Mechanical Ventilation in Adults [two special issues]. Respir Care 47:247-347, 416-518, 2002.

MacIntyre NR, Cook DJ, Guyatt GH (eds): Evidence-based guidelines for weaning and discontinuing ventilatory support. American College of Chest Physicians, American Association for Respiratory Care, and American College of Critical Care Medicine. Chest 120(6 Suppl):375S-484S, 2001.

Pauwels RA, Buist AS, Calverley PM, et al: Global strategy for the diagnosis, management, and prevention of chronic obstructive pulmonary disease. NHLBI/WHO Global Initiative for Chronic Obstructive Lung Disease (GOLD) Workshop summary. Am J Respir Crit Care Med 163:1256-1276, 2001.

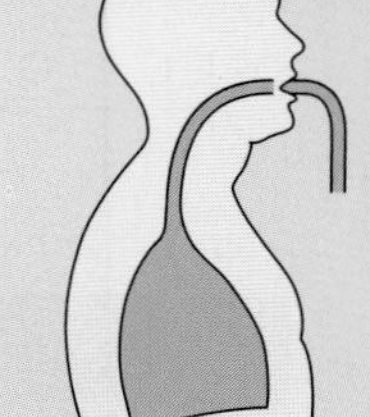

CHAPTER 15 Noninvasive Mechanical Ventilation

Nicholas S. Hill

Noninvasive ventilation is mechanical ventilation administered without an invasive artificial airway. Since the first description of a prototype negative pressure "tank" ventilator 150 years ago, many types of noninvasive ventilators have been developed. Tank ventilators, like the iron lung, were the mainstay of mechanical ventilatory assistance during the polio epidemics that occurred from the 1920s to the 1950s. By the 1960s, invasive positive pressure ventilation became the preferred treatment of acute respiratory failure. Noninvasive ventilators, mainly of the negative pressure type, continued to be used sporadically for chronic respiratory failure until the early 1980s. Following the introduction of nasal ventilation during the late 1980s, however, noninvasive positive pressure ventilation became the preferred mode for assisting patients with respiratory failure.

RATIONALE FOR THE USE OF NONINVASIVE VENTILATION

Invasive mechanical ventilation has proved to be effective and reliable, but use of an endotracheal airway involves potential complications. These complications may be categorized as:

1. Traumatic complications (e.g., hemorrhage, tracheal laceration, vocal cord paralysis)
2. Complications related to bypassing the airway defense system (interfering with cough, mucociliary action)
3. Discomfort (e.g., pain, interference with communication and swallowing)

These complications apply to acute translaryngeal intubations as well as chronic tracheostomies. Further, airway invasion serves as a continual irritant, increasing mucus production and necessitating intermittent suctioning. By avoiding these complications, noninvasive ventilation has the potential of improving patient outcomes, enhancing patient satisfaction, and reducing the cost of care. It must be emphasized, however, that patients who receive noninvasive ventilation must be selected carefully (see later).

TECHNIQUES AND EQUIPMENT

Noninvasive Positive Pressure Ventilation

Noninvasive positive pressure ventilation (NPPV) consists of a positive pressure ventilator connected by tubing to a mask or an "interface" that applies positive air pressure to the nose, mouth, or both.

INTERFACES

Nasal Masks

Nasal masks are the most commonly used interfaces for treating chronic respiratory failure because they are convenient and permit normal speech and swallowing. Manufacturers offer numerous modifications of the three basic types of nasal mask:

- Standard nasal continuous positive airway pressure (CPAP) masks
- Nasal "pillows" or "seals"
- Custom-fitted masks

Standard nasal CPAP masks consist of clear plastic triangular domes that fit over the nose (Fig. 15.1). A soft cuff makes contact with the skin around the perimeter of the nose to form an air seal. These masks must be properly fitted to minimize pressure over the bridge of the nose, which may cause redness, skin irritation, and occasionally ulceration. Thin silicone flaps are used to create an effective air seal with minimal strap tension, and forehead "spacers" are used to minimize pressure on the bridge of the nose. Strap systems that hold the masks in place are also important for patient comfort. "Mini-masks" that fit over the tip of the nose and nostrils are designed to minimize claustrophobia, and gel-containing seals have been introduced in recent years to enhance patient comfort.

Nasal pillows or seals consist of small rubber cones that are inserted directly into the nostrils (Fig. 15.2). These are useful for patients with nasal bridge irritation or ulceration because they make no contact with the bridge of the nose. Some patients alternate between different types of masks as a way of minimizing discomfort.

Although kits for custom molding are available commercially, they require time and skill for successful application and are rarely used because a suitable commercially available mask can almost always be found.

Oronasal Masks

Oronasal (full face) masks cover both the nose and the mouth (Fig. 15.3) and can reduce the amount of air leaking through the mouth, which may limit the efficacy of nasal masks. For this reason, they are the preferred interface for treating acute respiratory failure, but they interfere with speech and eating more than nasal masks do, have more dead space, and are less comfortable than nasal masks for chronic use. Concerns have been raised about the risk of aspiration if the patient vomits or asphyxiation if the ventilator fails, so recommended masks come with quick-release straps and anti-asphyxia (non-rebreathing) valves.

Oral Interfaces

Commercially available oral interfaces use a mouthpiece inserted into a lip seal that is strapped tautly around the head to minimize air leakage; there is also a strapless type that has

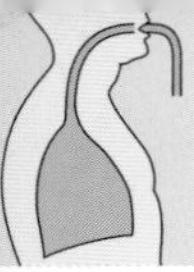

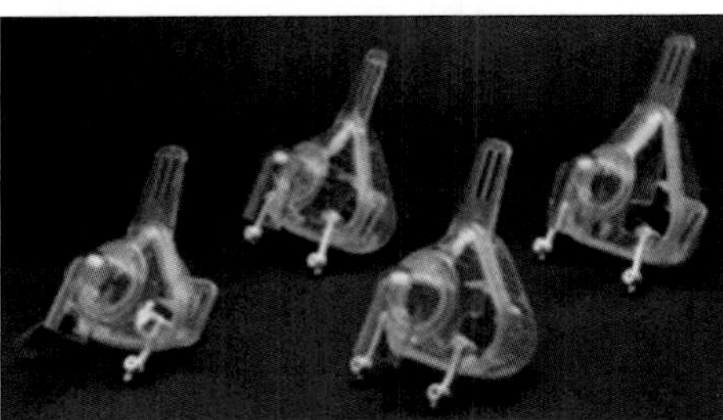

Figure 15.1 Standard nasal masks. Various sizes of standard nasal mask are available, ranging from small (left) to large (right).

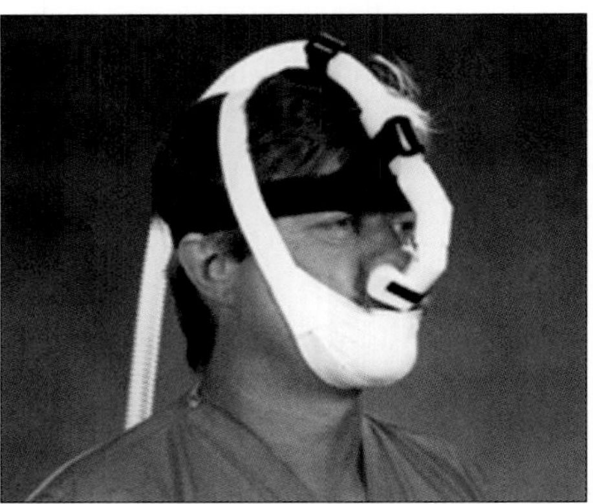

Figure 15.2 Nasal pillows. These avoid placing pressure on the bridge of the nose. The chin strap helps keep the mouth closed, reducing air leakage.

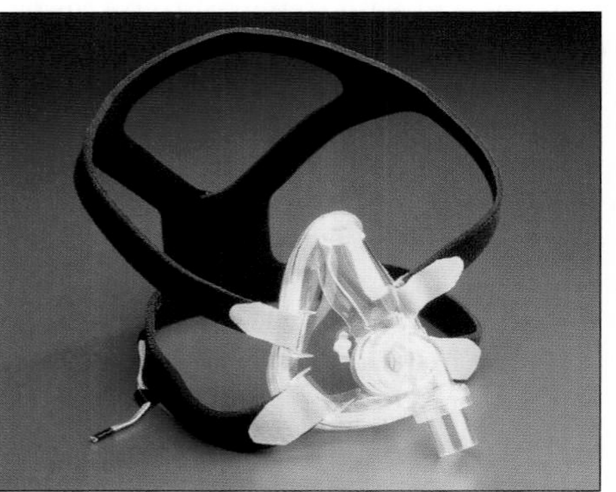

Figure 15.3 Oronasal face mask. The headgear (consisting of straps) is shown as though it were wrapped around the head. This mask has a very soft silicone seal and a rapid-release mechanism, and the exhalation valve is in the upper portion of the mask to minimize rebreathing.

flanges that fit inside and outside the lips. For daytime use, the mouthpiece can be mounted on a gooseneck device on a wheelchair, permitting patients to remain mobile while receiving ventilatory assistance. Strapless mouthpieces that are custom fitted by an orthodontist can be easily expectorated if necessary, even by patients with severe neuromuscular disease. These devices have been used for 24-hour ventilatory support in patients with neuromuscular disease, some of whom have little or no measurable vital capacity.

VENTILATORS

NPPV may be administered using volume-limited or pressure-limited modes on critical care ventilators (i.e., those designed mainly for invasive ventilation in the acute setting), ventilators designed specifically for acute applications of noninvasive ventilation, or portable positive pressure ventilators designed mainly for noninvasive ventilation in the home. The choice of ventilator depends largely on practitioner preferences and patient needs. For example, simple, portable, pressure-limited ventilators are frequently preferred because they lack sophisticated alarm systems that may needlessly interrupt sleep in patients requiring only nocturnal ventilatory assistance at home. In other situations, the enhanced alarm and monitoring capabilities of critical care ventilators may be preferred for acute applications. For chronic use in the home, simplicity and portability are important features.

Critical Care Ventilators

Many of the microprocessor-controlled ventilators currently used in critical care units can be adapted for noninvasive ventilation. Either volume-limited or pressure-limited modes may be selected, although most practitioners prefer pressure support ventilation, which has been rated by clinicians as better tolerated. The responses of these ventilators to the air leaks that inevitably occur with NPPV may be problematic, sometimes necessitating modifications in the masks or disabling of the alarms. Some newer critical care ventilators have noninvasive ventilation modes that automatically improve leak tolerance, disable alarms, and permit adjustments to limit inspiratory time. As long as the patient is critically ill, however, alarms should be disabled only in a closely monitored setting such as a critical care or step-down unit.

Portable Volume-Limited and Hybrid Ventilators

Portable volume-limited ventilators (Fig. 15.4) are commonly used to administer NPPV to patients with chronic respiratory failure. The ventilators are usually set in the assist/control mode to allow for spontaneous patient triggering, and the backup rate is usually set slightly below the spontaneous patient breathing rate. Currently available volume-limited ventilators have more alarm and pressure-generating capabilities than do most portable pressure-limited ventilators, and they may be better suited to patients who need continuous ventilation or those with severe chest wall deformities or obesity who need high inflation pressures. So-called hybrid ventilators have recently been introduced that offer both pressure- and volume-limited modes, some no larger than a laptop computer.

Pressure-Limited Ventilators

The use of portable ventilators that deliver pressure assist or pressure support ventilation (often referred to as bilevel devices) has increased in recent years. These deliver a preset inspiratory

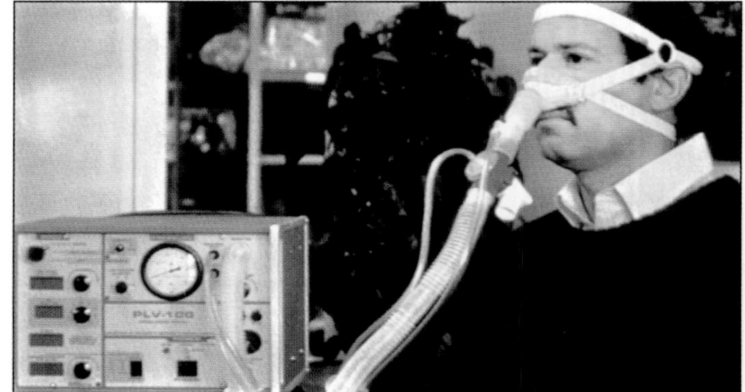

Figure 15.4 Typical volume-limited portable ventilator configured to deliver nasal ventilation.

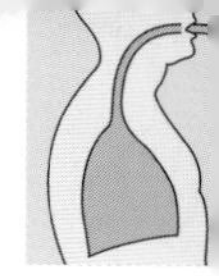

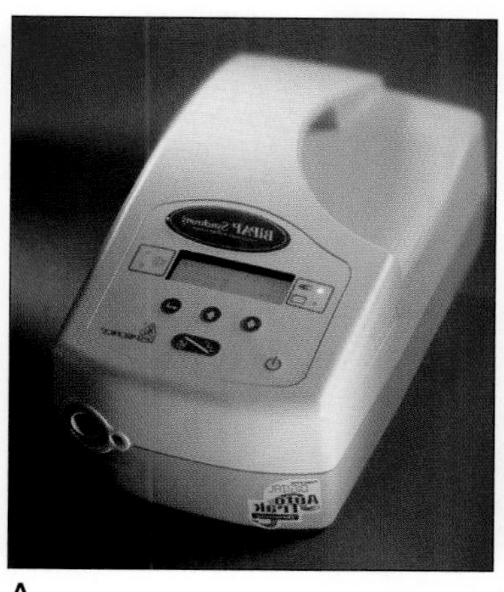

A

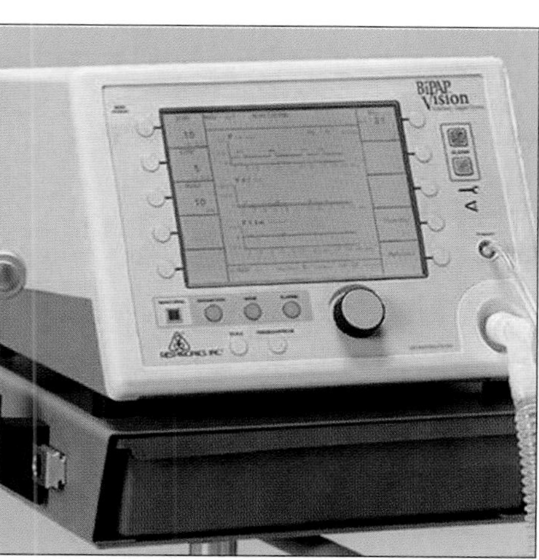

B

Figure 15.5 Typical bilevel-type portable pressure-limited ventilators. A, This device is designed for portability and convenience in the home. **B,** This device has an oxygen blender and graphics screen to facilitate in-hospital acute applications.

positive airway pressure (IPAP) that can be combined with positive end-expiratory pressure (PEEP) (Fig. 15.5). The difference between the IPAP and PEEP is the level of inspiratory assistance, or pressure support. Pressure support modes provide sensitive inspiratory triggering and expiratory cycling mechanisms, potentially allowing excellent patient-ventilator synchrony, reducing diaphragmatic work, and improving patient comfort. Because these devices are lighter (2 to 10 kg), are more compact ($<0.025\,m^3$), and have fewer alarms than critical care or portable volume-limited ventilators, they are preferred for patients requiring only nocturnal support in the home. Most have limited IPAP and oxygenation capabilities (up to 20 to 35 cmH_2O, depending on the ventilator) and lack alarms or battery backup systems. Unless appropriately modified, they have limited utility in the acute setting, although newer versions designed specifically for acute applications have sophisticated alarms and oxygen blenders.

Unlike volume-limited ventilators, bilevel devices are able to adjust inspiratory airflow to compensate for air leaks, potentially providing better support of gas exchange during leakage. Because they use a single tube with a passive exhalation valve, however, rebreathing can interfere with the ability to augment alveolar ventilation. This rebreathing problem can be minimized by using masks with in-mask exhalation valves, non-rebreathing valves, or PEEP pressures of 4 cmH_2O or greater; the last option ensures higher bias flows during exhalation.

Negative Pressure Ventilation

Negative pressure ventilators are used much less commonly today than in the past, but some centers in Italy and Spain still use them, mainly for patients with acute exacerbations of chronic obstructive pulmonary disease (COPD). Negative pressure ventilators include tank ventilators (like the iron lung; Fig. 15.6) and the smaller, more portable wrap or jacket ventilators (Fig. 15.7) and cuirass or shell ventilators (Fig. 15.8). The wrap ventilator consists of an impermeable nylon jacket suspended by a rigid chest piece that fits over the chest and abdomen. The cuirass ventilator is a rigid plastic or metal dome fitted over the chest and abdomen. Negative pressure ventilators expand the lungs by intermittently applying a subatmospheric pressure to the chest wall and abdomen, and expiration occurs passively by elastic recoil of the lung and chest wall. The tank is the most efficient and the cuirass the least efficient of these ventilators. Although these ventilators were commonly used to support patients with chronic respiratory failure in the past, this is no longer the case because of their tendency to exacerbate or even induce obstructive sleep apnea in patients with neuromuscular disease.

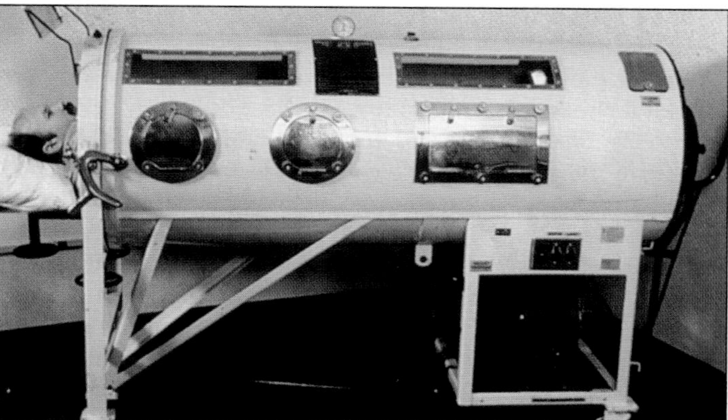

Figure 15.6 Iron lung. Tank-type negative pressure ventilator that was widely used during the polio epidemics.

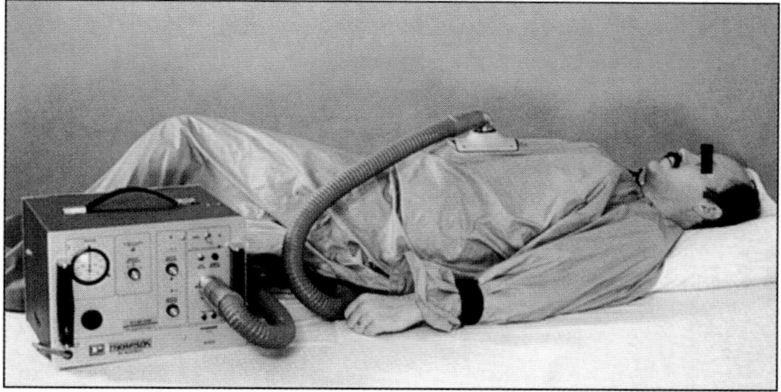

Figure 15.7 Wrap ventilator attached to a negative pressure generator. Note the contour of the rigid plastic chest piece, which suspends the wrap above the chest and abdomen.

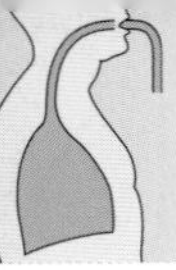

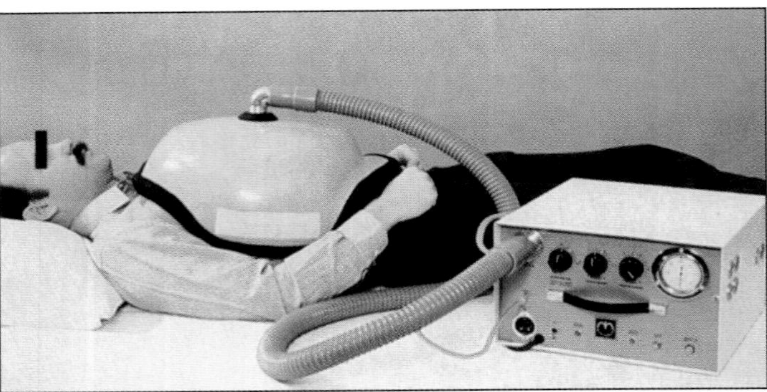

Figure 15.8 Chest cuirass attached to a negative pressure generator.

Abdominal Displacement Ventilation

The rocking bed and the intermittent abdominal pressure respirator, or "pneumobelt," both rely on displacement of the abdominal contents to assist ventilation. The rocking bed (Fig. 15.9) consists of a mattress on a motorized platform that rocks in an arc of approximately 40 degrees. When the patient is supine and the head rocks down, the abdominal viscera and diaphragm slide toward the head, assisting exhalation. As the head rocks up, the viscera and diaphragm slide toward the feet, assisting inhalation. The chief advantages of the rocking bed are ease of operation, lack of encumbrances, and patient comfort. Disadvantages include bulkiness, noisiness, lack of portability, and limited efficacy.

The pneumobelt uses a corset wrapped around the patient's midsection to hold an inflatable rubber bladder firmly against the anterior abdomen (Fig. 15.10). Intermittent inflation of the rubber bladder by a positive pressure ventilator compresses the abdomen, forcing the diaphragm upward and actively assisting exhalation. With bladder deflation, gravity returns the diaphragm to its original position, assisting inhalation. The pneumobelt is highly portable, can be mounted on a wheelchair to facilitate mobility, is easily hidden under clothing, and leaves the hands and face unencumbered. Because gravity is necessary to pull the diaphragm down during bladder deflation, nocturnal use is limited to patients who can learn to sleep while sitting.

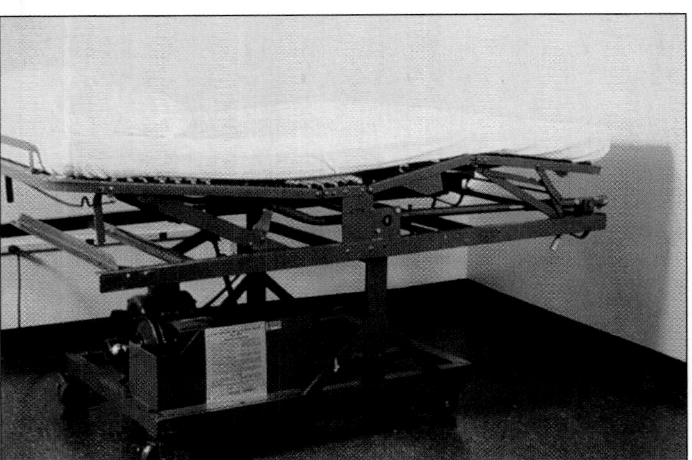

Figure 15.9 Rocking bed ventilator. At usual settings, the head rocks down approximately 10 degrees and the feet approximately 27 degrees. Sliding of the abdominal viscera assists diaphragm motion.

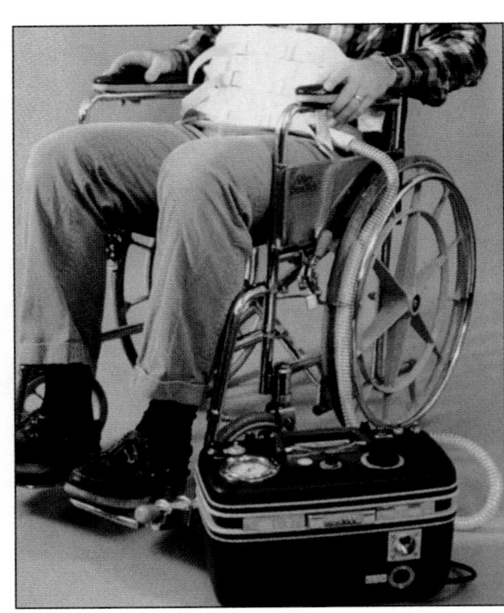

Figure 15.10 Intermittent abdominal pressure respirator, or "pneumobelt." This consists of a rubber bladder within the corset strapped to the patient's abdomen and attached to a portable positive pressure ventilator.

Like negative pressure ventilators, the pneumobelt and rocking bed have numerous disadvantages compared with NPPV and are used infrequently today. They are well suited to support patients with bilateral diaphragmatic paralysis, however, and are sometimes used for daytime assistance in patients with quadriplegia due to high spinal cord lesions.

Other Types of Ventilatory Assistance

Although technically not forms of "mechanical" ventilation, diaphragm pacing and glossopharyngeal breathing are ventilatory methods used in selected patients to enhance independence from mechanical ventilation. Diaphragm pacers consist of a radiofrequency transmitter and antenna that signal a surgically implanted receiver and electrode to stimulate the phrenic nerve. An intact phrenic nerve and diaphragm are usually required for successful application, but intercostal nerve implantation can be used when the phrenic nerves are damaged. Patients with high spinal cord quadriplegia, especially children, are the main users of pacers, allowing them freedom from invasive positive pressure ventilation.

Glossopharyngeal, or "frog," breathing uses intermittent gulping motions of the tongue and pharyngeal muscles to force air into the trachea. The technique can be used to provide freedom from mechanical ventilation for up to several hours, even in severely compromised patients. Use is limited to patients who have intact upper airway musculature, normal (or near normal) lungs and chest walls, and the ability to learn the technique. Good candidates include those with high spinal cord injuries, those with postpolio syndrome, and selected patients with other neuromuscular diseases.

ACUTE APPLICATIONS OF NONINVASIVE VENTILATION

Established Indications

CHRONIC OBSTRUCTIVE PULMONARY DISEASE

Earlier observations that NPPV reduces the work of breathing in patients with respiratory disease led investigators to hypothesize that it would be useful for ventilatory support of patients

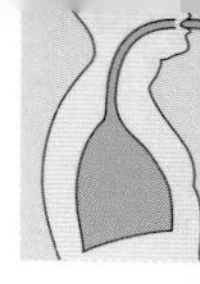

with acute respiratory deterioration who were developing respiratory muscle fatigue. This hypothesis has now been confirmed in patients with COPD. Two recent meta-analyses of multiple randomized, controlled trials confirmed that NPPV reduces respiratory rate, improves dyspnea and gas exchange, and lowers mortality compared with standard therapy. In these analyses, the intubation rate in those receiving NPPV was approximately 20%, down from the 50% rate seen in controls. European studies have demonstrated that NPPV also reduces hospital length of stay, but this has not been confirmed in North America, where length of stay tends to be much shorter than in Europe. Other studies have demonstrated that COPD complicated by pneumonia responds well to NPPV, that NPPV can be used to permit early extubation in selected COPD patients who require initial intubation, and that patients with mild exacerbations are not helped by NPPV, probably because they are not sufficiently ill to benefit from ventilatory assistance. The evidence is so strong for the initial use of NPPV for appropriately selected patients with COPD exacerbations that many now consider it a standard of care.

ACUTE PULMONARY EDEMA

The beneficial effects of positive pressure have long been known in patients with acute pulmonary edema. It improves compliance and oxygenation by increasing functional residual capacity and opening collapsed air spaces. At least four randomized, controlled trials have demonstrated that noninvasive CPAP alone improves dyspnea and oxygenation and lowers intubation rates in patients with acute pulmonary edema. One trial showed abbreviated intensive care unit stays compared with oxygen-treated controls, but no study has shown a reduction in mortality. More recently, several studies evaluated the efficacy of noninvasive ventilation (i.e., inspiratory assistance with pressure support superimposed on PEEP) compared with either oxygen therapy or CPAP alone. Although noninvasive ventilation has benefits similar to those previously demonstrated for CPAP, its superiority over CPAP alone has not been convincingly established, and one study raised the possibility that the myocardial infarction rate may be higher in those receiving noninvasive ventilation. Accordingly, CPAP alone is generally regarded as the initial noninvasive modality of choice, but noninvasive ventilation should be substituted if patients treated with CPAP remain dyspneic or manifest substantial carbon dioxide retention.

ACUTE RESPIRATORY FAILURE IN IMMUNOCOMPROMISED PATIENTS

Immunocompromised patients (those with *Pneumocystis jiroveci* pneumonia and those who have received solid-organ or bone marrow transplants) often have poor outcomes when they develop sufficient respiratory compromise to require invasive mechanical ventilation. Nosocomial infections and fatal bouts of septicemia are common complications in this setting, and those with hematologic malignancies may develop fatal airway hemorrhages due to thrombocytopenia and platelet dysfunction. Accordingly, avoiding intubation by using noninvasive ventilation is an attractive alternative. Randomized trials on patients with acute respiratory failure related to solid organ transplantation and hematologic malignancy have demonstrated reduced intubation and mortality rates compared with controls. Thus, noninvasive ventilation should be considered early during the development of respiratory failure in immunocompromised patients as a way to avoid intubation and its attendant mortality.

Other Possible Indications

Table 15.1 lists non-COPD causes of acute respiratory failure that may be treated with noninvasive ventilation in appropriately selected patients. As might be expected, other diseases with airflow limitation as an important manifestation (e.g., cystic fibrosis) appear to respond favorably, although randomized trials are lacking. A recent randomized trial treating acute asthma exacerbations in the emergency department indicated that noninvasive ventilation improves FEV_1 and lowers the hospitalization rate compared with sham ventilation.

Hypoxemic respiratory failure encompasses a diverse category of conditions, including acute respiratory distress syndrome, acute pneumonia, trauma, and acute pulmonary edema. With the exception of the last diagnosis and pneumonia in COPD or immunocompromised patients, however, evidence supporting the use of noninvasive ventilation is limited, and it should be applied selectively and with caution in these patients.

Other broad categories of respiratory failure that are increasingly being treated with noninvasive ventilation include postoperative patients, patients with extubation failure, and those in whom a decision has been made not to intubate. Although some randomized trials support the use of noninvasive ventilation in the first two categories, there are conflicting reports, and again, careful patient selection is mandatory. Although prophylactic use of noninvasive ventilation in patients at high risk for extubation failure has been proposed, available evidence suggests that it is not helpful and may even be harmful by delaying needed intubation. Noninvasive ventilation can be used with considerable success for do-not-intubate patients who have COPD exacerbations or acute pulmonary edema. It is less successful, however, in those with an underlying malignancy or acute pneumonia. Although noninvasive ventilation is generally reserved for patients with reversible diagnoses, it may occasion-

Table 15.1
Non-COPD causes of acute respiratory failure and general categories of patients treated with noninvasive positive pressure ventilation

Obstructive Diseases	**Hypoxemic Respiratory Failure**
Asthma (B)	ARDS (C)
Cystic Fibrosis (C)	Pneumonia (B*)
Upper airway obstruction (C)	Acute pulmonary edema (A†)
	Trauma (C)
Restrictive Diseases	**Others**
Kyphoscoliosis (C)	Immunocompromised patients (A)
Neuromuscular disease (C)	Postoperative respiratory failure (B)
Obesity Hypoventilation Syndrome (C)	Facilitation of extubation (A*)
	Extubation failure (B‡)
	Do-not-intubate patients (C)

Letters in parentheses indicate level of evidence: A, multiple controlled trials; B, single supportive controlled trial; C, uncontrolled trials, case reports.
*For COPD patients only.
†Strongest evidence for continuous positive airway pressure of 10 to 12 cmH_2O.
‡Conflicting data.
ARDS, acute respiratory distress syndrome; COPD, chronic obstructive pulmonary disease.

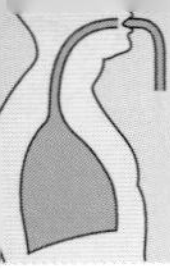

ally be appropriate for terminally ill patients to alleviate respiratory distress or to provide additional time to settle affairs. In these situations, patients and their families should be informed that it is being used as a form of life support.

Time Demands on Medical Personnel

The advantages of NPPV over conventional therapy for acute respiratory failure may be offset by excessive time demands on medical personnel. Earlier reports raised this as a potential problem, but it may have been related to a lack of experience with the technique. Nurses rate NPPV as no more demanding than conventional therapy, and they spend no more time with patients receiving NPPV than with controls. Respiratory therapists tend to spend more time with NPPV patients than with conventionally treated patients during the first 8 hours of use, but not subsequently. These findings indicate that NPPV initially requires more time to administer, but as patients and medical practitioners become familiar with the technique, time demands rapidly diminish.

Determinants of Success

Factors predicting the success of NPPV are shown in Table 15.2. In summary, these predictors indicate that patients most likely to benefit have advanced but not catastrophic respiratory failure. The predictors also suggest that there is a window of opportunity for the implementation of NPPV during which success is most likely. NPPV should be started when patients have evidence of acute respiratory distress and high Acute Physiology and Chronic Health Evaluation II (APACHE II) scores, but not too late, when they are approaching respiratory arrest, have advanced carbon dioxide retention and acidemia, have higher APACHE II scores, and are unable to cooperate.

Selection Guidelines

Selection guidelines for the use of NPPV in acute respiratory failure based on selection criteria used in randomized, controlled trials are shown in Table 15.3. In the two-step process, patients are identified as those at risk of needing ventilatory assistance (and possibly intubation) on the basis of clinical and blood gas indicators. Patients with mild respiratory distress are apt to do well without ventilatory assistance.

The second step is to exclude those who would be at higher risk of complications if they were managed noninvasively. Exclusions are listed in Table 15.3 and include patients who are too medically unstable or uncooperative, those with frank or imminent cardiopulmonary arrest, and those who cannot protect their airway. Obtundation is not necessarily an exclusion. Assiduous observation of the guidelines helps ensure the safe administration of noninvasive ventilation, but patients are still at risk for deterioration and should be monitored closely until stabilized. Delay of needed intubation by excessively prolonging failed attempts at noninvasive ventilation can add to morbidity and should be avoided.

The underlying cause and potential reversibility of the acute respiratory deterioration are also important considerations in patient selection. In this regard, NPPV may be viewed as a way to assist the patient during a critical interval of hours or days, allowing time for other therapies such as bronchodilators, corticosteroids, or diuretics to act. Severe, less reversible forms of respiratory failure that will likely require prolonged periods of ventilatory support, such as acute respiratory distress syndrome, should be managed with invasive ventilatory support. It might be argued that there is little to lose in trying noninvasive ventilation in a failing, do-not-intubate patient. NPPV should probably be used in this instance only if there is a reasonable expectation that the acute process can be reversed and the patient and his or her next of kin understand that NPPV is being used as a form of life support (albeit noninvasive).

Table 15.2
Characteristics of patients successfully treated with noninvasive positive pressure ventilation

Cooperative
Intact neurologic function
Able to coordinate breathing with ventilator
Moderately high (but not very high) APACHE II scores
Intact dentition
Less air leakage (often through the mouth) than in patients who fail
Able to control secretions
Hypercapnic, but not severely so
Acidemic, but not severely so (pH > 7.10)
Reduced respiratory rate and gas exchange within first 2 hours

Table 15.3
Selection guidelines for use of noninvasive positive pressure ventilation in patients with acute respiratory failure

Identify patients at risk of needing ventilatory assistance
Clinical criteria
Moderate to severe respiratory distress
Increased dyspnea
Tachypnea (respiratory rate >24/minute)
Use of accessory muscles
Paradoxical breathing pattern
Blood gas criteria
$PaCO_2$ > 45 mmHg (> 6.0 kPa) and pH < 7.35, or PaO_2/FIO_2 < 200
Exclude patients who would be more safely managed invasively
Respiratory arrest
Medically unstable
Shock states
Unstable cardiac status
Acute severe ischemia or infarction
Uncontrolled life-threatening arrhythmias
Active severe upper gastrointestinal bleeding
Uncooperative or agitated
Unable to protect airway
Excessive secretions
Severe cough or swallowing impairment
Severe facial trauma
Appropriate, reversible cause for respiratory failure (as in Table 15.1)

LONG-TERM APPLICATIONS OF NONINVASIVE VENTILATION

As recently as the mid-1980s, nocturnal negative pressure ventilation was used to reverse gas exchange abnormalities and symptoms in patients with chronic respiratory failure due to

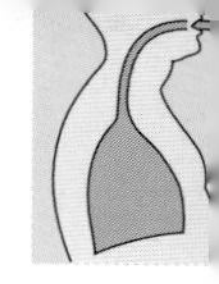

neuromuscular diseases and chest wall deformities. Because of the difficulty of application, limited efficacy, and tendency to aggravate or even induce upper airway obstructions, however, negative pressure and other "body" ventilators have been relegated to a second-line role in the management of chronic respiratory failure. On the basis of a number of uncontrolled studies published during the late 1980s and early 1990s, as well as widespread clinical experience, NPPV has become the ventilatory modality of first choice to treat these patients.

Restrictive Thoracic Disease

A few weeks of nocturnal nasal NPPV consistently improves gas exchange and symptoms in patients with chronic respiratory failure caused by restrictive thoracic disease (e.g., severe neuromuscular disease, kyphoscoliosis) and in patients with the obesity-hypoventilation syndrome. In addition, severe nocturnal oxygen desaturation is ameliorated when patients are switched from negative pressure ventilation to NPPV. Although no studies have compared nasal and mouthpiece NPPV, mouthpiece NPPV may be used for long-term ventilatory support in patients with severe neuromuscular disease who have virtually no measurable vital capacity.

Prospective, randomized trials to establish the efficacy of NPPV in patients with restrictive thoracic disease have not been done, largely for ethical reasons, but it is known that temporary withdrawal of nocturnal nasal ventilation from patients with chronic respiratory failure caused by restrictive thoracic disease results in worsening nocturnal gas exchange, daytime symptoms, and poorer sleep quality. These findings provide strong evidence that NPPV is effective in reversing nocturnal hypoventilation and improving symptoms in these patients. In addition, long-term follow-up studies on several hundred patients using NPPV for 3 to 5 years observed high rates of NPPV continuation (and hence survival) among patients with postpolio syndrome, most myopathies, and kyphoscoliosis. Survival is less favorable for patients with more rapidly progressive neuromuscular diseases such as amyotrophic lateral sclerosis, but NPPV appears to extend survival in these patients as well.

Although the long-term efficacy of NPPV for patients with restrictive thoracic disease appears to be well established, the optimal time for initiation is unclear. Most authorities recommend waiting for the onset of symptoms or daytime hypoventilation before initiating long-term NPPV. This is partly for pragmatic reasons, because patients comply better if motivated by the desire for symptom relief.

Chronic Obstructive Pulmonary Disease

The most controversial application of noninvasive ventilation has been in patients with severe but stable COPD. During the early 1980s, investigators theorized that the respiratory muscles in patients with severe COPD may be chronically fatigued and might benefit from intermittent rest. Early trials found that intermittent daytime sessions using negative pressure wrap ventilators improved daytime gas exchange and inspiratory and expiratory muscle strength in patients with severe COPD. Longer-term controlled studies failed to demonstrate the same favorable effects of intermittent negative pressure ventilation, however. In addition, COPD patients tolerated the wrap ventilators poorly, using them for less time daily than recommended, and they had trouble sleeping during ventilator use.

The disappointing results with negative pressure ventilators stimulated interest in the use of NPPV for severe COPD, but these studies have yielded conflicting results as well. In a 3-month crossover trial, only 7 of 19 patients with severe COPD improved, and this improvement was limited to tests of neuropsychological function; it was not apparent relative to nocturnal or daytime gas exchange, sleep quality, pulmonary function, exercise tolerance, or symptoms. In contrast, a similar study of 18 patients found that NPPV improved nocturnal and daytime gas exchange, total sleep time, and quality-of-life scores. The substantial difference in the baseline characteristics of patients entering these trials may explain the conflicting results. Patients entering the favorable study had greater hypercarbia ($Pa{CO_2}$ 56 mmHg versus 46 mmHg) and more nocturnal oxygen desaturation, despite having less severe airway obstruction (FEV_1 0.81 L versus 0.54 L), than did patients entering the unfavorable trial. These findings support the hypothesis that the subgroup of patients most likely to benefit from NPPV is that with substantial daytime carbon dioxide retention (>50 to 55 mmHg) and nocturnal oxygen desaturation. A recent controlled trial of COPD patients with chronic retention ($Pa{CO_2}$ > 50 mmHg) demonstrated less increase in $Pa{CO_2}$, less deterioration of quality of life, and a trend toward fewer hospital days after 2 years of nocturnal NPPV compared with oxygen-treated controls.

These studies suggest that, compared with oxygen therapy alone, NPPV maintains gas exchange and quality of life and probably reduces the need for hospitalization in patients with severe stable COPD who have substantial carbon dioxide retention. Adherence to the therapy remains a major challenge, however.

Selection Guidelines

A number of characteristics permit the selection of appropriate patients with chronic respiratory failure to receive NPPV (Table 15.4). The combination of mild to moderate daytime carbon dioxide retention (usually an indication of more severe nocturnal retention) and symptoms attributable to hypoventilation and associated poor sleep quality is a clear indication, as is symptomatic nocturnal hypoventilation even in the absence of daytime carbon dioxide retention. Secondary considerations include a history of repeated hospitalizations for bouts of respiratory failure.

Patients should be excluded from consideration if they are unable to protect their airway adequately because of swallowing impairment or excessive secretions, particularly if combined with a weakened cough mechanism. If such patients desire aggressive support, they are usually more safely managed with invasive ventilation.

The patient's diagnosis is also an important consideration. Those with stable or slowly progressive neuromuscular diseases or chest wall deformities are the best candidates. Others, such as those with central hypoventilation or obstructive sleep apnea who have failed a trial of nasal CPAP, are also acceptable candidates. Patients with rapidly progressive neuromuscular processes, particularly if there is upper airway involvement, are poor candidates. Selection criteria used by Medicare to guide reimbursement for patients with chronic airway obstruction are listed in Table 15.4. Because of the numerous studies showing

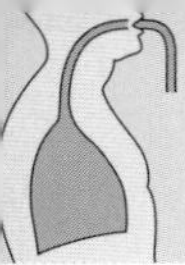

Table 15.4
Guidelines for initiating noninvasive ventilation in patients with chronic respiratory failure

Restrictive Thoracic Disorders

1. Symptomatic despite optimal medical therapy** (e.g., morning headaches, daytime hypersomnolence, chronic fatigue) and
2. Gas exchange disturbance:
   - Chronic CO_2 retention ($PaCO_2$ > 45 mmHg) or
   - Nocturnal hypoventilation (as evidenced by O_2 saturation < 88% for > 5 consecutive minutes while breathing room air), intact neurologically, or
3. Severe pulmonary dysfunction:
   - FVC < 50% predicted or
   - Maximal inspiratory pressure < 60 cmH_2O or
4. Other considerations:
   - Repeated hospital admissions for hypercapnic respiratory failure

Chronic Obstructive Pulmonary Disease

1. Symptomatic despite optimal medical therapy (including oxygen supplementation, if indicated) and
2. Gas exchange disturbance:
   - Chronic CO_2 retention ($PaCO_2 \geq 52$ mmHg) and
   - Nocturnal hypoventilation (as evidenced by O_2 saturation < 89% for ≥ 5 consecutive minutes while breathing usual FIO_2) and
3. Obstructive sleep apnea (OSA) excluded (on clinical grounds; sleep study needed only if clinically indicated); if OSA present, CPAP indicated initially
4. Other considerations:
   - Repeated hospital admissions for hypercapnic respiratory failure

* Based on Medicare guidelines for reimbursement of noninvasive ventilation. These guidelines do not recognize repeated hospital admissions as a reason for reimbursement, and appeal may be necessary if that is justification.
** Oxygen therapy alone may exacerbate CO_2 retention and should be avoided in hypercapnic patients with restrictive thoracic disorders.

no benefit among COPD patients with daytime carbon dioxide levels of 40 to 45 mmHg, the threshold for carbon dioxide retention is higher in these patients than in those with restrictive thoracic disease ($PaCO_2 \geq 52$ mmHg).

APPLICATION OF NONINVASIVE POSITIVE PRESSURE VENTILATION

Initiation

Techniques for initiating NPPV are similar in the acute and long-term settings, except that the level of urgency differs. Initiation must be tailored for each individual patient under both circumstances. In the acute setting, the interface and the ventilator must be selected rapidly. Accordingly, it is advisable to attach a "mask bag" containing a variety of types and sizes of nasal and oronasal masks and straps to a noninvasive ventilation cart or to initially use masks that will fit most individuals and can be rapidly applied. In the chronic setting, it is also useful to have a variety of interfaces readily available, but mask interchanges can be made over periods of days to weeks rather than minutes. In both settings, implementation by experienced practitioners who can impart a sense of confidence and reassurance is helpful.

Recent evidence and experience indicate that, in the acute setting, the oronasal mask is usually preferred because it has the advantage of controlling mouth leaks better than nose masks. The nasal mask is rated by patients as more comfortable for long-term application, so transitioning from an oronasal to a nasal mask should be contemplated after the first few days if NPPV is going to continue. Proper mask fit is also important. Selection of a mask that is too large should be avoided, because this necessitates excessive tightening of the straps to minimize air leakage. With regard to ventilator selection, both pressure-limited and volume-limited ventilators have been used with similar success rates. In the acute setting, pressure-limited ventilators specifically designed for noninvasive ventilation that offer oxygen blenders and display waveforms are gaining popularity; likewise, in the long-term setting, pressure-limited ventilators (bilevel type) have seen increasing use. Portable volume-limited ventilators are used mainly for patients with a continuous need for mechanical ventilation because of their enhanced alarm capabilities.

To begin NPPV, the mask should be placed on the patient's face and ventilation started. Cooperative patients may feel more comfortable if they hold the mask themselves. Initial ventilator settings should be relatively low to enhance patient comfort and acceptance, but inspiratory pressure or tidal volume should be adjusted upward as tolerated to provide adequate ventilatory assistance. Typical initial settings on pressure-limited ventilators are 8 to 12 cmH_2O for inspiratory and 4 to 5 cmH_2O for expiratory pressures (pressure support of 5 to 10 cmH_2O and PEEP of 4 to 5 cmH_2O), with subsequent adjustments as needed to alleviate respiratory distress (increased inspiratory pressure) or to counterbalance auto-PEEP, treat hypoxemia, or eliminate obstructive apnea (increased expiratory pressure). The difference between the two (pressure support) should be adequate to reduce ventilatory effort. In some patients, higher levels of IPAP or PEEP may be so effective in reducing the inspiratory work of breathing that the additional benefit of IPAP cannot be discerned. For volume ventilation, initial tidal volumes range from 10 to 15 mL/kg. The ventilator is usually set to allow patient triggering (assist/control mode). The ventilator backup rate is set at the spontaneous breathing rate if the aim is to assume the patient's breathing and minimize the work of respiratory muscles; it is set slightly below this level to encourage spontaneous breathing. Once the patient appears to be synchronizing with the ventilator, the head straps can be tightened. These should be adjusted to minimize air leakage, particularly into the eyes, but the practitioner should still be able to slip one or two fingers under the strap. Most manufacturers have developed ways to minimize facial trauma, such as forehead cushions and ultrathin silicon seals, and these should be used as recommended. Humidification is not needed in the acute setting for short-term use (<6 to 12 hours) but probably enhances comfort for longer-term applications. Oxygen supplementation is adjusted to maintain a desired oxygen saturation. It is administered via the blender on critical care ventilators and some bilevel ventilators, or directly via a cannula connected to the mask or T-connector in the ventilator tubing when using other bilevel ventilators.

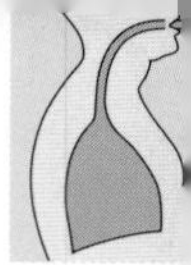

Adaptation and Monitoring

In the acute setting, the first 1 to 2 hours are critical in achieving successful adaptation. Coaching and encouragement are usually required to assist the patient in keeping the mouth shut during nasal ventilation and in adopting a breathing pattern that achieves synchronization with the ventilator and reduction of breathing effort. Instructions such as "Try to take slow, deep breaths and let the machine breathe for you" may be helpful. Also, judicious administration of low doses of sedatives such as midazolam may be helpful in enhancing patient acceptance.

Ventilators designed to administer noninvasive ventilation often lack sophisticated monitoring capabilities, but even when critical care ventilators are used for noninvasive ventilation in the acute setting, monitoring via the ventilator may be inaccurate or even misleading because of air leaks. Accordingly, close bedside monitoring is essential until the patient's respiratory status stabilizes. Although NPPV can easily be administered on general medical wards, the acuteness of the patient's illness and the need for close monitoring should dictate the site of administration. Acutely ill patients should be treated in an intensive care or step-down unit until their condition stabilizes, regardless of whether they are treated with invasive or noninvasive ventilation.

Achieving patient comfort (or at least minimizing discomfort), tolerance, and reduced respiratory effort is the most important initial goal, so frequent bedside assessments are obligatory. Oxygen saturation is monitored continuously, with oxygen supplementation titrated to achieve a target such as 92% or greater. Patient synchrony with the ventilator, respiratory and heart rates, and sternocleidomastoid muscle activity are monitored closely. Blood gases are also monitored as clinically indicated. Inspiratory pressures or tidal volumes are usually adjusted upward as tolerated to bring about desired improvements in $PaCO_2$. Some suggest that this is best achieved by increasing expiratory rather than inspiratory pressures, reducing the $PaCO_2$ by reducing the inspiratory work of breathing associated with auto-PEEP.

In the chronic setting, adaptation usually takes much longer than in the acute setting, mainly because the patient must learn to sleep using the ventilator. The patient is instructed to initiate noninvasive ventilation at home for 1- or 2-hour trial periods during the daytime and then try to fall asleep with the device at bedtime. The patient is encouraged to leave the equipment on as long as tolerated but is allowed to remove it if desired. During this period, frequent contact with an experienced home respiratory therapist helps ensure proper use and adjustment. Some patients successfully sleep through the night within days of initiation, but others require several months to become accustomed to the machine. Occasional patients are unable to adapt successfully to NPPV, usually because of mask intolerance. In these cases, trials with alternative noninvasive ventilators, such as negative pressure or abdominal ventilators, may be successful, as long as the patient has no more than mild obstructive sleep apnea.

Patients should be seen every few weeks by a physician during the initial adaptation period. At the time of office follow-up, symptoms and physical signs should be assessed for evidence of nocturnal hypoventilation or cor pulmonale. Spirometry is indicated, particularly in patients with progressive neuromuscular syndromes. Daytime arterial blood gases or pulse oximetry and end-tidal PCO_2 ($PetCO_2$) levels should be obtained at the time of visit or when symptoms worsen. Although there is no consensus on the ideal level, daytime $PetCO_2$ values ranging from about 40 to 55 mmHg are usually associated with good control of symptoms. Nocturnal monitoring using oximetry, multichannel recorders, or full polysomnography is also useful after adaptation to noninvasive ventilation to ensure the adequacy of oxygenation and ventilation.

Commonly Encountered Problems and Possible Remedies

NPPV is safe and well tolerated in most properly selected patients. The most commonly encountered problems are related to the interface or to air pressure or flow (Table 15.5). Patients often complain of mask discomfort, which can be alleviated by minimizing strap tension or trying different mask sizes or types. The most common error is to select a mask that is too large, necessitating excessive strap tension to minimize leaks. For acute applications, patients may be anxious and have difficulty synchronizing their breathing efforts with the ventilator. Adjustments in ventilator mode (to pressure support, which usually enhances synchrony) and in inspiratory and expiratory pressures, plus judicious use of sedation, may help. In patients with severe COPD who have intrinsic PEEP, increases in expiratory pressure may facilitate triggering.

Excessive air pressure leading to sinus or ear pain is another common complaint, alleviated by lowering the pressure temporarily and then gradually raising it again as tolerance improves. Patients may also complain of dryness or congestion of the nose or mouth. For dryness, nasal saline or gels or efforts to reduce air leaks may help. Heated, flow-by humidifiers may also be helpful, particularly in dry climates or during winter. For nasal congestion, inhaled corticosteroids or decongestants or oral antihistamine-decongestant combinations may be used.

Other commonly encountered problems include erythema, pain, and ulceration on the bridge of the nose related to pressure

Table 15.5
Adverse side effects and complications of noninvasive positive pressure ventilation

Mask-Related	Discomfort Nasal bridge redness, ulceration Anxiety, claustrophobia Acne-like skin rash
Related to Airflow or Pressure	Nasal or oral dryness or congestion Eye irritation Sinus or ear pain Gastric insufflation Air leakage Sleep arousals
Related to Ventilator Type	Asynchrony; inability to sense inspiration or expiration Inability to compensate for leaks Rebreathing
Major Complications	Failure to tolerate or ventilate, need for intubation (25–33%) Aspiration pneumonia Pneumothorax

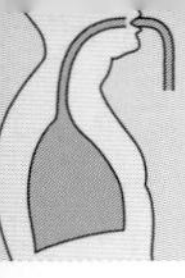

from the mask seal. Minimizing strap tension, using artificial skin, or switching to alternative masks such as nasal pillows can alleviate this problem. Gastric insufflation is common, but it is usually not severe, probably because inflation pressures are low compared with those used with invasive ventilation.

Air leaking through the mouth (with nasal masks), through the nose (with mouthpieces), or around the mask (with all interfaces) is inevitable during NPPV. Nasal and oronasal masks, particularly if too large, may leak air into the eyes, causing conjunctival irritation. Refitting or reseating the mask usually addresses this problem. Pressure-limited devices compensate for air leaks by maintaining inspiratory airflow during leaking; tidal volumes on volume-limited ventilators must be adjusted by the practitioner to compensate. To reduce air leaking through the mouth, patients are coached to keep the mouth shut or use chin straps or oronasal masks. Air leakage occurs during the majority of sleep in many patients, but fortunately, gas exchange is usually well maintained. Leaks may still contribute to arousals and poor sleep quality, however, and ventilatory assistance may occasionally be compromised. In this case, options include trials of alternative interfaces or ventilators or, if these fail, tracheostomy. Major complications of noninvasive ventilation, such as aspiration and pneumothorax, are unusual if patient selection guidelines are observed.

CONCLUSION

Noninvasive ventilation, mainly in the form of NPPV, has established itself as an important ventilator modality. In the acute setting, NPPV is preferred to invasive positive pressure ventilation for selected patients with COPD exacerbations because of reduced morbidity and mortality, the possibility of reduced costs, and enhanced patient comfort. NPPV is also suitable for initial mechanical ventilatory assistance in patients with a variety of other forms of acute respiratory failure, including those with acute pulmonary edema or an immunocompromised status, as long as selection guidelines are observed. These guidelines are designed to identify patients at risk of needing mechanical ventilatory assistance while excluding those who are too ill to be safely managed noninvasively. Also, the cause of the patient's respiratory failure should be one that is anticipated to be reversed within a few days.

NPPV is also considered the ventilatory modality of first choice for a variety of causes of chronic respiratory failure, including neuromuscular diseases, chest wall restrictive processes, and central hypoventilation. Here, NPPV offers comfort, convenience, and cost advantages over invasive positive pressure ventilation. Ideal candidates should require only intermittent ventilatory assistance and have intact upper airway function, but NPPV has been successfully applied even in patients requiring continuous assistance and those with bulbar dysfunction.

The efficacy of NPPV has not been firmly established in patients with chronic respiratory failure due to COPD, but patients with substantial hypercarbia and nocturnal oxygen desaturation appear to be the ones most likely to benefit.

If NPPV fails in patients with chronic respiratory failure, alternative forms of noninvasive ventilation, such as negative pressure ventilators, pneumobelts, or rocking beds, may still occasionally be effective.

SUGGESTED READINGS

Antonelli M, Conti G, Rocco M, et al: A comparison of noninvasive positive-pressure ventilation and conventional mechanical ventilation in patients with acute respiratory failure. N Engl J Med 339:429-435, 1998.

Hilbert G, Gruson D, Vargas F, et al: Noninvasive ventilation in immunosuppressed patients with pulmonary infiltrates, and acute respiratory failure. N Engl J Med 344:481-487, 2001.

Hill NS: Complications of noninvasive positive pressure ventilation. Respir Care 42:432-442, 1997.

Keenan S, Sinuff T, Cook DJ, Hill NS: Which patients with acute exacerbations of chronic obstructive pulmonary disease benefit from noninvasive positive pressure ventilation? A systematic review of the literature. Ann Intern Med 138:861-870, 2003.

Lightowler JV, Wedjicha JA, Elliott MW, Ram FS: Non-invasive positive pressure ventilation to treat respiratory failure resulting from exacerbations of chronic obstructive pulmonary disease: Cochrane systematic review and meta-analysis. BMJ 326:177-178, 2003.

Mehta S, Hill NS: Noninvasive ventilation—state of the art. Am J Respir Crit Care Med 163:540-577, 2001.

Wedjicha JA: Outcome of long-term noninvasive positive pressure ventilation. Respir Care Clin N Am 8:559-573, 2002.

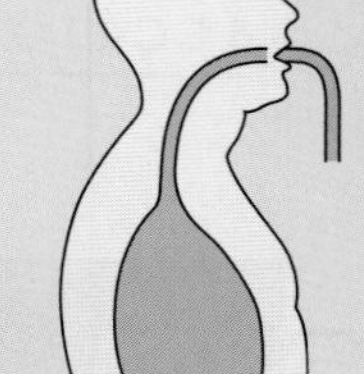

CHAPTER 16 Airway Management

Jeanine P. Wiener-Kronish and David W. Shimabukuro

The decision to intubate the airway is made in response to one or more of three circumstances:

1. Failure of oxygenation
2. Failure of ventilation
3. Airway protection

The medical practitioner responsible for securing the airway must know the advantages and problems associated with the techniques of airway management and rapidly integrate these concepts to treat a patient who needs immediate assistance. Adverse outcomes occur with failure to restore ventilation, failure to recognize an esophageal intubation, or massive aspiration by the patient around the time of intubation. Death or hypoxic brain damage occurs when airway management is poorly performed. Closed claim analyses have determined that, in many instances, there is an associated failure to recognize the scope of the clinical problem or a failure to act in a timely manner.

INDICATIONS AND CONTRAINDICATIONS

The most common indication for definitive airway management with endotracheal intubation is respiratory failure and the need to deliver positive pressure ventilation. This is generally manifested by hypoxia, hypercapnia, or an excessive work of breathing. Other indications include protecting the lungs from aspiration of gastric contents or blood in patients with neurologic compromise, leading to an inability to protect the airways; ensuring airway patency in cases of facial or airway trauma or swelling of upper airway structures; and administering deep sedation or general anesthesia for bedside procedures. The only contraindication to airway management is a patient's refusal.

TECHNIQUES

General Considerations

The initial approach to airway management is to obtain a history of any prior airway problems and to recognize situations that are associated with difficulty in securing an airway. Patients who have a restricted oral opening, small pharyngeal space, noncompliant submandibular tissue, limited atlanto-occipital flexion or extension, or partial airway obstruction from masses or redundant tissue can be difficult to manage. Mask ventilation may be particularly difficult in obese patients, edentulous patients, those with full beards, or those with partial airway obstruction.

Special Considerations

Patients with an increased risk of aspiration (those with nausea or vomiting; those who are postprandial, obese, or pregnant; and those with a hiatal hernia or a history of severe gastroesophageal reflux or intra-abdominal pathology) require the Sellick maneuver during direct laryngoscopy (Fig. 16.1). Alternatively, they can be intubated while awake or lightly sedated.

Hypotensive patients with acute myocardial ischemia or infarction, hypovolemia (hypovolemic shock), or sepsis requiring vasopressor therapy to maintain an adequate perfusion pressure have a higher incidence of peri-intubation death. These patients do not tolerate significant increases or decreases in heart rate or blood pressure. Accordingly, medications and techniques that maintain normal hemodynamics need to be employed.

Patients with aneurysms do not tolerate rapid alterations in their blood pressure, as this increases the risk of rupture. Therefore, as with those in shock, medications and techniques that maintain normal hemodynamics must be used.

Irrespective of the underlying disease, certain medications should be readily available before managing a patient's airway. These include, but are not limited to, sedatives, paralytics, vasopressors, and vasodilators.

Airway Management Paradigms

The six broad types of airway management are noninvasive ventilation, awake intubation, intubation with spontaneous ventilation, intubation with neuromuscular paralysis, emergent nonsurgical airway management, and surgical airway management.

NONINVASIVE VENTILATION

Patients may maintain adequate oxygenation and ventilation if assisted with continuous positive airway pressure or bilevel positive airway pressure. Both can be delivered either nasally or via a full face mask. Contraindications to these techniques include a depressed mental status, ventilatory or hemodynamic instability, requirement for sedation, inability to handle upper airway secretions, severe hypoxia, risk of aspiration, and inability to wear a tight mask.

AWAKE INTUBATION

Ideally, patients should be intubated while awake. However, most patients find the experience unpleasant and quite traumatic. Regardless, in those individuals with difficult airways, this is the preferred method because the patient can continue

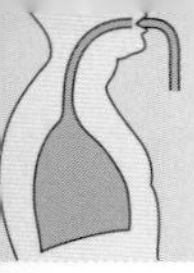

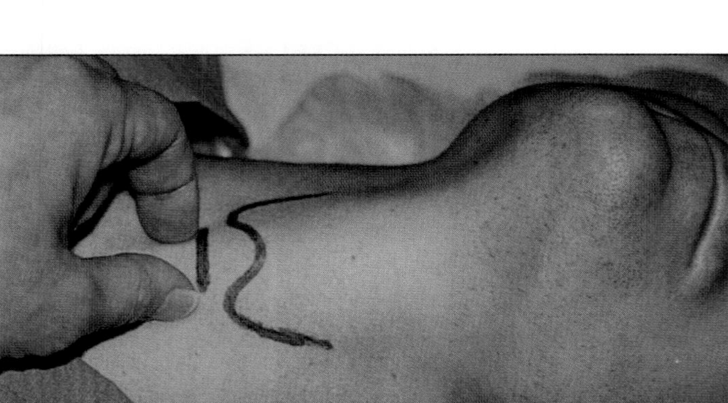

Figure 16.1 Sellick maneuver. The cricoid cartilage is identified by palpation below the thyroid cartilage. Firm pressure is placed on this structure to occlude the esophagus. Pressure is maintained until after intubation, and airway control is documented by auscultation of the lung fields and end-tidal CO_2.

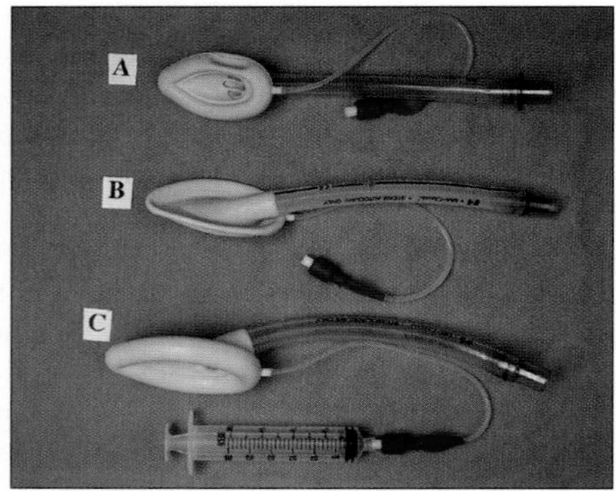

Figure 16.2 Laryngeal mask airway (LMA). Available in sizes 1 to 5. Note the slits to allow ventilation and placement of an endotracheal tube via a fiber-optic bronchoscope. There are several techniques for proper insertion. Commonly, the LMA is placed slightly inflated, with the tongue and mandible gently pulled anteriorly, with continuous pressure straight posteriorly until it "slides" in place. Position is confirmed after full inflation by the ability to ventilate the patient, as noted by chest rise and auscultation. Most adults will accept a size 4 or 5. *A*, Number 3, partially inflated. *B*, Number 4, completely deflated. *C*, Number 5, completely inflated.

to spontaneously ventilate and oxygenate. Approaches for awake intubation range from the blind nasal approach, which does not require laryngeal visualization, to direct laryngoscopy, which uses topical anesthesia and fiber-optic laryngoscopes or bronchoscopes.

INTUBATION WITH SPONTANEOUS VENTILATION

Sedative agents administered as a bolus can maintain spontaneous ventilation yet permit direct laryngoscopy or the placement of a laryngeal mask airway (LMA; Fig. 16.2). The LMA rests in the posterior hypopharynx, displacing the tongue anteriorly while keeping the glottis open. Once inflated, the LMA provides a seal to allow limited positive pressure ventilation, if needed. Because it sits above the larynx, it does not protect against aspiration of gastric contents. A fiber-optic bronchoscope can be passed through an LMA for placement of an endotracheal tube (Fig. 16.3).

INTUBATION WITH NEUROMUSCULAR PARALYSIS

Intubation with neuromuscular paralysis is the most common method used for direct laryngoscopy, because relaxation of the masseter muscle facilitates better visualization of the glottis (see Fig. 16.3). Loss of spontaneous respiration means that the practitioner must obtain immediate airway control or ensure adequate ventilation by mask. When this intubation option is selected, the provider must have an alternative plan, because the larynx is not always visualized.

A rapid-sequence approach is undertaken in patients thought to have airways that can be easily controlled by direct laryngoscopy and who are at significant risk for aspiration of gastric contents. Briefly, the patient is preoxygenated with 100% oxygen by full face mask to increase the alveolar PO_2. A sedative agent (hypnotic) and a short-acting muscle relaxant are administered sequentially (Table 16.1). At the same time, an assistant applies pressure to the cricoid cartilage (the only complete ring in the tracheobronchial tree) by means of the Sellick maneuver, which occludes the esophagus and decreases the risk of aspiration of gastric contents (see Fig. 16.1). This external pressure is maintained until the airway is secured by tracheal intubation. The goal is rapid, definitive airway control.

EMERGENT NONSURGICAL AIRWAY MANAGEMENT

Transtracheal catheter oxygenation or transtracheal jet ventilation is used in emergent situations when one or several approaches have failed and improvement in oxygenation is imperative (Fig. 16.4). This technique is usually able to achieve only minimally acceptable levels of oxygenation, but it allows time to perform more definitive measures to obtain an airway. Emergency cricothyroidotomy is not technically difficult (based on the Seldinger technique) and can be accomplished quickly with readily available equipment. Single-use sterile kits are commercially available. Percutaneous tracheotomy is also based on the Seldinger technique. Ideally, it should be done with the aid of direct visualization via a fiber-optic bronchoscope in the trachea. It is technically more difficult and requires more time than a cricothyroidotomy. Regardless, oxygenation and ventilation are easily achieved once the tracheotomy tube is properly placed (Fig. 16.5).

SURGICAL AIRWAY

Surgical access, emergent or nonemergent, is necessary when laryngeal visualization cannot be achieved and a definitive airway cannot be established. A surgical cricothyroidotomy requires more skill than a percutaneous approach, but it allows direct visualization of anatomy to ensure proper placement (see Fig. 16.4). An open surgical tracheotomy is not an option in an emergency because it is very time consuming. It should be performed only by physicians trained in this procedure. Surgical approaches can be performed with the patient awake using local anesthesia.

Choice of Airway Control

A number of considerations affect the choice of airway control. Regardless of whether all structures are seen by laryngoscopy or bronchoscopy, any visualization is preferable to blind techniques when placement of the endotracheal tube must be precise (i.e., when oxygenation is low, the patient is unstable, or the patient is soiling the airway).

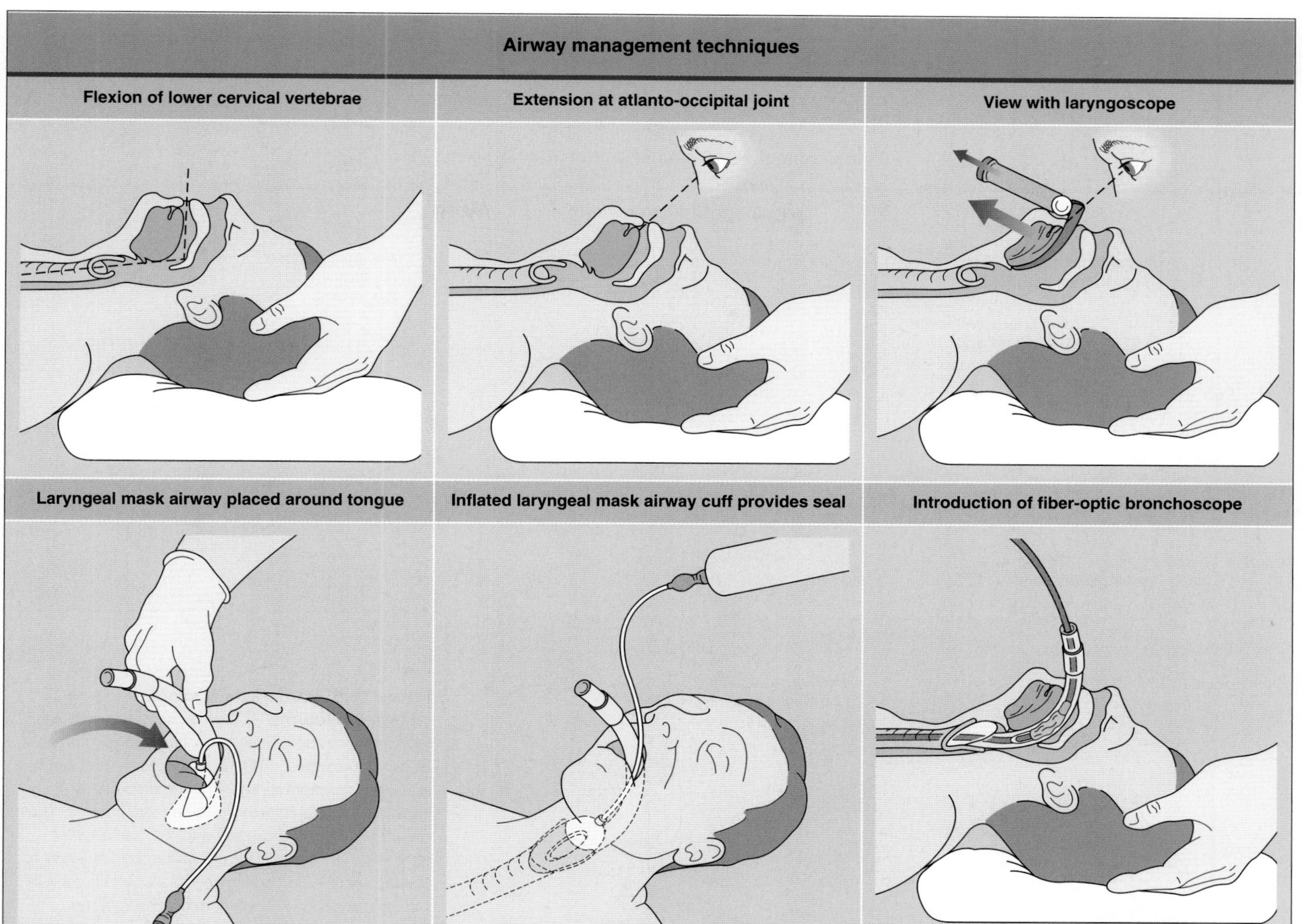

Figure 16.3 Airway management techniques. Correct positioning is important to optimize the view during direct laryngoscopy. Flexion of the lower cervical spine brings the trachea in line with the pharynx, and extension at the atlanto-occipital joint aligns the trachea with the oral cavity. The laryngoscope is usually introduced from the right side of the mouth. The tongue is displaced leftward into the mandible by traction in an anterocaudal direction *(arrow)* to reveal the glottis. The laryngeal mask airway (LMA) is placed manually around the tongue in an unconscious patient. The LMA cuff seats around the glottis and, when inflated, provides a seal to allow spontaneous or limited positive pressure ventilation. The LMA cuff also lies over the esophagus, which allows the possibility of gastric inflation, regurgitation, and pulmonary aspiration. A fiber-optic bronchoscope may be introduced via the mouth or nose and used to traverse the larynx. (A bronchoscope can also go through the LMA.) An endotracheal tube is then guided over the bronchoscope into the trachea.

Table 16.1
Common agents used for airway control

Drug		Dosage (mg/kg)	Comments
Sedative drugs	Thiopental	3-5	Cardiac depression, vasodilatation, can cause severe hypotension during hypovolemic states
	Propofol	1.5-2.5	Rapid onset and offset, vasodilates, easily contaminated, affirm sterility
	Etomidate	0.2-0.3	Hemodynamic stability, myoclonus, associated adrenal suppression
	Ketamine	0.5-2 mg IV 4-6 mg IM	Analgesic, sympathetic stimulant, bronchodilator, causes dysphoria
	Midazolam	0.5-0.25 mg	Vasodilatation, hypotension, dangerous in hypovolemic states
Neuromuscular blocking agents	Succinylcholine	1-2	Most rapid onset, lasts <5 minutes; contraindicated in hyperkalemia, burns, and chronic neural injuries; associated with malignant hyperthermia and masseter spasm in children
	Vecuronium	0.07-0.1	Clinical duration 30 minutes; higher dose required for rapid onset; associated with prolonged paralysis in corticosteroid-dependent patients
	Rocuronium	1-1.5	Rapid onset, but clinical duration 20 minutes; associated with prolonged paralysis in corticosteroid-dependent patients
	Cisatracurium	0.2-0.35	Slightly delayed onset, clinical duration 30 minutes; metabolism via plasma cholinesterase

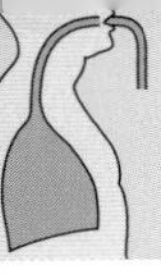

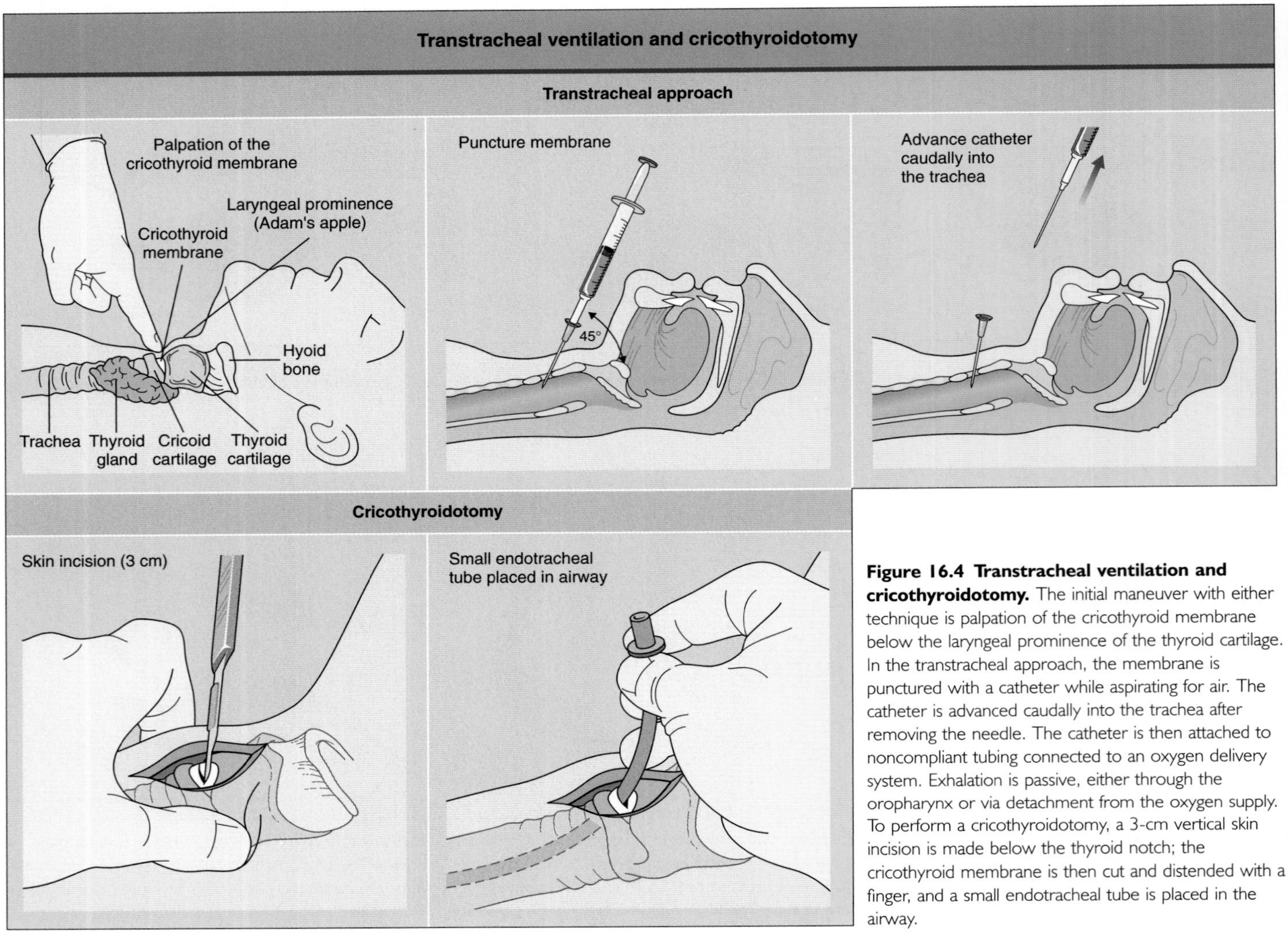

Transtracheal ventilation and cricothyroidotomy

Transtracheal approach

Palpation of the cricothyroid membrane
Laryngeal prominence (Adam's apple)
Cricothyroid membrane
Hyoid bone
Trachea
Thyroid gland
Cricoid cartilage
Thyroid cartilage

Puncture membrane
45°

Advance catheter caudally into the trachea

Cricothyroidotomy

Skin incision (3 cm)

Small endotracheal tube placed in airway

Figure 16.4 Transtracheal ventilation and cricothyroidotomy. The initial maneuver with either technique is palpation of the cricothyroid membrane below the laryngeal prominence of the thyroid cartilage. In the transtracheal approach, the membrane is punctured with a catheter while aspirating for air. The catheter is advanced caudally into the trachea after removing the needle. The catheter is then attached to noncompliant tubing connected to an oxygen delivery system. Exhalation is passive, either through the oropharynx or via detachment from the oxygen supply. To perform a cricothyroidotomy, a 3-cm vertical skin incision is made below the thyroid notch; the cricothyroid membrane is then cut and distended with a finger, and a small endotracheal tube is placed in the airway.

Techniques that maintain spontaneous ventilation give the clinician time, and the opportunity, to try different approaches. Practitioners must be able to achieve ventilation by mask if paralytic agents are being administered, but the relaxation of glottic structures that occurs with paralysis may make mask ventilation more difficult. Fiber-optic approaches usually take longer than 3 minutes and, accordingly, should not be the first choice in extremely emergent situations. When these approaches are selected, alternative methods, including LMAs, should be available to deal rapidly with acute deteriorations. New or unfamiliar techniques should not be tried in emergency situations that require immediate action or in situations that involve critically ill patients who have limited respiratory or ventilatory reserve.

If the approach selected is unsuccessful, proper judgment dictates abandoning the procedure, aiding the patient with mask ventilation as necessary, and either obtaining help or trying another approach. Once the patient stops breathing, one has only 3 minutes to achieve oxygenation. Transtracheal ventilation or cricothyroidotomy should be attempted instead of repeated attempts at laryngoscopy. Clinicians who instrument the airway must practice transtracheal ventilation or cricothyroidotomy until they can obtain an emergency airway in 3 minutes or less (Fig. 16.6).

COMPLICATIONS

The most serious complication is the inability to perform mask ventilation or to oxygenate a patient, leading to cardiac arrest and anoxic brain injury. Prolonged intervals of hypoxia can be caused by poor technique resulting in a lack of oxygen delivery.

In addition, there may be other serious complications. Oral and tracheal mucosal damage can arise from intubation attempts. Blades, stylets, and other objects in the airway can damage the airway mucosa and cause life-threatening hemorrhage. These risks are increased in patients with coagulopathies or friable mucosa (e.g., mucositis). Dental damage can also occur. Stylets should never protrude beyond the distal end of the endotracheal tube because they can tear the tracheal wall.

Transtracheal needles or catheters can lead to massive and life-threatening subcutaneous emphysema or pneumothorax. Tracheotomy tubes may be misplaced in nontracheal structures, resulting in subcutaneous emphysema and life-threatening

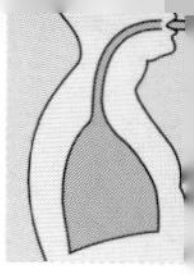

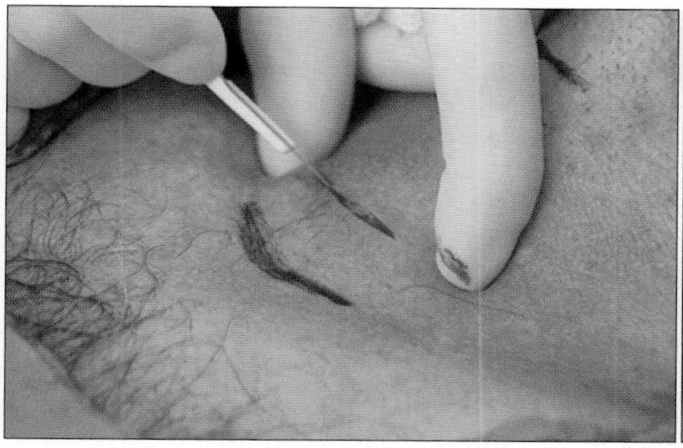

A

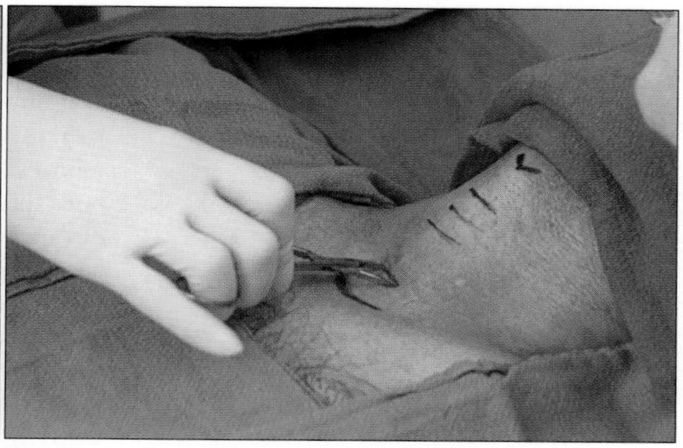

B

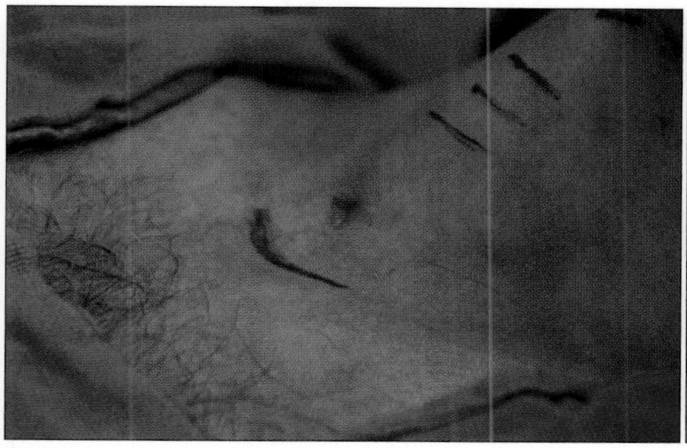

C

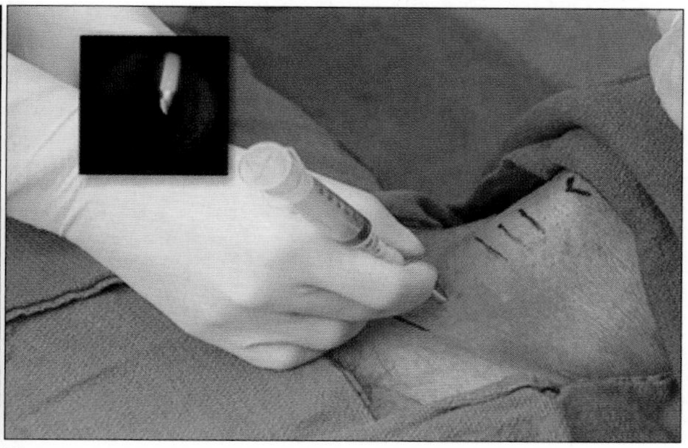

D

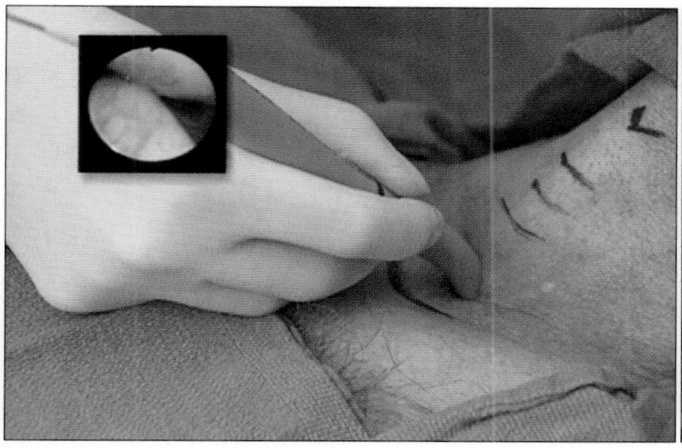

E

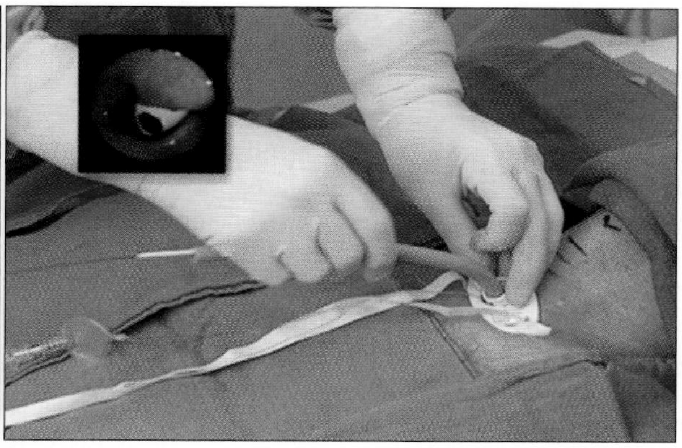

F

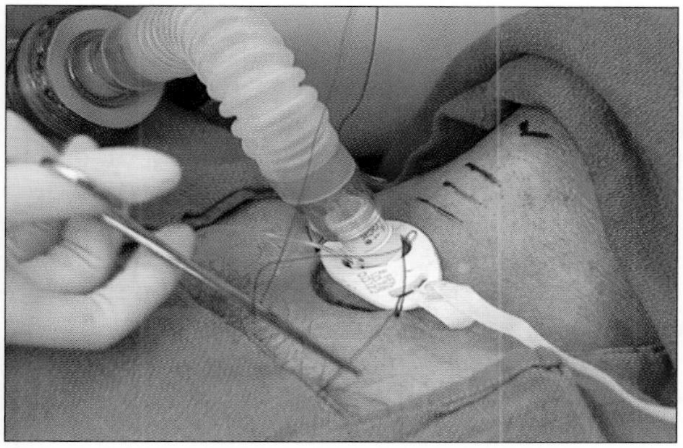

G

Figure 16.5 Bedside percutaneous dilatational tracheotomy. To perform a bedside percutaneous tracheotomy, a 1- to 2-cm horizontal skin incision is made at the level between the 1-2 or 2-3 tracheal rings **(A)**. Using a blunt clamp, the tissue is dissected to the level of the trachea **(B, C)**. An introducer needle with an attached syringe filled with fluid is placed into the trachea. Placement is confirmed by aspiration of air or bubbling of fluid in the syringe or by direct visualization with fiber-optic bronchoscopy **(D)**. The syringe is removed, and a J-tipped guide wire is advanced through the needle; the needle is then removed. Serial dilators are placed over the guide wire into the trachea to widen the opening **(E)**. The final dilator contains the tracheotomy tube. Once the tracheotomy tube is placed, the final dilator with guide wire is removed, and the tube is sutured and tied into place **(F, G)**. (Courtesy of Cook Critical Care, Bloomington, Indiana.)

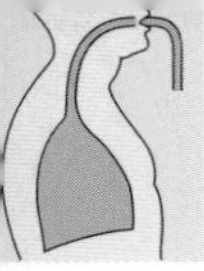

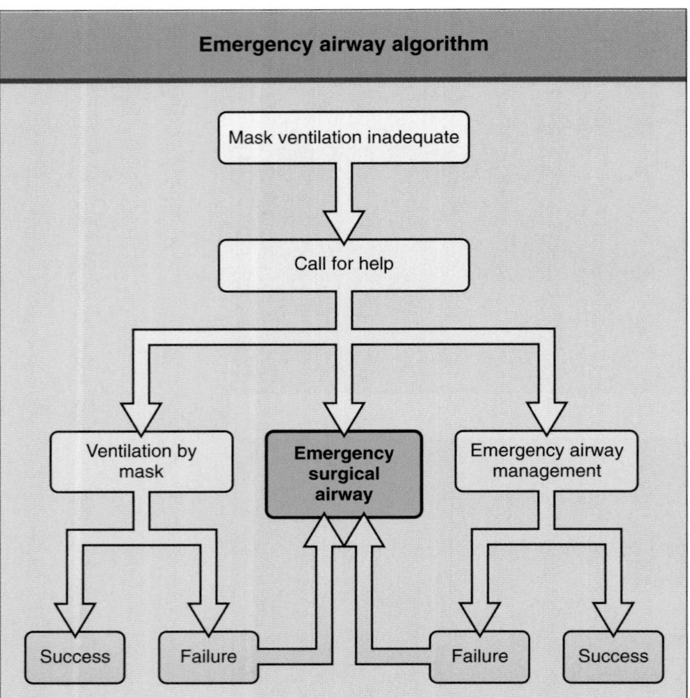

Figure 16.6 Emergency airway algorithm. If mask ventilation is insufficient, assistance from other personnel should be obtained to perform a jaw thrust and to place an oral airway. If these attempts fail, the provider must obtain an emergent airway (laryngeal mask airway, retrograde intubation techniques, transtracheal ventilation) or a surgical airway. (Adapted from the American Society of Anesthesiologists.)

hypoxemia. Also, the distal end of the endotracheal tube may inadvertently be placed in the right main-stem bronchus, with consequent single-lung ventilation. The position of all endotracheal and tracheotomy tubes should be confirmed by radiograph or by direct visualization and should be withdrawn sufficiently to sit above the carina.

Tracheotomies can lead to bilateral pneumothoraces secondary to the surgical site's proximity to the apices of the lungs. Damage to the veins in the neck can also occur, with the possibility of severe hemorrhage. Newly placed tracheotomy tubes should not be replaced by inexperienced clinicians because of the difficulty in finding the proper position in the trachea and the danger of creating a false passage. A reasonable option for the management of a dislodged fresh tracheotomy includes orotracheal intubation for airway control, followed by the elective replacement of the tracheotomy tube as a surgical procedure.

PITFALLS AND CONTROVERSIES

Oral versus Nasal Intubation

The nasal approach is somewhat easier than the oral because of the broader curve that the oral endotracheal tube must traverse before reaching the glottis. Nasal intubation usually requires smaller tubes and topical application of a local anesthetic mixed with a vasoconstrictor to the nasal mucosa to prevent bleeding. This approach should be avoided in patients who have coagulopathies or in those who have sustained midface trauma.

Stabilization of the Injured Cervical Spine

The risk of catastrophic neurologic injury makes it imperative that any lateral displacement of the cervical spine be avoided in patients who are suspected of having traumatic cervical spine injuries. Gentle manual stabilization may be all that is available, but this stabilization does not fully immobilize the head during the atlanto-occipital extension that occurs with direct laryngoscopy. The placement of a halo jacket on such a patient fully protects the cervical spine. Fiber-optic or blind nasal techniques should be used when full neck extension cannot be tolerated.

Ventilation after Failed Rapid Sequence Induction

When the trachea cannot be intubated during a rapid sequence maneuver, the external pressure on the cricoid cartilage should be maintained. Ventilation with small, rapid breaths maintains airway pressure at a low level, so that the pressure compressing the esophagus is not exceeded.

Management of Regurgitation during Mask Ventilation

Positive pressure in the airway forces regurgitated gastric contents from the hypopharynx into the trachea and can cause acute lung injury. Appropriate management includes maintenance of cricoid pressure and rapidly placing the patient in the Trendelenburg position. The bulk of the gastric contents is removed by manual clearance or by suctioning. If conditions allow, immediate direct laryngoscopy should be performed to inspect the vocal cords, with intubation of the trachea and suctioning of the airway before the resumption of positive pressure ventilation. If continued mask ventilation is necessary, small, gentle breaths are administered to limit gastric insufflation and the migration of gastric material into the distal airways.

Aspiration Prophylaxis

Aspiration prophylaxis is a prudent measure in high-risk patients (e.g., those with full stomachs, morbid obesity, gastroesophageal reflux; parturients). Antacids should be administered immediately before endotracheal intubation, because they rapidly increase the gastric pH above 2.5. Animal studies demonstrate that aspiration of particulate antacids is associated with the development of severe pneumonitis; thus, nonparticulate antacids, such as 10-30 mL of sodium citrate, are recommended. Although the administration of sodium citrate increases the gastric fluid volume, additional animal studies suggest that pulmonary injury is worse after the aspiration of small quantities of low-pH fluid than after the aspiration of larger quantities of high-pH fluid. H_2-receptor antagonists and proton pump inhibitors take longer to act and do not affect the preexisting gastric contents. They are of little value in the acute situation.

Endotracheal Tube Size

For the average adult male, an 8.0-mm internal diameter (ID) endotracheal tube is appropriate; a 7.5-mm ID tube is used for adult females. For pediatric patients, tube size is based on age, using the formula ID = (age + 16)/4. Depending on coexisting

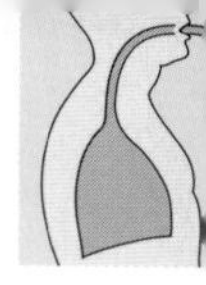

diseases and indications for endotracheal intubation, noncuffed endotracheal tubes may be preferable in children younger than 12 years. Tubes at least one size larger and smaller should always be available to accommodate individual anatomic variations.

Blade Type

Laryngoscope blades come in a variety of styles and sizes. The most commonly used blades include the curved Macintosh and the straight Miller blades. The curved blades are inserted into the vallecula, immediately anterior to the epiglottis, which is then flipped out of the visual axis to expose the larynx. The Miller blade is inserted past the epiglottis, which is simply lifted out of the way of the glottis. Many clinicians believe that the Macintosh blade is technically easier to use because the wider blade prevents intrusion of the tongue into the visual field. However, in difficult situations (e.g., anteriorly situated larynx, large epiglottis), the straight blade frequently affords improved visualization (Fig. 16.7).

Positioning the Obese Patient

The proper "sniff" position (neck flexion, head extension) should be achieved before attempts at direct laryngoscopy. In obese patients, this requires elevating and supporting the shoulders by the placement of towels or blankets. In addition to elevating the head to optimize the visual axis, this maneuver creates more room for head extension (Fig. 16.8).

Depth of Sedation

To avoid increasing bronchospasm, cardiac ischemia, or hypertension in a patient with a full stomach, a deep level of sedation or anesthesia should be achieved before laryngoscopy. Intubation attempts during "light" planes of anesthesia or sedation may cause dangerous sympathetic responses or intense bronchospasm. However, the risk of aspiration is increased with an increased depth of sedation.

An alternative approach is to test the ease of mask ventilation while administering cricoid pressure when the patient is awake. Small doses of sedation are then administered while gentle mask ventilation with cricoid pressure is continued. Tidal volumes are kept small to maintain low pharyngeal pressures. The depth of sedation can be titrated to maintain a stable heart rate and blood pressure. Muscle relaxation should be used. Laryngoscopy can be achieved in two stages. On the first view of the glottis, the cords and trachea are sprayed with lidocaine (lignocaine). Subsequent ventilation for 1 minute allows time for the local anesthetic to take effect. The patient's hemodynamic response is observed during the initial laryngoscopy to determine the adequacy of sedation. Marked sympathetic responses indicate the need for further sedation or for other autonomic agents before repeat laryngoscopy and placement of the endotracheal tube.

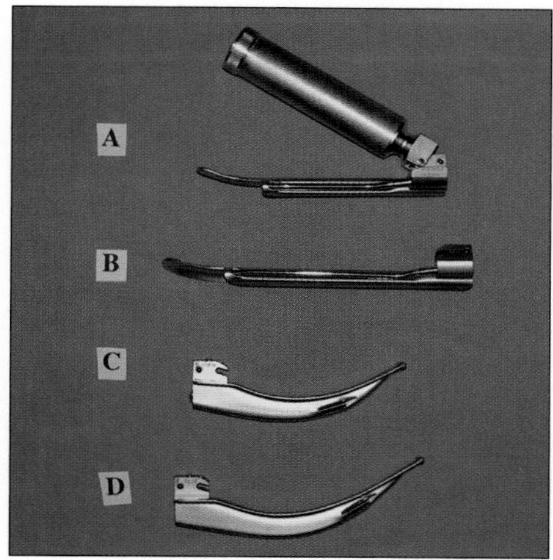

Figure 16.7 Laryngoscope blades. The most common laryngoscope blades are the Miller and Macintosh blades. **A**, Miller 2. **B**, Miller 3. **C**, Macintosh 3. **D**, Macintosh 4. In the average adult male, a Miller 2 or Macintosh 3 blade is best.

Positioning of the obese patient

Neck movement and access hindered by fat

Elevated shoulders and occiput improve access

Figure 16.8 Positioning the obese patient. With the obese patient in the supine position, neck movement and access with a laryngoscope are hindered by fat. When the same patient is positioned with the shoulders elevated and the occiput further elevated so that the head assumes a "sniffing" position, access to the airway is facilitated.

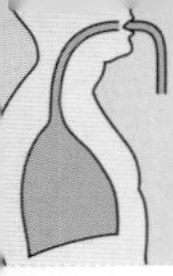

SUGGESTED READINGS

American Society of Anesthesiologists Task Force on Management of the Difficult Airway: Practice guidelines for management of the difficult airway. Anesthesiology 78:597-602, 1993.

Bainton C: Airway management: a perspective. Int Anesthesiol Clin 32:1-29, 1994.

Benumof JL: Laryngeal mask airway: indications and contraindications. Anesthesiology 77:843-846, 1992.

Hanowell L, Waldron R (eds): Airway Management. Philadelphia, Lippincott-Raven, 1996.

Miller RD (ed): Anesthesia, 5th ed. Philadelphia, Churchill Livingstone, 2000.

Schwartz DE, Matthay MA, Cohen NH: Death and other complications of emergency airway management in critically ill patients. Anesthesiology 82:367-376, 1995.

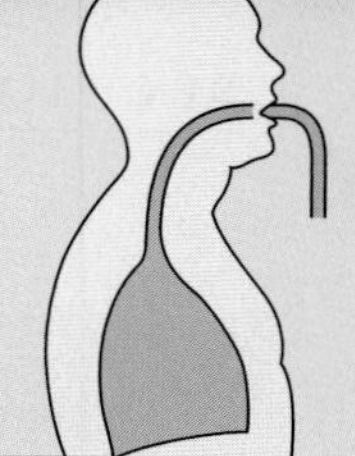

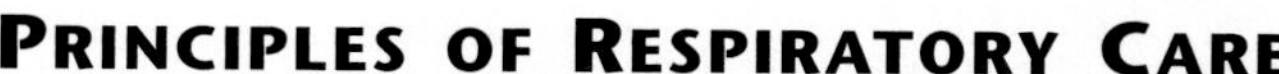

CHAPTER 17

Preoperative Pulmonary Evaluation

Erik R. Swenson and Edward W. Swenson

Short- and long-term pulmonary complications result in considerable morbidity and mortality in patients undergoing surgery for nonpulmonary disease or for lung resection. Pulmonary complications occur more often than cardiac complications and are responsible for longer hospitalizations. Predicting and managing the expected pulmonary complications depends on understanding the predictable changes and compromises in pulmonary function that take place in the perioperative period and, in the case of lung resection, the additional consequences of the permanent loss of some fraction of preoperative lung function. Evaluation and risk assessment begin with, and depend on, a careful history and physical examination, after which a variety of quantitative imaging and lung function tests can be obtained to select and prepare patients for successful lung resection surgery. This chapter reviews the changes in pulmonary function that occur with anesthesia and surgery; describes the typical complications arising from surgery, focusing on the risk factors that predict complications; and recommends a rational approach to evaluation and preoperative preparation.

PERIOPERATIVE PULMONARY PHYSIOLOGY

Pulmonary complications arising from surgery follow predictably from the decline in normal pulmonary function that occurs with surgery and anesthesia (Table 17.1). The restrictive changes following thoracic and abdominal surgery are characterized by moderate to severe reductions (≈50%) in vital capacity and somewhat larger, more important reductions (≈70%) in functional residual capacity (FRC), which may last as long as 1 week. With surgery that is more distant from the thorax, the loss in lung volume is less, such that operations on the extremities and head are associated with rather small losses of volume. Accordingly, it is not surprising that pulmonary complications are observed most commonly following thoracic and upper abdominal surgery. These changes occur without evident airway obstruction, so that the ratio of the forced expiratory volume in 1 second (FEV_1) to the forced vital capacity (FVC) remains unaltered.

General anesthesia may itself be responsible for some of the lung volume changes. The fact that these changes persist well after anesthesia is reversed, however, indicates that important changes in lung and chest wall mechanics occur as a result of the operation, with diaphragmatic dysfunction likely to be a major contributor (see later).

The reduction in FRC is most problematic because it is the relevant lung volume for gas exchange. As FRC falls, it converges on the closing capacity (CC), which is the lung volume at which small airways in dependent lung regions close during exhalation owing to loss of radial traction by surrounding parenchyma. At this point, regions of lung may become atelectatic (i.e., shunt units) or may open for only a portion of the tidal breath, so that they become relatively hypoventilated in proportion to their perfusion (i.e., low ventilation [$\dot{V}A$] to perfusion [$\dot{Q}c$] units), with consequent arterial hypoxemia. Factors that decrease the FRC include the supine position, obesity, pregnancy, general anesthesia, and pain; increasing age, smoking, edema, and chronic obstructive pulmonary disease (COPD) increase the CC.

The cause of diaphragmatic dysfunction with thoracic and upper abdominal surgery is not fully elucidated. Direct injury to the muscle during retraction for upper abdominal exposure has been proposed as a mechanism, but measurements of transdiaphragmatic pressure during maximal phrenic nerve stimulation also suggest that depressed central nervous system efferent traffic to the diaphragm occurs as a result of inhibitory reflexes involving pain and other stimuli to sympathetic, vagal, or splanchnic receptors.

Arterial hypoxemia and hypercapnia are commonly encountered postoperatively. Immediately following surgery, the residual effects of anesthesia are responsible and result in depression of normal $\dot{V}A/\dot{Q}c$ matching by impaired hypoxic pulmonary vasoconstriction, alveolar hypoventilation, low cardiac output, and increased metabolic rate. Beyond the first day, the restrictive changes noted earlier, especially the FRC-CC relationship, become important. The combination of hypoventilation, increased dead space ventilation with rapid or shallow breathing, and decreased mixed venous oxygen saturation due to low cardiac output, anemia, and arterial desaturation and increased peripheral oxygen consumption with pain, fever, and stress all contribute to the impairment of gas exchange.

Ventilatory depression is quite typical in the postoperative period. The residual effects of anesthetics include suppression of respiratory drive, with inhibition of the normal responses to hypoxia and hypercapnia. Narcotics and other analgesics and many sedatives are equally problematic. In higher doses, they may impair patients' ability to participate fully in their postoperative respiratory therapy efforts. Rarely, they may precipitate sleep apnea in patients with predisposing factors.

The lung defends itself from environmental injury and infectious agents by a wide variety of mechanisms, two of which may be greatly compromised by surgery: cough and mucociliary clearance. Cough is suppressed by both under- and overtreated pain. The shear stresses necessary to propel mucus upward depend on the force of the cough (expiratory muscle strength) as well as the inspired lung volume taken before the cough effort. These may be limited by the restrictive changes noted earlier and by

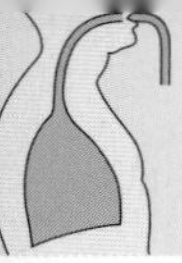

Table 17.1
Lung function changes with surgery and anesthesia

Reduction in lung volumes
Dysfunction of the diaphragm
Impairment of gas exchange
Depression of ventilatory control
Inhibition of cough and mucociliary clearance

Table 17.2
Postoperative pulmonary complications

General complications
Atelectasis
Infection
Bronchitis
Pneumonia
Bronchospasm
Pulmonary embolism
Exacerbation of underlying chronic lung disease
Respiratory failure and prolonged mechanical ventilation
Obstructive sleep apnea
Specific thoracic surgical complications
Phrenic nerve injury
Pleural effusion
Bronchopleural fistula and empyema
Sternal wound infection
Gastroesophageal anastomotic leak

the weakened inspiratory muscles. Apart from an ineffective cough, mucociliary clearance is compromised by atelectasis and ciliary damage and dysfunction from anesthetic gases and ventilation with dry hyperoxic gas, compounded by inadequate hydration.

POSTOPERATIVE PULMONARY COMPLICATIONS

Table 17.2 lists the variety of complications that are seen following surgery. The incidence of these complications varies widely, depending on the type of surgery and a number of patient characteristics. It can range from about 1% in young, healthy, nonobese, nonsmoking populations to more than 70% in high-risk groups.

Numerous preoperative and intraoperative risk factors have been identified that account for the majority of complications. Atelectasis is common following surgery but often has little or no morbidity beyond the need for additional oxygen. If persistent, however, atelectasis may be responsible for more serious problems. Many of the other complications arise from the expected declines in lung function that occur with surgery, especially if there is underlying chronic lung disease.

PREOPERATIVE RISK FACTORS

Special attention to well-established patient-related risk factors, as delineated in Table 17.3, will assist in decisions regarding surgery, anesthesia, preoperative preparation, and postoperative care. Effective communication about these issues with patients before surgery helps gain their active participation in early postoperative mobilization and respiratory therapy.

Table 17.3
Preoperative risk factors

Smoking
Heavy sputum production
Diminished health status
Older age
Obesity
Poor nutritional and metabolic status
Respiratory tract infection
Chronic lung disease

Smoking has long been recognized as a pulmonary risk factor, even in patients without underlying pulmonary disease. The relative risk for postsurgery complications in smokers is roughly 1.5- to 4-fold greater than that in nonsmokers and increases with as little as 10 pack-years of smoking. Although many smokers and recent quitters have normal pulmonary function or only minor abnormalities, the majority have hypersecretion of mucus and possibly an impairment in mucociliary clearance. In the setting of postoperative pain, analgesics, poor cough, atelectasis, and low lung volumes, the burden of uncleared secretions sets the stage for further gas exchange problems, local infection, and respiratory failure. In a recent study, the presence of mucus hypersecretion (defined by the presence of morning cough, frequent throat clearing, and sputum production) predicted an increased incidence of postoperative pneumonia or the need for mechanical ventilation far better than any lung function or gas exchange value in a multivariate model, with an odds ratio of 133 (2 to 10 times greater than any other variable).

Two retrospective studies examined preoperative smoking cessation and its impact on complications. Unfortunately, the data suggest that smoking cessation must occur as long as 4 to 8 weeks before surgery for the complication rate to fall to that of nonsmokers. This may represent the time for smoking-related airway irritation and sputum production to abate. Despite these data, however, every patient should be encouraged to stop smoking before surgery to reduce carbon monoxide levels. Nicotine replacement should be offered, if appropriate.

General health status, as reflected in the American Society of Anesthesiologists classification, is highly predictive of postoperative pulmonary complications. The Goldman cardiac risk index performs equally well for pulmonary complications, because cardiac and pulmonary disease share many common attributes. Older age often appears in univariate analyses as a moderate risk factor but drops out when confounding issues such as coexisting conditions are considered. Accordingly, age alone should not be given predictive weight in decision making, nor should it be grounds to withhold surgery. Conventional wisdom once held that obesity increased postoperative pulmonary complications, but a number of studies in the past decade, including reports on gastric bypass in morbidly obese patients, found no difference in pulmonary complication rates compared with those in the nonobese. With obese patients, however, obstructive sleep apnea may first appear or be worsened in the postoperative period.

Malnutrition adversely affects the respiratory system and contributes to a high rate of complications. Malnutrition reduces ventilatory drives to hypoxia and hypercapnia, contributes to respiratory muscle weakness, impairs humoral and cell-

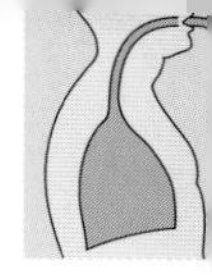

mediated host defenses, and alters lung elastic properties. Although preoperative nutritional support appears logical, only the most severely malnourished have a reduced rate of pulmonary complications after a 15-day course of total parenteral nutrition. Thus, beyond providing adequate nutrition during hospitalization, mild to moderate undernutrition need not be electively corrected.

Antecedent respiratory tract infections should be treated with appropriate antibiotics if a bacterial cause is suspected or documented, and surgery should be delayed to allow resolution of the accompanying airway hyperreactivity and mucus hypersecretion. Although there are published reports suggesting that it is safe to operate on patients with recent upper respiratory tract viral infections, it seems prudent to delay elective surgery.

Chronic lung disease, principally COPD, confers a three- to fivefold increased risk of pulmonary complications as a result of irreversible loss of lung function, decreased pulmonary reserve, ongoing airway hyperreactivity, and mucus hypersecretion. Because there is a definite correlation between baseline lung function and the rate and severity of pulmonary complications in patients with COPD (see later), attempts to improve lung function should be undertaken. Patients should receive aggressive preoperative bronchodilator therapy, antibiotics, smoking cessation education, and a short course of systemic corticosteroids. Elective surgery should be deferred if an acute exacerbation is present. Although an increased rate of postoperative pulmonary complications would be expected in patients with stable asthma, restrictive lung disease, or pulmonary vascular disease, no data exist to confirm this.

INTRAOPERATIVE RISK FACTORS

Table 17.4 lists the key intraoperative risk factors. The surgical site is the most important risk determinant, and complications increase with greater proximity to the diaphragm. Thus, upper abdominal and thoracic procedures have a 10% to 40 % incidence of postoperative problems. In the case of abdominal surgery, vertical incisions carry a greater morbidity than horizontal incisions. Video-assisted thoracoscopic and laparoscopic surgeries have approximately one tenth the pulmonary complication rates of open procedures.

Presumably because of the multiple adverse effects of general anesthesia on pulmonary function, there is a three- to fourfold increase in postoperative pulmonary complications in patients who undergo lengthy procedures (longer than 3 hours) compared with those having shorter operations. Although there is some debate, use of epidural and spinal anesthesia may reduce complication rates, because anesthesia to a T4 sensory level does not alter lung volume and gas exchange to the same extent as general anesthesia. Accordingly, epidural anesthesia should be strongly considered in marginal patients. Regional anesthetic blocks carry even less risk. Longer-acting neuromuscular blockers, such as pancuronium, are associated with more postoperative hypoventilation and should be replaced by shorter-acting vecuronium or atracurium in patients at high risk for pulmonary complications.

Table 17.4
Intraoperative Risk Factors

Surgical site
Type and duration of anesthesia
Type of neuromuscular blockade

MULTIFACTORIAL PULMONARY RISK INDICES

Multifactorial pulmonary risk indices have been developed along the lines previously undertaken for the prediction of postoperative cardiac complications. These indices include a number of the pre- and intraoperative factors already discussed, as well as laboratory assessment of renal function and nutrition (creatinine and albumin), but they do not rely on pulmonary function data or radiographs. The most ambitious are those developed by Arozullah and colleagues from a database of more than 150,000 patients and validated in separate groups for both postoperative pneumonia and respiratory failure. Five risk groups were identified by a scoring system (Table 17.5), with complication rates ranging from less than 1% in the lowest-risk group to 15% to 30% in the highest-risk group (Table 17.6). New risk factors identified included emergency surgery, impaired sensorium,

Table 17.5
Postoperative pneumonia and respiratory failure risk index scoring

Preoperative risk factor	Point value postoperative pneumonia	Respiratory failure
Type of surgery		
Abdominal aortic aneurysm repair	15	27
Thoracic	14	21
Upper abdominal	10	14
Neck	8	11
Neurosurgery	8	14
Vascular	3	14
Age		
>80 yr	17	6
70–79 yr	13	6
60–69 yr	9	6
50–59 yr	4	4
Functional status		
Totally dependent	10	7
Partially dependent	6	7
Weight loss >10% in past 6 mo	7	—
History of chronic obstructive pulmonary disease	5	6
General anesthesia	4	—
Impaired sensorium	4	—
History of cerebrovascular accident	4	—
Blood urea nitrogen level		
<2.86 mmol/L (<8 mg/dL)	4	—
2.87–7.85 mmol/L (8–21 mg/dL)	0	—
7.85–10.7 mmol/L (22–30 mg/dL)	2	—
>10.7 mmol/L (>30 mg/dL)	3	8
Transfusion >4 units	3	—
Emergency surgery	3	11
Steroid use for chronic condition	3	—
Current smoker within 1 yr	3	—
Alcohol intake >2 drinks/day in past 2 wk	2	—
Albumin	—	9

Adapted from Arozullah AM, Daley J, Henderson WG, Khuri SF: Multifactorial risk index for predicting postoperative respiratory failure in men after major non-cardiac surgery. Ann Surg 232:242-250, 2000; Arozullah AM, Khuri SF, Henderson WG, Daley J: Development and validation of a multifactorial risk index for predicting postoperative pneumonia after major noncardiac surgery. Ann Intern Med 135:847-857, 2001.

Table 17.6
Risk class assignment by postoperative pneumonia and respiratory failure risk index score

Risk Class	Postoperative Pneumonia Risk Index (Point Total)	Predicted Probability Pneumonia (%)	Respiratory Failure Risk Index (Point Total)	Predicted Probability Respiratory Failure (%)
1	0–15	0.2	0–10	0.5
2	16–25	1.2	11–19	2.2
3	26–40	4.0	20–27	5.0
4	41–55	9.4	28–40	11.6
5	>55	15.3	>40	30.5

Adapted from Arozullah AM, Daley J, Henderson WG, Khuri SF: Multifactorial risk index for predicting postoperative respiratory failure in men after major non-cardiac surgery. Ann Surg 232:242-250, 2000; Arozullah AM, Khuri SF, Henderson WG, Daley J: Development and validation of a multifactorial risk index for predicting postoperative pneumonia after major noncardiac surgery. Ann Intern Med 135:847-857, 2001.

reduced renal function, blood transfusion greater than 4 units, and recent alcohol intake.

PREOPERATIVE ASSESSMENT

Nonresectional Surgery

There is no substitute for a complete history directed at detecting and qualitatively assessing the severity of risk factors in each patient. Specifically, this should include a smoking history and status; respiratory symptoms of cough, sputum production, and dyspnea (rest and exertional); exercise capacity and tolerance; symptoms of sleep apnea; preexisting lung disease; and recent respiratory tract infection or exacerbation. The physical examination, although less helpful, should be aimed at eliciting signs of chronic lung disease, especially COPD, and deep venous thrombosis and providing a baseline against which postoperative examinations can be interpreted.

Full pulmonary function testing is commonly performed preoperatively, but whether this is truly cost effective and stratifies patient risk sufficiently to justify the cost remains controversial. Further, because COPD is the only chronic lung disease category that carries a higher risk, simple spirometry alone may be sufficient. Unlike the guidelines for lung resection, there is no level of pulmonary function below which surgery should be avoided solely because of a limited reserve. This extends even to disease that is severe enough to cause carbon dioxide retention and warrant chronic home oxygen therapy. The best that pulmonary function testing can offer with regard to risk assessment is that the worse the patient's function, the greater the risk that complications may develop due to limited reserve.

Guidelines for identifying patients who should be sent for preoperative spirometry and arterial blood gases include those undergoing coronary artery bypass surgery or upper abdominal surgery who have a history of smoking or dyspnea. For patients undergoing surgery at other sites with less impact on pulmonary function, spirometry should be obtained if there is a question of unexplained pulmonary disease and the possibility of prolonged or extensive surgery. Pulmonary function tests are recommended if it is unclear whether patients are at their best baseline and, if not, whether they might benefit from aggressive preoperative pulmonary therapy. Pulmonary function tests are also recommended for those with unexplained dyspnea or exercise intolerance when a finding of pulmonary compromise might change preoperative management.

Chest radiographs are usually unrevealing if the history and physical examination uncover no risk factors, and a preoperative chest radiograph rarely reveals a reason to postpone or reconsider surgery. A large meta-analysis of nearly 15,000 patients found that only 1% of radiographs yielded an unexpected abnormality, and only one tenth of those led to a change in management. Thus, a preoperative chest radiograph is indicated only if a patient has a new pulmonary symptom or there is unexplained worsening of a stable complaint in a patient with underlying lung disease, and there are no recent films available.

Lung Resection Surgery

Surgical resection for non–small-cell lung carcinoma remains the only effective cure. However, with steady improvements in radiation and chemotherapy and experience with their use, tumors previously deemed unresectable can now be removed. Because tobacco is the most important risk factor for lung cancer, many patients presenting with resectable lesions have underlying lung disease that, in combination with present or recent smoking, carries a higher risk for postoperative cardiac and pulmonary complications. Beyond the higher risks of transient pulmonary dysfunction and complications that occur with thoracic surgery, the loss of a portion of functional lung tissue adds to the problem. There is also the consequence of permanent lung function decline and possible disability. Accordingly, when evaluating patients for lung resection, two questions must be answered:

1. What is the surgical morbidity and mortality in those with underlying lung disease?
2. Will the patient have sufficient pulmonary reserve for normal activities?

In distinct contrast to the marginal utility of pulmonary function testing and imaging in the preoperative evaluation for surgery *not* involving lung resection, these modalities provide a solid quantitative foundation for predicting which patients will benefit from curative resection. For the most part, the thresholds of predicted postoperative function are appropriately conservative and underestimate the actual values at 6 months postoperatively by as much as 10% to 20%. An error in this direction is generally acceptable despite the probability of denying curative surgery to a few patients, because a cancer cure at the cost of functional disability is hardly a cure at all.

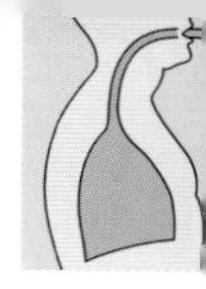

The usual evaluation involves pulmonary function tests, arterial blood gases, nuclide lung perfusion scans, and exercise testing. If there is preexisting pulmonary hypertension or concern about its development postoperatively, the evaluation should include echocardiography or pulmonary arterial catheterization (although two studies reported that the level of pulmonary arterial pressure measured during exercise did not predict perioperative complications).

Various spirometric values, such as the FEV_1, vital capacity, and maximum voluntary ventilation, are very useful. If they are above 80% of the predicted values, pneumonectomy can be tolerated. If they are below 80% but above 40% of the predicted values, after taking into account the expected volumetric loss of lung, surgery may still be recommended. Although predicted postoperative FEV_1 greater than 800 mL is often cited as a reliable threshold, it is better to use a threshold of greater than 40% predicted value, because women and smaller persons may be unfairly excluded. If the patient does not meet these thresholds by proportional volumetric estimation, it may be useful to consider whether the expected contribution of the involved segment, lobe, or lung is already compromised, such that its removal will have little or no effect on lung function. Chest radiographs and computed tomography scanning can readily detect causes such as endobronchial obstruction, atelectasis, or nonmalignant effusions that may allow the acceptance of an otherwise marginal functional value.

To extend the benefits of resection to more patients, one can use split lung function tests to better quantitate the functional contribution of the involved lung region. The simplest means of doing this is to perform quantitative perfusion scanning. This test has been well validated by more direct but invasive bronchial or pulmonary vascular studies, in which blood or airflow to the region is occluded to mimic the extent of functional loss anticipated as a result of the resection. Perfusion scanning takes advantage of the fact that blood flow is distributed preferentially to less impaired (better ventilated) regions owing to hypoxic pulmonary vasoconstriction and other $\dot{V}A/\dot{Q}c$ matching mechanisms. The quantitation of fractional regional blood flow can then be applied in a proportionate fashion to the planned area of resection and used to predict postoperative values.

Gas exchange measures such as arterial blood gases and diffusing capacity have been studied for their usefulness. Although arterial hypoxemia and hypercapnia generally denote marginal lung function and predict a higher incidence of postoperative respiratory failure, they are poor predictors of gas exchange after the operation, because resection of tumor-bearing lung may, in fact, remove the source of much shunting or low ventilation-perfusion mismatch. Predicted postoperative diffusing capacity below 40%, similar to volume and flow measurements, is a useful threshold, however.

Measurement of maximal oxygen consumption ($\dot{V}O_2max$) in a progressive, incremental cycle ergometry or treadmill test has proved helpful in risk assessment because the measurement integrates a number of relevant physiologic and functional aspects. Several studies have shown that patients with a $\dot{V}O_2max$ greater than 20 mL/kg per minute tolerate surgery, and that values of less than 10 mL/kg per minute are predictive of postoperative complications and disability. For patients who fall between these values, the predictive power is weak, and other considerations mentioned previously should be used.

Figure 17.1 presents an algorithm derived from a test series and then validated prospectively in a series of 167 consecutive patients. The approach uses a rigorous preoperative evaluation designed to clear as many patients as possible for surgery, yet achieve a low complication rate. The algorithm incorporates

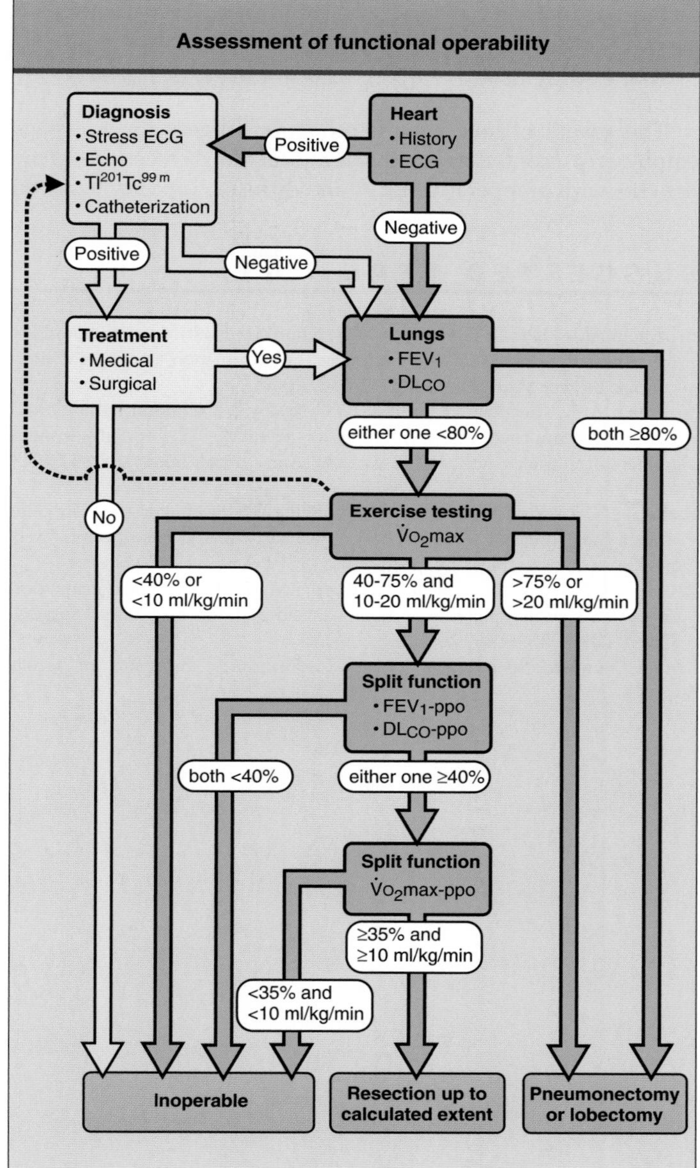

Figure 17.1 Proposed algorithm for the assessment of cardiorespiratory reserve in lung resection candidates. Patients undergo a successive stepwise evaluation until they either qualify for their intended surgery or are deemed inoperable. Split lung function testing by quantitative perfusion scanning allows a more accurate estimate of predicted postoperative (ppo) function. A safety loop for patients with possible cardiac disease detected on exercise testing (signs or symptoms of myocardial ischemia) is shown by the dashed line. DL_{CO}, diffusing capacity; ECG, electrocardiogram; FEV_1, forced expiratory volume at 1 second; $\dot{V}O_2max$, maximal oxygen consumption. Tl^{201}, thallium scan; Tc^{99m}, technicium scan. (From Wyser C, Stulz P, Soler M, et al: Prospective evaluation of an algorithm for the functional assessment of lung resection candidates. Am J Respir Crit Care Med 159:1450-1456, 1999.)

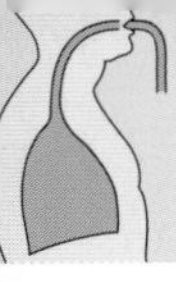

many of the tests described earlier and applies them in an economical and rational manner. Pulmonary function testing and exercise testing (both of which can be performed in a pulmonary function laboratory) are used to direct as many patients as possible to, or away from, surgery. Split lung function testing is then used in the remainder to determine their suitability for surgery by better estimating their predicted postoperative lung function or exercise tolerance. Exercise testing done as an early step for those with FEV_1 and diffusing capacity less than 80% of predicted adds another cardiac evaluation in those patients with normal resting electrocardiograms who, by their smoking history, are likely have a greater prevalence of coronary artery disease.

The advent of lung volume reduction surgery for end-stage emphysema has redefined the limits of lung resection. Many patients with preoperative FEV_1 and diffusing capacity between 20% and 40% of predicted have benefited from targeted removal of the most emphysematous lung regions. Postoperatively, pulmonary function improves, along with a reduction in dyspnea and greater exercise capacity. A number of these patients had small lung cancers detected in the resected areas, either preoperatively by computed tomography and positron emission tomography or by pathologic examination, and thus had tumor resection. This was not accompanied by the removal of regional nodes, however, as is standard in cancer resection surgery. The general tolerability of the procedure confirms the conservative nature of the previously mentioned thresholds and the fact that removal of the most diseased regions may permit better function of other regions as they expand to fill the new void. It remains to be determined whether tumor resection in conjunction with lung volume reduction surgery will be as successful as resection following conventional segmental approaches.

SUGGESTED READINGS

Arozullah AM, Daley J, Henderson WG, Khuri SF: Multifactorial risk index for predicting postoperative respiratory failure in men after major noncardiac surgery. Ann Surg 232:242-250, 2000.

Arozullah AM, Khuri SF, Henderson WG, Daley J: Development and validation of a multifactorial risk index for predicting postoperative pneumonia after major noncardiac surgery. Ann Intern Med 135:847-857, 2001.

Barisione G, Rovida S, Gassaniga GM, Fontana L: Upper abdominal surgery: does a lung function test exist to predict early severe postoperative respiratory complications? Eur Respir J 10:1301-1308, 1997.

Beckles MA, Spiro SG, Colice GL, Rudd RM: The physiologic evaluation of patients with lung cancer being considered for resectional surgery. Chest 123:105S-114S, 2003.

British Thoracic Society/Society of Cardiothoracic Surgeons of Great Britain and Ireland Working Party: Guidelines on the selection of patients with lung cancer for surgery. Thorax 56:89-108, 2001.

Lawrence VA, Hilsenbeck SG, Noveck H, et al: Incidence and hospital stay for cardiac and pulmonary complications after abdominal surgery. J Gen Intern Med 10:671-681, 1995.

Nakagawa M, Tanaka H, Tsukuma H, Kishi Y: Relationship between the duration of the preoperative smoke-free period and the incidence of postoperative pulmonary complications after pulmonary surgery. Chest 120:705-710, 2001.

Smetana GW: Preoperative pulmonary evaluation. N Engl J Med 340:937-944, 1999.

Wyser C, Stulz P, Soler M, et al: Prospective evaluation of an algorithm for the functional assessment of lung resection candidates. Am J Respir Crit Care Med 159:1450-1456, 1999.

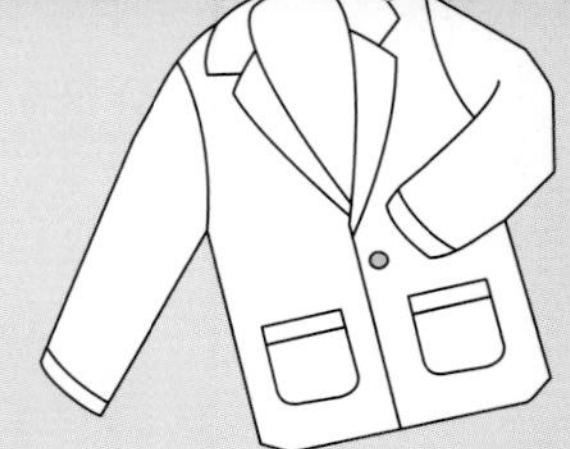

CHAPTER 18 Cough

Surinder S. Birring and Ian D. Pavord

Cough is an important defense mechanism that clears the airways of secretions and prevents entry of foreign bodies and irritants into the lower respiratory tract. It is a universal experience, but also a nonspecific presenting feature of a number of respiratory conditions. Cough is one of the most common presenting signs in patients seen by the general practitioner. Most cases result from viral and bacterial upper respiratory tract infection, are self-limiting, and do not require further evaluation, but a small proportion of patients have persistent cough that requires an evaluation by a specialist. Chronic cough is arbitrarily defined as a cough of longer than 3 weeks in duration. It is present in 3% of the general population and is responsible for between 5% and 10% of respiratory outpatient referrals. Chronic cough is often perceived as a trivial problem but can be a disabling symptom associated with impairment of quality of life and distressing associated symptoms such as musculoskeletal chest pains, syncope, incontinence, disturbed sleep, and social embarrassment.

One popular approach to establishing the cause of chronic cough is based on an understanding of the distribution of cough receptors and the physiology of the cough reflex, and particularly on the realization that most cases are due to disease of the upper respiratory tract, where cough receptors are most plentiful. Most cases of chronic cough are associated with heightened cough reflex sensitivity, particularly if the cough is dry. This can be assessed formally using cough challenge tests incorporating tussive substances such as capsaicin. A number of cough receptors have been described, but bronchial C fibers, activated via vanilloid cough receptors, and rapidly adapting receptors are probably the most important.

Sensitization of cough receptors has been shown to occur in experimental animals and in humans after administration of various inflammatory mediators such as prostaglandins. One plausible explanation for heightened cough reflex sensitivity and cough in patients with chronic cough is the presence of airway inflammation and increased concentrations of tussive mediators adjacent to cough receptors. Afferent nerve fibers pass to a central cough receptor in the medulla, triggering a forced expiratory maneuver against a closed glottis, followed by glottal opening and high-velocity expiration. Factors influencing activity of the central cough receptor are poorly understood, but opiates probably exert their antitussive effects here. Successful treatment of the underlying cause of the cough usually results in reduction in cough sensitivity.

The key to successful management is establishing a clear diagnosis and applying effective treatment for long enough to reset cough receptors at a more physiologic level. Important pitfalls include atypical presentations, the presence of multiple pathologies, and inadequate therapy of the underlying disorder. Further difficulty is presented by the fact that evidence for the efficacy of specific therapies in chronic cough is largely based on expert opinion or uncontrolled trials, and there is a paucity of randomized controlled trials with well-validated outcome measures to guide the clinician. Nevertheless, a systematic approach based on the so-called "anatomic diagnostic protocol" does seem to be successful, and various series have reported a high rate of treatment success even in tertiary referral populations. There is a general consensus that the cause of most cases of chronic cough in patients with normal spirometry and chest radiography is asthma, eosinophilic bronchitis, gastroesophageal reflux, rhinitis, or a combination of these. Many of these conditions can be recognized clinically, and successful diagnosis and management are often possible without recourse to expensive or invasive investigations. This review will primarily focus on chronic cough, because this is a common and difficult diagnostic problem for both primary care physicians and pulmonary specialists.

DIFFERENTIAL DIAGNOSIS

The manifestations of cough can be conveniently divided into acute and chronic (Table 18.1). An acute cough is arbitrarily defined as a cough of less than 3 weeks duration. Infectious and allergic conditions are by far the most common causes. Most acute coughs related to viral upper respiratory tract infection resolve within 3 weeks, but a small proportion become persistent and require further evaluation.

Most conditions implicated in causing chronic cough, such as chronic obstructive pulmonary disease, lung cancer, foreign bodies, pulmonary tuberculosis, sarcoidosis, idiopathic pulmonary fibrosis, and heart failure, are obvious after clinical assessment, spirometry, and chest radiography. The majority of patients referred for investigation of chronic cough are nonsmokers and have normal findings on physical examination and chest radiography. The most common causes in these patients are listed in Table 18.1. Chronic cough in 10% to 30% of patients has multiple causes.

EVALUATION OF PATIENTS

An initial assessment of a patient with chronic cough is directed at finding a specific cause, assessing severity, and initiating trials of treatment. A careful history and physical examination are paramount to the evaluation of a patient with chronic cough (Table 18.2). Details of the factors surrounding the onset of cough and associated symptoms and a careful assessment of the upper airways and the respiratory system are particularly important.

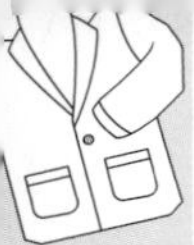

Table 18.1A
Common causes of acute cough

- Upper respiratory tract infections
- Acute sinusitis
- Allergic rhinitis
- Asthma

Table 18.1B
Common causes of chronic cough

Diagnosis	Approximate incidence (%)
Rhinitis	25-30
Asthma/eosinophilic bronchitis	20-25
Gastroesophageal reflux	15-20
Postviral cough	5-10
Chronic bronchitis	5-10
Bronchiectasis	5-10
ACE inhibitor induced cough	5-10
Unexplained	5-20

ACE, angiotensin-converting enzyme.

Table 18.2
An initial evaluation of a patient with chronic cough

History	Cough: onset, duration, character Sputum (volume, character) Smoking, occupation Upper respiratory tract infection Drug history (ACE inhibitors) Asthma: breathlessness, wheeze, nocturnal symptoms, atopy Gastroesophageal reflux: reflux-associated symptoms Rhinitis: postnasal drip, sinusitis, throat clearing, nasal congestion Adverse quality of life: musculoskeletal chest pains, incontinence, syncope, psychosocial issues, disturbed sleep
Examination	Clubbing External nasal: polyps Oropharyngeal: signs of post nasal drip Chest: signs of airflow obstruction, crackles
Investigations	Chest radiograph Spirometry ± bronchodilator reversibility Serial peak expiratory flow Full blood count and eosinophil differential cell count
Optional Investigations	Methacholine challenge test, induced sputum, allergen skin tests Sinus X-ray/CT sinus 24-hour esophageal pH and manometry CT chest/bronchoscopy in selected patients
Treatments	Directed at cause(s)

Basic initial investigations should include up-to-date chest radiograph, spirometry, and bronchodilator reversibility if appropriate. The history and physical examination are often unremarkable, in which case the evaluation of the patient focuses on the common upper airway conditions causing cough, namely, rhinitis, asthma, and gastroesophageal reflux. One approach

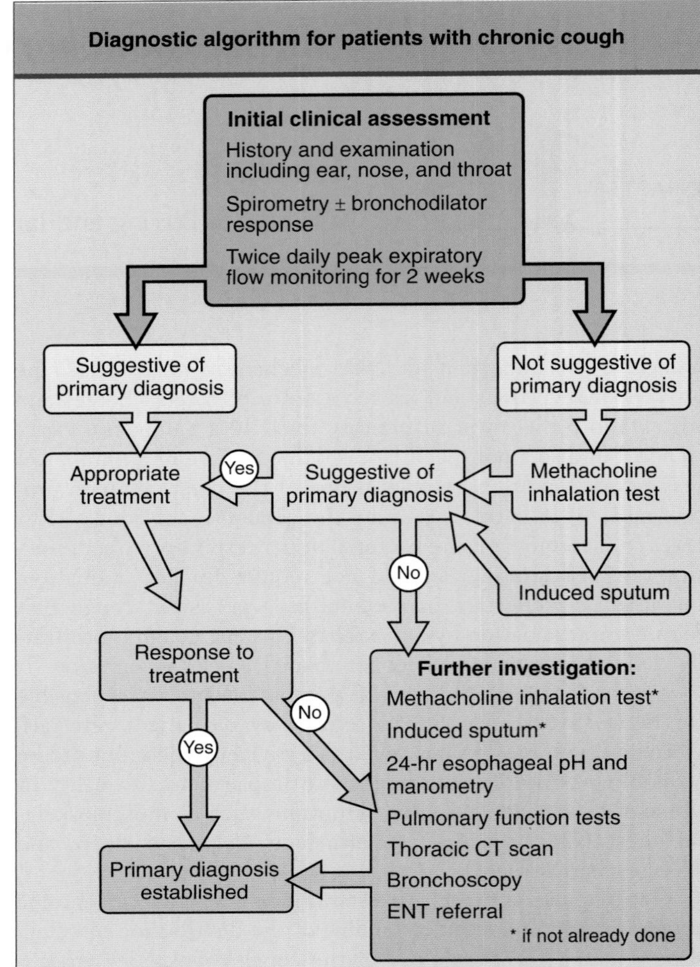

Figure 18.1 Diagnostic algorithm for patients with chronic cough.

based on the anatomic diagnostic protocol is suggested in Figure 18.1. It is important to emphasize the need to demonstrate objective evidence for the cause of cough in complex cases, especially if there are no suggestive features on initial evaluation. Multiple causes are common, particularly a combination of asthma, rhinitis, and/or gastroesophageal reflux. Once a cause has been established, the patient is reassessed for the presence and severity of cough after therapy. Treatment trials form an integral part of investigating a patient with chronic cough and are more easily interpreted when combined with attempts to validate the effects of treatment of the underlying cause and objective assessment of cough severity before and after treatment. Examples of the latter include cough visual analog scores (0 to 100 mm), cough-specific quality-of-life scores, and cough reflex sensitivity. Our approach is to regard a 15-mm change in visual analog score, a 2-point change in Leicester Cough Questionnaire quality-of-life score, and a 1.5 doubling dose change in C2 (concentration of capsaicin that causes two coughs) as significant. Further investigations depend on the patient's age, comorbid conditions, and local availability of tests and their costs (Fig. 18.1). The remainder of this section focuses on the evaluation of the more common causes of chronic cough.

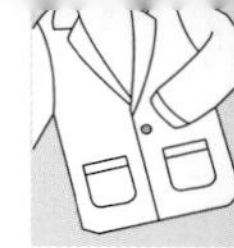

Rhinitis

Rhinitis, often associated with sinusitis and postnasal drip, is one of the most common causes of chronic cough. Allergy and infection are common causes of rhinitis and are thought to result in cough by mechanical stimulation from a postnasal drip and extension of local inflammation to the pharyngeal and laryngeal areas, where the cough receptors are most concentrated. Patients usually report nasal congestion, nasal discharge, and facial pain and may be aware of a postnasal drip and the need to clear the throat frequently. Careful examination of upper airways may reveal nasal quality to the voice, nasal polyps, sinus tenderness, and inflammation of the posterior pharyngeal wall with evidence of draining secretions. Investigations for rhinitis include nasal endoscopy and radiography or computed tomographic (CT) scan of the sinuses, which may reveal mucosal thickening and fluid levels. The opinion of an ear, nose, and throat specialist is helpful when there is diagnostic uncertainty or when severe disease is present.

Cough Variant Asthma and Eosinophilic Bronchitis

Asthma is a condition characterized by airway hyper-responsiveness and inflammation that presents with variable signs of cough, dyspnea, and wheeze. A subgroup can present with an isolated chronic cough, known as "cough variant asthma." Heightened cough reflex sensitivity is commonly seen in cough variant asthma but not in non–cough predominant asthma. The airway inflammation in cough variant asthma is essentially similar to that seen in classic asthma, and the reason for the different physiologic association is unclear. Typically the cough is dry or minimally productive, and it may occur nocturnally, after exercise, or after allergen or occupational exposure, although there are often no clinical clues. The key to diagnosing asthma is demonstrating variable airflow obstruction. Serial peak flow recordings and spirometry with bronchodilator response are routine first-line investigations but are often normal in cough variant asthma. Demonstration of airway hyper-responsiveness by methacholine bronchoprovocation testing is a more sensitive and specific index of variable airflow obstruction and can be the only abnormality seen. A blood eosinophilia and positive allergen skin-prick test result or presence of allergen-specific IgE provide supportive evidence for the presence of asthma. The diagnosis of cough variant asthma is usually confirmed by a reduction of cough with therapy.

Eosinophilic bronchitis is an increasingly recognized entity, that presents with a corticosteroid responsive cough, and is characterized by a sputum eosinophilia (Fig. 18.2) and heightened cough reflex sensitivity but no evidence of variable airflow obstruction or airway hyper-responsiveness. Studies suggest that it is responsible for 10% to 15% of cases of chronic cough. The airway inflammation is similar to that seen in asthma, although there is evidence that differences in airway physiology are due to the site of mast cell localization in the airway, with infiltration of the epithelium occurring in eosinophilic bronchitis and infiltration of the airway wall smooth muscle occurring in asthma. It is important to recognize eosinophilic bronchitis because it responds well to treatment with inhaled corticosteroids. An assessment of airway inflammation or, at the very least, a trial of corticosteroid therapy is indicated irrespective of the presence of airway hyper-responsiveness.

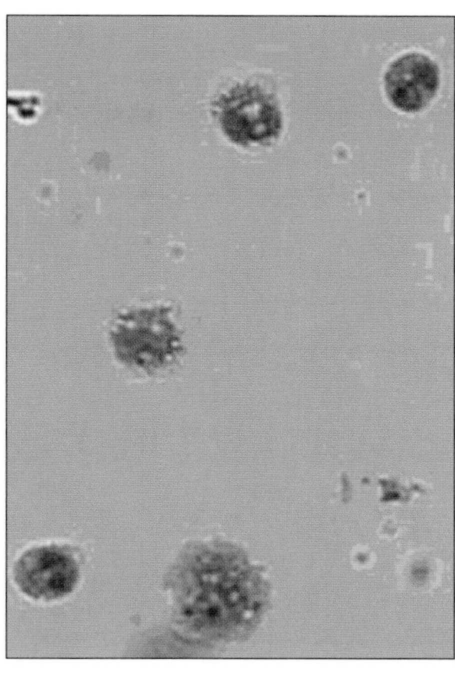

Figure 18.2 Sputum eosinophilia in eosinophilic bronchitis. Eosinophils are the cells with cytoplasmic granules stained bright red.

Gastroesophageal Reflux

Symptoms suggesting gastroesophageal reflux and abnormalities of esophageal function are common in patients with chronic cough of all age groups, and the frequent clinical observation that effective treatment of gastroesophageal reflux is associated with improvement of cough supports a causal association. The pathophysiology of gastroesophageal reflux–associated cough is poorly understood, but microaspiration of esophageal contents to the tracheobronchial tree and stimulation of neural esophageal-tracheobronchial reflexes are thought to be important. Gastroesophageal reflux–related cough is associated with the relaxation of the lower esophageal sphincter and often occurs during eating, talking, and on waking. Although most patients recognize heartburn, dysphagia, sore throat, globus, and dysphonia, up to one third of patients with gastroesophageal reflux–associated cough have no such symptoms.

Gastroesophageal reflux–associated cough is best diagnosed with 24-hour esophageal pH and manometry studies with simultaneous patient diary cards to record cough events. Esophageal pH monitoring may show evidence of abnormal standard parameters of gastroesophageal reflux. A temporal relationship between cough and reflux is particularly suggestive of gastroesophageal reflux–associated cough. The tracing in Figure 18.3 shows characteristic changes in the esophageal pressure due to cough shortly after episodes of gastroesophageal reflux. The alternative to esophageal studies, particularly indicated in patients with obvious gastroesophageal reflux symptoms, is a trial of a high-dose proton pump inhibitor for 3 months.

Angiotensin-Converting Enzyme Inhibitor–Associated Cough

Approximately 8% of patients taking angiotensin-converting enzyme inhibitors develop a persistent cough. The risk is higher in female patients and is similar with all types of angiotensin-converting enzyme inhibitors. Cough is not seen with

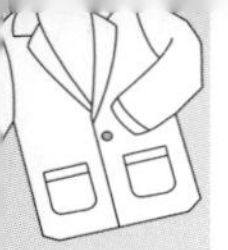

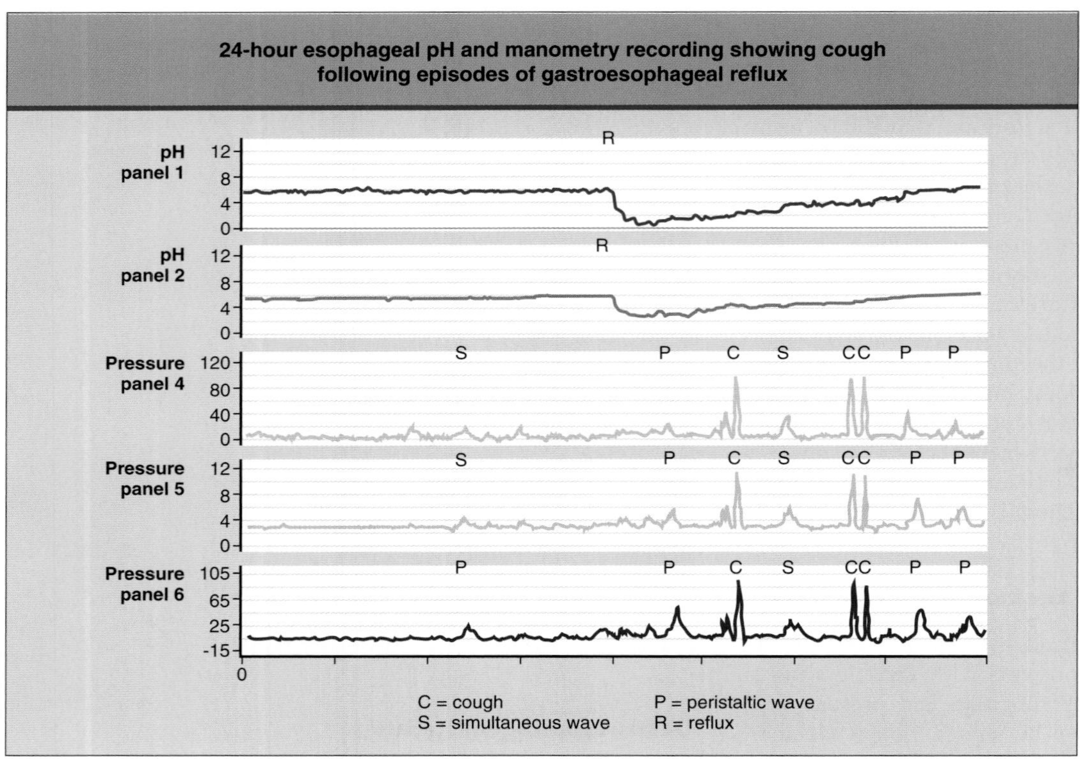

Figure 18.3 Twenty-four–hour esophageal pH and manometry recording showing cough following episodes of gastroesophageal reflux. *Panel 1*, Esophageal pH 5 cm above lower esophageal sphincter. *Panel 2*, Esophageal pH 10 cm above lower esophageal sphincter. *Panels 4, 5,* and *6*, Esophageal pressure 15, 10, and 5 cm above lower esophageal sphincter (mm Hg).

angiotensin-converting receptor antagonists. Increased airway concentrations of airway tussive mediators such as bradykinins and prostaglandins are thought to be responsible for heightened cough reflex sensitivity and cough in patients with angiotensin-converting enzyme inhibitor cough. The cough usually resolves promptly after treatment withdrawal. Persistence may suggest asthma, the onset of which has been linked to the use of angiotensin-converting enzyme inhibitors.

Other Causes of Cough

Community surveys suggest that most coughs related to upper respiratory tract infections resolve within 3 weeks. However, the cough can take several months to resolve in a small proportion of subjects. The infection in most cases remains unidentified, but respiratory viruses, *Mycoplasma pneumoniae*, *Chlamydia pneumoniae*, and *Bordetella pertussis* have been implicated in adults. Chronic bronchitis is a common cause of cough in smokers and may occur in nonsmokers who work in dusty environments. Typically patients have a productive morning cough.

Further Investigations

The use of fiber-optic bronchoscopy and high-resolution CT scanning should be reserved for patients with suggestive symptoms, signs, or chest radiographic findings or those with no objective evidence of more common causes of cough, as the investigations are invasive and expensive and the diagnostic yield is low. Cough reflex sensitivity measurement has limited value in the validation of the presence of chronic cough in clinical practice because of the wide overlap of cough sensitivity between healthy subjects and patients with chronic cough. Ambulatory cough monitors have the advantage of providing objective evidence of the presence and intensity of cough, but routine use is hampered by automation difficulty of analysis of the recordings.

TREATMENT

Treatment directed at the specific cause of chronic cough is summarized in Table 18.3. Using the anatomic diagnostic protocol, success rates of up to 95% in the management of chronic cough have been reported. The success rate goes down to approximately 80% in specialist cough clinics, possibly because of the complexity of cases referred. Reassessment of the patient after treatment and excluding additional aggravating factors or causes form an integral part of managing a patient with chronic cough. A common dilemma faced by physicians managing patients with chronic cough is that the diagnosis of cough often depends on successful trials of treatment; if treatment is unsuccessful, the difficult question arises as to whether the underlying condition has not responded or whether that condition is not responsible for the cough. However, the use of objective tests to make a diagnosis and careful validation of the effect of therapy for the underlying condition should minimize this problem.

Rhinitis

Topical corticosteroids are the mainstay of treatment for cough due to rhinitis. In cases in which nasal obstruction is prominent, initial additional treatment with topical decongestant sprays may be necessary, and antibiotics should be administered if infection is suspected. Topical ipratropium bromide is often helpful if rhinorrhea is prominent, and antihistamines are useful when sneeze and nasal itch are prominent and when there is

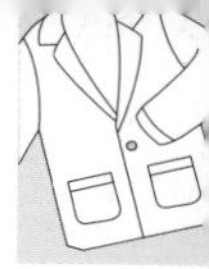

Table 18.3
Specific therapy for chronic cough

Cause	Treatment
Rhinitis	Nasal corticosteroids Selected patients: topical ipratropium, topical decongestants, oral antihistamines, surgery
Asthma	Inhaled corticosteroids, inhaled bronchodilators as required, leukotriene antagonists
Eosinophilic bronchitis	Inhaled corticosteroids, oral corticosteroids in selected cases
GERD-associated cough	Self-help measures: weight loss, smoking cessation, reduce alcohol intake, elevate head of bed, avoid eating within 2 hours of bedtime Acid suppression: proton pump inhibitors Prokinetic agents: metoclopramide in selected patients Surgery: laparoscopic fundoplication in selected patients
Chronic bronchitis	Smoking cessation
ACE cough	Drug withdrawal—substitution of alternative if appropriate
Postviral cough	Observation
Bronchiectasis	Chest physiotherapy and postural drainage, antibiotics
Idiopathic chronic cough	Antitussives (dextromethorphan, codeine), nebulized lidocaine

GERD: gastro-esophageal reflux; ACE: angiotensin converting enzyme.

coexisting atopy. Surgical treatment may be necessary when there are obvious anatomic abnormalities.

Cough Variant Asthma and Eosinophilic Bronchitis

Cough due to asthma responds well to bronchodilators and inhaled corticosteroids. A response typically occurs within 1 to 2 weeks of starting therapy and reaches a maximum after 8 to 10 weeks. Leukotriene antagonists are also helpful in cough variant asthma. The duration of asthma therapy remains unclear, but return of the cough on gradual withdrawal of therapy suggests long-term therapy may be necessary. Patients with cough variant asthma often have coexisting rhinitis or postnasal drip, and a complete response may not be seen until all potential aggravating factors are treated. Cough due to eosinophilic bronchitis is treated with inhaled corticosteroids. Rarely, oral corticosteroids are required to suppress eosinophilic airway inflammation and cough.

Gastroesophageal Reflux

Gastroesophageal reflux–associated cough is managed with self-help measures such as weight reduction, avoidance of tight clothing, elevation of headrest during sleep, reduced alcohol and tobacco intake, and drug therapy for acid suppression. Proton pump inhibitors are the most effective treatment for gastroesophageal reflux–associated cough. Anecdotal evidence suggests that high-dose therapy for at least 3 months is often required before the cough improves. Prokinetic agents such as metoclopramide may have a role in some cases. Antireflux surgery should be considered in gastroesophageal reflux–associated cough that has been diagnosed objectively and found to be unresponsive or only partially responsive to medical therapy.

Table 18.4
Common pitfalls in the management of chronic cough

- Incorrect diagnosis
- Not recognizing multiple causes of cough
- Lack of objective evidence for the diagnosis of asthma
- Prolonged and aggressive treatment may be required before cough improves
- Poor treatment compliance
- Postviral and gastroesophageal-associated cough may take many months to resolve
- Inappropriate labeling of psychogenic cough
- Failure to assess the impact of cough on quality of life

Idiopathic Chronic Cough

A proportion of cases, variously estimated at between 5% to 20% of referrals, remain unexplained after extensive investigations and treatment trials. These patients are predominantly middle-aged women with objective evidence of abnormality such as heightened cough reflex sensitivity and airway inflammation. They suffer considerable physical and psychological morbidity. Many patients with idiopathic chronic cough are labeled with a diagnosis of psychogenic cough, although there is little evidence to support this view, and it is perhaps more likely that any abnormal illness behavior is secondary to the adverse impact of cough

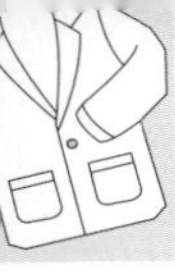

on psychosocial aspects of quality of life. When evaluating a patient with unexplained cough, it is important to use objective tests and recognize common pitfalls in managing chronic cough (Table 18.4). Therapy for idiopathic chronic cough is disappointing and is largely limited to nonspecific antitussive therapy such as dextromethorphan, codeine, and drugs with weak evidence of benefit such as baclofen and nebulized local anesthetics (lidocaine, mepivacaine). Referral to a physiotherapist for cough management advice may be of some help.

In conclusion, management of chronic cough with a careful history and physical examination and use of an anatomic diagnostic protocol can be rewarding in most cases. Successful treatment of the underlying disorder can achieve significant improvements in all aspects of quality of life.

SUGGESTED READINGS

Birring SS, Berry M, Brightling CE, Pavord ID: Eosinophilic bronchitis: clinical features, management and pathogenesis. Am J Respir Med 2:169-173, 2003.

Birring SS, Prudon B, Carr AJ, et al: Development of a symptom specific health status measure for patients with chronic cough: Leicester Cough Questionnaire (LCQ). Thorax 58:339-343, 2003.

Chung KF: Assessment and measurement of cough: the value of new tools. Pulm Pharmacol Ther 15:267-272, 2002.

Fuller RW, Jackson DM: Physiology and treatment of cough. Thorax 45:425-430, 1990.

Gibson PG, Dolovich J, Denburg J, et al: Chronic cough: eosinophilic bronchitis without asthma. Lancet 1:1346-1348, 1989.

Irwin RS, Boulet LP, Cloutier MM, et al: Managing cough as a defense mechanism and as a symptom. A consensus panel report of the American College of Chest Physicians. Chest 114(Suppl 2):33S-181S, 1998.

Irwin RS, Corrao WM, Pratter MR: Chronic persistent cough in the adult: the spectrum and frequency of causes and successful outcome of specific therapy. Am Rev Respir Dis 123:413-417, 1981.

Irwin RS, Madison JM: The diagnosis and treatment of cough. N Engl J Med 343:1715-1721, 2000.

Morice AH, Kastelik JA, Thompson R: Cough challenge in the assessment of cough reflex. Br J Clin Pharmacol 52:365-375, 2001.

Widdicombe JG: Neurophysiology of the cough reflex. Eur Respir J 8:1193-1202, 1995.

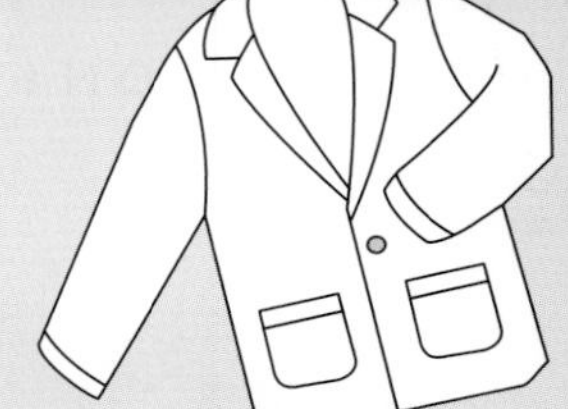

CHAPTER 19 Dyspnea

Dave Singh and Ashley Woodcock

Breathing is truly a strange phenomenon of life, caught midway between the conscious and the unconscious and peculiarly sensitive to both.

(DICKENSON RICHARDS, 1953)

Breathing is regulated by the brainstem, predominantly without conscious awareness. Patients use a variety of terms to describe an unusual awareness of breathing or the need to breathe more. Clinicians refer to this as dyspnea, which was defined by Means (1921) as "whenever the respiratory mechanisms cannot with ease [function] to the extent that the body processes require." This simple definition implies a disproportion between demand for and supply of ventilation. Thus, dyspnea may occur with increased demand (i.e., increased metabolic rate) or with reduced supply caused by cardiorespiratory disease. A more recent definition by the American Thoracic Society states that "dyspnea is a term used to characterize a subjective experience of breathing discomfort that consists of qualitatively distinct sensations that vary in intensity. The experience derives from interactions among multiple physiological, psychological, social, and environmental factors, and may induce secondary physiological and behavioral responses." This definition distinguishes between respiratory "sensations" from the activation of peripheral receptors and "perception," which is an individual's response to the sensation. Furthermore, individual perception is influenced by psychological and environmental factors, thus providing an explanation for why some patients perceive similar respiratory sensations in very different ways.

CONTROL OF BREATHING

Respiration is controlled by a motor efferent and a sensory afferent system (Fig. 19.1). Motor activity is initiated in the medulla, causing activation of the respiratory muscles responsible for ventilation. The consequent mechanical and biochemical changes are detected by a variety of sensory systems that send signals back to the brainstem. Sensory signals arise from chemoreceptors in the medulla, carotid and aortic bodies, pulmonary vagal receptors, and mechanoreceptors in the lung (pulmonary stretch receptors), chest wall (spindle muscle and joint receptors), and diaphragm (Golgi receptors). This afferent information is integrated into the higher centers and is used to regulate the motor system. Although breathing is predominantly controlled by these automatic mechanisms, signals originating from the cerebral cortex can voluntarily alter the pattern of respiration. Furthermore, any motor signals are also copied directly to the sensory cortex. This is known as central corollary discharge and results in a conscious awareness of respiratory motor activity.

MECHANISMS OF DYSPNEA

Campbell and Howell first introduced the concept of length tension inappropriateness as the underlying cause of dyspnea. They proposed that dyspnea occurs when the respiratory sense of effort translated as respiratory muscle tension is not matched by an appropriate change in respiratory muscle length detected by mechanoreceptors. This concept has since been extended to include all the afferent components of the respiratory sensory system; that is, dyspnea occurs when efferent motor activity is not matched by the integrated sensory afferent information arising from chemoreceptors, vagal signals, and mechanoreceptors. Afferent feedback is therefore a mechanism for the effectiveness of the response to ventilatory motor signals to be assessed, and the extent of dyspnea is dependent on the degree of imbalance between afferent feedback and efferent motor signals.

Respiratory disorders may alter afferent sensory feedback in different ways. For example, respiratory muscle weakness or fatigue detected by spindle receptors is a common cause of altered sensory feedback in neuromuscular disorders or patients with respiratory failure who have lost weight. In obstructive lung diseases such as asthma and chronic obstructive pulmonary disease (COPD), bronchoconstriction alters signaling from pulmonary stretch receptors. In addition, increased motor output is required to overcome increased airway resistance. This combination of increased motor output and decreased sensation of pulmonary expansion causes dyspnea. Similarly, in lung parenchymal diseases such as pulmonary fibrosis, sensory receptors detect decreased expansion relative to the motor output. In all of these cases the afferent sensory information is used by the higher centers to assess the current level of ventilation compared with the maximal achievable ventilation (that is, alveolar ventilation as a proportion of maximal voluntary ventilation, or VA/MVV). This ratio influences the severity of dyspnea. For example, although this ratio is increased in patients with lung disease because of an increase in VA, dyspnea will be more severe in patients who also have a reduced MVV (e.g., as a result of respiratory muscle weakness or restrictive lung disease). Furthermore, dyspnea occurs in both healthy subjects and patients with lung disease during exercise, because the increased motor output is not matched by sensory signals detecting adequate ventilation. In patients with a limited MVV, severe dyspnea may occur after minimal exertion, because a small increase in ventilation is still proportionally large relative to a reduced MVV.

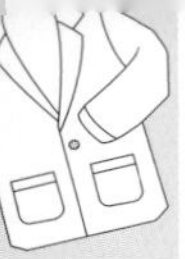

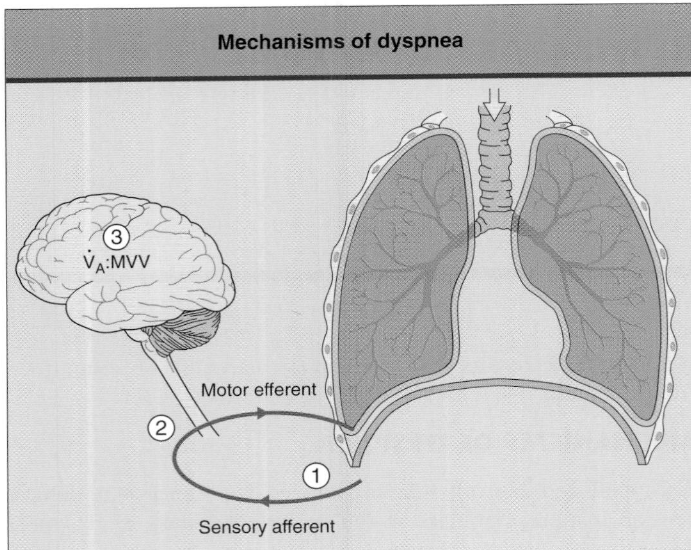

Figure 19.1 Mechanisms of dyspnea. (1) Sensory afferent information from chemoreceptors, vagal receptors, and mechanoreceptors (in the lung, chest wall, and diaphragm). Higher centers compare (2) sensory afferent and motor efferent activity and (3) alveolar ventilation (Va) to maximum voluntary ventilation (MVV).

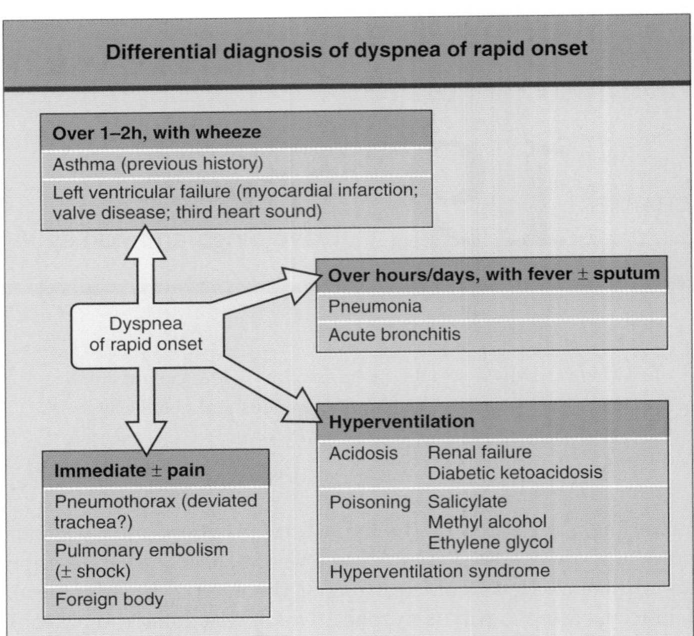

Figure 19.2 Differential diagnosis of dyspnea of rapid onset.

DIFFERENTIAL DIAGNOSIS

Pattern recognition can be lifesaving. Patients with dyspnea usually fit into a recognizable pattern in terms of the history of rate of onset and type of dyspnea, and the presence of associated symptoms. For example, dyspnea of sudden onset suggests an acute cardiopulmonary event (e.g., pneumothorax, massive pulmonary embolism, acute left ventricular failure). Patients who have these conditions either come to the hospital quickly or die, and they do not generally suffer long-standing dyspnea. Patients who have chronic dyspnea usually have respiratory disease (e.g., asthma, COPD, pulmonary fibrosis) or functional dyspnea (hyperventilation syndrome), but chronic dyspnea can be a feature of some chronic cardiac diseases with pulmonary venous congestion (e.g., poor left ventricular function, mitral stenosis, hypertrophic obstructive cardiomyopathy). Associated symptoms help complete a recognizable pattern. For example, dyspnea of sudden onset with pleuritic pain suggests pulmonary infarction or pneumothorax. Alternatively, the same symptoms, together with fever, cough, and sputum, suggest pneumonia. Figures 19.2, 19.3, and 19.4, although not mutually exclusive, give some idea of the range of diagnoses that depend on the rate of onset and the presence of additional symptoms.

Dyspnea of Rapid Onset

Dyspnea of abrupt onset (see Fig. 19.2) is a serious condition that requires urgent attention. The cause may be obvious, such as the inhalation of a foreign body, but more often associated symptoms, especially chest pain, give important clues. For example, if severe and associated with unilateral chest pain, dyspnea may indicate a large or even tension pneumothorax (Fig. 19.5). Absent breath sounds and deviation of the trachea to the opposite side may indicate the need for urgent pleural aspiration. The abrupt onset of dyspnea associated with severe central chest pain and hypotension suggests massive pulmonary

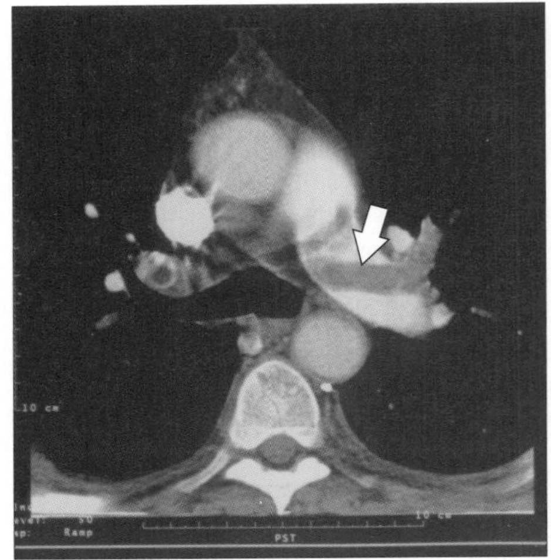

Figure 19.3 Massive pulmonary embolism. The patient had central chest pain and severe dyspnea of acute onset, associated with syncope and systemic hypotension. The contrast computed tomography (CT) scan shows a large embolus in the pulmonary trunk and both main pulmonary arteries. (Courtesy of Dr. A. Horrocks.)

embolism and the need for urgent pulmonary vascular imaging and anticoagulation (see Fig. 19.3).

The onset of breathlessness over 1 to 2 hours with wheeze usually suggests acute asthma but can be a feature of acute left ventricular failure. Differentiation in an elderly patient is often very difficult—a previous history of similar episodes suggests asthma, but a history of central chest pain and/or a third heart sound indicates cardiac disease (in practice, patients often receive initial treatment for both). Dyspnea that develops over hours or days usually indicates an acute respiratory problem. The association with fever, pleurisy, and sputum suggests pneumonia, whereas progressive wheezing in a smoker suggests acute on chronic bronchitis. A previous history of wheeze in a nonsmoker indicates asthma.

Hyperventilation is inappropriately high alveolar ventilation for the current metabolic rate, with lowered arterial $PaCO_2$. This can be secondary to poisoning (e.g., from salicylates, ethyl

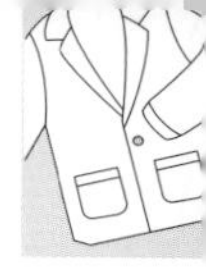

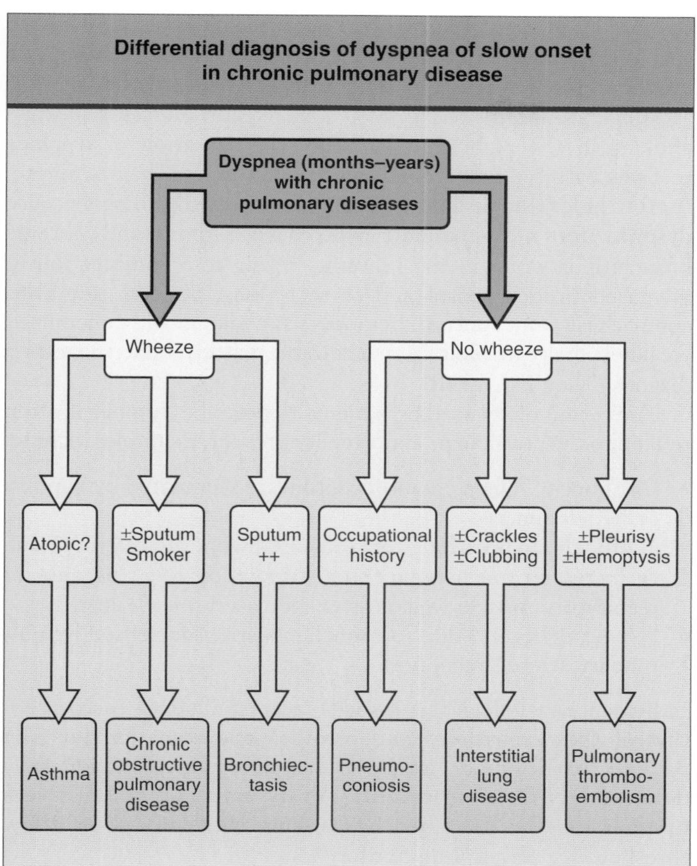

Figure 19.4 Differential diagnosis of dyspnea of slow onset in chronic pulmonary disease according to the presence or absence of wheeze.

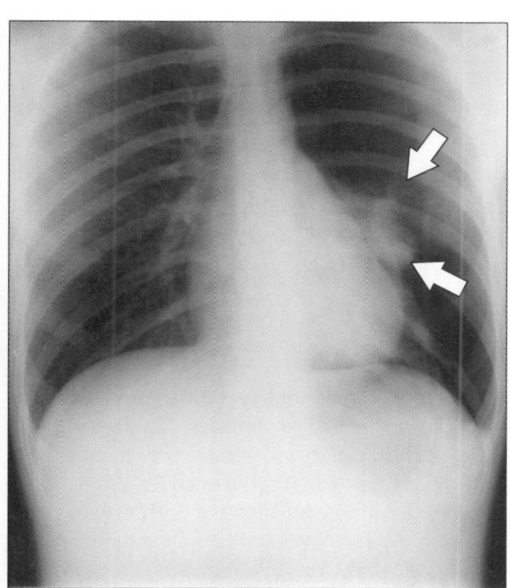

Figure 19.5 Pneumothorax. The patient had rapid onset of breathlessness that increased over 30 minutes, initially associated with left pleuritic pain. The chest radiograph shows a completely collapsed left lung. Although the mediastinum is central, at pleural aspiration an initial hiss of air indicated a degree of "tension" pneumothorax.

alcohol, ethylene glycol) or as a compensatory respiratory alkalosis to balance a metabolic acidosis (e.g., as in renal failure, diabetic ketoacidosis). Hyperventilation syndrome often occurs in young women who have no associated cardiopulmonary disease, although it can complicate other respiratory diseases, especially asthma. This should be a positive diagnosis rather than one of exclusion, as it has several characteristic clinical features.

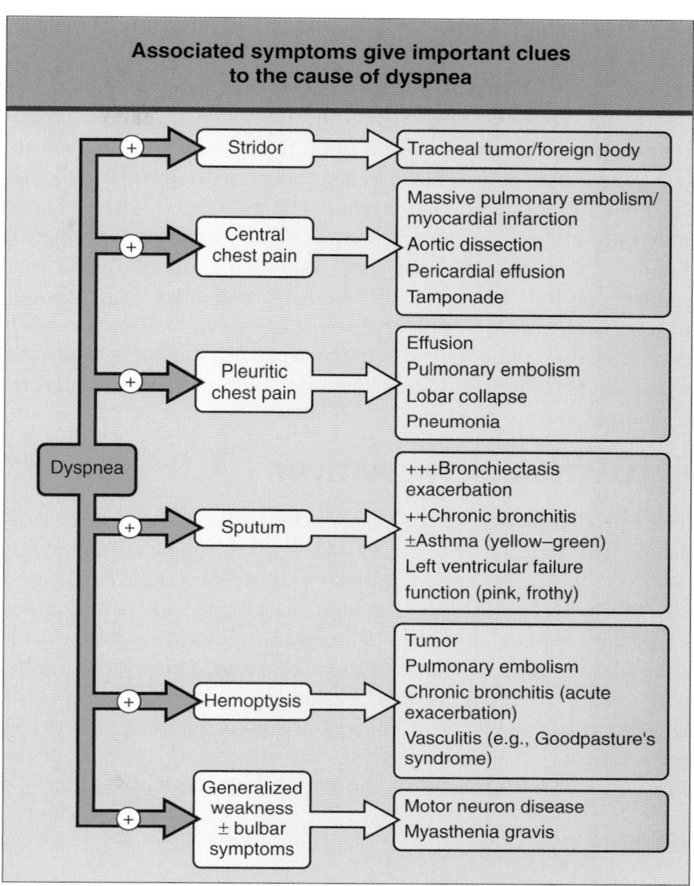

Figure 19.6 Symptoms that can be associated with dyspnea. Associated symptoms make a recognizable pattern of disease and give important clues to the cause of dyspnea.

Patients often complain that their breathing is somehow unsatisfactory and requires intermittent, deep inspirations with a chaotic respiratory pattern. Dizziness, peripheral paresthesias, a prickling sensation over the head and neck, and fatigue are common. Characteristically, it does not disturb sleep and is not present immediately on waking.

Chronic Dyspnea

Static or slowly progressive dyspnea is usually caused by more chronic pulmonary conditions (see Fig. 19.4). Wheezing indicates airway disease as opposed to parenchymal or pulmonary vascular disease. However, it can also be caused by chronic congestive cardiac failure, recurrent pulmonary emboli, anemia, and a variety of neuromuscular disorders.

Breathlessness associated with respiratory muscle weakness in myasthenia gravis and motor neuron disease is subtle, gradual, and often associated with choking on drinks because of bulbar weakness.

Breathlessness associated with diaphragm palsy tends to be static and worse when associated with obesity. When diaphragm paralysis is bilateral, it causes immediate and severe orthopnea, and typically patients cannot swim (during immersion the water pressure pushes the paralyzed diaphragm higher).

Detailed analysis of associated symptoms with chronic dyspnea is crucial to establish a likely cause (Fig. 19.6). Pleuritic chest pain is associated with pleural effusion, lobar collapse, pneumothorax, pneumonia, and pulmonary emboli. Purulent sputum in large volumes is associated with bronchiectasis, but in smaller amounts with chronic bronchitis, asthma, and pneumonia. Large volumes of often pink, frothy sputum can indicate left ventricular failure but can also occur with alveolar cell carcinoma. Patients who have hemoptysis associated with dyspnea may have a chest radiograph that shows a proximal lung cancer. Hemoptysis with a normal chest radiograph may indicate pulmonary emboli or, rarely, pulmonary vasculitis (e.g., Goodpasture's syndrome, polyarteritis). Dyspnea associated with generalized weakness, and particularly with bulbar symptoms, may indicate a neuromuscular disorder such as myasthenia gravis or motor neuron disease.

EVALUATION OF THE PATIENT

The initial approach to the patient depends on the clinical situation. The patient with rapid onset of dyspnea needs urgent clinical diagnosis, investigation, and treatment. Associated symptoms and rapidly elicited clinical signs provide useful clues. High-flow oxygen should be started to maintain oxygen saturation while urgent arterial blood gas tensions, chest radiographs, and electrocardiograms are obtained. Occasionally, specific treatment has to be started before any investigations take place, for example, pleural aspiration for suspected tension pneumothorax or nebulized bronchodilators for acute asthma.

Chronic Dyspnea

In patients who have chronic dyspnea, a more leisurely approach is possible, with the taking of a detailed history. An open question to a patient may elicit a wide range of descriptions of dyspnea, such as shortness of breath, difficulty with breathing in or breathing out, sense of suffocation, a sense of chest tightness, a sense of rapid breathing, the need to take added breaths, and so on. One key question is, "Do you wheeze?" because this differentiates airway diseases from other causes of dyspnea. A second specific question regards severity, that is, whether dyspnea occurs on exercise or at rest (if on exercise, at what level of exercise?). Third, it is important to determine whether breathlessness occurs when the patient is lying flat and whether it is eased by sitting upright (orthopnea), and whether it wakes the patient at night (paroxysmal nocturnal dyspnea). Although this is commonly associated with left ventricular failure, the most common cause of waking at night with breathlessness is asthma. Patients who have sleep apnea syndrome can also wake choking in the night, but typically the sensation of dyspnea resolves within a few seconds and always in less than a minute. It often helps establish how patients feel in the morning, because dyspnea for most patients who have asthma and chronic bronchitis is worst in the morning, owing to a combination of increased bronchospasm and/or secretions. Specific questions about chest pain, sputum, hemoptysis, choking, and generalized weakness help to build a recognizable pattern that suggests a diagnosis (see Fig. 19.6).

The terminology used by patients to describe dyspnea is often related to the physiologic abnormality present. Examples include:

- "Air hunger" when chemoreceptors are stimulated by hypoxia or hypercapnia
- "Difficulty in breathing" or "increased work of breathing" due to increased mechanoreceptor stimulation (e.g., because of respiratory muscle weakness or increased muscle load)
- "Chest tightness" due to bronchoconstriction sensed by pulmonary stretch receptors

Individual psychological and social factors influence the perception of these sensations and provide an explanation for why patients with similar levels of respiratory dysfunction may describe very different severities of dyspnea (e.g., more severe dyspnea may be described by patients with anxiety or a low threshold for physical discomfort).

PHYSICAL EXAMINATION

It is very important to be thorough, as occasionally the diagnosis may be apparent only on examination. To quantify the respiratory rate is mandatory. The patient may be distressed by shallow respiration associated with pleuritic chest pain in pneumonia or pulmonary infarction. Deep, sighing Kussmaul respirations (hissing through the teeth in apposition) may be caused by hyperventilation in patients who have renal failure, for example. In every patient who has dyspnea, the examiner must always establish whether the patient has stridor by listening at the open mouth (the history and chest radiograph may not be helpful; Fig. 19.7).

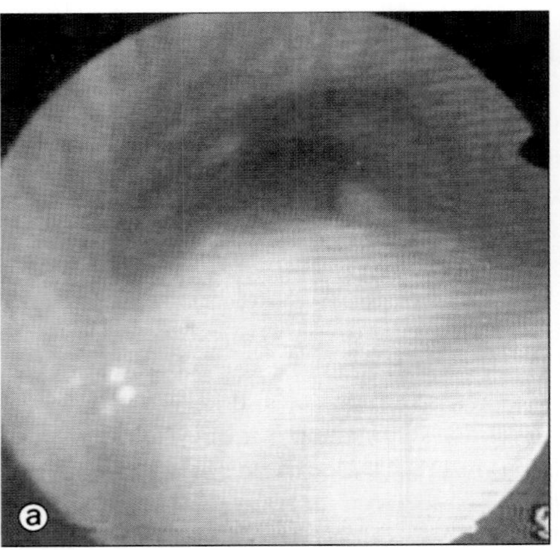

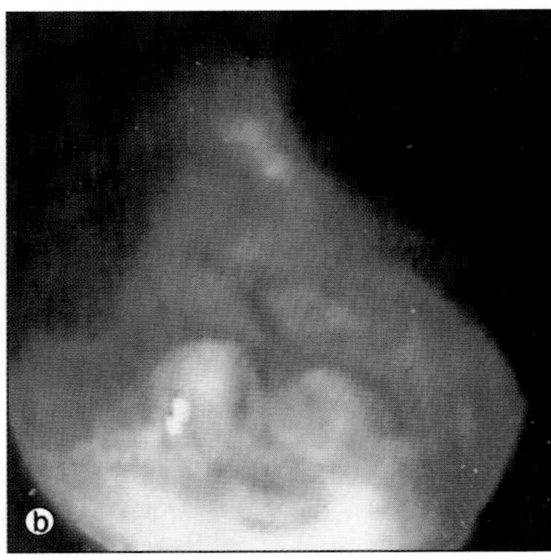

Figure 19.7 Adenoid cystic carcinoma of the trachea. This young nonsmoker had slowly progressive dyspnea and wheeze over the previous 12 months and was initially treated for asthma. Stridor (heard by listening at the open mouth) was present. **A,** The tumor just above the carina at presentation. **B,** After bulk removal. The patient's peak expiratory flow (150 L/min) was disproportionately low compared with the forced expiratory volume in 1 second (2.0 L), highly suggestive of upper airway obstruction. (Courtesy of Dr. P.V. Barber.)

The patient may appear to be in shock, that is, pale and clammy, with hypotension secondary to massive pulmonary embolism. Is the pattern of respiration that of the "pink and puffing" patient who has chronic airflow obstruction (that is, deep inspiration with a prolonged expiratory phase, while the patient sits with hands on knees to support the upper thorax to gain the best mechanical advantage)? Initial observation may demonstrate cyanosis, the flapping tremor of carbon dioxide retention, or the carpopedal spasm of acute hyperventilation. Central cyanosis indicates arterial hypoxemia, but peripheral cyanosis alone indicates a lowered cardiac output caused by pulmonary embolism or cardiac failure, for example. The presence of finger clubbing usually indicates chronic lung diseases (lung cancer, bronchiectasis, or fibrosis); it is associated rarely with a variety of other causes and is not usually associated with breathlessness. Lymphadenopathy (particularly cervical) may be associated with an obstructing lung carcinoma or lymphangitis carcinomatosa.

Examination of the cardiovascular system may reveal features of congestive cardiac failure such as an elevated jugular venous pressure, peripheral edema, and a third heart sound. Valve murmurs (e.g., mitral stenosis) may be audible. Unilateral edema may indicate a deep venous thrombosis and a potential source of emboli.

Examination of the respiratory system may reveal that the trachea is deviated, either away from a pneumothorax or effusion, or toward a lobar or lung collapse. The chest wall movements may be asymmetrical. The percussion note may be dull (pneumonia or collapse), stony dull (pleural effusion), or increased (pneumothorax). Auscultation may reveal focal abnormalities, such as absent breath sounds (e.g., pleural effusion or pneumothorax), or a diffuse abnormality, such as late inspiratory crackles (pulmonary fibrosis) or polyphonic wheezing (asthma or COPD). The importance of a localized, monophonic wheeze cannot be overemphasized. This may be the only feature of a partially obstructing, centrally located carcinoma at a stage when it is operable, and the chest radiograph may be completely normal. In the patient who has orthopnea, always observe the upper abdomen for paradoxical movement with the patient supine. Normally, the abdomen moves outward during inspiration as the diaphragm moves down, but in patients who have bilateral diaphragm paralysis, the diaphragm is sucked upward on inspiration and consequently the abdomen moves inward.

CHEST RADIOGRAPH

In the patient who has rapid onset of dyspnea, the chest radiograph can be diagnostic (e.g., pneumothorax, pneumonia, pulmonary edema), prompting immediate and specific treatment. In the patient who has more slowly progressive dyspnea, the chest radiograph more usually determines the diagnostic pathway (Fig. 19.8). For example, a normal chest radiograph can occur with airway diseases, neuromuscular disease, anemia, and recurrent pulmonary emboli and (together with the history) determines subsequent investigations. Cardiomegaly suggests the need for an echocardiogram. When the lung fields are focally or diffusely abnormal, the radiologic pattern suggests the most appropriate diagnostic pathway.

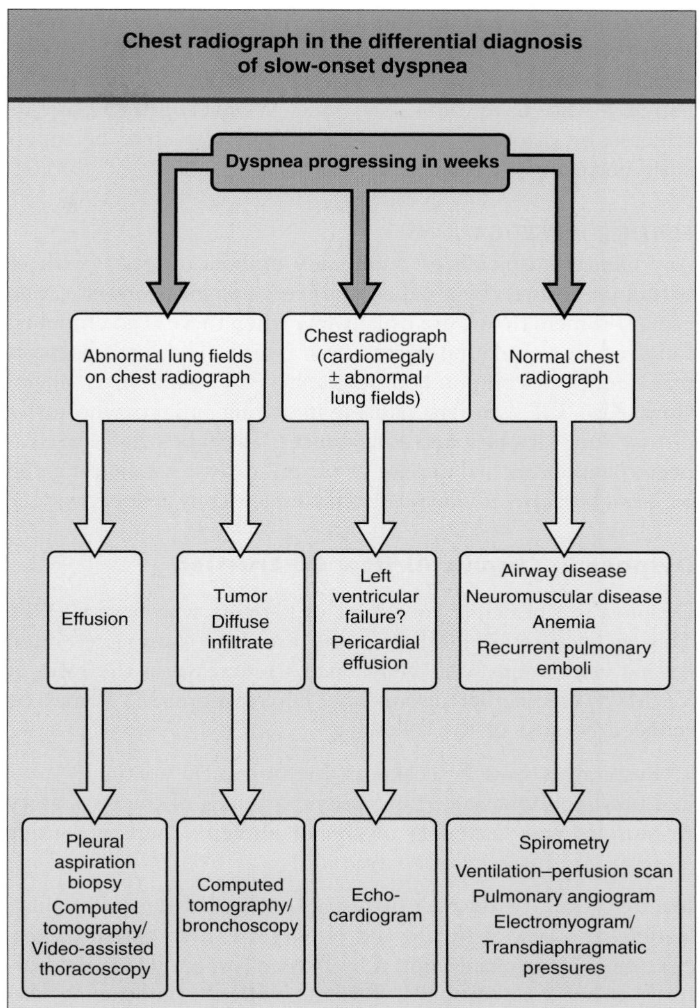

Figure 19.8 Value of the chest radiograph in the differential diagnosis of slow-onset dyspnea. The radiologic features fall into three broad groups—normal, abnormal lung fields with a normal heart size, and increased heart size with or without abnormal lung fields.

LUNG FUNCTION TESTS

Lung function tests are particularly important in patients who have slow-onset dyspnea. Simple spirometry in the clinic setting may show airflow obstruction, either irreversible in emphysema or reversible in asthma. More detailed investigation using flow-volume loops, gas transfer, and body plethysmography (lung volumes and airway resistance) helps to differentiate the chronic pulmonary conditions and stage the severity and rate of progression. If diaphragm weakness or a neuromuscular disorder is suspected, this can be screened for by videofluoroscopy or by maximal mouth or inspiratory sniff pressures, and assessed quantitatively by measurement of the transdiaphragmatic pressure. Arterial blood gas tensions may indicate type I (normocapnic) or type II (hypercapnic) respiratory failure. Oxygen desaturation on exercise may demonstrate an interstitial condition in patients who have a relatively normal chest radiograph (e.g., early pneumocystic pneumonia in human immunodeficiency virus patients). Simple exercise tests (e.g., shuttle or 6-minute walk) measure disability rate of progression and response

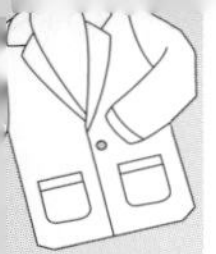

to treatment in patients who have chronic lung diseases. More complex cardiopulmonary exercise tests are valuable to differentiate severity of cardiovascular and respiratory diseases in patients who have both, and also in investigating patients affected by disproportionate breathlessness in spite of apparently normal cardiorespiratory function.

FURTHER INVESTIGATIONS

Any clinical suspicion of pulmonary embolic disease (with or without a normal chest radiograph) requires initial investigation using D-dimers (levels are usually low when there is no embolus) followed by ventilation-perfusion scanning. The final diagnosis may require a computed tomography (CT) pulmonary angiogram. Also, CT scans are valuable in staging patients who suffer diffuse lung diseases and lung cancer. Patients who have suspected endobronchial disease or pleural disease are investigated by bronchoscopy or video-assisted thoracoscopy, respectively.

Dyspnea in Chronic Airflow Obstruction

Dyspnea is a principle complaint of patients who have COPD. This is because of inefficient gas exchange causing elevated resting ventilation (VA), and hence an increase in the ratio of VA/MVV (see earlier discussion). Furthermore, MVV may be reduced because of the following:

1. Respiratory muscle weakness due to muscle wasting
2. Lung hyperinflation (this causes shortening of the inspiratory muscles and flattening of the diaphragm, thereby causing reduced efficiency of contraction)

Inactivity due to dyspnea may cause physical deconditioning, leading to a lack of fitness and obesity. In these patients exercise tolerance is often limited by fatigue (especially leg discomfort) rather than dyspnea. Patients with deconditioning also display increased lactic acid production by muscles during exercise. Lactic acid is a respiratory stimulus that increases motor output by the brain, thus worsening dyspnea. Limited exercise tolerance, due either to fatigue or dyspnea, can cause social isolation and depression. These social and physical factors all feed back adversely on the perception of dyspnea, which results in a vicious circle of deteriorating quality of life (Fig. 19.9).

Patients who have COPD may develop hypoxemia and hypercapnia because of inefficient gas exchange. Hypoxemia causes chemoreceptor-mediated respiratory motor stimulation. Acute hypercapnia also increases motor activity, probably through pH changes sensed in the brain. Additionally, the central interpretation of afferent signals may be directly influenced by hypercapnia, thereby increasing the severity of dyspnea. However, chronic hypercapnia results in metabolic compensation, which reduces respiratory sensitivity to pH changes. This relative insensitivity to variations in CO_2 concentrations explains why some COPD patients with respiratory failure have a reduced sensation of dyspnea compared with, for example, healthy subjects who have similar blood gas abnormalities.

It has long been suggested that a patient at one end of the clinical spectrum of COPD (i.e., the "pink puffer") is more dyspneic than the "blue bloater." Blue bloaters are in hypercapnic respiratory failure caused by a rapid, shallow pattern of breathing in response to increasing airflow obstruction. This results in alveolar hypoventilation, in spite of minute ventilation that is

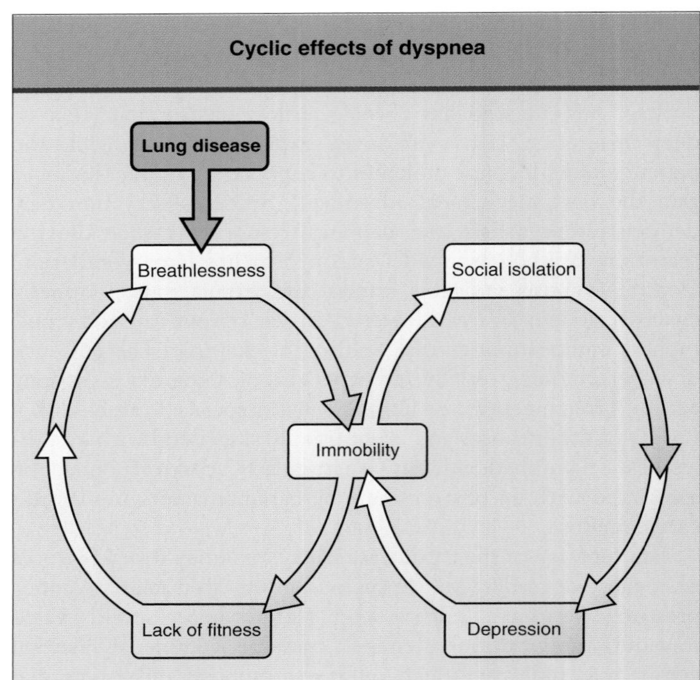

Figure 19.9 Vicious cycles in lung disease. Disability leads to lack of fitness, depression, and social isolation. Patients who suffer severe breathlessness because of chronic lung disease are frequently depressed.

comparable to that of pink puffers. This response to respiratory load is probably inherited. Exercise studies have shown no difference in dyspnea at rest or exercise between pink puffers and blue bloaters.

Measurement of Dyspnea

There are a variety of techniques for measuring dyspnea. Symptom rating scales such as the UK Medical Research Council dyspnea grade (Fig. 19.10) have been used in the clinical setting to assess the level of activity required to provoke dyspnea. Although this is a useful tool for assessing the severity of dyspnea, it is not sufficiently sensitive to evaluate changes within patients over time, for example, after pharmacologic treatment. This difficulty is overcome by the use of visual analog scales (VAS; Fig. 19.11). Usually, VAS are 10-cm lines, "anchored" by statements at either end, on which patients are asked to mark, for example, how breathless they feel at the moment. This gives quantitative measurements that can be used to assess changes within an individual over time. However, VAS cannot be used to compare different patients, as each individual uses them quantitatively differently.

The Baseline Dyspnea Index (BDI) allows not only the magnitude of the task causing dyspnea to be assessed ("unidimensional" assessment), but also allows two other dimensions to be quantified: the magnitude of effort exerted and the level of functional impairment (i.e., the physical impact of dyspnea). The BDI is administered by an interviewer who asks open-ended questions about each of the three dimensions. The interviewer grades the patient's dyspnea in each dimension on a scale from 0 (severe impairment) to 4 (no impairment) and calculates an overall score out of 12. The Transitional Dyspnea Index (TDI) can also be used to measure changes from the baseline score.

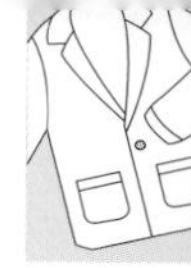

UK Medical Research Council dyspnea grade

Please mark the categories which most closely represent how you have been this week.

Breathless at rest or on minimal effort?	☐
Able to walk about 100 m (110 yards) on the level?	☐
Able to walk for 1.5 km (1 mile) on the level at own pace, but unable to keep up with people of similar age?	☑
Able to walk and keep up with people of similar age on the level, but not on hills or stairs?	☐
Normal?	☐

Exercise tolerance limited by other factors? Yes ☐ No ☑

If yes, please list factors ______________________

Figure 19.10 The UK Medical Research Council dyspnea grade. The dyspnea grade is useful for the initial assessment of patients' disability. The categories are generally too broad to help assess change in disability with treatment. The form is easily completed by a doctor, nurse, or health visitor.

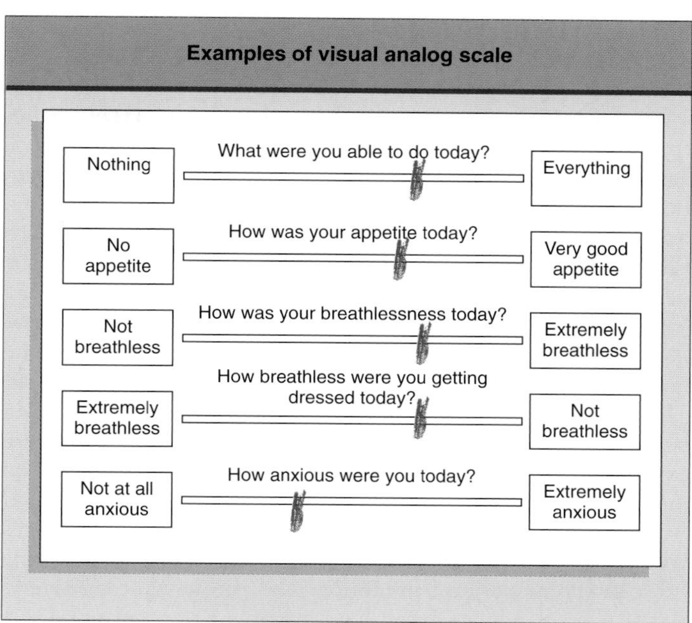

Figure 19.11 Example of a visual analog scale. Visual analog scales can be specific (e.g., "How breathless are you now?"); global (e.g., "How has your breathing been today?"); or applied (e.g., "How breathless were you when you dressed today?"). They are used to assess changes in breathlessness or disability with therapeutic intervention. The scale shown here can be used to assess changes in breathlessness in an individual patient who exercises at a fixed rate, on a treadmill, for example. The line is conventionally 10 cm long.

The techniques described rely on the patient's recollection of dyspnea in the recent past, which may lead to inaccuracies. This limitation can be overcome by assessing dyspnea during an exercise test, for example, by using the Borg Scale (Fig. 19.12) to measure the severity of dyspnea at a given level of ventilation or workload. This type of test, in which workload is fixed, is particularly valuable for assessing the responses of treatments specifically aimed at improving dyspnea. Simple walking tests are often used, as they are easy to perform in hospital corridors. Additionally, patients tend to walk at an even pace over 6 minutes, and this test is sufficiently discriminatory without being distressful even in very dyspneic patients. However, exercise tests can be affected by other physical factors (e.g., arthritis, angina). Furthermore, exercise tests such as bicycle tests performed in the laboratory may be of questionable relevance to daily activity.

The dyspnea rating systems described do not quantify and compare the different types of sensations experienced by patients (e.g., chest tightness, difficulty in breathing). Moreover, the results of rating scales are poorly correlated with disease severity, which is partly related to the different perception of dyspnea in patients with similar levels of respiratory dysfunction. It is for these reasons that history taking remains essential for assessing dyspnea in clinical practice; the tools described in this section provide supplementary information.

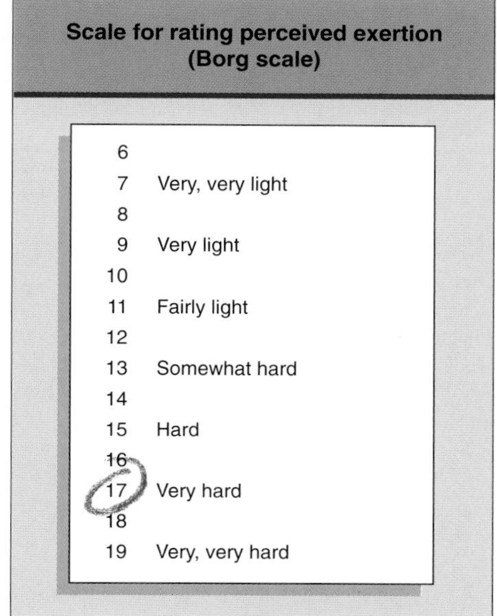

Figure 19.12 The scale for rating perceived exertion (Borg scale). The Borg scale for rating perceived exertion is used to assess the severity of tests that monitor exercise tolerance (e.g., 6-minute walking test). It is completed by the patient immediately on cessation of exercise.

TREATMENT

Treatment should be directed at specific conditions whenever possible (e.g., diuretics for cardiac failure, albuterol for asthma). However, the relationship between improvements in cardiorespiratory function and dyspnea is often unpredictable (e.g., an improvement of 5%, 10%, or 20% in lung function may not produce similar clinically important improvements in dyspnea). For the treatment of many respiratory diseases, inhaled bronchodilators are used empirically, but the therapeutic effect on dyspnea is variable and cannot be predicted from lung function tests. The use of theophyllines is limited, as they have smaller therapeutic effects and greater potential for adverse effects at higher serum levels.

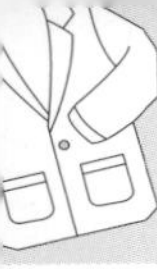

Despite maximal pharmacologic therapy for the underlying medical condition, many patients remain dyspneic. They require further treatments that objectively improve symptoms without necessarily changing lung function. Generally, further treatments for dyspnea reduce ventilatory demand, reduce ventilatory impedance, or improve respiratory muscle function. A widely used additional treatment is supplemental oxygen therapy, as it decreases ventilatory demand. This is achieved by reducing both chemoreceptor activity (thereby decreasing the hypoxic motor drive) and the metabolic load (by improving respiratory muscle function). Patients may also derive symptomatic benefit from the oxygen flow over the face, although the mechanism responsible for this is unclear. The use of oxygen has limitations, as individual responses can be very variable. Additionally, some patients cannot tolerate oxygen masks or find using oxygen cylinders during exercise too impractical.

Pulmonary rehabilitation involving exercise training reduces ventilatory demand by decreasing the metabolic load during exercise. Pulmonary rehabilitation may also have other beneficial effects; it reduces dyspnea by improving respiratory muscle function and can reduce disability by strengthening leg muscles, which may be important for patients with limited exercise tolerance because of fatigue. Noninvasive ventilatory support can be used to reduce ventilatory impedance. Partial ventilatory support can also improve respiratory muscle function by allowing the muscles to have intermittent periods of rest. However, some patients cannot tolerate ventilatory support devices or find their use too restrictive. Lung volume reduction surgery reduces ventilatory impedance. However, this treatment option benefits only a small proportion of emphysema patients.

Pharmacologic treatments have been sought for dyspnea. Opiates decrease ventilatory demand by altering the processing of central motor signals. This causes reduced central drive and respiratory depression. Additionally, opiates can alter the central perception of the sensation of dyspnea. However, side effects, tolerance, and the potential for addiction mean that opiates are not effective for all patients (e.g., mobile COPD patients). They are usually reserved for symptomatic relief of the desperately breathless and the terminally ill. Other pharmacologic treatments include alcohol, which has a small effect, probably because of bronchodilation, and anxiolytics. Initial data showing that anxiolytics may be a useful treatment for dyspnea have not been confirmed in controlled trials. However, these drugs are used on an individual basis in patients with the most potential for response (e.g., those with high levels of anxiety).

The treatment options already covered generally involve the modulation of physiologic abnormalities. However, altering the central perception of the sensation of dyspnea, such as by means of opioid or anxiolytic therapy, can also be an effective treatment. Perception may also be altered by psychological interventions. These include educational approaches, such as those used during pulmonary rehabilitation programs, and behavior modification, such as relaxation or distraction therapy to reduce anxiety during dyspnea. Patients with dyspnea often require a combination of the treatment approaches outlined in this section. For example, patients with COPD usually require pharmacologic treatments directed at the disease, such as bronchodilator therapy. They may also benefit from further treatments such as oxygen therapy or exercise training targeting the underlying pathophysiologic abnormalities, as well as educational approaches to alter the perception of dyspnea.

SUGGESTED READINGS

Ambrosino N, Scano G: Measurement and treatment of dyspnea. Respir Med 95:539-547, 2001.

American Thoracic Society. Dyspnea—mechanisms, assessment, and management: a consensus statement. Am J Respir Crit Care Med 159:321-340, 1999.

Jennings A-L, Davies AN, Higgins JPT, et al: A systematic review of the use of opioids in the management of dyspnoea. Thorax 57:939-944, 2002.

Johnson MA, Woodcock AA, Rehahn M, Geddes DM. Are pink puffers more breathless than blue bloaters? BMJ 286:179-182, 1983.

Mahler DA, Harver A, Lentine J, et al: Descriptors of breathlessness in cardiorespiratory diseases. Am J Respir Crit Care Med 154:1357-1363, 1996.

Mahler DA, Jones PW: Key outcomes in COPD: exacerbations and dyspnoea. Eur Respir J 12(Review 83):57-107, 2002.

Woodcock AA, Gross ER, Gellert A, et al: Effects of dihydrocodeine, alcohol, and caffeine on breathlessness and exercise tolerance in patients with chronic obstructive lung disease and normal blood gases. N Engl J Med 305:1611-1667, 1981.

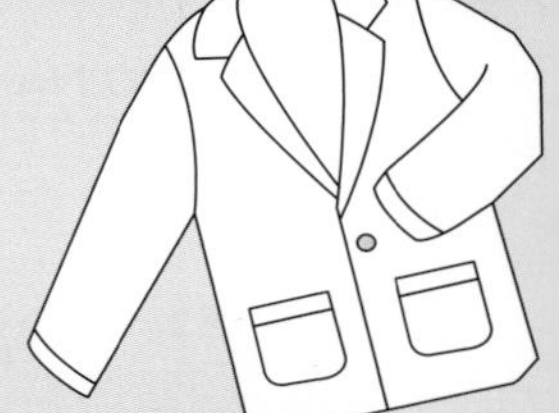

CHAPTER 20 Hemoptysis

John W. Kreit

Hemoptysis is defined as the expectoration of blood that results from hemorrhage into the lower respiratory tract. It can be caused by a wide variety of disorders and is a common reason for referral to a pulmonary specialist. The amount of blood expectorated can range from minimal streaking of the sputum to large volumes of pure blood and depends not only on the rate of bleeding but also on its location. For example, hemorrhage into the lung parenchyma or a distal airway may be accompanied by little or no hemoptysis, whereas even a relatively small amount of bleeding from a central airway may lead to a significant volume of expectorated blood.

Massive hemoptysis is an uncommon but potentially life-threatening event, because flooding of the airways and alveoli may lead to respiratory failure. It requires rapid evaluation and emergent and specific therapy, so massive hemoptysis is usually considered a distinct clinical entity and is discussed separately in a later section of this chapter.

Although hemoptysis is occasionally associated with a large, life-threatening hemorrhage, much more commonly it is important only as a sign of an underlying and often unrecognized disorder. Thus, hemoptysis is an extremely important symptom, and its cause must be determined by means of a thorough and orderly evaluation.

DIFFERENTIAL DIAGNOSIS

A large number of disorders have been reported to cause hemoptysis, and a rather extensive list is provided in Table 20.1. Of these, bronchogenic carcinoma, bronchiectasis, bronchitis, and bacterial pneumonia are responsible for the majority of cases. Table 20.2 lists the relative frequency of disorders causing hemoptysis in major series published since 1980. The significant variability, especially in the frequency of bronchiectasis, bronchitis, and tuberculosis, is due, in part, to the retrospective nature of most studies. It also reflects the fact that reported causes vary with the time of publication, the patient population studied, and the diagnostic tests and criteria employed. Figure 20.1 illustrates the percentage of patients with each diagnosis based on pooled data from these studies.

Neoplasms

In most series, malignancy is the most common cause of hemoptysis, and bronchogenic carcinoma accounts for the vast majority of these cases. In patients with hemoptysis, the tumor typically involves a central airway (i.e., a main, lobar, or segmental bronchus) and is most commonly a squamous cell carcinoma. Although most tumors are locally advanced or metastatic at the time of presentation, a significant percentage of patients have resectable disease. Much less commonly, hemoptysis is caused by other primary pulmonary neoplasms such as carcinoid tumor and hamartoma. Extrathoracic malignancies, especially melanoma and carcinoma of the breast, colon, and kidney, may also cause hemoptysis because of their propensity to metastasize to the bronchi and trachea.

Bronchiectasis

In studies published before the early 1960s, bronchiectasis was often the most common cause of hemoptysis and frequently accounted for 20% to 35% of cases. In the subsequent decades, this number dropped dramatically to less than 5%. Although this decline was correctly attributed to the greater availability and effectiveness of antibacterial and antituberculous therapy, it was probably also caused by a marked decrease in the use of bronchography, the principle diagnostic modality of that era. Since the advent of computed tomography (CT), bronchiectasis has been diagnosed with increasing frequency, and recent studies indicate that it remains a very important cause of hemoptysis.

Acute Bronchitis

Hemoptysis is often attributed to an acute infectious bronchitis based on compatible clinical or bronchoscopic findings, and this is a common final diagnosis in many series. Although acute bronchitis undoubtedly causes hemoptysis, the symptoms, signs, and bronchoscopic findings of this disorder are neither sensitive nor specific. In fact, several studies have demonstrated that the diagnosis of acute bronchitis is often made in patients with another source of bleeding. Thus, acute bronchitis must be considered a diagnosis of exclusion, and great care must be taken to search for other causes of hemoptysis.

Tuberculosis

Like bronchiectasis, tuberculosis was once a leading cause of hemoptysis. Although tuberculosis remains relatively common in certain patient populations and geographic regions, successful methods of treatment and prevention have markedly reduced both its incidence and its importance as a cause of hemoptysis. Although hemoptysis most commonly results from active disease, it may also be caused by the sequelae of infection, particularly bronchiectasis, parenchymal cavitation, and mycetoma formation.

Bacterial Pneumonia

Hemoptysis may result from virtually any type of bacterial pneumonia but most often accompanies infection with *Streptococcus*

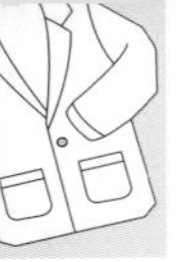

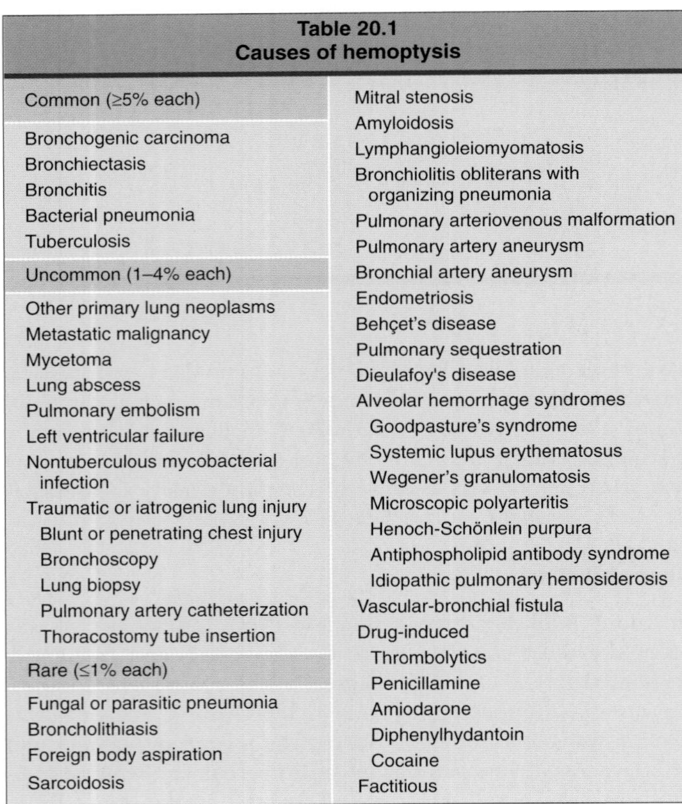

Table 20.1
Causes of hemoptysis

Common (≥5% each)	

Bronchogenic carcinoma
Bronchiectasis
Bronchitis
Bacterial pneumonia
Tuberculosis
	Mitral stenosis
	Amyloidosis
	Lymphangioleiomyomatosis
	Bronchiolitis obliterans with organizing pneumonia
	Pulmonary arteriovenous malformation
	Pulmonary artery aneurysm
	Bronchial artery aneurysm
	Endometriosis
	Behçet's disease
	Pulmonary sequestration
	Dieulafoy's disease
	Alveolar hemorrhage syndromes
	  Goodpasture's syndrome
	  Systemic lupus erythematosus
	  Wegener's granulomatosis
	  Microscopic polyarteritis
	  Henoch-Schönlein purpura
	  Antiphospholipid antibody syndrome
	  Idiopathic pulmonary hemosiderosis
	Vascular-bronchial fistula
	Drug-induced
	  Thrombolytics
	  Penicillamine
	  Amiodarone
	  Diphenylhydantoin
	  Cocaine
	Factitious

Uncommon (1–4% each)	

Other primary lung neoplasms
Metastatic malignancy
Mycetoma
Lung abscess
Pulmonary embolism
Left ventricular failure
Nontuberculous mycobacterial infection
Traumatic or iatrogenic lung injury
  Blunt or penetrating chest injury
  Bronchoscopy
  Lung biopsy
  Pulmonary artery catheterization
  Thoracostomy tube insertion	

Rare (≤1% each)	
Fungal or parasitic pneumonia Broncholithiasis Foreign body aspiration Sarcoidosis	

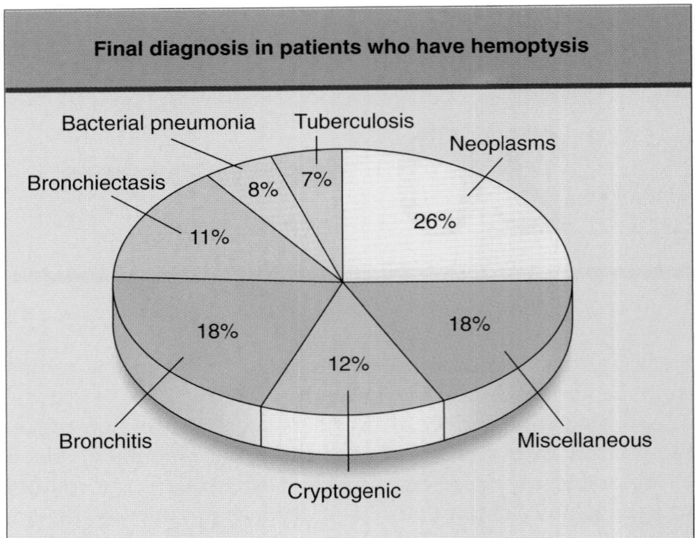

Figure 20.1 Final diagnosis in patients with hemoptysis. The approximate percentage of cases attributed to each diagnosis is shown.

pneumoniae. Other commonly implicated pathogens include *Klebsiella pneumoniae, Staphylococcus aureus, Pseudomonas aeruginosa,* and anaerobic organisms.

Miscellaneous Conditions

Only a few of the conditions listed in Table 20.1 account for most of the remaining specific diagnoses made in patients with hemoptysis. These disorders each account for 1% to 4% of cases and include pulmonary embolism, left ventricular (LV) failure, mycetoma, lung abscess, nontuberculous mycobacterial infection, and iatrogenic or traumatic lung injury.

Cryptogenic Hemoptysis

In almost all series, the cause of hemoptysis remains unknown in a significant percentage of patients. As shown in Table 20.2, the frequency of cryptogenic hemoptysis has varied widely, presumably because of differences in diagnostic criteria and the extent of evaluation.

PATIENT EVALUATION

When a patient reports a history of expectorating blood, the first step must be to determine if hemoptysis has actually occurred. That is, bleeding must be localized to the lower respiratory tract, and alternative sites, such as the nose, mouth, pharynx, larynx, and gastrointestinal tract, must be excluded. Few patients have difficulty distinguishing between vomiting and expectorating blood, although specific questions may be required to elicit a report of nausea and retching. Distinguishing between an upper and a lower airway source of bleeding is occasionally more

Table 20.2
Causes of hemoptysis in published series

Series	Gong et al.	Santiago et al.	Johnston et al.	McGuiness et al.	Hirshberg et al.	Fidan et al.
Year(s)	1975-80	1974-81	1977-85	1991-92	1980-95	2000
Location	Los Angeles	Los Angeles	Kansas City	New York	Jerusalem	Istanbul
No. of cases	129	264	148	57	208	108
Neoplasms (%)	24	31	19	12	19	34
Bronchiectasis (%)	40*	1	1	25	20	25
Bronchitis (%)	40*	23	37	7	18	0
Pneumonia (%)	3	6	5	0	16	10
Tuberculosis (%)**	3	6	7	16	1	18
Cryptogenic (%)	11	22	3	19	8	0
Other (%)	19	11	26	21	18	13

* Bronchiectasis and bronchitis were combined in this series. ** Active and inactive disease.

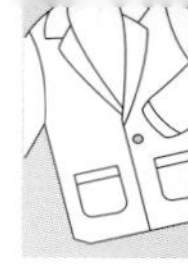

difficult, although this can usually be accomplished by a directed history and physical examination. Patients with hemoptysis almost always report that the expectoration of blood follows one or more episodes of coughing, whereas in those with an upper airway source it is typically preceded by a feeling of blood pooling in the mouth or the need to "clear the throat." A history of epistaxis is also an important indicator of upper airway hemorrhage. Routine examination of the nose, mouth, and pharynx is important to rule out an obvious site of bleeding. A thorough examination that includes rhinoscopy and laryngoscopy is indicated when an upper airway source cannot be reliably excluded.

Once hemoptysis has been confirmed, a search must be made for its cause. This process begins with an initial evaluation that consists of a complete history and physical examination and a chest radiograph. This information is then used to determine what, if any, additional testing is required to establish a specific diagnosis.

Initial Evaluation

A thorough history and physical examination are the first steps in identifying the cause of hemoptysis. Important symptoms, signs, and historical details that suggest one or more disorders are listed in Table 20.3. In some patients, such as those who have pulmonary embolism, LV failure, mitral stenosis, and traumatic or iatrogenic lung injury, the history and physical examination may provide the most important clues to the diagnosis.

Table 20.3
Important clinical features in patients with hemoptysis

Category	Feature	Disorder(s)
Historic	Cigarette smoking	Bronchogenic carcinoma
	Previously diagnosed malignancy	Metastatic malignancy
	Previously diagnosed pulmonary cardiac, pulmonary vascular, or systemic disease	
	Recent chest trauma or procedure	Traumatic/iatrogenic lung injury
	Risk factors for aspiration	Lung abscess, foreign body aspiration
Symptom	Purulent-appearing sputum	Bronchiectasis, bronchitis, pneumonia, lung abscess
	Pleuritic pain	Pneumonia, pulmonary embolism
	Paroxysmal nocturnal dyspnea, orthopnea	Left ventricular failure, mitral stenosis
	Fever	Pneumonia, lung abscess
	Weight loss	Bronchogenic carcinoma, other malignancy, tuberculosis, lung abscess
Sign	Bronchial breath sounds, egophony	Pneumonia
	Localized decrease in breath sounds, localized wheezing	Bronchogenic carcinoma, broncholithiasis, foreign body
	Coarse crackles, rhonchi	Bronchiectasis, bronchitis
	Pleural rub	Pneumonia, pulmonary embolism
	S3 gallop	Left ventricular failure
	Diastolic murmur	Mitral stenosis

Table 20.4
Important radiographic findings in patients who have hemoptysis

Radiographic finding	Disorder(s)
Nodule(s) or mass(es)	Bronchogenic carcinoma or other neoplasm, lung abscess, Wegener's granulomatosis, fungal infection
Atelectasis	Bronchogenic carcinoma or other endobronchial neoplasm, broncholithiasis, foreign body
Hilar/mediastinal adenopathy	Bronchogenic carcinoma or other neoplasm, mycobacterial or fungal infection, sarcoidosis
Dilated peripheral airways	Bronchiectasis
Air-space consolidation	Pneumonia, alveolar hemorrhage, pulmonary contusion
Reticulonodular densities	Sarcoidosis, lymphangitic carcinoma
Cavity/cavities	Mycobacterial or fungal infection, mycetoma, lung abscess, bronchogenic carcinoma
Hilar/mediastinal calcification	Previous mycobacterial or fungal infection, broncholithiasis

As shown in Table 20.4, the chest radiograph may also yield important information about the underlying cause of hemoptysis. In approximately 50% of patients, the chest radiograph is *localizing*—it demonstrates a mass, cavity, infiltrate, lobar atelectasis, or other finding that is likely to be directly related to the cause of hemoptysis. In the remainder, the chest radiograph is either normal or demonstrates abnormal but nonspecific findings such as emphysema, interstitial fibrosis, minor atelectasis, or pleural thickening, a category referred to as *nonlocalizing*. This radiographic classification has important diagnostic and prognostic implications. Malignancy is found in almost 40% of patients with hemoptysis who have localizing findings on the chest radiograph. On the other hand, cancer is diagnosed in only about 6% of patients with normal or nonlocalizing chest radiographs, and virtually all of these patients are current or former cigarette smokers over age 40 years.

Additional Testing

The history, physical examination, and chest radiograph are essential to reduce the number of possible causes of hemoptysis and often point toward specific disorders. This initial evaluation, however, yields a definite diagnosis in only a small percentage of patients, such as those who have bacterial pneumonia or an iatrogenic or traumatic lung injury. In the majority of cases, additional testing is required, which most commonly consists of fiber-optic bronchoscopy (FOB) and CT.

FIBER-OPTIC BRONCHOSCOPY

Since becoming widely available in the early 1970s, FOB has been used almost routinely in the evaluation of patients with unexplained hemoptysis. By combining endoscopic examination with brushings, washings, endobronchial and transbronchial biopsies, and transtracheal needle aspiration, FOB may be used to both identify the site of bleeding and determine a definitive diagnosis. FOB is most useful for diagnosing bronchogenic carcinoma and other endobronchial neoplasms (Fig. 20.2), but it is far less effective in detecting other causes of hemoptysis. It follows that the yield of FOB is relatively high in patients with localizing chest radiographs and very low in those whose chest

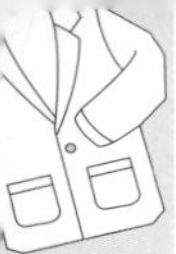

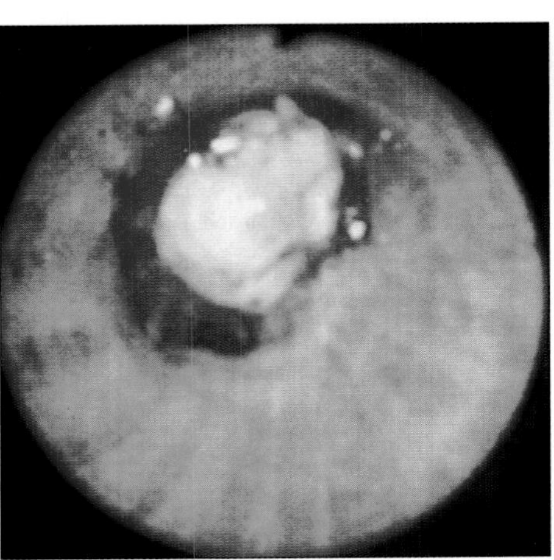

Figure 20.2 Bronchogenic carcinoma visualized through the fiberoptic bronchoscope. The tumor occludes the left upper lobe and is actively bleeding.

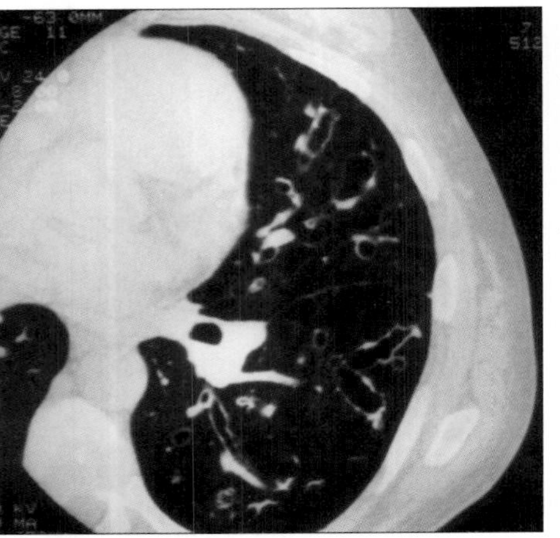

Figure 20.3 Computed tomography (CT) appearance of bronchiectasis. Dilated peripheral airways are clearly demonstrated by this high-resolution CT image.

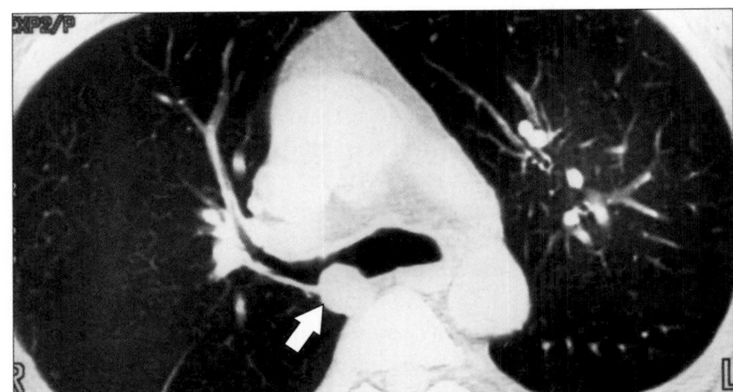

Figure 20.4 Computed tomography (CT) appearance of endobronchial mass. A bronchogenic carcinoma is clearly visible in the right main bronchus.

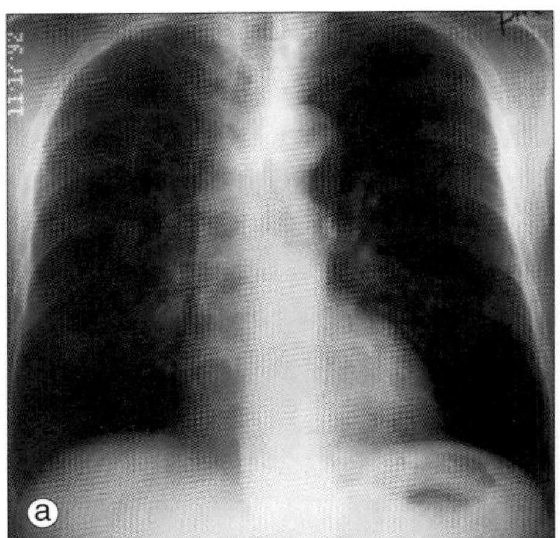

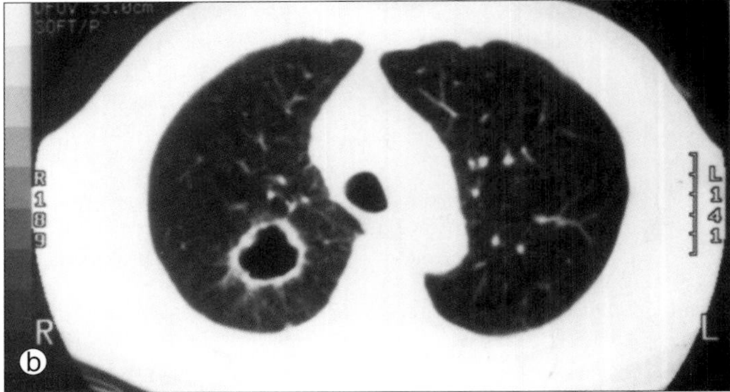

Figure 20.5 Chest radiograph and computed tomography (CT) in a patient who has a cavitary, squamous cell carcinoma. The cavitary lesion cannot be seen on the chest radiograph **(A)**, but is clearly demonstrated by the CT scan **(B)**.

radiographs are normal or nonlocalizing. The most common non-neoplastic diagnosis made by FOB is acute bronchitis, which is based on the presence of mucosal hyperemia and edema and purulent-appearing secretions. As previously discussed, however, these findings are nonspecific and are often unrelated to the actual cause of hemoptysis. When this diagnosis is excluded, a specific, non-neoplastic cause of hemoptysis is found by FOB in less than 10% of cases. In the remainder, FOB is either normal or reveals only blood in the airways. The timing of FOB appears to be of little importance. Although the detection of active bleeding is more likely when FOB is performed during or shortly after an episode of hemoptysis, a delay in the procedure does not affect the diagnostic yield or patient management.

COMPUTED TOMOGRAPHY

When compared with conventional chest radiography, CT is clearly superior for imaging the peripheral and central airways, mediastinum, and lung parenchyma. Thus, it is not surprising that CT has been shown to be very useful in the evaluation of patients with hemoptysis. In the presence of a normal or nonlocalizing chest radiograph, CT reveals an unsuspected cause of hemoptysis, most commonly bronchiectasis, in about one third of patients (Fig. 20.3). In addition, CT reveals an endobronchial lesion in approximately 6% of such patients (Fig. 20.4) and may also demonstrate an unsuspected parenchymal mass, nodule, or cavity (Fig. 20.5). CT is also useful in over one half of all patients who have a localizing chest radiograph, either by revealing a new source of hemoptysis or by providing additional information about a previously recognized abnormality.

Five studies have compared the sensitivities of CT and FOB for detecting bronchogenic carcinomas and other neoplasms in patients with hemoptysis. Most of these studies used a CT protocol that included high-resolution axial images through the central and peripheral airways. Out of a total of 83 patients with neoplasia, CT demonstrated all but one tumor found by FOB. Although it has not been studied, this high degree of sensitivity should be maintained or even improved using high-resolution helical images obtained with current-generation scanners. On the other hand, 12 patients in these studies (14%) had peripheral neoplasms that were evident only on CT and were not detectable with FOB.

Diagnostic Algorithm

Based on the information discussed in the preceding section, a suggested approach to the patient who has hemoptysis is shown in Figure 20.6. If the initial evaluation yields a firm diagnosis, such as bacterial pneumonia or iatrogenic or traumatic lung injury, appropriate therapy is instituted. Alternatively, the initial evaluation may suggest a cause of hemoptysis that requires one or more specific tests. For example, an echocardiogram may confirm the presence of LV failure or mitral stenosis, pulmonary embolism may be diagnosed by means of a ventilation-perfusion lung scan or CT angiogram, and sputum cultures may be diagnostic in patients with tuberculosis. In all other patients, CT, using a protocol that provides high-resolution images through the central and peripheral airways, is the most appropriate next step in the diagnostic evaluation. As discussed previously, CT often reveals an unsuspected cause of hemoptysis, even in patients whose chest radiographs are normal or nonlocalizing, and may provide important information in patients who already have a presumptive diagnosis. For example, in patients with suspected bronchogenic carcinoma, CT provides vital information for staging and also provides a "road map" for bronchoscopy by defining the exact location of a parenchymal mass and enlarged mediastinal lymph nodes.

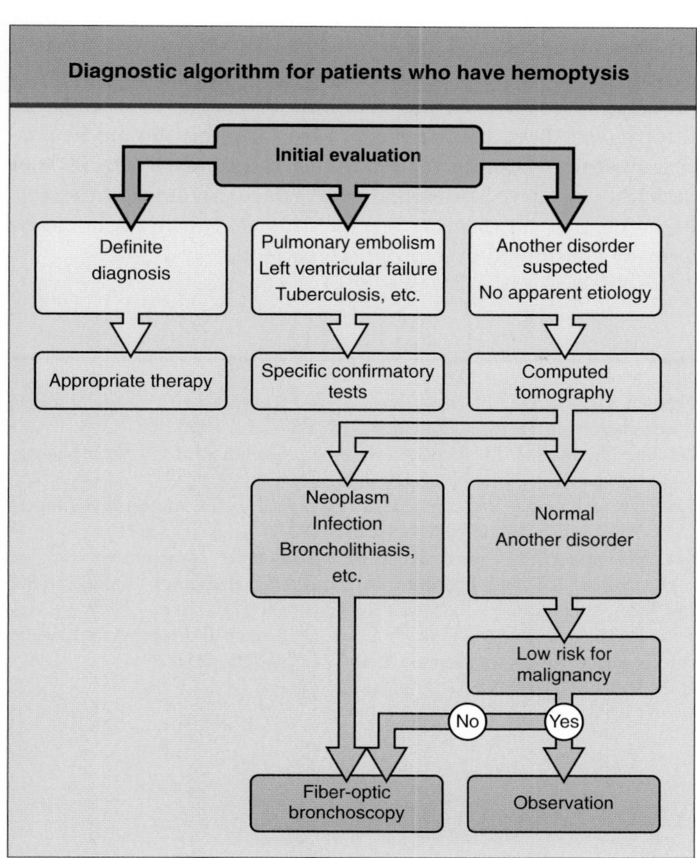

Figure 20.6 Diagnostic algorithm for patients who have hemoptysis.

If CT suggests a disorder that is amenable to bronchoscopic diagnosis, such as neoplasm, infection, or broncholithiasis, FOB is performed next in the diagnostic evaluation. Additional studies such as mediastinoscopy or surgical lung biopsy may be required if FOB is nondiagnostic. When CT either is normal or demonstrates another cause of hemoptysis, such as bronchiectasis, the role of FOB is less clearly defined. When appropriate imaging techniques are used, the absence of an endobronchial abnormality is associated with a low incidence of malignancy. Available data suggest that FOB may be safely omitted in nonsmokers younger than age 40 years. As CT occasionally fails to detect a small endobronchial lesion, FOB should probably be performed in all other patients.

TREATMENT

In most cases, hemoptysis requires no specific therapy. Instead, treatment must be directed at its underlying cause, and therapy of most of these disorders is discussed in detail in other chapters of this text. Patients in whom no cause of hemoptysis is found after CT and FOB have an excellent prognosis. Hemoptysis typically resolves within several days and is very rarely found to be caused by a serious pulmonary disorder.

MASSIVE HEMOPTYSIS

No definition of massive hemoptysis is generally accepted, although the most commonly used criteria require between 200 and 600 mL of blood over 24 hours. Any definition is, of course, arbitrary, especially because the amount of blood expectorated is often difficult to quantify. Because morbidity and mortality are dependent not only on the volume of expectorated blood, but also on the rate of bleeding, the ability of the patient to clear blood from the airways, and the extent and severity of any underlying lung disease, it is evident that a single definition is not applicable to all patients. Instead, for clinical purposes, it is more appropriate to define massive hemoptysis simply as bleeding that leads to impairment of respiratory function and gas exchange and that is, therefore, potentially life threatening. Overall, the risk of death from massive hemoptysis is approximately 20%, although reported mortality rates vary widely between 0% and 75%. Not surprisingly, the rate at which bleeding occurs appears to be the most important prognostic factor.

Massive hemoptysis is relatively uncommon and occurs in less than 5% of patients with lower respiratory tract bleeding. Although any of the disorders listed in Table 20.1 may potentially give rise to life-threatening hemorrhage, massive hemoptysis is most commonly caused by bronchiectasis, bronchogenic carcinoma, mycetoma, lung abscess, and tuberculosis (active or inactive).

Because of its associated morbidity and mortality, massive hemoptysis is a respiratory emergency and requires rapid evaluation and therapy. Unlike patients with small amounts of bleeding in whom the emphasis is placed on determining the underlying cause, in patients with massive hemoptysis the primary therapeutic goals are to maintain a patent airway and to localize and control the bleeding. Patients should be closely monitored in an intensive care unit, and elective endotracheal intubation is indicated when patients are unable to clear blood

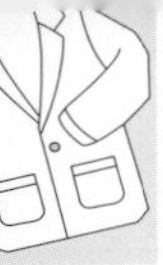

adequately from the airways. Bronchoscopy should be performed immediately in an effort to identify the source of bleeding, or at least to localize the bleeding to a specific segment, lobe, or lung. Bronchoscopy is often nondiagnostic in the absence of active hemorrhage, and repeated procedures during episodes of recurrent bleeding may be required. Either rigid bronchoscopy or FOB may be used, depending largely on the clinical circumstances. Rigid bronchoscopy, with its large lumen, affords excellent airway control and suctioning capability and is ideally suited for patients with very rapid bleeding. Disadvantages include relatively poor visualization of the segmental and lobar bronchi and the need for general anesthesia. In most patients, FOB is the procedure of choice, because it can be performed rapidly, requires only light sedation, and allows excellent airway visualization. All patients with massive hemoptysis should be intubated prior to FOB. This optimizes airway control, allows effective suctioning should the rate of bleeding increase, and permits the bronchoscope to be removed easily and reinserted if the suction channel becomes occluded.

Endoscopic localization of the bleeding site is important for two reasons. First, it provides a guide for therapy to control ongoing hemorrhage (see next paragraph). Second, in the setting of persistent, severe hemoptysis, it allows isolation of the bleeding site, which can be lifesaving by preventing aspiration of blood throughout the tracheobronchial tree. Guided by the FOB, a balloon catheter may be used to occlude a segmental or lobar airway. When bleeding can be localized only to one lung, a larger balloon may be inflated in a main-stem bronchus. Alternatively, the FOB can be used to selectively intubate and ventilate the nonbleeding lung. Double-lumen endotracheal tubes also allow unilateral lung ventilation through a cuffed bronchial lumen, which is placed in the left main bronchus, and a tracheal lumen, which is positioned above the carina. These endotracheal tubes have a number of significant drawbacks, however. They are difficult to insert, correct positioning is difficult to achieve and maintain, and suctioning is limited by the small diameter of each lumen.

Once the bleeding site has been localized and a stable airway has been achieved, therapy must be performed to control ongoing hemorrhage. Two options are available—arterial embolization and surgical resection. In over 90% of cases, massive hemoptysis originates from a bronchial artery or, less commonly, from a collateral vessel of the axillary, subclavian, internal mammary, or intercostal arteries. Guided by the results of bronchoscopy, abnormal vessels may be visualized using selective arteriography and occluded with embolized, nonabsorbable material, such as polyvinyl alcohol. Arterial embolization is successful for the acute control of hemorrhage in 73% to 98% of patients. Although complications are uncommon, unintentional arterial occlusion can have devastating consequences. For example, reflux of material from the bronchial artery into the aorta may lead to systemic embolization, and bronchial artery occlusion proximal to the origin of the anterior spinal artery may result in spinal cord infarction and paralysis. Arterial embolization is the initial therapy of choice in most patients with ongoing hemorrhage. It is ideally suited for patients who have bilateral disease, limited pulmonary reserve, or another contraindication to surgery and may be repeated as needed to control recurrent hemorrhage. Because surgical resection during active bleeding is accompanied by a mortality rate that approaches 30%, arterial embolization is also commonly performed in patients who would otherwise be surgical candidates. Elective surgery can then be performed, if necessary, once the patient's condition has been stabilized. Emergent surgery is reserved for patients in immediate danger of asphyxiation and for those in whom arterial embolization is unsuccessful.

Once bleeding has resolved, either spontaneously or following embolization therapy, its cause must be determined using the diagnostic algorithm (see Fig. 20.6). Specific treatment, such as antibacterial or antituberculous therapy, may successfully prevent further episodes of hemoptysis. When effective medical therapy is not available, recurrent bleeding is common. Approximately 35% of patients in whom bleeding spontaneously resolves will have recurrent and often life-threatening hemorrhage within 6 months, and bleeding recurs in 10% to 20% of patients who have undergone successful embolization therapy. Based on this information, elective surgical resection should be strongly considered in appropriate patients.

SUGGESTED READINGS

Eddy J: Clinical assessment and management of massive hemoptysis. Crit Care Med 28:1642-1647, 2000.

Goh P, Lin M, Teo N, et al: Embolization for hemoptysis: a six-year review. Cardiovasc Intervent Radiol 25:17-25, 2002.

Hirshberg B, Biran I, Glazer M, et al: Hemoptysis: etiology, evaluation, and outcome in a tertiary referral hospital. Chest 112:440-444, 1997.

Marshall TJ, Flower CDR, Jackson JE: The role of radiology in the investigation and management of patients with haemoptysis. Clin Radiol 51:391-400, 1996.

McGuinness G, Beacher JR, Harkin TJ, et al: Hemoptysis: prospective high-resolution CT/bronchoscopic correlation. Chest 105:1155-1162, 1994.

Naidich DP, Funt S, Ettenger NA, et al: Hemoptysis: CT-bronchoscopic correlations in 58 cases. Radiology 177:357-362, 1990.

Naidich DP, Harkin TJ: Airways and lung: correlation of CT with fiberoptic bronchoscopy. Radiology 197:1-12, 1995.

Santiago S, Tobias J, Williams AJ: A reappraisal of the causes of hemoptysis. Arch Intern Med 151:2449-2451, 1991.

Set PA, Flower CD, Smith IE, et al: Hemoptysis: comparative study of the role of CT and fiberoptic bronchoscopy. Radiology 189:677-680, 1993.

Swanson K, Johnson M, Prakash U, et al: Bronchial artery embolization: experience with 54 patients. Chest 121:789-795, 2002.

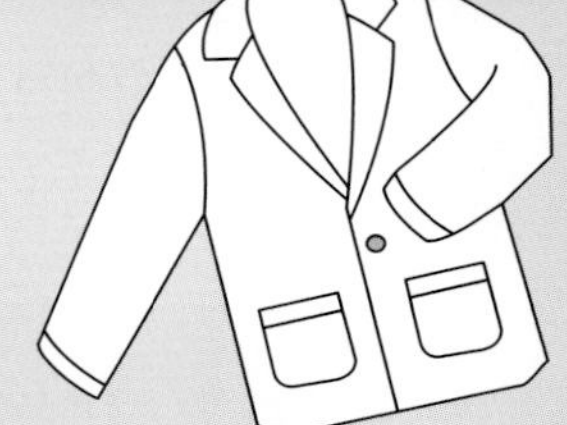

CHAPTER 21 Chest Pain

Richard K. Albert

Chest pain is the most frequent new symptom reported by patients seen in outpatient clinics. Although it is a remarkably nonspecific symptom (Table 21.1), it may be the presenting manifestation of a number of potentially life-threatening diseases. Accordingly, a complaint of chest pain always requires a thorough and careful investigation.

DIFFERENTIAL DIAGNOSIS

The pathophysiology of chest pain is understood for many, but not all, of the conditions with which it is associated.

Myocardial Ischemia

The chest pain associated with myocardial ischemia is attributed to an imbalance between myocardial oxygen (O_2) supply and demand. Most tissues can increase O_2 supply by increasing O_2 delivery, increasing O_2 extraction, or both. The O_2 extraction by the myocardium is much greater than that by other tissues, with the result that the O_2 content of coronary venous blood is normally much lower than that of blood coming from other muscles. Accordingly, the ability of the myocardium to increase O_2 extraction is limited (Table 21.2), and the primary mechanism by which the heart can increase O_2 delivery is to increase coronary blood flow.

Coronary blood flow is determined by the driving pressure (i.e., the aortic pressure minus the left ventricular end-diastolic pressure) and the resistance in the coronary arteries. Chest pain can therefore be caused by conditions that increase myocardial O_2 demand (e.g., hypertension, hyperthyroidism), decrease mean aortic pressure (e.g., aortic stenosis), decrease O_2 delivery (e.g., anemia, hypoxemia), or increase the downstream pressure for coronary arterial flow (e.g., aortic and mitral valve disease, cardiac hypertrophy or dilatation). The importance of coronary arterial diameter is emphasized by Poiseuille's law, which states that resistance is inversely related to the vessel radius taken to the fourth power and explains why anything that might result in even a small change in coronary arterial diameter (e.g., coronary arterial spasm, thrombosis, atherosclerosis) can result in chest pain.

Pericardial Pain

The visceral pericardium has no pain fibers, and the pain fibers in the parietal pericardium are localized to the caudal (i.e., diaphragmatic) region. The paucity of pericardial pain fibers may explain why various noninflammatory causes of pericardial effusions (e.g., myocardial infarction, uremia) are not associated with chest pain. Those effusions of infectious or other inflammatory causes may result in pain only when the inflammation spreads to the visceral pleura.

Mitral Valve Prolapse

Mitral valve prolapse has frequently been included as one of the causes of chest pain, but epidemiologic studies indicate that this might not be the case.

Pulmonary Pain

The lung parenchyma and the visceral pleura are insensitive to most painful stimuli. Pain can arise from the parietal pleura, the major airways, the chest wall, the diaphragm, and mediastinal structures. Inflammatory conditions affecting the lung periphery or the lateral portions of either hemidiaphragm cause chest wall pain when the process extends to the parietal pleura and stimulates the respective intercostal nerves. Inflammation of the parietal pleura that lines the more central portions of the diaphragm stimulates the phrenic nerves, with the result that the pain is referred to the ipsilateral neck or shoulder. The augmentation of pulmonary pain during inhalation is attributed to the stretching of the inflamed pleura.

Pulmonary Embolus

The pain associated with acute pulmonary embolus is thought to result from distention of the central pulmonary arteries. Pain occurring later in the illness is attributed to infarction of a peripheral segment of lung and inflammation of the adjacent pleura.

Pulmonary Hypertension

The pain of chronic pulmonary hypertension is attributed to the disparity between right ventricular myocardial O_2 supply and demand.

Musculoskeletal Pain

Costochondral and chondrosternal articulations are common sites of anterior and anterolateral chest pain. The articulations of the second, third, and fourth ribs are most commonly involved. When accompanied by swelling, redness, and heat, the condition is referred to as *Tietze's syndrome.* Coughing or trauma can result in dislocation of costochondral junctions (most commonly those of the tenth through twelfth ribs). The pain resulting from intercostal neuritis most frequently results

Table 21.1 Causes of chest pain
Cardiac system
Myocardial infarction
Myocardial ischemia
Angina pectoris
Variant angina
Syndrome X (microvascular angina in setting of non-insulin-dependent diabetes mellitus, dyslipidemia, and central obesity)
Myocarditis
Aortic dissection
Pericarditis (infections, Dressler's syndrome)
Aortic stenosis
Syphilitic aortitis
Takayasu's aortitis
Myocarditis
Hypertrophic cardiomyopathy
Pulmonary system
Pleurisy
Tracheobronchitis
Tumor
Pneumothorax
Pulmonary embolus (with or without infarction)
Pulmonary hypertension
Gastrointestinal system
Esophageal reflux
Esophageal dysmotility (i.e., spasm, achalasia, hyperactive lower sphincter)
Esophageal rupture
Peptic ulcer disease
Biliary colic
Pancreatitis
Splenic or hepatic flexure syndrome
Musculoskeletal conditions
Costochondritis
Subacromial bursitis
Biceps, supraspinitus, or deltoid tendinitis
Shoulder or spinal arthritis
Intercostal muscle cramps
Hyperabduction or strains of the anterior scalene or rectus abdominis muscles
Fibromyalgia
Slipping rib syndrome (pain at the costochondral junction, generally affecting the eighth, ninth, or tenth rib; may be post-traumatic)
Rib fractures
Sternal marrow pain (with acute leukemia)
Neurologic conditions
Neuritis–radiculitis (cervical compression, herpes zoster infection)
Brachial plexus involvement (cervical rib, spasm of the scalenus anterior, Pancoast's tumors)
Others
Breast inflammation
Chest wall tumors
Mondor's syndrome (thrombophlebitis of the superficial thoracic veins)
Diaphragm spasm
Mediastinal emphysema
Mediastinitis
Panic attacks
Hyperventilation syndrome

Table 21.2 Oxygen extraction at rest and maximum exercise

Rest	Body	Myocardium
Arterial oxygen content (mL/100 mL blood)	20	20
Venous oxygen content (mL/100 mL blood)	15	8
Oxygen extracted (mL/100 mL blood)	5	12
Extraction ratio	0.25	0.60
Maximum exercise		
Arterial oxygen content (mL/100 mL blood)	20	20
Venous oxygen content (mL/100 mL blood)	5	5
Oxygen extracted (mL/100 mL blood)	15	15
Extraction ratio	0.75	0.75
Increase in oxygen extraction (%)	300	125

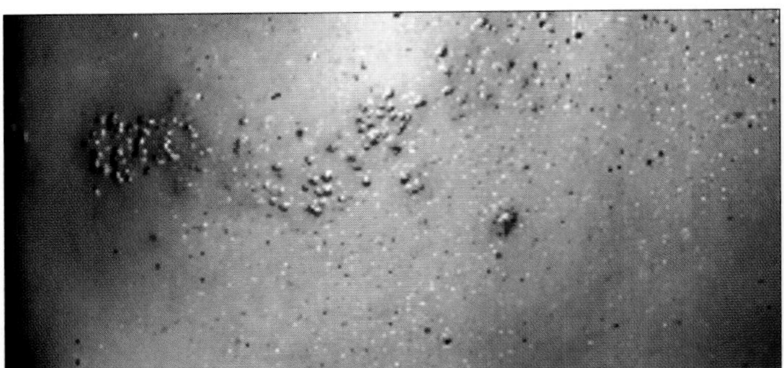

Figure 21.1 Herpes zoster infection affecting an intercostal nerve.

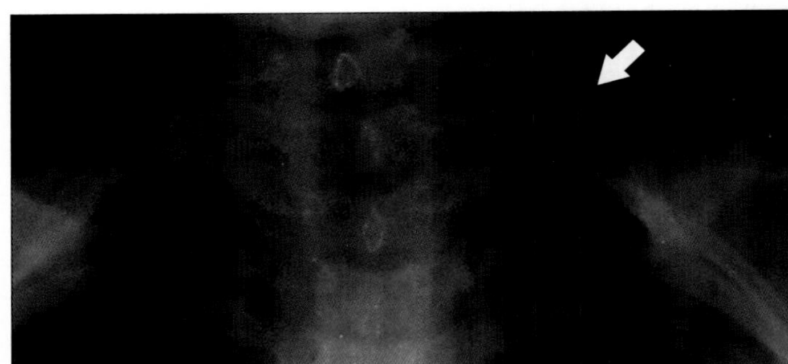

Figure 21.2 Chest radiograph showing compression of the left cervical nerve roots by a cervical rib *(arrow)*.

from cervical osteoarthritis. Intercostal neuritis is also seen with herpes zoster infection, in which the onset of pain may precede the typical rash by 1 or 2 days (Fig. 21.1). Thoracic roots are most commonly involved. Subacromial bursitis, biceps or deltoid tendinitis, and arthritis of the shoulder can manifest as chest pain with extension to the shoulder and arm. The brachial plexus and subclavian artery can be compressed by a cervical rib (i.e., the thoracic outlet syndrome; Fig. 21.2) or by spasm of the scalenus anticus muscle. The Pancoast syndrome (most commonly, but not exclusively, caused by bronchogenic carcinoma) may invade the C8, T1, and T2 nerve roots (Fig. 21.3).

Esophageal Reflux or Dysmotility

The chest pain resulting from esophageal reflux or dysmotility (i.e., esophageal spasm, achalasia, hyperactive lower sphincter) results from acid irritation of the esophageal mucosa. Esophageal reflux or dysmotility is found to explain a complaint of chest pain in as many as 30% of patients with normal coronary arteriograms.

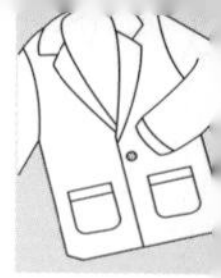

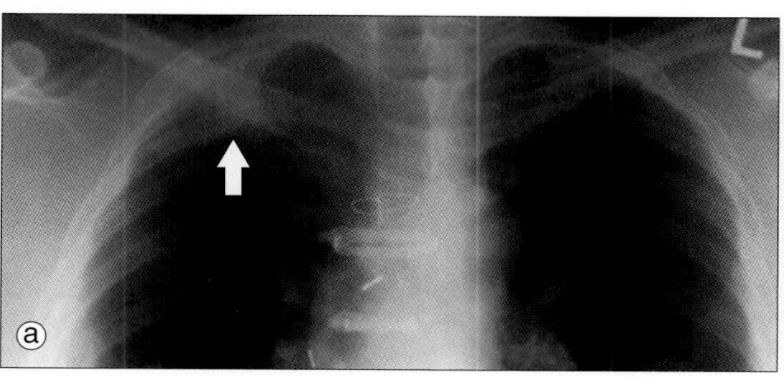

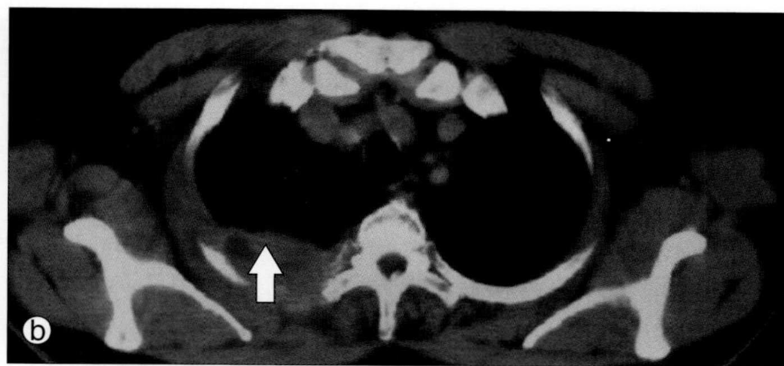

Figure 21.3 Pancoast tumor invading the C8, T1, and T2 nerve roots. A, Chest radiograph showing destruction of the posterior portion of the right second rib (*arrow*). **B,** Chest computed tomography (CT) scan showing necrotic tumor and rib destruction (*arrow*).

PATIENT EVALUATION

The approach to patients complaining of chest pain is directed by the approach needed to urgently diagnose the potentially lethal causes of the problem. Severe pain is more commonly associated with life-threatening causes, but all of these serious conditions may occur with minimal symptoms. Accordingly, patients are frequently treated as if the chest pain were life threatening until these conditions can be excluded by studies that offer information more specific than that obtained at the time of presentation.

Presentation

If symptoms are acute and the patient is hypotensive, myocardial infarction, pulmonary embolism, pericardial tamponade, dissecting aneurysm, and tension pneumothorax are considered and excluded (Fig. 21.4). Occasionally, a ruptured esophagus may also have this presentation. In other patients the approach is governed primarily by the history and physical examination, which are interpreted on the basis of actual or estimated prior probabilities for each of the conditions listed in Table 21.1. For example, a middle-aged man with one or more risk factors for coronary artery disease (e.g., hypercholesterolemia, diabetes, hypertension, obesity, smoking) who has exertional chest pain that abates with rest has a greater than 90% probability of having myocardial ischemia as the cause of his symptom. A similarly high risk is present for patients with exertional pain that occurs with ST depression, cardiac wall motion abnormalities, an increased or decreased blood pressure, an S4 gallop, or a systolic murmur indicative of ischemia-induced mitral regurgitation.

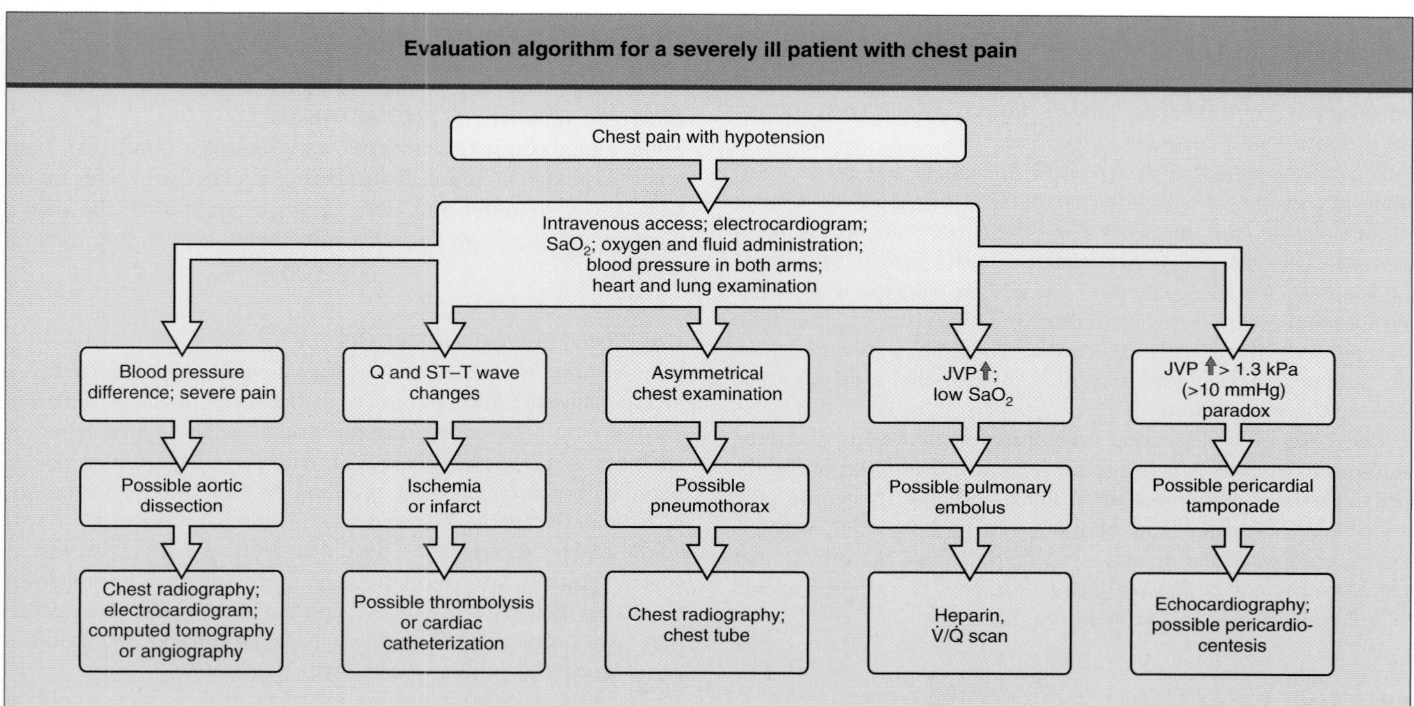

Figure 21.4 Evaluation algorithm for severely ill patient with chest pain. Therapeutic approach is determined by blood pressure and findings on brief examination of the neck, chest, and head. JVP, jugular venous pressure; SaO_2, arterial oxygen pressure.

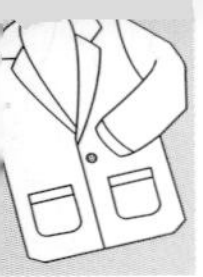

Chest pain may also be a presenting manifestation of myocardial ischemia in women with major or intermediate risk factors for coronary artery disease, including typical pain, postmenopausal state without hormone replacement therapy, smoking, diabetes mellitus, peripheral vascular disease, and hypertension or lipoprotein abnormalities.

History

The onset, duration, location, radiation pattern, character, and intensity of the pain should be determined, as should the factors that precipitate or diminish it. Unfortunately, both the sensitivity and specificity of the history is low for many of the conditions that must be considered. For example, most episodes of electrocardiographically documented ischemia in patients with stable angina are asymptomatic.

CARDIOVASCULAR DISORDERS

Myocardial ischemia is frequently described as a dull pain accompanied by a sensation of tightness, pressure, squeezing, or heaviness in the chest. It characteristically radiates down the ulnar aspect of the left arm, but radiation to the neck or jaw also occurs. The pain develops gradually; occurs in association with exertion, emotional distress, or large meals; and abates within 2 to 10 minutes after the stressful activity is curtailed or within 5 minutes of administration of nitroglycerin.

The pain associated with myocardial infarction is of greater intensity; lasts longer; can be associated with nausea (particularly with inferior infarctions), diaphoresis, hypotension, or arrhythmias; and is not relieved by nitroglycerin.

Variant or Prinzmetal's angina occurs in the early morning and at rest rather than during stress and results from coronary artery spasm. Patients with this type of angina frequently have other vasomotor symptoms such as migraine headaches or Raynaud's phenomenon. Angina that occurs with a progressively lower degree of exertion is considered unstable and is thought to be secondary to rupture of an atherosclerotic plaque with thrombin formation and coronary vasospasm.

Pericardial pain may be pleuritic in nature but more commonly is steady, worsens when the patient is recumbent or lying on the left side, and improves when the patient sits up and leans forward. The pain frequently radiates to the upper portion of the trapezius muscles. The pain can also be pleuritic if the adjacent parietal pleura is involved in the inflammatory process. Like the pain associated with myocardial ischemia, pericardial pain can radiate to the shoulder or neck. It can also radiate to the flank or the epigastrium.

The pain of a dissecting aortic aneurysm begins abruptly, becomes extremely severe within seconds or minutes, and radiates to the back, abdomen, neck, flank, and legs. It is commonly described as "tearing" and may be seen in association with an acute cerebrovascular event; a cold, pulseless extremity; and aortic insufficiency. Unusually large amounts of analgesic agents are generally needed to provide relief.

PULMONARY INFLAMMATION AND CHEST WALL PROBLEMS

Many adjectives have been used to describe the pain resulting from conditions that cause pulmonary inflammation or from chest wall problems (e.g., *sharp, dull, catching)*, but the pain is almost always pleuritic in nature in that it increases with forced inhalation or exhalation (e.g., during coughing or sneezing), during spontaneous breathing, and when pressure is applied to the chest wall by bending or lying down. In response to the pleuritic or positional character of the pain, patients frequently limit their depth of inhalation and, accordingly, may complain of dyspnea rather than pain.

Characterizing the development of the pain may be helpful. An abrupt onset suggests a rib fracture, pneumothorax, or pneumomediastinum; an onset of a few minutes or hours is seen with bacterial pneumonia and pulmonary emboli; and a gradual onset (e.g., days or weeks) is more compatible with chronic infections (e.g., tuberculosis, fungal infections) or tumor.

Patients with chronic obstructive pulmonary disease who develop an acute exacerbation of bronchitis frequently describe a burning type of chest pain that localizes in the substernal region. A similar symptom can occur in otherwise normal subjects in the setting of tracheobronchitis or during the hyperventilation that accompanies heavy exercise, particularly if the exercise is done in a cold environment.

In many instances, patients with costochondral pain or pain that results from muscle strains describe an episode of chest trauma or unusual upper extremity exercise (e.g., gardening, digging, scraping) that can result in a type of overuse syndrome. More commonly, no specific inciting event can be determined. The costosternal articulations are common "trigger sites" for the pain seen in fibromyalgia. Patients with this syndrome also have trigger sites in other locations. Musculoskeletal conditions are generally exacerbated by deep breathing and are frequently overlooked as causes of "pleuritic" or exercise-induced chest pain.

Intercostal neuritis is commonly described as being pleuritic. One potentially distinguishing characteristic is that patients may describe abrupt, shocklike sensations occurring in the same distribution as the pleuritic pain.

BURSITIS, TENDINITIS, AND ARTHRITIS

Subacromial bursitis, biceps and deltoid tendinitis, and arthritis of the shoulder can manifest as chest pain with extension to the shoulder and arm. In these conditions, the pain is worse with neck or shoulder movement but is not exercise related.

GASTROINTESTINAL DISORDERS

Like angina, the pain of esophageal reflux or dysmotility is located substernally; can radiate to the throat, neck, or left arm; and may be relieved by nitroglycerin. Unlike angina, however, the pain is rarely associated with exertion. Rather, it is exacerbated by bending, stooping, drinking alcohol, or lying supine and is frequently worse in the early morning in association with acidic gastric secretions. Chest pain from esophageal reflux or spasm typically lasts for 1 hour or more and may be improved by sitting upright or by ingesting antacids or food. The history may also be positive for odynophagia, dysphagia, regurgitation of undigested food, or weight loss.

The pain associated with peptic ulcer disease, biliary colic, or pancreatitis generally begins 1 or 2 hours after eating. Pain associated with peptic ulcer disease may improve or worsen with

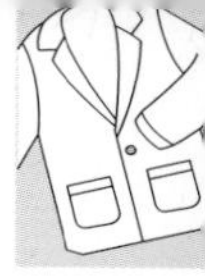

eating. The pain associated with biliary colic and pancreatitis is frequently accompanied by nausea and vomiting.

Physical Examination

Although the physical examination may provide a number of clues to the cause of chest pain, the clinician must recognize that the examination may be entirely normal even when the pain results from a life-threatening condition.

The initial observation of the patient may be helpful. Shallow, more rapid respirations may suggest pleural inflammation or a musculoskeletal cause of pain. Cyanosis may suggest hypoxemia from a variety of pulmonary or cardiac problems. Xanthelasma and tuberous xanthomas suggest the presence of coronary disease.

In addition to the standard vital signs, blood pressure should be measured in both upper extremities, as disparities suggest aortic dissection. Heart rate and rhythm abnormalities suggest acute ischemia or pulmonary embolism. Fever points away from musculoskeletal pain and suggests pneumonia, pulmonary embolus, pancreatitis, or biliary obstruction. Patients with myocardial infarctions may be febrile, but rarely does the temperature exceed 38° C.

Elevated jugular venous pressure, abnormalities in the carotid upstroke, crackles, a pleural or pericardial rub, signs of parenchymal consolidation, gallop rhythms, paradoxical or fixed splitting or an increased intensity of the pulmonary component of the second heart sound, and cardiac murmurs have a high specificity for many of the cardiopulmonary disorders associated with chest pain, but the sensitivity of these physical findings is probably low, because the physical examination may be entirely normal in patients with severe ischemia, pulmonary emboli, and many of the gastrointestinal causes of pain. The reduction in ventricular compliance that accompanies myocardial ischemia may be associated with an increase in left ventricular end-diastolic pressure sufficient to cause pulmonary edema.

Attempts should be made to reproduce or exacerbate the pain by moving the arms and shoulders and by thoroughly palpating the chest wall, particularly the peristernal region, the costochondral junctions, the subacromial bursae, the deltoid tendons, the shoulders, and the abdomen.

Intercostal neuritis is frequently associated with hyperalgesia or anesthesia over the distribution of affected intercostal nerves. Biliary colic and pancreatitis are frequently associated with right upper quadrant and midline abdominal tenderness, respectively.

Diagnostic Tests

Patients without a previous diagnosis of coronary artery disease are not likely to have an acute myocardial infarction as the explanation for the acute onset of chest pain if the pain does not radiate to the neck, left shoulder, or arm and if the electrocardiogram is normal. Although the finding of flat or down-sloping ST-segment depressions greater than 0.1 mV increases the likelihood that an episode of chest pain is caused by myocardial ischemia, the tracing may be normal at rest, between attacks, or even in the presence of active ischemia. Up to 80% of patients with coronary disease have these ST changes during exercise, but they may also be found in up to 15% of patients with no evidence of disease at catheterization. Nonspecific ST-T wave changes have been documented in the setting of acute cholecystitis and esophageal spasm, as well as other conditions for which chest pain is a presenting symptom (Table 21.3).

Table 21.3
Electrocardiographic findings in conditions presenting with chest pain

Condition	Electrocardiographic finding
Acute cholecystitis	Inferior ST elevation
Pulmonary embolism	Inferior ST elevation
Dissecting aortic aneurysm	ST elevation ST depression
Pneumothorax	Poor R-wave progression Acute QRS axis shift
Pericarditis	ST elevation (generally diffuse)
Myocarditis	ST elevation

Myocardial infarctions may be documented by ST elevations and the appearance of Q waves. Unfortunately, as many as 35% of patients who subsequently develop a myocardial infarction may have normal electrocardiograms at the time of presentation. Accordingly, more specific testing may be needed.

Exercise thallium scintigraphy and radionuclide ventriculography demonstrate abnormalities in approximately 80% of patients with angina and in as many as 10% of patients who have normal coronary arteries. Other studies shown to be useful in the diagnosis of coronary artery disease include exercise two-dimensional echocardiography and dipyridamole thallium stress testing, but coronary arteriography continues to be the definitive study.

Chest radiographs should be obtained in all patients with chest pain unless a clear-cut musculoskeletal cause of the pain is evident on clinical evaluation. With myocardial ischemia or infarction the chest radiograph may be entirely normal. Alternatively, it may reveal pulmonary edema, upper lobe vascular redistribution, valvular disease, or pericardial disease.

Radiographs may be normal in the setting of acute pulmonary emboli, although minor degrees of atelectasis, small effusions, a convex appearance of fluid in the costophrenic angle (i.e., Hampton's hump; Fig. 21.5), or distentior of the central pulmonary vessels may be seen.

A widened mediastinum or an apical effusion in films taken with the patient in the supine position (Fig. 21.6) suggests the possibility of a ruptured aortic aneurysm.

Arterial blood gas tensions may be normal in the setting of myocardial ischemia, but respiratory alkalemia and respiratory or metabolic acidemia can occur in as many as 30% of patients with pulmonary edema, along with an increase in the alveolar-arterial oxygen tension difference (A-aDO_2). The large majority of patients with pulmonary emboli have acute respiratory alkalemia, and most have an increased A-aDO_2.

A complete blood count should be obtained, with evidence of anemia (in the setting of possible angina) or leukocytosis sought in support of a diagnosis of pneumonia or other infectious cause of nonanginal chest pain.

Troponin T increases 4 to 12 hours after myocardial infarction and is a better predictor of acute infarction than creatine

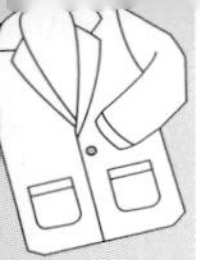

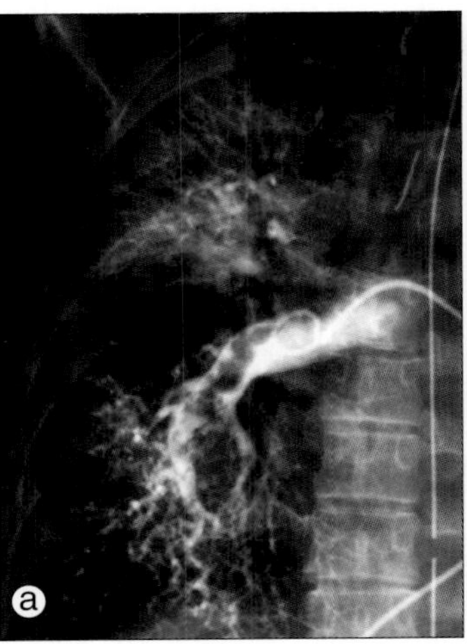

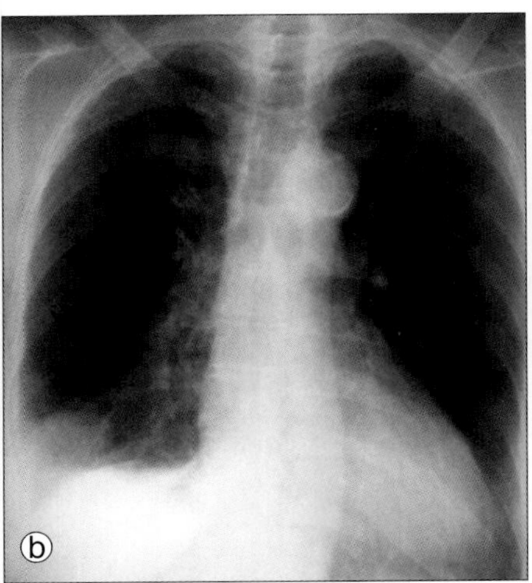

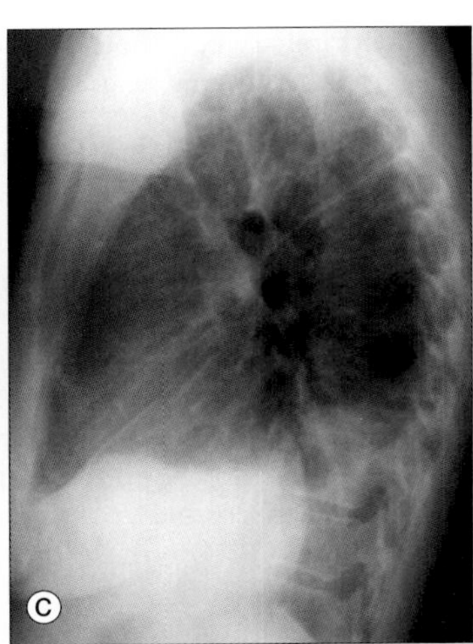

Figure 21.5 Hampton's hump. A, Pulmonary arteriogram of a patient with a pulmonary embolism showing a large thrombus in the right pulmonary artery. **B** and **C,** Chest radiographs of the same patient, showing a Hampton hump (i.e., lower lobe atelectasis taking a concave shape).

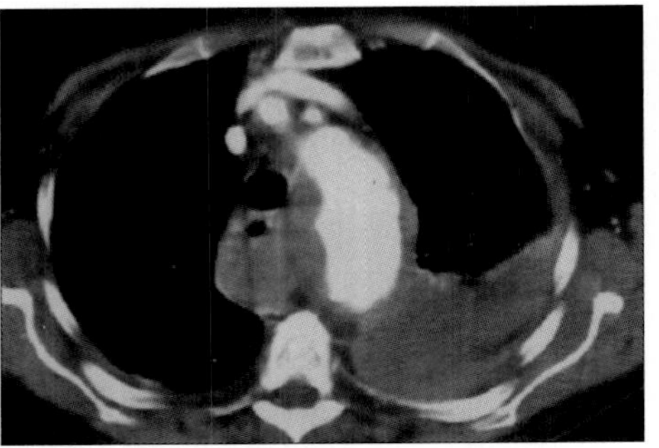

Figure 21.6 Aortic aneurysm. Chest computed tomography (CT) scan showing a dissecting aortic aneurysm.

kinase-MB, because the latter increases in both infarction and ischemia.

TREATMENT

The treatment of chest pain obviously depends on the cause.

Pharmacotherapy for patients with myocardial infarctions or acute coronary syndromes (e.g., patients with unstable angina and those with myocardial infarctions but without non–ST-segment elevations) includes aspirin, nitrates, β-adrenergic blockers, and low-molecular-weight heparin. In patients with infarctions or with high risk of infarction (ST-segment depression, increased troponins, persistent chest pain, hemodynamic instability), a glycoprotein IIb/IIIa inhibitor is added. In some patients angina may be improved by correction of anemia or treatment of hyperthyroidism. Relief of pain has been associated with reductions in oxygen consumption and circulating catecholamines. Invasive therapy includes percutaneous coronary stenting, balloon dilatation, thrombolytic therapy (in patients with infarctions only), and coronary arterial bypass grafting (CABG). Stenting is now used in the large majority of patients, and newer drug-eluting stents will likely increase their relative efficacy, because stent occlusion will be reduced.

The acute pericarditis occurring in the setting of large myocardial infarctions generally responds to aspirin. Nonsteroidal anti-inflammatory agents or corticosteroids may be contraindicated, as these agents slow the rate at which myocardial scar formation occurs and therefore may be associated with an increased frequency of myocardial rupture. The pain associated with Dressler's syndrome (i.e., pericarditis developing 1 or 2 months after an infarction in association with fever, leukocytosis, and elevations of antimyocardial antibodies) is treated with nonsteroidal anti-inflammatory agents. Systemic corticosteroids may be needed in more severe cases.

The pain associated with pulmonary inflammation may respond to nonsteroidal anti-inflammatory agents, although narcotics are occasionally needed. Right ventricular angina may be lessened by unloading the right ventricle through use of prostacyclin, prostacyclin analogs, endothelin-receptor antagonists, or calcium-channel blockers to dilate the pulmonary circulation. The pain associated with pneumothorax may be quickly replaced by that associated with the chest tube, and narcotics may be needed to circumvent limited chest wall excursions.

In addition to elevating the head of the bed, other ways of reducing the pain associated with esophageal reflux include avoiding food or liquid intake before reclining, eliminating substances known to reduce the lower esophageal sphincter pressure (e.g., coffee, chocolate, alcohol, mint, and use of antacids, calcium-channel blockers, H_2-receptor antagonists, metoclopramide, nitroglycerin, and/or proton-pump inhibitors). Endoscopic gastroplasty is being evaluated. Esophageal dysmotility has been treated with long-acting nitrates and calcium-channel blockers. Antacids, proton-pump inhibitors, H_2-antagonists, sulcralfate, and treatment for *Helicobacter pylori* may be needed to eliminate the pain associated with peptic ulcer disease. The pain of pancreatitis generally requires narcotics. Meperidine is favored over other opiates, as it does not contract the sphincter of Oddi. Intractable pain is a common indication for surgical or invasive endoscopic approaches.

Patients with musculoskeletal pain can be treated with nonsteroidal anti-inflammatory agents or the stretching exercises that are employed in physical therapy. The chest pain associated with fibromyalgia may be improved by use of amitriptyline.

The pain associated with herpes zoster infections may be so severe as to require narcotics. Amitriptyline and fluphenazine have also been used, as have systemic corticosteroids.

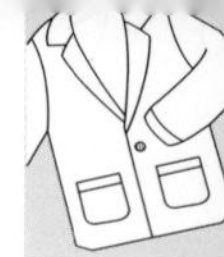

SELECTED READINGS

Bass C, Mayou R: Chest pain. BMJ 325:588-591, 2002.

Bonomo L, Di Fabio F, Rita Larici A, et al: Non-traumatic thoracic emergencies. Acute chest pain: Diagnostic strategies. Eur Radiol 12:1872-1885, 2002.

de Caestecker J: Diagnosis and management of gastrointestinal causes of chest pain of uncertain origin. Clin Med 2:402-405, 2002.

Dori G, Denekamp Y, Fishman S, Bitterman H: Exercise stress testing, myocardial perfusion imaging and stress echocardiography for detecting restenosis after successful percutaneous transluminal coronary angioplasty: A review of performance. J Intern Med 253:253-262, 2003.

Douglas PS, Ginsburg GS: The evaluation of chest pain in women. N Engl J Med 334:1311-1315, 1996.

Goldman L: Using prediction models and cost-effectiveness analysis to improve clinical decisions: Emergency department patients with acute chest pain. Proc Assoc Am Physician 107:329-333, 1995.

Goyle KK, Walling AD: Diagnosing pericarditis. Am Fam Physician 66:1695-1702, 2002.

Limacher M, Handberg E: Evaluating women with chest pain for the diagnosis of coronary artery disease. Dis Mon 48:647-658, 2002.

CHAPTER 22 An Approach to the Diagnosis of Pulmonary Infection

Mark A. Woodhead

Through its interface with the environment, the respiratory tract (like the skin and the gastrointestinal tract) is continuously exposed to huge numbers of microorganisms that have the potential to cause disease. Despite the multiplicity of host defenses (see Chapter 8), infections of the respiratory tract are extremely common and range from mild and usually self-limited illnesses to those associated with morbidity and mortality. Any part of the respiratory tract, from the nose and sinuses to the alveoli and pleural space, can be involved.

The spectrum of microorganisms known to cause respiratory infections is broad and constantly changing as new pathogens are identified, "old" pathogens change their resistance patterns, and the host immune response is altered by medications or other diseases or exposures. Because most such infections cannot currently be prevented, the aims of management are to prevent death and minimize morbidity. To accomplish these objectives, infections need to be identified correctly and the causal pathogen targeted with appropriate therapy.

Chapters 23 through 26 describe in detail aspects of pneumonia caused by specific pathogens. The purpose of this chapter is to provide a framework from which to approach an individual patient who may have pulmonary infection. Such a patient may be assessed by posing a number of questions (Table 22.1). In this section each of these steps is examined in turn, although in clinical practice a number of steps may be approached in parallel.

THE APPROACH

Is It Infection?

First, it is necessary to differentiate lung infection from other conditions. A careful history and physical examination are the essential starting points. Symptoms of fever, rigors, cough with purulent sputum production, and focal signs in the chest make infection the likely cause, but many infections have less specific presenting features. In some situations, to separate infection from noninfective causes of respiratory tract disease may not be possible. This is especially difficult in the community setting, in patients in whom cough is the predominant symptom (Fig. 22.1). It is also difficult in those who do not manifest the common signs of infection, such as the elderly, the immunocompromised, the severely ill, or patients in whom chronic lung disease (such as asthma, chronic obstructive pulmonary disease [COPD], or pulmonary fibrosis) makes differentiation from preexisting symptoms and signs difficult.

Investigations may help to separate infection from other causes, but although this is easy in the hospital setting, it may be impractical in the community. The finding of new parenchymal lung shadowing on the chest radiograph usually indicates infection (pneumonia), although there are many other causes of such lung shadowing (Table 22.2). The unconscious patient who is intubated and receiving assisted ventilation and develops lung shadowing is a common and difficult diagnostic problem. Signs and symptoms, such as fever and deterioration in gas exchange, are often nonspecific. A raised peripheral blood white blood cell count (WBC) is common in systemic bacterial infections; however, other inflammatory pathologies, such as lung infarction or pulmonary eosinophilia, may also cause this, as can drugs such as corticosteroids. Conversely, in many infections the WBC may be normal or reduced (e.g., viral infection and severe bacterial infection). Usually, C-reactive protein is elevated in bacterial infection and normal in other infections and noninfective pathologies. However, it is elevated in other inflammatory disorders.

Identification of a microorganism should be the best way to confirm infection, but this, too, has a number of limitations.

What Type of Infection Is It?

CLASSIFICATION OF PULMONARY INFECTIONS

The traditional anatomic classification of lung infection (see Fig. 22.1) forms a useful, but far from perfect, template on which to base this discussion. For various reasons, this classification schema must be used with some flexibility. Respiratory tract pathology can cause only a limited number of symptoms and signs. Although some may be quite specific (e.g., pleuritic pain as an indicator of pleural pathology), the majority are nonspecific (e.g., cough with purulent sputum as a feature of rhinosinusitis, airway infection, and/or pneumonia; see Table 22.2). This is a particularly important problem in the evaluation of outpatients when access to additional laboratory or radiologic investigations is limited. Localization of the site of infection may also be confused by underlying lung disease. For example, a patient who has pulmonary fibrosis and bronchitis may be wrongly diagnosed as having pneumonia because of the crackles heard over the lung fields, which result from pulmonary fibrosis. Finally, while many infections are limited by anatomic boundaries (e.g., a lobar pneumonia; Fig. 22.2), others do not fit easily into this classification schema (e.g., influenza virus infection).

The two main groups of acute pulmonary infections encountered in hospital practice are acute exacerbations of chronic bronchitis (see Chapter 35) and pneumonia (Chapter 23). A chest radiograph is the key to separating these two, as it is the

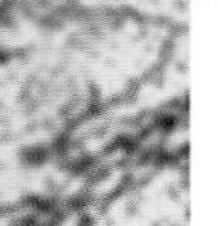

Table 22.1
How to approach the patient who may have pulmonary infection

1. Is it infection?
2. What type of infection is it?
3. How severe is the illness?
4. What is the likely pathogen?
5. How do I identify the causative pathogen?
6. Is pathogen identification necessary?

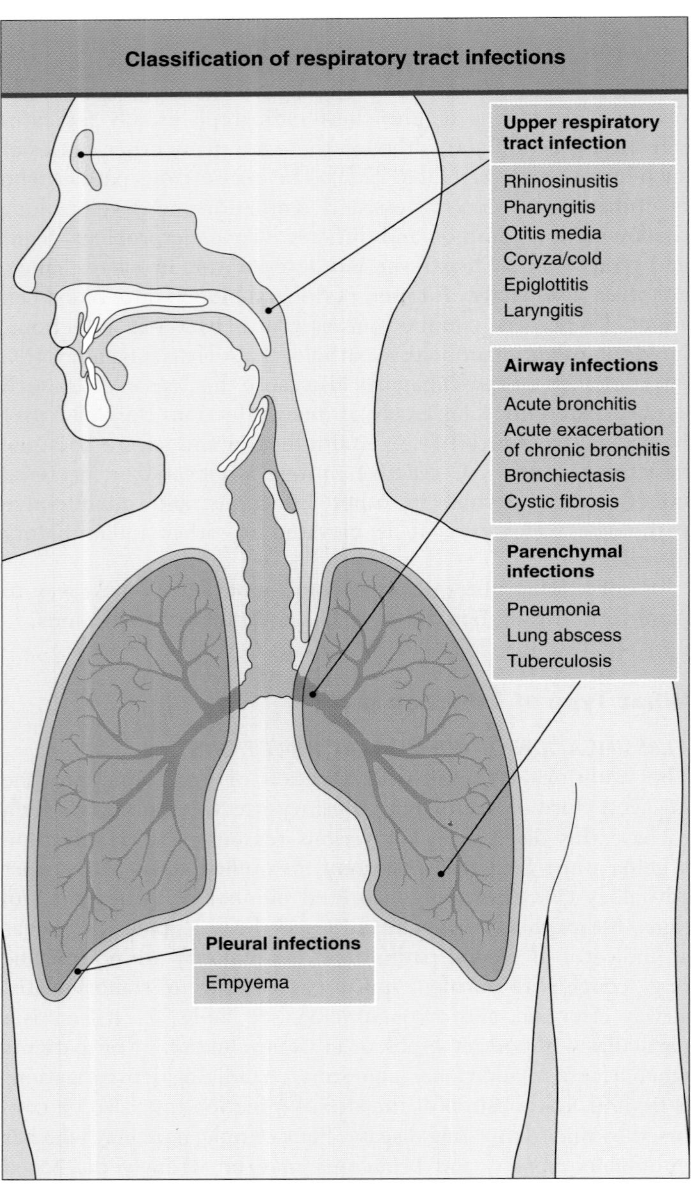

Figure 22.1 Classification of respiratory tract infections. The traditional approach based on anatomic site.

Table 22.2
Some alternative causes of respiratory symptoms

Feature	Noninfectious causes
Cough	Asthma Bronchial carcinoma Chronic bronchitis Parenchymal lung disease Drugs (e.g., captopril)
Purulent sputum	Asthma (caused by eosinophils)
Hemoptysis	Pulmonary infarction Bronchial carcinoma
Wheeze	Airway diseases Bronchial carcinoma
Pleuritic pain	Pulmonary infarction
Breathlessness	Airway diseases Parenchymal lung disease Pulmonary vascular disease
Fever	Inflammatory diseases (e.g., autoimmune disease)
Radiographic shadowing	Pulmonary edema Parenchymal lung disease Bronchial carcinoma Pulmonary infarction Pulmonary hemorrhage
Peripheral blood leukocytosis	Asthma Eosinophilia Steroid therapy

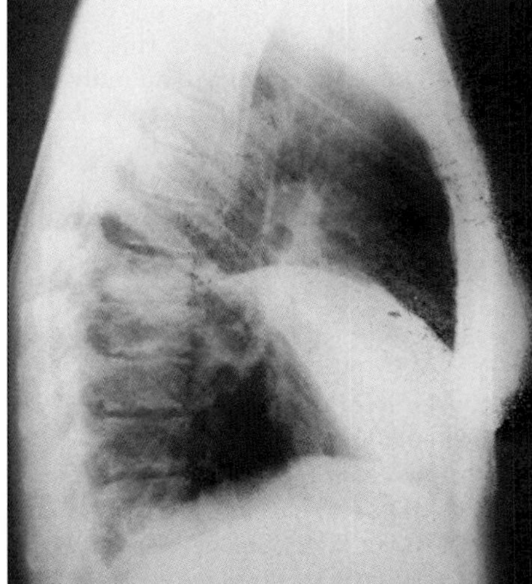

Figure 22.2 Mycoplasmal pneumonia. "Classic" homogeneous consolidation of the right middle lobe caused by a serologically confirmed infection of *Mycoplasma pneumoniae*.

most sensitive screening method for detecting pulmonary consolidation. The presence of focal crackles is the most common feature of underlying consolidation, as dullness to percussion, bronchial breathing, whispering pectoriloquy, and egophony, although more specific, are present in only one third of patients admitted to the hospital. A pleural rub, or features of pleural effusion, may coexist. Other less common features include diarrhea, hypotension, and, in the elderly, mental confusion, hypothermia, and urinary incontinence. When pneumonia is clinically suspected and the chest radiograph is normal, a chest CT scan may show changes in the lung parenchyma. However, other pathologies may mimic pneumonia (Figs. 22.3 through 22.5). In community-acquired infections these are rare and usually need not be considered, unless the clinical features are

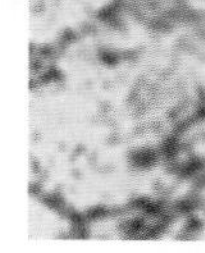

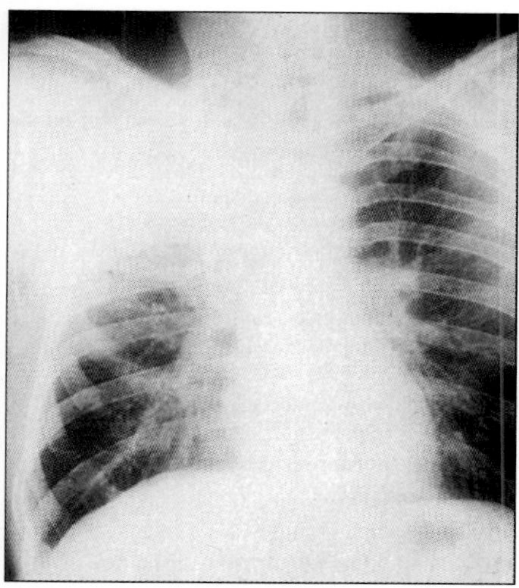

Figure 22.3 Pulmonary eosinophilia. Right upper lobe consolidation that mimics pneumonia.

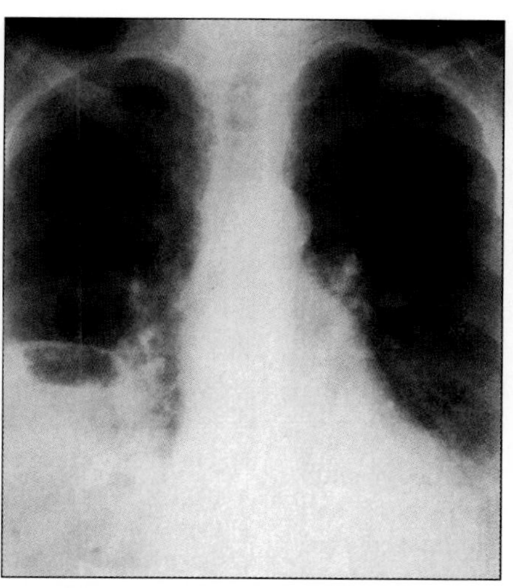

Figure 22.4 Pulmonary infarction. Cavitating right lower zone consolidation secondary to pulmonary infarction.

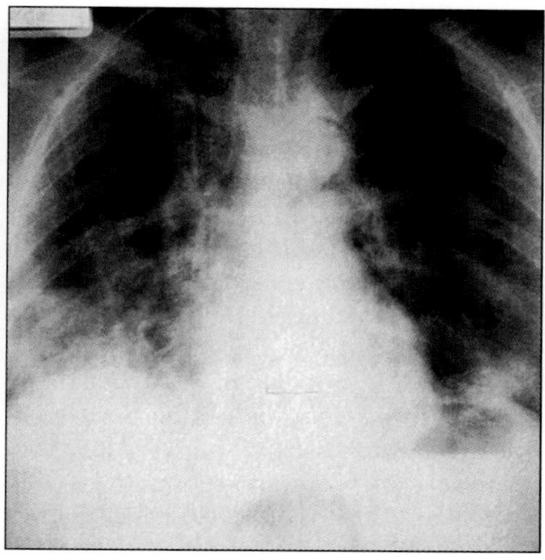

Figure 22.5 Drug-induced lung disease. Bilateral, patchy, predominantly basal consolidation secondary to bleomycin administration.

unusual or the patient fails to respond to appropriate therapy. More caution is needed in the evaluation of patients for nosocomial infections and for immunocompromised patients in whom such alterna-tive causes of consolidation are more common and clinical features may be less specific. In this setting a Clinical Illness Score (see Chapter 26) may be useful in the prediction of infection.

Other roles for the chest radiograph include an enhanced ability to assess the extent of disease, to detect complications (e.g., cavitation, abscess, pneumothorax, pleural effusion), to detect additional or alternative diagnoses (e.g., bronchiectasis, pulmonary fibrosis, bronchial neoplasm), and sometimes to guide invasive investigation. Its value in predicting the causative pathogen is considered later in this chapter.

How Severe Is the Illness?

The answer to this question guides the decisions about where to manage the patient (home or hospital; general ward or intensive care unit) and may also guide specific investigations and treatment strategies.

In the patient with an exacerbation of COPD, measures of respiratory distress (e.g., respiratory rate) and gas exchange are the best markers of illness severity.

For patients with community-acquired pneumonia (CAP), those who die are usually severely ill at presentation, so the correct interpretation of presenting features is important. This information should be supplemented by the results of investigations as they emerge. Features known to be markers of severe illness are given in Table 22.3. Early severity prediction can be based on immediately available information such as the presence of mental confusion, raised respiratory rate, and low blood pressure. The presence of any one feature is a marker of severity, and, in general, the more markers present the more severe the illness. Combinations of these features have been formulated to produce illness scores that give an objective measure of severity (see Chapter 23). The role of such scores in clinical practice is currently being evaluated.

Table 22.3
Features of severe community-acquired pneumonia

Time available	Factors
Immediately available	Increasing age Comorbid illness Alcoholism Respiratory rate ≥ 30 breaths per minute Systolic blood pressure ≤ 90 mm Hg Diastolic blood pressure ≤ 8.0 kPa (≤ 60 mm Hg) Cyanosis Mental confusion
Available soon after admission	Leukocyte count < 4 or > 20^9 cells/mm^3 Blood urea > 7 mmo/L (< 19.6 mg/dL) Pao_2 < 7.9 kPa (< 60 mmHg) Acidosis Bilateral lung shadowing
Available later	Bacteremia Hypoalbuminemia Abnormal liver function Progressive radiographic shadowing

Many of the features in Table 22.3 can also be applied to nosocomial pneumonia (NP) and pneumonia in the immunocompromised patient, although the importance of presenting features as opposed to features that develop during the course of the illness is less clearly defined for those who have CAP. Prior or inappropriate antibiotic therapy, renal failure, prolonged mechanical ventilation, coma, shock, and infection with *Pseudomonas aeruginosa*, *Acinetobacter* species, and methicillin-resistant *Staphylococcus aureus* (MRSA) are additional markers of severe NP (Table 22.4). High levels of lactate dehydrogenase that persist in peripheral blood, alveolar-arterial oxygen gradient greater than 4 kPa (>30 mm Hg) and greater than 5% neutrophils in bronchoalveolar lavage (BAL) are markers of severe *Pneumocystis jiroveci* (formerly *Pneumocystis carinii*) infection in patients who have autoimmune deficiency syndrome.

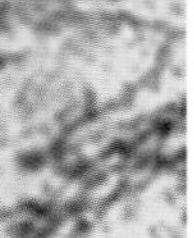

Table 22.4
Severe nosocomial pneumonia

Admission to the intensive care unit

Respiratory failure (mechanical ventilation or the need for > 35% oxygen to maintain an artificial oxygen saturation > 90%)

Rapid radiographic progression, multilobar pneumonia, or cavitating pneumonia

Severe sepsis with hypotension and/or end-organ dysfunction:

- Shock [systolic blood pressure < 12.0 kPa (< 90 mmHg) or diastolic blood pressure < 7.9 kPa (< 60 mmHg)]
- Requirement for vasopressors for > 4h
- Urine output < 20 ml/h or total urine output < 80 ml/h in 4h (without other explanation)
- Acute renal failure that requires dialysis

What Is the Likely Pathogen?

A wide range of microbial pathogens can cause pulmonary infection, which potentially makes management difficult without knowledge of the cause in an individual patient. In most patients the cause of the infection is never identified. In those in whom a pathogen is found, a delay always occurs between the patient's presentation and the availability of culture results. Because therapy should be started immediately, it is helpful to identify markers that may help to determine the cause of infection and hence to direct therapy. Generally, information obtained at presentation may point to potential groups of pathogens rather than to individual pathogens, since few features are pathogen specific.

Airway infections are often of viral origin. When bacteria are present, *Haemophilus influenzae*, *Streptococcus pneumoniae*, and *Moraxella catarrhalis* are most frequently found, although such organisms may simply represent colonization rather than pathogens. Nevertheless, when antibiotics are indicated (see Chapter 35) the initial empirical therapy is directed against these organisms. These bacteria are important in bronchiectasis, in which for some patients *S. aureus* and *P. aeruginosa* may also be important. The latter two organisms are particularly important in patients who have cystic fibrosis. In all patients who suffer bronchiectasis, knowledge of previous sputum culture results may be helpful (see Chapter 40).

The range of potentially treatable pathogens that may cause pneumonia is much more diverse. Classification of the pneumonia according to the immune status of the patient and the likely origin of the infection (Table 22.5) is helpful. Risk factors for unusual exposures (e.g., birds for psittacosis, grazing animals for Q fever) and immune/compromise (e.g., unsuspected intravenous drug abuse or sexual contact for human immunodeficiency virus risk) must always be sought.

The most frequent cause of CAP is *S. pneumoniae*, but a number of other pathogens are regularly encountered (see Table 22.5). Clinical and epidemiologic features are rarely specific and should be used with caution (Table 22.6). The widespread skin rash of varicella-zoster virus in a patient who has pneumonia is one of the few clinical features specific to a particular pathogen.

In general, the same pathogens are important in different age groups, with the exception of a lower incidence of *Mycoplasma* infection in the elderly. Gram-negative *Enterobacteriaceae* (e.g., *Escherichia coli, Proteus mirabilis*) may be more frequent in pneumonias in some elderly nursing home populations, and MRSA is now being recognized as a community pathogen in this setting. All the pathogens encountered in the community setting can produce illnesses of varying severity, although legionellal,

Table 22.5
Classification of the pneumonias according to likely origin and immune status

Pneumonia group	Likely pathogens
Community-acquired	Gram-positive bacteria *Mycoplasma, Chlamydia, Coxiella* Common viruses (e.g., influenza)
Nosocomial, early	As for community-acquired
Nosocomial, late	Gram-negative enterobacteria *Staphylococcus aureus* Antibiotic-resistant bacteria
Immunocompromised	Opportunistic organisms

Table 22.6
Prediction of microbial etiology in community-acquired pneumonia

Microorganism	Features that occur more frequently in community-acquired pneumonia caused by this organism
Streptococcus pneumoniae	Abrupt illness onset
Haemophilus influenzae	Preexisting lung disease
Staphylococcus aureus	Concurrent influenza epidemic Radiographic cavitation Severe illness Intravenous drug abuse
Legionella species	Recent foreign travel Concurrent epidemic Countries that border the Mediterranean
Mycoplasma pneumoniae	Age < 65 years
Chlamydia psittaci	Recent bird contact At-risk occupation
Coxiella burnetii	Animal contact (hoofed animals, cats, rabbits) At-risk occupation
Franciscella tularensis	Tick bites Rabbit contact
Brucella abortus	Cattle, sheep, goat, pig contact At-risk occupation (abattoirs, farming, veterinary work)
Gram-negative *Enterobacteriaceae*	Nursing home resident South Africa
Burkholderia pseudomallei	Southeast Asia, northern Australia
Hantavirus pulmonary syndrome	Rodent contact
Tuberculosis	Non-industrialized countries
Pneumocystis jiroveci	Risk factors for HIV Iatrogenic immune compromise

staphylococcal, and gram-negative enterobacterial infections are more commonly found in severely ill patients.

It is common clinical practice to attempt to differentiate "atypical" from "typical" pneumonias. It may be helpful to retain these terms to describe groups of pathogens (*atypical* referring to intracellular pathogens such as *Mycoplasma pneumoniae, Chlamydia pneumoniae,* and *Coxiella burnetii,* and *typical* referring to conventional bacteria such as *S. pneumoniae and H. influenzae*), but recent studies have shown that this clinical distinction may be helpful only for patients at the extreme ends of the spectrum of clinical presentation found in pneumonia; for the majority of patients, it does not work. *Legionella* pneumonia has been included in the "atypical" pneumonia group. In fact, the clinical features of this illness have much more in common with severe pneumococcal infection. When this disease was first described, a number of features, such as diarrhea, cerebral dysfunction, hyponatremia, and abnormal liver function tests, were thought to be associated specifically with this organism. These features are more frequent in legionellal pneumonia but occur commonly in severe pneumonia from any cause, and it appears to be the severity of the illness rather than the causative organism that relates to these features.

Radiographic features also usually do not help to differentiate causative pathogens; however, cavitation occurs most commonly in staphylococcal, anaerobic (Fig. 22.6), fungal, and tuberculous infections, and rarely with other pathogens.

It is helpful to distinguish NPs that develop within the first 5 days of hospitalization from those that develop thereafter. *S. pneumoniae* and *H. influenzae* are not uncommon within the first 5 days, but are rarely found after 5 days, after which *S. aureus* (both methicillin-sensitive and methicillin-resistant strains), *Acinetobacter* species, and *P. aeruginosa* are the most commonly seen. No specific clinical or laboratory features allow an accurate prediction of the causative pathogen in NP; however, *P. aeruginosa* is less common in patients who have NP that developed outside the intensive care unit.

Bacterial antibiotic resistance is becoming increasingly important in both community-acquired and nosocomial pathogens, although the individual frequency varies widely geographically and among institutions. In areas where antibiotic resistance is common, a history of prior antibiotic therapy predicts a higher risk of infection with resistant organisms. The clinical value of this information varies among institutions for the reasons previously cited, and it is therefore important to know the local resistance patterns of common pathogens.

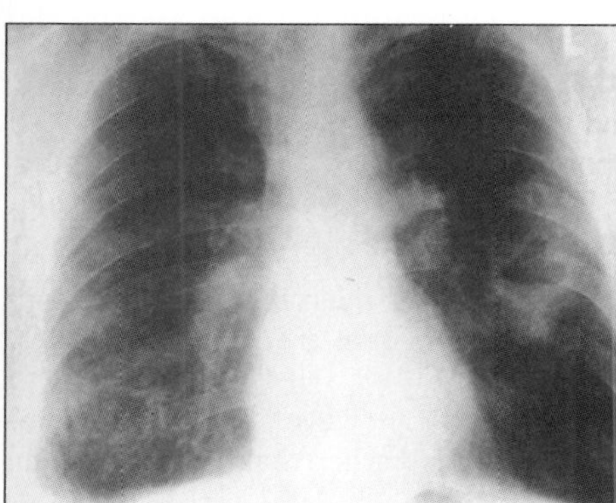

Figure 22.6 Cavitating pneumonia. Left midzone consolidation caused by anaerobic infection.

The range of pathogens that cause pneumonia in the immunocompromised patient is very broad and, in addition to routine bacterial and viral infections, also includes infections by opportunistic organisms that are usually nonpathogenic in the immunocompetent host. Polymicrobial infections also occur more commonly in these patients. Prediction of likely pathogens is again imprecise, but attention should be paid to the nature and degree of the immunosuppression, time course of events, cytomegalovirus (CMV) status of donor and recipient, use of prophylactic therapies, and radiographic features (Table 22.7). Symptoms and signs, as in NP, are seldom helpful, although pancytopenia commonly accompanies CMV infections.

How Can the Causative Pathogen Be Identified?

MINIMALLY INVASIVE TESTS

Throat Swab

A throat swab may be used to identify some predominantly intracellular pathogens such as viruses, *Mycoplasma*, and *Chlamydia*. Organisms can be identified by direct immunofluorescence (*Chlamydia*, viruses) or cell culture. The yields are low and the methodologies often labor intensive, which means that in adults this is usually impractical, other than for research. In children, detection of respiratory syncytial virus by this method may be helpful.

Table 22.7
Predicting microbial etiology in pneumonia in an immunocomprimised host

Feature	Criteria	Organism
Nature of immunosuppression	B-cell dysfunction	Bacterial
	T-cell dysfunction	Opportunist
	Neutropenia	Bacteria Fungi
Severity on HIV infection	CD4 > 200	Bacteria Tuberculosis
	CD4 < 200	*Pneumocystis jiroveci* pneumonia (PCP)
		Other opportunists
Time course of events	0-1 month post-transplant	Bacterial infection
	1-6 months post-transplant	Opportunist
Cytomegalovirus (CMV) status	CMV^+ donor to CMV^- recipent	CMV
Prophylactic therapy	PCP prophylaxis	PCP less likely + atypical presentations
Radiology	Focal consolidation	Bacterial infection
	Nodule	Lung abscess Fungi
	Diffuse shadowing	PCP CMV (transplants only)

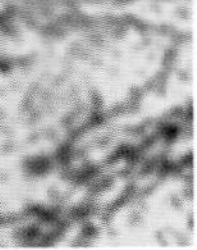

Sputum

In many patients who have respiratory infection this is easy to obtain. When not available, sputum production may be induced by administration of nebulized hypertonic saline—this is probably of value only for the detection of *Mycobacterium tuberculosis* or of *P. jiroveci* in immunocompromised patients. The value of examining sputum has been studied exhaustively, and its utility remains controversial. The main problems are that airway secretions have to pass through the oropharynx, which may be colonized by a variety of microorganisms, such that organisms identified in sputum may not be representative of what is happening in the lung. Second, bacteria may colonize the normally sterile airways when host defenses are compromised (e.g., by chronic bronchitis or intubation). The clinical illness may be attributed to these organisms when found in sputum even though another process (e.g., viral infection) is responsible.

Because some organisms are always pathogens (e.g., *Mycobacteria*, *Pneumocystis*, *Legionella*), their identification in sputum is always helpful. For other organisms, determination of the quality of the sputum sample is essential. Samples that contain 25 neutrophils and 10 or fewer squamous epithelial cells per high power microscope field are considered to be representative of the lower respiratory tract. Other samples should be discarded unless the pathogens listed previously are being sought.

Various tests can be performed on sputum; Gram stain and routine culture are the best known (Fig. 22.7). Visualization of an organism on Gram stain is more specific than culture but is less sensitive. In a patient who has CAP in which a predominant organism is identified within a purulent sputum sample, that organism is usually the cause of the pneumonia. As a result of their specific growth requirements, some organisms are identified in sputum only if appropriate stains are applied (e.g., *Pneumocystis*) or if culture is performed on specific media (e.g., *Legionella*, fungi); such practices are not routinely used in many laboratories.

Tracheal Aspirate

In NP, a tracheal aspirate can be obtained from the endotracheal tube. Even though the upper respiratory tract is bypassed, the frequency of colonization means that, as for sputum, microbiologic results from such a sample should be treated with caution. Culture results are often polymicrobial. Recent studies suggest that quantitative culture of tracheal aspirates may be as accurate as and less harmful than bronchoscopy in NP (see "Bronchoscopy," later in this chapter). Some authors suggest the use of serial quantitative cultures of tracheal aspirates as the best way to detect NP.

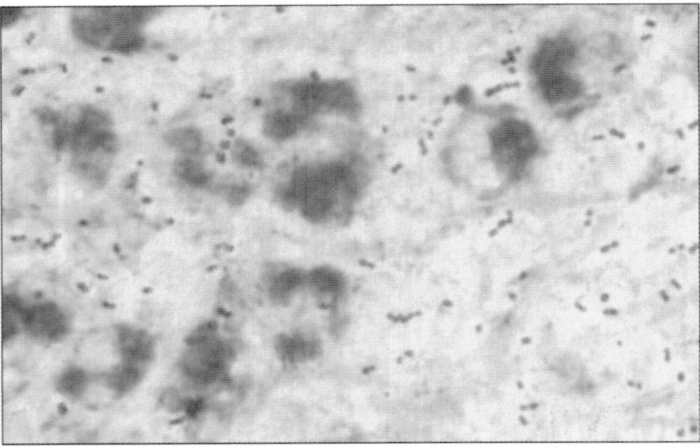

Figure 22.7 Sputum Gram stain. Gram-positive diplococci surrounded by degenerate neutrophils, which suggests pneumococcal infection.

Blood Culture

Blood culture is readily available and highly specific if positive. Its drawback is its relative insensitivity, being positive in only 10% to 20% of hospitalized adult patients who have CAP. Its yield is even less in NP and very low in children.

Pleural Fluid

When present, pleural fluid should be sampled, because the results are highly specific, as in blood cultures, and possibly more sensitive. Lymphocytosis suggests the possibility of tuberculosis. Pleural pH as well as cell content may help in the diagnosis of empyema. Pleural biopsy for histology and culture may help in this circumstance.

Urine

Enzyme-linked immunosorbent assay (ELISA) testing of urine for *Legionella* antigen is now the most rapid test for the diagnosis of *Legionella* infection. Its specificity approaches 100%, and its sensitivity is 70% to 80%. Minor drawbacks are that it is positive only in *Legionella pneumophila* serogroup I infection (>90% of cases of *Legionella* infection), that it may be negative if performed too early (antigen excretion begins around day 3 of clinical illness), and that antigen excretion may persist for up to 1 year after the clinical illness.

Serology

Many of the organisms that cause respiratory infection are difficult to identify or isolate, and their involvement can be assessed only indirectly by measurement of the response of the specific host antibody to the agent. This approach does not usually help in immunocompromised hosts or in patients affected by nosocomial infections, unless *Legionella* is specifically suspected (e.g., during an ongoing epidemic). In CAP, this is often the only method of diagnosis available for *Mycoplasma*, *Chlamydia*, *Coxiella*, *Legionella*, and viral infections. To establish such diagnoses, with certain exceptions, it is necessary to identify a fourfold rise in specific antibody titers to a titer of at least 1:128 between acute and convalescent samples. A single, high titer of 1:256 is presumptive evidence of infection. The need to wait for the second sample (often at least 10 days and in some situations up to 1 month) limits the clinical value of this method. Most methods seek complement-fixing antibodies, but for some organisms other techniques are required. For *Legionella* infection, indirect immunofluorescent, microagglutination, or ELISA techniques are necessary, and for C. *pneumoniae*, for which less than 30% of infections give rise to a positive complement-fixing test result, a microimmunofluorescent method is usually used. These techniques are not always widely available.

Most tests detect IgG antibodies; however, because the temporal rise in IgM antibodies occurs earlier than IgG, detection

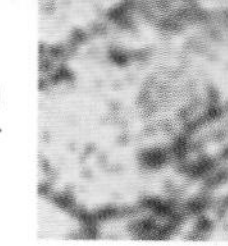

of such antibodies could be used for early diagnosis. This technique is used to detect *Mycoplasma* infection.

INVASIVE TESTS

Transtracheal Aspirate

The transtracheal aspirate technique enables a relatively uncontaminated lower airway sample to be obtained by the passing of a catheter through the cricothyroid membrane. The technique was employed quite frequently in the past, but the risks of hemorrhage and subcutaneous emphysema have rendered it hardly used today.

Bronchoscopy

Bronchoscopy allows direct sampling from the lungs, but because the bronchoscope passes through the nasopharynx and upper airway, it is important to use an approach that minimizes contamination. Other drawbacks are that the procedure and the associated local anesthetic and sedation may further compromise the patient's already altered ventilatory status; transbronchial biopsy may cause hemorrhage or pneumothorax; and the bronchoscope may also introduce infection. An advantage of BAL is that a wider area of the lung is sampled, but the risk of contamination is increased. Protected specimen brush (PSB) may be more specific, but it is less sensitive, as only a small area is sampled. Bronchoscopy has been the most commonly used technique for immunocompromised patients and those who have NP; it is most strongly validated in the former. In these patients, BAL or PSB may be the only investigations that reliably provide microbiologic information. Also, BAL has been especially well evaluated in the detection of *P. jiroveci* infection, where it approaches 100% specificity and has a sensitivity of up to 80% to 90% when coupled with silver or immunofluorescent staining of the BAL sample. The latter technique is more sensitive, but less specific for *P. jiroveci* pneumonia. Usually, BAL is the only sample required in such patients, but for those who have received *Pneumocystis* prophylaxis, interstitial *Pneumocystis* infection may occur that may be missed by BAL and only detected by transbronchial biopsy (TBBx).

The use of bronchoscopic samples in the management of NP remains unclear; PSB sampling is probably better than BAL. Apart from tracheal aspirates, this approach is most likely to identify a bacterium in such patients, but even when performed with great care and according to strict protocol using quantitative cultures and specific, predetermined thresholds for infection ($>10^3$ colony forming units [cfu] for PSB and $>10^4$ cfu for BAL), recent research suggests significant false-positive and false-negative rates. Some workers have, in addition, found the detection of intracellular bacteria in BAL to be a specific marker of NP, but this needs to be confirmed. No outcome benefit has been conclusively shown in those so investigated compared with patients managed without invasive sampling, and the technique cannot at present be recommended routinely.

In CAP no evidence supports the routine addition of bronchoscopy to noninvasive sampling. It may be of value in the patient whose initial therapy fails.

Percutaneous Fine-needle Aspiration

Percutaneous fine-needle aspiration is performed by inserting a 22-gauge needle percutaneously into consolidated lung tissue via an 18-gauge needle in the chest wall. A number of authors have suggested that this is a sensitive way to obtain evidence of a microbial cause, particularly in CAP. However, it carries a risk of pneumothorax and lung hemorrhage, and it cannot be recommended other than for research purposes in the hands of those experienced in the technique.

Open Lung Biopsy

The value of open lung biopsy has not been systematically evaluated because of the potential risks. Anecdotally, it has helped in all three types of pneumonia when the patient has failed to respond to empirical therapy and when other tests have been unhelpful.

OTHER TECHNIQUES

Methods that are currently experimental may become routine in the future. The techniques with the most promise are the molecular biologic methods, especially polymerase chain reaction (PCR). The potential of this technique lies in its exquisite sensitivity; the test can detect the DNA of a single microorganism. This may also limit its potential, however, because the separation of commensal organisms from pathogens may not be possible. In the respiratory tract its likely use is to detect noncommensal organisms in respiratory samples and commensal organisms in normally sterile sites (e.g., blood, pleural fluid). Its other roles may be to detect different organisms at the same time in a single sample (so-called "multiplex PCR") and to identify antibiotic resistance by detection of the specific gene defect that determines such resistance. Commercial kits are already available for detection of mycobacteria, although sensitivity and specificity are suboptimal.

The polysaccharide capsule of the pneumococcus and pneumococcal proteins are released into solution, especially by dividing organisms. These can be detected by a number of methods, which include countercurrent immunoelectrophoresis and latex agglutination. These techniques have the advantage that they do not depend on the presence of an intact organism and may therefore be positive after antibiotics have been given. Also advantageous is that they can be used on multiple specimens, which include (in descending order of likelihood of a positive result) sputum, urine, blood, pleural fluid, and bronchoscopic samples. Such techniques have been widely used in research studies in Europe, but not in North America. Their value outside the research setting has not been determined.

Serologic methods to identify pneumococcal infection are also being studied, including the detection of antibodies to pneumococcal products (e.g., pneumolysin) and immune complexes, but none are in clinical use at present.

Is It Necessary to Identify the Causative Pathogen?

In some patients it may be inappropriate to seek the causative pathogen because it is impractical, it is not cost effective, and/or the potential risk to the patient outweighs any benefit. In the community 95% or more of respiratory infections are managed empirically without investigation. The role for microbial investigations in this setting has yet to be determined, but these may be needed only when the patient fails to respond to initial therapy.

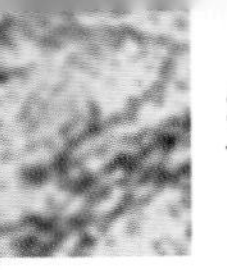

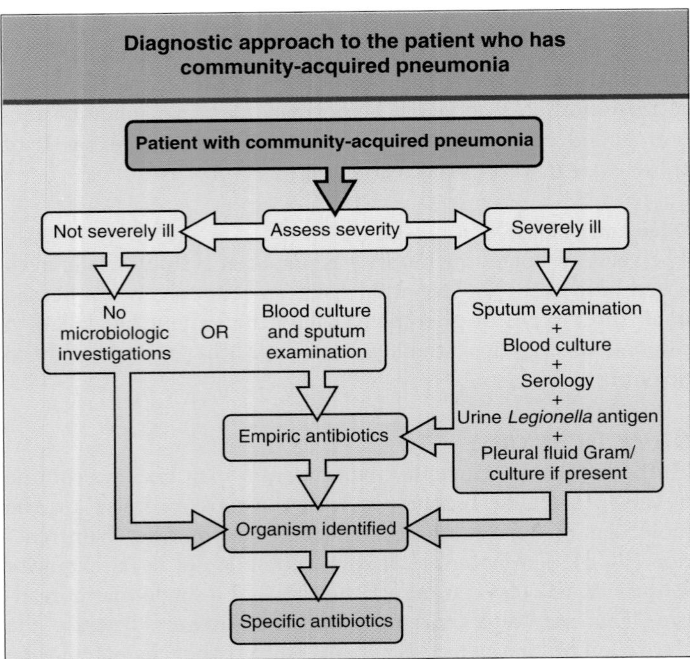

Figure 22.8 Diagnostic approach to the patient who has community-acquired pneumonia (CAP). A suggested algorithm to guide microbial investigation in CAP.

Microbial investigations on hospitalized patients are routine. However, in prospective studies of CAP in which intensive investigation is undertaken, pathogens are detected only in approximately 25% to 50% of patients, and the impact on treatment is small. Outcome benefit for bronchoscopic investigations in NP remains controversial. The reasons for the poor yield are multiple and relate to prior antibiotic therapy, inadequate sample collection, transport delays, and the use of insensitive laboratory methods that often depend on the presence of intact and viable organisms for a positive result. This may all change with the advent of newer microbiologic methods, but because empirical, broad-spectrum antibiotics are easy to give and patients who are not severely ill usually recover, it can be argued that airway infections or CAP microbial investigations should be limited (or not performed) in the mildly ill and used extensively only in the severely ill patient. In NP and the immunocompromised patient, microbial investigation may be more important, because it is often necessary to differentiate infective from non-infective pathology. Possible approaches in CAP, NP, and the immunocompromised patient are shown in Figures 22.8, 22.9, and 22.10, respectively.

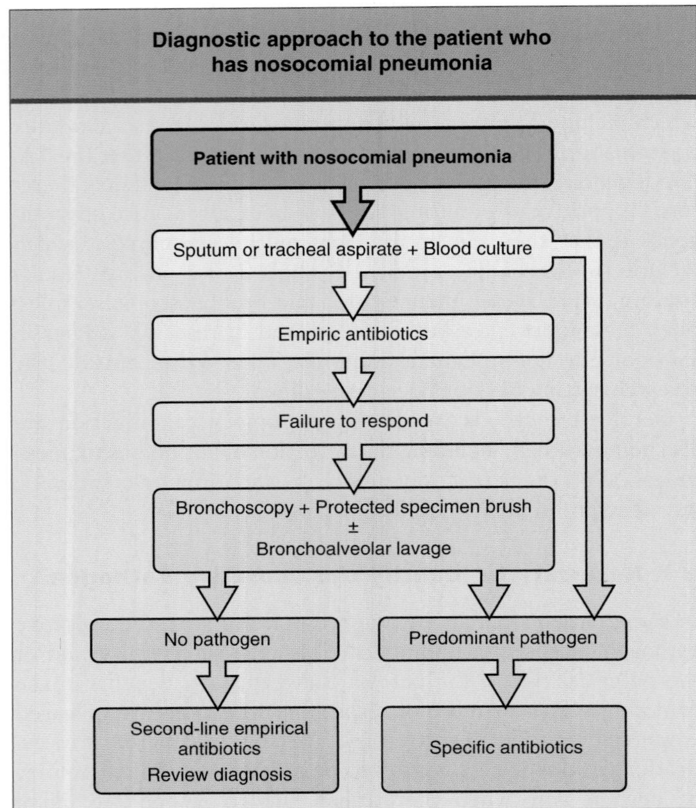

Figure 22.9 Diagnostic approach to the patient who has nosocomial pneumonia (NP). A suggested algorithm to guide microbial investigation in NP.

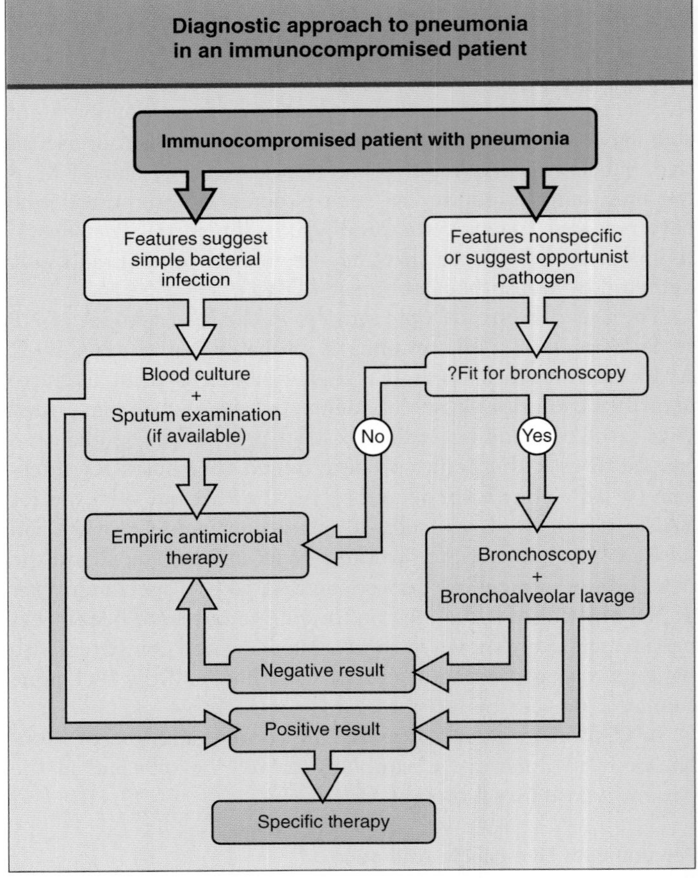

Figure 22.10 Diagnostic approach to pneumonia in an immunocompromised patient (ICP). A suggested algorithm to guide microbial investigation in ICP.

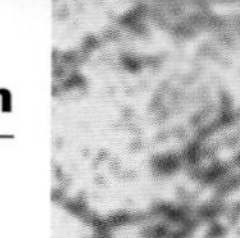

SUGGESTED READINGS

Bartlett JG, Dowell SF, Mandell LA, et al: Practice guidelines for the management of community-acquired pneumonia in adults. Infectious Diseases Society of America. Clin Infect Dis 31:347-382, 2000.

BTS Guidelines for the Management of Community Acquired Pneumonia in Adults. Thorax 56(suppl 4):IV1-IV64, 2001.

Campbell GD, Niederman MS, Broughton WA, et al: Guidelines for the initial empiric management of adults with hospital-acquired pneumonia: Diagnosis, assessment of severity, initial antimicrobial therapy and prevention strategies. Am J Respir Crit Care Med 153:1711-1725, 1996.

European Study on Community-acquired Pneumonia Committee: Guidelines for management of adult community-acquired lower respiratory tract infections. Eur Respir J 11:986-991, 1998.

Niederman MS, Mandell LA, Anzueto A, et al: Guidelines for the management of adults with community-acquired pneumonia. Diagnosis, assessment of severity, antimicrobial therapy, and prevention. Am J Respir Crit Care Med 163:1730-1754, 2001.

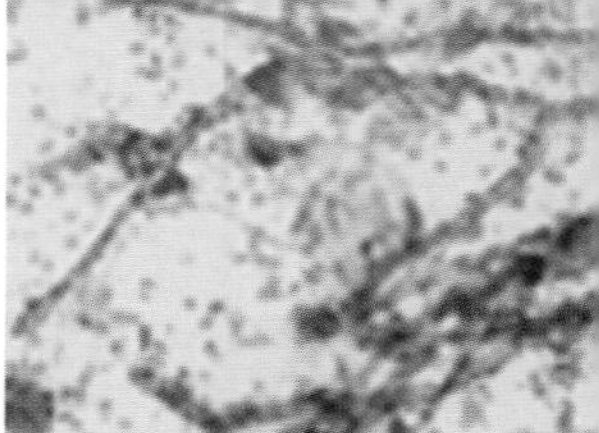

CHAPTER 23

Bacterial Pneumonia

Antoine Rabbat and Gérard J. Huchon

EPIDEMIOLOGY AND RISK FACTORS

Community-acquired pneumonias (CAPs) are a major health care and economic problem owing to their high morbidity and mortality and to the direct and indirect costs of their management. Most patients with community-acquired bacterial pneumonia are managed in the community by general practitioners; the clinical diagnosis is usually uncertain for various reasons, including the difficulty of identifying CAP in patients presenting with clinical findings indicative of a lower respiratory tract infection (LRTI) and the lack of sensitivity and specificity of laboratory and radiologic investigations. This uncertainty has an important clinical implication. CAP is often bacterial in origin and needs to be treated rapidly with an antibiotic, whereas other LRTIs are usually self-limited illnesses that do not require antibiotics. Because of the difficulty of excluding the diagnosis of CAP, however, most patients with LRTIs are given antibiotics. This results in excessive use of these drugs, which contributes to the resistance of bacteria to antibiotics.

Only a few studies have tried to document the frequency of CAP, and they suggest an incidence of 4.7 to 11.6 per 1000 and an association with increasing age. Hospital admission rates for pneumonia vary from 22% to 51%. The mortality is higher in less-developed countries, in the young, and in the elderly, varying from 10 to 40 per 100,000 inhabitants in some Western European countries between 1985 and 1990. European prospective studies indicate an average mortality of 7% for patients admitted to hospital, rising to 29% for those with severe pneumonia.

Infection develops when defense mechanisms that enable the lower respiratory tract to remain sterile are overwhelmed, when there is an increase in the virulence of the infecting agent or the volume of the inoculum, or when systemic host defenses fail. Risk factors for the occurrence of pneumonia should not be confused with risk factors for the severity of pneumonia, even though many factors may be significant for both.

Age

Age is a risk factor for pneumonia independent of other risk factors; every year over 65 increases the risk of contracting pneumonia. The annual incidence of CAP in noninstitutionalized elderly people is estimated to be 25 to 44 per 1000, compared with 4.7 to 11.6 per 1000 in the general population. The risk of pneumonia due to *Streptococcus pneumoniae* is higher in the elderly than in the general population. The frequency of hospital admissions as a result of severe infection also increases markedly with age, ranging from 1.6 per 1000 adults between 55 and 64 years to 11.6 per 1000 after 75. Age appears to be one of the main factors predictive of mortality due to CAP: mortality due to pneumonia or influenza has been evaluated at 9 per 100,000 in the elderly, rising to 217 per 100,000 in patients with one associated risk factor and to 979 per 100,000 in those with more than one. This high mortality rate is associated with coexisting heart failure, cerebrovascular disease, cancer, diabetes mellitus, or chronic obstructive pulmonary disease (COPD).

Institutionalization

Both the frequency and the severity of pneumonia increase in institutionalized patients. Oropharyngeal colonization by gram-negative bacilli or *Staphylococcus aureus* may play a major role here, because the pathophysiology of pneumonia is attributed to contamination of the lower respiratory tract from microaspiration. Epidemics of viral infections are also frequent in this population. The main microorganisms isolated in institutionalized patients with pneumonia are, in decreasing frequency, *S. pneumoniae*, *S. aureus*, gram-negative bacilli, and *Haemophilus influenzae*.

Alcoholism

Alcohol adversely affects many properties of the respiratory tract defense mechanism. It facilitates bacterial colonization of the oropharynx with gram-negative bacilli, impairs coughing reflexes, alters swallowing and mucociliary transport, and impairs the function of lymphocytes, neutrophils, monocytes, and alveolar macrophages. Each of these factors contributes to the reduced bacterial clearance from the airways found in these patients. The risks of alcoholism are compounded by the additional risks in the elderly, discussed earlier.

Infections caused by gram-negative bacilli and *Legionella pneumophila* occur more frequently in heavy drinkers. Bacteremia also seems to be more frequently associated with alcoholism. However, alcoholism is not a risk factor for pneumonia severity, except in the case of pneumococcal infection with leukopenia.

Nutrition

Susceptibility to infection is increased by a number of malnutrition-related phenomena, such as a decreased level of secretory immunoglobulin A, a failure in macrophage recruitment, and alterations in cellular immunity. As a result, the frequency of respiratory tract colonization by gram-negative bacilli is increased in patients with malnutrition, and the incidence and severity of respiratory infections are increased. Malnutrition acts in association with other comorbid conditions frequently found in patients with pneumonia, such as alcohol consumption, COPD, chronic respiratory failure, neurologic disease.

Smoking

Smoking alters mucociliary transport, humoral and cellular defenses, and epithelial cell function and increases adhesion of *S. pneumoniae* and *H. influenzae* to the oropharyngeal epithelium. Accordingly, an increased proportion of patients admitted to hospital with pneumonia are current smokers. Moreover, smoking predisposes to infection by influenza, *L. pneumophila*, and *S. pneumoniae*. However, smoking itself is not a risk factor for pneumonia severity.

Aspiration

The risk factors that predispose to aspiration are summarized in Table 23.1. Up to 50% of normal subjects aspirate oropharyngeal secretions during sleep. The prevalence increases to as much as 70% when consciousness is impaired by medications or neurologic disorders, or when patients are intubated or have a tracheostomy. In normal subjects, the volume of material aspirated is small, the host is protected by the pulmonary defense mechanisms, and the episodes have no clinically detectable consequence. Even in urgent intubations, clinically apparent aspiration is as low as 3.5%.

Aspiration of gastric contents initially causes a chemical pneumonitis due to the low pH of the fluid. Pneumonitis may be observed, however, even when the pH is relatively high (6 or higher). When this occurs, the lung injury is transient; when the pH is lower (<2.5), more persistent inflammatory and hemorrhagic bronchial damage may occur. Animal experiments suggest that the volume of material must exceed 1 to 4 mL/kg to cause inflammation. Atelectasis is frequent, occurs early, and likely arises from the deleterious effect of gastric acid on surfactant.

The diagnosis of aspiration pneumonia is generally restricted to patients who have a bacterial lung infection that occurs in association with a condition predisposing them to aspiration (see Table 23.1). Organisms encountered include a number of anaerobic bacteria (e.g., anaerobic streptococci and *Fusobacterium* and *Bacteroides* species) and gram-negative enteric bacilli. Periodontal disease is found in many of these patients, and these pockets of gingivitis are thought to be the source of these pathogens.

Table 23.1
Conditions that predispose to aspiration pneumonias

Cause	Intrinsic	Extrinsic including iatrogenic
Neurologic disorders	Seizures, stroke, trauma, multiple sclerosis, Parkinson's disease, myasthenia gravis, pseudobulbar palsy, amyotrophic lateral sclerosis	Trauma, alcoholism, drug abuse, general anesthesia
Gastrointestinal disorders	Esophageal achalasia, stricture, tumor, diverticula, tracheoesophageal fistula, cardiac sphincter incompetency, protracted vomiting, bowel obstruction, gastric distention or delayed emptying	Upper gastrointestinal endoscopy, nasogastric tube
Respiratory disorders	Larynx incompetency (vocal cord paralysis), impairment of tracheobronchial mucociliary clearance	Endotracheal intubation, tracheostomy, pharyngeal anesthesia

Associated Diseases

Associated diseases are frequent in patients hospitalized with CAP, with rates ranging from 46% to 80%. Conditions encountered include COPD (13% to 53%), cardiovascular diseases (6% to 30%), neurologic diseases (5% to 24%), and diabetes mellitus (5% to 16%). Pneumonia due to *S. pneumoniae*, *S. aureus*, streptococcus B, and *H. influenzae* may occur after a viral infection (influenza), as well as in patients with COPD, neurologic diseases, and diabetes mellitus, which also favor the occurrence of pneumonia due to gram-negative bacilli. Although associated diseases do not increase mortality in most studies, up to 70% of fatalities due to pneumonia had a comorbid condition, versus 40% among survivors, and the risk of death is multiplied 5-fold in association with cardiac disease.

Miscellaneous Factors

An increased frequency of *S. pneumoniae* pneumonia has been reported among soldiers (12 per 1000), painters (42 per 1000), and South African gold miners, and after hospital admission within the preceding year. Previous hospital stay increases the risk of pneumonia due to *S. pneumoniae* in particular. Being exposed to stagnant water or to domestic water supply systems may favor the development of legionnaires' disease. A variety of medications may contribute to the development of pneumonia in elderly people, especially when associated with other risk factors: morphine and atropine interfere with mucociliary clearance, sedatives alter coughing and epiglottic function, and corticosteroids and the salicylates act on phagocytosis.

CLINICAL FEATURES

Diagnosis

The symptoms of pneumonia are not specific but generally include fever, possibly chills, and general uneasiness associated with a variety of respiratory and nonrespiratory symptoms such as cough, purulent sputum production, thoracic pain, dyspnea, coryza, pharyngitis, vomiting, myalgia, and headache. The classic signs of consolidation (dullness to percussion, crackles, increased tactile fremitus, and bronchial breathing) are found in only 33% of adults admitted to the hospital with radiographically confirmed CAP and in only 5% to 10% of adults with CAP in the community. Accordingly, radiographic consolidation is required for the diagnosis of pneumonia. Such a feature is present in about 40% of patients with LRTI and focal chest signs, in contrast to almost none when there are no focal signs. Because a chest radiograph is sometimes difficult to obtain rapidly, a clinical diagnosis is usual in the community, despite the lack of an agreed clinical definition of CAP. However, radiography has to be performed if there are risk factors for complications or if resolution does not begin after 2 or 3 days. There is usually an increase in the white cell count and erythrocyte sedimentation rate during the course of CAP. Table 23.2 suggests when to perform chest radiography, microbiologic examination of the sputum, blood white cell counts, other laboratory investigations,

Table 23.2
Investigations in community-acquired lower respiratory tract infections managed at home

Risk factors	Chest radiography	Microbiologic examination of sputum	Blood white cell count, C-reactive protein, blood cultures, serologies, detection of pneumococcal and legionellal antigens
Patient with no risk factors of severity or of unusual microorganisms	Not recommended	Not recommended	Not recommended
Risk factors for unusual microorganisms (see Table 23.3)	Not recommended	Recommended	Not recommended
Risk factors for potential severity (see Figure 23.7)	To be considered	Not recommended	To be considered
Failure of first-line empiric therapy	Recommended	Recommended	To be considered
Focal chest signs	Recommended	Not recommended	Not recommended
Wheeze, atopy	Not recommended	Not recommended	Not recommended

Adapted from Huchon GJ, Woodhead MA, Gialdroni-Grassi G, et al: Guidelines for management of adult community-acquired lower respiratory tract infections. Eur Respir Rev 11:986-991, 1998.

Table 23.3
Risk factors for pneumonia occurrence, severity, and particular microorganisms in community-acquired lower respiratory tract infections

Risk factor	Microorganisms
Age >65 years	*Streptococcus pneumoniae*
Institutionalized patients	*Strep. pneumoniae*, Gram-negative enteric bacilli, *Staphylococcus aureus*, and anaerobic bacteria in nonambulatory elderly people
Alcoholism	Gram-negative bacilli and *Legionella* spp.
Comorbidity (chronic obstructive pulmonary disease, cardiovascular disease, neurologic diseases, diabetes mellitus, chronic liver or renal failure, recent viral infection)	*Strep. pneumoniae, Staph. aureus, Haemophilus influenzae*, Gram-negative enteric bacilli
Hospital admission	
Within the previous year	*Strep. pneumoniae* (especially penicillin-resistant strains in some areas)
Within the previous 2–4 weeks	Gram-negative enteric bacilli
Recent treatment with penicillin or other antibiotics	*Strep. pneumoniae* (especially penicillin-resistant strains in some areas), resistant microorganisms
Aspiration	Gram-negative bacilli, *Staph. aureus*, anaerobes

Adapted from Huchon GJ, Woodhead MA, Gialdroni-Grassi G, et al: Guidelines for management of adult community-acquired lower respiratory tract infections. Eur Respir Rev 11:986-991, 1998.

and blood cultures. Risk factors for unusual microorganisms are summarized in Table 23.3.

Typical versus Atypical Pneumonia

A traditional approach divides patients with pneumonia into those with typical and those with atypical manifestations, leading to the prescription of different antibiotics for each of these conditions. Typical pneumonia is characterized by an abrupt onset, high fever, chills, productive cough, thoracic pain, focal clinical signs, lobar or segmental radiographic findings, leukocytosis, and sputum Gram stain that is positive for bacteria, frequently of a single predominant type. Typical pneumonias are generally thought to be due to extracellular bacteria such as *S. pneumoniae*, *Streptococcus pyogenes*, and *H. influenzae*.

Atypical pneumonias are characterized by a progressive onset, fever without chills, dry cough, headache, myalgia, diffuse crackles, modest leukocytosis, interstitial infiltrates on chest radiograph, sputum Gram stain (and possibly culture) that is negative for bacteria, and possibly an upper respiratory tract infection. Atypical pneumonias are thought to be due to intracellular bacteria or to viruses. Unfortunately, pneumonia due to viruses and intracellular bacteria may also present with symptoms and signs consistent with typical pneumonia, and vice versa. Accordingly, many suggest that this classification scheme is of minor value.

Aspiration Pneumonia

Mendelson originally described the syndrome of aspiration of gastric contents in 1946 in 61 obstetric patients who developed aspiration pneumonia after ether anesthesia. Manifestations begin very rapidly after the event and include cough (dry or with pink sputum because of bronchoalveolar hemorrhage), tachypnea, tachycardia, fever, diffuse crackles, cyanosis, and bronchospasm in some cases. Chest radiographs show extensive atelectasis and infiltrates, and arterial blood gas tensions show hypoxemia and normo- or hypocapnia. In the most severe cases, the $PaCO_2$ may be elevated, and a metabolic acidosis may be present.

A number of clinical features help distinguish aspiration pneumonia from other CAPs. Aspiration pneumonia tends to have a more insidious course, such that the patient may have an empyema, lung abscess, or necrotizing pneumonia at the time medical care is first sought. The sputum may be putrid because of anaerobic bacteria, and weight loss is common. Chest imaging commonly shows necrotizing infiltrates or multiple abscesses, typically located in dependent regions (Figure 23.1).

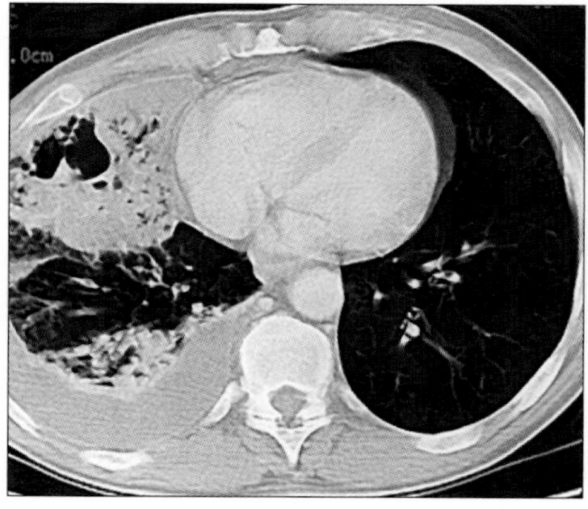

Figure 23.1 Necrotizing aspiration pneumonia. Chest computed tomography demonstrates involvement of the entire right middle lobe (which suggests pulmonary gangrene) and an effusion, which was found to be an empyema.

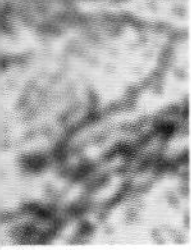

Lung Abscess

The incidence of pulmonary abscess has decreased over the last decade. Lung abscess is associated with several conditions, including poor dental status or periodontal disease, chronic alcoholism, intravenous drug use, and head and neck cancer. Lung abscess may complicate bronchiectasis (Figure 23.2) and the course of aspiration pneumonia in those with impaired consciousness, dysphagia and gastroesophageal reflux, or acute or chronic neurologic diseases, but it may also occur with bronchial obstruction by a foreign body or bronchial carcinoma.

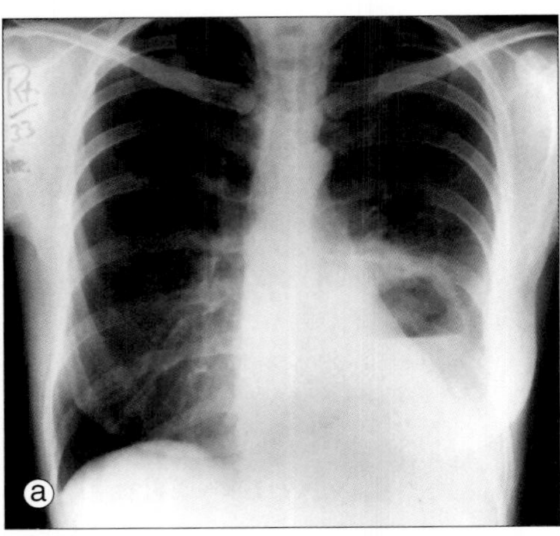

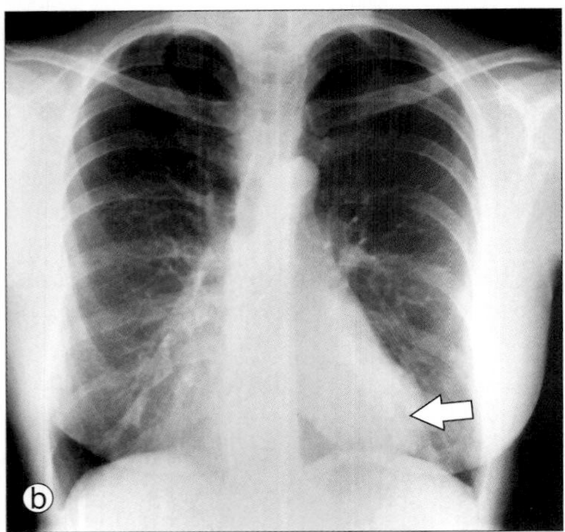

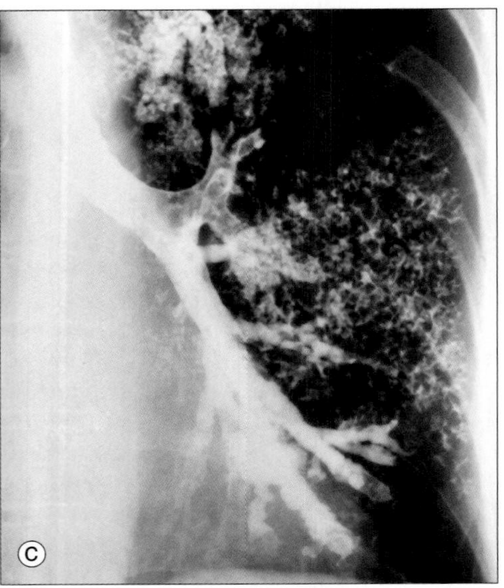

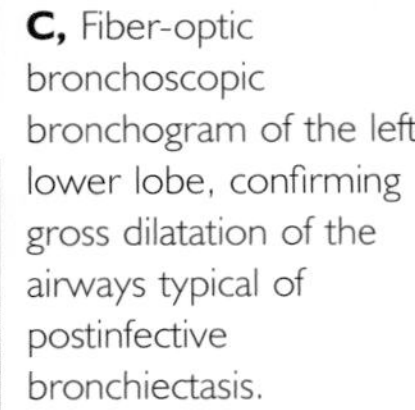

Figure 23.2 Left lower lobe pneumonia. A, Lung abscess associated with lower lobe pneumonia. **B,** Chest radiograph 3 months after resolution of the lung abscess, showing widened airways with thickened walls in the left lower lobe *(arrow)*. These bronchiectatic changes were consequent to the pneumonia. **C,** Fiber-optic bronchoscopic bronchogram of the left lower lobe, confirming gross dilatation of the airways typical of postinfective bronchiectasis.

Pulmonary abscesses are usually polymicrobial, with a predominant anaerobic flora such as *Streptococcus intermedius, Streptococcus salivarius, Streptococcus constellatus, Fusobacterium* species, *Prevotella* species, or *Bacteroides* species.

Clinical manifestations usually develop insidiously, particularly before necrosis develops. This period may last several weeks after an initial aspiration. When the lung abscess is diagnosed, patients may have lost weight and have a high fever, chills, putrid expectoration, and chest pain. Pleural involvement with an empyema is a frequent complication of lung abscess. Laboratory findings include a very high white cell count and considerable elevation of inflammatory and catabolic markers.

Radiologic features of lung abscess are typically a peripheral cavity more than 2 cm in diameter in the dependent lung regions. Computed tomography (CT) is useful to distinguish empyema with bronchopleural fistula from lung abscess.

Sputum Gram stain is often misleading. Bronchoscopic sampling such as bronchial aspirate, protected specimen brush, or bronchoalveolar lavage (BAL) should be performed onto anaerobic media. Percutaneous fluoroscopic or ultrasound- or CT-guided fine-needle aspiration may be a useful diagnostic technique. Aspirates should be grown on anaerobic media, and samples should be sent rapidly to the laboratory for specific anaerobic cultures.

Specific Pathogens

STREPTOCOCCUS *SPECIES*

S. pneumoniae is the most common bacterium isolated from patients with CAP. It is a saprophyte of the respiratory tract, which can easily proliferate as soon as natural defenses decline (as with increasing age, alcoholism, diabetes, smoking, immunosuppression). Classically, the onset is abrupt, characterized by intense and prolonged chills and considerable thoracic pain. Symptoms are rapidly progressive, with fever close to 40°C (104°F), tachycardia, and tachypnea; cough is common, as are oliguria and cyanosis. At this stage, a nasolabial herpes simplex lesion may develop, crackles are heard, and chest radiographs show homogeneous lobar or segmental consolidation. Without antibiotic treatment, cough persists and leads to rust-colored sputum. Leukocytosis is frequent, and blood cultures are positive in 10% to 20% of patients if these are obtained before antibiotic therapy. Arterial blood gas tensions show decreases in PaO_2 and $PaCO_2$. A symptom recrudescence can occur after a few days; then the body temperature falls abruptly to 37°C (98.6°F) and an abundant diuresis occurs. Radiologic and physical signs characteristically improve rapidly and considerably. The rapid rate of multiplication of *S. pneumoniae*, together with the high risk of secondary complications (e.g., empyema, meningitis, septicemia), make any *S. pneumoniae* pneumonia a medical emergency.

Streptococcus species other than *S. pneumoniae* rarely cause pneumonia, but among these, *S. pyogenes* is most often involved, more in the young than in the elderly. Pneumonia caused by *S. pyogenes* occurs after viral infections such as measles, varicella, or rubella in infants and following influenza, measles, or varicella in adults. The clinical presentation is that of typical pneumonia.

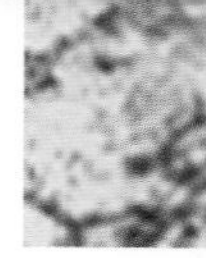

Pleural effusion and empyema frequently develop, and other complications include pneumothorax, pericarditis, mediastinitis, and bronchopleural fistula.

HAEMOPHILUS INFLUENZAE

Most invasive infections of *H. influenzae* result from encapsulated, typeable strains rather than from nonencapsulated, nontypeable strains. A history of upper respiratory tract infection is common. Small pleural effusions can occur, but empyema and cavitation are rare.

MYCOPLASMA PNEUMONIAE

Mycoplasma pneumoniae pneumonias usually occur in small epidemics, particularly in closed populations. The clinical presentation is commonly that of an atypical pneumonia, as described earlier. *M. pneumoniae* infections mimic, to some extent, the presentation of viral respiratory infections, but the incubation period is longer (10 to 20 days) than for viruses, and the fever is generally less than 39°C (102.2°F). Within a few days most symptoms improve, although the low-grade fever and cough frequently persist. A history of a preceding upper respiratory tract infection may be found in up to 50% of patients. A variety of extrapulmonary manifestations may be encountered, including arthralgia, cervical lymphadenopathy, bullous myringitis, diarrhea, immune hemolytic anemia, meningitis, meningoencephalitis, myalgia, myocarditis, hepatitis, nausea, pericarditis, skin eruptions, and vomiting. Diffuse crackles are occasionally heard. Infiltrates are usually localized in the lower lobes and regress very slowly over 4 to 6 weeks. Pleural effusions and mediastinal lymphadenopathy are rare.

CHLAMYDIA *SPECIES*

Psittacosis is a pneumonia caused by an intracellular bacterium, *Chlamydia psittaci*, which is responsible for ornithosis in the domestic fowl. *C. psittaci* can be transmitted to humans by inhalation from infected birds, including canaries, parakeets, parrots, pigeons, and turkeys. The clinical presentation is that of an atypical pneumonia. After 7 to 14 days' incubation, the onset might be abrupt. Fever of 38°C to 40°C (100.4°F to 104.0°F), possibly with chills, is associated with arthralgia, headache, myalgia, dyspnea, and thoracic pain. Cough may be severe, and sputum, if any, is usually mucoid. Splenomegaly and a macular rash are evocative of psittacosis. The radiologic appearance is variable but typically shows lower lobe infiltration. Hepatitis, phlebitis, encephalitis, myocarditis, renal failure, and intravascular coagulation are unusual complications. Despite the efficiency of antibiotics such as tetracycline and erythromycin, psittacosis is associated with a mortality of approximately 1%. Relapse is prevented by 2 weeks' treatment after return to a normal temperature.

Previously known as the TWAR agent, *Chlamydia pneumoniae* has been recognized as a pathogen responsible for pneumonia since 1985. The incidence of pneumonia due to *C. pneumoniae* is uncertain. The clinical presentation is that of an atypical pneumonia in young adults; in the elderly, the course may be severe, particularly if comorbidities are present. Sore throat may precede the appearance of fever (37.7°C to 39°C [100°F to 102.2°F]) and a nonproductive cough. The chest radiograph shows subsegmental infiltrates, which usually clear over 2 to 4 weeks.

LEGIONELLA PNEUMOPHILA

Legionella species are aerobic gram-negative intracellular bacilli; approximately 30 species have been identified, the most common being *L. pneumophila*. Water and air-conditioning systems are their natural reservoirs; spreading of the bacilli occurs by air, but no transmission between human beings has been reported. *L. pneumophila* infection may cause an asymptomatic seroconversion, a single episode of pyrexia, and mild to severe pneumonia. Pontiac fever has been associated with fever, chills, headache, and upper respiratory tract symptoms. Pneumonia occurs either sporadically or in small epidemics and is more likely to occur in immunocompromised hosts. After 2 to 8 days of incubation, headache, myalgia, high fever, and chills precede pneumonia by a few days. Initially there is a nonproductive cough that may become productive of watery or even purulent sputum. Dyspnea, hemoptysis, and chest pain frequently occur. Extrapulmonary symptoms and signs are numerous and include abdominal pain, agitation, watery diarrhea, arthralgia, confusion, skin rash, headache, hematuria, hyponatremia, hypophosphatemia, myalgia, nausea, oliguria, proteinuria, renal failure, seizures, splenomegaly, and vomiting. Leukocytosis, neutropenia, lymphopenia, and hepatic inflammation may be observed. The chest radiograph shows consolidation, often unilateral and dense, initially localized and then spreading gradually. Pleural effusion is frequently present; cavitation is rare. The outcome depends on the early clinical recognition and treatment and on comorbidities. Mortality is increased in immunosuppressed patients and in those who develop complications of the infection.

GRAM-NEGATIVE BACILLI

Gram-negative bacilli include various Enterobacteriaceae and Pseudomonadaceae, in particular *Klebsiella pneumoniae*, *Escherichia coli*, *Pseudomonas aeruginosa*, and *Acinetobacter* species. Gram-negative bacilli are more often responsible for nosocomial pneumonia than for CAP, but CAP attributable to these agents may result from their colonization of the oropharynx followed by inhalation or microaspiration of the organisms. Comorbidity is usual in patients acquiring these pneumonias. The clinical presentation is that of a typical pneumonia. The prognosis is poor, particularly in cases of immunodepression, alcoholism, neutropenia, and old age.

Friedländer's pneumonia *(K. pneumoniae)* typically occurs in men older than 40 years; alcoholism, diabetes mellitus, and chronic lung disease are predisposing factors. Historically, patients were thought to produce particularly large volumes of thick and bloody sputum; they were likely to present with prostration and hypotension and to have multiple patches of consolidation, particularly in the upper lobes, with bulging fissures (Figure 23.3) and multicavitation on chest radiographs (i.e., an expanding pneumonia).

E. coli pneumonia and *P. aeruginosa* pneumonia usually occur in chronically ill patients; hemoptysis is rare, and pneumonia usually involves the lower lobes. Abscess and empyema occur frequently. *Acinetobacter* pneumonia progresses very quickly, leading to severe hypoxemia, shock, bilateral consolidation, empyema, and even death within a few days.

Pseudomonas pseudomallei, which causes melioidosis, is an aerobic, gram-negative bacillus found in soil, vegetation, and water in tropical regions. Infection of the lung occurs more com-

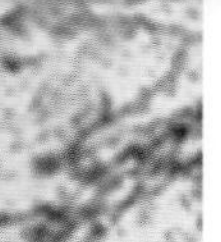

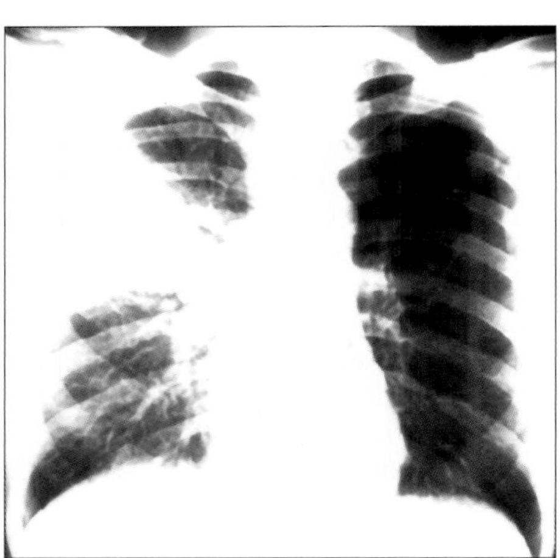

Figure 23.3 *Klebsiella* pneumonia. Chest radiograph showing a bulging fissure.

monly as a result of spread through the bloodstream after cutaneous infection than as a result of inhalation. The clinical presentation may be either acute or chronic. Acute melioidosis presents with high fever, dyspnea, chest pain, cough with purulent sputum, and hemoptysis. Local cellulitis and lymphangitis may be seen at the place of cutaneous inoculation. The chest radiograph shows diffuse miliary nodules, infiltrations, or cavitations. Chronic melioidosis may occur years after contracting the infection in the endemic area. Symptoms are either absent or may resemble those of pulmonary tuberculosis: asthenia, anorexia, weight loss, low-grade fever, productive cough, and hemoptysis. Chest radiographs show apical infiltrates, possibly with cavitations.

ANAEROBIC BACTERIA

Anaerobic bacterial pneumonia results from aspiration; therefore, it typically occurs in situations involving alcoholism, coma, seizure, and general anesthesia. Chronic dental infection; head, neck, and lung cancer; and bronchiectasis are additional risk factors. Anaerobic pneumonia begins as a typical pneumonia with pleuritic pain; pulmonary infiltrations preferentially involve the lower lobes, particularly the right lower lobe. If patients aspirate while lying supine, the segments involved are typically the posterior segment of the right upper lobe and the apical segment of the right lower lobe. Necrosis and suppuration follow, and fever higher than 39°C (102.2°F), dyspnea, and pleuritic pain persist. Sputum is purulent and fetid, which is often obvious on entering the patient's room. Leukocytosis is high, and segmental infiltrations with small transparent areas of necrosis are seen. Abscess and empyema occur frequently. The outcome is closely related to treatment—delay in antibiotic treatment or inappropriate antibiotic choice will probably result in necrotizing pneumonia, abscess, and empyema, which increases the fatality rate.

COXIELLA BURNETII

Coxiella burnetii is the causative agent of Q fever and is the most frequent pathogen responsible for pneumonia among the Rickettsiaceae. Ticks are vector agents, and various wild and domestic animals (cattle, sheep, goats) are infected with no evidence of disease; C. *burnetii* multiplies in the placenta of pregnant animals and spreads during parturition. Although C. *burnetii* is present in numerous species of ticks, the main route of transmission is by inhalation of infectious aerosols. C. *burnetii* is particularly resistant to chemical and physical agents. The clinical presentation is that of an atypical pneumonia. The onset occurs following a 2- to 4-week incubation period. Patients present with high fever (40°C [104°F]), chills, myalgia, and headache, all of which appear abruptly; cough is usually nonproductive. Abdominal and thoracic pain, pharyngitis, and bradycardia may also occur. There is usually no rash, in contrast with other rickettsial infections. Hepatomegaly and splenomegaly may be found on physical examination. The chest radiograph shows dense nodular infiltrates; pleural effusion and linear atelectasis may be seen. There is no leukocytosis, and mild hepatitis may be found. The course is usually benign.

STAPHYLOCOCCUS *SPECIES*

The severity of *Staphylococcus* infection is due to the prevalence of its resistance to multiple antibiotics and to lung tissue lysis as part of the infection, leading to bullae, rupture of bullae into the pleura (pneumothorax, pneumopyothorax), serious ventilatory defects, and septicemia. Staphylococcal infection occurs via the airways (inhalation, aspiration) or by hematogenous spread. Airborne contamination may follow a viral infection such as influenza or measles, or it may be linked to comorbidity (COPD, carcinoma, laryngectomy, seizure); hematogenous spread is the result of bacteremia (endocarditis, infective foci flowing into the bloodstream). Direct bloodstream infection due to intravenous drug abuse is the most common cause in many inner-city hospital emergency departments. The clinical presentation may be unusual compared with typical pneumonia when the infection develops via vascular dissemination (e.g., dyspnea, cough, and purulent sputum might be masked by symptoms of endocarditis or the primary infective focus) or when the infection is causing a pleural effusion, empyema, or lung abscess. The chest radiograph may show two possible features: central or segmental consolidation secondary to aspiration, or multiple infiltrates that are generally nodular early on and can subsequently progress to parenchymal consolidation with or without cavitation after vascular spread of the infection. Abscess, pleural effusion, and empyema are frequent, as well as septicemia. Overall outcome depends on associated diseases, spread of infection, and resistance of *Staphylococcus* to antibiotics.

NOCARDIA *SPECIES*

Nocardia asteroides and, to a lesser extent, *Nocardia brasiliensis* are responsible for most cases of *Nocardia* pneumonia. *Nocardia* are aerobic, gram-positive bacilli present mainly in soil. Approximately 50% of patients have no underlying disease. The others tend to have predisposing problems such as immunosuppression, malignancy, or long-term corticosteroid therapy. The onset of the infection is usually subacute, but it can be fulminant; in the latter case, there is a high fatality rate. Symptoms include fever, asthenia, anorexia, productive cough, and chest pain. Multiple subcutaneous abscesses may be present, as well as neurologic signs when there is central nervous system involvement. Chest radiograph abnormalities vary from infiltration to lobar consolidation; cavitation, nodules, abscesses, and pleural effusion may also be seen. The prognosis depends on whether the infection disseminates, but it is usually good in the case of isolated lung disease. Metastatic infection may occur anywhere but is particularly common in the central nervous system

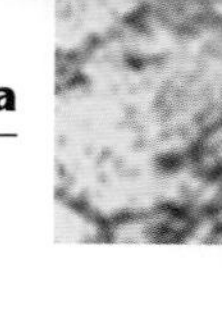

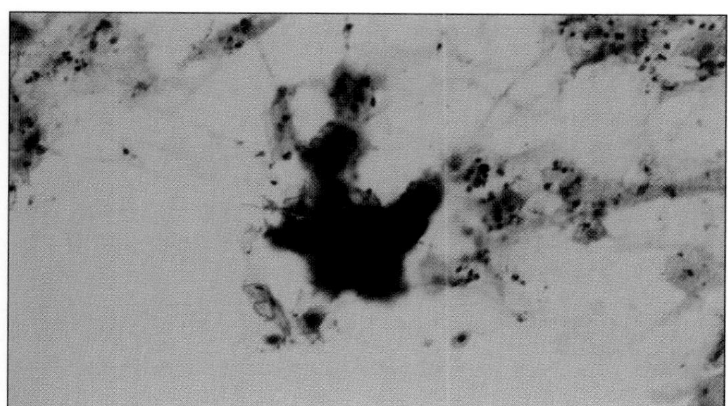

Figure 23.4 Sputum Gram stain showing actinomycetes (center).

and the skin. Infection may also reach the pleura and the chest wall.

ACTINOMYCES ISRAELII

Both *Actinomyces* species and *Arachnia* species can cause actinomycosis, but *Actinomyces israelii* is the main responsible organism. These are anaerobic, gram-positive, filamentous, branching bacilli (Figure 23.4) that were incorrectly thought to be fungi for many years. They normally reside in the oropharynx and become invasive pathogens when there is a defect in the anatomic barrier or when they are inhaled, at which time the infection may extend directly from one place to an adjacent area. Bad dentition, bronchiectasis, and COPD are risk factors for pulmonary infection. Men are far more frequently affected than women. The clinical presentation suggests tuberculosis, carcinoma, or chronic fungal infection; asthenia, anorexia, weight loss, and low-grade fever may precede cough and chest pain by months. Cervicofacial and thoracic involvement coexists rarely. When infection progresses to the pleural space and chest wall, the opening of a sinus tract may disclose pus. Radiographic features are variable and include small cavitary nodules confined to one segment; cavitary infiltration; extension of infection to the interlobar fissure, chest wall, bone, or pleura; and empyema.

PASTEURELLA MULTOCIDA

Pasteurella multocida is a gram-negative coccobacillus present in the oropharynx of mammals. It causes cutaneous infection in humans after animal bites. Pneumonia has been reported in patients with chronic pulmonary diseases. The clinical presentation is nonspecific and includes fever, cough, purulent sputum, and dyspnea. Chest radiographs show lower lobe infiltrates; pleural effusion and empyema may occur.

FRANCISELLA TULARENSIS

Francisella tularensis is a gram-negative bacillus found in various mammals and insects of the Northern Hemisphere. Tularemia occurs after the bite of, or contact with, an infected animal. The onset of pneumonia is abrupt; fever, chills and malaise precede dyspnea, cough, and chest pain. Painful ulceroglandular infection with adenopathy may be found at the site of bacterial inoculation. The chest radiograph shows signs of pneumonia, possibly with hilar adenopathy or pleural effusion.

YERSINIA PESTIS

Yersinia pestis or *Pasteurella pestis* is a short gram-negative rod that causes plague. It is a disease of rodents (squirrels, rabbits, rats) that is transmitted to humans by flea bites or by person-to-person contact via aerosol inhalation. Initial symptoms are chills, fever, prostration, delirium, headache, vomiting, and diarrhea. There are three forms of plague: bubonic, septicemic, and pneumonic. Bubonic plague consists of lymphadenopathy, with palpable masses forming in the cervical, axillary, femoral, and inguinal areas. Signs of septicemia are those of shock and petechial hemorrhages. Plague pneumonia results from either metastatic infection or inhalation of the pathogen. Pneumonia occurs within a week of initial exposure and is characterized by chest pain, productive cough, dyspnea, and hemoptysis. The chest radiograph shows lower lobe infiltrates, possibly nodules, lymphadenopathy, and pleural effusions.

BACILLUS ANTHRACIS

Bacillus anthracis is a large gram-positive rod that causes anthrax. *B. anthracis* is found in the soil, water, and vegetation and infects cows, sheep, and horses, which in turn infect humans after contact with contaminated materials. Fever and malaise usually appear progressively. Three forms of anthrax are found: cutaneous, intestinal, and pneumonic. Inoculation of *B. anthracis* into superficial wounds or skin abrasions causes cutaneous anthrax, which is characterized by a black crusted pustule on a large area of edema. Intestinal anthrax results from ingestion of contaminated material, and it can be severe. Pneumonic anthrax is due to inhalation of the contaminated material. Nonproductive cough and chest pain precede dyspnea, stridor, tachypnea, cyanosis, and edema of the neck and anterior chest. Peribronchovascular edema, enlargement of the mediastinum, and pleural effusions are usually seen on the chest radiograph.

BRUCELLA *SPECIES*

Brucella species are gram-negative coccobacilli found in the genitourinary tract of cows, pigs, goats, and dogs. Brucellosis results from contact with infected animals or from ingestion of unpasteurized milk products. The pathogen then spreads through the body via the bloodstream. General symptoms include fever, malaise, and headache. Hepatic enlargement and splenomegaly are common, as is lower back pain. Respiratory symptoms are less frequent than abnormalities on the chest radiograph, which include nodules, miliary infiltrates, and lymphadenopathy.

MORAXELLA CATARRHALIS

Moraxella catarrhalis, formerly named *Branhamella catarrhalis*, is a gram-negative diplococcus that is commonly found in the oropharynx of normal subjects. *M. catarrhalis* pneumonia is seen in patients with underlying chronic diseases such as COPD, congestive heart disease, or malignancy. Symptoms and radiographic findings are nonspecific. Leukocytosis is common, and the course is usually favorable.

DIAGNOSIS

History

The approach to the diagnosis of patients with CAP depends almost entirely on a careful history and physical examination that focus on the possibility that the infection may be the result

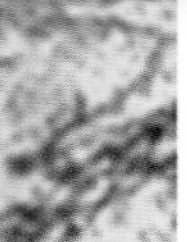

of unusual pathogens (e.g., exposure to birds or parturient animals, recent foreign travel). The infection must also be considered in the context of the individual patient (e.g., recent influenza or varicella infection, oropharyngeal colonization with gram-negative rods in nursing home patients, occupations or hobbies involving animal exposures). Finally, the chest radiograph must be examined for findings that suggest other than common pathogens (e.g., abscess, effusion, adenopathy, cavitation). When the clinical presentation suggests an unusual pathogen, every attempt should be made to obtain a bacteriologic diagnosis. In the absence of this suspicion, the value of bacteriologic studies is unclear.

Bacteriology

There are various ways to obtain an etiologic diagnosis. Blood culture specimens (with more than two needle sticks performed at separate sites) should be obtained from patients who require hospital admission for acute pneumonia. If a pleural effusion is present, pleural fluid should be collected for examination and culture. The value of Gram staining of expectorated sputum is controversial, but it is recommended in consensus statements on inpatient care. A sputum specimen should be obtained by a deep cough before antibiotic therapy; it should then be rapidly transported and processed in the laboratory within a few hours of collection.

Routine laboratory tests should include Gram staining, cytologic screening, and aerobic culture of specimens that satisfy cytologic criteria. Cytologic criteria for judging the acceptability of specimens include the relative number of polymorphonuclear cells (PMN) and squamous epithelial cells (SEC) in patients with normal or elevated white blood cell counts, determined by a low-power-field (LPF) examination; the acceptable values range from >25 PMN + <10 SEC/LPF to <25 SEC/LPF. Cultures should be performed rapidly. Interpretation of expectorated sputum cultures should include clinical correlations and semiquantitative results.

Numerous studies support the use of routine microscopic examination of Gram-stained sputum samples, with lancet-shaped, gram-positive diplococci suggestive of *S. pneumoniae.* Most show that the sensitivity of sputum Gram staining for patients with pneumococcal pneumonia is 50% to 60%, and the specificity is greater than 80%.

Routine cultures of expectorated sputum are neither sensitive nor specific when the common bacteriologic methods of many laboratories are used. The most likely explanation for unreliable microbiologic data is that the patient is unable to cough up a reliable specimen. Other reasons include prior administration of antibiotics, delays in processing the specimen, insufficient attention to separating sputum from saliva before smearing slides or culture plates, and difficulty with interpretation because of contamination by flora of the oral cavity and upper airways. In cases of bacteremic pneumococcal pneumonia, *S. pneumoniae* may be isolated in sputum culture in only 40% to 50% of cases when standard microbiologic techniques are used. The yield of *S. pneumoniae* is substantially higher from transtracheal aspirates, transthoracic needle aspirates, and quantitative cultures of BAL aspirates .

The utility of induced sputum specimens for detecting pulmonary pathogens other than *Pneumocystis jiroveci, L. pneumophila,* or *Mycobacterium tuberculosis* is poorly established.

Serologic tests are usually not helpful for the initial evaluation of patients with CAP but may provide useful data for epidemiologic surveillance. Most laboratories request a follow-up (paired) serum sample 10 to 14 days later.

Cold agglutinins in a titer greater than 1:64 support the diagnosis of *M. pneumoniae* infection with a sensitivity of 30% to 60%, but this test has poor specificity. Immunoglobulin M antibodies to *M. pneumoniae* require up to 1 week to reach diagnostic titers; reported results for sensitivity are variable. The serologic responses to *Chlamydia* and *Legionella* species take even longer, and the acute antibody test for *Legionella* in legionnaires' disease is usually negative or demonstrates a low titer only.

There are numerous reasons for not routinely undertaking a sputum examination in patients with LRTI:

- The study is difficult to perform in the outpatient setting.
- Results are nonspecific and of questionable sensitivity.
- Antibiotic treatment, if needed, has to be started before the result are obtained, based on the pathogens that are likely to be responsible for pneumonia in the community.

In most studies, no microorganisms are found in up to 50% of outpatients investigated for CAP. Viruses are found in approximately 10%; *S. pneumoniae* in 25%; *H. influenzae* in 7%; *Mycoplasma, Legionella,* and *Chlamydia* species in 10%; and gram-negative bacteria and *S. aureus* in only 1%. In hospitalized patients with CAP, gram-negative bacteria and *S. aureus* strains are more frequent (Figure 23.5).

SPECIFIC PATHOGENS

Chest radiographs in patients with *H. influenzae* pneumonia often show a peribronchial distribution of infiltrates (e.g., bronchopneumonia), as opposed to the more peripheral lobar or segmental consolidations seen with *S. pneumoniae*. The sensitivity and specificity of this distinction are low, however.

In *M. pneumoniae* infections, the leukocyte count is usually normal, although mild to moderate leukocytosis can occur. Cold

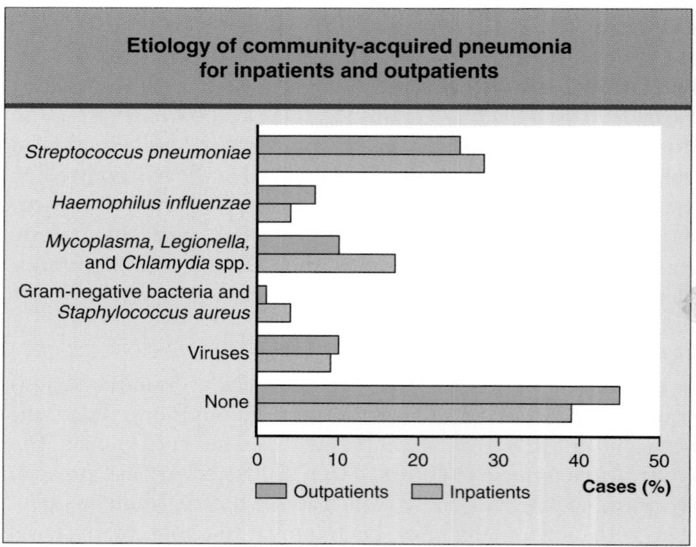

Figure 23.5 Community-acquired pneumonia. Cause in outpatients and in those requiring hospital admission.

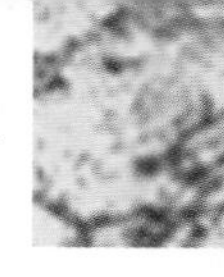

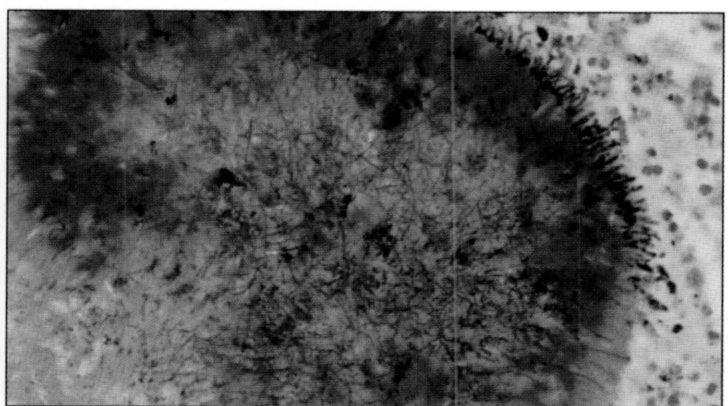

Figure 23.6 Sulfur granule seen in actinomycosis. Gram stain of sputum sample.

agglutinins are frequently present. The diagnosis can be made by acute and convalescent blood serologic testing. Despite a favorable response to therapy, *M. pneumoniae* may persist in the oropharynx for 1 to 3 months, during which time it may be transmissible to others.

The diagnosis of C. *pneumoniae*, C. *psittaci*, and Q fever is based on acute and convalescent blood serologies obtained 2 to 6 weeks apart.

Legionella pneumonia may be diagnosed within a few hours by direct immunofluorescence studies on respiratory tract specimens (e.g., sputum or tracheobronchial aspirates) or on urine; respiratory tract specimens can be analyzed by a DNA probe and can be cultured. A fourfold increase in the antibody titers can be seen on two samples obtained within 2 months.

Bacteriologic diagnosis of anaerobic infections depends on the type of specimen and the quality of the anaerobic transport medium; various gram-negative and gram-positive agents are found, sometimes in conjunction with aerobic pathogens.

The pus in sinus tracts caused by *Actinomyces* contains sulfur granules that are made up of mineralized 2-mm yellow granules composed of *Actinomyces* or *Arachnia*. When examined by Gram stain, these appear as dense aggregates of the organism (Figure 23.6). Microbiologic diagnosis relies on the characterization of the pathogens in specimens from biopsy, exudate, or pus, using histopathologic evaluation and culture in anaerobic conditions.

Tularemia is diagnosed by serologic testing on paired serum specimens.

Microbiologic diagnosis of *Y. pestis* and *B. anthracis* is made on blood, sputum, or lymph node aspirate culture, using routine bacteriologic or fluorescent antibody staining techniques.

A titer of *Brucella* agglutinins equal to or greater than 1:160 indicates active brucellosis.

A diagnosis of *P. pseudomallei* is made when the organism is cultured from respiratory tract secretions, cutaneous lesions, or blood or when serologic tests are positive.

TREATMENT

Severity and Admission to Hospital

When a diagnosis of pneumonia is suspected, one of the important first steps is to evaluate severity and determine whether the patient needs hospital care.

Severe CAP is defined as the presence of one of two major criteria, or the presence of two of three minor criteria. The major criteria are:

- Need for mechanical ventilation
- Septic shock

The minor criteria are:

- Systolic blood pressure 90 mmHg (12 kPa) or lower
- Multilobar disease
- PaO_2/FIO_2 ratio 250 or lower

Patients who have two of the four criteria from the 2001 British Thoracic Society guidelines also have more severe illness and should be considered for admission to the intensive care unit. These criteria are:

- Respiratory rate 30 breaths/minute or higher
- Diastolic blood pressure 60 mmHg (7.9 kPa) or lower
- Blood urea nitrogen 7.0 mM (19.1 mg/dL) or greater
- Confusion

Criteria suggested by the European Respiratory and American Thoracic Societies are shown in Figure 23.7.

Empirical Antibiotic Therapy

The initial antibiotic choice for CAP is empirical for the following reasons:

- In at least half the cases, responsible organisms will not be isolated using even the most sophisticated methods.
- All the guidelines for the management of patients presenting with CAP suggest that antibiotic treatment should be started as early as possible, without waiting for microbiologic results (if such investigations are performed). Delaying treatment increases the risk of complications and mortality, whereas correctly chosen empirical therapy improves outcome.
- Studies have shown that clinical data and radiologic findings, together with an assessment of comorbidity, risk factors for complications, and the severity of CAP, are sufficient for appropriate decisions regarding the choice of antibiotics and the necessity of hospital admission.

ANTIBIOTIC SELECTION

Table 23.4 summarizes antibiotic activity against bacteria that cause CAP. For patients with no risk factors who do not require hospitalization, an oral beta-lactam antibiotic should be prescribed when the clinical presentation is consistent with *S. pneumoniae* or other bacteria associated with typical pneumonias. When the clinical presentation is consistent with an atypical pneumonia, a macrolide is recommended. Aminopenicillins have the advantage of being active against most extracellular bacteria, including *S. pneumoniae*, and against a few intracellular bacteria.

In patients with risk factors, an aminopenicillin associated with a beta-lactamase inhibitor, or a second-generation cephalosporin, is indicated, possibly in conjunction with a macrolide or a fluoroquinolone (if there is a possibility of infection by intracellular agents). New quinolones are likely to be of great benefit because they are active against *S. pneumoniae*, including penicillin-resistant strains and most intra- and extracellular pathogens causing CAP.

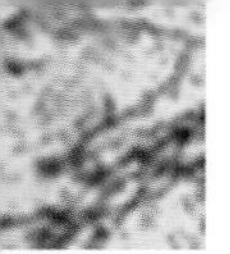

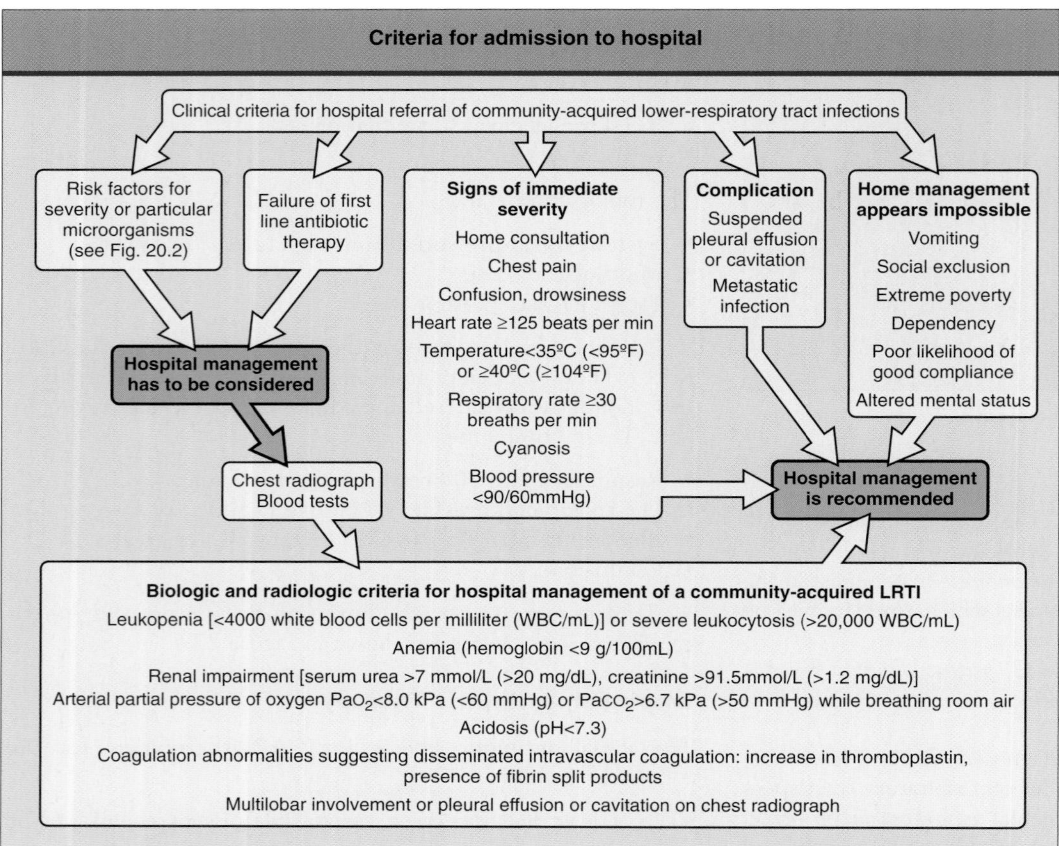

Figure 23.7 Criteria for admission to hospital. Biologic and radiologic investigations may be performed in patients referred to the hospital or in outpatients (depending, in part, on the local health care system and facilities), according to the criteria listed in Table 23.2. (Adapted from Huchon GJ, Woodhead MA, Gialdroni-Grassi G, et al: Guidelines for management of adult community-acquired lower respiratory tract infections. Eur Respir Rev 11:986-991, 1998.)

Local resistance patterns of microorganisms to antibiotics obviously must be taken into account when choosing the appropriate medication, and studies document that patterns of resistance can vary markedly. A decrease in the sensitivity of *S. pneumoniae* to penicillin was found in 41% of strains isolated in France in 1999, in 33% of strains in Spain in 1992, and in 25% to 35% of strains in the United States in 1997. Resistance of *S. pneumoniae* to macrolides was present in 42% of strains in France in 1999 and 14% of strains in Spain in 1992. In the United States, the proportion of isolates resistant to three or more classes of antibiotics increased from 9% to 14% between 1995 and 1998; there were also increases in the proportions of isolates that were resistant to penicillin (from 21% to 25%), cefotaxime (from 10% to 14%), erythromycin (from 11% to 15%), and trimethoprim-sulfamethoxazole (from 25 % to 29%).

The recommended strategy for choosing first-line antibiotics is summarized in Figure 23.8.

The recommended duration of antibiotic treatment for CAP is 1 week when the infection is due to extracellular organisms and 2 weeks when it is thought to be due to intracellular infection. Because they have a prolonged effect, macrolides such as azithromycin could be used for a shorter period; however, there is currently no definitive answer about the possible risk associated with shortening the duration of treatment.

Severe Bacterial Pneumonia

Bacterial pneumonia is also considered to be severe when it is accompanied by extension outside the lung parenchyma, when lung necrosis or septicemia develops, or when it occurs in patients with comorbid diseases. In these instances, it is much more important to establish a specific bacteriologic diagnosis. Antibiotic should initially be administered intravenously, and the choice of medication should include a consideration of the drug's diffusion into lung parenchyma, iatrogenic risks, and contraindications related to hepatic or renal function. Because *L. pneumophila* pneumonias may be severe and are frequently associated with diarrhea, they need to be treated with intravenous regimens that provide good intracellular penetration (e.g., erythromycin 3 to 4 g/24 hours, pefloxacin 800 mg/24 hours, and rifampicin 1200 mg/24 hours).

Patients with *Actinomyces* infections should be treated for prolonged periods (up to 6 months). The choice of antibiotics to treat *Nocardia* should be based on in vitro susceptibility testing. Duration of treatment (usually not less than 6 weeks) and drainage of purulent collections are critical factors affecting outcome.

Mendelson's Syndrome (Aspiration of Gastric Contents)

The lower airways are suctioned as soon as possible after aspiration has occurred. When solid material is aspirated, fiber-optic bronchoscopy is useful in an attempt to remove as much of the material as possible by direct suctioning. The rigid bronchoscope may be more effective. Tracheobronchial lavage with buffering solutions has little effect on the course of the disease, because aspirated acids are rapidly neutralized by the outpouring of plasma that occurs in response to the chemical injury. Intravascular volume support may be needed. Fever, purulent secretions,

Table 23.4
Antibiotics active against bacteria responsible for pneumonia

Bacteria	Antibiotics
Acinetobacter spp.	Aminoglycosides and piperacillin Aminoglycosides and imipenem
Actinomyces spp.	Penicillins
Anaerobes	Clindamycin Penicillin and metronidazole Cefoxitin Aminopenicillin and penicillinase inhibitor Imipenem
Bacillus anthracis	Penicillins Chloramphenicol Erythromycin Tetracyclines
Brucella	Streptomycin Trimethoprim–sulfamethoxazole
Chlamydia burnetii	Tetracyclines Chloramphenicol
Chlamydia pneumoniae	Tetracyclines Macrolides Quinolones
Chlamydia psittaci	Tetracyclines Chloramphenicol
Chlamydia trachomatis	Macrolides Sulfisoxazole
Coxiella burnetii	Tetracyclines Chloramphenicol
Francisella tularensis	Aminoglycosides Tetracyclines Chloramphenicol

Bacteria	Antibiotics
Gram-negative enterobacteria, including *Klebsiella pneumoniae* and *Haemophilus influenzae*	Aminoglycosides and cephalosporins Aminoglycosides and aminopenicillins Cephalosporins (third generation) Clarithromycin Azithromycin Quinolones Aminopenicillin and penicillinase inhibitor Chloramphenicol Trimethoprim–sulfamethoxazole
Legionella	Macrolides Trimethoprim–sulfamethoxazole Tetracyclines Quinolones
Moraxella catarrhalis	Cephalosporins Aminopenicillin and penicillinase inhibitor Erythromycin Tetracyclines Quinolones Trimethoprim–sulfamethoxazole
Mycoplasma pneumoniae	Macrolides Tetracyclines Quinolones
Neisseria meningitidis	Penicillin Cephalosporins (third generation) Chloramphenicol

Bacteria	Antibiotics
Nocardia	Trimethoprim–sulfamethoxazole Aminopenicillins Amikacin
Pasteurella multocida	Penicillins Tetracyclines Chloramphenicol
Pseudomonas aeruginosa	Aminoglycosides and piperacillin Aminoglycosides and ceftazidime Aminoglycosides and aztreonam Aminoglycosides and cefoperazone
Pseud. pseudomallei	Tetracyclines Ceftazidime Sulfonamides Chloramphenicol Kanamycin
Rhodococcus equi	Vancomycin Erythromycin Chloramphenicol Rifampin (rifampicin)
Staphylococcus aureus	Oxacillin Cephalosporins (first generation) Methicillin Vancomycin and rifampin
Streptococcus spp.	Penicillins Macrolides Cephalosporins (first generation) Vancomycin
Streptococcus pneumoniae	Penicillins Macrolides Cephalosporins (first generation)
Yersinia pestis	Streptomycin Tetracyclines

leukocytosis, and new pulmonary infiltrates may develop in the absence of infection. Accordingly, prophylactic antibiotics are not generally used; they do not appear to modify the course of the disease and may predispose to resistant bacteria. The decision when to begin antibiotics is based on clinical suspicion that a secondary bacterial infection has developed. Trials of corticosteroids have been disappointing.

Aspiration Pneumonia

Antibiotics are selected for their activity against anaerobic bacteria. Choices include amoxicillin plus clavulanate (because up to 40% of anaerobic bacteria produce beta-lactamase), penicillin or amoxicillin plus metronidazole, or clindamycin. The increased risk of *Clostridium difficile* infection with clindamycin has led some investigators to suggest that it be given only to patients who have evidence of necrotizing pneumonia; in this group, the benefit of clindamycin over other treatments has been demonstrated.

When the areas of necrosis progress to involve the entire lobe, pulmonary gangrene must be considered. This condition is thought to result from thrombosis of the lobar pulmonary artery, such that the major blood supply to the lobe is lost. Older literature suggests that pulmonary gangrene should be treated with lobar resection or open drainage, because conservative treatment has been associated with increased mortality. There are, however, no studies to validate a surgical approach, which should probably only be recommended if sepsis and necrosis persist despite antibiotic therapy.

CLINICAL COURSE

The course of CAP is favorable in the large majority of cases. Fever declines over a few days, and the abnormalities seen on the chest radiograph generally begin to resolve in 1 to 3 weeks. Persistence of fever should prompt concern about the presence of a resistant organism, a complication such as cavitation or empyema, the development of a nosocomial pneumonia caused by a resistant organism, or drug-related fever. An additional concern is that poor resolution may be caused by the presence of a coexistent problem such as lung cancer, bronchial foreign body, bronchiectasis, or chronic infection of the upper respiratory tract.

Regarding gastric content aspiration, all the patients reported by Mendelson recovered rapidly, whereas subsequent studies demonstrated mortality rates as high as 60%. The discrepancy is probably because Mendelson's patients were healthy young

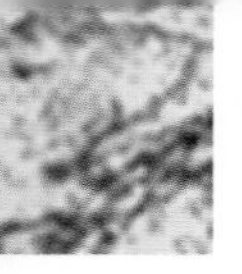

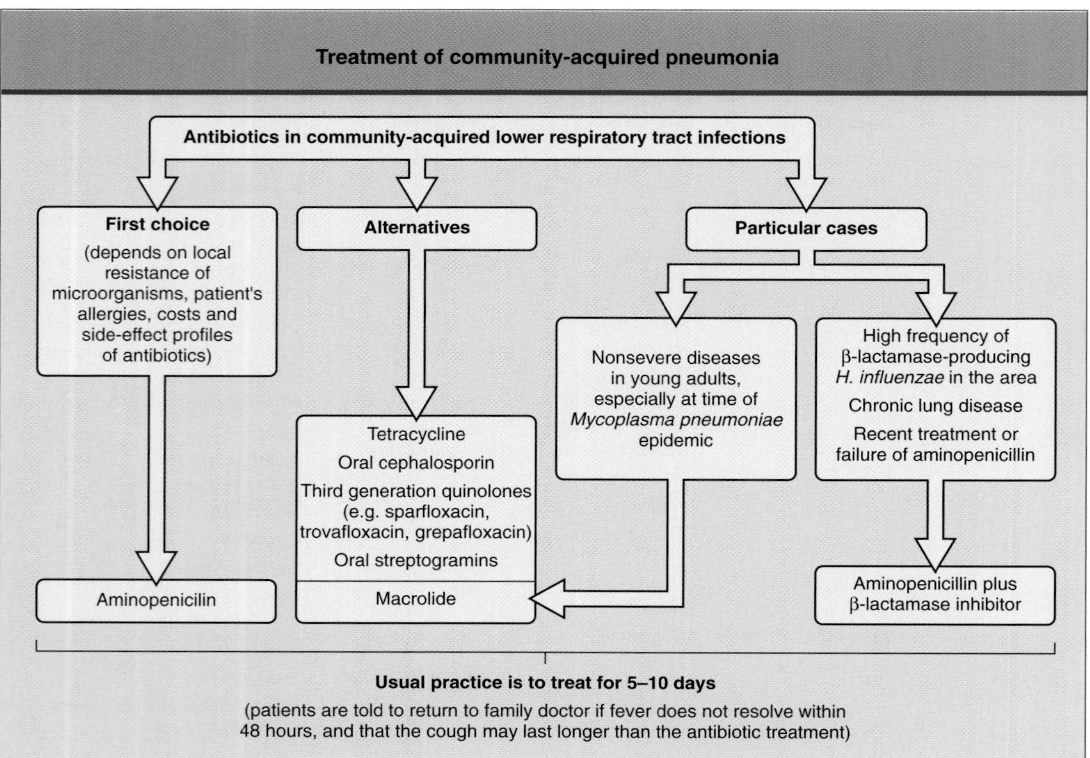

Figure 23.8 Treatment of community-acquired pneumonia. Choice of a first-line strategy should depend on the local resistance of microorganisms, the patient's allergies, and the costs and side-effect profiles of antibiotics. Patients should be told to return to the physician if the fever does not resolve within 48 hours. They should also be informed that the cough may last longer than the duration of antibiotic treatment. (Adapted from Huchon GJ, Woodhead MA, Gialdroni-Grassi G, et al: Guidelines for management of adult community-acquired lower respiratory tract infections. Eur Respir Rev 11:986-991, 1998.)

women, whereas later reports included patients who were older and had numerous comorbid illnesses. There are three patterns of response to gastric aspiration:

1. Rapid recovery (62%).
2. Rapid deterioration into acute respiratory distress syndrome (ARDS), with death within 24 hours (12%).
3. Initial recovery with subsequent development of fever and new infiltrates (26%), which suggests pulmonary superinfection, which may progress to ARDS.

When bacterial infection is demonstrated, the mortality increases by a factor of three.

COMPLICATIONS

Most cases of pneumonia resolve completely with appropriate antibiotic treatment and supportive care. However, a number of important complications may occur that require specific management. These include:

- Parapneumonic effusion
- Empyema
- Bronchopleural fistula
- Organizing pneumonia
- Bronchiectasis

Frequently, the diagnosis of these complications is delayed. Acute infective complications commonly present with a continuing pyrexia despite appropriate antibiotic therapy, but they may be more insidious, with or without a fever but with general ill health and continuing debility. The critical initial investigation is the chest radiograph. If an empyema or lung abscess is discovered, further imaging with CT or ultrasonography is often necessary.

Parapneumonic Effusion and Empyema

Pleural infection is a common disorder, with more than 65,000 cases in the United States and United Kingdom combined each year. It can be diagnostically challenging and carries an overall mortality of up to 20%, with a similar percentage requiring surgical intervention.

EPIDEMIOLOGY

Pleural infection affects patients of all ages but has a bimodal distribution, with peaks in childhood and old age. Men are affected twice as often as women. Its incidence is higher in those with diabetes, alcoholism and substance abuse, rheumatoid arthritis, and coincidental chronic lung disease. Diabetes is present in approximately 10% of patients, five times the background prevalence of this disease.

Three quarters of cases of complicated parapneumonic effusion and empyema follow CAP. The remainder result from hospital-acquired pneumonia, surgery, trauma, or iatrogenic insults. When the pleural infection is acquired in the hospital, the prognosis is worse. Hospital-acquired infections exhibit a microbiology that is strikingly different from that of community-acquired empyema and should probably be considered a different entity from both epidemiologic and therapeutic standpoints.

PATHOPHYSIOLOGY

There are three stages. The first is the exudative stage, in which an initial effusion is formed due to increased permeability of the pleural membranes. The accumulating pleural fluid has a normal glucose and pH level. No bacteria are detectable, and the effusion usually resolves spontaneously with antibiotic therapy for the underlying pneumonia.

The second, or fibropurulent, stage occurs when there is secondary bacterial invasion of the pleural space. The normal high levels of fibrinolytic activity are depressed, leading to fibrin deposition over the visceral and parietal pleura, with division of the pleural space by fibrinous septae. Bacterial metabolism and neutrophil phagocytic activity lead to increased lactic acid production and glucose utilization. A fall in pleural fluid pH and glucose level is the clinical hallmark of early transition to the infected state.

Finally, in the organizing stage, there is proliferation of fibroblasts and the evolution of pleural scarring. An inelastic peel forms on both pleural surfaces, with dense fibrous septations across the pleural cavity. As this solid fibrous peel replaces the soft fibrin, lung re-expansion is prevented, impairing lung function. In this stage, the only effective treatment is surgery.

PRESENTATION

The symptoms suggestive of a parapneumonic collection are increased breathlessness, swinging pyrexia, and raised inflammatory markers. The chest radiograph usually demonstrates the collection of fluid. A lateral chest radiograph or ultrasonography is useful to confirm the presence of fluid.

All pleural fluid should undergo Gram stain and culture, because the identification of significant bacterial cultures confirms the diagnosis of infection and aids in antibiotic choice. Unfortunately, about 40% of infected pleural effusions are culture negative, and in this situation, biochemical pleural fluid markers (pH, lactate dehydrogenase [LDH], white cell count [WCC], and glucose) are central to establishing a diagnosis. Based on a large meta-analysis, a pleural pH less than 7.2 is helpful in identifying pleural infection. This test should be performed routinely on any potentially infected pleural fluid.

BACTERIOLOGY

Approximately 40% of pleural infections are culture negative. Blood cultures are often the only source of positive culture and must be taken in all suspected cases. Pleural fluid is culture positive in half the cases, and the yield (particularly for anaerobic organisms) is substantially increased if blood culture bottles are used. Care must be taken, however, to ensure that the laboratory has a separate pleural fluid specimen to enable a Gram stain to be performed.

Hospital-acquired infections have a microbiology that is different from that of community-acquired empyema. Common organisms in community-acquired infection include, in order of frequency, *Streptococcus milleri* group, *S. pneumoniae*, *S. aureus*, Enterobacteriaceae, and anaerobes. In hospital-acquired infection, the most common cultured organism is *S. aureus*, with most of these being multiresistant *S. aureus*; *Enterococcus* species and Enterobacteriaceae are also commonly implicated.

Decisions about the length of treatment can be guided by repeated measurements of serum markers of the acute-phase reaction, such as C-reactive protein. The monitoring of fever lysis is also valuable, although elderly patients and those with indolent, often anaerobic empyema frequently fail to mount a fever; here, indices such as C-reactive protein are particularly helpful.

ANTIBIOTICS

The patient's clinical setting and the underlying cause of the empyema should inform the initial choice of antibiotic therapy. Antibiotics need to be given empirically while awaiting culture results. If the pleural infection is secondary to a community-acquired infection, community-acquired bacterial pathogens and anaerobic organisms should be covered. Suggested antibiotics in this setting include cefuroxime with metronidazole, or clindamycin with ciprofloxacin in penicillin- and cephalosporin-allergic individuals. In cases of hospital-acquired empyema, a broader spectrum of coverage is required for both gram-positive (including multiresistant *S. aureus*) and gram-negative aerobes, as well as anaerobes. Suggested antibiotics in this setting include vancomycin, cefuroxime, and metronidazole or vancomycin and meropenem.

NUTRITION

Adequate nutrition from the time of diagnosis is vital. Empyema patients characteristically suffer the protracted catabolic consequences of chronic infection, including immunodeficiency and slow recovery. In one series of 80 patients with infected pleural fluid, a low blood albumin level was the most important determinant of a fatal outcome. It is therefore essential to provide adequate nutritional support, which often requires nasogastric feeding.

DIFFERENTIAL DIAGNOSIS

Not all patients with a fever and an acidic, turbid pleural effusion have pleural infection. Pleural involvement occurs in up to 5% of patients with rheumatoid arthritis. They often present with pleuritis, raised inflammatory markers, and a markedly acidic pleural fluid with a low glucose level.

Pleural malignancy may also present with fever and an acidic pleural effusion. Here, the systemic inflammatory response is probably related to tumor-induced cytokine production. It may be impossible to resolve this differential diagnosis with certainty at presentation, and the patient should be treated for presumed infection until the correct diagnosis is established. Urgent cytology with or without pleural biopsy is appropriate in this setting.

In a patient with thick, opaque pleural fluid that is not malodorous, chylothorax and pseudochylous effusion enter the differential diagnosis. The diagnosis can usually be established by bench centrifuge of the pleural fluid. This leaves a clear supernatant in empyema, as the cell debris is separated; chylous and pseudochylous effusions remain milky. The diagnosis is confirmed by the measurement of pleural fluid triglyceride and cholesterol levels and by microscopy for cholesterol crystals.

Occasionally, pleural sepsis secondary to esophageal rupture can be confused with primary empyema, especially in the elderly, in whom the rupture may not be associated with a clear history of vomiting or chest pain. In these circumstances, the diagnostic clues include the presence of food particles in the pleural fluid, a raised pleural fluid amylase of salivary origin, and possibly the presence of a hydropneumothorax on the chest radiograph.

CHEST CATHETER DRAINAGE

The optimal catheter size for drainage of an infected pleural space remains contentious. Many consider a large-bore catheter

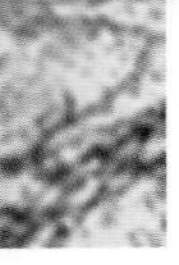

mandatory to enable high-viscosity pus to drain. However, smaller-bore catheters are less traumatic to insert and more comfortable for the patient.

A recent study suggests that children with pleural infection may leave the hospital more quickly if a flexible, small-bore catheter is used. In another study with more than 400 adult patients, there was no difference in outcome between the use of a large-bore tube versus drainage via a small flexible tube. However, in neither of these studies were the subjects randomized by drain size, so this debate will continue until randomized data are available to properly address this issue.

INTRAPLEURAL FIBRINOLYTICS

Introducing a fibrinolytic agent into the pleural space of a patient with a loculated pleural collection may improve drainage by breaking down the fibrin septae. Published randomized trials to date have shown that the use of these agents improves chest radiographs, but they have not shown whether there is less need for surgery or reduced mortality with this therapy. However, a large UK-based multicenter trial recently reported no reduction in mortality or need for surgery in patients given intrapleural streptokinase. Importantly, it should be noted that when streptokinase is given intrapleurally, streptokinase antibodies are produced systemically. Therefore, any patient who has received streptokinase intrapleurally should carry a card alerting physicians that if a fibrinolytic is needed to treat a subsequent myocardial infarction, intravenous streptokinase should be avoided.

SURGERY

Patients with late fibropurulent or organizing empyema often require surgery to establish complete drainage and adequate lung re-expansion. There are currently a number of surgical options available to achieve these goals, including open thoracotomy with decortication, mini-thoracotomy, video-assisted thoracoscopic surgery, and rib resection with open drainage.

Bronchopleural Fistula

A bronchopleural fistula is caused by a connection between the pleural space and the consolidated lung; it can complicate either an empyema or a lung abscess. The bronchopleural fistula causes a pyopneumothorax (i.e., air-fluid level in the pleural space), so that, on drainage of an empyema, not only pus but also air comes out through the chest drain. A bronchopleural fistula will not seal unless infection is controlled. Initial treatment is conservative, with antibiotics and tube drainage, to allow the fistula to seal. If this fails, surgery may be necessary to attempt primary closure of the fistula or closure of the potential space with other living tissues, such as muscle flaps. The management of bronchopleural fistulas that do not close with conservative treatment requires the surgical skills of a thoracic specialist.

Organizing Pneumonia

Organizing pneumonia, sometimes known as cryptogenic organizing pneumonia or bronchiolitis obliterans organizing pneumonia (BOOP), is a condition in which an organizing inflammatory exudate with fibroblast proliferation occurs after an episode of pneumonia. The consolidation is often patchy and may be fleeting. Organizing pneumonia following a bacterial infection is suggested when a residual consolidation (often fleeting) remains despite adequate antibiotic treatment. Investigation includes examination of sputum or bronchial washings to exclude infection. CT may help to visualize the consolidation and exclude other causes. The definitive investigation is an open lung biopsy showing the typical histologic appearance. If suspicion is great enough and the physician is confident of the diagnosis, a course of steroids usually leads to resolution. When the steroids are stopped, however, there may be a relapse; in this case, treatment for several months may be necessary (see Chapter 46).

Bronchiectasis

Permanent dilatation of the bronchus can occur following severe pneumonia, causing localized bronchiectasis. CT scanning during or after an episode of acute pneumonia may show bronchial dilatation, so the diagnosis cannot be made with confidence until after the pneumonia has completely resolved. The presence of bronchiectasis is suggested by continual cough productive of sputum or recurrent infections in one part of the lung. Investigation consists of sputum examination, when organisms associated with bronchiectasis such as *H. influenzae* or *P. aeruginosa* may be isolated. The diagnostic test of choice is a thin-section, high-resolution CT scan. Management consists of postural drainage of the infected lobe and antibiotic treatment for any acute infection. In patients who have coexisting airflow obstruction, treatment with bronchodilators or inhaled steroids may be helpful.

PREVENTION

There are various ways to prevent bacterial pneumonia, including the elimination of risk factors such as smoking and alcoholism and the use of vaccinations. Influenza vaccine is used in subjects older than 65 years, in those with chronic diseases, and in medical practitioners and nursing home employees. Pneumococcal vaccine is recommended in subjects older than 65 years and in younger patients with cardiovascular or pulmonary diseases, diabetes mellitus, alcoholism, cirrhosis, cerebrospinal fluid

Table 23.5
Prevention of aspiration pneumonias

Position (elevation of the head of the bed)
Prefer jejunostomy to nasogastric tube for enteral feeding
Monitoring gastric residue
H_2 blockers, gastric acid pump inhibitors (avoid antacids which may increase gastric fluid volume and cause pulmonary injury if aspirated)
Prokinetic agents (no conclusive data)?
Digestive decontamination in mechanically ventilated patients
Frequent upper airway suctioning in patients who have endotracheal tubes or tracheostomies
Gastric aspiration and awake endotracheal intubation for emergency general anesthetic?

Data from Pachon J, Prados MD, Capote F, et al: Severe community-acquired pneumonia: aetiology, prognosis and treatment. Rev Respir Dis 142:369-373, 1990; Fine MJ, Smith DN, Singer DE: Hospitalization in patients with community-acquired pneumonia: a prospective cohort study. Am J Med 89:713-721, 1990.

leak, and immunodepression (e.g., caused by HIV infection, chronic renal failure, organ transplantation, hematologic and lymphatic malignancies, asplenia, sickle-cell disease).

Steps for the prevention of aspiration pneumonia are summarized in Table 23.5 and should be applied in patients who have predisposing conditions. A number of surgical techniques have been advocated for patients who have anatomic abnormalities of the larynx or hypopharynx, including tracheostomy, cricopharyngeal myotomy, laryngeal suspension, cricoid resection, and vocal cord medialization. Aspiration of tube-fed patients can be detected by adding a food dye to the feeding formula and seeking evidence of its presence in tracheobronchial secretions, or by measuring the glucose content of the secretions. Neither of these approaches appears to be cost effective, however. Measuring the volume of residual gastric contents may help identify patients at risk (residual >100 to 200 mL).

(The section on parapneumonic effusion and empyema was written by R.N. Maskell.)

SUGGESTED READING

Bartlett JG, Dowell SF, Mandell LA, et al: Practice guidelines for the management of community-acquired pneumonia in adults. Guidelines from the Infectious Diseases Society of America. Clin Infect Dis 31:347-382, 2000.

British Thoracic Society: Guidelines for the management of community acquired pneumonia in adults. Thorax 56(S4):1-64, 2001.

Garau J, Gomez L: *Pseudomonas aeruginosa* pneumonia. Curr Opin Infect Dis 16:35-143, 2003.

Huchon GJ, Woodhead MA, Gialdroni-Grassi G, et al: Guidelines for management of adult community-acquired lower respiratory tract infections. Eur Respir Rev 11:986-991, 1998.

Johnson JL, Hirsch CS: Aspiration pneumonia. Recognizing and managing a potentially growing disorder. Postgrad Med 113:99-102, 105-106, 111-112, 2003.

Moss PJ, Finch RG: The next generation: fluoroquinolones in the management of acute lower respiratory infection in adults. Thorax 55:83-85, 2000.

Niederman MS, Ahmed OD: Community-acquired pneumonia in elderly patients. Clin Geriatr Med 19:101-120, 2003.

Niederman MS, Mandell LA, Anzueto A, et al: Guidelines for the management of adults with community-acquired pneumonia: diagnosis, assessment of severity, antimicrobial therapy, and prevention. Am J Respir Crit Care Med 163:1730-1754, 2001.

Reimer LG, Carroll KC: Role of the microbiology laboratory in the diagnosis of lower respiratory tract infections. Clin Infect Dis 26:742-748, 1998.

Stout JE, Yu VL: Legionellosis. N Engl J Med 377:682-687, 1997.

CHAPTER 24 Nonbacterial Pneumonia

Antoine Rabbat and Gérard J. Huchon

VIRAL PNEUMONIA

Although viral infections of the upper respiratory tract are common, viral pneumonia is rare in patients who are not immunocompromised, except for children and the elderly. Four major groups of viruses account for the large majority of viral pneumonias in immunocompetent children (Table 24.1).

Pneumonia accounts for 20% to 40% of viral lower respiratory tract infections in children. In adults, influenza is the most frequent cause of viral pneumonia, although respiratory syncytial virus (RSV) is also seen, and pneumonia may occur as part of systemic viral infections such as measles, chickenpox, and the hantaviruses. For each agent, epidemiology, risk factors, clinical features, diagnosis, treatment, clinical course, and prevention are considered.

Influenza Virus

Three types of influenza virus have been identified: A, B, and C. Type A is responsible for the most severe and widespread disease, and type C does not appear to be pathogenic. Major antigens of the virus envelope are hemagglutinin and neuraminidase (sialidase). In influenza A viruses, the former undergoes periodic changes, which may be major (resulting in antigenic shifts because of reassortments between strains, leading to an entirely new gene) or minor (resulting in antigenic drifts because of point mutations). Most of the host immune response is directed against hemagglutinin.

Influenza A and B viruses are responsible for at least 50% of the viral pneumonias encountered in immunocompetent adult subjects. Antigenic shifts are associated with pandemics when antigenic modifications lead to a decrease in the immunity of the community, whereas antigenic drifts are commonly associated with more limited epidemics. Outbreaks of severe disease occur every 10 to 30 years. During an outbreak, children are usually infected before adults (attack rates may reach 50% to 75%). The excess mortality because of influenza may be as high as 10,000 patients per year, and the economic consequences of outbreaks are considerable.

The host immune response involves both cellular and humoral defenses, as well as local antibody responses because of secretory immunoglobulin A (IgA). The result is mucosal inflammation that consists of hyperemia, edema, and, in severe cases, hemorrhage. Transmission is by respiratory secretions.

Pneumonia may occur directly after the acute illness (termed *primary pneumonia*, which is caused by the virus itself), or it may occur after a period of clinical improvement (*secondary pneumonia*, which results from bacterial superinfection, most commonly with *Streptococcus pneumoniae, Haemophilus influenzae*, or *Staphylococcus aureus*). Primary pneumonia seems to occur more commonly in association with conditions that result in increased left atrial pressure, whereas secondary pneumonia occurs mainly in older adults or in patients who have comorbid conditions, such as chronic cardiovascular or respiratory disease, diabetes mellitus, or chronic hepatic or renal failure.

A typical presentation includes the acute onset of cough, sore throat, conjunctival hyperemia, nasal discharge and congestion, fever, myalgia, headache, and malaise. Symptoms and findings of pneumonia are infrequent, and the disease is usually self-limited. Reappearance or worsening of respiratory symptoms and signs suggests pneumonia, but radiographic evidence of pneumonia may be found in the absence of such findings.

The typical radiographic findings of primary pneumonia are diffuse, interstitial, or patchy infiltrates. Secondary pneumonia may have a more segmental or lobar pattern. Primary and secondary pneumonia may occur in the same patient at the same time.

Indirect diagnosis is used primarily for epidemiologic purposes, as it requires two serologic assays performed 10 to 14 days apart. Direct diagnosis can be made by:

- Culture of respiratory secretions or lung tissue, a process that takes 2 to 5 days (less if antigen detection techniques are used).
- Immunofluorescence or enzyme-linked immunosorbent assay (ELISA) techniques on nasal or pharyngeal cells obtained by brushing or washing, a process that takes approximately 15 minutes.
- Antigen detection in respiratory secretions, a less sensitive but more rapid technique.

In addition to supportive care, treatment with specific antiviral therapy such as amantadine (100 mg/kg per day for 5 days) or rimantadine may be beneficial if administered early in the course of the disease (within 48 hours of symptom onset). Zanamivir and oseltamivir are related antiviral drugs with a similar mechanism of action and a similar rate of effectiveness against both influenza A and B viruses. Both are neuraminidase inhibitors; zanamivir is inhaled, and oseltamivir is given orally. Both drugs are approved for the treatment of influenza only in persons who have been symptomatic for less than 2 days. Clinical studies showed that the symptoms of influenza disappeared 1 to 1.5 days sooner in the drug-treated groups than in the placebo groups. Antibiotics active against *S. pneumoniae, H. influenzae*, and *S. aureus* are needed to treat patients who have secondary pneumonia.

The morbidity and mortality of influenza pneumonia are high, and patients can deteriorate to the point of developing acute res-

Table 24.1
Respiratory viruses that cause pneumonias in nonimmunocompromised hosts

	Influenza	Parainfluenza	Respiratory Syncytial Virus	Adenovirus
Family	Orthomyxoviridae	Paramyxoviridae	Paramyxoviridae	Adenoviridae
Genome	Single-stranded RNA	Single-stranded RNA	Single-stranded RNA	Double-stranded DNA
Envelope antigens	Hemagglutinin Sialidase	Hemagglutinin Sialidase Fusion Glycoprotein	Fusion glycoprotein Glycoprotein	250 capsomeres
Serotypes	Three (pathogenic in humans: A and B)	Four (pathogenic in humans: 1, 2, and 3)	Two (A and B)	50
Infected cells	Epithelial cells	Epithelial cells	Epithelial cells	Epithelial cells Lymphoid cells
Frequency among lower respiratory tract infections	Type A: 1–13% Type B: 1–9%	4–41%	6–63%	2–35%

Table 24.2
Epidemiologic and clinical characteristics of parainfluenza infection depending on the serotype

	Serotypes	
	1 and 2	**3**
Epidemiology	Epidemics during the fall	Endemic with increases during fall, winter, or spring
Clinical features	Croup (laryngotracheobronchitis); less severe with type 2	Bronchiolitis Pneumonia

piratory distress syndrome (ARDS). In such cases, the likelihood of developing a secondary pneumonia is high.

Inactivated influenza vaccines are modified each year to follow the antigenic modifications of influenza A strains. They provide 50% to 80% protection against influenza-related illnesses and 30% to 65% protection against influenza-related hospital admissions and deaths in the elderly. Accordingly, vaccination is recommended for all patients older than 65 years, all patients who have chronic comorbid conditions (regardless of age), patients who reside in chronic care facilities, and health care workers (because of their increased risk of contacting patients who have influenza and spreading it to other noninfected patients). Preventive administration of amantadine or rimantadine for 2 weeks after vaccination has been recommended in very high-risk patients to provide protection during the period required to develop an effective immunologic response.

Parainfluenza Virus

Four serotypes have been identified, with types 1, 2, and 3 being responsible for most infections in humans. Parainfluenza viruses are responsible for up to 20% of the respiratory infections that occur in children but are found infrequently in immunocompetent adults. The epidemiologic and clinical characteristics depend on the serotype and are summarized in Table 24.2.

As with influenza, parainfluenza viruses are transmitted between humans via respiratory secretions. The incubation period lasts 2 to 6 days, and humoral, local, and cellular immunities generate neutralizing circulating antibodies, local secretory IgA, and cytotoxic and helper T lymphocytes, respectively.

In adults, the disease may be completely asymptomatic or may present as a common upper respiratory tract infection with rhinitis and pharyngitis. Fever is unusual, as is the progression to pneumonia. When pneumonia does occur, the symptoms and signs are nonspecific, and the chest radiograph shows diffuse, interstitial infiltrates consistent with any type of atypical or viral pneumonia.

Although treatment with ribavirin (tribavirin) has some in vitro activity, it is only supportive. Corticosteroids have been reported anecdotally to accelerate recovery in patients who have severe involvement. No vaccine is yet available.

Respiratory Syncytial Virus

The leading cause of respiratory tract infection in young children, RSV is responsible for 25% of hospital admissions for pneumonia and 75% of bronchiolitis in children younger than 6 months old. The incubation period lasts 4 to 6 days; epidemics occur in the late fall and spring and usually last 1 to 5 months. Almost all children older than 5 years have anti-RSV antibodies.

Transmittal of RSV is by contaminated skin followed by autoinoculation in the conjunctiva or nose, or by aerosols produced by coughing or sneezing.

Immunity involves mainly local and serum antibodies, but cell-mediated immunity also develops. Infection by RSV induces IgE production, the magnitude of which predicts the risk of subsequent wheezing episodes.

Usually, RSV infection begins in the upper respiratory tract with nasal congestion and pharyngitis and is associated with fever of variable intensity. The lower respiratory tract rapidly becomes involved in 25% to 40% of cases, which leads to worsening cough, dyspnea, wheezing, and rhonchi. Hypoxemia is common. Two types of lower respiratory tract involvement occur—pneumonia and bronchiolitis. Both are associated with interstitial infiltrates, the former from lung inflammation and the latter from peripheral atelectasis or hyperinflation. In older adults who have chronic cardiopulmonary disease, RSV may cause severe bronchitis, pneumonia, or both.

Serologic diagnosis can be made, but the tests may be less reliable in children younger than 4 months. Direct diagnosis requires cultures from respiratory secretions, nasopharyngeal washings, or throat swabs; virus detection is possible after 2 to 7 days. Immunofluorescence techniques are frequently used, and they allow a reliable and more rapid detection in nasal scrapings or washings. The ELISA assay is less sensitive.

Treatment with aerosolized ribavirin improves the clinical course and should be administered for 12 to 18 hours/day for 2 to 5 days to patients who have severe disease. Systemic corticosteroids are also given to those who suffer the most severe involvement.

Table 24.3 Preventive measures against nosocomial respiratory syncytial virus infections
Isolation or cohorting of hospital-admitted infected infants in specific areas
Surface decontamination of objects and furniture
Isolation measures
Handwashing
Use of gowns, gloves, and eye–nose goggles

Because RSV may spread among hospitalized children and hospital staff, prevention of nosocomial infection is recommended (Table 24.3). No vaccine is available.

Adenovirus

Adenoviruses are responsible for up to 5% of respiratory infections in children but account for less than 2% of those in adults; an exception is military recruit populations, in which epidemics have been reported. Almost all adults have serum antibodies against adenoviruses (usually against several serotypes).

Adenovirus respiratory infection may be the consequence of airborne or of fecal-oral contamination. The incubation period lasts 4 to 7 days. Latent infection may develop and has even been implicated in the pathogenesis of chronic airway diseases such as asthma or chronic obstructive pulmonary disease. In children and military recruits, adenoviruses can cause bronchiolitis and pneumonia of variable severity.

Rapid diagnosis requires antigen detection or histopathologic examination of biopsy specimens (which show intranuclear basophilic inclusions). Virus isolation requires 3 days to several weeks, and serodiagnosis requires both acute and convalescent sera.

Treatment is supportive (e.g., analgesics, cough suppressants). Effective, enteric-coated live vaccines have been developed for military recruits, but they are not used in other settings.

Rubeola (Measles)

Measles virus belongs to the Paramyxoviridae family and is therefore similar to parainfluenza virus and RSV. Portals of entry are the respiratory tract and conjunctiva. Lower respiratory tract manifestations affect up to 50% of patients who have measles and include mainly bronchitis and pneumonia (which may be complicated by bacterial superinfection in up to 50% of cases). In the United States, pneumonia is the cause of 60% of measles-related deaths in children.

Patients who have measles show a typical viral prodrome that consists of fever, rhinitis, malaise, and anorexia and lasts for approximately 1 week before the onset of the rash. The maculopapular rash begins on the face and neck and progresses to the trunk and extremities. Leukopenia is seen early. Measles pneumonia can cause hilar lymphadenopathy and pleural effusions, in addition to reticulonodular parenchymal infiltrates. Secondary bacterial pneumonia also occurs.

Treatment is supportive, and antibiotics are required when bacterial secondary infection occurs. No consistent data are available on the effects of corticosteroids.

The measles vaccine has reduced the incidence of disease by 98% in developed countries and has shifted the median age of onset to the teenage years.

Varicella

Varicella causes pneumonia in adults, but this complication is unusual in immunocompetent children. Epidemics occur in the winter and spring, with infectivity rates that exceed 90% within the first 2 to 3 weeks following exposure.

Initially, a rash appears on the face and head, with subsequent spread to the thorax, abdomen, and extremities. The rash has a rather orderly progression, beginning with erythematous macules that progress to vesicles within hours to days. These subsequently become pustular and finally crust over. Lesions may also be found on mucosal surfaces (e.g., pharynx, vagina). When pneumonia occurs, it generally presents within the first 4 to 5 days after the onset of the rash. Cough is common, and pleuritic chest pain and hemoptysis may occur. Other organs such as the liver, kidney, heart, and brain may also be involved. Diffuse, small nodular infiltrates are the characteristic radiographic abnormality, and hilar adenopathy and effusions are common. With resolution, the nodules may calcify and persist for life (Fig. 24.1).

Varicella infections can be diagnosed by a cytologic examination of scrapings from the lesions (e.g., the Tzanck smear, seeking multinucleated giant cells), although the sensitivity of this test is low. The virus may be cultured or found by polymerase chain reaction. A number of serologic tests are available, including the fluorescent antibody to membrane antigen test and ELISA.

Treatment with early administration of acyclovir (10 to 12.5 mg/kg intravenously every 8 hours for 7 days) is recommended for immunocompromised hosts who have varicella and for immunocompetent patients who suffer pneumonia. Preventive administration of oral acyclovir in adults who have varicella may be prudent, especially in elderly subjects, pregnant women, or patients with chronic obstructive pulmonary disease. Zoster immune globulin is recommended to reduce the severity of illness in immunocompromised patients exposed to varicella.

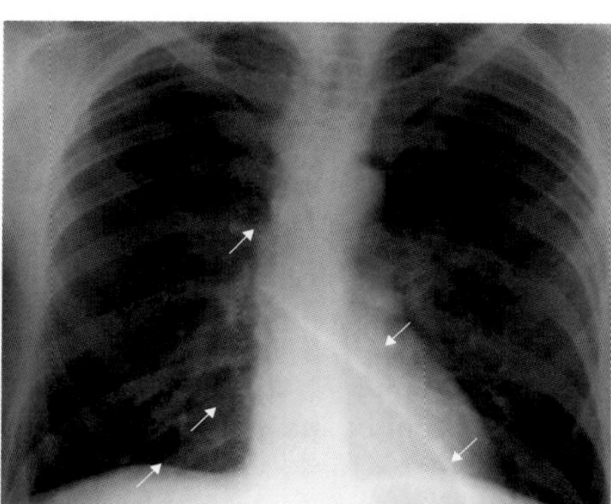

Figure 24.1 Calcific varicella nodules. Radiograph shows multiple 3- to 5-mm calcified nodules in the upper and lower lobes of a patient who had varicella pneumonia as a child.

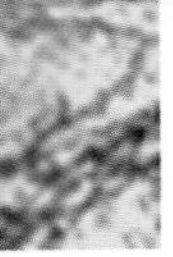

The infection can spread readily in the hospital setting, so strict isolation must be instituted until all lesions have crusted over.

Hantavirus

The hantavirus pulmonary syndrome was first recognized in the United States in 1983, but the disease was retrospectively identified using serologic testing in patients who had a similar illness in 1959. The syndrome can result from several hantaviruses, such as Sin Nombre virus. Almost all cases have been reported in North and South America. Rodents (e.g., field mice, voles, chipmunks) serve as the reservoir, and transmission to humans results from aerosolization of viruses contained in their feces. Person-to-person spread rarely, if ever, occurs.

The initial presentation is that of a flulike syndrome of fever, myalgia, nausea, vomiting, and gastrointestinal pain suggestive of gastroenteritis. These are followed by a dry cough that portends diffuse noncardiogenic pulmonary edema (sometimes associated with bilateral pleural effusion), which may lead to ARDS and shock in severe cases. Hematologic examination usually demonstrates neutrophilic leukocytosis, hemoconcentration, thrombocytopenia, and circulating immunoblasts. Renal failure may occur but is uncommon.

The diagnosis can be made by serologic or immunohistochemical techniques.

Treatment is mainly supportive, but the results of controlled trials of intravenous ribavirin are pending. Although in vitro effects of ribavirin have been demonstrated, preliminary results from an open-label trial are not impressive.

Avoidance of areas in which infected rodents reside is the only recognized preventive measure.

Severe Acute Respiratory Syndrome (SARS)

An outbreak of SARS was recently reported, mainly in Asian countries and Canada. The origin of the epidemic was believed to be Guangdong province in China. None of the previously described respiratory pathogens was consistently identified, and a new coronavirus isolated from patients with SARS is thought to be the responsible pathogen.

The incubation period ranges from 2 to 11 days. The clinical presentation and radiologic features of SARS are those of atypical pneumonia.

No effective treatment is available, despite the use of antiviral therapy such as ribavirin or steroids in many cases.

SARS is a serious respiratory illness that can lead to significant morbidity, with 10% to 25% of patients requiring admission to an intensive care unit and a mortality rate of about 10%. Factors associated with a poor outcome are age older than 60 years, significant comorbidities, diabetes mellitus, and initially elevated lactate dehydrogenase levels and elevated polymorphonuclear counts.

Because SARS is highly transmissible, it is recommended that patients be isolated in a single room (with negative pressure, if possible). Health care personnel should wear gloves, gown, mask, and eye protection and should wash their hands carefully after removing their gloves. The number of health care workers in contact with SARS patients should be limited. All suspected or confirmed cases should be reported to local health authorities and the World Health Organization.

FUNGAL PNEUMONIA

The most commonly encountered fungal and parasitic pulmonary infections are summarized in Table 24.4. The differential diagnosis in any given patient depends on his or her immunologic status, geographic locale, and travel history. A number of the fungal pneumonias occur almost exclusively in North America (e.g., histoplasmosis, blastomycosis, coccidioidomycosis). Although fungal and parasitic pulmonary infections are frequently self-limited, recurrent or severe disease is common when cell-mediated immunity is impaired. Infections in immunocompromised patients are covered in Chapter 25. Although amphotericin B remains the most effective medication for the majority of fungal infections, treatment is now facilitated by a number of new agents that are easier to administer and better tolerated. Therapeutic options are summarized in Table 24.5.

Aspergillosis

Aspergillus species are ubiquitous saprophytic fungi that produce several toxic substances (e.g., endotoxin, proteases). Airway colonization by *Aspergillus* is usually seen in patients with chronic lung lesions, such as bronchiectatic cavities, pulmonary fibrosis, or tuberculosis sequelae, and local host defense impairment. Invasive aspergillosis is an unusual finding in non-

Table 24.4
Agents of fungal and parasitic pneumonia, classified according to the immunologic status of the host

Type of Pathogen	Mainly in Normal Host	in Both Immunocompromised and Normal Host	Mainly in Immunocompromised Host
Fungi	*Histoplasma capsulatum* *Blastomyces dermatitidis* *Coccidioides immitis* *Paracoccidioides braziliensis*	*Cryptococcus neoformans* *Aspergillus* spp. *Sporothrix schenckii* *Penicillium marneffei* *Geotrichum* spp.	*Zygomycetes* *Candida* spp. *Trichosporon* spp. *Fusarium* spp. *Penicillium* spp. *Hansenula* spp. *Mucor, Rhizopus,* and *Absidia* genera (mucormycosis) *Pseudoallescheria boydii* *Pneumocystis jiroveci*
Parasites			
Protozoa	*Plasmodium* spp. (malaria) *Entamoeba histolytica* (amebiasis)	–	*Toxoplasma gondii* *Cryptosporidium* spp. *Babesia* spp.
Nematodes	*Ascaris* spp. Hookworm *Toxocara canis* (visceral larva migrans) *Dirofilaria immitis* *Wuchereria bancrofti,* *Brugia malayi* (tropical eosinophilia)	*Strongyloides stercoralis*	–
Platyhelminths	*Paragonimus* spp. *Schistosoma* spp. *Echinococcus* spp.	–	–

Table 24.5
Therapeutic options in fungal pneumonias of the nonimmunocompromised host

Disease		First-line treatment	Alternatives
Allergic bronchopulmonary aspergillosis		Corticosteroids plus itraconazole	–
Aspergilloma		Surgical resection	Embolization Itraconazole Intracavitary instillation of amphotericin B
Histoplasmosis	Acute	No treatment	Itraconazole
	Chronic	Itraconazole	Ketoconazole Amphotericin B
	Disseminated	–	Amphotericin B
Blastomycosis	Acute	Itraconazole	–
	Chronic	Itraconazole	Amphotericin B
Coccidioidomycosis	Acute	Itraconazole	Ketoconazole
	Chronic	Itraconazole	Ketoconazole Amphotericin B
Paracoccidioidomycosis	Mild	Itraconazole	–
	Chronic	Amphotericin B ± sulfadiazine	Itraconazole
Cryptococcosis		Fluconazole	Itraconazole Amphotericin B

neutropenic patients but has been described in patients with chronic obstructive pulmonary disease on long-term steroid therapy.

In nonimmunocompromised patients, *Aspergillus* species cause hypersensitivity pneumonitis (generally from *Aspergillus fumigatus*) and Löffler's syndrome (discussed in Chapters 39 and 46, respectively), allergic bronchopulmonary aspergillosis (covered in Chapter 39), and aspergillomas. Chronic necrotizing pneumonia has been described in non-neutropenic patients with preexisting lung disease or on chronic steroid therapy.

Amphotericin B is the most effective medication for the majority of fungal infections. Treatment is now facilitated, however, by a number of new agents that are easier to administer and better tolerated, such as itraconazole, voriconazole, and caspofungin.

Histoplasmosis

Histoplasma capsulatum is frequently isolated from soil that has been contaminated by bird or bat feces, which provide the organic nitrogen necessary for its growth. The disease occurs in the central United States (where the estimated prevalence and incidence of infection are $50/10^6$ and $500/10^3$, respectively), Mexico, and Puerto Rico. The disease was initially seen only in rural communities but is now found in patients who reside in urban settings as well, particularly in association with construction projects that involve moving contaminated soil. Numerous occupations have an increased risk of exposure.

The inhaled spores are contained in infective particles 2 to 5 μm in diameter, an ideal size to reach the airways and alveoli. After inhalation, multiplication converts the spores into yeasts, which are phagocytosed by macrophages in which they are able to survive, proliferate, and disseminate to metastatic sites such as the liver and spleen. A lymphocyte-mediated, delayed-type hypersensitivity reaction occurs and results in the formation of granulomas that resemble those found in mycobacterial diseases; the necrotic material may become caseous and calcify. The granulomas may be found in the lung as well as in a number of sites of metastatic infection. Patients affected by compromised cellular immunity (such as those who have AIDS or lymphoma) are more susceptible to histoplasmosis and may develop more severe disease.

The great majority of patients who have acute primary infections are undiagnosed because histoplasmosis remains subclinical. Those who inhale larger numbers of spores (frequently as a result of exposure in a closed space) develop a syndrome approximately 14 days later that has an abrupt onset and resembles influenza, bacterial pneumonia, or tuberculosis (Table 24.6). When the inoculum is particularly large, patients may develop ARDS.

The growth of *Histoplasma* species is slow, such that several weeks are needed for cultures to become positive. Giemsa staining of blood or bone marrow smears may be diagnostic when the fungus load is high, but this is unusual in immunocompetent patients. Tissue samples can demonstrate the organisms with

Table 24.6
Clinical presentations of acute histoplasmosis

	Mild acute pneumonitis	Pneumonic histoplasmosis	Progressive disseminating primary infection
Symptoms and physical signs	None or acute, influenza-like symptoms Arthralgia–erythema nodosum–erythema multiforme complex	Fever, chills, sweat, anorexia, weakness, cough with mucopurulent sputum, pleuritic chest pain Sometimes consolidation, rarely pleural effusion	Severe acute illness, often in immunocompromised patients Weight loss, low-grade fever, abdominal complaints, cough Sometimes mucosal ulcers, adrenal involvement
Chest radiography	Normal or consolidation 6 lymph node enlargement	Infiltrates of varying density, often with hilar lymph node enlargement, sometimes with pericarditis	Normal, or multiple nodules, linear opacities 6 lymph node involvement, or miliary aspect
Blood examination	–	–	In severe disease, leukopenia, thrombocytopenia, disseminated intravascular coagulation
Diagnosis	–	–	Few granulomas and many organisms in the most severe disease, the opposite in less severe forms
Clinical course	Spontaneous resolution; residual calcified nodules and lymph nodes	–	–

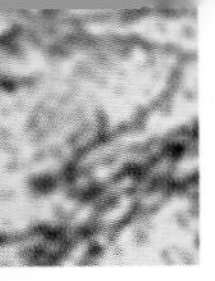

silver or periodic acid–Schiff (PAS) staining. Indirect diagnosis may be provided by several serologic techniques, including complement fixation, immunodiffusion, or radioimmunoassay, all of which may require several weeks to become positive.

Treatment is needed only for patients who suffer chronic, progressive histoplasmosis or for those who have dissemination. The use of amphotericin B is limited by the need for intravenous administration and the frequent development of renal toxicity, febrile reactions, and phlebitis. Renal toxicity may be reduced by the coadministration of large volumes of intravenous fluids. Side effects may also be reduced by use of the newly developed, but considerably more expensive, liposomal form of amphotericin. Ketoconazole has frequent gastrointestinal and antitestosterone effects. Fluconazole and itraconazole (200 to 400 mg/day) are as effective as amphotericin or ketoconazole in patients who have mild illness. Thus, amphotericin B should be reserved for patients who have more severe or disseminated disease.

Most acute primary infections are self-limited, require no treatment, and do not come to medical attention. Recurrent infiltrates may occur in some patients in association with eosinophilia, mimicking Löffler's syndrome. Evidence of calcified granulomas may be present in the lung (Fig. 24.2) and the spleen. On occasion, marked hilar lymphadenopathy or focal or diffuse mediastinal fibrosis may compress the central structures (e.g., airways, arteries, veins, esophagus).

Chronic, progressive disease occurs rarely, with symptoms of cough, hemoptysis, dyspnea, and fever. Chest radiographs usually show upper lobe or peripheral areas of consolidation, which evolve into cavities that mimic healed tuberculosis. Empyemas may occur, as may broncholithiasis, which has been associated with hemoptysis and bronchial obstruction. Chronic infection of the meninges, brain, or heart may occur rarely.

Blastomycosis

Blastomycosis is found in North America (in areas largely overlapping those where histoplasmosis occurs), Mexico, the Middle East, Africa, and India and results from inhalation of *Blastomyces dermatitidis*. The fungus grows in the soil, and the spores become airborne and are inhaled before converting to the yeast form in the lung. *B. dermatitidis* infection may occur sporadically or in epidemics. The initial defense mechanism involves polymorphonuclear cells, followed by macrophages and giant cells; epithelioid granulomas often develop. Depending on the type of predominant inflammatory response (pyogenic or granulomatous), the histopathologic pattern can mimic that of a bacterial infection, sarcoidosis, or mycobacterial disease. After multiplication of the yeast in the lungs, it may spread to the skin, bones, brain, peripheral lymph nodes, or other organs, and extrapulmonary manifestations may occur many years after the initial infection.

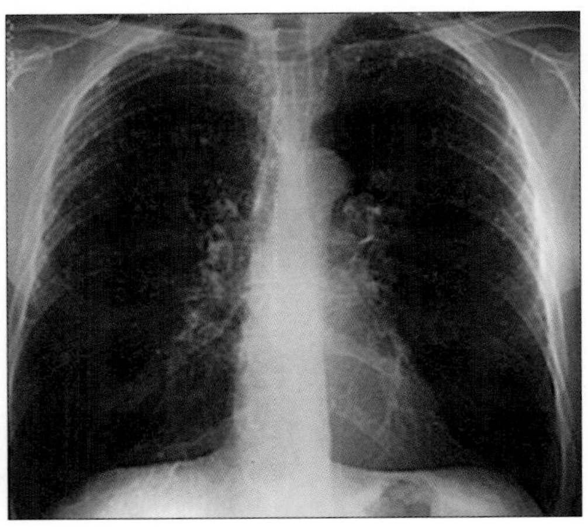

Figure 24.2 Calcified granulomas in the lung of a patient who has histoplasmosis.

The clinical manifestations of blastomycosis differ from one country to another. In North America, acute epidemic blastomycosis mimics bacterial pneumonia, with the abrupt onset of fever, chills, arthralgia and myalgia, cough with purulent sputum, and pleuritic chest pain. In milder cases, which are more frequent, the presentation is that of a more chronic disease, resembling tuberculosis; low-grade fever, cough, anorexia, and weight loss develop insidiously. Physical examination sometimes demonstrates erythema nodosum or findings of pulmonary consolidation, but it may be normal. The radiographic manifestations are nonspecific and include cavities, infiltrates, rounded densities, consolidation with air bronchograms, perihilar masses, or even a miliary pattern.

Mediastinal lymph node involvement is rare (<10% in most studies), and pleural effusions are quite uncommon. In the most severe cases, infection with *B. dermatitidis* can cause ARDS, even in immunocompetent hosts. Patients who suffer cutaneous blastomycosis frequently have a history of a self-limited pulmonary syndrome that occurred some years in the past.

The diagnosis of blastomycosis is made by microscopic examination of respiratory secretions digested by potassium hydroxide, or by histopathologic examination of tissue samples after silver or PAS staining. In culture of respiratory samples, detectable growth takes up to 1 week.

Because blastomycosis is often self-limited, treatment is restricted to those who suffer chronic disease and those who have severe acute infections. Itraconazole has the best ratio of efficacy to side effects, but amphotericin B is preferred in the most severe cases. Ketoconazole is an alternative in slowly progressive disease.

Coccidioidomycosis

Coccidioidomycosis results from another soil-dwelling fungus, *Coccidioides immitis*. It is endemic in the southwestern United States and northern Mexico and occurs mainly during hot, dry summers. Inhalation of airborne spores leads to polymorphonuclear-mediated suppurative and cell-mediated granulomatous inflammatory responses. The incubation period is 10 to 16 days.

Patients who have coccidioidomycosis may complain of fever, chills, arthralgia, myalgia, and headache in addition to cough, pleuritic chest pain, dyspnea, and, on occasion, hemoptysis (which results from areas of lung necrosis manifested by cavitation). Physical examination may reveal a macular rash, erythema nodosum, or erythema multiforme, as well as rhonchi, wheezes, or signs of consolidation or pleural effusion. In many patients, the physical examination is normal. Chest radiographs initially show one or more areas of consolidation, which may cavitate. Hilar lymphadenopathy may be found. Cavities or multiple calcified nodules may persist for life. Occasionally, patients develop progressive primary coccidioidomycosis, a condition in which the infiltrates and lymphadenopathy progress in association with fever, cough, and weight loss. Several months after the primary pulmonary infection, disseminated coccidioidomycosis may become manifest (affecting skin, bones, joints, genitourinary system, meninges), particularly but not exclusively in immunocompromised patients.

The diagnosis of coccidioidomycosis may be made by serologic or skin testing, both of which are most useful for epidemiologic purposes. Direct diagnosis can be made by microscopic examination of sputum or pus after potassium hydroxide digestion or Papanicolaou staining, by histopathologic examination of tissue biopsies after silver staining, or by cultures, which may demonstrate fungal growth after 5 days but pose an inhalation risk for laboratory personnel.

The treatment of coccidioidomycosis is similar to that of histoplasmosis and blastomycosis and relies on fluconazole and itraconazole, with amphotericin B and ketoconazole as alternatives. For the large majority of patients, no specific therapy is required.

Coccidioidomycosis is usually mild and self-limited, except in rare cases when it progresses or spreads hematogenously. Dissemination, which may be more common in dark-skinned races and in those who are immunocompromised, is associated with a high risk of meningitis and has a poor prognosis.

Paracoccidioidomycosis

Paracoccidioidomycosis results from inhalation of a soil fungus that is found mainly in South and Central America and in Mexico. In nonimmunocompromised patients, paracoccidioidomycosis presents as a chronic or subacute lung infection that is usually self-limited. In immunocompromised subjects, the clinical manifestations are those of an acute, severe disseminated infection.

The diagnosis of paracoccidioidomycosis relies on the same techniques used for coccidioidomycosis.

In severe or disseminated cases of paracoccidioidomycosis, treatment is similar to that of coccidioidomycosis but should be continued for up to 6 months.

Cryptococcosis

Cryptococcus neoformans is found throughout the world in bird guano. Cryptococcosis is a rare infection and is usually asymptomatic and self-limited in immunocompetent patients. In those who have impaired cell-mediated immunity, it may cause lung infection and meningitis. Symptoms of pulmonary infection include fever, malaise, cough, and chest pain. The chest radiograph may show large, nonspecific nodules (Fig. 24.3) or infiltrates, sometimes associated with lymphadenopathy.

C. *neoformans* can colonize the airways of immunocompromised patients and those who have chronic bronchitis without causing illness. Accordingly, culture of fungus from sputum does not always indicate disease.

Because cryptococcosis resolves spontaneously in normal hosts, and because patients who have chronic mucopurulent pulmonary conditions may be colonized by *Cryptococcus* species, positive cultures do not, in and of themselves, denote a specific indication for treatment. For patients who have progressive disease, amphotericin B or ketoconazole, fluconazole, or itraconazole is recommended.

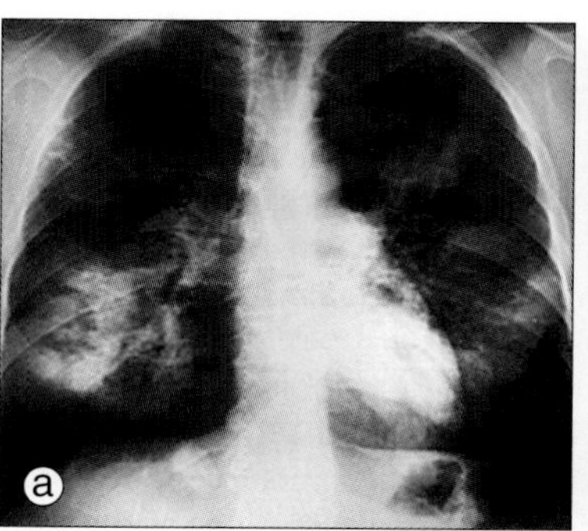

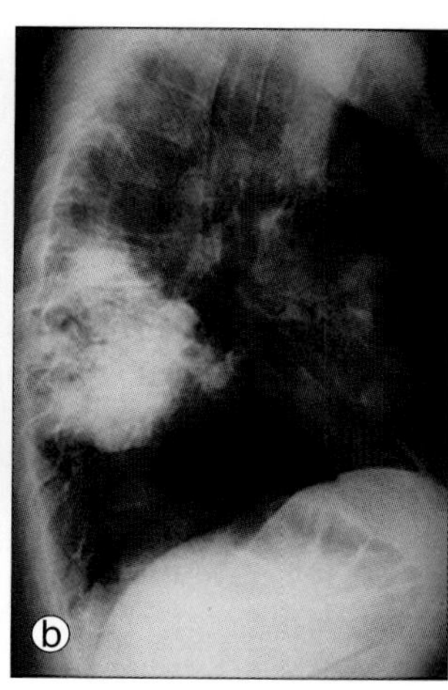

Figure 24.3 Cryptococcal lung infection. Chest radiographs of an immunocompetent patient show bilateral, large nodular densities.

PARASITIC PNEUMONIA

Pulmonary infections that result from parasites are infrequent in immunocompetent hosts but must be included in the differential diagnosis when patients have lived in endemic areas.

Amebiasis

Entamoeba histolytica is endemic in West and South Africa, South and Southeast Asia, South America, and Mexico. The disease is transmitted by ingestion of contaminated food or water, and sexual transmission has been reported in homosexual men.

The parasite disseminates from the intestine to the liver or, much less frequently, to the lung (in <5% of those with intestinal infection) or brain. Pleuropulmonary complications occur in up to 50% of patients who have liver abscesses as a result of either direct spread from the liver or hematogenous dissemination.

The main features of the disease are intestinal, ranging from diarrhea and abdominal cramps to dysentery or even intestinal perforation because of mucosal ulcerations. Pleuropulmonary symptoms include cough, dyspnea, and pleuritic pain (usually right-sided) associated with fever and chills, diaphoresis, and weight loss. The chest radiograph may show elevation of the right hemidiaphragm, pleural effusion, atelectasis, lung consolidation (which usually affects the right lower lobe), or lung abscess. Hepatobronchial fistulas have been reported in 47% of patients who have pleuropulmonary complications of amebiasis; this finding is associated with the production of copious volumes of chocolate-colored sputum. Pericardial involvement may be observed in up to 10% of such patients.

The diagnosis can be made by microscopic examination of stool, which has a sensitivity of less than 30%, or by serologic techniques, which have sensitivities and specificities as high as 95% in invasive disease. Antigen may be detected on pleural fluid or respiratory secretions. Needle aspiration of lung or of liver abscesses is seldom necessary.

The drug of choice for treating invasive amebiasis is metronidazole (750 mg every 8 hours for 10 days), in addition to agents that are active against intraluminal protozoa such as iodoquinol, diloxanide, or paromomycin.

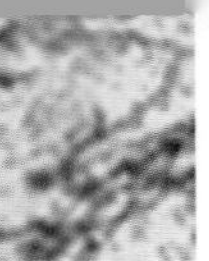

Malarial Lung

Pleuropulmonary complications result from *Plasmodium falciparum*, the agent of the most severe form of malaria. Mild respiratory involvement is probably underdiagnosed and may affect up to 20% of patients who have falciparum malaria. Pulmonary involvement is commonly associated with cerebral disease and marked parasitemia. Histopathologic features include capillary congestion, pulmonary edema, alveolar hemorrhage, and endothelial cell injury.

The pulmonary manifestations of malaria include mild cough associated with pleural effusion, lung consolidation, or interstitial infiltrates. Severe respiratory involvement can occur as a result of lung edema and pleural effusions, and patients may present with ARDS.

The diagnosis is made by examination of thin or thick blood smears stained with Giemsa or Wright stain.

Besides supportive and respiratory care, treatment of severe disease requires intravenous quinidine, and exchange transfusion in the most severe cases. Depending on the region of origin, drug-resistant strains must be considered, and alternative treatments offered. Despite these measures, prognosis for the malarial lung remains poor.

Pulmonary Ascariasis

The estimated worldwide prevalence of infection with the nematode *Ascaris lumbricoides* is 25%. The normal habitat of the adult worm is the jejunum, and infection follows ingestion of embryonated eggs. Maturation occurs during pulmonary migration and may be responsible for ascaris pneumonia, a self-limited disease that occurs 4 to 16 days after ingestion and lasts for 10 days to several weeks.

Ascariasis is responsible for a Löffler-like syndrome in approximately 20% of cases. Symptoms are dominated by cough (sometimes with hemoptysis), wheezing, dyspnea, and high-grade fever. Abdominal pain, nausea and vomiting, and hepatomegaly may be present, as well as a variety of cutaneous reactions (e.g., urticaria, angioedema). The chest radiograph shows unilateral or bilateral patchy, migratory peribronchial infiltrates; eosinophilia may be present, and (on occasion) IgE elevation may be found.

Sputum analysis reveals eosinophils and Charcot-Leyden crystals. Stool examination may be negative at this early stage of ascariasis.

The pneumonia does not require any specific treatment, as it is usually self-limited. Bronchodilators and corticosteroids may be useful when bronchospasm is present. Antihelminthic therapy is necessary to eradicate intestinal adult worms (Table 24.7).

Table 24.7
First-choice antihelminthic drugs active against *Ascaris lumbricoides* and hookworms

Drug	Dose and duration	Common side effects
Pyrantel pamoate	11mg/kg, single dose	Anorexia, nausea, abdominal pain, diarrhea
Mebendazole	100mg q12h for 3 days	Abdominal pain, diarrhea
Albendazole	400mg, single dose	Abdominal discomfort, diarrhea

Strongyloidiasis and Ancylostomiasis

Although *Strongyloides stercoralis* is endemic in tropical and subtropical areas, strongyloidiasis is less frequent than ascariasis and ancylostomiasis. The life cycle of the parasite is the same as that of ascaris and hookworm. Ancylostomiasis, or hookworm infection, may be caused by two nematodes: *Ancylostoma duodenale* and *Necator americanus*. The prevalence and life cycles are similar to those of *Ascaris lumbricoides* and *Strongyloides stercoralis*.

Patients may be asymptomatic or experience a Löffler-like syndrome following transient urticaria in association with abdominal symptoms. In some cases, massive invasion (which is favored by abnormal cell-mediated immunity and malnutrition-related immunosuppression) leads to a much more severe disease, termed the hyperinfection syndrome, which develops from disseminated disease (Table 24.8).

The diagnosis can be made by sputum or stool examination or by duodenal or pleural aspiration. Serologic techniques may be of help in chronic cases.

The preferred treatment is thiabendazole 25 mg/kg every 12 hours for 2 days (longer in disseminated disease), which may have to be repeated. Alternative agents are ivermectin and albendazole.

Visceral Larva Migrans

Human visceral larva migrans is caused by *Toxocara canis* or, less frequently, *Toxocara catis*. All canine species are hosts of the nematode, and the prevalence of the infection in dogs has been estimated at approximately 3%. Contamination of humans occurs after ingestion of eggs in contaminated food or soil. Larvae migrate to the liver and lungs through lymphatics and blood vessels and induce an IgE-mediated immune response. In rare cases, other organs may be involved, such as the heart or the central nervous system. Cells that infiltrate invaded tissues are mainly eosinophils and, to a lesser extent, lymphocytes.

Clinically apparent pulmonary involvement is common (20% to 85% of cases) and manifests as cough, wheezing, bronchiolitis, or pneumonia that may result in acute respiratory failure. Radiographic manifestations are usually mild migratory infiltrates, which are found in 50% of those who have respiratory symptoms. Systemic symptoms include weakness, malaise, anorexia, nausea, vomiting, weight loss, abdominal pain, or behavioral impairment. Overall, the severity of the clinical illness reflects the extent of the infestation.

Table 24.8
Clinical presentation of the hyperinfection syndrome or disseminated strongyloidiasis

Manifestation	Presentation
Abdominal	Anorexia, nausea, vomiting, diarrhea, abdominal pain ileus
Pulmonary	Cough, hemoptysis, wheezing, dyspnea Adult respiratory distress syndrome Bacterial superinfection
Other	Invasion of liver, skin, central nervous system Bacterial meningitidis Sepsis caused by secondary bacterial infection (usually gram-negative bacilli)

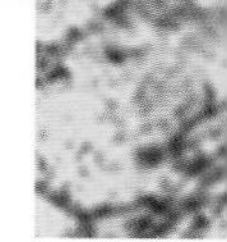

Table 24.9
Preventive measures to limit visceral larva migrans in humans

Behavioral measures	Veterinary measures	Environmental measures
Avoid geophagia Limit close contact between children and canine species	Deworming of cats and dogs	Keep children's sandbox dry

Because *Toxocara* larvae do not mature in humans, the diagnosis can be made only by serology or histologic examination of invaded tissues.

In mild cases, the disease is self-limited, so no treatment is required. In more severely affected patients, corticosteroids seem to improve the prognosis. Preventive measures are important to limit the spread of the disease (Table 24.9).

Dirofilariasis

Human dirofilariasis is the consequence of infestation by the nematode *Dirofilaria immitis,* which is a dog parasite transmitted by mosquitoes. In rare cases, larvae injected by mosquitoes into humans are transported by blood vessels to the pulmonary circulation, where they can cause thrombosis.

Clinical signs of cough, hemoptysis, chest pain, and fever are present in half of affected patients. Chest radiographs may show peripheral nodules of 1 to 5 cm in diameter, which may calcify. A minority of patients exhibit peripheral eosinophilia.

The diagnosis can be made by serology or histologic examination of lung tissues. No treatment is required.

Tropical Pulmonary Eosinophilia

Tropical pulmonary eosinophilia results from infection with *Wuchereria bancrofti* or *Brugia malayi,* which are lymphatic-dwelling filariae found in tropical and subtropical areas. Pulmonary manifestations are the consequence of a hypersensitivity reaction following the discharge of microfilariae into the circulation by gravid female filariae. Transmission is by mosquitoes that ingest the microfilariae and inject larvae when they bite humans. Of the patients who have tropical eosinophilia, 80% are men, and the lungs are involved in more than 90% of cases.

Clinical manifestations include fever, weakness, anorexia, weight loss, cough, wheezing, and dyspnea. Chest radiographs usually show bilateral basal, interstitial infiltrates and increased bronchovascular markings. Lymph node involvement and consolidation are infrequent.

The parasites may be found on histologic examination of affected organs, but the diagnosis is generally made by finding high levels of IgE and high titers of antibodies to filariae and by clinical improvement following treatment.

Standard treatment is diethylcarbamazine, 6 to 12 mg/kg body weight for up to 3 weeks. Alternatives are mebendazole and levamisole. New agents such as ivermectin are being evaluated. Corticosteroids or antihistamines may be used when patients exhibit allergic reactions to dying filariae. Some patients (10% to 20%) require repeated courses of treatment because the adult parasites may be relatively resistant. Response to treatment is inversely related to the duration of symptoms.

Paragonimiasis

Paragonimus species (most frequently *Paragonimus westermani)* are hermaphroditic flukes that are endemic in Southeast Asia, South America, and South Africa and are transmitted to humans by ingestion of insufficiently cooked crabs or crayfish that contain the encysted parasite. These go to the lung through the intestinal wall, peritoneal cavity, diaphragm, and pleura.

The illness may occur during the first weeks of infection, during the parasite's migration from the intestine to the lung. When this occurs, symptoms may include abdominal pain, diarrhea, hypersensitivity reactions (urticaria, eosinophilia, fever), chest pain, cough, and hemoptysis. In most cases, however, no symptoms appear until the adult parasite begins to produce eggs in the lung, which induces cough and hemoptysis. Chest radiographs usually show patchy infiltrates, which may progress to cavities surrounded by a rim of infiltration (ring cysts). Areas of fibrosis or pleural thickening are common. Pleural effusions are infrequent, except in some series of South Asian patients. The chest radiograph may be normal in up to 20% of cases.

The diagnosis is based on demonstrating eggs in bronchial secretions, pleural fluid, or feces. A number of serologic tests are also available.

The preferred treatment is praziquantel (25 mg/kg every 8 hours for 3 days), which is effective in more than 90% of cases. Bithionol (40 mg/kg every other day for 2 weeks) is a less effective alternative.

Schistosomiasis

Several *Schistosoma* species may be pathogenic for humans. The most frequently encountered are described in Table 24.10. The parasite forms released by snails (in which asexual reproduction occurs) penetrate the skin and transform into immature parasites, which are transported in the blood, where they mature in venous plexuses (see Table 24.10) and reproduce. Eggs are deposited in the intestine or bladder, depending on the site of the infected venous plexus. The eggs, in turn, induce overwhelming granulomatous reactions; they may migrate to the liver and cause portal hypertension, with subsequent migration to the lung via portosystemic collaterals.

Table 24.10
Pathogenic *Schistosoma* species

Species	Area	Predominant venous plexuses in which mature parasites develop	Treatment: doses of praziquantel
Schistosoma mansoni	Arabia, South America, Caribbean	Inferior mesenteric veins	20 mg/kg body weight x 2, for 1 day
Schist. japonicum	China, Japan, Philippines	Superior mesenteric plexus	20 mg/kg body weight x 3, for 1 day
Schist. haematobium	Africa, Middle East	Vesical plexus	20 mg/kg body weight x 2, for 1 day

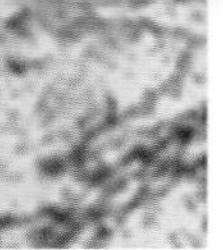

As shown in Table 24.11, symptoms depend on the stage of the disease. The most frequent pulmonary manifestation is pulmonary hypertension, which occurs in the chronic stages of infection with *Schistosoma mansoni* or *Schistosoma japonicum*. Nodular lesions can also develop, and this infestation should be included in the differential diagnosis of pulmonary nodules (Fig. 24.4).

The direct diagnosis may be based on examination of the stool (Kato thick smear), urine, or rectal biopsies. Several serologic techniques have been developed.

The most effective treatment is praziquantel. Doses depend on the *Schistosoma* species (see Table 24.10).

Hydatidosis

Cystic hydatid disease (CHD) is caused by larvae of *Echinococcus granulosus*, and alveolar hydatid disease (AHD) is caused by *Echinococcus multilocularis*. Both are platyhelminths that infect humans through the ingestion of eggs. The parasite is transported by the blood or lymphatics to other sites, mainly the liver and lungs. Whereas CHD is the manifestation of the growth of larvae, which form spherical cysts, AHD results from persistent invasion by and destructive proliferation of the parasite. Of human hydatidosis cases, 90% of patients have CHD (with respiratory involvement in 25% of these), and 9% have AHD.

In CHD, symptoms occur in approximately 70% of cases and are related to compression of adjacent structures or to complications such as rupture or secondary infection. Accordingly, symptoms include chest pain, cough, expectoration of cyst contents (e.g., grape skins), dyspnea, hemoptysis, or even near drowning in cyst fluid. Rupture may also lead to dissemination of cysts within the lungs, hypersensitivity reactions, or pleural effusion. In rare instances (<10%), hydatid cysts may develop in the pleural space itself after the rupture of a pulmonary cyst. Chest radiographs typically show rounded opacities (called cannonballs), the borders of which can calcify. Sharply demarcated cysts, which may contain smaller daughter cysts, are shown by computed tomography scans. This finding allows CHD to be differentiated from AHD; in the latter, computed tomography shows less well-demarcated masses that have necrotic centers. Eosinophilia is frequent.

The diagnosis relies on the demonstration of associated hepatic cysts, serologic tests, and, in some cases, the presence of cyst material in sputum. Aspiration of the cyst should be avoided to limit the possibility of dissemination and hypersensitivity reactions.

The treatment of choice is surgical resection of the cysts. When surgery cannot be done, or when the cysts rupture and the parasite disseminates, the preferred treatment is albendazole 400 mg every 12 hours (10 to 15 mg/kg per day) for 4 weeks. Treatment courses may be repeated.

Table 24.11
Clinical presentations of Schistosomiasis

Stage of disease	Involved species	Clinical signs
Skin penetration	All	Transient cutaneous symptoms ("swimming itch")
Tissue migration (immature parasite)	Mainly *Schistosoma japonicum*	Katayama fever: fever, chills, headache, myalgia, arthralgia, abdominal pain, diarrhea, weight loss, cough, wheezing, pulmonary infiltrates (sometimes with a miliary aspect), hepatosplenomegaly, lymphadenopathy, leukocytosis, eosinophilia, immune complexes
Chronic infection (mature reproducing parasites)	*Schistosoma mansoni* and *S. japonicum*	Abdominal pain, diarrhea, fatigue, portal hypertension, hepatic failure (presinusoidal hepatic fibrosis) Pulmonary hypertension Hypoxemia without pulmonary hypertension (intrapulmonary arteriovenous fistulas) Lung granulomas
	Schistosoma haematobium	Chronic bladder disease
Response to treatment	–	Transient and self-limited cough, wheezing, lung infiltrates, eosinophilia

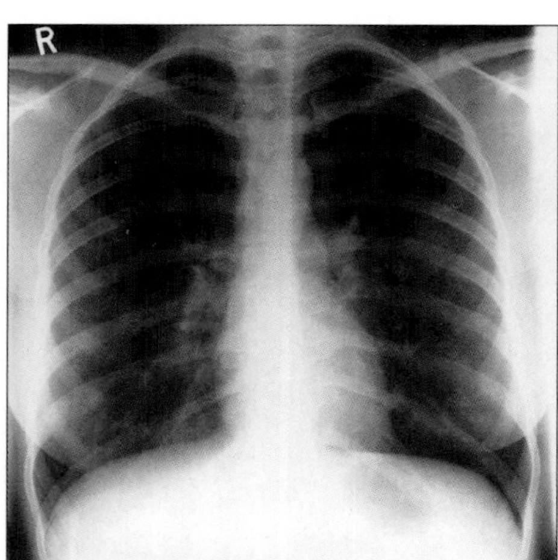

Figure 24.4 Multiple pulmonary nodules on the chest radiograph of a patient with schistosomiasis.

LIPOID PNEUMONIA

Lipoid pneumonia results from the aspiration of exogenous lipids contained in orally administered laxatives or nasal decongestants. The histology is that of giant-cell inflammation with oil-containing vacuoles and phagocytes, type II cell metaplasia, degeneration of arteriolar or bronchial walls, necrosis, and fibrosis. Oil droplets or lipophages may be transported by lymphatics or via the blood to the liver, spleen, kidney, or other organs. Special stains allow exogenous lipoid pneumonia to be distinguished from conditions that arise from the accumulation of endogenous lipids, as occasionally occurs in the setting of chronic primary lung inflammation (Table 24.12).

Symptoms include cough, dyspnea, fever, chest pain, and hemoptysis. The onset may be acute, but more commonly it is chronic and is accompanied by weight loss. In 50% of cases, the disease is clinically silent and is discovered on a chest radiograph. A number of radiologic presentations may be found (Table 24.13; Fig. 24.5). Computed tomography or magnetic resonance imaging scans may be useful when they demonstrate attenuation values of −30 to −150 Hounsfield units or high-intensity T1 signals with a slow decrease on T2-weighed images, respec-

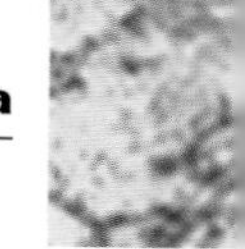

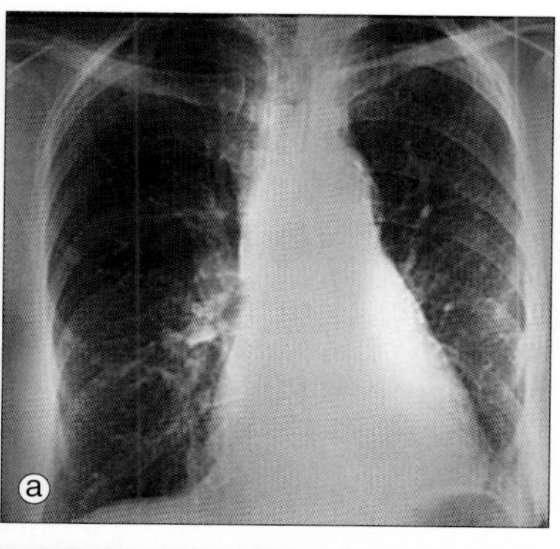

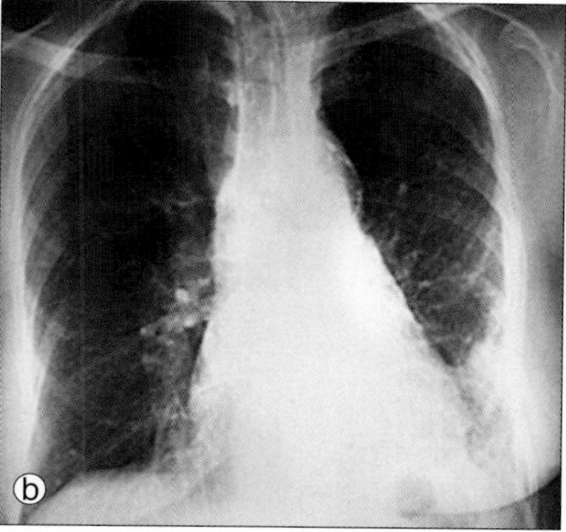

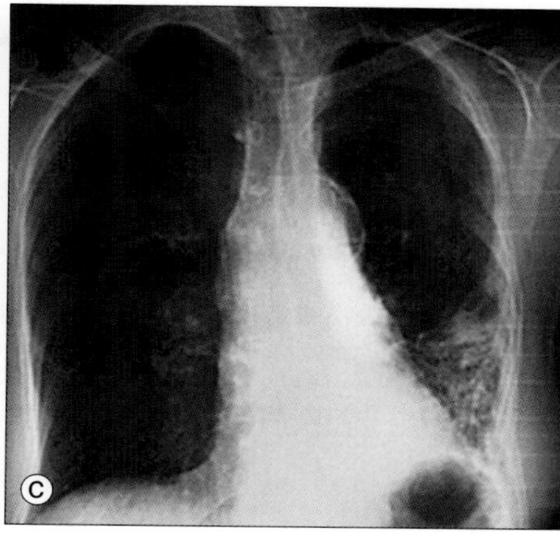

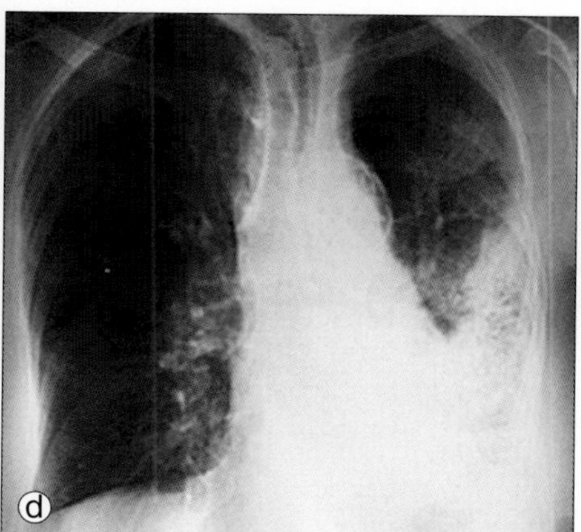

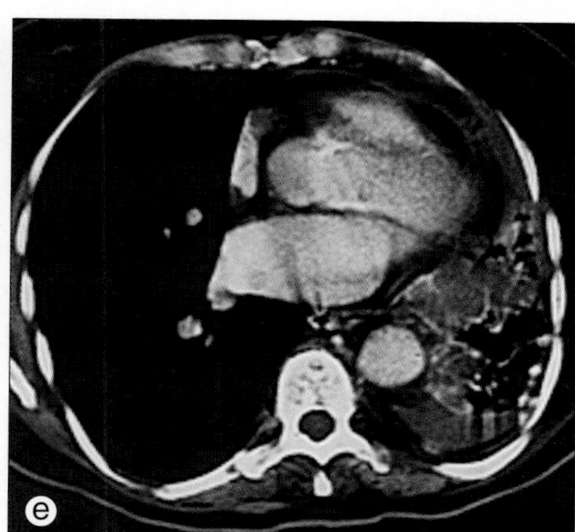

Figure 24.5 Lipoid pneumonia. This series of radiographs demonstrates infiltration of the left lower lobe that progressed slowly over 19 years—from 1974 **(A)** to 1993 **(D)**. The patient liberally applied a mentholatum-containing nasal grease each night before bed, and her husband documented that the patient routinely slept on her left side. The computed tomography scan shows low-density consolidation of the left lower lobe and a small left pleural effusion.

Table 24.12
Histopathologic differences between exogenous and endogenous lipoid pneumonias

Characteristic	Exogenous lipids	Endogenous lipids
Fat	Large droplets	Small droplets
Foreign body granulomas	Present	Absent
Birefringence under polarized light	Absent	Present
Special stainings		
Periodic acid–Schiff	Negative	Positive
Sudan black	Light blue	Black
Sudan IV	Orange	Red
Oil red O	Orange	Red
Nile blue sulfate	Negative	Light violet
Osmium tetroxide	Negative	Positive

Table 24.13
Findings in exogenous lipoid pneumonia on chest radiography

Dense consolidation with air bronchograms
Ground glass infiltrates
Cavitation
Interstitial infiltrate
Fibrotic infiltrates
Nodules, masses
Atelectasis
Emphysema
Pleural effusion

tively, as a result of the low density of fat. Sputum, bronchoalveolar lavage fluid, or transbronchial biopsies can be examined for fat-containing macrophages after the application of special stains.

The most important intervention is to stop the administration of the causative agent. Corticosteroids do not appear to be beneficial.

Exogenous lipoid pneumonia usually follows a benign course. The most frequently encountered complications are bacterial, fungal, or mycobacterial superinfections. Respiratory insufficiency occurs infrequently, unless the condition is far advanced (e.g., years of chronic aspiration), and neoplasm is uncommon. The use of oil-containing laxatives and decongestants should be discouraged.

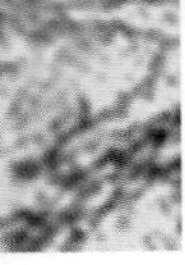

SUGGESTED READINGS

Batra P, Batra RS: Thoracic coccidioidomycosis. Semin Roentgenol 31:28-44, 1996.

Chapman SW, Bradsher RW Jr, Campbell GD Jr, et al: Infectious Diseases Society of America. Practice guidelines for the management of patients with blastomycosis. Clin Infect Dis 30:679–683, 2000.

Chitkara RK, Sarinas PS: Dirofilaria, visceral larva migrans, and tropical pulmonary eosinophilia. Semin Respir Infect 12:138–148, 1997.

Clancy CJ, Nguyen MH: Acute community-acquired pneumonia due to *Aspergillus* in presumably immunocompetent hosts: clues for recognition of a rare but fatal disease. Chest 114:629–634, 1998.

Couch RB: Drug therapy: prevention and treatment of influenza. N Engl J Med 343:1778–1787, 2000.

Ksiazek TG, Erdman D, Goldsmith CS, et al: A novel coronavirus associated with severe acute respiratory syndrome. N Engl J Med 348:1953–1966, 2003.

Lortholary O, Denning DW, Dupont B: Endemic mycosis: a treatment update. J Antimicrob Chemother 43:321–331, 1999.

Sarinas PS, Chitkara RK: Ascariasis and hookworm. Semin Respir Infect 32:130–137, 1997.

Spickard A 3rd, Hirschmann JV: Exogenous lipoid pneumonia. Arch Intern Med 154:686–692, 1994.

Wheat J, Sarosi G, McKinsey D, et al: Practice guidelines for the management of patients with histoplasmosis. Clin Infect Dis 30:688–695, 2000.

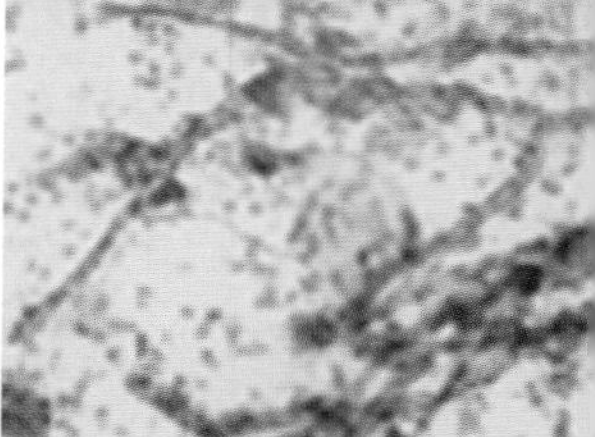

CHAPTER 25 Pneumonia in the Non-HIV Immunocompromised Host

Jim Egan

BACTERIAL PNEUMONIA

Bacterial infection is the most common cause of pneumonia in immunocompromised patients. These patients include those rendered neutropenic from cytotoxic chemotherapy, recovering from organ transplantation, or receiving prolonged immunotherapy for systemic disease. HIV-related infections are discussed in Chapter 30. The specific organism is dependent on the time after induction of immunosuppression (Table 25.1). Initially, nosocomial infection occurs with skin and gastrointestinal tract organisms such as *Escherichia coli*, *Klebsiella pneumoniae*, *Pseudomonas aeruginosa*, *Stenotrophomonas maltophilia*, and *Acinetobacter calcoaceticus*. Later, community-acquired capsulated bacteria (streptococci) may result in pneumonia.

Epidemiology and Risk Factors

Fifty percent of neutropenic patients experience bacterial infection, and 20% of patients with a neutrophil count of less than 100 cells/mm^3 demonstrate evidence of bacteremia. Bacterial pneumonia is reported to occur in 10% to 25% of patients after liver, heart, and kidney transplantation, and in up to 60% after lung transplantation.

In the 1980s, multiple organisms, especially gram-negative ones (*E. coli*, *Klebsiella*, and *Pseudomonas*), caused most pneumonias and were the targets for prophylaxis and treatment. As a consequence, gram-positive organisms now cause 60% to 70% of bacteremic episodes in neutropenic patients. Emerging resistance in gram-positive organisms is now increasingly common. Enterococci are relatively resistant organisms that require combination treatment with penicillin and aminoglycosides. Up to 42% of patients with vancomycin-resistant enterococci septicemia have underlying hematologic malignancies, and 35% have respiratory failure.

Risk factors for the development of bacterial pneumonia include the extent of immunosuppression, interruption of mucosal membranes, deep vein access, prior colonizing organisms (*Burkholderia cepacia*), gastrointestinal function, and cytomegalovirus infection. The pattern of bacterial infection is influenced by the impact and timing of immunosuppression. Chemoradiotherapy for hematologic malignancies and hematopoietic cell transplantation result in neutropenia with cellular and humoral immunodeficiency. Corticosteroids impair neutrophil and macrophage function; azathioprine and cyclophosphamide impair both neutrophil and lymphocyte production; cyclosporin, tacrolimus, and mycophenolate mofetil modify T-cell activity.

Poor nutrition and hypoalbuminemia in particular encourage pneumonia by promoting the adherence of gram-negative bacilli to epithelial cells and impairing neutrophil function. Abnormal colonization of the oropharynx by gram-negative bacilli, often from the sinuses and stomach, is associated with nosocomial pulmonary infection. Antibiotic therapy itself contributes to oropharyngeal and gastric colonization, and 30% of patients admitted to intensive care show evidence of gastric bacterial colonization. Prior antibiotic exposure may contribute to this phenomenon. Enteral feeding alkalizes the gastrointestinal tract and facilitates bacterial overgrowth in the stomach. Intermittent enteral feeding may be less harmful than continuous; however, treatment and prophylaxis with H_2-blockers against erosive gastritis may contribute to gastric bacterial overgrowth. Aspiration is an important risk factor for bacterial infection. The clinical spectrum of aspiration ranges from recurrent microaspiration that promotes inocula of gram-negative bacilli to food particle and chemical inhalation.

Certain factors can identify some neutropenic patients as being at low risk of severe infection, allowing oral antibiotic therapy. Factors determining this risk stratification include an absolute neutrophil count greater than 100 cells/mm^3, a short duration of neutropenia that is expected to resolve, disease remission, absence of organ-specific symptoms, normotension, age younger than 60 years, peak temperature less than 39°C (102.2°F), and normal renal and liver function.

Clinical Features

The classic symptoms and signs of pulmonary infection observed in an immunocompetent host, which include sputum production, pyrexia, and leukocytosis, are commonly absent in immunocompromised patients. Neutropenic patients may not generate sufficient leukocytes to produce sputum, and signs of infection may be subtle, including unexplained tachypnea, increased fluid requirements, or unexplained acidosis.

Diagnosis

Speed in making an accurate diagnosis influences a successful outcome, as this allows prompt, specific treatment; however, concurrent diagnoses need to be considered. For example, methicillin-resistant *Staphylococcus aureus* is often identified in conjunction with *P. aeruginosa*, and acute lung injury is seen in association with *Streptococcus viridans* infection. Bacterial pneumonia can be difficult to discriminate from candidemia-related sepsis and noncardiogenic pulmonary edema. Therefore, sputum

Table 25.1
Differential diagnosis of respiratory infections in the immunocomromised host in relation to time after transplantation

Time	Organism/diagnosis	Transplant	Comment
Early postoperative, 0–40 days	Nosocomial bacterial infection	All	–
	Aspiration	Lung, liver, hematopoietic cell	Mucositis and gastric paresis
During engraftment, 0–40 days	Fungal infection *Aspergillus* spp. *Candida* spp.	–	–
	Pulmonary edema Cardiogenic Noncardiogenic	Renal, hematopoietic cell Hematopoietic cell, lung, liver	–
Early post-transplant, 40–120 days	Nosocomial bacterial infection	–	–
	Cytomegalovirus	All	Donor cytomegalovirus seropositive Recipient cytomegalovirus seronegative
	Herpes simplex virus	–	–
Post engraftment (hematopoietic cell transplant), 40–120 days	*Aspergillus jiroveci*	Hematopoietic cell, lung, liver	–
	Pneumocystis pneumonia	–	Rare with trimethoprim–sulfamethoxazole prophylaxis
	Community-acquired viral infection Adenovirus Respiratory syncytial virus Influenza	Hematopoietic cell, lung	–
Late post-transplant, >120 days	Cytomegalovirus	–	Donor cytomegalovirus seropositive Recipient cytomegalovirus seropositive
Late post hematopoietic cell transplant, >120 days	*Pneumocystis jiroveci* pneumonia	–	Rare with trimethoprim–sulfamethoxazole prophylaxis; patients may be noncompliant
	Aspergillus spp.	–	Associated with cytomegalovirus
	Encapsulated bacteria (*Streptococcus viridans, Streptococcus pneumoniae*)	Graft-versus-host disease, splenectomy	Penicillin prophylaxis for 2 years
	Enterobacter spp.	–	–

culture, blood culture, chest radiographs, and bronchoscopy with bronchoalveolar lavage (BAL) and protected brush specimens are essential to achieve a diagnosis of bacterial pneumonia in the immunocompromised host.

Despite intense culture surveillance, specific organisms may not be identified in up to 40% of cases of pneumonia. This may occur because of partial prior treatment in the community, inefficient handling of culture specimens, or concurrent antibiotic therapy.

The chest radiograph may demonstrate little change in patients who are unable to mount an inflammatory response and may not be in synchrony with the clinical state.

High-resolution computed tomography (HRCT) scanning does not provide a bacteriologic or histologic diagnosis, but it may identify coexisting nodular disease and lymphadenopathy, suggesting either another opportunistic infection or persistent primary neoplastic disease. HRCT may facilitate targeted bronchoscopy and BAL.

Bronchoscopy has a vital role in the evaluation of immunocompromised patients, allowing a diagnosis in 60% of those with pulmonary infiltrates. Simple fiber-optic bronchial aspiration secures a diagnosis in 57% of cases, compared with 24% for protected brush specimens. Bronchoscopy-derived information leads to a change in antibiotics in 43% of cases.

Treatment

Because a bacterial organism is often not identified, early empirical therapy, particularly in febrile neutropenic patients, should still be targeted at gram-negative organisms, including *P. aeruginosa* and Enterobacteriaceae. Monotherapy in low-risk patients is acceptable. However, dual therapy, including an antipseudomonas penicillin with an aminoglycoside or an antipseudomonas cephalosporin with an aminoglycoside, is generally recommended. Quinolone-based dual therapy is comparable.

Rapidity and accuracy in providing antibiotic therapy are important. Inaccurate antibiotic therapy in ventilated patients leads to a 20% increase in mortality. Clinicians should be aware of the organism profiles in individual institutions to facilitate early, targeted empirical treatment and high bacterial kill rates, which may reduce pneumonia rates by 20%. However, the required surveillance programs are time consuming and costly.

Aminoglycosides have both direct and synergistic activity against gram-negative and gram-positive organisms. Dosages given every 12 or 8 hours have greater toxicity than once-daily therapy. A meta-analysis of 3091 patients who had bacterial infection showed that once-daily aminoglycoside therapy in neutropenic patients resulted in a trend toward improved outcome and reduced the risk of nephrotoxicity by 26%. In neutropenic patients, vancomycin is generally not required as initial empirical therapy, because infections due to coagulase-negative staphylococci and vancomycin-resistant enterococci are generally indolent. However, if there is clinical suspicion of a catheter-related infection or known colonization with methicillin-resistant *S. aureus*, vancomycin should be instituted. Teicoplanin is more active against enterococci than vancomycin and less nephrotoxic, but it is more expensive, and assays for teicoplanin levels are not widely available. Linezolid, an oxazolidinone, can be administered both intravenously and orally and is effective against resistant gram-positive organisms; however, its use may be limited by associated myelosuppression. After the initiation of antibiotic treatment, patients with febrile neutropenia should be reassessed in 3 to 5 days. If there is no deterioration, the chosen antibiotic regimen can be continued. If the clinical picture has deteriorated, the antibiotics should be changed and antifungal therapy initiated.

Appropriate supportive care is important. Optimal fluid management to minimize pulmonary edema is critical, as fluid overload is a frequent cause of rapidly deteriorating radiographs (Fig. 25.1). Many patients require high inspiratory flows (>10 L/minute) of oxygen. The early institution of intermittent noninvasive positive pressure ventilation may attenuate the need for mechanical ventilation. The improved survival in immunocompromised patients supported with noninvasive positive pressure ventilation may be the consequence of reducing the risk of secondary nosocomial infection associated with mechanical ventilation. In contrast, continuous positive airway pressure does not appear to be effective in preventing mechanical ventilation in immunocompromised patients.

Clinical Course and Prevention

Ideal antibiotic prophylaxis involves an inexpensive agent that is easily administered and of adequate potency that does not promote microbial antibiotic resistance. Oral quinolones and co-trimoxazole are potential candidates and have been shown to reduce the incidence of infection but not to improve survival rates. Selective decontamination of the gastrointestinal tract with nonabsorbable antibiotics to prevent colonization by gram-negative bacilli and *Candida*, while sparing anaerobic bacteria, has reduced the incidence of pulmonary infection. However, overall mortality has not been affected, and gram-positive infections have increased. Therefore, prophylaxis can be detrimental in terms of the emergence of antibiotic resistance and fungemia and cannot be recommended.

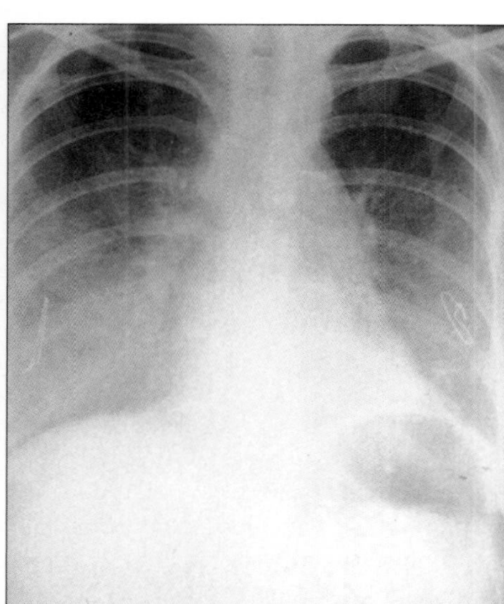

Figure 25.1 Aspiration pneumonia. Chest radiograph of a 22-year-old woman who underwent a double sequential lung transplant but, after 18 days, suffered an episode of aspiration with the development of noncardiogenic pulmonary edema. The radiograph shows a bilateral interstitial and alveolar infiltrate in association with a dilated stomach, which contains a bezoar.

Pneumococcus is an important pathogen in hematopoietic cell transplant recipients, particularly those who have graft-versus-host disease or have undergone splenectomy. Penicillin 250 mg twice daily is recommended for up to 2 years after BMT, and potentially longer in patients who have graft-versus-host disease. Despite this, pneumococcal pneumonia still occurs and should always be considered in the differential diagnosis because of patient noncompliance and penicillin-resistant strains. Many immunodeficient patients receive co-trimoxazole prophylaxis for *Pneumocystis jiroveci* pneumonia, which affects pneumococcal infection rates. Vaccination is widely recommended to prevent pneumococcal infection, but it is difficult to assess its impact, and data suggest that high-risk immunocompromised patients are not adequately protected.

Hematopoietic growth factors can shorten the duration of neutropenia. However, they have not been demonstrated to decrease infection-related mortality, so routine use is not recommended. In complicated, prolonged neutropenia, their use is acceptable. Hand washing by medical personnel is important and underemphasized, particularly for those being nursed outside protected environments.

VIRAL PNEUMONIA

Efficient T-cell immunosuppression, with the advent of cyclosporin, has heralded the era of successful organ transplantation. However, T-cell immunosuppression places patients at risk for opportunistic viral infection, of which human cytomegalovirus (CMV) is the most common. All transplant populations are at risk for CMV infection, with reported rates of infection ranging from 40% to 75%. Until the development of the antiviral agent ganciclovir, the direct mortality from CMV pneumonia approached 100%. Immunocompromised patients are also at risk for community-acquired viral infections caused by Paramyxoviridae, Orthomyxoviridae, and Adenoviridae.

Epidemiology

Immunocompetent hosts acquire CMV from others via body fluids and, at most, experience a mononucleosis-like syndrome. After acute infection, CMV assumes a latent state. Prior exposure to CMV may be assessed by the detection of host CMV immunoglobulin (IgG, seropositive). The rate of CMV seropositivity in the general population increases by approximately 10% for every decade of life; older patients who require heart and kidney transplantation are generally CMV seropositive, whereas younger patients (with acute lymphatic leukemia or cystic fibrosis) are often seronegative.

Seronegative immunocompromised patients are at risk for primary CMV infection if they acquire an organ from a CMV-seropositive donor. Other modes of acquisition include transmission by blood transfusion products, but this generally requires a substantial volume of leukocytes containing the virus to be transfused. Transmission of the virus via the transplanted

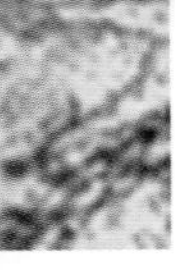

organ invariably results in a primary CMV infection, which is usually severe.

Secondary CMV infection occurs in a seropositive transplant recipient and is either a reactivation of endogenous virus or a superinfection from the donor's virus. The infection is generally less severe than primary infection because of the presence of both cytotoxic T cells specific to CMV and endogenous CMV immunoglobulin.

The risk in allograft hematopoietic cell transplant recipients is dependent on the recovery of T-cell-specific immunity, and graft-versus-host disease significantly increases the risk of CMV infection. Autologous hematopoietic cell transplant recipients experience less CMV-related infection, and it is usually milder.

Therefore, the risk of CMV infection is dependent on the patient's CMV serostatus, the level of immunosuppression, and the time of greatest risk following intensive immunosuppression, which is generally in the first 120 days after transplantation.

After allogeneic hematopoietic cell transplantation, 30% to 50% of patients develop idiopathic pneumonitis. Possible causes include viral pathogens in conjunction with radiation pneumonitis, a drug reaction, or human herpesvirus.

Community-acquired viral infections are also part of the differential diagnosis of pneumonitis and include the Orthomyxoviridae (influenza A, B, and C), Paramyxoviridae (parainfluenza 1 to 4, respiratory syncytial virus [RSV], and measles), and DNA (adenovirus) viruses, of which RSV, parainfluenza 3, and adenovirus have particularly high mortality rates. These viruses have a short incubation period with a seasonal distribution and are associated with nosocomial outbreaks. Transmission is from skin to skin, with subsequent inoculation to the upper respiratory tract. Lung transplant recipients, adult hematopoietic cell transplant recipients (9%), and pediatric hematopoietic cell transplant recipients (30%) in particular appear to be at increased risk (Fig. 25.2).

Clinical Features

The clinical features of CMV pneumonia in immunocompromised patients are nonspecific and include general malaise and lethargy, similar to graft rejection and graft-versus-host disease. Influenza and RSV infection cause respiratory tract symptoms and are seasonal. Coexisting bacterial infection is common, and the most consistent sign is pyrexia, but this can also be absent.

A useful surrogate for CMV infection is the development of leukopenia and abnormal liver function tests. Symptomatic CMV infection includes a mononucleosis-like syndrome of varying severity, with or without pyrexia, in conjunction with laboratory evidence of infection. Specifically, *CMV syndrome* refers to pyrexia related to CMV infection in conjunction with a 50% fall in leukocyte count and a 2.5-fold increase in serum transaminases; the definition of *CMV disease* includes tissue-based evidence of end-organ damage caused by the virus. Many consider patients to have CMV disease if they are clinically unwell with laboratory evidence of infection, even though tissue samples may not be available.

Diagnosis

No typical radiologic pattern is associated with CMV pneumonia. Indeed, a normal chest radiograph is common. An abnormal chest radiograph implies a large viral load with an intense inflammatory reaction. Radiographic changes may be asymmetrical and diffuse or nodular. Nodular changes in the presence of CMV pneumonia should prompt further investigations for aspergillosis.

Acquisition of lung tissue by transbronchial biopsy and demonstration of viral inclusion bodies with an inflammatory infiltrate constitute the gold standard for the diagnosis of CMV pneumonia. Typically, CMV appears as "owl eye" intranuclear inclusion bodies with hematoxylin-eosin staining of lung tissue (Fig. 25.3). Every effort must be made to acquire lung tissue for a firm diagnosis, but for patients who have a coagulopathy, this is not always possible. Therefore, the laboratory assessment of CMV infection is important to determine the probability and risk of CMV pneumonia. The tests available are summarized in Table 25.2.

The starting point for the laboratory characterization of viral infection, particularly CMV, is the use of serologic assessment. The direct early-antigen fluorescent foci test (shell vial assay) can be applied to BAL but is dependent on cell culture techniques.

CMV antigenemia and polymerase chain reaction (PCR) for CMV are diagnostic techniques with high (≈100%) negative

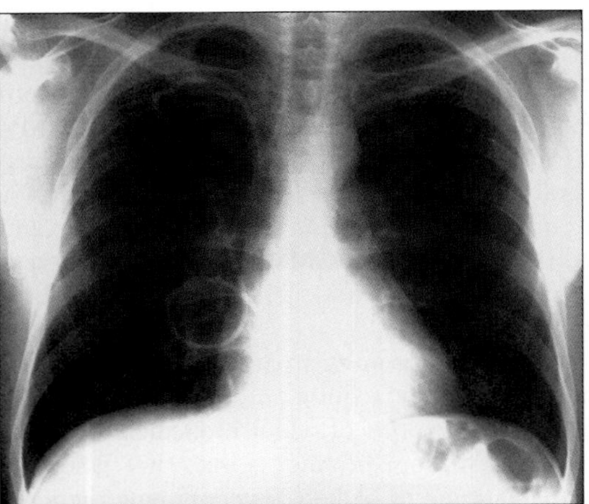

A

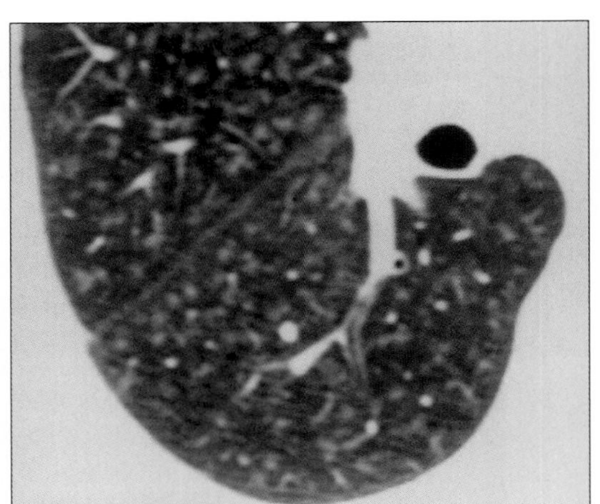

B

Figure 25.2 A, Normal chest radiograph in a man with acute lymphoblastic leukemia, increasing breathlessness, and fever. **B,** Computed tomography scan showing bronchial wall thickening of terminal bronchioles due to respiratory syncytial virus infection.

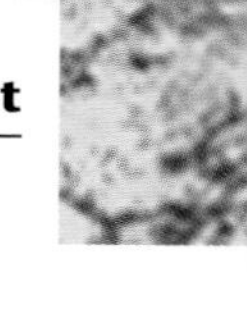

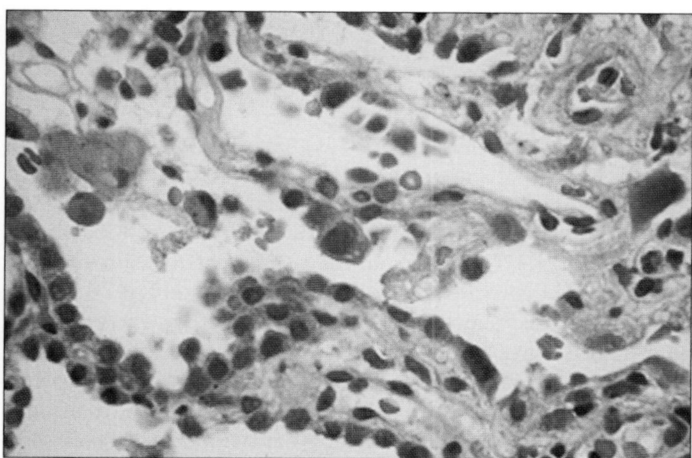

Figure 25.3 Cytomegalovirus pneumonitis. This transbronchial lung biopsy demonstrates "owl eye" intranuclear inclusion bodies in the center of the slide, with an associated inflammatory infiltrate.

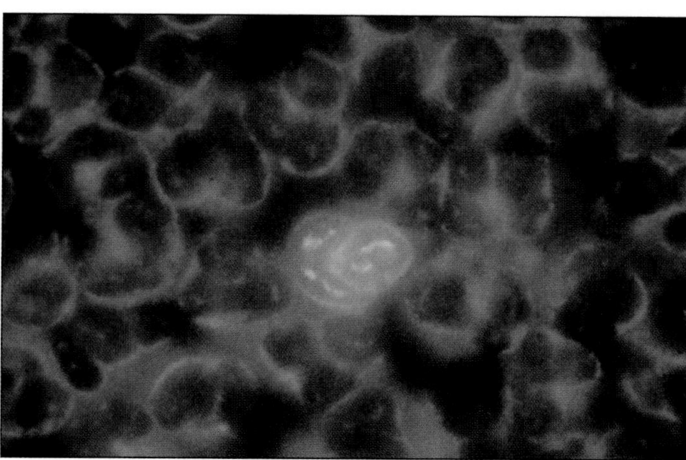

Figure 25.4 Cytomegalovirus antigenemia. This example demonstrates a polymorphonuclear leukocyte with positive immunofluorescent staining using a commercially available monoclonal antibody directed against pp65 low-matrix phosphoprotein.

predictive values (Fig. 25.4). A negative qualitative PCR assay virtually excludes the possibility of CMV pneumonia. However, sensitive qualitative PCR assays are commonly positive and do not discriminate between latent and replicating virus. Quantitative techniques, which include CMV antigenemia, quantitative PCR, and the detection of CMV mRNA, can differentiate between latent and replicating CMV.

In the absence of tissue, estimation of the probability of CMV pneumonia is dependent on three factors: (1) quantifying the replicating viral load, (2) the rate of change in viral load (viral kinetics), and (3) the circumstance of immunosuppression. For example, with an initial CMV load of $5\log_{10}$ genomes/mL and a rate of change of $0.1\log_{10}$ genomes/day, there is a 33% risk of disease; however, if the rate of change is $0.4\log_{10}$ genomes/mL

Table 25.2
Diagnostic tests for cytomegalovirus infection

Test	Sample	Method	Time	Comment
Culture	Blood, broncho-alveolar lavage	Suspension is added to human embryonic fibroblast culture medium Cytomegalovirus culture positive = cytopathic effect	2-6 weeks	Slow with low sensitivity and low specificity, of little practical application
Serology	Blood	Cytomegalovirus-specific IgM and IgG enzyme-linked immunosorbent assay	24-72 hours	Slow and change in IgG or IgM postdates clinical event
Shell vial assay or direct early antigen fluorescent foci test	Blood, bronchoalveolar lavage	Suspension is added to fibroblast culture medium and stained with monoclonal antibody at 24 and 48 hours	24-48 hours	Popular and relatively rapid; high sensitivity, but depends on the use of culture medium; low specificity
Antigenemia	EDTA blood (neutrophils)	Cytospin preparation of neutrophils with immunofluorescent staining by antibody against pp65 low-matrix phosphoprotein (see Fig. 25.4)	6 hours	Rapid and quantitative; high negative predictive value; however, demands rapid processing in the laboratory
Qualitative polymerase chain reaction (PCR)	Blood, bronchoalveolar lavage	Following DNA extraction, PCR assay using primers against a variety of targets – gp58, IE1, or pp150	24 hours	High negative predictive value, very low positive predictive value; virtually all seropositive patients are PCR positive
Quantitative PCR	Blood, bronchoalveolar lavage	Competitive PCR – applies a calculated ratio between a known quantity of internal standard competitor versus an unknown quantity in the patient's sample. Real-time PCR is a detection assay providing quantitation during the amplification process	24 hours	Different quantitative assays available; high negative value, relatively high positive predictive value. Kinetics are important
Immunocytochemistry	Bronchoalveolar lavage, dewaxed tissue	Monoclonal antibodies directed against cytomegalovirus	6 hours	Requires tissue; can be used as an adjunct to histology
Cytology	Bronchoalveolar lavage	–	6 hours	High specificity, low sensitivity
Histology	Tissue	Tissue stored in formalin, and fixed and stained with hematoxylin–eosin; infected cells are enlarged and contain intranuclear inclusions ("owl-eye" cells)	6 hours	Gold standard, may be superseded by quantitative PCR

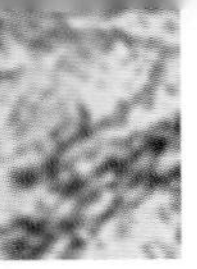

per day, the risk is 64%. Then, viral levels have to be interpreted in the context of different clinical settings or in different transplant populations. For instance, in hematopoietic cell transplant recipients, more than 3 CMV antigen-positive cells per polymorphonuclear leukocyte per slide is considered to represent high-level viral replication. In contrast, in heart transplant recipients, more than 50 antigen-positive cells per 2×10^5 polymorphonuclear leukocytes represents high-level viremia.

Progress in achieving the diagnosis of community-acquired viral pneumonia (RSV, adenovirus, influenza) is less satisfactory. A high index of suspicion and a proactive approach toward the diagnosis may explain why some groups have demonstrated that these viruses are important causes of infection and mortality in immunocompromised patients. The diagnosis in critically ill patients needs to be rapid, and because this is difficult, many infections may go unrecognized. Culture of upper respiratory tract specimens by BAL is the gold standard, but culture is confounded by a 6- to 12-day wait for results. Potentially superior techniques for diagnosis include immunofluorescent staining of culture specimens and antigen detection using enzyme-linked immunosorbent assay (ELISA). Detection of RSV antigen has a high sensitivity (88%) for the identification of RSV in BAL from adult BMT recipients. This contrasts with relatively low sensitivity for the identification of RSV from upper respiratory tract specimens, but this may reflect a lower viral load in the upper airway and emphasizes the importance of obtaining BAL specimens in patients with suspected RSV infection.

Treatment

GANCICLOVIR

Ganciclovir is the cornerstone of treatment for CMV pneumonia. The drug undergoes intracellular phosphorylation to ganciclovir trisphosphate, which is concentrated in virus-infected cells and competitively inhibits viral DNA polymerase metabolism of deoxyguanine triphosphate. Ganciclovir is administered at dosages of 5 mg/kg twice daily for 14 to 21 days. Dosage adjustment is required with renal impairment and the major side effects of leukopenia and thrombocytopenia. Hematopoietic growth factors (granulocyte colony-stimulating factor) can be administered for leukopenia, and because of the mutagenic effects of ganciclovir, effective contraception is advised.

The combination of ganciclovir and hyperimmunoglobulin has been reasonably successful in hematopoietic cell transplant recipients affected by CMV pneumonia, but treatment failure may occur if therapy is commenced late in the disease process. In recipients of solid organ transplants who have CMV pneumonia, ganciclovir alone is very effective. However, in those with CMV pneumonia as a consequence of primary infection, the use of CMV hyperimmunoglobulin for passive immunization must be considered.

FOSCARNET

Foscarnet is a virustatic agent effective against herpesviruses. It acts by the inhibition of herpesvirus-specific DNA polymerase and is usually reserved if ganciclovir treatment fails or if CMV-ganciclovir resistance is a concern. Foscarnet is given as intermittent infusions every 8 hours at a dose of 60 mg/kg in patients who have normal renal function. The dose has to be titrated according to the patient's creatinine level. A drug concentration of 150 mg/L is ideal. Foscarnet is directly nephrotoxic—30% of patients experience renal toxicity.

RIBAVIRIN

Ribavirin (tribavirin) is a synthetic guanosine nucleoside with a broad spectrum of antiviral activity. It has in vitro activity against RSV and influenza virus and is believed to interfere with the protein translation by mRNA of the RNA virus. Ribavirin is administered for 12 to 24 hours as a small-particle aerosol from a solution that contains the drug at a concentration of 20 mg/mL for 7 to 14 days. Shorter-dose treatments with a water solution of 60 mg/mL given over 2 hours three times per day compare favorably with standard treatment. Administration of ribavirin via a ventilator using a high-dose, short-duration treatment results in minimal or no detection of ribavirin in the room, and it has not been detected in the erythrocytes of exposed health care workers. Alternatively, ribavirin can be given intravenously at 25 mg/kg on day 1 followed by 15 mg/kg per day.

Prophylaxis

The advent of antiviral therapy, in conjunction with the morbidity and mortality of CMV infection, has resulted in the development of drug strategies aimed at preventing CMV infection and disease. The goal of prophylaxis is to suppress viral load during the period of greatest risk, up to 120 days after transplantation, until immune recovery occurs.

ACYCLOVIR

Acyclovir was the first safe and widely available antiviral therapy used as prophylaxis against CMV. It is a guanine nucleoside analog and inhibits viral DNA polymerase. Acyclovir preferentially inhibits herpes simplex and varicella-zoster, but CMV is less sensitive. Therefore, it is not sufficiently potent to treat CMV pneumonia. However, its high-dose administration as a prophylactic agent against CMV has been widely studied and appears to prevent CMV infection in renal transplant recipients. In high-risk patients, intravenous acyclovir maximizes its potency against CMV and compensates for variable oral bioavailability. In hematopoietic cell transplant recipients, intravenous acyclovir for 1 month, followed by oral therapy, reduced CMV infection and improved survival. However, oral prophylaxis is clearly preferential to intravenous. Valacyclovir, the valine ester of acyclovir, has improved oral bioavailability. Studies suggest that valacyclovir prevents CMV infection in hematopoietic cell transplant recipients and heart transplant recipients and also improves survival in renal transplant recipients.

GANCICLOVIR

Ganciclovir, which has greater potency against CMV than acyclovir, has also been widely studied in all transplant populations. Intravenous ganciclovir prevents CMV infection and disease in transplant recipients. Allogeneic hematopoietic cell transplant recipients who received various schedules of intravenous ganciclovir had a significantly reduced incidence of CMV infection, but there was no survival advantage compared with placebo; in addition, there was an increased incidence of leukopenia in patients who received ganciclovir compared with placebo. Therefore, widespread prophylaxis to all at-risk patients would result in some patients receiving unnecessary exposure to antiviral therapy, which is potentially hazardous and expensive and risks the emergence of ganciclovir resistance. Thus, preemptive treatment directed by diagnostic tests for CMV has been advocated.

Preemptive intravenous ganciclovir therapy in allograft BMT recipients directed by BAL surveillance on day 35 after transplantation resulted in improved survival for BAL CMV-positive patients who received 90 days of antiviral therapy. A second strategy in hematopoietic cell transplant recipients using peripheral blood culture for CMV also resulted in improved survival, but with this approach, 12% of patients developed CMV disease in advance of being blood-culture positive. With preemptive ganciclovir directed by CMV antigenemia in hematopoietic cell transplant recipients, patients experienced significantly more CMV infection compared with those who received intravenous ganciclovir prophylaxis. However, there was no difference in survival between the two groups, possibly because the patients who received indiscriminate ganciclovir prophylaxis had a significantly greater incidence of fungal infection. In heart and lung transplant recipients, preemptive treatment directed by CMV antigenemia has resulted in a significant reduction in CMV disease. These observations suggest that preemptive treatment directed by CMV antigenemia does not eliminate CMV infection but facilitates control, with reduced ganciclovir exposure and fewer complications.

Oral ganciclovir prophylaxis (1 g every 8 hours) is an alternative strategy, but randomized studies of oral ganciclovir versus placebo showed no difference in survival, despite less CMV disease with ganciclovir. The valine ester of ganciclovir, valganciclovir, at a dose of 900 mg orally once daily, has comparable bioavailabilty to 5 mg of intravenous ganciclovir.

The role for vaccination in the prevention of CMV and influenza infection is uncertain. In the setting of an influenza outbreak, amantadine or rimantadine (anti-influenza drugs) may be given to high-risk immunocompromised patients.

A number of strategies are available for the control of viral infection in immunocompromised patients. Optimal control of CMV includes the application of acyclovir or valacyclovir for prophylaxis, with surveillance for CMV infection by CMV antigenemia or qualitative PCR and ganciclovir for preemptive treatment in the presence of an increasing viral load.

FUNGAL PNEUMONIA

Fungal infection is a major hazard in immunocompromised patients because of the difficulty in achieving a diagnosis and the limitations of treatment. Increasingly sophisticated and intense immunosuppression, in conjunction with interventions that result in disruption of the host's mucosal integrity, predisposes patients to fungal infection. Inevitably, the lung is the key target organ for invasive fungal disease.

Epidemiology and Risk Factors

Aspergillus fumigatus, an inhaled environmental pathogen, is the most common cause of invasive pulmonary disease and is an increasing problem, with the infection rate increasing from 2.2% to 5.1% over a 14-year period in one autopsy study. *Candida albicans* is the most common cause of fungal infection in immunocompromised patients, but it rarely causes invasive pulmonary disease. *Candida* is endogenous in origin, emanating from the gastrointestinal tract, and usually results in mucocutaneous candidiasis. Nevertheless, in an immunocompromised host, candidemia commonly results in septicemia, and in conjunction with gram-positive or gram-negative organisms, *Candida* may be a pathogen that results in pneumonia (Fig. 25.5).

The incidence of fungal infection, including candidemia, approaches 50% in hematopoietic cell transplant recipients and 35% in lymphoma patients. The incidence of invasive pulmonary aspergillosis (IPA) in hematopoietic cell transplant recipients ranges from 6% to 15%, with a bimodal incidence occurring early (<40 days) and late (>40 days) after transplantation (post engraftment). A 5-year study of 1682 patients receiving allogeneic stem cell transplants suggests that there is a shift in the timing of IPA, occurring most commonly (53%) postengraftment. Factors associated with early IPA include the receipt of cord blood transplants, aplastic anemia, and myelodysplastic syndrome. Protection against IPA is conferred by the use of matched, related peripheral blood compared with matched, related bone marrow. Factors associated with increased postengraftment IPA include receipt of T-cell-depleted or CD34-selected stem cell products, corticosteroids, graft-versus-host disease, CMV, and viral respiratory infection.

In liver transplant recipients, IPA has an incidence of 1% to 10%. Isolated lung and heart-lung transplant recipients are commonly colonized with *Aspergillus* (25% to 40%), with an incidence of invasive disease of 15% to 25%. Heart transplant and renal transplant recipients have a rate of infection that is less than 10%. But the reported rates of infection, particularly in solid organ transplant recipients, are often influenced by outbreaks associated with local environmental factors. The overall mortality is on the order of 80% to 100%.

Aspergilli have a small spore size with the capacity to be inhaled. Pathogenicity is promoted by the ability to adhere to epithelial cells and also to survive over a wide temperature range, up to 50°C (122°F). *Aspergillus* includes a number of species, of which *A. fumigatus* is the most common, causing approximately 80% of invasive infections. *Aspergillus flavus* causes 5% to 10% of infections and particularly affects the sinuses.

The clinical patterns of IPA contrast with those of saprophytic infection, in which aspergilli colonize cavities to form an

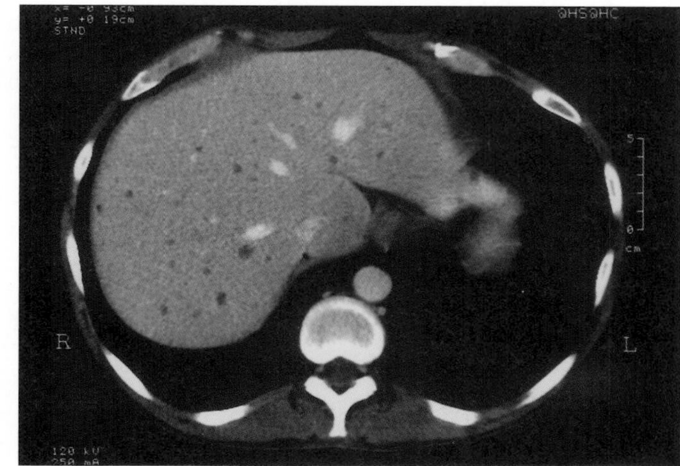

Figure 25.5 Computed tomography scan of the liver showing multiple abscesses due to *Candida* septicemia.

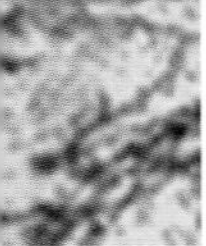

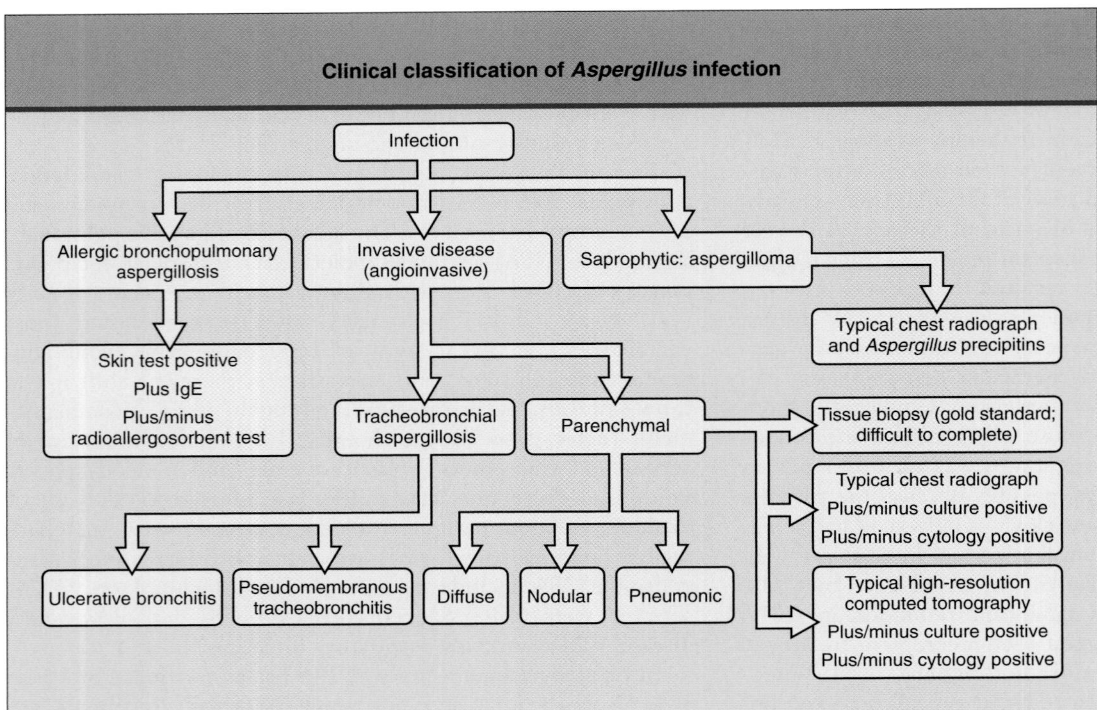

Figure 25.6 Classification of *Aspergillus* disease. Flow chart demonstrating the clinical classification of *Aspergillus* infection and disease.

aspergilloma, and that of allergic reactions to aspergillus (allergic bronchopulmonary aspergillosis). The pathology of IPA results from the spectrum of adherence, destructive invasion, and ultimately infarction of pulmonary tissue with systemic embolization and fungemia. Localization of IPA can be peripheral within the lung parenchyma or central with a tracheobronchial distribution (Fig. 25.6).

Some patients, particularly lung transplant recipients with impaired mucociliary clearance and poor cough reflex, develop tracheobronchial aspergillosis. This begins with *Aspergillus* colonization, progressing to tracheobronchitis, more severe ulceration, and ultimately an increasingly severe inflammatory response that culminates in membrane formation with mucus and necrotic tissue (Fig. 25.7).

Fungi, including *Cryptococcus* and *Mucorales*, are uncommon causes of invasive pulmonary disease in immunocompromised patients; mucormycosis carries a worse prognosis than aspergillosis. Other fungi have a geographic distribution: *Coccidioides* in southwestern North America and in South America, and *Histoplasma* in central North America and in South America. These fungi are associated with acute and chronic illnesses, and their clinical effects mirror acute sarcoidosis and chronic mycobacterial infection, respectively.

P. jiroveci is a widely distributed, eukaryotic pathogen that affects immunocompromised patients. Traditionally, *Pneumocystis* was classified as a protozoal organism. However, taxonomy has shown that it is more closely related genetically to fungi (see Chapter 30).

Clinical Features

Invasive pulmonary aspergillosis does not have specific clinical features with a high predictive value for clinical diagnosis. Diffuse, nodular, central, and peripheral patterns of infection

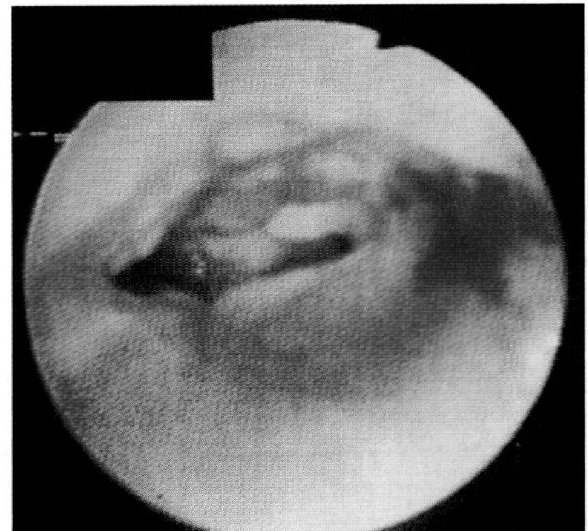

Figure 25.7 Tracheobronchial aspergillosis. Bronchoscopic finding of bronchial aspergillosis with ulceration of the right lower-lobe bronchus with membrane formation.

occur. The clinical diagnosis is dependent on a high index of suspicion in susceptible patients.

In febrile, neutropenic patients, pyrexia unresponsive to broad-spectrum antibiotics prompts further investigation. In other immunocompromised patients, fever may not be present. Clinical examination of the respiratory tract is often normal, and other organs subject to metastatic infection by fungi need to be examined, including the eye, skin, central nervous system, and urinary tract.

Diagnosis

Three levels of probability—proven, probable, and possible—have been agreed on for the diagnosis of fungal pneumonia. The gold standard of a proven diagnosis of invasive aspergillosis is based on histopathologic examination of lung tissue. However, this is rarely achieved, particularly in complex thrombocytopenic, immunocompromised patients. A probable diagnosis refers to both microbiologic evidence and clinical or radiologic evidence of pulmonary or sinus disease in a host at risk (neutropenia). Proven and probable diagnoses are accepted end points for treatment studies. A possible diagnosis of fungal infection is either microbiologic or radiologic evidence of fungal infection in an at-risk host. In clinical practice, a possible diagnosis should prompt empirical antifungal treatment. Despite the protean, heterogeneous clinical manifestations of invasive aspergillosis, a clinical-radiologic classification can be applied (see Fig. 25.6), which prompts an ordered strategy of investigation and treatment (Fig. 25.8).

The sensitivity of sputum culture for fungus is increased by collecting at least three consecutive samples and using specialized fungal media, such as Sabouraud dextrose agar. Nasal culture specimens have demonstrated encouraging positive predictive values for invasive aspergillosis in hematopoietic cell transplant recipients. All culture-positive specimens should be sent to a reference laboratory for identification. It is difficult to determine whether sputum positive to *Aspergillus* culture represents colonization or invasive disease. A positive culture for *Aspergillus* is associated with disease in 64% of hematopoietic cell transplant recipients and in 17% of solid organ transplant recipients. Microscopy of sputum and BAL is a key investigation in suspected cases of fungal disease. Microscopy is 20% more sensitive than culture for identifying fungus and provides a rapid result within 2 to 4 hours.

The isolation of fungemia from blood in neutropenic patients is rare and, if positive, is often thought to reflect contamination. Nevertheless, candidemia does occur, and its identification should prompt further investigation. The sensitivity of blood culture surveillance for fungemia can be increased by collecting a minimum of 20 mL of blood in aerobic culture. Surveillance for *Aspergillus* antigenemia has improved and supports a diagnosis of proven aspergillosis. A sandwich ELISA technique using a monoclonal antibody to galactomannan (Bio-Rad Laboratories) has a sensitivity and specificity greater than 90%. Two positive results are required because of the risk of false positives. Diagnostic PCR assays, using primers targeting a 135–base pair fragment in the mitochondrial region of *Aspergillus*, are important developments, but the routine use of PCR for the diagnosis of IPA cannot be recommended.

In invasive mycosis, the chest radiograph may be normal or abnormal and may demonstrate a nodular or diffuse pattern (Fig. 25.9). An abnormal chest radiograph demands targeted bronchoscopy and BAL. Nodular disease is highly suggestive of invasive aspergillosis or of nocardial or pneumocystic infection. A diffuse infiltrate also demands a bronchoscopy and BAL, because such a pattern may be CMV, *Pneumocystis*, or bacterial infection. Wedge-shaped shadowing can be caused by an *Aspergillus*-induced pulmonary infarction.

HRCT scanning is more sensitive and specific than plain radiology for the diagnosis of invasive aspergillosis. HRCT should be undertaken within 48 hours of microbiologic evidence of *Aspergillus* and after 7 days of unresolved pyrexia in neutropenic patients. Abnormalities on HRCT can be categorized as nodular or diffuse. Nodular disease is highly characteristic of invasive aspergillosis and reflects the pathologic process. In neutropenic patients who have invasive aspergillosis, a nodule surrounded by an area of increased attenuation (ground glass) relative to normal lung is highly specific for IPA, and this is much better seen on HRCT than on plain chest radiographs (Fig. 25.10). This pattern is referred to as the "halo sign." Pathologically, the area of increased attenuation that surrounds the nodule represents hemorrhage. Also, HRCT may identify another characteristic sign of invasive aspergillosis—a "crescent" formation. Infarction of the lung tissue occurs with vascular invasion, and tissue necrosis and repair result in a collection of air between normal and abnormal pulmonary tissue, which manifests as a crescent of air (see Figs. 25.9 and 25.10). HRCT is commonly used to exclude IPA because of the specificity of the halo and crescent signs, although a negative HRCT does not necessarily obviate the need for other investigations for IPA.

Fiber-optic bronchoscopy and BAL are important for the diagnosis of invasive aspergillosis, particularly in *Aspergillus* tracheobronchial disease, in which the chest radiograph is commonly normal (see Fig. 25.7). Here, sampling of the area is usually culture positive for *Aspergillus*, and stains of the sample for cytologic examination are also positive. Nevertheless, in the absence of a coagulopathy, such lesions should be biopsied.

In peripheral, localized, nodular aspergillosis, bronchoscopy is of limited value for the diagnosis of IPA, and percutaneous CT-guided biopsy is preferable. However, with peripheral disease, a negative BAL excluding other diagnoses is important before proceeding to more invasive diagnostic techniques. Bronchoscopy is more useful in diffuse radiologic disease and allows culture and cytologic examination. In addition to isolating *Aspergillus*, BAL may identify coexisting infection with other organisms, including *Pseudomonas* and CMV (Fig. 25.11).

Transbronchial lung biopsy is often not possible in patients who have suspected IPA, because many of them have a coagulopathy. There is often a reluctance to proceed to more invasive diagnostic techniques in complex immunocompromised patients, particularly because many centers do not have thoracic surgical expertise available on site. Open lung biopsies were reported to have acceptable morbidity rates with a high diagnostic yield compared with fiber-optic bronchoscopy and BAL in 13 febrile, neutropenic patients. Clearly, this strategy should be reserved for selected patients for whom a diagnostic dilemma exists. Nevertheless, the importance of an accurate diagnosis in an immunocompromised patient cannot be overstated. Anything less than intensive, targeted treatment carries immeasurable morbidity.

As a diagnostic technique, surgery competes with CT-guided percutaneous biopsy. The latter is less invasive and has a high yield in experienced hands. In thrombocytopenic patients, the risk of hemorrhage is reduced with platelet cover. However, sampling error is a potential problem, with the pathologist reporting the presence of necrotic tissue but no organism being identified.

Treatment

The successful treatment of invasive aspergillosis is confounded by the difficulty in achieving an early diagnosis. Therapy must be initiated either on the basis of proven disease or empirically in a high-risk patient with probable or possible IPA.

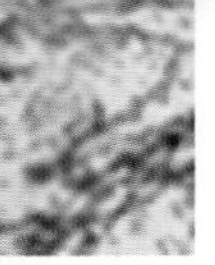

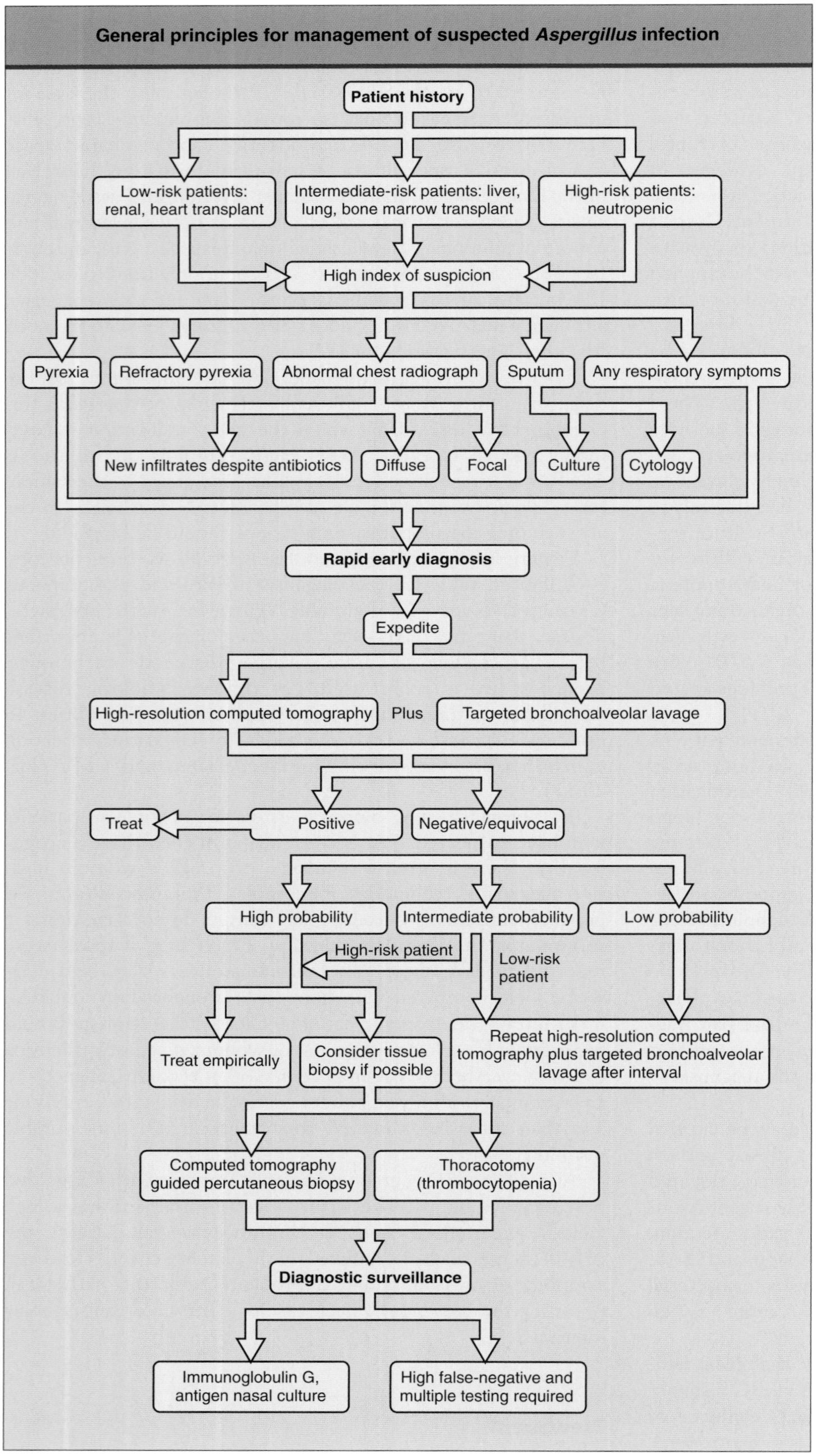

Figure 25.8 Principles for the management of suspected *Aspergillus* infection. A pulmonologist must understand the kinetics of risk factors, prevalence, and level of immunosuppression against the background of prophylaxis duration and timing of empirical therapy.

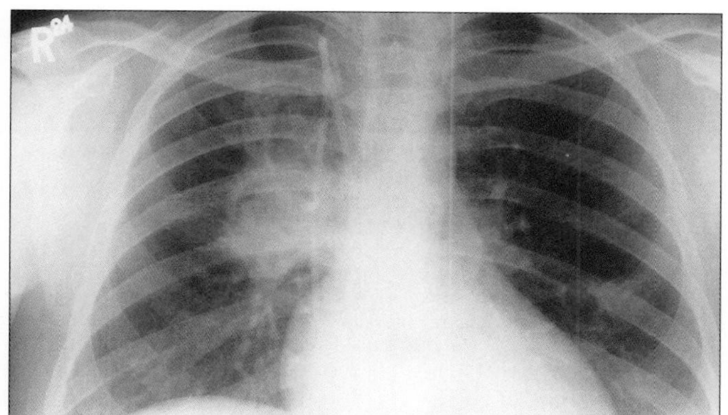

Figure 25.9 Chest radiograph of invasive aspergillosis showing the "crescent" sign, due to air in the cavity caused by a contracting, infarcted area of lung.

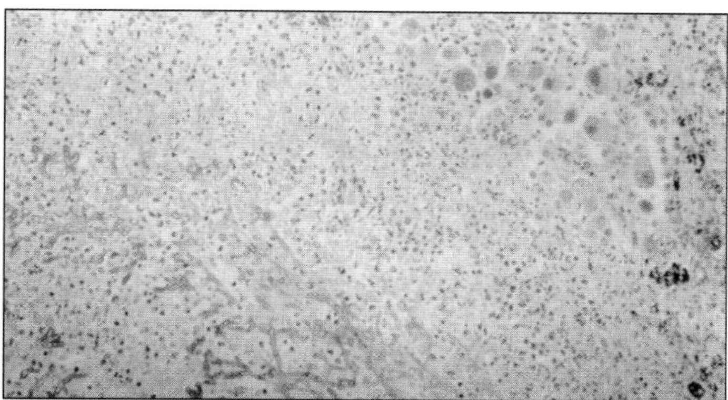

Figure 25.11 ***Aspergillus* and cytomegalovirus as copathogens.** Low-magnification light microscopy of lung tissue demonstrates invasive aspergillosis (filamentous hyphae, lower left) combined with cytomegalovirus "owl eye" intranuclear inclusion bodies (upper right).

Amphotericin B was the traditional gold standard. Amphotericin is a fungistatic, macrocyclic, polyene antibiotic derived from *Streptomyces nodosus* and is thought to bind to ergosterol (the principal sterol that makes up the fungal cell membrane), resulting in loss of cell membrane function. It has a broad range of activity against *Aspergillus* and *Candida*, as well as against the less common organisms *Mucorales* and *Histoplasma*. The choice of therapy often depends on renal function, gastrointestinal function, and expense. The major factor in favor of amphotericin B is its low cost, but the key limiting factor is the inevitable renal toxicity and systemic reactions to the drug. Because of the alternatives that are now available, there is a compelling case to avoid amphotericin B in patients who suffer impaired or reversible renal dysfunction. Amphotericin B is given in a dose of 0.1 to 1 mg/kg. A test dose of 1 mg in 20 mL over 30 minutes is advised, and subsequent doses should be given over 6 hours. Rapid escalation is reserved for critically ill patients, in whom four doses are administered over 40 hours, each dose totaling 50 mg or 1 mg/kg per 6 hours of infusion, whichever is less. Pretreatment with acetaminophen (paracetamol) and chlorpheniramine may ameliorate systemic reactions, which, if severe, can be treated with hydrocortisone. Renal dysfunction is inevitable, with 90% of patients developing uremia and an elevated creatinine level, in addition to renal tubular acidosis. A treatment gap is advised if this happens, but drug withdrawal in a patient who has invasive mycosis is hazardous.

Because of its improved safety profile, the delivery of amphotericin in a lipid complex form—liposomal amphotericin—has gained popularity. Different preparations are available (Table 25.3). Currently, animal and human data demonstrate that such preparations have minimal nephrotoxicity in comparison to amphotericin B. However, liposomal preparations should be administered at three times the dose of conventional amphotericin B. AmBisome is the only "true" liposomal preparation, being composed of small lipid spheres that contain amphotericin, which is inherently lipophilic and has minimal nephrotoxicity. Systemic reactions are uncommon, but some patients complain of back pain, which can be resolved by reducing the rate of infusion in conjunction with simple analgesia. Thrombocytopenia is another side effect.

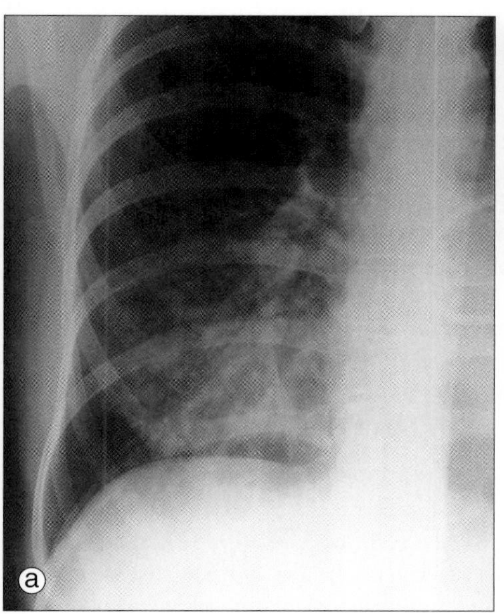

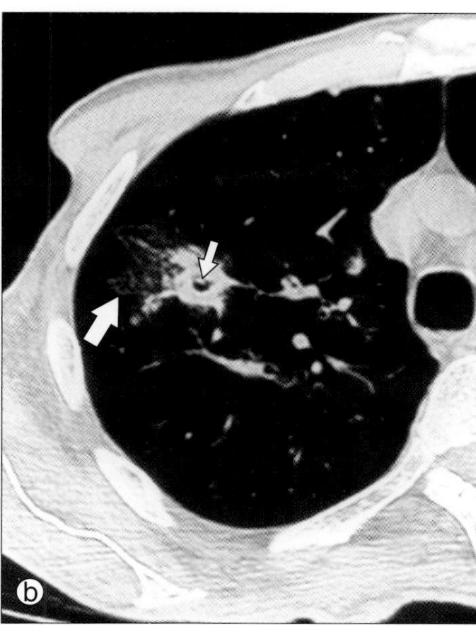

Figure 25.10 A, Chest radiograph of a neutropenic patient showing nonspecific nodular shadowing at the right base. **B,** High-resolution computed tomography clearly shows a nodule of invasive aspergillosis surrounded by a ground-glass infiltration—the "halo" sign *(large arrow)*. Within the nodule is a crescent of air and an area of opacification—the "crescent" sign *(small arrow)*. None of these features was visible on the radiograph.

Table 25.3
Treatment for invasive aspergillosis

Preparation	Administration	Structure	Relative Cost	Dose	Minimum Infusion	Duration of Infusion	Adverse Effects/Comments
AmBisome	Intravenous	Liposomes of amphotericin phospholipids	+ + + + +	1 mg/kg per day increasing to 1-3 mg/kg per day	25 ml for 50 mg	30-60 minutes	Low back pain
Amphocil	Intravenous	Disc-like colloidal dispersion of amphotericin with sodium cholesteryl sulfate	+ + +	1-4 mg/kg per day	80 ml for 50 mg	1-2 mg/kg per h (manufacturer), in practice 3-4 h	Systemic reactions easily controlled with acetaminophen and chlorpheniramine
Abelcet	Intravenous	Ribbon-like complex of amphotericin with phospholipids	+ + + +	5 mg/kg/day	Concentration 1mg/ml, dose dependent, e.g., 60 kg = 300 mg in 300 mL	2 h	Similar to other preparations
Amphotericin B	Intravenous	–	+	0.1 mg/kg per day or max. dose 50 mg	0.5 mg/mL, therefore 60 kg = 300 mL	6 h	Frequent systemic side effects, fever, and chills; treat with intravenous chlorpheniramine and hydrocortisone Nephrotoxicity the major limiting factor
Itraconazole	Oral	Imidazole	+	200 mg q8h for 4 days reducing to 200 mg/day	–	–	Poor absorption that is further inhibited by H_2-antagonist Inhibits P-450, interacts with cyclosporin, corticosteroids, cisapride; awaiting intravenous preparation
Voriconazole	Oral	Tirazole	+	6 mg/kg x 2 4 mg/kg/7 days	200 mg BID orally x 12 weeks	–	Visual disturbance
Caspofungin	Intravenous	Echinocandin	+	70 mg IV loaded 50 mg IV daily	–	–	Well tolerated

Oral itraconazole is a synthetic dioxolane triazole compound effective against both *Candida* and *Aspergillus* and is an attractive option for treatment and prophylaxis. Itraconazole interferes with the P-450–dependent enzyme 14a-demethlase, which leads to ergosterol depletion of the cell membrane, alteration in cell membrane function, and cell death. Its efficacy, however, is entirely dependent on achieving therapeutic levels, which is problematic because of erratic absorption. Clinically, this is a problem in patients who have bowel disturbance and malabsorption, such as hematopoietic cell transplant recipients and patients with graft-versus-host disease or cystic fibrosis. Absorption is also impaired by alkalization of the stomach (H_2-blockers and proton pump inhibitors). Oral syrup and intravenous preparations have improved bioavailability. The patient requires a loading dose of 200 mg every 8 hours for 4 days, followed by dose reduction to 200 mg every 12 hours and measurements of drug levels. A random itraconazole level of 1 mg/L is generally considered appropriate.

Itraconazole, because of its ability to inhibit the P-450 cytochrome system, interacts with a vast number of other medications, including antihistamines, midazolam, digoxin, and warfarin. This interaction is particularly important to immunocompromised patients who receive cyclosporin and tacrolimus, because itraconazole augments the levels of both drugs and increases the potential for nephrotoxicity. When itraconazole and cyclosporin must be administered concurrently, the dose of cyclosporin should be reduced to one third. In common with fluconazole, itraconazole should not be given with cisapride because of the risk of cardiac toxicity (torsades de pointes). Itraconazole has also been reported to augment the effects of corticosteroids.

Voriconazole is a new second-generation triazole derivative that is effective against both *Candida* and *Aspergillus*. It has reliable oral bioavailability, negating the need for drug-level monitoring. Twelve weeks' treatment of invasive aspergillosis with voriconazole significantly improves survival (71%) compared with conventional amphotericin B (58%). It is administered as a loading dose of 6 mg/kg every 12 hours for two doses, followed by 4 mg/kg every 12 hours for 7 days; then the patient can be switched to oral therapy 200 mg BID. Transient visual disturbances are common, occurring in 44% of patients.

Caspofungin is the first member of a new class of antifungal agents—the echinocandins—that inhibit fungal cell wall synthesis by glucan synthase inhibition. Caspofungin is effective in patients with invasive aspergillosis and *Candida* esophagitis. It is given intravenously as a loading dose of 70 mg, followed by 50 mg/day.

As in the case of bacterial infection, hematopoietic growth factors for neutropenia have not been shown to reduce the incidence of fungal infection; therefore, routine use is not recommended.

Surgical Treatment

Surgical therapy has only a limited role in IPA, and success depends on careful case selection. For diffuse disease caused by IPA, surgery has no role unless vascular invasion has occurred, in which case surgery must be considered to prevent life-threatening hemoptysis. In the case of localized disease in a patient who will receive intensive immunosuppression, surgery to excise a source of potentially fatal infection should be considered. Ultimately, surgery carries important risks, including hemorrhage and pleural contamination, and dissection can be difficult because of edematous tissues and reactive lymphadenopathy. Intensification of medical therapy is an accepted alternative to surgery.

Prophylaxis

The first step in prophylaxis is the application of high-efficiency particulate air filters and laminar flow rooms; avoidance of organic, uncooked food; and judicious use of broad-spectrum antibiotics and corticosteroids. Every hospital inevitably has ongoing expansion or refurbishment that may release fungal spores. Environmental surveillance by air sampling with fungal culture is important. A single fungal colony of growth in a hospital area with air filtration systems demands further investigation of the environment.

For oral therapy, the imidazoles and triazoles are potentially ideal candidates for prophylaxis. Fluconazole, a synthetic triazole active against *Candida*, is widely used as prophylaxis against candidemia. However, in a controlled study of 356 hematopoietic cell transplant recipients who received 400 mg of fluconazole per day during neutropenia, C. *albicans*–related infections were reduced, but no difference in survival was observed. The use of fluconazole as prophylaxis has seen increasing colonization with *Candida kruzi* and *Torulopsis glabrata*, yeasts inherently resistant to fluconazole. Similarly, *Aspergillus* resistance to itraconazole has been described.

The choice and circumstance of prophylaxis against *Aspergillus* vary among centers. Local prophylaxis in the form of intranasal or nebulized amphotericin has been used because the sinuses are an important reservoir for *Aspergillus* in hematopoietic cell transplant recipients. Nebulized amphotericin in lung transplant recipients is also used to augment local defenses against an inhaled pathogen in patients who have impaired mucociliary function.

In allogeneic hematopoietic cell transplant recipients, low-dose (20 mg/day) intravenous amphotericin B may be an effective preventive regimen, compared with historical controls, but this effect has not been reported consistently. A study in autologous hematopoietic cell transplant recipients failed to show a benefit with low-dose amphotericin B. The use of inexpensive but potentially nephrotoxic prophylaxis has to be balanced against the absolute requirement for other nephrotoxic drugs, including aminoglycosides, cyclosporin, and tacrolimus.

Cost efficacy of prophylaxis is important, particularly because the use of liposomal amphotericin is increasing. The potential advantages of intravenous liposomal formulations of amphotericin have been emphasized by a randomized comparison between liposomal amphotericin (1 and 3 mg/kg per day) versus conventional amphotericin B. This study evaluated the effect of amphotericin in the treatment of antibiotic-resistant febrile neutropenia. The end point was resolution of the pyrexia during the period of neutropenia. Both doses of liposomal amphotericin were significantly safer than conventional amphotericin B, and 3 mg/kg of liposomal amphotericin was significantly more efficacious than either 1 mg/kg of liposomal amphotericin and conventional amphotericin B for lysis of the pyrexia (64% versus 49%). Meta-analysis of prophylaxis or empirical antifungal treatment has shown that amphotericin-based treatment results in improved outcomes. However, on average, 73 patients (range, 48 to 158) had to be treated to prevent one case of invasive fungal disease.

SUGGESTED READINGS

Ascioglu S, Rex JH, de Pauw B, et al: Defining opportunistic invasive fungal infections in immunocompromised patients with cancer and hematopoietic stem cell transplants: an international consensus. Clin Infect Dis 34:7-14, 2002.

Denning DW, Kibbler CC, Barnes RA: British Society for Medical Mycology proposed standards of care for patients with invasive fungal infections. Lancet 3:230-240, 2003.

Emery VC, Sabin CA, Cope AV, et al: Application of viral-load kinetics to identify patients who develop cytomegalovirus disease after transplantation. Lancet 355:2032-2036, 2000.

Gavin PJ, Katz BZ: Intravenous ribavirin treatment for severe adenovirus disease in immunocompromised children. Paediatrics 110:1-8, 2002.

Gotzsche PC, Johansen HK: Meta-analysis of prophylactic or empirical antifungal treatment versus placebo or no treatment in patients with cancer complicated by neutropenia. BMJ 314:1238-1244, 1997.

Herbrecht R, Denning DW, Patterson TF, et al: Voriconazole versus amphotericin B for primary therapy of invasive aspergillosis. N Engl J Med 347:408-415, 2002.

Hilbert G, Gruson D, Vargas F, et al: Noninvasive ventilation in immunocompromised patients with pulmonary infiltrates, fever, and acute respiratory failure. N Engl J Med 344:481-487, 2001.

Hughes WT, Armstrong D, Bodey GP, et al: 2002 Guidelines for the use of antimicrobial agents in neutropenic patients with cancer. Clin Infect Dis 34:730-751, 2002.

Marr KA, Carter RA, Boeckh M, et al: Invasive aspergillosis in allogeneic stem cell transplant recipients: changes in epidemiology and risk factors. Blood 100:4358-4366, 2002.

Rano A, Agusti C, Jimenez P, et al: Pulmonary infiltrates in non-HIV immunocompromised patients: a diagnostic approach using non-invasive and bronchoscopic procedures. Thorax 56:379-387, 2001.

CHAPTER 26 Hospital-Acquired Pneumonia

Antoni Torres

EPIDEMIOLOGY

After urinary tract infections, pneumonia is the second most common nosocomial infection, accounting for approximately 10% to 15% of all hospital-acquired infections. The overall incidence of nosocomial pneumonia is approximately 6.0 to 8.6 per 1000 admissions, but the risk is greatly increased for all patients in intensive care units, where the incidence has ranged from 12% to 29%, making it the most frequent type of nosocomial infection encountered. The incidence in patients who receive mechanical ventilation ranges from 25% to 70%. Several risk factors have been associated with nosocomial pneumonia, the most important of which are the presence of an artificial airway, prior antibiotic treatment, predispositions to aspiration of oropharyngeal or gastric contents, and host factors that may impair the mechanical, humoral, or cellular defenses.

As many as 15% of all deaths that occur in hospitalized patients are directly related to nosocomial pneumonia. The crude mortality of hospital-acquired pneumonia ranges from 25% to 50%. Age, underlying disease, specific microbe, severity of disease, shock, and initial antibiotic selection are factors related to prognosis. It is important to distinguish early- from late-onset pneumonia with regard to prognosis and treatment. Early-onset pneumonia (i.e., occurring within 5 days of hospitalization) is caused by microorganisms that are already carried by the host—that is, "community" flora (e.g., *Streptococcus pneumoniae*, *Haemophilus influenzae*, *Staphylococcus aureus*, and anaerobes). Late-onset pneumonia occurs after 5 days of hospitalization and is caused by hospital-acquired flora, such as enteric gram-negative bacilli, *Pseudomonas aeruginosa*, and methicillin-resistant *S. aureus*.

ETIOLOGY

Enteric gram-negative bacilli and *S. aureus* (methicillin-resistant or methicillin-sensitive) are the most frequent microorganisms causing hospital-acquired pneumonia (Table 26.1). Overall, these microorganisms are those responsible for late-onset pneumonia, although methicillin-sensitive *S. aureus* is common in patients with early-onset pneumonia, particularly those admitted with coma. Microorganisms causing pneumonia in the community, such as *S. pneumoniae* and *H. influenzae*, are also responsible for some hospital-acquired pneumonias of early onset. The incidence and role of fungi are not well known, but one postmortem study found a prevalence of *Candida* spp of 8%. *Aspergillus* spp may cause pneumonia in immunosuppressed patients, particularly those receiving corticosteroids. Occasionally, immunocompetent patients can acquire *Aspergillus* spp as a result of local epidemics. Anaerobes are infrequent, and *Legionella pneumophila* may be endemic or epidemic.

In patients who require prolonged mechanical ventilation, enteric gram-negative bacilli (e.g., *Enterobacter* spp, *Serratia* spp, *Klebsiella* spp, *Proteus* spp), and, very importantly, *Pseudomonas aeruginosa* and methicillin-resistant *Staphylococcus aureus* are the most frequent etiologies. Currently, nonfermenting gram-negative bacilli such as *Acinetobacter* spp and *Stenotrophomonas maltophilia* have gained importance. The etiology of nosocomial pneumonia is polymicrobial in approximately 30% of cases. Microorganisms causing hospital-acquired pneumonia are frequently resistant to multiple antibiotics. The most important risk factors for antibiotic resistance are prolonged mechanical ventilation and prior antibiotic treatment.

Viral hospital-acquired pneumonias are more important in the pediatric population, with respiratory syncytial and parainfluenza viruses being the most frequently reported

CLINICAL FEATURES

The clinical features that are suspicious for nosocomial pneumonia include the presence of new and persistent pulmonary infiltrates, temperature greater than 38.3°C or less than 36°C, a white blood cell count greater than 12,000/mm^3 or less than 4000/mm^3, and purulent secretions. As a general rule, the existence of pulmonary infiltrates plus one of the remaining criteria should raise a suspicion for hospital-acquired pneumonia.

Although these criteria are well accepted for establishing a diagnosis in spontaneously breathing patients, a number of studies suggest that they are less reliable in diagnosing pneumonia in patients who require mechanical ventilation. Clinical criteria result in a false-positive diagnosis of pneumonia in up to 29% of patients with the acute respiratory distress syndrome when compared with autopsy findings as the gold standard. Radiographic criteria alone have a 32% incidence of misdiagnosis. In mechanically ventilated patients other entities may result in pulmonary infiltrates and fever (see the following section).

As a result of these difficulties, a diagnostic scoring system called the clinical pulmonary infection score (CPIs) was developed several years ago. A patient's score can range from 0 to 12 based on the following variables: temperature, blood leukocyte count, macroscopic evaluation of tracheal secretions, oxygenation (PaO_2/FIO_2 ratio), chest radiograph, and semiquantitative culture of tracheal aspirates. A score greater than 6 has a good correlation with a diagnosis of pneumonia on the basis of quantitative cultures of bronchoalveolar lavage (BAL) fluid (Table 26.2). Recently, some authors have used a modified clinical

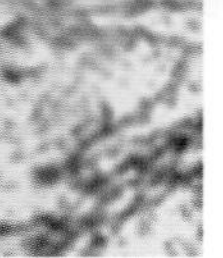

Table 26.1
Microbial etiology of hospital-acquired pneumonia

Microorganism	%
Pseudomonas aeruginosa	30
Staphylococcus aureus (including MRSA)	25
Gram negative enteric bacilli	25
Streptococcus pneumoniae	5
Haemophilus influenzae	5
Fungi (*Aspergillus* and *Candida* spp.)	5
Legionella pneumophila	5
Polymicrobial	30

Table 26.2
Clinical pulmonary infection score

Variable	Criterion	Points
Temperature	≥36.5 to ≤38.4°C	0
	≥38.5 to ≤38.9°C	1
	≥39 to ≤36°C	2
Leukocyte count	≥4000 to ≤11,000	0
	<4000 to >11,000	1
	Band forms	1+
Tracheal secretions	<14+ aspirations	0
	≥14+ aspirations	1
	Purulent secretions	1+
Oxygenation (PaO_2/FIO_2 ratio)	>240 or acute respiratory distress syndrome	0
	≤240	2
Chest radiograph	No infiltrate	0
	Diffuse	1
	Localized	2
Semiquantitative tracheal aspirate cultures (0, 1, 2, or 3+)	Pathogenic bacteria ≤1+ or no growth	0
	Pathogenic bacteria >1+	1
	Same pathogenic bacteria on Gram's stain	1+

This score ranges from 0 to 12 and includes six variables. A clinical score higher than 6 has a good correlation with pulmonary infection.

pulmonary infection score to start or stop antibiotics in patients with suspected hospital-acquired pneumonia. Overall, the sensitivity of the clinical pulmonary infection score is high, but the specificity is moderate and needs to be complemented by microbiologic information for the management of patients.

MICROBIOLOGICAL DIAGNOSIS

Although the initiation of antibiotics is empirical in most of the cases, it is imperative to obtain samples for culturing to confirm or exclude the diagnosis of pneumonia in some cases and to adjust antibiotics in others. Samples for microbiologic diagnosis can be obtained by means of noninvasive or invasive methods.

Noninvasive Methods

BLOOD CULTURES

Blood cultures are obligatory when considering a diagnosis of nosocomial pneumonia. Unfortunately, the sensitivity is low (10%-25%), and the specificity is reduced in critically ill patients who are at risk of bacteremia from multiple infectious foci. Accordingly, microorganisms isolated in blood cultures can only be considered as the definitive etiologic cause of nosocomial pneumonia when they coincide with the microbiologic results of respiratory secretions.

SAMPLING OF THE PROXIMAL AIRWAYS

In patients breathing spontaneously, respiratory secretions can be obtained by expectoration. A valid sample for microbiologic processing requires more than 25 polymorphonuclear cells and less than 10 epithelial squamous cells per field. The operative values of Gram stain and cultures of sputum in hospital-acquired pneumonia are not well known. Qualitative culturing of endotracheal aspirates (in mechanically ventilated patients) is not an accurate way to diagnose nosocomial pneumonia. Although the sensitivity of this technique is high (60% to 90%), the specificity seems to be very low (0% to 33%) because the oropharynx and upper airways of intubated patients are frequently contaminated by flora that do not cause pneumonia. In the absence of prior antibiotic treatment, however, the negative predictive value of these techniques (i.e., negative cultures indicating absence of bacteria pneumonia) is high. Several studies suggest that quantitative cultures of endotracheal aspirates using 10^5 to 10^6 colony-forming units (cfu)/mL as the cutoff point may be comparable in sensitivity and specificity with that obtained by bronchoscopic techniques.

Invasive Methods

Fiberoptic bronchoscopy provides direct access to the lower airways for sampling the bronchi and lung parenchyma. To reach the bronchial tree, however, the bronchoscope has to traverse the endotracheal tube, where it can become contaminated by colonizing flora. Several devices have been developed to allow uncontaminated sampling of the lower airway and parenchyma. The most popular of these is the protected specimen brush (PSB).

PROTECTED SPECIMEN BRUSH

The utility of the PSB was demonstrated nearly 25 years ago (Figure 26.1). This technique involves positioning the bronchoscope just above the orifice from which secretions are to be sampled and advancing the PSB catheter 3 cm from the end of the bronchoscope to avoid collecting secretions that may have accumulated on the bronchoscope tip. An inner cannula is extended, which results in ejection of a carbon-wax plug from the distal end of the catheter into the airway. The catheter is advanced to the desired subsegment. If purulent secretions are visualized, the brush is rotated into them. After sampling, the brush is retracted into the inner cannula, the inner cannula is retracted into the outer cannula, and the catheter is removed

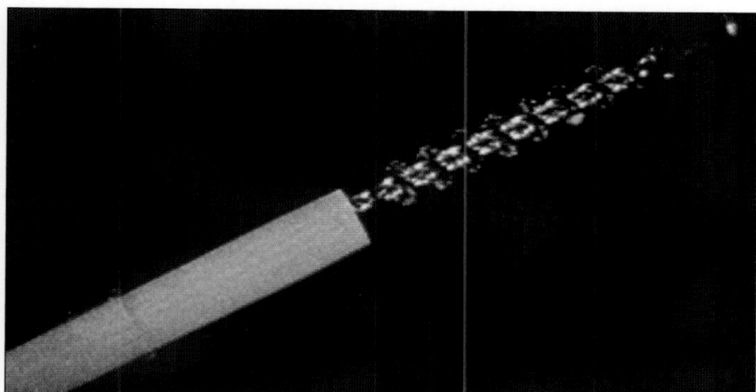

Figure 26.1 The protected specimen brush. The outer sheath has the carbon-wax plug intact; the inner sheath can be seen inside the outer one. The microbiologic brush and the inner sheath protrude outside the outer sheath.

from the bronchoscope. A small quantity of brushed secretions may be used for Gram stain. After wiping the cannula with 70% alcohol and cutting the catheter with sterile scissors, the brush is placed in 1 mL of diluent and immediately submitted for quantitative bacterial culture.

The volume of lower respiratory secretions retrieved is approximately 0.001 mL (range 0.01-0.001) and, as a result of dilution in the holding medium, the colony count on the culture plate represents the result of a 100- to 1000-fold dilution.

Although a large body of work strongly supports the utility of performing quantitative cultures on the material retrieved by PSB to differentiate colonization from infection, questions persist regarding the true "gold standard" with which these data can be compared, as do concerns regarding the effects of antibiotics and the utility of the information obtained. The currently accepted threshold to separate "colonization" from "infection" is greater than 10^3 cfu/mL.

BRONCHOALVEOLAR LAVAGE

The BAL technique was developed to sample a larger portion of lung parenchyma (approximately 10^6 alveoli) than was available with the PSB. Although BAL's sensitivity is generally considered to be high (again with reservations about the true "gold standard" and the effects of antibiotics), the specificity has been limited in part by contamination with upper airway bacteria in up to one fourth of specimens. To perform BAL is necessary to instill 100 to 150 mL in aliquots and then to pool the fluid retrieved for quantitative cultures. Quantitative cultures greater than 10^4 cfu/mL correlate with the presence of pneumonia. The detection of intracellular organisms in greater than 2% of the polymorphonuclear cells or macrophages of centrifugated BAL fluid is a very sensitive and specific marker of pneumonia.

In the last few years, several devices to perform protected BAL (to avoid contamination) have been as reliable or better than conventional BAL. One of the advantages of these techniques is that they can be used with less amount of fluid instilled to lower airways.

BLIND METHODS

Several investigators have examined the utility of blindly sampling the lower airway secretions in mechanically ventilated patients (i.e., without the help of the fiberoptic bronchoscope). Several studies have shown that PSB performed in this fashion has a similar accuracy to that done via bronchoscopy. Blind BAL has also been studied by a number of groups using different approaches (e.g., mini-BAL via protected catheters, Swan-Ganz catheters, or, more recently, protected catheters that can be directed to one or other side of the lungs depending on the location of the infiltrate in question). In summary, when a blind system is used, the results obtained are similar to those obtained using guided, more invasive methods with the general advantage of having fewer side effects.

DIAGNOSTIC STRATEGIES

If possible, it is important to obtain all samples *before* a new antibiotic treatment is started.

In nonventilated patients who have presumed nosocomial pneumonia, antibiotic treatment is started empirically after obtaining blood and sputum samples. If the patient does not respond within 72 hours (using standard clinical criteria of temperature, respiratory rate, oxygen saturation, physical examination, and white blood cell count and differential to evaluate the lack of response), many physicians recommend obtaining a PSB or a BAL via fiberoptic bronchoscopy and modifying the antibiotic regimen accordingly. In ventilated patients, the recommended approach is to obtain an endotracheal aspirate or bronchoscopic or blind samples for quantitative cultures when there is clinical suspicion of nosocomial pneumonia before any new antibiotics are started. Antibiotic therapy is started as soon as possible and continued for 48 hours (assuming the patient remains stable). Adjustments in the regimen can be made on the basis of the quantitative microbiologic cultures and the subsequent sensitivities. Although a number of randomized studies have explored the potential cost-effectiveness of invasive methods over noninvasive diagnostic methods, current recommendations leave it to the expertise of each clinician to choose the diagnostic method to be employed.

TREATMENT

Early and adequate initial antibiotic treatment is clearly related to a better prognosis, as are clinical pathways and treatment guidelines.

Empiric antibiotic treatment for nosocomial pneumonia is based on a number of studies that have documented the likely pathogens, as summarized in the 1996 American Thoracic Guidelines. The spectrum of potential pathogens can be classified according to three variables:

1. Is the extent of nosocomial pneumonia mild-to-moderate versus severe (Table 26.3)?
2. Are specific host or therapeutic factors present that predispose to specific pathogens?
3. Is the pneumonia early or late onset (occurring within or after the fifth hospital day)?

Using these variables, patients can be classified into three groups:

Group 1 patients are those who have no associated risk factors and who present with either mild-to-moderate nosocomial pneumonia at any time during hospitalization or who have severe pneumonia of early onset.

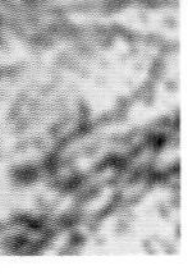

Table 26.3 Criteria for defining severity of nosocomial pneumonia	
Severe if any two of these criteria are present	**Admit to intensive care unit if one of these criteria is present**
Respiratory rate >30/min while receiving supplemental oxygen	Need for mechanical ventilation
PaO_2 <7.8kPa (<60mmHg) while receiving >35% oxygen, $PaCO_2$ >6.4kPa (>48mmHg), and pH <7.30	Patient suffering from shock (systolic blood pressure <90mmHg, or diastolic blood pressure <60mmHg)
Urine output <80mL/4h, unless other explanation exists, or the patient is on dialysis	Pharmacologic blood pressure support >4h
Change in mental status (delirium)	–

Group 2 patients have mild-to-moderate nosocomial pneumonia in the setting of associated risk factors that are present at the time of their hospitalization or develop during it.

Group 3 patients have severe, early-onset pneumonia with no risk factors, or have severe pneumonia at any time during their hospitalization in the presence of associated risk factors.

Figure 26.2 illustrates how patients are classified, the microorganisms that are most likely to be present, and the recommended antibiotic regimens. Group 1 patients should be treated with a second or nonpseudomonal, third-generation cephalosporin. A β-lactam/β-lactamase inhibitor combination is an acceptable alternative. In patients who are allergic to penicillin, fluoroquinolones, clindamycin, or aztreonam may be given. Monotherapy is usually appropriate in this setting.

Patients in Group 2 can be infected with the standard organisms seen in patients who have nosocomial pneumonia, but they have a higher likelihood of being infected with anaerobes, *S. aureus*, *Legionella* spp, and *P. aeruginosa* according to the presence or absence of specific risk factors for these organisms. Accordingly, these patients should receive not only empiric therapy directed at the standard organisms, but also additional antimicrobials directed at likely additional organisms. For example, clindamycin or metronidazole could be added to the second- or third-generation cephalosporin when anaerobes are suspected, as in the setting of a witnessed aspiration (a β-lactam/β-lactamase inhibitor combination would also provide sufficient anaerobic coverage). Vancomycin should be added in cases with associated coma or head trauma until methicillin-resistant *S. aureus* is excluded.

For Group 3 patients, treatment is directed against the standard organisms as well as against more resistant and virulent gram-negative bacilli, such as *Acinetobacter* spp and *P. aeruginosa*. Drugs active against these pathogens include anti-

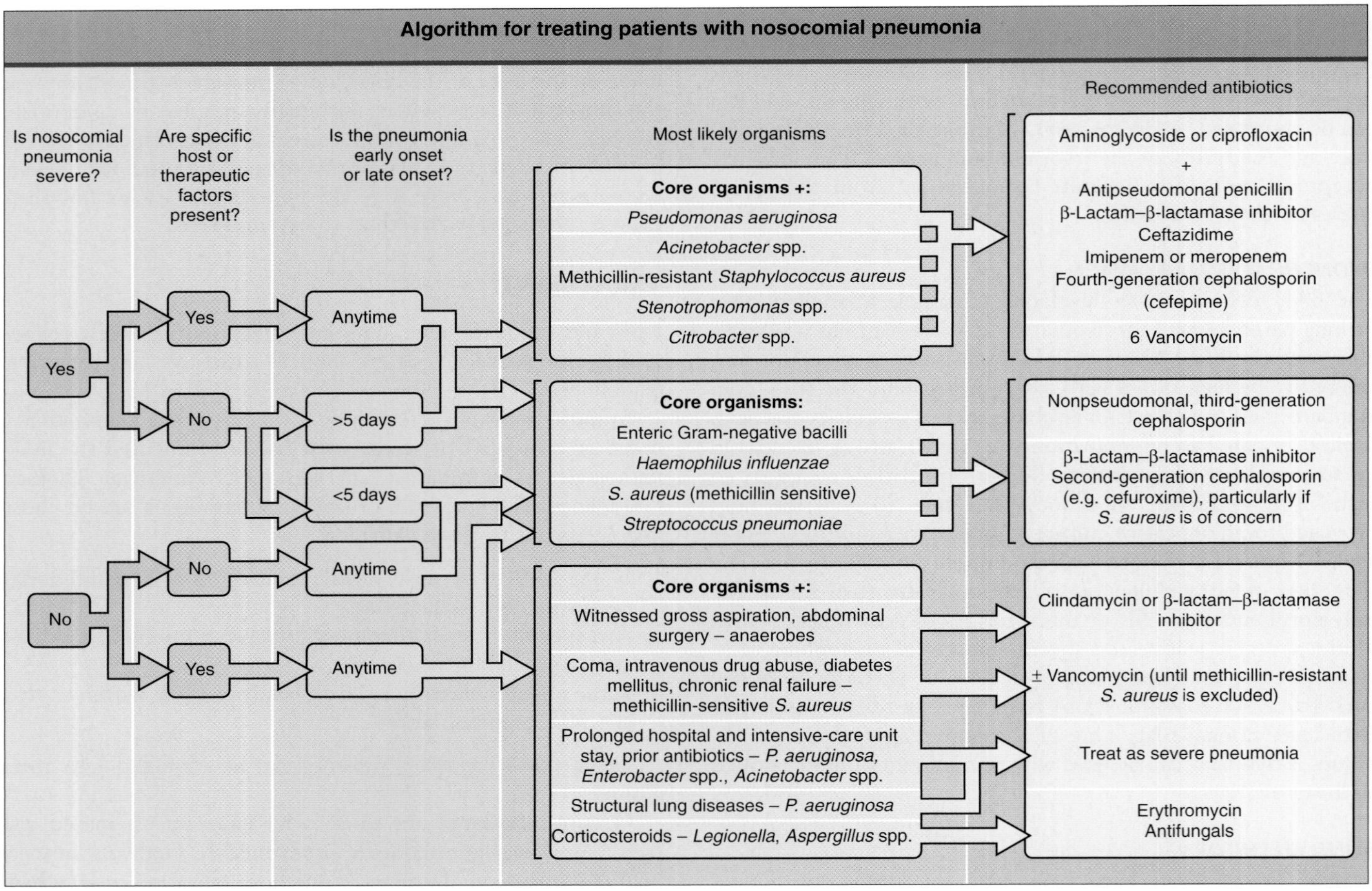

Algorithm for treating patients with nosocomial pneumonia

Is nosocomial pneumonia severe?
Are specific host or therapeutic factors present?
Is the pneumonia early onset or late onset?
Most likely organisms
Recommended antibiotics

Yes → Yes → Anytime
Yes → No → >5 days
Yes → No → <5 days
No → No → Anytime
No → Yes → Anytime

Core organisms +:
Pseudomonas aeruginosa
Acinetobacter spp.
Methicillin-resistant *Staphylococcus aureus*
Stenotrophomonas spp.
Citrobacter spp.

Aminoglycoside or ciprofloxacin
+
Antipseudomonal penicillin
β-Lactam–β-lactamase inhibitor
Ceftazidime
Imipenem or meropenem
Fourth-generation cephalosporin (cefepime)
6 Vancomycin

Core organisms:
Enteric Gram-negative bacilli
Haemophilus influenzae
S. aureus (methicillin sensitive)
Streptococcus pneumoniae

Nonpseudomonal, third-generation cephalosporin
β-Lactam–β-lactamase inhibitor
Second-generation cephalosporin (e.g. cefuroxime), particularly if *S. aureus* is of concern

Core organisms +:
Witnessed gross aspiration, abdominal surgery – anaerobes → Clindamycin or β-lactam–β-lactamase inhibitor
Coma, intravenous drug abuse, diabetes mellitus, chronic renal failure – methicillin-sensitive *S. aureus* → ± Vancomycin (until methicillin-resistant *S. aureus* is excluded)
Prolonged hospital and intensive-care unit stay, prior antibiotics – *P. aeruginosa*, *Enterobacter* spp., *Acinetobacter* spp. → Treat as severe pneumonia
Structural lung diseases – *P. aeruginosa* → Treat as severe pneumonia
Corticosteroids – *Legionella*, *Aspergillus* spp. → Erythromycin, Antifungals

Figure 26.2 Algorithm for treating patients who have nosocomial pneumonia.

pseudomonal penicillins, some third-generation cephalosporins (such as ceftazidime and cefoperazone), aztreonam, carbapenems (such as imipenem and meropenem), antipseudomonal β-lactam/β-lactamase inhibitor combination, aminoglycosides, and fluoroquinolones. When methicillin resistant *S. aureus* is endemic in the hospital, vancomycin should be added.

Obviously, guideline recommendations have to be adapted to the local hospital flora and patterns of antibiotic sensitivity. For some microorganisms such as *Enterobacter* spp, *P. aeruginosa,* and nonfermenting gram-negative bacilli, a combination of antibiotics is recommended. The advantages of antibiotic combination over monotherapy are to obtain a synergistic effect and avoid the emergence of resistances, which, in turn, is related to reduced mortality and morbidity. In patients with difficult-to-treat microorganisms such as *P. aeruginosa,* antibiotic dosing should be adjusted according to the minimal inhibitory concentrations observed in the laboratory.

The duration of antibiotic therapy is individualized depending on the severity of illness, the rapidity of the clinical response, and the specific infecting agent, if this can be determined. In general, pneumonia caused by *S. pneumoniae, H. influenzae,* and *S. aureus* requires a somewhat shorter duration of treatment (e.g., 7 to 10 days) than that caused by enteric gram-negative bacilli, methicillin-resistant *S. aureus* or *Legionella.* Recent information on the duration of antibiotic treatment confirms that there is no need to treat more than 7 to 10 days for most of the hospital-acquired pneumonias.

EVOLUTION

Thirty percent of patients do not respond to antibiotic therapy. This figure may be as high as 50% in ventilator-associated pneumonias. Recent studies have shown that most of the clinical and physiologic abnormalities resolve by day 6 after diagnosis is made in patients who receive adequate antibiotic therapy initially. Oxygenation is the first parameter to improve in this circumstance. In nonresponding patients there is a clear differentiation by day 3 in whom oxygenation is not improved or worsened. Other variables are not as useful for detecting treatment failure. When the patient fails to improve, or when rapid deterioration occurs, the possibility that the process is not pneumonia must be considered, and the patient should be reevaluated to assure that certain host, bacterial, or other therapeutic factors have not been overlooked. A number of noninfectious processes may be mistakenly labeled as nosocomial pneumonia, including atelectasis, congestive heart failure, pulmonary embolism with infarction, lung contusion (in trauma patients), chemical pneumonitis from aspiration, alveolar hemorrhage, and diffuse fibroproliferation in patients with acute respiratory distress syndrome. Any of these may mimic every clinical, laboratory, and radiographic sign of pneumonia. Host factors that are associated with failure to respond to appropriate treatment include the presence of other underlying diseases (e.g., endobronchial malignancy or foreign body), superinfections with organisms that are not sensitive to the antibiotics given, or any of a variety of types of immunosuppression. Bacterial factors associated with failure of initial therapy include primary or acquired resistance to the initial antibiotic(s) chosen. Pneumonia presenting in a nosocomial fashion can be caused by pathogens not commonly included in the differential diagnosis (e.g., *Mycobacterium tuberculosis,* a variety of fungi, viruses). Complications of the initial infection that may preclude the normal response to therapy include empyema or abscess formation. Finally, critically ill patients may have numerous other sources of fever, such as sinusitis, infections related to a vascular catheter, urinary tract infections, intraabdominal septic foci, and an allergic reaction to numerous medications.

PREVENTION

Understanding the pathogenesis and pathophysiology of nosocomial pneumonia is important to provide preventive and curative measures. Microorganisms can reach the lung by the following routes:

- Direct spread to the lung from the pleura or the mediastinum
- Hematogenous spread from distal foci (including the possibility of bacterial translocation from an ischemic gut in critically ill patients)
- Inoculation of aerosols
- Aspiration of oropharyngeal and gastric contents

Most episodes of pneumonia are attributed to aspiration of oropharyngeal secretions into the distal airways and subsequent bacterial proliferation that results from impaired mechanical, humoral, or cellular defense mechanisms, or as a result of an excessive bacterial load. Accordingly, attempts at prevention have focused on reducing cross transmission, the likelihood of aspiration (Table 26.4) and reducing the bacterial load in the oropharynx (Table 26.5).

Table 26.4
Measures to reduce the likelihood of aspiration

Maintain head elevation by positioning the patient in semirecumbency (i.e. at least 45° upright)
Use endotracheal tubes with cuffs and with supraglottic and glottic suction
Avoid emergency intubations and the need for reintubation whenever possible
Use non-invasive mechanical ventilation when possible
Perform extubations electively whenever possible
Minimize sedation
Limit enteral feeding to patients who require prolonged hospitalization and, when needed, administer the enteral feeding in small volumes, paying particular attention to body position and frequently checking the volume of residual liquid

Table 26.5
Methods to reduce the bacterial load in the oropharynx

Meticulous attention to hand washing after patient contact or wearing gloves prior to contact
Careful management and manipulation of respiratory therapy equipment
Individualized program to minimize the accumulation of pulmonary secretions in the lower airways
Adequate disinfection of bronchoscopes
Appropriate structure of wards and intensive care units
Appropriate use of postural drainage and chest percussion
Selective digestive decontamination or oral decontamination in selected populations

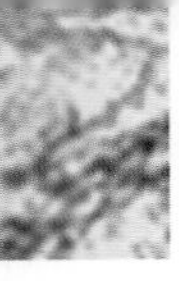

Currently, the most well-accepted and proven measures of prophylaxis include hand washing and adequate disinfection of respiratory therapy and diagnostic equipment to avoid cross-transmission, placing the patient in the semirecumbent position with the head elevated 15 degrees to 30 degrees (and careful enteral nutrition to avoid gastric aspiration), the use of endotracheal tubes with subglottic aspiration, and avoiding reintubation whenever possible.

Selective digestive decontamination should be reserved for specific populations of patients who are at high risk for nosocomial pneumonia (e.g., patients who are posttransplant or post-trauma). Systemic antibiotics have been shown effective in comatose patients to prevent early-onset pneumonia. Finally, antibiotics should always be used judiciously with the idea of reducing overuse.

SUGGESTED READINGS

Collard HR, Saint S, Matthay MA: Prevention of ventilator-associated pneumonia: An evidence-based systematic review. Ann Intern Med 138:494-501, 2003.

Craven DE, De Rosa FG, Thornton D: Nosocomial pneumonia: Emerging concepts in diagnosis, management, and prophylaxis. Curr Opin Crit Care 8:421-429, 2002.

Ewig S, Torres A: Prevention and management of ventilator-associated pneumonia. Curr Opin Crit Care 8:58-69, 2002.

Ewig S, Torres A: Flexible bronchoscopy in nosocomial pneumonia. Clin Chest Med 22:263-280, 2001.

Guidelines for the initial empiric management of adults with hospital-acquired pneumonia: Diagnosis, assessment of severity, initial antimicrobial therapy, and prevention strategies. Am J Respir Crit Care Med 153:1711-1725, 1996.

Mehta RM, Niederman MS: Nosocomial pneumonia. Curr Opin Infect Dis 15:387-394, 2002.

CHAPTER 27 Tuberculosis and Disease Caused by Atypical Mycobacteria

William A. Broughton, Rodrigo E. Morales, and John B. Bass, Jr.

The term tuberculosis (TB) describes an infectious disease that is believed to have plagued mankind since Neolithic times. It is caused by at least three species of *Mycobacterium*—*M. tuberculosis*, *M. bovis*, and *M. africanum*. This illness was called phthisis by physicians in ancient Greece to reflect its wasting character. In urban Europe during the 17th and 18th centuries, as many as 25% of deaths were caused by TB. Poor understanding of the contagious and progressive nature of the illness led to widespread fear and played a role in the development of a frightening mythology of revenants and vampires to explain the course of the illness in the community.

A more complete understanding of the illness began with Laennec's uniting of pulmonary and extrapulmonary tuberculous disease. The disease was verified as communicable by Villemin in 1865. When Koch isolated the tubercle bacillus in 1882, and reproduced the disease with the isolate, the microbiologic nature of the disease was established.

Despite this new understanding of the illness, fear and ignorance predominated. Without effective treatment, patients were isolated in sanatoria. Interventions such as pneumoperitoneum, therapeutic pneumothorax, plombage, and thoracoplasty (Figure 27.1) were carried out in attempts to decrease lung size and to close open tuberculous cavities. Despite the lack of a truly effective treatment, the use of sanatoria led to a decrease in death rate. It was not until streptomycin therapy for TB was introduced in 1946 and isoniazid became available in 1952 that realistic anti-infective therapy was available.

Although there is concern today about multidrug-resistant TB threatening our "control" of TB, it is important to recognize that an estimated 2 million people worldwide die from this disease every year. Our progress with TB is relatively recent—the last of the sanatoria in the United States closed in the mid-1970s. Unfortunately, the public's fear and ignorance about TB persists.

When the term *tubercle bacillus* is used, it refers to three species of the family of Mycobacteriaceae, Actinomycetales: *M. bovis*, *M. africanum*, and *M. tuberculosis*. *M. bovis* and *M. africanum* rarely cause disease now. Tubercle bacillus and *M. tuberculosis* are considered synonymous.

An obligate aerobe, *M. tuberculosis* is rod shaped and slow growing (12- to 18-hour generation time). Its cell wall has a high mycolic acid (long chain, cross-linked fatty acid) content and is quite hydrophobic. Thus, *M. tuberculosis* is impermeable to the common bacteriologic stains. The organism absorbs carbolfuchsin dye and maintains the resultant red color despite decolorization with acid alcohol. For this reason, it is referred to as acid fast (Figure 27.2). However, the term *acid-fast bacilli* (AFB) refers to mycobacteria in general, even though a few other organisms demonstrate acid-fast staining characteristics (e.g., *Nocardia* and *Cryptosporidium* spp).

The tubercle bacillus is quite a hearty organism and survives concentration and digestion techniques that would kill lesser organisms. It grows slowly and requires enriched media such as Löwenstein-Jensen egg-based media or synthetic Middlebrook 7H10/7H11 media. The colony appearance is buff colored and cordlike or heaped up. Because *M. tuberculosis* is the only mycobacterium to produce niacin, the presence of niacin as the product of a bacterial growth confirms identification. Today, the organism is grown in broth and rapidly identified with DNA probes.

EPIDEMIOLOGY AND PATHOGENESIS

Epidemiology

Disease caused by *M. tuberculosis* continues to kill millions of people yearly. Data from the World Health Organization indicate that 2 million deaths from TB occurred in 1995. As many as 8 million new cases of TB develop each year. More than 90% of these cases occur in developing nations that have poor resources and high numbers of individuals infected by the human immunodeficiency virus (HIV). Of the world's population, 20% to 40% is infected with *M. tuberculosis* and as many as 1% are newly infected each year. The tubercle bacillus may be responsible for up to 7% of annual global deaths.

In the United States the incidence of TB began to decline around 1900, which was thought to be the result of improved living conditions and the advent of sanatoria. With the addition of effective therapy, the incidence of tuberculous disease continued to decline until about 1985. At that time, HIV infection became common and cases related to it, as well as cases related to the increasing numbers of the homeless and foreign born, brought about a 20% increase in the incidence of TB. Since 1992, U.S. TB case rates are declining at an average of 5% per year.

Risk factors for TB in the United States include: U.S.-born non-Hispanic blacks, HIV positivity (such patients are 200 times more likely to contract TB than HIV-negative individuals), lower income strata, alcoholism, homelessness, those in crowded living conditions, those who have had gastrectomies in the past, the immunocompromised, and those who immigrate from a high-prevalence country. Health care workers are also at increased risk.

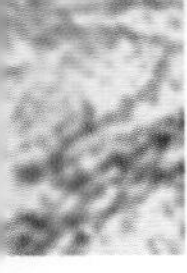

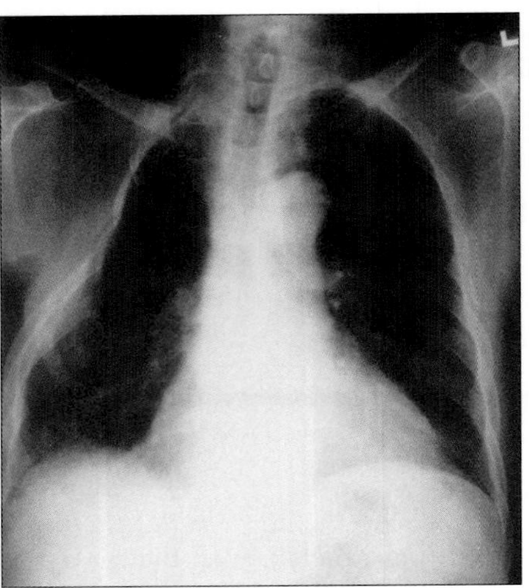

Figure 27.1 Thoracoplasty treatment for tuberculosis. Thoracoplasty was used to limit the size of the diseased lung and hopefully close tuberculous cavities. The procedure was intended to close apical cavities or near-completely obliterate the hemithorax.

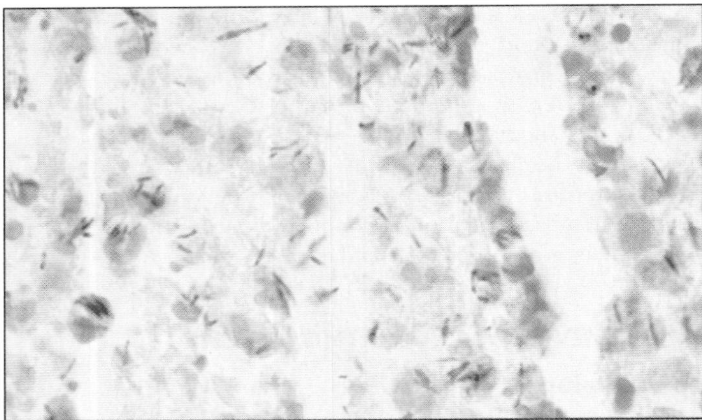

Figure 27.2 Acid-fast bacilli in tissue. Ziehl-Neelson stain of *Mycobacterium tuberculosis* in a tissue specimen.

In the mid-1990s, outbreaks of multidrug-resistant TB (MDR-TB) produced serious risk and high mortality in certain situations. These outbreaks primarily occurred in correctional facilities, hospitals, and homeless shelters. Because inadequate or incomplete therapy is the primary cause of MDR-TB, a push for directly observed therapy has reduced the incidence of MDR-TB isolates by about 50% in the United States.

Today, almost all cases of TB are acquired through person-to-person contact via droplet nuclei. These particles are originally tiny droplets of saliva that contain AFB organisms formed when individuals with TB phonate, cough, or sneeze. When these droplets of spit dry to or are the appropriate size, they can be held aloft by air currents. At diameters of 1 to 5 micrometers, they may contain two or three tubercle bacilli. This particular diameter is important because the inhalation of larger particles results in impaction of the droplet on the mucosal airway. Such impaction allows removal by the mucociliary system before infection can occur. Smaller particles reach the alveoli where infection begins, as outlined in the following section.

Prevention of transmission can be aided by combating the factors noted previously. When TB is recognized, effective therapy can rapidly decrease the number of organisms shed as droplet nuclei. Negative pressure rooms, ultraviolet radiation in the patient's room, and covering the mouth and nose of patients with tissue or a fine pore mask can reduce the number of droplets present in the patient's room. Because TB is not transmitted by fomites, no extreme measures need be taken with personal items used by the infected patient. Gloves and gowns are not required except where dictated by other illness. HIV-positive patients with TB do not transmit their disease to their contacts at a higher rate than do HIV-negative patients who have TB.

Pathogenesis: Infection versus Disease

For a droplet nucleus to cause an infection, it must successfully bypass the upper airway defenses. The infectious particle that reaches the alveolus is most likely to cause infection after macrophage ingestion of the bacterium. Depending on the virulence of the bacillus and the killing activity of the macrophage, the tubercle bacillus may or may not survive to create infection or disease.

When the tubercle bacillus deposited in the alveolus survives, it can multiply slowly within the macrophage. No immediate host response occurs. Bacterial numbers large enough to elicit a cellular response (approximately 10^3 to 10^4 organisms) requires 4 to 8 weeks of replication.

When sufficient bacterial growth has occurred, some of the macrophages may undergo lysis. Transmission of infected macrophages or free bacilli into lymphatics, and subsequently into the blood stream, allows hematogenous spread. Via the bloodstream, the tubercle bacillus reaches areas of high oxygen partial pressures, such as the apices of the lung, kidneys, brain, and bony areas, where further multiplication takes place prior to the restraining effects of developing cellular immunity. It is cell-mediated immunity (CMI) that controls the bacillus at its sites of deposition.

Containment of the initial areas of infection and sites of regional spread is accomplished by the compartmentalization of $CD4^+$ cells that release interferon-γ and activate macrophages producing protective cytokines (e.g., interleukin-12) and reactive oxygen species. Sometimes this process fails and infection progresses immediately. In most cases, tubercles are formed, and *M. tuberculosis* is further inhibited (Figure 27.3). Although the bacillus may survive, fibrosis and calcification of these tubercular lesions frequently occur, producing an isolated, calcified spot on the chest radiograph in the mid- to lower-lung field, which is called a *Ghon* complex. The combination of a Ghon complex with hilar calcification is referred to as a *Ranke* complex.

In a small fraction of infected patients, the initial lesion continues to enlarge and destroy surrounding structures. Cavities can be formed and bronchi destroyed in the process. Large numbers of bacilli live within the walls of cavities and, when a bronchus is violated, they can spread through the bronchial tree and into the environment. In a small portion of the population, the disseminated seeding stage may not be controlled, which can result in the seeding of multiple organs with the formation of

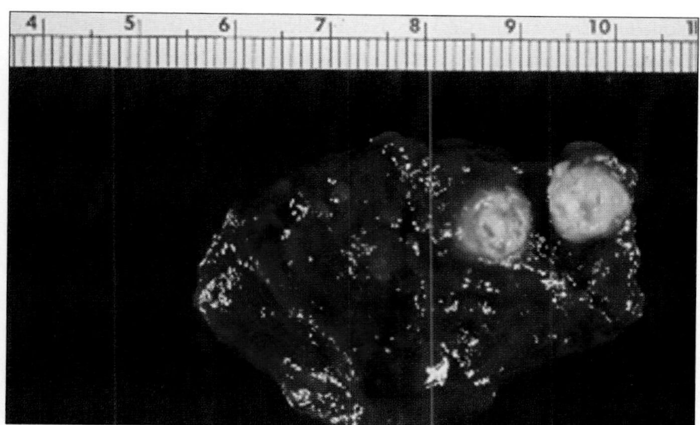

Figure 27.3 Tuberculoma—gross pathology. A specimen from lung resection revealing a small tuberculoma about 8 mm in diameter.

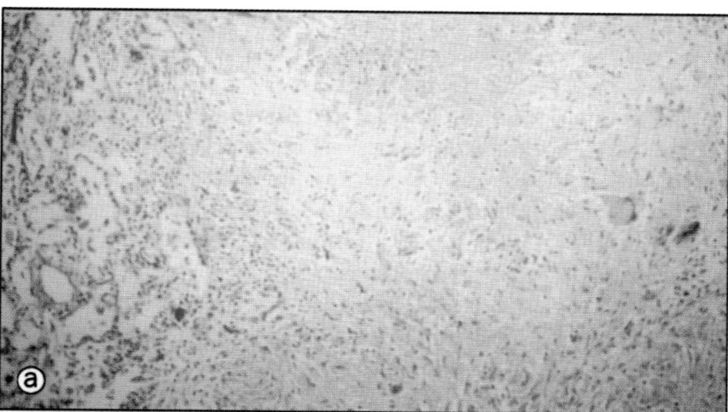

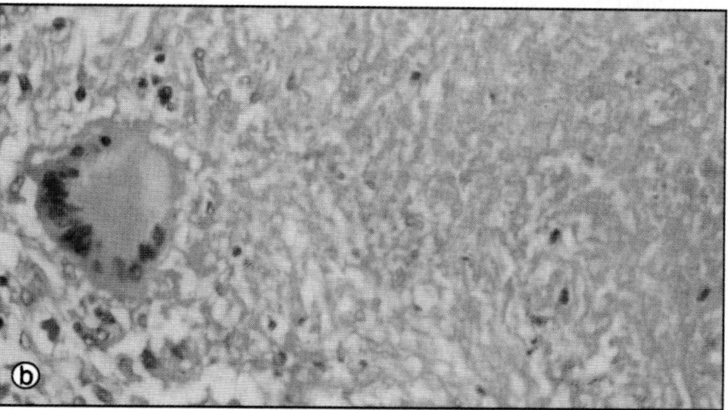

Figure 27.4 Histopathology of a caseous focus from lung. **A,** Lung is at the left margin and a caseous area is seen in the right upper and middle area of the view. A few Langerhans giant cells are seen (hematoxylin and eosin stain). **B,** A nearby area at higher magnification showing Langerhans cells and caseum.

numerous small granulomata. These can have the appearance of small nodules on the chest roentgenogram and suggest the presence of miliary TB ("miliary" from the resemblance of the small nodules to millet seed).

Another aspect of the development of CMI is the potential for tuberculin skin-test positivity. Such skin reactions recur as a result of delayed-type hypersensitivity (DTH). Sensitized T-helper ($CD4^+$) cells move to the site of antigen deposition and cytokines are released followed by tissue inflammation. This is the basis for the purified protein derivative (PPD) skin test (see the following section).

The nature of the pathologic findings of TB is dependent on the concentration of antigen and the degree of hypersensitivity that has developed. Where little antigen is present and hypersensitivity is active, the classic tubercle develops. The infiltration or development of organized lymphocytes, macrophages, giant cells (Langerhans), fibroblasts, and capillaries result in the formation of a classic granuloma. In some of these granulomata, incomplete necrosis occurs to produce a semisolid material much like cheese, called caseous necrosis. Caseating granulomata are common findings in TB (Figure 27.4). Although certain classic histopathologic findings are frequently associated with TB, histopathology alone cannot reliably distinguish disease caused by *M. tuberculosis* from that caused by other mycobacterial organisms. The fixing of tissue specimens reduces the identification of AFB by staining but studies of DNA and ribosomal RNA amplification in these situations are promising.

In those patients in whom the initial assault by the tubercle bacillus is controlled, their clinical status is referred to as latent tuberculosis infection (LTBI). They are asymptomatic, frequently have a positive PPD skin test, and cannot transmit the disease to others. When the tubercle bacillus causes clinically detectable disease, the individuals are said to have TB (tuberculous disease). About 3% to 5% of LTBI develops into active TB in the first year after infection and another 3% to 5% develop the disease over the remainder of their life.

CLINICAL MANIFESTATIONS

Only about 10% of people infected with *M. tuberculosis* ever develop tuberculous disease. Many of those who develop TB do so in the first few years after infection, but the bacillus may lie dormant in the body for decades. Clinical manifestations of TB are usually divided into the following categories: primary pulmonary TB, reactivation pulmonary TB, and extrapulmonary TB.

Primary Pulmonary Tuberculosis

Primary TB is by definition the result of progression of active disease directly from initial infection with *M. tuberculosis*. Although most initial infections are asymptomatic and controlled by CMI, some patients develop fever and nonproductive cough with characteristic abnormalities on chest radiographs. The usual appearance is of an inflammatory infiltrate that occupies the middle and lower lung fields. The infiltrates are commonly unilateral. Lymph node enlargement often occurs and may cause bronchial compression. Primary TB most frequently resolves spontaneously, but reactivation disease can occur in 50% to 60% of those patients who do not receive appropriate therapy.

The number of organisms present during active primary TB is thought to be low. Most of the findings noted are related to DTH, and smears are positive in less that 20% of patients with cultures positive in about 50%.

TUBERCULOUS PLEURITIS

A second manifestation of primary TB is tuberculous pleuritis, which occurs as the primary manifestation of TB in about 10% of patients who have the disease. The mechanism is believed to be a rupture of a subpleural caseous focus into the pleural space. It is primarily the tuberculous protein that gives rise to the DTH reaction responsible for the clinical features of tuberculous pleuritis. Despite the marked DTH that occurs in the pleural space, tuberculin skin testing can be negative. Symptoms of tuberculous pleuritis include nonproductive cough, chest pain (pleuritic), and fever. In past years, this manifestation of TB was more frequently seen in children and young adults, but in the latter part of the 20th century the affected population has been older (fifth and sixth decades). The natural history of tuberculous pleuritis is spontaneous resolution over 2 to 4 months with an incidence of reactivation TB as high as 65% within 5 years if not treated (Figure 27.5).

The fluid obtained by thoracentesis is initially a nonspecific, polymorphonuclear inflammatory exudate that soon gives rise to a lymphocytic exudative process. Glucose concentrations may be low. Cell counts are frequently in the range of 1000 to 6000 cells/mm, and are primarily made up of lymphocytes, which seem to be present after duration of the disease for 2 weeks or longer. The presence of more than 5% mesothelial cells virtually excludes the diagnosis of tuberculous pleural disease. The absence of mesothelial cells indicates only extensive pleural involvement; therefore, it is not diagnostic of TB by itself. The presence of more than 10% eosinophil cells excludes the diagnosis of TB unless prior thoracentesis or pneumothorax has occurred.

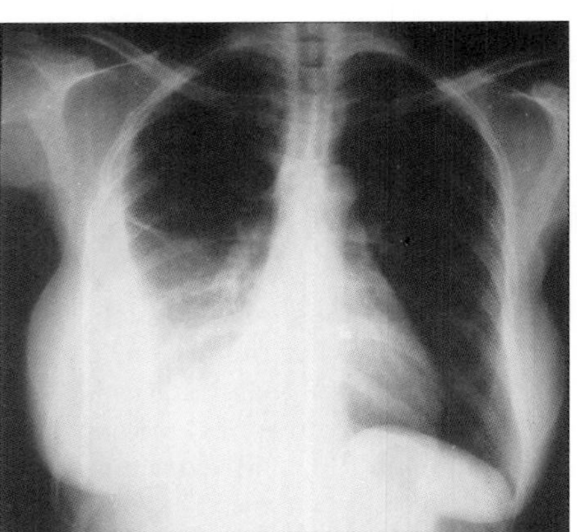

A

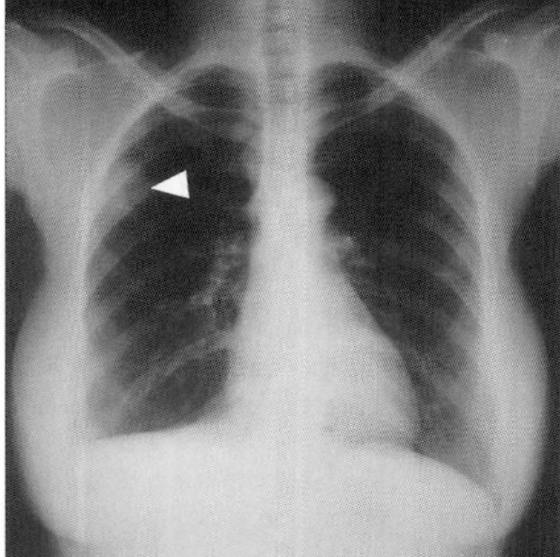

B

Figure 27.5 Tuberculous right pleural effusion followed by tuberculosis. **A,** A right pleural effusion diagnosed as tuberculous. Preventive therapy initiated but not maintained. **B,** Approximately 1 year later right upper lobe tuberculosis is seen (arrow).

Other tests for the diagnosis of tuberculous pleuritis are now available. Adenosine deaminase (ADA) is present in body fluid when CMI has been stimulated. A pleural fluid level of ADA greater than 40 IU (range 40 to 60 IU) is reasonably sensitive for the diagnosis of tuberculous pleuritis in the appropriate clinical circumstances.

Determination of the level of interferon-γ has also shown promising results in the diagnosis of tuberculous pleural effusion. What is considered a positive level varies by study and assay. Evaluation of pleural fluid for interferon-gamma to diagnose TB is not costly and has a sensitivity and specificity similar to ADA.

Other assays are also being studied. PCR of pleural fluid can be helpful but is complicated and expensive. The lysozyme:pleural fluid to serum ratio is also under investigation.

Pleural fluid cultures are positive in less than 25% of patients who have tuberculous pleuritis. Induced sputum cultures are positive in about 50% of patients even with a normal chest roentgenogram (except pleural effusion). Thus, negative cultures do not rule out involvement of the pleura with *M. tuberculosis*. Pleural biopsy is positive on the initial attempt in 60% of these patients. When three separate attempts at pleural biopsy are made, the yield increases to 80%. Thoracoscopy appears to be well-tolerated and superior to pleural biopsy in most pleural diseases but pleural adhesions lower its diagnostic value.

In the appropriate circumstances, a lymphocytic exudative pleural effusion and a positive PPD skin test (immediately or 6 weeks later) strongly suggest tuberculous pleuritis when no other diagnosis is evident. Pleural fluid testing for ADA and interferon-γ can help make the diagnosis more certain. The relatively benign nature of treatment for TB and the potential for prevention of reactivation disease make treatment with antituberculous agents in such circumstances very reasonable.

MILIARY TUBERCULOSIS

Miliary TB may develop as a result of primary or reactivation TB. As noted, miliary disease occurs as a result of unchecked, hematogenous dissemination in a minority of patients whose CMI is inadequate. The disease occurs most commonly in infants and children (younger than age 5 years), the elderly, alcoholics, patients who have neoplastic disease, HIV-infected patients, and other immunologically incompetent individuals.

The onset of miliary TB is insidious. Most patients experience fever, weakness, anorexia, and weight loss. Cough and dyspnea are less common. Headache and abdominal pain suggest involvement of the meninges and gastrointestinal tract, respectively. Rarely, adult respiratory distress syndrome and disseminated intravascular coagulation may be present in fulminant cases.

So-called cryptic miliary tuberculosis may also occur when the chest radiograph is normal and symptoms are atypical. Mortality with this cryptic form of the condition approaches 80%. Physical findings include pulmonary abnormalities, abnormalities of the retina, lymphadenopathy, splenomegaly, and hepatomegaly.

Diagnosis in miliary TB may be difficult because only 30% of patients have smears and sputum cultures that are positive for AFB. Bronchoscopy and transbronchial biopsy can help in about 70% of cases when the initial sputum specimens are negative. Reports indicate that liver biopsy is positive for granulomata in 60% of patients, with positive bone marrow results found in only about 30% of cases.

Miliary TB in the HIV-infected patient is associated with a tendency for a more severe degree of illness. Of acquired immunodeficiency syndrome (AIDS) patients who have extrapulmonary disease, up to 40% suffer disseminated tuberculous disease. A majority of patients show a typical chest radiographic appearance (see the following section). The occurrence of microbiologic positivity in this patient group breaks down as follows: sputum smear is positive in 25%, sputum culture is positive in 71%, and blood cultures are positive in 56%. Often, biopsy specimens are not helpful. The lack of immunocompetence can allow a "nonreactive" form of the disease, with overwhelming numbers of organisms and no granulomata. Despite standard treatment of miliary TB in AIDS, patient mortality remains greater than 30%.

Treatment of miliary TB involves the standard regimens and supportive care. Uncontrolled studies suggest that corticosteroids may help immunocompromised patients who have severe disease.

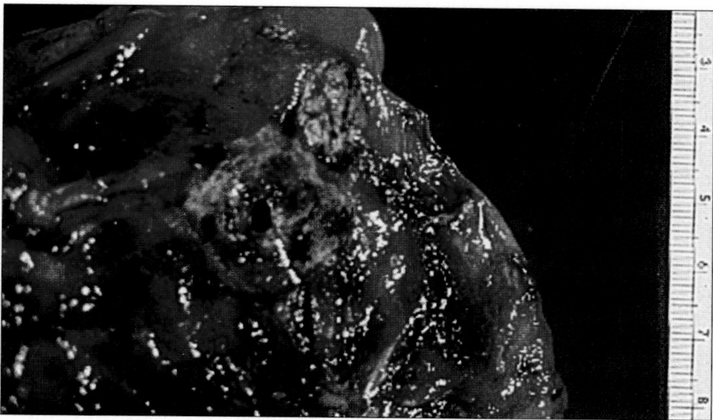

Figure 27.6 Gross pathology specimen of tuberculous upper lobe of lung. Close-up view of one tuberculous lesion showing cavitation.

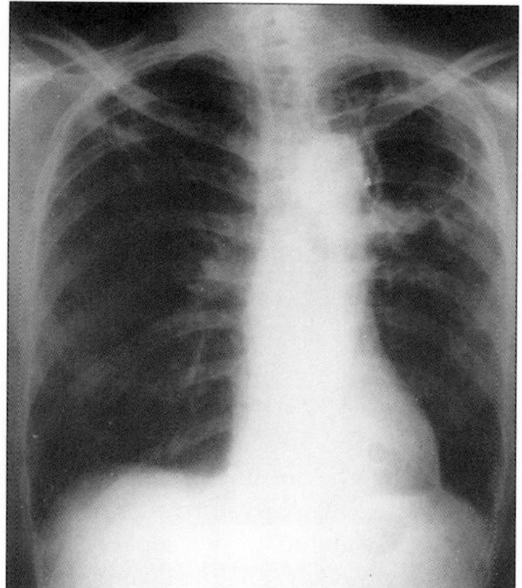

Figure 27.7 Roentgenographic appearance of "old" TB. Left upper lobe cavitation (later occupied by an aspergilloma) and scarring with significant left-sided volume loss. There is apical scarring on the right with compensatory hyperinflation.

Reactivation Tuberculosis

Reactivation TB is the most common form of the disease from a clinical standpoint. It represents activation of latent infection, usually in the upper lung zones, weeks to years after the primary infection. Reactivation TB is often called active TB. The nature of the illness involves reinitiation of bacterial multiplication and enlargement of a previously dormant lesion with resultant tissue destruction and caseation or liquefaction. This process further favors bacterial reproduction. Rupture of areas of liquid caseum into bronchi lead to endobronchial spread of tubercle bacilli and the creation of the cavity so often seen in classic TB pulmonary disease (Figure 27.6).

Reactivation TB begins insidiously over a period of weeks or months. Cough is common with a progressive increase in production of sputum. Constitutional symptoms such as fever, loss of appetite, weight loss, and night sweats are also frequent complaints (night sweats add little to diagnostic accuracy). Streaky hemoptysis is not uncommon. Dyspnea is unlikely unless there is underlying lung disease with marginal reserve or extensive tuberculous involvement of the lungs.

The appearance of the chest radiograph is very helpful in the diagnosis of TB. The typical findings include unilateral or bilateral apical inflammatory infiltration, often with cavity formation. The apical and posterior segments or subsegments of the upper lobes are typically involved. Volume loss may be apparent at the time of diagnosis. If an upper lobe abnormality is uncertain, an apical lordotic view of the chest may help. This view removes the clavicles from over the lung fields, so that the lung apices can be clearly seen. In HIV-infected patients, the appearance of the chest radiograph may be less typical, with cavities in the mid- and lower-lung fields, along with inflammatory infiltrates.

Old TB (i.e., previously treated or spontaneously resolved reactivation TB) is a common cause of hemoptysis (Figure 27.7). Blood in the sputum can be caused by bleeding from dilated vascular channels in areas of "dry bronchiectasis" related to old TB infection or from aspergilloma formation in an old tuberculous cavity. More significant hemoptysis from active TB occurred frequently before effective antituberculous therapy became available, and it was often a terminal event (usually because of the erosion of an expanding cavity into a pulmonary artery). The phenomenon was referred to as a Rasmussen aneurysm.

Extrapulmonary Tuberculosis

Hematogenous seeding of nonpulmonary organs by the tubercle bacillus is common. About 50% of patients who have active TB present with tuberculous disease in an extrapulmonary site. The sites most often involved include (in relative order of frequency): lymph nodes, pleural space, genitourinary tract, bone and joint sites, meninges, and in the peritoneum-gastrointestinal tract. The likelihood of extrapulmonary TB is increased in immunocompromised individuals. Though uncommon, the most

infectious form of TB is laryngeal involvement, which usually occurs as a result of lower airway disease. About 25% of patients diagnosed with extrapulmonary tuberculous disease usually have a history of TB, often with inadequate treatment.

TUBERCULOUS LYMPHADENITIS

Tuberculous infection of the lymph nodes is the most common form of the disease outside the lungs and is responsible for 25% of extrapulmonary disease. This manifestation of TB, when found in the neck, has been referred to as scrofula. This clinical presentation is assigned that name, whether caused by *M. tuberculosis* or *M. scrofulaceum*. It may result from a primary infection, reactivation, or extension from a contiguous site. The anterior and posterior cervical chain nodes are most commonly involved, although it may occur in any node or region of nodes.

When this form of disease comes to light in its early stage, it presents as a painless swelling of the lymph nodes. Initially, the nodes are discrete and firm, but without treatment become larger and may develop fistulous drainage. Needle biopsy or surgical specimens are frequently diagnostic, with reports that 50% of smears are positive and cultures are positive in 80% of cases. In older children and adults, this usual isolate is the tubercle bacillus. In patients younger than 5 years of age, non-tuberculous bacteria are more common. Antituberculous treatment and surgical intervention are often required when *M. tuberculosis* is implicated. Scarring from this form of TB can be profound.

GENITOURINARY TUBERCULOSIS

Genitourinary TB is responsible for 15% of cases of extrapulmonary disease. It used to be the most common form of TB—perhaps because of less effective early forms of therapy. Genitourinary tract TB is best considered as two separate entities—renal TB and genital TB—although renal involvement is a common accompanying phenomenon in patients who have the genital disease.

Renal TB commonly presents with local symptoms that include dysuria, hematuria, urinary frequency, and flank discomfort; less than 10% of patients present with fever and constitutional symptoms, and some patients may be asymptomatic. Renal disease is usually unilateral clinically, but bilateral granulomata can be demonstrated on biopsy. The characteristic laboratory finding of renal TB is sterile pyuria. With cultures of three morning urine specimens, growth of the tubercle bacillus can be demonstrated in about 90% of patients. Advanced imaging techniques can reveal multiple abnormalities, but these are nonspecific and not diagnostic of TB. Renal failure caused by TB is uncommon, but with antituberculous therapy the prognosis is excellent. Transmission of this form of the disease without concomitant pulmonary involvement is unlikely.

Genital TB is a frequent companion of renal TB—greater than 50% of patients who have genital manifestations also have renal infection. The reason for this is thought to be spread of TB via the urinary tract. In males, the presentation of genital TB is most commonly the development of a slowly progressive mass in the seminal vesicles, prostate, or epididymis. Usually, TB is not suspected until AFB are revealed in a surgical pathology specimen. Fine needle aspiration of these masses can reveal AFB. In females, the fallopian tube is a primary site of involvement. Presenting complaints include pelvic pain, pelvic inflammatory disease, abnormal uterine bleeding, irregular menses, amenorrhea, or infertility. Diagnosis can be best accomplished by urine culture and endometrial biopsy or curettage. Although treatment is effective, infertility is a common and untreatable outcome.

MUSCULOSKELETAL TUBERCULOSIS

About 6% of extrapulmonary TB affects the bones and joints, and TB is well known for causing spinal deformity. Pott's disease indicates tuberculous infection that collapses adjacent vertebral bodies (usually thoracic), to produce the classic gibbus deformity of the spine. In developed nations, this manifestation is now quite uncommon.

When involvement of the bony skeleton occurs now, it is most often found in middle-aged and HIV-infected patients. The lower spine and weight-bearing joints are most often affected, but sometimes the infection can track to the paravertebral soft-tissue areas and present as a "cold abscess." Abscess formation can also occur within the spinal canal, compress the spinal cord, and result in paraplegia. This form of TB also responds to antituberculous therapy, although sometimes surgical intervention may be required.

TUBERCULOUS MENINGITIS

Meningitis, which accounts for about 5% of extrapulmonary TB, is becoming increasingly less common and has shifted its predilection from children to elderly and HIV-infected patients. It probably results from rupture of a reactivated tubercle into the subarachnoid space. Tuberculous meningitis commonly presents with complaints of confusion, abnormal behavior, headache, fever, cranial nerve abnormalities, and sometimes seizures. It is the form of TB with the most rapid progression—50% of patients give a history of only 2 weeks of symptomatology.

Intracranial pressure may be elevated in this disease. Cerebrospinal fluid (CSF) evaluation is required to make the diagnosis; CSF protein is usually moderately elevated and glucose is almost always decreased. A moderate CSF pleocytosis is present with a white blood cell count of 100 to 1000 cells/cm. Differential analysis of the CSF cells usually shows predominantly lymphocytes, but polymorphonuclear cells can be dominant. In about 25% of patients, AFB smears of the CSF are positive and mycobacterial cultures are positive in 75% of cases. The mortality for tuberculous meningitis is reported at about 20%. Corticosteroids help when significant cerebral edema occurs or when blockage of CSF flow is present.

TUBERCULOUS PERICARDITIS

Tuberculous involvement of the pericardium usually results from prior hematogenous dissemination and latent reactivation of a pericardial focus, or because of spread from adjacent lung or mediastinal nodes. Presenting symptoms include fever, dyspnea or orthopnea, cough, and edema in 50% of patients. The usual constitutional symptoms are often seen, and a pericardial rub is absent in two thirds of the patients who have this illness.

A review of diagnostic testing suggests that skin testing with PPD is frequently positive in these patients. Diagnosis is dependent upon evaluation of pericardial fluid, which is often hemorrhagic with laboratory values similar to those of tuberculous

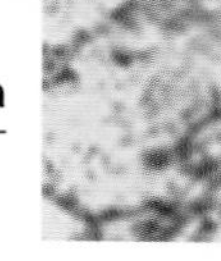

pleural fluid. Usually, lactate dehydrogenase and protein are significantly elevated and the glucose level is decreased. Cell analysis is usually lymphocyte predominant. In 50% of cases, AFB smears and cultures are positive. ADA (cutoff 30 IU) and interferon-γ (cutoff 200 pg/L) have recently been shown to be helpful in diagnosis. Pericardial biopsy with pathologic evaluation and culture offers the most specific results.

Without treatment, the mortality of tuberculous pericarditis is around 80%. All patients who suffer this illness require antituberculous therapy and the use of corticosteroids may reduce the incidence of constrictive pericarditis. Surgery is recommended if tamponade develops or recurs despite pericardiocentesis. Pericardial thickening and calcification of pericardium are not uncommon sequelae.

TUBERCULOUS GASTROINTESTINAL INVOLVEMENT

Gastrointestinal involvement is uncommon with TB, but when it occurs it can affect any area of the gastrointestinal tract. Ileocecal involvement and tuberculous peritonitis are the most frequent manifestations.

In the past, ileocecal TB was common, probably because of the ingestion of milk that contained the tubercle bacillus. Today, extension from nearby sites, swallowing infected secretions from pulmonary tuberculous, and hematogenous spread are more likely causes. The presenting clinical picture is that of symptoms consistent with appendicitis or Crohn's disease, diarrhea, and the usual constitutional symptoms. A fistula may develop, and surgery is often undertaken. The etiology of the illness is often unknown until pathologic specimens and cultures reveal the bacterial nature of the disease.

Tuberculous peritonitis is the result of direct spread from other infected sites or of hematogenous seeding. Abdominal pain, ascites, and a "doughy abdomen" can occur. The clinical impression of a mass is occasionally present. In these cases, the PPD skin test usually is positive and concurrent pulmonary involvement is not seen. The ascitic fluid samples again match the exudative description seen in pleural and pericardial fluid, with a cell analysis that indicates a predominantly lymphocytic nature. The protein content is usually greater than 3 g. Here, AFB smears are not particularly helpful, but cultures are positive in 80% of cases. Needle biopsy of the peritoneum that reveals caseating granulomata may help in culture-negative cases.

DIAGNOSIS OF TUBERCULOSIS

Chest Roentgenogram

The most common diagnostic test that leads to the suspicion of infection with the tubercle bacillus is a chest roentgenogram. Standard posteroanterior and lateral views are recommended, with apical lordotic views when the clavicles interfere with visualization of any questionable lesion in the lung apices. Computed tomography scanning is useful if cavity formation is unclear or if the location of the involvement is uncertain.

The chest radiographic appearance in primary TB most commonly demonstrates infiltrates of an inflammatory nature in the mid- and lower-lung fields. Most tidal ventilation goes to these areas and droplet nuclei are more likely to be carried there. Nodular infiltrates are common. Hilar and paratracheal adenopathy are seen in 15% of patients who have primary TB and may produce bronchial obstruction with atelectasis. Such findings are more frequent in children.

Reactivation TB commonly produces a classic chest radiographic appearance in the immunocompetent host (Figure 27.8). Infiltrates usually occur in the apical and posterior segments and subsegments of the upper lobes, and cavity formation is frequently seen. Upper lobe anterior segment involvement does not rule out TB, but strongly suggests another diagnosis. So-called "upstairs-downstairs disease" is seen as a result of rupture of a cavity full of liquefied material and bronchial spread of this material (Figure 27.9). In HIV-infected individuals, more atypical manifestations occur and cavities may not be seen or may occur in atypical locations. Other aspects of the radiographic appearance of reactivation TB include fibrotic scarring with atelectasis and volume loss in the upper lobes, tracheal deviation, and hilar traction.

Chest radiography of miliary TB has already been described (Figure 27.10). Diffuse nodular opacities of approximately 2 mm diameter are usually seen (though the size of the opacities can vary significantly). Infiltrates, cavities, and pleural effusions are sometimes noted.

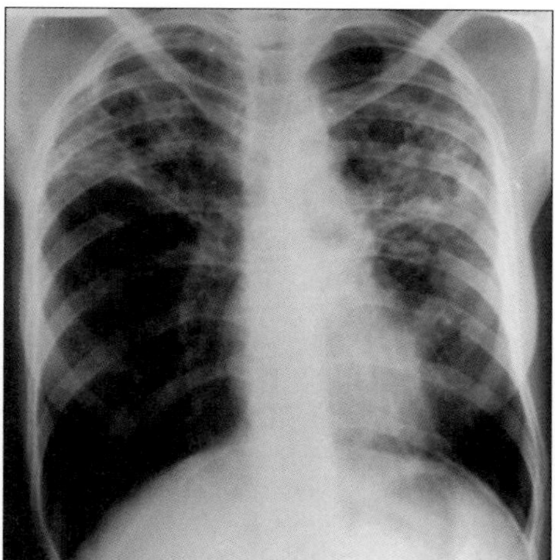

Figure 27.8 Chest roentgenogram of reactivation tuberculosis. Bilateral upper lobe involvement is noted and volume loss is already apparent in the right upper lobe. Note the numerous areas of cavitation.

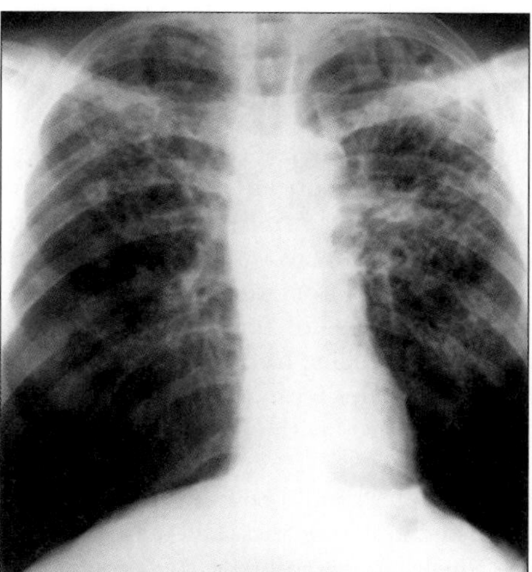

Figure 27.9 Chest roentgenogram of tuberculosis with bronchial spread of infection. What appears to be classic reactivation tuberculosis changes in the upper lobes bilaterally with additional involvement of the mid and lower lung fields. This is sometimes called "upstairs-downstairs disease."

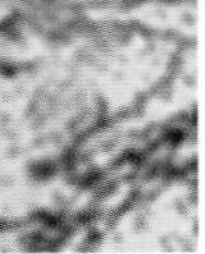

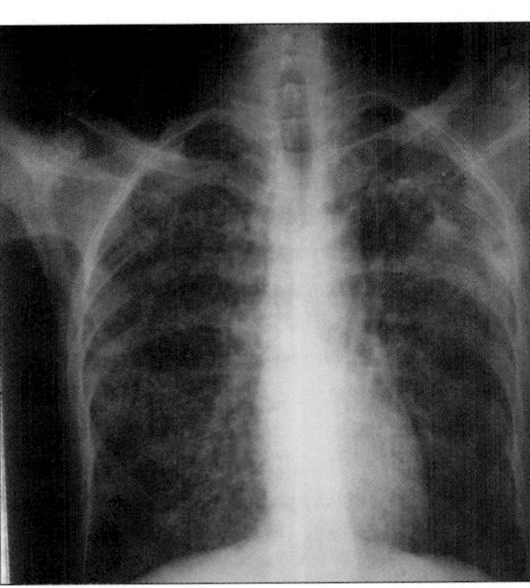

Figure 27.10 Miliary tuberculosis. Numerous miliary opacities seen in an adult with severe miliary tuberculosis.

Sputum Testing for AFB

Smear and culture results are most reliable when true sputum is obtained, although "spit" has been reported to be positive in as many as 30% of patients with cavitary disease. When copious sputum production is present, collection of specimens can be readily accomplished. When production of sputum is less voluminous, the collection of three deep sputum specimens taken in the morning is more likely to produce positive smears than are random specimens. This is based on the assumption that the respiratory tract has been relatively static through the night and the sputum is more likely to contain more organisms. In children, and those with very little sputum production, induction of sputum by inhalation of an aerosol of warm hypertonic saline may help to induce cough and sputum production.

When sputum is not available by the above means or remains negative in high-probability cases, there are other alternatives. Fiberoptic bronchoscopy can produce deep specimens but recent data suggest that it is no more useful than induced sputum. In children who cannot cooperate with sputum induction, samples of the early morning gastric aspirate (after nocturnal swallowing of secretions) have been reported positive in as many as 40% of patients.

On standard staining, *M. tuberculosis* is weakly gram-positive or colorless because of the hydrophobic nature of the cross-linked fatty acids in the cell wall, called mycocides. These cell-wall mycolic acids take up carbolfuchsin red dye that cannot be washed out by acid alcohol. The Kinyoun and Ziehl-Neelson stains were used routinely in the relatively recent past to identify AFB on smears. These stains produced a blue background for the classic beaded, corded-red organisms known as red snappers. Light microscopy of such specimens is still acceptable, but it is time-consuming. Current laboratory techniques use fluorescent staining to speed the process of organism recognition. These fluorescent stains are not specific for *M. tuberculosis*, but are merely modified AFB techniques with a fluorescent moiety. *Nocardia* spp can stain positive with current fluorescent techniques.

Smear positive sputum samples should be assayed with direct identification techniques such as nucleic acid amplification (NAA). This allows the quick confirmation of the presence of *M. tuberculosis* and appropriate treatment can be started. When the smear is negative and the clinical suspicion is high, NAA may identify up to 50% of smear-negative culture-positive cases of TB. Nucleic acid amplification is not recommended when the smear is negative and clinical suspicion is low.

Mycobacterial Culture

When a specimen stains positive for AFB, the underlying etiology may represent active TB or infection or colonization by a nontuberculous mycobacteria. For this reason, all specimens are submitted for culture. Because active tuberculous disease is potentially contagious, strong consideration is given to the initiation of antituberculous therapy at the time of culturing.

Clinical specimens should be processed as rapidly as possible. Specimens require liquefaction of organic components and a decontamination process to remove other microbial flora that might overgrow the slowly dividing tubercle bacillus in culture. This is usually accomplished by the treatment of specimens with a combination of a mucolytic agent (e.g., *N*-acetylcysteine) and 1% to 2% sodium hydroxide to limit other bacterial growth. Concentrating the specimen (e.g., centrifugation) increases culture sensitivity. *M. tuberculosis* organisms are reduced in number by the process of liquefaction and decontamination, but the procedure optimizes the likelihood of a positive result. Cultures obtained from normally sterile sites do not require digestion or decontamination.

Quantitative studies that examined the number of organisms necessary to produce positive smears indicate a need for 5000 to 10,000 organisms per milliliter to be present for an AFB smear to appear positive. Culture is a slower, but more sensitive method that requires only 10 to 100 organisms per milliliter for a positive result. Of specimens that have a positive smear, less than 1% have a negative culture when mycobacterial contamination is not present.

After appropriate handling, specimens are placed on or in media for culture. Current culture media include Löwenstein-Jensen media (egg), Middlebrook 7H10/7H11 (agar), and selective media. Growth is more rapid on agar media and specimens grow most rapidly in liquid media. Currently, automated culture systems have reduced the time necessary for positive culture detection from 3 to 8 weeks to 1 to 3 weeks. DNA probes can quickly identify *M. tuberculosis*. Cultures are usually held for 8 to 12 weeks before being reported as negative and discarded. Overall sensitivity of culture has been reported to be 80% to 85% with a specificity of 98%.

TREATMENT OF TUBERCULOSIS

Standard therapy for active TB in adults and children consists of a 6-month regimen, the first 2 months (initiation phase) with isoniazid (INH), rifampin/rifampicin (RIF), pyrazinamide (PZA), and ethambutol (EMB) followed by 18 weeks (continuation phase) of INH and RIF alone. Ethambutol can be omitted in situations where drug resistance is unlikely. Drug resistance is considered unlikely when the following situations occur:

- Less than 4% primary resistance to isoniazid in the community
- No prior history of treatment with antituberculous medications

- Patient is not from a country with a high prevalence of drug-resistant TB
- No known exposure to a drug-resistant case

Some general considerations for effective antituberculous therapy include:

- Multiple drugs are required in an effective therapeutic regimen to reduce the likelihood of the emergence of resistant organisms. The spontaneous occurrence of drug-resistant organisms is well-documented, but the likelihood of the spontaneous occurrence of a tubercle bacillus simultaneously resistant to two medications is statistically very low.
- A single new drug should **never** be added to a failing antituberculous regimen.
- Sensitivity testing for *M. tuberculosis* isolates must be performed in every case.
- Directly observed therapy should be considered for all cases of active TB.
- Individualized therapy in consultation with a TB expert is recommended in multidrug-resistant cases.
- Children are treated with the same considerations as noted for adults, with the appropriate adjustment of medication dosing.
- Extrapulmonary TB is treated along the standard treatment guidelines for pulmonary TB, except that children who have miliary TB, tuberculous meningitis, tuberculous arthritis, or tuberculous arthritis and bone disease should be treated for at least 12 months.

At times, individuals have an illness that resembles TB in clinical and radiographic appearance. For such individuals, treatment is frequently initiated in the face of negative AFB smears pending culture. This administration of appropriate treatment may seem to bring about an improvement in these patients' symptoms and chest radiographic appearance, but the cultures remain negative (Figure 27.11). This has been referred to as "culture-negative" TB. Tables 27.1 and 27.2 summarize dosing, activity, and side effects of first- and second-line anti-TB medications.

In pregnancy, the need to treat active TB outweighs the risk of therapy for mother and fetus. Pyrazinamide is used in pregnant women in many parts of the world, though few data about its potential teratogenic effects are available. In the United States, PZA is not recommended. Streptomycin is not recommended in pregnant women. Also, women on appropriate antituberculous therapy are not discouraged from breast feeding (nursing). Although INH, RIF, and EMB cross the placenta readily, antituberculous therapy is not toxic for the newborn. Supplemental pyridoxine is always recommended in pregnant women.

Although most of the principles for TB therapy also apply to HIV-seropositive patients, there are three considerations when dealing with these patients. First, there is a possibility of drug malabsorption and subsequent subtherapeutic serum levels. Monitoring of drug levels is expensive and of limited availability but should be considered in patients with an inadequate response to directly observed therapy or when treating MDR-TB. Second, a complex interaction between antiretroviral agents and rifamycins involving cytochrome P450-3A can decrease the effectiveness of the antiretroviral therapy or increase rifamycin toxicity. Because of the unpredictable consequences of this interaction, consulting an expert is recommended. Third, a clinical syndrome of transient worsening of treated TB after immune restoration by antiretroviral therapy in HIV patients has been described. The syndrome consists of the appearance of new signs, symptoms, or radiographic manifestations of TB after initiation of therapy. Because the reaction has been associated with low $CD4^+$ counts, high viral load, and burden of tuberculous bacilli, it is recommended to defer antiretroviral therapy for 1 to 2 months after initiating antituberculous therapy in patients with TB and an advanced stage of HIV. Prolonged antituberculous therapy is often necessary in the HIV-infected patient with TB.

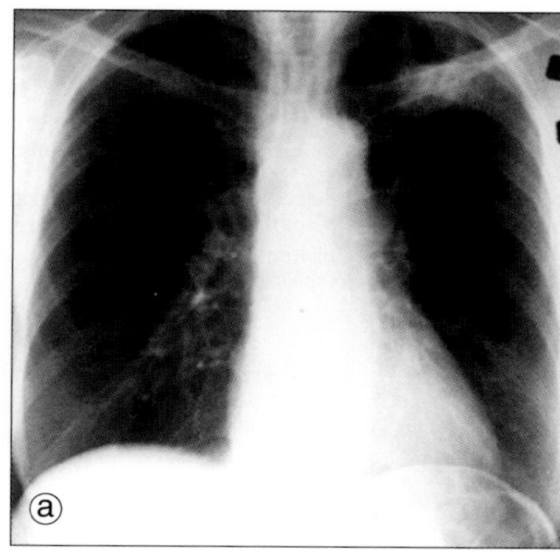

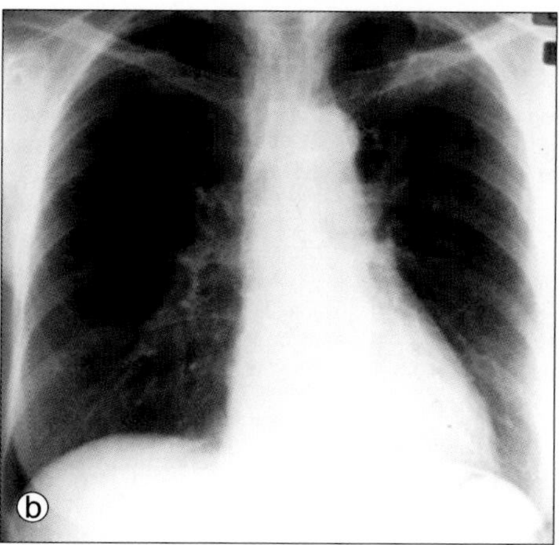

Figure 27.11 Chest roentgenograms in "culture-negative tuberculosis." **A,** Left upper lobe cavitary lesion with appropriate symptomology seen in a 64-year-old female with long history of a "very positive" tuberculin skin test 40 years ago. **B,** Same patient 8 weeks later with all smears and cultures negative and on appropriate antituberculous therapy. Left upper lobe cavity and infiltrate have almost resolved.

An overview of antituberculous regimens is given in Table 27.3.

PREVENTION OF TUBERCULOSIS

Bacille Calmette-Guerin

Bacille Calmette-Guerin (BCG) is named for two French researchers who developed the live, attenuated strain of *M. bovis* in 1921. It is currently used as a vaccination to prevent TB in areas of the world with high disease prevalence. Despite its use in millions of people globally, its efficacy is uncertain. Data suggest that it prevents disseminated TB and tuberculous meningitis in children, but protection against pulmonary TB has not been proven. Numerous trials have given unclear results, from suggestions of up to 80% protection from pulmonary TB with

Table 27.1
First-line drugs for the treatment of tuberculosis in adults and children

First-line drug	Dosage (daily dosing)	Dosage (weekly dosing)	Common side effects	Recommended follow-up tests	Special considerations
Isoniazid (INH)	Adults: 5 mg/kg with max dose of 300 mg/day (PO or IM) Children: 10-15 mg/kg with same max dose as adults	Adults: 15 mg/kg (PO or IM) 1,2 or 3/wk Children: 20-30 mg/kg in children 1,2 or 3/wk	Peripheral neuropathy Hepatotoxicity Hypersensitivity Drug interactions	Follow GOT/GPT in patients with symptoms of hepatitis	Bactericidal Pyridoxine 50 mg/day helpful for neuropathy Interacts with some anti-convulsants and ketoconazole
Rifampin (RIF)	Adults: 10 mg/kg with max dose of 600 mg/day (PO or IV) Children: 10–20 mg/kg	Adults and children: 10-20 mg/kg with a max dose of 600 mg (PO) 2 or 3/wk	Thrombocytopenia Leukopenia Hepatitis Fever Eosinophilia Interference with protease-inhibitor action and metabolism in patients infected by human immunodeficiency virus	In the appropriate situation: GOT/GPT and CBC and differential	Bactericidal Turns bodily secretions orange Interferes with: oral contraceptives quinidine oral anticoagulants methadone
Rifabutin	Adults: 5 mg/kg with max dose of 300 mg Children: unknown	Adults: 5 mg/kg with max dose of 300 mg 2 or 3/wk Children: unknown	Same as RIF Neutropenia in HIV pts. GI symptoms Pseudojaundice Uveitis Polyarthralgias	Same as RIF	Same as RIF Little data in pregnancy No dose change in renal failure Penetrates meninges
Rifapentin	Adults: no daily dosage recommended Children: not approved	Adults: 10 mg/kg with max dose of 600 mg 1/wk only in HIV sero-negative patients Children: unknown	Same as RIF and drug interactions via induction of hepatic enzymes	Same as RIF	Same as RIF CNS penetration uncertain Not approved in pregnancy Dosing adjustments unknown
Pyrazinamide (PZA)	Adults: 20-25 mg/kg/day Children: 15-30 mg/kg/day	Adults and children: 50-75 mg/kg with max dose of 4 grams (PO) 2 or 3/wk	Hyperuricemia Hepatotoxicity Hypersensitivity	Uric acid levels GOT/GPT when appropriate	Bactericidal Particularly active against dormant bacilli in the macrophage Not used in pregnancy (in the USA)
Ethambutol (EMB)	Adults and children: 15-20 mg/kg with no max dose (the lower range of dosing has less optic neuritis)(PO)	Adults and children: 50 mg/kg 2 or 3/wk	Optic neuritis (usually reverses with d/c of drug - 1st sign often loss of color vision) GI intolerance	Check red-green color discrimination and visual acuity	Renal excretion - may need drug levels checked in those with renal insufficiency May want to avoid EMB when eye testing not feasible (children)

Summary of first-line antituberculous medications. Includes dosing (daily and weekly therapy) for adults and children (age younger than 12 years), common adverse effects, appropriate clinical testing for adverse effects during therapy, and special considerations for each drug. Once-weekly therapy not recommended for patients with human immunodeficiency virus (HIV). Twice-weekly therapy is not recommended for HIV patients with $CD4^+$ counts less than 100/μL.

the administration of BCG to an increased susceptibility to active disease in those vaccinated.

In many people who receive the vaccination, BCG produces a positive tuberculin reaction that cannot be distinguished from a tuberculin reaction caused by exposure to other mycobacteria. Because BCG is used in areas of high prevalence of disease, it is best to evaluate every positive PPD skin test for the presence of tuberculous disease.

In the United States, BCG is not recommended. In other areas of the world, it may be useful in children and infants in the following situations:

- Continuous exposure to active TB
- Those who are frequently exposed to isoniazid- and rifampin-resistant tubercle bacilli
- Groups with a new infection rate greater than 1% per year

BCG is contraindicated in patients infected with HIV and those who might be otherwise immunocompromised.

Latent Tuberculosis Infection

The spread of TB is arrested in the presence of normal cell-mediated immunity through the formation of granulomata by activated T cells and macrophages. Within these granulomata, the tubercle bacilli remain viable but are unable to cause TB. This infected state is LTBI. Such patients are not infectious, but this state may progress to active TB if their immune function is compromised. Approximately 10% of patients with LTBI develop TB in their lifetime. In HIV-infected individuals with LTBI, as many as 50% develop TB in the first 2 years, with the risk increasing by as much as 10% per year.

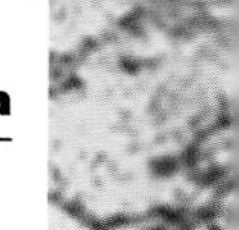

Table 27.2
Second-line drugs for the treatment of tuberculosis in adults and children

Second-line drug	Dosage (daily dosing)	Dosage (weekly dosing)	Common side effects	Recommended follow-up tests	Special considerations
Streptomycin (STM)	Adults: 15 mg/kg/d 5-7d/wk for first 2-8 weeks of therapy with max dose of 1 gram (IM) then 2-3x/wk Children: 20-40 mg/kg with same max dose as adults	Adults and children: 25-30 mg/kg with max dose of 1 gram (often given this way after first 2-8 weeks) 2x/wk	Auditory and vestibular dysfunction Nephrotoxicity	Check vestibular function and audiogram BUN/Cr	Bactericidal Avoid in elderly and those with renal impairment Not used in pregnancy
Ethionamide (ETH)	Adults and children: 15-20 mg/kg/d (PO) max dose 1 gram	Not recommended	GI intolerance Hepatotoxicity (2%) Neurotoxicity (1-2%) Impotence Alopecia Gynecomastia Metallic taste	None except when in doubt (hepatic enzymes and TSH)	Bacteriostatic If hepatic enzymes increase, a 5x increase is important even in the absence of symptoms Not used in pregnancy
Para-aminosalicylic acid (PAS)	Adults: 8-12 gm/d in 2-3 doses Children: 200–300 mg/kg/d (PO) with max dose of 12 grams	Not recommended	GI disturbance Hepatotoxicity (rare) Hypersensitivity Na^+ load Malabsorption	Hepatic enzymes TSH Coagulation studies	Bacteriostatic Should be given acidic drink (e.g., orange juice)
Capreomycin	Adults: 15 mg/kg/d (if >59 years 10 mg/kg/d) max dose 1 gm (IM/IV) Children: 15-30 mg/kg/d (IM/IV) with max dose of 1 gram	Adults and children: 15-30 mg/kg (IM) with max dose of 1 gram 2x/wk	Auditory Vestibular and renal toxicities	Audiogram Check vestibular function BUN/Cr	High frequency hearing loss in 3-9% Renal toxicity more common than STM Avoid in elderly and those with renal impairment Avoid in pregnancy
Kanamycin/ Amikacin	Adults: 15-30 mg/kg/d (IM/IV) with max dose of 1 gram Children: 15-30 mg/kg/d with max dose of 1 gram/d	Adults and children: 15-30 mg/kg (IM) with max dose of 1 gram 2/wk	Auditory and renal toxicity Vestibular toxicity rare	Audiogram monthly BUN/Cr	See capreomycin Contraindicated in pregnancy
Cycloserine	Adults and children: 15-25 mg/kg (PO) with max dose of 1 gram	Not recommended	Restlessness Convulsions Psychosis Rash Peripheral neuropathy especially when on INH	Assessment of mental status	Give with 150 mg of pyridoxine Avoid in those with history of psychological difficulties Interacts with phenytoin
Fluoro quinolones (levofloxacin - little data available on long-term use of gatifloxacin and moxifloxacin)	Adults: 500-1000 mg/d (PO) (moxifloxacin and gatifloxacin - 400 mg/day)	Not recommended	GI disturbance Mild neurological side effects Rash photosensitivity Pruritis	Not recommended	Not used in pregnancy Antacids hamper absorption May be considered in children with MDR

Summary of second-line antituberculous medications. Includes dosing (daily and weekly therapy) for adults and children (younger than age 12), common adverse effects, appropriate clinical testing for adverse effects during therapy, and special considerations for each drug. These drugs are reserved for difficult situations in the treatment of TB and are more difficult to use than first-line agents. If these drugs are thought to be necessary, the advice of an expert on the treatment of tuberculosis should be sought.

Skin testing for TB is currently the only effective way to identify individuals who have LTBI. This tuberculin skin test (TST) relies on DTH in which T cells sensitized by prior infection react to the applied tuberculin by producing skin induration. This test was first conceived by Sir Arthur Conan Doyle and came into being with Koch's discovery of "old tuberculin" in 1891. The substance consisted of components of *M. tuberculosis* from a liquid medium that, initially, was hoped to be a treatment for TB. In 1932, Seibert purified the protein substance and, in 1939, produced purified protein derivative-standard (PPD-S). This produced a skin reaction and later became an international standard. Current PPD is still bioassayed to demonstrate equal potency to PPD-S.

Purified protein derivative is best delivered by Mantoux testing, the intradermal injection of 0.1 mL (5 tuberculin units) of a substance bioequivalent to PPD-S. It is usually performed with a very small syringe (appropriately called a tuberculin syringe) and is delivered intradermally with the needle bevel up.

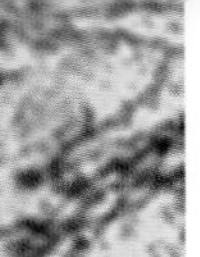

Table 27.3
Effective treatment regimens for tuberculosis

Indication	Drugs	Duration of therapy
New cases (smear +, culture + or suspected	INH/RIF/PZA/EMB*	2 mos INH/RIF/PZA followed by 4 mos INH/RIF (or 7 mos INH/RIF if positive culture at 2 mos or cavitary lung disease)
New cases in pregnancy	INH/RIF/EMB (PZA not approved for pregnancy)	9 mos INH/RIF
New "culture negative" case	INH/RIF/PZA*	2 mos INH/RIF/PZA 2 mos INH/RIF
INH resistance	RIF/EMB/PZA +/- FQN	2 mos RIF/EMB/PZA +/- FQN 4 mos RIF/EMB +/- PZA +/- FQN
RIF resistance	INH/PZA/EMB +/- FQN	2 mos INH/PZA/EMB +/- FQN +/- injectable agent 7-10 mos INH/PZA/EMB +/- FQN
MDR-TB	Use first-line agents if the isolate is susceptible, one injectable agent plus two additional oral agents	18-24 mos only if INH/RIF resistant 24 mos if more than only INH/RIF resistant
Re-treatment of standard case (while susceptability studies are pending or are unavailable)	INH/RIF/PZA/EMB plus two to three additional agents (one injectable agent)	Continuation of therapy should be tailored accordingly to susceptibility data

INH = isoniazid; RIF = rifampin; PZA = pyrazinamide; EMB = ethambutol; FQN = fluoroquinolone

* EMD should always be added to standard regimens when there is a high risk of INH-resistance (>4%) - see text for information regarding estimation of the degree of risk.

** If/when susceptibility data become available continuation of therapy should be tailored accordingly. Choices include, amikacin, kanamycin, or capreomycin. Duration of therapy should be 2-6 mos based on patient tolerance.

Effective treatment regimens for tuberculosis. These regimens are known to be effective under the circumstances listed above. In treatment failure or relapse, the opinion of an expert in tuberculosis should be sought. One should *never* add a single drug to a failing antituberculous regimen.

Other forms of skin testing (e.g., the "tyne test") are inferior, nonstandardized, and should not be used.

The tuberculin skin test is applied to the volar surface of the forearm in an area away from veins. When injected it raises a weal that appears pale and is 6 to 10 mm in diameter. After 48 to 72 hours, the site of injection is inspected for the size and induration produced by DTH. The best method of measurement is for the investigator to align perpendicularly to the long axis of the arm and draw a line with a ballpoint pen until it stops on the raised area on either side of the induration. The distance between the ink lines is then measured in millimeters. The likelihood that a positive test represents true infection depends on the prevalence of tuberculous infection in a determined population. Because tuberculin skin testing cross-reacts with other mycobacterial species, the specificity is low in areas with high prevalence of nontuberculous mycobacteria and low prevalence of tuberculous infection. The interpretation of the tuberculin skin test should take into consideration the size of the induration and the factors that identify patients at risk of recent infection and those who, regardless of the duration of the infection, are at increased risk for the progression to tuberculous disease.

The use of skin anergy testing (using an antigen control) to validate a negative PPD is inappropriate. A positive control skin test does not "prove" that a negative reaction to PPD is valid. The phenomenon of selective anergy to PPD is well known and, therefore, a negative reaction to PPD does not prove absence of tuberculous infection.

The identification of LTBI patients allows for the possibility of implementing prophylactic therapy for the prevention of TB. The efficacy of the treatment regimens for latent tuberculosis infection has been reported as high as 90%. The purpose of TST programs should be to identify this high-risk group of patients who will most benefit from preventative therapy.

Patients at risk for a recent infection or a high prevalence of LTBI can be identified at county health departments, jails, homeless shelters, methadone or drug rehabilitation clinics, and organizations serving foreign-born persons. It is recommended that a history of BCG vaccination be disregarded when interpreting a tuberculin skin test. Health care workers and people working in institutions caring for the previously named groups may also be considered at high risk for recent infection and annual testing has been recommended. LTBI patients with increased risk for progression to TB can be identified at HIV clinics and community health centers. Recently, therapy with antitumor necrosis factor antibody has been introduced for treatment of certain inflammatory diseases including rheumatoid arthritis, inflammatory bowel disease, and psoriasis. Case reports of associated TB development have begun to appear. The manufacturers of these medications recommend tuberculin skin

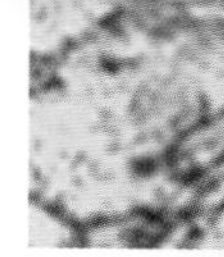

test for patients considered for antitumor necrosis factor therapy.

When interpreting a change in a repeated tuberculin skin test, four aspects need to be considered. First, random variability may result in differences of less than 6 mm and therefore an increase of at least 10 mm is considered significant in a previous positive TST. Second, skin test conversion is a new positive TST and represents a recent infection with *M. tuberculosis*. Third, a close contact to a patient with TB should be retested at least 8 to 10 weeks after last contact. Fourth, the booster phenomenon is a subsequent positive TST preceded by a negative TST by 1 to 5 weeks (up to 60 days). The reversion of a positive tuberculin skin test is recognized but the lack of epidemiologic data for TST underlies the axiom "once positive, no longer useful."

Because of the risk of development of drug resistance when TB is inadequately treated, active TB must be ruled out before instituting LTBI therapy. A history and physical examination (and in specific circumstances, radiographs and bacteriologic studies including final results of cultures) are often enough. Symptomatic patients with radiologic abnormalities should be considered for antituberculous therapy. Among TB case contacts, children younger than age 5 should be started on LTBI therapy even if initial TST is negative—therapy may be stopped if repeated TSTs remain negative. Immunosuppressed contacts to a TB case, including HIV patients, should receive complete LTBI therapy even if TSTs remain negative.

When suspecting TB, a positive TST should not replace a thorough attempt to isolate mycobacteria. A tuberculin skin test may, however, assist in the diagnosis of culture-negative cases or contribute in the diagnosis of a tuberculous pleural effusion.

The widely used regimens for LTBI therapy include: INH for 9 months or RIF for 4 months. A combination of RIF + PZA for 2 months has been shown to be effective, but the high risk of hepatotoxicity (and rarely death) associated with this regimen limits its use to very carefully selected patients. The risk of INH hepatotoxicity increases with age but monitoring of liver enzymes in asymptomatic patients is controversial and not recommended. Nonetheless, with the onset of abdominal symptoms or jaundice these medications must be stopped and the patient evaluated.

A new test based on the production of interferon-γ by patients' mononuclear cells when exposed to *M. tuberculosis* antigens is being evaluated in the diagnosis of LTBI. Presently it is not recommended in groups in whom a TST of 5 mm will be considered positive, in children younger than 17 years old, and for pregnant women.

DISEASES CAUSED BY ATYPICAL MYCOBACTERIA

Until the late 1950s, the mycobacteria other than TB represented a heterogeneous group of organisms that were thought to only occasionally cause disease in humans. In 1959, Runyon reported a classification system (Runyon Classification—Table 27.4) for these organisms that, for the first time, organized them according to microbiologic characteristics. Four groups were included in the schema based on tendencies toward the formation of pigmented colonies in various culture conditions and the speed of bacterial growth (*M. leprae* was excluded). Although Runyon's groups brought some order to the consideration of nontuberculous mycobacteria (NTM), as more and more species of mycobacteria were recognized the categorization became less useful. Of the more than 50 different species of *Mycobacterium*, approximately 40% appear to cause disease in humans. An American Thoracic Society (ATS) statement on NTM disease has provided a useful classification of disease-causing NTM based on the clinical diseases they produce. The disease groups presented are NTM pulmonary disease, NTM lymphadenitis, NTM cutaneous disease, and disseminated NTM disease.

Table 27.4
The Runyon Classification of nontuberculous mycobacteria

Runyon group	Pigment production	Representative organisms
I	Photochromogens – develop yellow pigment when exposed to light	*M. kansasii* *M. marinum*
II	Scotochromogens – develop yellow-orange pigment when exposed to light	*M. scrofulaceum* *M. szulgai*
III	Nonchromogens – no pigment develops when exposed to light	*M. gordonae* *M. terrae* *M. gastri*
IV	Rapid growers	*M. chelonae* *M. fortuitum* *M. smegmatis*

The Runyon classification. A classification system for nontuberculous mycobacteria based on the tendency to form pigment in the presence or absence of light, the lack of pigment formation, and speed of growth. Was more useful in previous years and newer classification schema are based on the type of disease the organisms cause in humans. These terms continue to be used today.

Epidemiology

Exposure to NTM primarily arises from the environment, specifically soil and water. It is not thought that transmission from animals or person-to-person spread represent significant aspect of transmission of the disease to humans. The reservoir for transmission of *M. avium-intracellulare* complex (MAC; a complex of *M. avium* and *M. intracellulare*) to the HIV-infected population is unclear, but MAC is frequently isolated from common tap water. Infections caused by rapidly growing NTM have been associated with exposure to various water sources, which include fish tanks, swimming pools, hot tubs, and salt or fresh water sites. Isolation of NTM from soil has been achieved, but some organisms such as *M. kansasii* cannot survive more than about 12 hours in the earth.

Based on the occurrence of geographic and specific clusters of infections, it is likely that certain local conditions favor disease development with particular organisms. Some general statements can be made regarding certain NTM organisms:

- *M. malmoense* has been recovered from waters in Finland and, not surprisingly, has emerged as a pathogen in Northern Europe
- *M. simiae* disease has been isolated and caused disease in the southwestern United States, Cuba, and Israel
- *M. xenopi*, a thermophilic organism, has been isolated from hot water sources in hospitals where it has been associated with the occurrence of cutaneous and pulmonary disease—

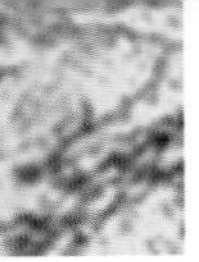

this organism is now reported as a common cause of insidious pulmonary disease in Western Europe.

Although consideration of the source of infection is important for epidemiologic reasons, geographic location and circumstance play little role in the diagnosis and management of disease caused by NTM. However, research continues in the hope of learning more about the geographic tendencies of these diseases. At present, the environment is thought to be the primary source of inoculation for NTM that cause disease.

Clinical Features

Because newer classifications deal with the general categorization of diseases caused by the various NTM, clinical presentation is discussed here by disease category: pulmonary disease, lymphadenitis, cutaneous disease, and disseminated disease.

PULMONARY DISEASE CAUSED BY NTM

The clinical presentation of pulmonary disease caused by NTM is nonspecific. Historical considerations are routinely unhelpful because common symptomatology consists of routine pulmonary and constitutional symptoms such as cough, production of sputum, and fatigue. Fever, malaise, weight loss, and hemoptysis are infrequently seen. The physical examination also may be unhelpful. Although crackles, decreased breath sounds, or amphoric breath sounds may be heard, physical findings are nonspecific with NTM lung infection, and these patients frequently have underlying chronic lung disease. Predisposing conditions are as follows: alcoholism, bronchiectasis, cyanotic heart disease, cystic fibrosis, prior mycobacterial disease (abnormal anatomy secondary to scarring), pulmonary fibrosis, smoking, chronic obstructive pulmonary disease, immunosuppression (including neoplastic and iatrogenic causes), and HIV disease with CD4 counts of less than 100.

The chest radiograph may be more helpful because NTM-induced pulmonary disease has a somewhat different appearance to that of pulmonary TB. The cavities formed with NTM-related pulmonary disease tend to have thin walls and little surrounding inflammatory process. Air-liquid interfaces in the cavities and pleural effusions are uncommon. Apical pleural reaction in the area of involvement may be intense, and these chronic, thickened pleural reactions are virtually pathognomonic of NTM infection. In many cases, single or numerous small pulmonary nodules may also be seen (Figure 27.12). Bronchiectasis is becoming a more frequent finding on high-resolution CT in NTM-related disease and is now being seen in patients without preexisting lung disease.

Mantoux testing for exposure to specific NTM is limited in utility by considerable cross-reactivity with *M. tuberculosis* and other NTM. Therefore, diagnosis usually rests on the demonstration of these atypical mycobacteria from culture of sputum and other fluids or tissue samples. The question of colonization with NTM, in the absence of primary NTM pulmonary disease, remains somewhat controversial. As a result, specific guidelines for the diagnosis of pulmonary disease caused by NTM have been recently published (see the following section).

In recent years, NTM have been responsible for a new pulmonary syndrome: "hot tub lung." This appears to be caused by aerosolized MAC. The illness appears to begin with vague flulike symptoms and progresses to cough and radiographic interstitial infiltrates or nodules. Biopsy material usually reveals granulomatous inflammation without necrosis. Antibiotics are often given but avoidance of the hot tub may be most important. This syndrome may represent hypersensitivity to MAC rather than infection.

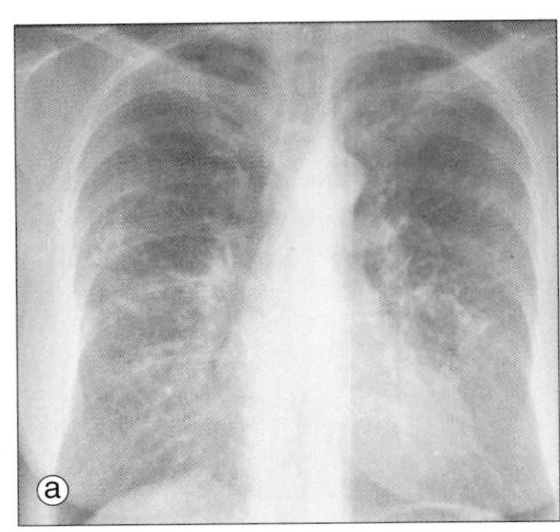

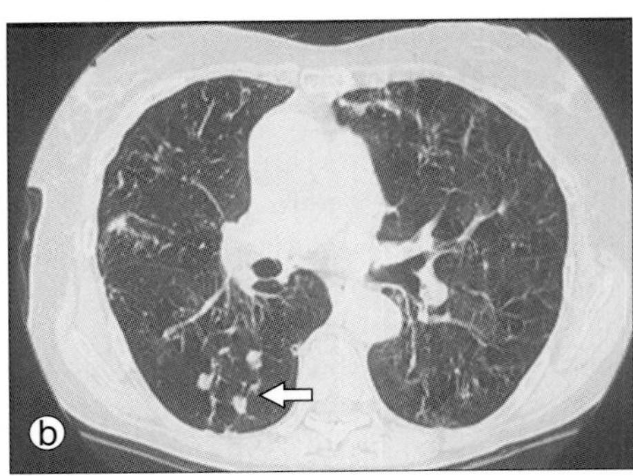

Figure 27.12 *Mycobacterium avium* complex. **A,** Posterior-anterior chest radiograph shows some patchy infiltrates in the mid-lung bilaterally. **B,** Computed tomography from a different patient shows the typical nodular lesions (arrow) associated with this organism.

The isolation of *M. abscessus* or *M. fortuitum* (rapid growers) should trigger suspicion of chronic aspiration. Further diagnostic investigation of swallowing may be necessary.

NONTUBERCULOUS LYMPHADENITIS (SCROFULODERMA)

While mycobacterial lymphadenitis can occur in all age groups, NTM is most commonly the cause in children between 1 and 5 years of age (95% of mycobacterial lymphadenitis seen in patients outside this age group is caused by *M. tuberculosis*). Insidious onset of nodal enlargement, usually unilateral and nontender, occurs primarily in the submandibular, submaxillary, cervical, or preauricular nodes (although any nodal group may be involved). Constitutional symptoms are uncommon. Rapid nodal enlargement is frequently seen and, at times, the involved nodes can rupture with a purulent discharge and consequent fistula formation. Histopathology, radiographic studies, and PPD skin studies are unhelpful in the younger, high-risk group. Specialized skin studies for specific species of NTM are not helpful.

In contrast to tuberculous lymphadenitis, which requires both surgery and antituberculous chemotherapy, treatment of lymphadenitis caused by NTM is primarily surgical. In most cases, the reason for pursuing a microbiologic diagnosis is the possibility of TB as the potential etiology.

Less invasive diagnostic techniques for lymphadenitis in the group at high risk for NTM are not very helpful. Incision and drainage of these lesions frequently results in the formation of fistulae, and needle aspiration of involved nodes is only positive in about 50% of cases. Although NTM-compatible histopathology (Figure 27.13) of excised nodes is common, microbiologic recovery of the organisms occurs in only 50% to 80% of cases. The most common pathogen varies by geographic region. In the United States, MAC causes the majority of disease with the remaining cases primarily caused by *M. scrofulaceum*. In Northern Europe, Scandinavia, and the United Kingdom, MAC is also the most common cause of NTM lymphadenitis, but *M. malmoense* is the second most common cause. In children, only about 10% of lymphadenitis caused by AFB results from *M. tuberculosis*.

CUTANEOUS AND SOFT-TISSUE DISEASE CAUSED BY NTM

Cutaneous infections caused by NTM usually result from direct inoculation of organisms into the skin. Virtually all atypical mycobacteria have been implicated in cutaneous involvement, but the most common organisms responsible are *M. abscessus*, *M. fortuitum*, *M. marinum*, and *M. ulcerans*. When the site of inoculation occurs where the skin has suffered trauma, *M. chelonae* is the prime suspect.

The most common cutaneous syndrome from NTM is infection with *M. marinum* to give "fish-tank" or "swimming-pool" granuloma, which presents as slowly enlarging papules or heaped up lesions that can ulcerate. Healing may be spontaneous, but is quite slow and the use of surgical excision and appropriate antimicrobial agents is recommended.

Skin disease caused by *M. ulcerans* is most commonly seen in Australia, Africa, and Mexico. The lesion it produces is known as the *Buruli ulcer*, which is progressive and destructive. It can result in severe, deforming changes in the extremities. Surgical excision and skin grafting are most helpful since single-drug therapy is of little utility. Cutaneous disease may also be caused by *M. malmoense*.

Bone and joint involvement with NTM can result in very significant illness. After cardiac surgery, *M. abscessus* and *M. fortuitum* have produced sternal wound infections with devastating results. Numerous other atypical mycobacteria can cause infections that involve the joint space, synovium, tendons, and bony tissue and produce a form of indolent chronic disease.

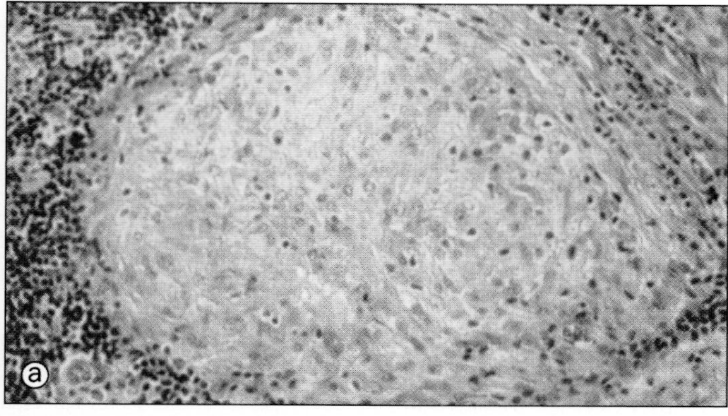

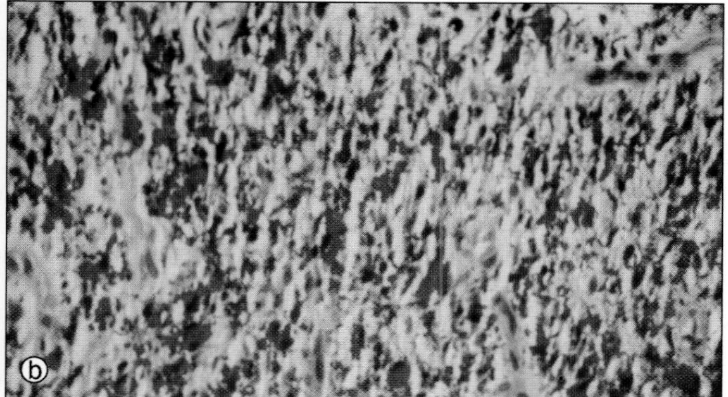

Figure 27.13 Histopathology of an infected lymph node related to *Mycobacterium avium* complex. **A,** Lymph node pathology revealing non-caseating granuloma (hematoxylin and eosin). **B,** Ziehl-Neelson stain over hematoxylin and eosin at higher magnification revealing numerous acid-fast (red staining) organisms.

DISSEMINATED INFECTION CAUSED BY NTM

In adults who do not have HIV infection, the dissemination of atypical mycobacteria is usually associated with some form of immunosuppression. Corticosteroid therapy, use of negative immunomodulating drugs, transplant patients, and those who have reticuloendothelial neoplasms are the most commonly afflicted. Mortality rates depend upon the degree of immunosuppression and clinical involvement. The most frequent offending NTM organisms are MAC, *M. fortuitum*, *M. kansasii*, and *M. chelonae*. Diagnosis requires isolation of the organism from a blood culture or sterile site (e.g., blood culture, bone marrow specimen).

In the HIV-infected patient, the likelihood of dissemination increases as the $CD4^+$ count drops below 100 cells/μL; MAC is the common causative organism (Figure 27.14). More than 90% of the time disseminated MAC infection in AIDS patients is associated with prolonged fever and night sweats. Diarrhea, abdominal pain, and weight loss are also common. These usually signal profound involvement of the bowel, the site from which dissemination is thought to occur, and the organism can commonly be isolated from stool or sputum specimens in AIDS patients. The diagnosis requires isolation of the organism from cultures of blood or a usually sterile site. When AFB-positive sputum specimens and abnormal chest radiographs are seen in an AIDS patient, the cause is more likely to be *M. tuberculosis* than MAC.

In AIDS patients, *M. avium* disease once occurred in those with $CD4^+$ counts of less than 100 cells/μL at a rate of about 20% per year. HAART (highly active antiretroviral therapy) has significantly reduced the incidence of NTM disease in AIDS. HAART usually raises the $CD4^+$ counts to levels greater than 100 cells/μL, a level at which NTM-related disease does not typically occur. The median $CD4^+$ lymphocyte count at the time of NTM diagnosis is around 10 cells/μL. If CD4+ lymphocyte counts cannot be raised, antimicrobial prophylaxis is indicated (macrolides, ethambutol, and rifabutin).

Diagnosis of Disease Caused by NTM

Handling of specimens, specimen staining, and culture techniques for NTM are similar to the techniques described for *M. tuberculosis*. When the AFB smear is positive, no staining property can reliably distinguish NTM from *M. tuberculosis*. As noted previously (Runyon classification), certain growth charac-

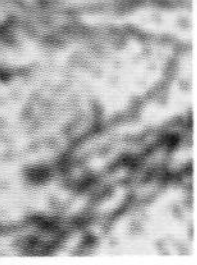

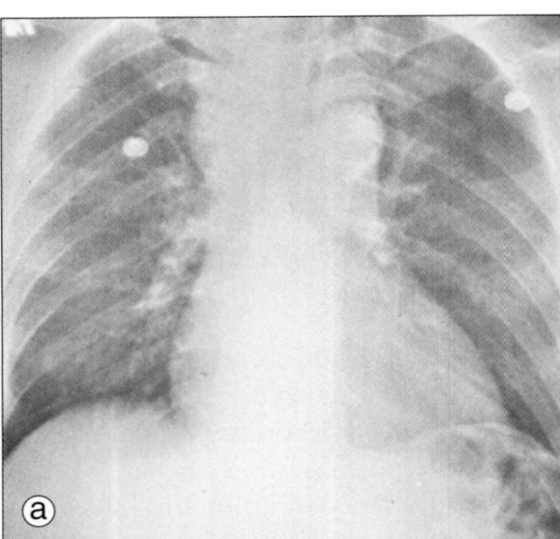

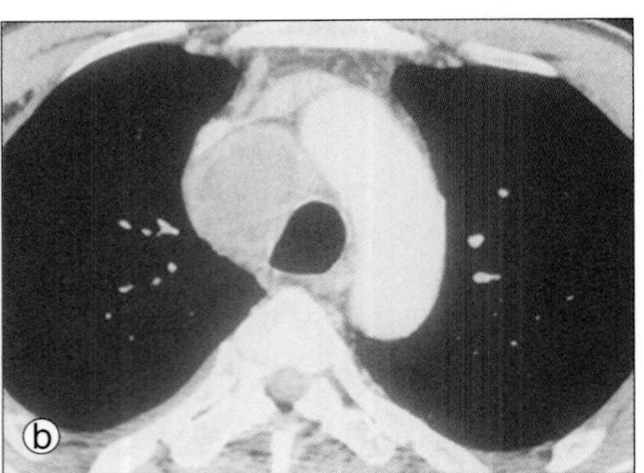

Figure 27.14 *Mycobacterium avium* complex infection in a patient with acquired immunodeficiency syndrome (AIDS). **A,** Chest radiograph and **B,** computed tomography show mediastinal adenopathy in a patient who has AIDS and active MAC disease. Isolated mediastinal adenopathy is a common manifestation of disseminated MAC in AIDS patients.

teristics, such as pigmentation under various culture conditions and speed of growth, may suggest a particular group of NTM, but final species identification is still likely to require biochemical testing, DNA probes, or high-pressure liquid chromatography. At present, reliable DNA probes for MAC, *M. kansasii*, and *M. gordonae* are available. Species of NTM can be highly suspected on the basis of growth patterns. For *M. genavense*, growth is often poor, but its growth characteristics are quite unusual, because it grows well on solid media but not in liquid media. Also, on an AFB stain it has a unique coccobacillary form.

The isolation of NTM in a culture does not in all cases constitute evidence of infection, especially when the culture is from the pulmonary system. For some organisms, isolation from cultures obtained on multiple occasions is necessary to establish diagnosis. A positive culture from a usually sterile site is usually diagnostic. DNA probes are now being used on various specimens to help identify some NTM (e.g., MAC). As a consequence of the frequent uncertainty associated with a culture positive for atypical mycobacteria, a new diagnostic system for the diagnosis of pulmonary disease caused by NTM has been proposed. The schema requires the fulfillment of clinical, radiographic, and bacteriologic confirmation of disease (Table 27.5).

Table 27.5
Criteria for the diagnosis of nontuberculous mycobacterial pulmonary disease

Category	Criteria
Clinical	Compatible signs and symptoms (cough, fatigue, fever, weight loss, hemoptysis, or dyspnea with documented deterioration in clinical status of underlying disease) Reasonable exclusion of other disease and/or treatment of other underlying diseases
Radiographic	Any of the following radiographic abnormalities: Evidence of progression if baseline films >1 year old Infiltrates with or without nodules Cavitation Multiple small nodules as a solitary finding Any of the following high-resolution computed tomography findings: Multiple small nodules Multifocal bronchiectasis with or without nodules
Bacteriologic	At least three sputum/bronchial wash specimens within previous year: Three positive cultures with negative acid-fast bacilli (AFB) smears [the presence of general, significant, immunosuppression not related to human immunodeficiency virus (HIV) requires positive culture with 1+ or greater growth; for HIV-infected individuals with CD4 cell count <200, positive culture with 1+ or greater growth is required (excludes *Mycobacterium avium* complex)] Two positive cultures and one positive AFB smear OR Inability to obtain sputum and one available bronchial wash: Positive culture with 2–4+ growth, or Positive culture with 2–4+ AFB smear OR Biopsy specimen, any of the following: Any growth from bronchopulmonary tissue biopsy Granulomata and/or AFB on lung biopsy pathology with at least one positive culture from sputum or bronchial wash Any growth from a usually sterile extrapulmonary site

Criteria for the diagnosis of pulmonary disease resulting from nontuberculous mycobacteria (NTM). To conclusively diagnose pulmonary disease resulting from NTM, all three criteria must be satisfied: clinical, radiographic, and bacteriologic. (Diagnosis and treatment of disease caused by nontuberculous mycobacteria. Am J Resp Crit Care Med 156 (suppl), Part 2, S1-S19,1997.

Treatment of Disease Caused by NTM

Although all the mycobacterial organisms share the same family and genus, their response to antimicrobial therapy is highly variable. Some respond to standard antibiotics, whereas others require specific regimens of antituberculous therapy. The need for adjunctive treatments, such as surgery, also varies from species to species and even according to the nature of the disease the organism appears to be causing. For this reason, no blanket statement can be made regarding the various treatments for the common causes of NTM disease. A summary of the various disease categories, causative organisms, and acceptable treatment measures is given in Table 27.6.

Sometimes it is not clear if the sporadic positive culture results for NTM organisms in the presence of a questionable pulmonary infiltrate represent identification of the cause of disease or not. In many cases cautious observation is acceptable, but in the face of clearly progressive illness it may be prudent to initiate treatment regardless of whether or not criteria for the diagnosis are met.

Recently, interleukin-12 and aerosolized interferon-γ have been used as adjunctive therapy in the treatment of severe nontuberculous mycobacteria pulmonary disease. These substances participate in mycobacterial killing at the cellular level.

Our understanding of disease related to NTM has progressed rapidly, given the general disregard for the category of organisms up until the 1950s, but we are still learning about the nature of

Table 27.6
Diseases caused by the nontuberculous mycobacteria and recommended therapy

Clinical disease	Common etiologies	Recommended antimicrobial therapy	Other etiologies
Pulmonary disease	1. *M. avium* complex (cavitary or bronchiectatic)	Clarithromycin 500 mg BID or azithromycin 250-500, rifabutin 300 mg or rifampin 600 mg, ethambutol 25 mg/kg and amikacin 15-20 mg/kg (for the first 2-3 mos) daily or thrice-weekly. Duration 6 to 24 mos depending on tolerance and risk relapsing.	1. *M. simiae* 2. *M. szulgai* 3. *M. celatum* 4. *M. asiaticum* 5. *M. haemophilum* 6. *M. smegmatis*
	2. *M. kansasii*	Isoniazid 900 mg/day, rifampin 600 mg/day, ethambutol 25 mg/kg/day x 2 mos followed by 15 mg/kg/day for 18 mos with at least 12 mos of negative sputum cultures. Note all *M. kansasii* isolates are resistant to pyrazinamide. Can add streptomycin in severe disease.	
3. Rapidly growing mycobacteria (consider chronic aspiration)	3.1. *M. abscessus*	Clarithromycin 500 mg BID, amikacin 15 mg/kg and cefoxitin 200 mg/kg/day (max 12 g/d divided in 3 to 4 doses/day) or imipenem 750 mg TID. Unknown duration. May require surgery.	
	3.2. *M. fortuitum*	Clarithromycin 500 mg BID plus one or two other agents (doxycycline 100 mg daily, trimethoprim sulfamethoxazole 1 DS BID or FQN daily) for 6 to 12 mos.	
	4. *M. xenopi*	Clarithromycin + rifampin or rifabutin + ethambutol ± initial streptomycin	
	5. *M. malmoense*	See treatment for *M. xenopi*	
Lymphadenitis	1. *M. avium* complex	Surgical excision of infected lymph nodes (mac only - a microlide + a rifamycin in recurrence and when excision is incomplete)	1. *M. fortuitum* 2. *M. chelonae* 3. *M. abscessus* 4. *M. kansasii* 5. *M. haemophilum*
	2. *M. fortuitum*	See *M. avium* complex	
	3. *M. chelonae*	See *M. avium* complex	
Cutaneous disease	1. *M. marinum*	Observation, excision, and/or antibiotics: ethambutol 15 mg/kg/day and any of the following for at least 3 mos: clarithromycin 500 mg BID, minocycline or doxycycline 100 mg BID, TM/SM 160/800 BID, or rifampin 600 mg/day	1. *M. ulcerans* 2. *M. avium* complex 3. *M. kansasii* 4. *M. nonchromo-genicum* 5. *M. smegmatis* 6. *M. haemophilum*
	2. *M. fortuitum*	Amikacin 5-7.5 mg IV BID (decrease dose over 50 years of age) and cefoxitin 12 grams/day IV for the first two weeks. Surgery required for extensive disease.	
	3. *M. chelonae*	Tobramycin IV (better activity *in vitro* than amikacin), clarithromycin, cefoxitin (or imipenem when isolate resistant to cefoxitin). Sometimes requires surgery.	
	4. *M. abscessus*	No studies available but: *in vitro* data suggest that clarithromycin, imipemen, cefoxitin, cefmetazole, and amikacin may be effective. For severe disease use clofazamine and clarithromycin and possible excision.	
Disseminated disease	1. *M. avium* complex	Three drugs are recommended: clarithromycin 500 mg BID or azithromycin, ethambutol 15 mg/kg/day (possibly 25 mg/kg/day for first 2 mos), and a rifamycin (rifabutin if using antiprotease re: drug interaction). Consider adding amikacin or streptomycin in severe disease.	1. *M. abscessus* 2. *M. xenopi* 3. *M. malmoense* 4. *M. genavense* 5. *M. simiae* 6. *M. conspicuum* 7. *M. marinum* 8. *M. fortuitum*
	2. *M. kansasii*	See *M. kansasii* in the pulmonary disease section	
	3. *M. chelonae*	Resistant to anti-tuberculous drugs. Consider combination from: tobramycin (sens. 100%), amikacin (sens. 100%), clarithromycin (sens. 100%), doxycycline (sens. 25%), ciprofloxacin (sens. 20%) and clofazamine.	
	4. *M. haemophilum*	Suggested drugs: ciprofloxacin, clarithromycin, and rifampin	

Diseases caused by the nontuberculous mycobacteria and recommended therapy. These diseases are relatively uncommon and the recommended therapies listed above are based on data available and expert opinion. If there is doubt about the appropriate regimen, an expert consultant should be sought.

infectious disease caused by the atypical mycobacteria. Medical progress is slowly enabling more rapid diagnosis and providing effective therapy in some NTM illness. In the interim, we continue to make our best efforts to standardize diagnosis and management and to watch carefully when the diagnosis is in doubt.

Pitfalls and Controversies

There are some important things to keep in mind when dealing with *M. tuberculosis* infections. First, TB will seldom be diagnosed if tuberculosis is not in the differential diagnosis. To avoid missing the diagnosis, always include TB as a possible causative agent. Second, when clinical suspicion is high and another diagnosis is not obvious, appropriate therapy for TB should be instituted. Antituberculous agents are generally well-tolerated. Third, treatment failures usually result from inadequate therapy or failure to comply with the treatment regimen. It is always appropriate to enlist the aid of experts when treating TB if one has any doubt about appropriate therapy. Last, making the diagnosis of TB and instituting appropriate therapy is only the beginning. To assure compliance and follow up of all potential contacts, most physicians will require the help of public health services. In many countries these services are well-qualified and provide invaluable assistance in controlling the spread of tuberculosis.

The length of time a patient remains contagious after initiation of therapy is still uncertain. Apparently the risk of household transmission after therapy is low with only mask-barrier precautions. The nosocomial spread of TB in low-prevalence countries is now being attributed to exposure because of a delay in diagnosis and treatment of TB in atypical presentations.

When dealing with a potential NTM infection, it is important to be certain that infection truly exists. An isolation of *M. kansasii* is indicative of a need for therapy. Isolating MAC in a situation that is consistent with MAC disease is likely enough

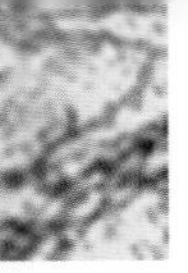

to warrant instituting therapy. Culturing an atypical mycobacterium from a sterile site is usually significant. In other situations, multiple repeat isolates are often necessary to distinguish NTM colonization from true infection.

SUGGESTED READINGS

American Thoracic Society: Control of tuberculosis in the United States. Am Rev Respir Dis 146:1623-1633, 1992.

American Thoracic Society: Diagnosis and treatment of disease caused by nontuberculous mycobacteria. Am J Respir Crit Care Med 156 (suppl 2):S1-S25, 1997.

American Thoracic Society/Centers for Disease Control and Prevention: Targeted tuberculin testing and treatment of latent tuberculosis infection. Am J Respir Crit Care Med 161 (suppl):S221-S247, 2000.

American Thoracic Society/Centers for Disease Control and Prevention/ Infectious Diseases Society of America: Treatment of tuberculosis. Am J Respir Crit Care Med 167:603-662, 2003.

Chan ED, Iseman MD: Current treatment of tuberculosis. BMJ 325;1282-1286, 2002.

Cantanzaro A, Daley C (eds): Nontuberculous mycobacterial infections. Clin Chest Med 23;#3 (September issue), 2002.

Lauzardo M, Ashkin D: Phthisiology at the dawn of the new century. Chest 117: 1445-1473, 2000.

Light RW: Tuberculous pleural effusions. In: Retford DC (ed): Pleural Effusions, 3rd ed. Baltimore, Williams and Wilkins, 1995:154-165.

Weir MR, Thornton GF: Extrapulmonary tuberculosis. Experience of a community hospital and review of the literature. Am J Med 79:467-478, 1985.

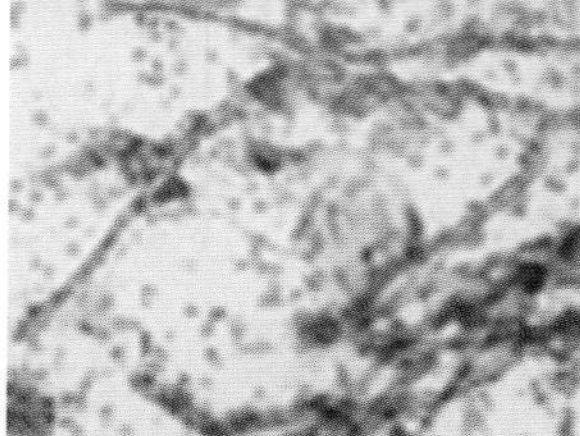

CHAPTER 28 Rhinitis and Sinusitis

Glenis Scadding and David Mitchell

EPIDEMIOLOGY, RISK FACTORS, AND PATHOPHYSIOLOGY

Rhinitis and sinusitis are terms that refer to inflammatory conditions of the nose and paranasal sinuses characterized by symptoms of:

- Rhinorrhea (anterior or posterior)
- Itching
- Sneezing
- Nasal obstruction

Secondary symptoms include:

- Headache
- Cough
- Facial pain
- Poor olfaction
- Disturbed sleep
- Pharyngitis
- Poor concentration
- Exacerbation of lower respiratory tract problems

In practice, inflammatory changes are usually continuous from nasal to sinus mucosa; therefore, the terminology *rhinosinusitis* is more accurate, but cumbersome—the two will be used interchangeably in this chapter. The condition has marked effects upon quality of life and is responsible for reduced school and workplace attendance (by 3% to 4%) and performance (by 30% to 40%). The resulting economic burden is high and rhinosinusitis and related conditions occupy around one third of primary care consultations.

The causes of rhinitis can be simply considered as:

- Allergy
- Infections
- Other causes or unknown.

The recent classification of rhinosinusitis taken from the ARIA (Allergic Rhinitis and its Impact on Asthma) guidelines is in Table 28.1, with the differential diagnosis in Table 28.2.

Considerable overlap between causes occurs; for example, allergic rhinitis characterized by sneezing, itching, and watery discharge results in considerable mucosal swelling, which may result in reduced sinus drainage and allow secondary infection to occur. Both allergic and infective inflammatory rhinosinusitis may be exacerbated by the presence of anatomic and mechanical defects, such as a deviated nasal septum or enlarged turbinates.

It is also important to consider the possibility of serious underlying conditions and their early recognition, which may be necessary to prevent later damage (e.g., defects of immunity, defects of cilial motility, vasculitic and granulomatous disease).

Rhinosinusitis is frequently associated with lower respiratory disease; for example, about one third of patients who have bronchiectasis also have chronic sinusitis, and patients who suffer cystic fibrosis invariably have sinusitis and frequently develop nasal polyps. Rhinitis is practically ubiquitous in asthmatics, with 10% of adults with late-onset asthma exhibiting aspirin hypersensitivity, often with nasal polyps (Samter's triad). Most asthma exacerbations begin with rhinitis, either infective, allergic, or both.

Rhinitis is a global problem with increasing prevalence. It is common in Westernized societies, with up to one third of the population affected (Figure 28.1).

Risk factors for allergic rhinitis are both genetic—with an affected parent or sibling being associated with increased risk—and environmental. Westernization appears to be associated with an increased prevalence of allergic disorders (asthma, eczema, rhinitis); the mechanisms involved are still under investigation, but several lines of evidence exist for a deviation of the immune response away from Th1 (protective immunoglobulin IgG immunity and delayed hypersensitivity) toward Th2 (atopy with IgE production) by decreased bacterial contact. Nasal polyposis also demonstrates a strong heritable component with a relative risk of 18 and 6 with an affected father and mother, respectively. The genetics of cystic fibrosis are discussed in Chapter 40. Primary ciliary dyskinesia is also genetic, with an incidence of around 1 in 20,000. Various structural ciliary defects have been described, but one common defect—a lack of inducible nitric oxide synthase in nasal mucosa—has recently been found.

Allergy

ALLERGIC RHINOSINUSITIS

Apart from viral colds, allergic rhinosinusitis is the most common cause of nasal symptoms; it affects 10% to 16% of the population and results from IgE-mediated immediate hypersensitivity reactions that occur in the mucous membranes of the nasal airways. Allergic rhinitis occurs in atopic individuals who have the genetic predisposition to produce IgE antibody responses to allergens, which are innocuous to normal individuals. The allergens responsible are usually airborne, so-called aeroallergens, and consist of plant pollen, fungal spores, insect aeroallergens (for example, from the house dust mite), and dander from domestic pets such as cats and dogs. Allergic rhinitis was formerly categorized as seasonal, perennial, and occupational; however, the recent World Health Organization ARIA guidelines suggest that intermittent

Table 28.1
Classification of rhinitis

Infectious	Viral Bacterial Other infectious agents
Allergic	Intermittent Persistent
Occupational (allergic and non-allergic)	Intermittent Persistent
Drug-induced	Aspirin Other medications
Hormonal	
Other causes	NARES Irritants Food Emotional Atrophic Gastroesophageal reflux
Idiopathic	

NARES, Nonallergic rhinitis with eosinophilia syndrome.

Table 28.2
Differential diagnosis of rhinitis

Polyps	
Mechanical factors	Deviated septum Adenoidal hypertrophy Foreign bodies Choanal atresia
Tumours	Benign Malignant
Granulomas	Wegener's granulomatosis Sarcoid Infectious Malignant-midline destructive granulomas
Ciliary defects	
Cerebrospinal rhinorrhoea	

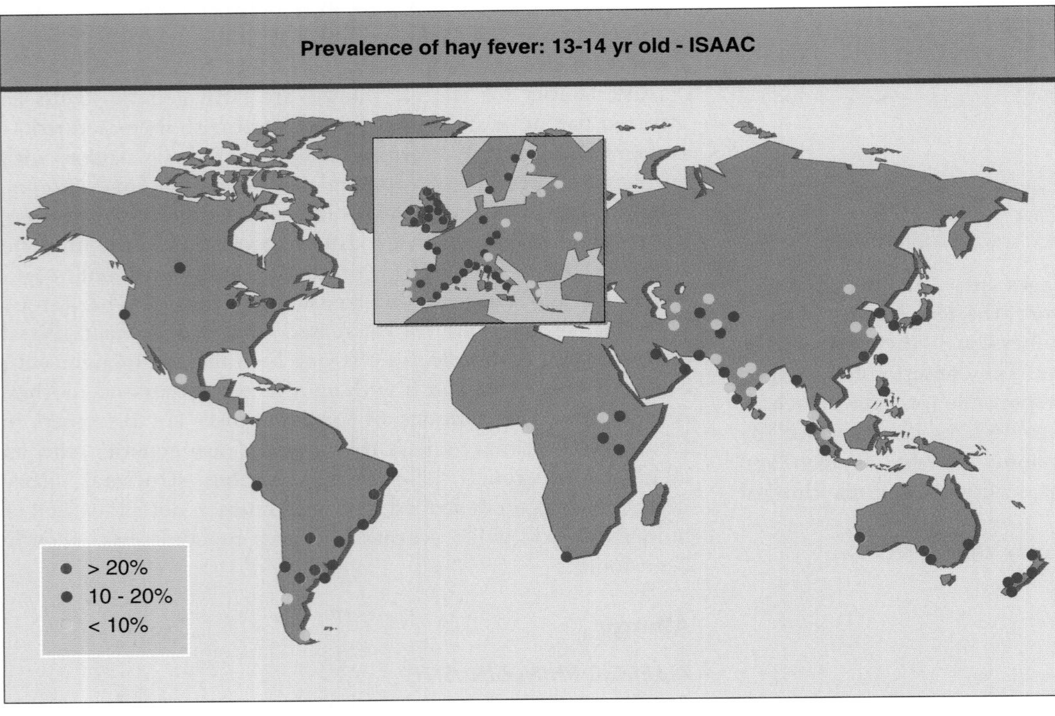

Figure 28.1 Global prevalence of hay fever in 13- to 14-year-olds—data from the International Study of Asthma and Allergies in Childhood. From Strachan D, Sibbald B, Weiland S, et al: Worldwide variations in prevalence of symptoms of allergic rhinoconjunctivitis in children: the International Study of Asthma and Allergies in Childhood (ISAAC). Pediatr Allergy Immunol, Nov 8(4):161-176, 1997.

and persistent are better divisions because they are globally applicable and influence treatment.

In the United Kingdom and other North European countries, symptoms in the spring are frequently caused by allergy to tree pollens such as birch, plane, ash, and hazel. In late spring and early summer—the classic hay fever season—allergic rhinitis results from allergy to grasses such as rye, timothy, and cocksfoot. In late summer, weed pollens, such as nettle and mugwort, are responsible, whereas in autumn the fungi *Cladosporium* spp, *Alternaria* spp, and *Aspergillus* spp provoke symptoms. In the United States, ragweed pollen allergy is a common cause of rhinitic symptoms, usually from mid-August to mid-September.

Allergy to grass pollen is probably the most common in the United Kingdom, and symptoms correlate with the presence of high airborne pollen counts. Perennial rhinitis—in which symptoms occur throughout the year—in the United Kingdom is most commonly caused by allergy to the fecal pellets of the house dust mite (*Dermatophagoides pteronyssinus*), which flourishes in warm, humid environments and lives in bedding and soft furnishings.

Allergy to dander from domestic pets (such as cats, dogs, rabbits, and hamsters) can account for perennial rhinitis,

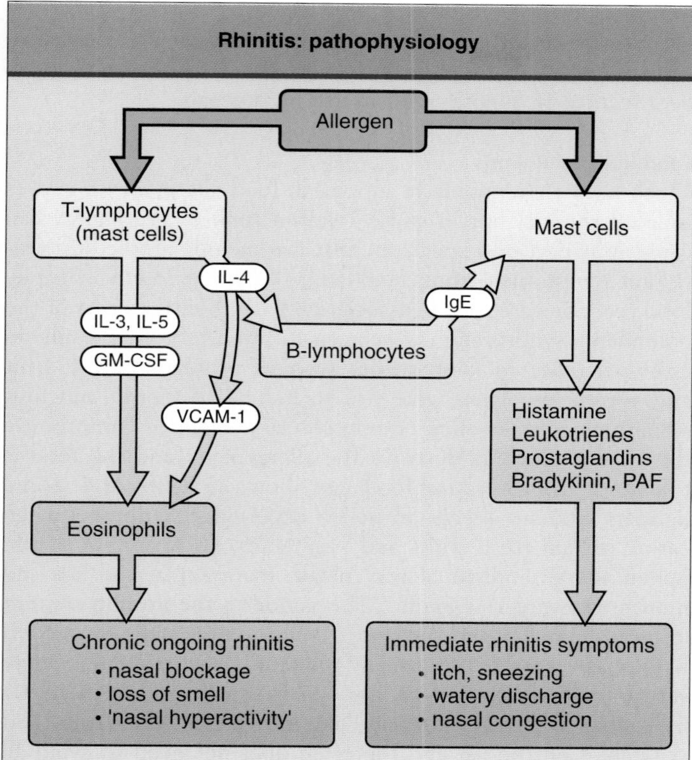

Figure 28.2 Immediate and late phases of the allergic rhinitis reaction. Mast cell degranulation leads to immediate symptoms, which are easily recognized. The late reaction, seen predominantly in persistent rhinitis, involves inflammation and produces nasal congestion and hyperreactivity, often unrecognized as allergic. (Courtesy of Professor Stephen Durham.)

whereas allergens encountered in the workplace are responsible for occupational rhinitis. Examples include sensitization to latex, flour, and grain (bakers); allergies to small mammals among laboratory workers; and allergy to wood dust, biologic products (such as antibiotic powder and enzyme-enhanced detergents), and rosin (colophony) from solder flux.

Allergic rhinitis is caused by a specific, immediate hypersensitivity reaction in the nasal mucosa that arises from IgE production to allergens. The allergic reaction can exhibit two phases: immediate and late (Figure 28.2). Mast cell degranulation with release of mediators such as histamine, leukotrienes, prostaglandins, bradykinin, and other mediators (platelet-activating factor, substance P, tachykinins), causes immediate symptoms of sneezing, itching, and running, typically seen where allergen contact is intermittent—for example, hay fever.

The late phase response involves ingress of inflammatory cells, particularly eosinophils, and is characterized by obstruction, decreased olfaction, and mucosal irritability—changes similar to those seen in chronic asthma. Similar but more marked inflammatory changes occur in aspirin-sensitive disease, without the involvement of interleukin-4 and IgE. Constant allergen contact or very high levels produce such symptoms, the allergic nature of which may not be recognized. Symptoms produced by consequent hyperreactivity to nonspecific irritants, such as inhaled fumes, dusts, and cold air may lead to an erroneous diagnosis of "vasomotor" rhinitis.

Table 28.3
Pathophysiology of rhinitis and asthma

Rhinitis	Asthma
Epithelium intact	Epithelium disrupted
Basement membrane normal	Basement membrane abnormal
No airway smooth muscle	Bronchial smooth muscle hypertrophy
Venous sinusoids	None
Submucosal glands	Less prominent
Antihistamine effective	Ineffective
β_2-agonists ineffective	Effective

Table 28.3 shows the similarities and differences between the pathophysiology of asthma and rhinitis.

Allergy to food may result in rhinitis, but this is nearly always accompanied by allergic reactions at other sites, such as oral itching, urticaria, asthma, and gastrointestinal symptoms. Rhinitic reactions in food allergy probably occur in less than 5% of cases overall. True allergic reactions occur most commonly to milk, egg, fish (cod), wheat, soy, and peanut. Less commonly, nuts, shellfish, and fruit may provoke allergic responses. Generally, food allergy is more common in children, often presenting as atopic dermatitis, which progresses to asthma as allergies switch from foods to inhalant allergens.

Allergy to food may be confused with food intolerance (in which IgE-mediated mechanisms are not involved). Some foods are rich in histamines (cheese, some fish, and some wines) that may result in flushing, headache, and rhinitis, and the same may occur with tyramine-rich foods (bananas). Food additives and coloring agents (such as sulfites, benzoates, and tartrazine) may also provoke reactions, especially in aspirin-sensitive subjects. Finally, alcohol or spicy, hot food may nonspecifically provoke rhinitic symptoms.

Nonallergic Rhinosinusitis

INFECTIOUS RHINOSINUSITIS

The nasal and sinus mucosa can be infected by all types of organisms: viruses, bacteria, fungi, and protozoa. Of these, viral infections are the most frequent.

Acute Coryza—The Common Cold

Most people have about three colds per year, but small children suffer from six to eight. Humans spend 2 years of their lives with colds, of which 50% result from rhinoviruses, a further 20% from corona viruses, and a further 20% from influenza, parainfluenza, adenoviruses, and respiratory syncytial virus; the remainder are caused by other viruses, including enteroviruses. Viral invasion occurs at the point of infection usually in the posterior nasopharynx and results in transient vasoconstriction of the mucous membrane followed by vasodilatation and edema with mucus production. A leukocytic inflammatory infiltrate develops, followed by desquamation of mucous epithelial cells. Initially, a clear watery secretion is produced, but it is followed by epithelial desquamation with opacification of secretions, which does not necessarily indicate bacterial infection, which

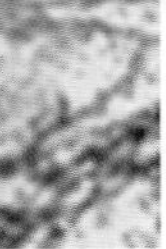

complicates only about 2% of colds. Resolution occurs in a few days in uncomplicated viral infections.

Acute Sinusitis

Although the nose harbors bacteria, the sinuses are normally largely sterile, possibly because of the nitric oxide concentrations therein and continuous mucociliary clearance. Acute sinusitis usually arises from the secondary bacterial infection of a common cold, but can also follow trauma, dental infections or procedures, and diving into polluted water. The mucous membranes of the nose and sinuses become swollen, which leads to blockage of the ostiomeatal complex and bacterial infection of the sinuses, particularly with *Haemophilus influenzae* and *Streptococcus pneumoniae*, with other causative bacteria being *Staphylococcus aureus*, *Moraxella catarrhalis*, *Streptococcus pyogenes*, and gram-negative bacteria such as *Klebsiella* spp and *Pseudomonas* spp. Anaerobic organisms may also be involved.

Chronic Sinusitis

Chronic sinusitis is defined as 8 or more weeks of continuous major symptoms, including nasal congestion or obstruction, nasal discharge, facial pain or pressure, headache, olfactory disturbance possibly plus minor symptoms of fever, and halitosis. Cough is a predominant symptom in children, leading to a possible misdiagnosis of asthma.

Chronic sinusitis can occur after failure of resolution of acute sinusitis after weeks with the same bacterial pathogens involved. However, there are often other factors present such as eosinophilic inflammation (allergic or nonallergic rhinosinusitis), immune deficiency (innate or adaptive), or structural abnormalities; the role of pathogens is disputed. One possibility is persistence of small numbers of organisms, which continually stimulate a damaging immune response.

Drug-induced Rhinitis

Antihypertensives, particularly β-blockers, can cause nasal obstruction by abrogation of the normal sympathetic tone, which maintains nasal patency. Exogenous estrogens in oral contraceptives or hormone replacement therapy also invoke rhinitis in some patients. Overuse of α-agonists results in rhinitis medicamentosa: a tachyphylaxis of α-receptors to extrinsic and intrinsic stimuli. The mucosa becomes swollen and reddened.

Aspirin hypersensitivity develops usually in adult life in patients with rhinitis (often nonallergic rhinitis with eosinophilia syndrome) with subsequent development of nasal polyps and asthma, in that order. Mast cell and eosinophil degranulation are seen in biopsies though IgE is not involved (pseudoallergy). Cox I inhibition by aspirin or nonsteroidal anti-inflammatory drugs appears to promote leukotriene production, whereas inhibiting that of prostaglandins, including PGE-2, a bronchodilator. Leukotrienes cause bronchoconstriction, mucosal swelling, and excess mucus production, and sensitivity to their effects is high in aspirin sensitivity, probably because of increased numbers of specific receptors. The clinical picture is often one of aggressive polyposis, severe asthma with life-threatening reactions to aspirin, nonsteroidal anti-inflammatory drugs, and frequent need for oral corticosteroids. A subgroup reacts also to E numbers, i.e., additives and preservatives (e.g., sulfites in wine), and high-salicylate foods such as herbs, spices, dried fruit, and jams.

Hormonal Rhinitis

Hormonal rhinitis is seen in pregnancy, occasionally in relation to menstruation, and at puberty. Chronic nasal obstruction can be a feature of hypothyroidism and acromegaly.

Food-induced Rhinitis

Much rarer than popularly supposed, food allergy rarely causes isolated rhinitis, but in small children milk or egg allergy can cause it as part of a spectrum that can include atopic dermatitis, gut symptoms, asthma, and failure to thrive. In older people, food reactions are seen in association with rhinitis as part of the oral allergy syndrome in which sensitization to pollen results in cross-reactivity to components such as profilin in fresh fruit and vegetables. These give rise to itching of mouth and lips, sometimes with swelling, rarely severe enough to compromise the airway. Cooking destroys the allergenicity and the food is tolerated. Cross-reacting foods are shown in Table 28.4. Some patients who are allergic to pollen experience symptoms when eating certain fresh fruits and vegetables. For example, a tree pollen allergic individual may notice irritation of the lips and mouth on eating raw apples. This is due to the profilin content of both the pollen and the fruit. Profilin is heat labile, so cooked fruits and vegetables are usually tolerated. The reaction is rarely severe and provision of an Epi-pen is usually unnecessary. An individual will react to only one or two of the fruits and vegetables on the list and therefore does not need to avoid all of them.

Food intolerance can give nasal symptoms: spicy foods such as peppers contain capsaicin, which irritates c fibers and leads to irritation and rhinorrhea. Frequent use results in desensitization and capsaicin has been used experimentally as a treatment for nonallergic rhinorrhea. Dyes, preservatives, and alcohol upset some noses—often in association with aspirin sensitivity.

Atrophic Rhinitis

Atrophic rhinitis is characterized by atrophy of mucosa plus the bone beneath. The nose is widely patent, but there is crusting and an unpleasant smell. *Klebsiella ozaenae* has been found in many patients, and cure with long courses of ciprofloxacin has been reported. However, it is uncertain whether this condition is primarily infective. It may follow extensive surgery, radiation, chronic granulomatous disease, or trauma. Possibly, the primary problem is failure of normal mucociliary clearance mechanisms.

Other Causes

Emotional stimuli such as sexual arousal and stress have powerful effects on the nasal mucosa via the autonomic system. Gastroesophageal reflux is thought to be a cause of rhinitis, especially in small children. Chronic exposure to dry air or occupational irritants—for example, those found in the shipbuilding industry—can lead to nasal mucosal changes, often with squamous cell abnormalities.

NONALLERGIC, NONINFECTIOUS RHINITIS

Patients with none of the aforementioned causes are usually divided according to the presence or absence of nasal eosinophilia.

Table 28.4 Oral allergy syndrome - cross reacting foods		
Plant material	**Cross-reacting foods**	
Silver birch pollen	Almond Anise seed Apple (raw) Apricot Caraway Carrot (raw) Celery (raw) Cherry Coriander Hazelnut Kiwi Lychee	Mango Nectarine Onion (raw) Orange Parsley Peach Pepper (capsicum) Plum Potato (raw) Tomato (raw) Walnut
Grass pollen	Kiwi Melon Peanut	Tomato (raw) Watermelon Wheat
Daisy family pollens	Lychee	Sunflower seeds
Mugwort (weed) pollen	Anise seed Carrot (raw) Celery (raw) Celery salt	Fennel Parsley Spices (some)
Latex (contact and/or inhaled allergy)	Avocado Banana Chestnut Kiwi Mango Melon Orange	Papaya Peach Peppers Pineapple Plum Tomato (raw)
Animal material	**Cross-reacting foods**	
House dust mite	Shellfish	Snails

NONALLERGIC RHINITIS WITH EOSINOPHILIA SYNDROME

The presence of eosinophils in nasal smears (more than 5% to 25% according to different authorities) characterizes a condition, which is probably the counterpart of intrinsic asthma and may precede nasal polyposis and aspirin sensitivity. It is usually responsive to topical nasal corticosteroids.

NONEOSINOPHILIC NONALLERGIC RHINITIS

Autonomic Rhinitis

In autonomic rhinitis, there is no evidence of nasal inflammation, but of autonomic dysfunction. Nasal and, in some patients, cardiovascular reflexes are abnormal, and there may be associated chronic fatigue syndrome. Topical ipratropium is useful in decreasing watery rhinorrhea; capsaicin applications may also relieve symptoms for several months after a few weeks of treatment.

The nasal mucosa receives a rich innervation from both the sympathetic and parasympathetic nervous system. Adrenaline and other sympathomimetics lead to vasoconstriction of the nasal mucosa, with increased nasal patency. Both α- and β-adrenergic blockers increase nasal resistance and can produce symptoms of nasal stuffiness. Stimulation of the parasympathetic system leads to an increase in nasal secretions. However, patients who have this condition also have increased responsiveness to both histamine and methacholine, which results in nasal blockage and rhinorrhea. It is also associated with hypertrophy of the inferior turbinates and nasal polyps are sometimes present. Certain stimuli result in rhinorrhea and other symptoms of rhinitis, such as cold air, exercise, mechanical or thermal stimuli, humidity changes, and a period of nasal hyperresponsiveness, often follow viral infection.

IDIOPATHIC OR INTRINSIC RHINITIS

Idiopathic or intrinsic rhinitis is a diagnosis of exclusion with no evidence for any of the aforementioned causes. Symptoms tend to be perennial and local allergy has been suggested as a cause, based on histologic findings of mast cells and eosinophils in resected turbinates and on positive responses to local nasal allergen challenge in a subgroup.

Direct release of mediators from mast cells or neurogenic mechanisms may be involved here.

Finally, emotional factors may play a part, ranging from stress that compounds nasal blockage and discharge to the patient emphatically or consistently complaining of gross nasal symptoms, yet with no abnormal findings on examination.

Structural Causes

Variant anatomy was thought to predispose to rhinosinusitis as a result of interference with normal drainage and aeration of the paranasal sinuses (Figure 28.3) at the ostiomeatal complex, the crucial point at which the maxillary, frontal, and anterior ethmoid sinuses drain into the nose. However, in three recent studies, patients with chronic rhinosinusitis showed no greater prevalence of structural abnormalities than did normal controls.

Neoplasms, foreign bodies, and trauma can all produce symptoms of obstruction, pain, purulent discharge, and epistaxis. In adults, the possibility of neoplasm is always considered in patients who have persistent symptoms, particularly if these are unilateral. In children, the presence of foreign bodies should be considered if nasal discharge is unilateral and foul-smelling. Local disease in the pharynx and larynx may also have an impact on the nose and paranasal sinuses (e.g., enlarged adenoids), as may dental disease (e.g., maxillary dental root infection), which may spread to the maxillary sinus.

Immune Defects

Panhypogammaglobulinemia is a severe condition with variable absence of all classes of immunoglobulin; it presents with bacterial and other infections at many sites. Initial presentation may be to the otorhinolaryngologist with symptoms of recurrent acute or chronic rhinosinusitis. It is important to make the diagnosis early before irreversible damage occurs at other sites (the lungs) and so that appropriate immunoglobulin therapy can be instituted. Total or relative absence of IgA may be present in the absence of any obvious clinical disease. However, IgA deficiency is now known to be associated in some patients with IgG_2 subclass deficiency, and such individuals may be more prone to episodes of sinusitis caused by capsulated bacteria such as *H. influenzae* and *S. pneumoniae*. Acute, chronic, and recurrent sinusitis are common in individuals who have human immunodeficiency virus infection, the most common organisms being *S. pneumoniae* and *H. influenzae*. A tendency to chronicity and to relapse is found, and in addition fungal (*Cryptococcus* spp, *Alternaria* spp, and *Aspergillus* spp) and viral (cytomegalovirus) sinusitis may occur.

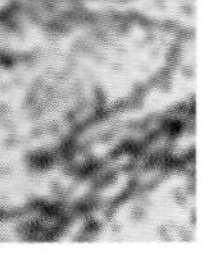

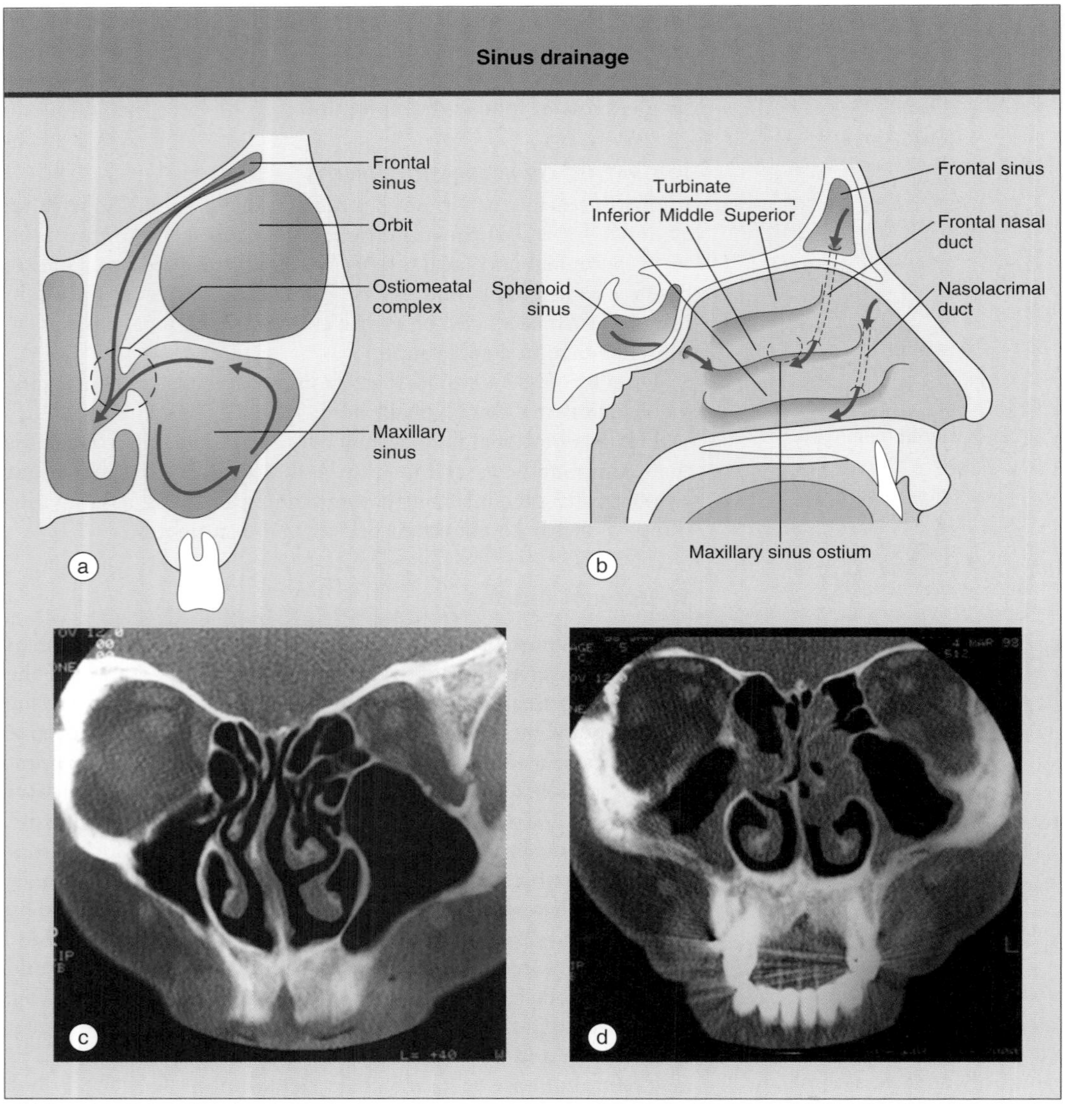

Figure 28.3 The top diagrams show sinus drainage pathways. In the left coronal diagram **(A),** the ostiomeatal complex is seen to drain the frontal, anterior ethmoid and maxillary sinuses. The right diagram **(B)** demonstrates these from the lateral view. Below the left coronal computed tomography (CT) scan, **(C)** shows clear paranasal sinuses in a patient with a deviated nasal septum. In the right scan **(D)** significant thickening of the mucosal lining is seen. CT changes do not correlate well with nasal symptoms, but do relate to eosinophil counts in blood and sputum and to pulmonary function in accompanying asthma. (CT scans courtesy of Mr. Ian Mackay.)

Mucus Clearance Defects

The nose and paranasal sinuses are lined with ciliated epithelium, which in a coordinated fashion moves a mucus blanket toward the nasopharynx. This mucus is important for the entrapment and removal of particulate material and toxic substances, which include bacteria and allergens. The integrity of the mucociliary clearance pathway is vital to the appropriate drainage and ventilation of the paranasal sinuses and the nose (see Figure 28.3). Primary ciliary dyskinesia is inherited as an autosomal recessive trait and is characterized by the presence of sinusitis, bronchiectasis, situs inversus (Kartagener's syndrome, present in 50% of these patients), and male infertility that results from dyskinetic sperm. Various ciliary structural defects have been described (e.g., absence of inner or outer dynein arms or both), but some cilia appear normal (Young's syndrome). Recent work suggests that deficiency of iNOS (inducible nitric oxide synthase) may be the common underlying abnormality. Presentation is with chronic sinusitis, bronchiectasis or bronchitis, and obstructive azoospermia.

Secondary ciliary defects may arise after viral or bacterial infections; a number of mechanisms are involved:

- Mucous membranes become swollen and inflamed, which may result in blockage of the sinus ostia and thus prevent clearance (this is particularly critical at the ostiomeatal complex)
- If viruses or bacteria damage the epithelial cell layer, the integrity of cilial clearance is destroyed
- Some bacteria produce toxins that inhibit cilial clearance mechanisms
- Mucus during infection becomes thick and difficult to clear

GRANULOMAS/VASCULITIS

A number of granulomatous diseases may involve the nose and sinuses as part of the generalized disease, or nasal symptoms may be the first manifestation. These include Wegener's granulomatosis, Churg-Strauss syndrome, and sarcoidosis, particularly in Afro-Caribbean individuals. Mucous membrane infiltration and thickening with granulomas may be present, and may

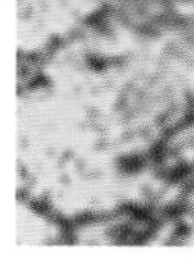

involve the septum, inferior turbinates, and occasionally the sinuses. Nasal congestion is a prominent symptom, sometimes with epistaxis and marked crusting. Sufferers feel unwell, with fatigue and malaise. Infective granulomatous disease may involve the nose and sinuses; examples are tuberculosis, leprosy, syphilis, blastomycosis, histoplasmosis, and aspergillosis.

NASAL POLYPS

Nasal polyps (Figure 28.4) result from prolapse of the mucous membrane that lines the nose and present as pale, grapelike protuberances arising predominantly from the middle meatus. They are insensitive to pain, but produce symptoms of nasal blockage and loss of sense of smell, and may be associated with aspirin hypersensitivity and asthma. Nasal polyps may also be related to infection and are common in patients who have cystic fibrosis. Nasal polyps are rare in children, but when they do occur are often associated with cystic fibrosis. Classification of nasal polyps is similar to that of rhinitis (Table 28.5).

OCCUPATIONAL RHINITIS

Occupational rhinitis can be allergic or nonallergic, with the former nearly always preceding occupational asthma.

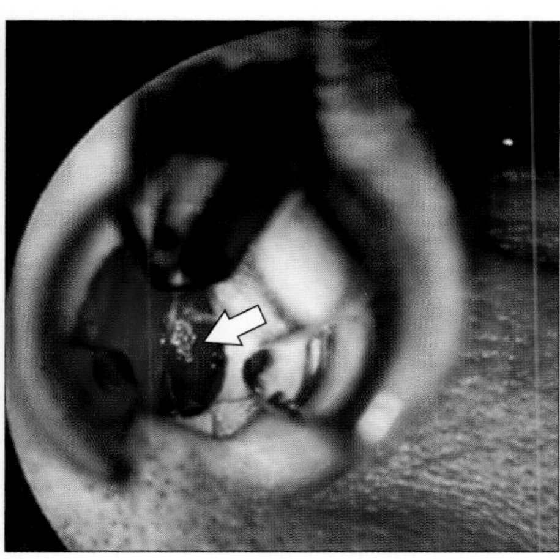

Figure 28.4 Speculum examination of nostril shows a pale watery polyp (arrow). Polyps are insensate and grayish, unlike turbinates that are sensitive and bluish-pink. (Courtesy of St. Mary's Hospital Audio-Visual Department.)

Table 28.5
Classification of nasal polyps

Allergic	Eosinophil rich Skin prick tests may be negative Allergic fungal Sinusitis Aspirin sensitive Churg-Strauss
Infective	Neutrophil-rich Cystic fibrosis Immune deficiency
Structural	Antrochoanal
Other	Malignancy

CLINICAL FEATURES

Allergy

ALLERGIC RHINITIS

This presents in two forms:

1. Runners/sneezers
2. Itchers

Symptoms tend to be intermittent and changeable, and are often closely related to allergen exposure during the day. Severity varies from trivial to extremely disabling. In addition, itching and injection of the conjunctivae may occur, with watery discharge and conjunctival swelling, and itching in the mouth, oropharynx, and ears. This form of allergic rhinitis tends to be a disorder of children and young adults, and up to one-third have associated asthma.

Blockers

The nose is chronically obstructed, with little in the way of immediate allergic symptoms.

Facial ache, headache, nasal hyperreactivity, and loss of sense of smell may also be present. Examination of the nose reveals pale or bluish mucosa, which is boggy and swollen, and a watery discharge may be present. Examination of the nose is important to exclude the concomitant presence of polyps, septal deviation, prominent turbinates, and evidence of other systemic disease and tumors.

Nonallergic Rhinosinusitis

INFECTIONS

Acute Coryza (The Common Cold)

The prodrome normally consists of a feeling of dryness, itching, and heat in the nose, which may last for a few hours and is often followed by a dry, sore throat, sneezing, watery discharge, and constitutional symptoms of feverishness and malaise. This phase is followed in a day or so, as a result of secondary infection, with symptoms of nasal obstruction and mucopurulent discharge, feverishness, and malaise, which may continue until resolution after 5 to 10 days. Initially, the symptoms of allergic rhinitis and coryza may be difficult to distinguish.

Acute Sinusitis

Acute maxillary sinusitis is characterized by facial pain, localized to the cheek, but also in the frontal area or the teeth, that is made worse by stooping down or straining. The pain can be unilateral or bilateral, and tenderness may overlie the sinus. Acute frontoethmoidal sinusitis may cause pain around the eye and in the frontal region, with overlying tenderness and erythema of the skin. There is usually fever, and toxemia may occur. Differential diagnosis of facial pain is wide and includes dental disease and the numerous causes of headache. Recently, all the accepted clinical signs and symptoms noted here have been shown to be unreliable as diagnostic aids to acute sinusitis, with the combination of erythrocyte sedimentation rate (ESR) and C-reactive protein (CRP) giving the best guide.

Chronic sinusitis is frequently pain free and presents with a sensation of congestion, poor concentration, tiredness, and

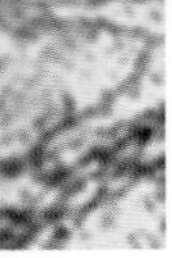

malaise. Other symptoms of chronic sinusitis include purulent nasal discharge (often postnasal), sore throat, and a productive cough, especially in children in whom misdiagnosis of asthma is not uncommon. Loss of smell and halitosis are additional features.

NONINFECTIVE RHINOSINUSITIS

Symptoms are similar to those of blockers, as mentioned previously. The differential diagnosis from allergic rhinitis depends upon skin prick or other allergy testing.

CLINICAL PRESENTATIONS THAT NEED PHYSICIAN REFERRAL

Unilateral symptoms, bloody discharge, polyps presenting for the first time, and systemically ill patients should be seen by a laryngologic surgeon. Orbital cellulitis demands urgent referral.

DIAGNOSIS, EVALUATION, AND TESTS

Examination

It is frequently possible to arrive at a diagnosis of rhinosinusitis based on a good detailed history. Physical examination should never be omitted and it is vitally important that chronic symptoms are appropriately investigated.

Observation of the patient's face may reveal an allergic crease or salute, a deviated nose, or more sinister collapse of the nasal bridge.

Anterior rhinoscopy with a bright light or head mirror using a Thudicum speculum allows simple examination of the anterior nasal cavity; also, the mucous membrane can be viewed and the presence of nasal polyps and disorders of the anterior part of the nasal septum can be seen.

Nasal endoscopy using either a rigid or fiberoptic flexible endoscope allows more detailed examination and assessment. Congenital defects, such as cleft palate and atresia, septal deviation and perforation, abnormalities of the turbinates, state of the mucous membranes, presence of purulent secretions, polyps, neoplasms, and foreign bodies can be determined.

DIAGNOSIS OF CORYZA

Coryza is normally diagnosed on the basis of a patient's history, and further investigations are rarely required. Viral culture or immunofluorescent techniques can identify specific viruses.

DIAGNOSIS OF ACUTE SINUSITIS

On examination, red, swollen nasal mucous membranes are present, and pus may be seen in the middle meatus. Endoscopy, together with imaging techniques, allows assessment of the severity and extent of involvement (diagnostic antral puncture and lavage are now rarely required). Middle meatal swabs provide material for bacteriologic culture. Immunoglobulin classes and subclasses are checked in cases of recurrent or chronic sinusitis.

Imaging Techniques

Radiography is rarely needed for diagnosis, unless a tumor is suspected. There is a high incidence of abnormalities in the general population: one third of unselected adults and 45% of children have abnormal scans. After a cold, computed tomography (CT) scans show changes for at least 6 weeks. The role of imaging is largely to provide a road map for the surgeon after failure of medical treatment.

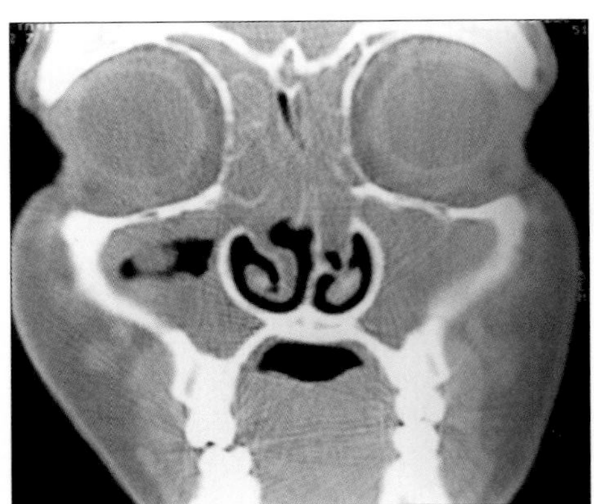

Figure 28.5 Coronal computed tomography scan of paranasal sinuses showing almost complete opacification of maxillary and ethmoid sinuses with polyps that obstruct the ostiomeatal complex. (Courtesy of Mr. Ian Mackay.)

Since the advent of computed tomography, plain sinus radiographs now have only a very limited role in acute rather than chronic sinusitis because opacification or a fluid level may be seen in a sinus or gross soft-tissue swelling may be evident. The imaging investigation of choice is CT, which is the best technique to demonstrate mucosal disease and underlying anatomic abnormalities (see Figure 28.3). The detailed anatomy of both bone and soft tissue is provided and axial and coronal sections can be obtained. The coronal cuts provide views of the ostiomeatal complex, important for planning surgery for acute and chronic sinusitis (Figure 28.5). Preoperatively, coronal sections at 3 to 4 mm give maximal anatomic detail, whereas axial views provide vital information regarding the relation of the optic nerve to the posterior ethmoidal and sphenoid sinuses. Magnetic resonance imaging is of very limited value, because bone is not well imaged. It is useful in distinguishing one soft tissue from another and has the advantage of avoiding irradiation.

Mucociliary Function Tests

SACCHARIN CLEARANCE

One quarter of a grain of saccharin is placed on the lateral nasal wall, 1 cm behind the anterior end of the inferior turbinate. A sweet taste is detected within 20 minutes if cilial function is normal—that is, the mucociliary mechanism is able to transport the particle to the nasopharynx and the pharynx, where taste is detected. If abnormal, more sophisticated tests of cilial activity using cells detached by brushings taken from the turbinate undertaken using phase contrast microscopy. Significant abnormalities on this test lead to electron microscopic examination of cilia.

Recent observations of very low nasal nitric oxide in primary ciliary dyskinesia and of lack of mucosal iNOS may simplify this process if confirmed.

Nasal Airway Tests

Dynamic tests include nasal inspiratory peak flow (using a mask attached to a peak flow meter, the patient sniffs hard with a closed mouth) and rhinomanometry. The technique is used to assess nasal airway resistance by measuring airflow across a pressure gradient with a pneumotachograph and face mask. Acoustic rhinometry uses a sound pulse to measure the nasal cross-sectional area.

Nasal resistance can change very dramatically within a few minutes. Congestion is produced by engorgement of venous erectile tissue within the nose; the mucous membrane receives dense, autonomic innovation. Nasal resistance falls with adrenaline and other sympathomimetic drugs, but also with exercise, rebreathing, and adoption of the erect posture. Nasal resistance increases in rhinitis and, in some individuals, with alcohol, aspirin, and other drugs, as well as when the supine posture is adopted.

Evaluation of Allergic Rhinitis

The diagnosis is usually obvious from a careful history and examination, but can easily be missed in chronic blockers; thus, skin prick tests should be performed in all rhinitis clinic patients. Skin tests using allergen extracts to elicit IgE-mediated immediate hypersensitivity responses can be used to confirm or exclude atopy. If all the skin tests are negative, it is unlikely that the rhinitis is allergic. However, positive tests do not confirm the diagnosis, because many asymptomatic individuals have positive skin tests to common allergens. Correlation between skin prick tests and history should be sought, because occasionally it is possible to identify an allergen that can be avoided. Measurement of total IgE is not helpful; however, measurement of specific IgE levels to common aeroallergens by means of radioallergosorbent testing may be useful and the results show a good correlation with skin test results. Very occasionally, particularly where occupational rhinitis may be a possibility, nasal challenge and provocation tests (with the offending allergen, histamine, aspirin, or methacholine) may be required.

Nasal Cytology

It may be of value to determine the presence or absence of eosinophils in patients who have perennial rhinitis, negative skin tests, and who are not atopic. A subset of these patients suffer nasal secretion eosinophilia, and are more likely to have allergic features such as sneezing and congestion; they may also respond to topical corticosteroids.

TREATMENT

Allergic Rhinitis

The basis of treatment for allergic rhinitis is:

1. Allergen avoidance
2. Pharmacotherapy
3. Immunotherapy
4. Rarely surgery
5. Patient education (vital)

IDENTIFY AND AVOID ALLERGENS

In practice, the identification and avoidance of allergens may be extremely difficult. House dust mites are responsible for much perennial allergic rhinitis. Mites flourish in temperatures around 15° C and 60% to 70% relative humidity, conditions present in many homes that contain central heating. They flourish particularly in soft furnishings, mattresses, pillows, and bed covers, as well as in carpets. Allergen avoidance and measures to reduce the load (i.e., wooden floors rather than carpets, regular vacuum cleaning, and barrier covers for mattresses and pillows) effectively reduce rhinitic symptoms. Acaricides that kill the mites do not eliminate the antigen, which is present in the fecal pellets. Removal of a pet may not remove symptoms because allergens may persist in rooms for many months, if not years. Avoidance of pollen is difficult, but vacationing or, failing that, staying indoors when the pollen count is high, closing windows, shutting car windows, and avoiding open grassy spaces, may help.

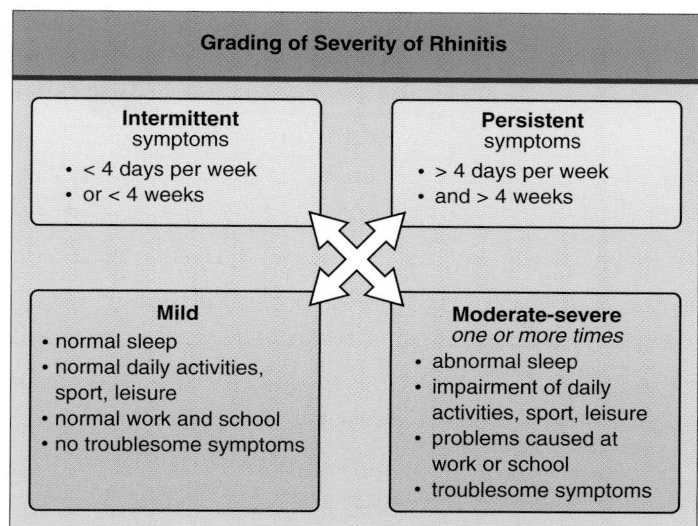

Figure 28.6 Division of rhinitis according to frequency and severity (taken from the Allergic Rhinitis and its Impact on Asthma guidelines).

MEDICAL SUPPRESSIVE THERAPY

The treatment plan for allergic rhinitis according to ARIA is shown in Figures 28.6 and 28.7.

Topical Corticosteroids

Meta-analysis has shown that these are the most effective treatment for allergic rhinitis. Regular use is needed and preseasonal dosing reduces development of seasonal rhinitis symptoms. For polyps or marked nasal blockage, betamethasone drops or oral corticosteroids for the first 2 weeks of therapy may be needed, followed by a nonabsorbed drop formulation, Flixonase nasules, in the long term for polyps. Side effects of topical corticosteroids include local irritation and minor epistaxis. Steroid absorption is low except for betamethasone and dexamethasone, which should be used only short term.

Sodium cromoglycate is less effective nasally, but may be suitable for small children, whereas severe conjunctival symptoms are best treated with sodium cromoglycate or nedocromil sodium. Corticosteroid eye drops are avoided.

Antihistamines

Antihistamines provide excellent relief of sneezing, itching, and rhinorrhea, but not congestion; oral ones have the advantage of being effective for mouth and eye symptoms. Chlorpheniramine is best avoided because it is sedating and reduces driving ability and academic performance. Newer H_1-antagonists are largely nonsedating. Certain molecules (terfenadine, astemizole, and diphenhydramine in particular) can produce QT prolongation and fatal cardiac arrhythmias, especially if blood levels are high because of overdosing or combining with other hepatically

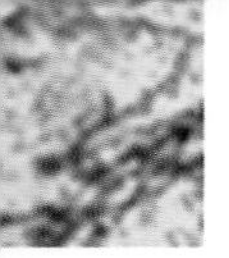

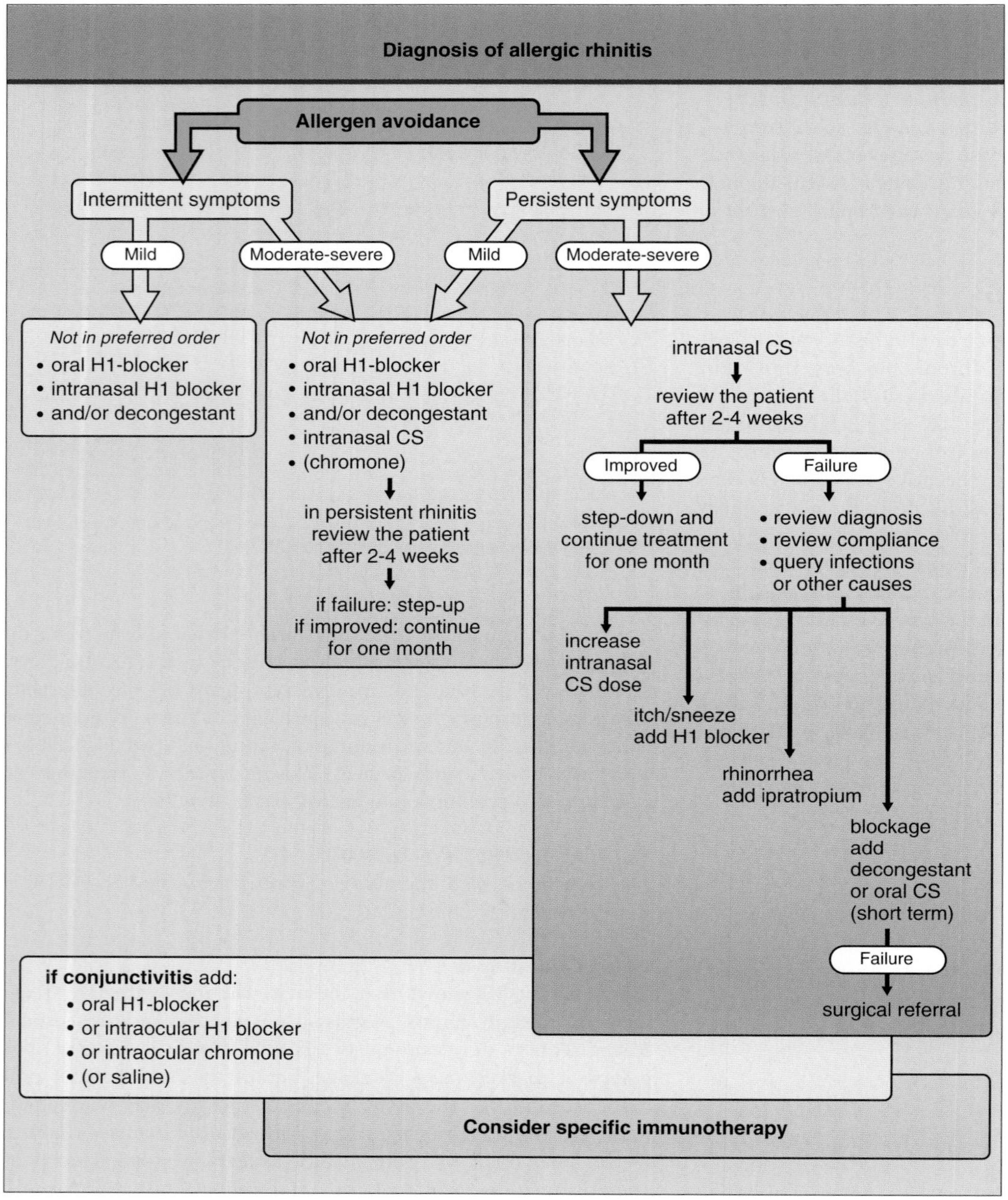

Figure 28.7 Rhinitis treatment based on the subdivision in Fig. 28.6 (taken from the Allergic Rhinitis and its Impact on Asthma guidelines).

metabolized drugs. Fexofenadine cetirizine, levocetirizine, and desloratadine appear safe in this respect. The latter two do have some measurable unblocking activity. Azelastine and levocabastine are useful topical antihistamines.

Other Agents

Vasoconstrictors are useful in the short term for marked congestion, but long-term use must be avoided because of the risk of rhinitis medicamentosa. Anticholinergics such as ipratropium bromide may be useful if extensive, watery secretion is a major problem.

Antileukotrienes are of similar efficacy to antihistamines in allergic rhinitis, with no major benefits from a combination of the two. However, in some polyp patients, they can reduce symptoms and polyp size when used with a topical steroid.

Douching the nose with isotonic saline can reduce symptoms of allergic rhinitis and improve endoscopic appearances and quality of life in chronic rhinosinusitis.

Immunotherapy

Desensitization involves the administration of increasing doses of relevant allergen extract by subcutaneous injection over a period of months and has been shown to effectively diminish symptoms of allergic seasonal rhinitis to grass pollen, ragweed, and birch pollen. Some studies also suggest efficacy to house dust mite and some animal danders. Desensitization has largely been superseded by the success of effective medical therapy in the suppression of allergic inflammation and so is reserved for nonresponders with severe disease. It is not always effective, and concerns have been raised regarding occasional anaphylactic reactions and deaths after the procedure, so it must be undertaken by well-trained individuals in a hospital setting with cardiorespiratory resuscitation facilities at hand. Safer sublingual approaches are being tried.

Surgical Intervention

Where medical treatment is only partially successful, a full otorhinolaryngologic assessment is performed because correction of a deviated nasal septum or reduction of hypertrophied mucosa may improve the symptoms. With coexistent chronic sinus infection, functional endoscopic sinus surgical techniques (FESS) may be necessary to facilitate sinus drainage, aeration, and access for medications.

Infections

CORYZA—THE COMMON COLD

Treatment is essentially symptomatic with analgesics, antipyretics, rest, and broad-spectrum antibiotics if secondary infection is present. Oral zinc may decrease symptoms and their duration.

ACUTE SINUSITIS

Most cases resolve spontaneously. Analgesics and antipyretics provide symptomatic relief, but aspirin must be avoided in those who may be hypersensitive. Acetaminophen (paracetamol) and codeine are satisfactory alternatives. Decongestants such as oxymetazoline and xylometazoline reduce edema and may improve sinus drainage. Broad-spectrum antibiotics are appropriate, but must have activity against the most common pathogens, namely *S. pneumoniae*, *H. influenzae*, and *M. catarrhalis*. Amoxicillin, trimethoprim-sulfamethoxazole (co-trimoxazole), or a macrolide such as clarithromycin are appropriate. Amoxicillin-clavulanate has the added advantage of activity against *S. aureus* and penicillin-resistant *H. influenzae*. If anaerobic infection is suspected, a combination of amoxicillin-clavulanate and metronidazole or clindamycin is appropriate.

CHRONIC SINUSITIS

The aims of treatment are to identify any underlying cause (e.g., immunologic defect, anatomic abnormality that prevents drainage) and to restore the integrity of the mucous membranes to allow normal ventilation of the sinuses and drainage (see Figure 28.3). Because chronic sinusitis frequently follows acute sinusitis, the same measures apply—namely analgesics and antipyretics, antibiotics, and decongestants. Topical corticosteroids may help to reduce mucous membrane swelling and improve drainage. Initially, betamethasone drops taken in the head-down position are used.

SURGICAL INTERVENTIONS FOR ACUTE AND CHRONIC SINUSITIS

Major changes have occurred in recent years as a result of the advent of high-resolution CT scans and FESS. Better demonstration of the nasal and sinus anatomy is achieved with CT scans, as well as of the important ostiomeatal complex, the vital region where sinus drainage by mucociliary clearance occurs. Obstruction in this zone is very important in the generation of chronic sinus disease. The main aim of FESS is to restore adequate drainage for the frontal, maxillary, and ethmoidal sinuses (see Figure 28.3). Where this fails, more radical sinus surgery may be needed, but complete investigation for underlying medical factors (e.g., immune deficiency) should be undertaken first.

Noninfectious Causes

INTRINSIC RHINITIS

Anticholinergics (ipratropium bromide) are useful for troublesome rhinorrhea, particularly when eosinophils are absent from nasal secretions. When eosinophilia is present, a response to topical corticosteroid therapy is usual. α-Agonist decongestants, such as pseudoephedrine and xylometazoline, are used sparingly. Surgical procedures may help if nasal obstruction is predominant.

STRUCTURAL DEFECTS

Occasionally topical corticosteroid therapy may ameliorate structural defects, but normally surgical correction is required.

IMMUNE DEFECTS

Therapy of immune defects is directed toward correction of the immunologic defect.

MUCUS CLEARANCE DEFECT

It is not possible to correct the underlying mucus clearance defect, so therapy relies on regular douching, improved drainage and aeration, and prevention of secondary infection.

GRANULOMAS

Appropriate, specific antimicrobial therapy is required for infectious causes of granulomatous disease. Sarcoidosis that involves the nose responds to either local or systemic glucocorticoid therapy.

DRUG-INDUCED DISEASE

A careful drug history must be taken and the incriminated drug excluded.

NASAL POLYPS

Where there are no contraindications and no suspicions about the nature of the polyp a medical polypectomy using prednisolone (0.5 mg/kg, enteric-coated) plus betamethasone drops (two in each nostril three times a day with the head upside down) for 5 days can prove as effective as surgery and is superior with respect to improvements in concomitant asthma. This should be followed by long-term corticosteroid drops—initially betamethasone for 2 weeks, then nonabsorbed fluticasone. Subsequently, a trial of a leukotriene receptor antagonist should be undertaken for 2 to 4 weeks, with continuation if beneficial. Other measures being evaluated include regular saline or antifungal douching and topical aspirin. Failure of medical treatment is an indication for surgery. Unilateral nasal polyps must be referred to exclude transitional cell papilloma, squamous cell carcinoma, encephalocele, or other sinister pathology.

CLINICAL COURSE AND PREVENTION

Allergic Rhinosinusitis

The clinical course is variable. With good compliance with allergen avoidance and regular pharmacotherapy, symptoms are usually minimal. Understandably, patients want a cure.

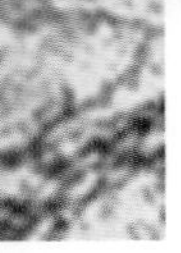

Immunotherapy remains of limited value, but with development in understanding of the mechanism of generation of IgE responses and of ways in which this can be modulated, may become more useful.

Infections

CORYZA—THE COMMON COLD

Unfortunately, avoidance of the common cold is virtually impossible and prevention by immunization has so far been a failure. However, colds are self-limiting, and normally last about 5 days. Complications include acute sinusitis, pharyngitis, otitis media, mastoiditis, and tonsillitis. The common cold frequently leads to lower respiratory infection, including laryngotracheitis, bronchitis, and occasionally pneumonia. Patients who have asthma in particular, but also those who suffer other cardiorespiratory diseases, may experience exacerbations.

ACUTE BACTERIAL SINUSITIS

Before the antibiotic era, acute sinusitis had a significant morbidity and mortality because of spread of bacterial sepsis beyond the sinuses. Osteolysis of the sinus wall occurred often, with abscess formation and direct spread to neighboring structures, in addition to local spread and thrombophlebitis. These local complications include orbital cellulitis with or without abscess formation, cavernous sinus thrombosis, sagittal sinus thrombosis, intracranial abscess, meningitis and encephalitis, osteomyelitis, and septicemia.

Complications are now rarely seen as most patients are prescribed broad-spectrum antibiotics.

INTRINSIC RHINITIS

Intrinsic rhinitis often has an onset in middle age or later and is often refractory to treatment. Combinations of therapy may prove helpful.

PITFALLS AND CONTROVERSIES

Points to consider in patients with rhinitis and sinusitis:

- Not all patients who have nasal symptoms have allergic rhinitis—neoplasm or foreign body could be present
- Unilateral discharge in children is probably a foreign body, but in adults it may be carcinoma
- Nasal decongestants must be used sparingly, if at all
- Most medical treatment failures result from poor compliance—once daily treatment is best, if possible
- Common cold, a cause of widespread morbidity, remains a major research challenge
- Intrinsic rhinitis can be troublesome to treat and further research is required
- Turbinates and polyps are difficult to distinguish—turbinates are rigid and pain-sensitive, polyps are mobile and insensitive to pain
- Unilateral lesions must be biopsied to exclude malignancy
- Facial pain in the absence of nasal symptoms is rarely caused by sinus disease, so other causes such as migraine, dental problems, and temporomandibular joint syndrome are considered
- Chronic refractory sinusitis stimulates investigation for underlying immune or other defects
- CT scan is the investigation of choice—plain radiographs or magnetic resonance imaging has a limited role.

SUGGESTED READINGS

Bousquet J, van Cauwenberge P, Khaltaev N: The ARIA Workshop Panel—Allergic rhinitis and its impact on asthma. J Allergy Clin Immunol 108(suppl):5147-5276, 2001.

Corrigan C: Immunotherapy in Allergy—The Way Forward. Clinical Focus 5. London: Rila Publications Ltd, 2002, pp 10-12.

Holgate S, Canonica W, Simons FE, et al: Consensus group on new-generation antihistamines (CONGA). Clin Exp Allergy 33:1305-1324, 2003.

Scadding GK: Non-allergic rhinitis: Diagnosis and management. Curr Opin Allergy Clin Immunol 1:15-20, 2001.

Scadding GK: Comparison of medical and surgical treatment of nasal polyposis. Curr Allergy Asthma Rep 2:494-499, 2002.

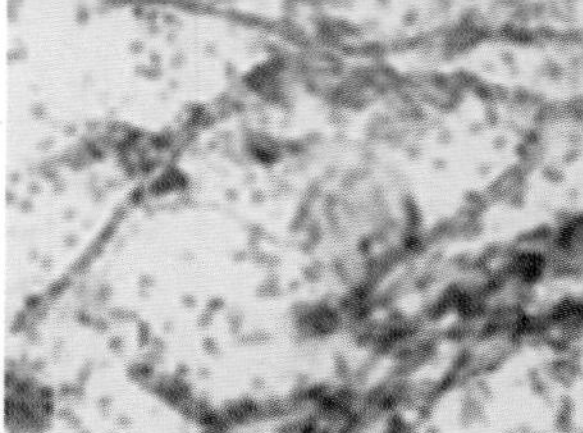

CHAPTER 29 **Bronchiectasis**

Alan F. Barker

DEFINITION

Bronchiectasis is a chronic respiratory disease involving repeated infection and inflammation of large and small airways. Based on careful examination of surgically resected or postmortem pathologic lung specimens and bronchography (contrast imaging of the airways), bronchiectasis has been defined as permanent dilatation of bronchi. Surgery is performed infrequently for this disease and bronchography has been replaced by chest computed tomography (CT) scanning. A modern clinical definition would include the daily production of mucopurulent phlegm and chest imaging that demonstrates dilated and thickened airways.

EPIDEMIOLOGY

There are no reliable estimates of the frequency of the disease. Susceptible populations include those with relatively poor access to health care and delayed treatment of respiratory infections. An increased prevalence has been reported in Native Americans from remote areas of Alaska, Maori in New Zealand, and from Nigeria and perhaps other sub-Saharan areas of Africa.

ETIOLOGY AND RISK FACTORS

Although 50% of individuals with bronchiectasis have no proven etiology, there are broad and specific categories of associations that merit attention (Table 29.1). Several of these associations warrant closer scrutiny.

Individuals with humoral immunodeficiencies of immunoglobulin IgG, IgM, and IgA are at risk for suppurative sinopulmonary infections, including recurrent sinusitis and bronchiectasis. Immunoglobulin replacement reduces the frequency of acute infectious exacerbations and probably reduces airway mucosal damage. Selective IgG subclass deficiency may also contribute to bronchiectasis.

The respiratory complications (bronchiectasis) of cystic fibrosis may not become apparent until adulthood or there be minimal pancreatic insufficiency. The clinical paradigm is sputum cultures growing *Pseudomonas aeruginosa* or *Staphylococcus aureus* and upper lobe infiltration on chest radiograph. Confirmatory testing includes sweat chloride levels above 50 to 60 mmol. Mutations of the cystic fibrosis transmembrane conductance regulator (delta F508) are most common but other mutations have been identified (See Chapter 40, Cystic Fibrosis).

Primary ciliary dyskinesia (PCD) is a condition in which poorly functioning cilia contribute to reduced clearance of airway secretions, foreign particles, and bacteria, leading to recurrent infections and bronchiectasis. Approximately one half of patients with PCD have classic Kartagener syndrome (bronchiectasis, sinusitis, situs inversus). The most common ciliary defect is an absence or shortening of the outer (dynein) arms that are responsible for propelling or moving mucus out of the respiratory tract (Figure 29.1).

Regarding infectious contributions and their sequelae, whooping cough and measles have been reduced, if not eliminated, in most parts of the world. Endemic tuberculosis is reduced and effectively treated in most developed nations. Primary *Mycobacterium avium* complex can cause an indolent respiratory syndrome in immunocompetent individuals. White women more than age 50 or 60 years are particularly recognized with unrelenting cough. The middle lobe or lingula on chest imaging shows changes of bronchiectasis. A major component of allergic bronchopulmonary aspergillosis is bronchiectasis. Individuals with asthma may have cough productive of mucus plugs. The aspergillus organism causes both allergic and perhaps infectious airway damage. Recognition of allergic bronchopulmonary aspergillosis (ABPA) in asthmatics will allow therapy with systemic steroids and antifungals to reduce the inflammatory and fungal load.

PATHOGENESIS

The induction of bronchiectasis requires an infectious insult, airway obstruction, or a defect in host defense. Some specific infectious insults were discussed in the previous paragraph. Episodes of acute bronchitis with bacterial pathogens such as *Pseudomonas* spp will perpetuate and worsen mucosal injury. This tissue injury is mediated by neutrophilic cellular infiltration and both host and organism inflammatory mediators including proteases, reactive oxygen intermediates, and cytokines such as interleukin-8. An impairment in host defense may be local as with ciliary dyskinesia or systemic with hypogammaglobulinemia or acquired immunodeficiency syndrome. Airway obstruction can be caused by a foreign body aspiration such as popcorn or a peanut in children or food particulate, crown, or fragmented tooth in an adult. Inebriation or altered mental status secondary to a stroke may delay recognition of the initial aspiration event. An intraluminal (partially) obstructing tumor such as carcinoid or fibroma (Figure 29.2) or extrinsic compression of an airway (enlarged lymph node) may interfere with proper drainage and lead to recurrent infections and bronchiectasis.

CLINICAL FEATURES

Daily cough and mucopurulent sputum production are cardinal features of almost every patient. More than half of affected patients will exhibit chronic and intermittent dyspnea, pleuritic

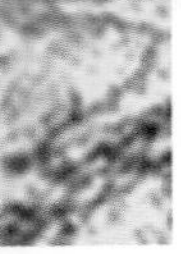

Table 29.1
Conditions associated with bronchiectasis

Focal bronchiectasis	Foreign body aspiration
	Benign tumors (fibroma, lipoma)
	Lymph node encroachment (middle lobe syndrome)
Diffuse bronchiectasis	**Post-infectious**
	Bacteria (pertussis)
	Virus (adenovirus, measles, human immunodeficiency)
	Fungi (*Aspergillus fumigatus, Coccidoides imitis, Histoplasma capsulatum*)
	Mycobacterium tuberculosis or *avium complex*
	Immunodeficiency
	Primary humoral (hypogammaglobulinemia)
	Secondary (CLL)
	Congenital
	Primary ciliary dyskinesia
	Alpha-one antitrypsin deficiency
	Cystic fibrosis
	Cartilage deficiency (Williams-Campbell syndrome)
	Tracheobronchomegaly (Mounier-Kuhn syndrome)
	Marfan syndrome
	Rheumatic and other
	Rheumatoid arthritis
	Inflammatory bowel disease

chest pain, and hemoptysis. The hemoptysis can vary from blood streaking to massive volume (greater than 300 mL in a day) during an acute exacerbation because of erosion of a mucosal neovascular arteriole. Physical findings noted on chest auscultation include crackles and rhonchi. Airway obstruction can produce wheezes that mimic findings in asthma. Layering of sputum in a container has distinctive features that yield a clue to the diagnosis (Figure 29.3). The older literature described a frequent finding of digital clubbing, but that probably occurs in fewer than 5% of patients currently seen. Pulmonary function tests provide a guide to impairment. Spirometry shows a normal or reduced FVC, reduced forced expiratory volume in 1 second (FEV_1), and reduced FEV_1/FVC consistent with obstructive impairment. Many patients will have an improved FEV_1 or FVC after aerosol bronchodilator.

Key confirmatory testing includes chest imaging. The chest X-ray is abnormal in most patients with bronchiectasis. Suspicious findings include linear atelectasis, dilated and thickened airways noted as ring shadows on cross section, and tram or parallel lines when seen in a longitudinal plane (Figure 29.4). Old granulomatous disease and cystic fibrosis have an upper lobe predominance of findings. A central distribution is typical of ABPA, and a middle lobe or lingular lobe distribution suggests *Mycobacterium avium* complex infection (MAC) as the genesis. Most other associations and idiopathic bronchiectasis present a lower lobe distribution of radiographic findings.

The high-resolution chest CT (HRCT) has become the defining tool, if not the gold standard, for confirmation of the diagnosis of bronchiectasis. Noncontrast studies are adequate with 1.0 to 1.5 mm sections and images obtained every 1 cm using a high spatial algorithm. The major HRCT findings are shown in Table 29.2 and Figure 29.5 and illustrated in the accompanying HRCTs. Confounding diagnoses occur when some of these radiographic findings are seen in other diseases. During an acute pneumonia and the resolution phase, airways may be seen as dilated and even thickened. Those findings would resolve. Individuals with asthma and even chronic bronchitis may have dilated areas and inspissated secretions that could be interpreted as bronchiectasis. Other diseases associated with parenchymal destruction can distort airways that mimic bronchiectasis. In pulmonary fibrosis, parenchymal scars contract and pull airways open leading to so-called traction bronchiectasis. In emphysema, small bullae may simulate the dilated airways of bronchiectasis but the walls are thin and often not complete.

The HRCT is complementary when the diagnosis is in doubt, location of changes may give a clue to an underlying association, bleeding needs to be localized, or a map is needed when surgical resection is considered.

DIAGNOSIS

Symptoms and sometimes chest findings will usually suggest the diagnosis. Chest imaging is always required to confirm the diagnosis. Sinus CT will be helpful and usually abnormal when there are upper respiratory complaints or host defenses are impaired affecting the whole respiratory system such as ciliary dyskinesia, humoral immunodeficiency, or cystic fibrosis. A complete blood count will not show specific changes, but eosinophilia may point to ABPA. IgG, IgM, and IgA quantitation should be performed because of therapeutic implications. Other blood tests such as rheumatoid factor, α-one-antitrypsin level, and precipitins for aspergillus are guided by clinical suspicion. Performance of sweat chloride iontophoresis will also depend on a suspicion of cystic fibrosis. Bronchoscopy is warranted when focal obstruction from a foreign body or tumor is suspected. Confirmation of ciliary dyskinesia requires a respiratory tract biopsy of the nasal mucosa or lower airway with examination of cilia by electron microscopy. Bacterial sputum cultures are not routinely helpful, but can point to a single or potentially resistant pathogen such as *Moraxella* or *Pseudomonas* spp. Cultures for fungus and mycobacteria can highlight problematic pathogens.

TREATMENT

Treatment of bronchiectasis includes seven principles:

1. Provide antibiotic therapy of acute exacerbations
2. Prevent acute exacerbations by reducing the burden of microbial pathogens with antibiotics
3. Treat resistant or problematic pathogens
4. Reduce inflammation with anti-inflammatory agents
5. Enhance secretion removal with bronchial hygiene
6. Surgically remove affected parts of the lung
7. Control hemoptysis

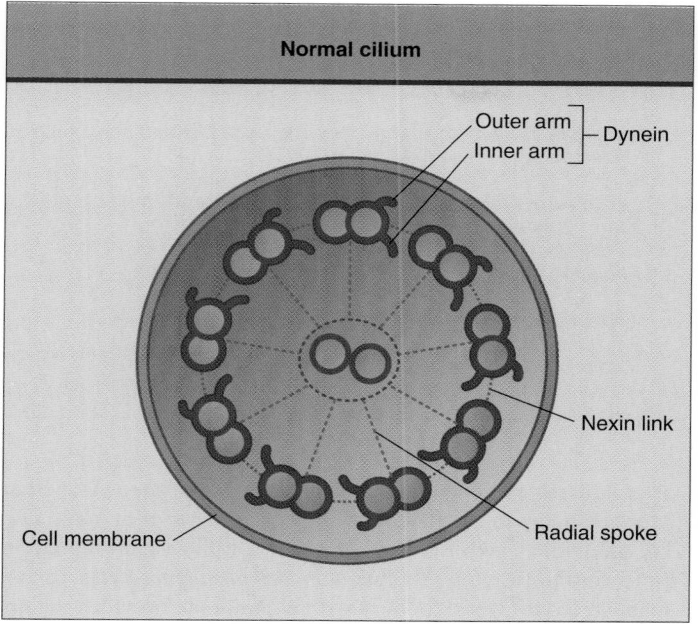

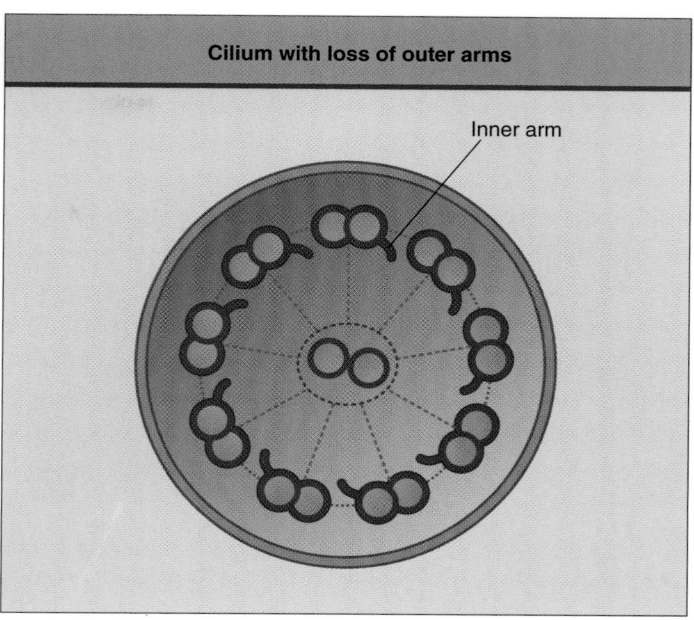

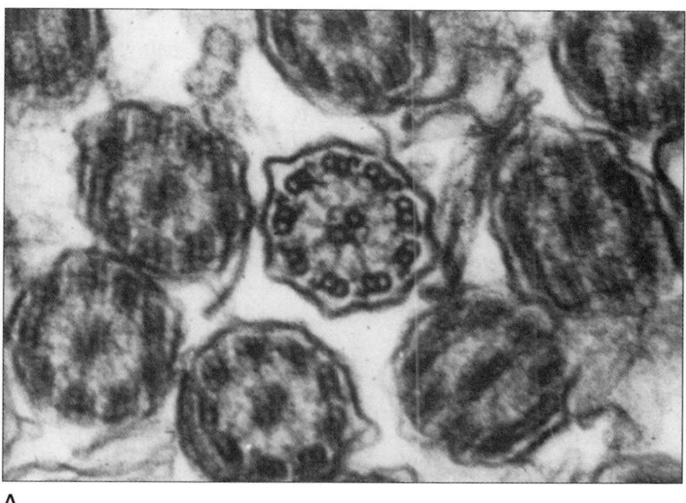
A

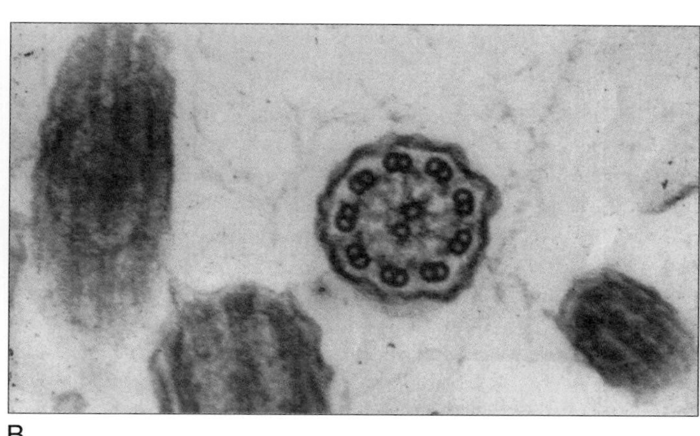
B

Figure 29.1 A. Electron micrograph of normal cilia and a stylized diagram noting inner and outer dynein arms. **B.** Electron micrograph of cilia of patient with the most common dyskinetic abnormality. The diagram illustrates the presence of inner arms and lack of outer arms.

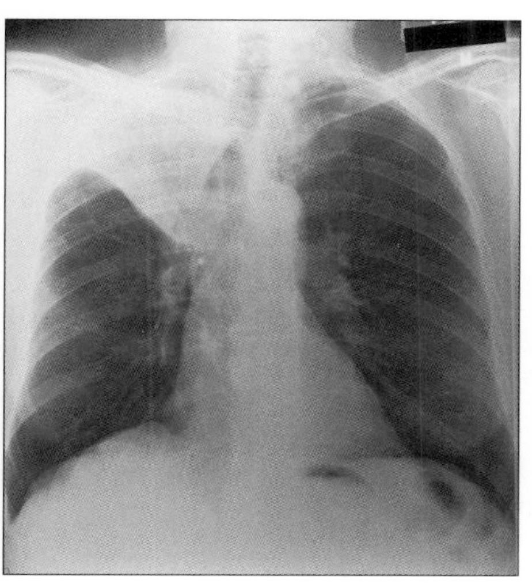

Figure 29.2 Chest radiograph of patient with lobar infiltrate and consolidation due to obstructing tumor.

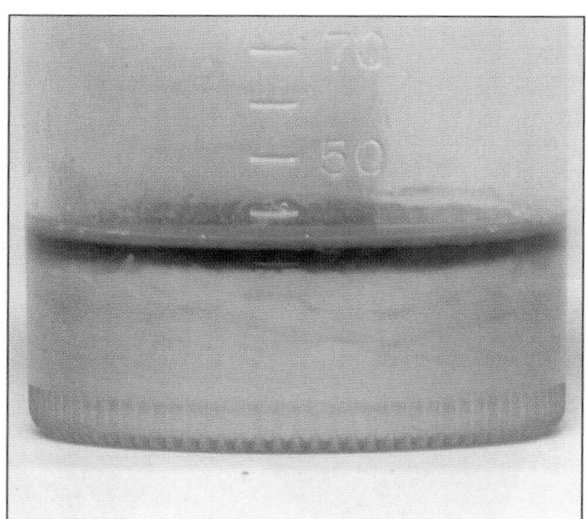

Figure 29.3 Sputum (in a cup) from a patient with bronchiectasis. The heavier cells, pigments, and debris sink to the bottom; there is a clear watery middle layer; airway mucus will foam or layer at the top.

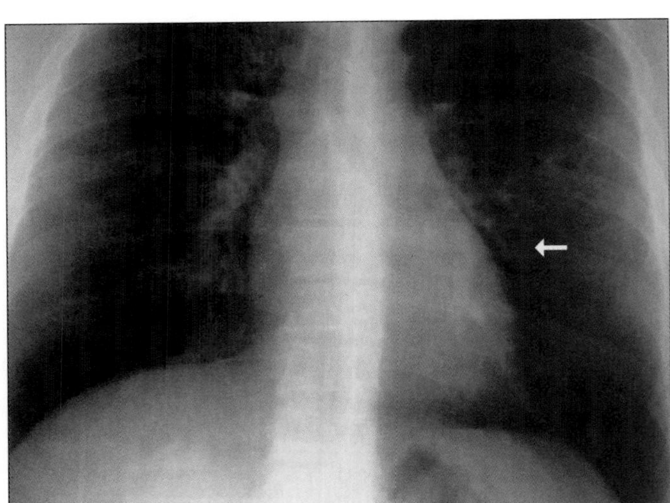

Figure 29.4 Chest radiograph of patient with bronchiectasis. Arrow points to dilated airways that appear as tram lines. In left mid-chest are other areas of dilated airways in cross section.

Table 29.2
High-resolution chest computed tomography findings in bronchiectasis

Failure of airways to taper as they approach the periphery of the chest (an early finding)
Dilated airways. An airway is dilated if the inner diameter is greater than 1.5 times the nearby vessel
Bronchial wall thickening; seen in the dilated airways
Distal mucous plugging; often seen as "tree-in-bud"
Dilated airways may cluster like grapes

ANTIBIOTIC THERAPY OF ACUTE EXACERBATIONS

Because cough and phlegm production are present most days for individuals with bronchiectasis, deciding when an acute exacerbation occurs is problematic. Reliance on respiratory symptom changes is useful. The sputum often increases in amount (although may be harder to expectorate), becomes more tenacious, and is darker in color. Hemoptysis may be an accompanying complaint. Other features include worsening dyspnea and pleuritic chest pain. Fatigue is usually present but fever and chills are lacking. Leukocytosis and new chest radiographic findings do not occur or are minimal.

The genesis of acute exacerbations must be suspected bacterial bronchitis. There is no evidence that viruses or atypical bacteria (e.g., *Mycoplasma* spp) play a role. Prompt antibacterial therapy is warranted. For ambulatory patients, choosing an antibiotic involves an educated guess unless recent sputum culture data are available. For individuals with no or few recent exacerbations, the colonizing flora can be presumed similar to individuals with chronic bronchitis. Coverage against *Streptococcus pneumoniae*, *Haemophilus influenzae*, and perhaps *Moraxella* spp is satisfactory. Choices are shown in Table 29.3. For individuals with longer duration of illness or failed previous antibiotic courses, *Pseudomonas aeruginosa* has to be a suspected pathogen. Therapy with a quinolone provides the only effective oral regimen. A choice would be ciprofloxacin 500 to 750 mg twice daily. Other quinolones such as levofloxacin 500 mg daily, moxifloxacin 400 mg daily, or gatifloxacin 400 mg daily may be reasonable alternatives. The duration of therapy is a minimum of 7 days but 10 to 14 days may be necessary when an initial antibiotic course fails. In any individual who fails a first course of antibiotics, sputum culture and sensitivity provide information to make an informed decision about subsequent therapy. Decisions about need for hospitalization involve systemic findings including hemodynamic or respiratory compromise, comorbid disease, or presence of a highly resistant organism that requires initiation of parenteral antibiotics.

PREVENTION OF ACUTE EXACERBATIONS AND REDUCTION OF BACTERIAL BURDEN

The strategy of reducing the bacterial load makes sense in patients with bronchiectasis but is not proven. There are several strategies that have been reported in small numbers of patients but have not shown efficacy based on clinical trials. The easiest strategy for patient administration involves an oral antibiotic

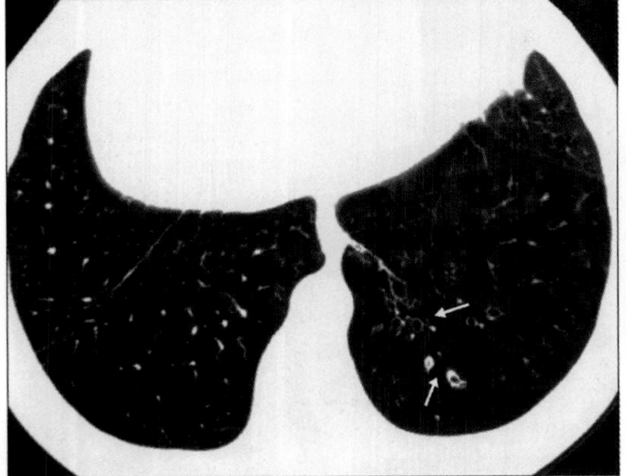

A

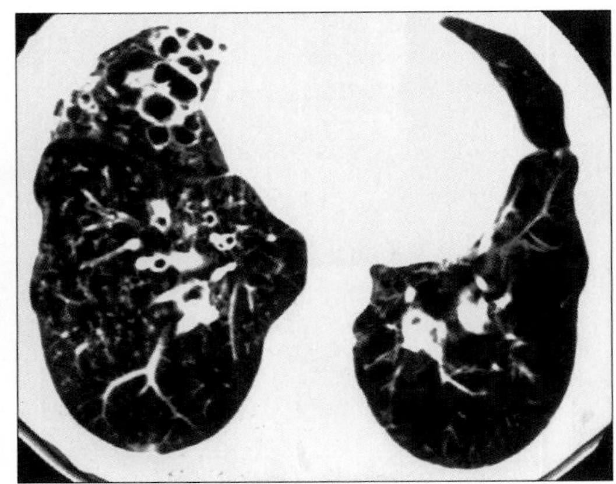

B

Figure 29.5 A. High-resolution chest computed tomography (HRCT) of patient with bronchiectasis. Upper arrow shows six or more very dilated airways. Lower arrow shows both dilated and thickened airways. **B.** HRCT of a patient with advanced bronchiectasis. There are multiple areas of dilated and thickened airways and peripheral small airways filled with mucus ("tree-in bud"). At the top on the right are hugely dilated cystic areas (grapelike clusters).

Table 29.3
Oral antibiotics for acute exacerbations of bronchiectasis

Category	Agents	Organisms
Penicillins	Amoxicillin 500mg, q8h Amoxicillin-clavulanate 875mg, q12h	*S. pneumoniae, H. influenzae* *S. pneumoniae, H. influenzae* *M. catarrhalis*
Cephalosporins	Cefaclor 500mg, q8h or Cefuroxime 500mg, q12h	*S. pneumoniae, H. influenzae* *M. catarrhalis* same
Macrolides	Azithromycin 500mg 1st day, then 250mg daily or Clarithromycin 500mg, q12h	
Quinolones	Ciprofloxacin 500-700mg, BID or Levofloxacin 500mg, qd or Moxifloxacin 400mg, qd or Gatifloxacin 400mg, qd	*P. aeruginosa* *S. pneumoniae, H. influenzae*
Other	Trimethoprim-sulfa 160-180mg, BID	*S. maltophilia*

Table 29.4
Prevention strategies for bronchiectasis

Strategy	Example
Intermittent or daily oral antibiotic	Ciprofloxacin 500-700mg, BID or Erythromycin 500mg, BID
High dose oral	Amoxicillin 3gm, sache qd*
Aerosol antibiotic (alternate months)	Tobramycin 300mg, BID* Colistin 150mg, BID*
Intermittent IV antibiotics (10-21 days)	Depends on bacterial flora in sputum

*Not approved USA

on an intermittent basis. Table 29.4 lists several such strategies.

TREATMENT OF RESISTANT OR PROBLEMATIC PATHOGENS

Expectorated (sometimes induced) sputum cultures or cultures obtained at bronchoscopy and lavage will be required to identify resistant pathogens. *Pseudomonas aeruginosa* is almost impossible to eradicate from patients with bronchiectasis. Strategies for suppression are noted in the previous paragraph. Treatment of ABPA includes augmentation or introduction of systemic steroids. Itraconazole 400 mg daily may reduce the burden of aspergillus but is less effective in individuals with bronchiectasis. Decisions about the diagnosis and therapy of *Mycobacterium avium* complex (MAC) are discussed in a statement of the American Thoracic Society. Therapy with a macrolide, rifampin or rifabutin, and ethambutol is required for many months.

TREATMENT WITH ANTI-INFLAMMATORY AGENTS

The neutrophilic influx into airways accompanying infection is presumed to be injurious and destructive. Systemic steroids at the time of an acute exacerbation (particularly with respiratory compromise) is a reasonable approach but has not been tested in a clinical trial. Short clinical trials have demonstrated utility of aerosol steroids to reduce inflammatory mediators and symptoms. Two agents that have been studied include beclomethasone and fluticasone. Nonsteroidal anti-inflammatory agents such as indomethacin (oral and aerosol) have been shown to reduce inflammatory mediators in bronchiectasis, but there are no clinical trials of efficacy.

ENHANCE SECRETION REMOVAL WITH BRONCHIAL HYGIENE

Because viscous secretions are part of the disease process, attention to bronchial hygiene is important. Strategies include hydration (systemic and airway), mucolytic agent administration, chest physiotherapy, and bronchodilator administration.

Oral liquids will usually maintain airway hydration, but nebulization of saline solutions will also reduce viscosity of tenacious secretions. Acetyl cysteine administered as a 20% solution by nebulizer is an effective mucolytic agent with its role

mainly confined to patients in whom saline nebulization is not effective. Acetyl cysteine may provoke bronchospasm and a bronchodilator can be delivered as adjunctive therapy. Recombinant DNAse is not effective in bronchiectasis. Osmotic- or ion-modifying agents such as hypertonic saline, mannitol, dextran, and uridine-5′-triphosphate improve some parameters, such as radiolabeled particulate clearance, but clinical trials are needed to show efficacy.

Chest physiotherapy involves a variety of mechanical measures to loosen tenacious secretions and enhance their removal from the airways. Chest clapping is effective for some individuals, but is time-intensive and requires an assistant. Mechanical percussors or vibrating vests applied to the chest, positive expiratory pressure valves, or flutter devices producing oscillatory positive airway pressures are modern approaches that are sometimes more comfortable and can be used or applied without an assistant. Postural chest drainage requires an individual to lie in multiple positions (to drain various affected lobes) on a bed, table, or couch and is often used in conjunction with chest clapping or mechanical percussors. Many patients find such positioning uncomfortable and time-intensive.

Response to bronchodilators, when tested in the pulmonary function laboratory, occurs in 30% to 50% of patients with bronchiectasis. Bronchodilators such as β-agonists or anticholinergics administered on an acute or chronic basis are probably effective, but a clinical trail has not been performed.

SURGICAL REMOVAL OF AFFECTED LUNG

The role of surgery has certainly declined over the past 3 to 4 decades. Because most individuals now have multiple affected areas of lung, total cure is not usually possible. There are several indications for which surgery should be considered: removal of a lobe or segment obstructed by a tumor or foreign body, reduction of an area of lung thought to be contributing to massive suppurative and tenacious secretions, removal of an airway subject to massive or recurrent hemorrhage, elimination of necrotic lung tissue thought to harbor resistant organisms such as MAC, multidrug resistant *Mycobacterium tuberculosis*, or aspergillus. Lung transplantation is now available for individuals with cystic fibrosis and some individuals with extensive bronchiectasis, but statistics on survival in non–cystic fibrosis bronchiectasis are not available.

CONTROL OF MASSIVE HEMORRHAGE

Hemoptysis in bronchiectasis can be blood-streaked or massive, causing respiratory compromise. Prompt identification of the location of hemorrhage with chest CT and bronchoscopy is warranted. Positioning of the patient in bed with affected side down and cough suppression may temporize the situation. Intubation with a divided endotracheal tube to protect the unaffected side is also a temporizing strategy. Definitive therapy includes aortography with bronchial or intercostal artery selective catheterization and potential embolization of a previously identified bleeding area or one with neovascularization. Thoracotomy and resection may be necessary when such efforts fail or proximal airways and vessels are involved.

CLINICAL COURSE

Although it is difficult to generalize about the course of patients with bronchiectasis, the number of acute exacerbations requiring antibiotics averages two to three per patient per year. The number of hospitalizations varies widely depending on severity of respiratory compromise, comorbid diseases, and practice patterns. In some locales hospitalization is necessary for intravenous antibiotics for most exacerbations. In other areas intravenous antibiotics can be administered in an ambulatory setting. Repeated exacerbations may lead to airway and parenchymal destruction, accelerated decline in pulmonary function, hypoxemia, and cor pulmonale. As noted previously, hemoptysis may be life-threatening. Concerning mortality, there are data from a hospital registry in Finland. Patients with bronchiectasis, asthma, and chronic obstructive pulmonary disease (COPD) were age matched (ages 35-74) and followed for 8 to 13 years. Twenty-eight percent of bronchiectasis patients, 20% of asthma patients, and 38% of COPD patients died. The underlying disease was the primary cause of death in the bronchiectasis and COPD patients. Cardiac disease was the primary cause of death in the asthma patients.

CONTROVERSIES

Bronchiectasis is an important but uncommon chronic respiratory disease using frequent medical resources. To facilitate diagnosis and help design clinical trials, a new disease definition needs agreement. The use of a combination of symptoms such as daily cough and purulent phlegm combined with chest CT imaging is probably the best direction, but no international consensus for any modern definition has been made. Treatment strategies are most often based on experiences at single institutions and referral centers. Their experiences may not reflect practice or disease conditions in a general pulmonary or even internal or family medicine practice. Virtually all treatment strategies have been adopted from practices and multicenter clinical trials in patients with cystic fibrosis. Because bronchiectasis is the main respiratory disease in cystic fibrosis, it would seem logical that cystic fibrosis treatment strategies should be effective in non–cystic fibrosis bronchiectasis. Such generalities are not always correct. Aerosolized DNAse is a proven effective mucolytic agent in cystic fibrosis. In the largest multi-center trial of a therapy in non–cystic fibrosis bronchiectasis, DNAse was found ineffective and may cause decline in pulmonary function.

SUGGESTED READINGS

Angrill J, Aguisti C, de Celis R, et al: Bacterial colonization in patients with bronchiectasis: Microbiologic pattern and risk factors. Thorax 57:15-19, 2002.

Barker AF: Medical progress: Bronchiectasis. N Engl J Med 346: 1383-1393, 2002.

Cohen M, Sahn SA: Bronchiectasis in systemic diseases. Chest 116:1063-1074, 1999.

Keistinen T, Saynajakangas O, Tuuponen T, et al: Bronchiectasis: an orphan disease with a poorly-understood prognosis. Eur Respir J 10:2784-2787, 1997.

O'Donnell AE, Barker AF, Ilowite JS, Fick RB: Treatment of idiopathic bronchiectasis with aerosolized recombinant Dnase I. Chest 113:1329-1334, 1998.

Pasteur MC, Helliwell SM, Houghton SJ, et al: An investigation into causative factors in patients with bronchiectasis. Am J Resp Crit Care Med 162:1277-1284, 2000.

Pryor JA: Physiotherapy for airway clearance in adults. Eur Respir J 14:1418-1424, 1999.

Wallace RJ Jr, Glassroth J, Griffith DE, et al: Diagnosis and treatment of disease caused by nontuberculous mycobacterial infection. Am J Resp Crit Care Med 156:S1-S25, 1997.

Webb WR, Muller NL, Naidich DP: Airway Diseases in High-Resolution CT of the Lung, 3rd ed. Philadelphia, Lippincott Williams and Wilkins, 2001, pp 467-546.

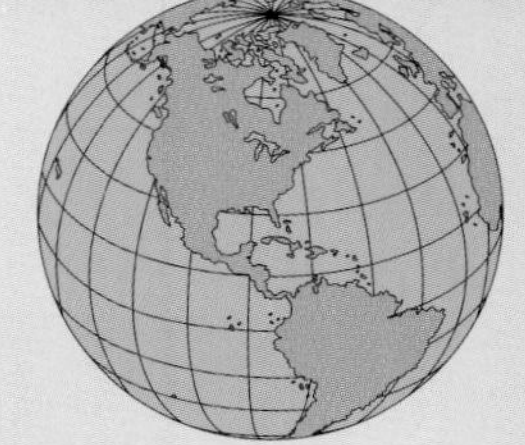

CHAPTER 30 Pulmonary Infections

Rob F. Miller and Marc C. I. Lipman

EPIDEMIOLOGY, RISK FACTORS, AND PATHOPHYSIOLOGY

Human Immunodeficiency Virus Infection—Background

It has been more than 20 years since the first reports of acquired immunodeficiency syndrome (AIDS). What are now regarded as common conditions, such as *Pneumocystis carinii* (now known as *Pneumocystis jiroveci*) pneumonia and Kaposi's sarcoma, were then almost unheard of. Initially confined largely to homosexual and bisexual men, it was soon apparent that the same clinical indicators of immunosuppression were present in injecting drug users, recipients of blood products, heterosexuals, and infants born to mothers with this illness. The isolation of human immunodeficiency virus (HIV) from patients with AIDS confirmed its infectious origin. However, despite enormous advances in terms of treatment, the question of how infection leads to immune dysfunction and clinical disease remains unclear.

The introduction in 1996, in the developed world, of highly active antiretroviral therapy (HAART) has altered the natural history of this extraordinary condition. Before HAART, defined as a combination of medications that usually includes at least three potent anti-HIV agents, treatment largely consisted of specific opportunistic infection management and less effective antiretroviral therapy. The clinical consequences of this change are enormous: The relative hazard for development of *Pneumocystis* pneumonia (PCP) in an HIV-infected individual has fallen by over 80%. Drug therapy does have a down side: It has significant unwanted effects as well as major interactions with other medication (e.g., rifamycins used in treating tuberculosis). The profound change in immunity induced by HAART may also lead to disease (the immune restoration inflammatory syndrome [IRIS]).

Notwithstanding HAART, respiratory disease remains an important cause of morbidity and mortality. Much of the world cannot afford such medication, and over two thirds of HIV-infected individuals have at least one respiratory episode during the course of their illness. In the early stages of HIV infection, when patients have relatively preserved immune responses, individuals have the same infections found in the general population, although at a greater incidence. With progressive HIV disease, subjects are at an increased risk of opportunistic disease. For example, the North American Prospective Study of Pulmonary Complications of HIV Infection (PSPC), a multicenter cohort drawn from all HIV risk groups at various stages of immunosuppression, revealed over an 18-month study period that of approximately 1000 subjects who were not using HAART:

- 33% reported an upper respiratory tract infection
- 16% had an episode of acute bronchitis
- 5% had acute sinusitis
- 5% had bacterial pneumonia
- 4% had PCP

The immune dysregulation that arises from HIV infection means that bacteria, mycobacteria, fungi, viruses, and protozoa can all cause disease in subjects with advanced infection. Table 30.1 shows the organisms that typically infect the lung in HIV disease. Of these, bacterial infections, tuberculosis, and PCP are the most important. In the West, 40% of AIDS diagnoses are due to PCP. This chapter provides a brief general overview of the epidemiology and pathogenesis of HIV infection before concentrating on HIV and its infectious pulmonary complications.

It is reported that by the end of 2002, up to 42 million individuals worldwide had acquired HIV infection (Fig. 30.1). Of these, over 40% are thought to have developed AIDS (for definition of AIDS, see Tables 30.2, 30.3, and 30.4). It is estimated that globally 5 million individuals acquired HIV infection in 2002, and over this time 3.1 million died of AIDS. The developing world has been most affected. Sub-Saharan Africa is the current epicenter of the pandemic (two thirds of all infections); here, one in five adults is HIV infected. South and Southeast Asia are responsible for 14% of the estimated HIV global burden. The biggest rise is in Central-Eastern Europe and Central Asia, where there has been an eightfold increase in HIV infection between 1997 and 2002, and there are currently 1.2 million HIV-infected individuals. In the developed world, North America and Western Europe account for approximately 980,000 and 575,000 infections, respectively. The vast majority of these are spread through sexual contact, although vertical (mother-to-child) and bloodborne infections are also common. In the developing world, heterosexual transmission is the norm; however, in North America and Europe homosexual and bisexual men constitute the largest group of infected individuals.

Virology and Immunology of the Human Immunodeficiency Virus

HIV was first isolated in 1983 from patients with symptoms and signs of immune dysfunction. Two subtypes (HIV-1 and HIV-2) have subsequently been identified. HIV-1 (hereafter referred to as HIV) is responsible for the majority of infections, has a more aggressive clinical course, and is the focus of this chapter.

HIV is a human retrovirus belonging to the lentivirus family. Cell-free or cell-associated HIV infects through attachment of

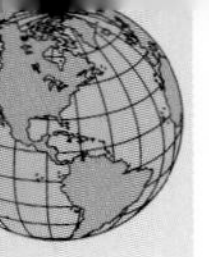

Table 30.1
Common etiologies of HIV-related pulmonary infections

Bacteria	Fungi	Parasites	Viruses
Streptococcus pneumoniae	*Pneumocystis jiroveci*	*Toxoplasma gondii*	*Cytomegalovirus*
Haemophilus influenzae	*Cryptococcus neoformans*	*Cryptosporidium* spp.	
Staphylococcus aureus	*Histoplasma capsulatum*	*Microsporidium* spp.	
Pseudomonas aeruginosa	*Candida albicans*	*Leishmania* spp.	
Nocardia asteroides	*Aspergillus* spp.	*Strongyloides stercoralis*	
Rochalimaea henselae	*Penicillium marneffei*		
Mycobacterium tuberculosis			
Mycobacterium avium-intracellulare			
Mycobacterium kansasii			

Table 30.2
Centers for Disease Control and Prevention classification

Group	Infection
I	Acute primary
II	Asymptomatic
III	Persistent generalized lymphadenopathy
IV	Other disease
Subgroup A	Constitutional disease (e.g. weight loss >10% of body weight or >4.5kg; fevers >38.5°C lasting >1 month; diarrhea lasting >1 month)
Subgroup B	Neurologic disease (e.g. HIV encephalopathy, myelopathy, peripheral neuropathy)
Subgroup C	Secondary infectious diseases
Subgroup C1	AIDS-defining secondary infectious disease (e.g. *Pneumocystis jiroveci* pneumonia, cerebral toxoplasmosis, cytomegalovirus retinitis)
Subgroup C2	Other specified secondary infectious diseases (e.g. oral candida, multidermatomal varicella zoster)
Subgroup D	Secondary cancers (e.g. Kaposi's sarcoma, non-Hodgkin's lymphoma)
Subgroup E	Other conditions (e.g. lymphoid interstitial pneumonitis)

its viral envelope protein (gp120) to the CD4 antigen complex on host cells. The CD4 receptor is found on several cell types, although the T-helper lymphocyte is the main site of HIV infection in the body. HIV gp120 must also bind to a cell surface protein coreceptor called chemokine receptor 5 (CCR5), or to other coreceptors, including CXCR4 and possibly CCR2, depending on the host cell type. Polymorphisms in genes for CCR5 may affect disease progression by reducing the ability of HIV to enter and infect cells.

Once HIV is inside the cell it can, using the enzyme reverse transcriptase (RNA-dependent DNA polymerase), transcribe its HIV RNA into a DNA copy that can translocate to the nucleus and integrate with host cell DNA using its viral integrase. The virus (as proviral DNA) remains latent in many cells until the cell itself becomes activated. This may arise from cytokine or antigen stimulation. The viral genetic material is then transcribed into new RNA, which, in the form of a newly created virion, buds from the cell surface and is free to infect other CD4-bearing cells.

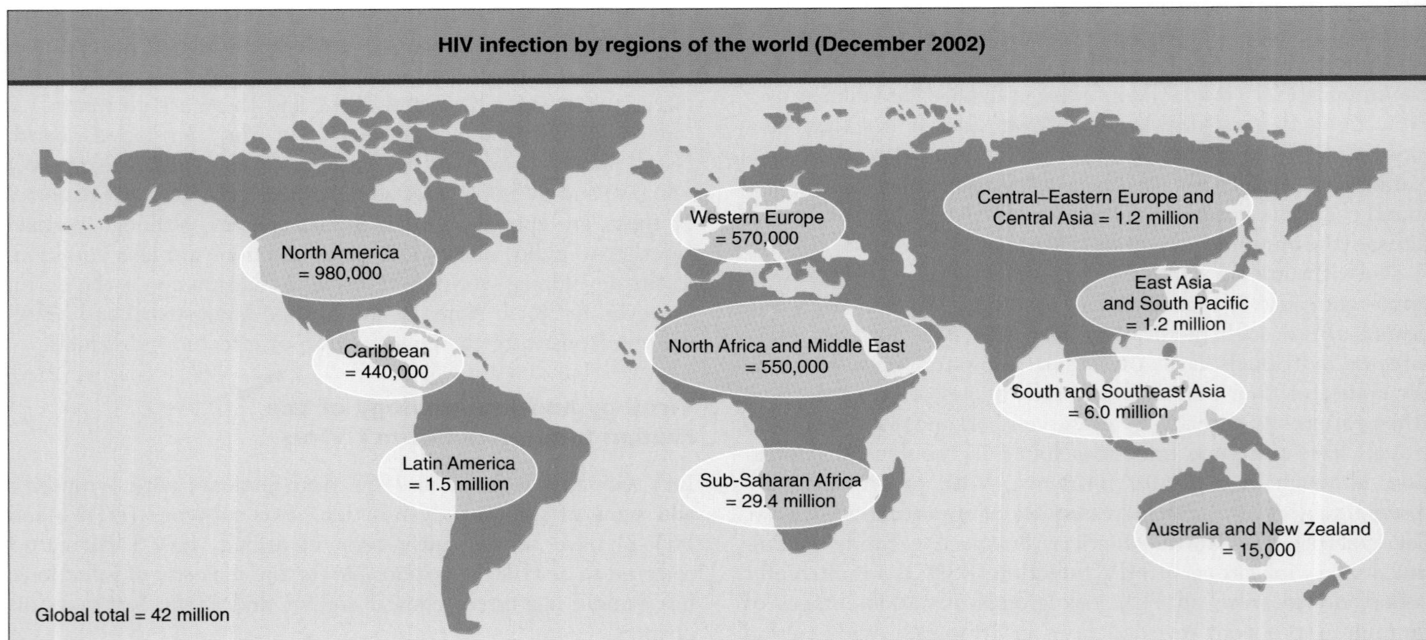

Figure 30.1 Estimated number of adults and children with human immunodeficiency virus (HIV) infection (to December 2002) by regions of the world. (Source: UNAIDS/WHO AIDS epidemic update: December 2002.)

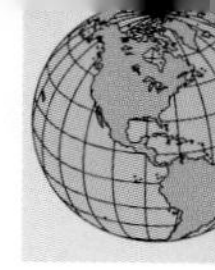

Table 30.3
Adult AIDS indicator diseases (1993)

Candidiasis of esophagus, trachea, bronchi, or lungs
Cervical carcinoma, invasive
Coccidioidomycosis, disseminated or extrapulmonary
Cryptococcosis, extrapulmonary
Cryptosporidiosis, with diarrhea for over 1 month
Cytomegalovirus disease (not in liver, spleen, or lymph nodes)
Encephalopathy caused by HIV (AIDS–dementia complex)
Herpes simplex: ulcers for 1 month or pneumonitis, esophagitis
Histoplasmosis, disseminated or extrapulmonary
Isosporiasis, with diarrhea for over 1 month
Kaposi's sarcoma
Lymphoma: Burkitt's or immunoblastic or primary in brain
Mycobacteriosis (including pulmonary tuberculosis)
Pneumocystis jiroveci pneumonia
Pneumonia recurrent within a 12-month period
Progressive multifocal leukoencephalopathy
Salmonellal (nontyphoid) septicemia, recurrent
Toxoplasmosis of brain
Wasting syndrome caused by HIV

Table 30.4
Revised (1993) CDC classification system for HIV infection – clinical categories

CD4 T-cell categories (cells/mL)	A: Acute (primary) HIV, asymptomatic or persistent generalized lymphadenopathy	B: Symptomatic (not A or C – see caption)	C: AIDS indicator conditions
≥500	A1	B1	C1
200–499	A2	B2	C2
<200	A3	B3	C3

HIV infection directly attacks the immune system and in particular the T-helper cells that are central to a coordinated immune response. This leads to progressive immune dysfunction and an inability to resist opportunistic disease. The pathogenic process is not well defined, although the picture that is emerging suggests that at the time of primary infection HIV spreads to the lymph nodes, circulating immune cells, and thymus. At this stage, a relatively potent immune response is present in most HIV-infected individuals. However, HIV replication is both very effective and error prone, such that the immune system has to try to control a rapidly moving target. Taken together with the direct cell killing caused by HIV, this ultimately leads in most individuals to progressive immune system destruction and dysfunction. The end results of this can be seen not only in the clinical diseases that indicate profound immunosuppression but in the gradual reduction in the circulating absolute CD4 cell count, the percentage of T cells expressing CD4 markers, and the CD4-to-CD8 T-cell ratio that occurs over time.

Natural History of Human Immunodeficiency Virus Infection

The use of HAART as well as prophylactic therapies for opportunistic infections has altered the "natural history" of HIV disease in countries where these interventions are available. Death rates have fallen to one sixth of their previous levels. However, in the absence of such treatments, the median interval between HIV seroconversion and progression to AIDS in the developed world has been estimated to be 10 years. Almost all individuals contract AIDS if untreated, and without HAART 95% of these will be dead within 5 years. In many parts of the world, the main causes of death in patients with HIV infection include bacterial pneumonia, tuberculosis, and PCP.

In practice, the course of HIV infection can be divided clinically into several distinct periods:

- Acquisition of the virus
- Seroconversion, with or without a clinical illness (primary HIV infection)
- Clinically silent period, lasting several months to years
- Development of symptoms and signs indicating some degree of immunosuppression
- AIDS (where the subject has opportunistic disease implying profound immunosuppression, e.g., PCP).

ACUTE PRIMARY HUMAN IMMUNODEFICIENCY VIRUS INFECTION

The time from primary HIV infection to the development of detectable antibodies (the "window" period) is usually approximately 6 to 8 weeks. Studies suggest that between 30% and 70% of individuals who become infected have a seroconversion illness. HIV antibody is normally detectable within 2 to 3 weeks of these symptoms. Tests that detect HIV RNA in peripheral blood may show evidence of HIV infection at an earlier stage.

The nonspecific features of primary HIV infection are almost always self-limiting, and typically seroconversion mimics glandular fever. The vast majority of individuals with primary HIV infection recover from the acute symptoms within 4 weeks. A proportion may have persistent symmetrical generalized lymphadenopathy. There is no difference in prognosis in this group compared with asymptomatic HIV-positive individuals.

CHRONIC HUMAN IMMUNODEFICIENCY VIRUS INFECTION

Although a proportion of individuals remain completely well without any treatment for an extended period (approximately 20% after 10 years), many HIV-infected individuals have minor symptoms and signs suggesting immune dysfunction. Examples of these include new or worsening rashes (including herpes simplex), tiredness, cough, and low-grade anemia. Certain clinical symptoms and signs provide important prognostic information. Most studies have shown that oral thrush and constitutional symptoms (e.g., malaise, idiopathic fever, night sweats, diarrhea, and weight loss) are the strongest clinical predictors of progression to AIDS.

AIDS itself is a surveillance definition and therefore has been modified to incorporate the expanding spectrum of recognized diseases affecting immunosuppressed individuals, such as

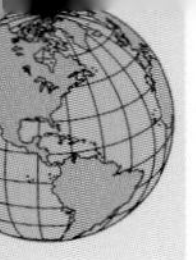

cervical carcinoma and recurrent bacterial pneumonia (see Table 30.3). The 1993 Centers for Disease Control classification included an immunologic criterion for AIDS (CD4 count <200 cells/μL or CD4 percentage <14% of total lymphocytes) regardless of clinical symptoms (see Table 30.4). These data are used to define a point at which the risk of severe opportunistic infection rises dramatically. An example of this can be seen in the Multicenter AIDS Cohort Study (MACS) of homosexual and bisexual men without AIDS, which found that the incidence of PCP in subjects not using prophylaxis rose from 0.5% at 6 months in men with a baseline CD4 count greater than 200 cells/μL to 8.4% in those with a CD4 count less than 200 cells/μL.

Apart from cervical carcinoma, AIDS indicator diseases differ little between men and women. Injecting drug users have a high incidence of wasting syndrome, recurrent bacterial pneumonia, and tuberculosis. Geographic differences in diseases occur that reflect the opportunistic pathogens present in the local environment (e.g., histoplasmosis or visceral leishmaniasis usually occur only in patients from endemic areas). In the developed world, sexual, racial, and HIV risk factor survival differences after an AIDS diagnosis mainly arise from differences in the ease with which medical care can be obtained.

In countries where HAART is available, the spectrum of HIV-related disease has changed. In the EuroSida cohort (a pan-European prospective study of HIV infection), opportunistic infections associated with very low CD4 counts (e.g., cytomegalovirus [CMV] retinitis and *Mycobacterium avium-intracellulare* complex [MAC] infection) are now far less common. Malignant disease such as non-Hodgkin's lymphoma has increased as a proportion of cases, from 4% of all AIDS-defining events in 1994 to 16% in 1998.

Although death rates have fallen in HAART-treated populations, there has been an increase in the proportion of non-AIDS deaths. In some series, this accounts for the majority of events. Causes include liver disease and cancer, as well as cardiovascular disease and drug-related toxicity. In such circumstances, AIDS deaths usually occur in patients who have not regularly accessed medical care and who present with advanced HIV disease.

A new manifestation of opportunistic infection has been described in patients commencing HAART. The immune reconstitution disease, IRIS, may cause severe, if temporary, clinical illness as the individual's immunity recovers, with acute symptoms of MAC infection, tuberculosis, hepatitis B, CMV retinitis, and herpes viral infection. Metabolic complications of HAART, such as ischemic heart disease and diabetes, are a potential problem in HIV practice in the developed world. A significant number of individuals taking HAART also experience drug toxicity. An increasing number of patients are also surviving to manifest symptoms associated with chronic infections such as hepatitis B and C.

Prognostic Markers

Laboratory markers and clinical symptoms (e.g., oral thrush) can independently reflect the immune changes that lead to serious disease. Staging systems have therefore been developed that can predict the risk of progression to AIDS. The fall in absolute blood CD4 T-lymphocyte count is the most widely used prognostic marker, although CD4 counts may be affected by a number of factors apart from HIV, including intercurrent infection, smoking, exercise, time of day, and laboratory variation. The percentage of CD4 cells and ratio of CD4 to CD8 cells are more stable measures, and may be used if the CD4 absolute counts appear to vary widely from visit to visit.

Measurement of plasma HIV RNA viral load provides important prognostic information that can both guide therapy and suggest long-term outcome. It has a particular value in subjects who are clinically well and have high CD4 counts because it can give some indication of the expected speed of clinical progression. The use of other prognostic markers (e.g., indicators of cellular activation) has, for the time being, been largely abandoned outside of the research setting.

Pulmonary Immune Response During Human Immunodeficiency Virus Infection

It is clear from the frequency with which HIV-related respiratory disease occurs that the pulmonary immune response is profoundly dysregulated. However, the mechanism underlying this has not been fully explained. In part, this is because the alterations that arise reflect the complex interplay between systemically derived HIV and other circulating antigens trafficking through the pulmonary vasculature, the local immune cells, and airborne antigen. Another problem is that most studies investigating the pulmonary immune response have used bronchoscopy and bronchoalveolar lavage (BAL) to recover lung cells. Until recently these have been performed on symptomatic patients who require bronchoscopy as a diagnostic procedure. These patients with pneumonitis in general have advanced HIV infection, and therefore are taking a number of different drugs (including antiretrovirals), and have any of a number of different pathogens causing their pulmonary disease—which in itself can influence the immune findings. Finally, the question of whether BAL fluid truly represents the site of the immune response (the lung parenchyma) is also germane.

Risk Factors for Respiratory Disease

A person's risk for respiratory disease is determined by their medical history (e.g., use of effective prophylactic or antiretroviral therapy), place of residence and travel history (e.g., the influence of geography on mycobacterial and fungal disease), and state of host immunity. Falling blood CD4 counts or high plasma RNA viral loads increase the chance of respiratory infection, with an increased spectrum of potential organisms responsible for infection in the more immunosuppressed individual. For example, HIV-infected individuals with a CD4 count less than 200 cells/μL are four times more likely to have one episode of bacterial pneumonia per year than those with higher CD4 cell counts. More exotic organisms are found in subjects with very low CD4 counts. These include bacteria such as *Rhodococcus equi* and *Nocardia asteroides* and fungi such as *Aspergillus* species and *Penicillium marneffei*. Just as with *P. jiroveci*, this reflects the importance of T-cell depletion and macrophage dysfunction in the loss of host immunity (a process that has been confirmed by animal experiments).

Among HIV-infected patients, injecting drug users are at greatest risk for development of bacterial pneumonia and tuberculosis. Individuals who have had previous respiratory episodes

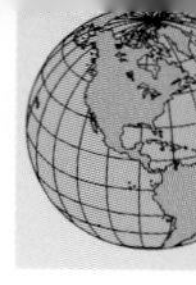

(PCP or bacterial pneumonia) appear to be at increased risk of further disease. Whether this relates to host or environmental factors is not certain, although it seems likely that structural lung damage and abnormal pulmonary physiology would in part contribute to this. This argument is supported by the increased rates of pneumonia in HIV-infected smokers compared with nonsmokers. Recent work has shown a high incidence of chronic pulmonary symptoms together with impaired respiratory function in HIV disease. These are more common in smokers and may presage the accelerated onset of severe respiratory illness that is not directly related to opportunistic disease, such as chronic obstructive pulmonary disease or lung cancer. Given that a large number of HIV-infected individuals smoke heavily, there is a pressing need to target this population for smoking cessation. This is reinforced by the association demonstrated in some (but not all) studies between smoking and a more rapid progression to first AIDS illness and death.

CLINICAL FEATURES

Bacterial Infection

BRONCHITIS

The presentation mimics bacterial exacerbations of chronic obstructive lung disease; most patients have a productive cough and fever. The pathogens commonly identified are similar to those in the general population (i.e., *Streptococcus pneumoniae* and *Haemophilus influenzae*). However, patients with advanced disease may be infected with *Pseudomonas aeruginosa* or *Staphylococcus aureus*. Response to appropriate antibiotic therapy in conventional doses is good, although relapses frequently occur.

BRONCHIECTASIS

Bronchiectasis is increasingly recognized in HIV-infected patients with advanced HIV disease and low CD4 lymphocyte counts. It probably arises secondary to recurrent bacterial or *P. jiroveci* infections. The diagnosis is most often made by high-resolution/fine-cut computed tomography (CT) scanning. Its prevalence has not been accurately determined, although with improved survival from both opportunistic infections and HIV disease it is likely that it will be increasingly common in clinical practice. The pathogens isolated in patients with bronchiectasis are those seen in bronchitis. In addition, *Pseudomonas cepacia* and *Moraxella catarrhalis* have been described.

PNEUMONIA

Community-acquired bacterial pneumonia occurs more frequently in HIV-infected patients than in the general population. It is especially common in HIV-infected injecting drug users. Recurrent bacterial pneumonia in an HIV-infected patient is an AIDS-defining diagnosis. The spectrum of bacterial pathogens is similar to that in non–HIV-infected individuals (see Table 30.1). *S. pneumoniae* is the commonest cause, followed by *H. influenzae*. HIV-infected individuals with *S. pneumoniae* pneumonia are frequently bacteremic. In one study, the rate of pneumococcal bacteremia in HIV-infected individuals was 100 times that of an HIV-negative population. More recent work has confirmed this to be the case for all causes of HIV-related bacterial pneumonia. Typically, blood cultures have a 40-fold increased pick-up rate in HIV-positive patients.

Bacterial pneumonia has a similar presentation in HIV-infected and uninfected individuals. Chest radiographs are frequently atypical, mimicking PCP in up to 50% of cases (Fig. 30.2). By contrast, radiographic lobar or segmental consolidation may also be seen in a wide range of bacterial infecting organisms (Fig. 30.3); these include *S. pneumoniae*, *P. aeruginosa*, *H. influenzae*, and *Mycobacterium tuberculosis*. PCP may also present with lobar or segmental consolidation.

In subjects with more advanced HIV disease and low CD4 lymphocyte counts, *P. aeruginosa* and *S. aureus* also cause pneumonia. Two patterns of presentation of *Pseudomonas* pulmonary infection have been described:

1. Acute pneumonia and "sepsis." This presentation is often nosocomially acquired, and patients are frequently neutropenic, receiving chemotherapy or glucocorticoid therapy, and may have indwelling intravenous catheters. Bacteremia is a frequent finding and the chest radiograph shows diffuse pulmonary infiltrates that may mimic PCP. The mortality rate here is high, and in bacteremic patients may be up to 40%.
2. Community-acquired indolent infection. Patients frequently have a subacute presentation without the risk factors listed previously. The mortality rate is low, though there is a high risk of relapse after treatment.

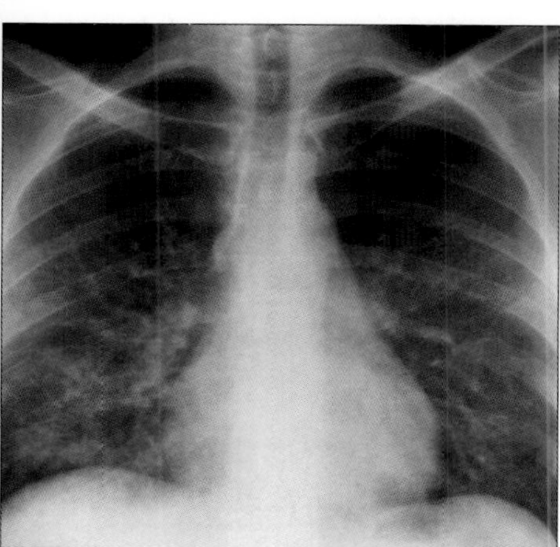

Figure 30.2 Chest radiograph showing bilateral, diffuse, interstitial infiltrates mimicking *Pneumocystis jiroveci* pneumonia. Etiology is *Streptococcus pneumoniae*.

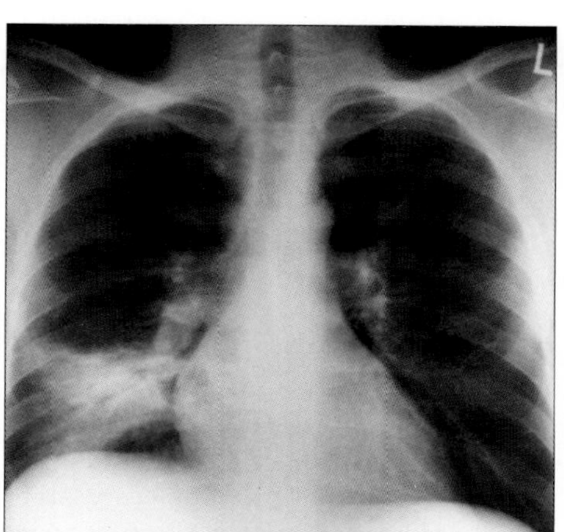

Figure 30.3 Chest radiograph showing lobar consolidation. Etiology is *Salmonella cholerae-suis*.

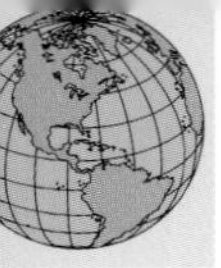

Complications of bacterial pneumonia frequently occur, and pleural effusions are twice as likely in HIV infection (often occurring with *S. aureus* infection); empyema and intrapulmonary abscess formation are present in up to 10% of patients. Inevitably, the mortality rate is high (approximately 10%).

OTHER BACTERIA

Nocardia asteroides **Infection**

This has been reported in patients with advanced HIV disease and low CD4 lymphocyte counts. The widespread use of trimethoprim/sulfamethoxazole (TMP/SMX) for prophylaxis of PCP may have reduced the incidence of infection. The clinical presentation is often indistinguishable from that of other bacterial infections. Chest radiographic appearances may mimic tuberculosis (see later), with upper lobe consolidation, cavitation, interstitial infiltrates, pleural effusion, and hilar lymphadenopathy. The diagnosis is made by identification of the organism in sputum/BAL fluid or lung tissue.

Rhodococcus equi

R. equi usually produces pneumonia in patients who have advanced HIV infection and have been in contact with farm animals or with soil from fields or barns where animals are housed. The presentation is subacute, with 2 to 3 weeks of cough, dyspnea, fever, and pleuritic chest pain. The chest radiograph typically shows consolidation with cavitation.

Pleural effusions are common. The diagnosis is usually made by culture of sputum or blood; fiberoptic bronchoscopy with BAL, or pleural aspiration may be necessary in some cases.

Bartonella henselae

B. henselae is a gram-negative bacillus that causes bacillary angiomatosis in HIV-infected patients. Clinically, the cutaneous lesions may mimic Kaposi's sarcoma, from which they may be distinguished by demonstration of organisms in tissue using Warthin-Starry silver stain. Bacillary angiomatosis may also infect the lungs, where it produces endobronchial red or violet polypoid angiomatous lesions, which may resemble Kaposi's sarcoma. Biopsy is necessary to confirm a diagnosis.

Mycobacterial Infections

TUBERCULOSIS

Tuberculosis is one of the most important diseases associated with HIV infection. Worldwide, HIV infection is the most important risk factor for the development of tuberculosis. It is estimated that there are at least 6 million individuals with HIV–tuberculosis coinfection. As such, tuberculosis is a major cause of HIV-related morbidity and mortality.

Many centers in the United Kingdom and United States routinely offer HIV antibody testing to all patients with tuberculosis, regardless of risk factors for HIV infection. The advantage of such a strategy is that individuals who are found to be HIV-infected can be offered HAART. Furthermore, counseling to modify high-risk behavior and reduce HIV transmission can be offered.

Tuberculosis may infect not only the immunosuppressed but the immunocompetent patient. Thus, clinical disease can occur at any stage of HIV infection, and unlike almost every other HIV-related infection, may do so despite effective antiretroviral therapy. In the United States, United Kingdom, and most European countries, reporting of tuberculosis in both HIV-infected and non–HIV-infected individuals is mandatory.

Clinical disease in HIV-infected patients may arise in several different ways: by reactivation of latent tuberculosis, by rapid progression of pulmonary infection, and by reinfection from an exogenous source. Studies using restriction fragment length polymorphisms show that up to 30% of HIV-associated tuberculosis in New York is due to exogenous reinfection.

Tuberculosis in HIV-infected persons presents as pulmonary disease in over two thirds of cases. The clinical manifestations are related to the level of an individual's cell-mediated immunity. Thus, those with early HIV disease have clinical features similar to "normal" adult postprimary disease (Table 30.5). Symptoms typically include weight loss, fever with sweats, cough, dyspnea, hemoptysis, and chest pain. These patients may have no clinical features to suggest associated HIV infection. The chest radiograph frequently shows upper lobe consolidation, and cavitary change is common (Fig. 30.4). The tuberculin skin test (purified protein derivative [PPD]) is usually positive, and the likelihood of spontaneously expectorated sputum or BAL fluid being smear positive for acid-fast bacilli is high.

Table 30.5
Tuberculosis and HIV infection

	Stage of HIV disease	
	Early	**Late**
Chest radiograph	Upper-lobe infiltrates and cavities (cf post primary infection)	Lymphadenopathy, effusions Miliary or diffuse infiltrates (cf primary infection) Normal
Sputum or bronchoalveolar lavage smear positive	Frequently	Less commonly
Tuberculin test positive	Frequently	Less commonly
Extrapulmonary disease	Less commonly	Frequently

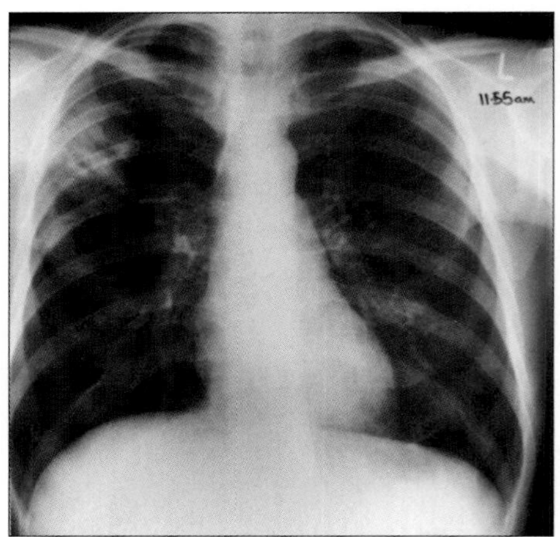

Figure 30.4 Chest radiograph of pulmonary tuberculosis in early-stage human immunodeficiency virus infection. Upper lobe infiltrates and cavities are shown.

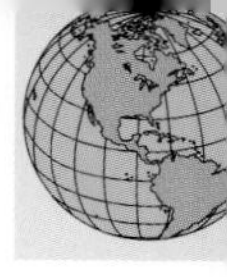

In individuals with advanced HIV disease (i.e., low CD4 lymphocyte counts and clinically apparent immunosuppression), it may be difficult to diagnose tuberculosis. The clinical presentation is often with nonspecific symptoms—fever, weight loss, fatigue, and malaise being mistakenly ascribed to HIV infection itself. In this context, pulmonary tuberculosis is often similar to primary infection, with the chest radiograph showing diffuse or miliary shadowing, hilar or mediastinal lymphadenopathy, or pleural effusion; cavitation is unusual. In up to 10% of patients the chest radiograph may be negative; in others, the pulmonary infiltrate may be bilateral, diffuse, and interstitial in pattern, thus mimicking PCP. Hilar lymphadenopathy and pleural effusion may also be produced by pulmonary Kaposi's sarcoma or lymphoma, with which *M. tuberculosis* may coexist. The tuberculin skin test is usually negative and spontaneously expectorated sputum and BAL fluid are often smear negative (but culture positive).

In addition to pulmonary tuberculosis, extrapulmonary disease occurs in a high proportion of HIV-infected individuals with low CD4 lymphocyte counts (<150 cells/μL). Mycobacteremia and lymph node infection are common, but involvement of bone marrow, liver, pericardium, meninges, and brain also occurs. Disseminated tuberculosis is an important factor in the development of "slim" disease in HIV-infected patients in Africa. This typically presents with fever, marked wasting, and diarrhea.

Evidence of extrapulmonary tuberculosis should be sought in any HIV-infected patient with suspected or confirmed pulmonary tuberculosis, by culture of stool, urine, and blood or bone marrow. Culture and speciation may take 6 to 10 weeks. Radiometric methods (e.g., Bactec, Becton Dickinson) that detect early growth may provide a diagnosis in only 2 to 3 weeks. Molecular diagnostic tests using *M. tuberculosis* genome detection (e.g., by polymerase chain reaction [PCR]) offer the possibility of yet more rapid diagnosis (within hours), but are not yet in widespread clinical use. Until the results of culture and speciation are known, acid-fast bacilli identified in respiratory samples, biopsy tissue, an aspirate, or blood in an HIV-infected individual, regardless of the CD4 lymphocyte count, should be regarded as being *M. tuberculosis* and conventional antituberculosis therapy should be commenced. If culture fails to demonstrate *M. tuberculosis* and instead another mycobacterium (see later) is identified, then treatment can be modified.

DRUG-RESISTANT TUBERCULOSIS

Multiple drug-resistant (MDR) tuberculosis—that is, *M. tuberculosis* that is resistant to isoniazid and rifampicin (rifampin), with or without other drugs, is now an important clinical problem in HIV-infected individuals in the United States, where it is responsible for approximately 3% of all tuberculosis in HIV-infected patients. Outbreaks of MDR tuberculosis have occurred in both HIV-infected and non–HIV-infected individuals in the United States in prison facilities, hostels, and hospitals. Similar outbreaks have also been documented among HIV-infected patients in Italy, Spain, and the United Kingdom. Inadequate treatment (including case management and supervision of medication) of tuberculosis and poor patient compliance with antituberculosis therapy are the most important risk factors for development of MDR tuberculosis. Other cases have arisen because of exogenous reinfection of profoundly immunosuppressed HIV-infected patients who are already receiving treatment for drug-sensitive disease.

Despite antituberculosis therapy, the median survival in HIV-infected individuals with MDR-tuberculosis was initially only 2 to 3 months. Recently this has improved, largely because of an increased awareness of the condition with early initiation of suitable therapy as determined by drug sensitivity testing.

MYCOBACTERIA OTHER THAN TUBERCULOSIS

Mycobacterium avium-intracellulare Complex

Before the widespread availability of HAART, disseminated MAC infection developed in up to 50% of HIV-infected patients. Disseminated MAC infection remains a problem in patients with very advanced HIV disease who are not receiving antiretroviral therapy and who have CD4 lymphocyte counts less than 50 cells/μL. Clinical presentation is nonspecific and may be confused with the effects of HIV itself. Fever, night sweats, weight loss, anorexia, and malaise are common. Anemia, hepatosplenomegaly, abdominal pain, and chronic diarrhea are frequent findings. The diagnosis of disseminated MAC infection is made by culture of the organism from blood, bone marrow, lymph node, or liver biopsy specimens. Also, MAC is frequently identified in BAL fluid, sputum, stool, and urine, but detection of the organism at these sites is not diagnostic of disseminated infection. Evidence of pulmonary MAC infection is not normally obtained from a chest radiograph, which may be negative or show nonspecific infiltrates. Rarely, focal consolidation, nodular infiltrates, and apical cavitation (resembling *M. tuberculosis*) have been reported.

Mycobacterium kansasii

Mycobacterium kansasii is the second most common nontuberculous opportunistic mycobacterial infection in HIV-infected individuals, and usually appears late in the course of HIV infection in patients with CD4 lymphocyte counts less than 100 cells/μL. The most frequent presentation is with fever, cough, and dyspnea. In approximately two thirds of those who have *M. kansasii* infection, the disease is localized to the lungs; the remainder have disseminated disease that affects bone marrow, lymph node, skin, and lungs. The diagnosis is made by culture of the organism from respiratory secretions or from bone marrow, lymph node aspirate, or skin biopsy. Focal upper lobe infiltrates with diffuse interstitial infiltrates are the most common radiographic abnormalities; thin-walled cavitary lesions and hilar adenopathy have also been reported.

Mycobacterium xenopi

Mycobacterium xenopi may occasionally be isolated from sputum or BAL fluid samples, but its significance is uncertain. Patients have low CD4 counts, and *M. xenopi* is usually accompanied by isolation of a copathogen, such as *P. jiroveci*. Treatment of the latter condition is associated in most cases with resolution of symptoms. There is some evidence that starting HAART prevents disease recurrence, provided there is an adequate immune response.

Pneumocystis jiroveci **Pneumonia**

The development of PCP is largely related to underlying states of immunosuppression induced by malignancy or treatment

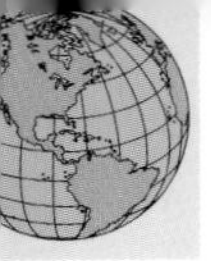

thereof, organ transplantation, or HIV infection. In 2003 in the United States, United Kingdom, Europe, and Australasia, PCP is largely seen only in HIV-infected individuals unaware of their serostatus or in those who are intolerant of, or noncompliant with, anti–*P. jiroveci* prophylaxis and HAART.

Until recently, *P. jiroveci* was regarded taxonomically as a protozoan, based on its morphology and the lack of response to antifungal agents such as amphotericin B. Use of molecular biologic techniques suggest, however, that *P. jiroveci* is a fungus. The demonstration of antibodies against *P. jiroveci* in most healthy children/adults suggests that organisms are acquired in childhood and persist in the lungs in a dormant phase. Subsequent immunosuppression (e.g., as a result of HIV infection) allows the fungus to propagate in the lung and cause clinical disease. This "latency" hypothesis is challenged by several observations:

- *P. jiroveci* cannot be identified in the lungs of immunocompetent individuals.
- "Case clusters" of PCP in health care facilities suggest recent transmission.
- Different genotypes of *P. jiroveci* are identified in each episode in HIV-infected patients who have recurrent PCP.
- Genotype of *P. jiroveci* in patients who have PCP correlates with place of diagnosis and not with their place of birth, suggesting infection has been recently acquired.

Taken together, these data suggest that PCP arises by reinfection from an exogenous source.

The clinical presentation of PCP is nonspecific, with an onset of progressive exertional dyspnea over days or weeks, together with a dry cough with or without expectoration of minimal quantities of mucoid sputum. Patients often complain of an inability to take a deep breath, which is not due to pleurisy (Table 30.6). Fever is common, yet patients rarely complain of temperatures or sweats. In HIV-infected patients, the presentation is usually more insidious than in patients receiving immunosuppressive therapy, with a median time to diagnosis from onset of symptoms of 25 days in those with AIDS compared with 5 days in non–HIV-infected patients. In a small proportion of HIV-positive individuals, the disease course of PCP is fulminant, with an interval of only 5 to 7 days between onset of symptoms and progression to development of respiratory failure. In others it may be much more indolent, with respiratory symptoms that worsen almost imperceptibly over several months. Rarely, PCP may present without respiratory symptoms as a fever of undetermined origin.

Clinical examination is usually remarkable only for the absence of physical signs; occasionally, fine, basal, end-inspiratory crackles are audible. Features atypical for a diagnosis of PCP that suggest an alternative diagnosis include a cough productive of purulent sputum or hemoptysis, chest pain (particularly pleural pain), and signs of focal consolidation or pleural effusion (see Table 30.6).

The chest radiograph in PCP is typically negative initially. Later, diffuse reticular shadowing, especially in the perihilar regions, is seen and may progress to diffuse alveolar consolidation that resembles pulmonary edema if untreated or if the patient presents late in disease. At this stage, the lung may be massively consolidated and almost airless (Fig. 30.5). Up to 20% of chest radiographs are atypical, showing lobar consolidation, honeycomb lung, multiple thin-walled cystic air space formation (pneumatoceles), intrapulmonary nodules, cavitary lesions, pneumothorax, and hilar and mediastinal lymphadenopathy. Predominantly apical changes, resembling tuberculosis, may occur in patients who develop PCP having received anti–*P. jiroveci* prophylaxis with nebulized pentamidine (Fig. 30.6). All these radiographic changes are nonspecific and similar changes occur with other pulmonary pathogens, including pyogenic bacterial, mycobacterial, and fungal infection, as well as Kaposi's sarcoma and nonspecific interstitial pneumonitis. Respiratory symptoms in an immunosuppressed, HIV-infected individual with a negative chest radiograph should not be discounted because over an interval of 2 to 3 days radiographic abnormalities may appear.

Table 30.6
Presentation of *Pneumocystis jiroveci* pneumonia

Examination	Typical presentation	Atypical presentation
Symptoms	Progressive exertional dyspnea over days or weeks	Sudden onset of dyspnea over hours or days
	Dry cough ± mucoid sputum	Cough productive of purulent sputum
	–	Hemoptysis
	Difficulty taking in a deep breath not because of pleuritic pain	Chest pain (pleuritic or crushing)
	Fever ± sweats	–
	Tachypnea	–
Chest	Normal breath sounds or fine end-inspiration basal crackles	Wheeze, signs of focal consolidation or pleural effusion
Chest radiograph	Early: normal, perihilar haze, or bilateral interstitial shadowing	–
	Late: alveolar-interstitial changes or 'white out' (marked alveolar consolidation with sparing of apices and costophrenic angles)	–
Arterial blood gases	PaO_2: early, normal; late, low	–
	$PaCO_2$: early, normal or low; late, normal or low	–

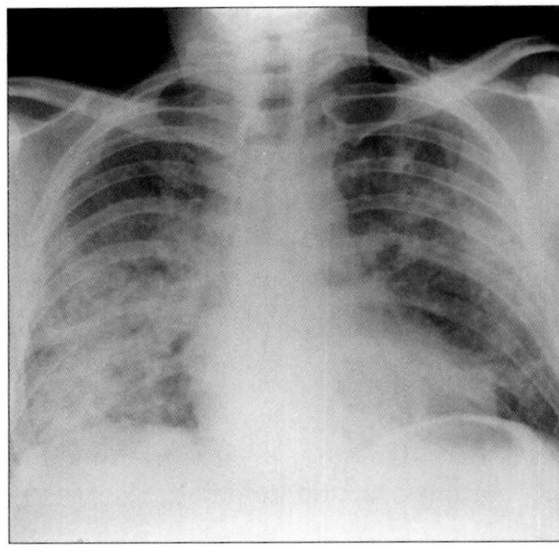

Figure 30.5 Chest radiograph of severe *Pneumocystis jiroveci* pneumonia. Diffuse bilateral interstitial infiltrates are shown.

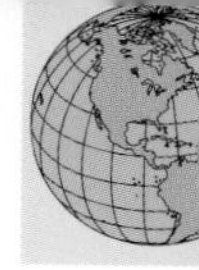

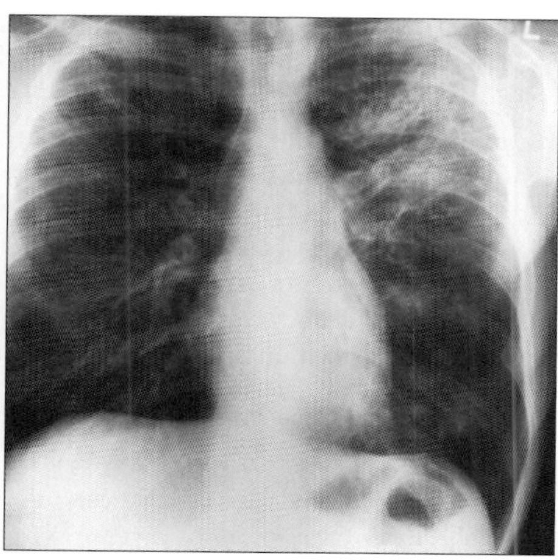

Figure 30.6 Chest radiograph of *Pneumocystis jiroveci* pneumonia. Upper lobe infiltrates are seen in this patient who had received nebulized pentamidine.

The diagnosis of PCP is made by demonstration of the organism in induced sputum, BAL fluid, or lung biopsy material using histochemical or immunofluorescence techniques.

Fungal Infections

Many fungal infections of the lung are confined to specific geographic regions, although with widespread travel they may present in patients outside these areas. *Candida, Aspergillus,* and *Cryptococcus* species are ubiquitous and occur worldwide.

CANDIDAL INFECTION

In contrast to infections of the oropharynx and esophagus, candidal infection of the trachea, bronchi, and lungs is rare in HIV-infected patients, as are candidemia, disseminated candidiasis, and deep focal candidiasis. The clinical presentation of pulmonary candidal infection has no specific features. Chest radiography is equally nonspecific—it may be negative or show patchy infiltrates. Isolation of *Candida* from sputum may simply represent colonization and does not mean the patient has candidal pneumonia. Indirect evidence may be obtained from positive cultures or rising antibody titers. However, in HIV-infected patients a high antibody titer alone is a less reliable indicator, and antibodies may be absent in proved cases of invasive candidal infection. Some correlation occurs between identification of large quantities of *Candida* species in BAL fluid and *Candida* species as the cause of pneumonia. Definitive diagnosis is made by lung biopsy.

ASPERGILLUS *INFECTION*

In contrast to patients immunosuppressed and made neutropenic by systemic chemotherapy, infection with *Aspergillus* species is relatively rare in HIV-positive individuals. Risk factors for aspergillosis are neutropenia (>50% cases) and the use of corticosteroids. Neutropenia is commonly induced by drug therapy such as zidovudine or ganciclovir. Fever, cough, and dyspnea are the most common presenting symptoms, but pleuritic chest pain and hemoptysis are found in approximately one third of patients.

Patterns of disease that involve the lung include cavitating upper lobe disease, focal radiographic opacities resembling bacterial pneumonia, bilateral opacities that are diffuse and patchy (being nodular or reticular-nodular in pattern), pseudomembranous aspergillosis, which may obstruct the lumen of airways, and tracheobronchitis. Diagnosis of pulmonary aspergillosis is made by the identification of fungus in sputum, sputum casts, or BAL fluid associated with respiratory tract tissue invasion (Fig. 30.7).

CRYPTOCOCCAL INFECTION

Infection may present in one of two ways: either as primary cryptococcosis or complicating cryptococcal meningitis as part of disseminated infection with cryptococcemia, pneumonia, and cutaneous disease (umbilicated papules mimicking molluscum contagiosum—Fig. 30.8). Primary pulmonary cryptococcosis presents in a very nonspecific way and is frequently indistinguishable from other pulmonary infections. In disseminated infection, the presentation is frequently overshadowed by headache, fever, and malaise (caused by meningitis). The duration of onset may range from only a few days to several weeks. Examination may reveal skin lesions, lymphadenopathy, and meningism. In the chest, signs may be absent or crackles may be audible. Arterial blood gas tensions may be normal or show hypoxemia. The most common abnormality on the chest

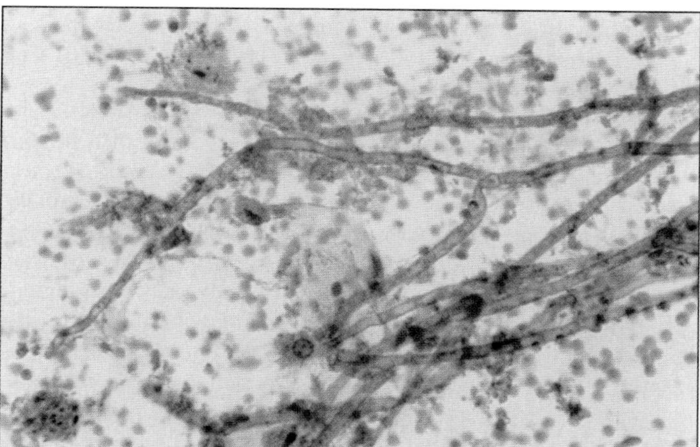

Figure 30.7 Bronchoalveolar lavage fluid with *Aspergillus fumigatus*.

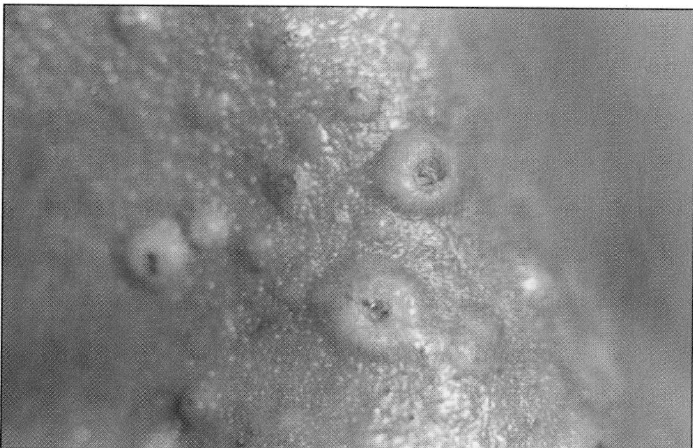

Figure 30.8 Skin in disseminated cryptococcosis. The multiple, umbilicated lesions resemble molluscum contagiosum.

radiograph is focal or diffuse interstitial infiltrates. Less frequently, masses, mediastinal or hilar lymphadenopathy, nodules, and effusion are seen.

The diagnosis of cryptococcal pulmonary infection (Fig. 30.9) is made by identification of *Cryptococcus neoformans* (by staining with India ink or mucicarmine, and by culture) in sputum, BAL fluid, pleural fluid, or lung biopsy. Cryptococcal antigen may be detected in serum using the cryptococcal latex agglutination (CrAg) test. Titers are usually high, but may be negative in primary pulmonary cryptococcosis, in which case BAL fluid (CrAg) is positive. In patients with disseminated infection, C. *neoformans* may also be cultured from blood and cerebrospinal fluid. The mortality rate is high in this disseminated form (up to 80%).

ENDEMIC MYCOSES

The endemic mycoses caused by *Histoplasma capsulatum*, *Coccidioides immitis*, and *Blastomyces dermatitidis* are found in HIV-infected patients living in North America (especially the Mississippi and Ohio River valleys). Histoplasmosis is also found in Southeast Asia, the Caribbean Islands, and South America. Coccidioidomycosis is endemic in the southwest United States (southern California), northern Mexico, and in parts of Argentina and Brazil. Blastomycosis has a similar distribution, with an extension north into Canada.

Histoplasmosis

Progressive, disseminated histoplasmosis in patients who have AIDS typically presents with a subacute onset of fever and weight loss; approximately 50% of patients have mild respiratory symptoms with a nonproductive cough and dyspnea. Hepatosplenomegaly is frequently found on examination and a skin rash (similar to that produced by *Cryptococcus* species) may be seen. Rarely, the presentation may be atypically fulminant, with clinical features of the sepsis syndrome with anemia or disseminated intravascular coagulation. The chest radiograph is negative in approximately one third of patients; characteristic abnormalities are bilateral, widespread nodules 2 to 4 mm in size. Other radiographic abnormalities are nonspecific and include interstitial infiltrates, reticular nodular shadowing, and alveolar consolidation. Histoplasmosis may disseminate to the central nervous system and produce meningoencephalitis or mass lesions. The diagnosis is made reliably by identification of the organism in Wright-stained peripheral blood or by Giemsa staining of bone marrow, lymph node, skin, sputum, BAL fluid, or lung tissue. It is essential that identification is confirmed by culture detection of *H. capsulatum* var. *capsulatum* polysaccharide antigen by radioimmunoassay, which has a high sensitivity. False-positive results may occur in patients infected with *Blastomycosis* and *Coccidioides* species. Tests for *Histoplasma* antibodies by complement fixation or immunodiffusion may be negative in immunosuppressed, HIV-positive patients.

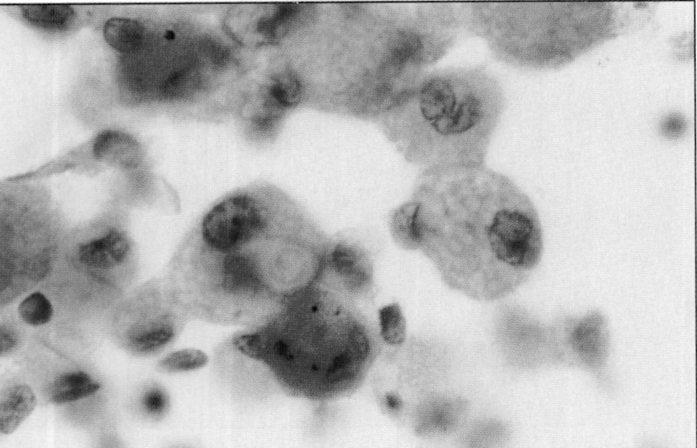

Figure 30.9 Bronchoalveolar lavage fluid with *Cryptococcus neoformans*.

Coccidioidomycosis

The clinical presentation of coccidioidomycosis is very variable. The chest radiograph may show focal pulmonary disease with focal alveolar infiltrates, adenopathy, and intrapulmonary cavities or, alternatively, diffuse reticular infiltrates. Diagnosis is made by isolation of the organism in sputum or BAL fluid. Disseminated disease is identified by isolating the fungus in blood, urine, or cerebrospinal fluid. Serologic tests may also be used for diagnosis.

Blastomycosis

Blastomycosis presents in patients who have advanced HIV infection, when CD4 lymphocyte counts are usually less than 200 cells/μL. Clinical symptoms include cough, fever, dyspnea, and weight loss. Patients may present late in respiratory failure. Disseminated disease may occur with both pulmonary and extrapulmonary features. There is frequently multiple involvement of the skin, liver, brain, and meninges. Chest radiographic abnormalities include focal pneumonic change, miliary shadowing, or diffuse interstitial infiltrates. Diagnosis is made by culture from BAL fluid, skin, and blood. In this infection, cytologic or histologic diagnosis is important for early diagnosis because culture of the organism may take 2 to 4 weeks. The mortality rate is high in patients who have disseminated infection.

PENICILLIUM MARNEFFEI *INFECTION*

P. marneffei infection is particularly common in Southeast Asia. Most HIV-infected patients present with disseminated infection and solitary skin or oral mucosal lesions, or with multiple infiltrates in the liver or spleen, or bone marrow (leading to presentation with pancytopenia). Pulmonary infection has no specific clinical features and chest radiographs may be negative or show diffuse, small nodular infiltrates. Diagnosis is made by identifying the organism in bone marrow, skin biopsies, blood films, or BAL fluid. The differential diagnosis of *P. marneffei* infection includes both PCP and tuberculosis.

Viral Infections

COMMUNITY-BASED RESPIRATORY VIRAL INFECTIONS

These occur with equal frequency in HIV-infected and non–HIV-infected patients; however, respiratory complications after influenza infection are increased in patients affected with underlying conditions such as cardiac or pulmonary disease and immunosuppression. In prospective studies of HIV-infected patients undergoing bronchoscopy for evaluation of suspected lower respiratory tract disease, the community-acquired

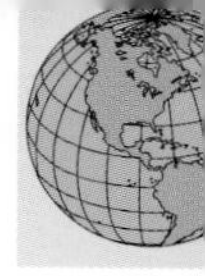

respiratory viral infections (i.e., influenza, parainfluenza, respiratory syncytial virus, rhinovirus, and adenovirus) are found only rarely, if at all.

Cytomegalovirus

CMV chronically infects most HIV-infected individuals, and up to 90% of homosexual HIV-infected men shed CMV intermittently in urine, semen, and saliva. Clinical disease may be caused by CMV in patients who have advanced HIV infection and CD4 counts less than 100 cells/μL, most frequently chorioretinitis but also encephalitis, adrenalitis, esophagitis, and colitis. Frequently, CMV is isolated from BAL fluid, being found in up to 40% of samples, although its role in causing disease is unclear (see later).

In patients who have CMV as the sole identified pathogen, the clinical presentation and chest radiographic abnormalities (usually diffuse interstitial infiltrates) are nonspecific. The diagnosis of CMV pneumonitis is made by identifying characteristic intranuclear and intracytoplasmic inclusions, not only in cells in BAL fluid but in lung biopsy specimens (Fig. 30.10).

Protozoal Infections

LEISHMANIASIS

Pulmonary involvement with *Leishmania* species may rarely occur as part of the syndrome of visceral leishmaniasis in HIV-infected patients. Patients usually have advanced HIV disease with CD4 lymphocyte counts less than 300 cells/μL and present with unexplained fever, splenomegaly, and leukopenia. Respiratory symptoms are often absent. Diagnosis of visceral leishmaniasis is most often made by staining a splenic or bone marrow aspirate and subsequent culture. Occasionally the parasite is found by chance in a skin or rectal biopsy or BAL fluid taken for other purposes. The chest radiograph may be negative or show reticular-nodular infiltrates.

TOXOPLASMOSIS

Toxoplasma gondii infection in patients who have AIDS usually occurs as a result of reactivation of latent, intracellular protozoa acquired in a primary infection. Patients are invariably systemically unwell, with malaise and pyrexia. Clinical disease in association with HIV infection is most commonly seen in the central nervous system, where it produces single or multiple abscesses. Multisystem infection with *T. gondii* is uncommon in patients who have HIV infection.

Toxoplasmic pneumonia is frequently difficult to distinguish from PCP. Nonproductive cough and dyspnea are the symptoms most commonly reported. Chest radiographic abnormalities include diffuse interstitial infiltrates indistinguishable from those of PCP (Fig. 30.11), as well as micronodular infiltrates, a coarse nodular infiltrate, cavitary change, and lobar consolidation. The diagnosis is made by hematoxylin-eosin or Giemsa staining of BAL fluid, which reveals cysts and trophozoites of *T. gondii*. Staining of BAL fluid is not always positive; the diagnostic yield is increased either by staining of transbronchial biopsy material or by performing nucleic acid amplification procedures such as PCR to detect *T. gondii* DNA in BAL fluid.

CRYPTOSPORIDIOSIS

The most frequent manifestation of infection with *Cryptosporidium* species in HIV infection is a noninflammatory diarrhea that may be of high volume, intractable, and life threatening. *Cryptosporidium* species may colonize epithelial surfaces, including the trachea and lungs, occasionally resulting in pulmonary infection. Most cases of pulmonary cryptosporidiosis have copathology such as PCP or bacterial pneumonia; ascertaining the exact role of cryptosporidiosis as the cause of respiratory symptoms may be difficult. Diagnosis is made by Ziehl-Neelsen or auramine-rhodamine staining of BAL fluid or transbronchial biopsy specimens.

MICROSPORIDIOSIS

Pulmonary *Microsporidia* infection may occur as part of systemic dissemination from gastrointestinal infection with *Septata intestinalis* or *Encephalitozoon hellem*. The organism may be identified by conventional staining in BAL fluid. Electron microscopy is necessary to distinguish the two species.

STRONGYLOIDIASIS

The nematode *Strongyloides stercoralis* is endemic in warm countries worldwide. In immunosuppressed patients, the organism has an increased ability to reproduce parthenogenetically in the gastrointestinal tract without the need for repeated exposure to new infection—so-called autoinfection. This results in a great increase in worm load and a hyperinfective state ensues; massive acute dissemination with *S. stercoralis* may occur in the

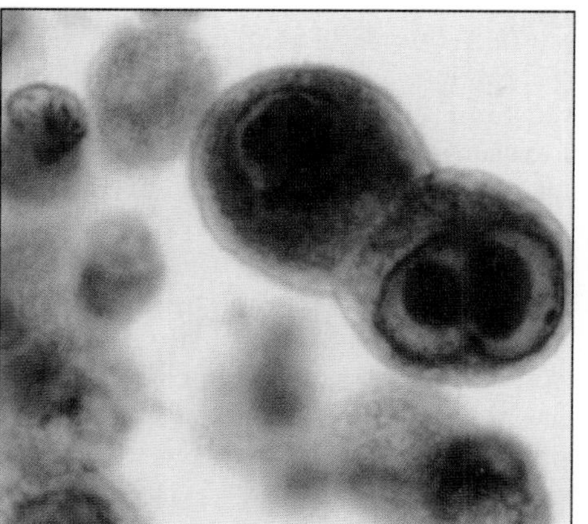

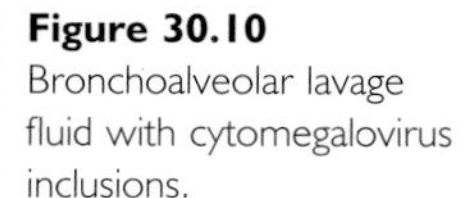

Figure 30.10 Bronchoalveolar lavage fluid with cytomegalovirus inclusions.

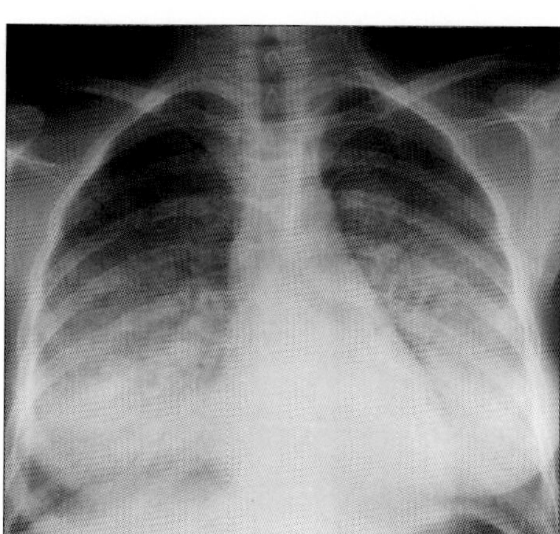

Figure 30.11 Chest radiograph of *Toxoplasma gondii* pneumonia. The diffuse bilateral infiltrates resemble *P. jiroveci* pneumonia. (Reproduced with permission from Miller RF, Lucas SB, Bateman NT: Disseminated *Toxoplasma gondii* infection presenting with a fulminant pneumonia. Genitourinary Med 72:139-143, 1996, BMJ Publishing Group.)

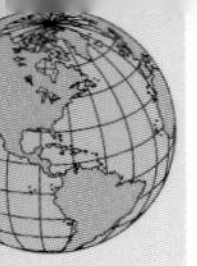

lungs, kidneys, pancreas, and brain. Although infection with *S. stercoralis* is more severe in immunocompromised patients, it is no more common in patients who have HIV infection. Presentation with hyperinfection may be with fever, hypotension secondary to bacterial sepsis, or disseminated intravascular coagulation. The clinical features of respiratory *S. stercoralis* infection are very nonspecific. *S. stercoralis* in sputum or BAL fluid (Fig. 30.12) may be identified in HIV-positive patients in the absence of symptoms elsewhere; this can predate disseminated infection and as such requires prompt treatment.

DIAGNOSIS

It is apparent from the foregoing discussion that HIV-related pneumonia of any cause may present in a very similar manner. A wide range of investigations are available to aid diagnosis. These are listed in Table 30.7. If the subject is producing sputum, it is important to obtain samples for bacterial and mycobacterial detection. In up to one third of cases these will assist in diagnosis. Three samples on consecutive days is the vital first step in the diagnosis of active (infectious) pulmonary tuberculosis. This is considerably easier and safer for health care personnel than obtaining hypertonic saline–induced sputum or BAL fluid. Blood cultures are also important because very high rates of bacteremia have been reported in both bacterial and mycobacterial disease (see earlier).

A patient who presents with symptoms and signs consistent with pneumonia should have chest radiography and arterial oxygen assessments performed at his or her first consultation. The question at this stage is usually whether this infectious episode is due to bacterial infection, tuberculosis, or PCP. In general, alveolar and interstitial shadowing is taken as evidence for PCP, although important caveats apply.

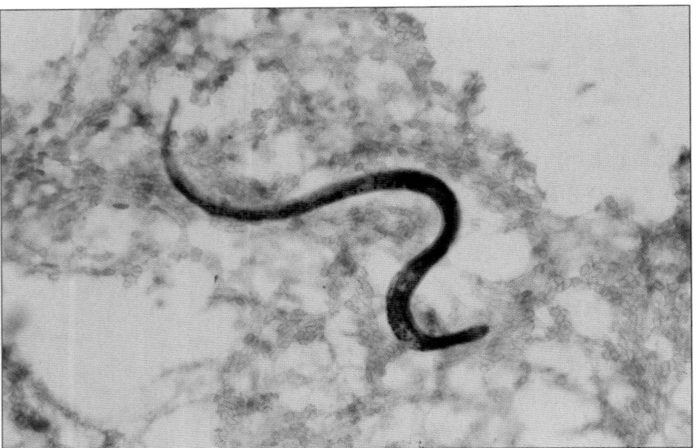

Figure 30.12 Bronchoalveolar lavage fluid with *Strongyloides stercoralis*.

Table 30.7
Tests available to aid the diagnosis of HIV-related pneumonia

Type	Test
Physiologic	Transcutaneous pulse oximetry Arterial blood gas analysis Lung function
Radiologic	Chest radiography Computed tomography of thorax
Pathologic	Serology (antigen or antibody testing) Serum lactate dehydrogenase enzyme measurement Microscopy and culture of body fluids/tissue (e.g. sputum, blood, bronchoalveolar lavage, lung tissue) obtained by Sputum induction Bronchoscopy and bronchoalveolar lavage Bronchoscopy and transbronchial biopsy Thoracoscopic biopsy Open-lung biopsy Nucleic acid detection of specific organisms (e.g. polymerase chain reaction for *Pneumocystis jiroveci* in sputum)

Arterial Oxygen Assessments

Transcutaneous pulse oximetry and arterial blood gas analysis are useful tests for hypoxemia. They can be used to distinguish an alveolar condition (i.e., PCP) from bacterial pneumonia. The alveolitis produces a greater impairment of oxygen transfer (especially during exercise), such that for a given clinical situation there will be more hypoxemia and a wider alveolar–arterial oxygen gradient ($PAO_2 - PaO_2$) in those who have PCP. With pulse oximetry this manifests as low oxygen saturations at rest that decrease further with exercise. In general, more information can be obtained from arterial blood gas analysis, although this advantage is offset by the need for direct arterial puncture.

Of patients with PCP, fewer than 10% have a normal PaO_2 and a normal $PAO_2 - PaO_2$. These measures are sensitive, although not particularly specific for PCP, and similar results may occur with bacterial pneumonia, pulmonary Kaposi's sarcoma, and *M. tuberculosis* infection. The diagnostic value of identifying exercise-induced desaturation, measured by transcutaneous oximetry, has been validated only in HIV-infected patients who have PCP and a normal, or "near normal" appearance on chest radiographs. The test's value has not been confirmed in patients with chest radiograph abnormalities caused by PCP or other pathogens. Exercise-induced desaturation may persist for many weeks after treatment and recovery from PCP, in the absence of active pulmonary disease.

Lung Function Testing

Abnormalities of lung function are well documented with HIV infection. However, most abnormalities manifest in those tests that measure gas exchange, rather than as changes in the conducting airways. In general, an overall reduction in diffusing capacity for carbon monoxide (DLco) occurs at all stages of HIV infection, with the largest changes found in HIV-infected patients with PCP. Thus, patients who have probable PCP can be differentiated and treatment guided. A normal DLco in an individual who has symptoms but a negative or unchanged chest radiograph makes the diagnosis of PCP extremely unlikely. Data from the North American PSPC cohort study suggest that individuals with rapid rates of decline in DLco are at an increased risk for development of PCP.

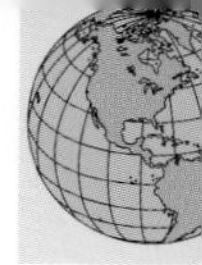

Computed Tomography Scanning

High resolution (fine-cut) CT scanning of the chest may be helpful when the chest radiograph is either negative, unchanged, or equivocal. The characteristic appearance of an alveolitis (i.e., areas of ground-glass attenuation through which the pulmonary vessels can be clearly identified) may be present, which indicates active pulmonary disease. This feature, however, is neither sensitive nor specific for PCP. A negative test result implies an alternative diagnosis.

Lactate Dehydrogenase Enzyme

In the context of an HIV-infected patient who presents with an acute or subacute pneumonitis, an elevated serum lactate dehydrogenase (LDH) enzyme level is strongly suggestive of PCP. When interpreting the finding of an elevated serum LDH, it is important to remember that other pulmonary disease processes (e.g., pulmonary embolism, nonspecific pneumonitis, and bacterial and mycobacterial pneumonia) and extrapulmonary disease (Castleman's disease and lymphoma) may also cause elevations of LDH. These processes should be excluded before ascribing the cause to PCP.

From the previous information, it is evident that noninvasive tests cannot reliably distinguish the different infecting agents from each other, but may be useful in excluding acute opportunistic disease. Thus, the clinician is left with either proceeding to diagnostic lung fluid or tissue sampling (using either induced sputum collection or bronchoscopy and BAL with or without transbronchial biopsy; Table 30.8), or treating an unknown condition empirically. HAART has also altered the investigation of respiratory disease. The numbers of invasive procedures performed are falling and tend to be in patients not taking antiretroviral drugs (usually to exclude PCP), or where there has been no response to empiric antibiotic therapy (regardless of the CD4 count).

Induced Sputum

Spontaneously expectorated sputum is inadequate for diagnosis of PCP. Sputum induction by inhalation of ultrasonically nebulized hypertonic saline for 20 to 60 minutes may provide a suitable specimen (see Table 30.8). The technique requires close attention to detail and is much less useful when samples are purulent. Sputum induction must be carried out away from other immunosuppressed patients and health care workers, ideally in a room with separate negative-pressure ventilation, to reduce the risk of nosocomial transmission of tuberculosis. Although very specific (>95%), the sensitivity of induced sputum varies widely (55% to 90%), and therefore a negative result for *P. jiroveci* prompts further diagnostic studies. The use of immunofluorescence staining appears to enhance the yield of induced sputum compared with standard cytochemistry.

Bronchoscopy

Fiberoptic bronchoscopy with BAL is commonly used to diagnose HIV-related pulmonary disease. When a good "wedged" sample is obtained, the test has a sensitivity of over 90% for detection of *P. jiroveci* (Fig. 30.13). Just as with induced sputum, fluorescent staining methods increase the diagnostic yield, which makes it the procedure of choice in most centers. More technically demanding (both of the patient and the operator) than induced sputum collection, bronchoscopy and BAL have the advantage that direct inspection of the upper airway and bronchial tree can be performed and, if necessary, biopsies taken. Transbronchial biopsies may marginally increase the diagnostic yield of the procedure. This is relevant for the diagnosis of mycobacterial disease, although the relatively high complication rate in HIV-infected individuals (pneumothorax in up to 10%) outweighs the advantages of the technique for routine purposes.

Samples of BAL fluid are examined for bacteria, mycobacteria, viruses, fungi, and protozoa. Inspection of the cellular component may also provide etiologic clues—cooperation of a pathology department with experience in opportunistic infection diagnosis is vital. The drug interactions associated with antiretroviral protease inhibitors (PIs) mean that special care should be exercised when using either benzodiazepine or opiate sedation during bronchoscopy in patients taking these drugs. Prolonged sedation and life-threatening arrhythmias have been reported.

Table 30.8
Induced sputum, bronchoalveolar lavage, and surgical biopsy in the diagnosis of *Pneumocystis jiroveci* pneumonia

Technique	Ease of procedure	Diagnostic sensitivity (%)	Cost	Notes
Induced sputum	Simple – once technique established	50–90	Low	Requires dedicated staff and facility Risk to staff from expectorated aerosol
Broncho-alveolar lavage	Moderate	90–>95	Moderate	Risk of deterioration post procedure Risk to staff from coughed secretions Sensitivity may be increased by two-lobe lavage
Surgical biopsy	Complex	>95	High	Requires staff with surgical expertise

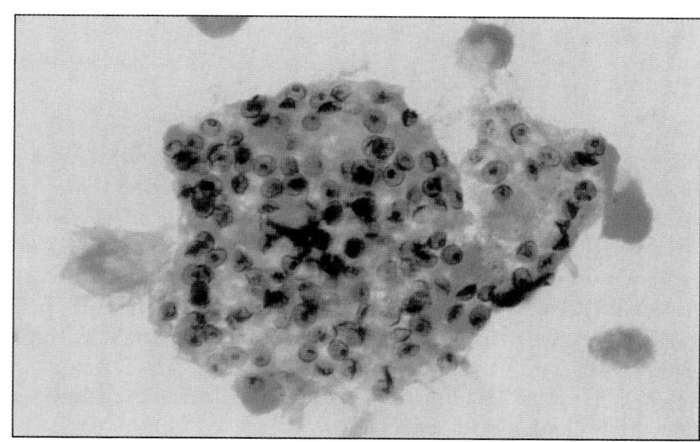

Figure 30.13 Bronchoalveolar lavage fluid with *Pneumocystis jiroveci* (Grocott silver staining).

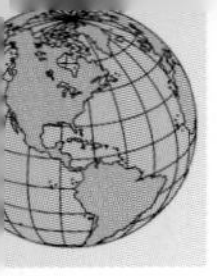

A diagnostic strategy therefore includes sputum induction and, if results are nondiagnostic or if the test is unavailable, bronchoscopy and BAL. If this does not yield a result, consideration is given to either a repeat bronchoscopy and BAL with transbronchial biopsies, or surgical biopsy. The latter can be performed as either an open lung or thoracoscopic procedure. Surgical biopsy has a high sensitivity.

Empirical Diagnosis and Therapy

Although empirical therapy is usually reserved for the management of presumed bacterial pneumonias, and at first sight may appear unwise when dealing with possible opportunistic infection, in reality PCP is almost invariably a diagnosis of exclusion, and certain clinical and laboratory features may guide the assessment of an HIV-infected individual's risk for this condition. The likelihood that *P. jiroveci* is the causative organism increases if the subject is not taking effective anti-*Pneumocystis* drug prophylaxis or has a previous medical history with clinical or laboratory features that suggest systemic immunosuppression (i.e., recurrent oral thrush, longstanding fever of unknown cause, clinical AIDS, or blood CD4 count <200 cells/μL). Hence, some centers advocate use of empirical therapy for HIV-infected patients who present with symptoms and chest radiographic and blood gas abnormalities typical of mild PCP, without the need for bronchoscopy. Invasive measures are reserved for those with an atypical radiographic presentation, those who fail to respond to empirical therapy by day 5, and those who deteriorate at any stage.

Most clinicians in North America and the United Kingdom would seek to obtain a confirmed diagnosis in every case of suspected PCP. In practice, both strategies appear to be equally effective, although a number of caveats should be borne in mind when empirical treatment is given for PCP. Patients who have PCP typically take 4 to 7 days to show clinical signs of improvement, so a bronchoscopically proved diagnosis ensures that the treatment is correct, particularly in the first few days of therapy, when it may not be well tolerated. In addition, the diagnosis of PCP has implications for the infected individual—it may be psychologically important for them to clarify whether they have an AIDS-defining illness, and it may also influence their decision to start either HAART or anti-*Pneumocystis* prophylaxis. Finally, empirical therapy requires the patient to be maximally adherent with treatment because nonresolution of the symptoms may be seen as failure of therapy, rather than of compliance.

Nucleic Acid Detection

The techniques of molecular biology (such as PCR) are increasingly used in the diagnosis of respiratory disease. Two examples of this are DNA amplification of loci of the *P. jiroveci* and *M. tuberculosis* genomes. The advantages of molecular methods are that the diagnosis may be made using samples that are more readily obtained than BAL fluid, (i.e., expectorated sputum or nasopharyngeal secretions), and also that these methods are rapid (the answer may be available within a working day, compared with conventional mycobacterial culture, which may take weeks). Despite encouraging results in the research setting (sensitivity and specificity have been reported as 60% to 100% and 70% to 100%, respectively), problems persist when these techniques are applied to routine diagnostic samples. These include extraction of nucleic acid from clinical material, cross-contamination with the products of previous assays, and clinical interpretation of a test result. It is expected that these difficulties will, within a short time, be overcome and that molecular methods will become a part of the standard diagnostic workup. The use of real-time PCR, which allows determination of whether a pathogen is alive or dead, is an exciting and important advance that will have major implications for rapid diagnostics in centers where it is available.

TREATMENT

Individuals infected with HIV, compared with the non–HIV-infected general population, have an increased likelihood of adverse reactions to therapy, not just to TMP/SMX (see later) but to other drugs, including antimycobacterial agents. In addition, there are complex drug interactions with other medications, particularly components of HAART. Before instituting therapy for any infectious complication in an HIV-infected individual, it is important to consult with a physician experienced in the care of patients with HIV infection and to seek advice from a specialist pharmacist.

Bacterial Pneumonia

The main organisms causing pneumonia in HIV-infected individuals are similar to those found in the general population with community-acquired pneumonia. Thus, bacterial pneumonia in HIV-infected patients should be treated in a similar manner to that in HIV-negative individuals, using published American Thoracic Society and British Thoracic Society guidelines. In addition, expert advice on local antibiotic resistance patterns should be sought from infectious disease or microbiology colleagues because treatment is usually begun on an empirical basis before the causative organism is identified and the antibiotic sensitivities are known. The same clinical and laboratory prognostic indices that are described for the general population apply to HIV-infected patients and should be documented on presentation.

Response to appropriate antibiotic therapy is usually rapid and is similar to that seen in the non–HIV-infected individual. Early relapse of infection after successful treatment is well described. Those HIV-infected patients who have presumed PCP, are being treated empirically with high-dose TMP/SMX, and who have infection with either *S. pneumoniae* or *H. influenzae* rather than *P. jiroveci*, may also improve. In addition, in those patients who are treated with benzylpenicillin for proved *S. pneumoniae* pneumonia but do not respond, and penicillin resistance can be discounted as the cause, it is important to consider whether there is a second pathologic process, such as PCP. Copathogens are reported in up to 20% of cases of pneumonia.

Pneumocystis jiroveci Pneumonia

Before instituting treatment, it is important to make an assessment of the severity of PCP using the history, findings on examination, arterial blood gas estimations, and chest radiographic abnormalities to stratify patients into those having mild, moderate, or severe disease (Table 30.9). This is necessary because some drugs are of unproven benefit and others are known to be ineffective for the treatment of severe disease. In

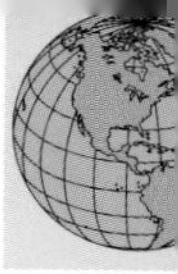

Table 30.9
Grading of severity of *Pneumocystis jiroveci* pneumonia

	Mild	Moderate	Severe
Symptoms and signs	Dyspnea on exertion with or without cough and sweats	Dyspnea on minimal exertion and occasionally at rest; cough and fever	Dyspnea and tachypnea at rest; persistent fever and cough
Oxygenation PaO_2, room air, at rest (kPa; mmHg)	>11.0; >83	8.1–11.0; 61–83	≤8.0; ≤60
SaO_2, room air, at rest (%)	>96	91–96	<91
SaO_2, on exercise (%)	>90	<90	<90
PAO_2–PaO_2 (kPa; mmHg)	<4.7; <35	4.7–6.0; 35–45	>6.0; >45
Chest radiograph	Normal or minor perihilar shadowing	Diffuse interstitial shadowing	Extensive interstitial shadowing with or without diffuse alveolar shadowing

Table 30.10
Treatment of *Pneumocystis jiroveci* pneumonia according to disease severity

	Mild	Moderate	Severe
First choice	Trimethoprim–sulfamethoxazole	Trimethoprim–sulfamethoxazole	Trimethoprim–sulfamethoxazole
Second choice	Clindamycin–primaquine	Clindamycin–primaquine	Clindamycin–primaquine
	Trimethoprim–dapsone	Trimethoprim–dapsone	Trimethoprim–dapsone
Third choice	Atovaquone	Trimetrexate–folinic acid	Trimetrexate–folinic acid
Fourth choice	Trimetrexate–folinic acid	Atovaquone	
	Intravenous pentamidine	Intravenous pentamidine	Intravenous pentamidine
Adjuvant corticosteroids	Benefit not proved	Benefit proved	Benefit proved

addition, adjuvant glucocorticoid therapy may be given to patients with moderate or severe pneumonia. Patients with glucose-6-phosphate dehydrogenase deficiency should not receive TMP/SMX, dapsone, or primaquine because these drugs increase the risk of hemolysis.

TRIMETHOPRIM-SULFAMETHOXAZOLE

Several drugs are effective in the treatment of PCP. TMP/SMX is the drug of first choice (Tables 30.10 and 30.11). Adverse reactions to TMP/SMX are common and usually become apparent between days 6 and 14 of treatment. Neutropenia and anemia (in up to 40% of patients), rash and fever (up to 30%), and biochemical abnormalities of liver function (up to 15%) are the most frequent adverse reactions. Hematologic toxicity induced by TMP/SMX is neither attenuated nor prevented by coadministration of folic or folinic acid, and use of these agents may be associated with increased therapeutic failure. During treatment with TMP/SMX, full blood count, liver function, and urea and electrolytes should be monitored at least twice weekly.

Table 30.11
Treatment schedules for *Pneumocystis jiroveci* pneumonia

Drug	Dosage	Notes
Trimethoprim–sulfamethoxazole	Trimethoprim 20mg/kg i.v. q24h and sulfamethoxazole 100mg/kg i.v. q24h in 2–4 doses for 3 days then reduced to trimethoprim 15mg/kg i.v. q24h and sulfamethoxazole 75mg/kg i.v. q24h for 14–18 further days	Dilute 1:25 in 0.9% saline infused over 90–120 minutes
	1920mg (co-trimoxazole tablets) p.o. q8h or q6h for 21 days	
Clindamycin–primaquine	Clindamycin 450–600mg i.v. or p.o. q6h and primaquine 15–30mg p.o. q24h for 21 days	Methemoglobinemia less likely if dose of 15mg p.o. q24h of dapsone is used
Pentamidine	4mg/kg i.v. q24h for 21 days	Dilute in 250mL 5% dextrose in water and infuse for 1–2h
Trimethoprim–dapsone	Trimethoprim 20mg/kg p.o. q24h in 2 or 3 divided doses and dapsone 100mg p.o. q24h for 21 days	
Trimetrexate–folinic acid	45mg/mm^2 i.v. q24h and 20mg/mm^2 i.v. p.o. q24h for 21 days	
Atovaquone	750mg p.o. q12h for 21 days	
Glucocorticoids		
Prednisolone	40mg p.o. q24h days, 1–5 40mg p.o. q24h, days 6–10 20mg p.o. q24h, days 11–21	Regimen recommended by the National Institutes of Health Consensus, widely used in the USA
Methylprednisolone	i.v., at 75% of dose given above for prednisolone	
Methylprednisolone	1g i.v. q24h, days 1–3 0.5g i.v. q24h, days 4–6 then	Regimen widely used in United Kingdom
Prednisolone	40mg p.o. q24h reducing to 0, days 7–16	
Hydrocortisone	200mg i.v. q6h, days 1–5	

NB: None of these regimens for adjuvant glucocorticoid therapy have been compared in prospective clinical trials.

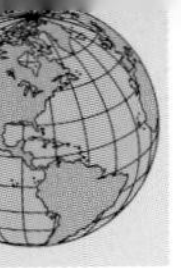

It is not known why HIV-infected individuals, especially those with higher CD4 counts, have such a high frequency of adverse reactions to TMP/SMX. Several hypotheses have been proposed, which include HIV-induced changes of acetylator status–dependent metabolism of TMP/SMX to toxic metabolites (such as hydroxylamines), alterations of immunoglobulin E synthesis or glutathione deficiency, and the immunopathogenetic effects of HIV and herpesviruses (such as Epstein-Barr virus or CMV). None of these has been confirmed in prospective studies. The optimum strategy for an HIV-infected patient who has PCP and who becomes intolerant of high-dose TMP/SMX has not been established. Many physicians "treat through" minor rash, often adding an antihistamine and a short course of oral prednisolone (30 mg every 24 hours, reducing to zero over 5 days). Desensitization has been successful in up to 75% of patients, usually with a 5- to 7-day graded increasing dosage.

OTHER THERAPY

If treatment with TMP/SMX fails, or is not tolerated by the patient, several alternative therapies are available (see Tables 30.10 and 30.11).

Clindamycin-Primaquine

The combination of clindamycin and primaquine is widely used for treatment of PCP whatever the severity, although there is no license in the United Kingdom or United States for this indication. The combination is as effective as oral TMP/SMX and oral trimethoprim-dapsone for the treatment of mild and moderate-severity disease. As a second-line treatment it is effective in up to 90% of patients. Methemoglobinemia due to primaquine occurs in up to 40% of patients. If 15 mg four times daily of primaquine is used, rather than 30 mg four times daily, the likelihood of methemoglobinemia is reduced. Diarrhea develops in up to 33% of patients receiving clindamycin; if this happens, stool samples should be analyzed for the presence of *Clostridium difficile* toxin.

Trimethoprim-Dapsone

This oral combination is as effective as oral TMP/SMX and oral clindamycin plus primaquine (see earlier) for treatment of mild and moderate-severity PCP. The combination has not been shown to be effective in patients who have severe PCP. Most patients experience methemoglobinemia (caused by dapsone), which is usually asymptomatic. Up to one half of patients have mild hyperkalemia (<6.1 mmol/L) caused by trimethoprim.

Trimetrexate

A methotrexate analog, trimetrexate, is given intravenously together with folinic acid "rescue" to protect human cells from trimetrexate-induced toxicity. In patients who have moderate to severe disease, trimetrexate-folinic acid is less effective than high-dose TMP/SMX, but serious treatment-limiting hematologic toxicity occurs less frequently with trimetrexate-folinic acid.

Atovaquone

Atovaquone is licensed for the treatment of mild and moderate-severity PCP in patients who are intolerant of TMP/SMX. In tablet formulation (no longer available), this drug was less effective, but was better tolerated than TMP/SMX or intravenous pentamidine for treatment of mild or moderate-severity PCP (see Tables 30.10 and 30.11). There are no data from prospective studies that compare the liquid formulation (which has better bioavailability) with other treatment regimens. Common adverse reactions include rash, fever, nausea and vomiting, and constipation. Absorption of atovaquone is increased if it is taken with food.

Intravenous Pentamidine

Intravenous pentamidine is now seldom used for the treatment of mild or moderate-severity PCP because of its toxicity. Intravenous pentamidine may be used in patients who have severe PCP, despite its toxicity, if other agents have failed (see Tables 30.10 and 30.11). Nephrotoxicity develops in almost 60% of patients given intravenous pentamidine (indicated by elevation in serum creatinine), leukopenia develops in approximately half, and up to 25% have symptomatic hypotension or nausea and vomiting. Hypoglycemia occurs in approximately 20% of patients. Given the long half-life of the drug, this may occur up to several days after the discontinuation of treatment. Pancreatitis is also a recognized side effect.

Adjuvant Glucocorticoids

For patients who have moderate and severe PCP, adjuvant glucocorticoid therapy reduces the risk of respiratory failure by up to half and the risk of death by up to one-third (see Tables 30.10 and 30.11). Glucocorticoids are given to HIV-infected patients with confirmed or suspected PCP who have a PaO_2 of less than 9.3 kPa (<70 mm Hg) or a $PAO_2 - PaO_2$ of greater than 4.7 kPa (>33 mm Hg). Oral or intravenous adjunctive therapy is given at the same time as (or within 72 hours of starting) specific anti–*P. jiroveci* therapy. Clearly, in some patients treatment is commenced on a presumptive basis, pending confirmation of the diagnosis as soon as possible. In prospective studies, adjuvant glucocorticoids have not been shown to be of benefit in patients with mild PCP. However, it would be difficult to demonstrate benefit because the outcome in mild disease with standard treatment is good.

GENERAL MANAGEMENT OF PNEUMOCYSTIS JIROVECI *PNEUMONIA*

Patients with mild PCP may be treated with oral TMP/SMX as outpatients if they are able to cope at home and willing to attend the outpatient clinic for regular review, and provided there is clinical and radiographic evidence of recovery. If the patient is intolerant of oral TMP/SMX despite clinical recovery, either the treatment is given intravenously or treatment may be changed to oral clindamycin plus primaquine. All patients with moderate and severe PCP should be hospitalized and given intravenous TMP/SMX or intravenous clindamycin and oral primaquine and adjuvant steroids. Patients with moderate or severe disease who show clinical and radiographic response by day 7 to 10 of therapy may be switched to oral TMP/SMX to complete the remaining 14 days of treatment. If the patient has failed to respond within 7 to 10 days or deteriorates before this time while receiving TMP/SMX, then treatment should be changed to clindamycin and primaquine, or trimetrexate plus folinic acid.

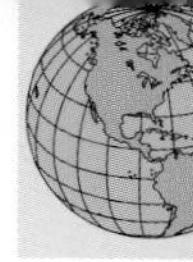

DETERIORATION IN THE PATIENT WITH PNEUMOCYSTIS JIROVECI PNEUMONIA

Deterioration in a patient who is receiving anti–*P. jiroveci* therapy may occur for several reasons (Table 30.12). Before ascribing a deterioration to treatment failure and considering a change in therapy, these alternatives should be evaluated carefully. It is also important to consider treating any copathogens present in BAL fluid, to perform bronchoscopy if the diagnosis was made empirically, to repeat the procedure, or to carry out open lung biopsy to confirm that the diagnosis is correct.

INTENSIVE CARE

Most centers advocate mechanical ventilation for first and second episodes of PCP and for acute severe deterioration after bronchoscopy. The important factors that discriminate between survivors and nonsurvivors among HIV-infected patients who have severe PCP and respiratory failure and require ventilation are the interval between starting specific anti–*P. jiroveci* therapy with adjuvant glucocorticoids and the start of mechanical ventilation, the duration of known HIV seropositivity, and the patient's CD4 lymphocyte count. Those with shorter HIV histories, CD4 counts greater than 200 cells/μL, and those who receive less than 5 days of therapy before commencing mechanical ventilation have high survival rates—approximately 50%. In contrast, those who are mechanically ventilated 5 or more days after starting treatment have mortality rates that approach 95%. Adjuvant glucocorticoid use has probably influenced the natural history of PCP-induced respiratory failure by "selecting out" a subgroup of patients with severe pneumonia in whom treatment has failed. Patients in whom pneumothoraces develop during ventilation also have a worse outcome. This reflects both the association between this complication and PCP, and also the subsequent difficulty in successful ventilation of such individuals.

Treatment of Mycobacterial Diseases

TREATMENT OF TUBERCULOSIS

The treatment of HIV-related mycobacterial disease is complicated. Not only do individuals have to take prolonged courses of relatively toxic agents, but these antimycobacterial drugs have side effects similar to those of other prescribed medications, especially HAART. Drug–drug interactions are also extremely common.

Overlapping Toxicity

Isoniazid-related peripheral neuropathy is rare in HIV-negative subjects taking pyridoxine. The nucleoside reverse transcriptase inhibitors (RTI) didanosine and stavudine can also cause a painful peripheral neuropathy. This complication develops in up to 30% of patients if stavudine and isoniazid are coadministered. Rash, fever, and biochemical hepatitis are common adverse events with rifamycins, pyrazinamide, and isoniazid (occurring more frequently in patients with tuberculosis who have HIV infection with hepatitis C coinfection). The non-nucleoside RTI drugs (e.g., nevirapine) have a similar toxicity profile. If treatment for both HIV and tuberculosis is coadministered, then ascribing a cause may be problematic.

Drug–Drug Interactions

Drug–drug interactions between medications used to treat tuberculosis and HIV infection occur because of their common pathway of metabolism, through the hepatic cytochrome P-450 enzyme system. Rifampin is a potent inducer of this enzyme (rifabutin less so), which may result in subtherapeutic levels of non-nucleoside RTI and PI antiretroviral drugs, with the potential for inadequate suppression of HIV replication and the development of resistance to HIV. In addition, the PI class of antiretroviral drugs inhibits the metabolism of rifamycins, which leads to increases in their plasma concentration and is associated with increased drug toxicity. The non-nucleoside RTI drugs are inducers of this enzyme pathway: Coadministration of rifabutin with efavirenz requires an increase in the dose of rifabutin to compensate for the increase in its metabolism induced by efavirenz (see later).

Type and Duration of Therapy for Tuberculosis

The optimal duration of treatment of tuberculosis, using a rifamycin-based regimen, in a patient who has HIV infection is unknown. Current recommendations (Joint Tuberculosis Committee of the British Thoracic Society and the American Thoracic Society) are to treat tuberculosis in HIV-infected patients in the same way as for the general population (i.e., for 6 months). The American Thoracic Society in addition recommends that treatment be extended to 9 months in those who have cavitation on the original radiograph, continuing signs, or a positive culture after 2 months of therapy.

Recent work has highlighted the increased risk for development of rifampin monoresistance in HIV-infected individuals on treatment. This is especially so if intermittent regimens are used, and may arise from a lack of efficacy of the other drugs present in the combination (e.g., intermittent isoniazid). Hence, daily medication regimens are recommended and should be closely supervised in all HIV-positive patients. Directly observed therapy (DOT) is an important although labor-intensive strategy that has the support of the World Health Organization.

When to Start Antiretroviral Therapy in a Patient with Tuberculosis

The best time to start therapy in patients being treated for tuberculosis is unknown. The clinician is faced with balancing a

Table 30.12
Causes of deterioration in an HIV-infected individual who has *Pneumocystis jiroveci* pneumonia

Cause	Notes
Severe progressive pneumonia	
Side effects of therapy	
Postbronchoscopy Pneumothorax	Sedation
Iatrogenic Drug-induced anemia	Left ventricular failure due to fluid overload
Copathology Bacterial infection	Pulmonary Kaposi's sarcoma
Wrong diagnosis	If diagnosis has been made empirically but diagnosis is really bacterial pneumonia and not *Pneumocystis jiroveci* pneumonia
Inadequate therapy	Wrong dose or route of administration Adjuvant glucocorticoids inadvertently omitted

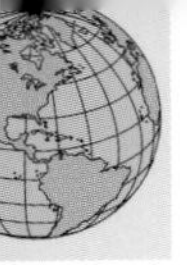

decision based on evidence that early institution of antiretroviral therapy is associated with a marked reduction in likelihood of HIV disease progression, and the risks of needing to discontinue antituberculosis therapy or HIV therapy because of drug toxicity or drug–drug interactions.

Pragmatically, delaying the start of antiretroviral therapy simplifies patient management and may reduce or prevent adverse drug reactions and drug–drug interactions, and may also reduce the risk of IRIS. Based on current evidence, patients with CD4 counts greater than 200 cells/μL have a low risk of HIV disease progression or death during 6 months of treatment for tuberculosis. In these patients, the CD4 count should be closely monitored, and antiretroviral therapy may be deferred until treatment for tuberculosis is completed. In patients who have CD4 counts from 199 to 100 cells/μL, many centers currently delay starting antiretroviral therapy until after the first 2 months of treatment for tuberculosis have been completed. In patients who have CD4 counts of less than 99 cells/μL, antiretroviral therapy is started as soon as possible after beginning treatment for tuberculosis. This is based on evidence that shows a significant short-term risk of HIV disease progression and death in this patient group if antiretroviral therapy is delayed.

Two options exist for starting antiretroviral therapy in a patient already being treated for tuberculosis. First, the rifampin-based regimen is continued and antiretroviral therapy is started with a combination of two nucleoside RTIs, and a non-nucleoside RTI, such as zidovudine and lamivudine, with efavirenz (if the patient weighs >50 kg, the efavirenz dose is increased to 800 mg once daily to compensate for rifampin-induced metabolism of efavirenz). An alternative regimen would be to use the nucleotide RTI tenofovir, with reduced-dose didanosine, and efavirenz. This regimen has the advantages of once-daily dosing and a low pill "burden." Alternatively, the rifampin is stopped and rifabutin is started: Antiretroviral therapy is given, with a combination of two nucleoside RTI drugs and either a single PI or a non-nucleoside RTI. If the latter option is chosen and efavirenz is used, then the dose of rifabutin is increased to 450 mg four times daily (see earlier).

Immune Reconstitution Inflammatory Syndrome

After initiation of antiretroviral therapy in a patient who is being treated for tuberculosis, there may be an IRIS, or "paradoxical reaction." This is characterized by development of new symptoms (fever, dyspnea), signs (lymphadenopathy, pleural effusion), or radiographic changes (parenchymal infiltrates, mediastinal adenopathy, effusion), or progression of existing abnormalities. These features are not due to failure of treatment of tuberculosis, or to another disease process. The mechanism for IRIS is thought to be antiretroviral therapy–induced partial immune reconstitution permitting an immune response to mycobacterial antigens (on both dead and alive organisms). IRIS develops in up to one third of HIV-infected patients being treated for tuberculosis when antiretroviral therapy is started. It appears to be more likely in patients who have disseminated tuberculosis, and possibly a lower baseline CD4 count. A rapid fall in HIV load as well as a large increase in CD4 counts in response to HAART also predict IRIS.

The median onset of IRIS is 15 days after antiretroviral therapy is started. Although IRIS is often self-limiting, it may persist for several months. In a patient with IRIS, it is important to exclude progressive or (multi) drug-resistant tuberculosis, poor drug adherence and drug absorption, or an alternative pathologic process as an explanation for the presentation. Glucocorticoids may be needed to control fever. Recurrent aspiration of lymph nodes or effusion may also be needed. Rarely, temporary discontinuation of antiretroviral therapy is required. In this situation there may be precipitous falls in CD4 counts and patients are at risk of other opportunistic infections.

TREATMENT OF DISSEMINATED MYCOBACTERIUM AVIUM-INTRACELLULARE *COMPLEX INFECTION*

Combination antimycobacterial therapy by itself does not cure MAC infection. A commonly used regimen is oral rifabutin (ansamycin) 300 mg once daily with oral ethambutol 15 mg/kg once daily and oral clarithromycin 500 mg once daily or every 12 hours. If clarithromycin is not used, oral rifabutin 600 mg once daily is given. Use of three drugs has no impact on overall outcome, although it reduces the risk of resistance and possibly enhances early mycobacterial killing. In patients severely compromised by symptoms, intravenous amikacin 7.5 mg/kg once daily for 2 to 4 weeks is also given. Trough blood levels must be measured to ensure toxic accumulation of amikacin does not occur. Fluoroquinolones such as moxifloxacin or ciprofloxacin may be extremely useful because they have good antimycobacterial activity with limited side effects. At present, many of these agents are not licensed for this indication.

MYCOBACTERIUM KANSASII *INFECTION*

A frequently used regimen includes rifampin, isoniazid, and ethambutol in conventional doses; all drugs are given by mouth.

Treatment of Fungal Infections

The treatment regimens for fungal infections complicating HIV infection are shown in Table 30.13.

CRYPTOCOCCOSIS

After initial treatment of cryptococcal infection there is a high likelihood of relapse of infection; hence, lifelong secondary preventative therapy is needed unless antiretroviral therapy is commenced and results in sustained improvements in CD4 counts and suppression of HIV load in peripheral blood. Secondary prophylaxis is most often oral fluconazole 200 to 400 mg four times daily.

HISTOPLASMOSIS

Oral itraconazole 100 to 200 mg four times daily is the suppressive therapy of choice. Fluconazole appears less effective as suppressive therapy. The same caveat applies as described for cryptococcosis.

COCCIDIOIDOMYCOSIS

Treatment of this infection is difficult. After initial treatment with amphotericin B, itraconazole or fluconazole may be given for long-term suppression. The overall prognosis is poor, with a 40% mortality rate despite therapy. There are no data on the impact of antiretroviral therapy on which to base decisions about secondary prophylaxis.

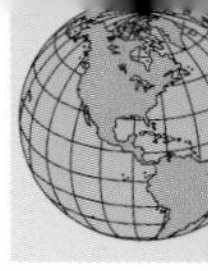

Table 30.13
Treatment of fungal pulmonary infection in HIV-infected individuals

Infectious cause	Drug	Notes
Candida spp.	Amphotericin B i.v. for 2–20 weeks	Continue until clinical/mycologic response is achieved
Aspergillus spp.	Amphotericin B 1mg/kg or Itraconazole 200mg p.o. q12h	Use for severely ill patients, monitor renal function
Cryptococcus neoformans	Amphotericin B 0.25–1.0mg/kg i.v. q24h for 2–4 weeks	Monitor renal function
	and 5-Flucytosine 25–50mg/kg	Infuse over 20–40 minutes
	or Fluconazole 200mg p.o. q12h or q8h for 2–4 weeks	
Histoplasma capsulatum	Itraconazole 200–400mg p.o. q24h for 4–6 weeks	
	or Amphotericin B 0.25–1.0mg/kg i.v. q24h	Use in severely ill patients; monitor renal function
Coccidioides immitis	Amphotericin B 0.25–1.0mg/kg i.v. q24h	Monitor renal function
Penicillium marneffei	Itraconazole 200–400mg p.o. q24h for 4–6 weeks	
	or Amphotericin B 0.25–1.0mg/kg i.v. q24h for 4–6 weeks	Use in severely ill patients

PENICILLIUM MARNEFFEI *INFECTION*

Oral itraconazole has now replaced amphotericin B as the treatment of choice for *P. marneffei* infection, apart from the subgroup who are acutely unwell. Fluconazole is less effective than itraconazole. After initial treatment, lifelong suppressive therapy with itraconazole is needed. There are no data on the impact of antiretroviral therapy on use of secondary prophylaxis.

Treatment of Parasitic Infections

The treatment regimens are shown in Table 30.14.

TOXOPLASMOSIS

A combination of sulfadiazine and pyrimethamine is the regimen of choice for *T. gondii* infection. The most frequent dose-limiting side effects are rash and fever. Adequate hydration must be maintained to avoid the risk of sulfadiazine crystalluria and obstructive uropathy. Alternative regimens are given in Table 30.14. Once treatment is completed, lifelong maintenance is necessary to prevent relapse unless antiretroviral therapy achieves adequate immune restoration.

CRYPTOSPORIDIUM *INFECTION*

This infection is often self-limiting and requires no specific therapy. Where *Cryptosporidium* species are identified with other organisms in respiratory samples, the copathologic process should be aggressively treated.

VISCERAL LEISHMANIASIS

Visceral leishmaniasis is best treated with liposomal amphotericin B. A high rate of relapse follows successful treatment. Second-line therapy (or first-line in cash-poor environments) is to use a pentavalent antimonal agent (see Table 30.14). Alternatively, the aminoglycoside paromomycin is cheap and relatively nontoxic.

Table 30.14
Treatment of parasitic pulmonary infections in HIV-infected individuals

Infectious cause	Drug	Notes
Toxoplasma gondii		
First choice	For 14–28 days: Sulfadiazine 2g p.o. q8h + Pyrimethamine 50mg p.o. q24h + Folinic acid 15mg p.o. q24h	Rash and fever are common
Second choice	For 14–28 days: Clindamycin 450–600mg p.o. q6h + Pyrimethamine 50mg p.o. q24h + Folinic acid 15 mg p.o. q24h	If diarrhea develops analyze stool for *Clostridium difficile* toxin
Third choice	For 14–28 days: Clarithromycin 2g p.o. q24h + Pyrimethamine 75mg p.o. q24h or Minocycline 100mg p.o. q12h	
Cryptosporidium spp.	Azithromycin 900mg p.o. q12h for 1 day then 600–1200mg p.o. q24h for 28 days	If nausea, vomiting, and diarrhea develop reduce the dose
Leishmania spp.		
First choice	Liposomal amphotericin B 2–3mg/kg i.v. q24h for 10 days	
Second choice	A pentavalent antimonial, either sodium stibogluconate (100mg of antimony/mL) or meglumine antimonate (85mg of antimony/mL): antimony 10–20mg/kg i.v. q24h for 3–4 weeks	
Third choice	Paromomycin 15mg/kg i.v. or i.m. q24h for 21 days	Monitor renal function
Strongyloides stercoralis	Thiabendazole 22mg/kg p.o. q12h for 2 days *or* Ivermectin 200mg/kg p.o. q24h x 4 doses over 16 days	Risk of treatment failure is higher than in non-HIV infected individuals

STRONGYLOIDES STERCORALIS *INFECTION*

The treatment of choice is thiabendazole, but risk of treatment failure with this agent in HIV-infected individuals is higher than that in patients immunosuppressed by other causes. Alternative therapy is ivermectin.

Treatment of Viral Infections

Cytomegalovirus pneumonitis is treated with intravenous ganciclovir 5 mg/kg every 12 hours, for 14 days. Drug-induced neutropenia is treated with granulocyte colony-stimulating factor. An oral formulation of ganciclovir, valganciclovir, is licensed for treatment of CMV retinitis. At a dose of 900 mg orally every 12 hours it is equivalent to intravenous ganciclovir (dose as previously). Some centers are using valganciclovir to treat CMV pneumonitis. Side effects and their management are as for ganciclovir. Phosphonoformate is now rarely used for treatment of CMV end-organ disease (e.g., pneumonitis) because of its toxicity. Cidofovir is second-line treatment for

CMV retinitis. There are no data demonstrating efficacy for cidofovir for treatment of CMV pneumonitis

CLINICAL COURSE AND PREVENTION

Within the last few years, drug therapy has radically altered the depressingly predictable nature of progressive HIV infection. Combinations of specific opportunistic infection prophylaxis and antiretroviral therapy can reduce both the incidence and the mortality associated with common conditions. The observational North American MACS cohort has demonstrated that the risk of PCP in individuals with blood CD4 counts of less than 100 cells/μL can be reduced almost fourfold if both specific prophylaxis and antiretrovirals are taken (from 47% to 13%). However, as common conditions are prevented, so other less treatable illnesses may arise.

The initial impact of *P. jiroveci* prophylaxis was to produce a reduction in incidence of PCP at the expense of an increase in cases of disseminated MAC infection, CMV infection, esophageal candidiasis, and wasting syndrome. New prophylactic therapies targeting those conditions associated with high morbidity and mortality (in particular MAC) have further improved survival. It has become apparent that specific infection prophylaxis may also confer protection against other agents. This "cross-prophylaxis" is particularly seen with the use of TMP/SMX for pneumocystosis, which also provides cover against cerebral toxoplasmosis and common bacterial infections; and with macrolides for MAC infection, which further reduce the incidence of bacterial disease and also possibly PCP. Use of large amounts of antibiotic raises the possibility of future widespread drug resistance. This is clearly of concern, and recent reports suggest that indeed in some parts of the world the incidence of pneumococcal TMP/SMX resistance is rising. Current preventive therapies pertinent to lung disease focus on *P. jiroveci*, MAC, *M. tuberculosis*, and certain bacteria (Table 30.15).

Pneumocystis jiroveci Prophylaxis

Numerous studies have demonstrated the greatly increased risk in subjects who do not take adequate drug therapy with blood CD4 counts less than 200 cells/μL. Clinical symptoms are also an independent risk factor for PCP, and hence the current guidelines recommend lifelong prophylaxis against *P. jiroveci* in HIV-infected adults who have had prior PCP, CD4 counts less than 200 cells/μL, constitutional symptoms (documented oral thrush or fever of unknown cause of >37.8°C that persists for more than 2 weeks), or clinical AIDS. The importance of secondary prophylaxis (i.e., used after an episode of PCP) becomes clear from historical data, which indicate a 60% risk of relapse in the first 12 months postinfection.

The increases in systemic and local immunity that occur with HAART have led to several studies evaluating the need for prolonged prophylaxis in individuals with sustained elevations in blood CD4 counts and low HIV RNA load. In summary, it appears that both primary and secondary PCP prophylaxis can be discontinued once CD4 counts are greater than 200 cells/μL for more than 3 months. An extra caveat that may be applied is that the patient should have a low or undetectable HIV RNA load and that the CD4 percentage is stable or rising and is greater than 14%.

The risk of PCP recurrence is real if the CD4 count falls below this level. If this does happen, PCP prophylaxis should be restarted. Similar algorithms have been successfully used for all the major infections except tuberculosis. They all rely on an estimation of the general blood CD4 count above which clinical disease is highly unlikely. For example, secondary prophylaxis of MAC may be discontinued once the blood CD4 count is consistently greater than 100 cells/μL. This is a "rule of thumb," however, and patients must be assessed on an individual basis.

TRIMETHOPRIM-SULFAMETHOXAZOLE

As with treatment strategies, TMP/SMX is the drug of choice for prophylaxis (Table 30.16). It has the advantages of being highly effective for both primary and secondary prophylaxis (with 1-year rates of PCP while on the drug being 1.5% and 3.5%, respectively). It is cheap, can be taken orally, acts systemically, and provides cross-prophylaxis against other infections, such as toxoplasmosis, *Salmonella* species, *Staphylococcus* species, and *H. influenzae*. Its main disadvantage is that adverse

Table 30.15
Prevention of respiratory infections in HIV-infected adults

Organism	Preventive method	Specific agent	Indications	Cost	Notes
Pneumocystis jiroveci	Regular drug	Trimethoprim–sulfamethoxazole (daily)	Persistent thrush, fever, AIDS, blood CD4 count <200 cells/μL	Cheap	Provides cross-protection May lead to resistance
Mycobacterium tuberculosis	Regular drug	Isoniazid (12 months)	Purified protein derivative positive Close contact with active case	Cheap	Compliance a potential problem, therefore resistance possible
Mycobacterium avium-intracellulare complex	Regular drug	Clarithromycin (daily) *or* azithromycin (weekly)	CD4 count <50 cells/μL	Expensive	Provides cross-protection May lead to resistance
Streptococcus pneumoniae	Immunization	23-Valent capsular polysaccharide (single dose)	All subjects at diagnosis	Cheap	Uncertain protection Transient increase in HIV load
Influenza virus	Immunization	Whole or split virus (yearly)	All subjects	Cheap	Uncertain protection Transient increase in HIV load

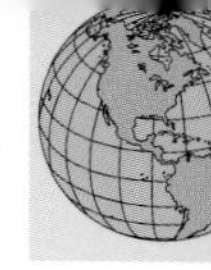

Table 30.16
Primary and secondary prophylaxis regimens for *Pneumocystis jiroveci*

Drug	Dose	Notes
Trimethoprim–sulfamethoxazole	1 double-strength[a] tablet p.o. q24h	Other options for primary prophylaxis: 1 double-strength[a] tablet p.o. q24h three times a week or 1 single-strength[b] tablet p.o. q24h
		Protects against toxoplasmosis and certain bacteria
Dapsone	100mg p.o. q24h	With pyrimethamine (25mg p.o. q24h three times a week) protects against toxoplasmosis
Pentamidine	300mg via Respirgard II (jet) nebulizer every 4 weeks	Less effective in subjects with CD4 <100 cells/μL
		Provides no cross-prophylaxis
	60mg via Fisoneb (ultrasonic) nebulizer every 2 weeks	Well tolerated (but see text)
Atovaquone suspension	750mg suspension p.o. q12h	Absorption increased if administered with food
		Protects against toxoplasmosis
Azithromycin	1250 mg p.o. once weekly	

[a]160mg trimethoprim, 800mg sulfamethoxazole
[b]80mg trimethoprim, 400mg sulfamethoxazole

reactions are common (see earlier), seen in up to 50% of individuals taking the prophylactic dose.

The standard dose of TMP/SMX is one double-strength tablet (160 mg trimethoprim, 800 mg sulfamethoxazole) per day. Other regimens have been tried; these include one "double-strength" tablet thrice weekly and one single-strength tablet per day. In general, when used for primary prophylaxis these regimens are tolerated well (if not better than the standard) and appear as efficacious as one double-strength tablet per day. The data are less clear in secondary prophylaxis, in which subjects are at a much higher risk of recurrent PCP. Attempts to desensitize patients who are intolerant of TMP/SMX have met with some success.

DAPSONE

In patients who cannot tolerate TMP/SMX, dapsone is a safe and inexpensive alternative. It has been studied in a number of trials as both primary and secondary prophylaxis, and is effective at an oral dose of 100 mg/day. When combined with pyrimethamine (25 mg thrice weekly), it provides a degree of cross-prophylaxis against toxoplasmosis. Before starting dapsone, patients are tested for glucose-6-phosphate dehydrogenase deficiency.

PENTAMIDINE

Nebulized pentamidine has largely fallen from use as a prophylactic agent. This is despite it being better tolerated and having a similar efficacy to TMP/SMX for primary preventive therapy. However, its breakthrough rate is higher in subjects who have lower CD4 counts (i.e., <100 cells/μL) and in those who take it as secondary prophylaxis. Other disadvantages include equipment costs and complexity (alveolar deposition is crucial), the risk of transmission of respiratory disease (e.g., tuberculosis) to other patients and staff during the nebulization procedure, an alteration in the clinical presentation of PCP while on pentamidine (increased frequency of radiographic upper zone shadowing, increased incidence of pneumothorax), and a lack of systemic protection against *Pneumocystis* and other infectious agents. There is also an acute bronchoconstriction effect during nebulization. Long-term follow-up studies have not demonstrated any significant negative effect on lung function.

ATOVAQUONE

Atovaquone oral suspension is used as a second-line prophylactic agent in subjects intolerant of TMP/SMX. It appears to have similar efficacy to dapsone (given together with weekly pyrimethamine), with a reduced incidence of side effects, of which the most frequent are rash, fever, and gastrointestinal disturbance.

AZITHROMYCIN

Azithromycin is used in many centers as a third-line prophylactic agent. It is given at a dose of 1250 mg once weekly, and may provide protection against some bacterial infections, as well as MAC.

PREDICTORS OF PNEUMOCYSTIS *PROPHYLAXIS FAILURE*

A low blood CD4 count (<50 cells/μL) is the current best laboratory predictor of prophylaxis failure (relative risk [RR] = 2.8 compared with blood CD4 counts of 100 to 200 cells/μL). Persistent fever of unknown cause is an important clinical risk factor for PCP (RR = 2.2). Used as preventive therapy, TMP/SMX significantly reduces the chance for development of pneumocystosis (RR = 0.5). It is therefore vital that subjects who are most vulnerable be encouraged to use this drug on a regular basis. The PSPC cohort study revealed that 21% of subjects with a CD4 count below 200 cells/μL were not receiving any form of PCP prophylaxis.

Bacterial Infection Prophylaxis

The effective and safe (i.e., replication incompetent) bacterial vaccines that are available would be expected to be widely used to prevent HIV-related disease. In fact, uptake of both the 23-valent pneumococcal and the *H. influenzae* type b (Hib) vaccines is poor (current estimates for the former are at most only 40% of the infected population). One reason for this may be because the protection conferred by vaccination (90%) in non–HIV-infected subjects is not seen in the immunosuppressed population, reflecting their inability to generate good memory B-cell responses (especially subjects with CD4 counts <200 cells/μL). However, in North America, the pneumococcal vaccine is recommended as a single dose as soon as HIV infection is diagnosed, with a booster at 5 years, or if an individual's blood CD4 count was less than 200 cells/μL and then increased on HAART. Several studies have shown that there is a benefit in this population in reducing the risk of invasive pneumococcal infection. This does not appear to be the case in a developing world setting, where not only was the 23-valent vaccine ineffective against both invasive and noninvasive pneumococcal disease, but the overall incidence of pneumonia was increased.

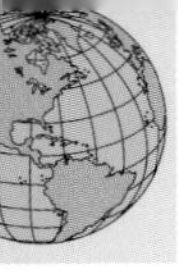

Infection with *H. influenzae* type b is much less common in HIV-infected adults and therefore immunization with Hib vaccine is not routinely recommended.

There is little evidence to suggest that the high frequency of bacterial infections in the HIV population is related to bacterial colonization. Therefore, continuous antibiotics are rarely indicated, although both TMP/SMX and the macrolides (clarithromycin and azithromycin) given as long-term prophylaxis for opportunistic infections have been shown to reduce the incidence of bacterial pneumonia, sinusitis/otitis media, and infectious diarrhea. There is little evidence, however, that TMP/SMX protects against pneumococcal infection.

Mycobacterium tuberculosis Prophylaxis

The interaction between HIV and tuberculosis is of fundamental importance because the annual risk for the development of clinical tuberculosis in a given individual is estimated to be 5% to 15% (i.e., similar to a non–HIV-infected subject's *lifetime* risk). HIV-infected individuals with pulmonary tuberculosis are less likely to be smear positive than their HIV-negative counterparts, although they can still transmit tuberculosis. Thus, within a community, tuberculosis prevention involves case-finding and treatment of active disease as well as specific prophylactic drug therapies for those exposed. If possible, HIV-positive subjects should make every effort to avoid encountering tuberculosis (e.g., at work, homeless shelter, health care facility).

One of the problems with standard methods of tuberculosis contact tracing in HIV infection is that both tuberculin skin test results and chest radiology may be unreliable. However, in the absence of bacillus Calmette-Guerin (BCG) immunization, a positive PPD (e.g., >5 mm induration with 5 tuberculin units) indicates a greatly increased risk (6- to 23-fold compared with nonanergic, PPD-negative, HIV-infected subjects) of future active disease. The chance that HIV-infected subjects may contract disseminated infection if given BCG means that (having excluded active infection) the only option in these circumstances is to use a prophylactic drug regimen. Options include 9 months of isoniazid (together with pyridoxine to prevent peripheral neuropathy). This is safe and well tolerated, although compliance is a problem and DOT may need to be instituted (e.g., 900 mg isoniazid twice weekly). There is little evidence to suggest that this single-agent regimen leads to isoniazid resistance, although the consequences of this could be catastrophic. Recent work has focused on the use of two drugs (rifampin and pyrazinamide) for short-course prophylaxis (2 months). This appears to be as effective as 12 months of isoniazid, although there have been reports of fatal hepatotoxicity (almost exclusively in the HIV-negative population). Liver function should be closely monitored and it is recommended that this regimen not be given to patients with preexisting liver disease (e.g., due to alcohol or viral hepatitis). Rifampin should not be used by subjects taking PIs. This may limit widespread application of the two-drug regimen. The same applies to combinations of isoniazid and rifampin, which are also effective in HIV-negative individuals. Alternative protocols also exist for subjects thought to be resistant to first-line prophylactic agents. These have not been widely clinically evaluated. It is recommended that HIV-infected subjects who have had close contact with an active case of tuberculosis should also receive prophylaxis. There is little evidence to suggest that anergy confers an increased risk for development of clinical disease. However, patients who have not had BCG, have a negative skin test, and have started HAART may benefit from regular skin tests because there is some evidence that cutaneous responses may return with increasing CD4 counts, and that this may help in identifying newly infected individuals requiring prophylaxis.

In populations where the prevalence of tuberculosis is low and BCG is routinely given during childhood or adolescence (e.g., the United Kingdom), the value of PPD testing is more limited. Here, an arbitrary cutoff of 10 mm for tuberculin reactions is used to define who should receive preventive therapy.

Secondary tuberculosis prophylaxis may be important because studies indicate a high rate of relapse in endemic areas. Here, no specific guidelines exist, although studies of 6 months of isoniazid and rifampin after a full treatment course show a greatly reduced risk of relapse within the subsequent 2 years. Whether this is enough to prevent clinical disease (which may also arise from reinfection in areas of high tuberculosis prevalence) without concomitant antiretroviral therapy is unclear. In the developed world, secondary prophylaxis is usually not recommended.

The use of HAART also can reduce the risk of tuberculosis in endemic areas. Work in South Africa indicates that this is most beneficial in patients with advanced disease, and leads to a reduction in RR of at least 80%.

Mycobacterium avium-intracellulare Complex Prophylaxis

Data from North America indicate that the prevention of disseminated MAC infection has an effect on survival (25% reduction in mortality rate in subjects taking clarithromycin). The U.S. guidelines advise prophylaxis with a macrolide (either clarithromycin 500 mg orally twice per day or azithromycin 1200 mg orally once a week) in all HIV-infected individuals with blood CD4 counts less than 50 cells/μL. In Europe, where the prevalence of disseminated MAC infection is probably lower (perhaps because of previous BCG vaccination), this may be less relevant. Here, surveillance cultures of blood may be more cost effective in the potentially at-risk HIV population with low CD4 counts. Routine stool and sputum cultures probably do not add much to this strategy because disseminated MAC is much more common than isolated organ disease.

Single-agent prophylaxis certainly produces a degree of antibiotic resistance (25% to 29% of subjects developed MAC while taking clarithromycin), which does not seem to be reduced by the addition of a second drug (rifabutin) to the prophylactic regimen. The latter drug is now a second-line prophylactic agent, largely as a result of its rather worse protective effect and its adverse interaction profile with PIs. As mentioned earlier, if an individual sustains a rise in CD4 count greater than 100 cells/μL for more than 6 months, it is safe to discontinue prophylaxis.

PROGNOSIS

Pneumocystis jiroveci

Several clinical and laboratory features have prognostic significance in HIV-infected individuals with PCP (Table 30.17). A severity score based on the serum LDH levels, the $PAO_2 - PaO_2$,

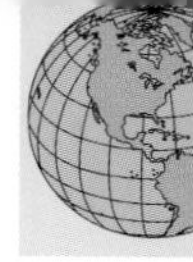

Table 30.17
Prognostic factors associated with poor outcome in *Pneumocystis jiroveci* pneumonia

On admission	No previous knowledge of HIV status
	Tachypnea (respiratory rate >30/min)
	Second or subsequent episode of *Pneumocystis jiroveci* pneumonia
	Poor oxygenation – PaO_2 <7.0kPa (<53mmHg) or PAO_2–PaO_2 >4.0kPa (>30mmHg)
	Low serum albumin (<35g/dL)
	Peripheral blood leukocytosis (>10.8 × 10^9/L)
	Marked chest radiographic abnormalities – diffuse bilateral interstitial infiltrates with or without alveolar consolidation
	Elevated serum lactate dehydrogenase levels (>300IU/L)
Following admission	Bacterial copathogen in bronchoalveolar lavage fluid or induced sputum
	Neutrophilia (>5%) in bronchoalveolar lavage fluid
	Serum lactate dehydrogenase levels that remain elevated despite specific antipneumocystis therapy.

and the percentage of neutrophils in the BAL fluid can predict survival reasonably accurately, with the highest scores indicating the worst outcome. Other workers have shown that increased age (>50 years) leads to a doubling of mortality rates—largely as a result of late, "unsuspected" diagnosis. Low blood CD4 counts of less than 25 cells/μL and CMV cultured in respiratory secretions have also been associated with poor prognosis. The overall mortality rate from an episode of PCP is currently under 10%. Recent work has suggested that patients who either are taking HAART on a regular basis at the time PCP develops or are started on antiretrovirals when unwell have a 60% reduction in mortality rate. The explanation for this is unclear but may reflect the improved immunity associated with HAART, which could either enable patients to clear their infection, or in fact could induce a transient deterioration as a result of their immune response (an IRIS effect), after which they recover from apparent PCP.

HAART has improved post-AIDS survival. In 1981, the median survival after PCP was 9 months. By 1995 this had risen to 20 months. The introduction of HAART led to a further increase, with a survival in the period up to year 2000 of 40 months.

Bacterial Infection

In general, mortality from bacterial respiratory infection in HIV-infected individuals is similar to that seen in the general population. Clinical and laboratory markers of disease severity that have been defined in the adult general population (e.g., those described in the American Thoracic Society, or the British Thoracic Society Guidelines for the management of community-acquired pneumonia in adults) apply to HIV-infected patients. These are confusion, raised respiratory rate, abnormal renal function, and low blood pressure. Recurrent pneumonias are common (reported in up to 55% of cases) and may lead to chronic pulmonary disease.

Mycobacterium tuberculosis

Although tuberculosis normally responds to standard multiple-drug therapy, work from Africa has highlighted the increased mortality rate in HIV-infected compared with non–HIV-infected individuals (RR = 17.1). A relationship has also been described between mortality and declining blood CD4 count: HIV-infected patients with CD4 counts less than 200 cells/μL have a mortality rate of 10% compared with 4% in those with CD4 counts 200 to 499 cells/μL. Compared with HIV-infected individuals without tuberculosis, the main effect on mortality is seen in patients with higher CD4 counts (>200 cells/μL), where the relative risk of death is three times that of the nontuberculous population.

Mycobacterium avium-intracellulare Complex

Several case–control studies have indicated that in the absence of effective treatments, MAC-infected patients have a reduced survival compared with blood CD4 level–matched control subjects (approximately 4 months versus 9 months, respectively). Currently available treatment regimens may reduce this difference, although severe anemia appears to be an independent predictor of mortality.

Cytomegalovirus

As mentioned previously, the presence of CMV in BAL fluid also containing *P. jiroveci* has been related to outcome. The mortality rate at 3 and 6 months after bronchoscopy is greater in those with CMV detected at bronchoscopy. However, CMV recovered as a sole pathogen does not have an impact on future survival.

PITFALLS AND CONTROVERSIES

The Effect of Antiretroviral Therapy on Opportunistic Infections

The introduction of HAART, together with the wide availability of accurate methods of determining plasma RNA viral load, has led to profound changes in both clinical practice and HIV outcome. Data indicate that clinical progression is rare in subjects who are able rigorously to adhere to at least 95% of their antiretroviral drug regimen. Mortality rates have fallen by 80% for almost all conditions, and it appears that a damaged immune system can be reconstituted. This translates to a situation where the clinician may be faced with patients whose presentation may be due to drug therapy rather than opportunistic infection or tumor. The side effect profile of HAART (e.g., metabolic and mitochondrial toxicities, liver damage, and neuropsychiatric disorders), as well the large number of drug–drug interactions, makes this a very complex area of management. The best example of this is HIV-related tuberculosis. Here, not only is there overlapping toxicity and pharmacologic interaction, but IRIS is very common. Research is needed to address this area. Studies should inform the decision on when to start HAART in patients already on antituberculosis medication.

Predictors of Disease

Despite the benefits of HAART, it is likely that in the long term many patients will progress to severe disease. There is currently little research in this area. Research should focus on

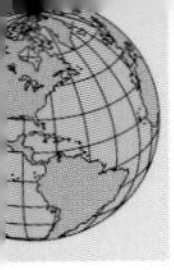

correlating clinical and laboratory findings. An example of this would be assessing the risk of an individual for development of active tuberculosis. It is clear that much of the excess mortality in HIV–tuberculosis coinfection occurs early in HIV infection. Thus, if tests can be devised that indicate who has latent tuberculosis infection (and who is therefore most likely to develop clinical disease), steps can be taken to prevent illness. The use of enzyme-linked immunospot (ELISPOT) blood tests, which measure specific CD4 cell reactivity against mycobacterial antigens, offers considerable promise. The difficulty here (apart from the cost) is that these rely on CD4 effects, which are diminished in HIV infection. Currently it is research laboratory based, and the test would need to work in a field setting if it were to be of value in the developing world. The advantages include its sensitivity (far greater than tuberculin skin tests) and the fact that it is unaffected by previous BCG immunization.

The other role for a test such as this would be in rapid diagnostics. It is common to be faced with a patient who has nonspecific symptoms and a wide differential diagnosis. Often treatment is multiple and empirical. A quantitative test would help resolve some of these dilemmas by indicating the chance of the condition being due to a particular disease. An example would be the patient from an endemic tuberculosis area, with low CD4 counts who has both pulmonary and central nervous system disease. Is this tuberculosis, toxoplasmosis, cryptococcosis, or viral or bacterial infection?

Rapid diagnostic assays that assess organism viability are also important. If a clinician can receive early feedback on whether treatment is producing a suitable killing effect, then therapy can be tailored to the individual. This enables regimens to be "dose adjusted" as needed and removes the element of concern that is often present when patients are slow to respond. Examples of this would be in the treatment of PCP or mycobacterial disease.

Pneumocystis jiroveci

Newer methods of diagnosis (e.g., PCR tests on saliva) may prove invaluable for quick and easy disease confirmation, although their applicability to routine samples needs further evaluation.

P. jiroveci prophylaxis was the first important HIV treatment widely available. However, despite the efficacy of TMP/SMX, compliance remains a problem. Regimens that use a gradual increase in dosage when starting prophylaxis may help. One concern with widespread use of prophylaxis is that resistance will start to occur to TMP/SMX. Reports have indicated that there are mutations in the *P. jiroveci* dihydropteroate synthetase gene that confer resistance. These seem to be increasing over time, although they do not appear to be present in many patients who fail treatment for PCP with TMP/SMX. The implications of this are uncertain, but are bound to affect the current policy in the developing world of using regular TMP/SMX as infection prophylaxis in large numbers of HIV-infected subjects. Presumably this also will have an impact on bacterial resistance patterns.

Bacterial Infections

The frequency of bacterial infection (often recurrent) with its attendant sequelae makes effective strategies for vaccination an important priority. It is uncertain why there is a differential response to vaccination—even in the United States, African Americans do not seem to derive the same benefit as whites. This needs further research, together with more emphasis on identifying the local immune response present in the lung in such individuals.

Bacterial infections may be clinically indistinguishable from other pathogens, and only two thirds of all respiratory infections are formally diagnosed. There is a need for improved methods to assist with this. The use of rapid antigen tests may be one way forward. This is especially the case given the high incidence of (potentially fatal) bacteremia present in such populations. For maximum benefit, this needs to use a system that is simple and cheap, in developing as well as developed countries.

Mycobacterial Diseases

M. tuberculosis is globally the most important HIV-related pathogen. Much of the preceding discussion has focused on this organism. Strategies of control and prevention are vital to ensure that millions of people do not become coinfected and that those who are do not go on to development of clinical disease. Beyond public health measures, such as DOT, fixed-dose combination drugs, case management, and education, research needs to improve on current drug therapy. Long-acting preparations such as rifapentine show promise but, as the problem with rifampicin monoresistance demonstrates, there is still much work to be done.

Vaccination against *M. tuberculosis* using BCG has understandably not been widely used in this immunosuppressed population. However, a safe vaccine may be the only affordable way to protect large parts of the world from tuberculosis. It was hoped that use of immunotherapy with heat-killed *Mycobacterium vaccae*, in combination with chemotherapy, would improve outcome. Unfortunately, a recent trial has shown no benefit over placebo when combined with standard treatment. However, this is an area needing urgent attention, and given the commitment shown by charities such as the Gates Foundation, it is hoped that research and progress will continue.

Smoking-Related Diseases

HIV-infected populations in the developed world have high rates of smoking. The evidence that this is harmful above those effects seen in the general population continues to accrue. The accelerated course of both obstructive lung disease and cancer, together with the increased risk of respiratory infection in smokers, persuasively argues the case for targeted smoking cessation. That HAART has profound (and probably negative) effects on blood lipids and insulin resistance further supports the need to reduce smoking rates in this population. It is predicted that there may soon be an epidemic of cardiovascular disease in "healthy" HIV-infected individuals.

The natural history of HIV-related respiratory disease continues to evolve. HAART and newer therapeutic strategies have made a significant impact on morbidity and mortality. Yet individuals continue to become HIV infected, progress, and die from an ever-expanding range of conditions. *P. jiroveci* remains the most common AIDS-defining event in the developed world, whereas *M. tuberculosis* is globally the most common cause of death. Bacterial respiratory infection is not far behind. Given the huge number of individuals with HIV infection, the only effective way to manage this disease is to find simple ways of treating HIV itself, and thus contain the worst ravages of this illness.

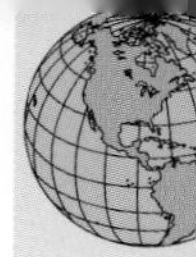

SUGGESTED READINGS

Burman WJ, Jones BE: Treatment of HIV-related tuberculosis in the era of effective antiretroviral therapy. Am J Respir Crit Care Med 164:7-12, 2001.

Castro M: Treatment and prophylaxis of *Pneumocystis carinii* pneumonia. Semin Respir Infect 13:296-303, 1998.

Masur H, Kaplan JE, Holmes K: Guidelines for preventing opportunistic infections among HIV-infected persons—2002. Recommendations of the U.S. Public Health Service and the Infectious Diseases Society of America. Ann Intern Med 137:435-478, 2002.

Miller RF: Prophylaxis of *Pneumocystis carinii* pneumonia: Too much of a good thing? Thorax 55(suppl 1):S15-S22, 2000.

Semple SJG, Miller RF (eds): AIDS and the Lung. Oxford, Blackwell Scientific, 1997.

Stringer JR, Beard CB, Miller RF, Wakefield AE: A new name (*Pneumocystis jiroveci*) for pneumocystis from humans. Emerg Infect Dis 8:891-896, 2002.

Zumla A, Johnson MA, Miller R (eds): AIDS and Respiratory Medicine. London, Chapman & Hall, 1997.

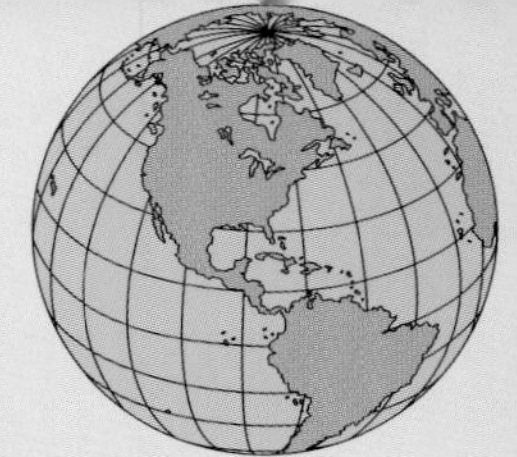

SECTION 8
Acquired Immunodeficiency Syndrome and the Lung

CHAPTER 31

Noninfectious Conditions

Gianpietro Semenzato, Carlo Agostini, Venerino Poletti

Although most lung complications that occur during the clinical course of human immunodeficiency virus (HIV) arise from infection, especially early in the disease, HIV-infected patients may present with mild respiratory complications related to alterations in local immune regulation (Table 31.1). A marked CD8 T-cell infiltration in the lung may be caused by HIV in both asymptomatic and symptomatic patients; the vast majority of pulmonary T cells are cytotoxic T lymphocytes (CTL) selectively directed against HIV-infected cells. In some HIV-infected individuals, macrophages may accumulate within the alveolar space and produce macrophage alveolitis, which presumably reflects specific immune responses. The effects of HIV on the pulmonary microenvironment include a progressive decline in local immunocompetence that results in failure to mount a protective immune response against opportunist infections (immunodeficiency). The spectrum of noninfectious complications associated with HIV infection encompasses other idiopathic conditions and pulmonary malignancies, which include Kaposi sarcoma (KS), Hodgkin's and non-Hodgkin's lymphomas (NHLs), and solid tumors (see Table 31.1). After the introduction of the highly active antiretroviral therapy (HAART), the clinical spectrum of HIV-associated pulmonary complications has extended because it has been reported that the partial restoration of immune function from HAART administration may lead to an unusual tissue response in the pulmonary microenvironment.

PATHOPHYSIOLOGY

Bronchoalveolar lavage (BAL) provides access to lung cell populations, bringing immunologic and virologic studies closer to the focus of inflammatory events and permits evaluation of cellular abnormalities that might represent the effects of retroviral infection on host lung defenses (Figure 31.1).

The several patterns in which HIV causes noninfective pulmonary infiltrations are described briefly here.

HIV Infection of the Lung

After primary infection, HIV disseminates throughout the body and is sequestered in secondary lymphoid tissues. Extracellular virions are trapped in the follicular dendritic cell network, which represents a continuous source of infection for lymphoid cells. With the onset of acquired immunodeficiency syndrome (AIDS), destruction of the follicular, dendritic cell network in the lymph nodes leads to an inability to trap extracellular virions and favors HIV redistribution beyond the secondary lymphoid tissues. Because the lung can be considered a classic tertiary lymphoid organ, it is not surprising that HIV spreads early to the resident cell populations of the lung. Alveolar and interstitial macrophages, pulmonary T lymphocytes (both $CD4^+$ and $CD8^+$), and lung fibroblasts can be infected by the etiologic agent of AIDS from the early phases of the infection. The intraalveolar presence of HIV-infected cells evokes a discrete CTL immune response, the principal by which retroviral infection is cleared from the pulmonary environment. Alveolar macrophages release a broad array of mediators of inflammation, such as monokines, proinflammatory cytokines, chemokines, and growth factors relevant to the development of effector mechanisms that account for the clearance of the virus.

Alveolitis Associated with HIV in Asymptomatic Patients Who Have No Respiratory Illness

The presence of HIV may cause marked increases in the number of immunocompetent cells in the lungs (lymphocytic and macrophagic alveolitis) of asymptomatic patients even when no infection is detectable. The alveolitis is observed in every HIV risk group and is mild in the majority of patients, but some cases may develop a true lymphoid interstitial pneumonitis (LIP, see following sections). The term *nonspecific interstitial pneumonitis* (NSIP) has been proposed for HIV patients who have clinical and functional signs of respiratory dysfunction in the absence of opportunistic infections or detectable lung neoplasms (see following sections).

Lymphocytic alveolitis results mainly from the oligoclonal expansion of major histocompatibility complex (MHC)-restricted $CD8^+$ CTLs, which recognize and attack HIV structural proteins on the surface of infected cells. The high number of HIV-specific CTLs confers a resistant state against the spread of HIV into the surrounding microenvironment. The persistence of lymphocytic alveolitis and a strong HIV-specific CTL activity is also observed in long-term nonprogressors. In contrast, when an impairment of CTL efficiency is demonstrated during the clinical course of HIV disease, the loss of lytic function is usually associated with progression of pulmonary disease and the development of opportunistic infections.

The mechanisms that result in the local accumulation of alveolar macrophages (macrophagic alveolitis) are also nonspecific, because the phenomenon has been demonstrated in both HIV-seropositive individuals who have and do not have lung infections or other respiratory diseases. Colony stimulating factors (CSFs) able to induce the replication of macrophages, such as granulocyte macrophage (GM)-CSF, and chemokines for monocyte macrophages are crucial in the control of infiltration of macrophages, and thus in macrophage alveolitis development. Acting as antigen-presenting cells (APC), alveolar macrophages

Table 31.1
Noninfectious pulmonary complications associated with human immunodeficiency virus infection

Idiopathic and immunologic manifestations	Malignancies
Alveolitis in asymptomatics associated with human immunodeficiency virus	Kaposi's sarcoma
Nonspecific interstitial pneumonitis	Non-Hodgkin's lymphomas
Lymphoid interstitial pneumonitis	Hodgkin's lymphoma
Local immunodeficiency	Lung cancer
Bronchiolitis obliterans organizing pneumonia	
Pulmonary hypertension	

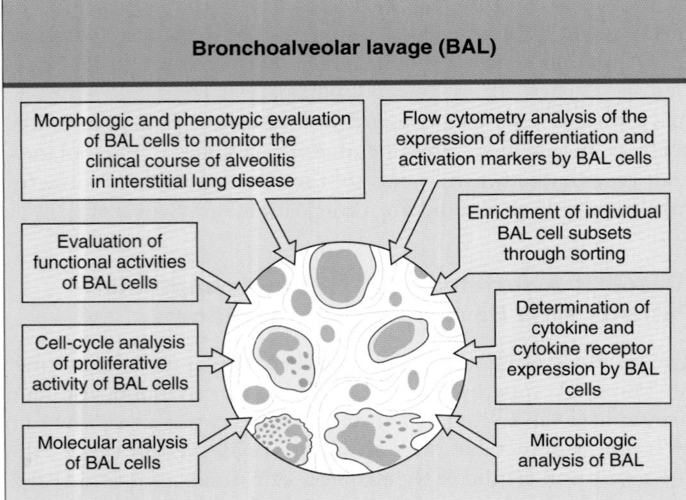

Figure 31.1 Bronchoalveolar lavage (BAL): an open window on the respiratory tract. This is a useful and safe way to sample cellular components from the respiratory tract. Modern molecular biology techniques have refined diagnostic tools used to detect infectious microorganisms and to evaluate human immunodeficiency virus (HIV) tropism for different BAL cell populations. With the availability of pure recombinant cytokines and molecular probes for cytokines and their receptors, it is possible to study the involvement of several cytokines in the pathologic changes associated with autoimmune deficiency syndrome. Also, BAL cells can be stained for flow cytometric analysis. This technique is used in clinical practice to study lung diseases characterized by a lymphocytic alveolitis, to provide information about the activation state of pulmonary immunocompetent cells, and to determine the expression of cytokines and cytokine receptors on BAL immunocompetent cells. A variety of tests are also available to determine pulmonary T, B, and natural killer lymphocyte functional activities during HIV disease.

also release biologic mediators relevant to the expansion of effector mechanisms that clear invading microorganisms. Thus, in an immunocompetent individual, an increased number of tissue macrophages may help trigger a relatively effective, cell-mediated immune response against single microorganisms or HIV itself.

Nonspecific Interstitial Pneumonitis

Those HIV-seropositive individuals who show evidence of lung disease may have a high-intensity alveolitis associated with a reduction in pulmonary function. It is likely that underlying infectious and noninfectious insults can trigger lung damage. Subclinical pneumonitis might induce the chronic release of macrophage-derived cytokines, including tumor necrosis factor-α (TNF-α). By inducing damage to alveolar epithelial cells, the release of the cytokine could also enhance the probability that opportunistic organisms colonize lung tissue, and result in a decline in pulmonary function. Finally, immune responses elicited by pathogens may trigger extracellular degranulation of neutrophils present in the respiratory tract, and thus significantly contribute to the injury of alveolar structures.

Lymphoid Interstitial Pneumonitis

The first reports to describe HIV with LIP in children appeared in 1983. Pulmonary lymphoid hyperplasia, follicular bronchitis or bronchiolitis, and widespread lymphoid infiltrate that extended to the alveolar interstitium were the characteristic histopathologic findings. In adults, the lymphoid infiltrate is milder and mainly peribronchiolar (lymphocyte bronchiolitis); as in NSIP, concomitant morphologic pulmonary lesions may be observed—areas of intraalveolar, loose fibrosis (bronchiolitis obliterans organizing pneumonia [BOOP] pattern), and honeycombing. Noncaseating granulomas have occasionally been reported in HIV-associated LIP.

Local Immunodeficiency Induced by HIV

Patients who have HIV infection that shows relatively intact local immunocompetence characteristically have HIV-related alveolitis, LIP, and NSIP. Nonetheless, with time, the majority of patients experience several infectious pulmonary complications that result from the local immunodeficiency induced by the retrovirus. In general, a close association is found between the development of pulmonary opportunistic infections and the progressive decline in lung $CD4^+$ T cells. Tissue CD4 T cells are needed to maintain an effective T-cell–mediated immune response against pathogens, which explains why HIV-induced impairment of CD4 T cells leads to an increased susceptibility to pulmonary infections.

Shifts in the helper T (TH) cells TH1-TH2 regulatory networks are also important in determining the progressive impairment of local immunocompetence (Figure 31.2).

Although pulmonary lymphocytes that express the CD4 receptor are the principal cell target for HIV, lung $CD8^+$ T cells of most patients who have AIDS present with an unexpected in vivo HIV infectivity. This has crucial implications for understanding a second mechanism that contributes to progressive immunodeficiency; that is, the progressive fall in lytic activity and effectiveness of pulmonary CTL. Repeated contacts that occur in the lung microenvironment between HIV-specific CTL and relevant targets and the recruitment of HIV-infected precursors ultimately results in the infection of the CD8 cell compartment (Figure 31.3).

Bronchiolitis Obliterans Organizing Pneumonia

The term BOOP defines a characteristic clinicopathologic condition characterized by a pneumonia-like syndrome that manifests with a nonspecific pattern of alveolar damage and formation of granulation tissue (Masson body) in alveoli, ducts, and small airways (Figure 31.4; see Chapter 46).

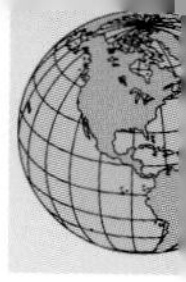

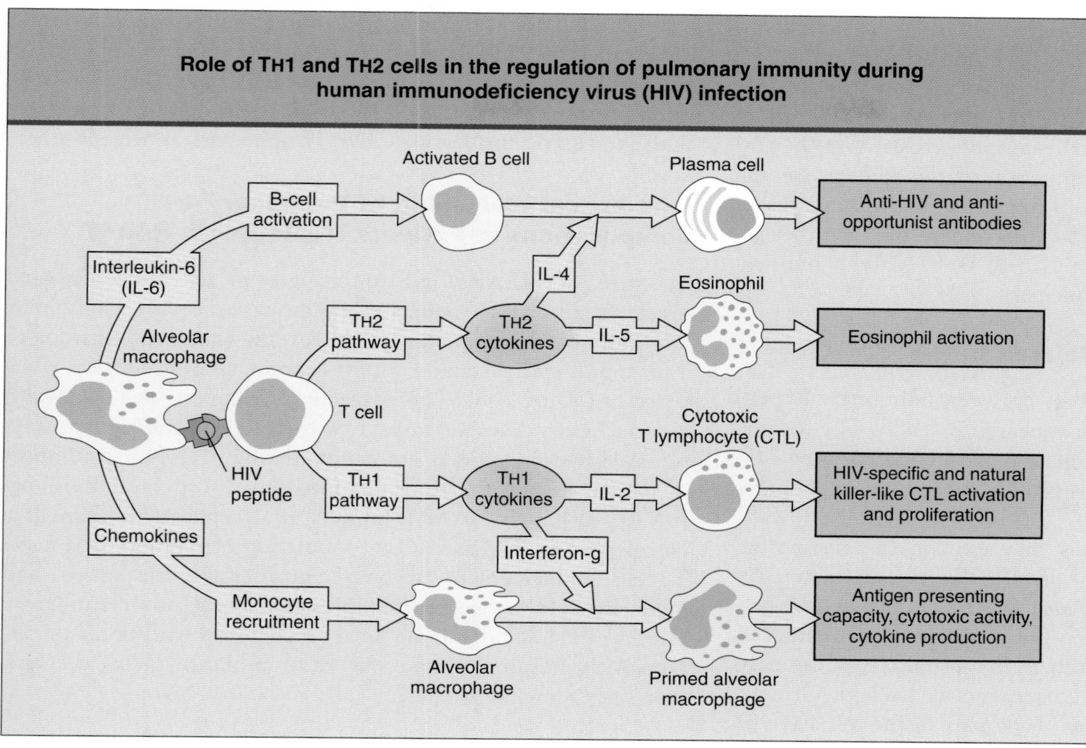

Figure 31.2 Helper T-cells 1 (TH1) and TH2 immune response in the human immunodeficiency virus (HIV) lung. At least in the early phases of HIV disease, pulmonary macrophage-derived cytokines promote a TH1-like pulmonary inflammatory response, which in turn favors the development of CD8 alveolitis and elicits further activation of the macrophage component of the alveolitis. As the disease progresses, a loss of the pulmonary TH1-like response occurs with relative preservation of the TH2-like function. This perturbation is likely to play a role in the loss of the local, protective cell-mediated responses to HIV and intracellular pathogens.

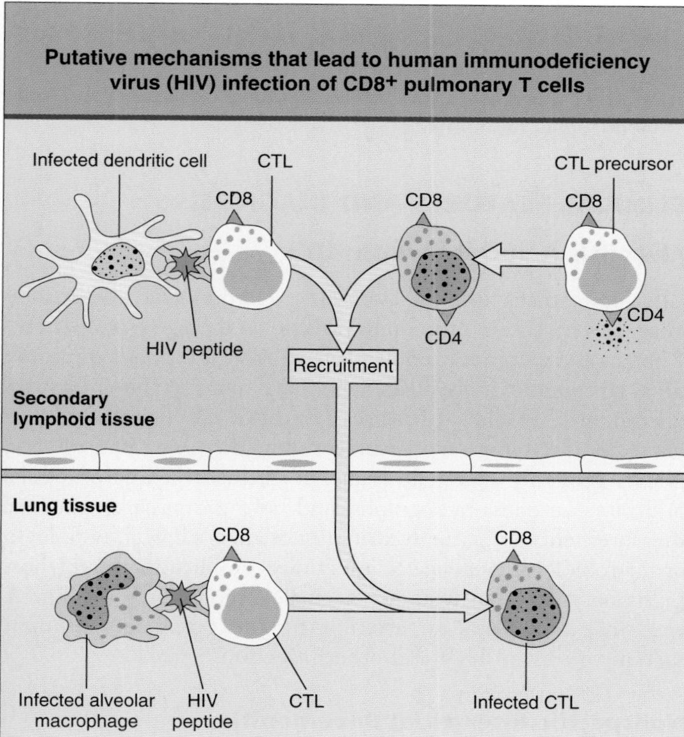

Figure 31.3 Mechanisms leading to the decrease in lytic activity of lung cytotoxic T lymphocytes (CTLs). Lung $CD8^+$ T cells may be infected by human immunodeficiency virus (HIV), which leads to the progressive loss of in situ cytotoxic activity and, ultimately, to the progression of pulmonary disease. The virus may be transmitted to CTLs through cell-to-cell contact between persistently infected CD4 cells and CD8 CTLs. An additional hypothesis is that pulmonary, HIV-specific CTLs derive from T-cell precursors that transiently coexpress both CD4 and CD8 determinants in secondary follicles in which trapped extracellular virions are present.

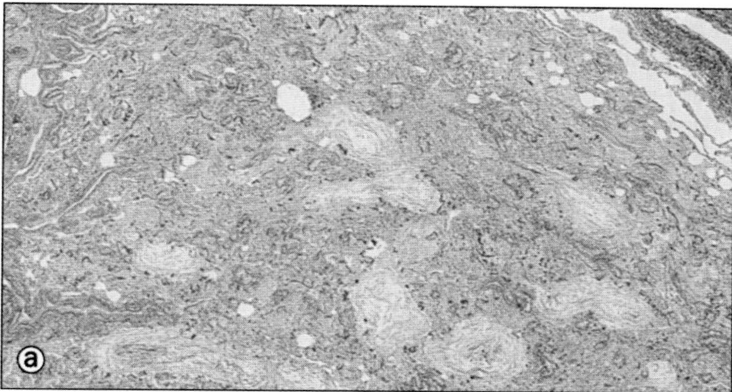

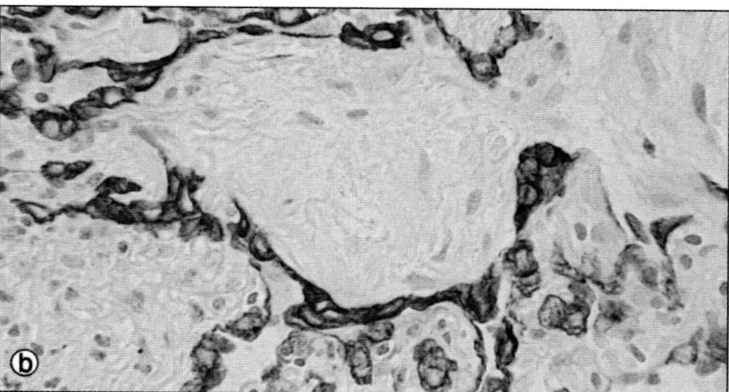

Figure 31.4 Histologic and immunohistochemical characteristics of bronchiolitis obliterans organizing pneumonia. **A.** Histopathologic evaluation reveals foci of intraalveolar fibrosis; note the variation in shape from round to oval, or serpiginous aspect. This phenomenon occurs because areas of fibrosis conform to the shape of alveolar ducts and alveoli (Van Gieson-elastic fibers). **B.** An intraalveolar fibrotic bud is surrounded by hyperplastic type II pneumocytes marked by positive immunostaining (peroxidase-antiperoxidase staining with anticytokeratin CK116 monoclonal antibody).

The pathogenesis of HIV-related BOOP is unknown. Although HIV-infected target cells have not been identified in BOOP lesions, it is possible that the retroviral infection of the respiratory airways may account for the excessive proliferation of granulation tissue and the $CD8^+$ lymphocytosis. Whether or not a latent or persistent HIV infection of the alveolar lumen may favor the epithelium injury together with the altered immune response characterized by the release of a number of cytokines (GM-CSF, interleukin [IL]-8, IL-6, platelet derived growth factor [PDGF]) is still unclear.

Pulmonary Hypertension Related to HIV

The first reports of the association between pulmonary hypertension (PH) and HIV infection appeared in 1987. The former may be associated with both idiopathic and HIV-associated LIP. An association with membranous proliferative glomerulonephritis has also been noted.

An immunologic pathogenesis may explain the distinctive proliferation of plexiform lesions of HIV-PH: this characteristic pattern might reflect a host response to HIV, determined by one or more human leukocyte antigen-DR alleles located within the MHC. However, how HIV induces hypertensive pulmonary vascular diseases in HIV-infected patients is unclear. Growth factors, in particular PDGF, may play a part in the initiation or progression of PH.

Histologically, plexiform pulmonary lesions are found more frequently in the small, muscular arteries of the lung, immediately distal to a site of ramification (Figure 31.5). They consist of local dilatation of arteries. The aneurysmal expansion contains a distinctive proliferation of tiny vascular channels lined by factor VIII positive cells. Less frequently, thrombotic arteriopathy or venoocclusive disease is the morphologic basis of HIV-related PH.

Airway Diseases

Airway disease and emphysema may be associated with HIV infection and opportunistic infections. In particular, an emphysema-like condition has been recognized in the lungs of young HIV-infected smokers, suggesting the presence of pathogenic synergies between HIV infection and smoking. There are also data indicating that cytotoxic T lymphocytes are implicated in the pathogenesis of airway disease in HIV disease, because computed tomographic studies show that emphysema correlates with increased numbers of $CD8^+$ lymphocytes in the alveoli.

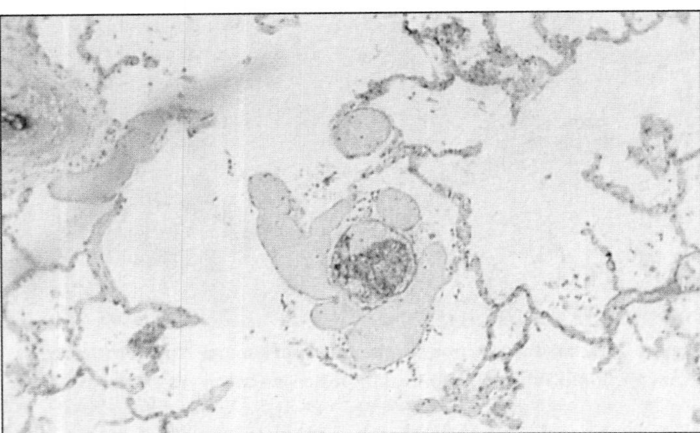

Figure 31.5 Histopathologic evaluation of pulmonary plexiform hypertension. Histopathologic evaluation shows an atypical plexiform lesion. An intraacinar artery is surrounded by a proliferation of aneurysmatic, thin-walled vascular channels (peroxidase-antiperoxidase staining with anti-CD34 monoclonal antibody).

Paradoxical Worsening of Pulmonary Complications in Patients Treated with HAART

The use of HAART led to changes in the incidence and presentation of HIV-associated pulmonary diseases. Combining inhibitors of HIV-1 protease and reverse transcriptase leads to a profound and sustained suppression of viral replication along a rise in CD4+ cells. This favors improvements in HIV health care and has a dramatic impact on the rates of pulmonary infections. However, reports are accumulating of growing numbers of patients suffering from inflammatory disorders of the lung. In fact, although HAART inhibits viral replication, there is a corresponding increase in the population of memory and naive T cells, enhancement of lymphoproliferative responses, and increased cytokine receptor expression. These proinflammatory effects of HAART underlie newly recognized syndromes associated with immunological reconstitution and involving the lung (see the following section).

Pulmonary Malignancies in HIV Infection

Pulmonary KS and intrathoracic manifestations of NHLs are relatively frequent complications of HIV infection. Other tumors have occasionally been reported to affect the lung in HIV-infected subjects, including Hodgkin's disease (HD) and bronchogenic carcinoma.

CLINICAL FEATURES AND DIAGNOSIS

Alveolitis Associated with HIV

Clinical features of HIV-associated lymphocytic and macrophagic alveolitis are extremely variable, and range from patients who are asymptomatic, and thus have no respiratory symptoms, to symptomatic individuals who have nonspecific interstitial pneumonitis or clinical features typical of LIP (see the following section). Asymptomatic subjects who do not have respiratory illness generally show no signs of diffuse or micro-nodular infiltrates on chest radiographs, and have normal arterial blood measurements. In patients who do not show clinical, radiologic, or microbiologic evidence of infectious complications and whose pulmonary function tests are normal, alveolitis may be beneficial since it reflects an attempt by the pulmonary immune system to control HIV and other infectious agents.

Nonspecific Interstitial Pneumonitis

Clinical experience suggests, however, that the development of an alveolitis is not always beneficial. Some HIV-infected patients who have no identifiable lung infections or neoplasms have reduced mean carbon monoxide transfer factor values and accelerated technetium-99m diethylenetriamine penta-acetic acid clearance. Histopathologic evaluation in these patients reveals mild, diffuse alveolar damage, a peribronchial infiltrate of CD8 T cells, and macrophages and patchy areas of fibrosis (Figure

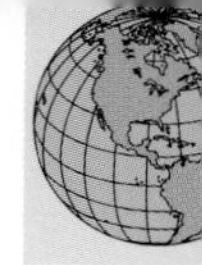

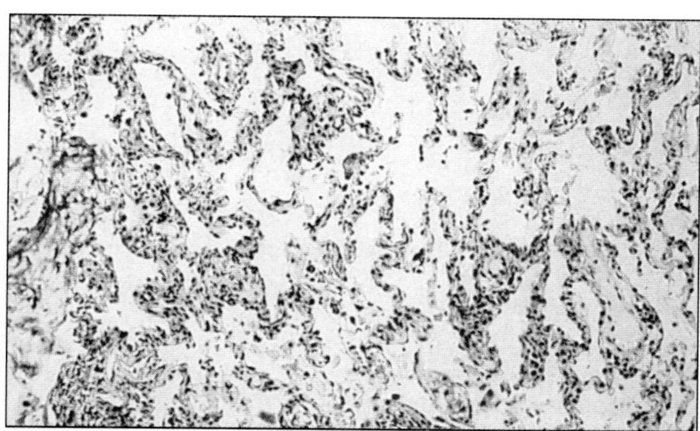

Figure 31.6 Transbronchial lung biopsy from a patient infected by human immunodeficiency virus who showed typical, nonspecific, interstitial pneumonitis. Histopathologic evaluation reveals a mild lymphoid interstitial infiltrate and scattered alveolar buds of granulation tissue rich in extracellular matrix (Giemsa).

31.6). The term *nonspecific interstitial pneumonitis* has been proposed for episodes of symptomatic interstitial pneumonitis in HIV-infected patients who have no evident infections or neoplasms.

Most patients who have NSIP show mild symptoms, which include nonproductive cough, mild dyspnea, and occasionally fever. Rales are often heard. Chest radiographs are either normal or show nonspecific, bilateral reticulonodular or interstitial infiltrates. Mild arterial hypoxemia may be present. Although NSIP may resolve spontaneously, in some individuals the alveolitis persists, which results in significant lung damage and chronic hypoxemia. Not all patients who have NSIP can be classified as having an HIV-related, infiltrative immune disorder. In individuals who present with progressive dyspnea, chronic productive cough, malaise, persistent fever, or diffuse interstitial infiltrates, the presence of an underlying infectious complication, such as *Pneumocystis jiroveci*, must be ruled out. Although symptoms, physical findings, and blood gas values may be quite similar, it is usually possible to differentiate NSIP from *P. jiroveci* pneumonia on the basis of the higher weight, serum albumin levels, and CD4 T-cell counts; furthermore, lactate dehydrogenase levels are usually normal in patients who have NSIP.

LIP

A clinicopathologic entity, LIP is characterized by massive, pulmonary alveolar-septal infiltration of small lymphocytes admixed with plasma cells, immunoblasts, histiocytes (sometimes aggregated in non-necrotizing granulomas), and other inflammatory cells (Figure 31.7). From a clinical point of view, LIP is characterized by fever, cough, dyspnea, and interstitial and consolidative infiltrates. In the pre-AIDS era, LIP was associated with autoimmune disorders or congenital immunodeficiency, and in the majority of these patients the lymphocytic infiltrate was predominantly sustained by polyclonal B cells in the lymphoid nodules and by T cells in the alveolar walls. Familial LIP has been described in some patients. There is also anecdotal evidence of progression from LIP to polyclonal or monoclonal B lymphomas.

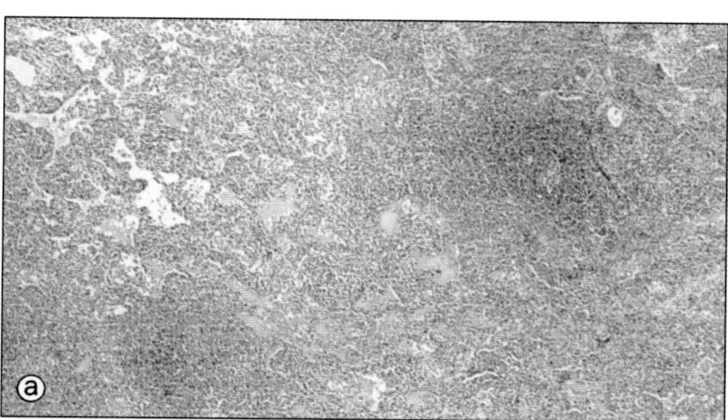

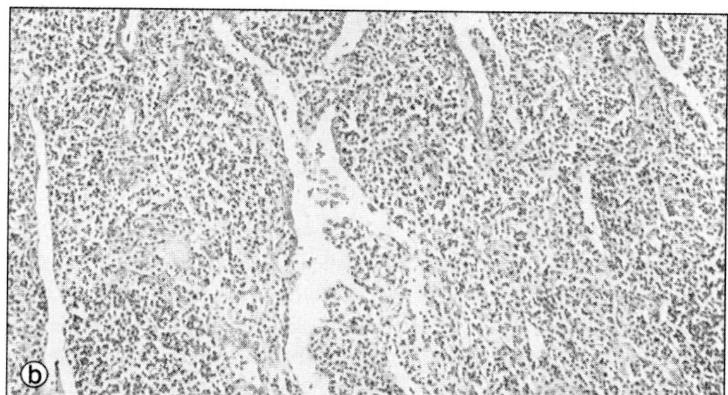

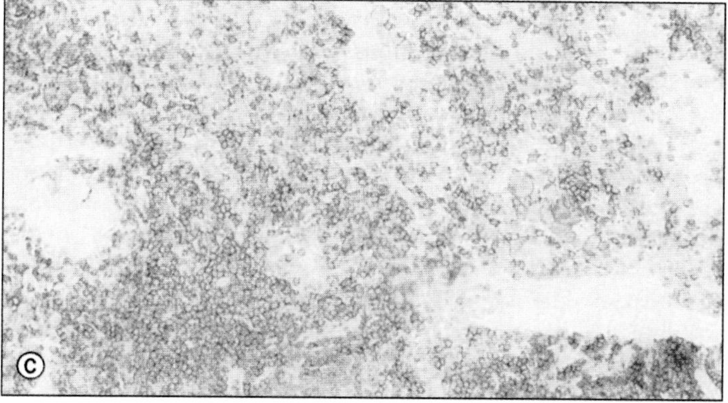

Figure 31.7 Open lung biopsy from a patient infected by human immunodeficiency virus showing the histologic and immunohistochemical characteristics of lymphoid interstitial pneumonitis. **A.** Histopathologic evaluation reveals a dense, diffuse lymphoid interstitial infiltrate with germinal centers (hematoxylin and eosin [H&E] stain). **B, C.** The vast majority of lymphoid cells are marked by a CD8 monoclonal antibody—**B.** H&E and **C.** peroxidase-antiperoxidase staining of CD8 positive cells.

The clinical manifestations are often nonspecific. Gradual, progressive dyspnea, cough, weight loss, and fever are frequent. In children and in a third of all adults, hepatosplenomegaly, systemic lymphadenopathy, and parotid enlargement may occur. Finger clubbing is a common feature in pediatric LIP, whereas rales are more frequent in adults. In most cases, especially atypical or rapidly progressing cases, the diagnosis is definitively made by histopathologic evaluation of open lung biopsies. Invasive approaches are often required to obtain a definitive diagnosis, because LIP may mimic pulmonary infections (e.g., *P. jiroveci* pneumonia or pulmonary tuberculosis), and in turn

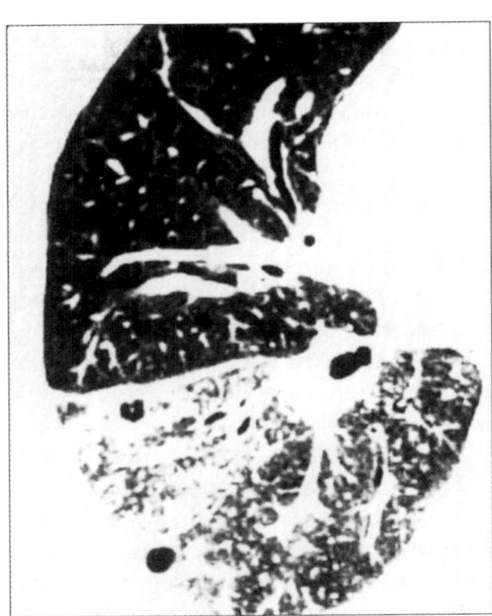

Figure 31.8 Lymphoid interstitial pneumonitis. High-resolution computed tomography demonstrates a reticulonodular pattern, more prominent in the lower right lobe. Some "holes," secondary to peripheral air trapping, are present.

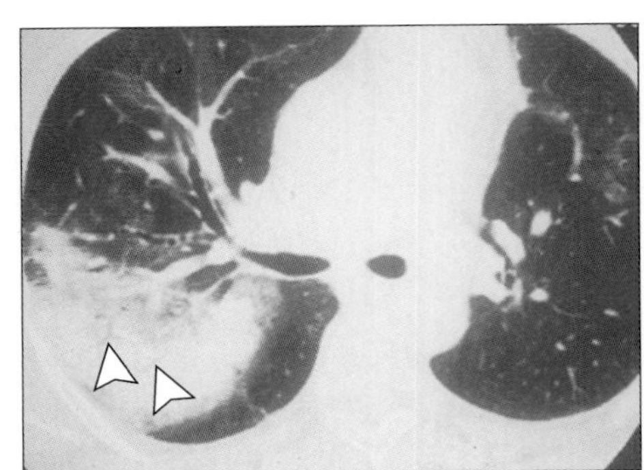

Figure 31.9 Bronchiolitis obliterans organizing pneumonia. High-resolution computed tomography shows alveolar opacifications (arrowheads); areas of patchy, ground-glass attenuation are evident in the left lung.

pulmonary infections may complicate the clinical course of patients who have LIP, who are particularly susceptible to bacterial infections. However, chest radiographs are frequently inconclusive—LIP patients may present with reticular or nodular opacities, or consolidation, which often predominate in the lower lobe. On high-resolution computed tomography (HRCT), patchy ground-glass attenuation or well-defined centrilobular nodules are seen frequently (Figure 31.8). Multiple cysts throughout the respiratory tract were described recently. In other patients, conventional chest radiographs and HRCT may demonstrate fibrotic changes and bronchiectasias after a protracted course of LIP. Abnormalities of pulmonary function are nonspecific—a restrictive pattern with a reduced or normal diffusion capacity is most common, but obstructive airway disease may also be observed. The risk of obstructive sleep apnea secondary to the adenoidal and tonsil hyperplasia is possible in children. Low partial pressure of arterial oxygen and an increase in the alveolar-arterial gradient may be present. An association of LIP and smooth muscle tumors has been reported in children.

Lymphoepithelial cysts (LEC) as manifestations of an HIV-induced autoimmune syndrome may occur in salivary glands and less frequently in thymus and lungs of patients with HIV infection. Pulmonary LEC are lined by pseudostratified columnar epithelium permeated by lymphoid cells and occur as infrahilar masses with an endobronchial component. The diagnosis of LEC, although rare, should be considered in patients with cystic lesions, particularly if they have parotid cysts or other unusual lymphoproliferative disorders.

BOOP

The presenting clinical features of BOOP in HIV-infected patients may be dramatic, with the development of a flulike illness with acute-subacute onset of symptoms (fever, malaise, anorexia, weight loss, nonproductive cough, and dyspnea). However, true cases of BOOP, although possible, are rare in previously asymptomatic, HIV-infected patients. More frequently, BOOP-like clinical and histologic patterns may be observed in immunocompromised patients who have infections or tumors.

Inspiratory crackles are frequently heard on chest examination of patients who have typical BOOP. Chest radiographs may be distinctive, with multiple, bilateral, patchy alveolar opacities. Linear or nodular interstitial infiltrates are rarely present, and neither is honeycombing. Usually, CT confirms the radiographic pattern or reveals unexpected, more extensive, diffuse air-space consolidations than do conventional chest radiographs (Figure 31.9). Pulmonary function tests are usually impaired, with a restrictive pattern and gas exchange abnormalities. In patients who have typical BOOP, BAL may demonstrate a mild alveolitis characterized by $CD8^+$ lymphocytosis, foamy macrophages, and a slight increase in the number of neutrophils, eosinophils, and mast cells.

PH Related to HIV

Dyspnea, hypoxemia, and peripheral edema may be observed in most patients. Pulmonary systolic pressures range from 6.5 to 15.7 kPa (49 to 118 mmHg). Clearly, the clinical features and chest radiograph of PH are not typical enough to diagnose an HIV-associated idiopathic form of the disease. Magnetic resonance, CT, and echocardiographic studies are ancillary tests. However, the final diagnosis is usually confirmed only in autopsy studies. Other causes of PH in patients who have HIV infection include emboli of foreign material (e.g., in drug abusers), chronic pulmonary thromboembolism, chronic hypoxemia, liver disease, and an antiphospholipid antibody syndrome. Primary PH observed in HIV seronegative patients is less rapidly progressive than HIV-related PH. Death is usually a direct consequence of PH.

Airway Diseases

The association of cigarette smoking with emphysema is well known; however, the percentage of HIV-seropositive smokers who develop emphysema is striking. As a result, smoking-related respiratory symptoms and impairment may assume increasing importance as part of the natural history of HIV, particularly in light of the prevalence of cigarette smoking in this population.

Paradoxical Worsening of Pulmonary Complications in Patients Treated with HAART

HAART regimens may be not without toxicity in patients with HIV infections and who have or had pulmonary diseases. As an example, immune reconstitution syndromes with paradoxical worsening of tuberculosis, cytomegalovirus, and *P. jiroveci* infections associated with beginning HAART have been reported in

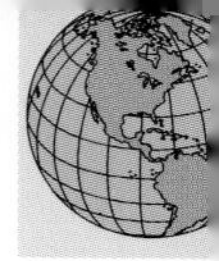

most HIV-infected patients. Some patients with latent or active infections may develop fever, lymphadenopathy, opacities on the chest radiograph, and respiratory failure after immune restoration with HAART (Figure 31.10). Others show reactivation of latent sarcoidosis and the development of a sarcoid-like illness with a CD4$^+$ alveolitis following the initiation of HAART and the raise of CD4$^+$ T-cell pool.

Kaposi Sarcoma

The most common neoplasm to occur in HIV-infected patients is KS, which in 1981 became one of the first AIDS-defining diagnoses. Although AIDS-associated KS is a multiorgan disease, skin involvement is the predominant clinical feature. Characteristically, the cutaneous lesions are pink, red, or violet multiple macules, often raised, and form plaques, which can ulcerate and bleed. Common sites of skin involvement are the face (especially the nose), oral cavity, periorbital and periauricular areas, lower extremities, and genitalia.

Most patients develop extra cutaneous KS. Lymph nodes, gastrointestinal tract, liver, and lungs are the most frequently involved organs. In particular, intrathoracic AIDS-associated KS may present as multifocal, interstitial infiltrates or nodular masses that have the potential to increase in size. Hemorrhagic pleural effusion may occur. Usually, pulmonary involvement follows the cutaneous disease. Nonetheless, rare cases initially present with AIDS-associated KS in the lung.

Some experimental data suggest that AIDS-associated KS is not a true malignancy. The majority of data suggests that KS-cell populations are polyclonal, and that KS lesions comprise cells of different histogenetic origin, such as endothelial cells of vascular and lymphatic origin, fibroblastoid cells, and dermal dendrocytes that proliferate in response to a number of cytokines (e.g., IL-1, IL-6, PDGF, TNF-α, fibroblast growth factor, GM-CSF, transforming growth factor [TGF-β], oncostatin M). The Tat protein of HIV is able to enhance the growth of these cells in concert with cytokines. It is also conceivable that agents of coinfection could initiate the angiogenesis. In particular, the recently discovered γ-2 herpesvirus HHV-8 has been related to the dysregulated cellular proliferation or differentiation that leads to the development of typical KS lesions.

The diagnosis of pulmonary AIDS-associated KS may be difficult. Clinical features and respiratory examination can be nonspecific. Chest radiographs may demonstrate the presence

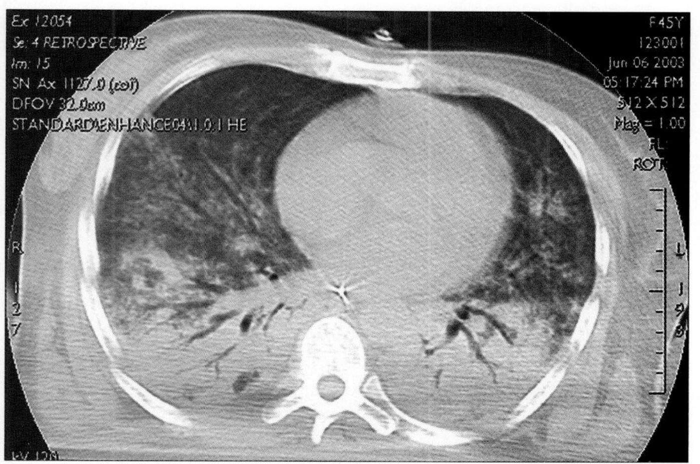

A

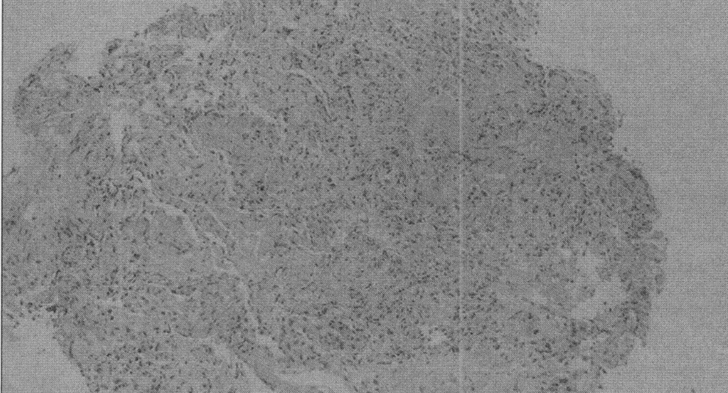

B

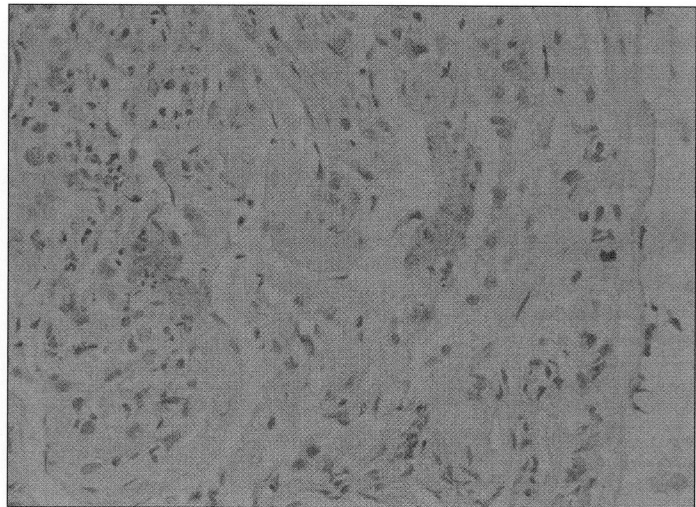

C

Figure 31.10 Acute respiratory failure after highly active antiretroviral therapy introduction in patient treated for *Pneumocystis jiroveci* pneumonia. **A.** High-resolution computed tomography. Alveolar opacities with bibasilar and subpleural distribution. **B.** Transbronchial lung biopsy. Interstitial and intraalveolar edema with granulation tissue, inflammatory infiltrates both interstitial and intraalveolar consisting mostly of mononuclear cell and type II cell hyperplasia (diffuse alveolar damage pattern in early proliferative phase) (hematoxylin and eosin, low power). **C.** Transbronchial lung biopsy. Small clusters of cysts of *P. jiroveci* are depicted by monoclonal antibodies (immunohistochemistry using monoclonal antibodies against *P. jiroveci*, high power).

of nodules, mediastinal adenopathy, and pleural effusion. Nuclear medicine can support the diagnosis of KS when gallium-67 and thallium scintigraphies are negative and positive, respectively. Given the peculiar lymphangitic growth pattern of AIDS-associated Kaposi sarcoma, CT is quite specific; typical findings include nodules, a peribronchovascular distribution of the disease, lymphadenopathy, interlobular septal thickening, consolidation or ground-glass opacity, and pleural effusions (Figure 31.11). A massive, hemorrhagic pleural effusion can occur when cysts are related to *P. jiroveci* pneumonia superimposed on the KS. In fact, AIDS-associated KS may mimic opportunistic infections and, in turn, infectious complications (such as *P. jiroveci* pneumonia) may occur in most patients who have pulmonary involvement of AIDS-associated KS.

Endobronchial KS is demonstrated if the distinctive lesions are seen in bronchoscopy (as flat or raised, bright red, violet plaques); in such cases biopsy is avoided because of the risk of bleeding. Parenchymal involvement is more difficult to confirm—transbronchial biopsy has a low yield (less than 10%) in patients who have parenchymal disease, and BAL is used only to rule out the presence of concomitant opportunistic infections. Large pieces of pulmonary tissue or pleura obtained with an open lung biopsy or a closed pleura biopsy can demonstrate the characteristic histologic pattern of AIDS-associated KS—spindle-shaped, cytokeratin-negative, vimentin-positive cells surround thin vascular channels, a variable infiltration of plasma cells and lymphocytes, and clefts formed by spindle cells that contain erythrocytes (Figure 31.12). Occasionally, examination of pleuritic, exudative effusions demonstrates the presence of atypical $CD34^+$ KS cells, which helps make the diagnosis.

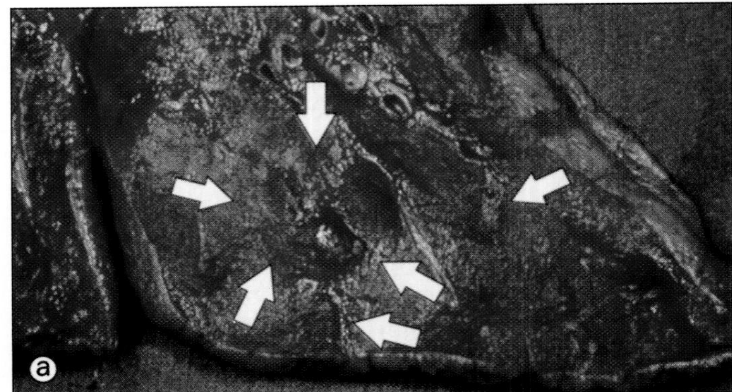

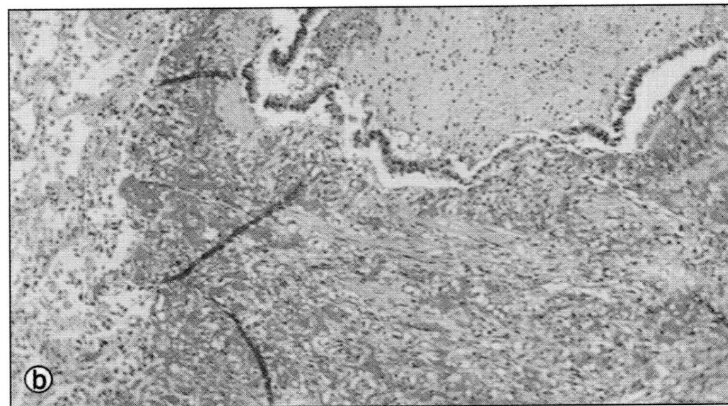

Figure 31.12 Autopsy specimens from a patient infected by human immunodeficiency virus and who has Kaposi sarcoma. **A.** Macroscopic evaluation reveals diffuse confluent patchy areas of red-brown hemorrhagic consolidations along lymphatic routes (arrowheads). **B.** Histopathologic evaluation shows peribronchiolar, dense, spindle-cell infiltration that contains clefts with red cells (hematoxylin and eosin).

Non-Hodgkin's Lymphomas

An intermediate or high-grade NHL is an AIDS-defining condition that occurs 60 times more often in HIV-infected patients than in the general population. Although rare cases of T-cell lymphomas have been described, HIV-associated NHLs are usually of B-cell origin as defined by the expression of B-cell associated antigens (CD19, CD20, or CD22) and the absence of T-cell–associated molecules. Three major histologic types are commonly observed—large-cell immunoblastic plasmacytoid, large-cell cleaved or noncleaved, and small, noncleaved cell (Burkitt and non-Burkitt lymphomas). Occasional cases of low-grade, B-cell lymphoma of mucosa-associated lymphoid tissue have been described. Most patients who have AIDS-associated NHL show widespread disease and extranodal involvement at the time of diagnosis. The gastrointestinal tract, liver, and central nervous system (CNS) are the more frequent sites of extranodal involvement. Pulmonary involvement or primary lung manifestations of AIDS-associated NHL are relatively rare (less than 10%), and are mostly large-cell lymphomas of the B-cell type.

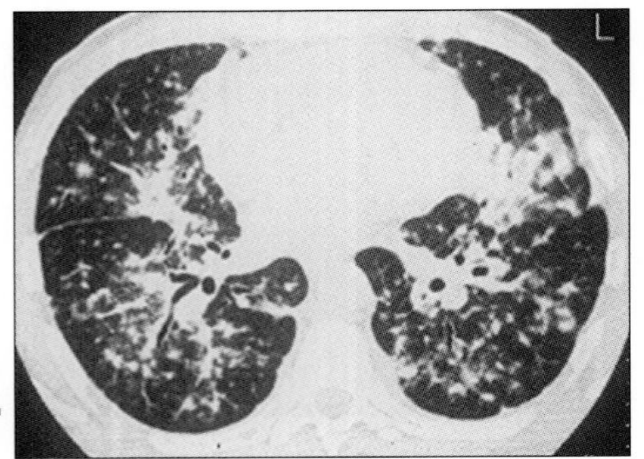

Figure 31.11 Kaposi sarcoma. High-resolution computed tomography shows peribronchovascular cuffing and nodules along lymphatic routes.

The molecular basis of lymphoma genesis in HIV-infected patients has been extensively evaluated. Data show an indirect role for HIV and HIV proteins in inducing a dysregulated production of certain cytokines, such as IL-6 and IL-10, which may cause chronic B-cell proliferation that is superimposed on the profound $CD4^+$ T-cell depletion characteristic of AIDS. Polyclonal B-cell activation may be induced by coinfecting viruses, which include Epstein-Barr virus (EBV) and its relative HHV-8; both viruses have been isolated in peripheral blood B cells, and in some B-cell lymphoma cell lines from patients who have HIV infection and a low number of $CD4^+$ T cells. There are data HHV-8 has been also found in a rare form of AIDS-associated B-cell lymphoma, the so-called "body cavity–associated lymphoma" characterized by bilateral pleural effusions, in some AIDS-associated primary CNS lymphomas, and in some patients who have HIV-related Castelman disease.

The putative role of viral coinfections in lymphomagenesis has been recently confirmed by a retrospective histopathologic review of lymphoid proliferations associated with HIV infection. It has been observed that EBV-driven polymorphic B-cell lymphoproliferative disorders comparable morphologically and mol-

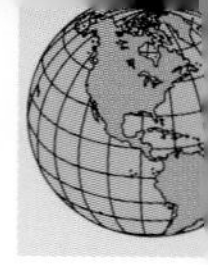

ecularly to those arising after solid organ transplantation can be shown in lymph nodes, lungs, the parotid gland, perineum, and skin of patients with HIV infection. Lymphoid proliferation exhibits a diffuse growth pattern and is composed of a polymorphic lymphoid cell population exhibiting a variable degree of plasmacytic differentiation, cytologic atypia, and numbers of atypical immunoblasts. The nongermline hybridizing bands are usually faint, suggesting that the clonal B-cell population represents only a subpopulation within the polymorphic lesion. Nonetheless, strong clonal rearrangement bands can be shown when there is a clear morphologic evidence of transformation to diffuse large cell lymphoma.

In most patients the diagnosis of pulmonary involvement by NHL is problematic. Radiography and nuclear scanning are rarely useful. In HIV-infected patients, NHL of the lung can mimic every pulmonary manifestation possible. Thus, pulmonary infiltrates by KS, bronchopneumonia of different etiologies, an atypical *P. jiroveci* pneumonia, and mass consolidations of other tumors must be considered in the differential diagnosis (Figure 31.13). In most patients, definitive information is obtained only by the histologic examination of bronchial or transbronchial biopsies, CT-guided percutaneous biopsies, transtracheobronchial needle biopsies, or open-lung biopsies. Thoracic lymphomas in HIV-positive patients can have a distinctive tracheal or bronchial involvement—exophytic growths in tracheal or bronchial lumen, patchy necrosis of the tracheal or bronchial wall, mucosal thickening, and extrinsic compression. The demonstration of clonal rearrangements confirms the neoplastic origin of the infiltrate.

Hodgkin's Lymphoma

Although Hodgkin disease has not been included in AIDS-defining conditions, it is five times more prevalent in patients who have AIDS than in HIV-negative individuals. An interesting association between EBV infection and HD has been demonstrated in HIV-infected patients. The majority of cases are of the mixed cellularity type and most patients show a poor prognosis. Pulmonary involvement by HD is rare in HIV-infected patients. It may occur with or without associated hilar and mediastinal lymphadenopathy.

Lung Cancer

The peculiar epidemiologic distribution of lung cancers in some ethnic populations and the demonstration that bronchogenic carcinoma may be documented in young patients (including intravenous drug users) raises the question whether frequency of pulmonary cancer increases during HIV infection. Those HIV patients who develop lung cancers are usually young, male smokers with a history of intravenous drug use. The predominant histologic type of lung tumor in HIV-infected individuals is adenocarcinoma, and an association between pulmonary tuberculosis and lung cancer has been reported in some series of patients. Recently, the occurrence of pseudomesotheliomatous adenocarcinoma was reported in HIV-infected subjects. The usual symptoms include cough, dyspnea, and hemoptysis, as in non–HIV-infected patients. The diagnosis is made using the same diagnostic procedures as for non–HIV-infected patients (see Chapter 41). The prognosis is poor.

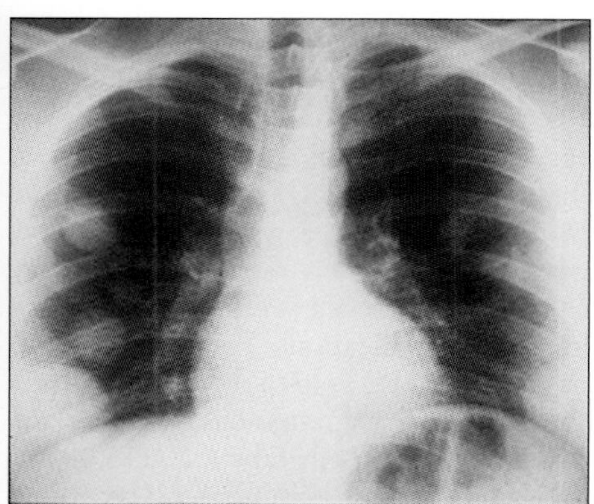

Figure 31.13 Non-Hodgkin's lymphoma of the lung. A posteroanterior chest film demonstrates nodules throughout both lungs.

TREATMENT

Alveolitis Associated with HIV in Asymptomatic Patients

Clinical action is not required in subjects who have lymphocytic or macrophagic alveolitis but no symptoms—most cases resolve spontaneously.

Nonspecific Interstitial Pneumonitis

The introduction of effective HAART regimens has had a dramatic impact in the decline of the episodes of interstitial lung diseases characterized by a histologic diagnosis of NSIP in patients with HIV infection. In any case, the patient is usually followed without therapy to evaluate whether NSIP spontaneously resolves or stabilizes. Corticosteroids may occasionally be used in patients who present with severe symptoms. Therapy with co-trimoxazole (trimethoprim-sulfamethoxazole) may have beneficial effects, even if infectious agents are not detected.

Lymphoid Interstitial Pneumonitis

Corticosteroids represent the specific, initial treatment for symptomatic patients who have LIP. Other immunosuppressants (chlorambucil) and antiviral therapy have been used in HIV-infected subjects who have LIP, but it is unclear whether immunosuppressive treatments should be used only until the patient shows improvement or whether they should be maintained for a longer period of time to avoid further recurrence of the disease.

Local Immunodeficiency Induced by HIV

Chapter 30 describes symptoms, and clinical and radiologic findings observed in the different infectious complications that affect the respiratory tract during HIV disease and their treatment. As previously reported, the rates of AIDS-related mortality and opportunistic infections have fallen drastically since the introduction of HAART in the therapy regimens.

Bronchiolitis Obliterans Organizing Pneumonia

In the majority of patients, glucocorticoid treatment results in a remission or stabilization of the disease. Treatment using macrolides is helpful in cases of cryptogenic organizing pneumonia. Nonetheless, BOOP may rapidly relapse when cortico-

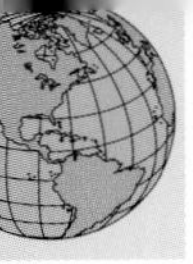

steroids are withdrawn, often within 1 month, but retreatment using corticosteroids re-establishes control of the condition in most.

Pulmonary Hypertension Related to HIV

Specific treatments do not exist, but highly active antiretroviral therapies may exert a beneficial effect on the pressure gradient.

Airway Diseases

The demonstration of airway disease in patients with HIV infection (chronic obstructive pulmonary disease, emphysema) may represent an indication for HAART treatment.

Worsening of Pulmonary Complications in Patients Treated with HAART

Atypical inflammatory lung disorders coincident with reconstitution of the $CD4^+$ lymphocyte pool may develop after initiation of HAART. Reconstitution of immune responses against opportunists explains in part the phenomenon of paradoxic reactions observed in patients concurrently being treated for tuberculosis or *P. jiroveci* infections.

Diagnostic criteria and standards of therapy for immune restoration syndromes are yet to be defined. There are data suggesting that steroid therapy may lead to dramatic improvement in patients who develop diffuse lung disease with recovery of $CD4^+$ lymphocyte population, including sarcoidosis.

Kaposi Sarcoma

The use of HAART is associated with a dramatic decrease in the incidence of AIDS-KS and with a regression of KS lesions. If KS develops, patients who have cutaneous KS may be observed or treated with interferon-α and antiviral therapy, whereas chemotherapy and radiotherapy are the therapeutic modalities employed in patients who have visceral involvement. In general, vincristine and bleomycin are employed both as single agents and in dual-agent chemotherapy. Low-dose, multiagent chemotherapy is also used in advanced KS and involves various combinations of drugs that are active in single-agent chemotherapy (doxorubicin, bleomycin, vinblastine, actinomycin D [dactinomycin], dacarbazine, and etoposide). Liposomal doxorubicin seems to improve survival and quality of life in patients who have disseminated AIDS-associated Kaposi sarcoma. Cases of regression of AIDS-associated KS after highly active antiretroviral therapy were reported recently. Unfortunately, concurrent opportunistic infections may be troublesome during chemotherapy. In addition, discontinuation of chemotherapy is associated with a high rate of relapse, and interferon-α does not prolong remission time.

Non-Hodgkin's Lymphoma

Overall, the prognosis is poor and the patients are usually managed using chemotherapy. In particular, no chemotherapy regimens are designed specifically for HIV-related NHL in which patients are subdivided into individualized groups according to the presence or absence of prognostic factors. Patients who have a previous history of opportunistic infection and poor performance status are treated using low-dose chemotherapy regimens (e.g., a cyclophosphamide, vincristine, doxorubicin, and prednisone regimen) and antiviral therapy. Low-risk patients are eligible for intensive treatment (e.g., methotrexate, doxorubicin, cyclophosphamide, vincristine, and prednisone or LNH-84 [doxorubicin, cyclophosphamide, vindesine, bleomycin, and prednisone]). For all patients, CNS and *P. jiroveci* prophylaxis are recommended.

Hodgkin's Lymphoma

Combinations of antineoplastic chemotherapy (nitrogen mustard, vincristine, procarbazine, and prednisone or doxorubicin, bleomycin, vinblastine, and dacarbazine) with and without antiretroviral therapy have been used to treat Hodgkin lymphomas in HIV-infected patients.

Lung Cancer

Surgery may be considered for resectable tumors. Chemotherapy is unlikely to help, and palliative measures are more appropriate in patients who have advanced disease.

CLINICAL COURSE AND PREVENTION

The development of respiratory failure may be observed in most patients who suffer noninfectious, HIV-related pulmonary complications, particularly in severely immunocompromised patients who have a $CD4^+$ T cell count of less than 200 cells/mm. Follow-up studies showed that superimposed opportunistic infections of the respiratory tract are the most important factors in the development of lung function abnormalities in patients who have idiopathic manifestations or lung neoplasms. Thus, preventive therapy for pulmonary infections is an important element in the management of HIV-infected patients who have noninfectious pulmonary complications.

Tuberculosis, *P. jiroveci*, and bacterial infections are the main targets of prophylaxis. Co-trimoxazole, pentamidine aerosols, and dapsone are used for the prophylaxis of pneumocystosis; specifically, *P. jiroveci* prophylaxis is indicated for all patients who receive chemotherapy, regardless of the $CD4^+$ T-cell count. Isoniazid remains the recommended drug to prevent disease progression in HIV-infected patients coinfected with *Mycobacterium tuberculosis*. Although bacterial infections are frequent in HIV-infected patients whose $CD4^+$ T-cell count is less than 200 cells/mm, clear guidelines for a preventive strategy of bacterial pneumonia do not exist; uncontrolled trials suggest the use of co-trimoxazole to protect against severe bacterial infections.

The frequency of fatal pulmonary complications that affect the clinical course of HIV infection has resulted in attempts to better define candidates for prophylaxis through an improved definition of risk factors for the development of respiratory failure. A number of abnormalities predict the clinical outcome of pulmonary involvement. The presence of gas-exchange abnormalities and the accumulation of neutrophils in BAL may strongly correlate with imminent mortality in HIV-seropositive patients who have pulmonary complications. Phenotypic evaluation of BAL cell populations may also help to define the natural history of HIV-associated pulmonary complications—in the multivariate model a low number of BAL $CD4^+$ T cells represents an adverse prognostic factor. The rate of $CD4^+$ T-cell

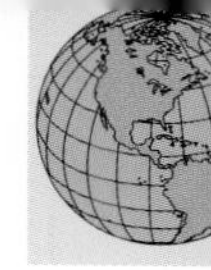

decline in peripheral blood also predicts survival, but only up to a CD4+ T-cell count of 100 cells/mm^3.

Recent findings suggest that HIV-infected individuals whose therapy involves potent antiretroviral drugs (double and triple regimens with protease inhibitors) have significantly lower mortality and longer AIDS-free survival. Inhibition of HIV replication using antiretroviral therapy may result in reduced infectiousness of the lung environment and improved local immune function. Indeed, in patients whose therapy involves protease inhibitors, the viral burden progressively reduces and the number of lung CD4+ T cells may increase. Favorable outcomes may result, with reductions in the incidence of infectious and noninfectious pulmonary complications.

PITFALLS AND CONTROVERSIES

Idiopathic and Immunologic Pulmonary Manifestations

The differential diagnosis of pulmonary idiopathic inflammatory manifestations may be difficult in HIV-positive patients. A diagnosis of NSIP should be considered only after a reasonable effort has been made to exclude opportunistic infections in the lung. In particular, *P. jiroveci* must be carefully sought in induced sputum and BAL fluid. In addition, a transbronchial lung biopsy through a flexible or rigid bronchoscope is considered a necessary diagnostic step. The appropriate management of this condition is still unclear—the role of co-trimoxazole is under review, and probably a prophylaxis strategy using this antibiotic should be initiated in any patient.

A diagnosis that should be considered in children who have respiratory complications is LIP. Clinical experience suggests that LIP is quite uncommon in adults, so adults who have suspected LIP require an open lung biopsy to obtain a definitive diagnosis, inasmuch as the diagnostic yield of the transbronchial lung biopsy is poor. Specific therapies for LIP are limited, and the role of new anti-HIV drugs in the treatment of LIP in children is unclear.

As reported previously, BOOP is a nonspecific histopathologic lung lesion. A number of infectious agents can give BOOP as their prevalent morphologic expression in immunocompromised hosts (e.g., *Mycoplasma pneumoniae*, *Chlamydia pneumoniae*, *Legionella pneumophila*, community-acquired pneumonias, *P. jiroveci*). Also, BOOP-like lesions occur as a manifestation of drug pulmonary toxicity or in tissues that surround neoplastic infiltration. Serologic tests, enzyme immunoabsorbent assays, immunofluorescence, immunohistochemical, and polymerase chain reaction tests on serum, BAL fluid, or lung tissue are recommended for the diagnosis of pulmonary infections. Exposure to drugs that are potentially toxic to the pulmonary tract or neoplastic involvement of the lung must be excluded. Some clinicians suggest that therapy with macrolides or rifampin (rifampicin) be used along with corticosteroids, even if the underlying infectious agents are not identified. Finally, because BOOP is a common lesion in both immunocompetent and immunocompromised individuals, its occurrence may be merely coincidental in an HIV-infected subject.

Because HIV-related PH is an incurable disease, clinicians should consider any alternative diagnostic hypothesis in which a specific treatment may help. A search for anticardiolipin and lupus anticoagulant antibodies and deep venous thromboses must be conducted, and a liver-related PH excluded.

The possible use of cytokines to modulate local immune responses is also unclear. The effect of cytokines on HIV viral replication in the pulmonary microenvironment needs to be specified. Several cytokines that could theoretically be used to restore the cell-mediated response in the lung of patients who have pulmonary opportunistic infections have been shown to upregulate viral expression in cells chronically or latently infected with HIV, which operatively prevents their therapeutic use. New biologic modifiers that may potentiate local antiviral mechanisms and avoid the risk of spread of HIV infection are needed.

Lung Neoplasms

Because KS is related to HHV-8, it is important to establish whether detection of this virus in BAL fluid could be a sensitive and specific method to diagnose tracheobronchial KS. Pitfalls in the diagnosis of AIDS-associated KS may arise because the differential diagnosis of granulation tissue in the lung or of bacillary angiomatosis (rarely reported in lung parenchyma of HIV-infected subjects) may be difficult.

A number of clinical trials using different chemotherapeutic agents for pulmonary malignancies linked to HIV infection are under way. However, comparison of the efficacy of the chemotherapeutic regimens being used is fraught with difficulties. Pitfalls present in many clinical trials often reflect the staging systems used to group patient populations. Naturally, partial remission rate differs between patients who belong to better or worse prognostic groups or between patients who have more or less limited neoplastic disease. Furthermore, it is unclear whether antiviral therapy should be started at the end of the chemotherapy regimen and, if so, which drug to use. The palliative therapy to use in HIV patients who have poor prognoses is also unclear.

Epidemiologically, the significance of lung cancer in young patients who have HIV infection needs to be established.

SUGGESTED READINGS

Agostini C, Zambello R, Trentin L, Semenzato G: HIV and pulmonary immune responses. Immunol Today 17:359-364, 1996.

Beck JM, Rosen MJ, Peavy HH: Pulmonary complications of HIV infection. Report of the Fourth NHLBI Workshop. Am J Respir Crit Care Med 164:2120-2126, 2001.

Biggar R, Rabkin S: The epidemiology of acquired immunodeficiency syndrome-related lymphoma. Curr Opinion Oncol 4:883-893, 1992.

Levine AM: Acquired immunodeficiency syndrome-related lymphoma. Blood 80:8-20, 1992.

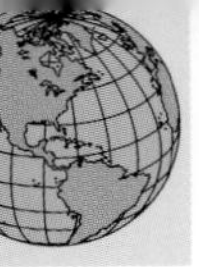
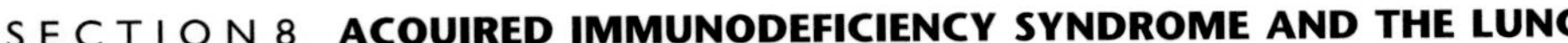

Levine AM: AIDS-related malignancies: The emerging epidemic. J Natl Cancer Inst 85:1382-1397, 1993.

Nador RG, Chadburn A, Gundappa G, et al: Human immunodeficiency virus (HIV)-associated polymorphic lymphoproliferative disorders. Am J Surg Pathol 27:293-302, 2003.

O'Neil KM: The changing landscape of HIV-related lung disease in the era of highly active antiretroviral therapy. Chest 122:768-771, 2002.

Saukkonen JJ, Farber HV: Lymphocytic interstitial pneumonitis. In: Zumla A, Johnson MA, Miller RF, eds. AIDS and Respiratory Medicine. Chapman & Hall, 1997, pp 331-343.

Semenzato G, ed: AIDS and the lung. Eur Respir Monogr 2:1-384, 1995.

White DA, Stover DE, eds: Pulmonary complications of HIV infection. London, Clin Chest Med 17:621-822, 1996.

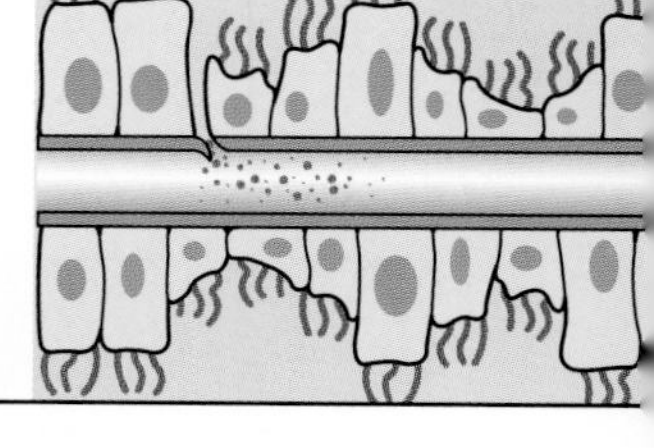

CHAPTER 32 β-Agonists, Anticholinergics, and Other Nonsteroid Drugs

Peter J. Barnes

Asthma therapy can be classified into two main types—bronchodilators (or relievers) that give rapid relief of asthma symptoms, and controllers that give long-term control of asthma symptoms either by suppression of the chronic inflammatory process (anti-inflammatory drugs), by inhibition of the release of bronchoconstrictors, or by some other mechanism that does not involve a direct relaxant effect on airway smooth muscle (Table 32.1). Chronic obstructive pulmonary disease (COPD) is treated predominantly by bronchodilators, because there is no evidence that controllers influence progression of the disease. In this chapter the mode of action and the clinical use of the main classes of drug used in asthma therapy are reviewed, apart from corticosteroids (see Chapter 33). Although drugs are traditionally classified as controllers and relievers, some drugs, such as theophylline and antileukotrienes, appear to have bronchodilator and anti-inflammatory properties.

β_2-AGONISTS

Inhaled β_2-agonists are the most effective bronchodilators and have minimal side effects when used correctly, and so they are the treatment of choice. Short-acting and nonselective β-agonists, such as isoproterenol (isoprenaline) and orciprenaline, have no place.

Mode of Action

β-Agonists produce bronchodilatation by directly stimulating β_2-receptors in airway smooth muscle, which leads to relaxation. This can be demonstrated in vitro by the relaxant effect of β-agonists on human bronchi and lung strips (indicating an effect on peripheral airways) and in vivo by a rapid decrease in airway resistance. β-Receptors have been demonstrated in airway smooth muscle by direct receptor-binding techniques, and autoradiographic studies indicate that β-receptors are localized to smooth muscle of all airways from the trachea to the terminal bronchioles.

Activation of β_2-receptors results in activation of adenylate cyclase and an increase of intracellular cyclic adenosine-3′,5′-monophosphate (cAMP) (Figure 32.1). This leads to activation of a specific kinase (protein kinase A) that phosphorylates several target proteins within the cell, resulting in:

- Lowered intracellular calcium ion (Ca^{2+}) concentration by active removal of Ca^{2+} from the cell into intracellular stores;
- Inhibitory effect on phosphoinositide hydrolysis;
- Direct inhibition of myosin light-chain kinase;
- Opening of large-conductance, calcium-activated potassium channels (K_{Ca}), which repolarize the smooth muscle cell and may stimulate the sequestration of Ca^{2+} into intracellular stores (β-agonists may be directly coupled to K_{Ca} and relaxation of airway smooth muscle may therefore occur independently of an increase in cAMP).

β-Agonists act as functional antagonists and reverse bronchoconstriction, irrespective of the contractile agent. This is an important property, because multiple bronchoconstrictor mediators (inflammatory mediators and neurotransmitters) are released in asthma.

β-Agonists may have additional effects on airways, and β-receptors are localized to several different airway cells (Table 32.2 and Figure 32.2):

- Inhibition of mediator release from mast cells and other inflammatory cells
- Reduction and prevention of microvascular leakage and thus the development of bronchial mucosal edema after exposure to mediators such as histamine and leukotrienes
- Increased mucus secretion from submucosal glands and ion transport across airway epithelium (effects that may enhance mucociliary clearance, and therefore reverse the defect in clearance found in asthma)
- Reduction in neurotransmitter release from airway cholinergic nerves, thus reducing cholinergic reflex bronchoconstriction
- Inhibition of the release of bronchoconstrictor and inflammatory peptides, such as substance P, from sensory nerves

Although these additional effects of β-agonists may be relevant to the prophylactic use of the drugs against various challenges, their rapid bronchodilator action is probably caused by a direct effect on airway smooth muscle.

Anti-inflammatory Effects?

The inhibitory effects of β-agonists on the release of mast-cell mediators and microvascular leakage are clearly anti-inflammatory, which suggests that β-agonists may modify acute inflammation. However, β-agonists do not have a significant inhibitory effect on the chronic inflammation of asthmatic airways, which is suppressed by corticosteroids. Bronchial biopsies in asthmatic patients who regularly take β-agonists show no significant reduction in the number of or activation in inflammatory cells in the airways, in contrast to suppression of inflammation which occurs with inhaled corticosteroids. This is

Table 32.1 Current therapy for asthma	
Relievers (bronchodilators)	**Controllers (anti-inflammatory treatments)**
β_2-Agonists	Corticosteroids
Theophylline	Cromones
Anticholinergics	Antileukotrienes
	Corticosteroid-sparing therapies: Methotrexate Gold Cyclosporin A

Table 32.2 Localization and function of airway β-adrenoreceptors		
Cell type	**Subtype**	**Function**
Smooth muscle	β_2	Relaxation (proximal = distal) Inhibition of proliferation
Epithelium	β_2	Increased ion transport Secretion of inhibitory factor Increased ciliary beating Increased mucociliary clearance
Submucosal glands	β_1/β_2	Increased secretion (mucus cells)
Clara cells	β_2	Increased secretion
Cholinergic nerves	β_2	Reduced acetylcholine release
Sensory nerves	β_2/β_3	Reduced neuropeptide release Reduced activation?
Bronchial vessels	β_2	Vasodilation Reduced plasma extravasation
Inflammatory cells:		
Mast cells	β_2	Reduced mediator release
Macrophages	β_2	No effect?
Eosinophils	β_2	Reduced mediator release?
T-lymphocytes	β_2	Reduced cytokine release?

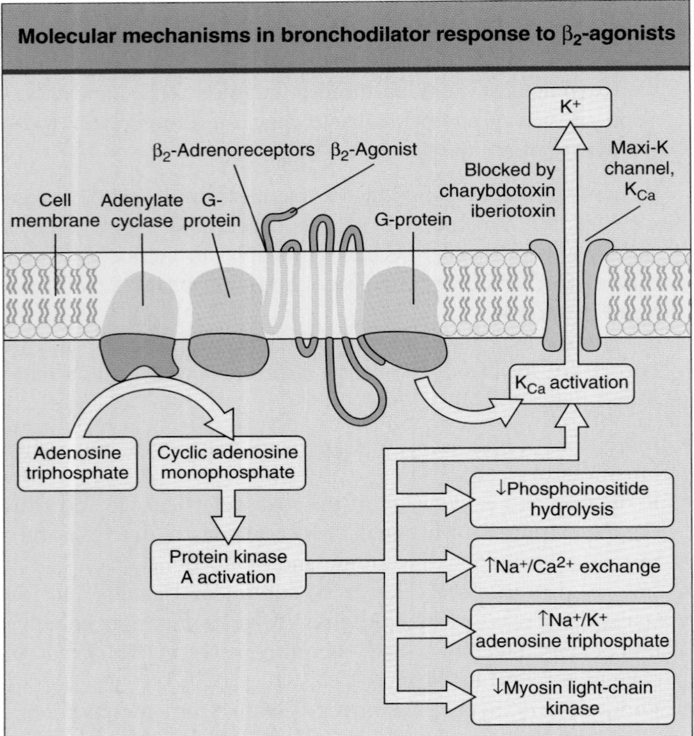

Figure 32.1 Molecular mechanisms involved in bronchodilator response to β_2-agonists. Activation of β_2-adrenoreceptors on airway smooth muscle cells is coupled via a G protein to adenylyl cyclase, which results in increased intracellular cyclic adenosine monophosphate formation. This activates protein kinase A, which phosphorylates a number of substrates, including large, conductance calcium-activated potassium channels (K_{Ca}), which can also be directly coupled to β_2-receptors.

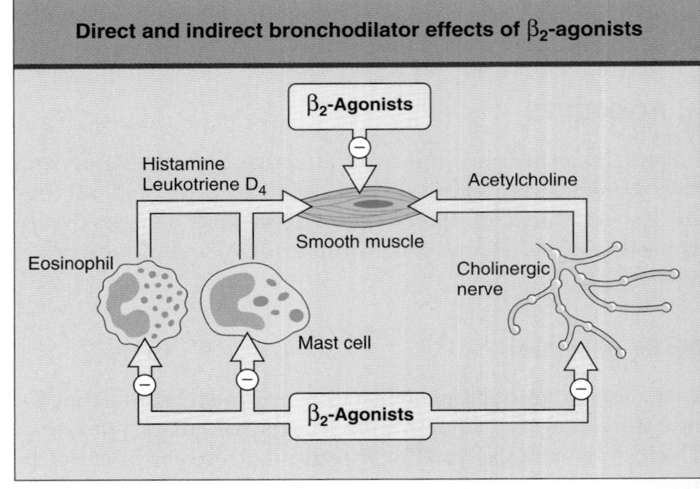

Figure 32.2 Direct and indirect bronchodilator effects of β_2-agonists. β_2-Agonists may cause bronchodilatation directly via activation of β_2-receptors on airway smooth muscle, and also indirectly via inhibition of mediator release from inflammatory cells and neurotransmitter release from nerve endings.

probably explained by the fact that β-agonists not having long-term inhibitory effect on macrophages, eosinophils, or T lymphocytes, the cells involved in chronic inflammation and airway hyperresponsiveness.

Clinical Use

Short-acting inhaled β_2-agonists, such as albuterol (salbutamol) and terbutaline, are the most widely used and effective bronchodilators for the treatment of asthma. When inhaled from metered-dose inhalers (MDIs) they are convenient, easy to use, rapid in onset, and without significant side effects. In addition to an acute bronchodilator effect, they effectively protect against various challenges, such as exercise, cold air, and allergen. They are the bronchodilators of choice for the treatment of acute severe asthma, for which the nebulized route of administration is as effective as intravenous use. The inhaled route of administration is preferable to the oral route because side effects are less common, and also because it may be more effective (better access to surface cells such as mast cells). Short-acting, inhaled β_2-agonists should not be used on a regular basis for the treatment of mild asthma, but should be used as required by symptoms. Increased usage is an indicator for the need for more

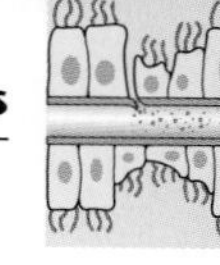

Structure of catecholamines	
Norepinephrine (noradrenaline)	HO, HO (ring) –CH(OH)–CH_2–NH_2
Epinephrine (adrenaline)	HO, HO (ring) –CH(OH)–CH_2–NH(CH_3)
Isoproterenol (isoprenaline)	HO, HO (ring) –CH(OH)–CH_2–NH($CH(CH_3)_2$)
Albuterol (salbutamol)	HOH_2C, HO (ring) –CH(OH)–CH_2–NH($C(CH_3)_3$)
Salmeterol	HOH_2C, HO (ring) –CH(OH)–CH_2–$NHCH_2(CH_2)_5OCH_2(CH_2)_3$–(ring)
Formoterol	HCONH, HO (ring) –CH(OH)–CH_2–NHCH(CH_3)–CH_2–(ring)–OCH_3

Figure 32.3 Structures of catecholamines showing the development of short- and long-acting selective β_2-agonists.

anti-inflammatory therapy; oral β-agonists are indicated as an additional bronchodilator. Slow-release preparations (such as slow-release albuterol and bambuterol) may be indicated in nocturnal asthma, but are less useful than inhaled β-agonists because of an increased risk of side effects. Long-acting inhaled β_2-agonists (LABA—salmeterol and formoterol) should be used twice daily as add-on therapy when patients are not controlled by low doses of inhaled corticosteroids (see the following section).

Therapeutic Choices

Several short-acting β_2-selective agonists are available (Figure 32.3). These drugs are as effective as nonselective agonists in their bronchodilator action, because airway effects are mediated only by β_2-receptors. However, they are less likely to produce cardiac stimulation than isoproterenol, because β_1-receptors are stimulated relatively less. With the exception of rimiterol (which retains the catechol ring structure and is therefore susceptible to rapid metabolism), their duration of action is longer because they are resistant to uptake and enzymatic degradation. There is choice between the various short-acting β-agonists currently available; all are usable by inhalation and orally and have similar duration of action (usually 3 to 4 hours, but less in severe asthma) and side effects. Differences in β_2-selectivity have been claimed, but are not clinically important. Drugs in clinical use include albuterol, terbutaline, fenoterol, tulobuterol, rimiterol, and pirbuterol. It has been claimed that fenoterol is less β_2-selective than albuterol and terbutaline, which results in increased cardiovascular side effects, but this evidence is controversial, because all of these effects are mediated via β_2-receptors. The increased incidence of cardiovascular effects is more likely to be related to the greater effective dose of fenoterol used and perhaps to more rapid absorption into the circulation.

Side Effects

Unwanted effects are dose-related and result from stimulation of extrapulmonary β-receptors. Side effects are not common with inhaled therapy, but more common with oral or intravenous administration:

- Muscle tremor caused by stimulation of β_2-receptors in the skeletal muscle is the most common side effect, and may be more troublesome for elderly patients;
- Tachycardia and palpitations caused by reflex cardiac stimulation secondary to peripheral vasodilatation, by direct stimulation of atrial β_2-receptors, and possibly also by stimulation of myocardial β_1-receptors as the doses of β_2-agonist increase;
- Metabolic effects (increase in free fatty acid, insulin, glucose, pyruvate, and lactate) seen only after large systemic doses;
- Hypokalemia caused by β_2-receptor stimulation of potassium entry into skeletal muscle (hypokalemia might be serious in the presence of hypoxia, as in acute asthma, when there may be a predisposition to cardiac dysrhythmias);
- Increased ventilation-perfusion mismatching by causing pulmonary vasodilatation in blood vessels previously constricted by hypoxia, which results in the shunting of blood to poorly ventilated areas and a fall in arterial oxygen tension—although in practice the effect of β-agonists on PaO_2 is usually very small, a fall of less than 0.7 kPa (less than 5 mmHg), occasionally in severe chronic airway obstruction it is large, but it may be prevented by giving additional inspired oxygen.

Tolerance

Continuous treatment with an agonist often leads to tolerance (subsensitivity, desensitization), which may be caused by uncoupling or downregulation of the receptor. Many studies of bronchial β-receptor function after prolonged therapy with β-agonists have been conducted. Tolerance of non-airway β-receptor responses, such as tremor, cardiovascular, and metabolic, is readily induced in normal and asthmatic subjects. Tolerance of human airway smooth muscle to β-agonists in vitro has been demonstrated, although the concentration of agonist necessary is high and the degree of desensitization is variable. Animal studies suggest that airway smooth muscle β-receptors may be more resistant to desensitization that β-receptors elsewhere, because of a high receptor reserve; it is necessary to reduce β-receptor number by 95% before the maximal bronchodilator response is reduced. In normal subjects, bronchodilator tolerance has been demonstrated in some studies after high-dose, inhaled albuterol, but not in others. In asthmatic patients, tolerance to the bronchodilator effects of β-agonists has not usually been found. However, tolerance develops to the bronchoprotective effects of β_2-agonists, which is more marked with indirect constrictors such as adenosine, allergen, and exercise (which activate mast cells) than with direct constrictors such as histamine and methacholine. The high level of β_2-receptor gene expression in airway smooth muscle compared with that of peripheral lung may also contribute to the resistance to development of tolerance, because a high rate of β-receptor synthesis is likely. Tolerance to the bronchodilator effects of the LABA formoterol but not to salmeterol has been reported.

Experimental studies have shown that corticosteroids prevent the development of tolerance in airway smooth muscle, and prevent and reverse the fall in pulmonary β-receptor density. However, inhaled corticosteroids do not appear to prevent the tolerance to the bronchoprotective effect of inhaled β_2-agonists.

Safety

A possible relationship between adrenergic drug therapy and the rise in asthma deaths in several countries during the early 1960s casts doubts on the safety of β-agonists. However, a causal relationship between β-agonist use and mortality has not been established. A particular β_2-agonist—fenoterol—has been linked to the rise in asthma deaths in New Zealand during the 1980s because significantly more fatal cases had been prescribed fenoterol than the case-matched control patients. This association was strengthened by subsequent studies and by a fall in asthma mortality when fenoterol was withdrawn. An epidemiologic study based in Saskatchewan, Canada, examined the links between death or near death from asthma attacks and drugs prescribed for asthma, based on computerized records of prescriptions. A marked increase in the risk of death was associated with high doses of all inhaled β-agonists. The risk was greater for fenoterol, but when the dose was adjusted to the equivalent dose of albuterol, no significant difference in the risk for these two drugs was found. The link between high β-agonist usage and increased asthma mortality does not prove a causal association, because patients with more severe and poorly controlled asthma, and who are therefore more likely to have an increased risk of fatal attacks, are more likely to be using higher doses of β-agonist inhalers and less likely to be using effective anti-inflammatory treatment. Indeed, in patients who regularly used inhaled corticosteroids there was no significant increase in the risk of death.

Regular use of inhaled β-agonists was also suggested to increase asthma morbidity. In a study carried out in New Zealand, the regular use of fenoterol was associated with worse control and an increase in airway hyperresponsiveness compared with patients using fenoterol on demand for symptom control over a 6-month period. However, this was not found in subsequent careful studies of albuterol. Some evidence suggests that regularly inhaled albuterol may increase exercise-induced asthma and inflammation in asthmatic airways.

Although it is unlikely that normally recommended doses of β_2-agonists worsen asthma, this may occur with larger doses. Furthermore, some patients may be more susceptible if they have polymorphisms of the β_2-receptor that more rapidly downregulate. Short-acting, inhaled β_2-agonists should only be used on demand for symptom control and if they are required frequently (more than three times weekly), an inhaled corticosteroid is indicated. An association occurs between increased risk of death from asthma and the use of high doses of inhaled β_2-agonists; although this may reflect severity, it is also possible that high-dose β-agonists have a deleterious effect on asthma. Patients on high doses of β-agonists (more than one canister per month) should be treated with inhaled corticosteroids and attempts should be made to reduce the daily dose of inhaled β-agonist.

Long-acting, Inhaled β_2-agonists

Salmeterol and formoterol have been a major advance in asthma therapy, and they are also useful bronchodilators in patients with COPD. Both drugs have a bronchodilator action of greater than 12 hours and also protect against bronchoconstriction for a similar period. They are particularly useful in treating nocturnal asthma. Both improve asthma control (when given twice daily) compared with regular treatment with short-acting β_2-agonists four times daily. Both drugs are well tolerated. Tolerance to the bronchodilator effect of formoterol and the bronchoprotective effects of formoterol and salmeterol have been demonstrated, but a loss of protection does not occur, the tolerance does not appear to be progressive and is of doubtful clinical significance.

Although both drugs have a similar duration of effect in clinical studies there are some differences. Formoterol has a more rapid onset of action and is a fuller agonist than salmeterol, which might confer a theoretical advantage in more severe asthma, whereas it may also make it more likely to induce tolerance. There are few studies where these drugs have been directly compared, however.

Recent studies suggest that LABA might be introduced earlier in therapy. In asthmatic patients not controlled on either 400 to 800 μg of inhaled corticosteroids, the addition of a LABA gives better control of asthma than does increasing the dose of inhaled corticosteroid and also reduces exacerbation frequency. This suggests that LABA may be added to low or moderate doses of inhaled corticosteroids if asthma is not controlled and this is preferable to increasing the dose of inhaled corticosteroids. It is recommended that LABA should be used only in patients who are also prescribed inhaled corticosteroids. Fixed-combination inhalers (e.g., salmeterol + fluticasone propionate, formoterol + budesonide) are now widely used and not only improve compliance and guard against continuation of the inhaled corticosteroids, but may also give better control of asthma, as the two drugs are delivered to the same areas of the lung to allow positive molecular interactions between these two classes of drug. Combination inhalers are also useful in COPD patients.

THEOPHYLLINE

Methylxanthines related to caffeine, such as theophylline, have been used in the treatment of asthma since 1930. Indeed, theophylline is still the most widely used antiasthma therapy worldwide because it is inexpensive. Theophylline became more useful with the availability of rapid plasma assays and the introduction of reliable slow-release preparations. However, the frequency of side effects and the relative low efficacy of theophylline have recently led to reduced usage, since β-agonists are far more effective as bronchodilators and inhaled corticosteroids have a greater anti-inflammatory effect. In patients who have severe asthma, it still remains a very useful drug, however. Evidence is increasing that theophylline has an anti-inflammatory or immunomodulatory effect and may be effective in combination with inhaled corticosteroids.

Mode of Action

Although theophylline has been in clinical use for more than 70 years, its mechanism of action is uncertain and several modes of action have been proposed (Table 32.3):

- Inhibition of phosphodiesterases, which break down cAMP in the cell, leads to an increase in intracellular cAMP concentrations (Figure 32.4)—theophylline is a nonselective phosphodiesterase inhibitor, but the degree of inhibition is minor at the concentrations of theophylline within the new therapeutic range. This is likely to account for the bronchodilator action of theophylline, however. Phosphodi-

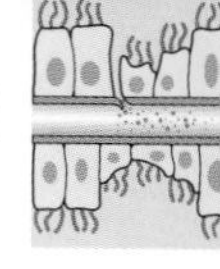

Table 32.3 Mechanisms of action of theophylline
Phosphodiesterase inhibition
Adenosine receptor antagonism
Stimulation of catecholamine release
Mediator inhibition
Inhibition of intracellular calcium release
Increased histone deacetylase activity

esterase inhibition may account for the most common side effects of theophylline, namely nausea and headaches
- Adenosine receptor antagonism, because adenosine is a bronchoconstrictor in asthmatic patients through activation of mast cells—adenosine antagonism may account for some of the side effects of theophylline, such as central nervous system stimulation, cardiac arrhythmias, and diuresis
- Increased secretion of adrenaline from the adrenal medulla, but the increase in plasma concentration is small and insufficient to account for any significant bronchodilator effect
- Recently a novel mechanism of action has been proposed to account for the anti-inflammatory actions of theophylline at low plasma concentrations; this involves activation of histone deacetylases, nuclear enzymes that are recruited by corticosteroids to switch off inflammatory gene expression. This mechanism also accounts for the synergistic interaction with the anti-inflammatory effect of corticosteroids.

It is possible that any beneficial effect in asthma is related to its action on other cells (such as T lymphocytes or macrophages) or on airway microvascular leak and edema (Figure 32.5). Theophylline is a relatively ineffective bronchodilator and its antiasthma effect is more likely to be explained by an anti-inflammatory action, particularly at low plasma concentrations now used clinically. Theophylline is ineffective when given by inhalation until a therapeutic plasma concentration is reached. A placebo-controlled theophylline withdrawal study indicates that it appears to have an immunomodulatory effect and decreases the number of activated T lymphocytes in the airways, probably by blocking their trafficking from the circulation. Theophylline also reduces eosinophils in bronchial biopsies and induced sputum at low plasma concentrations.

Clinical Use

In patients who have acute asthma, intravenous aminophylline is less effective than nebulized β-agonists, and is therefore reserved for the few patients who fail to respond to β-agonists. Theophylline should not be added routinely to nebulized β-agonists, because it does not increase the bronchodilator response and may only increase their side effects.

Theophylline has little or no effect on bronchomotor tone in normal airways, but reverses bronchoconstriction in asthmatic patients, although it is less effective than inhaled β-agonists and is more likely to have unwanted effects. Theophylline and β-agonists have additive effects, even if true synergy is not seen, and evidence exists that theophylline may provide an additional bronchodilator effect even when maximally effective doses of β-agonist have been given. Thus, if adequate bronchodilatation is not achieved using a β-agonist alone, theophylline may be added to the maintenance therapy with benefit. Theophylline may be useful in some patients who have nocturnal asthma, because slow-release preparations can provide therapeutic concentrations overnight and are more effective than slow-release β-agonists. Although theophylline is less effective than a β-agonist and corticosteroids, some asthmatic patients appear to derive particular benefit. Even patients on high-dose inhaled corticosteroids and oral corticosteroids may show a deterioration in lung function when theophylline is withdrawn. Addition of low-dose theophylline is as or more effective than doubling the dose of inhaled corticosteroids in patients not controlled on low doses of inhaled corticosteroids. However, it is less effective as an add-on therapy as LABA, although it is less expensive and so may be

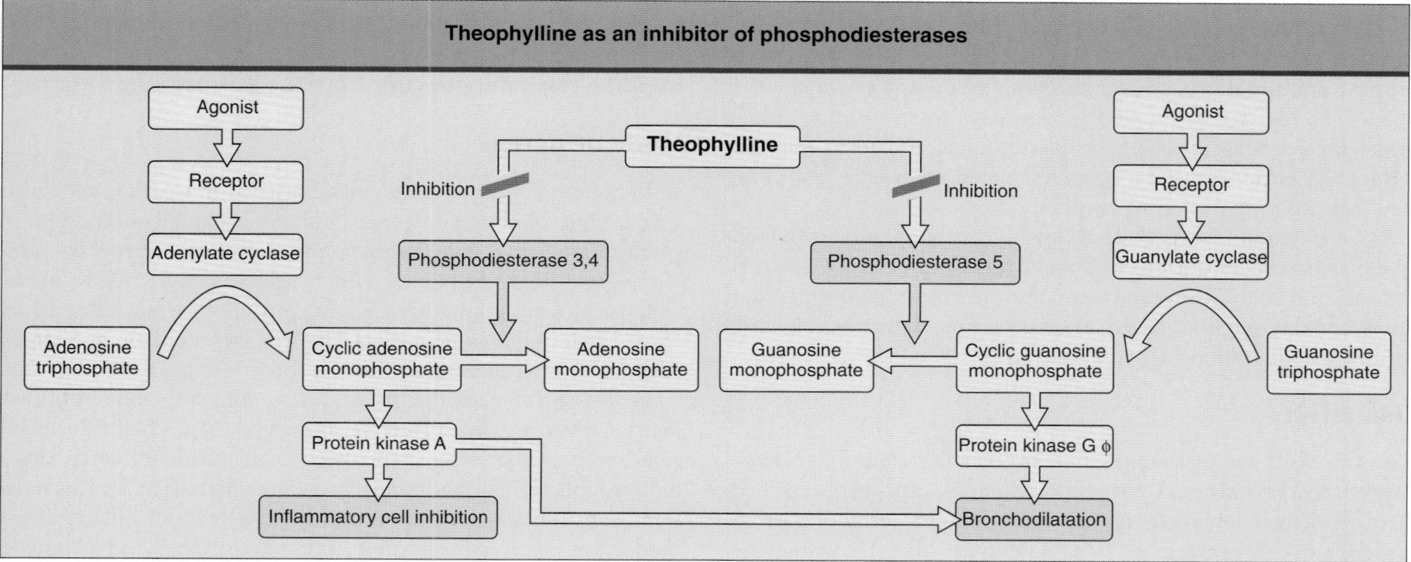

Figure 32.4 Theophylline as an inhibitor of phosphodiesterases. Theophylline is a weak phosphodiesterase inhibitor and increases the concentrations of cyclic adenosine monophosphate and cyclic guanosine monophosphate in airway cells, which results in bronchodilatation and inhibition of inflammatory cells.

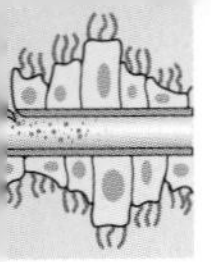

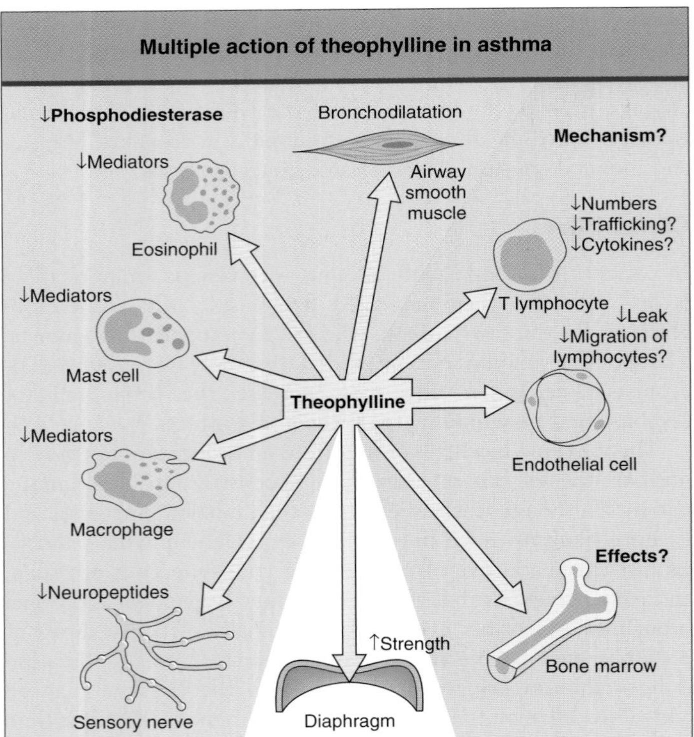

Figure 32.5 The multiple actions of theophylline in asthma. Some of these effects are probably mediated via phosphodiesterase inhibition, but others are so far unexplained.

a preferred option in countries where medication costs are limited.

Theophylline is readily and reliably absorbed from the gastrointestinal tract, but many factors affect plasma clearance, and therefore plasma concentration, so the drug is relatively difficult to use (Table 32.4).

Many different formulations of slow-release theophylline or aminophylline are available and differ in their pharmacokinetic profile. Several preparations are available for twice-daily administration, and also as once-daily preparations. Twice-daily administration may be preferable with a higher dose given at night to prevent nocturnal bronchoconstriction, whereas a lower dose is needed in the day as inhaled β-agonists may be used as additional bronchodilators. The frequency of side effects may be reduced. Caution must be observed when switching from one slow-release preparation to another.

Recent studies suggest that low-dose theophylline (which give plasma concentrations of 5 to 10 mg/L) effectively controls asthma, and such doses are below the previously recommended doses for theophylline based on plasma concentrations needed for bronchodilatation (10 to 20 mg/L).

Side Effects

Unwanted effects of theophylline are usually related to plasma concentration and tend to occur when plasma levels exceed 20 mg/L. However, some patients develop side effects even at low plasma concentrations. To some extent, side effects may be reduced by gradually increasing the dose until therapeutic concentrations are achieved. The most common side effects are

Table 32.4
Factors that affect clearance of theophylline

Increased clearance	Decreased clearance
Enzyme induction – rifampin (rifampicin), phenobarbital (phenobarbitone), ethanol	Enzyme inhibition – cimetidine, erythromycin, ciprofloxacin, allopurinol, zileuton
Smoking – tobacco, marijuana	Congestive heart failure
High-protein, low-carbohydrate diet	Liver disease
Barbecued meat	Pneumonia
Childhood	Viral infection and vaccination
	High carbohydrate diet
	Old age

Table 32.5
Side effects of theophylline

Side effects of theophylline
Nausea and vomiting
Headaches
Gastric discomfort
Diuresis
Behavioral disturbance (?)
Cardiac arrhythmias
Epileptic seizures

headache, nausea and vomiting, abdominal discomfort, and restlessness (Table 32.5). Increased acid secretion and diuresis may also occur. Concern that theophylline, even at therapeutic concentrations, may lead to behavioral disturbance and learning difficulties in school children is not supported by convincing evidence. At high concentrations, convulsions, cardiac arrhythmias, and death may occur.

ANTICHOLINERGICS

Atropine is a naturally occurring compound that was introduced for the treatment of asthma but, because of side effects (particularly drying of secretions), less soluble quaternary compounds (e.g., ipratropium bromide) were developed. These compounds are topically active and are not significantly absorbed from the respiratory tract or from the gastrointestinal tract.

Mode of Action

Anticholinergics are specific antagonists of muscarinic receptors and inhibit cholinergic nerve-induced bronchoconstriction. A small degree of resting bronchomotor tone is caused by tonic cholinergic nerve impulses, which release acetylcholine in the vicinity of airway smooth muscle, and cholinergic reflex bronchoconstriction may be initiated by irritants, cold air, and stress. Although anticholinergics afford protection against acute challenge by sulfur dioxide, inert dusts, cold air, and emotional factors, they are less effective against antigen challenge, exercise, and fog. This is not surprising, because anticholinergic drugs only inhibit reflex cholinergic bronchoconstriction and have no significant blocking effect on the direct effects of inflammatory mediators, such as histamine and leukotrienes, on bronchial smooth muscle (Figure 32.6). Furthermore, cholinergic antagonists probably have little or no effect on mast cells, microvas-

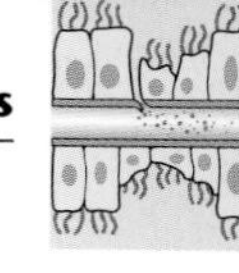

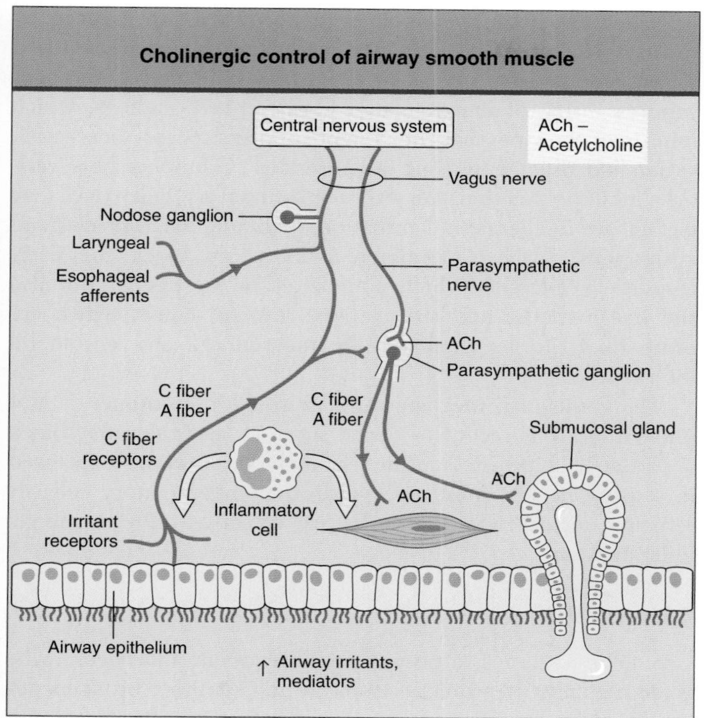

Figure 32.6 Cholinergic control of airway smooth muscle. Preganglionic and postganglionic parasympathetic nerves release acetylcholine (ACh) and can be activated by airway and extrapulmonary afferent nerves. Note that mediators released from inflammatory cells directly activate airway smooth-muscle cells, as well as a cholinergic reflex, so that anticholinergics are less effective than β_2-agonists as bronchodilators in asthma, because the latter counteract the effect of all bronchoconstrictors.

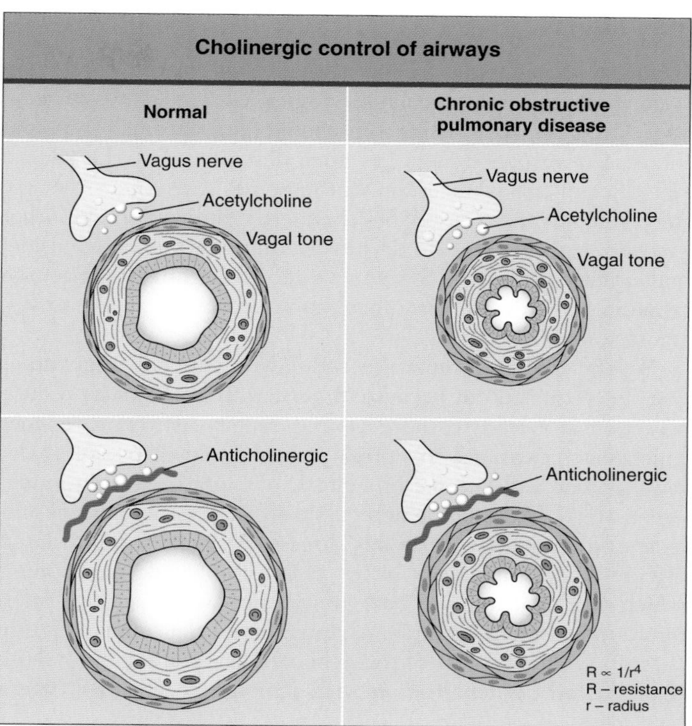

Figure 32.7 Cholinergic control of airways in patients who have chronic obstructive pulmonary disease (COPD). Normal airway has a certain degree of vagal cholinergic tone caused by tonic release of acetylcholine, which is blocked by muscarinic antagonists. This effect may be exaggerated in patients who have COPD because of fixed narrowing of the airways as a result of geometric factors. Thus, anticholinergic drugs have a greater bronchodilator effect in COPD than in normal airways.

cular leak, or the chronic inflammatory response. For these reasons, in patients who have asthma, anticholinergics are less effective as bronchodilators than β_2-agonists. By contrast, anticholinergics are the bronchodilators of choice in COPD.

Clinical Use

In asthmatic subjects, anticholinergic drugs are less effective as bronchodilators than β_2-agonists and offer less efficient protection against various bronchial challenges, although their duration of action is longer. These drugs may be more effective in older patients who have asthma and in whom an element of fixed airway obstruction is present. Nebulized anticholinergic drugs are effective in acute severe asthma, although they are less effective than β-agonists in this situation. Nevertheless, in the acute and chronic treatment of asthma, anticholinergic drugs may have an additive effect with β-agonists and should therefore be considered when control of asthma is not adequate with β-agonists, particularly if there are problems with theophylline, or inhaled β-agonists give troublesome tremor in elderly patients. The time course of bronchodilatation with anticholinergic drugs is slower than with β-agonists, reaching a peak only 1 hour after inhalation, but persists for more than 6 hours.

In COPD, anticholinergic drugs are even more effective than β-agonists. Their relatively greater effect in chronic obstructive airway disease than in asthma may be explained by an inhibitory effect on vagal tone which, although not necessarily being increased in COPD, may be the only reversible element of airway obstruction that is exaggerated by geometric factors in a narrowed airway (Figure 32.7).

Therapeutic Choices

IPRATROPIUM BROMIDE

Ipratropium bromide is the most widely used anticholinergic inhaler and is available as an MDI and nebulized preparation. The onset of bronchodilatation is relatively slow and is usually maximal 30 to 60 minutes after inhalation, but may persist for more than 6 hours. It is usually given by MDI three to four times daily on a regular basis, rather than intermittently for symptom relief, in view of its slow onset of action.

OXITROPIUM BROMIDE

Oxitropium bromide is a quaternary, anticholinergic bronchodilator that is similar to ipratropium bromide in terms of receptor blockade. It is available in higher doses by inhalation and its effect may therefore be more prolonged, so it may be useful in some patients who have nocturnal asthma.

TIOTROPIUM BROMIDE

Tiotropium bromide is a newly introduced anticholinergic with a much more prolonged duration of action caused by slow dissociation from muscarinic M_3 receptors. It is suitable for once-daily administration and is superior to four-times-daily ipratropium bromide. It is likely to become the bronchodilator of choice in COPD in the future.

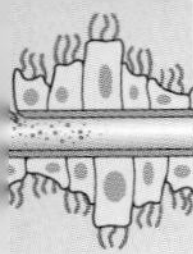

Side Effects

Inhaled anticholinergic drugs are usually well tolerated and there is no evidence for any decline in responsiveness with continued use. On stopping inhaled anticholinergics, a small rebound increase in responsiveness has been described, but the clinical relevance of this is uncertain. Atropine has side effects that are dose related and caused by cholinergic antagonism in other systems, and may lead to dryness of the mouth, blurred vision, and urinary retention. Systemic side effects after taking ipratropium bromide are very uncommon because virtually no systemic absorption occurs.

Several studies of mucus secretion with anticholinergic drugs have been carried out because of concern that they may reduce secretion and lead to more viscous mucus. Atropine reduces mucociliary clearance in normal subjects and in patients who have asthma and chronic bronchitis, but ipratropium bromide, even in high doses, has no detectable effect in either normal subjects or in patients with airway disease. A significant, unwanted effect is the unpleasant bitter taste of inhaled ipratropium, which may contribute to poor compliance with this drug. Nebulized ipratropium bromide may precipitate glaucoma in elderly patients, a direct effect of the nebulized drug on the eye, which is prevented by nebulization with a mouthpiece rather than a face mask.

Reports of paradoxic bronchoconstriction with ipratropium bromide, particularly when given by nebulizer, were largely explained by the hypotonicity of the nebulizer solution and by antibacterial additives, such as benzalkonium chloride. Nebulizer solutions free of these problems are less likely to cause bronchoconstriction. Occasionally, bronchoconstriction may occur with ipratropium bromide given by MDI. It is possible that this results from blockade of prejunctional M_2-receptors on airway cholinergic nerves, which normally inhibit acetylcholine release. The commonest side effect with tiotropium bromide is dryness of the mouth, which occurs in approximately 10% of patients.

Cromones

Cromones include cromolyn sodium (sodium cromoglycate) and nedocromil sodium. Cromolyn sodium is a derivative of khellin, an Egyptian herbal remedy that was found to protect against allergen challenge without bronchodilator effect. Nedocromil sodium is structurally related and has very similar clinical effects, although some evidence indicates that it is more potent.

Mode of Action

Initial investigations indicated that cromolyn sodium inhibited the release of mediators by allergen in passively sensitized human and animal lungs, and inhibited passive cutaneous anaphylaxis in the rat, although it had no effect in guinea pig. This activity was attributed to stabilization of the mast cell membrane and thus cromolyn sodium was classified as a mast-cell stabilizer. However, cromolyn sodium has a rather low potency in stabilizing mast cells of the human lung, and other drugs more potent in this respect have little or no effect in clinical asthma. This has raised doubts that mast-cell stabilization is the major mode of action of cromolyn sodium.

Cromones potently inhibit bronchoconstriction induced by sulfur dioxide, metabisulfite, and bradykinin, which are believed to activate sensory nerves in the airways. In dogs, cromones suppress firing of unmyelinated C-fiber nerve endings, which reinforces the view that they might suppress sensory nerve activation and thus neurogenic inflammation. Cromones have variable inhibitory actions on other inflammatory cells that may participate in allergic inflammation, including macrophages and eosinophils. In vivo cromolyn sodium can block the early response to allergen (which is mediated by mast cells), but also the late response and airway hyperresponsiveness, which are more likely to be mediated by macrophage and eosinophil interactions.

The molecular mechanism of action of cromones is not understood, but recent evidence suggests that they may block a particular type of chloride channel that may be expressed in sensory nerves, mast cells, and other inflammatory cells. It remains unclear why cromones are effective only in allergic inflammation.

Current Use

Cromolyn sodium is a prophylactic treatment and needs to be given regularly. It protects against various indirect bronchoconstrictor stimuli, such as exercise and fog. It is only effective in mild asthma, but does not appear to be effective in all patients and no sure way of predicting the patients are likely to respond has been established. Indeed, a systematic review of clinical studies of cromolyn in children concluded that it provided little benefit. One reason for the discrepancy between its beneficial effects in various indirect challenges and its poor efficacy in clinical practice is likely to be its short duration of action (approximately 2 hours) as it needs to be given at least 4 times daily. Because of its poor efficacy and high cost, it is now used less and less, particularly as low doses of inhaled corticosteroids have been shown to be much more effective and just as safe in children with mild asthma.

In clinical practice, nedocromil has a similar efficacy to cromolyn sodium and is therefore indicated in patients who have mild asthma, but the unpleasant taste makes cromolyn sodium preferable to many patients. No place exists for cromones in the management of COPD.

Side Effects

Cromolyn sodium is one of the safest drugs available and side effects are extremely rare. The dry powder inhaler may cause throat irritation, coughing, and (occasionally) wheezing, but this is usually prevented by prior administration of a β-agonist inhaler. Very rarely, a transient rash and urticaria are seen and a few cases of pulmonary eosinophilia have been reported, all of which arise from hypersensitivity. Side effects with nedocromil are not usually a problem, although some patients have noticed a sensation of flushing after using the inhaler. Many patients find the bitter taste unpleasant, but a menthol-flavored version is now available and seems to overcome this problem.

ANTILEUKOTRIENES

Antileukotrienes are a relatively new class of antiasthma agent.

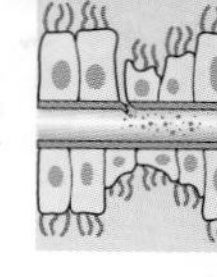

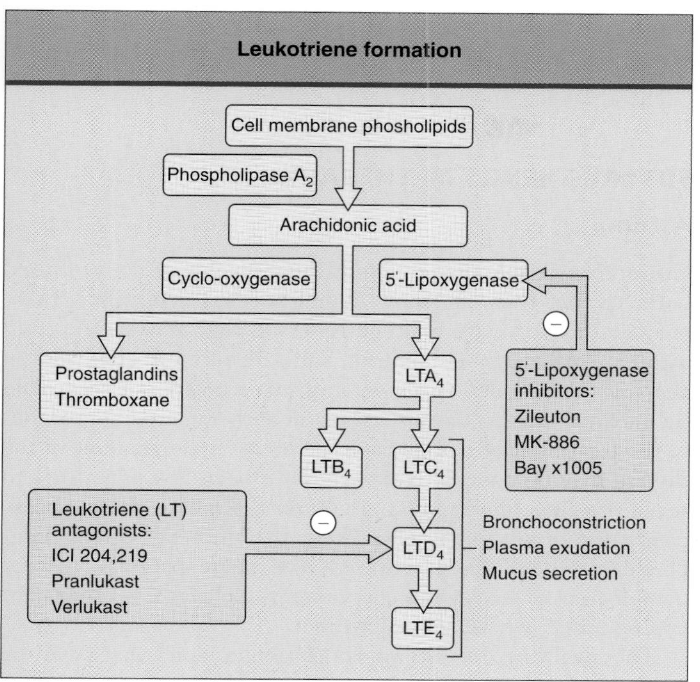

Figure 32.8 Leukotriene formation. Generation of cysteinyl-leukotrienes from arachidonic acid by 5′-lipoxygenase.

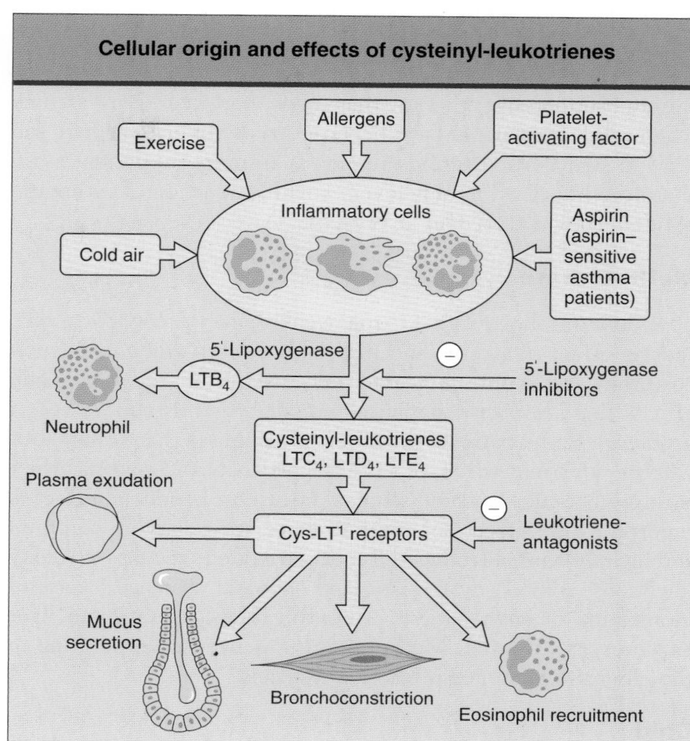

Figure 32.9 Cellular origin and effects of cysteinyl-leukotrienes.

Mode of Action

Elevated levels of cysteinyl-leukotrienes (cys-LTs: LTC_4, LTD_4, LTE_4) are detected in bronchoalveolar lavage fluid and elevated LTE_4 levels in the urine of asthmatic subjects. Cys-LTs are generated from arachidonic acid by the rate-limiting enzyme 5′-lipoxygenase (5-LO; Figure 32.8). Cys-LTs are potent constrictors of human airways in vitro and in vivo, cause airway microvascular leakage in animals, and stimulate airway mucus secretion (Figure 32.9). These effects are all mediated in human airways via cys-LT_1 receptors and potent cys-LT_1 antagonists (montelukast, zafirlukast, pranlukast) are now available. Antileukotrienes reduce allergen-induced, exercise-induced, and cold air–induced asthma by about 50% to 70%, and inhibit aspirin-induced responses in aspirin-sensitive asthmatics almost completely. The only 5-lipoxygenase inhibitor clinically available (only in the United States) is zileuton, the efficacy of which is similar to that of receptor antagonists. Antileukotrienes have also been shown to have weak anti-inflammatory effects and may reduce eosinophilic inflammation, which may be provoked by cys-LTs.

Clinical Use

Antileukotrienes may have a small and variable bronchodilator effect, indicating that leukotrienes may contribute to baseline bronchoconstriction in asthma. Long-term administration reduces asthma symptoms and the need for rescue β_2-agonists, and improves lung function. The effects are significantly less than with inhaled corticosteroids in terms of symptom control, improvement in lung function, and reduction in exacerbations. Antileukotrienes may be useful in patients whose asthma is not controlled on inhaled corticosteroids, and are as effective as doubling the dose of inhaled corticosteroids. They are effective in some but not all patients with aspirin-sensitive asthma. Patients differ in their response to anti-leukotrienes, and it is impossible to predict which patients will respond best.

A major advantage of antileukotrienes is that they are orally active, and this is likely to improve compliance with long-term therapy. However, they are expensive, and a trial of therapy is indicated to determine which patients will benefit most. Antileukotrienes have no place in the management of COPD.

Side Effects

Side effects are uncommon. Some drugs produce mild liver dysfunction, so liver function tests are important. Several cases of Churg-Strauss syndrome (systemic vasculitis with eosinophilia and asthma) have been observed in patients on antileukotrienes, but this may be because a concomitant reduction in oral corticosteroids (made possible by the antileukotriene) allows the vasculitis to flare up.

KETOTIFEN

Ketotifen is described as a prophylactic antiasthma compound. Its predominant effect is histamine H_1-receptor antagonism, which accounts for its sedative effect. Ketotifen has little effect in clinical asthma—in acute challenge, on airway hyperresponsiveness, or on clinical symptoms. A long-term placebo-controlled trial of oral ketotifen in children who had mild asthma showed no significant clinical benefit. It is claimed that ketotifen has disease-modifying effects if started early in asthma in children and that it may even prevent the development of asthma in atopic children. More carefully controlled studies are needed to assess the validity of these claims.

IMMUNOSUPPRESSIVE OR CORTICOSTEROID-SPARING THERAPY

Immunosuppressive therapy has been considered in asthma when other treatments have been unsuccessful or to reduce the dose of oral corticosteroids required. Immunosuppressives are therefore indicated in only a very small proportion of asthmatic patients (fewer than 1%) at present.

Methotrexate

Low-dose methotrexate (15 mg weekly) has a corticosteroid-sparing effect in asthma and may be indicated when oral corticosteroids are contraindicated because of unacceptable side effects (e.g., in postmenopausal women when osteoporosis is a problem). Some patients show better responses than others, but whether a patient will have a useful corticosteroid-sparing effect is unpredictable. In some studies, no useful beneficial effect is reported. Side effects of methotrexate are relatively common and include nausea (reduced if methotrexate is given as a weekly injection), blood dyscrasias, and hepatic damage. Careful monitoring of such patients (monthly blood counts and liver enzymes) is essential. Methotrexate has been disappointing in the clinical experience of most physicians.

Gold

Gold has long been used in the treatment of chronic arthritis. Anecdotal evidence suggests that it may also be useful in asthma, and it has been used in Japan for many years. A controlled trial of an oral gold preparation (auranofin) demonstrated some corticosteroid-sparing effect in chronic asthmatic patients maintained on oral corticosteroids. Side effects such as skin rashes and nephropathy are a limiting factor.

Cyclosporin A

Cyclosporin A is active against $CD4^+$ lymphocytes and is therefore potentially useful in asthma, in which these cells are implicated. A trial of low-dose oral cyclosporin A in patients who had corticosteroid-dependent asthma indicated that it can improve control of symptoms in patients who suffer severe asthma and are on oral corticosteroids, but other trials have been unimpressive. Its use is likely to be limited by severe side effects, such as nephrotoxicity and hypertension, which are common. In clinical practice it is very disappointing as a corticosteroid-sparing agent and has largely been abandoned.

Intravenous Immunoglobulin

When high doses were used (2 g/kg), intravenous immunoglobulin was reported to have corticosteroid-sparing effects in corticosteroid-dependent asthma, although in controlled trials at lower doses it is ineffective. This is an extremely expensive treatment that cannot be recommended

FUTURE TRENDS IN THERAPY

Asthma

Currently available therapy for asthma is highly effective if used correctly, but there are some unmet needs. For example, there is a need for effective oral controllers in the treatment of mild asthma, particularly in children, and for more effective add-on therapies in patients with severe asthma who are not controlled by maximal inhaled therapy. Many new therapeutic approaches to the treatment of asthma based on better understanding of the disease may be possible, yet there have been few new drugs to reach the clinic. β_2-Agonists are by far the most effective bronchodilator drugs and it is unlikely that more effective bronchodilators could be discovered. For many patients, a fixed combination of LABA and corticosteroid inhaler is a convenient and effective way to control asthma.

The ideal drug for asthma is probably a tablet that could be administered once daily to improve compliance. It should have no side effects, which means that it should be specific for the abnormality of asthma (or allergy). So far, inhibitors of specific cytokines have proved to be ineffective and a more generalized antiinflammatory treatment is needed. Phosphodiesterase-4 inhibitors may be promising and anti–immunoglobulin E antibodies appear to be useful in patients with severe asthma. The possibility of developing a cure for asthma seems remote, but when more is known about the genetic abnormalities of asthma, a search for such a therapy may be feasible.

COPD

Tiotropium bromide is a long-acting anticholinergic suitable for once-daily dosing and is likely to replace ipratropium bromide as the bronchodilator treatment of choice in COPD. No currently available therapy alters the progression of COPD, and there is no evidence that corticosteroids are effective. Future approaches may include drugs that inhibit the characteristic neutrophilic inflammation of COPD (LTB_4 antagonists, interleukin-8 antagonists, phosphodiesterase-4 inhibitors), more potent antioxidants (glutathione analogs), and drugs that inhibit proteases (neutrophil elastase inhibitors, matrix metalloproteinase inhibitors). The testing of these new drugs will be difficult, as long-term studies will be necessary to demonstrate a reduction in the progressive decline in lung function.

SUGGESTED READINGS

Barnes PJ: New directions in allergic disease: mechanism-based anti-inflammatory therapies. J Allergy Clin Immunol 106:5-16, 2000.

Barnes PJ: New treatments for COPD. Nature Rev Drug Disc 1:437-445, 2002.

Barnes PJ: Theophylline: New perspectives on an old drug. Am J Respir Crit Care Med 167:813-818, 2003.

Barnes PJ: Therapy of chronic obstructive pulmonary disease. Pharmacol Ther 97:87-94, 2003.

British Thoracic Society: British guideline on the management of asthma. Thorax 58(suppl 1):1-194, 2003.

Disse B: Antimuscarinic treatment for lung diseases from research to clinical practice. Life Sci 68:2557-2564, 2001.

Drazen JM, Israel E, O'Byrne PM: Treatment of asthma with drugs modifying the leukotriene pathway. N Engl J Med 340:197-206, 1999.

Kips JC, Pauwels RA: Long-acting inhaled β_2-agonist therapy in asthma. Am J Respir Crit Care Med 164:923-932, 2001.

CHAPTER 33 Corticosteroids

Paul M. O'Byrne

Corticosteroids have been used to treat a variety of lung diseases since the early 1950s, when benefits of oral cortisone were first reported on hay fever and asthma induced by ragweed pollen, and also from inhaled cortisone in a small group of patients who had allergic or nonallergic asthma. Subsequently, a multicenter trial run by the Medical Research Council in the United Kingdom in 1956 demonstrated improvement in acute, severe asthma, and a subsequent report described benefit in chronic asthma; thus, the unequivocal benefit of corticosteroids in asthma was demonstrated. Subsequently, both oral and inhaled corticosteroids have evolved into the most important drugs currently available to treat many lung diseases, especially asthma. Because inhaled corticosteroids are the most effective treatment for asthma and the most widely used regular treatment for airway disease, this review focuses on their pharmacology.

ANTI-INFLAMMATORY ACTIVITY OF CORTICOSTEROIDS

Most of the actions of corticosteroids, and almost certainly their anti-inflammatory activity, occurs through activation of the glucocorticosteroid receptor (GCSr), which is found in virtually all of the body's cells. Only one receptor type has been identified, and in the resting state it is bound to two molecules of heat shock protein-90 (HSP-90), and one molecule of the immunophilin p-59. Binding of the corticosteroid to the receptor disassociates the receptor from HSP-90, which results in a conformational change of the receptor complex. The corticosteroid-receptor complex binds to the promoter-enhancer regions of target genes, glucocorticosteroid response elements, which results in upregulation or downregulation of the gene, and thereby of the gene product (Figure 33.1).

The corticosteroid-receptor complex can regulate gene product in several other ways (see Fig. 33.1). First, the complex can bind directly (by protein-protein interaction) with the transcription factors, such as AP-1 (which is unregulated during inflammation), and thereby inhibit the proinflammatory effects of a variety of cytokines. Second, the complex can bind to a glucocorticosteroid response element that overlaps with the upregulatory site for another proinflammatory product (i.e., a cytokine). Third, the complex is known to reduce the availability of another important transcription factor for cytokine production, NFκB. Fourth, glucocorticosteroids can increase the levels of cell ribonucleases, and thereby reduce the levels of messenger RNA. Finally, corticosteroids have been shown to act by recruitment of histone deacetylases to the site of active inflammatory gene transcription. This inhibits the acetylation of histones needed for inflammatory gene transcription. It is likely that this multiplicity of action is the reason for the marked anti-inflammatory activity of corticosteroids in so many inflammatory diseases. However, their complexity of activity makes it very difficult to establish which of these actions is responsible for their marked efficacy in asthma.

Routes of Administration

Corticosteroids are administered either systemically (orally or intravenously) or topically (inhaled) to treat lung diseases. Systemic administration is generally reserved for patients who have severe asthma, or as a trial of therapy to attempt to optimize lung function in patients thought to have a component of fixed air-flow obstruction, or in patients with a mainly peripheral lung disease such as sarcoidosis. Corticosteroids, such as prednisone or methylprednisolone, are rapidly and completely absorbed across the gastrointestinal tract and have a very high oral bioavailability. Therefore, intravenous glucocorticosteroids need only be used to treat airway diseases in exceptional circumstances, such as for patients who cannot swallow or who are vomiting. The majority of severe exacerbations of asthma, however, can be treated adequately with oral prednisone (0.5 to 1 mg/kg per day, or its equivalent).

Inhaled corticosteroids are the preferred route to treat airway diseases because of the availability of topically potent corticosteroids, which are very effective, and which have much less unwanted systemic effects than systemically administered glucocorticosteroids. Inhaled glucocorticosteroids can be delivered to the airways by a wide variety of inhaler systems, each of which has inherent advantages and disadvantages. Because no currently available inhaler system is ideal in every clinical situation, each of these needs to be considered when making a choice of inhaler systems for a specific clinical circumstance.

Pharmacokinetics

ABSORPTION AND FATE OF GLUCOCORTICOSTEROIDS

Cortisone and prednisone are prodrugs, which require hydroxylation in the liver to the active compounds hydrocortisone and prednisolone. These glucocorticosteroids have less affinity for the mineralocorticosteroid receptor, and/or enhanced affinity for the GCSr, and/or improved uptake and metabolism when compared with the parent compound. For example, unsaturation of the 1-2 bond of the hydrocortisone skeleton produces prednisolone, which improves the stability in the liver and doubles its half-life. Also, the binding affinity for the GCSr for prednisolone is 12 times higher, and for dexamethasone it is 25 times higher than that for hydrocortisone. Most of these com-

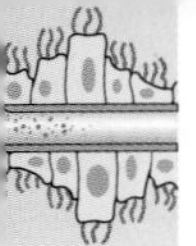

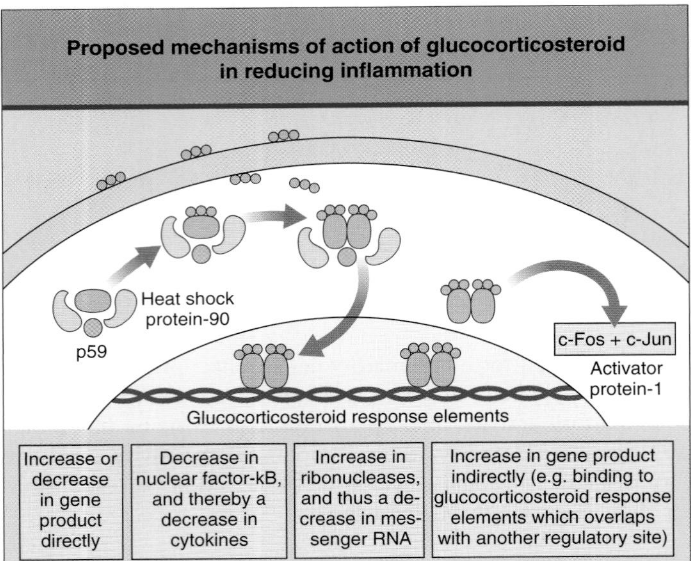

Figure 33.1 Proposed mechanisms of action of the complex of glucocorticosteroid and glucocorticosteroid receptor in reducing asthmatic inflammation.

pounds are still widely used as the systemic glucocorticosteroids of choice in a variety of inflammatory diseases.

All of these compounds are readily absorbed across epithelial lining by diffusion. No active transport systems are required for glucocorticosteroid absorption. The oral bioavailability of the systemic glucocorticosteroids ranges from 60% for hydrocortisone to 90% for methylprednisolone. This difference does not reflect the ability of the drug to be absorbed across the gut epithelium, but rather the efficiency of the first-pass metabolism through the liver. All the systemically available glucocorticosteroids are metabolized by p450 systems in the liver, and their clearance rates can be altered by severe liver diseases and liver cirrhosis. The systemic half-life also varies from 1.9 hours for hydrocortisone to 4.4 hours for dexamethasone.

In the 1960s, modification of the hydrocortisone skeleton produced glucocorticosteroids with topical selectivity for dermal application and the treatment of skin diseases. These compounds, betamethasone valerate and beclomethasone dipropionate (BDP) (highly lipophilic compounds, as are dexamethasone and triamcinolone), were tried by inhalation in the treatment of asthma in the early 1970s, and BDP has been a mainstay of asthma treatment since. Later, other lipophilic glucocorticosteroids [flunisolide, budesonide, fluticasone propionate (FP), mometasone and ciclesonide (Figure 33.2)] were developed for the treatment of asthma and allergic rhinitis.

Lipophilic glucocorticosteroids have two main advantages for topical use in the airways—a very high binding affinity for GCSr (at least 100 times greater than that of hydrocortisone) and a very efficient first-pass hepatic metabolism, which results in an extremely low oral bioavailability. The clearance rates for budesonide and fluticasone, for example, are very close to maximal hepatic clearance, and thus entirely limited by hepatic blood flow (approximately 1.5 L/min); the resultant oral bioavailability via gut absorption for budesonide is 11% and

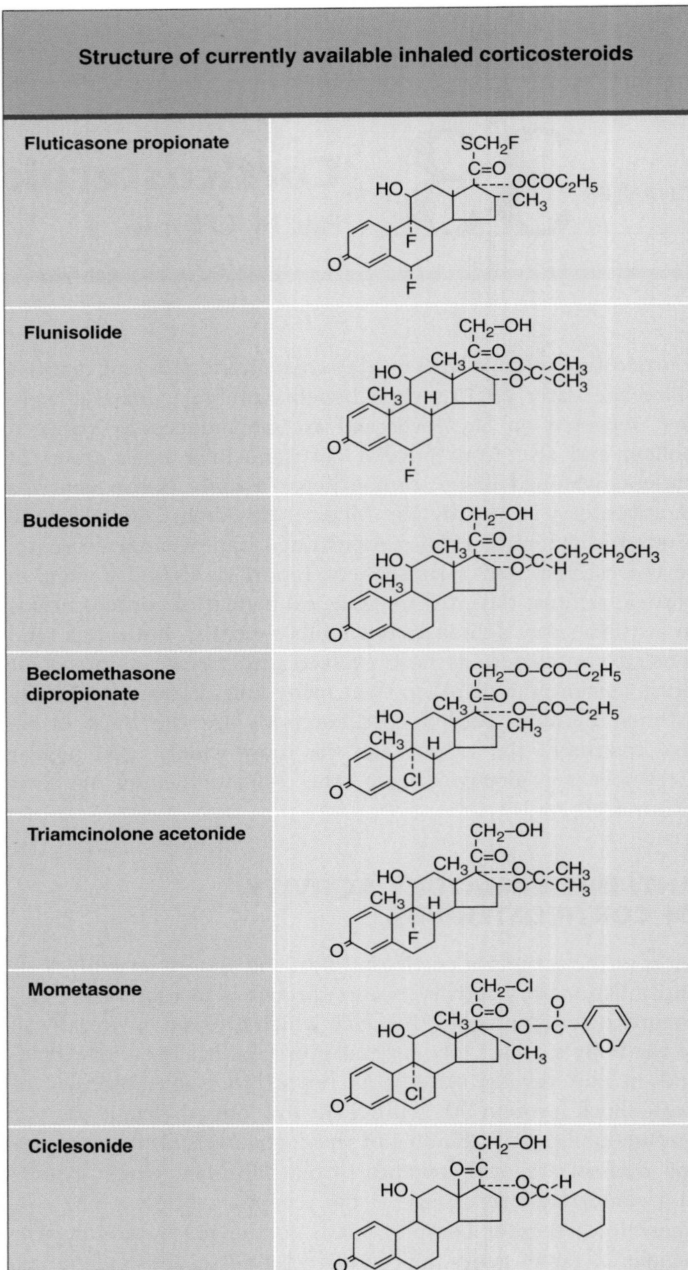

Figure 33.2 Structure of currently available inhaled corticosteroids.

for FP less than 1%. Thus, the systemic bioavailability of these compounds results almost entirely from absorption across the lung epithelium, rather than that from the gut epithelium.

CURRENTLY AVAILABLE INHALED CORTICOSTEROIDS

Currently, six topically active glucocorticosteroids are available by the inhaled route for the treatment of asthma—beclomethasone dipropionate, triamcinolone, flunisolide, budesonide, fluticasone propionate, and mometasone, with another, ciclesonide, in the final stages of clinical development (see Fig. 33.2). Their pharmacologic properties are given in Table 33.1.

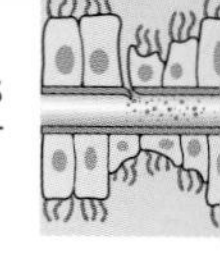

Table 33.1
Relative receptor affinity and basic pharmacokinetic parameters of inhaled corticosteroids

Corticosteroid	Relative binding affinity[1]	Half-life (h)	Volume of distribution (L/kg)	Clearance (L/min)	Water solubility (mg/mL)	Relative topical blanching potency	Oral availability (%)	Protein binding (%)
BDP	0.5/13	NA	NA	NA	0.1/10	0.6/0.4	NA	87
Budesonide	9.4	2–3	2.7–4.3	0.9–1.3	14	1	11	88
Flunisolide	1.9	1.6	1.8	10	100	3	21	80
Fluticasone	18	4–14	3.7–8.9	0.9–1.3	4	1–1.7	<1	90
Triamcinolone	3.6	1.5	1.5	7	40	4	23	71
Mometasone	12.4	4.5	4.5	0.89	NA	NA	<1	NA
Ciclesonide	12	3.4	10	3.8	1.7	NA	<1	99

NA: not available; [1]dexamethasone = 1

BECLOMETHASONE 17,21-DIPROPIONATE

Since 1972, BDP has been available by inhalation for the treatment of asthma. It has all of the properties of the other lipophilic glucocorticosteroids; however, because of its early development, very little pharmacokinetic information is available on this compound. Initially, BDP is biotransformed into its active metabolite, beclomethasone monopropionate, in the liver, but further metabolism of beclomethasone monopropionate appears to be slower than that of the newer, topically active glucocorticosteroids.

TRIAMCINOLONE

Triamcinolone has also not been fully characterized with regards to its pharmacokinetics. Its oral bioavailability is 22%, and plasma half-life is 1.5 hours after intravenous administration. Triamcinolone has a moderate affinity for GCSr, four times that of dexamethasone.

FLUNISOLIDE

Flunisolide has an oral bioavailability of 21%, but a lower affinity for GCSr, being five times lower than budesonide and ten times lower than FP in human lung tissues. Its plasma half-life after intravenous administration is 1.6 hours, which is almost identical to the half-life after inhalation of a single dose and indicates no lung metabolism.

BUDESONIDE

Budesonide is the most extensively studied inhaled glucocorticosteroid to date, in terms of its pharmacokinetics. Its oral bioavailability is 6% to 13%, which indicates a high first-pass liver metabolism, with a plasma clearance of 1.3 L/min, which is close to the maximal liver clearance. The plasma half-life after intravenous administration is 3 hours. After a single inhaled dose of 500 μgm, the peak plasma levels are achieved within 30 minutes, and the half-life is 2 hours, which suggests little lung metabolism occurs. Budesonide has a high binding affinity for GCSr, being 10 times that of dexamethasone. In vivo, after topical superperfusion of rat trachea, budesonide and FP were retained to a similar extent, and both were retained longer than BDP. During washing, the subsequent release was slower for budesonide than for the other steroids tested. This retention is associated with an intracellular formation of long-chain fatty acid conjugates (esterification) of budesonide. Intact budesonide is regained in a rate-limited fashion, and this appeared to prolong the pharmacologic effect of the drug.

FLUTICASONE PROPIONATE

Fluticasone propionate's oral bioavailability is less than 1%, which is the lowest of the available inhaled glucocorticosteroids. This is not only because of its rapid first-pass liver metabolism, which is 0.87 L/min per 1.73 m, but also because of poor absorption across the gut epithelium. The plasma half-life after intravenous administration varies from 3.7 to 14.4 hours. The prolonged plasma half-life may be because it is highly lipophilic, with retention in lipid stores. Also, FP has the highest binding affinity to the GCSr yet measured, being 18 times that of dexamethasone.

MOMETASONE

Mometasone is a newer inhaled corticosteroid, whose oral bioavailability is also less than 1%. It has a high receptor binding, being 12.4 times that of dexamethasone. Its plasma half-life is 4.5 hours, and it has a volume of distribution of 4.5 L/kg. It has a long duration of clinical activity, having been shown in many patients to be effective with once-daily dosing. No information is yet available to demonstrate whether this is due to intracellular esterification.

CICLESONIDE

Ciclesonide is another newly developed inhaled corticosteroid, which is a pro-drug when inhaled and is activated by esterases. This does not appear to occur in the mouth, but does in the lower airways. Ciclesonide has been shown to be effective in many patients when administered once daily, possibly because of intracellular esterification in the airways. Its oral bioavailability is less than 1%, with a receptor binging affinity of 12 times dexamethasone. It is the most lipophilic of the available corticosteroids, with a water solubility of 1.7 mg/mL and a volume of distribution of 10 L/kg. Interestingly, it has the highest protein binding, being 99% protein bound in the circulation.

Pharmacodynamics

DOSE-RESPONSE CHARACTERISTICS OF INHALED GLUCOCORTICOSTEROIDS

To establish the dose-response characteristics of inhaled corticosteroids has been very difficult, mainly because these vary greatly between patients, and even vary in the same patient when the disease is mild or more severe. Also, the outcome variable to measure is unclear, as is how long to wait after initiation of treatment at any specific dose before a response is measured. This is quite different from, for example, examining the dose-response of an inhaled β_2-agonist, for which the standard outcome variable of improvement is forced expiratory volume in 1 second or peak expiratory flow rate, and the response can be measured over minutes to hours. The maximal clinical benefit for symptoms or lung function for an inhaled glucocorticosteroid can take 6 to 8 weeks to be achieved (Figure 33.3), and for some physiologic parameters, such as improvements in airway hyperresponsiveness, improvements can continue for up to 1 to 2 years (Figure 33.4). Thus, the dose response characteristics of an individual inhaled corticosteroid depend not only on the pharmacology of the compound, but also on the outcome studied and the duration of treatment.

Most studies demonstrate a statistically significant and clinically useful benefit from increasing the inhaled doses by fourfold. However, no large and well-designed study has been able to demonstrate a difference between two-fold incremental doses for those outcome variables most often measured in clinical asthma studies (i.e., symptoms and lung function) in the type of patients (those who have mild or moderate asthma) most often studied (Figure 33.5). It appears, from examining these studies, that patients who have mild-to-moderate asthma have a very steep dose-response curve, and achieve maximal benefit from doses of inhaled glucocorticosteroids, such as budesonide or BDP, as low as 200 μgm/day. By contrast, patients who have more severe asthma often receive clinical benefit from higher inhaled doses of 800 to 1600 μgm/day. A dose-response effect may be more obvious if a different outcome variable is measured, as has been demonstrated for exercise bronchoconstriction in children (Figure 33.6). Recent studies also identify that, after asthma control is achieved, the doses of inhaled glucocorticosteroids needed to maintain control are lower.

The dose frequency of inhaled glucocorticosteroids has been addressed in several studies. These studies demonstrate that in patients who suffer moderate-to-severe asthma, an administra-

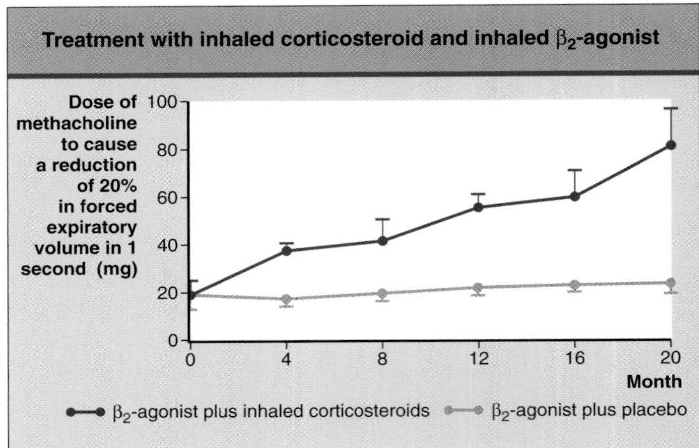

Figure 33.4 Effect of 20 months treatment with an inhaled corticosteroid plus an inhaled β_2-agonist or placebo plus an inhaled β_2-agonist on methacholine airway responsiveness in asthmatic children. The inhaled corticosteroid progressively improved methacholine airway responsiveness over time. (Reproduced with permission from van Essen-Zandvliet EE, Hughes MD, Waalkens HJ, et al: Effect of 22 months of treatment with inhaled corticosteroids and/or β_2-agonists on lung function, airway responsiveness and symptoms in patients with asthma. Am Rev Resp Dis 146:547-554, 1992.)

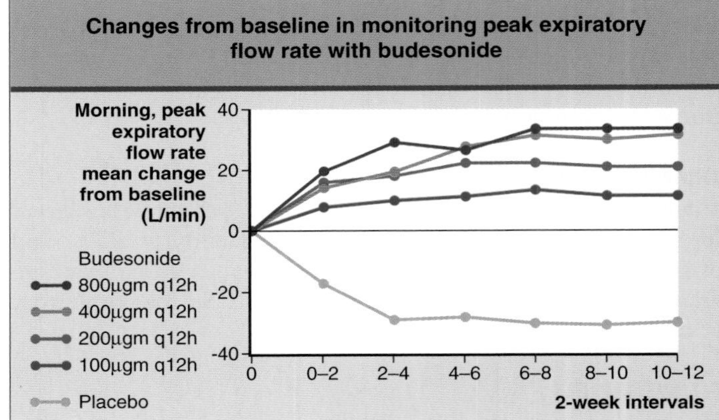

Figure 33.5 Mean changes from baseline in morning peak expiratory flow rate in patients treated with placebo or various doses of budesonide for 12 weeks of treatment. A significant dose-response is demonstrated; however, the difference between placebo and budesonide 100 μgm every 12 hours is greater than that between 100 and 800 μgm every 12 hours. (Drawn from data in Busse WW: Dose-related efficacy of Pulmicort Turbuhaler in moderate to severe asthma. J Allergy Clin Immunol 93:186A, 1994.)

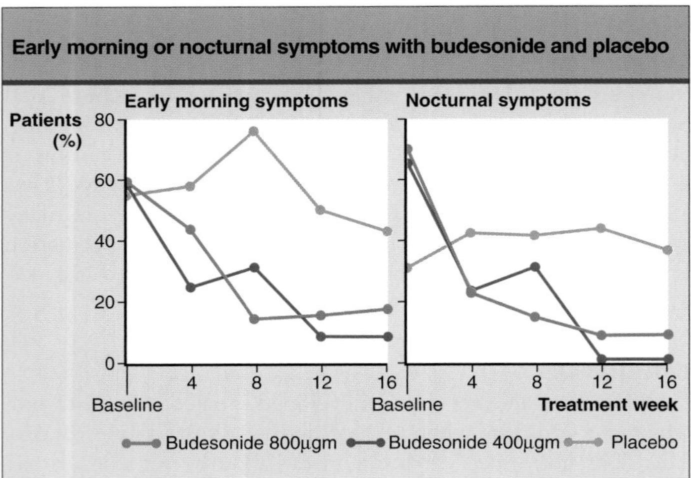

Figure 33.3 Proportion of patients who experience early morning symptoms or nocturnal symptoms with budesonide. Measurements taken in the month prior to evaluation at baseline and after treatment with inhaled budesonide at treatment weeks 4 to 16 for patients on placebo, budesonide 400 μgm/day and budesonide 800 μgm/day. The maximal benefit was achieved after 8 weeks of treatment. (Reproduced with permission from O'Byrne PM, Cuddy L, Taylor DW, et al: The clinical efficacy and cost benefit of inhaled corticosteroids as therapy in patients with mild asthma in primary care practice. Can Resp J 3:169-175, 1996.)

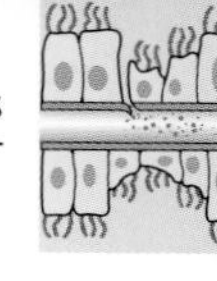

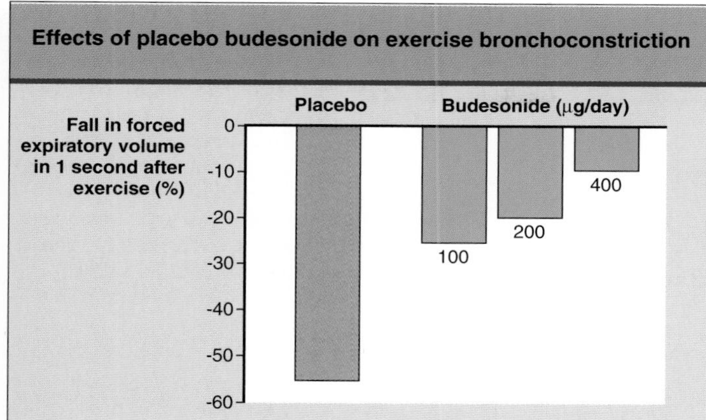

Figure 33.6 Effects of placebo or treatment with budesonide 100 μgm, 200 μgm, or 400 μgm daily on exercise bronchoconstriction. A significant dose-response effect was demonstrated between the different doses of budesonide. (Reproduced with permission from Pedersen S, Hansen OR: Budesonide treatment of moderate and severe asthma in children: A dose-response study. J Allergy Clin Immunol 95:29-33, 1995.)

tion of the inhaled glucocorticosteroids four times per day is better than the same total dose administered twice daily; however, this benefit is less obvious in patients who have milder asthma. An additional factor that must be considered is the compliance of the patient who takes doses four times a day. For these reasons, twice-daily dosing—morning and evening—is generally recommended for many asthmatics. In patients who have milder asthma, dosing once per day has been demonstrated to be effective for budesonide, mometasone, and ciclesonide.

SIDE EFFECTS OF CORTICOSTEROIDS

Inhaled corticosteroids are absorbed across the lung into the systemic circulation and do have effects beyond the lungs. Concerns about their systemic unwanted effects have greatly limited their use, especially in children. The side effects of inhaled glucocorticosteroids are dose related, with little or no evidence of clinically relevant, systemic, unwanted effects at doses of less than 400 μgm/day of beclomethasone or budesonide in children and of less than 1000 μgm/day in adults.

Local Side Effects

The main side effects that do occur with lower doses of inhaled corticosteroids are oral candidiasis, because of the oropharyngeal deposition of the inhaled corticosteroid, and dysphonia. Clinically obvious oral candidiasis occurs in 5% to 10% of adult asthmatics treated with inhaled corticosteroids, but in only 1% of children. However, positive oropharyngeal cultures for *Candida* spp have been demonstrated in up to 45% of children and 70% of adults using corticosteroids. The risk of clinically obvious oral candidiasis is increased by the concomitant use of antibiotics and inhaled corticosteroids, and is greatly reduced by the use of a large volume spacer or AeroChamber to deliver the inhaled corticosteroid, and by mouth rinsing after use.

Dysphonia is a more common topical side effect of inhaled corticosteroids, which may occur in up to 30% of patients. It is more common in patients who use their voice a lot, is sometimes temporary, and is only really troublesome in patients who use their voice to earn income.

Corticosteroids applied topically to the skin cause skin thinning and atrophy. This is because the corticosteroid remains on the skin for several hours. By contrast, inhaled corticosteroids are rapidly absorbed across the airway mucosa, and are unlikely to have this effect on the airway mucosa. Indeed, studies of airway biopsies of asthmatics who have used inhaled corticosteroids for months or years have not demonstrated any evidence of airway mucosal atrophy, but rather of repair of the epithelial damage so characteristic of asthma.

Systemic Side Effects

Doses of inhaled glucocorticosteroids of greater than 200 μgm/day in children and of greater than 1000 μgm/day in adults result in measurable systemic effects, such as changes in growth velocity in children, and biochemical changes indicated by effects on bones and the adrenal glands in adults. All physicians who treat asthmatics must be conscious that these types of adverse effects may develop in patients who use corticosteroids to treat asthma or other diseases. The potential adverse effects of corticosteroids are outlined in the following section.

EFFECTS ON THE HYPOTHALAMIC-PITUITARY-ADRENAL AXIS

The effects of corticosteroids on the hypothalamic-pituitary-adrenal (HPA) axis are measured in a number of different ways. The most commonly used and easiest to carry out, but also the least sensitive method is to measure early morning serum cortisol levels. Much more sensitive to the effects of excess glucocorticosteroids on the HPA axis are measurement of 24-hour urinary cortisol or the short tetracosactin (ACTH) stimulation test.

The different inhaled glucocorticosteroids are not equal in their effects on the HPA axis. For example, in children a dose-dependent effect of urinary cortisols has been demonstrated with doses of BDP from 200 to 800 μgm/day. By contrast, doses of budesonide of 400 μgm/day do not cause any effect on urinary cortisols, even when used for up to 1 year. In adults, many studies have examined the effects of inhaled glucocorticosteroids on HPA axis function, and no evidence convincingly shows any measurable effect on the HPA axis of doses of BDP less than 1500 μgm/day and budesonide less than 1600 μgm/day. The measurable effects seen at higher doses clearly indicate systemic activity of the inhaled glucocorticosteroid, but are of questionable clinical significance. Only a few reports exist of clinically evident adrenal insufficiency in patients treated only with inhaled glucocorticosteroids after the inhaled glucocorticosteroid has been withdrawn.

OSTEOPOROSIS

Osteoporosis is an important complication of the use of ingested glucocorticosteroids, particularly in high-risk patients, such as postmenopausal women. This occurs through an increase in bone resorption and a decrease in bone formation, and results in an increased risk of fractures, especially the hip and spine. Inhaled corticosteroids can affect the bone metabolism, but little evidence indicates that they cause osteoporosis or cause an increased risk of fractures at conventionally used doses. High

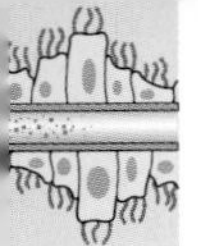

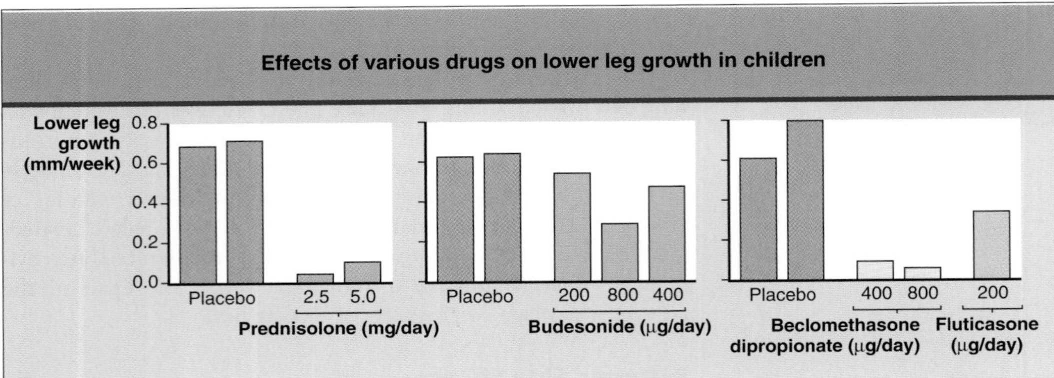

Figure 33.7 Effect of treatment with placebo, prednisone 2.5 or 5.0 mg for 1 week, or increasing inhaled doses of budesonide, BDP, or fluticasone on lower leg growth, measured by knemometry, in children. Prednisone and BDP 400 μg or 800 μg/day significantly reduced lower leg growth. (Reproduced with permission from Barnes PJ, Pedersen S: Efficacy and safety of inhaled corticosteroids in asthma. Am Rev Resp Dis 148:S1-26, 1993.)

doses of inhaled BDP (greater than 1000 μgm/day), used for several years, has been associated, in a case controlled study, with a slight increased risk of hip fractures in older patients.

The effects of inhaled glucocorticosteroids on bone metabolism were demonstrated by measuring serum osteocalcin, a measure of changes in bone formation, and urinary hydroxyproline, measured after a 12-hour fast, which increases with increased bone resorption. Pyridium cross-links in urine are measures of bone resorption that have the advantage over urinary hydroxyproline of not being dietary dependent; however, to date, the effects of inhaled glucocorticosteroids on this measure of bone resorption have not been reported.

The effects of BDP and budesonide on serum osteocalcin and urinary hydroxyproline have been studied in adults. Both drugs have been shown to influence serum osteocalcin levels in a dose-dependent manner, but only BDP increases urinary hydroxyproline excretion at doses up to 2000 μgm/day. In children, doses of budesonide of less than 800 μgm/day, and of FP of 200 μ/day have no effect on any biochemical marker of bone turnover.

Bone densitometry has been measured in adult asthmatics over 2 years while these patients were taking various doses of inhaled BDP (mean dose 630 μgm/day). This study suggests that these patients had no increase in bone loss. Also, to date, no studies have demonstrated that these biochemical markers of bone turnover are associated with an increased risk of bone fracture.

POSTERIOR SUBCAPSULAR CATARACTS

Posterior subcapsular cataracts occur more frequently in patients who take ingested corticosteroids, which complicates the issue of whether they occur with greater frequency in patients who use inhaled glucocorticosteroids. After the confounding effect of ingested glucocorticosteroids is removed, most studies in adults and children suggest that inhaled glucocorticosteroids do not increase the risk of developing posterior subcapsular cataracts. One recent study has, however, indicated that high inhaled doses of BDP are associated with a slightly greater risk of posterior subcapsular cataracts in older patients. This study did not, however, stratify for the confounding risk of allergy for cataract development in this population.

GROWTH RETARDATION IN CHILDREN

Concern about growth retardation in children as a result of inhaled corticosteroid use, is a major reason that these drugs are used very sparingly, perhaps even underused, to treat pediatric asthma. There is little doubt that systemic corticosteroids can stunt growth in children and that this effect is usually permanent. To resolve this issue for inhaled corticosteroids in asthmatic children has been exceedingly difficult, in part because asthmatic children do not have the same growth patterns as nonasthmatic children. Many asthmatic children have delayed onset of puberty, which appears more marked in children who have severe asthma. However, eventually these children do catch up with their nonasthmatic peers and achieve normal height, so comparing asthmatic children to nonasthmatic controls may not be appropriate. Also, studies that examine growth in children need to be continued over several years, because individual children have very different growth patterns.

A surrogate method to measure growth in children is knemometry, which measures short-term linear growth in the lower leg in children and is extremely sensitive to the systemic effects of glucocorticosteroids. Daily doses of prednisone of 2.5 mg can totally inhibit lower leg growth (Figure 33.7). By contrast, doses of inhaled budesonide of 400 μgm/day have no effect on knemometry measurements, while daily doses of 800 μgm/day of budesonide and 400 μgm/day of BDP and 200 μgm/day of FP do significantly inhibit it (see Fig. 33.7). All currently available inhaled corticosteroids can be demonstrated to have small effects on growth velocity, an effect which is greatest in the first year of use. Fortunately, however, the final height of children treated with inhaled budesonide, at a mean daily dose of greater than 400 μgm for more that 8 years, was normal when compared with their estimated height, indicating that catch up of the growth velocity does occur.

CORTICOSTEROID PSYCHOSIS

Corticosteroid psychosis may occur in as many as 2% of patients treated with systemic corticosteroids, and has been reported to occur very occasionally in patients who take inhaled corticosteroids. Thus far, eight patients have been reported who developed symptoms within days of being treated with either inhaled BDP or budesonide. The psychosis resolved promptly after stopping the inhaled glucocorticosteroid.

RISKS OF LUNG INFECTION

Risks of lung infection are not increased in patients who use inhaled glucocorticosteroids. Also, inhaled glucocorticosteroids do not increase the risks of reactivation of pulmonary tuberculosis, and therefore prophylactic isoniazid treatment is not

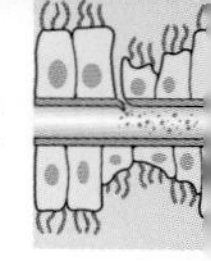

needed when inhaled glucocorticosteroids are used in patients who have inactive pulmonary tuberculosis.

SKIN BRUISING

Skin bruising does occur as a dose-dependent side effect of inhaled corticosteroid use. It is rare at daily doses of less than 1000 μg/day, and its incidence increases with age and duration of treatment. In one study of older patients on high doses of BDP, the prevalence of easy bruising was 47% for those on inhaled glucocorticosteroids and 22% for those who were not.

CONCLUSIONS

Corticosteroids are a valuable and widely used treatment for a variety of lung diseases. Inhaled corticosteroids are the mainstay of asthma treatment, and their pharmacokinetics, pharmacodynamics, and systemic unwanted effects have been the focus of extensive research since their introduction in 1972. The availability of topically potent corticosteroids, with effective first-pass metabolism in the liver, has ensured that the efficacy is obtained in almost all patients at doses not associated with clinically relevant unwanted effects.

SELECTED REFERENCES

Barnes PJ, Pedersen S, Busse WW: Efficacy and safety of inhaled corticosteroids: New developments. Am J Respir Crit Care Med 157:1-53, 1998.

Busse WW, Chervinsky P, Condemi J, et al: Budesonide delivered by Turbuhaler is effective in a dose-dependent fashion when used in the treatment of adult patients with chronic asthma. J Allergy Clin Immunol 101:457-463, 1998.

O'Byrne PM, Cuddy L, Taylor DW, et al: The clinical efficacy and cost benefit of inhaled corticosteroids as therapy in patients with mild asthma in primary care practice. Can Resp J 3:169-175, 1996.

Pauwels RA, Lofdahl C-G, Postma DS, et al: Effect of inhaled formoterol and budesonide on exacerbations of asthma. N Engl J Med 337:1405-1411, 1997.

Pauwels RA, Pedersen S, Busse WW, et al: Early intervention with budesonide in mild persistent asthma: A randomised, double-blind trial. Lancet 361:1071-1076, 2003.

Pedersen S, O'Byrne PM: A comparison of the efficacy and safety of inhaled corticosteroids in asthma. Allergy 52:1-34, 1997.

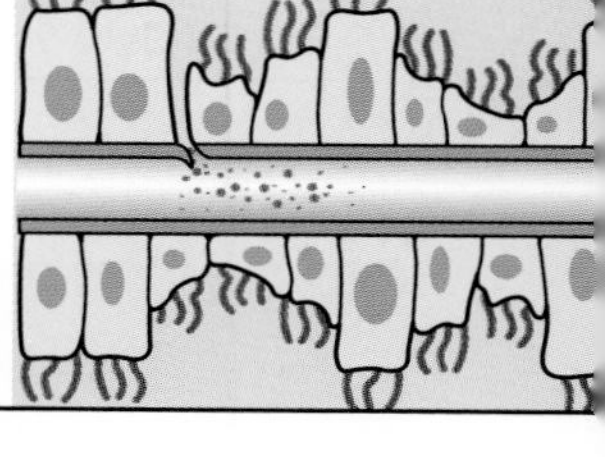

CHAPTER 34 Chronic Obstructive Pulmonary Disease: Epidemiology, Pathophysiology, and Clinical Evaluation

William MacNee

Chronic obstructive pulmonary disease (COPD) is a preventable and treatable condition that is characterized by airflow limitation that is not fully reversible. Although hidden by the generic term "COPD," the condition is a heterogeneous collection of syndromes with overlapping manifestations. This situation has led to major difficulties in obtaining an acceptable definition of the condition.

Our understanding of the pathogenesis, physiology, clinical features, and management of COPD has increased substantially in recent years. Although cigarette smoking is a major risk factor, COPD occurs in nonsmokers, and individuals vary greatly in their susceptibility to the effects of tobacco smoke.

COPD has a considerable morbidity and mortality. In 1990 it was the 12th leading cause of morbidity and the 6th leading cause of death worldwide. Of all the major diseases, COPD is the one whose burden is rising fastest, and it is projected to be the fifth leading cause of disability and the third leading cause of death by 2020 (Fig. 34.1).

Patients frequently attribute their symptoms of breathlessness, cough, and sputum production to aging or to their cigarette smoking. In addition, many health care providers consider the condition to be irreversible to the extent that treatment offers very little. Accordingly, COPD is markedly underdiagnosed despite the fact that it is an easy diagnosis to make, and is also frequently undermanaged.

It is now well recognized that COPD may be partially reversible and that clinically significant responses to treatment do occur. Whereas treatment was previously considered for patients at the severe end of the disease spectrum, recent guidelines recognize that diagnosis and treatment at an earlier stage can offer important benefits for patients. Although current treatments are unable to cure COPD, they reduce symptoms, improve function, and reduce exacerbations, and may decrease the enormous health care costs associated with COPD.

DEFINITIONS

Several problems have to be considered with regard to defining COPD. The first relates to the use of the term *chronic obstructive pulmonary disease* because this is not truly a disease but a group of diseases. The second problem relates to the terms *chronic bronchitis* and *emphysema*; these conditions comprise the syndrome of COPD, but the terms describe clinical or pathologic findings rather than pertaining to airflow limitation. A third major problem is the difficulty in differentiating this condition from asthma, particularly the persistent or poorly reversible airway obstruction of older patients with chronic asthma that is often difficult or even impossible to distinguish from COPD. A further difficulty is the considerable overlap between the physiologic mechanisms that underlie chronic asthma and the syndromes comprising COPD. Indeed, COPD may develop in some patients with asthma, or these two common conditions can coexist in the same individual (Fig. 34.2). Chronic bronchitis is defined clinically by the American Thoracic Society and the United Kingdom Medical Research Council as "the production of sputum on most days for at least 3 months in at least 2 consecutive years when another cause of chronic cough has been excluded." Chronic bronchitis has been classified into three forms: simple bronchitis, defined as mucus hypersecretion; chronic or recurrent mucopurulent bronchitis, defined as persistent or intermittent mucopurulent sputum; and obstructive bronchitis, when chronic sputum production is associated with airflow obstruction.

Emphysema is defined as abnormal, permanent enlargement of the air spaces distal to the terminal bronchioles, accompanied by destruction of their walls and without obvious fibrosis. As with chronic bronchitis, the definition of emphysema does not require the presence of airflow obstruction.

Bronchiolitis is a disease of the small airways, where the smaller bronchi and bronchioles less than 2 mm in diameter are the major sites of airway obstruction. Inflammation in the small airways is difficult to detect by physiologic measurements but is the earliest pathologic change found in asymptomatic smokers. Although relatively little is known of the natural history of this condition, it is considered to contribute increasingly, as it progresses, to the airflow limitation in COPD.

It is difficult to determine the relative contributions to airflow limitation in individual patients by airway abnormalities versus distal air space enlargement. Thus, the term *COPD* was introduced in the 1960s to describe patients with incompletely reversible airflow limitation due to a *combination* of airway

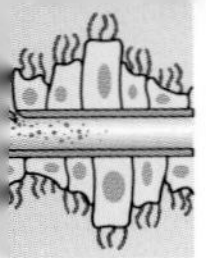

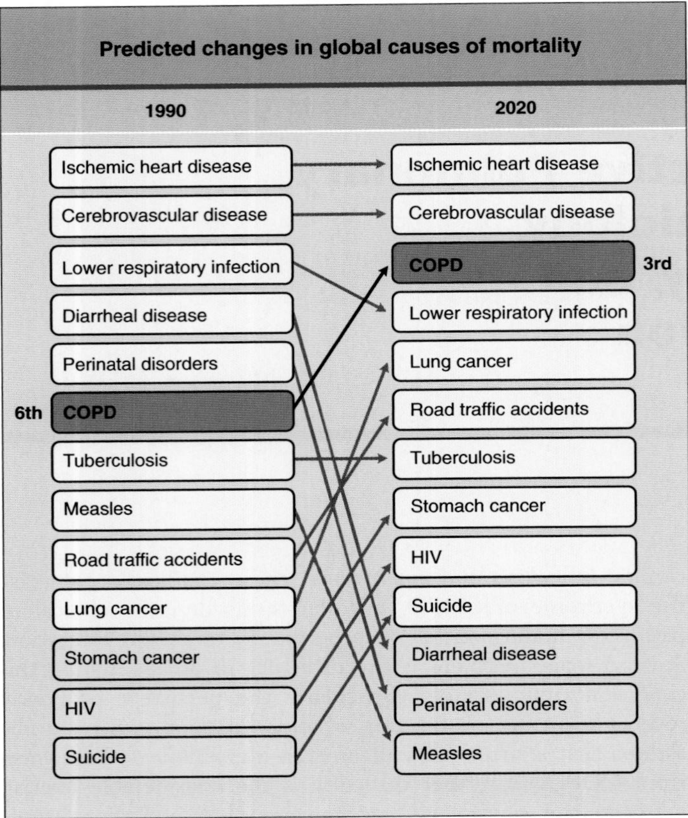

Figure 34.1 Predicted changes in global causes of mortality. (Data from Murray CJ, Lopez AD: Lancet 349:1269-1276, 1997.)

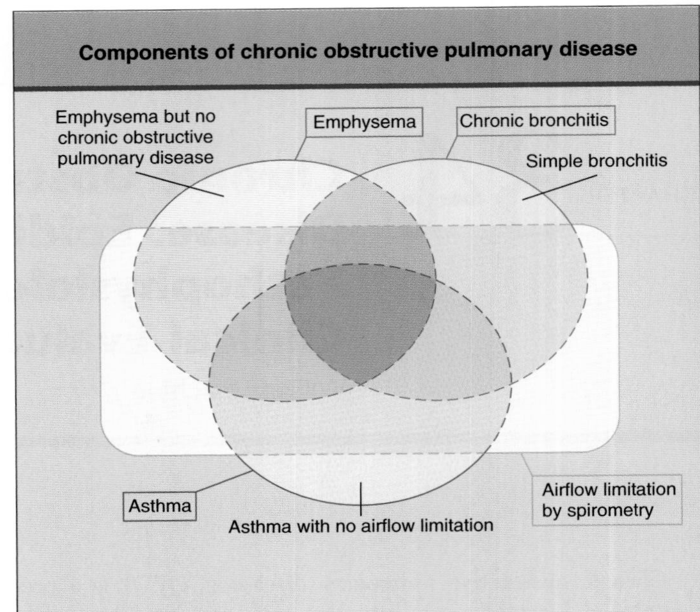

Figure 34.2 Components of chronic obstructive pulmonary disease (COPD). Each circle represents a nosologic entity. The rectangle represents airflow limitation as documented in a forced vital capacity maneuver. The shaded area corresponds to patients diagnosed as having COPD. Notice that a patient may present with emphysema but no COPD (e.g., a patient who has bullae on chest radiography but no airflow limitation). Similarly, a patient may present with sputum production and normal spirometry (with simple bronchitis). Finally, an asthmatic may present with no airflow limitation, and is only diagnosed after a positive bronchoprovocation test.

disease and emphysema, without defining the contribution of these conditions to the airflow limitation.

In their forthcoming statement on the standards for diagnosis and care of patients with COPD, the American Thoracic Society and European Respiratory Society define COPD as "a preventable and treatable disease state characterized by air flow limitation that is not fully reversible. The airflow limitation is usually progressive and is associated with an abnormal inflammatory response in the lungs to noxious particles or gases, primarily caused by cigarette smoking. Although COPD affects the lungs, it also produces significant systemic consequences." This is similar to the definition produced by the Global Initiative on Obstructive Lung Disease (GOLD), which first introduced the concept of COPD as an inflammatory disease into its definition.

The diagnosis of COPD should be considered in any person with:

- History of chronic progressive cough, wheeze, or breathlessness, with little variation in these symptoms
- Causative risk factors such as cigarette smoke or occupational and environmental dust and/or gaseous exposure

The diagnosis of COPD requires objective evidence of airflow limitation determined by spirometry. A forced expiratory volume in the first second (FEV_1)/forced vital capacity (FVC) less than 0.7 measured after inhaling a bronchodilator confirms the presence of airflow limitation that is not fully reversible.

A number of specific causes of airway obstruction such as cystic fibrosis, bronchiectasis, and bronchiolitis obliterans are not included in the definition of COPD and should be considered in its differential diagnosis.

PATHOLOGY

The pathologic changes in COPD are complex and occur in the central conducting airways, the peripheral airways, the lung parenchyma, and the pulmonary vasculature. The relative contributions of the pathologic changes in the airways versus those of emphysema to the airflow limitation observed have been the subject of considerable study. In general, pathologic changes correlate rather poorly with both clinical and functional patterns of disease.

Inflammation initiated by exposure to particles or gases underlies most of the pathologic lesions associated with COPD. Enhanced inflammation also contributes to the recurrent exacerbations in which acute inflammation is superimposed on the chronic disease. Good evidence exists suggesting that all smokers have inflammation in their lungs. There is individual susceptibility in the inflammatory response to tobacco smoking, however. The pathologic changes in the different lung compartments vary among individuals, resulting in the clinical and pathophysiologic heterogeneity that is seen in these patients.

Although the clinical and physiologic presentation of chronic asthma may be indistinguishable from COPD, the pathologic changes are distinct from those of patients with COPD due to

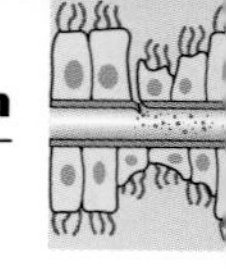

smoking. The histologic features of COPD in the 15% to 20% of patients with COPD who are nonsmokers have not yet been studied.

Chronic Bronchitis

Chronic hypersecretion of mucus results from changes in the central airways—the trachea, bronchi, and bronchioles greater than 2 to 4 mm in diameter. Mucus is produced by mucus glands in the larger airways and by goblet cells in the airway epithelium. Hypertrophy of the mucus glands occurs and the number of goblet cells increases and extends more peripherally. The volume of sputum production correlates with mucus gland area or volume. Bronchial biopsy studies confirm studies of resected lung material by showing bronchial wall inflammation in chronic bronchitis (Fig. 34.3). Activated T lymphocytes are prominent in the proximal airway walls. In contrast to asthma, however, macrophages are also prominent, and the CD8 suppressor T-lymphocyte subset predominates, rather than the CD4 subset, as occurs in asthma. Sputum volume also correlates with the degree of inflammation in the airway wall. Neutrophils are present, particularly in the mucus glands, and become more prominent as the disease progresses.

Several studies, previously using bronchoalveolar lavage (BAL) and more recently using spontaneous or induced sputum, demonstrate intraluminal inflammation in the air spaces of patients with chronic bronchitis, with or without airflow obstruction. In stable chronic bronchitis, the high percentage of intraluminal neutrophils is associated with the presence of neutrophil chemotactic factors, including interleukin (IL)-8 and leukotriene B 4. There is evidence that the air space inflammation in patients with chronic bronchitis persists after smoking cessation, particularly if the production of sputum persists, although cough and sputum production improve in most smokers who quit. Preliminary studies suggest that the inflammatory changes present in the large airways may reflect those present in the small airways and perhaps in the alveolar walls.

Airway wall changes include squamous metaplasia of the airway epithelium, loss of cilia and ciliary function, and increased smooth muscle and connective tissue. Bronchial biopsies taken from patients during mild exacerbations of chronic bronchitis indicate increased numbers of eosinophils in the bronchial wall, although far fewer than are present in exacerbations of asthma. Increased numbers of neutrophils are also observed. Eosinophils may not be predominant in severe exacerbations.

Small Airways Disease/Bronchiolitis

The smaller bronchi and bronchioles, less than 2 mm in diameter, are a major site of airflow obstruction in COPD. Small airway inflammation is one of the earliest changes to occur in asymptomatic cigarette smokers, and considerable changes can occur without giving rise to symptoms or altering spirometry results. The inflammatory cell changes in the small airways are similar to those in larger airways, including the predominance of CD8+ lymphocytes and the increase in the CD8:CD4 ratio. The increased peripheral airway resistance is a result of several processes:

1. Destruction of the alveolar support
2. Loss of elastic recoil in the parenchyma that provides this support consequent on a narrowing of the airways
3. Occlusion of the lumen by mucus and cells

Mucosal ulceration, goblet cell hyperplasia, and squamous cell metaplasia may be present. In addition, there may be mesenchymal cell accumulation and fibrosis. As the condition progresses, structural remodeling may occur, characterized by increased collagen content and scar tissue formation that narrows the airways and produces fixed airway obstruction (Fig. 34.4).

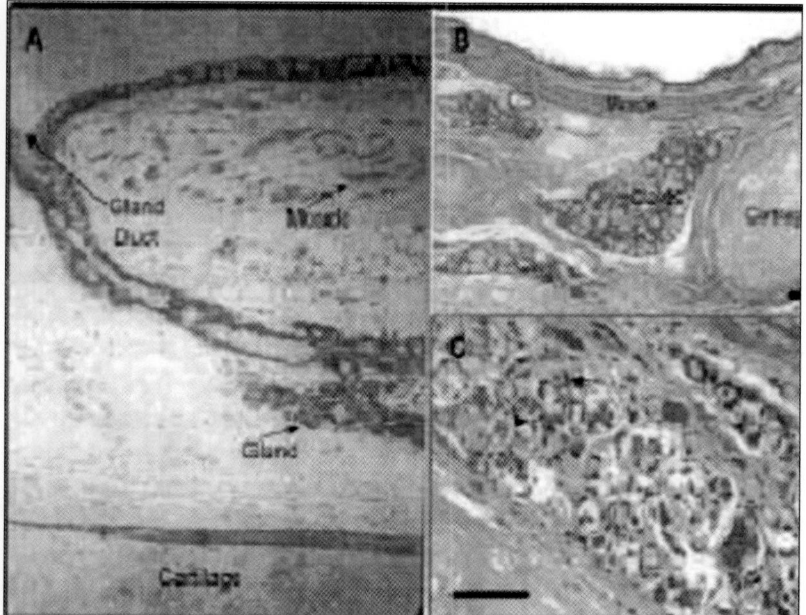

Figure 34.3 Pathologic changes in large airways. (Reproduced with the permission of Dr. James C. Hogg, St. Paul's Hospital, and Stuart Greene, University of British Columbia, Vancouver, British Columbia, Canada.)

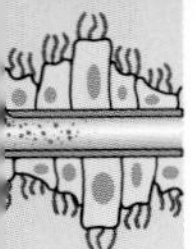

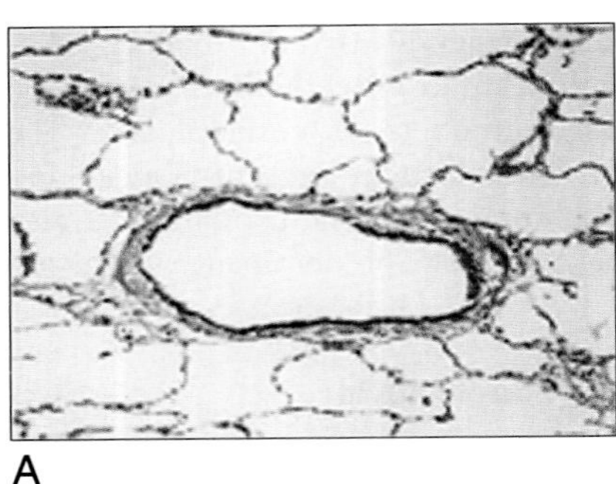

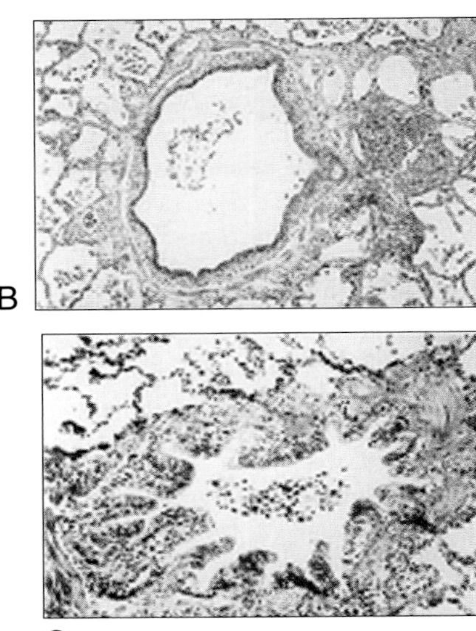

Figure 34.4 Histologic sections of peripheral airways. **A,** Section from a cigarette smoker with normal lung function, showing a nearly normal airway. **B,** Section from a patient with small airways disease, showing inflammatory exudates in the wall and the lumen of the airway. **C,** A more advanced case of small airways disease, with reduced lumen, structural reorganization of the airway wall, increased smooth muscle, and deposition of peribronchiolar connective tissue.

Emphysema

Pulmonary emphysema is defined as "abnormal permanent enlargement of airspaces distal to the terminal bronchioles accompanied by destruction of their walls." The major types of emphysema are recognized according to the distribution of enlarged air spaces in the acinar unit, the acinar being that part of the lung parenchyma supplied by a single terminal bronchiole:

- Centriacinar (i.e., centrilobular) emphysema, in which large air spaces are initially clustered around the terminal bronchiole
- Panacinar (i.e., panlobular) emphysema, where the large air spaces are distributed throughout the acinar unit (Fig. 34.5)

Air space enlargement can be identified macroscopically when the enlarged air space reaches 1 mm (Fig. 34.6). Although obvious fibrosis is, by definition, not present in emphysema, in the region of the terminal respiratory bronchioles fibrosis has been recognized as part of a respiratory bronchiolitis seen in smokers, and lung collagen content is increased in mild emphysema. Centriacinar and panacinar emphysema can occur alone or in combination. The association with cigarette smoking is clearer for centriacinar than panacinar emphysema, although both types can develop in smokers. Those with centriacinar emphysema appear to have more abnormalities in the small airways. Panacinar emphysema appears to be more severe in the lower lobes and is associated with alpha$_1$-proteinase inhibitor or alpha$_1$-antitrypsin deficiency but can also be found in cases where no genetic abnormality has been identified. Centriacinar emphysema usually predominates in the upper lobes.

Other types of emphysema also exist, such as periacinar (i.e., paraseptal or distal acinar) emphysema, which describes enlarged air spaces along the edge of the acinar unit, but only where it abuts against a fixed structure such as the pleura or a vessel (see Fig. 34.4). This type of emphysema is usually of little clinical significance except when it occurs extensively in a subpleural position, in association with pneumothorax. Scar or irregular emphysema describes enlarged air spaces around the

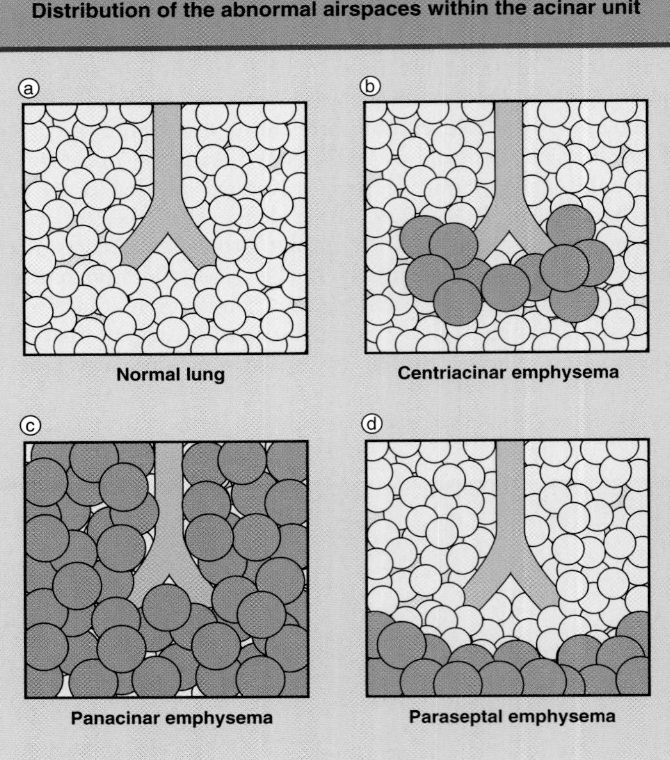

Figure 34.5 A diagrammatic representation of the distribution of the abnormal air spaces in the acinar unit in the three major types of emphysema. **A,** Acinar unit in a normal lung (although the illustration shows a clearly defined area for the purposes of clarity, adjacent acinar units intercommunicate and are not necessarily demarcated by septa). **B,** Centriacinar emphysema: focal enlargement of the air spaces around the respiratory bronchiole. **C,** Panacinar (panlobular) emphysema: confluent, even involvement of the acinar unit. **D,** Periacinar (paraseptal or distal acinar) emphysema: peripherally distributed, enlarged air spaces where the acinar unit butts against a fixed structure such as the pleura.

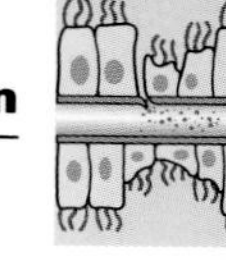

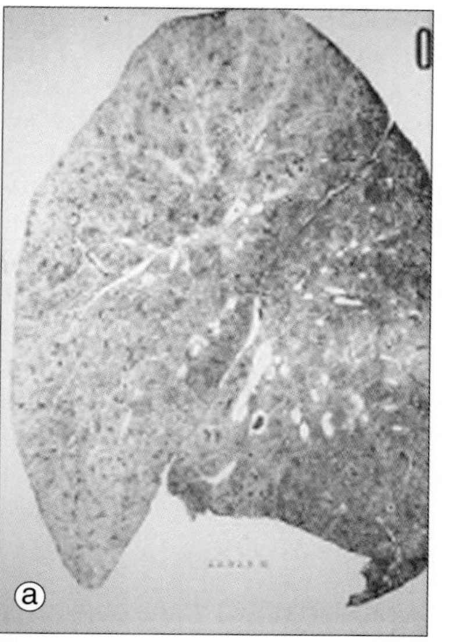

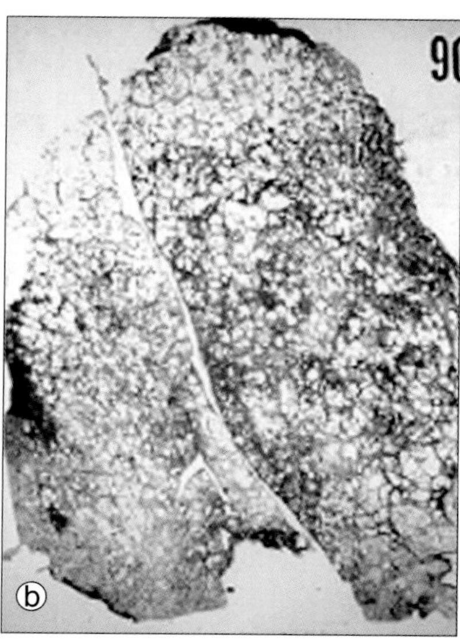

Figure 34.6 A, Paper-mounted whole-lung section of normal lung. **B,** Paper-mounted whole-lung section from a lung with severe centrilobular emphysema (note that the centrilobular form is more extensive in the upper regions of the lung).

margins of a scar unrelated to the structure of the acinus. This lesion is excluded from the current definition of emphysema. A bulla is a localized area of emphysema conventionally defined as being greater than 1 cm in size.

The bronchioles and small bronchi are supported by attachments to the outer aspect of their walls by adjacent alveolar walls. This arrangement maintains the tubular integrity of the airways. These attachments may distort the airways to the extent that the irregularities in the walls are sufficient to cause airflow limitation (Fig. 34.7).

The inflammatory cell profile in the alveolar walls is similar to that described in the airways and persists throughout the course of the disease.

Pulmonary Vasculature

Changes in the pulmonary arteries occur early in the course of COPD, the first of these being thickening of the intima, followed by an increase in smooth muscle and infiltration of the vessel wall with inflammatory cells, including macrophages and CD8+ T lymphocytes. As the disease progresses, greater amounts of smooth muscle, proteoglycans, and collagen are present in the arterial wall and cause it to thicken. The development of chronic alveolar hypoxia in patients with COPD results in hypoxic vasoconstriction and contributes to the structural changes, with resulting pulmonary hypertension and right ventricular hypertrophy and dilatation.

ETIOLOGY AND RISK FACTORS

Cigarette Smoking

Cigarette smoking is the single most important identifiable etiologic factor in COPD. In general, there is a correlative dose effect, with smokers having lower lung function the more and longer they smoke. There is, however, considerable variation (Fig. 34.8). Some nonsmokers have impaired lung function and as many as 20% of patients with COPD are lifelong nonsmokers. Conversely, some heavy smokers are able to maintain normal lung function, although the frequently quoted 10% to 20% of smokers in whom clinically significant COPD is thought to develop is probably an underestimate.

There is a trend toward an increased relative risk of chronic airflow limitation from passive smoking, but the effect is not

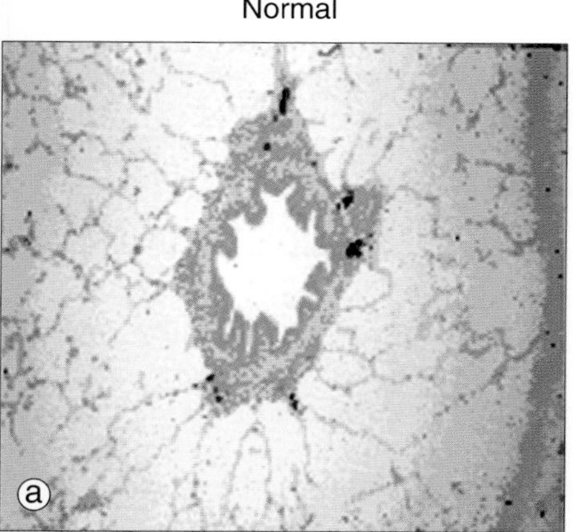

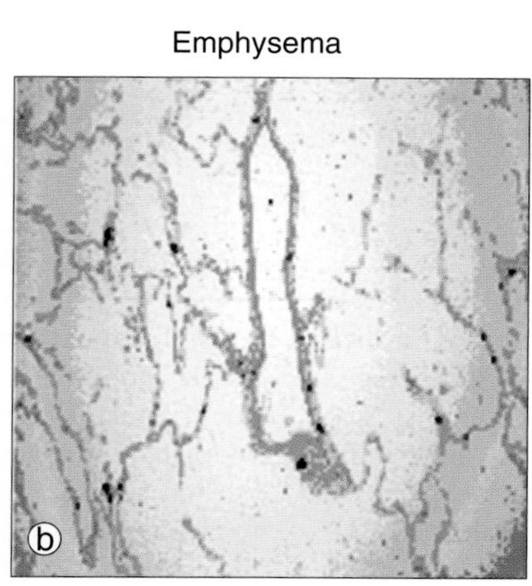

Figure 34.7 A, Histologic section of normal small airway and surrounding alveoli connecting with attached alveolar walls. **B,** Histologic section showing emphysema, with enlarged alveolar spaces, loss of alveolar wall and attachments, and collapsed airways.

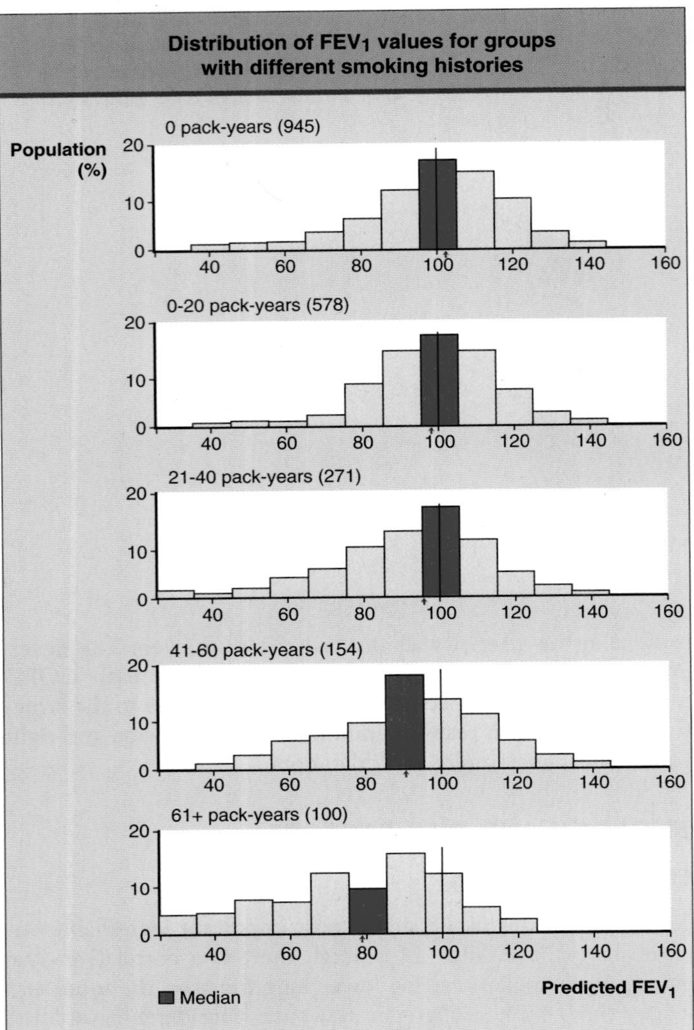

Figure 34.8 Distribution of forced expiratory volume in 1 second (FEV_1) values as a percentage of predicted value for groups with differing smoking histories. (From Traver GA, Cline MG, Burrows B: Predictors of mortality in chronic obstructive pulmonary disease. A 5-year follow-up study. Am Rev Respir Dis Jun;119(6):895-902, 1979.)

powerful enough to demonstrate clinical significance. Exposure to environmental tobacco smoke during childhood, however, is associated with a lower FEV_1 in adulthood. Furthermore, maternal smoking is associated with low birth weight, and smoking by either parent is associated with an increased frequency of respiratory illness in the first 3 years of life, and this may also result in airflow limitation in later life.

Air Pollution

Air pollution has been recognized as a risk factor in chronic respiratory disease as a result of various air pollution episodes, such as the London smog of December 1952 in which 4000 excess deaths from cardiorespiratory disease occurred.

The introduction of air quality standards in the 1950s and 1960s led to a decrease in smoke and sulfur dioxide levels, which resulted in less discernible associations between peaks of pollution and respiratory morbidity and mortality. More recent studies, however, show an association between respiratory symptoms, general practitioner consultations, and hospital admissions in patients with airway diseases, including COPD, and levels of particulates less than 100 μg/m^3, levels that are currently experienced in many urban areas in Western countries. The role of long-term exposure to outdoor air pollution as a risk factor for the development of COPD is still debated. Air pollution does appear to be a risk factor for mucus hypersecretion, although the association with airflow limitation and accelerated decline in FEV_1 is less clear. Air pollution may affect the growth of lung function in childhood, which may influence the risk of COPD in adulthood. It is also recognized that indoor air pollution, derived from the combustion of biomass fuel in fires and stoves, may be an important etiologic factor in the development of COPD and is a particular problem in women in developing countries.

There is a causal link between occupational dust exposure and the development of mucus hypersecretion. In addition, longitudinal studies in workers exposed to dust show an association between the exposure and a more rapid decline in FEV_1. Exposure to welding fumes or cadmium is also associated with a small but significant risk for development of COPD or emphysema, respectively.

Chronic Mucus Hypersecretion

Population studies indicate a higher prevalence of cough and sputum among smokers than nonsmokers. Cessation of smoking is associated with cessation of sputum production in 90% of patients. In studies of working men in London, Fletcher and Peto showed that smoking accelerated the decline in FEV_1, but they failed to show a correlation between the degree of mucus hypersecretion and an accelerated decline in FEV_1 or mortality. By contrast, mortality was strongly related to the development of a low FEV_1. Recent data from a more general population study in Copenhagen between 1976 and 1994, however, suggested that mucus hypersecretion was associated with increased risk of hospital admission and an accelerated decline in FEV_1. Moreover, as the FEV_1 decreases, the association between mucus hypersecretion and mortality becomes stronger.

Differences in the degree of airflow obstruction between the populations in these two studies may explain the different findings.

Chronic Bronchopulmonary Infection

Previous studies by Fletcher and Peto in the 1960s and 1970s in men with chronic bronchitis did not show a relationship between recurrent infective exacerbations of bronchitis and the decline in lung function. This has been challenged recently in the Lung Health Study, which showed an association in continued smokers between lower respiratory tract infection and a faster rate of decline in lung function. This is supported by newer population studies of patients with COPD.

Cough and sputum production in adulthood is more commonly reported in those with a history of chest illness in childhood. The association between childhood respiratory illness and ventilatory impairment in adulthood is probably multifactorial. Several factors, such as low economic status, greater exposure to passive smoking, poor diet and housing, and residence in areas of high pollution, may contribute to this finding.

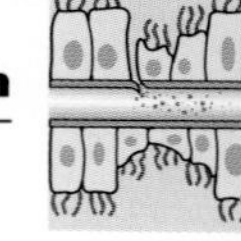

Growth and Nutrition

Several studies indicate that mortality from chronic respiratory diseases correlates inversely and adult ventilatory function correlates directly with birth weight and weight at 1 year of age. Thus, it appears that impaired growth in utero may be a risk factor for the development of chronic respiratory diseases, including COPD.

Diet may have an influence on the development of COPD. One study of British adults showed a direct correlation between consumption of fresh fruit and ventilatory function, a relationship which held both in smokers and in subjects who had never smoked. Dietary factors, particularly a low intake of vitamin C and low plasma levels of ascorbic acid, were related to a diagnosis of bronchitis in the U.S. National Health and Nutrition Examination Survey (NHANES).

Atopy and Airway Hyperresponsiveness

A hypothesis was proposed in the 1960s that smokers with chronic, largely irreversible airway obstruction and subjects with asthma shared a common constitutional predisposition to allergy, airway hyperresponsiveness, and eosinophilia—the "Dutch hypothesis." Smokers tend to have higher levels of immunoglobulin E and higher eosinophil counts than nonsmokers, but these are not as high as those found in asthmatic patients. Studies in middle-aged smokers with airflow limitation show a positive correlation between accelerated decline in FEV_1 and increased airway responsiveness to either methacholine or histamine. There is no increase in atopy in cigarette smokers (defined by positive skin tests), however. Whether airway hyperresponsiveness is a cause or consequence of COPD remains a subject of debate.

Genetic Factors

A number of candidate genes have been associated with the development of COPD. The associations are not consistent in different populations, however (Table 34.1). The only proven association is with $alpha_1$-antitrypsin ($alpha_1$-proteinase inhibitor) deficiency. $Alpha_1$-antitrypsin is the major inhibitor of serine proteinases, including neutrophil elastase. Over 75 biochemical variants of $alpha_1$-antitrypsin have been described in relation to their electrophoretic properties, giving rise to the phase inhibitor (Pi) nomenclature. The most common allele in all populations is PiM and the most common genotype is PiMM, which occurs in 86% of the population in the United Kingdom. PiMZ and PiS are the two next most common genotypes and are associated with $alpha_1$-proteinase inhibitor levels of between 15% to 75% of the mean levels of PiMM subjects. Similar levels occur in the much less common PiSS type. In the PiSZ genotype, basal $alpha_1$-proteinase inhibitor levels are 35% to 50% of normal. The threshold point for increased risk of emphysema is a level of approximately 80 mg/dL, which is approximately 30% of normal. The homozygous PiZZ type, in which serum levels are 10% to 20% of the average normal value, is the strongest genetic risk factor for the development of emphysema. Such individuals, particularly if they smoke, are likely to acquire COPD at an early age. The onset of disease occurs at a median age of 50 years in nonsmokers and 40 years in smokers.

Table 34.1
Case–Control Genetic Association Studies in Chronic Obstructive Pulmonary Disease

Category	Candidate Gene	Support Association	Do Not Support Association
Proteinase/ antiproteinase	PiMZ AIAT 3′ flanking region $Alpha_1$-antichymotrypsin	3	3
Oxidant/ antioxidant	Microsomal epoxide hydrolase Heme oxygenase-1 Glutathione S-transferase P1	3	1
Other candidates	CFTR ABO blood group ABH secretor status Vitamin D binding protein Tumor necrosis factor-α	5	5

The defect that results in $alpha_1$-antitrypsin deficiency has now been determined. In the PiZZ subject, $alpha_1$-antitrypsin protein accumulates in the endoplasmic reticulum of the liver. The structure of this protein indicates that the defect results in the development of abnormal polymers that prevent the $alpha_1$-antitrypsin from passing through the endoplasmic reticulum and being secreted. These polymers may also be chemotactic for inflammatory cells and may thus contribute to the increased elastase burden. It is postulated that a deficiency in $alpha_1$-proteinase inhibitor results in excess activity of neutrophil elastase and therefore in increased tissue destruction and emphysema.

Studies of blood donors in the United States identify a 1/2700 prevalence of PiZZ subjects, of whom most had normal results on spirometry. It is estimated that approximately 1/5000 children in the United Kingdom are born with the homozygous deficiency (PiZZ). The number of subjects identified with disease is, however, much fewer than has been predicted from the known prevalence of the deficiency. Accordingly, it is not inevitable that respiratory disease will develop in all individuals with the homozygous deficiency.

The life expectancy of $alpha_1$-deficient subjects is reduced, particularly if they smoke. In a prospective follow-up of PiZZ subjects there was a greatly accelerated decline in FEV_1 (albeit with large variations between individuals, particularly between index cases and affected family members).

Other Factors

An association between having a diagnosis of COPD, economic status, education, lung function, and COPD hospitalization has been shown in a Danish study, despite relatively small differences between social classes. It is likely, however, that social risk factors are multifactorial (e.g., intrauterine exposure, childhood infections, childhood environment, diet, housing conditions, and occupational factors).

The role of gender as a risk factor for COPD remains unclear. Although most previous studies have shown that COPD mortality is greater among men than women, more recent studies show a change in the prevalence of the disease, so that COPD is now almost equal in prevalence among men and women, probably reflecting the change in the prevalence of tobacco smoking in the sexes. Recent studies have suggested that women may be more susceptible to the effects of tobacco smoke than men, but this is still debated.

EPIDEMIOLOGY

COPD is a leading cause of morbidity and mortality worldwide. The prevalence of COPD and its morbidity and mortality vary across countries. The imprecise and variable definitions of COPD, and the lack of spirometry to confirm the diagnosis, have made it difficult to quantify the true morbidity and mortality of the disease. In addition, prevalence data underestimate the total disease burden because COPD is not usually diagnosed until it is clinically recognized, usually when it has already progressed to at least a moderately advanced stage. The mortality from this condition is also likely to be underestimated because it is often cited as a contributory, rather than a primary, cause of death.

Prevalence

Older studies reported a prevalence of cough and excessive sputum production of up to 50% in middle-aged men, and 20% in women of all ages. More recent studies, however, have shown a prevalence of 10% to 15% in men, with women continuing to have a prevalence of 20%.

Prevalence studies of COPD are normally based on abnormalities in FEV_1. In a population survey in the United Kingdom, 10% of men and 11% of women ranging in age from 18 to 64 years had an FEV_1 greater than two standard deviations below their predicted values, with the percentage of affected patients increasing with age, particularly in smokers. In current smokers versus nonsmokers from 40 to 65 years of age, 18% versus 7% of men and 14% versus 6% of women have an FEV_1 greater than two standard deviations below normal.

Approximately 14 million people in the United States have COPD, and the number has increased by 42% since 1982. The best data available come from the third NHANES study, a large national survey conducted in the United States between 1988 and 1994. For subjects 25 to 75 years of age, the prevalence of mild COPD (defined as FEV_1/FVC <70% predicted and FEV_1 >80% predicted) was 7% and of moderate COPD (defined as FEV_1/FVC <79% predicted and FEV_1 ≤80% predicted), 6%. The prevalence of both mild and moderate COPD was higher in men than women and in whites than in blacks, and increased steeply with age. Airflow limitation was estimated to be present in 14% of current white male smokers, 7% of ex-smokers, and 3% of never-smokers. In white female subjects, airflow limitation occurred in 14% of smokers, 7% of ex-smokers, and 3% of never-smokers. Interestingly, fewer than 50% of individuals with COPD based on the presence of airflow limitation had a physician's diagnosis of COPD.

Morbidity

Morbidity data in patients with COPD are less available and less reliable than mortality data, but the prevalence of physician visits, emergency department visits, and hospitalizations in COPD increases with age, is greater in men than women, and is likely to increase in the future with the aging of populations. A recent report from the United States indicates that patients with COPD had 1,464,000 hospital discharges, 12,002,000 physician office visits, 15,500 emergency department visits, and 7,349,700 visits by physicians in a hospital or nursing home setting in 1996.

Mortality

COPD is the fourth leading cause of death worldwide and is estimated to become the third leading cause of death by 2020. There are large international variations in the death rate for COPD that cannot be entirely explained by differences in diagnostic patterns, diagnostic labels, or smoking habits. Figures from death certification underestimate the mortality from COPD because COPD is often cited as a contributory factor to the cause of death. COPD death rates are very low under the age of 45 years and increase steeply with age. Although mortality from COPD in men has been falling slightly, there has been an increase in mortality in women. In 1991, COPD was the fourth leading cause of death in the United States (85,544 deaths) and was the most rapidly increasing cause of death between 1979 and 1991, with a 33% increase.

Natural History and Prognosis

The airway obstruction in susceptible smokers develops slowly as a result of an accelerated rate of decline in FEV_1 that continues for years. As noted previously, impaired growth of lung function during childhood and adolescence as a result of recurrent infections or exposure to tobacco smoke may lead to lower maximally attained lung function in adulthood. This failure in lung growth, often combined with a shortened plateau phase in teenage smokers, increases the risk of COPD. In never-smokers, the FEV_1 declines at a rate of 20 to 30 mL/year (Fig. 34.9). Smokers as a population have a faster rate of decline, and reported changes in FEV_1 in patients with COPD are greater

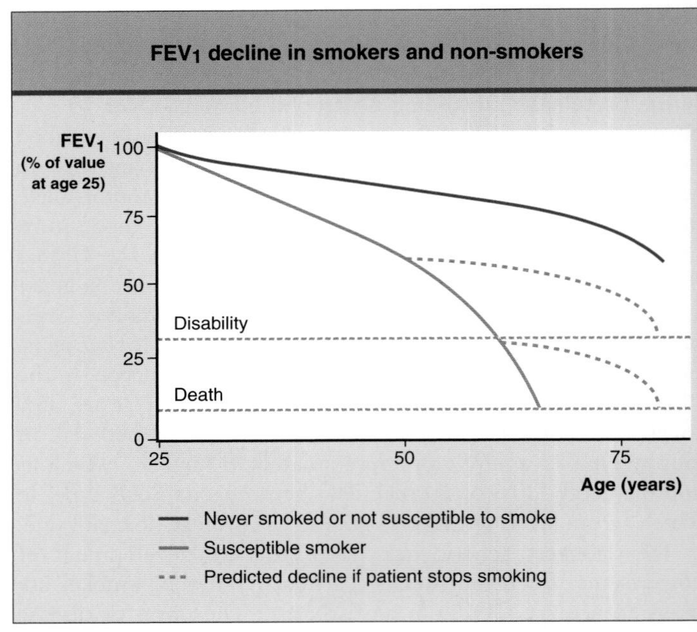

Figure 34.9 Decline in forced expiratory volume in 1 second (FEV_1) in smokers and nonsmokers.

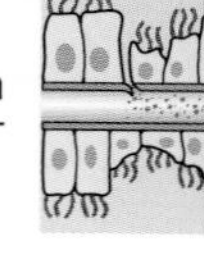

than 50 mL/year. There is a relationship between the initial level of FEV_1 and the annual rate of decline in FEV_1, and individuals in the highest or lowest FEV_1 percentiles remain in the same percentiles over subsequent years. This suggests that susceptible cigarette smokers can be identified in early middle age by a reduction in the FEV_1. There is a tendency for annual rates of decline in FEV_1 to be slower in advanced than in mild disease.

Longitudinal data from the Lung Health Study in the United States show that stopping smoking, even after significant airflow limitation is present, can result in some improvement in function, and will slow or even stop the progression of airflow limitation. Men who quit smoking at the beginning of the study had an FEV_1 decline of 30.2 mL/year, whereas in those who continued to smoke throughout the study, the decline was 66.1 mL/year. Similar findings were seen in women.

FEV_1 is a strong predictor of survival. Fewer than 50% of patients whose FEV_1 has fallen to below 30% of predicted are alive 5 years later. The best association between FEV_1 and survival is the postbronchodilator, rather than prebronchodilator FEV_1. Other clinical parameters have also been shown to be important prognostic indicators independent of FEV_1. Weight loss is a bad prognostic sign (Fig. 34.10). Other unfavorable prognostic factors include severe hypoxemia, raised pulmonary arterial pressure, and low carbon monoxide transfer, which become apparent in patients with severe disease.

PATHOGENESIS

Several processes are important in the pathogenesis of COPD. Central to the pathogenesis appears to be an enhanced inflammatory response to inhaled particles or gases. Several processes are involved in this response.

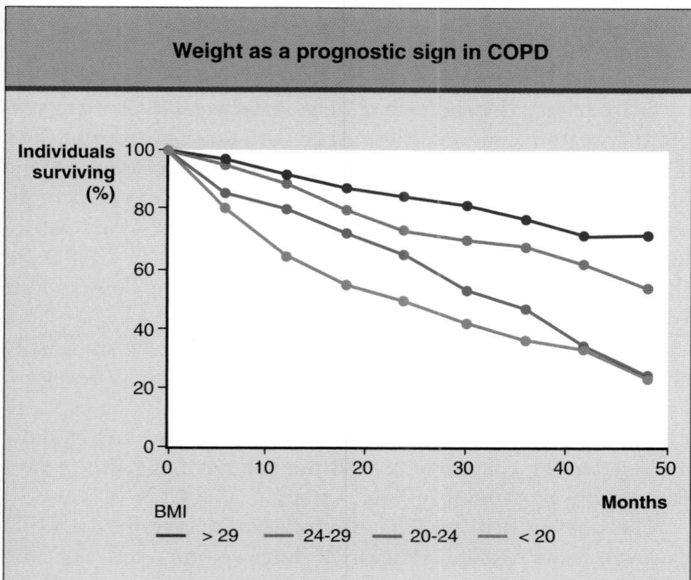

Figure 34.10 Weight as a prognostic sign in chronic obstructive pulmonary disease (COPD). Survival is inversely correlated with body mass index. The data represent 400 consecutive patients with COPD referred for rehabilitation, who received no special dietary intervention. BMI, body mass index (mass [kg]/height^2 [m^2]). (From Schols AM, Slangen J, Volovics L, Wouters EF: Weight loss is a reversible factor in the prognosis of chronic obstructive pulmonary disease. Am J Respir Crit Care Med 157:1791-1797, 1998.)

- Increased proteinase burden/decreased antiproteinase function
- Oxidant/antioxidant imbalance—oxidative stress
- Defective lung repair

Airway Inflammation

Both central and peripheral airways are inflamed in smokers with COPD. Smokers with chronic bronchitis have greater inflammation around gland ducts. Recent studies characterizing the inflammation show increased infiltration of mast cells, macrophages, and neutrophils in smokers with chronic bronchitis. An increase in T lymphocytes, mainly the CD8+ subset, is present, in contrast to the predominance of the CD4+ T-cell subset in asthma. CD8+ lymphocytes may have a role in apoptosis and destruction of alveolar wall epithelial cells through the release of perforins and tumor necrosis factor (TNF)-α. It is possible that an excessive recruitment of CD8+ T lymphocytes may occur in response to repeated viral infections damaging the lungs in susceptible smokers.

Although several studies indicate that smoking cessation has beneficial effects on pulmonary function, the few studies in which a direct assessment of airway inflammation was made after smoking cessation show persistence of the inflammatory response, suggesting that there are perpetuating mechanisms that maintain the chronic inflammatory process once it has become established despite the absence of direct smoke exposure.

A variety of inflammatory mediators is associated with the bronchopulmonary inflammation present in COPD. TNF-α and IL-8 are increased in the sputum of patients with COPD. IL-8 is an important chemoattractant and activator of neutrophils. Cigarette smoke can stimulate epithelial cells to release IL-8 through activation of the transcription nuclear factor κB (NF-κB), and this may be important for the neutrophil recruitment to the lungs.

TNF-α is present in high concentrations in sputum and is detectable in bronchial biopsies. TNF-α also activates NF-κB, which in turn activates the IL-8 gene in epithelial cells and macrophages. Leukotriene B 4 may also be involved in neutrophil recruitment to the lungs in COPD and is increased in sputum and BAL fluid of patients with COPD. Other chemoattractants such as monocyte chemoattractant protein are present in increased concentrations in BAL fluid in patients with COPD compared with healthy nonsmokers. There is also higher expression of transforming growth factor-β in bronchial epithelial cells.

Proteinase/Antiproteinase Imbalance

Important in understanding the pathogenesis of COPD was the observation of an association between alpha$_1$-antitrypsin deficiency and the development of early-onset emphysema. From these studies, a hypothesis was developed suggesting that, under normal circumstances, the proteolytic enzymes released from inflammatory cells that migrate to the lungs to fight infection, or in response to cigarette smoke inhalation, do *not* cause damage because they are inactivated by an excess of inhibitors. In conditions of excessive enzyme load, however, or where there is an absolute or functional deficiency of antiproteinases, such as may occur during cigarette smoking, an imbalance develops

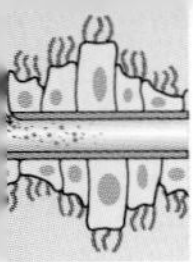

between proteinases and antiproteinases in favor of proteinases, leading to uncontrolled enzyme activity, degradation of lung connective tissue in alveolar walls, and emphysema.

This simplified proteinase/antiproteinase theory is complicated by the presence of other antiproteinases such as antileukoproteinase and other proteinases such as metalloproteases released from macrophages.

Elastase Synthesis and Repair

An abnormality of elastin synthesis and repair may be involved in the pathogenesis of emphysema. Severe starvation has been reported to cause COPD both in humans and animals; in addition, starvation can exacerbate proteinase-induced emphysema in animal models. An intriguing possibility is that starvation alters the quantity or quality of surfactant production, augmenting the tissue strains at the alveolar level. This might relate to the cystic changes seen in patients with *Pneumocystis* pneumonia who also have abnormalities in surfactant. Whether the milder malnutrition that occurs in emphysematous patients has a role in the pathogenesis of COPD is unknown.

Certain disorders of connective tissues, including Ehlers-Danlos syndrome and cutis laxa, have been associated with the development of emphysema. Emphysema also develops in some animal models with genetic defects in tissue metabolism.

Oxidant/Antioxidant Imbalance

There is considerable evidence supporting the presence of oxidative stress in patients with COPD as a result of an imbalance in the ratio of oxidants to antioxidants that favors the oxidants. Cigarette smoke itself produces a huge oxidant burden in the air spaces, and oxidants are released in increased amounts from the activated inflammatory cells that migrate into the air spaces in response to smoking. Important antioxidants such as glutathione may also be affected by inhalation of cigarette smoke. Smoking initially depletes glutathione but a subsequent rebound of levels occurs, presumably as a protective mechanism against the effects of cigarette smoking.

Several studies have measured activity of free radicals, such as products of lipid peroxidation reactions, in biologic fluids of patients with COPD as indirect measurements of reactive oxygen species activity. There is evidence of increased markers of oxidative stress in BAL fluid, sputum, exhaled breath, and breath condensate, and also systemically in the blood and skeletal muscle of patients with COPD. There is also evidence that molecules have been altered by oxidants to a greater extent in the lungs in patients with COPD compared with smokers in whom the disease has not developed, supporting a role for oxidative stress in the pathogenesis of this condition. Oxidative stress can directly damage cells, increase air space epithelial permeability, inactivate antiproteinases, and, importantly, trigger an enhanced inflammatory response by activating redox-sensitive transcription factors such as NF-κB and AP1, which are important in the regulation of proinflammatory genes.

Other Mechanisms

Both oxidants and proteinases such as elastase are important secretagogues for mucus and may therefore contribute to the hypersecretion of mucus in chronic bronchitis. Recent studies have shown that airway mucus synthesis is regulated by the epidermal growth factor receptor (EGFR) system. Cigarette smoke upregulates EGFR expression and activates EGFR tyrosine phosphorylation, causing mucus synthesis in epithelial cells by a mechanism probably involving oxidative stress.

Studies have shown that latent adenoviral infection might be associated with an enhanced susceptibility to development of COPD through the enhancement of transcriptional factor–activated proinflammatory gene expression. Apoptosis has also been shown to occur in alveolar walls in emphysema through a mechanism involving downregulation of the vascular endothelial growth factor receptor, in which oxidative stress may also play a role.

PATHOPHYSIOLOGY

Lung Mechanics

The characteristic physiologic abnormality in COPD is a decrease in maximum expiratory flow, which results from:

1. Loss of lung elasticity
2. Increase in airway resistance in small or large airways

In healthy young subjects, significant airway closure occurs only below the functional residual capacity (FRC). Enhanced airway closure occurs in the early stages of COPD, however, as demonstrated by the single-breath oxygen test. The "closing volume" so derived measures the lung volume at which some lung units close their airways and hence stop emptying, as manifested by abrupt increases in expired nitrogen concentrations. In healthy young nonsmokers, the closing volume is approximately 5% to 10% of vital capacity (VC), increasing to 25% to 35% of VC in old age. Compared with nonsmokers, young, asymptomatic adult smokers have an increase in closing volume (Fig. 34.11). As the airway disease progresses, the ability to define a closing volume decreases, and therefore the test is not useful in established disease.

Compared with nonsmokers, asymptomatic smokers also show frequency dependence of lung compliance (worsening respiratory system and lung compliance with rapid breathing). This abnormality results from inequality of time constants in the lungs, which in turn results from abnormalities in the compliance and resistance of parallel lung compartments. The pathologic changes that occur in the peripheral airways in COPD are thought to be reflected in changes in maximum flow at lung volumes below 50% of VC.

The FEV_1 and measurements of airway resistance are usually abnormal in patients with COPD when breathlessness develops. Residual volume, FRC, and (in some cases) total lung capacity (TLC) increase. Maximum expiratory flow–volume curves show a characteristic convexity toward the volume axis, with preservation of peak expiratory flow initially (Fig. 34.12).

The uneven distribution of ventilation in advanced COPD causes a reduction in "ventilated" lung volume, and thus the carbon monoxide transfer factor (TLCO) is almost always reduced, although the lung diffusing capacity for carbon monoxide (DLCO), normalized to ventilated alveolar volume (DLCO/VA/KCO), may remain relatively well preserved in those without emphysema.

The ability to draw air through the conducting airways during inspiration depends on the strength of the respiratory muscles

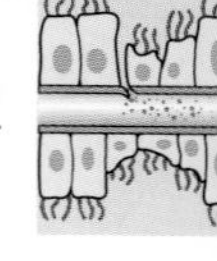

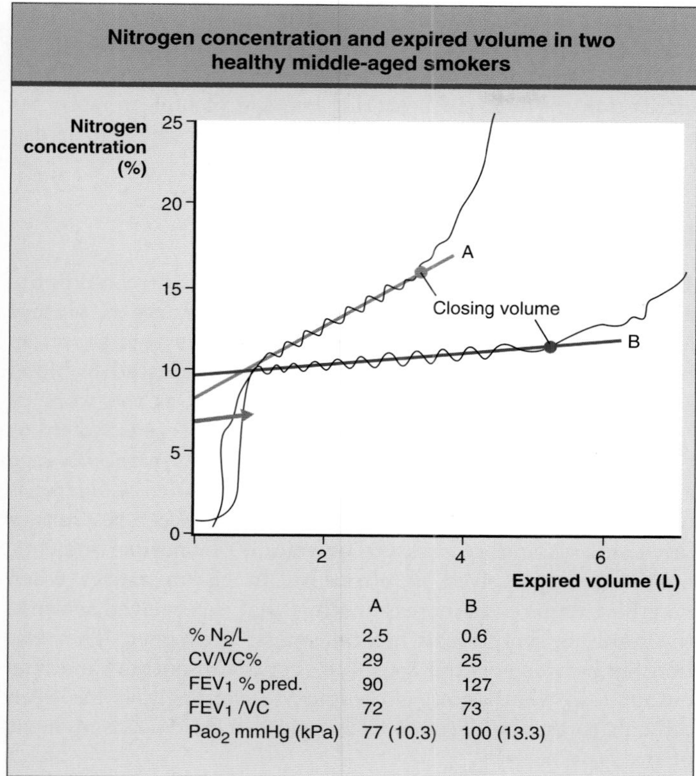

	A	B
% N_2/L	2.5	0.6
CV/VC%	29	25
FEV_1 % pred.	90	127
FEV_1 /VC	72	73
Pao_2 mmHg (kPa)	77 (10.3)	100 (13.3)

Figure 34.11 Nitrogen concentration plotted against expired volume after a single vital capacity breath of 100% oxygen for two healthy middle-aged smokers. Greater slope (percentage N_2/L) in subject A indicates more uneven distribution of ventilation and asynchronous emptying. Abrupt change of slope at the closing volume (CV) indicates the volume at which some lung units in the most dependent lung zones stop emptying. Note that arterial PO_2 (PaO_2) is lower in subject A, suggesting ventilation–perfusion mismatching on the basis of uneven distribution of ventilation. (After Pride NB, Milic-Emili J: Lung Mechanics. In Calverley PMA, MacNee W, Pride NB, Rennard SI [eds]: Chronic Obstructive Pulmonary Disease, 2nd ed. London, Chapman & Hall, 2003.)

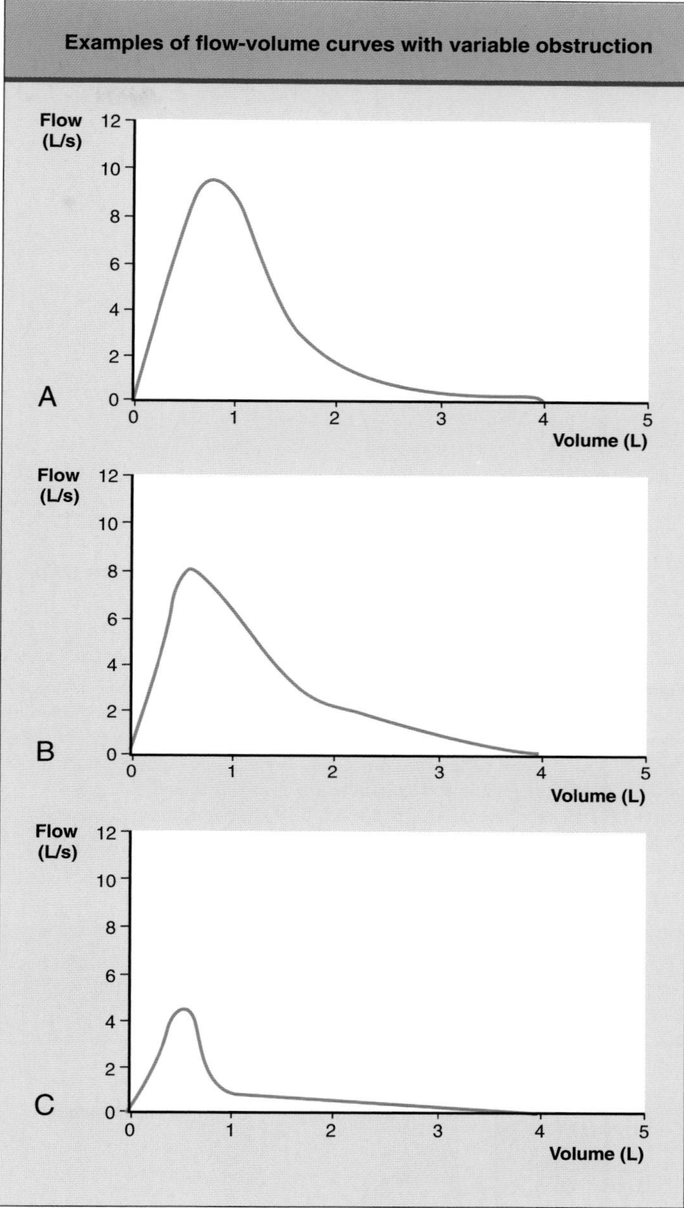

Figure 34.12 Examples of flow–volume curves. **A,** Mild obstruction. **B,** Moderate obstruction. **C,** Severe obstruction.

(which in turn depends on their resting length), the compliance of the respiratory system (i.e., lung and chest wall), and the resistance of the airways. Exhalation is normally passive and is a result of the elastic recoil of the lungs.

The characteristic changes in the static pressure–volume curve of the lungs in COPD are an increase in static compliance and a reduction in static transpulmonary pressure at any given lung volume (Fig. 34.13). These changes are generally thought to indicate emphysema.

The resistance to airflow depends on the length and diameter of the airways and the physical properties of the respirable gas. At a constant airway diameter, flow inhalation is proportional to the difference between the pressure of atmospheric gas and that in the alveolus. During exhalation, it depends on the difference between alveolar and atmospheric pressures. Throughout inhalation and during the initial portion of exhalation, this relationship is constant. However, at a certain point during exhalation, flow cannot increase despite further increases in alveolar pressure. This is a result of dynamic compression of the airways, which limits flow.

This is illustrated by the flow–volume loop (Fig. 34.14). During exhalation from TLC, flow increases to a point beyond which additional expiratory effort has no effect. During tidal breathing, expiratory flow is well below that attainable during maximum expiration. In COPD, however, the flow–volume loop is markedly different. The major site of the fixed airway narrowing in COPD is in peripheral airways that have a diameter less than 2 mm. Loss of lung elastic recoil pressure is also important in the mechanism of airway obstruction, as a result of a reduction in the distending force applied to the intrathoracic airways. Dynamic expiratory compression of the airways is enhanced by loss of lung recoil and by atrophic changes in the airways and loss of support from the surrounding alveolar walls, allowing flow limitation at lower driving pressures and flows.

In addition to a decrease in peak expiratory flow, the later expiratory portion of the flow–volume curve is markedly

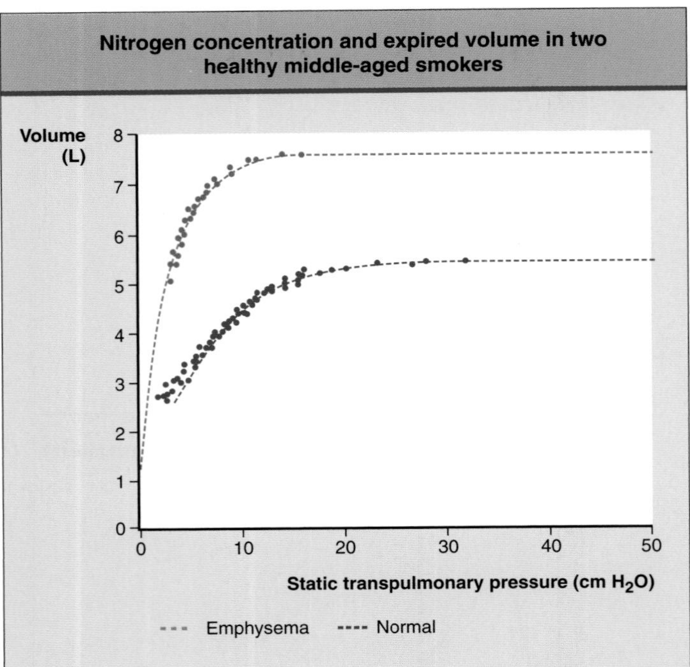

Figure 34.13 Representative static expiratory pressure–volume curves of lungs in a subject with severe emphysema compared with a normal subject. Lung volume measured by body plethysmography. Solid lines through experimental points were derived by exponential curve-fitting procedure. Broken lines indicate extrapolation of curve to infinite pressure and to volume axis at zero pressure. Values of k (cm H_2O^{-1}): for emphysema, 0.325; normal, 0.143. (Adapted from Gibson GJ, Pride NB, Davis J, Schroter RC: Exponential description of the static pressure-volume curve of normal and diseased lungs. Am Rev Respir Dis 120:799, 1979.)

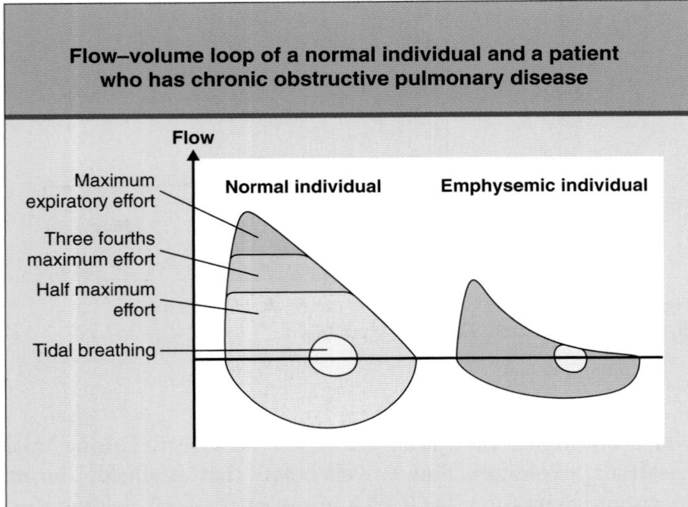

Figure 34.14 Flow–volume loop of a normal individual and a patient who has chronic obstructive pulmonary disease (COPD). Patients who have COPD may reach airflow limitation even during tidal breathing. (From Celli et al: In Comprehensive Respiratory Medicine. Elsevier Science 1999.)

concave relative to the volume axis in patients with COPD. In severe disease, the flow that is generated during tidal breathing may actually reach the maximum possible flow. Such patients, in response to the increased metabolic demands of exercise, for example, are unable to increase ventilation. Increases in respiratory rate result in gas trapping from incomplete alveolar emptying—so-called "dynamic overinflation." This increased lung volume increases the elastic recoil and is associated with an increase in the end-expiratory alveolar pressure. The result is an increase in the work of breathing because pleural pressure has to drop below alveolar pressure before inspiration of air can occur.

Ventilatory Control

The respiratory center that controls ventilation is located in the upper part of the medulla and integrates a variety of sensory inputs (e.g., mechanical from stretch receptors; neural factors from the resultant dyspnea; chemical factors related to blood gases and pH; and other sensory inputs such as the work of breathing). Output is through the peripheral nervous system to the respiratory muscles, which shorten to deform the rib cage and abdomen and generate intrathoracic pressures. *Coupling* is the term used to describe the relationship between respiratory drive and respiratory pressure or volume. In normal subjects, breathing is perceived as effortless. In circumstances when breathing requires an increased effort that is perceived as work, the resulting symptom is breathlessness or dyspnea. The relationship between central drive (i.e., control of output) and final output (i.e., ventilation) is complex. Accordingly, it has been difficult to ascribe dyspnea to any given individual component of the system.

Ventilation (V_E, $\dot{V}$) represents the final effectiveness of the ventilatory drive. V_E has two components, the tidal volume (V_T) and respiratory frequency. In COPD, as the disease progresses, adverse lung mechanics and changes in ventilation–perfusion ($\dot{V}/\dot{Q}$) relationships occur, and V_E increases as a response. The increase in V_E is affected initially by an increase in V_T, but as airflow limitation worsens and the consequent work increases, V_T decreases. The respiratory rate increases as the airflow limitation worsens.

V_E can be expressed in terms of the ratio of inspiratory time (T_I) to the total volume of inspiration (T_{TOT}) (T_I/T_{TOT}) and V_T. V_T/T_I reflects the respiratory drive, whereas T_I/T_{TOT} reflects respiratory timing. In COPD, T_I/T_{TOT} is reduced from the normal value of 0.38 by the increase in V_T, whereas V_T/T_I increases.

It is apparent from these measurements that as the degree of airflow limitation progresses, the central drive to breathing increases and is maximum in patients who suffer from respiratory failure. In the early stages of the disease, respiratory drive is effectively coupled to the increase in V_T. As the work of breathing increases, V_T drops, and when this occurs the only way to increase V_E is to increase the respiratory rate. However, the ability to increase respiratory rate to increase V_E is limited by a reduction in the elastic recoil, which limits expiratory flow and results in air trapping. Increases in lung volume may help dilate the airways, but this benefit is offset by a concurrent reduction in respiratory muscle strength and the development of auto-positive end-expiratory pressure.

Pulmonary Gas Exchange

$\dot{V}/\dot{Q}$ mismatching (as a result of decreased alveolar ventilation without a corresponding reduction in perfusion) is the most important cause of impaired pulmonary gas exchange in COPD.

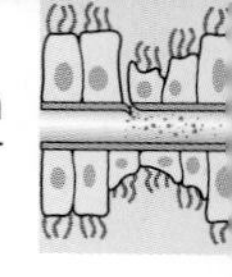

Other causes, such as impaired alveolar–capillary diffusion of oxygen and increased shunt, are of much less importance. The distribution of ventilation is very uneven in patients with COPD. A reduction of blood flow is produced by several mechanisms, including local destruction of vessels in alveolar walls as a result of emphysema, hypoxic vasoconstriction in areas of severe alveolar hypoxemia, and passive vascular obstruction as a result of increased alveolar pressure and distention (if cardiac output is reduced).

Respiratory Muscles

In patients with severe COPD, lung overinflation results in muscle weakness. In addition, the load against which the respiratory muscles need to act is increased because of the increase in airway resistance. Overinflation of the lungs leads to shortening and flattening of the diaphragm, thus impairing its ability to generate force to lower pleural pressure. During quiet tidal breathing in normal subjects, expiration is largely passive, and depends on the elastic recoil of the lungs and the chest wall. Patients with COPD increasingly need to use their rib cage muscles and inspiratory accessory muscles, such as the sternocleidomastoids, even during quiet breathing. During exercise, this pattern may be even more distorted and may result in paradoxical motion of the rib cage.

Breathlessness

Breathlessness limits exercise in patients with COPD. The symptom arises from increases in lung volume producing secondary respiratory muscle activation, and parallels the increased sensation of respiratory effort. The sensation of breathlessness increases as the ratio of the pressure needed to ventilate to the maximum possible inspiratory pressure increases, and also worsens in proportion to the duration of inspiration (i.e., T_I/T_{TOT}) and to the respiratory frequency. The respiratory muscles of patients with severe COPD function at a level that approaches the threshold of fatigue. Electromyographic evidence of fatigue has been shown during acute exacerbations of COPD. Respiratory muscle fatigue may also contribute to the carbon dioxide retention that occurs in some patients with COPD as the disease progresses. Because these circumstances also result in acute gas trapping, with the resulting increase in lung volume, it is difficult to distinguish decreased respiratory strength occurring as a result of fatigue from that attributable to weakness from the muscles having to work at their maximum length.

There is a good relationship between the sensation of breathlessness and the end-expiratory lung volume or the change in end-expiratory lung volume that occurs during exercise. Reducing the degree of overinflation by use of bronchodilators can reduce breathlessness at rest in more severe cases.

The changes in chest wall geometry that accompany these altered lung volumes reduce the capacity of the inspiratory muscles to develop pressure. Indeed, reduced maximum inspiratory pressure predicts those patients with COPD complaining of breathlessness. The importance of lung mechanical abnormalities, particularly elastic loading secondary to overinflation, has been confirmed by the effect of lung volume reduction surgery in reducing resting and exercise breathlessness. Reductions in lung volume are accompanied by an increased ability to develop inspiratory pressure and a decreased tension time index of the respiratory muscles. Thus, changes in lung mechanics seems to be the critical factor in generating breathlessness in COPD.

The role of blood gases in producing breathlessness has been difficult to establish. Patients with COPD do increase their perceived effort as the $PaCO_2$ rises, but hypoxia appears to be less important in producing breathlessness. Oxygen desaturation during exercise, for example, does not relate to subsequent intensity of breathlessness.

Cor Pulmonale

Pulmonary arterial hypertension occurs late in the course of COPD, concurrent with the development of hypoxemia and usually hypercapnia. Cor pulmonale is the major cardiovascular complication of COPD, is associated with the development of right ventricular hypertrophy, and carries a poor prognosis. Peripheral edema results from a combination of increased venous pressure and renal hormonal changes, leading to increased salt and water retention (Fig. 34.15).

Systemic Effects

Patients with COPD have skeletal muscle dysfunction and loss of body mass. The explanations for these effects are understudied but are presumed to relate to the effect of systemic oxidative stress and inflammation. Weight loss portends a poor prognosis and, accordingly, is a target for therapeutic intervention.

CLINICAL FEATURES

A summary of the clinical evaluation of patients with COPD is given in Table 34.2.

Symptoms

Patients with COPD characteristically complain of breathlessness on exertion, sometimes accompanied by wheeze and cough. The cough is often, but not invariably, productive. Patients often date the onset of their illness to an acute exacerbation of cough with sputum production, which leaves them with a degree of chronic breathlessness. Close questioning, however, usually reveals many years of a "smoker's cough" with the production of small amounts of mucoid sputum, often predominating in the morning.

A smoking history of at least 20 pack-years is usual.

Breathlessness is usually first noticed on climbing hills or stairs, or hurrying on level ground. It usually heralds the existence of at least moderate impairment of expiratory flow. When the FEV_1 has fallen to 30% or less of the predicted value, breathlessness is usually present on minimal exertion. Severe breathlessness is often triggered by changes in environmental temperature or occupational exposure to dust and fumes. Some patients have severe orthopnea, relieved by leaning forward, whereas others find greatest ease when lying flat. Breathlessness can be assessed using the Medical Research Council (MRC) Dyspnea Scale, the Borg Scale, and visual analog scales.

Nocturnal cough may also be increased in stable COPD. Paroxysms of coughing in the presence of severe airway obstruc-

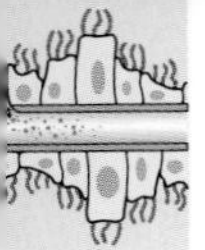

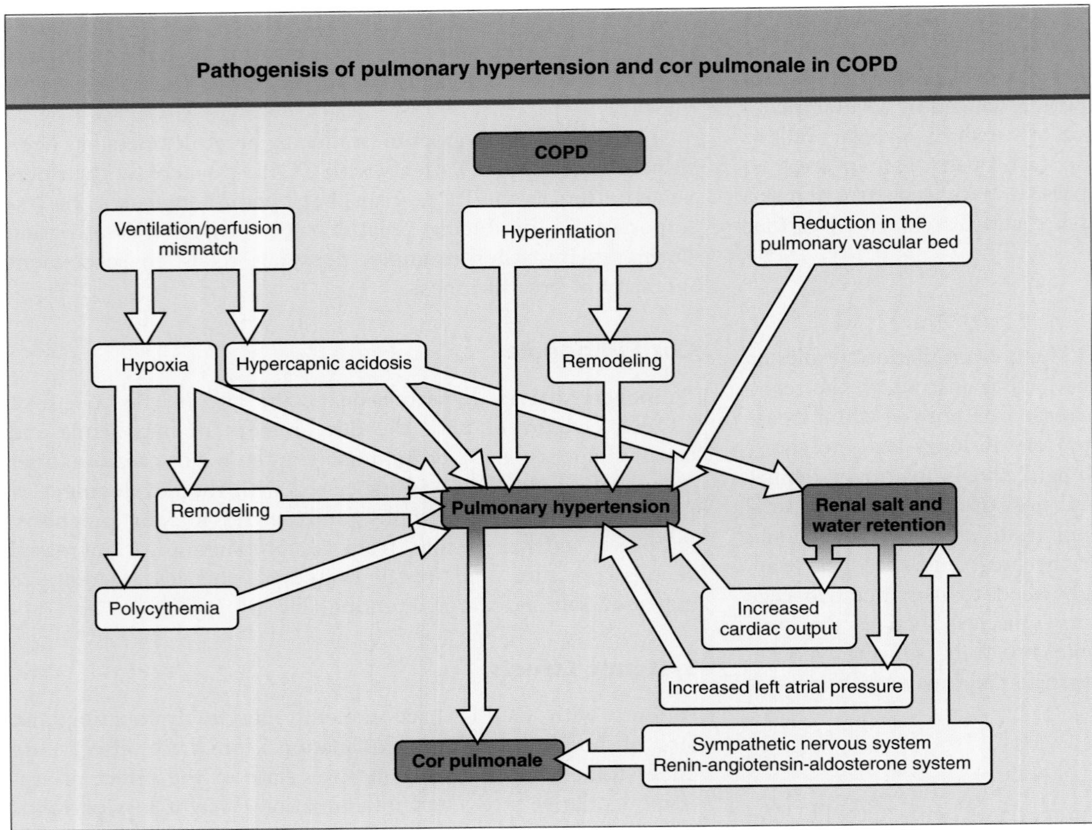

Figure 34.15 Pathogenesis of pulmonary hypertension and cor pulmonale in chronic obstructive pulmonary disease. (From Naeije R, MacNee W: Pulmonary Circulation. In Calverley PMA, MacNee W, Pride NB, Rennard SI [eds]: Chronic Obstructive Pulmonary Disease, 2nd ed. London, Chapman & Hall, Chapter 17, 2003, pp 228-242.)

Table 34.2
Clinical Evaluation of Chronic Obstructive Pulmonary Disease

History	Breathlessness Exercise intolerance Cough, sputum production Smoking history Occupational exposure Family history Weight changes
Examination	Increased respiratory rate Signs of overinflation Use of accessory respiratory muscles Retraction of the lower rib cage Intercostal indrawing Prolonged exhalation Wheeze Edema/raised jugular venous pressure
Investigations	Decreased FEV_1 and FEV_1/forced vital capacity Radiographic evidence of emphysema Decreased diffusing capacity for carbon monoxide Hypoxemia and hypercapnia

FEV_1, forced expiratory volume in 1 second.

tion generate high intrathoracic pressures, which can produce syncope and "cough fractures" of the ribs. Wheeze is common but not specific to COPD because it is due to turbulent airflow in large airways from any cause.

Substernal chest pain is common in patients with COPD. It may be a result of the COPD itself, or may result from underlying ischemic heart disease or gastroesophageal reflux. Chest tightness is a common complaint during periods of worsening breathlessness, particularly during exercise, and this is sometimes difficult to distinguish from ischemic pain. Pleuritic chest pain may suggest an intercurrent pneumothorax, pneumonia, or pulmonary infarction. Hemoptysis can be associated with purulent sputum and may be due to inflammation or infection. However, this symptom should also prompt consideration of the possibility of bronchial carcinoma.

Weight loss and anorexia are features of severe COPD and are thought to result from both decreased calorie intake and hypermetabolism.

Psychiatric morbidity, particularly depression, is common in patients with severe COPD. Sleep quality and sexual function are impaired, which may be contributing factors.

The history in COPD should also record:

- History of asthma, allergy, respiratory infections in childhood, or any other respiratory diseases such as tuberculosis
- Family history of COPD or other respiratory diseases
- Number of exacerbations or hospitalizations
- Comorbidities, particularly those that have the same risk factor (smoking), such as ischemia, heart disease, or peripheral vascular disease.

Exposure History

A detailed smoking history is important because the disease is rare in never-smokers. Although there is, in general, a dose response relating the number of cigarettes smoked and the level

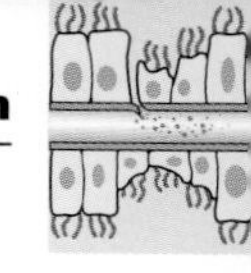

of the FEV_1, there are considerable individual variations, presumably reflecting variations in susceptibility to cigarette smoke. The typical patient has a smoking history of more than 20 pack-years. Those with less extensive smoking histories should be evaluated for $alpha_1$-antitrypsin deficiency, asthma, or the other exposures resulting in COPD (see earlier).

Clinical Signs

Patients typically present in the fifth decade of life. The physical examination may be completely negative early in the course of COPD. The physical signs are not specific and depend on the degree of airflow limitation and pulmonary overinflation. The sensitivity of the physical examination to detect or exclude moderately severe COPD is rather poor.

General Examination

The respiratory rate may be increased. A forced expiratory time greater than 5 seconds strongly suggests the presence of airflow limitation. The prolonged expiratory phase, with or without pursing of the lips, is characteristic of patients with COPD. Use of accessory muscles of respiration, particularly the sternocleidomastoids, is often seen in advanced disease and these patients often adopt a posture in which they lean forward, supporting themselves with their arms to fix the shoulder girdle. This allows use of the pectorals and the latissimus dorsi to increase chest wall movement.

Tar-stained fingers emphasize the smoking habit in many patients. In advanced disease, cyanosis may be present, indicating hypoxemia, but it may be diminished by anemia or accentuated by polycythemia, and is a fairly subjective sign. The flapping tremor, associated with hypercapnia, is neither sensitive nor specific, and papilledema associated with severe hypercapnia is rare.

Weight loss may also be apparent in advanced disease, as well as a reduction in muscle mass. Finger clubbing is not a feature of COPD and should suggest the possibility of complicating bronchial neoplasm or bronchiectasis.

Examination of the Chest

In the later stages of COPD the chest is often barrel-shaped in the setting of kyphosis, resulting in an increased anterior–posterior chest diameter, horizontal ribs, prominence of the sternal angle, and a wide subcostal angle. The distance between the suprasternal notch and the cricoid cartilage (normally three fingerbreadths) may be reduced owing to the elevation of the sternum. These are all signs of overinflation. An inspiratory tracheal tug may be detected, attributed to contraction of the low, flat diaphragm. The horizontal position of the diaphragm also acts to pull the lower ribs in during inspiration (i.e., Hoover's sign). Widening of the xiphosternal angle and abdominal protuberance occur, the latter due to forward displacement of the abdominal contents, giving the appearance of apparent weight gain. Increased intrathoracic pressure swings may result in indrawing of the suprasternal and supraclavicular fossae and of the intercostal muscles.

There is decreased hepatic and cardiac dullness on percussion, indicating overinflation. A useful sign of gross overinflation is the absence of a dull percussion note, normally due to the underlying heart, over the lower end of the sternum. Breath sounds may have a prolonged expiratory phase or may be uniformly diminished, particularly in the advanced stages of the disease. Wheeze may be present both on inspiration and expiration, but is not an invariable sign. Crackles may be heard, particularly at the lung bases, but are usually scant and vary with coughing.

Cardiovascular Examination

Air trapping decreases venous return and compresses the heart. Accordingly, tachycardia is common. The presence of positive alveolar pressure at the end of exhalation (i.e., auto- or intrinsic positive end-expiratory pressure) results in the need to create a more negative pleural pressure than usual, manifested by the presence of a paradoxical pulse. Overinflation makes it difficult to localize the apex beat and reduces the cardiac dullness. The characteristic signs that indicate the presence or consequences of pulmonary arterial hypertension may be detected in advanced cases. The heave of right ventricular hypertrophy may be palpable at the lower left sternal edge or in the subxiphoid regions. Heart sounds are usually soft, although the pulmonary component of the second heart sound may be exaggerated in the second left intercostal space. A right ventricular gallop rhythm may be detected (disappearing on exhalation) in the fourth intercostal space to the left of the sternum. The jugular venous pressure can be difficult to see in patients with COPD because it swings widely with respiration and is difficult to discern if there is prominent accessory muscle activity. There may be evidence of functional tricuspid incompetence, producing a pansystolic murmur at the left sternal edge. The liver may be tender and pulsatile, and a prominent "v" wave may be visible in the jugular venous pulse. The liver may also be palpable below the right costal margin as a result of overinflation of the lungs.

Peripheral vasodilatation accompanies hypercapnia, producing warm peripheries with a high-volume pulse. Pitting peripheral edema may also be present as a result of fluid retention.

CLINICAL INVESTIGATIONS

Physiologic Assessment

The degree of airflow limitation cannot be predicted from the symptoms and signs noted on the clinical evaluation. Accordingly, the degree of airflow limitation should be assessed in every patient. At an early stage of the disease, conventional spirometry may reveal no abnormality. Results of tests of small airway function, such as the frequency dependence of compliance and closing volume, may be abnormal, however. These tests are difficult to perform, have high coefficients of variation, and are valid only when lung elastic recoil is normal and there is no increase in airway resistance. They are therefore not recommended in normal clinical practice.

SPIROMETRY

Spirometry is the most robust test of airflow limitation in patients with COPD. Spirometric measurements have a well-defined range of normal values. A low FEV_1 with an FEV_1/FVC ratio below the normal range is a diagnostic criterion for COPD.

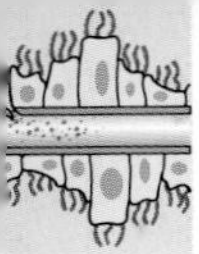

The rate of decline of the FEV_1 can be used to assess susceptibility in cigarette smokers and progression of the disease.

It is important that a volume plateau is reached when performing the FEV_1, which can take 15 seconds or more in patients with severe airway obstruction. If this maneuver is not carried out, the VC can be underestimated. The FEV_1 as a percentage of the predicted value can be used as part of the assessment of severity of the disease (Table 34.3). FEV_1 values within ±20% of the predicted value are considered to be within the normal range. Thus, an FEV_1 of 80% or more of the predicted value is considered to be normal. Under normal circumstances, 70% to 80% of the total volume of the air in the lungs (FVC) should be exhaled in the first second. When the FEV_1/FVC ratio falls below 70%, airflow limitation is present.

OTHER EXPIRATORY FLOWS

Expiratory flows measured at 75% or 50% of VC have also been used to identify patients with COPD. These measurements are less reproducible than the FEV_1, such that the measurement must fall below 50% of the predicted values. Flows at lung volumes less than 50% of VC were previously considered to be an indicator of small airways function, but probably provide no more clinically useful information than measurements of the FEV_1.

Peak expiratory flow can either be read directly from the flow–volume loop or measured with a hand-held peak flow meter. The latter is relatively easy to use and is particularly useful in subjects with asthma, who reveal variations in serial measurements. In patients with COPD, however, many of the variations are often within the error of the measurement. The peak expiratory flow may underestimate the degree of airflow limitation in COPD.

REVERSIBILITY TESTING

Assessment of reversibility to bronchodilators is recognized as an essential part of the investigation and management of patients with COPD. Reversibility tests are important to

- Help distinguish those patients with asthma
- Establish the postbronchodilator FEV_1, which is the best indicator of long-term prognosis
- Establish the best obtainable lung function

There is no agreement on a standardized method of assessing reversibility, but this is usually quantified on the basis of a change in the FEV_1 or the peak expiratory flow. There may be changes in other lung volumes after bronchodilators, however (e.g., inspiratory capacity, residual volume), which may explain why some symptoms improve in some patients after a bronchodilator without a change in spirometry results. An improvement in FEV_1 in response to a bronchodilator does not necessarily predict a symptomatic response.

Bronchodilator reversibility can vary from day to day, depending on the degree of bronchomotor tone. A change in FEV_1 that exceeds 200 mL is considered to be greater than random variation. Therefore, changes should be reported as significant only if they exceed 200 mL. In addition to this absolute change in FEV_1, a percentage change of 12% over baseline has been suggested as significant by the American Thoracic Society and GOLD Guidelines, whereas an improvement of 15% over baseline FEV_1 and a 200-mL absolute change has been suggested by the European Respiratory Society and British Thoracic Society Guidelines.

It is usually recommended that reversibility be assessed using a large bronchodilator dose, either using repeated doses from a metered-dose inhaler, or by nebulization, because this produces a larger number of patients with a significant response. In some cases, the addition of a second drug, such as an anticholinergic drug, to a β-agonist produces a further increase in FEV_1.

Reversibility testing with a bronchodilator is usually indicated only at the time of diagnosis. Approximately 30% of patients with COPD show significant reversibility of their airflow obstruction in response to a bronchodilator.

REVERSIBILITY TO CORTICOSTEROIDS

Whether all patients with symptomatic COPD should have a formal assessment of steroid reversibility remains controversial, but this practice is not included in the most recent guidelines for assessment and management of the disease. The most common method for doing this is to administer 30 mg of prednisone or prednisolone for a period of 2 weeks. Although patients who have previously shown a response to nebulized bronchodilators are more likely to show a response to steroids, it is not possible to predict the response to corticosteroids in an individual patient.

LUNG VOLUMES

Static lung volumes such as TLC, residual volume (RV), and FRC, and the ratio RV/TLC are measured in patients with COPD to assess the degree of overinflation and gas trapping, and are usually increased. These measurements are not necessary in every patient.

The standard method of measuring static lung volumes, using the helium dilution technique during rebreathing, may underestimate lung volumes in COPD, particularly in those patients with bullous disease, because the inspired helium may not have sufficient time to equilibrate properly in the air spaces. Body plethysmography uses Boyle's law to calculate lung volumes

Table 34.3
GOLD Classification of Severity of Chronic Obstructive Pulmonary Disease

Stage	Characteristics
0: At risk	• Normal spirometry • Chronic symptoms (cough, sputum production)
I: Mild COPD	• FEV_1 : FVC <70% • FEV_1 ≥80% predicted • With or without chronic symptoms (cough, sputum production)
II: Moderate COPD	• FEV_1 : FVC <70% • 30% ≤ FEV_1 < 80% predicted
IIA	50% ≤ FEV_1 < 80% predicted
IIB	30% ≤ FEV_1 < 80% predicted
III: Severe COPD	• FEV_1 : FVC <70% • FEV_1 <30% predicted or FEV_1 <50% predicted plus respiratory failure or clinical signs of right heart failure

COPD, chronic obstructive pulmonary disease; FEV_1, forced expiratory volume in 1 second; FVC, forced vital capacity; GOLD, Global Initiative on Obstructive Lung Disease.

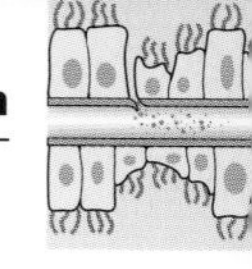

from changes in mouth and plethysmographic pressures. This technique measures trapped air in the thorax, including poorly ventilated areas, and therefore gives higher readings than the helium dilution technique.

GAS TRANSFER FOR CARBON MONOXIDE

A low DLCO is present in many patients with COPD. Although there is a relationship between DLCO and the extent of microscopic emphysema, the severity of the emphysema in an individual patient cannot be predicted from the DLCO, nor is a low DLCO specific for emphysema. The commonly used method is the single-breath technique, which uses alveolar volume calculated from the helium dilution during a single-breath test. This method underestimates alveolar volume in patients with severe COPD, producing a lower value for the DLCO. This test can be useful to distinguish patients with COPD from those with asthma because a low DLCO excludes asthma.

ARTERIAL BLOOD GASES

Arterial blood gases are needed to confirm the degree of hypoxemia and hypercapnia that develops in patients with COPD. Hypoxemia and hypercapnia are not usually observed until the FEV_1 falls below 40% of predicted. It is essential to record the inspired oxygen concentration when reporting blood gases. It is also important to note that it may take at least 30 minutes for a change in inspired oxygen concentration to have its full effect on the PaO_2 because of long time constants for alveolar gas equilibration in COPD, particularly during exacerbations. Pulse oximetry is increasingly used to measure the level of oxygenation, but it should not replace an assessment of blood gas tensions in patients with FEV_1s below 40% predicted, or in those with elevations of their serum bicarbonate concentrations, because measurements of $PaCO_2$ are often required.

Blood gas abnormalities may worsen during exercise and sleep and during acute exacerbations.

EXERCISE TESTS

Exercise increases oxygen consumption and carbon dioxide production from skeletal muscle. Patients with COPD may have considerably higher oxygen consumptions for a given workload than normal subjects as a result of the increased work of breathing they may experience. Dead space ventilation is higher and thus larger minute ventilations are also needed to maintain carbon dioxide at a constant level. Many patients with COPD have expiratory airflow limitation occurring in the normal tidal volume range. In these patients, the only way to increase minute ventilation is to increase inspiratory flow or shift the end-expiratory lung volume up so that flow can increase (Fig. 34.16). Both of these maneuvers are problematic in patients with COPD and require more work from already compromised inspiratory muscles, or result in progressive overinflation, which increases both the work of breathing and symptoms. The increased cardiac output that occurs with exercise may also lead to increased perfusion of poorly ventilated areas, worsening the $\dot{V}/\dot{Q}$ mismatching to the extent that arterial oxygenation may fall. Moreover, metabolic acidosis develops at lower work rates in patients with severe COPD. In patients with COPD, progressive cycle exercise is limited by dyspnea in 40% and by leg fatigue in 25%, reflecting skeletal muscle dysfunction.

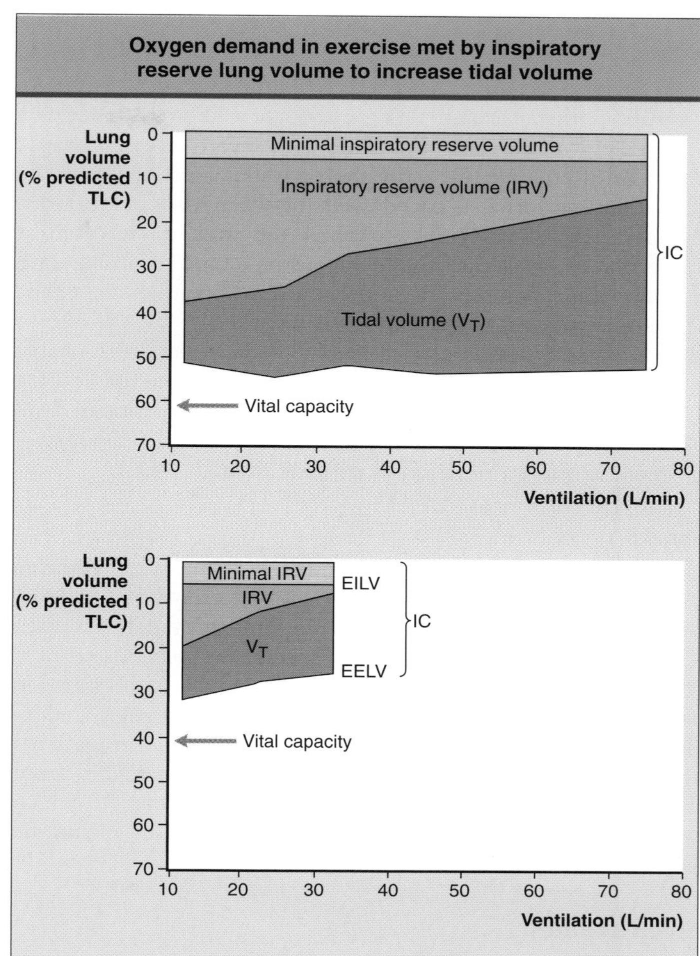

Figure 34.16 In good health, the body meets the increased oxygen demand produced by exercise by using some of the inspiratory reserve volume of the lungs to increase tidal volume. EELV, end-expiratory lung volume; EILV, end-inspiratory lung volume; IC, inspiratory capacity; IRV, inspiratory reserve volume; TLC, total lung capacity; VC, vital capacity.

Although exercise testing is rarely needed to diagnose COPD, useful information might accrue from doing any of three types of tests:

1. *Progressive symptom limited exercise* tests. This requires the patient to maintain exercise on a treadmill or a cycle until symptoms prevent him or her from continuing while the workload applied is continuously increased. A maximum test is usually defined as a heart rate of greater than 85% of predicted or a ventilation greater than 90% predicted. The results are particularly useful when simultaneous electrocardiography and blood pressure monitoring are performed to assess whether coexisting cardiac or psychological factors contribute to exercise limitation.
2. *Self-paced exercise* tests are simple to perform and give information on sustained exercise that may be more relevant to problems in daily life. The commonly used test is the 6-minute walk, which has a coefficient of variation of approximately 8%. A learning effect, however, may influence the result of repeated tests. This test is useful only in patients

with moderately severe COPD (FEV_1 <1.5 L) who would be expected to have an exercise tolerance of less than 600 m in 6 minutes. There is a weak relationship between 6-minute walking distance and FEV_1, although walking distance is a predictor of survival in patients with severe disease.

An alternative test is the shuttle walking test, in which the patient performs a paced walk between two points 10 m apart (the shuttle). The pace of the walk is increased at regular intervals dictated by bleeps on a tape recording until the patient is forced to stop because of breathlessness. The number of completed shuttles is recorded.

3. *Steady-state exercise* tests involve exercise at a sustainable percentage of maximum capacity for 3 to 6 minutes during which blood gases are measured, enabling calculation of dead space–tidal volume ratio (V_D/V_T) and shunt. This assessment is seldom required in patients with COPD.

OTHER TESTS

Lung pressure–volume curves are difficult to measure, requiring assessment of esophageal pressure with an esophageal balloon, and are not part of the routine assessment of patients with COPD. They may be necessary in special circumstances.

Measurements of small airway function with nitrogen washout test, helium flow–volume loops, or frequency dependence of compliance have poor reproducibility in patients with COPD. Although they can differentiate smokers from nonsmokers, they are not useful for predicting in which smokers COPD will develop, and thus are not used in routine practice.

Sleep Studies

Selected patients should be assessed for the presence of nocturnal hypoxemia. Finding nocturnal hypoxemia does not, however, provide any further prognostic or clinically useful information in the assessment of patients with COPD unless coexisting sleep apnea syndrome is suspected. Individuals who desaturate at night may be candidates for oxygen therapy.

Assessment of Breathlessness

Symptomatic improvement, particularly in breathlessness, is one of the important goals of treatment in COPD. Breathlessness is a subjective feature but can be quantified. The appearance of breathlessness heralds moderate to severe impairment of airway function. By the time patients seek medical advice, the FEV_1 has usually fallen to approximately 1 to 1.5 L in an average man (30% to 45% of the predicted value). Patients with COPD may adapt their breathing pattern and their behavior to minimize the sensation of breathlessness, usually by greatly restricted activity.

The perception of breathlessness varies greatly between individuals with the same degree of ventilatory capacity. It can be assessed using a modified Borg Scale (Table 34.4), a visual analog scale, or the MRC Dyspnea Scale (Table 34.5). The oxygen-cost diagram is more sensitive to change than the MRC scale and allows the patient to mark a 10-cm line to represent the point beyond which he or she becomes breathless (Fig. 34.17). The distance in centimeters from the zero point can be used to obtain a score.

Table 34.4
The Modified Borg Scale for Assessing Breathlessness

Scale	Severity Experienced by Patient
0	Nothing at all
0.5	Very, very slight (just noticeable)
1	Very slight
2	Slight (light)
3	Moderate
4	Somewhat severe
5	Severe (heavy)
6	
7	Very severe
8	
9	Very, very severe (almost maximal)
10	Maximal

Table 34.5
The Medical Research Council Dyspnea Scale for Assessing Breathlessness

Grade	Degree of Breathlessness Related to Activities
0	Not troubled by breathlessness except on strenuous exercise
1	Short of breath when hurrying or walking up a slight hill
2	Walks slower than contemporaries on the level because of breathlessness, or has to stop for breath when walking at own pace
3	Stops for breath after walking about 100 m or after a few minutes on the level
4	Too breathless to leave the house, or breathless when dressing or undressing
5	Breathless at rest

Health Status

Quality of life is a measure of the impact of the disease on daily life and well-being. Breathlessness in patients with COPD limits exercise, reduces expectations, diminishes daily activity, restricts social activities, disturbs mood, and impairs the sense of well being. Several questionnaires are available to assess health status. These are commonly used in hospital rehabilitation programs and in research. The Chronic Respiratory Disease Index Questionnaire is sensitive to change, but is very time-consuming and requires training to administer properly. The St. George's Respiratory Questionnaire is a self-completed questionnaire with three components: symptoms, which measures distress due to respiratory symptoms; activity, which measures disturbance of daily activities; and impact, which measures psychosocial function. The three components are summed to give a total score of overall health status. The Breathing Problems Questionnaire is a self-completed questionnaire that is easy to complete but relatively insensitive to change. The St. George's Respiratory Questionnaire is the most validated in COPD.

There is a rather poor relationship between the St. George's Respiratory Questionnaire and the FEV_1. It is clear from a

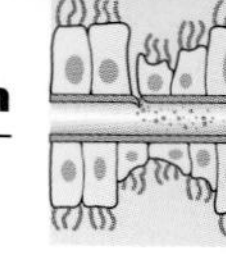

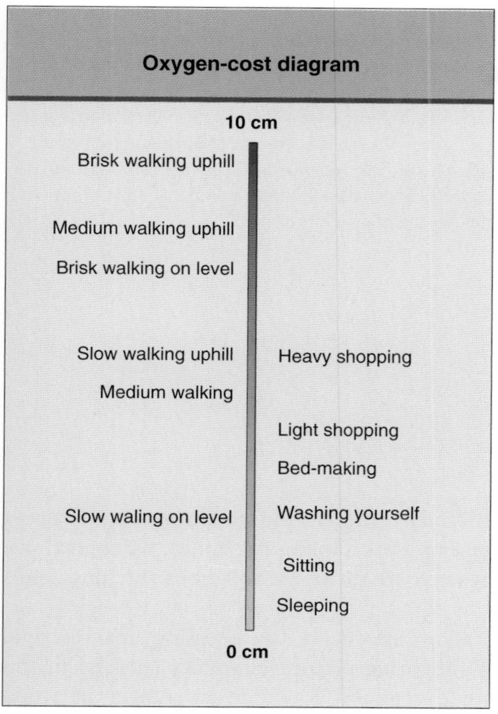

Figure 34.17 Oxygen-cost diagram.

number of studies that there can be improvement in health status without any improvement in FEV_1 in response to drugs. The threshold of clinical improvement is a change of four units in the St. George's Respiratory Questionnaire. Exacerbations of COPD have a clear detrimental effect on health status.

Other Measurements

Erythrocythemia is important to identify in patients with COPD because it predisposes to peripheral vascular, cardiovascular, and cerebrovascular events. Erythrocythemia/polycythemia does not develop until there is clinically important hypoxemia (PaO_2 <7.2 kPa, 55 mm Hg) and is not an inevitable occurrence even at this level.

Alpha$_1$-antitrypsin screening with measurements of the level and determination of allelic phenotype is indicated for patients with an early onset of emphysema (<45 years of age) and in those with a family history of premature emphysema. Because of the potential importance for other family members, some experts recommend that all patients with COPD be screened. In the United States, replacement therapy is reimbursed by insurers for patients with homozygous deficiency. Intravenous infusions every 2 to 4 weeks are costly and are not reimbursed in many countries. The effectiveness of replacement therapy in delaying the progression of COPD has not been confirmed in a randomized, controlled trial because of the projected cost and complexity of such an investigation.

Echocardiography is not routinely required in the assessment of patients with COPD except where coexisting cardiac morbidity is suspected. It is an insensitive technique for the diagnosis of cor pulmonale. Overinflation of the chest increases the retrosternal air space, which transmits sound waves poorly, making echocardiography difficult in patients with COPD. Thus, an adequate examination can be achieved in only 65% to 85% of patients with COPD.

Two-dimensional echocardiography has been used in the investigation of right ventricular dimensions. Pulsed-wave Doppler echocardiography is used to assess ejection flow dynamics of the right ventricle in patients with pulmonary hypertension. The tricuspid gradient can be used to calculate the right ventricular systolic pressure. The technique estimates the pressure gradient across the tricuspid regurgitant jet recorded by Doppler ultrasonography. The maximum velocity of the regurgitant jet is measured from the continuous-wave Doppler recordings, and the simplified Bernoulli equation is used to calculate the maximum pressure gradient between the right ventricle and the right atrium as $P_{RV} - P_{RA} = 4v^2$, where P_{RV} and P_{RA} are the right ventricular and right atrial pressures and v is the maximum velocity. The right atrial pressure is estimated from clinical examination of the jugular venous pressure.

Imaging

PLAIN CHEST RADIOGRAPHY

COPD does not produce any specific features on a plain chest radiograph unless features of emphysema are present. There may be no abnormalities, however, even in patients with severe disability. The most reliable radiographic signs of emphysema can be divided into those due to overinflation, vascular changes, and bullae.

The following radiologic features are indicative of overinflation:

- A low, flattened diaphragm (i.e., the border of the diaphragm in the mid-clavicular line on the posterior–anterior film is at or below the anterior end of the seventh rib, and is flattened if the perpendicular height from a line drawn between the costal and cardiophrenic angles to the border of the diaphragm is less than 1.5 cm; Fig. 34.18).
- Increased retrosternal air space, visible on the lateral film at a point 3 cm below the manubrium, is present when the horizontal distance from the posterior surface of the aorta to the sternum exceeds 4.5 cm (see Fig. 34.17).
- An obtuse costophrenic angle on the posterior–anterior or lateral chest radiograph
- An inferior margin of the retrosternal air space 3 cm or less from the anterior aspect of the diaphragm

The *vascular changes* associated with emphysema result from loss of alveolar walls and are shown on the plain chest radiograph by

- Reduction in the number and size of pulmonary vessels, particularly at the periphery of the lung
- Vessel distortion, producing increased branching angles and excess straightening or bowing of vessels
- Areas of increased lucency

Critical to the assessment of vascular loss in emphysema is the quality of the chest radiograph because increased translucency may simply be due to overexposure.

The accuracy of diagnosing emphysema on plain chest radiography increases with severity of the disease and has been reported to be 50% to 80% in patients with moderate to severe disease. However, the sensitivity has been reported to be as low as 24% in patients with mild to moderate disease.

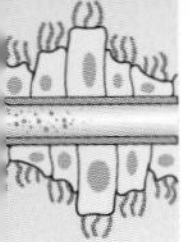

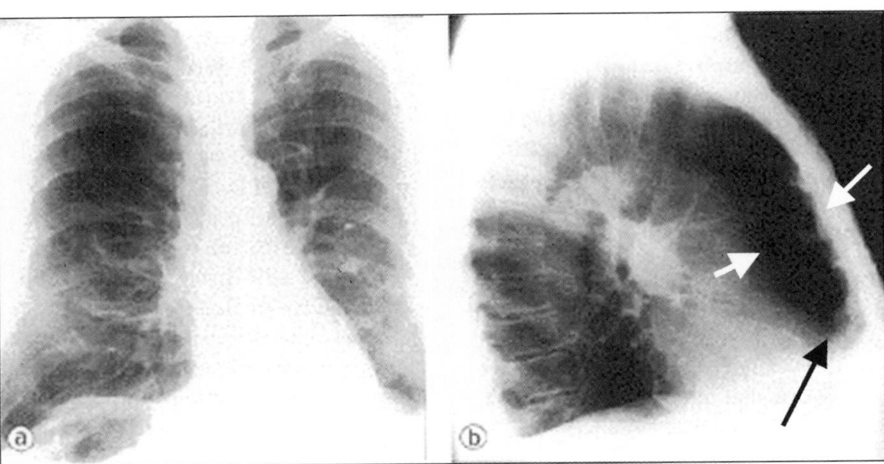

Figure 34.18 Plain chest radiographs of generalized emphysema particularly affecting the lower zones. **A,** Posterior–anterior radiograph showing a low, flat diaphragm (below the anterior ends of the seventh ribs), obtuse costophrenic angles, and reduced vessel markings in lower zones, which are transradiant. **B,** Lateral radiograph showing a low, flat, and inverted diaphragm and widened retrosternal transradiancy (*white arrows*) that approaches the diaphragm inferiorly (*black arrows*).

Right ventricular hypertrophy or enlargement produces nonspecific cardiac enlargement on the plain chest radiograph. The plain chest radiograph can be used as a screening tool to assess pulmonary hypertension. The width of the right descending pulmonary artery, measured just below the right hilum, where the borders of the artery are delineated against air in the lungs laterally and the right main stem bronchus medially, is normally up to 16mm in men and 15mm in women. Measurements greater than this can predict the presence, but not the level, of the pulmonary arterial hypertension.

COMPUTED TOMOGRAPHY

Computed tomography (CT) scanning has been used to detect and quantify emphysema. Techniques can be divided into those that provide a visual assessment of low-density areas on the CT scan, which can be either semiquantitative or quantitative, or those that use CT lung density to quantify areas of low x-ray attenuation. These techniques are used to measure macroscopic or microscopic emphysema, respectively.

A visual assessment of emphysema on CT scanning shows

- Areas of low attenuation without obvious margins or walls
- Attenuation and pruning of the vascular tree
- Abnormal vascular configurations

Areas of low attenuation correlate best with areas of macroscopic emphysema. Visual inspection of the CT scan can be used to locate macroscopic emphysema, although assessing the extent is insensitive and subject to high intraobserver and interobserver variability. The CT scan can be used to assess different types of emphysema—centrilobular emphysema produces patchy areas of low attenuation prominent in the upper zones, whereas those of panlobular emphysema are diffuse throughout the lung zones (Fig. 34.19).

A more quantitative approach to assessing macroscopic emphysema is by highlighting picture elements (pixels) in the lung fields in a predetermined low density range, between −910 and −1000 Hounsfield units, the so-called "density mask" technique.

Although the choice of the density range is fairly arbitrary, there is a good correlation between the pathologic emphysema score and the CT density score. This technique may still miss areas of mild emphysema, however.

Microscopic emphysema can be quantified by measuring CT lung density. CT density is measured on a linear scale in Hounsfield units (water = 0, air = −1000). CT lung density is a direct measure of physical density and, thus, as emphysema develops, a decrease in alveolar surface area occurs as alveolar walls are lost, associated with an increase in distal air space size, which would decrease lung CT density.

More studies are required before CT lung density can be used as a standardized technique to quantify microscopic emphysema.

A bulla is defined arbitrarily as an emphysematous space greater than 1cm in diameter. On the plain chest radiograph, a bulla appears as a localized avascular area of increased lucency, usually separated from the rest of the lung by a thin, curvilinear wall. Marked compression of the surrounding lung may be seen and bullae may also depress the diaphragm.

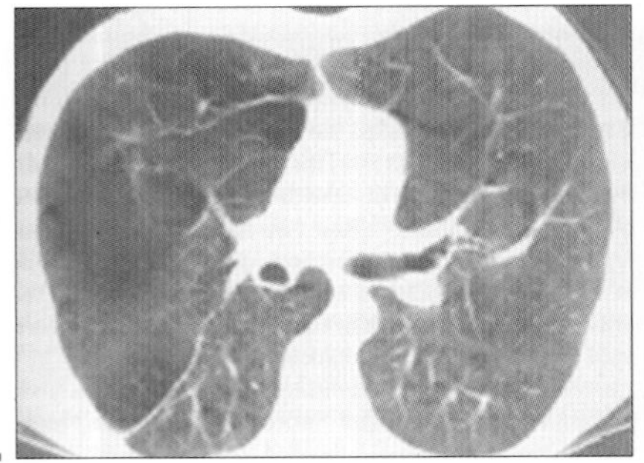

A

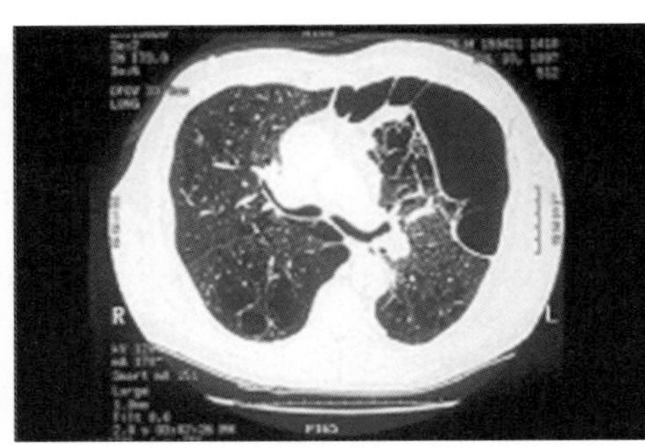

B

Figure 34.19 High-resolution computed tomography scans of the lungs. **A,** Diffuse panlobular emphysema. **B,** More patchy centrilobular emphysema with bullae.

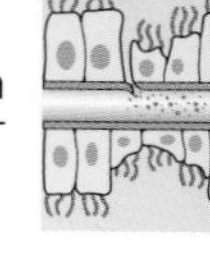

CT scanning is much more sensitive than plain chest radiography at detecting bullae and can be used to determine their number, size, and position.

CT scanning has been used to quantify the extent and distribution of emphysema as part of the assessment for surgery in bullous disease and for lung volume reduction surgery.

PITFALLS AND CONTROVERSIES

Differentiating COPD from asthma may be difficult because of the overlap in pathophysiology, clinical presentation, pulmonary function test results, and treatment. This differentiation is important, however, because treatment options now differ for both conditions (e.g., importance of anticholinergics versus β-agonist therapy, use of corticosteroids, use of pulmonary rehabilitation).

Underdiagnosis of COPD is another common problem because the disease is usually far advanced before patients present with related symptoms. Screening spirometry is, accordingly, needed in every smoking patient, regardless of age or degree of symptoms.

SUGGESTED READINGS

Barnes P, Drazen J, Rennard S, Thomson N (eds): Asthma and COPD: Basic Mechanisms and Clinical Management. London, Academic Press, 2002.

Calverley PMA, MacNee W, Pride NB, Rennard SI (eds): Chronic Obstructive Pulmonary Disease, 2nd ed. London, Chapman & Hall, 2003.

MacNee W (ed): Oxidants/Antioxidants and Chronic Obstructive Pulmonary Disease: Pathogenesis to Therapy. Novartis Found Symp 234:169-185, 2001.

Pauwels RA, Buist AS, Calverley PM, et al: Global strategy for the diagnosis, management, and prevention of chronic obstructive pulmonary disease. NHLBI/WHO Global Initiative for Chronic Obstructive Lung Disease (GOLD) Workshop summary. Am J Respir Crit Care Med Apr;163(5):1256-1276, 2001.

Voelkel NF, MacNee W (eds): Chronic Obstructive Lung Disease. London, BC Decker, 2002.

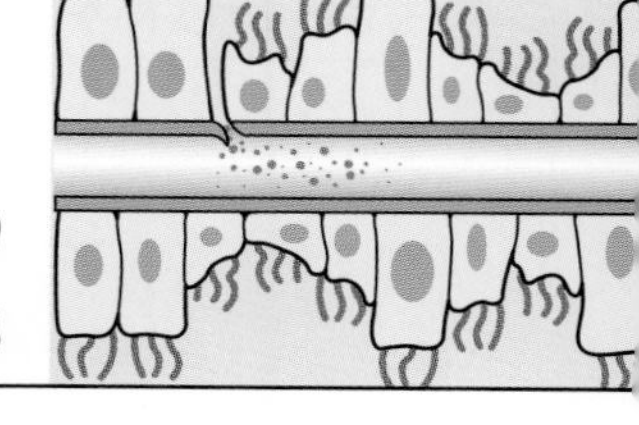

CHAPTER 35 Management of Exacerbations in Chronic Obstructive Pulmonary Disease

Jadwiga A. Wedzicha and Peter R. Mills

EPIDEMIOLOGY

Exacerbations of chronic obstructive pulmonary disease (COPD) are a major cause of morbidity and mortality found in this condition and impairment of health-related quality of life. They lead to frequent hospital admissions and readmissions and contribute greatly to the cost of managing patients who have COPD. Approximately 30,000 deaths result from exacerbations of COPD per year in the United Kingdom. In 1986, nearly 2 million Americans were hospitalized for COPD exacerbations, and this represented the fifth most frequent cause of death.

Although there is no standardized definition of a COPD exacerbation, an exacerbation is often described as an acute worsening of respiratory symptoms. The most important symptoms are dyspnea, increased sputum volume, and purulence.

A classical study from Canada defined exacerbations as Type 1 if they had all three of these symptoms, Type 2 exacerbations with two of the above symptoms, and Type 3 when one of the symptoms was combined with cough, wheeze, or symptoms of an upper respiratory tract infection. Others have proposed definitions based on health care utilization (e.g., unscheduled physician visits, use of oral steroids or antibiotics, and hospital admission).

Exacerbations have been associated with a number of precipitating factors (Table 35.1). Exacerbations occur more frequently with increasing severity of COPD. Many seem to be associated with bacterial infection or viruses, particularly rhinovirus, the cause of the common cold. That COPD exacerbations are more common in the winter months has been attributed to an increased seasonal viral load. Patients who suffer COPD may have increased airflow obstruction during the winter, and thus may become even more susceptible to those factors that cause acute exacerbations. Environmental factors, such as atmospheric pollutants, may also be important and may interact with respiratory viruses to precipitate exacerbation rather than acting alone.

Recent studies have shown that around half of COPD exacerbations are associated with viral infections, and that the majority of these were due to rhinovirus. Exacerbations triggered by respiratory viruses are associated with symptomatic colds and prolonged recovery, compared with those exacerbations where viruses were not detected. There are also suggestions that rhinovirus can infect the lower airway and thus directly contribute to inflammatory changes at exacerbation. Exacerbations associated with the presence of rhinovirus in induced sputum have larger increases in airway inflammatory markers, suggesting that viruses increase the severity of airway inflammation at exacerbation.

Bacteria also play a role at exacerbation and the common bacteria involved are *Haemophilus influenzae* and *Streptococcus pneumoniae*. Exacerbations associated with purulent sputum have a high chance of showing bacteria in the sputum. Antibiotic therapy is effective when purulent sputum occurs during the exacerbation. The airways of patients with COPD also have bacteria colonizing in the stable state, however, and there is still some controversy about the exact relationship between airway bacterial colonization in the stable state and detection of bacteria at exacerbation. Recently a study has suggested that isolation of a new bacterial strain was associated with an increased risk of an exacerbation, although important criticisms were raised.

Some patients are prone to frequent exacerbations and these are the COPD patients that are most likely to require hospital admission. The number of past exacerbations is a predictor of exacerbation frequency, which suggests that some patients may have a particular susceptibility. Patients with a history of frequent exacerbations (e.g., three or more per year) have a significantly worse health-related quality of life than patients with a history of infrequent exacerbations. Thus, exacerbation frequency is an important determinant of health status in these patients and is now regarded as one of the most useful outcome measures in COPD patients.

Some patients may not recover from an acute exacerbation to their basal symptoms or lung function. The reasons for the incomplete recovery are not clear, but may involve inadequate treatment or persistence of the causative agent. The incomplete physiologic recovery after an exacerbation could contribute to the decline in lung function with time though there is no direct evidence to support this hypothesis. There is now evidence, however, that in COPD patients who are smokers, exacerbations are associated with more lung function decline. In another study, patients with a history of frequent exacerbations had a faster decline of forced expiratory volume in 1 second (FEV_1) compared with patients without such a history. Patients with a history of frequent exacerbations have increased airway inflammatory markers and the increased inflammation may also contribute to the accelerated lung function decline.

Table 35.1 Causes of Chronic Obstructive Pulmonary Disease exacerbations	
Viruses	Rhinovirus (common cold) Influenza Parainfluenza Coronavirus Adenovirus RSV
Atypical bacteria	*Chlamydia pneumoniae* *Mycoplasma pneumoniae*
Bacteria	*Haemophilus influenzae* *Streptococcus pneumoniae* *Branhamella cattarhalis* *Staphylococcus aureus* *Pseudomonas aeruginosa*
Common pollutants	Nitrogen dioxide Particulates Sulphur dioxide Ozone

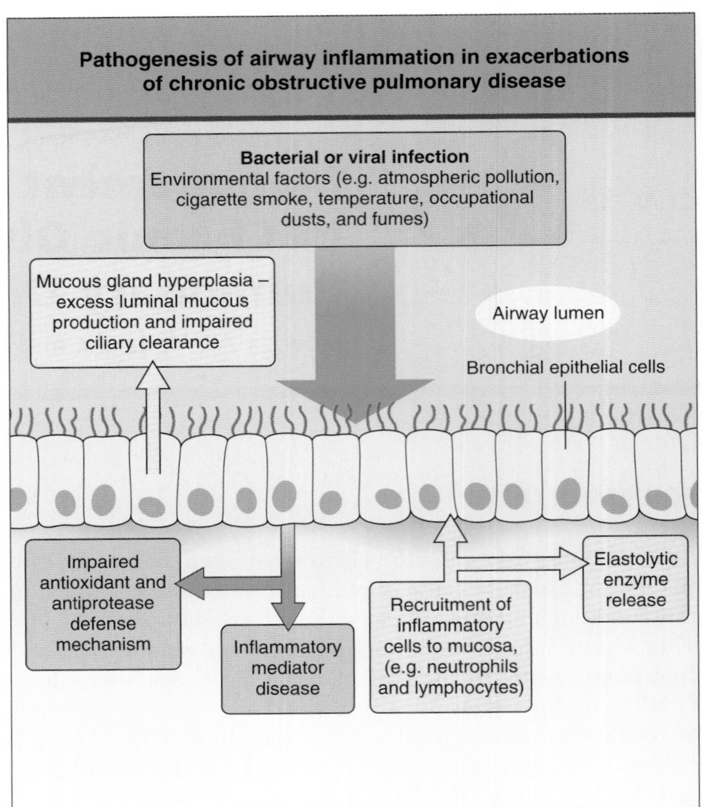

Figure 35.1 Pathogenesis of airway inflammation in exacerbations of chronic obstructive pulmonary disease (COPD). The interplay of different factors involved in the pathogenesis of airway inflammation in exacerbations of COPD.

PATHOPHYSIOLOGY

Relatively little information is available on the pathologic changes that occur in the airway during a COPD exacerbation. Airway inflammation increases during exacerbations, and this produces a variable increase in airflow obstruction as a result of mucosal and submucosal edema, mucus accumulation in the airway, or bronchospasm that develops in response to release of a variety of inflammatory mediators (Figure 35.1). The resultant air-trapping increases the work of breathing, as both chest wall and lung parenchymal compliance are reduced, and the development of air trapping requires that the patient generate a more negative pleural pressure to initiate inspiratory flow (to overcome the positive alveolar pressure at the end of exhalation). The adverse effects of the increased work are magnified by the reduction in the mechanical performance of the respiratory muscles as they lengthen in response to the air trapping, and exceed their optimal length-tension relationship.

Minute ventilation may be normal during an acute exacerbation, but the respiratory rate is generally increased while the tidal volume is decreased. Although this breathing pattern may be optimal with regard to reducing the work of breathing, the associated increase in physiologic dead space impairs carbon dioxide elimination, and the resulting acidemia can further reduce inspiratory muscle function. Tidal volume may fall as a result of the gas trapping as the respiratory system moves closer to its total capacity at end-exhalation.

The hypoxemia seen in acute COPD exacerbations results from a combination of alveolar hypoventilation and an increase in ventilation-perfusion (V/Q) heterogeneity. The reduction in alveolar ventilation occurs because of the factors summarized above. Increases in V/Q heterogeneity are attributed to:

- Reduction in the efficiency of hypoxic vasoconstriction as a result of an increase in pulmonary artery pressure (which develops in response to the alveolar hypoxia) or the release of vasodilating inflammatory mediators;
- Inability to redirect perfusion away from poorly ventilating alveoli because of diffuse disease or a reduction in the pulmonary vascular bed, which occurs as part of the emphysematous process.

Acidemia is an important prognostic factor for the survival of a COPD exacerbation, and thus early correction of acidemia is considered as an essential goal of therapy.

CLINICAL FEATURES

Exacerbations of COPD most frequently present with increasing sputum production, an increase in the purulence and viscosity of the sputum, increasing cough, and a worsening of dyspnea. There may be a recent history of upper respiratory tract infection or a common cold, and exacerbations associated with recent viral infections are often more severe. Patients who have more severe exacerbations may have nocturnal hypoxemia or carbon dioxide retention and may report morning headaches or even confusion. Associated symptoms may include an increase in orthopnea, and a deterioration in sleep duration and quality.

Patients generally appear in distress, especially those with more severe COPD. Accessory muscle use is seen with increasing severity of the exacerbation and purse-lip breathing may be observed. Wheezing may be audible without a stethoscope. In the most severely affected patients air movement may be so poor that breath sounds are inaudible.

Vital signs show tachypnea and tachycardia. Cyanosis is an insensitive physical finding but, when observed, commonly indicates respiratory failure. Finger or earlobe oximetry may frequently indicate hypoxemia, but a normal or low-normal oxygen saturation does not exclude the possibility of carbon dioxide retention and acute respiratory acidemia. The vasodilatation associated with hypercapnia causes warm, flushed skin, papilledema, and a strong peripheral pulse. Patients who have severe, acute carbon dioxide retention may present in coma. If cor pulmonale is present, peripheral edema is observed, as is an elevated jugular venous pressure, hepatomegaly, or ascites. Cardiac sounds may be difficult to hear because of the wheezing and air-trapping. A right ventricular gallop may be heard in the setting of pulmonary hypertension. Low-grade fever is common.

DIAGNOSIS

No additional investigations are required in patients affected by mild-to-moderate exacerbations, and are deemed to be candidates for outpatient therapy. Patients who suffer more severe exacerbations and require admission need a careful evaluation for conditions that might mimic, or be associated with, the acute respiratory decompensation. The decision to admit a patient is made on the basis of a number of factors, which include the patient's living and social circumstances, mental status, degree of hypoxemia or hypercapnia, and routinely taken medications. Those who are too dyspneic to manage their activities of daily living independently, or who have confusion or a deterioration of their arterial blood gases, require admission. Patients may require admission to hospital if they are already on a maximal outpatient medical regimen that includes systemic corticosteroids.

When respiratory decompensation is observed in the absence of a history of COPD or acute bronchitis, and if the patient does not have clinical or radiographic evidence of pneumonia, it is important to search for another cause of such a presentation. Other conditions associated with respiratory failure may require a completely different therapeutic approach (e.g., pulmonary embolus, pneumothorax, pulmonary edema).

Any patient admitted to the hospital with an exacerbation of COPD must have arterial blood gases obtained, with care taken to record the inspired oxygen concentration at the time the blood is obtained. Hypoxemia should be corrected, but an arterial saturation greater than 90% to 92% is not needed, and may be detrimental (see the following section). A chest radiograph should be performed. Some suggest obtaining a daily measurement of airflow (e.g., an FEV_1 or peak flow), but the utility of this practice has not been established and patients may provide suboptimal effort early in the exacerbation. Sputum culture has not been found useful.

Other investigations are summarized in (Table 35.2).

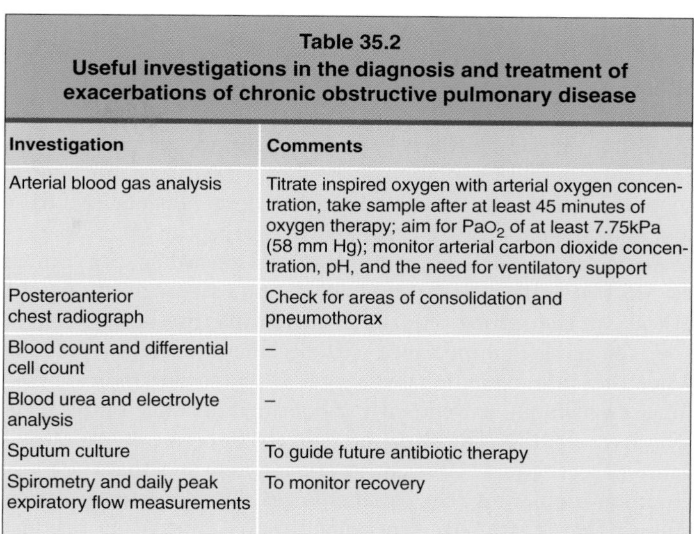

Table 35.2
Useful investigations in the diagnosis and treatment of exacerbations of chronic obstructive pulmonary disease

Investigation	Comments
Arterial blood gas analysis	Titrate inspired oxygen with arterial oxygen concentration, take sample after at least 45 minutes of oxygen therapy; aim for PaO_2 of at least 7.75kPa (58 mm Hg); monitor arterial carbon dioxide concentration, pH, and the need for ventilatory support
Posteroanterior chest radiograph	Check for areas of consolidation and pneumothorax
Blood count and differential cell count	–
Blood urea and electrolyte analysis	–
Sputum culture	To guide future antibiotic therapy
Spirometry and daily peak expiratory flow measurements	To monitor recovery

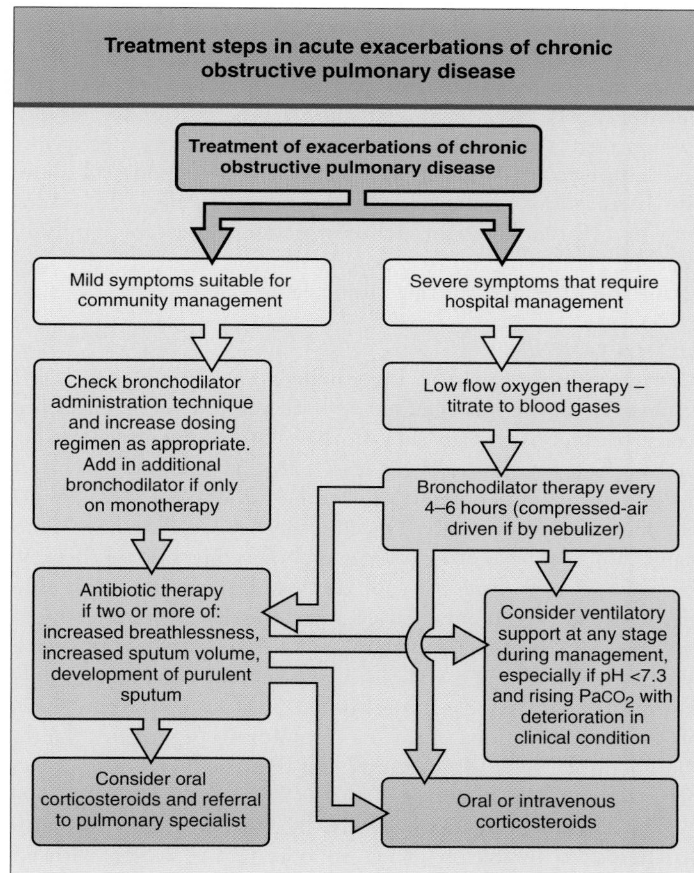

Figure 35.2 Treatment of exacerbations of chronic obstructive pulmonary disease.

TREATMENT

Treatment of exacerbations of COPD is given in Figure 35.2.

Pharmacological Therapy

INHALED BRONCHODILATOR THERAPY

Both β_2-agonists (e.g., albuterol [salbutamol]) and anticholinergic agents (e.g., ipratropium bromide) are generally administered. Although both have bronchodilating activity, symptomatic improvement can be attained without marked changes in spirometry, probably as a result of reduced air trapping. Studies in stable COPD have found that anticholinergic agents produce a greater bronchodilator response than that seen with β_2-agonists, presumably because of the excessive, cholinergic, neuronal bronchoconstrictor tone seen in this condition or loss

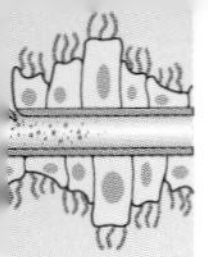

or downregulation of β_2-receptors. When the two agents are given in combination there seems to be an additive effect, although this point is still unclear in the setting of acute exacerbations.

Although many physicians routinely administer bronchodilators via a nebulizer, numerous studies have found no benefit to nebulization over simple, metered dose inhalers (MDI)—assuming the patients are capable of activating the MDI. Spacers seem to allow patients more freedom regarding the timing of MDI activation and actual inhalation, although studies of efficacy in the setting of acute exacerbations are lacking.

Of far greater importance is the technique used by patients when they administer inhaled agents. Many studies indicate that inhaler technique is frequently suboptimal in stable outpatients who have COPD. The situation is likely to be far worse during acute exacerbations. Clinical experience indicates that the most common problem is that patients begin the inhalation at a lung volume that is far above functional residual capacity or residual volume. Accordingly, the vital capacity is so small that a minimal amount of medication actually reaches the lower airway. When the medications are delivered by nebulization most patients simply perform repeated tidal breathing, with no attempt to reach maximum inspiratory capacity. Additional errors frequently encountered include inhaling the medication too rapidly (which results in excess deposition on the posterior pharynx) and failure to hold the inspiration for a few seconds (to allow the medication to deposit on the airway walls). To assure maximum bronchodilator delivery, patients must be carefully coached and prompted to exhale to near maximum before triggering the MDI and starting an inhalation.

METHYLXANTHINES

Methylxanthines such as theophylline were previously used extensively in the management of both stable COPD and acute exacerbations. Although they do have bronchodilating effects, the degree of response is far less than that seen after inhaled β_2-agonists or anticholinergics. Studies of intravenous aminophylline therapy in acute exacerbations of COPD showed no significant beneficial effect over and above conventional therapy. In addition, the propensity of methylxanthines to cause side effects (most commonly nausea and difficulty sleeping) is high, and many medications and acute and chronic illnesses interfere with methylxanthine metabolism, and thereby raise blood levels to toxic concentrations. If methylxanthines are used, then levels of these medications must be monitored to ensure that a therapeutic dose is administered and that the levels are not too high to risk toxic side effects.

The therapeutic action of methylxanthines was formerly attributed to inhibition of phosphodiesterase, which allowed higher intracellular concentrations of cyclic adenosine monophosphate with resultant bronchodilatation. More recently, numerous phosphodiesterases have been discovered, some of which interact with the G-protein signaling system and have generalized anti-inflammatory effects. As opposed to theophylline, which is a weak and nonspecific phosphodiesterase inhibitor, specific inhibitors for each of the newly described phosphodiesterases are being developed and some may come to clinical use in the near future as anti-inflammatory agents. Methylxanthines cause mild stimulation of ventilatory drive and, as such, may actually increase the sensation of breathlessness in patients who are unable to increase their alveolar ventilation. Although some investigators suggest that theophylline strengthens diaphragmatic contractions and possibly improves cardiac function, these effects are unclear and have not been shown to have any substantive clinical utility.

CORTICOSTEROIDS

There are now numerous studies indicating that corticosteroids are beneficial for patients with acute exacerbations. The first randomized, controlled trial found that patients receiving 3 days' corticosteroids had larger improvements in pre- and post-bronchodilator FEV_1. A second randomized trial confirmed these results through day 5. The largest controlled trial again confirmed the benefit of corticosteroids and also found that the rates of treatment failure were higher in the placebo group at 30 days, compared with the combined 2- and 8-week prednisolone groups. No difference in the results was seen in groups that receive a 2- versus an 8-week treatment protocol. Accordingly, steroids should be used at COPD exacerbation in short courses of no more than 2 weeks' duration to avoid risk of complications. Recent studies also demonstrate that oral corticosteroids are beneficial in milder exacerbations as well.

ANTIBIOTICS

Exacerbations of COPD often present with increased sputum purulence and volume, and antibiotics have traditionally been used as first-line therapy. This approach has been questioned, however, because viral infections seem to be the precipitating factor in many instances. A recent meta-analysis identified only nine randomized, controlled trials of significant duration to address the question and concluded that antibiotic therapy offered a small, but significant, benefit in exacerbations.

The choice of antibiotic is based on the susceptibility of the most likely pathogens, which are *Streptococcus pneumoniae*, *Haemophilus influenzae*, and *Moraxella catarrhalis*. Local resistance patterns should be reviewed with regard to *Staphylococcus aureus* and gram-negative organisms, as these may cause infection in patients who have severe COPD. Most centers tend to use more cost-effective agents such as amoxicillin for first-line therapy. For more severe exacerbations, or inadequate response results from first-line agents, a broad-spectrum cephalosporin, macrolide, or quinolone can be used.

OXYGEN THERAPY

Hypoxemia occurs with more severe exacerbations and usually requires hospital admission. During acute exacerbations caution is needed when supplemental oxygen is administered, because an increase in carbon dioxide ($PaCO_2$) can occur. Classic teaching has been that patients who have COPD with $PaCO_2$ elevations have blunted their ventilatory responses to $PaCO_2$ such that raising PaO_2 with supplemental oxygen satisfies the hypoxic ventilatory drive at a lower minute ventilation, which increases $PaCO_2$. With marked increases, CO_2 narcosis may develop.

A number of studies suggest that the mechanism by which oxygen administration increases $PaCO_2$ may not involve ventilatory drive, but rather, by increasing alveolar oxygen tension, it decreases hypoxic vasoconstriction such that perfusion of poorly ventilating alveoli increases, which raises $PaCO_2$. The reason acute $PaCO_2$ elevations are generally only seen during acute exacerbations is that, during this period, resting minute ventilation approaches the maximum possible such that patients are not able to compensate for the increase in $PaCO_2$ by augmenting their ventilation. Because the hypoxemia in COPD results from increased V/Q heterogeneity, small increases in alveolar oxygen tension are generally sufficient to raise PaO_2 to an acceptable level. Accordingly, supplemental oxygen should be delivered at an initial flow rate of only 1 to 2 L/min using a nasal cannula, or 24% to 28% inspired oxygen using a venturimeter mask, with repeat blood gas analysis after 30 to 45 minutes. Further adjustments to oxygen therapy are made to keep PaO_2 greater than 7.5 kPa (>55 mm Hg). If $PaCO_2$ rises and pH falls, other interventions may be needed.

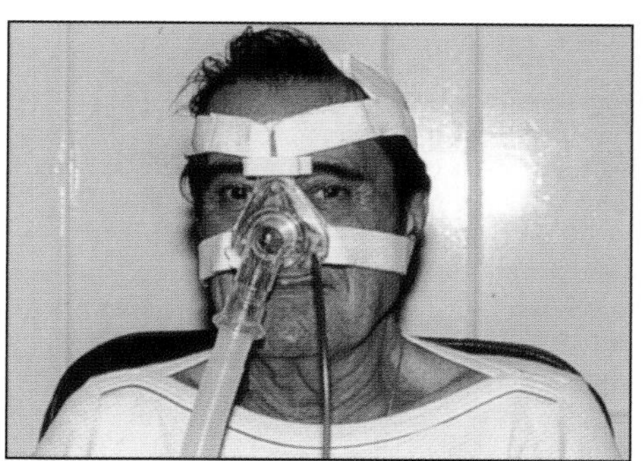

Figure 35.3 Patient who has chronic obstructive pulmonary disease receives noninvasive ventilation via a nasal mask. Note the port for the delivery of supplemental oxygen.

RESPIRATORY STIMULANTS AND OTHER THERAPIES

Hypercapnia during COPD exacerbations may be managed initially with the use of respiratory stimulants. The most commonly used is doxapram, which acts centrally to increase respiratory drive and respiratory muscle activity. Its effect is probably only appreciable for 24 to 48 hours; the main factor limiting its use is side effects that can lead to agitation and are often not tolerated by the patient. Only a few studies of the clinical efficacy of doxapram have been carried out, and short-term investigations suggest that improvements in acidosis and arterial carbon dioxide tension can be attained. A small study that compared doxapram with noninvasive positive pressure ventilation (NPPV) in acute exacerbations of COPD suggested that therapy with NPPV was superior with regard to correction of blood gases during the initial treatment phase. More information is required to assess the exact role doxapram should have in the acute management of hypercapnic respiratory failure in COPD, especially now that the use of NPPV has become more widespread. It seems that an important role of respiratory stimulants may be in reversing hypercapnia associated with excess supplemental oxygen use and before NPPV can be set up and administered.

Increases in pulmonary artery pressure during exacerbations of COPD can result in right-sided cardiac dysfunction and development of peripheral edema. Diuretic therapy may thus be necessary if edema or a rise in jugular venous pressure occurs. Vasodilators have been used with limited success in the treatment of pulmonary hypertension in chronic, stable COPD; the effects on pulmonary hemodynamics appear to be short lived and probably do not translate to improvements in symptoms or outcome. Thus, at present, no evidence advocates vasodilator therapy in COPD exacerbations.

The value of chest physical therapy in exacerbations of COPD lies in the potential benefit gained from clearance of retained secretions and hence alleviation of dyspnea. Although arterial oxygen desaturation during physical therapy could potentially be problematic, the use of guided breathing techniques reduces this substantially. Thus, it seems appropriate to provide physical therapy for those patients who have large volumes of retained sputum during the acute phase, together with instruction regarding breathing control.

Ventilatory Support

NONINVASIVE VENTILATION

The introduction of NPPV using nasal or face masks has had a major impact on the management of exacerbations of COPD and has enabled acidosis to be corrected at an early stage. Studies have shown that NPPV can produce improvements in pH relatively rapidly, at one hour after instituting ventilation. This allows time for other conventional therapy to work, such as oxygen therapy, bronchodilators, corticosteroids, and antibiotics, and thus reverse the progression of respiratory failure and reduce mortality. With NPPV, improvements occur with work of breathing and in minute ventilation.

With the use of NPPV, patient comfort is improved; also, sedation is not required, which enables preservation of speech and swallowing (Figure 35.3). Intensive care is unnecessary and the technique can be applied in a high-dependency unit or on a specialist respiratory ward, though full staff training in the technique of NPPV and its limitations is essential for the service to run well. Patient cooperation is important in the application of NPPV and excessive secretions can be troublesome, as there is no direct access to the airway. The main advantage of the use of NPPV is avoidance of tracheal intubation and the ability to offer ventilatory support to patients who have respiratory failure caused by severe COPD, and who would be considered unsuitable for intubation.

Following a number of uncontrolled studies, randomized, controlled trials have shown benefit of NPPV in COPD exacerbations. Randomized controlled trials have demonstrated that NPPV corrects the pH more rapidly, improves breathlessness over the initial 3 days of ventilation, and reduces the intubation rate and mortality compared with a control standard therapy group. Complications, which were specifically associated with the use of mechanical ventilation, were also reduced. The difference in mortality disappeared after adjustment for intubation, which suggests that the benefits with NPPVs result from fewer patients who require intubation.

These studies have treated patients in whom the pH was less than 7.35, rather than just below 7.26, when the prognosis of COPD worsens. A number of these patients may have improved without NPPV, though it seems that the major effect of NPPV is the earlier correction of acidosis and thus avoidance of tracheal intubation, with all its associated complications. Studies have shown that NPPV can be successfully implemented in up to 80% of cases. However, NPPV is less successful in patients who have worse blood gases at baseline before ventilation, are underweight, have a higher incidence of pneumonia, have a greater level of neurologic deterioration, higher Acute Physiologic and Chronic Health Evaluation (APACHE) II scores, and in whom compliance with the ventilation is poor (Table 35.3).

If NPPV is unavailable, continuous positive airway pressure (CPAP) masks can be used as the CPAP provided will counter

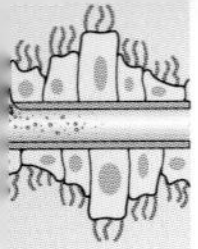

Table 35.3 Factors associated with a poor outcome with noninvasive positive pressure ventilatory support

Pneumonia
Severe acidosis
Neurologic impairment
Low body weight
High APACHE II scores
Poor compliance with noninvasive positive pressure ventilatory support

auto-positive end-expiratory pressure (PEEP) and thereby reduce the work of breathing and the resulting carbon dioxide production which, in turn, will improve the pH irrespective of the effect on minute ventilation.

INDICATIONS FOR INVASIVE VENTILATION

If NPPV fails, invasive ventilation may be required in the presence of increasing acidosis and should be considered for any patient in whom the pH falls below 7.26. Decisions to ventilate these patients may be difficult, though with improved modes of invasive ventilatory support and better weaning techniques, the outlook for the COPD patient is improved.

Patients are suitable for tracheal intubation if this is the first presentation of COPD exacerbation or respiratory failure, or there is a treatable cause of respiratory failure, such as pneumonia. Information is required on the past history and quality of life, especially the ability to perform daily activities. Patients who have severe disabling and progressive COPD may be less suitable, but it is important that adequate and appropriate therapy be used in these patients, with documented progression. The patient's wishes and those of any close relatives must be considered in any decision to institute or withhold life-supporting therapy.

Supported Discharge Schemes

Patients can be discharged early in their exacerbation if the appropriate level of outpatient care has been arranged. This might include domiciliary visits made to these patients after discharge by trained respiratory therapists or nurses. Benefits obtained include reductions in hospital stay and cost savings. Only about 25% of patients presenting for hospital admission with a COPD exacerbation are actually suitable for home therapy, however, and thus selection is required.

CLINICAL COURSE AND PREVENTION

Most community exacerbations of COPD resolve within 5 to 10 days and have no long-term sequelae. The mortality of COPD patients who have developed respiratory failure and been admitted to hospital with exacerbations varies in different series. Prognosis depends on a number of factors, which include the severity of acidosis with an increased mortality observed in patients who have a pH less than 7.26. Outcome also depends on the severity of the underlying COPD and on the nature of the factor that precipitates the exacerbation. Although the long-term prognosis of these patients is poor it does not seem to be worse than for patients with comparable degrees of airflow limitation who do not suffer acute exacerbations.

Relatively little attention has been paid to aspects of prevention of exacerbations in patients who have COPD. Influenza and pneumococcal vaccinations are recommended for all patients with COPD. Long-term antibiotic therapy has been used in patients with very frequent exacerbations, though there is little evidence of effectiveness. There seems to be an association between airway bacterial colonization and exacerbation frequency such that long-term antibiotics may prevent or reduce the severity of exacerbations. With newer antibiotics available that have more specific targets, further study of the effects of long-term antibiotic therapy will be warranted.

A recent study of long-term inhaled steroids in patients with moderate to severe COPD is presented as showing a reduction in exacerbations around 25%, and the effect was greater in patients with more impaired lung function. Many patients with acute exacerbations were excluded from this study at entry, however. The new long-acting anticholinergic agent tiotropium may reduce exacerbations.

Increased patient education is necessary about detecting and treating exacerbations. More specific written treatment plans for the at-risk COPD patients may be useful (as are produced for asthmatics), though such an approach requires testing. After an exacerbation, the COPD patient's condition should be reviewed and attention given to risk factors and compliance with therapy.

PITFALLS AND CONSIDERATIONS

Patients with COPD tend to under report exacerbations, and many of the exacerbations in the community are self-limiting. Patients who have COPD accept their chronic disability and may not notice warning symptoms of deterioration in their clinical condition. It is possible that earlier presentation to the doctor with the exacerbation could prevent complications, though this has not been investigated. Not only should COPD patients receive education about their disease, but also instruction on the need to recognize symptoms of exacerbation at an early stage.

A number of inhaled therapies can be useful to reduce the frequency of COPD exacerbations—for example, inhaled steroids, long-acting beta agonists and long-acting anticholinergic agents. However it is interesting that all these therapies individually have a similar action in reducing exacerbations by around 25%. Future studies will need to address whether combinations of inhaled therapies have more effects on exacerbations and which of the pharmacological therapies in combination are most effective.

A number of randomized trials have shown NPPV to be effective in the management of acute exacerbations with respiratory failure. However, most of the studies recruited patients with pH levels of less than 7.35, and few of these studies included patients with pH less than 7.26, when the prognosis is reduced. It is possible that a number of these patients would have improved spontaneously, and more studies are needed on the use of NPPV in patients with pH levels of 7.27 to 7.35, as opposed to patients with pH levels less than 7.26. The main value of NPPV seems to be in early correction of acidosis and

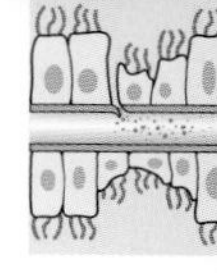

further prevention of deterioration, yet few centers can provide NPPV on arrival in the emergency room. It is possible that the early use of the respiratory stimulant doxapram could play a role in the control of acidosis, before the institution of NPPV. Administration of NPPV requires skilled staff that must be available on a 24-hour basis. The result of studies on ventilatory support during exacerbation emphasizes the important principle of early diagnosis, referral, and intervention in this high-risk patient group. Only then will a significant impact be made on mortality in COPD.

SUGGESTED READINGS

Burge PS, Calverley PMA, Jones PW, et al: Randomised, double blind, placebo controlled study of fluticasone propionate in patients with moderate to severe chronic obstructive pulmonary disease: The ISOLDE trial. BMJ 320:1297-1303, 2000.

Burge PS, Calverley PMA, Jones PW, et al: Prednisolone response in patients with chronic obstructive pulmonary disease. Thorax, in press.

Connors AF, Dawson NV, Thomas C, et al: Outcomes following acute exacerbation of severe chronic obstructive pulmonary disease. Am J Respir Crit Care Med 154:959-967, 1996.

Davies L, Angus RM, Calverley PMA: Oral corticosteroids in patients admitted to hospital with exacerbations of chronic obstructive pulmonary disease: A prospective randomized controlled trial. Lancet 354:456-460, 1999.

Greenberg SB, Allen M, Wilson J, Atmar RL: Respiratory viral infections in adults with and without chronic obstructive pulmonary disease. Am J Respir Crit Care Med 162:167-173, 2000.

Kanner RE, Anthonisen, NR, Connett JE: Lower respiratory illnesses promote FEV_1 decline in current smokers but not ex-smokers with mild chronic obstructive pulmonary disease. Am J Respir Crit Care Med 164:358-364, 2001.

Niewoehner DE, Erbland ML, Deupree RH, et al: Effect of systemic glucocorticoids on exacerbations of chronic obstructive pulmonary disease. N Engl J Med 340:1941-1947, 1999.

Saint S, Bent S, Vittinghoff E, Grady D: Antibiotics in chronic obstructive pulmonary disease exacerbations. A meta-analysis. JAMA 273:957-960, 1995.

Seemungal TAR, Harper-Owen R, Bhowmik A, et al: Respiratory viruses, symptoms and inflammatory markers in acute exacerbations and stable chronic obstructive pulmonary disease. Am J Respir Crit Care Med 164:1618-1623, 2001.

Seemungal TAR, Donaldson GC, Bhowmik A, et al: Time course and recovery of exacerbations in patients with chronic obstructive pulmonary disease. Am J Respir Crit Care Med 161:1608-1613, 2000.

Seemungal TAR, Donaldson GC, Paul EA, et al: Effect of exacerbation on quality of life in patients with chronic obstructive pulmonary disease. Am J Respir Crit Care Med 151:1418-1422, 1998.

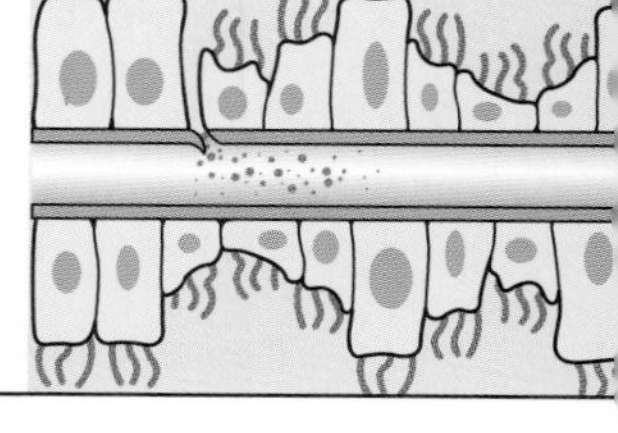

CHAPTER 36

Chronic Obstructive Pulmonary Disease: Management of Chronic Disease

Ronald Balkissoon and Barry Make

Chronic obstructive pulmonary disease (COPD) is a chronic disorder that causes severe physiologic and functional impairment in patients with advanced disease.

Early identification of patients with COPD and secondary prevention by encouraging smoking cessation or changing an occupation where indicated should be the primary goals of treatment. Unfortunately, far too few individuals are routinely screened for early evidence of COPD; more often, patients with COPD present with symptoms of cough and phlegm, or with dyspnea on exertion, suggesting that significant lung damage has already occurred, much of which may be largely irreversible. Only after the diagnosis is confirmed and the severity of the patient's disease has been established can appropriate therapy be determined.

Although COPD is not curable, available therapies do reduce the impact of the disease on patients. Beneficial outcomes can be obtained with appropriate use of medications, ambulatory oxygen, selected surgical interventions, and comprehensive management programs (i.e., pulmonary rehabilitation). Management of COPD requires a multifaceted, multidisciplinary approach to ensure optimal patient outcomes.

GOALS OF MANAGEMENT OF STABLE COPD

The goals of management of patients with COPD are to:

1. Establish a correct diagnosis and assess severity of disease with spirometry
2. Reduce the risk for progression by encouraging smoking cessation and avoidance of other causative agents
3. Reduce dyspnea by appropriate administration of bronchodilators
4. Prevent and treat complications such as hypoxia and acute exacerbations

Table 36.1 outlines the goals of management and the therapeutic strategies to achieve those goals.

REDUCE RISK WITH SMOKING CESSATION

All patients who are current or former smokers or have occupational or other risk factors for development of COPD should be strongly and repeatedly encouraged to discontinue smoking. A clear, concise smoking cessation message should be provided during *every visit* with any health care provider. *Smoking cessation is the most effective tool* to preserve lung function and functional capacity.

As depicted graphically in Figure 36.1, patients who are susceptible to the adverse effects of cigarettes have a more rapid decline in lung function than nonsmokers. Discontinuing smoking markedly reduces the rate of decline in FEV_1, essentially to that of a nonsmoker or nonsusceptible smoker, but it does not *reverse* the damage that has already occurred. Studies have shown, however, that pulmonary function improves slightly in the year after smoking cessation (Fig. 36.2). These concepts may be useful in educating patients about the benefits of smoking cessation.

The key features of a successful smoking cessation program are vigilance in inquiring about smoking status of patients who smoke and assessing their preparedness or motivation to quit. Direct physician inquiry and advice to discontinue smoking can lead to a 10% to 20% cessation rate at 1 year. Many smokers require repeated attempts at smoking cessation before they are successful.

A useful approach to smoking cessation is the "five A's" (Table 36.2):

Ask if the patient is still smoking every visit.
Advise the patient about the advantages and reasons to quit.
Assess the patient's willingness to quit.
Assist in quitting by educating the patient about nicotine withdrawal and addictive behavior, providing follow-up counseling and support, and prescribing nicotine replacement therapy (NRT) and bupropion as needed.
Arrange for regularly scheduled follow-up contact, either in person or by telephone, to check on status.

Patients smoking less than 10 cigarettes per day should be put on NRT with caution and should be monitored for signs of nicotine toxicity. Pregnant women, adolescents, and patients with unstable coronary artery disease, recent myocardial infarction, or untreated peptic ulcer disease should be considered for NRT only with caution and reservation. NRT is available in several formulations: patches, gum, inhaler, and nasal spray. Physicians should understand the method for using each of these formulations and educate patients on the appropriate technique of administration. The combination of (1) nicotine replacement therapy, (2) bupropion, and (3) behavioral counseling provides the highest smoking cessation rates.

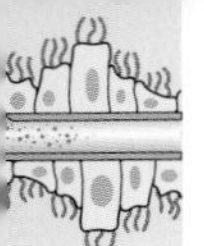

Table 36.1
Goals of management for patients with stable chronic Obstructive Pulmonary Disease

Goal		Method		Means
Diagnose	⇨	*Education*	⇨	Spirometry
⇩				
Reduce risk	⇨	*Education*	⇨	Smoking cessation Immunize Reduce other exposures
⇩				
Reduce symptoms	⇨	*Education*	⇨	Bronchodilators Consider inhaled steroids Pulmonary rehabilitation
⇩				
Reduce complications	⇨	*Education*	⇨	Consider oxygen Treat exacerbations

The goals of management suggested by the Global Initiative for Chronic Obstructive Pulmonary Disease (GOLD) guidelines are noted on the left side and the methods to achieve those goals are outlined on the right.
From Pauwels R, Anthonisen N, Bailey WC, et al: Global strategy for the diagnosis, management, and prevention of chronic obstructive pulmonary disease: NHLBI/WHO workshop [update, 2003]. Available at www.goldcopd.com; accessed August 2, 2003.

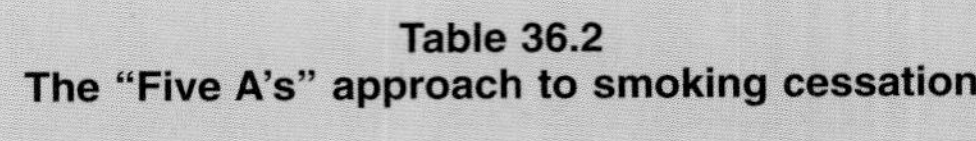

Table 36.2
The "Five A's" approach to smoking cessation

1. ASK if smoking at every visit
2. ADVISE to quit at every visit
3. ASSESS readiness to quit
4. ASSIST in smoking cessation
5. ARRANGE for follow-up

This easy-to-remember algorithm has been promoted in a clinical practice guideline published in the United States.
From Fiore MC, Bailey WC, Cohen SJ, et al: Clinical Practice Guideline: Treating Tobacco Use and Dependence. Bethesda, Md, U.S. Department of Health and Human Services, Public Health Service, June, 2000.
Tobacco Use and Dependence Clinical Practice Guideline Panel. JAMA 283:3244, 2000.

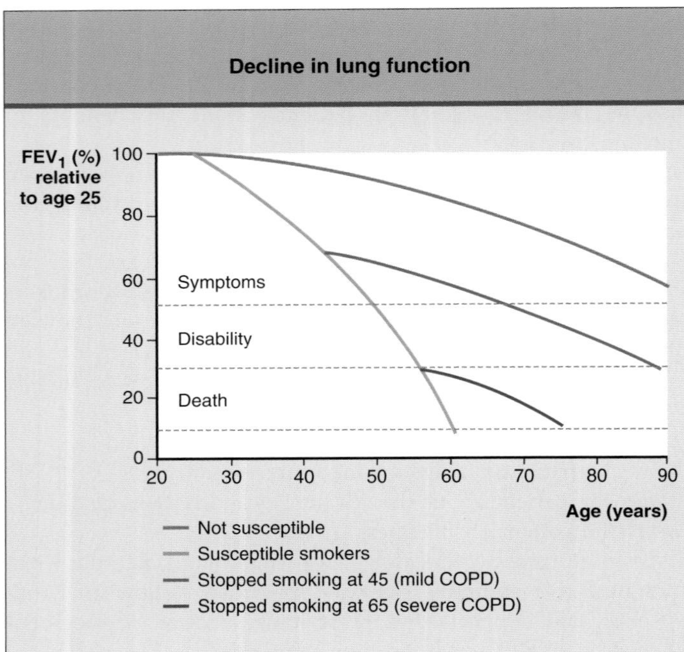

Figure 36.1 Graphic depiction of decline in lung function in cigarette smokers and the effects of smoking cessation. Lung function declines more rapidly in smokers who are susceptible to the adverse effects of cigarettes compared with nonsmokers. Discontinuing smoking in both a 45-year-old patient with mild disease and in a 65-year-old with more severe disease reduces the accelerated decline in lung function and delays progression of symptoms. COPD, chronic obstructive pulmonary disease. (Modified from Fletcher C, Peto R: The natural history of chronic airflow obstruction. BMJ 1:1645-1648, 1977.)

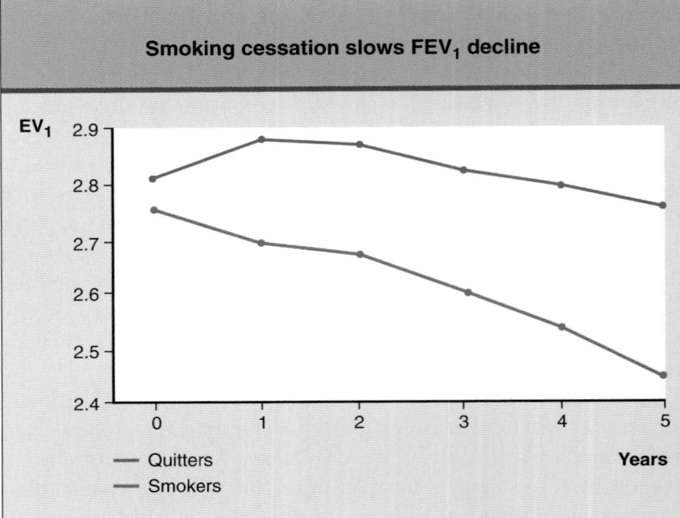

Figure 36.2 Effect of smoking cessation on lung function. In this study, the forced expired volume in 1 second (FEV_1) improved in the year after smoking cessation. The decline in lung function in later years was less in former smokers compared with continuing cigarette smokers. (From Anthonisen N, Connett JE, Kiley JP, et al: Effects of smoking intervention and the use of an inhaled anticholinergic bronchodilator on the rate of decline of FEV_1: The Lung Health Study. JAMA 272:1497-1505, 1994.)

REDUCE SYMPTOMS WITH BRONCHODILATORS

COPD is characterized by airflow obstruction due to chronic inflammation and airway remodeling. In addition, there is the loss of small airway support because of destruction of the alveolar architecture leading to airway collapse, air trapping, and hyperinflation and an increased work of breathing. To date, there are no pharmacologic interventions that have been shown to alter the disease process or progression. Bronchodilators remain the mainstay of pharmacologic therapy for most patients because they provide symptomatic relief and improve exercise capacity. The increase in functional capacity is due to reductions in gas trapping and hyperinflation, increased airflow, and improvement in inspiratory capacity, allowing patients to perform activities with a greater degree of comfort. Although the need for bronchodilators can generally be *suggested* by the degree of airflow limitation as assessed by the FEV_1, the actual prescription should be tailored to the dyspnea experienced by each individual patient.

Inhaled bronchodilators are currently considered the most effective and therefore the first line of treatment. Nebulized bronchodilators have not been shown to provide any benefit over metered-dose inhalers (MDI) or dry powder inhaler (DPI) delivery devices. The choice of which bronchodilator to use should be based on availability, effectiveness in achieving the desired outcomes, and adverse effects. Combining bronchodilators of different classes may improve their effectiveness and lessen the side effects compared with use of higher doses of a single class of agents. Long-acting agents are more convenient for patients and their use may increase compliance with the prescribed regimen.

Anticholinergic Bronchodilators

Ipratropium bromide is a quaternary ammonium derivative of atropine sulfate that is delivered by inhalation and results in bronchodilatation in patients with COPD. There are muscarinic (M) receptors on airway smooth muscle and submucosal gland cells. Agents such as ipratropium bromide are relatively nonselective and block the effect of acetylcholine on M_1 receptors in parasympathetic ganglia, M_2 receptors on cholinergic nerve endings, and M_3 postganglionic muscarinic receptors. Figure 36.3 demonstrates the sites of action of anticholinergic and β-agonist bronchodilators. Preganglionic blockade of M_2 receptors can actually *increase* acetylcholine release because cholinergic stimulation of the M_2 receptors leads to inhibition of the release of acetylcholine (negative feedback). This seems to be of less importance in terms of the actions of ipratropium bromide compared with M_3 stimulation on airway smooth muscle, which is the primary site leading to reductions in bronchomotor tone. Cholinergic stimulation of the muscarinic receptors causes bronchoconstriction and mucus secretion, but no significant changes in mucus secretion occur with the use of anticholinergic bronchodilators. The duration of action of short-acting anticholinergics is similar to that of the short acting $β_2$-agonists (i.e., 4 to 6 hours). Ipratropium bromide is available in the United States in an MDI dispensing 18 μg/dose. Typical dosing is 2 puffs 4 times per day (maximum recommended daily dose, 12 puffs), but higher doses are recommended in patients with more severe disease. Increased doses can cause clinically important adverse effects, but these are uncommon. Ipratropium bromide is also available as a nebulized 0.02% solution (500 μg/2.5-mL unit dose), and patients typically receive a unit dose of 500 μg three or four times daily. Atropine-like side effects of the anticholinergics are relatively few because they are not systemically absorbed but include hypertension, skin rashes, urinary retention, constipation, and headache. Dry mouth is the most common side effect. There is no evidence that individuals develop tachyphylaxis to ipratropium bromide.

The bronchodilator effects of ipratropium bromide are equal, if not superior, to those of $β_2$-agonists in COPD. Regular use of ipratropium bromide reduces symptoms and improves health status.

Oxytropium bromide is similar to ipratropium bromide, with the same duration of action and side effect profile, and is available in MDI form (100 μg) and as a nebulized solution of 1.5 mg/mL. It is reported to have a slightly longer duration of action than ipratropium. This drug is not available in the United States.

Tiotropium is a new, long-acting anticholinergic bronchodilator that requires only once-daily dosing because its effects last over 24 hours. Tiotropium binds with equal avidity to M_1, M_2, and M_3 receptors but dissociates fairly rapidly from the M_2 receptors, whereas it dissociates more slowly from M_1 and M_3 receptors. It is available as an 18-μg formulation DPI. Reports of side effects indicate they are no greater than those seen with the short-acting anticholinergics. Use of the long-acting anticholinergic is more convenient for patients with COPD but may be more expensive. This drug is available in many countries, but U.S. Food and Drug Administration (FDA) approval is pending in the United States.

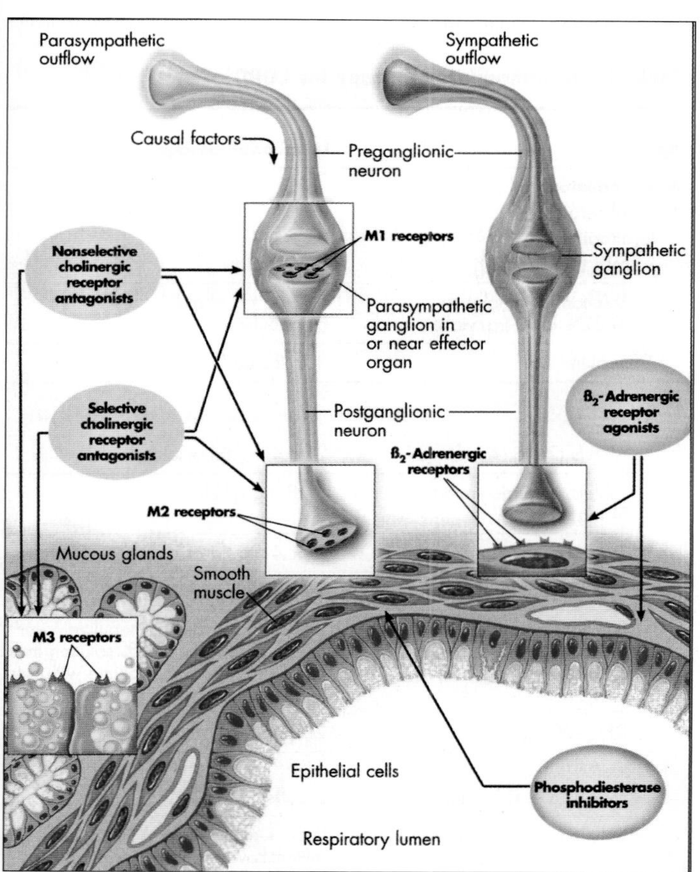

Figure 36.3 Sites of action of β-agonist and anticholinergic bronchodilators. (From Manda W, Rennard SI: COPD: New treatments. Consultant 43:953-965, 2003.)

$β_2$-Agonist Bronchodilators

Short-acting $β_2$-specific agonists (SABAs) cause smooth muscle relaxation by direct stimulation of $β_2$ receptors as mimics of endogenous adrenergic neurotransmitters. $β_2$ stimulation activates adenylate cyclase and increases concentrations of intracellular cyclic adenosine monophosphate. SABAs have minimal binding to the $β_1$ receptors of the heart. They preferentially bind to the hydrophilic site of the $β_2$ receptor and have a rapid onset of action, reaching peak bronchodilation within 5 to 15 minutes. Their effects abate within 4 to 6 hours, however, requiring redosing at least four times per day. Dose-response relationships for SABAs are relatively flat for many patients with COPD, with only modest changes in FEV_1 despite increasing doses of medication. Albuterol (or salbutamol) is a SABA that is available for inhalation as a DPI, 200 μg/dose, as an MDI, 100 μg/dose, and as a solution for nebulization (0.5% [5 mg/mL] and 0.083% [0.83 mg/mL]). Typical dosing with a nebulized solution is 2.5 mg, or a 3-mL unit dose of the 0.083% solution. It is also available orally as a long-acting pill and as a syrup (0.024% 2 mg/5 mL). Dosing of the MDI devices is typically two puffs four times per day when used on a regular basis or as a "rescue" medication for intermittent dyspnea.

SABAs can downregulate the β_2 receptors, leading to tachyphylaxis. Accordingly, overzealous rescue use (more than six times total per day) should be discouraged. Toxicity of SABAs is somewhat greater than with ipratropium bromide because they are systemically absorbed. Side effects include tachycardia, palpitations, nervousness and shakiness, gastrointestinal (GI) upset and promotion of reflux, and hypokalemia.

Other available formulations include fenoterol, 100 to 200 μg/dose (MDI, DPI) and terbutaline, 400 or 500 μg/dose (DPI). Fenoterol is also available as an oral syrup (0.05%). Terbutaline is available as pills (2.5 and 5 mg) and as an injectable (0.2 or 0.25 mg/vial).

There are two long-acting β-agonists (LABA) available for use. Salmeterol preferentially binds to the lipophilic site of the β receptor, takes 30 to 60 minutes to reach maximum bronchodilation, and lasts for up to 12 hours. Formoterol is amphililic and binds with equal avidity to the hydrophilic and lipophilic sites on the β receptors. This provides a relatively rapid onset of action, from 5 to 15 minutes, and a 12-hour duration of action. The LABAs share the same properties of the SABAs, causing smooth muscle relaxation by direct stimulation of adrenergic receptors. The LABAs are both available as DPIs. Both SABAs and LABAs have similar benefits. Although the LABAs are more expensive, they are more convenient.

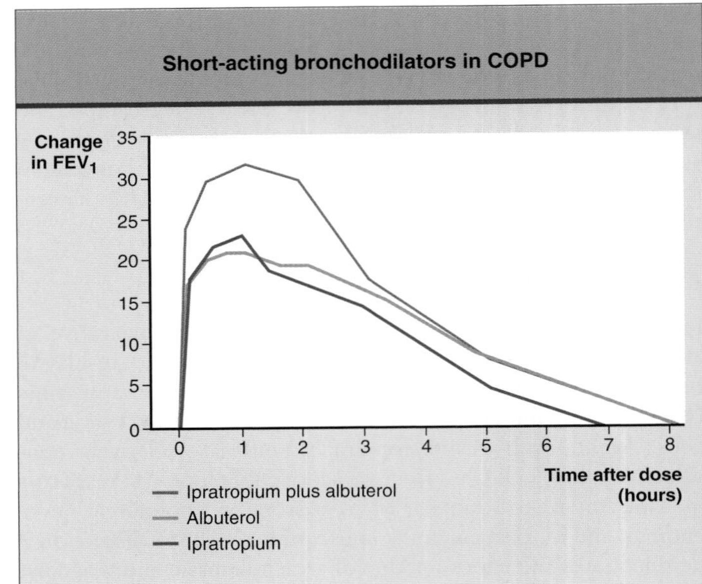

Figure 36.4 Effects of short-acting β_2-agonist and anticholinergic bronchodilators on airflow in chronic obstructive pulmonary disease. Combining a short-acting β_2-agonist and a short-acting anticholinergic bronchodilator results in more improvement in forced expired volume in 1 second (FEV_1) than the use of either agent alone. (From Combivent Inhalation Study Group: In chronic obstructive pulmonary disease, a combination of ipratropium and albuterol is more effective than either agent alone: An 85-day multicenter trial. COMBIVENT Inhalation Aerosol Study Group. Chest 105:1411-1419, 1994.)

Combining β-Agonist and Anticholinergic Bronchodilators

The combination of β_2-agonists and anticholinergic agents has proven to provide superior bronchodilation and improvement in health status compared with using either of these agents individually. These benefits are seen both with the use of SABAs (Fig. 36.4) and LABAs (Fig. 36.5).

In patients who remain symptomatic with persistent dyspnea despite the use of a single class of bronchodilators, a combination of β-agonist and anticholinergic bronchodilators can be used simultaneously on an intermittent or regularly scheduled basis.

Theophylline

The methylxanthines, such as theophylline, are modest bronchodilators but have other properties that improve breathing in patients with COPD. There is considerable potential for side effects, however, and the necessity for monitoring blood levels, together with their inferior bronchodilating ability, have relegated them to second-line therapy. The mechanisms of action and the exact role of methylxanthines in treatment of COPD remain areas of active debate, but they are known to be nonspecific inhibitors of phosphodiesterase enzymes. Theophylline is the most commonly used methylxanthine and has both bronchodilator and anti-inflammatory effects. It also has mild diuretic properties, stimulates the central respiratory drive, improves diaphragm function, and reduces diaphragm fatigue. Theophylline is metabolized by the cytochrome P-450 mixed-function oxidases. The toxic–therapeutic ratio for this class of drugs is low. Maintaining levels less than 15 mcg/mL will limit side effects, but physicians and patients should be alert to the fact that many other medications interfere with theophylline metabolism. Typical dosing for theophylline is 100 to 900 mg/day in a pill formulation. Side effects include nausea, vomiting, diarrhea, abdominal pain, gastroesophageal reflux (by inhibiting contraction of the lower esophageal sphincter), nervousness, headache, sleep disorders, muscle cramps, arrhythmias, including sinus and ventricular tachycardia and premature ventricular contractions, and seizures.

Unfortunately, development of these side effects does not always correlate with elevated serum levels, and more serious problems (e.g., arrhythmia and seizures) may occur without being preceded by other symptoms.

Theophylline should be considered for patients who remain symptomatic despite the use of inhaled bronchodilators because the drug improves airflow when added to inhaled LABAs (Fig. 36.6). Discontinuing the medication has decreased exercise capacity and increased symptoms in patients with severe COPD.

Second-generation inhibitors of phosphodiesterase-4 have shown some promise in preliminary studies. Newer formulations under study that maintain the bronchodilator and anti-inflammatory properties but have fewer GI side effects include cilomilast, piclamilast, and roflumilast.

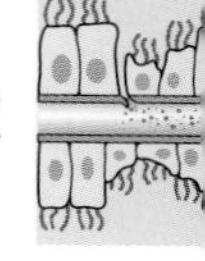

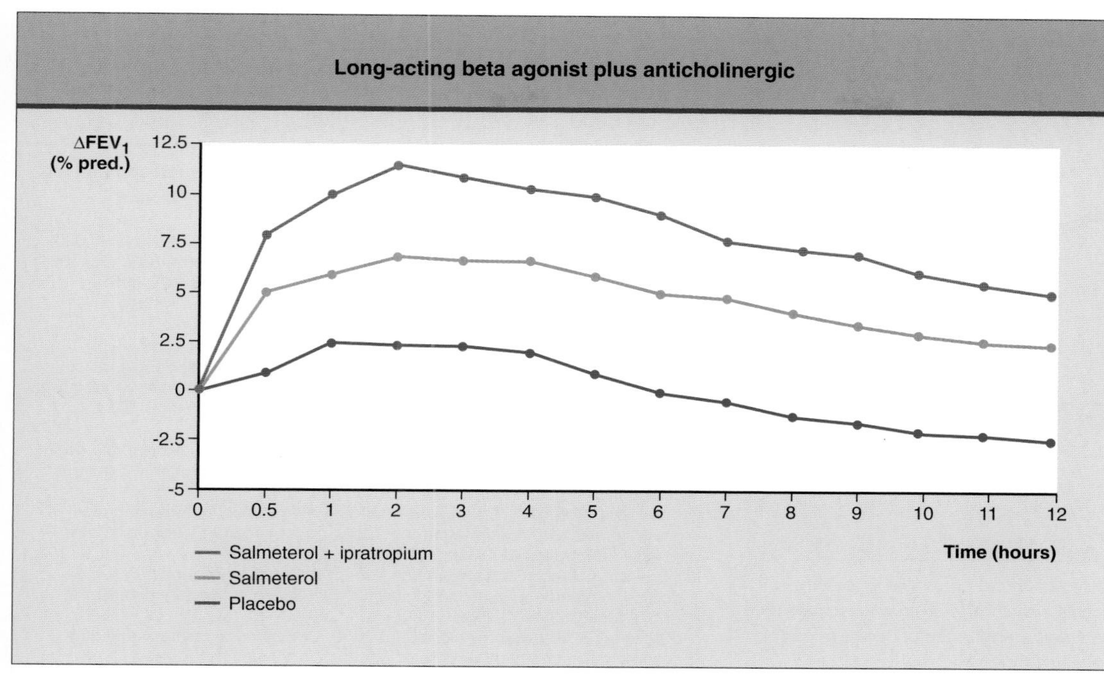

Figure 36.5 Effects of long-acting β_2-agonist and anticholinergic bronchodilators on airflow in chronic obstructive pulmonary disease. Combining a long-acting β_2-agonist and a short-acting anticholinergic bronchodilator results in more improvement in forced expired volume in 1 second (FEV_1) than the use of either agent alone. (From Van Noord JA, de Munck DR, Bantje TA, Hop WC: Long-term treatment of chronic obstructive pulmonary disease with salmeterol and the additive effect of ipratropium. Eur Respir J 15:878-885, 2000.)

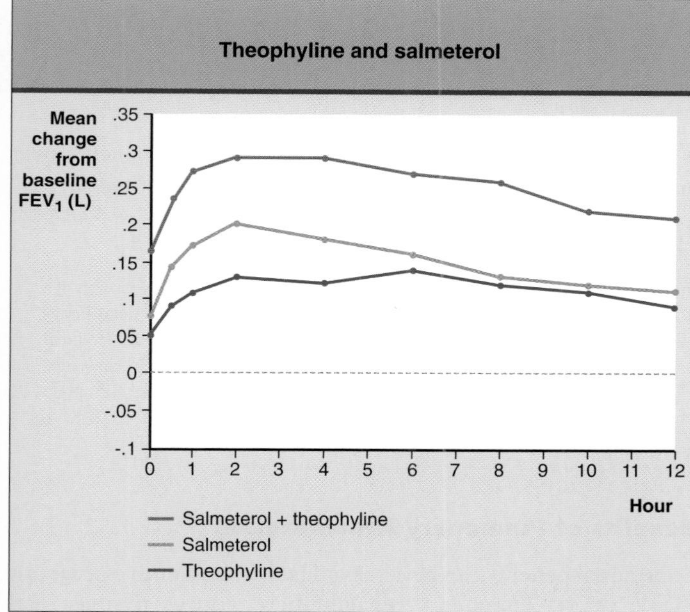

Figure 36.6 Effects of theophylline and salmeterol on forced expired volume in 1 second (FEV_1) in patients with chronic obstructive pulmonary disease. There is improved airflow (FEV_1) with the combination of a long-acting β-agonist bronchodilator and theophylline (From ZuWallack RL, Mahler DA, Reilly D, et al: Salmeterol plus theophylline combination therapy in the treatment of COPD. Chest 119:1661-1670, 2001.)

CORTICOSTEROIDS

Corticosteroids act by inhibiting the transcription of a large number of mediators from a number of inflammatory cells. Although the nature of the chronic inflammation in COPD (i.e., macrophage, neutrophil, and CD8 lymphocyte predominance) has led to the opinion that COPD is not a steroid-responsive condition, corticosteroids have been shown to be effective in selected patients and settings.

Both oral and systemic steroids given for no longer than 2 weeks are effective in increasing the rate of recovery and reducing the frequency of treatment failure in patients with acute COPD exacerbations. Long-term oral steroids do not appear to have a role in the chronic management of COPD because of their significant side effects.

Several large studies have demonstrated that chronic use of inhaled corticosteroids does not preserve lung function or retard the rate of decline in FEV_1 over time (Fig. 36.7). Approximately 10% of patients with stable COPD but no bronchial hyperresponsiveness, however, have marked increases in their FEV_1 (i.e., >30% improvement) after a 2-week course of oral steroids.

A number of trials suggest that chronic use of inhaled steroids reduces the frequency of acute exacerbations, particularly for patients with an FEV_1 of less than 50% predicted (Table 36.3). In some studies, respiratory symptoms were reduced. Unfortunately, there are no good predictors of which patients will be steroid responsive. Current international guidelines suggest that inhaled steroids should be considered for patients with an FEV_1 less than 50% predicted who have frequent exacerbations. Oral steroid trials may not accurately predict the response to inhaled corticosteroids and hence are not recommended to assess the efficacy of inhaled corticosteroids as maintenance therapy. Inhaled corticosteroids come in a variety of formulations; fluticasone and budesonide are the most potent, and other formulations include beclomethasone, triamcinolone, and flunisolide. The most common side effects are a bitter taste in the mouth, oral thrush, and hoarseness. Concerns have also been

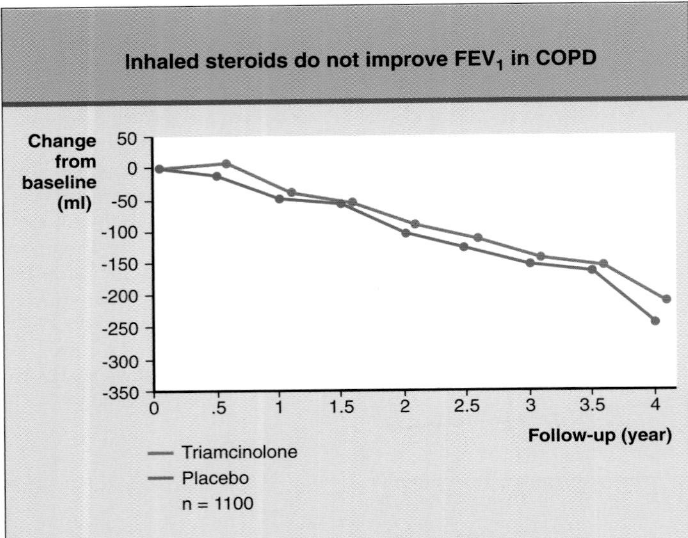

Figure 36.7 Lack of effect of an inhaled corticosteroid on decline in forced expired volume in 1 second (FEV_1) in patients with chronic obstructive pulmonary disease. In this 4-year, controlled trial, there was a similar rate of decline in FEV_1 in patients who received inhaled triamcinolone and those who received placebo. (From The Lung Health Study Research Group: Effect of triamcinolone on the decline in pulmonary function in chronic obstructive pulmonary disease. N Engl J Med 343:1902-1909, 2000.)

Table 36.3
Selected large recent studies of the effect of inhaled corticosteroids on exacerbations in patients with Chronic Obstructive Pulmonary Disease

Author	Treatment (μg/day)	Patients	Exacerbation Effect vs. Placebo
Burge et al.*	FP 1000	751	↓ Ex 25% (*P* = .026)
Paggiaro et al.†	FP 1000	281	↓ 60%-86% (*P* = .001)
Vestbo et al.‡	BUD (800)	290	↓ Ex 4% (NS)
LHSRG§	TAA (1200)	1100	↓ Ex (*P* NA)
Calverley et al.ll	FP (1000)	1465	↓ Ex 25% (*P* = .0)

*Burge PS, Calverley PMA, Spencer JS, et al: Randomised, double blind, placebo controlled study of fluticasone propionate in patients with moderate to severe chronic obstructive pulmonary disease: The ISOLDE trial. BMJ 320:1297-1303, 2000.
†Paggiaro PL, Dahl R, Bakran I, et al: Multicentre randomised placebo controlled trial of inhaled fluticasone propionate in patients with chronic obstructive pulmonary disease. Lancet 351:773-780, 1998.
‡Vestbo J, Sorensen T, Lange P, et al: Long-term effect of inhaled budesonide in mild and moderate chronic obstructive pulmonary disease: A randomised controlled trial. Lancet 353:1819-1823, 1999.
§The Lung Health Study Research Group: Effect of triamcinolone on the decline in pulmonary function in chronic obstructive pulmonary disease. N Engl J Med 343:1902-1909, 2000.
llCalverley P, Pauwels RA, Vestbo J, et al: Combined salmeterol and fluticasone in the treatment of chronic obstructive pulmonary disease: A randomised controlled trial. Lancet 361:449-456, 2003.
BUD, budesonide; FP, fluticasone propionate; NA, not applicable; NS, not significant; TAA, triamcinolone.

raised about osteoporosis and cataracts as long-term adverse effects in older subjects. Inhaled steroids have not been approved by the FDA for use in COPD.

Inhaled corticosteroids may be used in combination with LABA. Studies have generally suggested improved benefits with administration of both agents compared with use of either agent alone.

OTHER AGENTS

Mucolytics

There does not appear to be a role for routine use of mucolytics (guaifenesin). Orally administered *N*-acetylcysteine has been shown in uncontrolled or small European studies to reduce exacerbations, but this is attributed to its antioxidant rather than its mucolytic effects. *N*-acetylcysteine can cause some minor GI upset. It is not approved for use in the United States by the FDA and is not currently recommended by international guideline statements. DNase was shown to reduce the frequency and duration of acute exacerbations of acute bronchitis in patients with cystic fibrosis but is ineffective in treating acute or chronic bronchitis in patients with COPD.

PULMONARY REHABILITATION

Even after a maximal medication program as described previously, many patients with COPD still have disabling symptoms, particularly dyspnea, which limit their daily activities and impair their quality of life. In such situations pulmonary rehabilitation is an effective therapeutic program that provides benefits over and above those that can be achieved with medications alone.

Pulmonary rehabilitation has been defined by a National Heart, Lung, and Blood Institute workshop as:

> A multidimensional continuum of services directed to persons with pulmonary disease and their families, usually by an interdisciplinary team of specialists, with a goal of achieving and maintaining the individual's maximum level of independence and functioning in the community. (Fishman AP: Pulmonary rehabilitation research: NIH workshop summary. Am J Respir Crit Care Med 149:825-833, 1994.)

Benefits of Pulmonary Rehabilitation

Substantial benefits can be achieved by comprehensive programs (Table 36.4). Pulmonary rehabilitation reduces dyspnea and improves exercise capacity. The improvement in symptoms leads to an increased ability to perform daily activities with associated improvement in health-related quality of life (Fig. 36.8).

A clear and concise description of the expected outcomes of rehabilitation should be used to convey the benefits to patients considering participating, physicians referring patients, and insurers providing payment for medical care. Pulmonary rehabilitation does not alter the underlying physiology of COPD, the spirometric indices of airflow limitation, or the degree of oxygenation. The education provided during a pulmonary rehabilitation program should improve compliance with prescribed medications and, accordingly, lead to an additional reduction in symptoms.

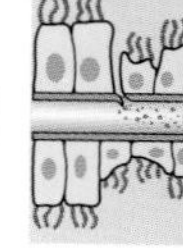

Table 36.4
Outcomes of pulmonary rehabilitation

Symptom/Therapy/Outcome	Outcome	Grade*	Recommendation
Dyspnea	Reduced dyspnea	A	Dyspnea outcomes should be routinely measured
Lower extremity exercise	Improved exercise tolerance	A	Exercise training of muscles of ambulation is recommended
Upper extremity exercise	Improved arm function with strength and endurance training	B	Arm exercise is recommended
Ventilatory muscle training	Improved respiratory muscle strength, but improved dyspnea and exercise tolerance only in some studies	B	Not an essential component of pulmonary rehabilitation; may be considered in selected patients with decreased respiratory muscle strength and dyspnea who remain symptomatic despite optimal therapy
Psychosocial and education	Decreased affective distress	C	Recommended based on expert opinion; cognitive and behavioral intervention enhance exercise adherence
Quality of life	Improved quality of life	A	
Health care utilization	Reduced hospitalizations in some uncontrolled studies	B	
Survival	Survival may be improved	C	

*Grade of evidence supporting recommendation:
A: Evidence provided by controlled trials with statistically significant, consistent results.
B: Evidence provided by observational studies or controlled trials with less consistent results.
C: Expert opinion because of results or lack of controlled trials.

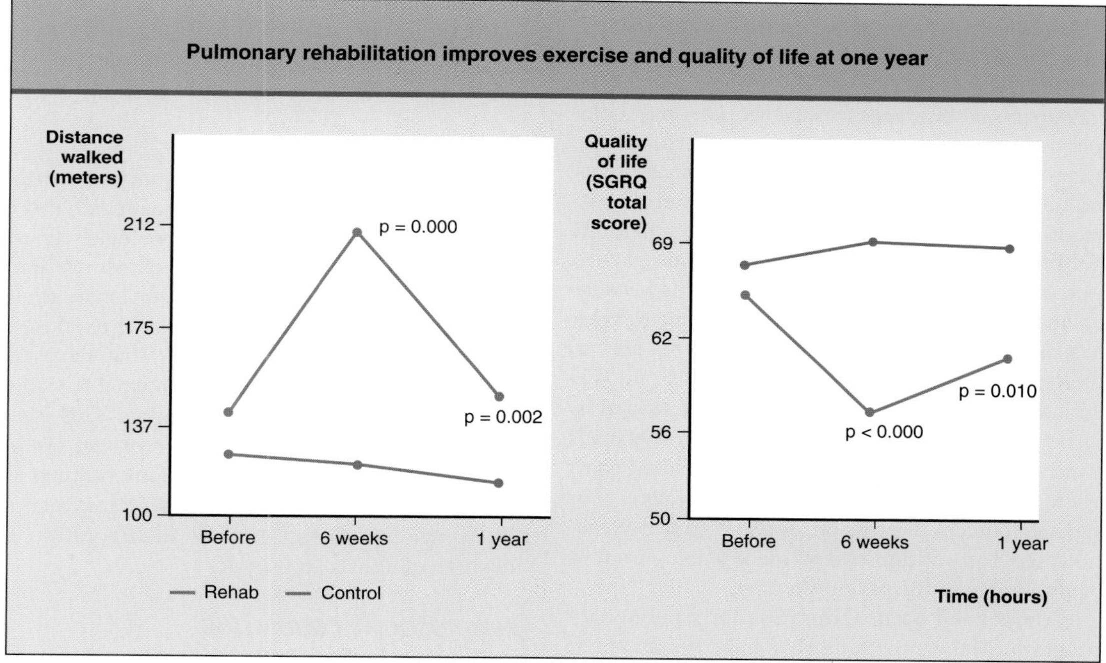

Figure 36.8 Outcomes of pulmonary rehabilitation. *Left,* Exercise (as measured by the shuttle walk distance) is increased immediately after rehabilitation (6 weeks) and at 1 year in patients with chronic obstructive pulmonary disease (COPD) randomized to receive comprehensive pulmonary rehabilitation compared with patients receiving standard medical management. *Right,* Disease-specific quality of life (measured by the St. George's Respiratory Questionnaire [SGRQ] Total Score) is improved immediately after rehabilitation (6 weeks) and at 1 year in patients with COPD randomized to receive comprehensive pulmonary rehabilitation compared with patients receiving standard medical management. Note that lower scores indicate improved health status. (Based on data from Griffiths TL, Burr ML, Campbell IA, et al: Results at 1 year of outpatient multidisciplinary pulmonary rehabilitation: A randomized controlled trial. Lancet 355:362-368, 2000.)

Principles of Pulmonary Rehabilitation

Two key principles guide the application of pulmonary rehabilitation:

1. The program should be tailored to meet the needs of each individual.
2. Multiple therapeutic components should be included.

Although comprehensive pulmonary rehabilitation programs usually have defined components that are carried out over a defined time period for all participants, all forms of rehabilitation are tailored to the unique needs of each individual. This requires that the patient have input into designing the goals and directions of the program. An initial session conducted by the program coordinator should be devoted to assessing

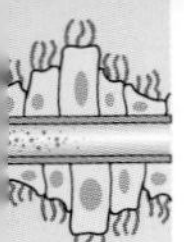

Table 36.5
Key Components of Comprehensive Pulmonary Rehabilitation

Medical evaluation and management
Assessment and goal setting
Therapeutic modalities
Exercise training
Education
Psychosocial counseling
Breathing retraining
Daily activity performance and energy management
Nutritional counseling
Outcome evaluation
Long-term continuation

the individual's needs and desires. Goal setting with realistic and achievable goals enhances participation and optimal outcomes.

The components of pulmonary rehabilitation are listed in Table 36.5. As can be seen, multiple personnel with experience in each modality are most often integrated into a multidisciplinary team to provide a coordinated program. Programs may include one or more of the following health professionals: physical therapist, occupational therapist, social worker, psychologist, nurse, respiratory therapist, psychiatrist, and dietitian. The types of health care professional employed in pulmonary rehabilitation depend on the expertise available, the program's structure, and the needs of the patients. For example, many patients with severe COPD and marked functional limitations experience some degree of anxiety and depressive symptoms because of their dyspnea and issues related to their adjustment to their diminished physical role. Because these symptoms are so common, psychological counseling for individuals with COPD is routinely included in most pulmonary rehabilitation programs. Counseling may be performed by nurses or other professionals who are skilled and experienced in this area, or by mental health professionals such as social workers or psychologists. For patients with signs of clinical depression, referral to a psychiatrist may be indicated for antidepressant medications, or to a social worker or psychologist for psychotherapy.

There is no clearly defined optimal duration for a pulmonary rehabilitation program. Many programs that have documented beneficial patient outcomes are conducted 2 or 3 days each week for a duration of 6 to 12 weeks, and more effective results are encountered with increasing program duration. In addition to supervised training sessions, patients are encouraged to exercise on their own for a total of four to five sessions a week until optimal exercise level is achieved. After the formal program, patients should exercise three to four times each week to maintain the gains in performance.

Role of the Physician and Patient Selection

Pulmonary rehabilitation must be ordered for appropriate patients by a physician. Patients are candidates if they have severe dyspnea and reduced quality of life even with a maximal medical program. Other markers indicating the potential need for rehabilitation include frequent hospitalizations or emergency visits due to respiratory disease, frequent office visits, and suboptimal adherence to medical treatment or oxygen therapy. The degree of airflow limitation is an imprecise criterion for pulmonary rehabilitation because the FEV_1 may not provide an accurate estimate of the patient's symptoms or quality of life. Nevertheless, the presence of severe airflow limitation (FEV_1 $\leq$35% of predicted) should alert the physician to the potential need for pulmonary rehabilitation. Many programs require that patients be nonsmokers before beginning therapy, as evidence that they are committed to adhering with the recommended program. Significant comorbidities that may preclude exercise, such as coronary artery disease, should be excluded before referral, and comorbidities that may impair exercise training, such as arthritis, should be maximally treated.

Although most commonly applied to patients with COPD, the principles of pulmonary rehabilitation can also be applied to patients with other respiratory disorders such as asthma.

Pulmonary Rehabilitation Components

INITIAL ASSESSMENT

The coordinator of the pulmonary rehabilitation program should enlist the cooperation of the patient in the development of specific patient-centered goals. Achievement of short-term goals is useful to enhance patient motivation and participation.

EXERCISE TRAINING

Exercise training is the most important component. Although even low-level exercise may be beneficial, more intensive training as tolerated improves physiologic function and lessens dyspnea. Exercise includes lower extremity aerobic training that most often consists of walking or stationary cycling. Training programs should follow the principles of exercise duration, session frequency, and exercise intensity that have been shown to be useful in healthy individuals. A formal maximum exercise test is usually performed before training. This is useful to exclude significant coronary artery disease or exercise-induced arrhythmias that would preclude strenuous training and to determine if the patient will need supplemental oxygen during the training program. Exercise that incorporates upper extremity strengthening is also useful.

PSYCHOSOCIAL COUNSELING

Depression and anxiety are frequently seen in patients with COPD. Psychological assessment and counseling are designed to assist the patient and family in managing the psychological stresses of the illness.

CONTROL OF DYSPNEA

Breathing retraining can assist the patient in controlling and managing his or her shortness of breath without overuse of medications. Pursed-lip breathing, diaphragmatic breathing, and controlled breathing also improve oxygenation, slow the respiratory rate, increase tidal volume, decrease air trapping, and reduce the work of breathing.

Instruction in daily activity performance is also useful to reduce dyspnea. Coordinating breathing with specific activities, avoiding breathholding, and exhaling while doing tasks that require unusual effort all reduce dyspnea. Pacing breathing with

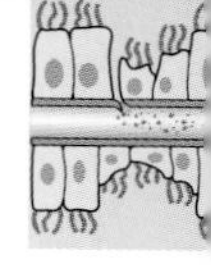

activities such as stair climbing can also reduce dyspnea and improve performance of physical tasks.

Reducing energy requirements can enhance performance of activities in patients with limited respiratory reserve. Techniques such as using proper body mechanics, pacing of activities, and planning sufficient rest periods are useful.

EDUCATION

Education should be undertaken with the goal of improving patient adherence with the most effective health-enhancing behaviors. A behavioral approach requires education about specific details of the techniques and timing of medication use that can be successfully incorporated into the patient's daily schedule of activities to allow maintenance of a more normal lifestyle. Individual education for each patient about his or her medical program, combined with group education, are key components of comprehensive rehabilitation programs.

NUTRITIONAL COUNSELING

Having a body weight less than 90% of ideal weight is a marker for increased mortality in COPD. Nutritional counseling in such patients may play a role in improving muscle mass necessary for normal daily activities. In overweight patients, weight loss may improve exercise. A diet adequate to meet caloric needs is required during exercise training. Accordingly, nutritional assessment and counseling are commonly provided during pulmonary rehabilitation.

OXYGEN THERAPY

The goals of oxygen therapy in patients with COPD are to:

1. Improve survival
2. Reduce dyspnea
3. Allow more exercise by eliminating exercise-induced hypoxemia

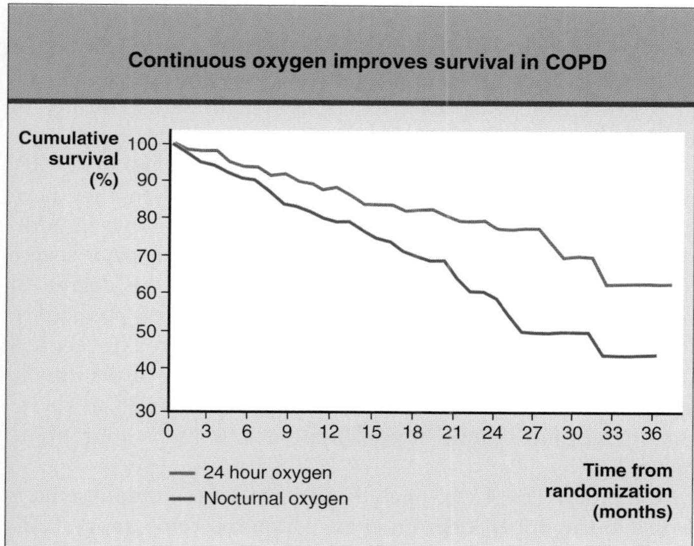

Figure 36.9 Survival in patients with chronic obstructive pulmonary disease and hypoxia randomized to either continuous oxygen therapy or nocturnal oxygen therapy. Patients receiving continuous oxygen therapy during the day and night have better survival than those receiving oxygen only at night. (From Nocturnal Oxygen Therapy Trial Group: Continuous or nocturnal oxygen therapy in hypoxemic chronic obstructive lung disease: A clinical trial. Ann Intern Med 93:391-398, 1980.)

Table 36.6
Indications for Ambulatory Continuous Oxygen Therapy in Patients with Chronic Obstructive Pulmonary Disease

Stable chronic obstructive pulmonary disease on optimal medical therapy and:
$PaO_2 \leq 55$ mm Hg ($SaO_2 \leq 88\%$) seated at rest
or
$PaO_2 = 56$-59 mm Hg
plus
Erythrocytosis: hematocrit ≥ 56%
Right heart dysfunction: P pulmonale, edema

These indications are based on the entry criteria for the Nocturnal Oxygen Therapy Trial (Nocturnal Oxygen Therapy Trial Group: Continuous or nocturnal oxygen therapy in hypoxemic chronic obstructive lung disease: A clinical trial. Ann Intern Med 93:391-398, 1980), and are accepted by Medicare and most health care insurers.
PaO_2, partial pressure of arterial oxygen; SaO_2, arterial oxygen saturation.

Studies reported in the 1980s conclusively demonstrated the survival benefit of long-term oxygen therapy in patients with hypoxia and COPD (Fig. 36.9). The inclusion criteria for these studies have been adopted as the indications for oxygen therapy by most health care insurers, including Medicare (Table 36.6). The indications for continuous oxygen therapy to improve survival are a PaO_2 ≤50 mm Hg or a PaO_2 of 56 to 59 mm Hg when there is also evidence of end-organ dysfunction secondary to chronic hypoxia (e.g., peripheral edema without another cause, pulmonary hypertension, or erythrocytosis [hematocrit ≥56%]). With the advent of pulse oximetry, the need for oxygen can also be suggested by oxygen saturation measurements (i.e., a saturation of ≤88% with the patient seated at rest or a saturation of 89% with other evidence of chronic hypoxemia). Oximetry is less invasive and more easily performed in an office setting than arterial blood gas analysis. However, oximetry readings are less accurate and reproducible than arterial blood gas analysis, and oximetry results can be affected by factors such as poor vascular circulation, motion artifact, ambient light, and nail polish. In patients who meet these criteria, oxygen should be used continuously (during the day, with activity, and nocturnally), and not only when patients experience dyspnea.

The assessment for long-term oxygen therapy should be performed with patients seated, at rest, and breathing room air when they are in optimal medical condition rather than during an acute exacerbation. Patients should be using appropriate medications for COPD, including bronchodilators.

Other beneficial effects of continuous oxygen therapy in hypoxemic patients with COPD include improvements in the degree of pulmonary hypertension, improved neuropsychological function, increased exercise capacity, and reduced dyspnea.

The goal of chronic oxygen therapy is to increase the PaO_2 to above 60 mm Hg (an oxygen saturation of ≥90%). Pulse oximetry is useful while titrating the oxygen flow rate to achieve this result. Oxygen flows should be adjusted both at rest and during activity to achieve oxygen saturations of 90% or greater.

Many patients with COPD require higher flows of oxygen with exercise to maintain the desired saturation. In the Nocturnal Oxygen Therapy Trial, which demonstrated a survival benefit from long-term oxygen in COPD, the oxygen flow rate was increased at night by 1 L above that required at rest during the day. The prescription for oxygen should include flow rates at rest, during activity, and with sleep.

Oxygen prescriptions should include the number of hours of daily use, the need for oxygen required for ambulation, the type of oxygen system to use, and the method of delivery. In patients who meet the aforementioned criteria, oxygen should be prescribed for use 24 hours each day. Many patients with COPD do not meet the criteria for oxygen at rest, however, but do have desaturation with activity. Oxygen therapy provided during activity in patients with desaturation to 88% or less with activity decreases dyspnea during the activity and improves exercise capacity. Such patients may be prescribed oxygen only during activity.

Oxygen sources include concentrators, compressed gaseous oxygen, and liquid oxygen. Electrically powered concentrators obtain oxygen by concentrating air and are the least expensive way of providing oxygen supplementation. Concentrators are not adaptable to use outside the home, however, and they also generate considerable heat and noise. Compressed gas cylinders are heavy but are available in various sizes and may be used as a stationary oxygen source. Liquid oxygen is the most costly supply system because it requires personnel visiting the patient's home, usually weekly, to refill the containers. Only two of these systems are available for use during ambulation—compressed gas oxygen and liquid oxygen. Compressed gaseous cylinders are bulky and smaller cylinders may not contain sufficient oxygen for longer periods of use. Very small, lightweight, convenient liquid systems are now available (Fig. 36.10).

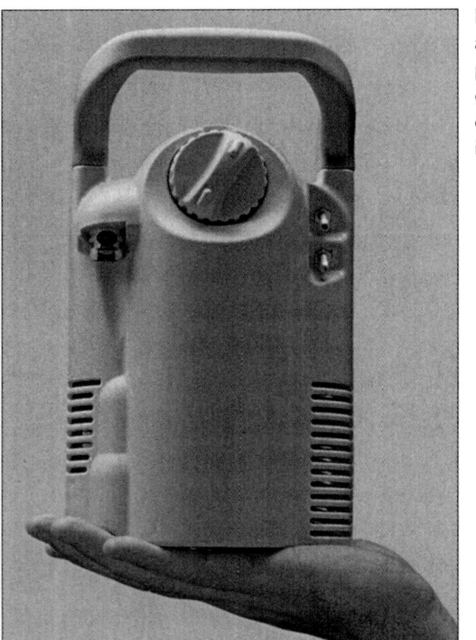

Figure 36.10 Example of a small, lightweight, portable liquid oxygen canister that incorporates demand delivery during inspiration only.

Oxygen has been most commonly delivered as a continuous flow of gas. However, oxygen reaches the lung only when the patient inhales; oxygen delivered during exhalation is wasted. Oxygen conservation devices have used this principle to reduce the amount of oxygen required and increase the duration of portable supply systems. Demand delivery devices (also called pulse-dose systems) are available that administer a bolus of oxygen during the initial period of inhalation. Demand delivery devices sense when patients begin to inhale and then trigger the delivery of oxygen. Flow ceases during exhalation, thereby reducing oxygen wastage. Demand delivery devices have been incorporated into portable gaseous and liquid oxygen systems. Oxygenation using demand or pulse-dose oxygen delivery systems, however, is not always equivalent to continuous oxygen flow delivery. Accordingly, the appropriate oxygen flow rate for each patient should be determined with the specific delivery system the patient actually uses over the long term.

Patients frequently do not understand the role of supplemental oxygen. Some of the more common misunderstandings are that oxygen is required only for control of dyspnea, and that using higher doses will eliminate dyspnea. Thus, patient education is a prerequisite for proper use and adherence to therapy. Other barriers include patient vanity over appearance, denial of the illness, difficulty of use during ambulation, and fear that oxygen use will impair quality of life. Education and pulmonary rehabilitation can address these issues.

LUNG VOLUME REDUCTION SURGERY

It seems counterintuitive that removing part of the lung might be an effective therapy for patients with severe emphysema. However, publications from individual centers and results from a large, randomized, controlled, multicenter trial have established the benefits of this type of surgery in carefully selected patients. In these selected patients, LVRS improves survival, increases exercise capacity, enhances health status (quality of life), and improves oxygenation and pulmonary function.

Because of the morbidity, mortality, and cost of LVRS, however, patients should be considered only when they have significant dyspnea despite maximal medical therapy. In addition, LVRS is usually reserved for patients who have severe disease based not only on symptoms, but on the degree of physiologic abnormality (i.e., an FEV_1 <40% to 45% predicted). Potential candidates for LVRS should be referred to centers that have experience with the procedure. Such centers usually are also experienced with lung transplantation and can therefore determine if lung transplantation is a more appropriate option.

Candidates for LVRS include patients whose emphysema is worse in the upper lobes on chest computed tomography (CT) scan (Fig. 36.11). Those with severe airflow limitation (FEV_1 ≤25% predicted) who also have either a very low diffusing capacity (≤25% predicted) or diffuse emphysema on chest CT scan are *not* candidates for LVRS because they have increased mortality. Figure 36.12 provides information on the survival, exercise capacity, and quality-of-life outcomes of LVRS in subgroups identified by the National Emphysema Treatment Trial.

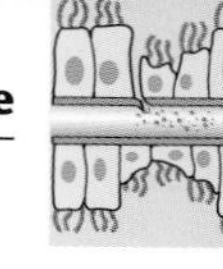

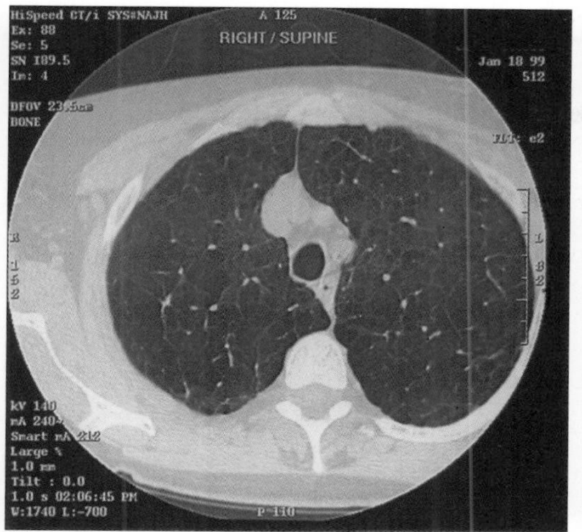

A

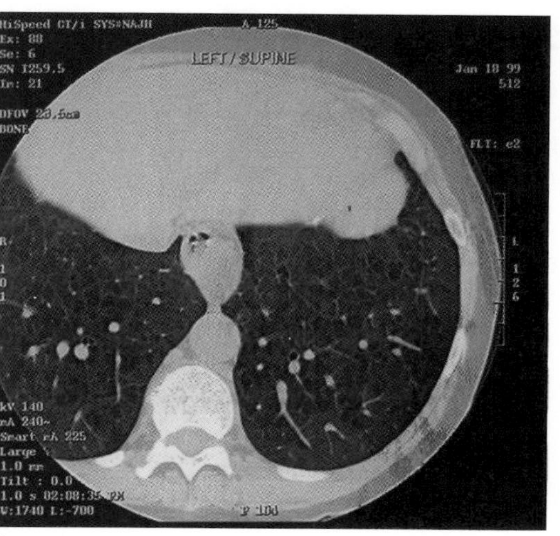

B

Figure 36.11 Chest computed tomography scans demonstrating severe emphysema. **A,** Severe emphysema is seen in the upper lobes bilaterally. **B,** Emphysema is less severe in the lower lung zones.

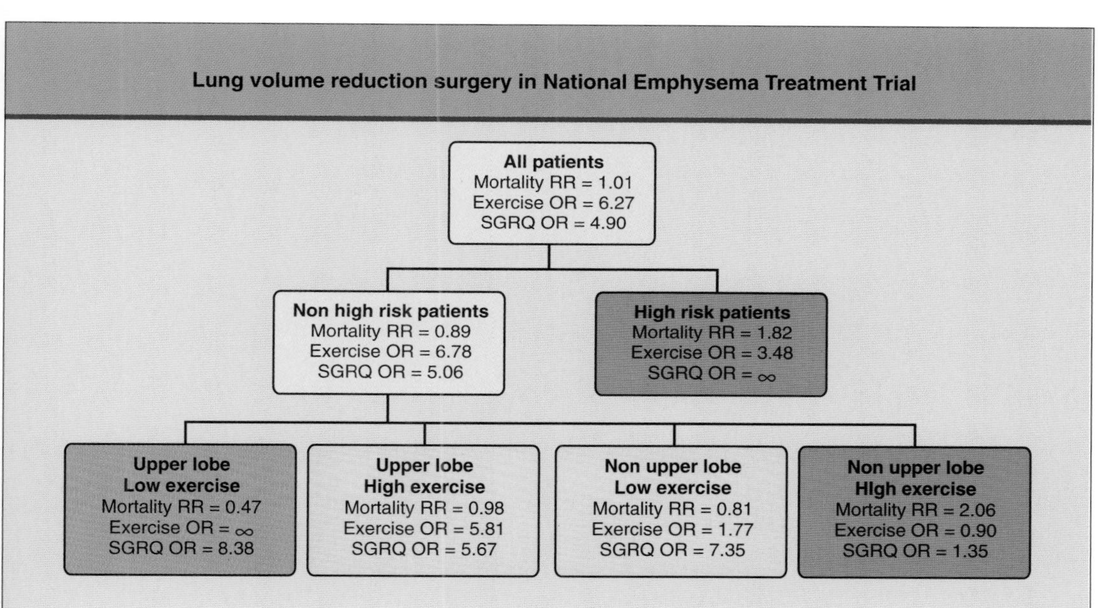

Figure 36.12 Results of the lung volume reduction surgery from the National Emphysema Treatment Trial, a controlled, randomized clinical trial of 1218 patients with severe emphysema. The green box identifies characteristics and outcomes of patients with a positive outcome (mortality, exercise, and quality of life). The red boxes identify subsets of patients with poor outcomes. The yellow boxes highlight patients with intermediate outcomes. OR, odds ratio; RR, relative risk; SGRQ, St. George's Respiratory Questionnaire. (Courtesy of the National Emphysema Treatment Trial.)

SUMMARY

Smoking cessation has an important role in preventing progression of COPD and should be aggressively pursued in all smokers.

Currently, bronchodilator therapy remains central to the management of symptomatic patients. The choice of bronchodilators allows physicians and patients to make decisions based on many factors, such as effectiveness, cost, ease of use, and convenience. Ultimately, the best selections are those that optimize adherence. It is important to appreciate that the mechanisms of action of many of these drugs are complementary and that additional benefits may be obtained when they are used in combination.

For selected patients with severe disease, other therapies are effective. For those with a history of exacerbations, the addition of inhaled corticosteroids may prove beneficial. Long-term ambulatory oxygen therapy improves survival and reduces dyspnea in patients with documented hypoxia. LVRS is an option for carefully selected patients with CT evidence of emphysema.

Newer drugs will augment bronchodilation even further, but more importantly will retard the long-term decline in FEV_1, a feature that no current therapy is able to claim. As we gain greater insights into the underlying pathophysiologic process of COPD we will be able to design and study therapies that target the underlying disease process more directly rather than simply palliate its end effects.

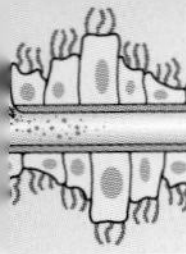

SUGGESTED READINGS

American Thoracic Society: Pulmonary rehabilitation, 1999. Am J Respir Crit Care Med 159:1666-1682, 1999.

Fiore MC, Bailey WC, Cohen SJ, et al: Clinical Practice Guideline: Treating Tobacco Use and Dependence. Bethesda, Md, U.S. Department of Health and Human Services, Public Health Service, June, 2000.

National Emphysema Treatment Trial Research Group. A randomized trial comparing lung-volume-reduction surgery with medical therapy for severe emphysema. N Engl J Med 348:2059-2073, 2003.

Pauwels R, Anthonisen N, Bailey WC, et al: Global strategy for the diagnosis, management, and prevention of chronic obstructive pulmonary disease: NHLBI/WHO workshop [update, 2003]. Available at www.goldcopd.com; accessed August 2, 2003.

Similowski T, Derenne J-P, Whitelaw WA (eds): Lung Biology in Health and Disease. In Clinical Management of Chronic Obstructive Pulmonary Disease. New York, Marcel Dekker, 2002.

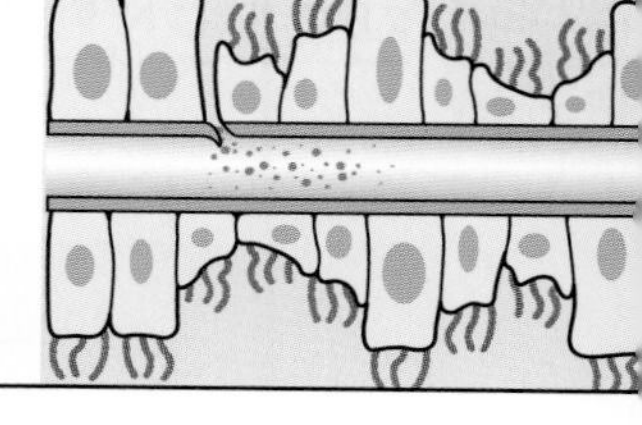

CHAPTER 37 Asthma: Epidemiology and Risk Factors

Dirkje S. Postma, Huib A.M. Kerstjens, and Nick H.T. Ten Hacken

Asthma is one of the most common diseases encountered in clinical medicine in both children and adults. It is one of the classic diseases recognized by Hippocrates more than 2000 years ago, yet today it is still underdiagnosed. Its prevalence and pathogenesis have been extensively studied, but the factors that cause the disease and the interplay between these are still unclear. By most criteria used for a diagnosis, asthma is a major health problem that affects 2% to 30% of the population. In this chapter, the epidemiology of asthma is discussed. Overall, the consensus is that the prevalence of asthma is increasing worldwide, especially in children. Epidemiologic studies to establish the prevalence of asthma in different communities are complicated by several methodologic problems. The disease has periods of remission of symptoms, and signs may not be present when patients are interviewed or investigated. Many surveys do not include lung function measurements for logistic reasons—and often objective validation of the diagnosis has not been performed. One study in which airway function in asthmatics was investigated found that 62% of the asthmatics had significant airway obstruction on the day of testing, whereas 38% had normal airway functions. However, on another day, abnormal flow might be present again. Therefore, all prevalence rates should be interpreted with caution.

Current data on the epidemiology of asthma and the putative risk factors for the disease that have been obtained from epidemiologic studies are reviewed herein.

EPIDEMIOLOGY AND RISK FACTORS

Incidence of Asthma

Incidence of asthma serves as the epidemiologic measure of disease onset. For all age groups, incidence varies between countries from 2.65 to 4 per 1000 individuals per year. For children younger than age 5 years in whom a firm diagnosis is difficult, incidence rates of 8 to 14 in 1000 and 4.3 to 9 in 1000 per year have been reported for boys and girls, respectively. The incidence of asthma after age 25 years has been estimated at 2.1 of 1000 individuals per year. New asthma in adulthood is not uncommon. Among a Tasmanian cohort followed for more than 20 years, one in nine children not reported as having asthma at 7 years of age developed asthma by age 30 years. Risk factors for new asthma included female sex, maternal hay fever, and lower lung function in childhood. Figure 37.1 gives the age and sex distribution of individuals who attended their family practitioner for asthma. It is clear that asthma increases both in early childhood and later in life.

Only one study has investigated the trend in incidence. Over 20 years' time, the incidence, which was age- and sex-adjusted, for combined definite and probable asthma increased from 183 to 284 per 100,000 in Minnesota. This increase was fully explained by increases localized in the 1- to 14-year age group.

Prevalence of Childhood Asthma

Prevalence reflects both the incidence and the duration of a disease. Clearly, asthma and wheezing illness are frequently present in children and young adults. The diagnosis of asthma is partly culturally dependent and related to a population's access to medical care. Furthermore, the prevalence can vary threefold in the same population depending on the definition used. Therefore, all studies have to be interpreted cautiously when prevalence values for asthma are given. Prevalences that vary between 3.3% and 34% have been reported. It is not possible to list here all the studies on the prevalence of asthma in the world during the past 30 years; overviews have shown that the prevalence of childhood asthma in most affluent countries is 2% to 5%. In 1998, data became available from a worldwide study on asthma, the International Study of Asthma and Allergies in Childhood (ISAAC). The study investigated 463,801 children ages 13 to 14 in 56 countries. The results showed considerable variability between countries in the prevalence of childhood self-reported asthma (Figure 37.2). The highest prevalence was about 20 times higher than the lowest. For instance, the highest 12-month prevalences of asthma were from centers in the United Kingdom, Australia, New Zealand, and Republic of Ireland (the highest being 36.8%), followed by centers in North, Central, and South America. The lowest prevalences were from participating centers in several Eastern European countries, Indonesia, China, Taiwan, Uzbekistan, India, and Ethiopia (the lowest in these countries being 1.6%). Although the prevalences were quite similar generally in centers in any one country, differences were large between different countries. Analysis of this difference might ultimately result in the discovery of different risk factors, as has been the case for the development of cancer in epidemiologic studies.

The prevalence of wheezing in childhood has increased over the past decades. However, differences in methodology, definitions, and use of the label asthma may have exaggerated the true increase in prevalence. Awareness of asthma in the population may have increased because of widespread publicity. Therefore, the authors carefully examined the data to prevent bias, and some studies still showed an increase in prevalence. Analyses of

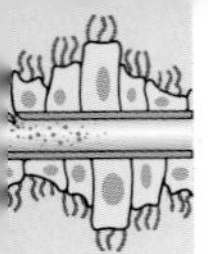

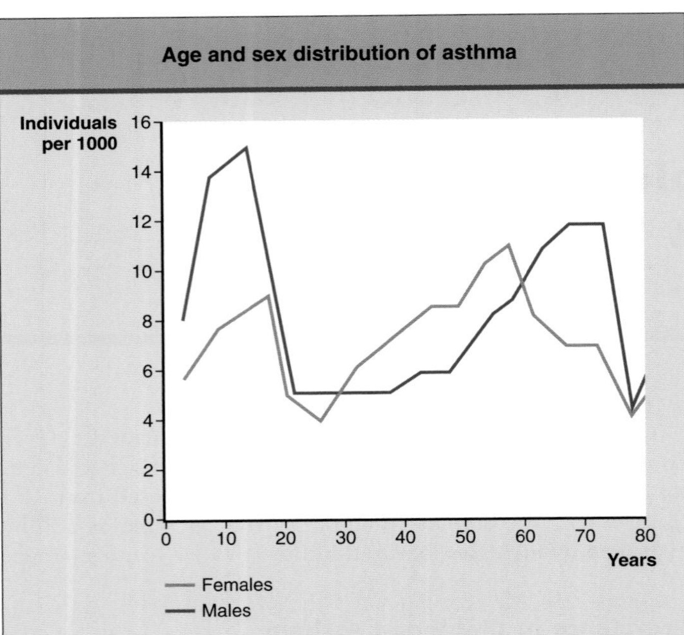

Figure 37.1 Age and sex distribution of patients who visit their family practitioner for asthma. (Adapted with permission from Weeke ER, Pedersen PA: Allergic rhinitis in a Danish general practice. Allergy 36:375-379, 1981.)

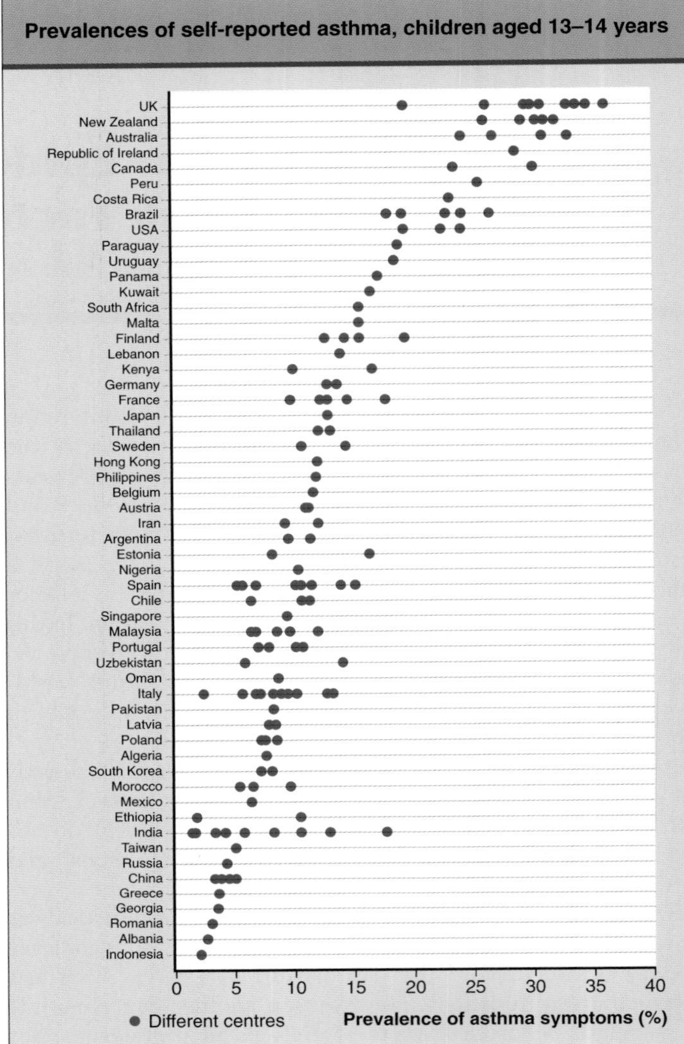

Figure 37.2 Twelve-month prevalences of self-reported asthma with a written questionnaire, for children ages 13 to 14 years. (Adapted with permission from The International Study of Asthma and Allergies in Childhood [ISAAC] Steering Committee: Worldwide variation in prevalence of symptoms of asthma, allergic rhinoconjunctivitis, and atopic eczema: ISAAC. Lancet 351:1225-1232, 1998.)

the available data suggest an increase in asthma prevalence from 1970 onward.

In Australia in 1969, 19.2% of 7-year-old children experienced recurrent episodes of wheezing; in New Zealand in 1973, 23% of 9-year-old children had a history of one or more attacks of wheezing. These were cross-sectional studies, and therefore they do not simply reflect an increase in prevalence. In a UK population study in which 36 regions were investigated in 1982 and again in 1992 using the same methodology, a threefold increase in asthma attacks in children ages 5 to 11 years occurred, with a 30% to 60% increase in occasional wheeze and a 30% to 40% increase in persistent wheeze, which suggests a real increase in asthma prevalence. In the United States, reported prevalence of wheeze among children ages 6 to 11 years increased significantly from 4.8% between 1971 and 1974 to 7.6% between 1976 and 1980. In addition, childhood asthma was rare in Africa up to the late 1970s; yet, recent studies suggest that the current prevalence is in the highest range.

Prevalence of Adult Asthma

Few data are available on adults, and it is unclear whether the prevalence of asthma is increasing in adults as well. The same considerations in interpreting the results of different studies as noted for childhood asthma apply for adult asthma. The European Community Respiratory Health Study showed considerable variation between countries for adult asthma. Wheezing during the past 12 months was present in 20% to 27% of the different populations, with more variability for nocturnal dyspnea and attacks of asthma. When airway hyperresponsiveness was taken as a measure of asthma, the prevalence was high in New Zealand, Australia, United States, Britain, France, Denmark, and Germany, whereas it was low in Sweden, Italy, and Spain.

Early data from inhabitants of Tristan da Cunha suggest that current asthma has increased from 11% in 1974 to more than 20% in 1995. In Sweden, the prevalence of asthma in 18-year-old military conscripts increased by 47% (from 1.8% to 2.8%) between 1971 and 1981. In Finland, investigations in 19-year-old conscripts showed an increase in adult asthma from 0.08% in 1961 to 1.29% in 1966 and then up to 1.79% in 1989. It seems unlikely that a rise of this kind relates only to diagnosis, because this would imply that 95% of the cases were undiagnosed in 1966.

A 1996 study in Greenwich, United Kingdom, showed that the prevalence of asthma among adults (16 to 50 years old) has increased since a similar survey in 1986, although with a lower amount of increase.

Most studies report that asthma prevalence diminishes with age. Curiously, in some developing countries the prevalence of asthma in adults is higher than that in children. For instance, in

Papua New Guinea, the point prevalence of asthma in children in the 1970s was nil and the adult prevalence was only 0.28%. A decade later, the prevalence was 0.6% in children and 7.3% in adults. Severe asthma now also occurs in these adults, especially when exposed to high levels of house dust mites. The striking rise in asthma was not observed in a similar village, in which a fourfold lower mite density in blanket dust occurred. No good explanation exists for this higher asthma prevalence occurring in adults than in children in Papua New Guinea as opposed to almost all other countries.

Asthma Mortality

Asthma rarely leads to death, as reflected in the mortality rates, which are measured in deaths per 100,000 subjects. For many countries, asthma deaths are less than a few hundred per annum. According to World Health Organization data, revised in 2000, asthma deaths numbered 1,800,000 persons per year worldwide. Decreasing accuracy in asthma diagnosis and hence mortality rates occurs in decedents older than 35 years of age, and only a low percentage of asthma deaths are validated by autopsy. In spite of these and other limitations, much has been learned about mortality rate changes. A large variability in asthma mortality occurs between countries, similar to the large variation of its prevalence. Mortality rates vary from 9 in 100,000 in Germany to 1.5 of 100,000 in Hong Kong for persons of all ages (Figure 37.3). A recent Dutch study showed that asthma mortality in the age group 5 to 34 years decreased between 1980 and 1994, from 3.1 deaths per million people to 1.1, one of the lowest reported in the literature. A history of severe disease, lack of access to medical care, suboptimal pharmacotherapy, emotional depression, and family disturbance have all been suggested as risk factors for asthma mortality.

On two occasions in the past three decades, a substantial increase in mortality in England, Wales, Australia, and New Zealand occurred. This was attributed to a direct toxic effect of high-dose sympathicomimetic bronchodilator use, delay in obtaining medical care, and increased exposure to aeroallergens. Whether inhaled β_2-agonists are associated with or alternatively cause subsequent mortality remains unclear.

In a Danish follow-up study in adults, it appeared that cigarette smoking, age, presence of blood eosinophilia, degree of impairment of lung function, and degree of reversibility to β_2-agonists contributed to asthma mortality. Greater reversibility was a risk factor in contrast to expectations. It might be that this signifies that asthma was undertreated in these individuals, which supports other data that the outcome of asthma is improved when inhaled corticosteroids are instituted as early as possible.

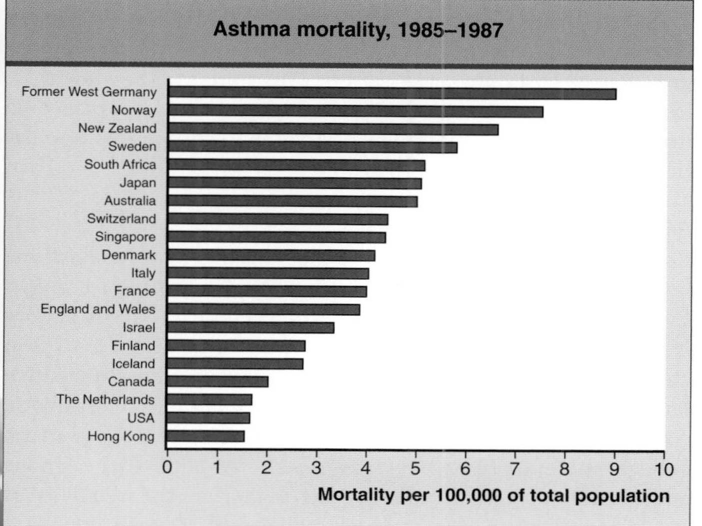

Figure 37.3 Asthma mortality (total population) rate per 100,000, measured from 1985 to 1987. (From Sears MR: Worldwide trends in asthma mortality. Bull Int Lung Dis 66:79-83, 1991.)

Risk Factors for Development of Asthma

Because asthma prevalence and mortality are increasing, it seems important to determine which risk factors cause this increase. Many studies have tried to assess risk factors and found evidence that, for example, atopy, hyperresponsiveness, (passive) smoking, and diet, could be considered as single risk factors for the presence of asthma. Until recently, only a few studies had assessed the risk for development of asthma using logistic regression analyses. Only in this way can one interpret the relative risks of different factors that all ultimately contribute to the development of disease. These studies are addressed in the following sections.

A distinction can be made between inherent factors (atopy, genetic predisposition, sex), causal factors (smoking), and contributing factors (e.g., the load of allergen exposure) as risk factors in the development of asthma (Table 37.1).

ATOPY

Atopy is characterized by elevated levels of total serum immunoglobulin (Ig)E, presence of specific IgE against common aeroallergens, or positive skin tests to common aeroallergens. In many countries, atopy is the greatest risk factor for asthma in childhood and adulthood (Figure 37.4). Asthmatics tend to be more atopic than nonasthmatics. In children, the odds ratios for the association between increased airway responsiveness, thought to be almost a prerequisite for the diagnosis of asthma, and skin-test reactivity range between 1.5 and 9.2, and in adults from 0.6 to 2.6, which suggests that atopy plays a more prominent role in asthmatic children than in adults. This is supported

Table 37.1
Factors that contribute to asthma

Inherent factors	Causal factors	Contributing factors
Atopy	Smoking	Indoor allergens (domestic mites, animal allergens, cockroach allergens, fungi)
Gender	Respiratory infections	Outdoor allergens (pollens, fungi)
Hyperresponsiveness	Low birth weight	Occupational sensitizers
Genetic abnormalities	Diet	
	Air pollution	
	Level of lung function	

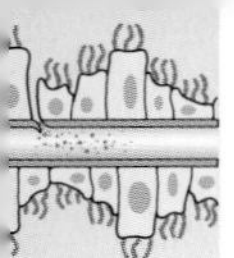

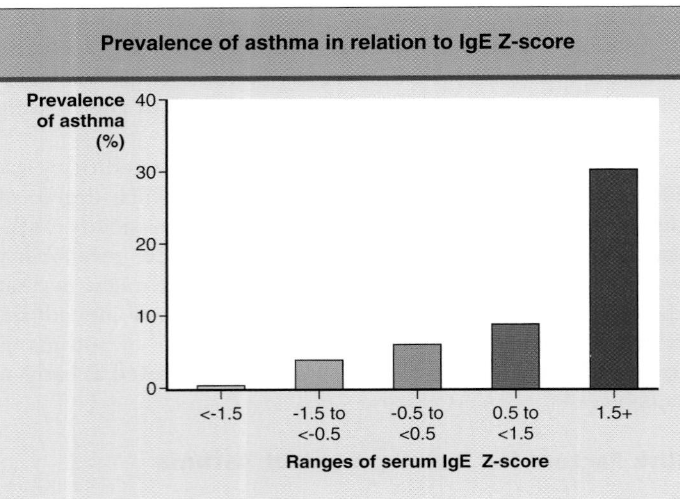

Figure 37.4 Prevalences of asthma in relation to immunoglobulin E Z-scores (standardized for age and sex) in 1662 Tucson persons who had completely negative skin tests to house dust. (From Burrows B, Martinez FD, Halonen M, et al: Association of asthma with serum IgE levels and skin-test reactivity to allergens. N Engl J Med 320:271-277, 1989.)

by the observation that the prevalence of positive skin tests to allergen peaks in those ages 20 to 25 years and (just as the IgE levels) declines with age thereafter. Most childhood asthmatics are thus reported to be atopic, whereas 50% to 70% of adults who have asthma show positive skin tests, although IgE may be elevated with negative skin tests. The reason for this is unknown.

The likelihood that asthma is diagnosed is increased not only by the presence of atopy, but also by the intensity of atopy as assessed with the size of the wheals to relevant allergens. The type of allergen that plays a role in the development of asthma appears to differ between countries. House dust mites are considered to be the most common risk factor. Sears showed in a New Zealand cohort that, next to house dust mites, the cat is an important risk factor, but *Alternaria* spp. and pollens, depending on the environment, have been identified as well. House dust mite and cat sensitivity are major predictors not only for diagnosed asthma, but also for the presence of airway hyperresponsiveness to methacholine.

Allergen exposure and allergen load are also important factors for the development of atopy and asthma. In the United Kingdom, children exposed to furry pets are at twice the risk for symptoms of asthma. Furthermore, the home environment contains other risk factors for asthma apart from mites and pets. Dampness in the home increases the risks of asthma associated with passive smoking to an odds ratio of 1.3, and increases the risks associated with cat or dog exposure in combination with smoke exposure to an odds ratio of 8.0. Dampness in the child's bedroom in combination with rugs or a carpet in the bedroom increases the risk of asthma development in children in Kenya to odds ratios greater than 2.5. An association between the levels of house dust mites in the bedrooms of babies during the first year of life and clinical asthma at 8 years of age has been demonstrated. Studies have also shown an increased atopy to birch and grass pollens in those children born in the spring. Living at high altitude, where levels of mites and pollen are negligible, is associated with decreased sensitization to these agents and reduced asthma symptoms. Increasing evidence indicates a critical age in early infancy at which sensitization to environmental allergens occurs, rather than the development of immunologic tolerance that would normally be expected with immunologic maturation. In an animal model, protective antibodies were not developed when allergens were inhaled during the first 2 weeks after birth, but they were made when inhaled for 3 weeks. This supports the concept of a window for the induction of atopy and probably of asthma.

Furthermore, at least two reports suggest that an early age of onset of atopy may be predictive not only of the development of asthma, but also of the persistence of airway hyperresponsiveness and asthma. These observations have led to several ongoing studies to assess whether intervention in house dust mite exposure at an early age might prevent the development of asthma.

Several surveys in Eastern Europe carried out immediately after the fall of the communist system showed that the prevalence of atopic disease in children and adults was low compared with that in Western countries. Lower prevalences of asthma, hay fever, and airway hyperresponsiveness were reported among schoolchildren ages 9 to 11 years who lived in Leipzig, East Germany, than in children of the same age who lived in Munich, West Germany. The discovery of this striking difference in prevalence has been attributed to smaller family size, higher socioeconomic lifestyle, Western diet, and increasing allergen exposure attributable to insulated housing conditions. A recent study in Leipzig showed that during the time that drastic changes toward a Western lifestyle occurred, the frequencies of asthma and airway hyperresponsiveness remained virtually unchanged, whereas hay fever increased. The children surveyed were born about 3 years before the end of communism and were therefore exposed to changing living conditions after the age of 3 years. This may suggest that only factors that operate in early life are important for early childhood asthma and that the development of atopy and hay fever is affected more by environmental factors that occur after infancy, in addition to early-life factors.

Studies from China and Africa show that striking differences in asthma prevalences may exist in populations, despite similar prevalences of atopic sensitization. This supports the view that, in addition to atopic sensitization, other risk factors may be important in the development of asthma in susceptible populations. These are discussed below.

FAMILY HISTORY AND GENETICS

Logistic regression analysis shows that parental history of asthma is an important risk factor for asthma after adjusting for atopy. Even in nonatopic children with asthma, a positive family history is a risk factor for disease, the risk ratio being about 2 to 3 in children who have a parent who suffers from asthma. A positive family history of asthma or hay fever in the families of asthmatic college students is twice that of the families of nonasthmatic college students (41.5% versus 22.2%, respectively). Among adults, the increase in allergy was higher in the relatives of extrinsic asthmatics (onset before the age of 20 years and skin-test positive) than among intrinsic asthmatics (onset after the age of 30 years and skin-test negative). The prevalence of asthma among siblings of extrinsic asthmatics tends to increase if both

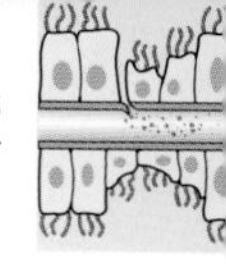

parents suffer asthma. The prevalence in subjects whose parents are not atopic was 8%, 15.8% when one parent was atopic, and when both parents were atopic 28.6%. It is, however, not possible to determine how much can be attributed to genetic predisposition and how much to environment.

Several studies suggest a genetic risk for the development of asthma. Twin studies have shown a 19% concordance for asthma in monozygotic twins and 4.8% for dizygotic twins. Another study of 3808 pairs of twins in Australia found that approximately 60% of asthma was due to genetic effects, and other studies suggest a genetic heritability of airway hyperresponsiveness, even when there is no clinical concordance for asthma. In the past decade, numerous studies confirmed the hereditary component in asthma. With atopy, Koppelman and colleagues reported the highest heritability for specific IgE to derP1 (0.57), followed by an estimate of 0.41 for a positive Phadiatop assay, 0.30 for log eosinophil count, and 0.29 for a positive skin test response to house dust mites (Figure 37.5).

The human genome is composed of approximately 3 billion base pairs and is estimated to contain 60,000 to 80,000 genes. There are two main approaches to identify genes predisposing to disease. The first is termed a *genome scan* in which the entire genome is screened using a panel of polymorphic DNA markers spaced across the genome to identify specific regions linked to specific phenotypes. This is followed by the identification of the gene (or genes) within this region, and polymorphisms within these genes that contribute to the development of the disease. The second of these is the candidate gene approach in which genes, selected for their relevance to the pathophysiology of the disease, are directly tested for their involvement by linkage or association with the disease. This is then followed by the identification of causative mutations or polymorphisms. Performing linkage analysis requires pedigree data of multiple families and knowledge of the mode of inheritance, penetrance, and allele frequencies.

Genome-wide searches have shown evidence that genetic variants associated with asthma and asthma-related traits are present on chromosomes 3, 5, 6, 11, 12, and 20. Interestingly, many of these chromosomes harbor genes that are relevant to the pathogenesis of asthma and atopy. Recent studies have shown that polymorphisms in interleukin (IL)-13, located on chromosome 5q, are associated with an increased risk to have high IgE and airway hyperresponsiveness. IL-13 exerts its effect on IgE production by B cells via the IL-4 receptor. Polymorphisms in the IL-4R have been shown to be associated with airway hyperresponsiveness. It is an interesting observation that interaction of polymorphisms in the IL-13 gene and the IL-4R gene are associated with a fivefold increased risk to the presence of asthma. Recently, chromosome 20p13 was significantly linked to asthma and airway hyperresponsiveness in families with asthma from the United Kingdom and the United States. ADAM33 was identified in this chromosomal region as a candidate gene for asthma and airway hyperresponsiveness. ADAM33 is a member of the family of proteins known as ADAMs (A Disintegrin And Metalloproteinase). ADAM proteins play a role in cell fusion, cell adhesion, cell signaling, and proteolysis. The latter includes the shedding of cytokines, growth factors, or their receptors from the cell surface. Because ADAM33 is expressed in airway smooth muscle cells and lung fibroblasts, it seems a plausible candidate for airway remodeling. This was the first gene discovered in asthma by genome screen and further fine mapping of the chromosomal region. Nevertheless, it is clear that asthma is not a single-gene disease. Therefore, many combinations of small changes in the genome may lead to asthma, with determinants becoming even more complicated with incomplete penetrance. It has still not been determined which genes contribute to the development of asthma, but eventually they will be found. This may result in a better understanding of human physiology and hopefully lead to successful preventive strategies (Figure 37.6).

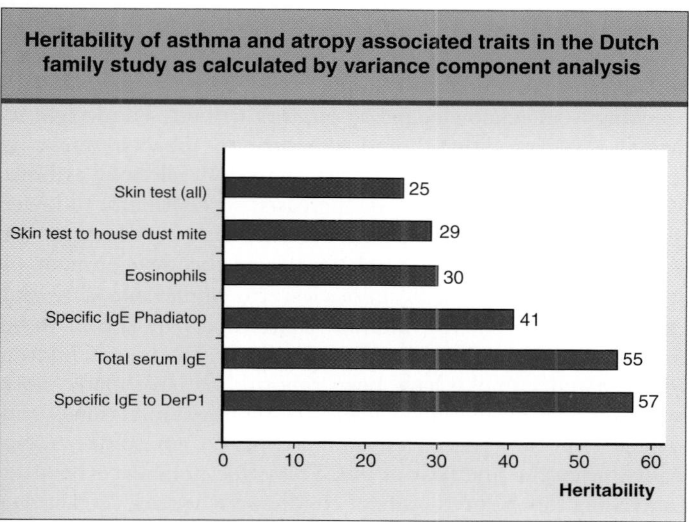

Figure 37.5 Heritability of asthma and atopy associated traits in the Dutch Family study. (From Koppelman G, Stine O, Xu J, et al: Genome-wide search for atopy susceptibility genes in Dutch families with asthma. J Allergy Clin Immunol 109:489-506, 2002.)

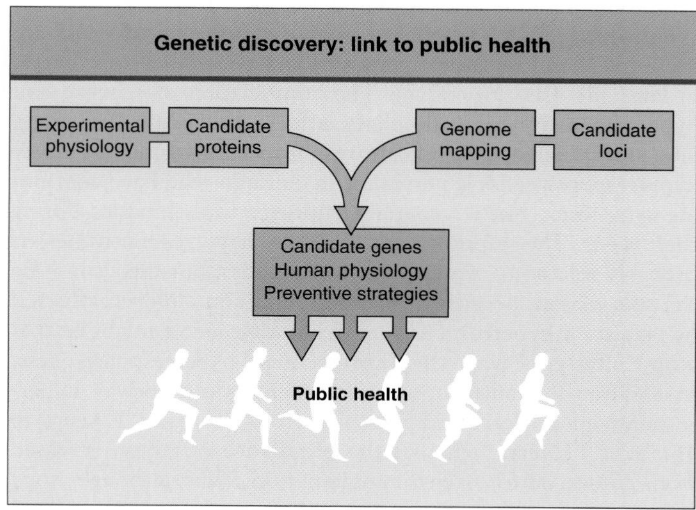

Figure 37.6 Relationship between mapping of the full genome for genes for asthma, whereupon candidate loci are found, and increased knowledge of the physiology, which will lead to the discovery of new proteins. These two lines of research may result in finding the candidate genes of asthma. Thereafter, human physiology has to decipher their role in the development and progression of asthma and finally in the development of new therapeutic strategies.

SEX

Gender affects many aspects associated with the epidemiology of asthma, from birth onward to established asthma. The incidence and prevalence of asthma is higher in boys than girls in childhood and throughout puberty. At adult age the incidence of asthma is higher among females, and specific factors that are associated with female reproduction affect the course and severity of asthma throughout this phase of life. Boys are more susceptible to *in utero* smoke exposure, and have a lower maximal expiratory flow rate at functional residual capacity (FRC) than girls in the first year of life, even with a similar antenatal exposure to cigarettes. This effect seems to persist in the phase of lung function growth during childhood. Furthermore, boys have higher IgE levels at 6 months of age, a known risk factor for asthma, which persists to ages 2 through 4. Lower expiratory flow rates in boys between birth and early adolescence suggest that boys have smaller airways relative to their lung size than girls up to puberty. Similarly, boys have increased muscle tone in the airways as compared with girls. Hospitalization rates from asthma reflect the difference in asthma prevalence as observed between boys and girls. At age 1 year, the hospital admission rate is 5.3 in 1000 for boys and 2.9 in 1000 for girls. At puberty the admission rate begins to equalize and remains similar throughout the teens. The underlying mechanisms of gender differences both in childhood and adult asthma remain unclear.

HYPERRESPONSIVENESS

Both children and adults who have frequent symptoms of asthma invariably show airway hyperresponsiveness to histamine or methacholine, and increased airway responsiveness usually precedes the development of asthma. This has not only been observed in children and young adults, but also in middle-age men not selected for an allergic history. More severe hyperresponsiveness is associated with development of symptoms (Figure 37.7) or of more severe symptoms, and a steeper fall in forced expiratory volume in 1 second (FEV_1). Furthermore, in symptomatic individuals in the population affected by hyperresponsiveness, those who have milder hyperresponsiveness are more likely to lose these symptoms and become asymptomatic in later life (see Fig. 37.7). The combination of wheeze and hyperresponsiveness particularly affects the asthmatic group who suffers ongoing significant respiratory impairment. Airway hyperresponsiveness is persistent in children who have continuing symptoms, but it generally improves in asthmatics during their teens. The improvement in airway hyperresponsiveness is probably related to growing airway diameter, but this cannot be the sole reason, because airways also grow in children affected by persistent hyperresponsiveness. Another factor might be that atopy interferes with the expression of hyperresponsiveness. In children in Southampton, United Kingdom, airway hyperresponsiveness decreased with age from 29.1% at 7 years to 16.5% at 11 years, whereas the prevalence of atopy increased from 26% to 31.6% over the same period. Thus, although atopy is associated with hyperresponsiveness, and the presence of atopy is a risk factor for its development, it does not fully explain its presence. Finally, the importance of persistent airway hyperresponsiveness in predicting ongoing respiratory symptoms has been demonstrated in two long-term epidemiologic studies.

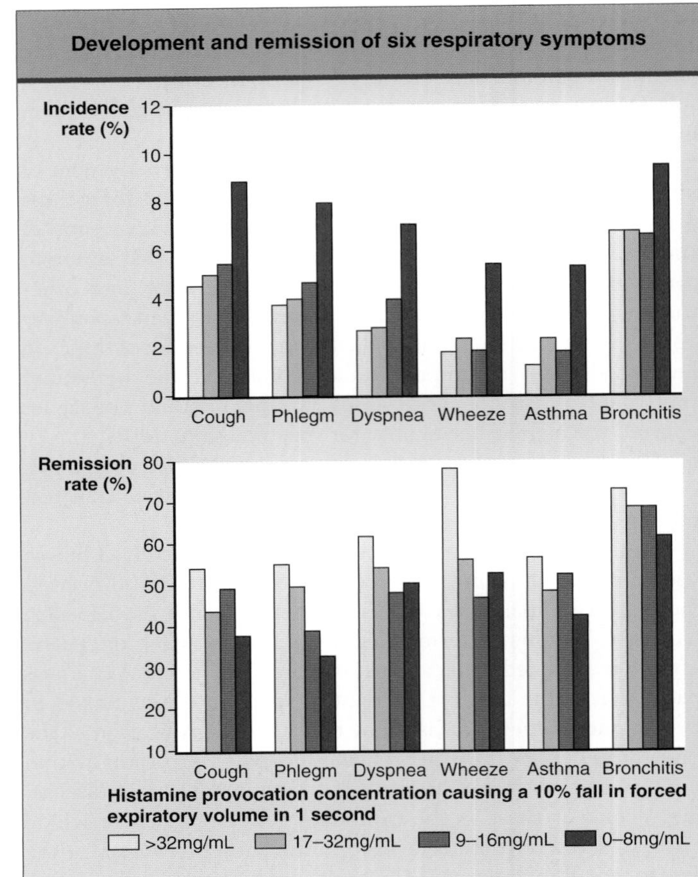

Figure 37.7 Development and remission of six respiratory symptoms. Hyperresponsiveness as a determinant of the development of respiratory symptoms in those who did not have respiratory symptoms. Less severe hyperresponsiveness in individuals who had symptoms predicted a higher likelihood of loss of symptoms (remission). (From Xu X, Rijcken B, Schouten JP, Weiss ST: Airways responsiveness and development and remission of chronic respiratory systems in adults. Lancet 350:1431-1434, 1997.)

SMOKING

Smoking is an acknowledged respiratory irritant. The weight of evidence suggests that home exposure to tobacco smoke is second only to atopy as a major risk factor for childhood asthma. Mechanisms suggested include increased susceptibility to lower respiratory tract infections and increased risk for development of atopy. Thus, parental smoking affects the development of atopy and asthma, and *in utero* cigarette smoke exposure and exposure in the first few months of life especially appear to be risk factors for the development of atopy and asthma. Children whose parents smoke have been reported to have many more problems with wheezing, lower respiratory infections, and asthma than do children of parents who do not smoke, especially during the first year of life. This effect remains even after controlling for the predictors of childhood wheezing such as day care, season of birth, sharing a bedroom, or parental history of childhood respiratory trouble. In Tucson, Arizona exposure to smoke of more than 10 cigarettes a day was associated with a 2.5 times increased risk of development of asthma before the age of 12 years, as was a lower maximal midexpiratory flow among children of women with 12 years or less of education; this association was not present in women with higher education.

The observation that active smoking during adolescence is associated with shortening of the plateau phase of FEV_1—which generally occurs between 20 and 35 years—does suggest an overall negative effect of smoking in adolescence, which may also be present in asthmatics. Further observations show that smoking cessation during adolescence has a positive impact on lung growth.

EARLY RESPIRATORY TRACT INFECTIONS

The relationship between respiratory tract infections and the development of asthma is complex. A number of mechanisms have been proposed to explain how viral infections may induce asthma symptoms. Viral infections damage airway epithelium, cause reflex bronchoconstriction from upper airway inflammation, and cause local airway generation of proinflammatory cytokines; enhanced recruitment of inflammatory cells to the airways accompanied by enhanced mediator release and virus-specific IgE antibody generation may follow. Asthmatic individuals have been reported to have viral infections more frequently. However, atopic infants (eczema and/or positive skin test) have not been reported to have more respiratory infections than nonatopic infants during the first year of life. In a prospective study to investigate risk factors for the development of asthma in childhood, respiratory infections appeared to be important. They had a lasting effect on respiratory symptoms as well as lung function in childhood. Those children whose bronchiolitis was caused by respiratory syncytial virus (RSV) had greater exercise lability than did control children who had the same degree of atopy. Wheeze and airway hyperresponsiveness were also increased in children after RSV bronchiolitis, although the prevalences of recognized and treated asthma, and of atopy, were similar in a control group. Sensitization to the viral agent has been reported to play a role, because production of virus-specific IgE is associated with wheeze for RSV and parainfluenza virus. In addition, viral respiratory tract infections cause exacerbations in asthmatics.

In contrast, some circumstantial evidence also indicates that early respiratory tract infections may be a protective factor. Those who have fewer infections early in life may be prone to increased prevalence of atopic disease, a risk factor for the development of asthma in itself. An inverse relationship between the prevalence of atopy and the number of siblings has been reported. This could be related to increased infections in those who have a large number of older siblings, which thus reduces the tendency to develop atopy—further investigation is required.

ENVIRONMENTAL EXPOSURE

It is now well established that episodes of air pollution increase morbidity from asthma. Prevalence of asthma is increased in polluted areas compared with unpolluted areas in Israel. Among several key studies on air pollution and the development of asthma, one study compared respiratory illness in the former East and West Germany. Children in the more-polluted city of Munich had higher rates of wheezing (20% versus 17%), diagnosed asthma (9.3% versus 7.3%), and hay fever (8.6 versus 2.4%) compared with children in Leipzig. The latter group of children had more bronchitis, 30.9%, versus 15.9% in Munich. These results may be interpreted as air pollution being a risk factor for atopy and asthma, although other explanations for these data have been given (see section on atopy as a risk factor). However, the study is a cross-sectional one. It may well be that environmental air pollution does not increase the prevalence of atopic status, but enhances the development and duration of clinical symptoms among already sensitized subjects. Another risk factor that might interact with exposure to air pollution is hyperresponsiveness. Both factors were found to be of importance in a recent study in The Netherlands, in which children who had both airway hyperresponsiveness and above-median levels of serum total IgE were especially susceptible to air pollution. The effects of air pollution are, however, thought to be smaller than those of indoor environment, because the ISAAC study found no consistent evidence for an effect of industrial air pollution in an area of New Zealand exposed to emissions from paper mills and sulfur fumes.

LEVEL OF PULMONARY FUNCTION

Reduced lung function appears to be a predisposing factor for a first wheezing illness in infants. Martinez and colleagues prospectively studied 124 newborn infants and found that the risk of a wheezing illness was 3.7 times higher among infants whose airway conductance was in the lowest third compared with those in the highest two thirds. Children who had transient wheezing that resolved by the age of 6 years were more likely to have had initially reduced lung function, whereas children in whom asthma persisted were more likely to be atopic and reduced lung function was not a significant factor. Thus, respiratory tract infection may be a risk factor for wheeze, but not for the development of asthma. Both in children and in adults, low levels of FEV_1 appear to be predictive for continuation of wheezing into adulthood and reduced level of lung function in adulthood, as well as for more rapid decline of FEV_1.

BIRTH WEIGHT

With the increasing survival of premature infants and the associated pulmonary problems, the role of prematurity in asthma has come under increasing scrutiny. Prematurity has been reported to be a risk factor for the development of respiratory symptoms later in life. Mothers of premature infants have a higher prevalence of hyperresponsiveness than do mothers of full-term infants. Thus, a genetic or familial factor may have induced respiratory symptoms in premature infants, but prematurity itself was not the cause. A family history of asthma, but not of nonasthmatic allergies, was identified as a predictor for children who have respiratory distress syndrome developing bronchopulmonary dysplasia in one study, but not in another. Other investigators reported that low birth weight and prematurity, regardless of neonatal respiratory disease, are associated with decreased flow rates and airway conductance in childhood. A recent study in Austria reported that low birth weight, a low level of maternal education, and a larger family size predicted a decrease in level of most lung function parameters in children between ages 7.5 and 11 years, which confirmed results obtained in the United Kingdom in 1993. This effect could result from gestational age itself, but even after adjustment for

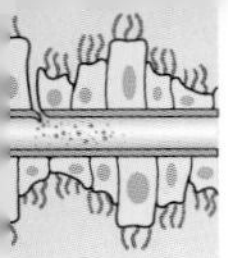

this, birth weight remained a major risk factor for reduced lung function. Below a birth weight of 2 kg (4.4 lb), children had more problems with cough but not wheeze compared with age-matched schoolmates.

DIET

Eating fish more than once a week had a protective effect on the development of asthma in Australian children. After adjusting for gender, country of birth, ethnicity, atopy, respiratory infection in the first 21 years of life, and a parental history of asthma, children who ate fresh oily fish with greater than 2% fat had a reduced risk for current asthma. Furthermore, an increased prevalence of methacholine responsiveness was reported in children and adults who had a higher salt intake. Studies on salt intake in adults are less consistent, and the influence of sodium in the development of asthma remains unclear.

In a prospective study in more than 77,000 women, vitamin E appeared to be protective against asthma, but only when increased intake was part of a diet and not when given as a supplement, which suggests that other factors might be responsible for the observed protective effect.

OCCUPATIONAL EXPOSURE

Some studies show that toluene diisocyanate exposure may induce asthma, and that the longer the exposure, the less likely is the asthma to remit after stopping exposure. Occupational asthma may account for a considerable part of the total burden of asthma in a population—some 15% of all cases of asthma in Japan are attributed to occupational causes. However, in Western countries, the numbers are far lower. In some industries more than 30% of the workers develop asthma; in others, the numbers are low or even zero. The level of allergen exposure and the presence of atopy appear to be risk factors in animal workers.

PROTECTIVE FACTORS AGAINST ASTHMA

A study investigated East German children (5 to 14 years old) in 1992 and found that the later children went into day care before the age of 2, the higher the prevalence of atopy. Since then many studies have investigated the so-called "hygiene hypothesis" (i.e., whether protective effects exist by early infectious exposure for the development of asthma). It has been shown many times that the development of atopy and asthma is less common among children with more exposure to other children at home or in day care during the first 6 months of life. This has been extended in that children living in farming families had less atopy than those in nonfarming families in the same area of the country. These observations have been reconciled in the hypothesis that a child's exposure to concentrations of bacterial components that are present in stables or come about with respiratory infections, such as endotoxins, may stimulate the immune system into a Th1 direction (i.e., a protective way to allergy development).

Pitfalls and Controversies

Asthma is like love. Everyone knows what it is, but its definition is difficult. This brings about the big pitfall in epidemiologic studies on asthma. A simple statement that wheeze equals asthma would provide an overrepresentation of wheezers in childhood under the heading of asthma. It has been clearly shown in epidemiologic longitudinal studies that many children younger than 5 years of age lose their wheeze and do not represent asthmatics. However, at an older age, asthma is likely to be overdiagnosed in females, because doctors label older smoking females less commonly as having chronic obstructive pulmonary disease. Furthermore, asthma characteristically has periods of symptom remission, and signs may not be present when patients are interviewed or investigated. Many surveys do not include lung function measurements for logistic reasons, and, often, objective validation of the diagnosis has not been performed. Only with objective measures can one establish the incidence and prevalence of asthma. Yet one has to realize that even lung function tests do not detect ongoing airway inflammation in subjects who have lost their asthma symptoms.

There is still uncertainty as to which genes are involved in the development of asthma. However, the same pitfalls that exist for asthma prevalence and incidence exist for genetic studies. This is why one prefers not only an overall diagnosis of asthma in genetic studies, but also an association with objective phenotypes closely linked to asthma.

There is agreement that allergen and smoke exposure may contribute to the development of atopy and asthma. For many factors mentioned previously, it is unclear whether they contribute similarly to the development of atopy as of asthma. Controversy exists whether preventive measures directed at allergen avoidance will change the prevalence of asthma. Furthermore, there is uncertainty whether early exposure to endotoxin indeed has a causal chain with prevention of asthma and atopy. Future studies have also to elucidate whether preventive environmental measures with or without early institution of anti-inflammatory treatment will prevent the development of asthma and the persistence of asthma into adulthood. Studies are under way and are eagerly awaited.

SUGGESTED READINGS

Gregg I: Epidemiological aspects. In Clark TJH, Godfrey S (eds): Asthma. London, Chapman and Hall, 1983, pp 242-284.

Grol MH, Gerritsen J, Postma DS: Asthma: From childhood to adulthood. Allergy 51:855-869, 1996.

Landau LI: Risks of developing asthma. Pediatr Pulmonology 22:314-318, 1996.

Martinez FD, Morgan WJ, Wright AL, et al: Diminished lung function as a predisposing factor for wheezing respiratory illness in infants. N Engl J Med 319:1112-1117, 1988.

Meijer B, Bleecker ER, Postma DS: Genetics. In Barnes PJ, Rodger IW, Thomson NC (eds): Asthma. Basic mechanisms and clinical management. London, Academic Press, 1998, pp 35-46.

Peat JK: The rising trend in allergic illness: Which environmental factors are important? Clin Exp Allergy 24:797-800, 1994.

Sears MR: Worldwide trend in asthma mortality. Bull Int Lung Dis 166:79-83, 1991.

Strachan DP, Cook DG: Parental smoking and childhood asthma: Longitudinal and case-control studies. Thorax 53:204-212, 1998.

The International Study of Asthma and Allergies in Childhood (ISAAC) Steering Committee: Worldwide variation in prevalence of symptoms of asthma, allergic rhinoconjunctivitis, and atopic eczema: ISAAC. Lancet 351:1225-1232, 1998.

Weeke ER, Pedersen PA: Allergic rhinitis in a Danish general practice. Allergy 36:375-379, 1981.

Xu X, Rijcken B, Schouten JP, Weiss ST: Airways responsiveness and development and remission of chronic respiratory symptoms in adults. Lancet 350:1431-1434, 1997.

CHAPTER 38 Asthma: Cell Biology

Sandra van Wetering, Pieter S. Hiemstra, and Klaus F. Rabe

Since the first clinical definition of bronchial asthma by Henry Salter in 1859, the perception of and knowledge about asthma have changed dramatically. Pathology studies as early as 1922 by Huber and Koessler indicated that asthma is an inflammatory disorder, and with the recognition of the role of airway hyperreactivity, more insight has been gained into the cell biology of this disease. It is now widely recognized that gene–environment interactions lead to the early development of inflammatory changes in the susceptible individual. Early events involve dendritic cells (DCs) and T cells. At later stages, leukocytes such as eosinophils and possibly neutrophils orchestrate inflammation, whereas subsequently myofibroblasts and smooth muscle cells predominate and become functionally more relevant, particularly in more severe disease. In this chapter, we describe the current knowledge and concepts surrounding the progression from early events to chronic disease.

EARLY EVENTS

Dendritic Cells

DCs are the most potent antigen-presenting cells and are strategically located at places where maximal exposure to allergen occurs, such as the skin, gut, and airways. Studies in humans have shown an extensive network of DCs residing in the epithelial layer of the upper and lower airways and in the alveoli. When DCs enter the lung, they display an immature phenotype that is geared toward uptake of inhaled antigen, such as allergens, viruses, and bacteria (Fig. 38.1). Subsequently, the migratory capacity of DCs allows them to transport ingested antigens to the T-cell area of the draining lymph nodes. DCs that reach the lymph nodes are fully matured and display the unique capacity to stimulate naive T-helper (Th) cells and subsequently induce polarization into either a Th1 or Th2 phenotype. In addition, they can activate resting or memory T cells that have previously encountered antigen. Two subsets of DCs are distinguished that, because of the release of mediators during antigen presentation, determine the polarization of naive Th cells. Type I, or myeloid, DCs release interleukin (IL)-12, which preferentially causes naive T cells to differentiate into Th1 cells, and type II, or plasmacytoid, DCs release IL-10, which favors differentiation into Th2 cells.

In asthma, it appears that the number of DCs is increased, which may contribute to the Th2-dominant phenotype. Elevated numbers of plasmacytoid DC have been described in blood, the epithelium, and the subepithelial lamina propria of both atopic and nonatopic asthmatic subjects. There is also evidence that significant numbers of DCs migrate to the airway epithelium during an inflammatory response induced by a broad spectrum of stimuli, and that they are involved in the development of chronic eosinophilia in response to inhaled allergens. There are a few possible explanations as to why DCs are increased in asthma, and especially in atopic asthma. Elevated levels of chemokines and mediators such as RANTES (regulated upon activation, normal T-cell expressed and secreted), monocyte chemoattractant proteins (MCP) 1 through 4, eotaxin, and platelet-activating factor have been described in the asthmatic airway. These agents attract not only inflammatory cells but also DCs. In addition, monocytes appear in the airways and may be able to differentiate into DCs in response to IL-4 and granulocyte–macrophage colony-stimulating factor (GM-CSF), cytokines that are increased in asthma.

The question remains as to what determines the DCs to induce a specific T-cell response. Although it is recognized that microbial products such as lipopolysaccharides stimulate DCs to induce a Th1 response, the factors that are involved in inducing a Th2 response are still unclear. One possibility is that atopic patients are (genetically) deficient in IL-12 production or IL-12 responsiveness. Another explanation might be that the local environment of the lung favors Th2 development because epithelial cells secrete IL-10 and prostaglandin E_2 (PGE_2), which are known to downregulate IL-12 production. Finally, recent experimental studies raise the possibility that, owing to exposure to allergens at low concentrations, fewer numbers of DCs reach the lymph nodes. As a result, a low T-cell–DC interaction may occur, thereby modulating the Th2 response.

T Cells

T-helper cells are activated in response to antigen presentation with the relevant major histocompatibility complex class II molecules and costimulatory signals. Depending on their cytokine profile induced by antigenic stimulation, they are divided into two subtypes: CD4+ Th1 cells, which predominantly express interferon (IFN)-γ and IL-2, and CD4+ Th2 cells, which preferentially express IL-4 and IL-5. Recently, a third CD4+ subtype has been identified, designated the Th3 cell or regulatory T cell, that secretes high levels of immunosuppressive cytokines, such as transforming growth factor (TGF)-β and IL-10. For asthma pathogenesis, a central role is attributed to the CD4+ Th2 cell. Activated Th2 cells, as well as elevated levels of IL-4, IL-5, and IL-13, are present in bronchial biopsies and bronchoalveolar lavage (BAL) samples obtained from both atopic and nonatopic asthmatic subjects. Also, various studies report increased T-cell activation in intrinsic and occupational asthma. In general, T-cell activation and the preferential production of IL-4 and IL-5 are

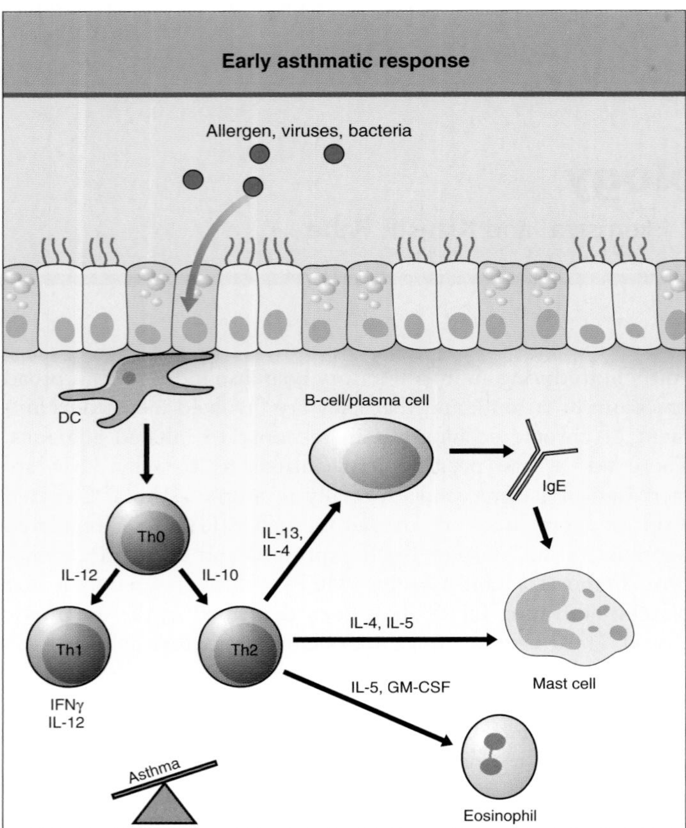

Figure 38.1 Early inflammatory events in asthma. On antigen encounter, dendritic cells (DC) are activated and induce the differentiation of T-helper 0 (Th0) cells into either Th1 or Th2 cells. In asthmatic subjects, this process leads to a preferential differentiation into a Th2 phenotype. These Th2 cells may mediate a wide range of events that contribute to the (allergic) inflammatory response, such as immunoglobulin E (IgE) production, mast cell development, and maturation and activation of eosinophils. GM-CSF, granulocyte–macrophage colony-stimulating factor; IFN, interferon; IL, interleukin.

found to correlate with eosinophil influx, asthma severity, and airway hyperreactivity. The elevated numbers of T cells and their secreted products are able to influence a wide range of events that contribute to the chronic (allergic) inflammatory response. These include immunoglobulin (Ig) E production, mast cell development, activation and maturation of eosinophils, airway hyperreactivity, and mucus hypersecretion.

In normal subjects, inhalation of allergens may result in production of IFN-γ, which characterizes the Th1 response. However, in (allergic) asthmatic subjects, inhalation of allergens results in a typical Th2 response. The reasons for this dominant Th2 response in asthma are still unclear. However, a shift from Th1 to Th2 could be the result of an increase in factors stimulating and/or a decrease in factors inhibiting this skewing process. This has been put forward as the rationale for the so-called "hygiene hypothesis". This hypothesis is based on the proposition that the increase in allergy and asthma in the past few decades is due to the Western lifestyle (e.g., clean environment, vaccinations, and antibiotics), where there is a limited exposure to bacterial and viral antigens during early childhood. This may lead to insufficient stimulation of Th1 cells, which in turn cannot counterbalance the expansion of Th2 cells, thus predisposing to allergy. This hypothesis is supported by observations such as those showing that bacterial colonization prevents atopic sensitization in 1-year-old infants, and that atopy and asthma are less common in people frequently exposed to fungi and viruses. This may also explain why an agricultural lifestyle, with increased exposure to microbial products that stimulate Th1 responses, is protective against the development of hay fever and allergic asthma. Although this explanation for the hygiene hypothesis is attractive, it does not explain the general increase in autoimmune disorders over the past few decades that has occurred in parallel with the increase in allergy and asthma. This is important because autoimmune disorders, which have also been associated with the hygiene hypothesis, are associated more closely with Th1 than Th2 responses. Alternative explanations come from observations such as those showing that asthma is quite uncommon in people who have worm infestations, despite the fact that the helminth parasite induces a Th2 response. However, the infection also induces high levels of IL-10, which is known to inhibit T-cell activation and switches B cells from IgE to IgG production. Indeed, various studies demonstrated that administration of IL-10 in mice models reduces airway eosinophilia and infiltration of DCs and lowers the levels of Th2 cytokines. This points to a role for the recently discovered regulatory T-cell subset that is known to secrete IL-10 and TGF-β, which may act to suppress inflammatory responses in allergy and asthma, as well as in autoimmune disorders.

Macrophages

Macrophages are released from the bone marrow as monocytes and continue to differentiate in tissue. They migrate to the lung in response to inhaled substances that are ingested and—if possible—destroyed. Macrophages are the most prominent cell type recovered by BAL in both nonasthmatic and asthmatic subjects. The role of macrophages in asthma is incompletely understood, but their role as antigen-presenting cells is probably limited, and alveolar macrophages have even been suggested to suppress immune responses to inhaled antigens because of their ability to release IL-10. Alveolar macrophages express the low-affinity IgE receptor that appears to be increased in patients with asthma. Furthermore, macrophages secrete a large variety of mediators that can induce bronchoconstriction, cell recruitment, and activation of other cell types, including mast cells.

INFLAMMATORY EVENTS

Recruitment of inflammatory cells is one of the first essential steps in perpetuating the inflammatory response. Inflammatory cells contribute to the pathologic process of asthma either directly, by releasing mediators that stimulate other cells to proliferate or release components such as extracellular matrix (ECM) proteins, or indirectly by stimulating other local inflammatory cells. Furthermore, inflammatory cells are capable of directly damaging surrounding tissue because of their cytotoxic potential (Fig. 38.2).

Eosinophils

A defining characteristic of asthma is the presence of eosinophils, which for a long time were considered to be the critical effector cell in the pathogenesis of asthma. A large

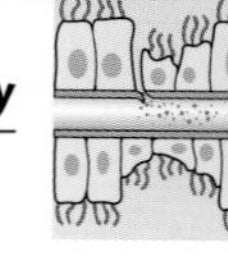

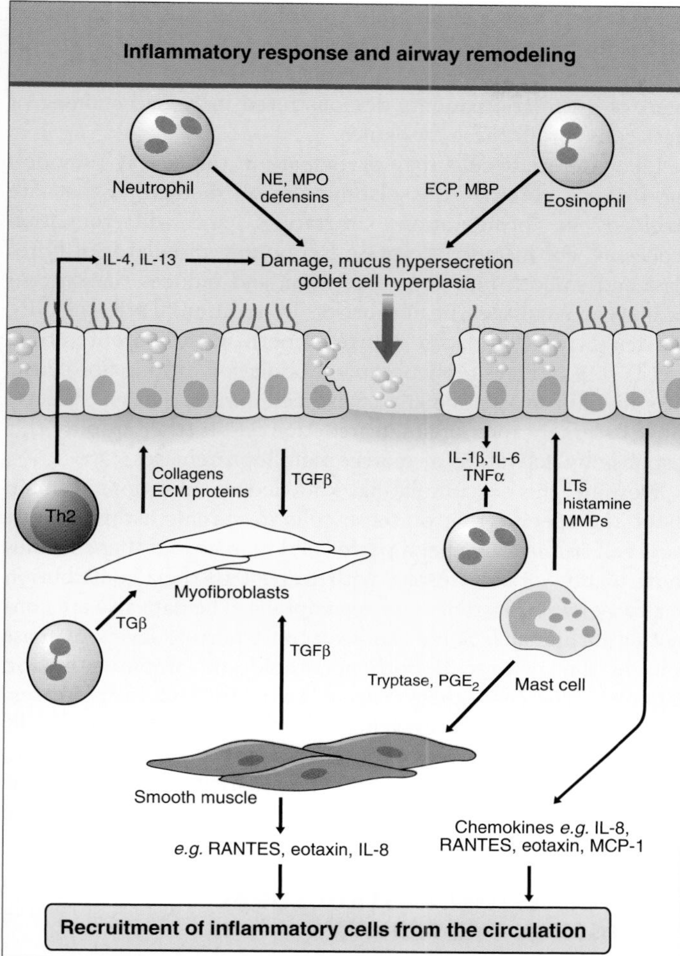

Figure 38.2 Inflammatory response and airway remodeling in asthma. Schematic representation showing the complex interaction between inflammatory cells and resident cells, resulting in enhanced airway inflammation and airway remodeling. The latter process is characterized by processes such as extracellular matrix (ECM) production, epithelial damage, and mucous differentiation. ECP, eosinophilic cationic protein; IL, interleukin; LT, leukotriene; MBP, major basic protein; MCP, monocyte chemoattractant protein; MMP, matrix metalloproteinase; MPO, myeloperoxidase; NE, neutrophil elastase; PGE_2, prostaglandin E_2; RANTES, regulated upon activation, normal T-cell expressed and secreted; TGF, transforming growth factor; TNF, tumor necrosis factor.

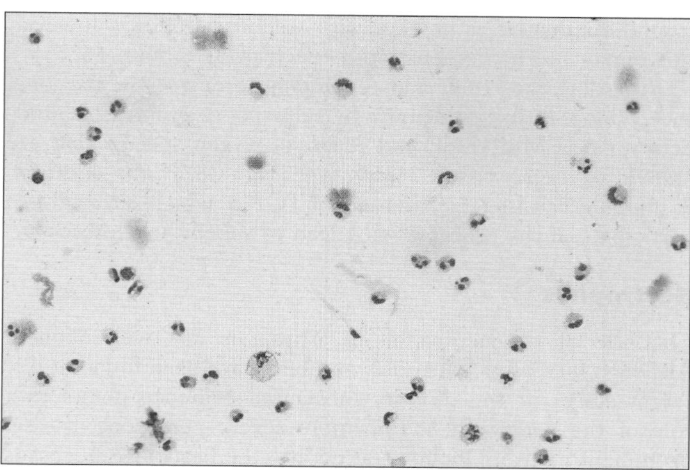

Figure 38.3 Sputum of asthmatic subjects obtained after sputum induction by hypertonic saline (a noninvasive method to study airway inflammation) contains high numbers of eosinophils.

number of studies have demonstrated increased numbers of eosinophils in BAL, peripheral blood, and bronchial biopsies obtained from asthmatic subjects, and these were found to correlate with disease severity and airway hyperreactivity. Elevated levels of toxic cationic eosinophil degranulation products, such as eosinophilic cationic protein (ECP) and major basic protein (MBP), have been found in bronchial biopsies and BAL of asthmatic subjects, indicating that the eosinophils are in an activated state. Finally, increased eosinophil numbers have been described in the late asthmatic response. To demonstrate airway inflammation with eosinophilia in asthma, standardized noninvasive methods such as sputum induction (sputum production induced by inhalation of hypertonic saline) are now available (Fig. 38.3). Eosinophils mature in the bone marrow under influence of cytokines released by Th2 cells, such as IL-2, IL-3, IL-4, IL-5, and GM-CSF. In atopic patients with asthma, elevated levels of these cytokines in both BAL and bronchial biopsies have been found, in particular during the late-phase response to allergen challenge. In this context, IL-5 was found to be the key cytokine responsible for the recruitment, survival, and activation of eosinophils. Recent evidence suggests also that the family of chemokines that specifically bind to the CCR3 receptor are involved in causing eosinophilia. Members of this family include eotaxins 1, 2, and 3, MCP-2, -3, and -4, RANTES, and macrophage inflammatory protein-1α. Eotaxins are of special interest because they are the only chemokines specific for eosinophils and their levels are increased in allergen-induced eosinophilia.

Despite the classic view of asthma as an eosinophil-dominated disease, a growing body of evidence questions the direct causal association between eosinophilic inflammation and airway responsiveness. Large observational studies have shown only a weak correlation between induced sputum eosinophilia and airway responsiveness to methacholine in atopic subjects. Furthermore, studies with anti–IL-5 monoclonal antibodies have shown an effective reduction in eosinophil counts in peripheral blood and sputum, without any effect on the late response or on the severity of asthma reactivity. Similarly, administration of IL-12, which preferentially drives T-cell differentiation to a Th1 rather than a Th2 phenotype, reduces eosinophil numbers without affecting the increased response of the airways to contractile stimuli. These observations suggest that there is an "eosinophil-independent" component of airway hyperreactivity or that other, yet unknown, components of the inflammatory response that are closely linked to the eosinophilic response are involved.

Although eosinophilia is a characteristic of asthma, not all asthmatic subjects display eosinophilic inflammation. In 10% to 20% of patients with asthma, there is no increase in sputum eosinophilia, but these patients have elevated numbers of neutrophils in their sputum. The reason for this is unclear, but because eosinophil inflammation is closely related to a Th2 pattern of cytokine production, it is suggested that in "neu-

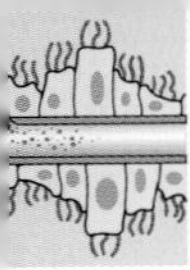

trophil-dominated asthma" a Th1 response occurs. However, this remains to be demonstrated conclusively in humans.

Regarding the repair and remodeling processes in the lung, the eosinophil may contribute by releasing degranulation products such as MBP, ECP, and reactive oxygen species that are known to cause tissue injury (see Fig. 38.2). In addition, eosinophils release large amounts of TGF-β, which is thought to participate in the processes that lead to subepithelial fibrosis.

Neutrophils

The role of the neutrophil in asthma is less well defined. Although increased neutrophil numbers have been found at different stages of the disease, substantial evidence points to a role of the neutrophil in the more severe persistent disease. Prominent neutrophilic infiltration into the bronchial mucosa is reported in fatal asthma and during exacerbations. Elevated numbers of neutrophils as well as increased levels of the neutrophil chemoattractant chemokine IL-8 also have been found in the BAL of patients with chronic severe asthma, which suggests that in this condition IL-8 is involved in neutrophil recruitment and activation. The significance of this neutrophilia is still poorly understood. One hypothesis is that neutrophil-dominated inflammation is resistant to corticosteroid treatment, which is explained by the sustained elevation of IL-8 and neutrophils in severe persistent asthma, despite treatment. On the other hand, it might be possible that, in severe asthma, steroid treatment enhances neutrophilia because of the inhibitory effect of steroids on neutrophil apoptosis. Finally, it has been suggested that the increased influx of neutrophils is due to ongoing inflammation, which starts with epithelial injury and release of IL-8 by various cell types, leading to subsequent attraction and activation of neutrophils. In turn, neutrophils can contribute to the inflammatory response and remodeling process based on their ability to release proteolytic enzymes or peptides (matrix metalloproteinases, elastase, defensins), lipid mediators (leukotriene B 4), reactive oxygen species, and proinflammatory cytokines (tumor necrosis factor [TNF]-α, IL-1β, IL-6). Indeed, release of neutrophil-derived mediators such as neutrophil elastase is associated with increasing asthma severity and suggests a role for neutrophils in airway injury in chronic persistent asthma.

Mast Cells

Mast cells are important secretory cells distributed widely throughout the bodily tissues, particularly near epithelial surfaces. Mast cells represent only a small proportion of the cells recovered by BAL, but comprise 20% of the inflammatory cells localized in airway tissue. They play an important role in innate and specific immunity, including IgE-mediated allergy and inflammation. Because they express the high-affinity Fc receptor for IgE, mast cells play a key role in the early events that follow allergen inhalation in asthma. Interaction of (allergen-specific) IgE with mast cells occurs predominantly through these receptors. Exposure to allergen then leads to rapid (within minutes) release of prestored or newly synthesized mediators such as histamine, tryptase, cytokines, leukotrienes, and prostaglandins. This initiates and maintains a series of cellular events, including bronchoconstriction and activation of other inflammatory and resident cells.

Mast cells may also directly contribute to the chronicity of asthma by the release of cytokines, such as IL-3, IL-4, IL-5, IL-6, and TNF-α. Immunohistochemical analysis of biopsy specimens of asthmatic patients demonstrated increased staining of mast cells for all these cytokines.

Likewise, mast cells may participate in the airway remodeling process through the elaboration of mediators that are involved in proliferation, migration, and differentiation processes. For instance, tryptase is a potent stimulator of fibroblast and smooth muscle proliferation and induces the synthesis of type I collagen in fibroblasts. In addition, TNF-α, PGE_2, and leukotriene D 4 can induce smooth muscle proliferation, and TGF-β induces a phenotypic modulation of lung fibroblasts into myofibroblasts. Finally, mast cell proteases can directly cause basement membrane degradation and further amplify this response by activation of matrix metalloproteinases.

Despite this accumulating knowledge, questions remain about the specific role of these cells in chronic asthma. Most mast cell studies have been performed in mice and these studies show highly variable results with respect to their contribution to airway hyperreactivity and eosinophilia. The data also are conflicting in humans. Some studies report normal levels of mast cells in the airways of both nonatopic and atopic asthmatic patients, whereas others report two- to sixfold increases. However, there is also evidence that the number of mast cells is increased in the airways of both asthmatic adults and children, which correlates with bronchial hyperreactivity. Furthermore, it appears that in chronic asthma mast cell degranulation is more pronounced compared with nonasthmatic subjects.

CHRONIC ASTHMA—STRUCTURAL CHANGES IN THE AIRWAYS

During the development of asthma, structural changes in the airways and adjacent tissue occur. These changes, which are referred to in general as *airway remodeling*, are described in the following section. Although the pathophysiologic consequences of airway remodeling remain to be fully established, clinically it leads to an increased thickness of the airway wall, contributing to exaggerated airway narrowing, hyperreactivity, and reduced baseline caliber.

Bronchial Epithelium

The bronchial epithelium forms a physical barrier between the external environment and the inner milieu of the lung, and therefore its integrity is essential for airway defense. In asthma, epithelial desquamation is historically considered to be a hallmark of the disease. Evidence of epithelial damage and shedding has been reported in bronchial biopsies and in postmortem studies. Furthermore, extensive loss of columnar cells, shown as clumps in sputum (Creola bodies), and increased presence of epithelial cells in BAL fluid have been described. Evidence is accumulating that in asthma epithelial cells exhibit a more "fragile" phenotype, resulting in increased injury. Nevertheless, it has been suggested that the epithelial disruption observed in bronchial biopsies in asthma is due to the bronchoscopic procedure itself causing epithelial injury to the fragile epithelium.

A major cause of epithelial damage in asthma is thought to result from the release of products by eosinophils and macrophages, although other inflammatory cells also can induce tissue injury. In addition, environmental agents such as cigarette smoke and air pollutants may cause tissue injury. In response to injury, the epithelium normally reacts with a mitotic response that leads to repair and restoration of normal structure and function. Among the signals that regulate epithelial repair, the epidermal growth factor (EGF) family of growth factors (including EGF, heparin-binding EGF-like growth factor, and TGF-α) and their receptors (e.g., EGF receptor [EGFR]) are of particular importance. In asthma, there is some evidence that, despite the enhanced expression of EGF and EGFR in the asthmatic airway, the mitogenic response is disturbed. It is thought that, as a consequence, the epithelium remains in a repair and proinflammatory phenotype. This is demonstrated by increased activation of transcription factors (signal transducer and activator of transcription-1 [STAT1], activator protein-1 [AP-1], nuclear factor [NF]-κB) and enhanced release of proinflammatory cytokines, chemokines, and growth factors. These mediators may either directly or indirectly influence the behavior of cells located on or directly underneath the basement membrane, such as fibroblasts and myofibroblasts, and may induce recruitment of inflammatory cells. Communication between epithelial cells and these mesenchymal cells is reminiscent of airway "remodeling" during embryonic development and has led to the proposal of the epithelial–mesenchymal trophic unit (EMTU). It has been suggested that in the asthmatic airways, the EMTU either remains activated after birth, or is reactivated again during the onset of asthma and drives the airway remodeling process.

Another epithelial remodeling response that is frequently observed in asthma is goblet cell hyperplasia and mucus hypersecretion. Mucins, produced by goblet cells of the surface epithelium and submucosal glands, contribute to the host defense by trapping inhaled particles that are subsequently removed from the airways by ciliary clearance and the cough reflex. However, when secreted in excess, mucins may also be an important cause of airway narrowing. Most asthmatic patients produce sputum, especially during or after an exacerbation, and mucus plugs are almost always found in patients with fatal asthma (Fig. 38.4). As can be expected, the increased mucus release is associated with goblet cell hyperplasia. Although goblet cell hyperplasia is a prominent feature in fatal asthma, it is not restricted to severe disease because recent studies in bronchial biopsies from patients with mild to moderate asthma also show a threefold increase in goblet cell number and stored mucin volume compared with control subjects.

The mechanisms underlying goblet cell hyperplasia and mucus hypersecretion are not precisely understood. Animal studies, predominantly in mice, are now beginning to delineate the involvement of Th2 cytokines (IL-4, IL-9, and IL-13), which, when overexpressed in vivo, can induce goblet cell hyperplasia and mucus hypersecretion. Also, the EGFR is proposed as a key player in goblet cell hyperplasia and mucus hypersecretion because of its ability to initiate intracellular signaling pathways that lead to increased mucin synthesis and elevated numbers of goblet cells.

Subepithelial Membrane

Thickening of the subepithelial reticular basement membrane (also called the lamina reticularis) is a characteristic feature of the asthmatic lung and occurs early in the disease process, presumably as early as childhood in early-onset asthma. The thickening is due to an increased deposition of collagens (types I and III) and fibronectin and leads to so-called subepithelial fibrosis. The cellular origin of these matrix components is incompletely understood, but the myofibroblasts, which form a specialized network underneath the lamina reticularis and have increased numbers in asthma, are probably involved (see Fig. 38-2). Despite the increased thickening of the lamina reticularis, the significance of this event in asthma is unclear. Some studies report a correlation between subepithelial fibrosis and severity and duration of the disease, whereas others do not find such a correlation. Subepithelial fibrosis has also been observed in patients with nonasthmatic rhinitis who present with eosinophilia, and this supports a possible link between eosinophils and subepithelial fibrosis. A recent study in children (ages 5 to 14 years) demonstrated increased collagen deposition in the lamina reticularis that was associated with increased activation of fibroblasts. Because at the time of this study these children (except for one) lacked an eosinophilic infiltrate, it was suggested that subepithelial fibrosis could be used as a diagnostic marker for the early onset of the disease. This was supported by another study showing a thickening of the lamina reticularis several years before asthma could be diagnosed.

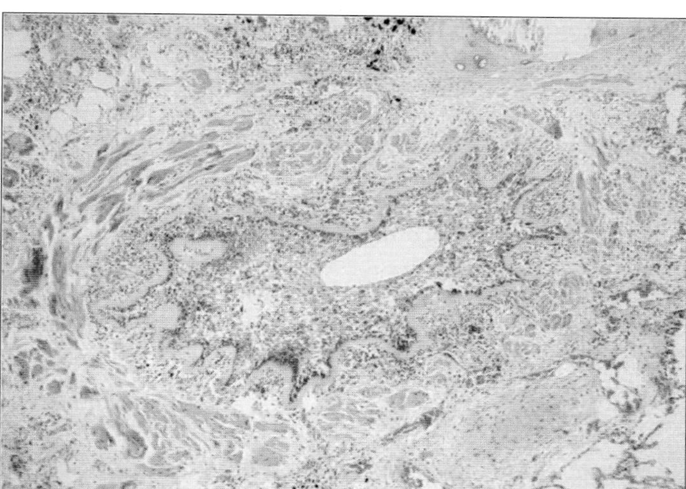

Figure 38.4 Histologic section of a constricted airway of a patient who died from asthma showing sloughing of the epithelium, prominent thickening of the subepithelial basement membrane, infiltration of the mucosa by inflammatory cells, and enlargement of the bronchial smooth muscle area. The airway lumen is filled with cell detritus and mucus plugs obstructing the airways.

Airway Smooth Muscle Cells

Human airway smooth muscle cells (HASM) have been recognized for a long time as being fundamental to asthma and the key effector cells for bronchoconstriction and bronchial hyperreactivity. The first study describing increased smooth muscle layer thickness was published as early as 1922, an observation that was subsequently confirmed by a large number of investigations in both fatal and nonfatal asthma. Smooth muscle cells are generally thought to play a role in airway hyperreactivity and narrowing, both important features in asthma. This is because, in addition to their increased mass, HASM ex vivo also display a more contractile response reflected by an increased sensitivity to bronchospasmogenic stimuli such as histamine, methacholine, and leukotrienes. A recent study further underscores this notion, demonstrating that HASM mass and markers of contractility are increased in severe asthma (Fig. 38.5). The reason for this increase in mass and contractility is still unclear. Various in vitro studies demonstrate smooth muscle cell proliferation in response to a wide range of soluble factors, including growth factors such as EGF. It has been suggested that HASM from asthmatic subjects are more responsive to these mitogenic stimuli. Furthermore, inflammatory cells such as T cells and mast cells may interact with HASM to induce proliferation. Finally, it is suggested that the increased mass can also be due to the increased numbers of myofibroblasts that "adopt" the contractile phenotype (see later).

An additional factor positioning HASM centrally in the process of asthma is their recently discovered synthetic functions. HASM have the potential to participate actively in the inflammatory process by synthesizing chemokines (RANTES, eotaxins, IL-8), cytokines (GM-CSF, IL-11), and prostaglandins, and expressing adhesion molecules (intercellular adhesion molecule-1, vascular cell adhesion molecule-1). In turn, this can lead to attraction and activation of other inflammatory cells, such as T cells, eosinophils, and macrophages. Most of these conclusions are based on in vitro studies. There is only a limited amount of data supporting the immunoregulatory role of HASM in vivo. RANTES expression has been demonstrated in HASM in biopsies from both asthmatic patients and healthy volunteers. Furthermore, increased eotaxin staining is reported in HASM from asthmatic compared with control subjects.

Fibroblasts and Myofibroblasts

Fibroblasts are thought to play an important role in the remodeling process. They are able to form and deposit collagen and other matrix components that make up elastic and reticular fibers. Although they are regarded as fixed cells, they retain the capacity for growth and regeneration and are pluripotent. Increased numbers of fibroblasts are found in the asthmatic airways. They express a more differentiated phenotype and are suggested to be highly responsive to TGF-β, elevated levels of which are found in BAL of asthmatic subjects. This growth factor is known to stimulate fibroblasts to release various ECM proteins, such as collagens, and induces the transformation of fibroblasts into myofibroblasts. It is recognized that myofibroblasts have a higher capacity for collagen synthesis than fibroblasts.

Myofibroblasts were originally discovered in granulation tissue and found to be important for normal wound healing. Later, increased numbers of myofibroblasts were identified in a variety of pathologic conditions, including asthma and pulmonary fibrosis. In asthma, the number of myofibroblasts is increased in the lamina reticularis and is found to correlate with the thickness of the reticular basement membrane and the duration of asthma. The number of myofibroblasts also increases after allergen challenge, and the cells follow a differentiation process that makes them structurally similar to smooth muscle cells.

Despite their increase in asthmatic airways, the contribution of myofibroblasts to asthma is not well understood. Myofibroblasts are suggested to be involved in wound healing because of their ability to cause tissue contraction and release matrix components, both essential for wound closure. It is supposed that the myofibroblasts are important for propagating and amplifying signals from the bronchial epithelium into the deeper layers of the submucosa, through release of various mediators. These include matrix components such as laminin, elastin, and fibronectin, as well as growth factors.

CONCLUSIONS

Increasing knowledge of the cellular biology of bronchial asthma has enabled research into specific interventions to alter the cause of the disease. For example, the recognition of IL-5 as an important component in the recruitment and survival of eosinophils has led to the development of monoclonal antibody strategies.

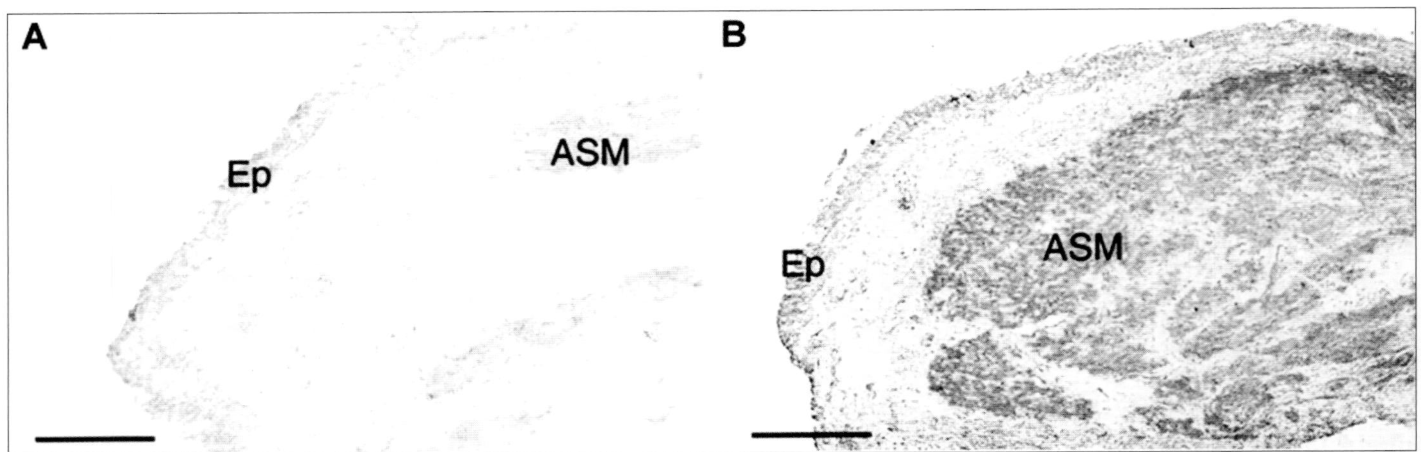

Figure 38.5 Airway remodeling in bronchial biopsies of a control subject (**A**) and a patient with severe asthma (**B**). Biopsy from the control subject shows normal epithelial (Ep) integrity and airway smooth muscle (ASM) area, whereas that of the asthmatic patient shows enlargement of the subepithelial basement membrane and increased ASM content. Scale bar = 200 μm. (Adapted with permission from Benayoun L, Druilhe A, Dombret M, et al: Airway structural alterations selectively associated with severe asthma. Am J Respir Crit Care Med 167:1360-1368, 2003.)

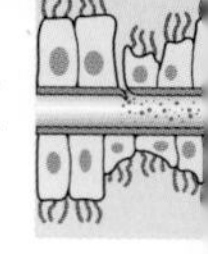

These novel tools have indeed further contributed to the understanding of molecular mechanisms of asthma because blocking of IL-5 has—as predicted—led to the decrease of eosinophils in peripheral blood and sputum of patients with asthma. Very much to the disappointment of researchers, this has so far not translated into significant clinical improvements in patients. These approaches, however, have made possible the introduction of monoclonal antibody therapy into the armamentarium for treatment of asthma; this is further documented by the recent registration of a humanized antibody against IgE for the treatment of this condition.

Several important questions remain with regard to the processes of remodeling in children with asthma. Our conceptual view of remodeling processes taking part only later in the course of the disease probably needs to be questioned. We are still uncertain whether specific processes that we collectively call *remodeling* might occur very early in the disease, and further studies are needed. Equally, our understanding of the role of matrix deposition in the lungs of patients with asthma is also incomplete. Recent studies suggest that deposition of matrix might also have beneficial effects. Inhaled corticosteroids, for example—undoubtedly an effective treatment for asthma—might result in an unexpected increased deposition of selected matrix components, a finding that needs to be elucidated.

Finally, conceptual links between cell biology and clinical asthma have to be made. Atopy, although recognized and described in detail for patients with milder disease and at younger age, might play much less of a role in chronic disease and in older patients. Also, our clinical definition of severity of this disease is not truly reflected in a more severe form of inflammation. It appears that different cellular mechanisms are operative in early disease and in patients with mild forms, whereas more severe asthma might even represent a different disease entity that is predominantly linked to structural changes in which smooth muscle cells, fibroblasts, and myofibroblasts play a significant role.

SUGGESTED READINGS

Bach JF: The effect of infections on susceptibility to autoimmune and allergic diseases. N Engl J Med 347:911-920, 2002.

Benayoun L, Druilhe A, Dombret M, et al: Airway structural alterations selectively associated with severe asthma. Am J Respir Crit Care Med 167:1360-1368, 2003.

Herrick CA, Bottomly K: To respond or not to respond: T cells in allergic asthma. Nat Rev Immunol 3:405-417, 2003.

Huber HL, Koessler KK: The pathology of bronchial asthma. Arch Intern Med 30:687, 1922.

Kay AB: Advances in immunology: Allergy and allergic diseases—first of two parts and Advances in immunology: Allergy and allergic diseases—second of two parts. N Engl J Med 344:30-37 and 109-113, 2001.

Lambrecht BN, Hammad H: The other cells in asthma: Dendritic cell and epithelial cell crosstalk. Curr Opin Pulm Med 9:34-41, 2003.

Leckie MJ, ten Brinke A, Khan J, et al: Effects of an interleukin-5 blocking monoclonal antibody on eosinophils, airway hyper-responsiveness, and the late asthmatic response. Lancet 356:2144-2148, 2000.

Payne DN, Rogers AV, Adelroth E, et al: Early thickening of the reticular basement membrane in children with difficult asthma. Am J Respir Crit Care Med 167:78-82, 2003.

Yazdanbakhsh M, Kremsner PG, van Ree R: Allergy, parasites and the hygiene hypothesis. Science 296:490-494, 2002.

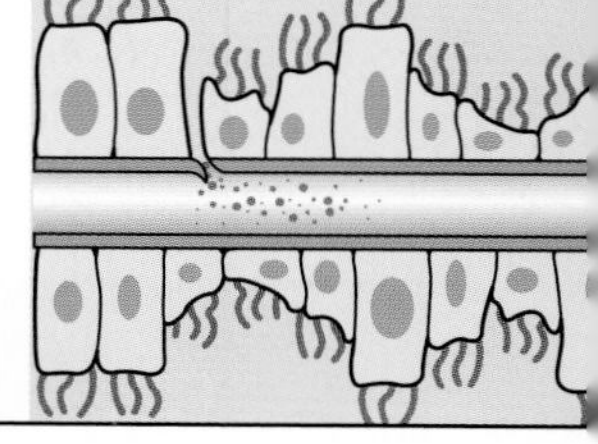

CHAPTER 39 Asthma: Clinical Features, Diagnosis, and Treatment

Martyn R. Partridge

Asthma is a common condition. The clinical features associated with it, however, are not exclusive to it, and objective diagnostic tests are not practical in the very young. Both overdiagnosis and underdiagnosis are likely to be common. Effective treatments for the condition exist, but even if correctly prescribed they are often not taken. As with many long-term medical conditions, asthma represents a challenge to the clinician, but one most likely to be successfully tackled if managed in a partnership with the patient.

The rising prevalence of asthma (see Chapter 37) appears to be associated in some way with civilization, Westernization, or modern living. The population's genetic constitution cannot have changed over the past 20 to 30 years, and so environmental factors must be activating the inherited predisposition to asthma and other atopic diseases in more people now than ever. Studies in Zimbabwe and Ghana show increased frequencies of asthma in richer urban areas compared with rural areas, and in the Far East much higher rates of asthma are found in children who live in Hong Kong than among those of similar genetic constitution who live in the neighboring provinces of Southern China. Although prevalence appears to vary widely from country to country, in no country is the importance of asthma insignificant. In Pakistan, for example, 9% of children of school age have asthma, and health services therefore have to tackle a rising prevalence of this and other "developed country" diseases, while still facing the burden of traditional infectious diseases.

The reasons asthma prevalence is increasing remains unclear. Maternal smoking is associated with an increased risk of the offspring developing a wheezing illness, but there are many other hypothetical causes. Higher rates of asthma occur in populations that take less magnesium and less oily fish in the diet, among those exposed to fewer infections in early life (e.g., the first born in a family), and in those who exhibit less tuberculin skin-test reactivity. Dietary factors, less breastfeeding, and a lack of early life exposure to infections may thus render a genetically susceptible individual more prone to asthma; this enhanced tendency may then be activated by other recent changes in our environment. These might include changes in our homes—in many countries more "closed," less well-ventilated housing allows increased concentrations of allergens or the exhaust gases associated with cooking. Other environmental changes may be those associated with poverty (increased exposure to cockroach allergen in poor housing), chlorine breakdown products in swimming pools, or increased traffic pollution.

The major challenge is that of primary prevention of the condition—that is, to identify what activates asthma in increasing numbers of those born with a genetic susceptibility. Once identified, the hope is that suitable environmental avoidance procedures or vaccines can be used to reduce the prevalence. There is increasing evidence that there might be windows of opportunity for such primary prevention interventions; for example, exposure to domestic pets may be protective against asthma at one stage of fetal or neonatal life and have an adverse effect at a later age. Because primary prevention is not yet possible, the current aim remains restricted to that of secondary prevention—to ensure that those who have asthma benefit from current knowledge and from the treatments available. This involves well-educated health professionals working in a well-organized, adequately funded system, and offering treatment in a manner that makes that treatment likely to be taken. An overview of the scope for both primary and secondary prevention and of the basis of the clinical features of asthma is shown in Figure 39.1.

CLINICAL FEATURES

Asthma is defined in physiologic terms as "a generalized narrowing of the airways, which varies over short periods of time either spontaneously or as a result of treatment." As an airway disorder, asthma's clinical features are common to other airway disorders and may include cough, wheezing, tightness in the chest, and breathlessness, but the key feature is the variability of these symptoms and the tendency for them to be worse at night or in the early morning and to be worse after exercise (Table 39.1). The wheeze arises from vibration of the airway walls, the chest tightness and breathlessness reflect reduced airway caliber, and all of these and the cough reflect underlying airway inflammation and airway hyperresponsiveness (AHR). The factors that underlie the development of inflammation and AHR are shown in Figure 39.1. Characteristic pathologic features include the presence in the airway of inflammatory cells, plasma exudation, edema, smooth muscle hypertrophy, mucus plugging, and shedding of epithelium. Such features may be present even in those who have mild asthma, and the characteristic pathologic changes are frequently present even when no symptoms are found. Not only does the presence of these basic changes mean that clinical symptoms can develop at any time, but increasing indirect evidence also shows that the persistence of such untreated inflammatory change may lead to the airway narrowing becoming "fixed" with time. It is possible that such irreversible change may occur relatively early in the course of the disease.

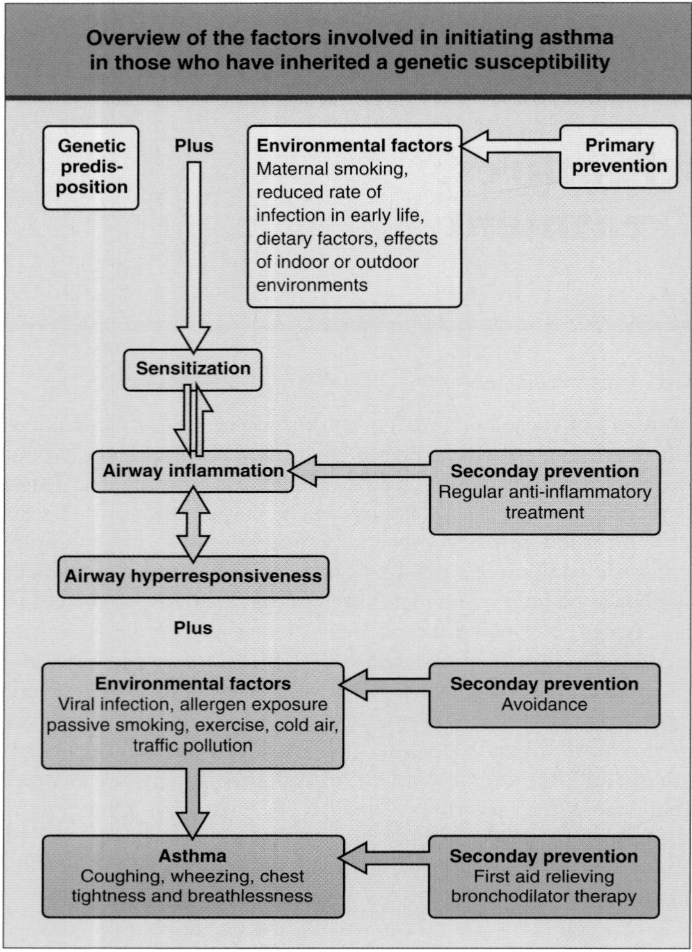

Figure 39.1 Overview of the factors involved in initiating asthma in those who have inherited a genetic susceptibility. The scope is shown for potential primary and secondary interventions.

Table 39.1
Clinical features suggestive of asthma
(Adapted from National Heart, Lung, and Blood Institute.)

Investigation	Outcome
Medical history	Episodic wheezing, chest tightness, shortness of breath, cough Symptoms worsen in presence of aeroallergens, irritants, or exercise Symptoms occur or worsen at night, awakening the patient Patient has allergic rhinitis or atopic dermatitis Close relations have asthma, allergy, sinusitis, or rhinitis
Physical examination	Hyperexpansion of the thorax Sounds of wheezing during normal breathing or a prolonged phase of forced exhalation Increased nasal secretions, mucosal swelling, sinusitis, rhinitis, or nasal polyps Atopic dermatitis/eczema or other signs of allergic skin problem

Table 39.2
Factors that may exacerbate asthma (trigger factors)

Factor	Comment
Smoking	Active and passive
Infections	Especially rhinoviruses, respiratory syncytial virus, influenza virus
Exercise	Especially on cold dry days
Changes in the weather	Thunderstorms
Pollution	Ozone and sulfur dioxide
Allergens	Pet allergens, house dust and house dust mite, cockroach allergens, pollens
Drugs	Aspirin, nonsteroidal anti-inflammatory agents, β-blockers (oral and ophthalmic)
Occupational factors	Dusty work places, 'cold rooms'

Exacerbating Factors (Triggers)

The important risk factors for predisposition to asthma are detailed in Chapter 37. Several of these, and others, can also exacerbate or trigger asthma at some stage; a list is given in Table 39.2.

INFECTIONS

In children, viral infections (especially rhinoviruses, respiratory syncytial virus, and influenza virus) are some of the most common triggers of asthma, and the same most likely applies to adults. The adverse effects of such viruses are likely to be through the release from lung cells of similar chemical mediators as those that occur in asthma and through enhancement of the allergic response. Even in normal subjects, it is possible to demonstrate enhanced airway irritability for several weeks after viral infections, and it is not difficult to imagine how the addition of postviral AHR to the intrinsic AHR of asthma leads to enhanced symptoms.

ALLERGIC TRIGGERS

After an individual is sensitized to an allergen, subsequent re-exposure is likely to worsen that individual's asthma. Common allergens are grass or tree pollen, pets, house dust, and mites. Exposure to only small quantities is sufficient to exacerbate the clinical condition. Although avoidance of allergens is a logical approach attractive to patient and health professional alike, it is, in reality, difficult to achieve. Cat allergen travels widely on other peoples' clothing and is found in circumstances in which cats are not found (e.g., on public transport, in hospital outpatient departments, or in a cinema). Other pet allergens include dogs and small mammals, which may be found not only in the home, but also at school and in the workplace.

Indoor allergens include house dust mites and cockroaches. The former are globally distributed, but it is possible that changes in home design have enhanced exposure in some countries. House dust contains multiple organic and inorganic materials, but the most common domestic mite is the *Dermatophagoides* spp., which feed on human scales. The mites live in soft furnishings and especially thrive in warm, moist surroundings. In other environments, sensitization to cockroach allergen is more common and lifestyle changes (e.g., increased use of central heating) have increased the number of environments in which cockroaches survive and thus enhanced the population's potential exposure to them.

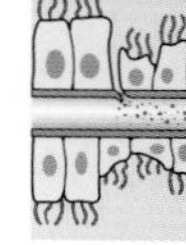

AIR POLLUTION

Most people spend more than 95% of their lives indoors; therefore, the adverse effects of pollutants on the clinical features of asthma involve both indoor and outdoor pollution. Indoor pollutants include nitric oxide, nitrogen oxides, carbon monoxide, sulfur dioxide, carbon dioxide, and volatile organic compounds, which may arise from cooking, heating, or the use of insulation materials and paints. Outdoor pollutants may include visible smog or invisible agents that can damage respiratory epithelium, such as nitrogen oxides, ozone, sulfur dioxide, or particulate matter. The magnitude of the role of these agents in triggering attacks of asthma is unclear. Although they can certainly make asthma worse, the likelihood is that these triggers have significant effects only in those affected by more severe disease. However, it is possible that pollutants have an adverse synergistic effect, such that exposure to atmospheric pollution may enhance the risk of sensitization to allergens to which an individual is simultaneously exposed.

EXERCISE

Exercise is likely to exacerbate or provoke asthma at all ages and in all patients. How prominently exercise is quoted as a trigger depends on the intensity of the exercise and on whether the person with asthma has adjusted his or her lifestyle to avoid this trigger. Exercise-induced asthma is more likely to occur in cold, dry environments (e.g., cross-country running on frosty days) than in a heated indoor swimming pool, and this reflects its likely mechanism—water loss from the airway wall that results in increased osmolarity of surface liquid, which induces mediator release. Knowledge that exercise easily induces asthma has led to its frequent use as a diagnostic test (see the following section).

OCCUPATIONS

Occupational sensitizing agents may be responsible for the initiation of asthma, but certain occupational environments may also worsen the condition in those who already have it, as discussed in Chapter 60. It is essential that the possibility of occupational asthma is considered in all adults presenting for the first time with the disease and in those with unexplained worsening of their condition. Important questions to ask include enquiry as to whether their condition is better when away from work, at weekends, or on holidays.

DRUGS

Some drugs may trigger attacks of asthma. The most severe reactions can be those with β-blocker tablets—topical β-blockers are also used in the treatment of glaucoma and enough may be absorbed from this site to have severe or even fatal effects on airway function. Some studies have shown that just one drop of timolol to each eye may halve spirometry.

Up to 3% of those who suffer asthma may be aspirin sensitive, and aspirin (as well as other nonsteroidal anti-inflammatory agents and possibly biphosphonates) may cause severe attacks. The patient may have previously taken aspirin with impunity, but within minutes to hours of a subsequent ingestion, fatal asthma may occur. Such adverse reactions may be more common in women than men and in those who have nasal polyps, but it can affect anyone who has asthma. However, use of aspirin as a preventive agent in cardiac and cerebrovascular disease is increasingly recognized to be of value. Those with asthma should not in general be denied its use, but any suggestion of worsening of asthma after aspirin use should be taken seriously and further use avoided. Occasionally desensitization to aspirin can be undertaken. It is important to note that aspirin sensitivity is often a marker of more severe asthma, in the same way as is fungal hypersensitivity. Typically patients have rhinosinusitis and nasal polyps with loss of sense of smell and taste and the severity of their asthma often necessitates long-term oral steroid therapy. In one study of more than 145 patients who had required mechanical ventilation for severe asthma, a quarter of them were subsequently shown to be aspirin-sensitive. An additional problem may be cross-reactivity between aspirin sensitivity and use of parenteral hydrocortisone; aspirin-sensitive asthmatics may develop increased airway narrowing if given intravenous hydrocortisone for the treatment of an exacerbation of asthma. Because there is no evidence that parenteral steroids confer any advantage over steroid tablets, use of intravenous steroids should be restricted to those who are unconscious or who may be vomiting or unable to swallow.

PREMENSTRUAL ASTHMA AND ASTHMA IN PREGNANCY

Worsening of symptoms of asthma may occur in women in the premenstrual and menstrual phases. The peak of worsening symptoms occurs 2 to 3 days before menstruation begins and correlates with the late luteal phase of ovarian activity, when circulating progesterone and estrogen levels are at their lowest. Such an association may be overlooked by the patient or doctor unless specifically questioned, and in severe cases hospitalization has been shown to have always occurred around this time in an individual's cycle. For most patients, treatment remains of the standard type, if necessary increased in quantity, but progesterone supplementation (orally and by pessary) is necessary in a minority of patients.

Asthma may worsen, stay the same, or improve during pregnancy. The pattern may be repetitive in subsequent pregnancies. For those who experience a worsening of asthma, this is likeliest in the second and third trimester—but problems during labor are extremely unusual. Treatment for asthma should be the same during pregnancy as in the nonpregnant state, except that leukotriene antagonists should not be initiated during pregnancy. In the absence of appropriate advice, those with asthma may stop their medication on discovering they are pregnant, and it is important that pregnant women are reassured as to the safety of usual asthma therapies—both routine and those used for treatment of exacerbations. After delivery, breastfeeding should be encouraged; none of the commonly used asthma medications are secreted in breast milk to the degree that any alteration in treatment is necessary.

ASSOCIATED CLINICAL CONDITIONS

Several important conditions may exacerbate asthma or cause chronic deterioration or occur in association with it.

Rhinosinusitis

Asthma frequently coexists with rhinosinusitis; the latter may make asthma worse but also impair the patient's and health professional's assessment of the severity of the asthma. Allergic rhinitis often coexists not only with asthma but also with sinusitis, otitis media, and allergic conjunctivitis. The main features

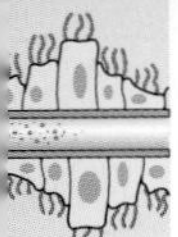

are of rhinorrhea, nasal obstruction, nasal itching, and sneezing. Correct diagnosis and management are essential and can lead to improvements in accompanying asthma (see Chapter 28). Nasal corticosteroids represent the most effective treatment for patients with persistent or moderate to severe rhinitis, but in those with milder or intermittent disease antihistamines or chromones may have a role.

Churg-Strauss Syndrome

Originally described in 1951, this syndrome was characterized initially on the basis of histologic appearances that included vasculitis and extravascular granulomas occurring in patients with asthma and allergic rhinitis. Such a dependence on histologic characterization has the potential to delay diagnosis, and more recent understanding of the syndrome emphasizes the necessity for prompt diagnosis based largely upon clinical suspicion.

The criteria for diagnosis of Churg-Strauss syndrome (CSS) has been described as:

1. Presence of asthma
2. Peripheral blood eosinophilia (more than 1500 cells per microliter), and
3. Systemic vasculitis involving two or more extrapulmonary organs

Others have also included in their definition the presence of pulmonary infiltrates, sinus abnormalities, and demonstration of histopathologic changes. Those suggesting biopsy confirmation have done so because of a realization that rarely does CSS predate asthma or occur without marked eosinophilia. Although such biopsy of easily accessible affected tissue can be helpful, it should not delay institution of treatment (Figure 39.2). Antineutrophilic cytoplasmic antibodies are present in two thirds of cases but are not specific for CSS. The key to prompt diagnosis of CSS is to think of the condition especially when faced with an adult who presents with allergic rhinitis, sinusitis, and worsening asthma followed by odd systemic features such as fever, rash (especially lower limb purpura), weight loss, or arthralgia. Other features include pulmonary infiltrates, peripheral neuropathy, cranial and other isolated nerve palsies, cerebrovascular incidents, abdominal pain, bloody diarrhea, and, occasionally, intestinal perforation. Renal disease occurs in a minority of patients and can be associated with hematuria, proteinuria, and hypertension. Cardiac involvement is one of the most feared and serious manifestations of CSS, with granulomatous eosinophilic infiltration of the myocardium and coronary vasculitis leading to heart failure and a risk of sudden death. These manifestations of disease may develop over a short period. In other cases adult onset of upper airway problems is followed some time later by the onset of asthma, which later becomes severe, and, after a further variable time, systemic symptoms develop and other organs become involved. The differential diagnosis clearly depends on the manifestation of CSS occurring in that individual but pulmonary manifestations may need differentiating from allergic bronchopulmonary aspergillosis (ABPA), other pulmonary eosinophilias, or pulmonary sarcoidosis. If and when vasculitis develops, differentiation is necessary from Wegener's granulomatosis, microscopic polyangiitis, and polyarteritis nodosa.

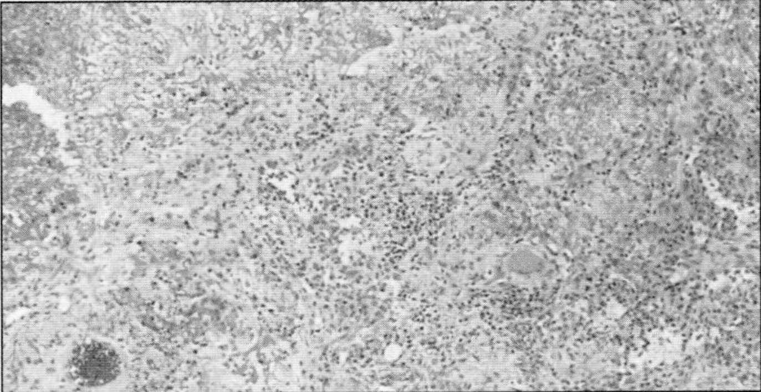

Figure 39.2 Histopathology of Churg-Strauss syndrome (CSS). This photomicrograph shows a combination of parenchymal necrosis and focally marked tissue eosinophilia in CSS. The inflammatory infiltrate includes a combination of eosinophils and variable numbers of epithelioid histocytes in a vaguely granulomatous appearance.

In the early stages of disease and with limited manifestations, the response to steroids alone may be very good. In others with more aggressive disease, additional treatment with cyclophosphamide is necessary. Prognosis reflects the degree of severity of the disease and its manifestations, with the worst outcomes being in cases in which cardiac decompensation or cerebrovascular manifestations develop.

The association of CSS with treatment of asthma using leukotriene antagonists has recently attracted attention. Although theoretically it is possible that any drug could induce a hypersensitivity vasculitis, the likeliest reason some have developed CSS after starting a leukotriene antagonist is that improved control of their asthma has led to a reduction in oral steroid dose and the unmasking of a previously inapparent systemic condition. In anyone with a history of difficult asthma in whom steroids are being reduced or tailed off, one should be alert to a risk of unmasking CSS, and inflammatory markers and eosinophil counts should be monitored.

Bronchopulmonary Aspergillosis

The fungus *Aspergillus* is globally distributed and found in soil and decaying leaf mold and vegetable matter. Fungal spores are dispersed by the wind, and peak levels are found during the winter. The size of the spores enhances inhalation and deposition within the lung, where body temperature is optimal for growth. The fungus can easily be found in sputum samples from those patients with a variety of lung conditions. Some patients with asthma develop hypersensitivity to *Aspergillus* on repeated exposure. These patients are likely to have other demonstrable sensitivities to common inhaled allergens such as house dust mite and pollen, but *Aspergillus* hypersensitivity may be associated with longer duration of disease and more severe disease. Other patients develop the condition known as allergic pulmonary aspergillosis wherein, in addition to having asthma and *Aspergillus* hypersensitivity, they develop pulmonary eosinophilia and infiltration with an intense allergic reaction in the proximal airways. This can result in bronchial occlusion, which may give rise to segmental or lobar collapse visible on the chest radiograph, predominantly in the upper lobes. Such episodes are manifest clinically as fever, worsening asthma, or

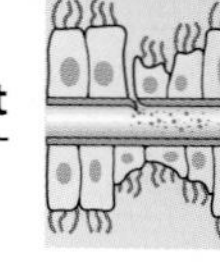

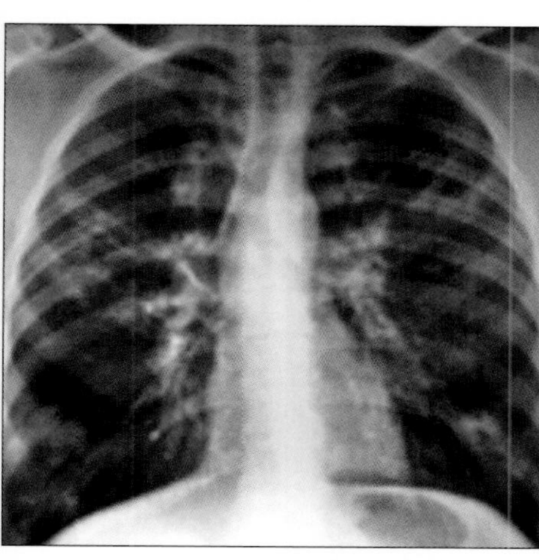

Figure 39.3 Allergic bronchopulmonary aspergillosis. Chest radiograph of a 21-year-old woman with asthma showing interstitial markings suggestive of bronchiectasis and patchy opacities (mucoid plugging) bilaterally.

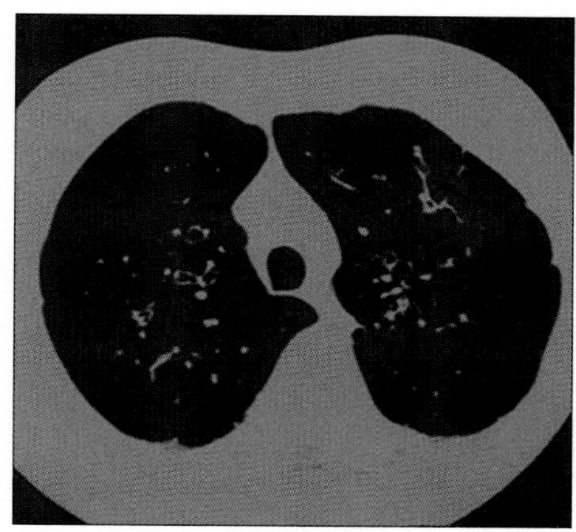

Figure 39.4 Computed tomography scan performed on a patient who has bronchopulmonary aspergillosis. Significant proximal airway bronchiectasis is shown.

chest pain. If untreated, such episodes can result in significant bronchial wall damage and the development of bronchiectasis of the proximal airways (Figure 39.3). Investigation of suspected ABPA includes:

1. Measurement of peripheral blood and sputum eosinophilia
2. Demonstration of a positive immediate skin prick test to *Aspergillus fumigatus*
3. Positive precipitins to *Aspergillus fumigatus*, and
4. A raised total immunoglobulin E level

Computed tomography scanning of the thorax can demonstrate the proximal bronchiectasis (Figure 39.4). Although the acute syndrome associated with pulmonary infiltration is undoubtedly helped by oral corticosteroid therapy, the exact indication for long-term steroids is less clear. In most cases it is preferable to treat episodes with courses of oral steroids and maintenance inhaled steroids in between attacks. If the episodes of infiltration are very frequent and severe, long-term maintenance corticosteroid therapy may be necessary. In such cases, a 4-month trial of the oral triazole antifungal agent Itraconazole may decrease oral steroid requirements and improve asthma control.

Cryptogenic Eosinophilic Pneumonia

Eosinophilic pneumonia may occur as a complication of bronchopulmonary aspergillosis, as a result of the usage of certain drugs (e.g., nitrofurantoin, sulfasalazine), as a complication of parasitic infections, or represent a cryptogenic eosinophilic pneumonia (see Chapter 46). Although termed *cryptogenic*, this last condition is one that has a characteristic and consistent clinical presentation and has been recognized as a distinctive syndrome for more than 30 years. At least 50% of patients who have cryptogenic eosinophilic pneumonia already have asthma, and many develop it subsequent to the pneumonia. The characteristic presentation is of fever, breathlessness, weight loss, and profound and drenching night sweats; the chest radiograph shows a classic photographic negative of that seen in pulmonary edema, with peripheral shadowing most marked in the upper zones (Figure 39.5). The condition is sometimes mistaken for

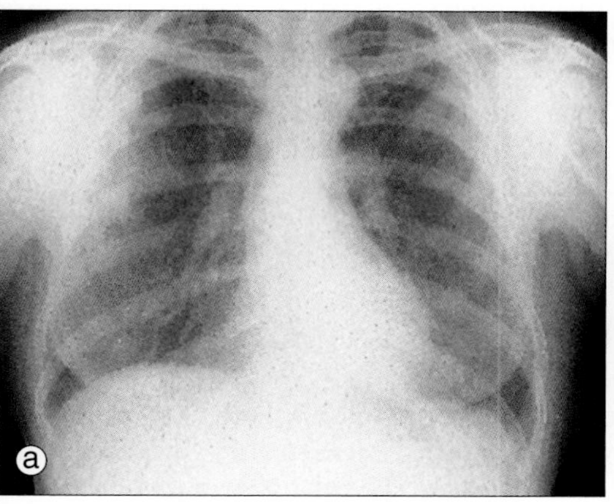

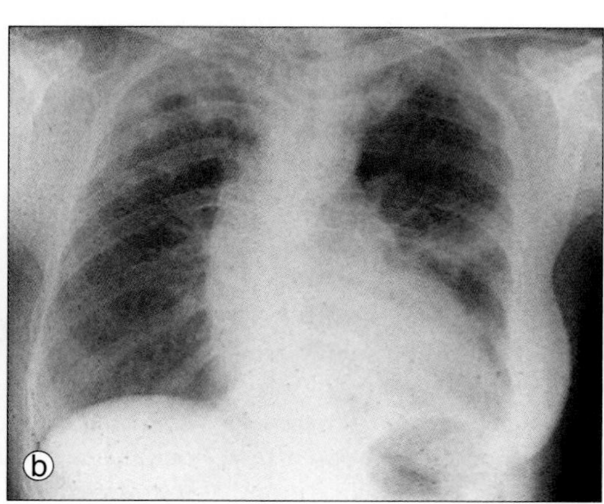

Figure 39.5 Chest radiographs of cryptogenic eosinophilic pneumonia. **A,** Predominantly peripheral upper zone shadowing. **B,** In this example, it is easier to see how cryptogenic eosinophilic pneumonia may be mistaken for tuberculosis unless the appropriate tests are performed.

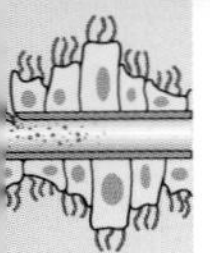

Table 39.3 Differential diagnosis of airway diseases in the consideration of asthma

Airway diseases	
Localized	**Generalized**
Vocal cord paresis	Asthma
Laryngeal carcinoma	Chronic obstructive pulmonary disease
Thyroid enlargement	Bronchiectasis
Relapsing polychondritis	Cystic fibrosis
Tracheal carcinoma	Obliterative bronchiolitis
Bronchial carcinoma	
Bronchial carcinoid	
Post-tracheostomy stenosis	
Foreign bodies	
Bronchopulmonary dysplasia	
Obstructive sleep apnea	

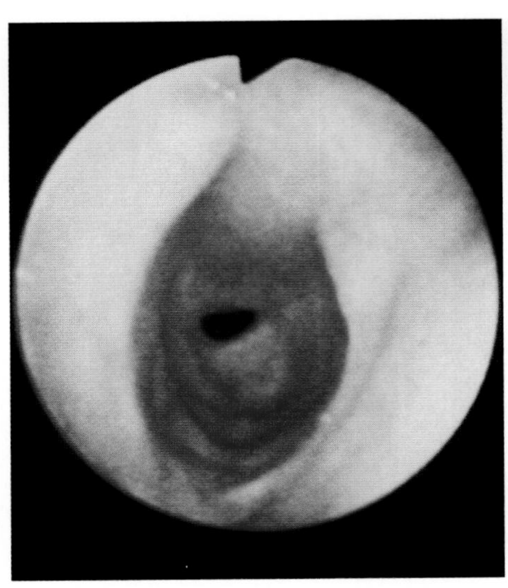

Figure 39.6 Severe tracheal narrowing secondary to prolonged previous endotracheal intubation and mechanical ventilation. The localized nature of this man's airway obstruction was overlooked for some time and he was mistakenly treated for asthma using bronchodilators and inhaled corticosteroids.

pulmonary tuberculosis; the important diagnostic differentiation is to measure the peripheral blood eosinophil count especially when someone with asthma presents in this way.

Gastroesophageal Reflux

In some studies, one third of the population has been demonstrated to have gastroesophageal reflux at some stage. It may be more common in asthma and may make asthma worse, and some asthma therapies such as theophyllines may enhance reflux of acid into the esophagus. There is no evidence that treatment of gastroesophageal reflux influences control of asthma (see Chapter 18).

DIAGNOSIS, DIFFERENTIAL DIAGNOSIS, AND ASSESSMENT OF SEVERITY

Asthma is a common disease with a high profile and awareness among both the general public and health professionals. This can lead to the potential for overdiagnosis. It is but one of many common respiratory conditions, but symptoms of respiratory diseases may be shared with disorders of other systems—breathlessness can be caused not only by lung disease, but also by heart disease, pulmonary vascular disease, diaphragm weakness, and systemic disorders such as anemia, obesity, or hyperthyroidism. A cough may similarly reflect an airway disorder but may also be due to diffuse parenchymal lung disease or treatment with an angiotensin-converting enzyme inhibitor. Even if one is relatively confident that a patient's symptomatology reflects an airway disorder, remember that they are many in number (Table 39.3) and that airway obstruction may be localized (Figure 39.6) or generalized. Clinically, clues to the presence of a localized airway obstruction may be that the wheezing is asymmetrical, monophonic rather than polyphonic, or there may be stridor emanating from the upper airways. Even when the wheezing and airway narrowing appears to be generalized, the list of differential diagnosis must be considered (see Table 39.3). Obliterative bronchiolitis is a rare cause of unexplained, generalized airway narrowing that can occur especially in women who have rheumatoid arthritis; it also occurs as a complication of rejection after lung transplantation. In patients who produce large quantities of sputum, the alternate diagnosis of bronchiectasis is considered, and patients who suffer cystic fibrosis occasionally have late presentations and may be misdiagnosed as having asthma. After all of these diagnoses have been considered, in adults the final differentiation in many cases is that from chronic obstructive pulmonary disease (COPD).

Differentiation of Asthma from Chronic Obstructive Pulmonary Disease

Some may argue that these conditions are a spectrum in which reversible airway obstruction occurs at one end and fixed narrowing at the other. Furthermore, many patients who have COPD exhibit some reversibility, and many who have asthma develop a fixed component to the airway narrowing. Some of the treatments are also common to the two disorders. However, a more satisfactory approach seems to be to separate the two conditions, as in the Venn diagram shown in Chapter 34.

The reasons for differentiation are that the cause of the two conditions is dissimilar (COPD being essentially from smoking), the pathologic processes can be quite different (emphysema does not occur in asthma), the natural history is different (progressive decline in airway caliber is likely in those patients who have COPD who continue to smoke), and the response to treatments is dissimilar in terms of both magnitude and type. Taking a "prescription-oriented approach" to COPD can often cause harm (e.g., from side effects of corticosteroid therapies that have only a limited beneficial effect in COPD compared with asthma) and by deflection away from other issues that can help those who suffer COPD (e.g., correct selection of the right type of supplementary oxygen, attention to depression and social factors, and smoking cessation support). A summary of the key points of differentiation is shown in Table 39.4.

Vocal Cord Dysfunction

Vocal cord or glottic dysfunction is an important condition that can cause serious diagnostic difficulty in both adolescents and adults and, if not recognized, unnecessary overtreatment. Glottic wheezing or vocal cord dysfunction can occur within a

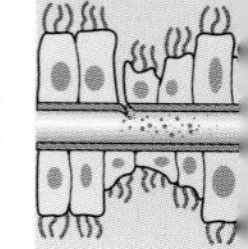

Table 39.4
Differentiation of asthma from chronic obstructive pulmonary disease

	COPD	Asthma
Age	Develops in 4th, 5th, and 6th decades	Often a history of childhood asthma (or wheezing in childhood, childhood bronchitis, or inability to take part in sports)
Symptoms	Shortness of breath is usually confined to exertion	Shortness of breath can occur at rest, or on exertion, and frequently awakens the patient in the early hours of the morning
Natural history	Progressive decline in exercise capacity especially if continues smoking	If treatment is adequate and instituted early in the course of the disease, normal lung function should be maintained in between attacks
Smoking history	History of current or previous smoking	May or may not be or have been a smoker
Atopic diseases	May or may not have a personal or family history of asthma, hay fever or eczema	Likely to have a personal history of other atopic diseases, or a family history of asthma, hay fever or eczema
Markers of inflammation		Likely to have increased exhaled NO levels, more eosinophils in blood, sputum or airway samples than in those with COPD
Lung function	Likely to have higher residual volume and lower diffusing capacity than those with asthma, and flow volume curves may show pressure-dependent airway collapse	
Response to treatment	Limited reversibility with inhaled bronchodilators and steroids	Good reversibility with inhaled bronchodilators and steroids

spectrum of severity—at one extreme complicating genuinely troublesome asthma and at the other representing a conversion symptom or Munchausen syndrome. A diagnosis of vocal cord dysfunction is made with considerable care, and in acute cases of wheezing the diagnosis and treatment must always be regarded as that of pure asthma until that diagnosis is disproved.

Wheezing that arises from the glottis is heard throughout the lung fields when auscultation is performed using a stethoscope, but in cases of vocal cord dysfunction the glottic origin can often be determined by removing the stethoscope from the ears, and standing behind the patient and listening at neck level. The glottic origin of the noise (which often sounds more forced than usual wheezing) then becomes apparent. Direct visualization of the glottis by laryngoscopy may reveal the characteristic inspiratory apposition of the cords.

Sometimes those who have asthma make this noise because they subconsciously feel the need to impress upon the doctor the severity of their condition. In other patients the noise occurs for purely psychological reasons and no evidence of asthma is found. Patients may be of either sex, but are often women in the age range of 16 to 50 years who may have a paramedical background. Their "asthma" appears "resistant" to standard treatments and often they have been admitted to a hospital on many occasions and been treated with large doses of corticosteroids and other treatments.

Home peak-flow readings and attempts at spirometry may be variable, but show little correlation with attacks or treatment. Flow-volume curves may show a characteristic "fluttering" of the inspiratory curve. Measurement of total airway resistance in a body plethysmograph may be diagnostic, because the panting maneuver necessary for such measurement abolishes the vocal cord adduction and airway resistance can be shown to be normal. Occasionally patients end up being mechanically ventilated because of "severe" asthma, but once paralyzed it can be seen that airway resistance is normal and there is no necessity for high inflation pressures.

Vocal cord dysfunction is probably much more common than appreciated and if underdiagnosed or mistaken for asthma, overtreatment is likely. Correct diagnosis is essential, and if vocal cord dysfunction is the sole or major part of the wheezing disorder, speech therapy can be helpful. As with other "conversion" symptoms confrontation or challenge is best avoided and attempts should be made to help the patient deflect stress away from the throat.

Investigations Used in the Diagnosis and Assessment of Asthma

PEAK EXPIRATORY FLOW RATE

Because asthma is defined in physiologic terms, physiologic tests are required to make the diagnosis. Many of the differential diagnoses listed previously have characteristic clinical features, but in other cases asthma is only excluded or confirmed as a diagnosis by establishing whether the patient fulfills the definition of "generalized airway narrowing that varies over short periods of time either spontaneously or as a result of treatment." In the great majority of cases, this definition may be fulfilled by measurement of peak expiratory flow rate (PEFR) on more than one occasion in the clinic or surgery, by the use of a meter for recording two to three times daily at home, or, in cases of occupational asthma, at work (Figure 39.7). Variability may be quantified and asthma diagnosed when there is greater than 20%

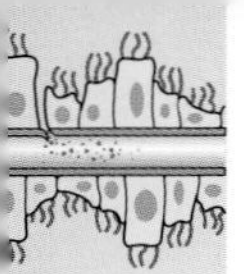

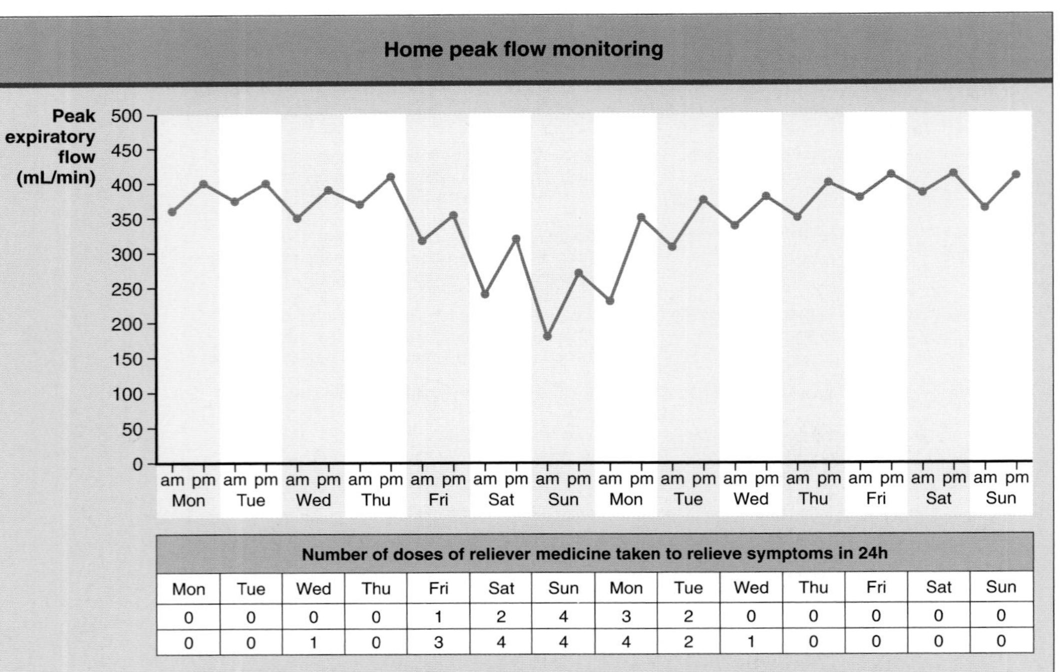

Mon	Tue	Wed	Thu	Fri	Sat	Sun	Mon	Tue	Wed	Thu	Fri	Sat	Sun
0	0	0	0	1	2	4	3	2	0	0	0	0	0
0	0	1	0	3	4	4	4	2	1	0	0	0	0

Figure 39.7 Peak flow readings made twice daily at home by a middle-aged man. The diurnal variation and the day-to-day variation in readings is of such magnitude that there can be no doubt that the patient's airway narrowing fulfilled the diagnostic definition of asthma. (The daily readings are the best of three blows morning and evening.)

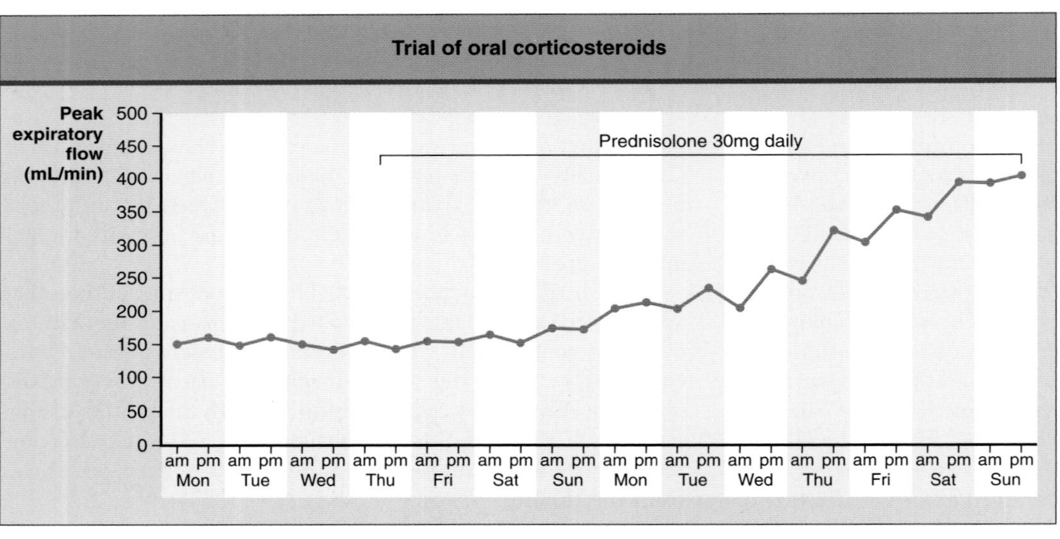

Figure 39.8 Trial of oral corticosteroids. Home peak-flow recordings showed little initial variability. However, after corticosteroids were instituted (within bracket), significant improvement in peak flow occurred, which confirmed a diagnosis of asthma. (The daily readings are the best of three blows morning and evening.)

diurnal variation on 3 or more days in a week for 2 weeks on a peak flow diary. Amplitude of peak flow variability is calculated as: highest PEFR – lowest PEFR/highest PEFR × 100%.

SPIROMETRY

Although less generally available, spirometry is used as the standard measurement of dynamic airflow to detect the presence of airway obstruction and to test for reversibility of flow. Airflow obstruction is established if the forced expiratory volume in 1 second (FEV_1) is less than 80% predicted, or the ratio of FEV_1 to forced vital capacity is less than 75% or below the lower limit of normal. If evidence of airway narrowing is detected, response to a bronchodilator must be established, and if positive (greater than 15% response), a diagnosis of asthma is made. In other cases, little spontaneous variation of peak flow may occur over the period of observation, and the response to inhaled bronchodilators may be slight; in these cases, differentiation from COPD, for example, is difficult unless a trial of corticosteroid tablets (Figure 39.8) is given. In some cases a prolonged course of high-dose, inhaled corticosteroids (ICSs) can be used as an alternative test of corticosteroid responsiveness.

In some patients, additional tests are needed when asthma is suspected and spirometry normal, when coexisting conditions

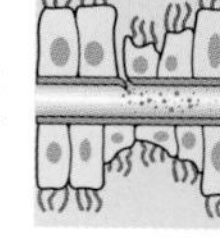

Table 39.5
Additional tests for suspected asthma if the diagnosis is uncertain

Reason	Test
Patient has symptoms, but spirometry is normal or near normal	Assess diurnal variation of peak flow over 1–2 weeks Consider bronchoprovocation with methacholine, histamine, or exercise
Suspect infection, large airway lesions, heart disease, or obstruction by foreign body	Chest radiograph and consider bronchoscopy
Suspect coexisting chronic obstructive pulmonary disease, restrictive defect, or central airway obstruction	Additional pulmonary function tests (e.g., diffusing capacity)
Suspect other factors that contribute to asthma	Allergy tests – skin or in vitro Nasal examination Gastroesophageal reflux assessment

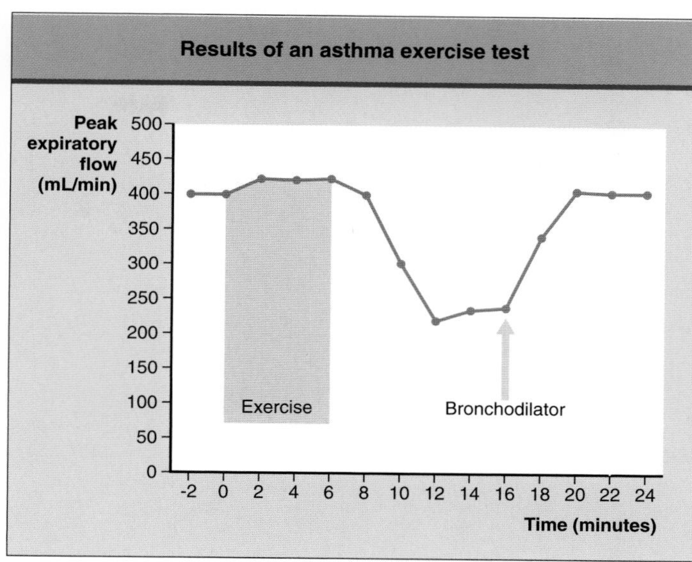

Figure 39.9 Results of an asthma exercise test. Here, 6 minutes of free running induced severe asthma in an adolescent who had normal peak flow when first tested.

are suspected, or for other reasons (Table 39.5). If no airway narrowing is apparent at the time of consultation and if the history is unclear, it may help to observe the PEFR at home for 1 to 2 weeks, as described previously. An alternative is to establish whether the airway narrowing can be induced and fulfill the diagnostic definition of asthma in that way. In some suspected cases of occupational asthma, disease may be induced by careful exposure to small quantities of the probable incriminating agent (i.e., challenge testing).

More commonly, airway narrowing and a positive diagnosis of asthma are induced by means of exercise, which can be performed simply and is applicable to both adults and children old enough to use a peak flow meter. It is best carried out by asking the patient suspected of having asthma to make some baseline peak-flow readings and then to undertake 6 minutes of free running (Figure 39.9). Any postexercise fall in peak flow is abnormal, but a fall of greater than 15% is regarded as diagnostic of asthma. Peak flow readings are made at 2-minute intervals for up to 20 minutes after exercise, and, if significant asthma is induced, bronchodilators are given. False-positive tests do not occur, but a false-negative result can happen; therefore, a negative exercise test does not exclude the possibility of asthma at other times.

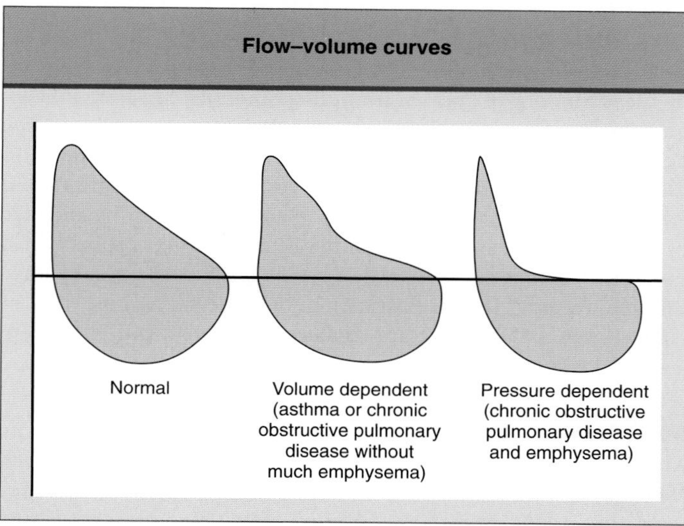

Figure 39.10 Flow-volume curves in some common diseases and their (limited) use in differentiating asthma from some other conditions.

OTHER LUNG FUNCTION TESTS

Detailed lung function may help in the differentiation of other conditions from asthma. The expiratory flow–volume curve is useful to identify pressure-dependent reduction in expiratory flows—because of loss of elastic recoil forces seen in emphysema (Figure 39.10). The maneuver is also excellent for identifying upper airway problems. However, if the differential diagnosis is from chronic obstructive bronchitis (i.e., pure airway disease, with no emphysema), the expiratory flow–volume curve has a volume-dependent shape (see Fig. 39.10) and is similar in both COPD and asthma. In general, measurements of lung volume tend to show an increase in total lung capacity with COPD, but both COPD and asthma patients can show increased levels of functional residual capacity and residual volume, the values in asthma increasing with the severity of the disease.

The measurement of the single-breath gas transfer factor is normal in asthma, but can be reduced in COPD, and is reduced in emphysema.

Lung function tests are rarely diagnostic, but the demonstration of restrictive spirometry and a reduction in lung volumes, for example, excludes asthma and introduces the differential diagnosis of restrictive (small) lung disorders.

CHEST RADIOGRAPH

The radiograph in asthma can show airway wall thickening, best seen in the larger proximal airways. The lungs can appear larger than normal because of gas trapping, with flattened diaphragms and horizontal ribs—they appear quite distinct from those of

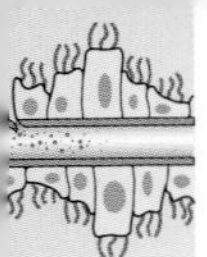

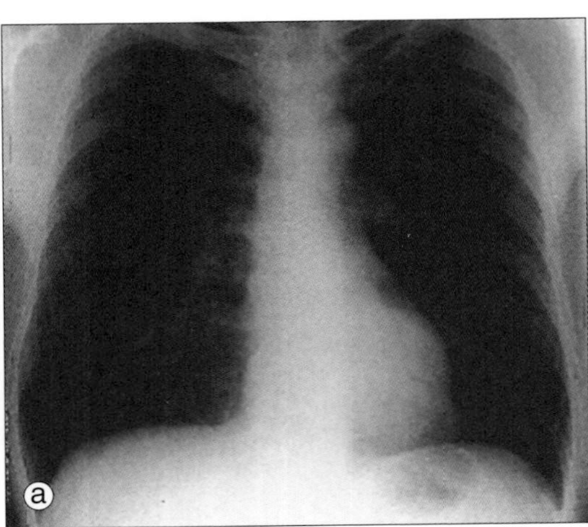

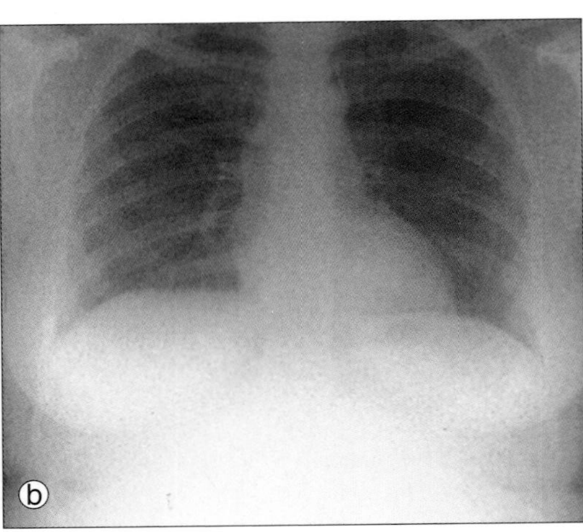

Figure 39.11 Comparative lung sizes on chest radiograph. **A,** Radiograph of a man who has hyperinflation secondary to severe airway narrowing. **B,** The small lungs (restrictive disorder) often seen in the very obese.

restrictive disorders (Figure 39.11). The chest radiograph can also alert the physician to complications of asthma such as bronchopulmonary aspergillosis, infection, pulmonary eosinophilia, or pneumothorax.

SKIN PRICK TESTING

The demonstration of an allergic state by skin prick testing (or by measurement of specific immunoglobulin E) can help in diagnosis by characterizing an individual as being atopic, and this may be useful in some unclear situations. Such testing may also identify possible trigger factors for an individual's asthma and advice regarding environmental manipulation or avoidance procedures, such as removing a family cat, should probably not be given without demonstrating sensitization. Allergen-specific immunotherapy (hyposensitization or desensitization) can of course only be given if appropriate allergens—mites, pollen, animal dander, or molds—have been identified.

MEASUREMENT OF AIRWAY HYPERRESPONSIVENESS

Measurement of airway hyperresponsiveness is a state in which there is an abnormal increase in airflow obstruction after exposure to a stimulus. Stimuli may be directly acting stimuli such as histamine, cholinergic agonists, leukotrienes, or prostaglandins, or indirectly acting agents such as exercise, fog, metabisulphate, or cold air hyperventilation. Airway hyperresponsiveness is a cardinal feature of asthma, but it is not specific to it. It may also occur in a general population or in those with COPD but failure to demonstrate airway hyperresponsiveness in someone with suspected asthma should lead to reconsideration of the diagnosis. It is usually measured by use of histamine or methacholine. FEV_1 is initially measured and then remeasured after administration of saline to obtain a baseline value. Increasing doses of a constricting agent such as histamine or methacholine are then administered and FEV_1 measured after each increase in dose and the test is stopped once a 20% fall in FEV_1 has been achieved. The result is expressed as the provocative dose or concentration that produces a 20% fall in FEV_1. In those with asthma, measurement reflects the degree of sensitivity of the airways and can reflect severity. Measurement is useful for research reasons and occasionally to clarify whether a diagnosis of asthma is or is not likely.

SPUTUM EXAMINATION AND MEASUREMENT OF EXHALED NITRIC OXIDE AND NONINVASIVE MARKERS OF INFLAMMATION

The recent understanding of asthma as a chronic inflammatory disease came about over the last two decades, largely as a result of bronchial mucosal biopsies being taken from small numbers of individuals both when well and when troubled by asthma. Subsequently, other methods of assessing the degree of inflammation in the airways have been developed or refined and are now beginning to find a place in both the diagnosis and in the assessment of severity and, more recently, as a tool against which treatment may be titrated. These newer tools include assessment of airway inflammation by measurement of exhaled nitric oxide and by estimation of inflammatory cells in induced sputum samples. Correlation of these markers with measured airway hyperresponsiveness may occur in the untreated state but not necessarily in the treated state. Their exact role in the diagnosis and management of asthma remains unclear.

Nitric oxide is the most extensively studied exhaled marker of inflammation and may be elevated in a variety of lung diseases, but especially in asthma. An elevated level, therefore, is not specific for asthma but it may be useful, for example, in determining the cause of a cough when an elevated level might suggest asthma as the cause, and it might be useful to monitor the course of disease and response to therapy. Nitric oxide may not necessarily correlate with other external markers of inflammation and each marker may reflect the site of inflammation as well as type of inflammation present within the airway. Changes in sputum eosinophil counts may be a good marker of airway inflammation and rises may predict imminent loss of asthma control. Treatment is currently adjusted according to symptoms or measurements that reflect airway caliber and the relationship of these to the basic degree of inflammation present in the airways is tenuous. Recent work using sputum eosinophil counts to direct the dosing of inhaled steroid therapy has shown promise in terms of reduced asthma exacerbations and better asthma control without any overall greater use of therapy.

Grading of Severity of Asthma

The diagnosis of asthma is made by hearing a cough, wheeze, or breathlessness that is worse at night or in the early morning, and

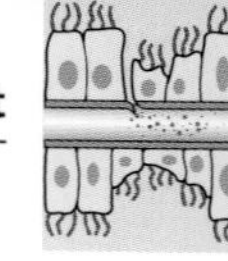

Table 39.6
Classification of asthma severity: clinical factors before treatment (Adapted from National Heart, Lung, and Blood Institute.)

Step	Days with symptoms	Nights with symptoms	Peak expiratory flow (%)	Peak expiratory flow variability (%)
4 – severe, persistent	Continual	Frequent	≤60	>30
3 – moderate, persistent	Daily	≥5 per month	>60 to <80	>30
2 – mild, persistent	3–6 per week	3–4 per month	≥80	20–30
1 – mild, intermittent	≤2 per week	≤2 per week	≥80	<20

by demonstrating evidence of a reduced peak flow or obstructive spirometry that varies with time or after treatment. The same parameters may be used to assess severity, poor control, and the need for more treatment. These symptoms may be paralleled by peak-flow recordings that show severe morning "dips" (see Fig. 39-7). The normal (or predicted normal) peak-flow rate depends upon an individual's age, sex, and height; it is therefore important to relate assessment of severity to the predicted value (or to relate it to that individual's previous best reading where known). Advice for management in accident and emergency departments, for example, can then be based upon relating an individual peak-flow rate to predicted values, so that a peak flow, say, greater than 75% of predicted is regarded as reflecting mild asthma, 50% to 75% as moderate, 33% to 50% severe, and less than 33% life threatening. Several other classifications of asthma severity are available, most of which are based on PEFR or FEV_1 values plus symptoms. The National Institutes of Health (NIH) classification is summarized in Table 39.6. However, in anyone who has asthma, the presence of fatigue, exhaustion, or cyanosis represents critical severity. Measurements of oxygen saturation and blood gas partial pressures, although of no value in the routine management of asthma, are of greater importance in the management of acute severe asthma (see the following section). One problem in assessing the control of an individual's asthma is that the doctor/patient interaction occurs only at one point in time. All too often a patient's recall of his or her condition expressed as "I am fine" does not reflect the true situation over the preceding days or weeks. This may lead to an underestimation of the severity of an individual's asthma and persisting unnecessary morbidity which, if detected, could have led to a change in therapy and better asthma control. This is why the British Guidelines on Asthma Management have adopted the recommendation of the Royal College of Physicians of London and suggested that at every consultation with a person with asthma, the following questions should be asked and the answers recorded in the notes.

Three questions to be asked at every consultation:
In the last week or month,

1. Have you had any difficulty sleeping because of your asthma symptoms (including cough)?
2. Have you had your usual asthma symptoms during the day (cough, wheeze, chest tightness, or breathlessness)?
3. Has your asthma interfered with your usual activities (e.g., housework, work/school)?

MANAGEMENT AND TREATMENT

In this section, drug treatments for asthma, environmental manipulations, immunotherapy, and complementary therapies are considered, with a brief description of the common inhalational devices available for use.

Other aspects of management, which include education and self-management, are considered in the section on prevention and organization of care.

The medicines available for the routine management of asthma are best divided into:

- Those taken to relieve symptoms when they occur and
- Those that need to be taken regularly.

The pharmacology of these interventions has been extensively reviewed in Chapters 32 and 33 and only clinical aspects are discussed here.

Inhaler devices may include:

- Pressurized metered-dose inhalers (pMDI)
- pMDIs plus a spacer device
- Breath-activated MDIs
- Breath-activated dry powder devices
- Nebulizers

Aerosols

Some knowledge of the properties of aerosols will aid understanding of their use. The size of aerosol particles and their distribution are expressed as if the aerosol were composed of a suspension of spheres with different diameters. The mass median diameter of the aerosol is the diameter about which 50% of the total particle mass resides. The mass median aerodynamic diameter (MMAD) is the product of the mass median diameter and the square root of the particle density. The MMAD of an aerosol has a profound effect on where the majority of particles entering the lung will land and thereby act. Particle deposition is influenced by inspiratory flow—the higher the entry flow, the more central will be the deposition—because of inertial impaction, particularly of large particles (greater than 6 mm). Smaller particles (less than 5 mm) will reach smaller airways and those of 2- to 3-mm size reach the alveoli. Small particles may not settle and will be expired. The relationship of site of deposition and particle size is shown in Figure 39.12. Deposition is also greatly affected by turbulent flow, and the deposition at airway bifurcations can be up to 100 times more than elsewhere. In general, inertial impaction of aerosols occurs with large particles in large airways where flow is high (i.e., nose, pharynx, larynx, trachea, and carina). Deposition is enhanced by turbulent flow that predominates in these central passages. Gravitational sedimentation is time-dependent and affects the small particles. These settle in small airways, provided time is sufficient (i.e., slow breathing or breath-holding). The combination of small particles, low flow, and short distances favors sedimentation. Thus, the mode of inhalation and type of breathing influences deposition. Fast inhalation enhances central inertial impaction and slow inhalation with breath-holding favors peripheral sedimentation.

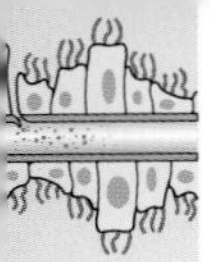

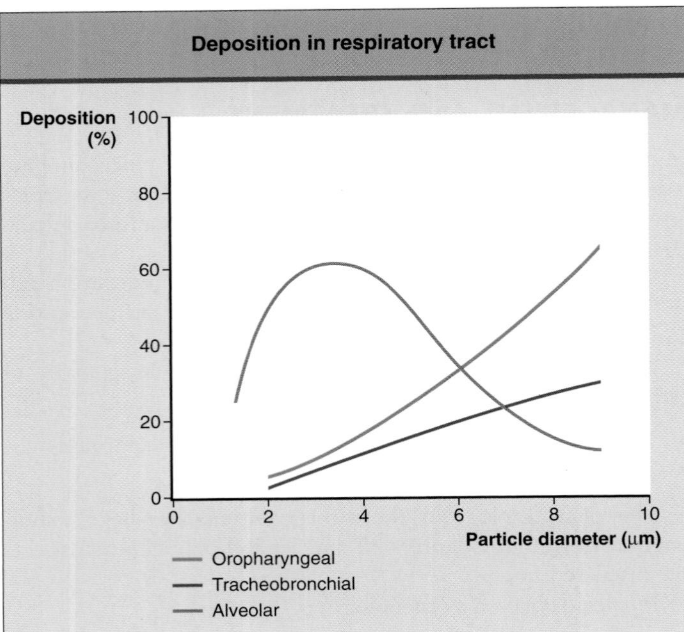

Figure 39.12 Relationship between percentage deposition in the respiratory tract and the diameter of the aerosol particles.

AEROSOL PRODUCTION, DELIVERY, AND EFFICACY

Pressurized Metered-dose Inhalers

The pMDI has been widely used in clinical practice since the early 1960s. It comprises a canister and a plastic actuator. The drug is contained in the small canister either dissolved or suspended as crystals in a liquid propellant mixture of chloroflourocarbons (CFCs) with low boiling points. To prevent aggregation of the small particles, a low concentration of a surfactant is included to act as a lubricant. The aerosol released from the pMDI consists of large droplets of propellant enclosing the drug particles. The propellants boil off as soon as they leave the canister, and this breaks the liquid stream up into droplets that continue to evaporate as they move away at an initial velocity of 30 m/sec. Because of the high velocity of the drug particles, the effects of the evaporating propellants and the hygroscopicity of the drug itself, together with the curved anatomy of the upper respiratory tract, means that most of the drug impacts in the oropharynx and less than 25% of the released dose reaches the lungs. However, it is important to note that, because different drugs have different characteristics of hygroscopicity and electrostatic charge, although a pMDI will reproducibly emit a constant dose of a drug, it cannot be assumed that the same quantity of every drug administered by this system will reach the lungs. The same is true for the dry powder system. A recent change is the international agreement (Montreal Protocol) to introduce a ban on CFC-containing pMDIs. Formulation with non–CFC propellants (hydrofluoroalkane; HFA) has proved to be difficult. Some HFA formulations use ethanol to make the drug soluble rather than a suspension stabilized by surfactants. Furthermore, the mean particle size (i.e., MMAD) of some of the newer non–CFC-containing pMDIs is around 2 mm compared with 3 to 4 mm for the CFC aerosols, making it likely that more drug may be delivered peripherally, with not as much to the bronchial tree. (Clinical aspects of the transition to non-CFC pMDIs is discussed on page 497.)

USE AND COMPLIANCE

The most efficient way of using a pMDI is:

1. Shake the canister thoroughly and remove the cap.
2. Place mouthpiece of the actuator between the lips.
3. Breathe out steadily, taking care not to actuate the canister during exhalation.
4. Release the dose while taking a slow deep breath in.
5. Hold in the breath and count to 10.
6. Wait 1 minute before repeating.

These instructions, although simple, are followed incorrectly in some way or another by the majority prescribed this device. There are pros and cons for the use of pMDIs (Table 39.7).

LARGE VOLUME SPACERS

Increasing the distance from the actuator to the mouth allows the particles to evaporate and slow down before inhalation. The spacer device allows large particles of drug to impact on the surfaces of the chamber, minimizing oropharyngeal deposition and increasing the respirable fraction, nearly doubling drug deposition below the larynx. The large volume spacers also decrease the incidence of oropharyngeal candidiasis that occurs with pMDIs containing corticosteroids. The spacer causes little inconvenience when used twice daily with ICSs and long-acting bronchodilator devices. It would be less convenient for bronchodilator therapy taken on an as-required basis. The spacers are particularly useful in treating young children and are an alternative to nebulizers in chronic and severe acute asthma.

Tube spacers—tubelike attachments to the pMDI—with a much smaller internal volume than the large volume spacers are also available to permit slowing down of the aerosol before reaching the mouth.

Attempts have been made to facilitate the use of the pMDI by making it breath actuated, as the commonest problem is coordination of inspiration with the dose actuation. When primed, the valve is actuated by an inspiratory flow of above 30 L/min

Table 39.7
The pros and cons of using a pressurized metered-dose inhaler

Pros	Cons
Small doses	Difficult (young, elderly, arthritic)
Topically very active	Education needed
Stores up to 200 doses	Poor compliance
Easy to use	Hard-to-monitor compliance
Minimal side effects	Dose and deposition uncertain
Portable	Less effective with increased airway obstruction
Unobtrusive	Requires high inspiratory flow or deep breath
	Wide variation in particle size
	Oropharyngeal impaction
	Cough in up to 30% of users
	Can be difficult to know when cannister is empty

and is easier to use than the conventional pMDI. A further problem is the canister is enclosed within the device, making "shaking" useless for guessing the amount of drug remaining—a potential hazard when the patient needs "rescue" medication.

Drug Powder Inhalers

The drug powder inhaler (DPI) systems depend entirely on the patient's inspiratory effort and are generally easier to use than the pMDIs. They inherently require faster inspiratory flows to disimpact the powder and allow the inhaled fraction to be less than 5 μm. They now come as reservoir inhalers containing multiple doses, usually designed for use through 1 month.

Reservoir Drug Powder Inhalers. These devices are breath-actuated by breathing in as fast and as deeply as possible. Patients are sometimes disconcerted that, because only micronized drug is released, the dose is so tiny that they feel nothing. The two common devices are the Turbuhaler, which is a 50- to 200-dose DPI, and the Accuhaler or Diskus, which contains a ribbon of blisters containing micronized drug and lactose. It contains up to 120 doses, with a counter visible; the drug is released by pressing a "trigger" to puncture the blister and then inspiring deeply from the mouthpiece.

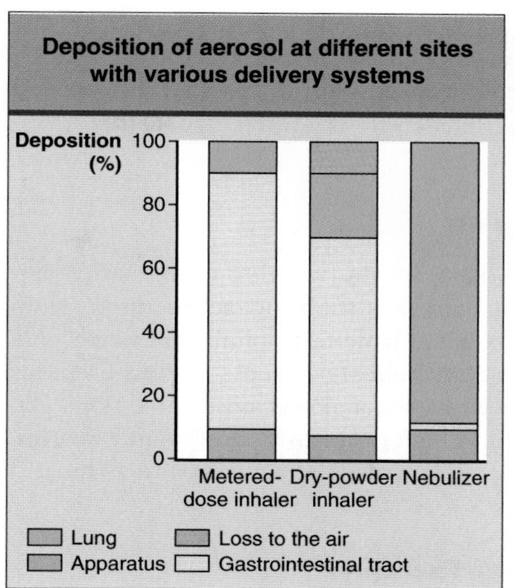

Figure 39.13 Deposition of aerosol delivered by pressurized metered-dose inhaler, dry-powder inhaler, and a nebulizer to different sites. (Adapted from Zainuddin et al, with permission of BMJ Publishing Group.)

Nebulizers

There are two types of nebulizers: jet and ultrasonic. The latter produces quite large particles (3-10 mm) from high-frequency (1-2 mHz) sound waves induced by the vibration of a piezoelectric crystal, which, when focused on the surface of a liquid, creates a fountain of droplets. The mean particle size is inversely proportional to the frequency of the ultrasonic vibrations of the crystal. It has less clinical use than the jet nebulizer.

The jet nebulizer achieves its particulate mist from a stream of compressed air or oxygen that draws up the liquid drug through a capillary by the Venturi effect and then atomizes it into tiny fragments. More than 99% of these initial droplets are large particles that impinge on suitable baffles and drop back into the reservoir for further nebulization, leaving just small particles in the aerosol leaving the nebulizer. Approximately 1 mL of the original drug solution (usual 2 mL) is left on the baffles after completion of nebulization and constitutes dead volume that cannot be used. This inefficient characteristic can be improved by increasing the fill to 4 to 6 mL, but the period of nebulization is then considerably prolonged.

DEPOSITION AND EFFICACY

All three systems (pMDI, DPI, and jet nebulizer) are relatively inefficient, with only about 8% to 15% drug reaching the lung (Figure 39.13).The nebulizer system is also extremely wasteful because the stream of aerosol mist is continuous, causing wastage during expiration, which in airway obstruction is often two thirds of the respiratory cycle. In general, therefore, nebulizers are, dose for dose, no more efficient than the pMDI or DPI systems.

Medicines Taken to Relieve Symptoms ("Relievers" or "Rescue Medications")

Medicines taken to relieve symptoms are of two main types: β_2-agonists and anticholinergic agents. The former are the most important and most widely used.

β_2-AGONISTS

β_2-Agonists are advances upon epinephrine (adrenaline) and isoproterenol (isoprenaline), and the two most commonly used are albuterol (salbutamol) and terbutaline. Classified as having β_2-selectivity, all members of these classes have the potential to be beneficial bronchodilators, but may also cause cardiac effects (tachycardia, increased cardiac output, peripheral vasodilatation and arrhythmia) and systemic effects (hypokalemia, hyperglycemia, tremor, uterine relaxation). Such effects are dose-related and related to the method of administration—inhaled, ingested, or parenteral (subcutaneous, intramuscular, or intravenous). For routine use these drugs are always recommended to be administered by the inhaled route wherever possible, so that high concentrations reach the airways where needed and systemic side effects are minimized or avoided. The onset of action is also quicker by the inhaled route compared with that of tablet administration. Short-acting β-agonist relief inhalers are used only to relieve symptoms; the need for such medication on a regular basis reflects poorly controlled asthma and the need for more regular preventive therapy of different types. Increased use of these medicines thus indicates to the physician that a change in routine medication is needed, but is also a guide to the patient that change is needed; this advice is best given within the context of a written personal asthma action plan.

In acute attacks of severe asthma, the dose of albuterol (salbutamol) or terbutaline may be increased and administered either from the routine inhaler, from the routine inhaler plus a large volume-spacer device, or by nebulization. There is no evidence that nebulization has any advantage over the standard inhaler plus spacer device. Persistent use of nebulizers within secondary care probably reflects a perception that it is quicker for a nurse or therapist to start a patient on a nebulizer than to supervise multiple actuations from an inhaler through a spacer. However, availability of nebulization in hospitals may encourage patients to bypass primary care or to wrongly assume that self-treatment at home according to a written personal asthma action plan may lead to them omitting a useful medication.

With all inhaled medications, it is important that the cheapest, most effective device (or combination of devices) with which the patient is comfortable is used, and that instructions as to correct use of the inhaler are reinforced frequently.

Anticholinergic Agents

The most common of these agents (whether called anticholinergic or antimuscarinic agents) is the short-acting ipratropium bromide, but there is now available tiotropium that needs only to be taken once daily. Anticholinergic agents are less effective in asthma than β-agonists having a slower onset of action. The addition of ipratropium in high doses to β-agonists is, however, synergistic in the initial management of acute severe asthma.

Regular (Preventive) Therapies

Regular preventive therapy for asthma involves the use of either specific anti-inflammatory agents (ICSs, cromones, and leukotriene modifiers) or regular bronchodilators (oral and inhaled long-acting β-agonists, and theophyllines).

INHALED CORTICOSTEROIDS

The exact mechanism of action of ICSs remains unclear (see Chapter 33), but they are potent anti-inflammatory agents that interfere with arachidonic acid metabolism and synthesis of leukotrienes and prostaglandins and inhibit cytokine production and secretion. This results in less inflammatory cell infiltration, reduced vascular leakage and permeability, and increased responsiveness of airway smooth muscle β-receptors. Their use increases lung function, reduces ARH, symptoms, frequency of attacks of asthma, the need for courses of corticosteroid tablets, and improves quality of life. Serial bronchial mucosal biopsies show that they also reduce markers of airway inflammation. Commonly used ICSs include beclomethasone, budesonide, flunisolide, triamcinolone, fluticasone, and mometasone, and all are available in the inhaled form from a similar range of inhaler devices as for the inhaled β-agonists. Flunisolide and triamcinolone are little used outside the United States. Comparative daily doses of different inhaled steroids in the United States and the United Kingdom are shown in Table 39.8.

Differences between the various formulations of ICSs in terms of efficacy, absorption, metabolism, and side effect profile are frequently claimed. Although such differences may be demonstrated according to the particular parameter or outcome studied, it seems unlikely that, for the vast majority of patients who have asthma, there is much difference between the drugs. The exceptions are that inhaled fluticasone is as effective as beclomethasone and budesonide at half the dose when given by equipotent delivery systems. It is therefore advised to be given at half the dose recommended for beclomethasone and budesonide. Also, budesonide given via a Turbuhaler device delivers approximately twice as much ICS to the lung and doses should probably be halved when this device is used. One manufacturer's reformulation of beclomethasone with a non–CFC propellant is also claimed to enhance pulmonary deposition of the inhaled steroid necessitating a similar halving of dosage.

Intervention with inhaled steroids early in the course of the disease probably improves the chances of maintaining good lung function. In one seminal study, in adults who had mild asthma and who had been treated for 2 years with either ICSs or an inhaled β-agonist, significant reduction in the need for rescue bronchodilation occurred. The β-agonist–treated group were then given ICSs and the former either a lower dose of ICSs or placebo. Placebo was ineffective, but low-dose ICSs moderately effective at maintaining bronchial responsiveness at the level achieved with the previous higher dose ICS. In the group who had previously received bronchodilators alone, a significant improvement occurred in spirometry and peak flow, but to a lesser degree than in those who had been treated with ICSs from the beginning of the study.

CROMOGLYCATE AND NEDOCROMIL

These two medicines represent alternative anti-inflammatory agents. Both are taken by the inhaled route—the former needs a four times daily medication regimen, the latter twice daily. The mechanism of action is unclear, but the medications inhibit activation of, and mediator release from, several types of inflam-

Table 39.8
Estimated comparative daily doses of different inhaled corticosteroids and comparisons of low, medium, and high doses in the United States and the United Kingdom

Inhaled corticosteroid	Units of drug available (μg)		Low dose (μg)		Medium dose (μg)		High dose (μg)	
	USA	UK	USA	UK	USA	UK	USA	UK
Beclomethasone dipropionate	42, 84	50, 100, 200, 250	168–504	100–400	504–840	400-800	>840	800–2000
Budesonide	200, 400	100, 200, 400	200–400	100–400	400–600	–	>600	800–2000
Flunisolide	250	N/A	500–1000	N/A	1000–2000	N/A	>2000	N/A
Fluticasone	44, 110, 220	50, 125, 250, 500	88–264	50–200	264–660	200-400	>660	400–1000
Triamcinolone acetonide	100	N/A	400–1000	N/A	1000–2000	N/A	>2000	

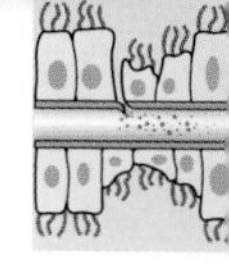

matory cells and may inhibit neuronal pathways. Both preparations reduce symptoms and improve lung function in those people who have asthma, but their effectiveness is usually much less than that of ICSs and their role in adults is extremely limited. In children who have mild asthma, although less effective than ICSs, these medications remain an alternate anti-inflammatory treatment.

LEUKOTRIENE MODIFYING AGENTS

Leukotrienes are inflammatory mediators that play a significant role in the causation of asthma. They are formed from arachidonic acid in the cell membrane by the action of an enzyme called 5-lipoxygenase. Leukotrienes that contain a cysteinyl molecule (cysteinyl leukotrienes) cause constriction of smooth muscle in the airway wall; swelling, edema, and leakage from blood vessels in the airway walls; mucus gland stimulation; and secretion of mucus. They also attract eosinophils into the airways.

Leukotriene modifiers work either by inhibiting 5-lipoxygenase (e.g., Zileuton) or by acting as a leukotriene receptor antagonist (e.g., Zafirlukast, Montelukast). Leukotriene modifiers represent a medication worth trying in people whose asthma remains troublesome despite the use of ICSs and long-acting inhaled bronchodilators, and also as an alternative to low doses of inhaled steroids for a minority of people.

Regular Bronchodilators

Regular bronchodilators include oral and inhaled longer-acting β-agonists, and theophyllines.

THEOPHYLLINES

Theophyllines have been available for many years and have bronchodilator effects. They can improve lung function and reduce symptoms, and when given in addition to anti-inflammatory agents in slow-release form, they may help cases of persistent nocturnal asthma. However, at bronchodilator levels side effects such as nausea and vomiting (and less likely seizure and tachycardia) are frequent occurrences in up to 50% of users. Recent studies suggest that levels of theophylline traditionally thought to be below those needed to achieve bronchodilation may increase asthma control when added to low-dose ICSs. This suggests that at these low doses theophylline may have some other nonbronchodilator anti-inflammatory effect. Two such studies show that for patients who are poorly controlled on low-dose ICSs, the addition of low doses of theophyllines may prove as effective as the alternative strategy of using high doses of ICSs.

LONG-ACTING β-AGONISTS

Long-acting β-agonists include oral products such as slow-release albuterol or bambuterol, or inhaled long-acting β-agonists such as salmeterol or formoterol. They have no anti-inflammatory action and must not be used alone to treat asthma. Two high-dose ICSs versus low-dose ICSs plus salmeterol studies in adults showed that not only do both options work, but also that the salmeterol-containing option was slightly better in terms of both lung function and reduction in symptoms.

Formoterol, another long-acting, inhaled β-agonist with a similar duration of action to salmeterol, but a quicker onset of action, has also been shown to reduce symptoms and improve lung function when added to modest doses of ICSs. Whether in children or adults, inhaled, long-acting β-agonists are useful when taken with low-dose inhaled steroids as an alternative to high-dose inhaled steroids, but also as an adjunct to high-dose ICSs when treatment with these alone is not sufficient.

CORTICOSTEROID TABLETS

Corticosteroid tablets may be lifesaving in the treatment of acute attacks of asthma. For a very tiny proportion of patients, corticosteroid tablets are needed in the long term to control the condition. In short courses, the side effects are usually negligible (indigestion, weight gain), but in the longer term they may typically cause osteoporosis, hypertension, skin thinning, muscle weakness, obesity, cataracts, and hypothalamic-pituitary-adrenal axis suppression. Maximal use of ICSs and other therapies should reduce the need for corticosteroid tablets, but, when essential, the dose must always be kept as low as possible and must be taken first thing in the morning. In those patients being started on regular oral steroids and in those taking frequent courses of steroid tablets, consideration of bone protection is important. Use of systemic steroids is associated with a significantly increased risk of hip and vertebral fracture. The higher the dose, the higher the risk, but the risk is significant even at daily doses of 7.5 mg of prednisolone. Loss of bone mineral density occurs maximally soon after starting steroid tablets, and steroid-induced osteoporosis is more prone to be associated with bone fracture than age-related, postmenopausal osteoporosis. Measurement of bone mineral density should therefore be undertaken when starting most patients with asthma on regular oral steroid therapy, and good nutrition, adequate dietary calcium intake, and physical activity encouraged. Tobacco use and excess alcohol should be avoided. In the elderly and in those with a history of previous fractures, bone protective therapy should be started at the time of institution of oral steroid therapy. In others a decision regarding the need for bone protective agents will need to be made according to the results of bone densitometry estimations.

Trends in the Usage of Medications

Inhaled steroids were introduced for the management of asthma more than 30 years ago. Seminal work, much of it in Finland in the 1980s, emphasized the presence of persistent inflammation within the airways of those with asthma even at times when they had little in the way of symptoms. Early guidelines on the management of asthma were therefore able to adopt a rather simplistic approach to the routine management of asthma that suggested that if bronchodilators were needed more than occasionally, one should take regular low-dose inhaled steroids. If, despite their use, asthma was not well-controlled, high-dose inhaled steroids should be used. If these did not effect adequate asthma control, any other available medication should be added to the high-dose inhaled steroids; if the patient was still symptomatic, he or she should be treated with regular steroid tablets. Approximately 10 years ago, new studies emerged that suggested that the guidelines might be promoting a suboptimal strategy, and a plethora of trials showed that the use of long-acting β-agonists (whether salmeterol or formoterol) in addition to low-dose inhaled steroids could achieve results equal to or

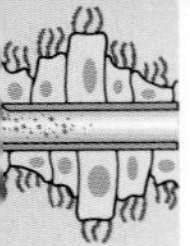

better than that obtained with high-dose inhaled steroids. This was true both for improvement in lung function and in terms of more days free of symptoms. Similar results were obtained for salmeterol and formoterol added to beclomethasone, budesonide, or fluticasone, but also to a lesser extent with the addition of theophylline or bambuterol to low-dose inhaled steroids. Some studies suggested that the higher dose of inhaled steroids were still necessary for those suffering frequent exacerbations. These studies have led to a trend toward guidelines suggesting that for those not well-controlled on low-dose inhaled steroids, a long-acting bronchodilator (usually an inhaled β-agonist) should be added before increasing the dose of inhaled steroids. An additional factor in this change in emphasis has been the recognition that the dose-response curve with inhaled steroids is rather flat and, although additional doses achieve only small increments in terms of benefit, they may increase the risk of side effects. Although the latter are negligible compared with those with steroid tablets or compared with the risk of poorly controlled asthma, high-dose inhaled steroids can be associated with skin purpura and possibly an excess of cataracts and glaucoma. Their long-term safety with regard to an effect on bone mineral density requires ongoing study. In children, excessive doses outside the licensed range can undoubtedly affect the hypothalamic-pituitary-adrenal axis. The trend is therefore downward in doses of inhaled steroids used, and by the addition of alternative agents where necessary. More recently, in addition to long-acting inhaled β-agonists, leukotriene modifying agents have become more widely used, usually as an adjunct to inhaled steroids, but in some countries as an alternative to low-dose inhaled steroids, although all guidelines suggest low-dose inhaled steroids as the preferred optimal treatment.

All guidelines have always recommended the stepping down of treatment when asthma control is maintained and achieved. Unfortunately, human nature being what it is, a patient telling a doctor that he or she is "fine" leaves a health professional with a subconscious tendency not to risk altering a satisfactory situation with the result that many may be on higher doses of inhaled steroids than are necessary. Recent studies have emphasized that an active step-down approach can lead to significant reduction in dosages of inhaled steroids used without any increase in exacerbation rates. Other recent studies have shown similarly that teaching patients to vary their dose themselves can achieve significant reductions in doses of steroids used compared with those on fixed dosage regimens. Such advice can and should be incorporated into written personal asthma action plans (see page 495).

Environmental Manipulation

Clearly, wherever possible, those people who have asthma must avoid identifiable triggers. The difficulty is that many are not identifiable or not avoidable (e.g., the common cold). Avoidance of animal allergens is practical; if a child is shown to have developed symptoms after acquiring a cat and shown to have positive skin-prick test reactions to cat allergens, removal of the cat is obviously preferable to drug therapy. Reducing exposure to cockroach allergens can be achieved by clearing infested homes and careful use of pesticides. Reducing the quantity of house dust mite exposure by having as few soft furnishings as possible, use of good ventilation, intermittent deep freezing of soft toys, and barrier bedding may improve the control of asthma in some individuals sensitive to house dust mites. Avoidance of drugs or occupational agents known to affect the individual adversely is essential. Avoidance of passive smoking is helpful to all. However, despite the logic behind environmental manipulation and the patients desire to do it, it is often of only limited benefit and an adjunct to drug therapy; only rarely is it a substitute for drugs.

Immunotherapy

Widely used some years ago, and still used in some countries, the role of specific immunotherapy in asthma remains unclear and is a subject that merits further study. Aimed at treatment of the underlying allergy, even when well-performed it can be associated with unexpected side effects, and most guidelines no longer recommend its routine use in asthma. However, refinements in technique and patient selection are redefining a limited role for immunotherapy in allergic rhinitis, and for asthma it may appear as an adjunctive therapy for a few specific instances when given by a specialist. The opinion of the NIH expert panel is that immunotherapy be considered when:

- Clear evidence is found of a relationship between symptoms and exposure to an unavoidable allergen to which the patient is sensitive
- Symptoms occur all year or during a major portion of the year
- Difficulty occurs with the control of symptoms using pharmacologic management because multiple medications are required or medications are ineffective or not accepted by the patient

The course of allergen immunotherapy is typically of 3 to 5 years' duration.

Complementary Therapies

Six percent of patients with asthma reported current use of complementary therapies in one recent study. Such therapies may include homeopathy, acupuncture, breathing techniques, herbal therapies, and ionizers. Not all are free of side effects; pneumothoraces and hepatitis have been reported after acupuncture, and use of ionizers may increase nocturnal cough. The taking of Royal Jelly (propolis) has been claimed as being beneficial for those with asthma but deaths from severe reactions have been reported after its use. Many studies of Chinese medicines and acupuncture have been reported but design of appropriate trials is difficult and no definite evidence of benefit can be concluded. Similarly, homeopathy has been assessed in several trials with conflicting results and no recommendations for use can be made on the available information. Breathing exercises including yoga and the Buteyko technique have attracted much interest. Pranayama breathing can be associated with reduced airway hyperresponsiveness and the Buteyko technique associated with a reduced need for bronchodilators.

Perhaps of greater importance than the efficacy or lack of efficacy of complementary therapies is the reason why they remain popular amongst those with asthma. Studies have suggested that this often reflects dissatisfaction with the relationship of the patient with those offering traditional medicine. Complaints include those reflecting the quality of the doctor-patient relationship and a lack of time. Other reasons include dissatisfaction with treatment, "distrust" of drugs, dislike of regular medication, and a desire for a cure.

Management Strategies for the Use of Medicines in the Day-to-Day Management of Asthma

The short-term aims of asthma management can be defined as:

- Rapid resolution of symptoms
- Restoration of quality of life
- Reduction in risk of attacks

The long-term aims of asthma management can be defined as:

- Best possible lung function
- Minimal side effects from treatment

To achieve these two sets of aims, most guidelines support a stepwise approach to therapy, which is summarized in Figure 39.14 and Table 39.9. Two sets of guidelines apply to the management of chronic asthma in adults—one from the British Thoracic Society (UK; see Fig. 39.14) and the other from the NIH (US; see Table 39.9)—and both are very similar to the recommendations of the Global Initiative for Asthma. They follow very similar principles of therapy, albeit with a different number of steps. Both sets aim at a gradual increase in ICS and emphasize the importance of stepping down the intensity of therapy once control has been achieved.

It is important to stress that these are guidelines as to how to manage asthma over the weeks and months—a more acute self-management plan may be administered in a zone fashion as a self-treatment plan (see the following section). When using the stepwise approach, doctors must start at the step most appropriate to the severity of the individual's asthma at the time of consultation and subsequently step up or step down to control the condition. At any time it may be necessary for the patient to take a short course of corticosteroid tablets to regain control. After control is achieved, the emphasis of management remains on stepping treatment down to the minimum levels needed to maintain control.

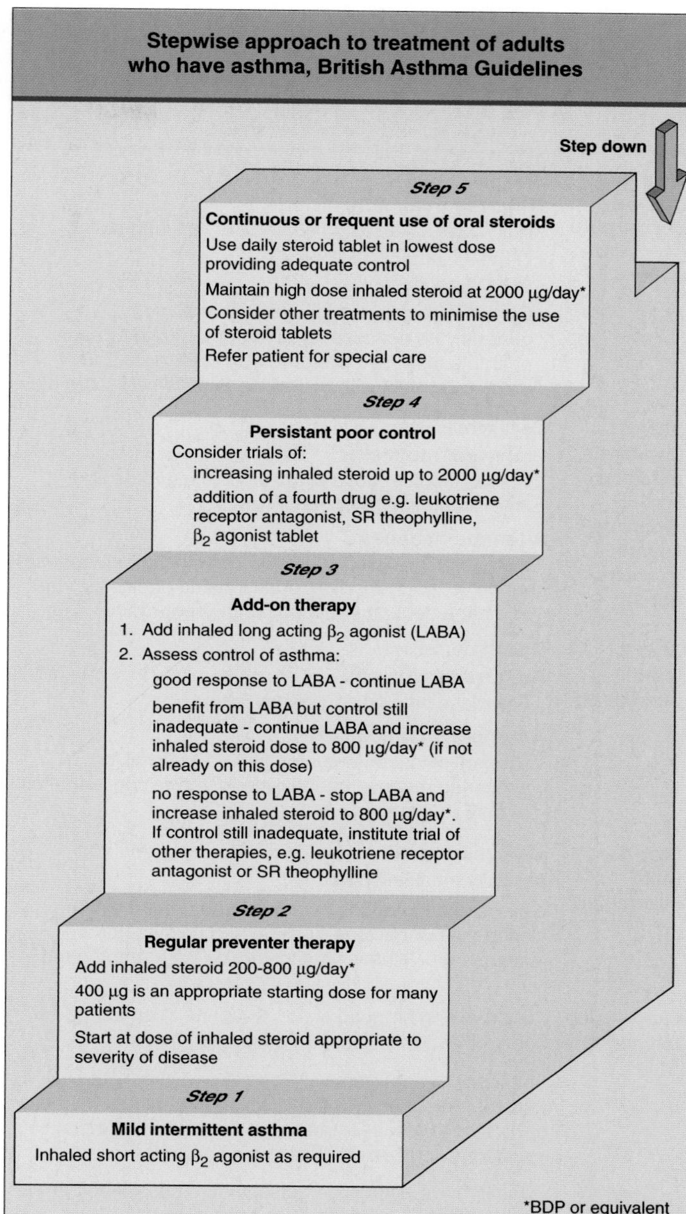

Figure 39.14 Stepwise approach to treatment of adults who have asthma—British Asthma Guidelines. (Adapted with permission from British Thoracic Society.)

MANAGEMENT OF ACUTE ASTHMA

Most acute asthma is not actually acute. Although it may be severe, the asthma "attack" suffered by many children and adults has often been developing for some time. In one study, 53% of adult patients admitted to hospital with severe asthma had been waking because of asthma for at least 5 nights before admission. Half of these patients had sought advice from their primary care physician in the week before admission because of deteriorating asthma, but too often they received antibiotics or more bronchodilators rather than the corticosteroid tablets they probably needed. In another national survey of all patients who attended emergency departments because of asthma, one fifth had been waking because of "acute" asthma for 3 nights before attendance, and in a further Canadian study a fifth of those being admitted to hospital with asthma were shown to have had symptoms of deteriorating asthma for at least 3 weeks before admission. Figures such as these suggest that many patients had adequate time to alter their treatment to prevent deterioration to crisis levels. Thus, undertreatment or inappropriate therapy is a major contributor to asthma morbidity and mortality. As a consequence, asthma is the third leading cause of preventable admissions to hospital and more than 5000 deaths per year in the United States, and 1500 deaths per year in the United Kingdom are from asthma.

People who have asthma die because either they, their loved ones, or their doctors underestimate the severity because of delays in seeking medical treatment and because of underuse of oxygen and corticosteroid tablets. The severity of an exacerbation therefore must be carefully assessed, and the outcome determines the treatment given and where it is given. Of children and adults seen in the accident and emergency departments who had asthma, fewer than half in one study received anti-inflammatory therapy and only few adults admitted had written plans to manage their asthma and control an exacerbation

Table 39.9
Stepwise approach for the management of asthma in adults and children—National Institutes of Health. Preferred treatments are given in bold (Adapted from National Heart, Lung, and Blood Institute)

Step 4 (severe persistent)	Daily medication: **Preferred treatment:** High-dose inhaled corticosteroids and long-acting inhaled β_2-agonists AND, if necessary Corticosteroid tablets or syrup (2 mg/kg/day, generally do not exceed 60 mg/day). (Make repeat attempts to reduce systemic corticosteroids and maintain control with high-dose inhaled corticosteroids)
Step 3 (moderate persistent and recurring severe exacerba-tions)	Daily medication: **Preferred treatment:** Low-to-medium dose inhaled corticosteroids and long-acting inhaled β_2-agonists **Alternate treatment:** Increased inhaled corticosteroids within medium-dose range or low-to-medium dose inhaled corticosteroids and either leukotriene modifier or theophylline
Step 2 (mild persistent)	Daily medication: **Preferred treatment:** Low-dose inhaled corticosteroids **Alternate treatment:** Cromolyn, leukotriene modifier, nedocromil, or sustained release theophylline to serum concentration of 5-15 mcg/mL.
Step 1 (mild intermittent)	Daily medication: No daily medication needed Severe exacerbations may occur, separated by long periods of normal lung function and no symptoms. A course of systemic corticosteroids is recommended.
Quick relief (all patients)	Short-acting bronchodilator: 2-4 puffs short-acting inhaled β_2-agonists as needed for symptoms. Intensity of treatment will depend on severity of exacerbation; up to 3 treatments at 20-minute intervals or a single nebulizer treatment as needed. Course of systemic corticosteroids may be needed. Use of short-acting β_2-agonists > 2 times a week in intermittent asthma (daily, or increasing use in persistent asthma) may indicate the need to initiate (increase) long-term-control therapy.

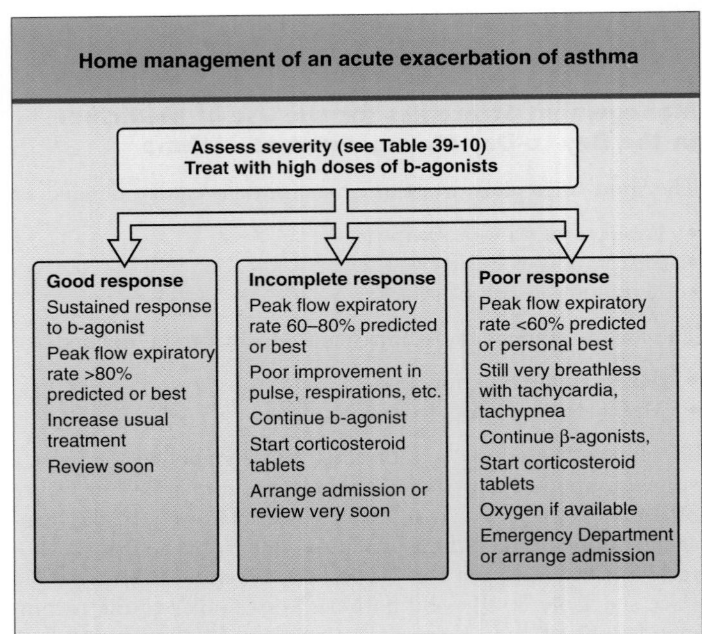

Figure 39.15 Home management of an acute exacerbation of asthma.

(Figure 39.15). Table 39.10 shows features associated with exacerbations of asthma of mild, moderate, severe, or critical nature. All but the mildest attacks require treatment with bronchodilators, corticosteroids, and oxygen, and careful follow up and assessment of responses to each intervention (see Fig. 39.15).

The criteria for admission to an intensive care unit include exhaustion; the most common reason those who have severe asthma require mechanical ventilation is that of exhaustion. The first warning of this may be a normal or raised arterial partial pressure of carbon dioxide ($PaCO_2$) on blood gas sampling—the normal picture in acute asthma being one of a low PaO_2 and a high $PaCO_2$.

The recognition and assessment of severe acute asthma begins at home, where it is often underestimated, sometimes by the patient, the caregiver, or the attending physician (Table 39.11; see also Fig. 39.15 and Table 39.10). Symptoms and PEFR must be assessed immediately and the severity graded. Treatment is with high doses of β-agonists (e.g., nebulized albuterol [salbutamol] 5 mg, or 2 to 4 puffs via MDI and large volume spacer every 10 to 15 minutes). A good response (e.g., PEFR greater than 80% predicted or best) with symptom relief is followed by continuing regular β-agonists every 4 hours for 24 to 48 hours, increase the dose of ICS for 7 days, and review the patient within days.

An incomplete response (PEFR 50% to 80% predicted or best) with persistent symptoms requires continuation of β-agonists every 2 to 4 hours and prompt addition of oral corticosteroids. Either admission is arranged or the patient is seen again urgently (same day or next morning).

With a poor response (PEFR less than 60% predicted or best) with signs of distress, the patient is instructed to continue β-agonists (MDI or nebulizer), start oral corticosteroids, use oxygen if available, and proceed to the emergency department or call emergency services.

ACUTE ASTHMA IN THE EMERGENCY ROOM

Proper recognition and assessment is vital (Table 39.11)—an algorithm for further management is given in Figure 39.16—and severity must be assessed (see Tables 39.10 and 39.11). Treatment is begun with nebulized β-agonists, high-flow oxygen, and systemic corticosteroids (e.g., prednisolone 30 to 60 mg orally daily) (see Fig. 39.16). The aim is to achieve an arterial oxygen saturation (SaO_2) of greater than 92%. Ipratropium bromide (500 mg) can be added to albuterol (salbutamol). No sedatives of any kind can be given. A chest radiograph is indicated if a pneumothorax or consolidation is suspected in life-threatening cases, if there is a failure to respond to initial treatment, or if

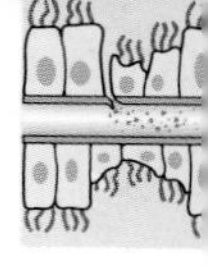

Table 39.10
Guide to the severity of asthma exacerbations (Adapted from National Heart, Lung, and Blood Institute/World Health Organization Workshop)

Symptoms	Mild	Moderate	Severe	Respiratory arrest imminent
Breathless	Walking Can lie down	Talking Prefers sitting	At rest Hunched forward	
Talks in	Sentences	Phrases	Words	
Alertness	May be agitated	Usually agitated	Usually agitated	Drowsy or confused
Respiratory rate	Increased	Increased	Often >30 breaths per minute	
Accessory muscles and suprasternal retractions	Usually not	Usually	Usually	Paradoxic thoracoabdominal movement
Wheeze	Moderate, often only end expiratory	Loud	Usually loud	Absence of wheeze
Pulse per minute	<100	100–120	>120	Bradycardia
Peak expiratory flow rate after initial bronchodilator (% predicted or % personal best)	Over 80	ca. 60–80	<60 (<100L/min adults) or response lasts <2h	
Arterial pressure of oxygen (PaO_2; on air)	Normal Test not usually necessary	>8.5kPa (>60 mm Hg)	<8.0kPa (<60 mm Hg) Possible cyanosis	
$PaCO_2$	<6kPa (<45 mm Hg)	<6kPa (<45 mm Hg)	>6kPa (>45 mm Hg) Possible respiratory failure (see text)	
Arterial oxygen saturation (%; on air)	>95	91–95	<90	
Hypercapnia (hypoventilation) develops more readily in young children than in adults and adolescents				

Table 39.11
The recognition and assessment in hospital of acute severe asthma

Features of acute severe asthma
Peak expiratory flow rate (PEFR) ≤50% of predicted or best Cannot complete sentences in one breath Respirations ≥25 breaths per minute Pulse >110 beats per minute
Life-threatening features
PEFR <33% of predicted or best Silent chest, cyanosis, or feeble respiratory effort Bradycardia or hypotension Exhaustion, confusion, or coma If arterial saturation of oxygen <92% or a patient has any life-threatening features, measure arterial blood gases
Blood gas markers of a very severe, life-threatening attack
Normal [5–6 kPa (36–45 mm Hg)] or high arterial partial pressure of carbon dioxide ($Paco_2$) Severe hypoxia, Pao_2 <8.0 kPa (60 mm Hg) irrespective of treatment with oxygen A low pH (or high H^1)
No other investigations are needed for immediate management
Caution: patients who have severe or life-threatening attacks may not be distressed and may not have all these abnormalities – the presence of any should alert the doctor.

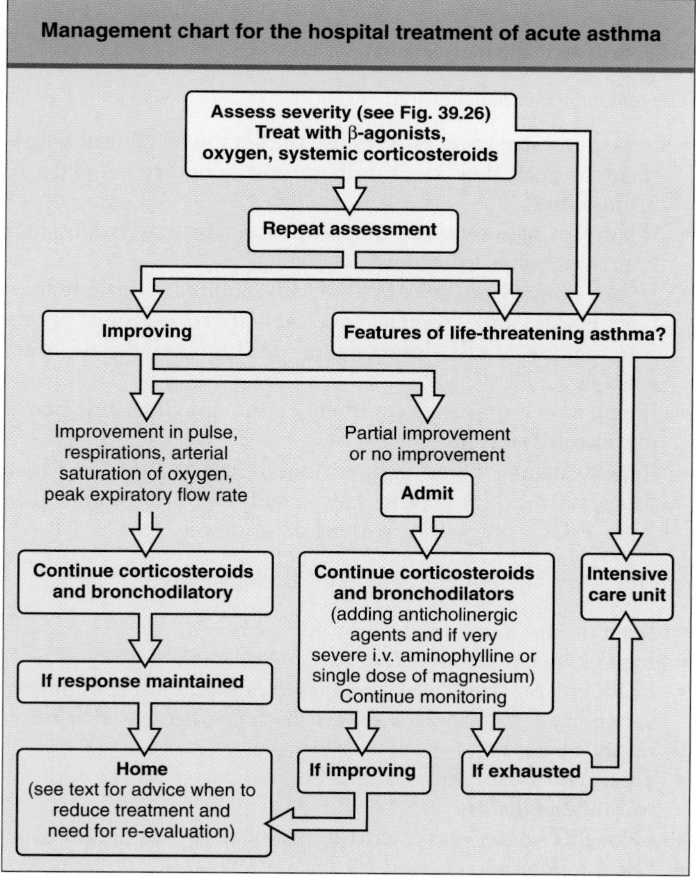

Figure 39.16 Management chart for the hospital treatment of acute severe asthma.

Table 39.12
Features of potentially fatal asthma

Any of the following:
1. An episode of respiratory failure requiring intubation
2. Respiratory acidosis associated with an attack of asthma not requiring intubation
3. Two or more hospital admissions for asthma despite chronic use of oral steroids
4. Two episodes of pneumothorax (or pneumomediastinum) associated with an asthma attack

there is a requirement for mechanical ventilatory support. If the SaO_2 does not reach 92% on high-flow oxygen or the PEFR is less than 100 L/min, arterial blood gas pressures are measured. If life-threatening features are present (Table 39.11), the patient is transferred to the intensive care unit accompanied by a doctor prepared to intubate if any of the following occur:

- Deteriorating PEFR
- Worsening or persistent hypoxia or hypercapnia
- Exhaustion, feeble respirations, confusion, or drowsiness
- Coma or respiratory arrest

Intravenous aminophylline 250 mg over 20 minutes can be given if the patient is not taking regular oral theophyllines, followed by or starting with—if on oral theophylline—aminophylline 0.5 mg/kg/hr as an infusion. A single dose of magnesium sulphate (1.2 to 2 g intravenous infusion over 20 minutes) has also been shown to be safe and effective in acute severe asthma.

Subsequent Management

Thereafter, the management includes:

- Repeated estimation of response to therapy by clinical assessment of peak flow measurement and oximetry every 15 to 30 minutes
- If improving, continue oxygen, oral corticosteroids four hourly, nebulized β-agonist
- If not improving after 15 to 30 minutes, continue corticosteroids and oxygen, give nebulized β-agonist every 30 minutes, add ipratropium 500 μg nebulized every 6 hours
- If still not improving, commence aminophylline infusion if not already started
- Repeat arterial blood gas tensions if initial PaO_2 less than 8 kPa (60 mmHg) unless subsequent SaO_2 is greater than 92%, $PaCO_2$ normal, or patient deteriorates.

On recovery, the patient should at discharge have:

- Been on discharge medication for 24 hours
- Inhaler technique checked
- PEFR greater than 75% of predicted or best and PEFR diurnal variability less than 25% unless discharge agreed with respiratory physician
- Treatment with oral and inhaled corticosteroids in addition to bronchodilators
- Own PEF meter and a written personal asthma action plan
- Local follow-up arranged for within a week
- Follow-up appointment in chest clinic within 4 weeks

Table 39.13
The emergency management of asthma

Checklist for use after an emergency attendance or admission because of asthma
• Was this potentially fatal asthma? (see Table 39.12)
• Was the patient's inhaler technique satisfactory?
• Prior to the attack were they on, and were they taking, sufficient preventative therapy?
• Was there an avoidable precipitating cause, e.g., aspirin use, premenstrual worsening, alcohol, allergen exposure or occupational cause?
• Was this a genuine sudden severe (brittle) attack and do they need to be taught the special first aid measures needed by this group?
• Is the patient a poor perceiver of severity?
• Did the patient react appropriately to the impending attack, and did they have a written personal asthma action plan?
Note that every episode of severe asthma represents a potential failure of our previous management.

The reason(s) for the exacerbation and admission must be determined (Table 39.13) and details sent to the local physician, together with a discharge plan and potential best PEF.

The advice at discharge is most important. Patients need to be given clear advice as to how long to continue corticosteroid tablets, which should be continued in full dose until the patient is better and then either stopped suddenly (if the patient was not previously on corticosteroids and has taken them for less than 2 weeks) or tapered off. The length of course needed often reflects the length of deterioration of asthma before initiation of treatment; a short period of worsening asthma tends to respond more quickly than does an attack that followed a long period of poor control. For those patients treated with high doses of bronchodilators (whether from a nebulizer or a spacer device), it is important that they are not discharged from observation until the dose is reduced, for fear that the bronchodilator may mask signs of suboptimal control.

Every attack of severe asthma and every hospital admission or emergency room attendance must be regarded as a sign of failure of that patient's previous asthma management. After successful medical management of the attack comes the more important part—a review of the circumstances that led up to the attack. It is important to assess the patient's inhaler technique and self-monitoring skills. Was this a potentially life-threatening attack (see Table 39.12)? What was the prodromal use and dose of anti-inflammatory therapy? If a patient has been taking a regular preventive therapy, an attack of asthma generally indicates the need for at least a temporary increase in dose. Was there an avoidable cause for the attack (e.g., running out of inhalers), an occupational cause, premenstrual worsening, or a potentially life-threatening inadvertent use of a β-blocker? Finally, did the patient react appropriately to the deteriorating control of his or her asthma, and, if a self-management plan was available, had it been used? These issues are summarized in Table 39.13.

Prevention and Organization of Care

Not only must therapeutic methods of prevention be considered, but so must the nonpharmacologic aspects of the management of

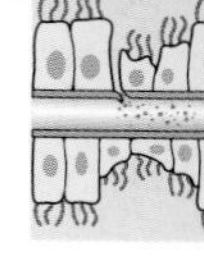

Table 39.14
Factors associated with noncompliance in asthma

Type of factor	Factor
Pharmacologic	Difficult multiple-drug, multiple-dose regimens Real or perceived side effects Inadequate instruction in use of inhaler devices
Nonpharmacologic	Misunderstanding Lack of information Dislike of regular medications Unexpressed fears or concerns Denial of diagnosis Denial of severity/risk Poor communication between patient and health professional

Table 39.15
Suggested content for an asthma educational discussion

- Nature of the disease
- Nature of the treatment - differences between relievers and preventers
- Identify areas where patient wants treatment to have its effect
- How to use the treatment
- Acquisition of skills necessary to recognize worsening asthma
- Self monitoring
- Negotiation of goals and discussion regarding the future
- Appropriate allergen avoidance and environmental manipulation
- Receipt of a written personal asthma action plan

what is, for most patients who have asthma, a long-term condition. This involves consideration of the important subjects of communication, patient education, and self-management.

Writing the correct prescription is only one small part of the treatment of asthma, but in a high proportion of cases the treatment is not taken in the way suggested by the doctor. The reasons for noncompliance (nonadherence) are given in Table 39.14; it is important to understand that often the reason is a simple failure of understanding or lack of information. Of patients who suffer asthma, 50% complain of lack of information, and in only a minority of cases do doctors write down for the patient or parent simple instructions as to which medication to use when. Such written advice is capable of dramatically increasing the proportion of patients, both children and adults, who can correctly describe their drug regimen—and writing down instructions for patients takes only a few seconds, especially if partially preprinted forms are used. However, up to 15% of adults attending hospital clinics and emergency rooms are functionally illiterate, and this has been shown to be associated with increased use of health service resources and with diminished ability to cope with inhaler techniques. Pictorial representation of the medication regimen may be helpful for these patients.

Reinforcement of spoken messages and acquisition of skills and techniques in inhaler use and in peak-flow monitoring can also be undertaken using written materials, loan of videotapes and audiotapes, and subsequent consultation with respiratory trained nurses. The messages offered to the patient by the whole health professional team need to be consistent and uniform, for nothing confuses a patient more than to be given apparently different messages from different people. The use of guidelines on asthma management provides a common text from which to teach patients. Even with a common text, however, it must be recognized that every person who has asthma is an individual and that the starting point for subsequent good communication and patient education is to recognize that each patient has a different set of needs and a different set of fears and concerns regarding the condition, as well as different expectations. A basic education regarding asthma should be offered to all and the ground to be covered is shown in Table 39.15.

The importance of the effect of good communication on subsequent compliance cannot be underestimated. Many patients exhibit denial of either the diagnosis or its implications, and many have concerns regarding perceived or real side effects of treatment which need adequate airing if they are to feel happy taking treatment. Many express concerns at the unpredictable nature of asthma and express irritation at this uncertainty and the effect on quality of life.

Self-management education and the receipt of a written personal asthma action plan is one way of reducing patients' feelings of uncertainty and feelings of dependency. The patient or parent receives written advice from the health professionals as to how to adjust treatment in a variety of circumstances and when and from whom more urgent medical advice should be sought. These plans may be based upon symptoms, or in adults on symptoms and objective monitoring of peak flow; a typical plan is given in Figure 39.17.

Most published studies on successful self-management education have involved patients monitoring their condition and detecting worsening using a combination of symptoms and peak-flow levels. However, results of other studies have suggested that subjective monitoring achieves similar results to objective monitoring. Yet another study showed that in 60% of patients there is no significant correlation between how they feel and measurements of airflow, and there is also evidence to suggest that those with the most severe asthma may be less able to perceive deterioration in airway caliber. Further studies may therefore be needed to better define the role of home peak-flow monitoring, but currently the decision should be to discuss objective monitoring with patients and to recommend it, as a minimum, for those with moderate to severe disease.

Self-management may mean any of the following:

- Using a relieving bronchodilator as required and seeking medical attention if its use becomes more frequent or exceeds, for example, every 4 to 6 hours
- Requesting an early consultation if night-time symptoms develop
- Increasing preventive therapy at the first sign of cold
- Increasing preventive therapy when bronchodilator usage increases or night-time symptoms occur
- Starting a course of corticosteroid tablets in response to deteriorating symptoms or falling peak flow

Most published plans suggest that suitable thresholds for therapeutic change based upon peak-flow readings would be:

- Peak flow greater than 85% of usual best: Continue normal therapy
- Peak flow 70% to 85% of usual best: Increase inhaled steroid

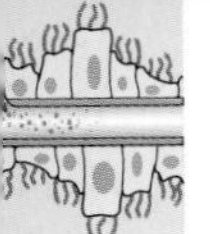

Typical partially preprinted self-treatment plan

ZONE 1*

Your asthma is under control if

It does not disturb your sleep

It does not restrict your usual activities **and**

Your peak flow readings are above ______

ACTION

Continue your normal medicines

Your preventer is ______

You should normally take ______ puffs/doses ______ times every day (using a spacer), even when you are feeling well

Your reliever is ______

You should normally only take it when you are short of breath, coughing or wheezing, or before exercise

Your other medicines are ______

ZONE 2

Your asthma is getting worse if

You are having to use your ______ (reliever inhaler) more than usual

You are waking at night with asthma symptoms

and

Your peak flow readings have fallen to between ______ and ______

ACTION

Increase your usual medicines

Increase your ______ (preventer inhaler) to ______

Continue to take your ______ (reliever inhaler) to relieve your asthma symptoms

ZONE 3

Your asthma is severe if

You are getting increasingly breathless

You are having to use your ______ (reliever inhaler) every ______ hours or more often

and

Your peak flow readings have fallen to between ______ and ______

ACTION

Start a course of corticosteroid tablets

Take ______ prednisolone (corticosteroid) tablets strength ______ (mg each) and then ______

Discuss with your doctor how and when to stop taking the tablets

Continue to take your ______ (reliever and preventer inhalers) as prescribed

ZONE 4

It is a medical emergency if

Your symptoms continue to get worse

and

Your peak flow readings have fallen to below ______

Do not be afraid of causing a fuss. Your doctor will want to see you urgently.

ACTION

Get help immediately

Telephone your doctor straightaway on ______ or call an ambulance

Take ______ prednisolone (corticosteroid) tablets strength ______ (mg each) immediately

Continue to take your ______ (reliever inhaler) as needed, or every 5–10 minutes until the ambulance arrives

* If you persistently in this zone, your doctor may reduce your usual medication

Figure 39.17 Typical partially preprinted self-treatment plan.

- Peak flow 50% to 70% of usual best: Start a course of steroid tablets
- Peak flow less than 50% of usual best: Seek urgent medical attention

Many recent studies and systematic reviews support the use of self-management. Two controlled studies recruited outpatients who had moderately severe asthma and followed them up for 6 or 12 months after being given self-management advice. In each case the intervention group had less need for emergency medical care, less time off work, and a better quality of life than did the control group. In one of the studies, the self-management group not only had better-controlled asthma, but achieved it using lower overall doses of corticosteroid tablets over a 12-month period compared with the control group. This implies either that increasing ICSs at the first sign of deterioration is an important therapeutic step or that giving patients control of their condition enhances compliance so that they take their ICSs and are less likely to deteriorate to a point where they need corticosteroid tablets. Compliance with the self-management plans was remarkably high—on 77% of the occasions when circumstances suggested that patients needed to start corticosteroid tablets, they did so. Another study has shown that the collecting of prescriptions for inhaled steroids was significantly greater in a group of patients who had received self-management education and a written personal asthma action plan than in a group of control asthmatics.

There is some controversy regarding whether doubling inhaled steroids at the first sign of deterioration is beneficial. Although one study in which that was the only variable did not show a reduction in those subsequently needing steroid tablets or hospitalization, all of the self-management studies that have shown beneficial outcomes have included that action. It may be that including that action within a four-zone plan prompts some to restart the inhaled steroids they may not have been taking as prescribed. Other studies suggest that perhaps a simple doubling of inhaled steroids may be insufficient, and one study showed benefit of quadrupling the dose. Clearly, this depends upon the initial starting dose, and advice needs to be tailored to the individual. If the basic principle of always using the lowest dose of

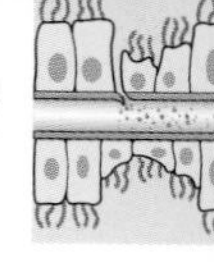

medication that controls the disease is adopted, it is possible that patients may routinely be on very low doses of maintenance inhaled steroids (where necessary by the addition of long-acting inhaled β-agonists) but triple or quadruple the dose at the first sign of deterioration. Controversy regarding exact details of the intervention described on a personal asthma action plan should not be an excuse for not implementing the principle, especially in the face of more than 36 randomized control trials showing benefits from self-management education.

Asthma is an increasingly common condition. The challenge for the future is to prevent more people from developing it, but in the meantime excellent therapies are available to control it. However, these have to be offered to the patient in a manner that makes it likely they will be used to maximal benefit.

PITFALLS AND CONTROVERSIES

Accurate Diagnosis

Until a patient carries the correct diagnosis, he or she is unlikely to receive the correct treatment—repeated chest infections usually are not such and should raise the suspicion of asthma. Persistent coughs in adults and children may also be the most prominent features of undiagnosed asthma, so persistent cough merits investigation and a trial of asthma therapy. An occupational cause should always be considered in an adult presenting for the first time with asthma. Overdiagnosis must also be avoided; unfortunately, publicity regarding asthma has led to a situation in which every respiratory symptom (and some cardiac ones) is treated for asthma until proved otherwise. Constant reminders that asthma is only one of numerous respiratory diseases are necessary.

Self-management Education

Doctors are good at writing prescriptions. They are often not as good at implementing nonpharmacologic interventions that may be of equal or greater benefit. Good communication, self-management education, and the offering of a written personal asthma action plan to all with asthma should become normal practice.

Use of Inhaled Steroids

There is little doubt that the single chemical entity that has most improved the situation for 300 million people with asthma worldwide over the last 30 years has been the introduction of inhaled steroids. However, for many with asthma in the less prosperous countries of the world, these basic medicines are either not available, not prescribed, cannot be afforded, or not used because of cultural misconceptions or barriers. In other countries where inhaled steroids are easily available, they may be used suboptimally because of steroid phobia and less efficient medications used in their place. In other cases, inhaled steroids may be misused, with excessive doses being used and "step down" not being practiced.

Transition to Chlorofluorocarbon-free Metered Dose Inhalers

Withdrawal of CFC propellants from MDIs under the Montreal Protocol means that most patients are now in the process of being changed to CFC-free MDIs. Patients need to be forewarned that reformulation of their inhaled medicines with new HFA propellants may lead to the inhaler feeling or weighing differently from their predecessors, and the impact of the aerosolized medicines on the oropharynx is likely to be less. A difference in taste may also occur. For some products, reformulation involves a change in dose of the medicine administered. Patients need to be reassured that:

- Treatment is as safe as it was previously
- Treatment is as effective as it was previously
- Previous propellants were environmentally, and not individually, damaging
- New inhalers are very similar
- The active ingredient is the same

More trials have been undertaken with the new products than were ever undertaken with the original inhalers.

Successful Management

To offer treatment in a manner that makes it likely it will be taken involves:

- Eliciting the patients' understanding of the condition
- Eliciting their fears, concerns, and information needs
- Discussing common goals and clarifying the risks versus benefits of treatment or no treatment
- Giving control of the condition to the patient by means of a written personal asthma action plan
- Reinforcing the spoken word with personalized written information
- Offering regular follow-up during which reinforcement of these messages is given, as is further opportunity for discussion, and reduction of therapy to the minimum necessary to control the condition.

SUGGESTED READINGS

British Thoracic Society/Scottish Intercollegiate Guideline Network: British guideline on the management of asthma. Thorax 58:1-94, 2003.

National Asthma Education and Prevention Program. NAEPP Expert Panel Report: Guidelines for the diagnosis and management of asthma—update on selected topics (NIH Publication No. 02-5075). Bethesda, Md, National Institutes of Health, 2002.

National Institutes of Health. National Heart, Lung and Blood Institute: Global Strategy for Asthma Management and Prevention (update from NIH Publication No. 02-3659). Bethesda, Md, Global Initiative for Asthma (GINA), 2002.

CHAPTER 40 Cystic Fibrosis

Daniel V. Schidlow and Stanley B. Fiel

EPIDEMIOLOGY

Cystic fibrosis (CF) is the most common genetically inherited disease in white people. The mode of inheritance is autosomal recessive. The estimated frequency of occurrence is approximately 1 in 3300 live births among whites, 1 in 15,000 African Americans, 1 in 9500 Hispanics, and 1 in 32,000 live births of individuals of Asian origin in the United States.

HISTORICAL PERSPECTIVE

Already in the Middle Ages, folk writings propounded that young infants and children whose skin tasted salty had a high risk of dying young. In 1938, Dr. Dorothy Anderson coined the term *cystic fibrosis of the pancreas*, which established the concept of CF as a multisystem disease of genetic origin. Later, Sidney Farber coined the term *mucoviscidosis* to reflect the presence of thick and tenacious mucus in various organ bodies. In 1946, Dr. Anderson again proposed that the mode of inheritance indeed followed an autosomal recessive pattern. In the early 1950s, sweat electrolyte abnormalities that consisted of excessive secretion of sodium and chloride were observed by DiSant'Agnese. This clinician and his collaborators treated several children who were admitted with hypotonic dehydration to the Babies' Hospital in New York during a heat wave, and confirmed that the cause of this dehydration and metabolic alkalosis was excessive secretion of sodium and chloride through the skin. This observation gave rise to the sweat test, which has served until recently as the only diagnostic laboratory study to confirm the diagnosis of CF.

It took more than 30 years to begin to gain further insights into the cause and pathogenesis of CF. In the 1980s, several investigators, including Quinton, Knowles, and Boucher, described abnormal ion conductance in epithelia of patients with CF. In 1989, a multinational team of investigators based in Michigan and Toronto (Collins, Toohey, and Riordan) successfully identified and cloned the CF gene. Since then, research efforts have been directed at enhancing our knowledge of the relationship between the genetic defect, disease mechanisms, and clinical manifestations. Currently, research efforts are aimed at correcting the genetic defect and its cellular consequences.

GENETICS

The origin of CF is a mutation on the long arm of chromosome 7 that encodes for a protein product called the CF transmembrane conductance regulator, or CFTR. This protein acts as a chloride channel that also has regulatory functions over sodium channels located in epithelial cell membranes (Fig. 40.1). The CF gene is approximately 250,000 base pairs in length, and more than 1000 mutations of the gene have been reported to date. The most common mutation, ΔF508, is characterized by the absence of a single phenylalanine from the protein gene product. This mutation arises from a deletion of three bases in the encoding exon.

Five different classes of mutations have been described and grouped (Fig. 40.2). Class I mutations are those in which the synthesis of CFTR is defective. These mutations prevent transcription of *CFTR* into full-length messenger RNA (mRNA), which leads to a defect in protein production and a loss of CFTR function. Abnormal transcription is caused by the omission of an exon or abnormal splicing as a consequence of nonsense, splice site, and frame shift mutations.

Class II mutations are those in which defective processing of protein occurs. A typical example of these mutations is ΔF508, wherein the CFTR protein fails to undergo appropriate folding required for its trafficking to the correct position in the cell membrane. As a result, the protein is degraded and entrapped in the endoplasmic reticulum. An interesting feature of this mutation of potential therapeutic relevance is that ΔF508 undergoes folding and improper processing, and achieves function at very low (i.e., $<30°$ C) temperatures.

Class III mutations affect the regulation and activation of CFTR at the cell surface, in which abnormal CFTR proteins arrive at the site of function unable to activate or function normally as ion channels. Some of these mutations affect binding sites and the regulatory (or "R") domain of CFTR, and consequently disrupt the binding of adenosine triphosphate (ATP) and hydrolysis.

Class IV mutations interfere with the conductance of the chloride channel, which results in a reduction of ion flow and induces changes while the ion channel remains open.

Class V mutations result in decreased production of CFTR. The latter two mutations result in somewhat preserved CFTR function and tend to be associated with milder or incomplete clinical expression of the disease (i.e., normal pancreatic function).

Some authors also have described a class V mutation in which decreased, attenuated production of CFTR and attenuated conductance occur (see Fig. 40.2).

PATHOPHYSIOLOGY

Defense Mechanisms

Although CFTR is a cyclic adenosine monophosphate–regulated chloride channel, it also has other functions, which include the regulation of other membrane proteins, such as the outward

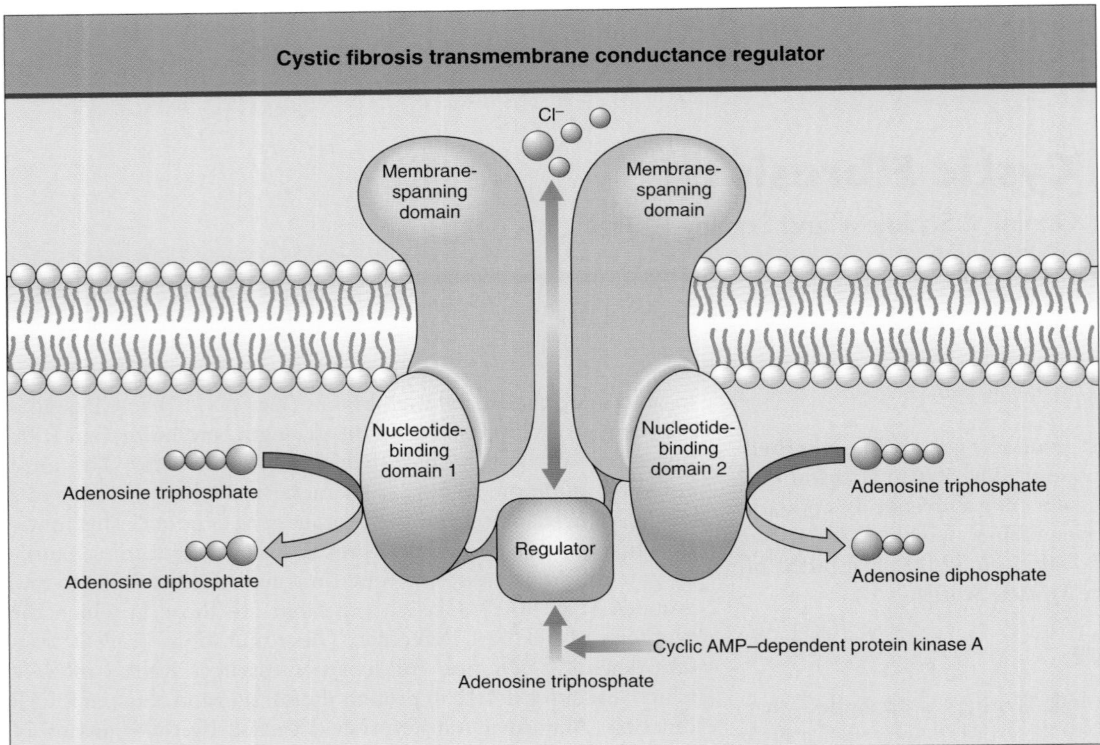

Figure 40.1 Cystic fibrosis transmembrane conductance regulator. AMP, adenosine monophosphate.

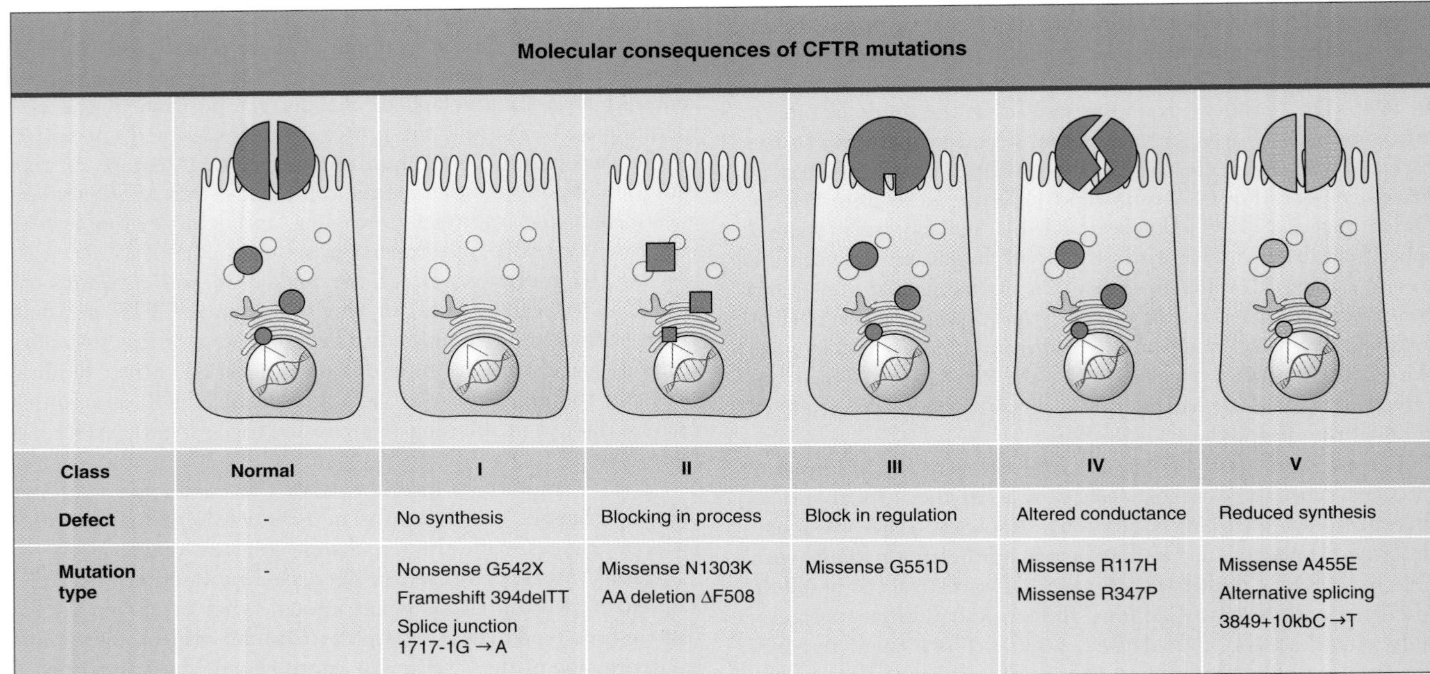

Figure 40.2 Major classes and molecular consequences of cystic fibrosis transmembrane conductance regulator (CFTR) mutations.

rectifying chloride channel and sodium channels, and it may possibly have an impact on other ion conductances.

The cardinal problem in CF relates to the presence of abnormal, highly adherent, viscous mucus in all epithelium-lined organs. The ion channel abnormality, caused by the defective protein, leads to formation of the thick mucus characteristically observed in CF. The mechanisms of this stepwise defect are not completely understood; however, knowledge of the process has facilitated understanding of the multiorgan involvement of CF and the variety of clinical manifestations observed.

Abnormal secretions in the lung appear to engender an inflammatory response despite the absence of demonstrable infection. The abnormal epithelial fluid present in the respiratory tract of patients with CF inhibits or inactivates microbial

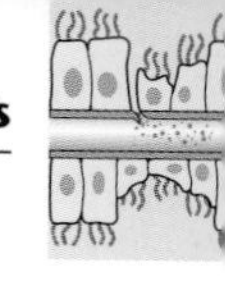

clearance mechanisms, such as the β-defensins, as described by Wilson and others. Microbial colonization and persistence is favored by the abnormal adherence between microorganisms in the respiratory tract (particularly *Pseudomonas aeruginosa*), which gives rise to a progressively severe cycle of infection and inflammation over the person's life span. The first organisms to invade the respiratory tract, frequently during early childhood, are gram-negative, nontypeable nonfermenters (i.e., *Haemophilus influenzae* and *Staphylococcus aureus*). As patients with CF age, *P. aeruginosa* eventually invades the airway and binds to the cell surface, which results in permanent colonization and chronic infection. A mucoid variant of *P. aeruginosa* colonizes and infects the lungs, and is considered pathognomonic for CF. This variant has not been observed in any other disease or in patients who do not have CF.

The endobronchial inflammatory process of CF is characterized by spontaneous antigenic stimulation, T-cell activation, and the release of cytokines (including tissue necrosis factor and various interleukins [ILs], particularly IL-8) that result in a strong immunologic response and the recruitment of neutrophils (Fig. 40.3). Bacterial binding and subsequent neutrophil degradation liberate oxidizing compounds such as superoxide, hydrogen peroxide, and hydroxyl ions. Concurrently, neutrophils stimulate the release of different chemicals that cause inflammation to attack and destroy the bacteria. Unfortunately, these mediators of inflammation (which include proteases such as elastase) interfere with normal, complement-mediated, phagocytic host defense, and result in tissue inflammation and destruction. Although such an immunologic response is anticipated and normal, in individuals who have CF the respiratory tract is overwhelmed by the magnitude of elastase release. This antiprotease response results in a deficit of neutralizing protein and the presence of free elastase in the respiratory fluid of these patients. This lung environment, unique to CF, promotes mucus secretion that leads to secretory metaplasia, as well as interference with and cleavage of normal neutralizing proteins.

Goblet cell and submucosal gland hypertrophy quickly supervene. Left unchecked, airway walls weaken and become dilated over time. In the presence of increasingly thickened, tenacious mucus, the bronchi become obstructed. Small airway obstruction progresses, and bronchiolectasis and subsequent bronchiectasis occur as the patient matures. The gradual, yet relentless, progression of lung damage diminishes and eventually destroys healthy lung tissue, which renders the intake of sufficient oxygen and elimination of carbon dioxide impossible.

PATHOLOGY

Airways

At autopsy, the typical gross appearance of the lung is one of consolidation. Numerous areas of bronchiectasis filled with mucopurulent material, mucus plugging of the smaller airways, thickening and fibrosis of the airway walls, and the presence of fibrinous pleuritis can be observed in areas where infection has bored through to the pleural surface (Fig. 40.4). Microscopically, obliteration of bronchioles, dilatation of air spaces with destruction of interalveolar septa, diffuse airway occupation by eosinophilic materials, and diffuse interstitial fibrosis are common. In some patients, subpleural blebs and large bronchiectatic cysts may be present. In patients who have experienced prolonged hypoxemia, the vascular changes of pulmonary hypertension also may be evident.

Pancreas

Approximately 95% of patients with CF exhibit some degree of exocrine pancreas dysfunction. Enzyme insufficiency leads to maldigestion of protein and fat, by which the normal structure of the pancreas is replaced. Microscopically, a loss of normal anatomy occurs, fibrous fatty tissue diffusely occupies the parenchyma, and small cysts develop from dilated ducts present throughout the organ (hence the term "CF of the pancreas"; Fig. 40.5).

Hepatobiliary System

In a large number of individuals, the liver appears abnormal microscopically on autopsy. Secretions and bile become inspissated, bile duct proliferation occurs, and an inflammatory reaction is present in approximately 30% of patients with CF. Overt nodular cirrhosis is rare and is associated with death in only a small minority (i.e., 1% to 5%) of patients with CF (Fig. 40.6). The gallbladder is commonly hypoplastic (i.e., microbladder) and contains inspissated bile, viscous material, or bile stones.

Intestines

Goblet cell hyperplasia and accumulation of eosinophilic secretions in the crypts in the lumen of the intestine are characteristic in CF. Mucus abnormality may be a factor in the increased tendency of stools to adhere to the walls of the organ.

Reproductive System

Although spermatogenesis can be demonstrated by testicular biopsy, greater than 99% of male patients with CF are sterile because of incomplete development of the wolffian ducts. The epididymis and vas deferens are either partially or completely absent; seminal vesicles may be very small or absent as well. Many women are anovulatory secondary to chronic lung disease, although the fertility rate may be as high as 20%. Further, viscous and inspissated cervical mucus may plug the cervical canal and prevent conception.

Upper Respiratory Tract

Virtually all patients with CF experience increased production of secretions and thickening of the mucosal lining of the sinuses. Nasal polyposis occurs in up to 30% of patients with CF. Upper respiratory manifestations range from small formations that cause increased posterior nasal drainage to large tumors that completely obstruct the nasal passages. In rare instances, mucoceles and ballooning of the sinus cavity may compress the orbit. Infraorbital edema with widening of the nasal bridge should increase clinical suspicion of polyps and more significant sinus disease in patients with CF (Fig. 40.7).

Lower Respiratory Tract

Chronic or recurrent bronchiolitis, in the presence of cough, wheezing, tachypnea, and prolonged expiration, is commonly

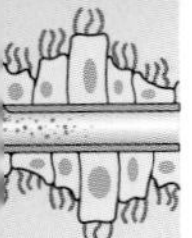

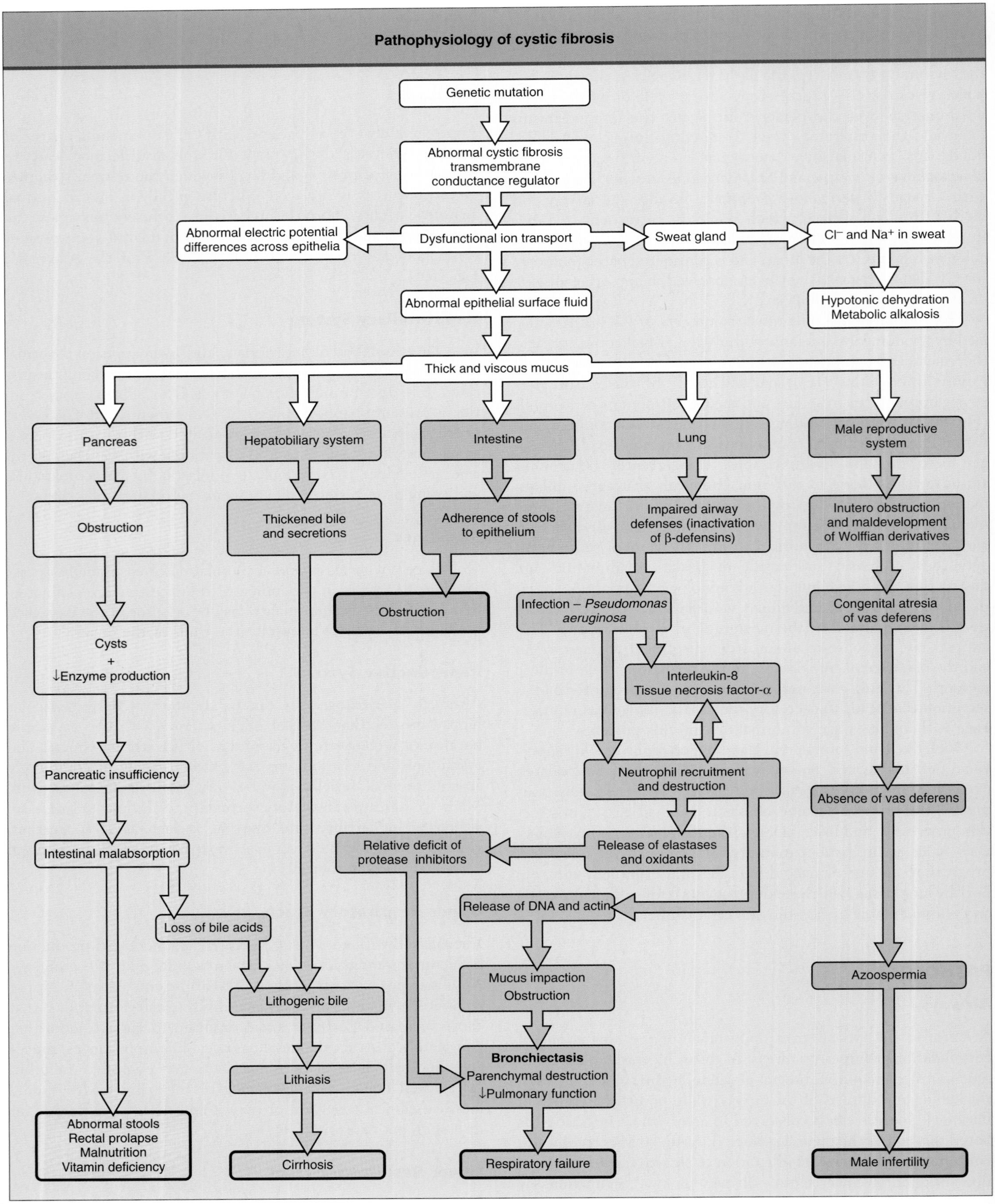

Pathophysiology of cystic fibrosis

Figure 40.3 Pathophysiology of cystic fibrosis.

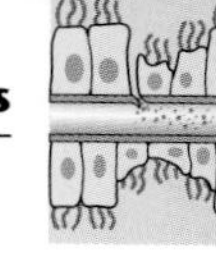

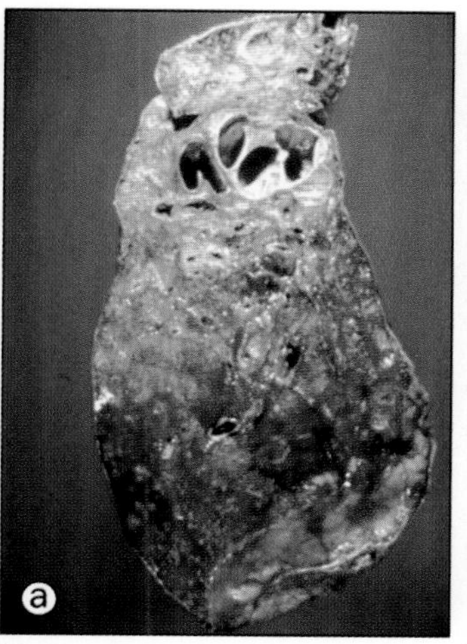

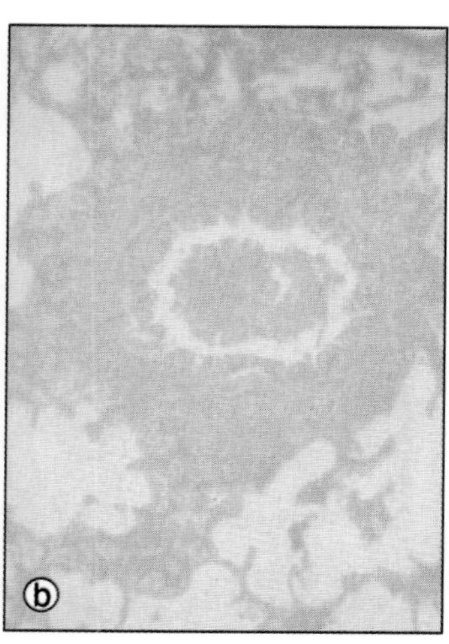

Figure 40.4 Lung pathology. **A,** Gross abnormal lung showing bronchiectatic cysts. **B,** Microscopic view of a cystic fibrosis lung with small bronchus showing occupation of the lumen. (Courtesy of J. Palmer.)

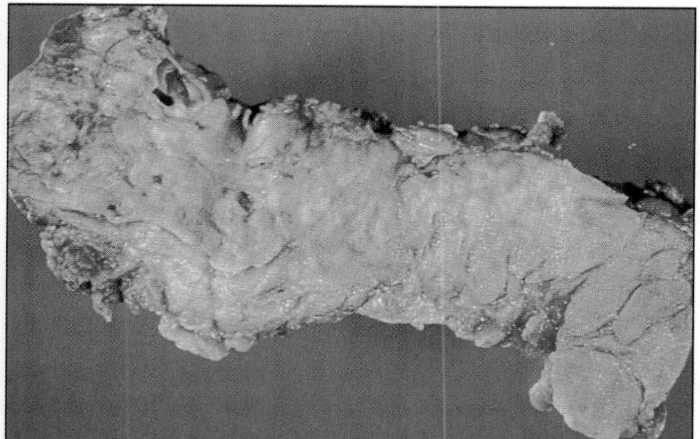

Figure 40.5 Gross cystic fibrosis pancreas pathology.

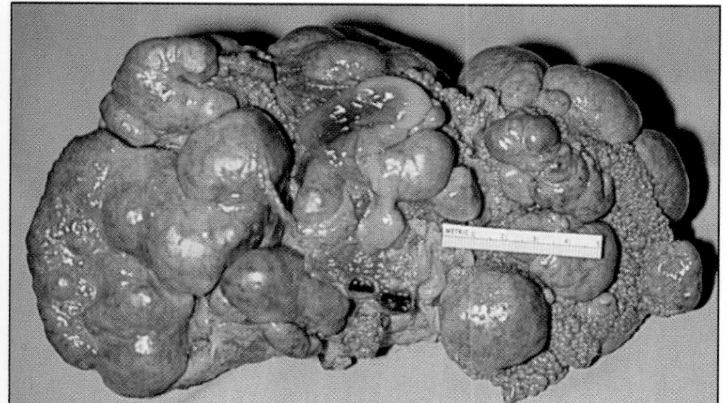

Figure 40.6 Gross cystic fibrosis liver showing nodular cirrhosis. The patient died from hepatic failure.

observed in infants who have CF. As growth and aging progress, the contribution of small airways to the overall airway diminishes resistance. Classically, CF is characterized by periodic flare-ups of chronic bronchitis. An increase in daily cough, increased lung mucus production, and an increase in sputum become common features in most patients. Sputum ranges from light yellow to deep green and is usually thick and tenacious (Fig. 40.8). Exacerbations are usually triggered by infection with viruses or mycoplasma. During these episodes, cough and expectoration increase, and sputum becomes thicker and more abundant. Patients also may run a low-grade fever, experience increased fatigue (sometimes accompanied by shortness of breath), and exhibit a decrease in or loss of appetite (coupled with weight loss). Wheezing in the presence of crackles in additional lung areas, prolonged expiration, and suprasternal (and occasionally intercostal) retractions also can be present. Chest radiographs may show hyperinflation, increased mucus plugging, and obstruction of the airways.

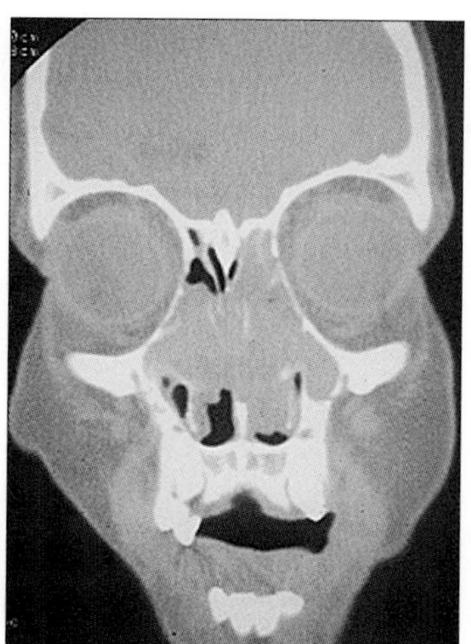

Figure 40.7 Sinus disease in cystic fibrosis. Computed tomography scan shows opacification of the ethmoid sinuses and large nasal polyps in a patient with cystic fibrosis.

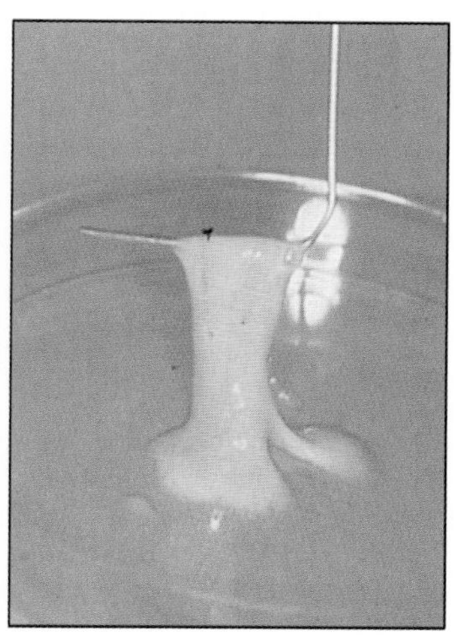

Figure 40.8 Thick, tenacious sputum from a patient with cystic fibrosis. (Courtesy of J. Palmer.)

CLINICAL FEATURES

The abnormal physiology associated with CF affects many body systems; thus, it is not surprising that a variety of complications may be seen in patients who have the disease, although pulmonary abnormalities comprise the major focus of concern. The most common primary clinical manifestations of CF include endobronchial inflammation (i.e., chronic, recurrent airway obstruction and infection), pancreatic insufficiency with intestinal malabsorption, and congenital bilateral absence of the vas deferens in male patients. Nonpulmonary manifestations also are

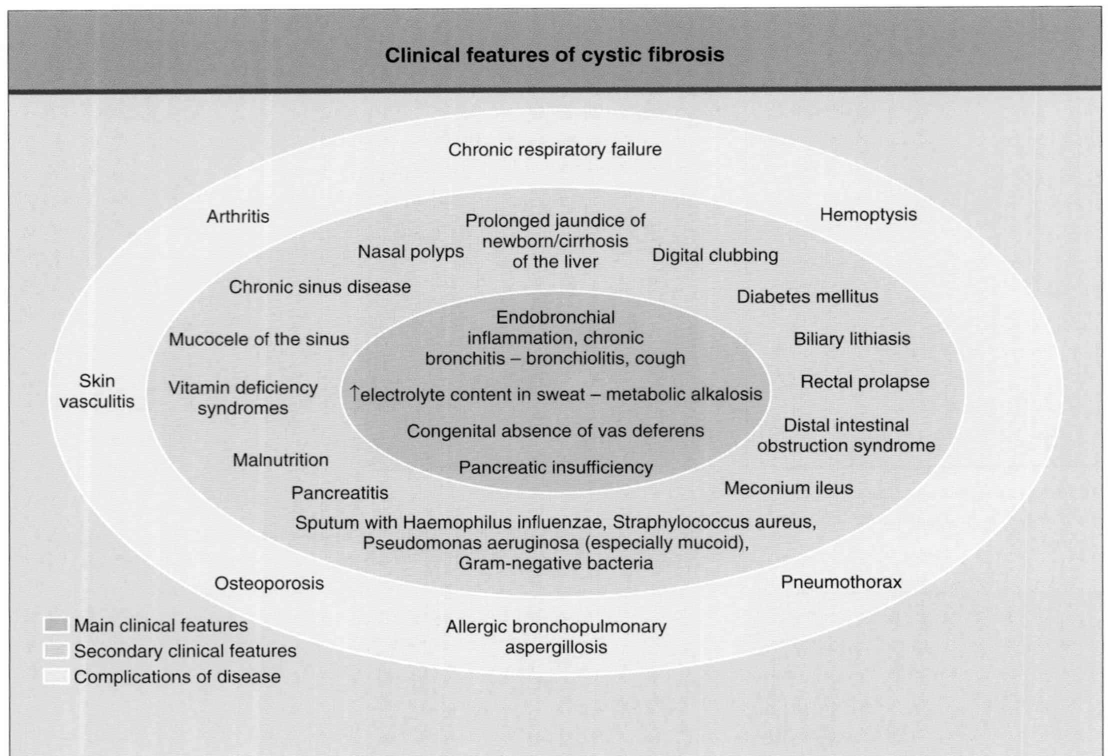

Figure 40.9 Clinical features of cystic fibrosis.

common and include meconium ileus, malabsorption, fatty infiltration of the liver, focal biliary cirrhosis, glucose intolerance, and a predilection for heat prostration because of severe salt depletion (Fig. 40.9).

Bacterial Colonization and Infection

Endobronchial infection occurs very early in life in patients with CF. The initial microorganisms to colonize the lungs are gram-negative bacteria such as *Escherichia coli*, protease and *Klebsiella* variants. Also, *H. influenzae* and *S. aureus* are recovered on initial encounter in many patients. There appear to be regional differences in the reported incidence of microorganisms, particularly with *H. influenzae*. By the age of 15 to 16 years, over 60% of patients with CF acquire *P. aeruginosa*. The mucoid variant of *P. aeruginosa* is considered pathognomonic for CF. An alginate confers this variant with its mucoid characteristics.

In the past several years, clinicians have witnessed the emergence of multiresistant strains of *P. aeruginosa* along with other multiresistant species such as *Stenotrophomonas maltophilia*, *Achromobacter xylosoxidans*, *Ralstonia* species, and various *Burkholderia* species, including *Burkholderia cepacia* complex and *Burkholderia gladioli*. The exact reason for the development of resistance is not well understood, but environmental factors, such as an increased presence of these microorganisms, coupled with the aggressive use of several antimicrobial agents in CF therapy have been postulated. The transmission mechanisms of *B. cepacia* complex in the CF population are not well understood; however, evidence suggests that acquisition may occur both from direct patient-to-patient contact and through the environment. Recent findings suggest that the initial infecting strain of *B. cepacia* complex may be replaced by another, potentially more virulent strain, placing patients at even higher risk. Further, research suggests that phenotypes of the *B. cepacia* complex may influence chronic human infection by intrinsically contributing to a broad range of resistance to antimicrobial agents as well as nonoxidative killing by human phagocytic cells. Some factors identified to affect virulence include pili and adhesins that mediate bacterial adherence to the epithelial cells, lipopolysaccharides and exopolysaccharides, lipases, proteases, phosphatases, hemolysins, and siderophores. The adverse prognosis in patients who become infected, together with these data, demand strenuous efforts to prevent new acquisitions. This has prompted the implementation of rigorous infection control measures in CF centers in which patients who are known to be colonized with *Burkholderia* species are treated.

Advances in the taxonomy of *B. cepacia* have identified nine distinct bacterial species of the complex—all of which have now received formal binomial designations, confronting clinicians with an array of evolving species names and adding to the confusion in definitive species designation. Misidentification rates as high as 10% have been observed when *B. cepacia* species are confused with other nonfermenting gram-negative bacteria (i.e., *Stenotrophomonas*, *Alcaligenes*, *Pandoraea*, and *Ralstonia*). This may be attributed to the variability in adherence to microbiology laboratory protocols, use of commercial systems not well suited to the task, or the difficult and complex taxonomy of the *B. cepacia* species. In the CF patient population, the prevalence of patients infected with *B. cepacia* is approximately 3% to 4%, and it is believed to affect 1 in 10 adults with CF. The most frequently recovered species include *Burkholderia multivorans* and *Burkholderia cenocepacia*, accounting for approximately 80% of the infected population of patients with CF. Research is under way to investigate effects of multiple antibiotic regimens targeted to specific genomovars in an effort to reduce mortality in these populations. Researchers continue to investigate the virulence of specific genomovars in patients with CF and CF subgroup populations (i.e., transplant recipients).

Aspergillus fumigatus and other fungi such as *Candida albicans* also are recovered frequently from the respiratory tracts of patients who have CF. The significance of this is unclear because these fungi are relatively ubiquitous. On occasion, allergic bronchopulmonary reactions to *Aspergillus* species have been observed in patients with CF, as well as allergy to other fungi that have produced severe respiratory exacerbations in some (particularly older) patients with CF. Although the significance of this finding is as yet unclear, it appears that, in some cases, these microorganisms may be pathogenic; however, a cause-and-effect relationship between the presence of these microbacteria in the sputum and signs or symptoms of disease has not been fully elucidated.

There is an increasing prevalence of nontuberculous mycobacterial (NTM) pulmonary infection in patients with CF; however, researchers and clinicians remain unclear regarding the implications of NTM disease in patients with CF, how to distinguish clinically significant infection from colonization, and whether treatment alters the clinical course of the disease. Guidelines issued by the American Thoracic Society for all patients for the diagnosis of NTM pulmonary disease recommend that patients must meet the following clinical, radiographic, and bacteriologic criteria:

1. *Clinical criteria*: signs and symptoms compatible with reasonable exclusion of other disease (i.e., cough, fatigue, fever, weight loss, hemoptysis, dyspnea)
2. *Radiographic criteria*: by chest radiography or high-resolution computed tomography scan abnormalities (persistent or progressive infiltrates or nodules, cavitation, multiple nodules, or multifocal bronchiectasis with or without small nodules)
3. *Microbiologic criteria*: three positive cultures with negative smears, two positive cultures with one positive smear, or growth from tissue biopsy with granuloma/acid-fast bacilli or growth from a sterile site. The degree of growth required varies with risk factors.

Applying these strict criteria to patients with CF and NTM presents a quandary. Although the clinical symptoms in patients with CF and NTM are relatively compatible with bacterial exacerbations of CF lung disease, radiographic findings may be difficult to distinguish from those of non–NTM-infected patients with CF. Culture results also may be difficult to interpret in the absence of credible clinical and radiographic evidence. Thus, it remains unclear whether there are additional factors that could distinguish a population of NTM-infected patients with CF in whom treatment of NTM may improve clinical outcomes.

Pulmonary Features

Airway hyperreactivity is quite common in CF, such that the incidence surpasses that of asthma in the general population. It is present very early in life and remains so throughout adulthood in patients with CF. Frequently, airway hyperreactivity becomes apparent during the adolescent years, but the cause is not well understood. It has been postulated that this is because of the presence of "true" asthma and atopy, exposure to increased endobronchial levels of mediators of inflammation and bronchopulmonary *Aspergillosis* species, and other, less well-defined factors.

Pulmonary function is one of the most important outcome criteria in the clinical evaluation of patients who have CF. Loss of pulmonary function occurs with the progression of CF disease, evidenced by a decline in forced expiration volume in 1 second (FEV_1) values. Very early in life, signs of small airways obstruction become evident. In those institutions in which pulmonary function tests can be performed in infants, increased airways resistance and decreased compliance have been demonstrated (particularly during episodes of exacerbation) even in infants who have normal pulmonary function test values. Characteristic pulmonary function patterns in patients with CF indicate an initial mild obstruction of the small airways that progressively worsens, coupled with progressive increases in functional residual capacity and residual volume. With increasing tissue destruction and fibrotic scarring, this pattern escalates to severe obstructive and restrictive lung disease. Remarkably, hypoxemia does not usually occur until significant deterioration of pulmonary function has taken place. Hypercapnia occurs as a late event in CF disease progression and carries a very poor prognosis.

Radiographic Evidence

Radiographic evidence of hyperinflation in infants who have CF provides one of the earliest signs of lung deterioration. In addition, right upper lobe atelectasis has been described as a characteristic complication of early disease. As CF progresses, peribronchial cuffing and interstitial disease become increasingly prominent. Nodular cystic lesions (characteristic of bronchiectatic changes and inflammation) are also commonly observed. Radiographic hallmarks of severe disease include diffuse interstitial markings, nodular cystic lesions, areas of sub-segmental atelectasis, and large bronchiectasis cysts (Fig. 40.10). Several numeric scoring systems for radiographic findings in CF have been devised to assess the degree of disease severity. The most popular system is the Birmingham Score, developed by Brasfield and colleagues.

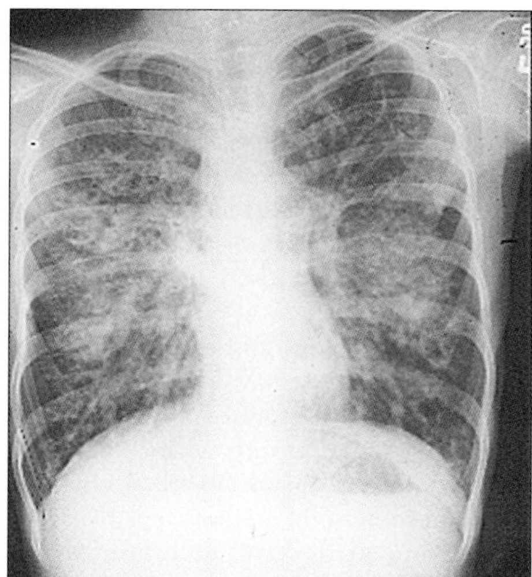

Figure 40.10 Chest radiograph of advanced pulmonary disease in cystic fibrosis. Shown are hyperinflation, interstitial fibrosis, peribronchial thickening, and a bronchiectatic cyst in the upper left lobe. (Adapted with permission from Rosenstein BJ, Cutting GR: The diagnosis of cystic fibrosis: A consensus statement. J Pediatr 32:589-595, 1998.)

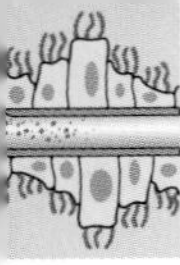

Complementary Imaging Modalities

Computed tomography of the chest can help to assess the early signs of bronchiectasis, particularly for infants, in whom radiographic findings may appear relatively normal.

OTHER SYSTEMIC COMPLICATIONS OF CYSTIC FIBROSIS

Pancreatic Disease

Long considered one of the hallmarks of CF, pancreatic insufficiency is present in approximately 95% of patients with CF. The presence of this abnormality is genetically endowed and can be traced back to the presence of specific mutations (see later section on Genotype–Phenotype Relationship). The occlusion of pancreatic ducts results in insufficient or absent secretion of enzymes into the duodenum, and the consequent maldigestion of all foodstuffs. As a result of lack of absorption of fat and protein, patients experience symptoms that include abdominal distention and very bulky, frequent, and greasy stools that have a characteristic, sui generis offensive odor. If left uncorrected, intestinal malabsorption can result in severe malnutrition and vitamin deficiency states, particularly of the liposoluble vitamins.

In some young infants, lack of vitamin A can cause pseudotumor cerebri and other neurologic problems. Lack of vitamin D can result in rickets, and vitamin K deficiency may produce hypoprothrombinemia and bleeding. Although such conditions of vitamin deficiency are rare, clinicians need to remain alert to these complications in infants who have CF to ensure that appropriate and timely management is implemented. Osteoporosis and pathologic fractures, two conditions that are now beginning to be reported in adults who have CF, are likely associated with a history of insufficient intake of vitamin D and calcium, or poor compliance with enzyme supplementation prescribed for the management of intestinal malabsorption. Pancreatitis is diagnosed in a very small fraction of patients who have CF and occurs most commonly during late adolescence or in adulthood.

Intestinal Manifestations

Meconium ileus, an intestinal obstruction that occurs in utero, is present in approximately 15% to 20% of neonates who have CF. With the advent of ultrasonography, however, it is common for intestinal obstruction to be identified in utero. In such cases, it is often the initial clue to a CF diagnosis.

In meconium ileus, severe abdominal distention develops in the neonate, usually within the first 2 days of birth, and surgical intervention is required in most cases. The meconium obstruction occurs at the level of the ileocecal valve. Frequently, the colon is quite small (i.e., microcolon) and concretions may be present. Occasionally, the intestines may become so filled because of the blockage that the wall perforates and meconium peritonitis ensues. In addition, as some patients with CF become older, they may experience recurrent distal intestinal obstruction syndrome (DIOS)—or meconium ileus equivalent (MIE)—as a result of stools that adhere to the wall of the intestine. Fortunately, surgical intervention is rarely, if ever, required for this complication in adults, and medical management is sufficient to resolve the blockage.

Both MIE and DIOS occur in patients who have pancreatic insufficiency. Intussusception occurs with a slightly greater frequency in patients with CF and can present as an intestinal obstruction that is nearly indistinguishable from DIOS. In general, patients who present with intestinal obstruction later in life require a contrast enema to make the diagnosis.

Biliary Tree—Liver

Although cholestasis is common in CF, approximately 30% of patients have only elevated levels of liver enzymes and alkaline phosphatase. In a small number of patients, however, cirrhosis of the liver, accompanied by portal hypertension and liver failure, occurs. Severely malnourished young infants may present with a fatty liver. In this condition, the liver appears hyperlucent on radiography. Fatty liver in infants is corrected with proper nutrition.

Cholelithiasis is being increasingly detected in patients who have CF. Most of these patients may have gallbladder stones, whereas biliary colic and symptomatic biliary disease occur in few patients. When these are present, surgical intervention may be required.

Reproductive System

Infertility is a nearly universal feature of men who have CF. Congenital bilateral absence of the vas deferens and, less commonly, atresia of the vas deferens result in azoospermia. Only approximately 1% of men with CF are fertile, and these individuals usually have very mild disease manifestations. Further, although spermatogenesis is normal in these men, the incidence of abnormal spermatozoa is higher than that observed in the non-CF population. Recently, surgical retrieval of sperm from the epididymis and assisted reproductive techniques have facilitated biologic fatherhood for a small number of men with CF.

Women who have CF are more prone to infertility because of the characteristic inspissated mucus that covers the cervix. Concomitant malnutrition and severe lung disease also contribute to infertility, and failure to ovulate is not uncommon. Although initial reports of pregnancy in women who have CF documented a high rate of complications and risk, recent prospective studies showed that, in women who have CF who carried to term, pregnancy did not modify health risks. In general terms, the impact of pregnancy on the health of the woman who has CF (and the fetus she carries) depends greatly on her pulmonary function and nutritional status at baseline (i.e., impregnation), and her success in maintaining optimal health throughout the full course of the pregnancy. Relatively mild airflow obstruction, excellent nutritional status, intact pancreatic function, and diagnosis at a later age all were shown to contribute to a more favorable prognosis.

OTHER COMPLICATIONS

Sweat Gland

The abnormality in the sweat gland is characteristic and diagnostic of CF. Patients eliminate abnormal amounts of chloride and sodium in sweat, which predisposes them to hypotonic

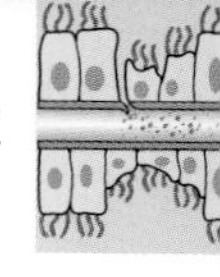

dehydration and metabolic alkalosis, particularly in hot climates. This condition can be life threatening in young infants, in whom rapid loss of water and electrolytes can produce circulatory collapse. In older individuals, CF sweat abnormalities more commonly cause weakness and asthenia.

Diabetes Mellitus

Diabetes mellitus and glucose intolerance occur commonly in patients with CF. The diagnosis and management of these problems are especially challenging and unique in CF. The risk profile for the CF population extends beyond those patients who have confirmed diabetes. In patients with CF, a prediabetic, insulin-deficient state is associated with increased risk for weight loss, impaired pulmonary function, and death. There is a spectrum of glucose tolerance in CF that ranges from normal glucose tolerance to varying degrees of impaired glucose tolerance to overt diabetes. At which point an individual falls along this continuum depends primarily on volume of insulin secretion and degree of insulin sensitivity. In CF, several other distinct factors influence glucose tolerance, including:

- Glucagon deficiency
- Inadequate nutrition or malabsorption
- Abnormal intestinal transit time
- Liver dysfunction
- Pulmonary-related factors such as the presence of chronic or acute infection and increased energy expenditure

Most challenging, because these factors are not static, is that an individual's status is likely to shift along this spectrum of glucose tolerance. Reports of the incidence of diabetes in CF vary and depend on the criteria used to establish the diagnosis and the age distribution of the patients studied. The Cystic Fibrosis Foundation Patient Registry reports that approximately 5% of patients of all ages followed in the United States and Canada receive insulin therapy.

Skin and Joints

Vascular purpura and arthritis have been reported in a few severely ill patients with CF. Characteristically, rashes are circumscribed to the lower extremities and appear to worsen when the patient is standing. In addition, polyarticular pain and joint swelling can occur without an apparent trigger in patients with CF who have advanced disease. In some individuals, these conditions may present concomitantly. Although the pathogenesis of skin and joint disorders in CF is poorly understood, these conditions presumably arise from an immune complex phenomenon. Circulating immune complexes and hypergammaglobulinemia are recognized to occur in association with several skin and joint disorders, and similar clinical findings have been described in such conditions as Waldenström's hypergammaglobulinemia and intestinal bypass syndrome.

Digital Clubbing

Digital clubbing occurs in most patients who have CF and is often present early in the course of pulmonary manifestations of this disease. Severity appears to correlate with the degree of pulmonary dysfunction, but this is not universal. Digital clubbing is also seen in patients who have mild pulmonary disease accompanied by liver disease or other concomitant conditions.

DIAGNOSIS

In the United States, CF is diagnosed in approximately 71% of patients by the age of 1 year. In another 8% of patients, the diagnosis is confirmed by the age of 10 years. With the advent of new diagnostic techniques, an increasing number of patients are being diagnosed after the age of 18 years. Clinicians agree that it is important to confirm or promptly exclude the diagnosis of CF to avoid unnecessary testing, to provide appropriate treatment and counseling to the family and patient, and to ensure that specialized medical services are made available to patients.

In most cases, CF is suspected based on the presence of one or more typical clinical features (Table 40.1). The diagnosis of CF is based on the presence of one or more of these phenotypic features, or a history of CF in a sibling, or a positive newborn screening test plus laboratory evidence of a CFTR abnormality that has been documented by an elevated sweat chloride concentration (Fig. 40.11). Other criteria recently identified by a consensus panel of the Cystic Fibrosis Foundation include the identification of two CF mutations or in vivo demonstration of characteristic abnormalities in ion transport across the nasal epithelium. Also, CF may be considered in the absence of clinical features (i.e., individual has an affected sibling) when suspicion is appreciable (Table 40.2)

The ability to detect CF gene mutations and to measure transepithelial bioelectric properties has expanded the CF clinical spectrum. These technologies enable clinicians to identify and confirm diagnoses in patients who have atypical presentations (i.e., borderline or normal sweat chloride concentrations in the presence of several characteristic phenotypic features). As a more recent development, when suspicion is high and circumstances warrant, prenatal screening can facilitate accurate in utero CF diagnosis.

In patients who have an atypical phenotype and in whom a CF diagnosis has been confirmed (see Fig. 40.11), it is of great

Table 40.1
Phenotypic features consistent with a cystic fibrosis diagnosis (Adapted with permission from Cystic Fibrosis Foundation.)

Chronic sinopulmonary disease
Persistent bacterial colonization and infection with typical cystic fibrosis pathogens
Chronic cough and sputum production
Nasal polyps
Digital clubbing
Gastrointestinal and nutritional abnormalities
Meconium ileus
Distal intestinal obstruction syndrome
Pancreatic insufficiency
Focal biliary cirrhosis
Failure to thrive
Salt loss syndromes
Chronic metabolic alkalosis
Urogenital abnormalities in males that result in azoospermia
Congenital bilateral absence of the vas deferens
Atresia of the vas deferens

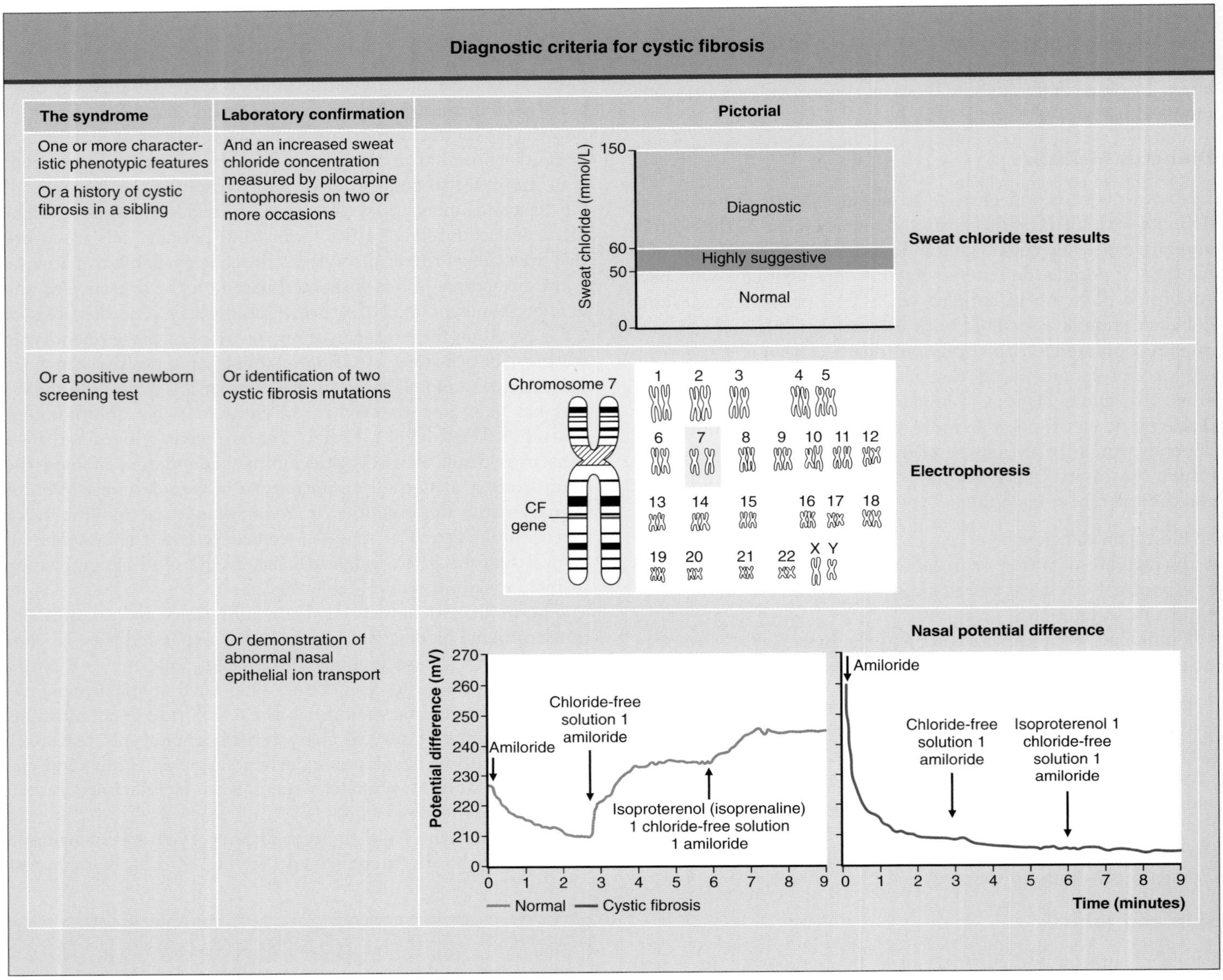

Diagnostic criteria for cystic fibrosis

The syndrome	Laboratory confirmation	Pictorial
One or more characteristic phenotypic features Or a history of cystic fibrosis in a sibling	And an increased sweat chloride concentration measured by pilocarpine iontophoresis on two or more occasions	Sweat chloride test results
Or a positive newborn screening test	Or identification of two cystic fibrosis mutations	Electrophoresis
	Or demonstration of abnormal nasal epithelial ion transport	Nasal potential difference

Figure 40.11 Diagnostic criteria for cystic fibrosis. (Adapted with permission from Rosenstein BJ, Cutting GR: The diagnosis of cystic fibrosis: A consensus statement. J Pediatr 32:589-595, 1998.)

benefit to perform a comprehensive clinical, radiographic, and laboratory evaluation. This enables assessment for features known to be consistent with CF. Such an assessment should include exocrine pancreatic function, respiratory tract microbiology, and a urogenital evaluation.

Assessment of these features is clinically useful in development and optimization of care plans for patients with CF, particularly infants and young children. Early diagnosis and aggressive therapeutic intervention are associated with improved nutritional status, decreased morbidity, and decreased deterioration in lung function.

TREATMENT

More than 98% of patients with CF die because of respiratory failure or pulmonary complications (Fig. 40.12). Most treatment in CF is aimed at combating the clinical consequences of the basic defect. New delivery systems and advanced formulations of antimicrobial, anti-inflammatory, and mucus-modifying agents, in combination with standard chest physical therapy and improved nutritional supplementation, have contributed to an increase in median survival and quality of life for individuals who have CF. These advances, however, are simply management tools; they cannot normalize the disrupted cellular function caused by abnormal CFTR (i.e., the basic defect).

The goals of general CF care are to prevent or slow the decline of lung function, improve nutritional status, and optimize quality of life. Because CF is a disease that affects multiple body systems, a multidisciplinary team can be highly effective in providing continuity of care as patients mature. Cystic fibrosis centers throughout North America and Europe provide a framework of specialized health care sites focused on providing early and aggressive treatment of deterioration and complications, as well as patient education and family support.

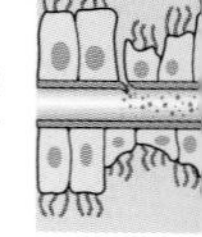

Table 40.2 Cystic fibrosis diagnosis and complications at birth		
Complications at birth	**% Newly Diagnosed in 2001** (n = 1031)	**% All CF Patients** (n = 22,732)
Meconium ileus or intestinal obstruction	18.2	20.0
Diagnosis suggested by*:		
Respiratory symptoms	43.8	51.5
Nasal polyps/sinus disease	4.2	2.8
Electrolyte imbalance	1.8	5.5
Failure to thrive/malnutrition	29.3	43.1
Steatorrhea/abnormal stools	24.4	35.0
Meconium ileus/intestinal obstruction	18.5	20.8
Rectal prolapse	3.5	3.8
Liver problems	1.2	1.2
Family history	14.2	17.2
Genotype	6.3	2.6
Prenatal diagnosis	3.9	1.5
Neonatal screening	9.1	3.8
Edema and/or hypoproteinemia/ hypoalbuminemia	1.5	0.6
Other	2.6	1.1
Unknown	1.1	2.3

*Not mutually exclusive.
(Source: Cystic Fibrosis Foundation Patient Registry Annual Data Report to the Center Directors, 2001. September 2002.)

In addition, the central gathering of data into national and international registries has expanded our understanding of the epidemiologic characteristics of this condition and facilitated therapeutic advances.

Pulmonary Exacerbations

Although no criteria to define a pulmonary exacerbation are universally accepted, a recent consensus panel developed a list of signs and symptoms that are recognized by clinicians experienced in the management of CF to be commonly associated with pulmonary exacerbation (Table 40.3 and Fig. 40.12). Pulmonary function invariably declines during an exacerbation, and it is the single most important objective marker by which to assess the severity of an exacerbation and the patient's response to treatment. Sputum cultures and bacterial sensitivities are performed routinely at the onset of an exacerbation, and treatment decisions are based on these laboratory results. Oral or inhaled antibiotic therapies are commonly used when symptoms, signs, and pulmonary function decrements are mild (Table 40.4); however, it is important to monitor the patient's progress to ensure clinical improvement. When an exacerbation is severe (or when sputum cultures fail to identify a microbial susceptibility to an oral agent), intravenous antibiotics are administered to the patient (Table 40.5). Similarly, should the clinician determine that home care is suitable, close monitoring of the patient's progress and condition is critical.

In addition to choosing an agent to which the organism is sensitive, patients with CF require adequate antibiotic dosages (to achieve bactericidal levels) administered for a sufficient period to achieve a clinical response. Although a 2-week course of

Pulmonary complications of cystic fibrosis					
Complication	**Cause**	**Management**	**Complication**	**Cause**	**Management**
Pneumothorax	Bursting of sub-pleural blebs	Thoracotomy and chest tube insertion. If no resolution within 48 hours, limited pleural abrasion via thoracoscopy or thoracotomy	Atelectasis	Mucus plugging of proximal bronchus	Antibiotic therapy, energetic chest physical therapy, endoscopy

Figure 40.12 Pulmonary complications of cystic fibrosis. These radiographs show two complications of cystic fibrosis. Not shown are hemoptysis and allergic bronchopulmonary aspergillosis.

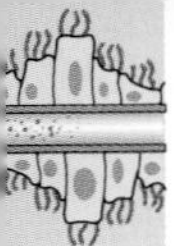

therapy usually suffices for the patient who has not undergone multiple courses of treatment, longer intervals may be necessary for those patients with CF who do not achieve a complete response at 14 days or for those patients who have more severe disease. Routinely, patients with CF require high-dose antibiotic therapy, which must also be administered in a considerably higher concentration than required for a patient without CF. This requirement for dosage adjustment results from the metabolic impact of CF on rate of absorption and whole-body clearance of antibiotics. Pharmacokinetic studies in patients with CF during antibiotic administration have clearly demonstrated that metabolic alterations, unique to the CF population, result in reduced antibiotic concentrations and activity in the sputum when standard doses are administered. To compound this, the properties of *P. aeruginosa* that relate to coexistent populations of varying drug sensitivities and alginate product (mucoid strains) render the organism more difficult to treat. Further, other agents, such as tobramycin, may be inactivated because of binding to free DNA in the infected CF airway secretions.

The goal of therapy is to return the patient to baseline, or pre-exacerbation status. Symptoms, sputum product, and lung function must be evaluated at presentation, midpoint in the treatment course, and when treatment is terminated. Alone, radiographic chest films (which may remain unchanged during an exacerbation) are insufficiently sensitive for the evaluation of therapeutic outcomes. Significant declines in FEV_1 and forced vital capacity can frequently occur, and spirometry is routinely used to assess the treatment response in a patient with CF. However, the timing for initiation of treatment in patients with CF poses some problems. Certainly in the presence of an exacerbation, treatment is required; however, the issue of treating inflammation or documented bacterial colonization is less clear. Data suggest that coupled with frequent monitoring, aggressive intervention may delay declines in pulmonary function—a major factor in mortality—in patients with CF.

The goal of CF management is to prevent pulmonary deterioration through:

- Use of antibacterial prophylaxis to avoid chronic pulmonary infection
- Eradication of newly identified pulmonary infection

Table 40.3
Signs and symptoms of pulmonary exacerbation
(Adapted with permission from Cystic Fibrosis Foundations.)

Signs and symptoms
Increased cough
Increased sputum production and/or a change in appearance of expectorated sputum
Fever (≥ 100.5° F [≥ 38° C] for at least 4 h in a 24 h period) on more than one occasion in the previous week
Weight loss ≥1 kg or 5 % of body weight associated with anorexia and decreased dietary intake or growth failure in an infant or child
School or work absenteeism (because of illness) in the previous week
Increased respiratory rate and/or work of breathing
New findings on chest examination (e.g., rales, wheezing, crackles)
Decreased exercise tolerance
Decrease in forced expiration volume in 1 second of ≥ 10% from previous baseline study within past 3 months
Decrease in hemoglobin saturation (as measured by oximetry) of ≥ 10% from baseline value within past 3 months
New finding(s) on chest radiograph

Table 40.4
Oral antibiotic treatment in cystic fibrosis
(Adapted from Ramsey and Varlotta and Schidlow.)

Antibiotic		Standard adult dose for cystic fibrosis	Organisms targeted
Penicillins	Amoxicillin–clavulanate	500 mg q8h or 875 mg q12h	*Staphylococcus aureus, Haemophilus influenzae*
	Dicloxacillin	500 mg q6h	*S. aureus*
Cephalosporins	Cefaclor	500 mg q8h	*S. aureus, H. influenzae*
	Cephalexin	500 mg q6h	*S. aureus*
	Cefuroxime	500 mg q12h	*S. aureus, H. influenzae*
Others	Azithromycin	500 mg on day 1, followed by 250 mg/day on days 2–5; TIW >40 kg = 500 g, <40 kg = 250 g	*S. aureus, H. influenzae*
	Chloramphenicol	500 mg q6h	*Burkholderia cepacia, H. influenzae*
	Clarithromycin	500 mg q12h	*S. aureus*
	Doxycycline or minocycline	100 mg q12h	*H. influenzae*
	Erythromycin	500 mg q6h–q8h	*S. aureus*
	Trimethoprim–sulfamethoxazole	160 mg q12h/800 mg q12h	*S. aureus, H. influenzae, B. cepacia*
Quinolones	Ciprofloxacin (not indicated for use in patients <18 years of age)	500–750 mg q12h	*Pseudomonas aeruginosa, S. aureus, H. influenzae*
	Levofloxacin	500 mg once daily	*S. aureus, H. influenzae, P. aeruginosa*
	Gatifloxacin	400 mg qd	*S. aureus, H. influenzae, Streptococcus pneumoniae*

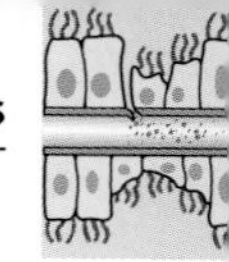

Table 40.5
Intravenous antibiotic treatment in cystic fibrosis
(Adapted from Ramsey and Varlotta and Schidlow)

Antibiotic		Standard adult dose for cystic fibrosis	Organisms targeted
Aminoglycosides (dosages given are starting doses; guided by peak and trough serum levels, as indicatd)			
	Amikacin	20–30 mg/kg per day in 2–3 divided doses	*Pseudomonas aeruginosa, Haemophilus influenzae*
	Gentamicin	6–15 mg/kg per day in 2–3 divided doses	*P. aeruginosa, H. influenzae*
	Tobramycin	6–15 mg/kg per day in 2–3 divided doses	*P. aeruginosa, H. influenzae*
Cephalosporins	Cefepine	2g IV q8	*P. aeruginosa*
	Ceftazidime	2 g q8h	*P. aeruginosa, H. influenzae, Burkholderia cepacia*
	Cefuroxime	0.75–1.5 g q8h	*H. influenzae*
Penicillins	Ampicillin–sulbactam	1.5–2.0 g q6h	*Staphylococcus aureus, H. influenzae*
	Nafcillin	1.0–2.0 g q6h	*S. aureus*
	Piperacillin, piperacillin–tazobactam	3.0–4.0 g q4h–q6h	*P. aeruginosa, H. influenzae*
	Ticarcillin, ticarcillin–clavulanate	3.0 g q4h–6qh	*P. aeruginosa, H. influenzae*
	Oxacillin	1.0–2.0 g q6h	*S. aureus*
Other	Aztreonam	1.0–2.0 g q6h	*P. aeruginosa, H. influenzae*
	Chloramphenicol	50 mg/kg per day in 4 divided doses	*B. cepacia, H. influenzae*
	Ciprofloxacin (not indicated for patients <18 years of age)	400 mg q12h	*P. aeruginosa, H. influenzae, S. aureus*
	Clindamycin	600–900 mg q8h	*S. aureus*
	Imipenem–cilastatin	0.5–1.0 g q6h	*P. aeruginosa, H. influenzae, S. aureus*
	Meropenam	2 g IV q8	*P. aeruginosa*
	Trimethoprim–sulfamethoxazole	12.0–20.0 mg/kg per day in 2–4 divided doses	*B. cepacia, H. influenzae, S. aureus*
	Vancomycin	500 mg q6h	*S. aureus*

- Reduction of symptoms associated with acute exacerbation of pulmonary infection
- Suppression of chronic bacterial pulmonary infection

In a large observational study, using data collected in the Epidemiologic Study of Cystic Fibrosis database (Johnson et al.), researchers reviewed the management of more than 18,000 patients with CF, aged 6 to more than 18 years, collected over a 2-year period. The purpose of the review was to assess whether differences in the lung health of patients with CF, treated at different CF care sites, was associated with differences in monitoring and interventions. The authors reported substantial differences in lung health across different CF care sites, attributing improved outcomes to more frequent monitoring (including spirometry) and the increased use of appropriate medications in the management of CF. Importantly, another potential factor cited in relation to improved outcome was nutritional support, as has been observed in Danish data (Frederiksen et al.).

For patients who have end-stage disease, bilateral lung transplantation is the only therapeutic alternative. Both organ demand (which far exceeds the number of suitable organs available for transplantation) and advance preparation of the patient and family (which routinely includes a waiting period of 18 to 24 months) preclude lung transplantation as an emergency procedure. Several other factors, such as portal hypertension, severe malnutrition, and lung colonization with *B. cepacia*, may negate transplant surgery for patients in some centers. Transplant survival data show a 73% survival rate at 1 year post-transplantation, 63% at 2 years, and 57% at 3 years, with patients generally enjoying a good quality of life.

Nonpulmonary Management

As a result of increased metabolic demands created by the work of breathing, battling chronic infection, and imbalances in digestion and nutritional absorption, patients with CF may require 120% to 140% of the recommended daily allowance for caloric intake. Maintaining an unrestricted-fat, high-calorie diet, with liberal salt intake and vitamin plus mineral supplementation, is encouraged. Patients affected by exocrine pancreatic deficiency are aided by enzyme replacement therapy; however, the administration of high doses of lipase has been associated with fibrosing colonopathy, and close monitoring is prudent. Children who experience growth failure because of inadequate nutritional intake may benefit from enteral supplemental feedings at night, commonly accomplished by gastrostomy.

PROGNOSIS

Despite the research and technological advances available in the new millennium, CF is still considered a chronic, progressive, lethal disease. Increased understanding of the

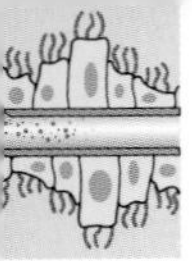

pathophysiology of this disease, coupled with earlier diagnosis and improved management, have resulted in steady increases in median survival. With the increased detection of patients who show milder disease expression, the development of new therapies to correct the basic ion transport defect, and the advent of lung transplantation, it is reasonable to expect this trend to continue.

Currently, survival among male patients is slightly better than that among female patients, although the reasons for this remain unclear. These differences in male and female survival rates occur during the age range 1 to 20 years. No significant predictive difference between men and women has been clearly established for pulmonary function, nutritional status, and airway microbiology, although each of these factors is closely associated with mortality. Factors positively linked to improved longevity include pancreatic sufficiency, male sex, absence of colonization with mucoid *P. aeruginosa*, a predominant presentation of gastrointestinal symptoms, appropriate and supportive family functioning and coping, and compliance with treatment regimens. To date, no definitive research has established a link between early diagnosis and improved survival.

Genotype–Phenotype Relationship

Correlation of genotype–phenotype expression in CF is confounded by the identification of approximately 1000 CF mutations (and the factorial potential for genotypic permutations). Further, individual variability in compensatory homeostatic mechanisms, environmental factors, and other genetic modifiers increases the challenge of identifying these relationships in CF. Several factors, such as age at diagnosis, diversity in presentation, disease severity, and rate of progression appear to be directed by the specific gene mutation.

The high frequency of the ΔF508 mutation has facilitated research to establish genotype–phenotype correlations with this genotype; however, other mutations occur so infrequently that to perform statistically relevant studies is extremely difficult. Knowledge of these more than 1000 CF mutations has, however, facilitated the development of functional classifications on the basis of CFTR protein alterations (see Fig. 40.2).

Pancreatic status has been demonstrated to have the strongest genotype–phenotype correlation yet identified. For example, a strong concordance of pancreatic function status (phenotype) among affected individuals in the same family (genotype) has been documented. The relationship between the phenotypic expression of pulmonary manifestations in CF and genotype is less clear.

Investigational Therapeutic Approaches

Although research continues to elucidate the role of CFTR in the progression of CF, efforts are also underway to identify new antimicrobial agents that will enhance the management of the disease. Some recent data regarding azithromycin, a macrolide antibiotic with anti-inflammatory activity against *P. aeruginosa* in CF respiratory tract infections, suggests that short-term use in patients with CF may improve clinical and quality-of-life parameters. It is thought that the drug may act synergistically with other antimicrobial agents, resulting in increased in vitro activity; however, its clinical efficacy has yet to be demonstrated. Azithromycin is usually well tolerated, with rash reported as the main adverse event.

In 1989, a group of U.S. and Canadian scientists cloned and sequenced the *CFTR* gene. Since that time, an intensive effort has been under way to develop a vector to facilitate correction of the faulty gene. In an attempt to identify a mechanism that can deliver a functional *CFTR* gene, several vector types are being researched. These include three types of viral vectors:

- Adenoviral vectors (or Ad vectors)
- Adeno-associated viral vectors (AAV)
- Retroviral vectors (lentiviruses)

Research is also being carried out on the use of nonviral vectors (liposomes). All of these vectors can be broadly grouped by mechanism of action into two categories. The Ad vectors, liposomes, and molecular conjugates lead to transient expression of the CFTR protein, in which the *CFTR* gene functions as extrachromosomal (or episomal) DNA in the nucleus. The AAV and retroviral vectors integrate or insert into the host cell genome. Studies are under way with naturally occurring viruses as well as recombinant vectors, while such issues as efficacy, delivery site, duration of function, immune response, and general safety are being explored.

Gene-Assist Therapy

Gene-assist therapy focuses on the abnormal gene product, CFTR, and seeks to normalize chloride concentrations in the airway surface fluids (i.e., trafficking), either by repairing the defective protein or by bypassing the cellular defect and opening alternative chloride channels. Early research efforts demonstrated that partial correction of chloride ion transport to the nasal tissues may be possible with the drug CPX (8-cyclopentyl-1,3-dipropylxanthine), which essentially promotes chloride ion transport and improves CFTR trafficking. Another investigational agent, UTP (uridine phosphatidylglycerol), bypasses the cellular defect and opens alternative chloride channels. The objective of gene-assist therapy is to restore the normal ionic composition of the airway fluid and thereby the activity of endogenous antimicrobial substances that protect against infection.

Protein Repair Therapy

Recent research has enhanced our understanding of *CFTR* gene mutations, and protein repair therapy (a relatively new concept) is aimed at manipulating the class mutation defects in CFTR production, folding, trafficking, or chloride conduction. For example, class I mutations decrease the production of CFTR protein through stop codons, which prematurely terminate *CFTR* mRNA. This results in truncated mRNA transcripts that are unstable and usually not translated into proteins. Based on genotype, patients known to carry two class I mutant alleles can be given an agent (aminoglycoside antibiotic) to suppress the "nonsense" mutations (and thereby prevent the early termination of *CFTR* mRNA) and permit production of full-length *CFTR* protein (see Fig. 40.2).

Class II mutations result in accumulation of the mutant CFTR protein in the endoplasmic reticulum, where the protein is degraded. The ΔF508 mutation, a single–amino acid deletion of phenylalanine at position 508, is the prototype of this class.

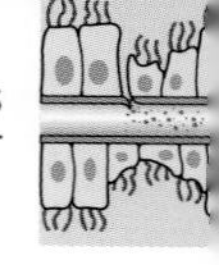

It is thought that the premature destruction of ΔF508 results from a block in protein trafficking or from misfolding during translation. The ΔF508 protein is nearly completely degraded (i.e., 99%) by the quality-control mechanisms in the endoplasmic reticulum, the role of which is to degrade misfolded or mutant protein. Interestingly, this protein can be recovered by growing cells at subphysiologic temperatures (23° to 27°C [73.5° to 80.5°F]), which has led to the development of a number of new therapeutic approaches (see Fig. 40.2). These mutations are severe and associated with pancreatic insufficiency.

Class III mutations are completely defective in regulation and activation of chloride channel activity. So far, no clinical trials have been announced specifically to address the class III mutations, although compounds that affect the interaction of the nucleotide-binding folds with ATP may prove to be useful in future trials. Further, because several of the class III and IV mutations may prove unresponsive to direct stimulation, it is reasonable to explore the use of gene therapy, rather than protein repair alone, for some of these mutations.

Class IV mutations, associated with milder forms of CF that are characterized by pancreatic sufficiency, comprise CFTR proteins that have reduced conductance for chloride. Although a few agents are under investigation, no therapeutic agents for class IV mutations have been announced.

CONCLUSION

Achievements in patient management and traditional therapeutic agents, coupled with advances in our understanding of the pulmonary biology and pathophysiology of CF, have significantly improved the clinical prognosis and quality of life for patients with CF. As scientists continue with ongoing molecular and genetics research, the promise of novel therapeutics and strategies using gene therapy and protein repair techniques offers renewed hope in the battle with this most challenging foe.

SUGGESTED READINGS

Coenye T, Vandamme P, Govan JRW, LiPuma JJ: Taxonomy and identification of the *Burkholderia cepacia* complex. J Clin Microbiol 39:3427-3436, 2001.

Equi A, Balfour-Lynn IM, Bush A, Rosenthal M: Long-term azithromycin in children with cystic fibrosis: A randomized, placebo-controlled crossover trial. Lancet 360:978-984, 2002.

Fuchs HJ, Borowitz DS, Christiansen DH, et al: Effect of aerosolized recombinant human DNase on exacerbations of respiratory symptoms and on pulmonary function in patients with cystic fibrosis: The Pulmozyme Study Group. N Engl J Med 331:637, 1994.

Johnson C, Butler SM, Knostan MW, et al: Factors influencing outcomes in cystic fibrosis: A center-based analysis. Chest 123:20-27, 2003; and accompanying editorial: Fiel SB: Early aggressive intervention in cystic fibrosis: Is it time to redefine our "best practice" strategies? Chest 123:1-2, 2003.

Konstan MW, Byard PJ, Hoppel CL, Davis PB: Effect of high-dose ibuprofen in patients with cystic fibrosis. N Engl J Med 332:848, 1995.

Liou TG, Adler FR, Fitzsimmons SC, Cahill BC: Predictive 5-year survivorship model of cystic fibrosis. Am J Epidemiol 153:345, 2001.

Moss RB: Long-term benefits of inhaled tobramycin in adolescent patients with cystic fibrosis. Chest 121:55, 2002.

Olivier KN, Weber DJ, Wallace RJ Jr, et al: Nontuberculous mycobacteria: I. Multicenter prevalence study in cystic fibrosis. Am J Respir Crit Care Med 167:828, 2003.

Ramsey BW: Management of pulmonary disease in patients with cystic fibrosis. N Engl J Med 335:179, 1996.

Rosenstein BJ, Cutting GR: The diagnosis of cystic fibrosis: A consensus statement. J Pediatr 32:589-595, 1998.

Rosenstein BJ, Zeitlin PL: Cystic fibrosis. Lancet 351:277, 1998.

Yankaskas JR, Mallory GB Jr: Lung transplantation in cystic fibrosis: Consensus conference statement. Chest 113:217, 1998.

Zeitlin PL: Therapies directed at the basic defect. Clin Chest Med 19:6.1-6.11, 1998.

CHAPTER 41 Lung Tumors

David E. Midthun and James R. Jett

Lung cancer is the leading cause of cancer death in both women and men in Canada, China, and the United States (Fig. 41.1). In Australia, France, Germany, Scandinavia, Spain, and the United Kingdom, lung cancer is the number one cause of cancer death in men and the second or third cause in women. The prevalence is particularly alarming given that, at the turn of the twentieth century, lung cancer was a rare malignancy. Because the 5-year survival for lung cancer in the United States and Europe is currently about 14%, the devastation caused by this single cancer type is alarming. The frequent presence and lethal nature of lung cancer has maintained its position in the forefront of problems in pulmonary medicine.

The term *lung cancer* is used to describe cancer that arises in the airways or pulmonary parenchyma. Lung cancer is classified into primarily two subgroups: small-cell lung cancer (SCLC) and non–small-cell lung cancer (NSCLC). The distinction in subgroups is essential with regard to treatment and prognosis. Approximately 95% of all lung cancers fall into either small-cell or non–small-cell categories (Table 41.1). Although lung cancer and bronchogenic carcinoma are terms often used synonymously, tumors of other rare cell types compose the other 5% of cancers that originate in the lung. The majority of this chapter is devoted to a discussion of SCLC and NSCLC. Carcinoid tumor, lymphoma, mucoepidermoid carcinoma, adenoid cystic carcinoma, hamartoma, and lung metastasis are discussed at the end of the chapter.

EPIDEMIOLOGY, PATHOGENESIS, AND PATHOLOGY

Epidemiology

Cigarette smoke is by far the number one cause of lung cancer. The relationship between smoking and lung cancer was initially reported in the 1940s and was further established from epidemiologic research in the 1950s. The first US Surgeon General's *Report on Smoking and Health* was published in 1964 and concluded that cigarette smoking was causally related to lung cancer.

In 1965, 52% of men and 34% of women in the United States older than age 18 years were cigarette smokers. By 2001, the percentages had declined to 26% for men and 21% for women. Smoking rates in many countries in Europe and Asia have been equivalent to or higher than in the United States. According to 2002 data from the World Health Organization, rates for men were more than 60% in China and Russia, and 30% to 39% in most of Europe. However, smoking prevalence rates for women were less than 10% in China and Russia; 30% to 39% in France, Germany, and Norway; and 20% to 29% for the United Kingdom, Spain, and Poland. Each day in the United States, approximately 3000 teenagers start to smoke. Approximately 1 of every 5 deaths results from smoking, and long-term studies estimate that about half of all regular smokers are eventually killed by their habit.

According to most reported series, approximately 85% to 90% of lung cancer occurs in smokers or former smokers. This may be an under estimation; the Edinburgh Lung Cancer Group reported that of 3070 new patients who had lung cancer, only 74 (2%) were lifelong never smokers. Cigarette smoking is identified as the major cause of each of the histologic types of lung cancer: small cell, squamous cell, large cell, and adenocarcinoma. The risk of developing lung cancer increases with the number of cigarettes smoked, earlier age at which smoking started, and longer duration of smoking. Cigarette smoke contains more than 4000 chemical constituents, some of which have been identified as carcinogens. Smoking is also associated with the formation of cancers of the larynx, pharynx, mouth, esophagus, pancreas, and bladder. Current smokers of one pack a day for 20 years have a rate of lung cancer 10 to 15 times that of someone who has never smoked. The risk increases to 20 to 25 times if two or more packs per day of cigarettes are consumed for a similar duration (Fig. 41.2). The British physician study showed the risk of lung cancer remains elevated long after smoking cessation and takes 15 years to approach that of someone who has never smoked. Results of the Multiple Risk Factor Intervention Trial were similar. After 10.5 years of follow-up, 119 men who were smokers or former smokers at entry died of lung cancer compared with no lung cancer deaths among men who reported never smoking. The lag time for a significant reduction in lung cancer death from smoking cessation was many years. Even if cigarette consumption ceased today, the current epidemic of lung cancer would persist for decades.

Passive smoking is sidestream smoke that is unintentionally inhaled by someone in the presence of a smoker. A number of epidemiologic studies have evaluated passive smoking and the risk of lung cancer. Studies that involved women who never smoked but who lived with a smoking husband suggest a 1.2 to 2 times increase in lung cancer risk compared with nonsmoking women in smoke-free homes. There does not appear to be a threshold for tobacco carcinogenesis. Passive smoking is estimated to account for approximately 3000 new cases of lung cancer per year in the United States.

Radon exposure is perhaps the greatest element of lung cancer risk for nonsmokers who have not been exposed to asbestos. Radon is a decay product of naturally occurring radium, which, in turn, is a breakdown product of uranium. Radon is present in indoor and outdoor air, and the relative risk

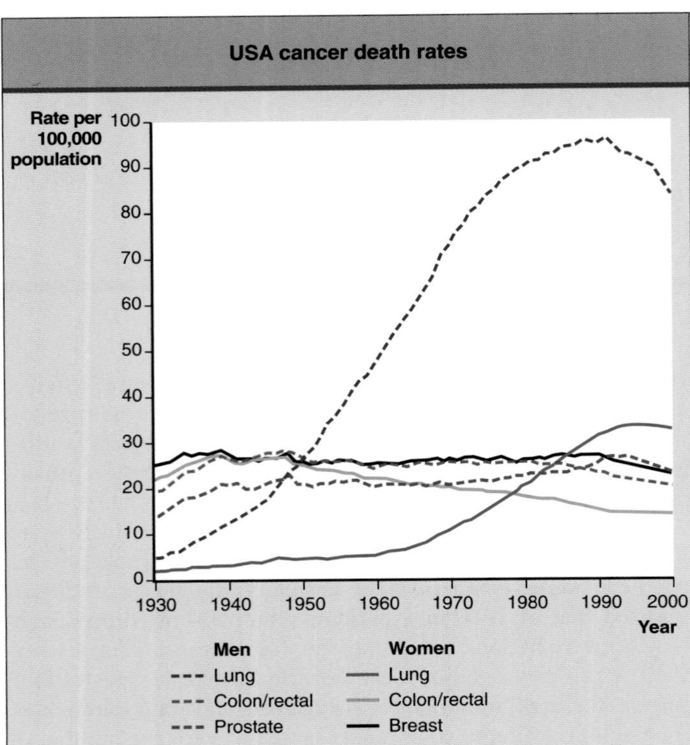

Figure 41.1 United States cancer death rates. (From Jemal A, Murray T, Samuels A, et al: Cancer statistics, 2003. CA, Cancer J Clin 53:5-26, 2003.)

Table 41.1 Lung cancer classification

Category	Incidence (%)
Small-cell lung cancer	20
Non–small-cell lung cancer	75
Adenocarcinoma	35
Squamous cell carcinoma	30
Large-cell carcinoma	10
Others	5
Carcinoid tumors	–
Pulmonary lymphoma	–
Mucoepidermoid carcinoma	–
Adenoid cystic carcinoma	–
Sarcomas	–

of lung cancer appears to increase linearly with exposure. The Committee on Biological Effects of Ionizing Radiation reported that radon in the general environment is responsible for 10% of all lung cancers in the United States, placing it as the second most frequent cause of lung cancer. The US Environmental Protection Agency has established acceptable levels for annual exposure to radon and has advised that most houses be tested for radon.

Air pollution from motor vehicles, factory emissions, and wood and coal burning heaters has been shown to contain carcinogens. The degree of risk related to air pollution is difficult to quantify, but it is estimated to cause 1% to 2% of all lung cancer.

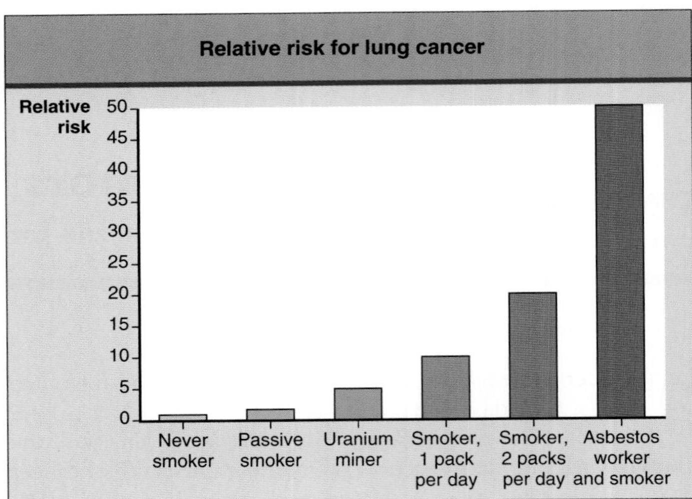

Figure 41.2 Approximate relative risk factors for lung cancer.

A clear association exists between asbestos exposure and lung cancer, although the increased risk is generally not observed until 20 or more years after the initial exposure. A naturally occurring, fibrous silicate ubiquitous in the soil, asbestos was commercially used in the construction industry and for its fire-retardant properties. There are different types of asbestos fibers and some are more carcinogenic than others. A combination of asbestos exposure and cigarette smoking results in an approximate 50-fold increase in the risk of lung cancer compared with someone who has never smoked and has not been exposed to asbestos. Exposures to other materials that have been shown to cause lung cancer include chromium, nickel, and arsenic.

Dietary factors also appear to play a role in the eventual development of lung cancer. In retrospective case control studies, fruit consumption was suggested to be protective, though results of prospective studies have been mixed. Vegetable consumption has been associated with decreased lung cancer risk. No protective role has been found for retinol but studies support a protective role for beta-carotene and vitamin C. However, three randomized controlled trials failed to show a protective effect of supplementation with beta-carotene—an increased risk for lung cancer was found among heavy smokers in the alpha-Tocopherol beta-Carotene Cancer Prevention Study.

Although no specific, inherited lung cancer gene has been identified, a family history of lung cancer does predict increased risk after controlling for smoking. Squamous cell carcinoma appears to be most associated with familial clustering of lung cancer. Women may be at greater risk than men who have an equivalent smoking history. An increasing number of genetic abnormalities are recognized in resected lung cancers. Genetic predisposition may result from a difference in carcinogen metabolism, genetic instability of DNA repair processes, or altered oncogene expression.

Studies have shown that chronic obstructive pulmonary disease is a risk factor for lung cancer over and above the risk from cigarette smoking. Presence of airflow obstruction on pulmonary function testing was associated with a 4 to 6 times' greater risk of lung cancer when controlled for cigarette smoking. The association of airflow obstruction and lung cancer

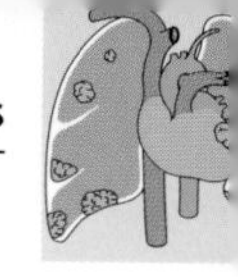

was further supported by the Lung Health Study, in which 5800 patients who had mild airway obstruction and a history of smoking were assessed for effectiveness of smoking cessation and anticholinergic therapy. Lung cancer was the leading cause of death during the 5 years of follow-up for this study. Whether airflow obstruction predisposes to lung cancer or whether both arise from a common factor is unclear.

PATHOGENESIS

The current understanding of the pathogenesis of lung cancer is that of a multistep process of carcinogen-induced genetic damage to cells that proceeds through the stages of initiation, promotion, and progression. The increased incidence of lung cancer with aging and the pathologic change of bronchial epithelium from dysplasia to carcinoma in situ in smokers are consistent with a multistep process. The mechanism by which smoking causes lung cancer is not completely understood. Components of cigarette smoke have been shown to initiate and promote the process of carcinogenesis. Genetic changes have also been demonstrated in histologically respiratory epithelial cells of normal appearance obtained from smokers.

Greater recognition of the genetic changes that occur in lung cancer will lead to a better understanding of its pathogenicity. Gene expression arrays have shown gene expression patterns in lung cancer are highly variable and upregulation or downregulation of genes is inconsistent. Early-stage cancers have shown a number of genetic and molecular alterations including mutations in the p53 tumor suppressor gene and K-ras proto-oncogene, hypermethylation of the p16 tumor suppressor gene, and loss of chromosome heterozygosity. Both SCLC and NSCLC have been shown to contain certain chromosomal abnormalities. K-ras mutations are present in about 30% of adenocarcinomas and are uncommon in other cell types. Mutations of p-53 tumor suppressor gene are present in about 50% of NSCLC and 70% of SCLC. Overexpression of epidermal growth factor and its receptor is present in about 60% of NSCLC. Identification of critical, early molecular alterations may allow early detection of cancer through analysis of sputum, blood, or stool.

Although survival with lung cancer correlates best to the stage of disease, large survival discrepancies among patients within a single stage of disease are unexplained and may reflect a specific tumor biology. Research in cancer biology has revealed a number of markers that may be significant in tumor behavior. Predictions of a good or bad outcome have been attempted on the basis of oncogene amplification; level of tumor-associated antigens, specific enzymes, and growth factors; rate of cell proliferation; and other biologic factors. Clarification of these tumor biologic factors may help focus the estimation of specific patient prognosis and lead to tumor-specific treatment.

Pathology

Histopathologic designation of lung cancer is based on the World Health Organization Classification System. Differing cell types are designated by their appearance under light microscopy. A correct histologic distinction between small cell and non–small cell is imperative to determine treatment and prognosis. An agreement between pathologists in the separation of SCLC and NSCLC occurs in greater than 95% of cases. NSCLC is further subdivided into squamous cell, adenocarcinoma, and large-cell carcinoma. Considerable variation in histologic differentiation in individual cases leads to differences in interpretation. Interobserver variation among pathologists in the recognition of NSCLC subtypes ranges as high as 25% to 40% of cases. However, this difficulty does not appear to be clinically significant, because subtypes of NSCLC within the same stage have similar treatment and prognosis.

Adenocarcinoma is the most frequent histologic cell type of lung cancer and it composes 30% to 35% of lung cancer series. Adenocarcinoma is the most common cell type among smokers and accounts for nearly all of lung cancer identified in patients who have never smoked. The most frequent location of adenocarcinoma is in the peripheral aspects of the lung parenchyma as a solitary nodule or mass (Fig. 41.3). The histologic identification of adenocarcinoma requires evidence of neoplastic gland formation or the presence of intracytoplasmic mucin. Bronchoalveolar cell is a subtype of adenocarcinoma and may present as a nodule or mass as well as a pneumonia-like infiltrate (Fig. 41.4). Histologic features of bronchoalveolar cell carcinoma include origin distal to grossly recognizable bronchi, well-differentiated cytologic features, and growth along intact alveolar septa.

Squamous cell carcinoma is the second most common cell type, composes about 30% of lung cancer, and is highly correlated to smoking. Squamous cell type correlates highly with smoking history and originates most often in association with central airways (Fig. 41.5). Patients who have squamous cell carcinoma often have symptoms of airway involvement such as cough and hemoptysis. Radiographic presence of squamous cell

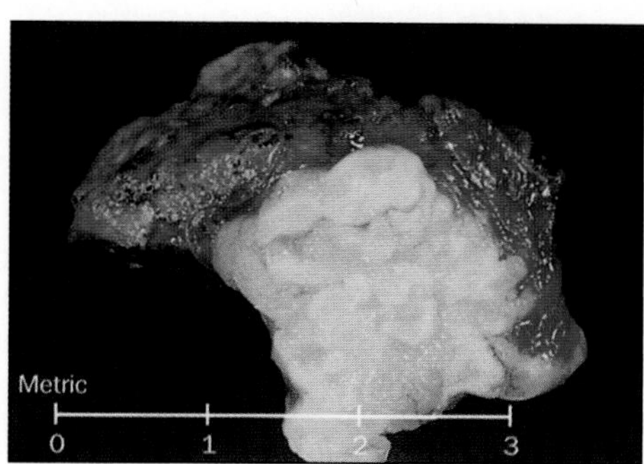

Figure 41.3 Peripheral adenocarcinoma. This wedge resection gross specimen of a peripheral nodule showed grade 2 adenocarcinoma. The patient underwent a lobectomy with formal lymph node dissection.

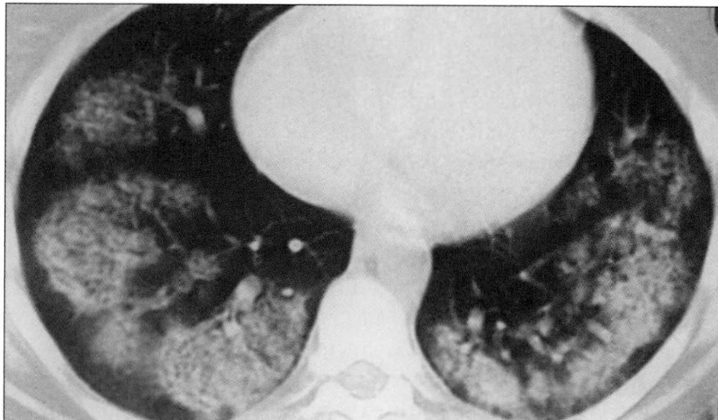

Figure 41.4 Bronchoalveolar cell carcinoma. Computed tomography scan of the chest in a patient who has unresolving pneumonia, showing bilateral alveolar infiltrates. Transbronchoscopic biopsy revealed bronchoalveolar cell carcinoma.

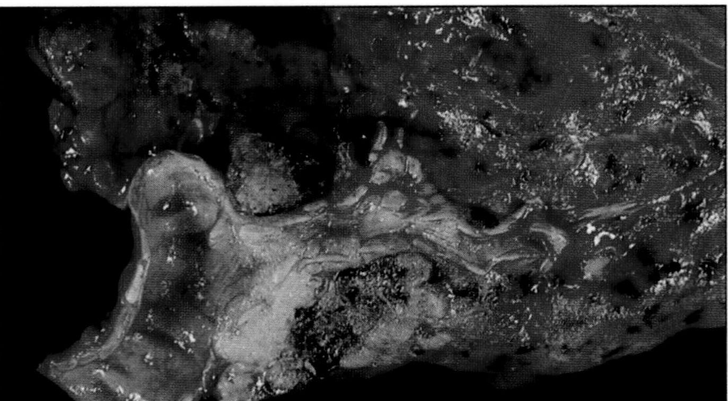

Figure 41.5 Squamous cell lung cancer. Gross specimen of the left lung showing obstruction of the left upper lobe bronchus by tumor and peribronchial extension. Histology showed grade 2 squamous cell carcinoma.

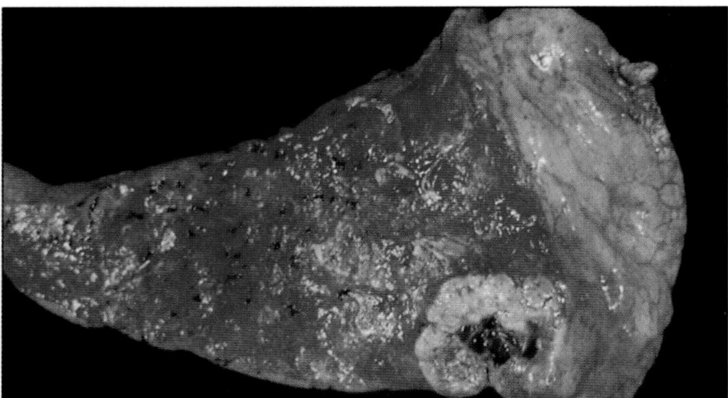

Figure 41.6 Cavitating squamous cell carcinoma. Gross specimen of the right lower lung showing a peripheral, thick-walled cavity with central necrosis. Histology revealed squamous cell carcinoma.

carcinoma may be suggested by evidence of airway obstruction such as a lobar collapse or postobstructive pneumonia. Due to the central location, the tumor may be radiographically occult and even inapparent in early stage on computed tomography (CT). Squamous cell may present as a peripheral mass, and cavitation may be seen as it may in other types of NSCLC (Fig. 41.6). The diagnosis of squamous cell carcinoma requires histologic evidence of squamous cell differentiation in the form of visible keratinization or desmosomes.

Large-cell, undifferentiated carcinoma is a cell type that is less well-differentiated under light microscopy and lacks glandular or squamous differentiation. Large-cell tumors compose about 10% of most series, but considerable variability may occur between centers, dependent on the nuances of the pathologist's interpretation of poorly differentiated carcinomas. Large-cell, undifferentiated carcinoma usually presents as a peripheral mass, and necrosis is often prominent.

Small-cell type accounts for approximately 20% of most series of lung cancer; SCLC is most highly associated with smoking and tends to occur in areas of the chest adjacent to the major airways and often with extensive adenopathy (Fig. 41.7). SCLC is the most common lung cancer to present with evidence of distant metastasis and is considered a systemic disease even in limited stage—the sole exception being SCLC presenting as

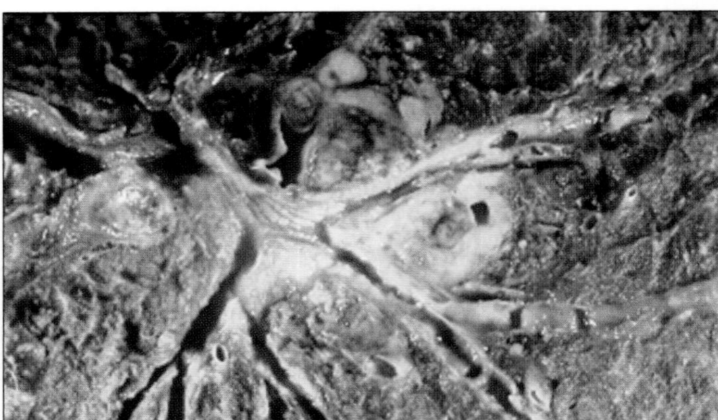

Figure 41.7 Small-cell lung cancer. Right lung gross specimen showing a lung mass with lymphadenopathy and extrinsic bronchial compression.

a peripheral nodule with no adenopathy. SCLC is the most frequent cell type to exhibit one of the distinct paraneoplastic syndromes. Histologic features include a pleomorphic population of small cells, which may be round, oval, or angulated and contain variable amounts of cytoplasm. The nuclei are typically hyperchromatic and have dispersed chromatin.

CLINICAL FEATURES

The clinical presentation of lung cancer is, unfortunately, a frequent occurrence. Prompt and thorough evaluation of a patient who has lung cancer may reveal an early-stage lesion and lead to curative treatment. Physicians need to maintain a high index of suspicion for this disease, particularly among smokers or former smokers.

Asymptomatic Presentation

One fourth of patients who have lung cancer present with no symptoms at the time of diagnosis. The desired situation is to detect a lesion early at a curable stage and before the onset of symptoms, though this discovery is often serendipitous. A nodule or mass may be identified on a chest radiograph carried out as part of a preoperative evaluation for unrelated surgery. Alternatively, a nodule noted on imaging carried out in pursuit of other concerns, such as the spine or abdomen, in which part of the lungs are included (Fig. 41.8). To date, screening sputum cytology and chest radiography have shown an ability to detect lung cancer at an earlier stage, but have not proved a role in reducing mortality. As a result, the American Cancer Society, the American College of Radiology, and the National Cancer Institute have not recommended screening for lung cancer. CT screening for lung cancer has shown promise and may be a means to detect lung cancer while it is still asymptomatic.

Symptomatic Presentation

Approximately three fourths of patients who have lung cancer present with symptoms at the time of diagnosis. Local extension, metastasis, or paraneoplastic effects may cause symptoms from lung cancer. The majority of patients who present with symptoms show evidence of metastasis at the time of presentation and are unresectable.

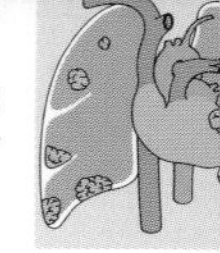

LOCAL EFFECTS

Symptoms that stem from local effects of malignancy include cough, hemoptysis, chest pain, and dyspnea. Cough is present in 50% to 75% of patients who present with lung cancer and occurs most frequently with squamous cell and small-cell types. New onset of cough in a smoker or former smoker raises concern for airway disease as well as cancer. Lung cancer is uncommonly the cause of chronic cough because of rate of disease progression. Slow-growing neoplasms such as carcinoid tumor or hamartoma may present in this way. Bronchorrhea or cough productive of large volumes of thin, mucoid secretions may be a feature of bronchoalveolar cell carcinoma and usually indicates advanced disease. Although bronchitis is the most common cause of hemoptysis, hemoptysis occurs in 25% to 50% of patients who present with lung cancer. Bronchoscopic series reveal bronchogenic carcinoma with incidences in the range of 2.5% to 9% in patients who had hemoptysis and an unsuspicious or normal chest radiograph. Any amount of hemoptysis can be alarming to the patient and, when in large enough volume, may be lethal. Death from hemoptysis results from asphyxiation from occlusion of the major airways rather than from exsanguination.

Chest pain is present in approximately one fourth of patients who present with lung cancer and can be quite variable in character. Dull, aching, persistent pain may occur from mediastinal, pleural, or chest wall extension (Fig. 41.9). Pleuritic pain may be the result of pleural involvement, obstructive pneumonitis, or a pulmonary embolus. Pain is more often present on the side of the chest that contains the neoplasm and, importantly, the presence of pain may not preclude resectability. Patients with carcinomas that involve the chest wall in the absence of lymph node involvement have a favorable survival after surgery.

Approximately 25% of patients have dyspnea when they present with lung cancer. Dyspnea may be due to extrinsic or intrinsic airway obstruction, obstructive pneumonitis or atelectasis, pleural effusion, lymphangitic metastasis, tumor emboli, pneumothorax, or pericardial effusion with tamponade (Fig. 41.10). Partial obstruction of a bronchus may cause a local wheeze, heard by the patient or by the physician on auscultation. Larger airway obstruction may cause stridor. Flow-volume loop abnormalities on pulmonary function testing may arise from presence of tumor in the trachea itself, from extrinsic compression, or from vocal cord paralysis.

METASTATIC EFFECTS

Hardly any body tissue is immune from the metastatic presence or effects of lung cancer. Lung cancer may spread by direct extension, through lymphatics, or hematogenously.

Liver

The liver is a frequent site of spread from lung cancer. Autopsy studies have shown evidence of hepatic metastasis in greater

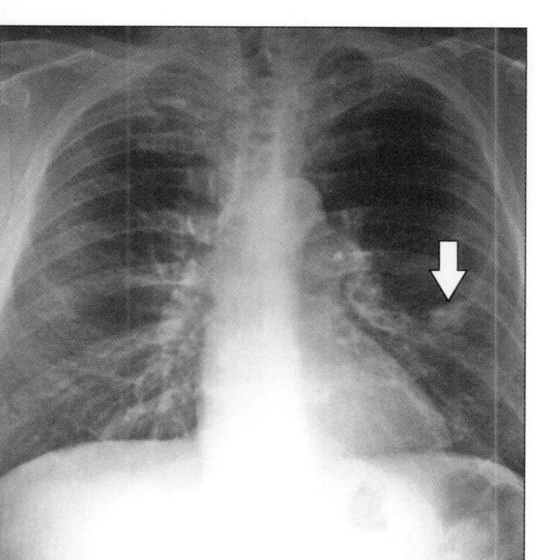

Figure 41.8 Solitary pulmonary nodule (SPN). The chest radiograph shows a 2-cm long left, midlung SPN (*arrow*); resection revealed small-cell carcinoma.

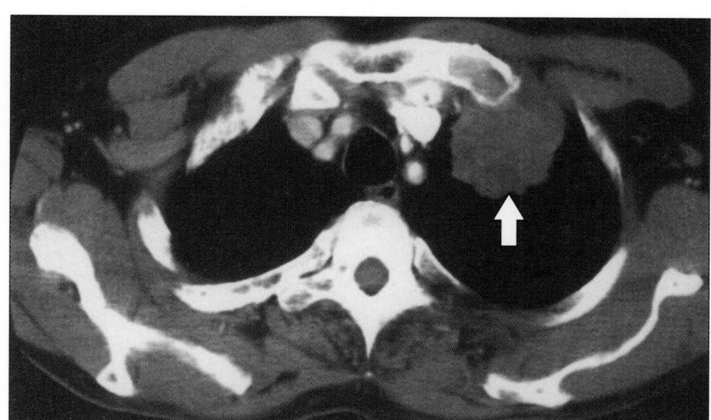

Figure 41.9 Stage IIB squamous cell carcinoma. Computed tomography scan showing a 4-cm diameter, left upper lobe mass (*arrow*) adjacent to the chest wall. Resection included aspects of the first and second rib, as histologic evidence of chest wall involvement was found. No lymph node involvement was found (T3N0M0, see text).

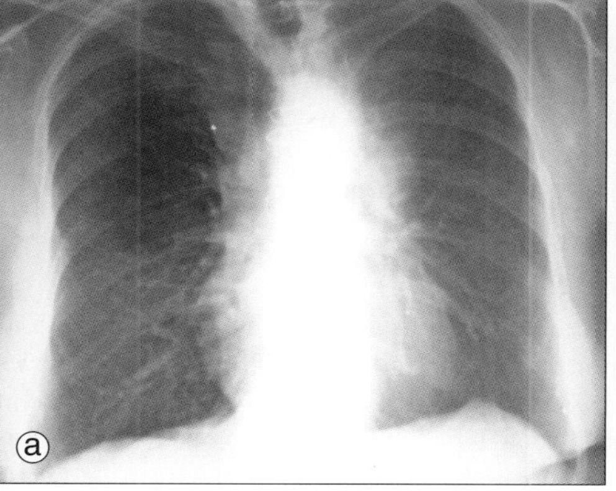

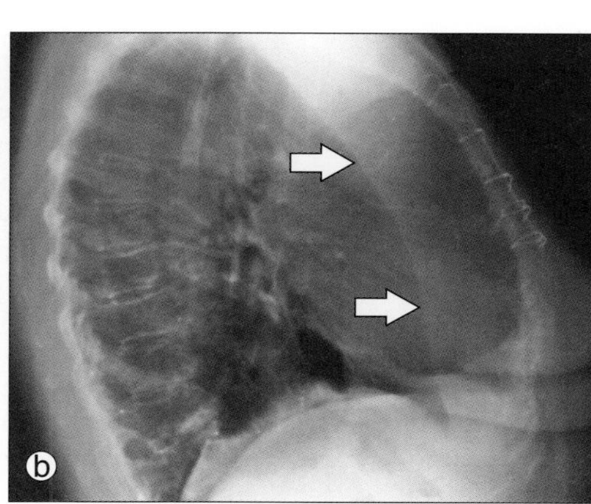

Figure 41.10 Squamous cell carcinoma causing lobar collapse. The posteroanterior **A,** and lateral chest **B,** radiographs show a left upper-lobe collapse (*arrows*) in a patient who presented with cough. Bronchoscopy revealed a squamous cell carcinoma that occluded the left upper-lobe bronchus.

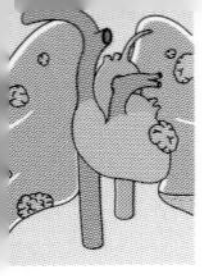

than 60% of patients who have small cell type and about 30% of those who have squamous cell carcinoma of the lung (Fig. 41.11). The presence of hepatic metastasis at presentation is much less common. Among patients diagnosed to have operable NSCLC in the chest, approximately 5% show CT evidence of liver metastasis. Involvement of the liver is shown by CT in about 25% of patients who have SCLC at initial staging. Patients who have liver involvement are often asymptomatic at initial presentation.

Adrenal

Metastasis to an adrenal gland is present at autopsy in 25% to 40% of patients who have lung cancer (Fig. 41.12). The usual scenario in the concern for adrenal metastasis is a unilateral adrenal mass found during staging CT for lung cancer. One series found that, of 330 patients who have operable NSCLC, 25 (7.5%) had isolated adrenal masses and 8 (2.4%) proved malignant. Even in the setting of initial evaluation for lung cancer, most of the adrenal masses are benign and usually caused by adenomas, nodular hyperplasia, or hemorrhagic cysts. The finding of a unilateral adrenal mass in a patient who has otherwise resectable disease requires a negative positron emission tomography (PET) scan or a needle biopsy guided by CT to confirm the absence of metastasis.

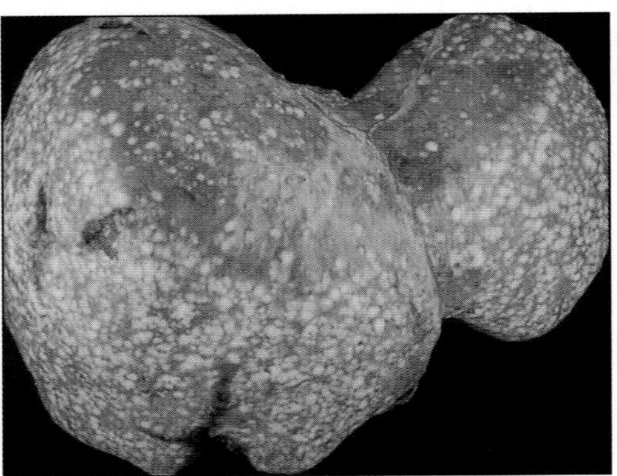

Figure 41.11 Liver metastases from small-cell carcinoma of the lung. The gross autopsy liver specimen from a 50-year-old male smoker shows innumerable metastatic foci of small-cell carcinoma.

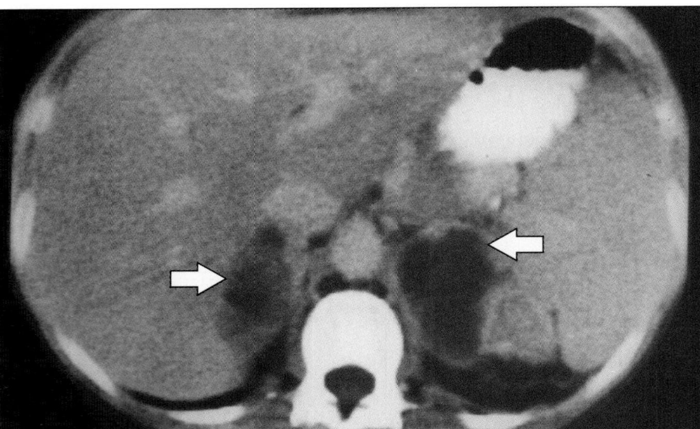

Figure 41.12 Adrenal metastases. Computed tomography scan of the abdomen showing large adrenal metastases (*arrows*) in a patient who has a lung mass and mediastinal adenopathy. Fine-needle aspirate of the adrenals showed adenocarcinoma.

Bone

Bone metastasis from lung cancer is most common in the small-cell type, but is also frequent in nonsmall types. An osteolytic radiographic appearance is more frequent than an osteoblastic one, and vertebral bodies are the most common bones involved. Approximately 30% to 40% of patients initially stage for SCLC with a bone scan, and bone marrow provides evidence of metastasis. Chest pain, skeletal pain, bone tenderness, and elevated levels of serum calcium or alkaline phosphatase are usually present in patients who have bony metastasis caused by NSCLC. Bone pain and elevated levels of serum calcium or alkaline phosphatase are often absent in patients who have SCLC and bone marrow involvement. PET scanning has improved the ability to identify metastases to many organs, including bone, with greater sensitivity than CT or bone scanning.

Nervous System

Neurologic manifestations of lung cancer include direct metastatic effects and paraneoplastic syndromes; the latter are discussed in the next section. The presence of central nervous system metastasis may be asymptomatic or cause headache, vomiting, seizures, hemiparesis, cranial nerve deficit, or visual field loss. Autopsy series have shown brain metastasis in the range of 25% to 40% for patients who had lung cancer. Squamous cell carcinoma has the least tendency to metastasize to the central nervous system and SCLC the greatest. Sequential resection may be feasible in selected cases that have operable NSCLC in the chest and a solitary brain metastasis. Various surgical series have shown 2-year survival rates of 25% to 45% in this setting.

Isolated nerve dysfunction may be the result of regional extension of bronchogenic carcinoma. Neoplasm is the most common cause of unilateral vocal cord paralysis, and lung cancer is the most common malignancy. The presence of hoarseness in a smoker raises concern for lung cancer. Extension of lung cancer into the phrenic nerve may result in diaphragm paralysis; patients may report dyspnea or be asymptomatic.

Superior Vena Cava Syndrome

Bronchogenic carcinoma accounts for 65% to 80% of superior vena cava (SVC) syndrome in reported cases. A sensation of fullness in the head and dyspnea are the most common presenting features of SVC syndrome. Cough, pain, and dysphagia are less frequent symptoms. Physical findings include dilated neck veins, a prominent venous pattern on the chest, facial edema, and a plethoric appearance (Fig. 41.13). The chest radiograph typically shows widening of the mediastinum or a right hilar mass, but may be normal. For most patients who have SVC syndrome secondary to lung cancer, the symptoms resolve after radiation or chemotherapy. Occasionally surgical palliation or vascular stenting is necessary.

Pleural

Presence of carcinoma cells in the pleural fluid establishes the lung cancer as unresectable (T4 or stage IIIB). Of patients who have lung cancer, less than 10% have pleural involvement at presentation. Dyspnea and cough are common symptoms that occur

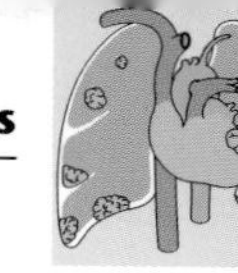

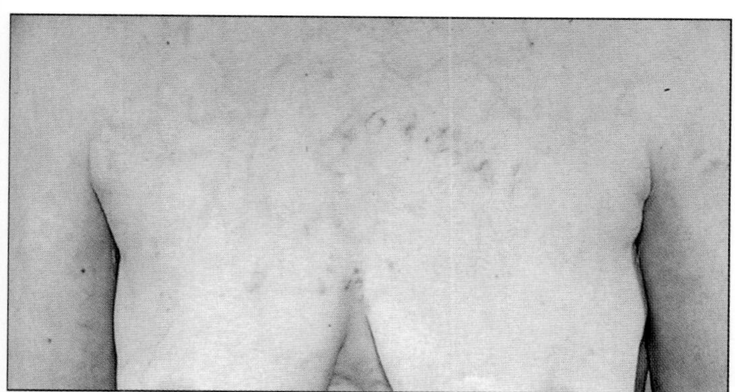

Figure 41.13 Superior vena cava (SVC) syndrome. The prominent venous pattern on this woman's chest arose from SVC obstruction caused by lung cancer.

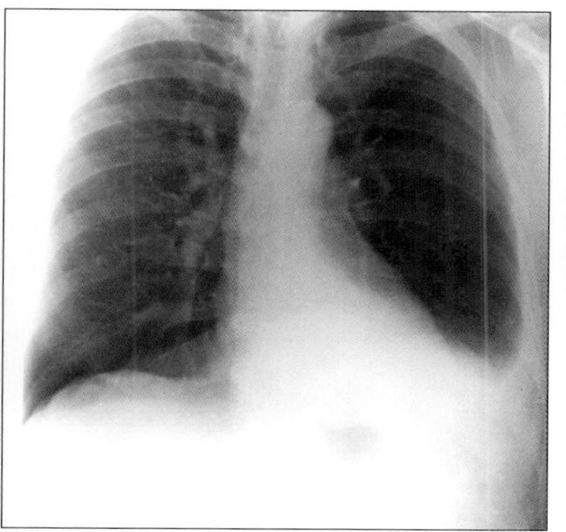

Figure 41.14 Malignant pleural effusion. Chest radiograph showing a left pleural effusion; thoracentesis revealed adenocarcinoma consistent with a lung primary tumor.

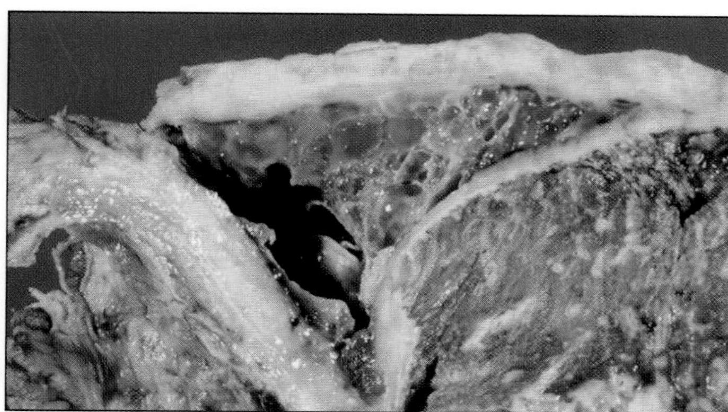

Figure 41.15 Pleural involvement by adenocarcinoma. The gross specimen shows malignant pleural involvement similar to the appearance of mesothelioma. Histology revealed adenocarcinoma.

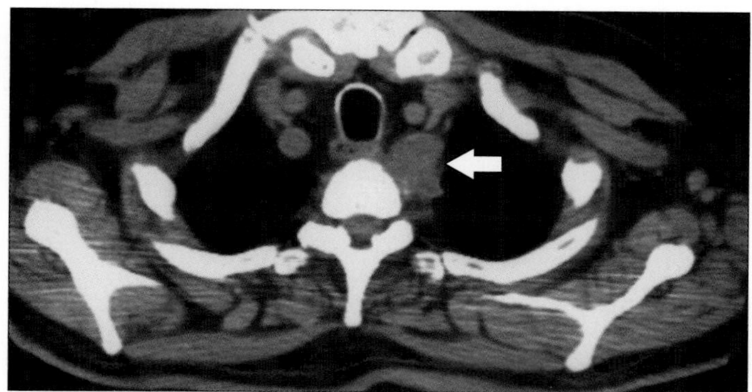

Figure 41.16 Superior sulcus tumor. Computed tomography scan from an 81-year-old man who presented with left scapular pain shows a superior sulcus mass (*arrow*) in the left lung apex. Ptosis and myosis were also present. Transbronchoscopic biopsy revealed grade IV non–small-cell carcinoma.

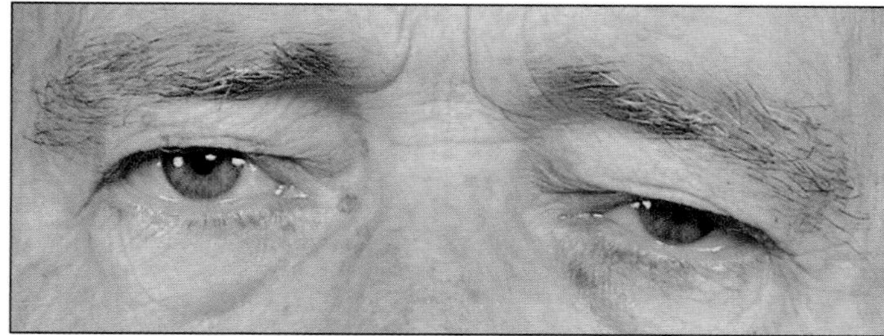

Figure 41.17 Ptosis as part of Pancoast syndrome. Drooping of this man's left eye is evident as part of Pancoast syndrome, and meiosis was also present. His computed tomography scan is shown in Fig. 41.16.

with malignant pleural effusions; approximately one fourth of patients who have lung cancer and pleural metastases are asymptomatic (Fig. 41.14). Malignant effusions are typically exudates and may be serous, serosanguineous, or grossly bloody. The simple presence of a pleural effusion in the setting of bronchogenic carcinoma does not establish unresectability. A benign pleural effusion may result from lymphatic obstruction, postobstructive pneumonitis, or atelectasis in the presence of a resectable lung cancer. The presence of pleural metastasis needs to be confirmed so that a chance for curative resection is not overlooked (Fig. 41.15). Documented cases of malignancy have shown the yield of pleural fluid cytology to be about 65%. Pleural biopsy adds little to the yield of cytologic examination. In a patient suspected to have malignancy, repeat pleural fluid cytology with or without pleural biopsy is appropriate if the initial study is negative.

Superior Sulcus Tumor

The superior sulcus is a groove created by the subclavian artery in the rounded vault of the pleura and apices of the upper lobes of the lungs. The resulting syndrome of characteristic pain, Horner syndrome, bony destruction, and atrophy of hand muscles in the setting of a superior sulcus tumor was first described by Dr. Pancoast (Figs. 41.16 and 41.17). Pancoast syndrome is most commonly caused by NSCLC and only rarely by small-cell carcinoma. Pain results from superior sulcus tumors and is most commonly located in the shoulder, followed by the forearm, scapula, and fingers. Patients often seek a chiropractor or orthopedist before proper diagnosis.

PARANEOPLASTIC SYNDROMES

The remote effects of cancer are those not related to the direct invasion, obstruction, or metastatic effects of tumor, and are generally termed paraneoplastic. Paraneoplastic syndromes related to bronchogenic carcinoma occur in 10% to 20% of patients (Table 41.2).

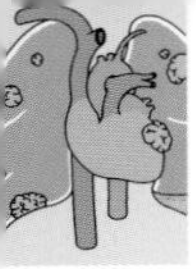

Table 41.2
Paraneoplastic syndromes

System	Paraneoplastic syndrome	System	Paraneoplastic syndrome
Musculoskeletal	Hypertrophic osteoarthropathy Polymyositis Osteomalacia Myopathy	Neurologic	Lambert–Eaton syndrome Peripheral neuropathy Encephalopathy Myelopathy Cerebellar degeneration Psychosis Dementia
Cutaneous	Clubbing Dermatomyositis Acanthosis nigricans Pruritus Erythema multiforme Hyperpigmentation Urticaria Scleroderma	Vascular/hematologic	Thrombophlebitis Arterial thrombosis Nonbacterial thrombotic endocarditis Thrombocytosis Polycythemia Hemolytic anemia Red cell aplasia Dysproteinemia Leukemoid reaction Eosinophilia Thrombocytopenic purpura Hypercoagulable state
Endocrinologic	Cushing's syndrome Syndrome of inappropriate antidiuretic hormone secretion Hypercalcemia Carcinoid syndrome Hyperglycemia/hypoglycemia Gynecomastia Galactorrhea Growth hormone excess Calcitonin secretion Thyroid-stimulating hormone	Miscellaneous	Cachexia Hyperuricemia Nephrotic syndrome

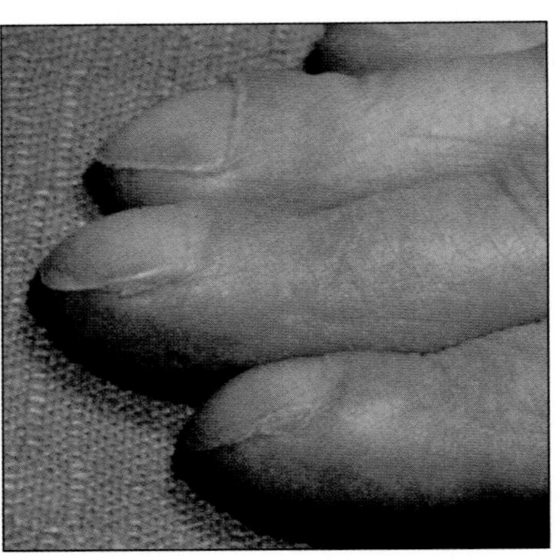

Figure 41.18 Clubbing. Hypertrophy of the connective tissue in the terminal phalanges of this patient who has lung cancer.

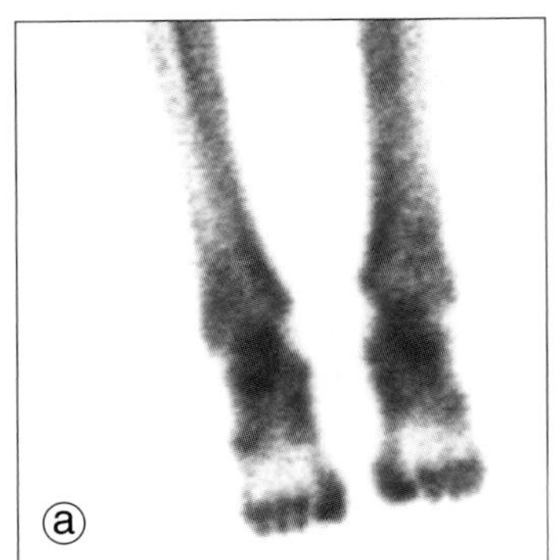

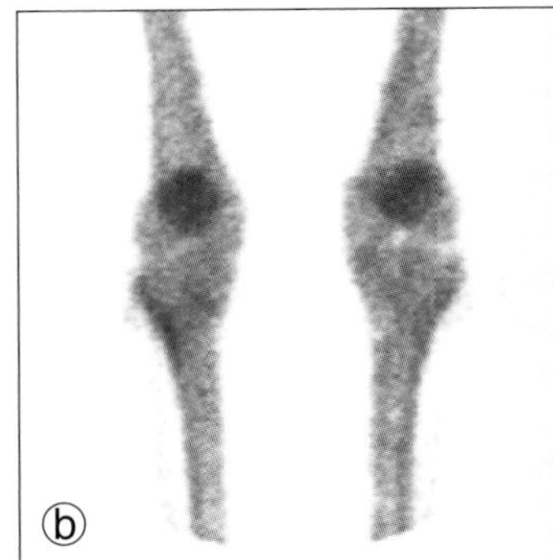

Figure 41.19 Hypertrophic pulmonary osteoarthropathy. The bone scan shows diffuse uptake of the ankles **(A)** and long bones **(B)** in this patient who had lung cancer.

Musculoskeletal

Clubbing of the digits may be a manifestation of lung cancer or other diseases. Clubbing may involve the fingers and toes and consists of selective enlargement of the connective tissue in the terminal phalanges (Fig. 41.18). Physical findings include loss of the angle between the base of the nail bed and cuticle, rounded nails, and enlarged fingertips. Clubbing is an isolated finding and is usually asymptomatic. Nonmalignant causes of clubbing include pulmonary fibrosis, congenital heart disease, and bronchiectasis.

Hypertrophic pulmonary osteoarthropathy (HPO) is an uncommon process associated with lung cancer. HPO is characterized by painful arthropathy that usually involves the ankles, knees, wrists, and elbows and is most often symmetric. The pain and arthropathy are caused by proliferative periostitis that involves the long bones, but may also involve metacarpal, metatarsal, and phalangeal bones. Patients may have clubbing of fingers and toes in addition to the painful arthralgia. The pathogenesis of HPO is uncertain, but may arise from a humoral agent. For patients who smoke and have a new onset of arthralgias, HPO must be considered. A radiograph of the long bones (i.e., tibia and fibula) usually shows characteristic, periosteal new bone formation. An isotope bone scan typically demonstrates diffuse uptake by the long bones (Fig. 41.19). Large cell and adenocarcinoma are the most common histologic types associated with HPO. The symptoms of HPO may resolve after thoracotomy, whether the primary cancer is resected or not. For patients who are not operable, the best treatment is with nonsteroidal anti-inflammatory agents.

Although still a topic of debate, population-based studies from Scandinavia suggest a frequency of malignancy of 15% to

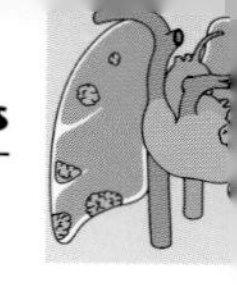

25% in patients with dermatomyositis-polymyositis. The highest risk of malignancy is in the first 2 years after the diagnosis of dermatomyositis-polymyositis. A reasonable approach to cancer surveillance in these patients is a careful history and physical examination, chest radiograph, basic laboratory tests, and age-appropriate cancer screening exams. Other tests should be based on abnormalities detected during the basic evaluation.

Hematologic

Anemia frequently occurs in patients who have lung cancer and may be caused by iron deficiency, chronic disease, or bone marrow infiltration. Anemia is also a frequent consequence of chemotherapy. Eosinophilia is more commonly associated with Hodgkin's disease but may occur in patients who have lung cancer. Production of various cytokines by neoplastic cells may result in eosinophilia, leukocytosis, or thrombocytosis, of which thrombocytosis is by far the most common.

The association of deep venous thrombosis and malignancy was described by Trousseau more than a century ago, and lung cancer is the most common malignancy associated with Trousseau syndrome. The causes of the hypercoagulable state remain poorly understood. One large study documented clinically significant association of idiopathic thrombosis and the subsequent development of overt cancer; however, other investigators concluded that the literature does not enable firm recommendations about whether to screen for a malignant neoplasm in patients who have unexplained venous thromboembolism. A careful clinical evaluation that includes history, physical examination, routine laboratory tests, chest radiograph, and age-appropriate screening tests appears appropriate. Routine CT scans of the chest and abdomen are not generally accepted as being cost-effective. Thromboembolism in the patient who has malignancy is often refractory to warfarin treatment. Treatment with low-molecular-weight heparin on a chronic basis may be effective, but this can be associated with significant cost, and the patient should be monitored for thrombocytopenia.

Hypercalcemia

Hypercalcemia in association with malignancy may arise from a bony metastasis or, less commonly, secretion of a parathyroid hormone-related protein (PTHrP) or other bone-resorbing cytokine secreted by the tumor. The most common cancers to cause hypercalcemia are those of the kidney, lung, breast, head and neck, and myeloma and lymphoma. In one study of 690 consecutive lung cancers, 2.5% had tumor-induced hypercalcemia. Squamous cell histology is the most common cell type associated with hypercalcemia, and generally patients have advanced disease (stage III or IV) and are seldom resectable. The median survival in patients who have hypercalcemia resulting from NSCLC is approximately 1 month. Symptoms of hypercalcemia include anorexia, nausea, vomiting, constipation, lethargy, polyuria, polydipsia, and dehydration. Confusion and coma are late manifestations, as are renal failure and nephrocalcinosis. Cardiovascular effects include shortened QT interval, broad T wave, heart block, ventricular arrhythmia, or asystole. Individual patients may manifest any combination of these signs and symptoms in various degrees.

Hypercalcemia of malignancy that is not caused by bony metastases results from accelerated bone resorption, decreased bone deposition, or increased renal tubular reabsorption of calcium. Accelerated bone resorption is caused by activation of osteoclasts by cytokines or PTHrP in most cases. Serum parathyroid hormone levels are usually normal or low, but an elevated level of PTHrP can be detected in the serum in approximately one half of these patients. Cytokines or PTHrP are secreted autonomously by the tumor. Not only does PTHrP cause calcium readsorption, but also it interferes with renal mechanisms for readsorption of sodium and water with resultant polyuria. Polyuria and vomiting result in dehydration; decreases in glomerular filtration further aggravate the hypercalcemia.

Mild elevation of serum calcium may not require treatment, so the decision is based on the patient's symptoms. For patients who have widely metastatic and incurable malignancy, it may be most appropriate to give supportive care only and not treat the hypercalcemia. The average life expectancy in this situation is 30 to 45 days, even with aggressive treatment.

Most patients who have a serum calcium of 12 to 13 mg/dL (3 to 3.25 mmol/L) or higher are treated. The corrected serum calcium in such individuals who have low albumins is calculated by: measured serum calcium + 0.8 × [4 g/dL (or 40 g/L) – measured serum albumin] = corrected serum calcium.

The four basic goals of treatment are:

1. Correct dehydration
2. Increase renal excretion of calcium
3. Inhibit bone resorption
4. Treat the underlying malignancy

Because of the polyuria, patients with hypercalcemia are volume-contracted. Initial treatment is with intravenous normal saline, using 3 to 6 L per 24 hours as tolerated, with careful attention to volume status. After hydration, a loop diuretic such as furosemide (frusemide) or ethacrynic acid should be added. Thiazide diuretics are not used because they increase calcium resorption in the distal tubule. Fluids and diuretics generally result in only a mild decrease of the calcium; additional treatment is needed to inhibit the accelerated bone resorption. The bisphosphonates have a high affinity for bone and inhibit osteoclast activity. Zoledronate, a newer bisphosphonate, is the most effective; the usual dose is 4 mg given intravenously over 15 minutes. Normal calcium levels are achieved within 4 to 10 days in 85% of patients and last a median of 30 to 40 days. Adverse effects are generally mild and transient, and include fever, hypophosphatemia, and asymptomatic hypocalcemia. Occasional renal adverse events may occur with elevation of serum creatinine. Calcitonin inhibits bone resorption, increases renal calcium excretion, and has a rapid onset of action, but the duration of action is short-lived. Calcitonin is a relatively weak agent and, when used alone, does not usually normalize the serum calcium of patients who have marked hypercalcemia. Use of calcitonin is appropriate when the calcium needs to be lowered urgently (onset of action 4 to 6 hours) while waiting for the more effective but slower-acting agents to take effect or when relief of bony pain is desired. The effects of calcitonin and bisphosphonates are additive. Other agents such as gallium nitrate or plicamycin have been used to treat hypercalcemia, but have not generally been adopted as front-line therapies because of inconvenience of administration schedules or associated toxicities.

Syndrome of Inappropriate Antidiuretic Hormone Secretion

Causes of hyponatremia include tumors, pulmonary infections, central nervous system disorders, and drugs. Approximately 10% of patients who have SCLC exhibit the syndrome of inappropriate antidiuretic hormone secretion (SIADH); however, SCLC accounts for approximately 75% of cases of SIADH. Antidiuretic hormone (vasopressin) is secreted in the anterior hypothalamus and exerts its action on the renal collecting ducts by enhancing the flow of water from the lumen into the medullary interstitium, which results in the concentration of urine. The criteria for the diagnosis of SIADH include:

- Hyponatremia associated with serum hypo-osmolality (<275 mOsm/kg)
- Inappropriately elevated urine osmolality (>200 mOsm/kg) relative to serum osmolality
- Elevated urine sodium (>20 mEq/L)
- Clinical euvolemia without edema
- Normal renal (creatinine <1.5 times the upper limit of normal), adrenal, and thyroid function.

The serum uric acid is usually low, and the urine osmolality : serum osmolality ratio is frequently greater than 2.

The severity of symptoms is related to the degree of hyponatremia and the rapidity of the fall in serum sodium. In one large series of SIADH patients, only 27% had signs or symptoms of hyponatremia despite a median sodium level of 117 mEq/L (range 101 to 129 mEq/L). Symptoms of hyponatremia include anorexia, nausea, and vomiting. With rapid onset of hyponatremia, symptoms caused by cerebral edema may include irritability, restlessness, personality changes, confusion, coma, seizures, and respiratory arrest. In minimally symptomatic or asymptomatic patients, fluid restriction of 500 to 1000 mL per 24 hours is the initial treatment of choice. If further treatment is needed, oral demeclocycline 900 to 1200 mg/day is considered. Demeclocycline induces a nephrogenic diabetes insipidus and blocks the action of antidiuretic hormone on the renal tubule, thereby increasing water excretion. The onset of action varies from a few hours to a few weeks, so this drug is not recommended for acute emergency treatment. In patients who have more severe or life-threatening symptoms (serum sodium of less than 115 mEq/L), treatment consists of intravenous fluids with 0.9% saline and supplemental potassium and diuresis with loop diuretics such as furosemide or ethacrynic acid. With severe confusion, convulsions, or coma, it may be appropriate to treat with 300 mL of 3% saline given over 3 to 4 hours in combination with a loop diuretic. Saline with no diuretic ultimately does not raise the sodium concentration. Rapid correction of the sodium may have life-threatening consequences, and caution is advised. The rate of correction of the sodium is best limited to 2 mEq/L/hour or a maximum of 20 mEq/L/day until a level of 120 to 130 mEq/L is reached. Faster correction has been associated with the development of central pontine myelinolysis, which may result in quadriplegia, cranial nerve abnormalities that manifest as pseudobulbar palsy, alteration in mental status, and subsequent death. Accordingly, in the course of treating hyponatremia, serum sodium must be monitored frequently to ensure that correction is not too rapid. For patients with SIADH resulting from SCLC, treatment with chemotherapy should be initiated as soon as possible, and is likely to result in improvement in the hyponatremia within a few weeks. After an initial response to chemotherapy, SIADH may recur after disease relapse.

Ectopic Corticotropin Syndrome

Ectopic production of corticotropin or corticotropin-releasing hormone with associated Cushing syndrome has been identified in patients who have SCLC; carcinoid tumors of the lung, thymus, or pancreas; and neurocrest tumors such as pheochromocytoma, neuroblastoma, and medullary carcinoma of the thyroid. In ectopic corticotropin secretion, SCLC accounts for 75% of cases. Cushing syndrome is seldom caused by NSCLC.

Classic features of Cushing syndrome include truncal obesity, striae, rounded (moon) face, dorsocervical fat pad (buffalo hump), myopathy and weakness, osteoporosis, diabetes mellitus, hypertension, and personality changes. However, the rapid growth of SCLC means that patients are more likely to present with edema, hypertension, and muscular weakness rather than with the classic symptoms. Hypokalemic alkalosis and hyperglycemia are usually present. Of patients who have SCLC, 2% to 5% develop Cushing syndrome. Patients who suffer SCLC and Cushing syndrome appear to have a shortened survival period than do patients who have SCLC without the syndrome, and this may be because of more frequent opportunistic infections. The best screen for Cushing syndrome is the 24-hour urine free-cortisol measurement. Elevation of cortisol production and lack of suppression with high-dose dexamethasone and plasma corticotropin levels greater than 200 pg/mL (40 pmol/L) are highly suggestive of ectopic corticotropin as the cause of Cushing syndrome in the absence of a pituitary adenoma (negative imaging study). The plasma level of adrenocorticotropin hormone (ACTH) is elevated in many, but not all patients.

Treatment of Cushing syndrome because of ectopic corticotropin has included adrenal enzyme inhibitors such as metyrapone, aminoglutethimide, or ketoconazole, given alone or in combination. Ketoconazole given orally at a dosage of 400 to 1200 mg/day may control hypercortisolism within a few days to weeks, but the response is variable. Dose adjustments are based on the urinary free cortisol levels. Symptomatic hypoadrenalism may result from treatment, and some authorities recommend a replacement dose of glucocorticoid when an enzyme inhibitor is started. When Cushing syndrome arises from SCLC, it is advisable to proceed with appropriate chemotherapy and carefully watch for superimposed infections, as is necessary for any patient who takes high-dose corticosteroids. Cushing syndrome related to a bronchial carcinoid is best treated by surgical resection of the tumor.

Neurologic

The paraneoplastic neurologic syndromes associated with lung cancer, mostly small-cell type, are quite variable. They include Lambert-Eaton myasthenic syndrome (LEMS), subacute sensory neuropathy, encephalomyelopathy, cerebellar degeneration, autonomic neuropathy, retinal degeneration, and opsoclonus. The frequency of any of these neurologic syndromes in SCLC is approximately 5%, and neurologic symptoms may

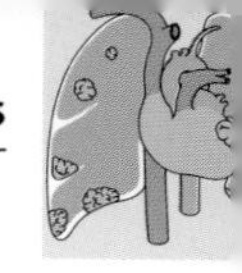

precede the diagnosis by months to years. Most patients who have SCLC and an associated paraneoplastic syndrome have limited stage disease that may or may not be obvious on initial evaluation. Careful radiographic evaluation of the lungs and mediastinum is indicated in a smoker who has a suspected paraneoplastic neurologic syndrome. In this setting, even subtle abnormalities of the mediastinum require a biopsy. A positive PET scan may help identify the lesion to facilitate biopsy confirmation of the diagnosis.

These paraneoplastic neurologic syndromes are thought to be immune-mediated based on the identification of a number of autoantibodies. The literature is confusing because of different names employed by various investigators. The anti-Hu antibody is the same as the antineuronal nuclear-antibody type I (ANNA-1), and the anti-Ri antibody is identical to ANNA-2. Both of these antibodies, predominantly ANNA-1, have been associated with SCLC. Such antibodies should not be confused with the anti-Purkinje antibody (anti-yo), which is characteristically found in patients who have subacute cerebellar degeneration as a manifestation of gynecologic malignancy or breast cancer. The newly described CRMP-5 antibody, also known as CV-2, has been associated with SCLC and thymomas.

In a review of 162 sequential patients who had ANNA-1, 142 (88%) were proved to have cancer, 132 of which were SCLC (Table 41.3). In 97% of these cases, the diagnosis of SCLC followed the onset of the associated neurologic syndrome, usually by less than 6 months, but in 20% the period was more than 6 months. Of special note is that 90% of cases had disease limited to the lung or mediastinum (limited stage disease). In one large series, ANNA-1 antibodies were identified in 16% of SCLC cases. These antibodies were associated with limited stage disease, complete response to therapy, and longer survival as compared with patients who had SCLC and no ANNA-1 antibody. These neurologic syndromes almost seldom improve with treatment, so the goal is to prevent progression of the disease process.

Less common manifestations of neurologic paraneoplastic syndromes are orthostatic hypotension and intestinal dysmotility. The ANNA-1 binds to the nucleus of all neurons in the central and peripheral nervous system, including the sensory and autonomic ganglia, myenteric plexus, and cells of the adrenal medulla. The gastrointestinal symptoms may present as nausea, vomiting, abdominal discomfort, or altered bowel habits suggestive of intestinal pseudo-obstruction. Many of these patients present with gastrointestinal symptoms and significant weight loss before the diagnosis of SCLC.

Table 41.3
Neurologic manifestations in 162 patients positive for antineuronal nuclear antibody type I (From Luchinetti CF, Kimmel DE, Lennon VA: Paraneoplastic and oncological profiles of patients seropositive for Type I anti-neuronal nuclear antibodies. Neurology 50:652-657, 1998.)

Manifestation	Frequency (%)
Neuropathy	90
Sensory	40
Sensorimotor	30
Autonomic	18
Motor	2
Cerebellar	18
Limbic encephalitis (cognitive dysfunction with or without seizures)	14
Cranial neuropathy	15
Lambert–Eaton myasthenic syndrome	6

Proximal muscle weakness, hyporeflexia, and autonomic dysfunction characterize LEMS. Cranial nerve involvement may be present and does not differentiate LEMS from myasthenia gravis. LEMS has been strongly associated with antibodies directed against P/Q-type presynaptic voltage gaited calcium channels of peripheral cholinergic nerve terminals. These antibodies have been identified in more than 90% of patients who have LEMS and block the normal release of acetylcholine at the neuromuscular junction. In contrast, myasthenia gravis is associated with antiacetylcholine receptor antibodies, which are present in approximately 90% of patients. Malignancy is present in approximately one half of patients who have LEMS, and SCLC is by far the most common histologic type. Of all patients who suffer SCLC, only 2% to 4% have LEMS. Calcium channel autoantibodies have also been identified in 25% of SCLC patients who are not affected by neurologic problems. The diagnosis of LEMS is based on characteristic electromyographic findings that show a small amplitude of the resting compound muscle-action potential and facilitation with rapid, repetitive, supramaximal nerve stimulation or after brief exercise of the muscle. A single-fiber electromyograph is optimal for making the diagnosis.

Treatment of SCLC that induces remission of the cancer may result in attenuation or remission of the LEMS in some patients. LEMS is the predominant paraneoplastic neurologic syndrome that may improve with successful treatment of the associated lung cancer. The use of acetylcholinesterase inhibitors is of limited benefit in LEMS. Diaminopyridine enhances the release of acetylcholine and has been used with mixed results for treatment of both motor and autonomic deficits.

DIAGNOSIS AND STAGING

Diagnosis

Although most lung cancers are initially detected when patients present with symptoms and abnormalities are noted on a plain chest radiograph, the diagnosis of bronchogenic carcinoma requires histology or cytology. The presence of a solitary pulmonary nodule (SPN) leads to diagnostic controversy (Fig. 41.20). By definition, an SPN is a solitary lesion surrounded by normal lung and not involved with atelectasis or hilar enlargement. The overall goal in evaluating an SPN is promptly to resect potentially curable cancers and avoid removal of benign nodules. The likelihood that a nodule is malignant increases with advancing age of the patient, history of smoking, and prior history of malignancy, and is determined by nodule size. Review of prior chest radiographs is critically important to identify whether the nodule is new, stable, or enlarging. Nodules shown to diminish in size are benign, and nodules shown to be stable in size over a 2-year period are highly likely to be benign. Evidence of nodule enlargement is a reliable indicator of malignancy, though growth may occasionally be seen in a granuloma.

Evaluation of focal pulmonary opacities has greatly improved with CT scans. Thin-section CT is more sensitive than plain film or plain tomography in the detection of calcium, and multiple

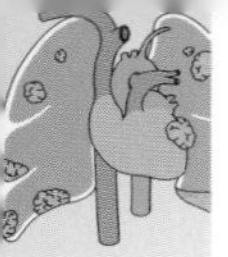

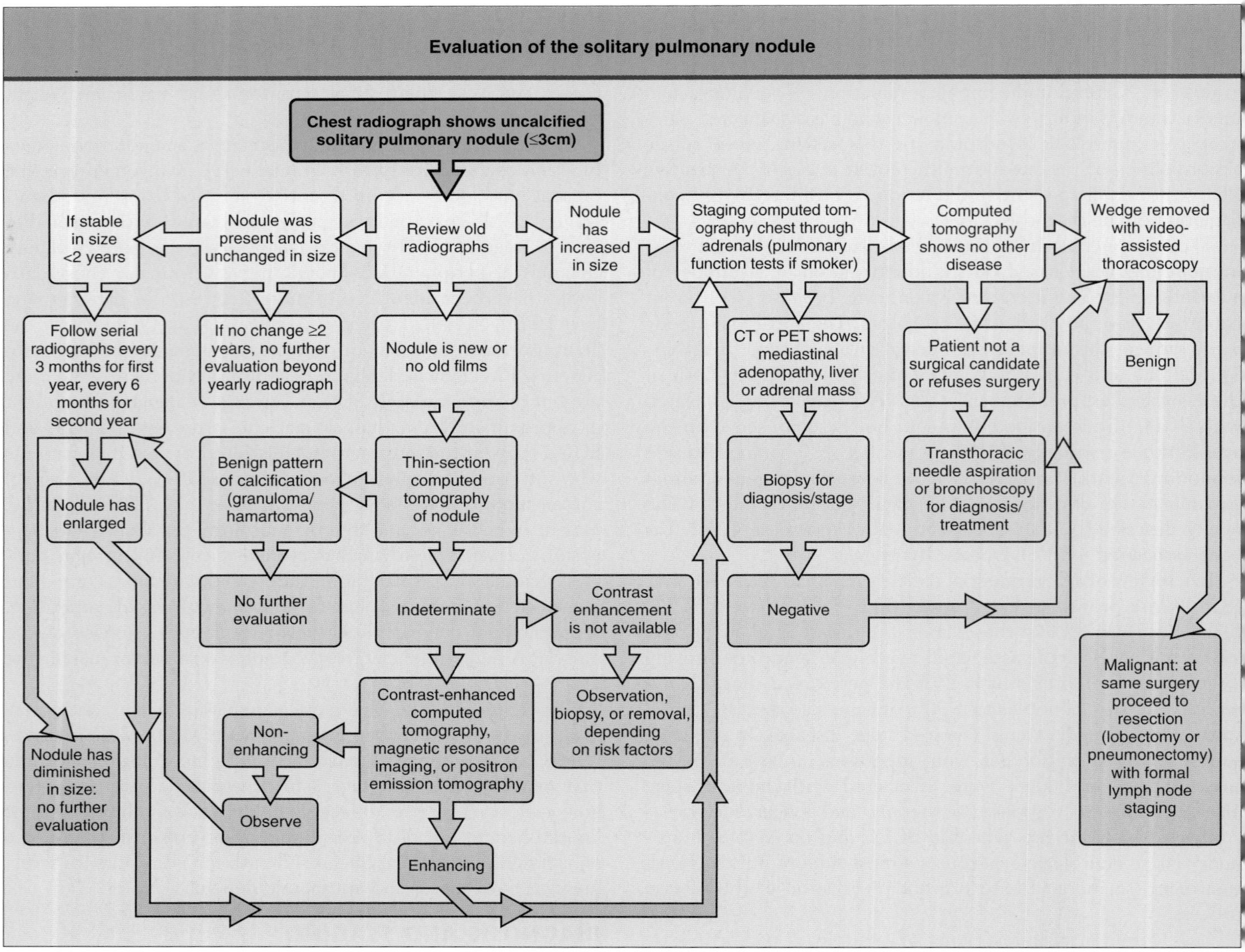

Evaluation of the solitary pulmonary nodule

Chest radiograph shows uncalcified solitary pulmonary nodule (≤3cm)
Review old radiographs
Nodule was present and is unchanged in size
If stable in size <2 years
Follow serial radiographs every 3 months for first year, every 6 months for second year
Nodule has enlarged
Nodule has diminished in size: no further evaluation
If no change ≥2 years, no further evaluation beyond yearly radiograph
Nodule is new or no old films
Thin-section computed tomography of nodule
Benign pattern of calcification (granuloma/ hamartoma)
No further evaluation
Indeterminate
Contrast enhancement is not available
Observation, biopsy, or removal, depending on risk factors
Contrast-enhanced computed tomography, magnetic resonance imaging, or positron emission tomography
Non-enhancing
Observe
Enhancing
Nodule has increased in size
Staging computed tomography chest through adrenals (pulmonary function tests if smoker)
CT or PET shows: mediastinal adenopathy, liver or adrenal mass
Biopsy for diagnosis/stage
Negative
Computed tomography shows no other disease
Patient not a surgical candidate or refuses surgery
Transthoracic needle aspiration or bronchoscopy for diagnosis/ treatment
Wedge removed with video-assisted thoracoscopy
Benign
Malignant: at same surgery proceed to resection (lobectomy or pneumonectomy) with formal lymph node staging

Figure 41.20 Evaluation algorithm for the solitary pulmonary nodule. Thin-section computed tomography (CT), contrast-enhanced CT, and staging CT may be carried out as a single study.

nodules may be identified. The presence of calcification within a nodule is a reliable indicator that the nodule is benign, unless the calcification is eccentric. Nodules that are indeterminate after radiographic assessment require a decision between observation, biopsy, or removal. A decision for close observation requires serial radiographs approximately every 3 months for 1 year and every 6 months for a second year, looking to establish benignancy by lack of growth or reduction in size. Plain chest radiograph may be used to follow the nodule if it is well seen. CT may be required for follow up of nodules too small to be seen on a chest radiograph. Nodules of a few millimeters in size may be followed at intervals of 6 or 12 months.

Bronchoscopy and transthoracic needle aspiration are the two methods available for biopsy. Bronchoscopy is not appropriate for the evaluation of most SPNs. For nodules 2 cm or less in diameter, the yield from bronchoscopy is in the range of 10% to 20%. Bronchoscopy in the setting of an SPN rarely alters stage or identifies a synchronous tumor and is not needed for routine preoperative assessment. Presence of an air-bronchogram or bronchus leading into the nodule greatly increases the likelihood of diagnosis with bronchoscopy. Transthoracic needle aspiration has a 60% to 80% yield in nodules 2 cm or smaller. Both procedures are limited by the frequent inability to make a specific benign diagnosis. Bronchoscopic biopsy and transthoracic needle aspiration are techniques discussed elsewhere in this chapter. A new spiculated nodule in a smoker may be best managed by proceeding to staging evaluation or to surgical resection without biopsy. The best management of an indeterminate SPN can be difficult, and it is important to inform and involve patients in the decision-making process.

Establishing cell type may be accomplished through bronchoscopy, needle aspiration, sputum cytology, or surgery. Sputum cytology is inexpensive and carries a high diagnostic specificity. Sputum cytology in patients who have larger tumors, or tumors that are centrally located, has higher likelihood of being positive. Sensitivity of a single sputum specimen for the detection of lung cancer is about 50% and increases with repeated specimens. Sputum cytology is not often positive in

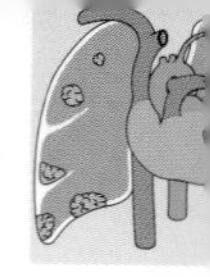

patients who have small peripheral tumors. Radiographically occult squamous cell carcinomas may be detected at an early stage by sputum cytology; however, positive sputum cytology in the setting of adenocarcinoma is usually a poor prognostic sign.

Staging

The finding of a lung mass in a smoker presents less of a diagnostic challenge than finding an SPN. After lung cancer is strongly suspected, two main questions need to be answered: what is the cell type and what is the stage of the disease? The clinical evaluation for suspected lung cancer requires a careful history and physical examination, as well as complete blood count and serum chemistry panel that includes liver function tests. Localized pain, lymphadenopathy, or specific laboratory abnormalities direct the physician in further testing. In a patient who has radiographically suspected lung cancer and an otherwise negative careful clinical evaluation, the likelihood of finding metastatic disease from a head CT scan or radionuclide bone scan is very low. Various series have found brain metastasis in 4%, bony metastasis in 3%, and liver metastasis in 1.5% after a negative careful clinical evaluation. The American Thoracic Society and European Respiratory Society recommend that all patients who have lung cancer have a careful history and physical examination, basic blood parameters, and a CT scan of the chest that extends through the liver and adrenal glands. Pursuing tumor markers in the serum is not recommended. Pulmonary function testing should be obtained in patients who are considered for surgical resection. Quantitative ventilation-perfusion lung scan or cardiopulmonary exercise testing may assist in the selection of surgical candidates among patients who have borderline pulmonary function.

The role of PET in the evaluation of patients with known or suspected lung cancer is being defined. PET is based on the principle that cancer cells have a high rate of glycolysis and an increased cellular uptake of glucose because of an increased number of transport proteins as compared to non-neoplastic cells. The PET tracer 18-fluoro-deoxyglucose (18-FDG) is taken up into cells, metabolically trapped, and accumulates. 18-FDG is a positron emitter and therefore can be measured. PET has been used been used to evaluate SPNs and has a sensitivity of approximately 90% and a specificity of 85% for determining malignancy. These data are based on nodules of 1 cm or larger. The resolution limit of nodules for PET evaluation is approximately 7 to 8 mm. False-positive PET scans have been reported with tuberculosis, fungal diseases, other infections, and sarcoidosis. Inflammatory disorders such as a rheumatoid nodule or cryptogenic organizing pneumonia may also cause false-positive PET scans. False-negative PET scans may occur with low-grade tumors such as bronchoalveolar cell carcinoma or carcinoid tumor and tumors less than 1 cm in size. Hyperglycemia interferes with 18-FDG uptake and may result in a false negative scan.

For evaluation of mediastinal lymph node metastasis, PET has a sensitivity and specificity of approximately 90% and 85% to 90%, respectively, based on a meta-analysis of the literature. This compares very favorably with the use of CT scan staging of the mediastinum where there is an approximately 30% to 40% rate of both false positives and false negatives. PET has also been shown to detect distant metastases in 10% to 15% of patients who are thought to be operable (Fig. 41.21). Because of the 10% to 15% rate of false-positive PET scans, it is absolutely necessary to obtain biopsy or other imaging proof of distant metastasis before deciding that the patient is inoperable.

An important aspect of the clinical evaluation is to establish both resectability and operability. The history, physical examination, laboratory tests, and chest CT through the adrenals are used to try to establish whether or not resectable disease is present. Resectability is determined by stage: whether or not the tumor may be removed surgically and result in a survival benefit.

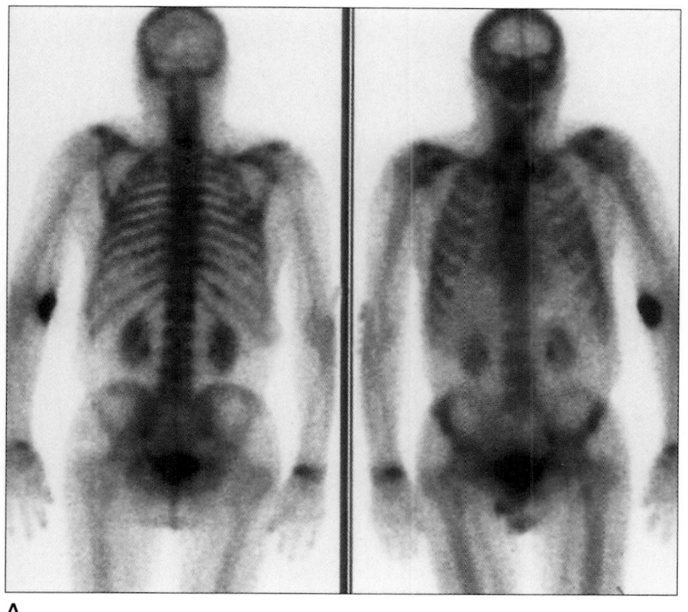

A

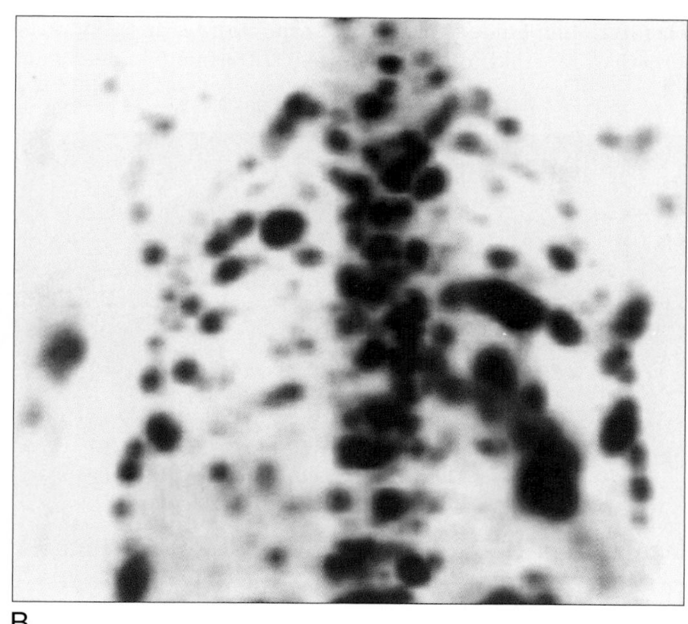

B

Figure 41.21 Negative bone scan and positive positron emission tomography (PET) scan indicating metastatic disease. **A,** Bone scan in a patient with limited-stage small-cell lung cancer. **B,** PET scan done within one week in the same patient indicating extensive bone metastases.

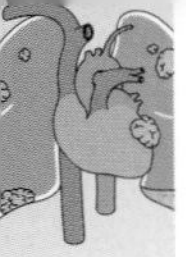

The specifics of resectability are discussed in the section following on staging and in the section on treatment. Operability is determined by whether or not the patient can withstand the operation. In other words, stage I peripheral nodule may be resectable, but if the patient's pulmonary function is too poor, then he or she may not be operable. Multiple factors are involved in operability, including functional status, pulmonary function, cardiac and other medical problems, and willingness to undergo surgery. Some of these are more quantifiable than others and some may be modifiable. Regarding pulmonary function, the ability to tolerate resection is estimated by the predicted postoperative lung function (preoperative function minus resected function). Patients who have normal pulmonary function can be anticipated to tolerate pneumonectomy or a lesser resection. A quantitative lung scan may assist the prediction of postoperative lung function. If the postoperative predicted forced expiratory volume in 1 second and diffusing capacity are greater than 40%, surgery is generally well-tolerated. Additional exercise assessment, specifically aerobic capacity, may help predict the appropriateness of surgery in patients who have less than 40% predicted function. Some patients refuse to undergo surgery even when a good outcome is predicted.

Diagnosis and staging of bronchogenic carcinoma presenting as a large mass or central lesion is often easily accomplished through bronchoscopy. Diagnostic yield approaches 100% with bronchial biopsy when the malignant lesion is present endobronchially. The visual extent of the tumor can guide surgical resection. Transbronchial needle aspiration through the flexible bronchoscope may be used to sample lymph nodes in the paratracheal, subcarinal, hilar, and aorticopulmonic window positions (Fig. 41.22). Bronchoscopic needle aspiration may allow mediastinal lymph node sampling and result in simultaneous diagnosis and staging of lung cancer. Care must be taken not to contaminate the needle specimen with airway secretions, which may contain cancer cells and lead to a false-positive sample. Needle aspiration at the time of bronchoscopy is an underused technique. Sampling of mediastinal nodes via esophagoscopy with ultrasound-guided fine needle aspiration is an additional alternative for diagnosis and stage. Ultrasound-guided fine needle aspiration is particularly effective for stations 4 (left paratracheal) 7 (subcarinal), and 8 (paraesophageal) node groups. Diagnosis and stage may also be accomplished by cytologic examination of a pleural effusion or by needle aspiration of a liver or adrenal metastasis.

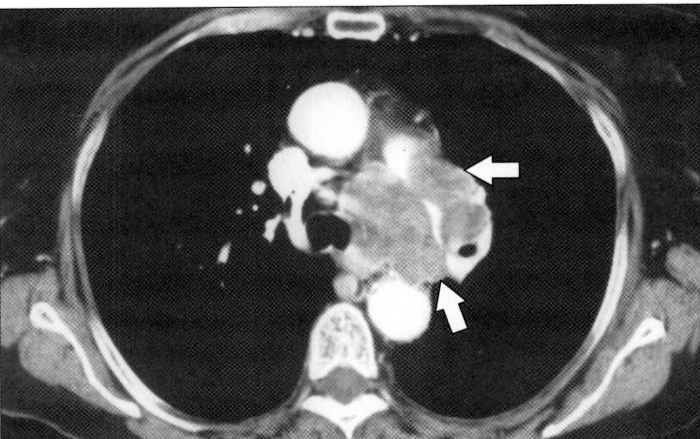

Figure 41.22 Small-cell lung cancer with mediastinal adenopathy. Computed tomography scan of the chest shows a large, left upper-lobe mass with extensive left hilar and mediastinal adenopathy (*arrows*), and extrinsic compression of the left main stem bronchus. Transbronchial needle aspiration revealed small-cell carcinoma.

Staging: Non–small-cell Lung Cancer

Staging of lung cancer is the most accurate means to estimate prognosis and guide treatment decisions. The characteristics of the primary tumor (T) (Figs. 41.23 and 41.24), regional lymph nodes (N) (Fig. 41.25), and metastatic involvement (M) (Fig. 41.26) are used to stage NSCLC according to the TNM system. Descriptors of the staging classifications are provided (Table 41.4), and the stage groupings are outlined (Table 41.5). Changes have occurred in the staging system as of 1997 and include the splitting of both stages I and II into A and B, as well as moving a T3N0M0 lesion from stage IIIA to IIB. A satellite tumor nodule within the ipsilateral primary-tumor–bearing lobe is classified as T4, and a metastatic tumor nodule in an ipsilateral nonprimary-tumor–bearing lobe is classified as M1. Tracheobronchial lymph nodes are classified as N1 hilar nodes. The importance of this staging system is to improve uniformity and allow appropriate comparison of prognosis and treatment studies between institutions and between countries.

Staging: Small-cell Lung Cancer

The TNM staging system discussed previously is primarily used to stage NSCLC, but it can be applied to SCLC; however, the limitation is that less differentiation in survival is available for

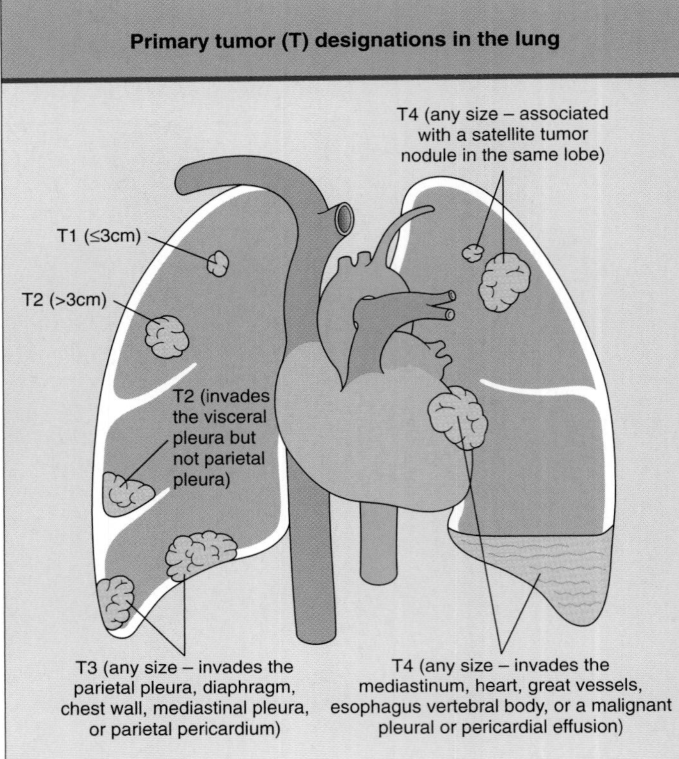

Figure 41.23 Primary tumor (T) staging classification in the lung.

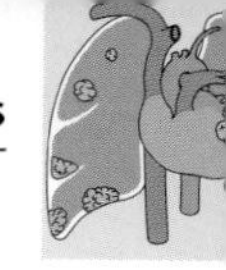

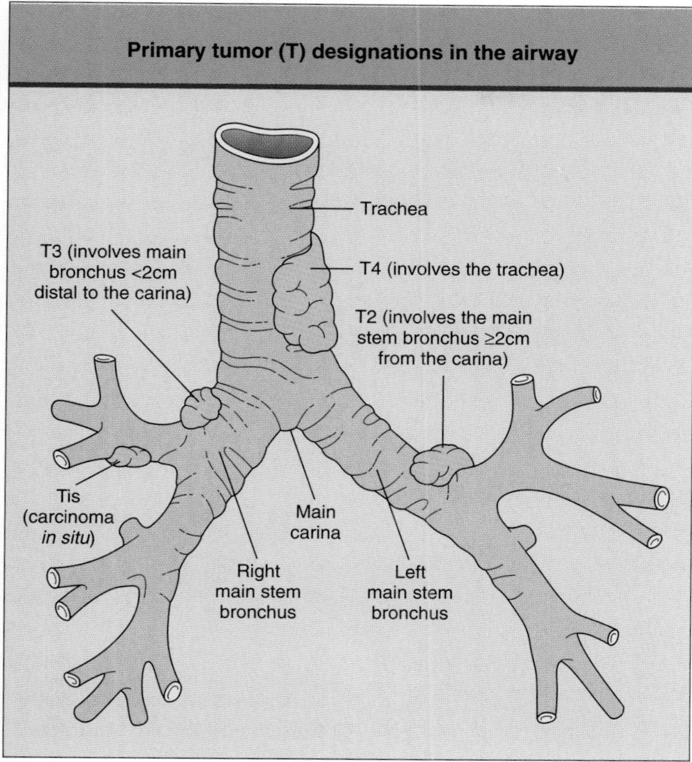

Figure 41.24 Primary tumor (T) staging classification in the airway.

the various stages. Accordingly, most physicians use the old Veterans Administration staging system of "limited" and "extensive"' disease categories (Fig. 41.27). Limited disease is defined as disease confined to one hemithorax and the ipsilateral supraclavicular nodes. This stage of disease can be encompassed within one radiation portal. Extensive stage disease is defined as disease that has spread beyond these confines and cannot be encompassed in one radiation portal. Contralateral hilar lymph nodes, cervical lymph nodes, or distant organ metastasis is considered extensive stage disease. A pleural effusion that is cytologically positive for malignant cells or a bloody effusion in the setting of known SCLC is usually classified as extensive stage disease.

TREATMENT AND PROGNOSIS

Non–small-cell Lung Cancer

STAGES 0, IA/B, AND IIA/B

At initial presentation, only 15% to 25% of patients have resectable disease. Patients who have asymptomatic lung cancer at the time of diagnosis have a significantly better prognosis. The treatment of choice for stage 0 (carcinoma in situ), IA/B, or IIA/B NSCLC is surgical resection, provided the patient is medically fit. The 30-day operative mortality with lobectomy is 2% to 3% and 5% to 7% for pneumonectomy. The primary causes of operative mortality include pneumonia, respiratory failure, bronchopleural fistula, empyema, myocardial infarction, and pulmonary embolus.

In the 1990s, video-assisted thoracoscopic surgery developed rapidly and is now commonly used at most thoracic surgical centers. This method is useful for lung biopsies and removal of

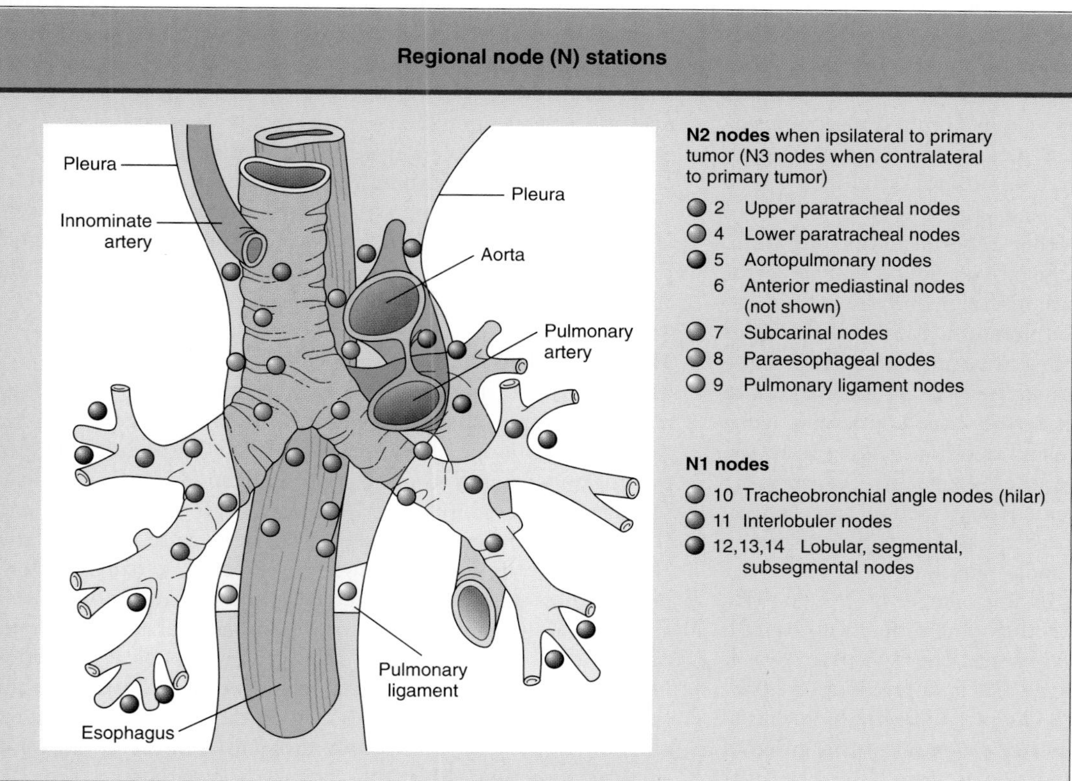

Figure 41.25 Lymph node stations (N) for lung cancer staging. (From Mountain CF, Dresler CM: Regional lymph node classification for lung cancer staging. Chest 111:1718-1723, 1997.)

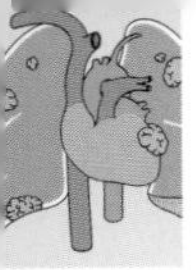

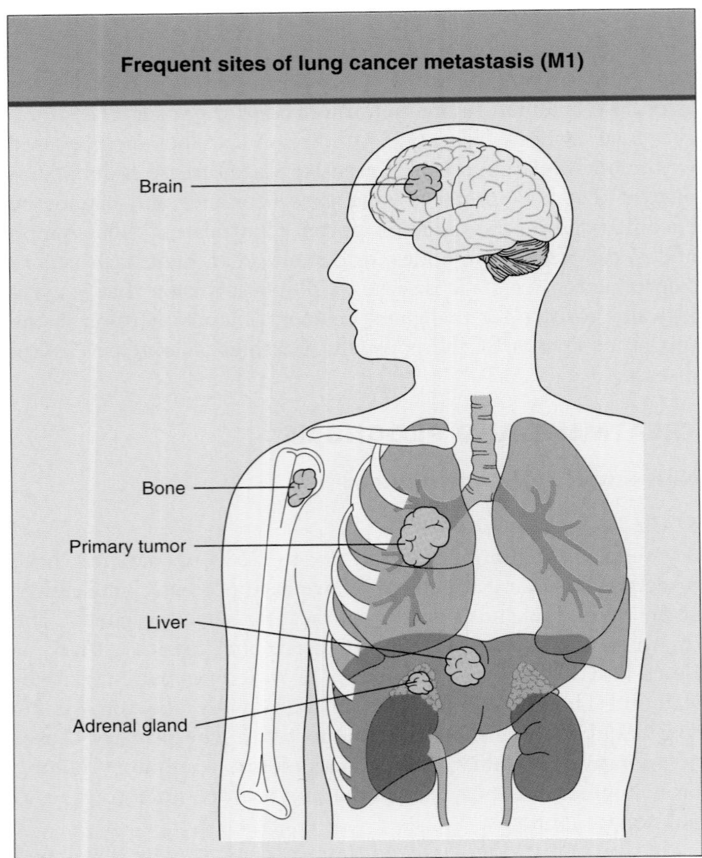

Figure 41.26 Metastases (M) in lung cancer staging.

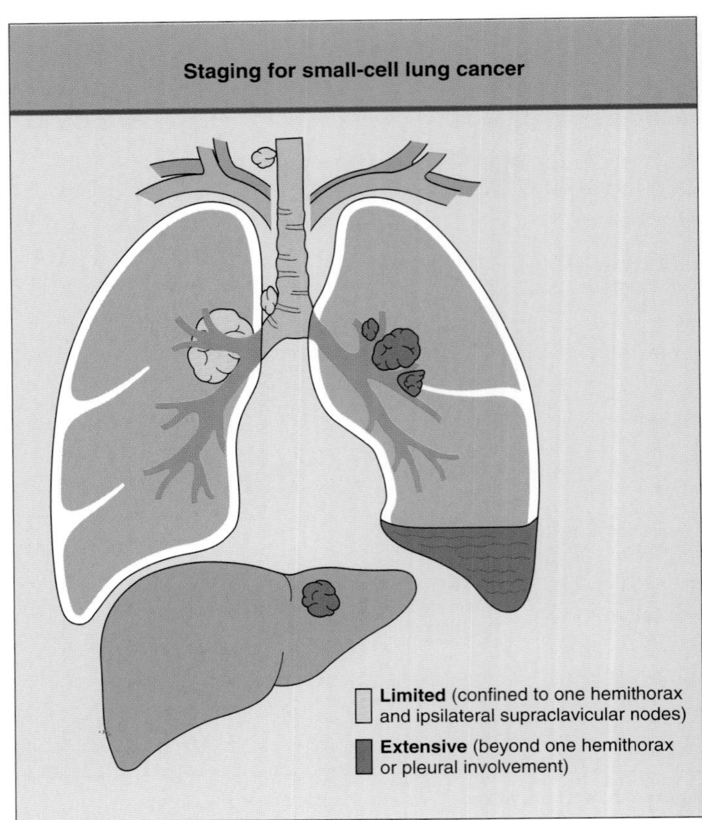

Figure 41.27 Staging classification for small-cell lung cancer.

nodules, but has not been accepted as standard treatment for lung cancer. A prospective trial by the Lung Cancer Study Group in North America randomized patients with lesions 3 cm in diameter or smaller to resection by lobectomy or a more limited resection (segmentectomy or wedge)—all patients underwent thoracotomy. Patients who had limited resection suffered three times as many local recurrences compared with those who underwent lobectomy. The survival difference was of borderline significance (P = .08, one-sided) in favor of lobectomy. Based on this trial and other reports in the literature, lobectomy is considered the surgical procedure of choice for lung cancer if it yields an adequate resection and the patient has sufficient pulmonary function to tolerate it. Ideally, lung cancer surgery is accompanied by sampling of lymph nodes from three or four different mediastinal stations (see Fig. 41.25). Failure to biopsy mediastinal lymph nodes results in suboptimal staging, which impedes adequate staging and decision-making as to the need for additional therapy. In the twenty-first century, no patient should have lung cancer surgery without mediastinal lymph node sampling. Many surgeons advocate radical lymph node resection rather than just nodal sampling.

The 5-year survival for stage IA lung cancer is 70% to 80%; for stage IB, it is 50% to 60% in different series (Fig. 41.28). For patients who have stage IIA disease, the 5-year survival is 40% to 55% and survival for stage IIB is approximately 40%. Stage IIB includes the patient who has a T3N0M0 lesion caused by chest wall involvement. The better prognosis of this group of patients prompted their reclassification as stage IIB in the 1997 revision of the staging system, and they are best treated by surgical resection. From 40% to 60% of patients who have stage IB, IIA, or IIB NSCLC suffer recurrences within the first 5 years of surgical resection. Postoperative thoracic radiotherapy has not improved survival in these patients. Recently a large randomized trial from Europe demonstrated a 5% absolute survival advantage at 5 years in patients with totally resected stage I, II, and IIA disease who received three to four cycles of adjuvant cisplatin–based chemotherapy versus those who received no chemotherapy. Current trials are evaluating preoperative chemotherapy followed by surgical resection, but the results are too preliminary to make any conclusions other than that this approach be considered investigational at this time.

STAGES IIIA AND IIIB

The presence of metastasis to an ipsilateral mediastinal lymph node (N2) establishes stage IIIA disease and was generally considered to be inoperable disease, but N2 lymph node involvement is no longer an absolute contraindication to surgery. In two recent randomized, prospective trials of carefully selected stage IIIA patients, patients were treated with preoperative chemotherapy followed by surgical resection or surgery alone. Both of these small, randomized trials showed highly statistically and clinically significant differences in survival in favor of the preoperative chemotherapy followed by surgical resection. Numerous other phase II trials employed neoadjuvant therapy (preoperative treatment) with two or three cycles of systemic chemotherapy with or without thoracic radiotherapy prior to surgical resection. Most of these trials enrolled stage IIIA

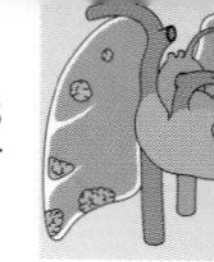

Table 41.4
The TNM (primary tumor, regional lymph nodes, and distant metastasis) lung cancer staging descriptions. (From Mountain CF: Revisions in the international system for staging lung cancer. Chest 111:1710-1717, 1997.)

Aspect	Descriptor	Description
Primary tumor (T)	TX	Primary tumor cannot be assessed, or tumor is proved by the presence of malignant cells in sputum or bronchial washings but not visualized by imaging or bronchoscopy
	T0	No evidence of primary tumor
	Tis	Carcinoma *in situ*
	T1	Tumor ≤3cm in greatest dimension, surrounded by lung or visceral pleura, without bronchoscopic evidence of invasion more proximal than the lobar bronchus (i.e., not in the main bronchus); the uncommon superficial tumor of any size with its invasive component limited to the bronchial wall, which may extend proximal to the main bronchus, is also classified T1
	T2	Tumor with any of the following features of size or extent: >3cm in greatest dimension Involves main bronchus, ≥2cm distal to the carina Invades the visceral pleura Associated with atelectasis or obstructive pneumonitis that extends to the hilar region, but does not involve the entire lung
	T3	Tumor of any size that directly invades any of the following: chest wall (including superior sulcus tumors), diaphragm, mediastinal pleura, parietal pericardium Tumor in the main bronchus <2cm distal to the carina, but with no involvement of the carina Associated atelectasis or obstructive pneumonitis of the entire lung
	T4	Tumor of any size that invades any of the following: mediastinum, heart, great vessels, trachea, esophagus, vertebral body, carina Tumor with a malignant pleural or pericardial effusion, or with satellite tumor nodule(s) within the ipsilateral primary tumor lobe of the lung
Regional lymph nodes (N)	NX	Regional lymph nodes cannot be assessed
	N0	No regional lymph node metastasis
	N1	Metastasis to ipsilateral peribronchial and/or ipsilateral hilar lymph nodes, and intrapulmonary nodes involved by direct extension of the primary tumor
	N2	Metastasis to ipsilateral mediastinal and/or subcarinal lymph node(s)
	N3	Metastasis to contralateral mediastinal, contralateral hilar, ipsilateral or contralateral scalene, or supraclavicular lymph node(s)
Distant metastasis (M)	MX	Presence of distant metastasis cannot be assessed
	M0	No distant metastasis
	M1	Distant metastasis present; (separate metastatic tumor nodule(s) in the ipsilateral nonprimary tumor lobe(s) of the lung also are classified M1)

Table 41.5
The TNM (primary tumor, regional lymph nodes, and distant metastasis) lung cancer stage groupings (From Mountain CF, Dresler CM: Regional lymph node clasification for lung cancer staging. Chest 111:1718-1723, 1997.)

Stage	TNM subset
0	Carcinoma *in situ*
IA	T1N0M0
IB	T2N0M0
IIA	T1N1M0
IIB	T2N1M0 T3N0M0
IIIA	T3N1M0 T1N2M0 T2N2M0 T3N2M0
IIIB	T4N0M0; T4N1M0 T4N2M0 T1N3M0; T2N3M0 T3N3M0; T4N3M0
IV	Any T; Any N; M1

patients, but some included carefully selected stage IIIB patients. The 3-year survival in these trials was generally 25% to 35%. The potential negative aspects of the neoadjuvant approach in advanced stage disease are a higher rate of pneumonectomy and a 10% to 15% treatment-related mortality rate. Recently, investigators completed a randomized phase III trial that compared the neoadjuvant treatment followed by surgery versus treatment with chemotherapy and thoracic radiation without surgery. An early report did not show any difference in survival between the two approaches, but maturation of the data will show a more definitive answer.

Pancoast tumors or superior sulcus tumors are usually stage IIB, IIIA, or IIIB. Unresectable Pancoast tumors have been treated with thoracic radiotherapy alone, but, more recently, a combination of chemotherapy and concurrent thoracic radiation was shown to be superior to thoracic radiotherapy alone for lung cancer. When potentially resectable, Pancoast tumors have been treated using preoperative radiotherapy of 30 to 50 Gy (3000 to 5000 rads), followed by surgical resection. Higher doses of preoperative radiotherapy increase postoperative complications. The 5-year survival of Pancoast tumors treated using radiotherapy and surgical resection is 25% to 35%. Based on a recent multicenter trial, concurrent chemoradiotherapy following surgical resection has become standard treatment for resectable cases.

In patients who have unresectable stage IIIA or IIIB NSCLC, thoracic radiotherapy alone has been the standard treatment. The 5-year survival using radiotherapy alone is 3% to 5%; 70% of treatment failures occur within the field of radiation and a 50% to 70% rate of distant metastasis occurs within the first 2 years. Accordingly, investigators conducted randomized trials of thoracic radiotherapy alone versus combination chemotherapy and thoracic radiotherapy. Using cisplatin-based chemotherapy, a number of multicenter trials demonstrated the superiority of combined modality therapy. Results are most favorable in patients who have better performance status and minimal weight loss. Meta-analyses of these trials show an approximate

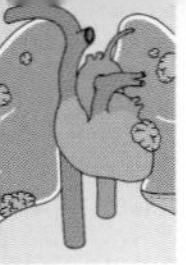

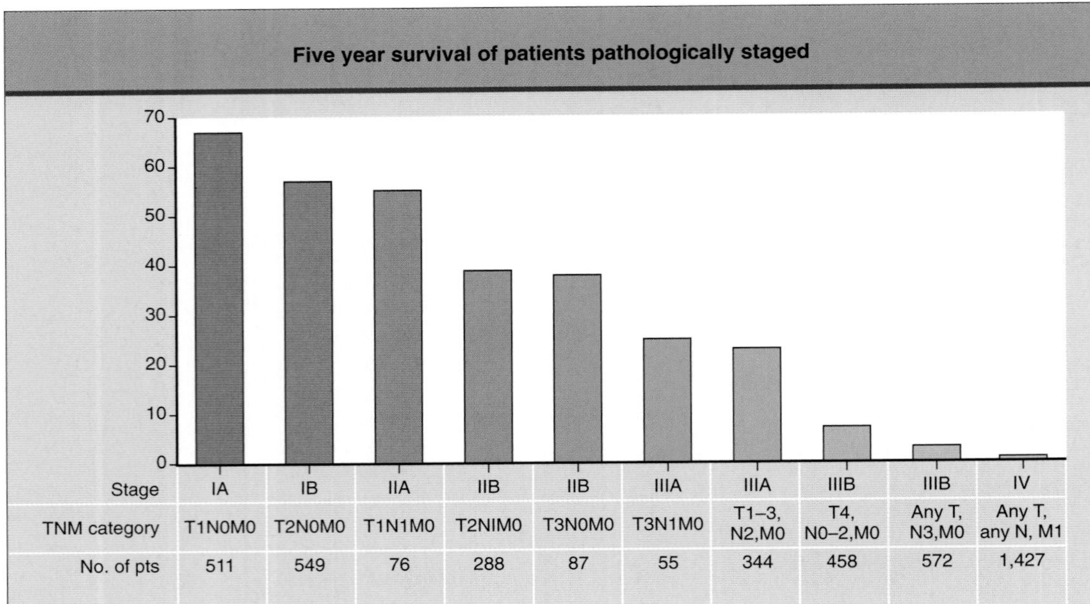

Stage	IA	IB	IIA	IIB	IIB	IIIA	IIIA	IIIB	IIIB	IV
TNM category	T1NOMO	T2NOMO	T1N1MO	T2NIMO	T3NOMO	T3N1MO	T1–3, N2,MO	T4, NO–2,MO	Any T, N3,MO	Any T, any N, M1
No. of pts	511	549	76	288	87	55	344	458	572	1,427

Figure 41.28 Prognosis in non–small-cell lung cancer. (From Mountain CF: Revisions in the international system for staging lung cancer. Chest 111:1710-1717, 1997.)

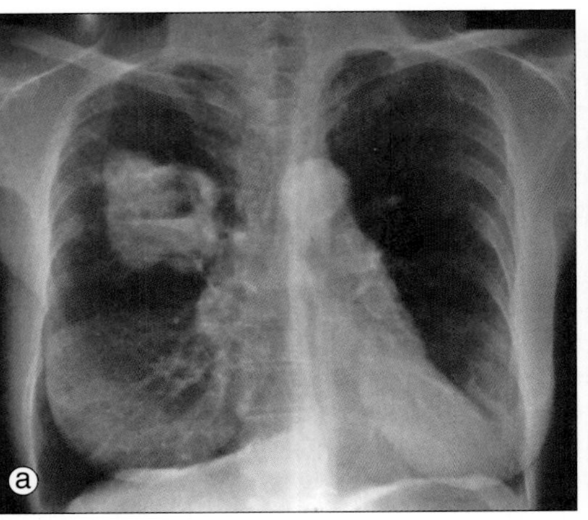

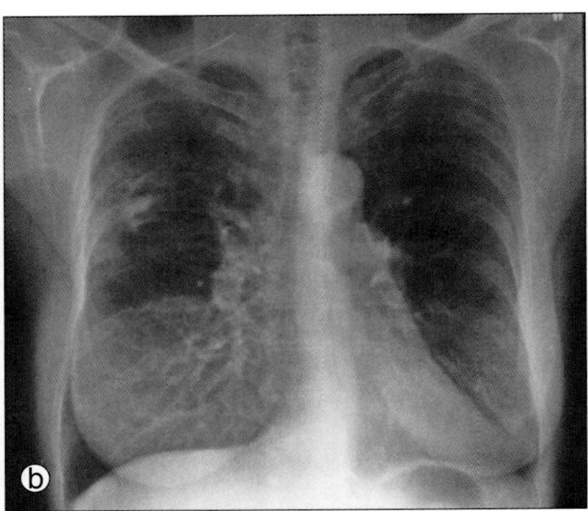

Figure 41.29 Response to chemotherapy in stage IIIB lung cancer. **A,** Chest radiograph showing a cavitary squamous cell carcinoma of the right lung. The patient had mediastinal lymph node involvement. **B,** Chest radiograph showing tumor regression following four cycles of chemotherapy with paclitaxel and carboplatin.

10% absolute superiority in survival at 3 to 5 years using combination chemoradiotherapy. One of the North American Cooperative Groups reported a 7-year follow-up of their trial. The 5-year survival was 6% for radiotherapy alone versus 17% for the combined modality therapy. In the United States alone, this improvement in survival translates into a saving of 4000 to 6000 additional lives per year. The current recommended treatment for unresectable stage IIIA or IIIB NSCLC is combination chemotherapy and thoracic radiation if the patient is physically fit enough to tolerate this approach.

Radiotherapy alone may be indicated in the more debilitated patient. The most commonly employed treatment schedule of radiotherapy when it is being given for curative intent is 60 to 65 Gy (6000 to 6500 rads) given in single daily fractions. Recent trials have evaluated the role of concurrent chemoradiotherapy versus sequential therapy and have demonstrated superior results with concurrent therapy. Trials evaluating multiple daily fractions of thoracic radiotherapy with concurrent chemotherapy have not demonstrated superior survival to the once-daily fractions of radiotherapy with concurrent chemotherapy. Concurrent chemoradiotherapy is associated with modest increases in esophagitis and not likely to be tolerated in patients with poor performance scores. The chemotherapy is platinum bases, but no one regimen has been proven to be superior.

STAGE IV

Approximately 50% of all patients who have NSCLC have distant metastasis (M1) at the time of initial diagnosis. No curative treatment is available for these individuals. The goal of therapy is to try to control their disease and palliate symptoms. Major response rates (more than 50% tumor shrinkage) of 20% to 30% have been reported with numerous combination chemotherapy regimens in patients who have this stage of disease. Almost all responses to treatment are partial; complete clinical remission is achieved in less than 5% of patients (Fig. 41.29). Patients who respond to chemotherapy gain, on the average, an additional 6 to 9 months of life, but eventually relapse and die of their disease. The median survival time for stage IV NSCLC is 3 to 4 months, with a 1-year survival of approximately 15%.

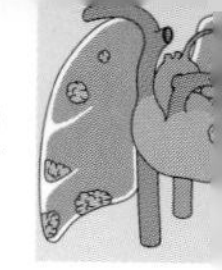

As a result of the toxicity and lack of curative therapy, therapeutic nihilism has been prevalent among physicians responsible for the care of these patients. A recent meta-analysis evaluated eight trials that enrolled more than 700 patients and each of the trials randomized patients to best supportive care versus chemotherapy using a cisplatin-based regimen. This analysis showed a benefit in survival to patients treated with chemotherapy. A reduction in the risk of death of 27% and an absolute improvement in survival of 10% at 1 year occurred in the chemotherapy-treated group. In the 1990s, a number of promising new chemotherapeutic agents were developed and used in patients who had stage IV NSCLC. These agents include paclitaxel, docetaxel, irinotecan, vinorelbine, and gemcitabine. Numerous phase III trials have been completed evaluating platinum bases combinations (cisplatin or carboplatin) with these newer chemotherapy agents. No one platinum doublet of chemotherapy has been shown to be superior. However, using platinum bases doublets, the median survival time is 8 to 9 months, and the 1-year survival is 30% to 35%. The results have been consistent in North America, Europe, and Japan.

Patients who are going to respond to systemic chemotherapy generally do so after the first two to three cycles of therapy. Randomized clinical trials have demonstrated that there is no advantage to treatment beyond four to six cycles of chemotherapy. Accordingly, it is reasonable to offer patients initial treatment with systemic chemotherapy and to treat for a maximum of four to six cycles, as long as no evidence of disease progression occurs. After the initial therapy, it is reasonable to observe until the patients develop progressive disease. When progressive disease is evident, the risks and benefits of additional therapy using alternative agents need to be weighed. Docetaxel has been shown to prolong survival in patients who have failed initial therapy. In 2003, gefitinib (Iressa) was approved in the United States for third-line therapy of patients with NSCLC. Whenever possible, patients who have stage IV NSCLC should be treated on prospective clinical trials. These studies offer the patient the optimal chance of benefit and add to the scientific knowledge about the role of new therapies. No progress can be made without enrolling patients onto prospective clinical trials.

Quality of life (QOL) is difficult to evaluate and quantify. A number of questionnaires have been developed as QOL tools for cancer, including the Functional Living Index-Cancer Instrument, Functional Assessment of Cancer Therapy, and the Quality of Life Index. A positive correlation occurs between the baseline QOL score and survival in lung cancer patients. Trials have shown that patients who maintain or improve their QOL scores, based on serial measurements, have superior survival to those whose QOL scores decrease. To date, no trials have shown serial QOL measurements in randomized trials of treatment versus supportive care only in patients who have advanced-stage lung cancer. In general, QOL decreases as the disease progresses even without any associated toxicity from chemotherapy. Numerous trials using chemotherapy have documented improvement of disease-related symptoms in those patients who achieve a disease regression as well as in some patients who show no evidence of an objective tumor response. Improvement in symptoms such as cough, dyspnea, or pain undoubtedly results in improvement in the patient's QOL.

BRONCHOSCOPIC TREATMENT

In addition to its role in the diagnosis and staging of lung cancer, bronchoscopy is used to treat lung cancer in the form of photodynamic therapy (PDT), laser therapy, brachytherapy, and implantation of airway stents.

Of these, PDT is appropriate for superficial NSCLC, and the other bronchoscopic interventions may be applied to either NSCLC or SCLC. In PDT, photosensitivity is used to form toxic oxygen radicals, which results in cancer cell death. After peripheral injection of hematoporphyrin derivatives, photosensitization is achieved by exposure to an argon-pumped dye laser carried by an optical fiber through the working channel of the flexible bronchoscope. Light energy is absorbed by the photosensitizer and produces cytotoxic tissue effects that are apparent over the next 6 to 48 hours. The patient may expectorate the necrotic tissue. Only cancers within the reach of the flexible bronchoscope and those that do not penetrate more than 4 to 5 mm into the bronchial wall have been treated effectively by PDT. Superficial squamous cell carcinomas that are radiographically occult appear to be most appropriate for this form of therapy. Studies to date include patients who are not surgical candidates for reasons other than tumor stage, as well as some patients who have potentially resectable tumors. After one or two PDT applications, 70% to 80% of patients achieve complete response rates with subsequent recurrence rates of 10% to 15%. Generally, surgical excision is still deemed most appropriate for those lesions that are surgically resectable. However, early, superficial squamous cell carcinomas may be managed successfully using bronchoscopic PDT alone if they are smaller than 3 cm in surface area, are in situ, or have only a few millimeters of microinvasion and are located within the reach of the flexible bronchoscope.

Various lasers have been used for palliative resection of endobronchial tumors, through both rigid and flexible bronchoscopes. The greatest clinical experience for this purpose is with the neodymium:yttrium aluminum garnet (Nd:YAG) laser, though lasers of other wave lengths are applied. Tissue effects from laser application include both photocoagulation and thermal necrosis. Initial experience with the Nd:YAG laser was at a power of 90 W, which occasionally resulted in significant hemorrhage and death. Subsequent use has reduced complications by employing power in the range of 30 to 40 W with pulses of 0.5 to 1.0 seconds. Appropriate patients for consideration of Nd:YAG laser endobronchial malignant resection include those who are unresponsive to other treatment modalities, have lesions that involve the bronchial wall but do not obviously extend through the cartilage, have an identifiable bronchial lumen, and show evidence of functioning lung tissue beyond the level of the endobronchial obstruction. The success of Nd:YAG laser treatment is greatest in proximal lesions of the trachea and main stem bronchi, because these are most easily accessible and provide the opportunity to regain the largest quantities of distal lung function. Palliation of symptoms is often immediate, though temporary, and median survival after laser resection is approximately 6 months. Survival improvement has been shown only in patients who undergo emergency Nd:YAG laser therapy when compared with similar patients who receive only external beam radiation.

Brachytherapy provides a means of intraluminal application of radiation in patients who have previously received maximal

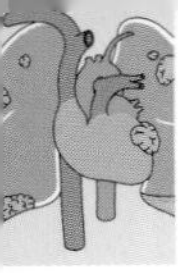

doses of external beam radiation. Brachytherapy is appropriate for both intrinsic and extrinsic malignant airway obstruction when functioning lung may be maintained or regained by achieving airway patency. Radiation applications of low- and high-dose rate have been used successfully. The radiation is applied through a nylon catheter placed through the lesion endoscopically. Response rates range from 30% to 80%, with success more likely in those patients who had favorable response to previous external beam radiation. Median survival after brachytherapy is in the range of 4 months. Hemorrhage or fistula formations are the most frequent complications and occur in approximately 15% of patients.

Bronchoscopic placement of prosthetic airway stents has become popular for palliation of both intrinsic and extrinsic malignant obstruction. The largest international experience has been with a silastic stent, though metal stents, and combinations of metal and silastic, as well as other, materials are being used for stent composition. Stent insertion may be accomplished using either the rigid or flexible bronchoscope, depending on the composition and delivery method of the prosthesis. Symptomatic improvement from regaining airway patency may be immediate and impressive. An attractive feature of the silastic stent is that it can be removed. Complications with the silastic stents include migration, mucus obstruction, and granulation tissue formation. The metal stents become incorporated into the bronchial wall and may be irretrievable or removed with great difficulty, and the formation of granulation tissue is more prevalent. Malignant growth may occur through the wall of the uncoated metal stents, or proximal or distal to either type of stent.

Small-cell Lung Cancer

Approximately 15% to 20% of all lung cancer is SCLC. This cell type has the strongest association with cigarette smoking, and SCLC is rarely observed in an individual who has never smoked. Accordingly, if this diagnosis is made in an individual who has never smoked or has a minimal smoking history, a careful pathologic review should be undertaken to consider alternative diagnosis such as bronchial carcinoid tumor or lymphoma. This histologic type of cancer contains neuroendocrine granules identified by electron microscopy and is the cell type most commonly associated with ectopic hormone production and also is associated with many of the paraneoplastic syndromes.

LIMITED-STAGE SCLC

Approximately one third of patients who have SCLC have limited stage disease at diagnosis. Limited stage is highly responsive to treatment, with 80% to 90% response rates to conventional therapy. A complete clinical remission is obtained in 50% to 60% of limited stage patients. The median survival time varies from 18 to 20 months in recent trials, with 2-year survival rates of 30% to 40% and 5-year survival of 15% to 25%.

Role of Surgery

Before the discovery of chemotherapeutic agents active against SCLC, surgery was employed against this malignancy. The 5-year survival after surgery only was 1% to 2%. A randomized trial by the British Medical Research Council evaluated surgery versus thoracic radiotherapy alone for limited-stage disease and noted a median survival time of 199 days with surgical treatment versus 300 days with radiotherapy. This report, along with the discovery of active chemotherapeutic agents, resulted in the abandonment of surgical treatment for SCLC in the 1960s.

In the past decade, the role of surgery for very limited SCLC has been reexamined. Reports of highly selected, nonrandomized trials noted 5-year survival rates of 25% to 35% after surgical resection of SCLC that presented as a solitary nodule. The Lung Cancer Study Group in the United States has evaluated the role of surgery in a randomized prospective trial of patients who had limited stage SCLCs. All patients received five cycles of cyclophosphamide, doxorubicin, and vincristine (CAV). Patients who show at least a partial response were randomized to either thoracotomy and resection or no surgery. All patients received identical thoracic radiotherapy. Survival rates on the two arms were identical (P = .91), which proved no survival advantage in treating the usual patient with limited-stage SCLC surgically.

The substantial 5-year survival rates after surgery in patients who have SCLC that presented as a pulmonary nodule indicate that it is advisable to treat these patients with surgical resection after appropriate staging to rule out distant metastasis. Occasionally, nodules diagnosed as SCLC after transthoracic needle aspiration or bronchoscopic biopsy are reclassified as a carcinoid tumor after resection. Patients who have SCLC that is completely resected should be treated with four cycles of adjuvant standard chemotherapy and thoracic radiotherapy. Preoperative evaluation of a peripheral SCLC should include magnetic resonance imaging of the brain or CT scan of the head with contrast, CT scan of the chest and upper abdomen, and PET scan or isotope bone scan to rule out distant metastasis. Ideally, such patients should undergo mediastinoscopy, and the lymph nodes should be negative for metastasis before proceeding to resection. Of all SCLC patients, less than 5% present as a peripheral nodule.

Chemotherapy and Radiation

In the 1970s, the treatment of choice was CAV chemotherapy. Subsequent randomized trials have shown similar survival, but less toxicity, using cisplatin and etoposide. The most common treatment regimens now are etoposide and cisplatin or etoposide and carboplatin. These regimens yield similar response rates and survival. The etoposide and carboplatin regimen is generally well tolerated, has been associated with less toxicity, and can be used in elderly patients.

Randomized trials in patients who have limited-stage disease compared chemotherapy alone versus combination chemotherapy and thoracic radiotherapy. A meta-analysis of 13 randomized trials that included more than 2000 patients showed that combined modality therapy resulted in a 14% decrease in the risk of death. The benefit in terms of absolute survival at 3 years was 5.4%. Accordingly, combined modality therapy with chemotherapy and thoracic radiation is considered standard for limited-stage SCLC.

The timing of thoracic radiotherapy is unclear. In a randomized trial from Canada, patients who received thoracic radio-

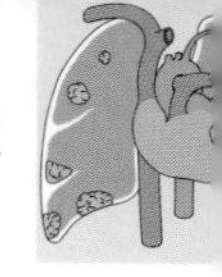

therapy with cycle two of chemotherapy had a significantly better survival rate than those who received the radiotherapy with cycle six. The authors concluded that early radiotherapy was superior to delayed radiotherapy. At this time, it is generally thought that radiotherapy should be given earlier in the treatment course rather than later. Trials with concurrent chemotherapy and thoracic radiation have resulted in superior survival versus sequential therapy, and are now the standard of care in North America.

The best treatment approach for limited-stage SCLC is combined chemotherapy using etoposide and cisplatin or etoposide and carboplatin and concurrent radiotherapy with radiotherapy being administered early in the treatment program. With this approach, 50% to 60% of patients achieve a complete remission with 2-year and 5-year survivals of 40% and 20% to 25%, respectively. Unfortunately, 70% of the complete remissions relapse within 2 years. Second-line therapies for relapse SCLC yield only modest results.

There have been only modest improvements in survival for SCLC patients in the past 20 years. First, the beneficial role of thoracic radiotherapy in addition to chemotherapy has been substantiated. Second, concurrent chemotherapy and thoracic radiotherapy for limited-stage disease has resulted in improved survival as compared with sequential therapy. Third, the number of chemotherapy cycles has decreased to 4 to 6 cycles (from the previous treatment using 12 or more cycles). Randomized trials showed that additional chemotherapy beyond four to six cycles does not improve long-term survival, but adds to toxicity of the treatment. The proliferation of new treatments with novel mechanisms of action is the hope of the future.

EXTENSIVE-STAGE SMALL-CELL LUNG CANCER

Two thirds of all SCLC patients have extensive-stage disease at diagnosis. Their response to chemotherapy is 60% to 80%, with a median survival time of 9 to 10 months and a 2-year survival of less than 10%. Virtually no patients survive for 5 years (see Figs. 41.21A and B).

Approximately 20% of patients experience a complete clinical remission with treatment. The chemotherapeutic agents used are identical to those used for limited-stage disease. Virtually identical response rates and survival rates have been observed with regimens of etoposide and cisplatin; etoposide and carboplatin; etoposide, ifosfamide, and cisplatin; or cyclophosphamide, doxorubicin, and etoposide. Despite the high initial response rates using standard chemotherapy, the dismal 2-year survival rates emphasize the need to develop new active agents against this disease. Some of the cooperative oncology groups treat patients who have extensive-stage SCLC on phase II trials using promising new agents. In these trials, the major end point is response rate. The design of the trials allows for a rapid crossover of nonresponding or progressive-disease patients to standard therapy using the agents mentioned previously. This approach has not resulted in a significant survival disadvantage compared with initial treatment with standard chemotherapeutic regimens. Two newer agents for SCLC are paclitaxel and topotecan. Both of these agents showed good single-agent activity in previously untreated patients who had SCLC. The combination of paclitaxel and topotecan has yielded response rates and survival similar, but not superior, to standard chemotherapy.

Relapse

The median survival of SCLC patients after relapse from prior therapy is 3 to 4 months. No cures have occurred using second-line therapy. The chance of responding to second-line therapy is worse if the patient has not responded to first-line therapy with a platinum-containing agent, or if the relapse interval is less than 90 days since the prior therapy. If the patient's first-line therapy did not include a platinum-based regimen, the patient should be treated with etoposide and cisplatin or etoposide and carboplatin, in which case the chance of response to second-line therapy is 50% or greater. If patients show a good response to first-line therapy and have been in remission for 6 months or longer, it is reasonable to retreat them with the same chemotherapeutic agents that they received initially; the chance of response again is 50% or greater.

If patients relapse within 6 months of therapy using a platinum-based regimen or if they fail to respond to initial therapy, second-line treatment decisions are more difficult. Response rates to second-line CAV have generally been poor and are 25% or less. Early studies reported response rates of 25% to 35% for single-agent topotecan or paclitaxel in relapse SCLC. The chance of responding to these agents as second-line therapy is increased significantly if the patients responded to initial therapy and if they have been off this prior therapy for 3 months or longer. As no standard second-line therapy is established for SCLC, these patients should, whenever possible, be enrolled in prospective clinical trials to evaluate new therapies.

CLINICAL COURSE AND PREVENTION

Among patients who have lung cancer, the overall 5-year survival is 14%. Taking this into account, the clinical course of most patients who have lung cancer is unpleasantly predictable. The best efforts of the physician, surgeon, and medical and radiation oncologist uncommonly result in cure or a greatly prolonged survival. The two most important prognostic factors are tumor stage and performance scores. Resected stage IA NSCLC has a 5-year survival of approximately 70% compared with 10% for stage I tumors in patients who are not surgical candidates because of medical problems or refusal to undergo surgery. Long-term survival in patients at various stages of lung cancer detected in the absence of symptoms is 35% versus 10% among those detected in the presence of symptoms. To identify patients in the preclinical phase of lung cancer is desirable, but a clearly effective screening tool has not been identified. Younger patients and those who have squamous cell type carry a better prognosis among those patients who have operable disease. The prognosis is poor for patients who have NSCLC beyond surgical resectability and in those who suffer SCLC.

After resection and possible cure for any stage of disease, the risk of developing a second primary lung cancer is 2% to 3% per year. Accordingly, patients are followed at intervals of 3 to 4 months for the first 2 years after treatment for the development of recurrent disease. Most lung cancers recur within the first 2 years. After this, patients are followed every 6 to 12 months for the possible development of late recurrence or a new primary lung cancer. No specific follow-up protocol has been shown to be effective in improving survival. In addition, no adjuvant therapy has proved to prolong survival after curative resection, but studies are under way.

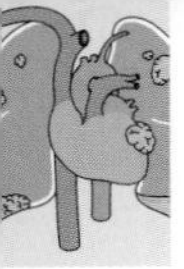

Functional status has been shown to be an important predictor of survival. The Karnofsky Performance Status assesses activity and ability for self-care on a scale from 100 to 0. A performance status 70 or less (one who is unable to work or pursue normal activities, but who lives at home and carries out self-care) is recognized as an independent predictor of shortened survival. Other performance status scales are in use and have shown the ability to predict survival. These measures help to both focus the estimation of prognosis and determine when treatment is appropriate in advanced stage disease.

Weight loss of more than 10% of body weight and male sex are also independent predictors of shortened survival among patients who have unresectable disease. Poor prognosis is also associated with the presence of distant metastasis to liver, bone, and brain, as is an elevated lactate dehydrogenase level. Within a single stage of lung cancer, considerable discrepancies arise in survival between patients, which suggests that other biologic factors are involved in prognosis. Research into cancer biology has identified a number of markers that may play a role in tumor behavior but, at this point, the role is unclear.

Recurrence or progression of disease occurs in the vast majority of patients who have lung cancer, which eventually results in death. Patients who suffer squamous cell carcinoma have a higher rate of local failure and a lower rate of distant metastasis when compared with those who have adenocarcinoma or large-cell carcinoma. Patients who suffer small-cell carcinoma have a higher rate of distant spread, and approximately 25% die of local tumor complications and the remainder show evidence of carcinomatosis. An investigation of terminally ill patients who had lung cancer gave insight into the role of palliative care. In one series hyperalimentation was administered in 90% of the patients, oxygen therapy in 78%, and morphine in 40%. The most frequent cause of death was respiratory failure caused by progression of cancer followed by infection and effusions of the pleura or pericardium. Hospice care can extremely effectively ensure the patient receives adequate pain control and other palliative measures, while it allows the patient to reside at home. Autopsy series show that approximately one half of patients who have cancer of various cell types have brain metastasis at the time of their demise.

Lung cancer remains a highly preventable disease, because approximately 85% of lung cancers occur in smokers or former smokers, and so primary prevention remains the avoidance of the cigarette. Efforts at early detection and treatment should not diminish the energy devoted to help patients quit smoking. Smoking rates have fallen in the United States and are showing signs of diminishing elsewhere in the world. Unfortunately, cigarette smoking is highly addictive, and smoking cessation often proves difficult. Physicians may be important motivators to help patients quit smoking. A 3-minute interview session with a physician can lead to a 5% success rate in smoking cessation when combined with antismoking reading materials and a follow-up visit. Use of supplemental nicotine, group therapy, behavioral training, hypnosis, or acupuncture achieves 1-year abstinence rates of around 20% in controlled trials. A sustained-release form of the antidepressant bupropion showed cessation rates of 44% after 7 weeks of treatment and 23% at 1-year follow-up in a placebo controlled trial. Interestingly, the mean weight gain among patients was 1.5 kg compared with 2.9 kg in the control group (P = .02) at the end of 7 weeks of therapy. Clearly, primary prevention by avoidance of smoking or through smoking cessation is the best way to prevent the devastating grip of this disease. Home radon testing may also play a role in reducing an individual's risk for lung cancer.

OTHER LUNG NEOPLASMS AND LUNG METASTASES

Carcinoid Tumor

Bronchial carcinoid tumors are low-grade malignant neoplasms comprising neuroendocrine cells and account for 1% to 2% of all tumors of the lung. Patients may present with hemoptysis, have evidence of bronchial obstruction, or be asymptomatic (Fig. 41.30). The association of carcinoid syndrome with bronchial carcinoid tumor is rare, as is ectopic production of adrenocorticotropic hormone and Cushing syndrome. Because carcinoid tumors are often endobronchial, bronchoscopy is an effective means to establish a diagnosis, but this is a relatively vascular tumor so caution in sampling is appropriate. Surgical resection is often curative, and in the absence of nodal metastasis, 10-year survival is greater than 90% for typical carcinoids. Prognosis is lessened in tumors larger than 3 cm or in the presence of nodal metastasis.

When histologic evidence of increased mitotic activity, nuclear pleomorphism, and disorganization is present, lesions are designated as atypical carcinoids, which tend to have a higher rate of metastasis and be larger at the time of diagnosis than typical carcinoid tumors. The 5-year survival with atypical carcinoid tumors is approximately 60% to 70%, and surgical treatment is desired when feasible.

Pulmonary Lymphoma

Primary pulmonary lymphomas account for less than 1% of all lung cancer and are uniformly non-Hodgkin's lymphomas. In one series of 33 patients, 22 patients had small-cell lymphoma, 6 had large-cell lymphoma, and 5 had mixed-cell lymphoma. In these patients treated with surgery, surgery plus chemotherapy, or chemotherapy alone, 5-year survival was 77%. Surgical resection of a localized, primary non-Hodgkin's lymphoma may be

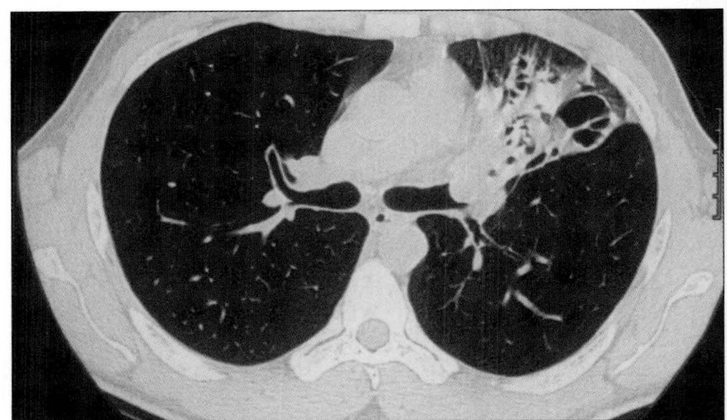

Figure 41.30 Carcinoid tumor. Computed tomography of the chest in a 34-year-old man with a 1-year history of recurrent left upper-lobe pneumonia and hemoptysis. Tumor obstructs the left upper-lobe bronchus with associated focal bronchiectasis. Bronchoscopy and subsequent resection revealed carcinoid tumor.

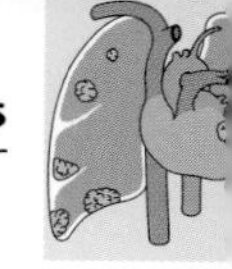

curative, and chemotherapy appears effective in patients who have bilateral or disseminated disease.

Mucoepidermoid Carcinomas

Mucoepidermoid carcinoma is another rare airway neoplasm derived from minor salivary gland tissue in the proximal tracheobronchial tree. As a result of the central airway location, patients usually present with cough, hemoptysis, or obstructive pneumonia. Surgical resection remains the treatment of choice when feasible, and complete resection portends an excellent prognosis. Lesions of low-grade histology are uncommonly associated with nodal metastases.

Adenoid Cystic Carcinoma

Adenoid cystic carcinoma is the most common salivary gland-like tumor to occur in the lower respiratory tract and accounts for less than 1% of all primary lung cancers. Adenoid cystic carcinomas usually arise in the lower trachea, main stem, or lobar bronchi and are rarely peripheral. Presenting symptoms are usually cough, hemoptysis, or evidence of airway obstruction. Surgical resection is preferred; however, this cell type has a propensity to recur locally and metastasize and is often incompletely resected. Delayed recurrence as long as 15 to 20 years after initial resection has been reported.

Hamartoma

Hamartomas are the most common benign neoplasm to occur in the lung. Histologically, the lesions consist of a combination of cartilage, connective tissue, smooth muscle, fat, and respiratory epithelium. Most hamartomas are detected when patients are asymptomatic, and the highest incidence is in the sixth or seventh decade. A series of 215 patients reported that only 4 patients had symptoms related to the hamartoma. The classic radiographic appearance of popcorn-ball calcification occurs in only about 25% of hamartomas. Approximately 15% show evidence of fat on thin-section CT scanning (Fig. 41.31). Radiographic recognition allows for simple observation in most instances; radiographically indeterminate lesions may be resected for confirmation. Multiple pulmonary hamartomas have been reported rarely.

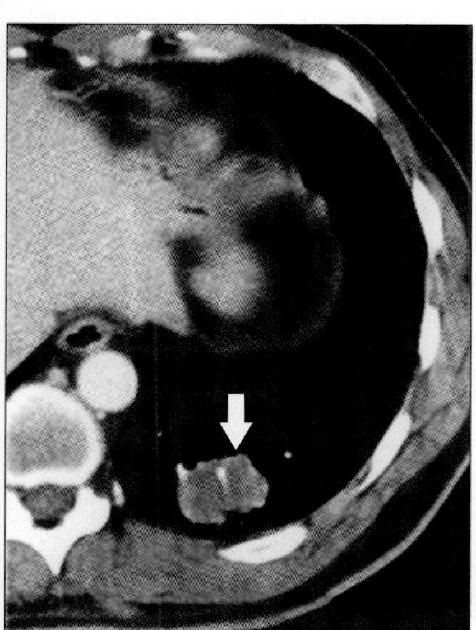

Figure 41.31 Hamartoma. Thin-section computed tomography through this solitary pulmonary nodule reveals evidence of calcification and fat consistent (*arrow*) with a hamartoma.

Lung Metastases

The lung is a frequent site of metastasis from a variety of extrathoracic malignancies. Carcinomas recognized as frequent sources for pulmonary metastases include those of the head and neck, colon, kidney, breast, and thyroid, and melanoma. Approximately 10% to 30% of all malignant nodules resected are metastases. In addition to solitary or multiple nodules, metastatic patterns include lymphangitic, endobronchial, pleural, and embolic. The finding of multiple or innumerable nodules is the most common clinical situation (Fig. 41.32). Depending on the size and location of the nodules, a diagnosis may be obtained by transthoracic needle aspiration or bronchoscopy. Surgical resection may be appropriate in the setting of a solitary pulmonary metastasis when evidence of other sites of metastatic disease have been excluded. Although randomized studies have not been performed, some evidence suggests improved survival in some patients who have solitary pulmonary metastasis from sarcomas, renal cell carcinoma, breast cancer, and colon cancer.

PITFALLS AND CONTROVERSIES

Screening for Lung Cancer

Chest radiography or sputum cytology to screen for lung cancer has not proved to reduce mortality; however, it is unclear whether or not the use of such screening has been disproved. In the 1970s, the National Cancer Institute sponsored three large, randomized trials. Participants were men age 45 years or older who had smoked one pack of cigarettes per day or more within the year before enrollment. The Mayo Lung Project randomized patients to a chest radiograph and 3-day pooled sputum cytology every 4 months in the screened group, and the control group was advised to have an annual chest radiograph and sputum cytology, but had no scheduled follow-up. Johns Hopkins and Memorial Sloan-Kettering were the other two participating centers, and both randomized patients to a dual screen with an annual chest radiograph and 3-day pooled sputum cytology every 4 months versus an annual chest radiograph. None of these trials demonstrated a decrease in lung cancer mortality in the screened group, but none of the three centers had an untested control group. In each, the 5-year survival from lung cancer in the screened group was approximately 35%, which is more than

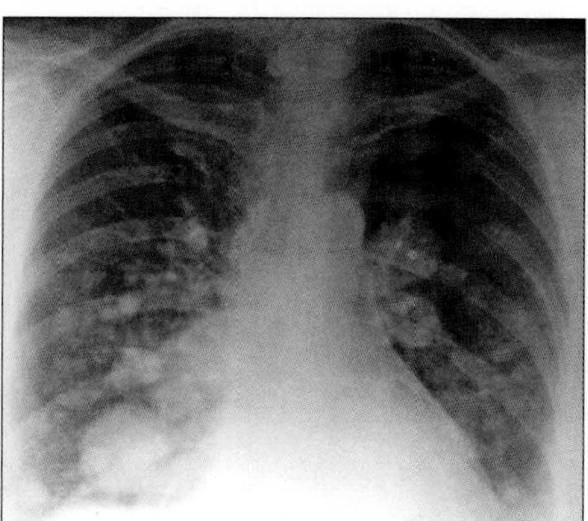

Figure 41.32 Pulmonary metastases. Chest radiograph of a 64-year-old woman showing innumerable nodules from metastatic adenocarcinoma of the thyroid.

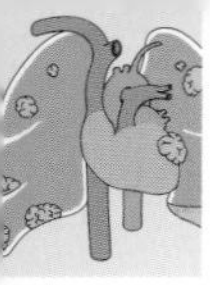

double the historical precedent. Mortality remains the only measure free of bias; however, in the absence of a no-screen control group in the studies, the question remains unanswered.

Computed Tomography Screening

The most sensitive image modality currently available for detecting pulmonary nodules is CT. Conventional chest CT requires radiation dosage and image-acquisition time that is impractical for screening purposes. The development of low-dose, fast-spiral CT greatly reduced the radiation dose and the scan time, making screening feasible. Conventional CT images are obtained at 140 to 300 milliamperes (mA) and are performed over many minutes using multiple breath holds. In contrast, low-dose, fast-spiral CT images may be obtained at 20 to 50 mA and the entire scan completed in 15 seconds during a single breath hold.

Initial studies from Japan created excitement in suggesting the viability of low-dose spiral CT as a tool for early lung cancer detection. The first report in the compared low-dose spiral CT scanning with chest radiography in screening a high-risk population for lung cancer. CT detected 15 cases of peripheral lung cancer; 11 of these were missed on chest radiography. An amazing 93% of the non–small-cell carcinomas identified were stage IA. In the United States, CT screening efforts were led by the Early Lung Cancer Action Project. Enrollment included 1000 current or former smokers age 60 years or greater and screened with low-dose spiral CT and chest x-ray CT detected a total of 27 prevalence lung cancers; 23 of the 27 (85%) malignancies were surgical stage IA. A total of 559 noncalcified nodules were detected in 233 participants (23%). In the Mayo CT Screening study, 1520 participants age 50 years or greater who were current or former smokers of more than 20 pack-years were enrolled and screened within 1 year. Baseline scanning revealed one or more noncalcified nodules in 51% of the participants. Results of baseline and 1- and 2-year follow-up scanning revealed 60% of NSCLC cases detected were stage 1A. The high rate of nodule detection (false-positive scans) in these studies raises concern.

Single-arm studies suggest that low-dose spiral CT has the potential to shift identification of a lung cancer to stage I or II from a more advanced stage. A shift in stage at diagnosis would be an anticipated finding of a screening tool that expected to reduce mortality. A randomized controlled trial of CT screening versus chest radiograph is currently under way in the United States.

Evaluation of the Solitary Nodule

The optimal evaluation of an SPN is unclear (see Fig. 41.20). Nodules that are indeterminate after radiographic investigations call for a decision between observation, biopsy, or removal. Newer radiologic techniques will, hopefully, ease the decision making and reduce the incision making. Contrast-enhanced CT, PET, and magnetic resonance imaging are useful to identify malignancy in the setting of an SPN. A multicenter study has reported that CT enhancement has a sensitivity of 98% and a specificity of 73% in the identification of malignant neoplasms. The test involves the administration of conventional, iodinated contrast material at a specific rate with thin-section CT assessments through the nodule at 1-minute intervals (Fig. 41.33). Malignant neoplasms enhance significantly more (more than 15 Hounsfield units) than do granulomas and benign neoplasms. The overall accuracy of 93% establishes CT contrast enhancement as a valuable tool in the evaluation of indeterminate SPNs. PET scanning with ^{18}F-fluorodeoxyglucose identifies malignant lesions with a sensitivity of 95% to 100% and a specificity of 80% to 89%. PET is becoming more widely available and provides additional staging information.

Treatment: Stage IIIA

One important area that is unclear is the most appropriate treatment for stage IIIA NSCLC. The literature strongly suggests that surgery alone or radiotherapy alone is not an optimal treatment. If the patient has a negative mediastinoscopy or CT scan of the chest for adenopathy and is found to have stage IIIA disease at the time of thoracotomy, consideration should be given to postoperative therapy. A recent trial of adjuvant chemotherapy with cisplatin-based treatment demonstrated an absolute 5-year survival advantage of 5% versus no adjuvant treatment. With surgery alone the 5-year survival is approximately 25%. In patients who are not operative candidates, the combination of concurrent chemotherapy and radiotherapy has been shown to be superior in those of good performance status and minimal weight loss.

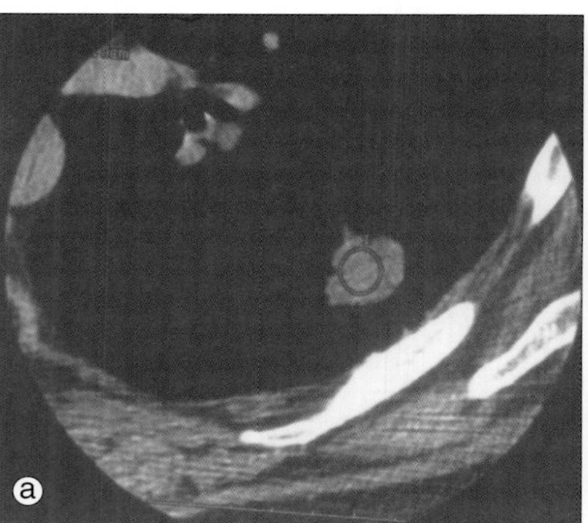

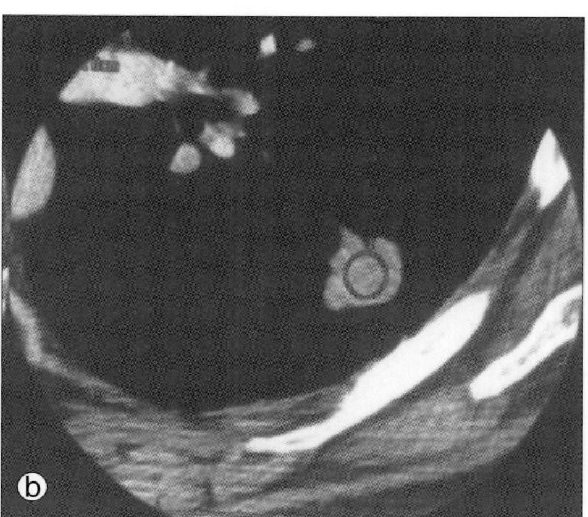

Figure 41.33 Evaluation of a solitary pulmonary nodule with computed tomography (CT) contrast enhancement. **A,** Before contrast injection. **B,** After injection of contrast according to protocol, CT scanning is carried out at 1-minute intervals and shows an increase in nodule density of 63 Hounsfield units (HU). Enhancement by >15 HU indicates a higher likelihood of malignancy. Resection revealed stage IA (T1N0M0) NSCLC.

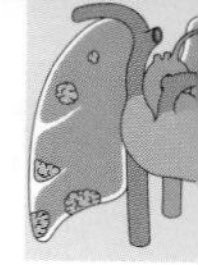

Prophylactic Cranial Irradiation: Small-cell Lung Cancer

Randomized trials have clearly documented that prophylactic cranial irradiation (PCI) reduces the rate of brain metastasis in patients who have SCLC. A large meta-analysis of PCI versus no PCI has shown a significant survival advantage with PCI. Ataxia, difficulty with concentration, memory problems, and dementia are occasionally observed in patients treated with cranial irradiation. Recent trials have employed lower dose and fraction regimens, and preliminary reports have not noted any significant detrimental neurologic sequelae. Most medical and radiation oncologists now recommend PCI for patients in complete remission. PCI is inappropriate for a patient who is not in complete clinical remission.

SUGGESTED READINGS

Alberg AJ, Samet JM: Epidemiology of lung cancer. Chest 123:21S-49S, 2003.

Anderson JE, Jorenby DE, Scott WJ, Fiore MC: Treating tobacco use and dependence: An evidence based clinical practice guideline for tobacco cessation. Chest 121:932-941, 2002.

Bach PB, Kelly MJ, Tate RC, McCrory DC: Screening for lung cancer: A review of the current literature. Chest 123:72S-82S, 2003.

Dewamena BA, Sonnad SS, Angobaldo JO, Wahl RL: Metastases from non-small cell lung cancer: Mediastinal staging in the 1990s meta-analytic comparison of PET and CT. Radiology 213:530-536, 1999.

Jemal A, Murray T, Samuels A, et al: Cancer statistics, 2003. Cancer J Clin 53:5-26, 2003.

Mao L: Recent advances in the molecular diagnosis of lung cancer. Oncogene 21:6960-6969, 2002.

Mountain CF: Revisions in the international system for staging lung cancer. Chest 111:1710-1717, 1997.

Schiller JH, Harrington D, Balance CP, et al: Comparison of four chemotherapy regimens for advanced non-small cell lung cancer. N Engl J Med 346:92-98, 2002.

Spiro SG, Porter JC: Lung cancer—where are we today? Current advances in staging and nonsurgical treatment. Am J Respir Crit Care Med 166:1166-1196, 2002.

Toloza EM, Harpole L, McCrory DC: Noninvasive staging of non-small cell lung cancer: A review of the current evidence. Chest 123:137S-146S, 2003.

CHAPTER 42 Approach to Diagnosis of Diffuse Lung Disease

Athol Wells

The term *diffuse lung disease* (DLD) covers infiltrative lung processes that involve the alveolar spaces or lung interstitium. This definition is fundamentally unsatisfactory because it groups together a wide variety of diverse disorders, some of which (such as cryptogenic organizing pneumonia) are not diffuse, strictly speaking, but patchy and sometimes limited in extent. Furthermore, many secondary infiltrative abnormalities, including bacterial infection and malignancy, are excluded, whereas others, such as pulmonary involvement in connective tissue disease, are retained in most DLD classifications. The DLDs are grouped for historical reasons; in early series, they presented most frequently with widespread clinical and chest radiographic abnormalities. However, with increasing clinician awareness of the possibility of DLD, the diagnosis is often made when chest radiographic findings are limited, or disease is apparent only on high-resolution computed tomography (HRCT).

The diagnostic difficulties resulting from the wide diversity of disorders contained within the DLDs are exacerbated by semantic confusion. Synonymous terms abound for some of the more frequently encountered DLDs, such as:

- Cryptogenic organizing pneumonia (bronchiolitis obliterans organizing pneumonia, proliferative bronchiolitis)
- Idiopathic pulmonary fibrosis ([IPF] cryptogenic fibrosing alveolitis)
- Hypersensitivity pneumonitis (extrinsic allergic alveolitis)

Moreover, in some disorders, such as hypersensitivity pneumonitis, the natural history and treated course are highly variable, ranging from self-limited inflammation to inexorably progressive fibrotic disease. In routine clinical practice, a simplified pragmatic approach to diagnosis is essential; consideration of a checklist of the more commonly encountered diseases is often useful. The classification of DLDs by their disease burden was addressed most definitively in a study from Bernalillo County, New Mexico, in which the incidence and prevalence of individual DLDs was quantified using a variety of methods (Table 42.1). New cases were estimated to occur in 32/100,000 person-years in men and 26/100,000 person-years in women; thus, although less common than lung infection, malignant disease, or obstructive airways disease, the DLDs are responsible for a considerable disease burden. Moreover, the workload for the pulmonary physician is disproportionate because the diagnosis of individual DLDs is often uncertain despite more intensive investigation than is usually required in obstructive airways disease or lung infection.

A consideration of the differential diagnosis of DLD, based on prevalence alone, is merely a starting point, for two reasons. First, clinical information at initial evaluation profoundly alters diagnostic probabilities; therefore, a lengthier checklist of the DLDs, based on the possible underlying cause, is indispensable. Second, the lengths to which a specific diagnosis is pursued, with particular reference to surgical biopsy, is critically dependent on the importance of discriminating between likely differential diagnoses in individual cases. This crucial point is discussed in detail in the concluding section of the chapter.

INITIAL CLINICAL EVALUATION

Even before chest radiography and HRCT findings are considered, a wealth of diagnostic information can be obtained from initial evaluation. A possible underlying cause is often apparent, although environmental and drug exposures occurring many years earlier and apparently limited exposures are difficult to interpret in isolation, in many cases. A great deal of information can often be obtained on the longitudinal behavior of disease from the evolution of symptoms, serial chest radiographic data, and, less frequently, serial spirometric volumes. The presence of associated systemic disease or prominent airway-centered symptoms may both provide essential diagnostic clues. Less frequently, physical examination may serve to broaden the differential diagnosis. In addition to chest radiography and HRCT (considered in separate sections), certain noninvasive ancillary tests should be performed in selected cases, including autoimmune serology, measurement of precipitins, and echocardiography.

Clinical History

The identification of an underlying cause is the single most important contribution made by clinical evaluation. A checklist of the more important causes of DLD is provided in Table 42.2. A careful occupational history is essential and should include details of all previous occupations, including short-term employment. Asbestos exposure is often extensive in railway rolling-stock construction workers, shipyard workers, power station construction and maintenance workers, naval boilermen, garage workers (working with brake lining), and other occupations in which asbestos exposure is obvious. In general, workers in these occupations are well aware of their asbestos exposure; however, other workers, including joiners, electricians, carpenters, and manual workers in the building trade who handle asbestos in the

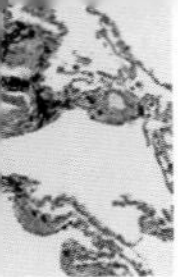

Table 42.1
Prevalence and incidence of interstitial lung diseases in Bernalillo County, New Mexico

Cause	Interstitial lung disease	Prevalent cases, n (%)	Incident cases, n (%)
Occupational and environmental	Pneumoconiosis	8 (3.1)	–
	Anthracosis	3 (1.1)	–
	Asbestosis	17 (6.6)	15 (7.4)
	Silicosis	8 (3.1)	6 (3.0)
	Hypersensitivity pneumonitis	–	3 (1.5)
Drug/radiation	Drug-induced interstitial lung disease	5 (1.9)	7 (3.5)
	Radiation fibrosis	1 (0.4)	3 (1.5)
Pulmonary hemorrhage syndromes	Goodpasture's syndrome	–	1 (0.5)
	Vasculitis	–	1 (0.5)
	Hemosiderosis	2 (0.8)	–
	Wegener's granulomatosis	2 (1.2)	6 (3.0)
Connective tissue disease	Mixed connective tissue disease	2 (0.8)	2 (1.0)
	Systemic lupus erythematosus	6 (2.3)	1 (0.5)
	Rheumatoid arthritis	14 (5.4)	10 (5.0)
	Scleroderma	9 (3.5)	3 (1.5)
	Sjögren's syndrome	–	1 (0.5)
	Dermatomyositis/polymyositis	2 (0.8)	1 (0.5)
	Ankylosing spondylitis	–	–
Pulmonary fibrosis	Pulmonary (chronic) Fibrosis/postinflammatory	43 (16.7)	28 (13.9)
	Idiopathic/interstitial fibrosis	58 (22.5)	63 (31.2)
	Interstitial pneumonitis	8 (3.1)	12 (5.9)
Sarcoidosis		30 (11.6)	16 (7.8)
Other	Alveolar proteinosis	1 (0.4)	–
	Amyloidosis	–	–
	Bronchiolitis obliterans	–	1 (0.5)
	Chronic eosinophilic pneumonia	3 (1.2)	1 (0.5)
	Eosinophilic (granuloma) infiltration	2 (0.8)	–
	Infectious/postinfectious interstitial lung disease	3 (1.2)	1 (0.5)
	Lymphocytic infiltrative lung disease	1 (0.4)	–
	Interstitial lung disease, not otherwise specified	29 (11.1)	20 (9.8)
Total		**258**	**202**

form of roofing and insulation material are often unaware of significant exposure. Other occupations associated with DLD include coal mining (coal worker's pneumoconiosis), metal polishing (hard-metal disease), and sandblasting (silicosis).

A careful history also discloses exposure to organic antigens known to cause hypersensitivity pneumonitis. The two most prevalent forms of hypersensitivity pneumonitis are farmer's lung (in which the offending antigen, thermophilic actinomycetes, is contained in moldy hay) and bird fancier's lung, in which avian proteins are inhaled by those breeding birds or, more commonly, those who keep birds as domestic pets. However, a wide range of other exposures also cause hypersensitivity pneumonitis, and particular attention should be paid to molds (often arising in sites of water damage); bathroom molds (as in "basement shower syndrome" and "hot-tub lung") are easily overlooked. Hobbies should also be considered (e.g., "cheese-maker's lung," "wine-maker's lung"). There are now over 100 known causes of hypersensitivity pneumonitis, and because it is unrealistic to hope to memorize these, an up-to-date list of the 50 more frequent causes of hypersensitivity pneumonitis, such as that provided by Bertorelli and colleagues, is highly useful.

Table 42.2
Frequently encountered diffuse lung diseases with identifiable underlying cause

Cause	Differential diagnosis	
Occupational or other inhalant-related, inorganic	Coal worker's pneumoconiosis	Metal polisher's lung/hard metal fibrosis
	Asbestosis	Berylliosis
	Silicosis	Baritosis (barium)
	Talc pneumoconiosis	Siderosis (iron oxide)
	Aluminum oxide fibrosis	Stannosis
Occupational or other inhalant-related, organic	Bird fancier's lung	Mushroom worker's lung
	Farmer's lung	Maple bark stripper's lung
	Bagassosis (sugar cane)	Malt worker's lung
	Coffee worker's lung	Tea grower's lung
	Tobacco grower's lung	Pituitary snuff-taker's lung
	Fishmeal worker's lung	
Collagen vascular disease related	Systemic lupus erythematosus	Ankylosing spondylitis
	Rheumatoid arthritis	Mixed connective tissue disease
	Scleroderma	Primary Sjögren's syndrome
	Polymyositis	Behçet's syndrome
	Dermatomyositis	Goodpasture's syndrome
Drug related	Amiodarone	Bleomycin
	Propranolol	Busulfan
	Tocainide	Cyclophosphamide
	Nitrofurantoin	Chlorambucil
	Sulfasalazine	Melphalan
	Cephalosporins	Methotrexate
	Gold	Azathioprine
	Penicillamine	Cytosine arabinoside
	Phenytoin	Carmustine
	Mitomycin	Lomustine
	Bromocryptine	
Physical agents/ toxins	Radiation/radiotherapy	Cocaine inhalation
	High concentration oxygen	Intravenous drug abuse
	Paraquat toxicity	
Neoplastic disease	Lymphangitis carcinomatosis	
	Bronchoalveolar cell carcinoma	
Vasculitis related	Wegener's granulomatosis	
	Giant cell arteritis	
	Churg–Strauss syndrome	
Disorders of circulation	Pulmonary edema	
	Pulmonary veno-occlusive disease	
Chronic infection	Tuberculosis	Viruses
	Aspergillosis	Parasites
	Histoplasmosis	
Smoking induced	Emphysema	Desquamative interstitial pneumonia
	Langerhans cell histiocytosis	Respiratory bronchiolitis
	Alveolar cell carcinoma	Non-specific interstitial pneumonia
	Respiratory bronchiolitis with associated interstitial lung disease	

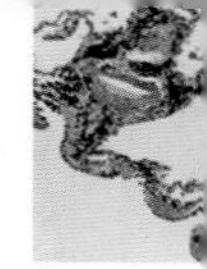

A detailed drug history is also essential. The drugs most frequently causing DLD are probably amiodarone, methotrexate (at doses used in connective tissue disease), and antineoplastic agents, especially bleomycin. However, a wide variety of other agents (over 100 at present) cause DLD, although often in only a small number of cases, and the list increases year by year. Fortunately, there is now an international Web site devoted to drug-induced lung disease (www.pneumotox.com), through which all medications should be routinely checked in patients with DLD. Other therapeutic modalities causing DLD include radiation therapy and exposure to high concentrations of oxygen (especially in those previously receiving bleomycin). Paraquat ingestion (causing acute or delayed proliferative bronchiolitis), inhalation of crack cocaine or heroin (causing eosinophilic pneumonia, diffuse alveolar hemorrhage, organizing pneumonia, or pulmonary edema), and intravenous drug abuse (causing veno-occlusive disease) are also relevant.

Smoking-related DLD is increasingly diagnosed; diseases other than chronic obstructive pulmonary disease that are caused by smoking include Langerhans cell histiocytosis, respiratory bronchiolitis–associated interstitial lung disease (RBILD), desquamative interstitial pneumonia, and nonspecific interstitial pneumonia (NSIP). Recently, HRCT evaluation has made it clear that all these processes may coexist in the same patient. Furthermore, both sarcoidosis and hypersensitivity pneumonitis are very rare in current smokers. Because RBILD and hypersensitivity pneumonitis often have overlapping clinical and HRCT features, the smoking history is an important discriminator between these two disorders.

A great deal of information on likely longitudinal behavior is often available. The distinction between acute and chronic disease is important because acute infection, heart failure, and disseminated malignancy may all simulate DLD clinically and radiologically. The duration of dyspnea and cough, pattern of symptomatic progression, and previous responsiveness (or non-responsiveness) to corticosteroid therapy may provide valuable diagnostic clues. Variable dyspnea and cough over a number of years, responding to steroid therapy, is compatible with hypersensitivity pneumonitis or sarcoidosis, whereas inexorably progressive dyspnea for 2 to 3 years, not responding to steroid therapy, is typical of IPF. A perusal of previous chest radiographs may be highly useful, with unchanging appearances over many years a frequent finding in sarcoidosis, but not in IPF. Previous detailed pulmonary function tests are seldom available, but serial spirometry is sometimes performed in general practice (because asthma is often suspected when the first symptoms of DLD occur); thus, it is sometimes possible to draw useful conclusions from the rapidity of decline (or, conversely, the duration of stability) of spirometric volumes.

Relevant systemic diseases associated with DLD include malignancy (lymphangitis carcinomatosis or multiple metastases) and connective tissue diseases complicated by DLD, especially rheumatoid arthritis, systemic sclerosis, systemic lupus erythematosus, polymyositis/dermatomyositis, and Sjögren's syndrome. Lung disease may precede systemic manifestations in all the connective tissue diseases (most frequently in polymyositis/dermatomyositis) or may develop concurrently with the onset of systemic manifestations. Thus, a full history should include details of arthritis/arthralgia, myositis, skin disorders, Raynaud's phenomenon, and dryness of the eyes or mouth. In a subgroup of patients with autoimmune disease who fail to meet formal criteria for an individual disorder and are considered to have "undifferentiated connective tissue disease," DLD may nonetheless develop.

Airway-centered symptoms may help to refine the differential diagnosis. Cough occurs frequently in IPF, but prominent wheeze is more suggestive of hypersensitivity pneumonitis or, less frequently, sarcoidosis. Wheeze is also an important feature of some of the pulmonary vasculitides, especially Churg-Strauss syndrome and, occasionally, Wegener's granulomatosis. Hemoptysis is the most frequent pulmonary symptom at presentation in Goodpasture's syndrome; however, the volume of hemoptysis is not a good guide to disease severity because hemoptysis may be trivial or even absent, despite considerable alveolar hemorrhage.

Clinical Examination

Physical examination tends to be less fruitful than the history and HRCT findings in refining the differential diagnosis of DLD. Bilateral, predominantly basal crackles on auscultation are a defining feature of IPF and are very frequent in other forms of idiopathic interstitial pneumonia and asbestosis, but are seldom present in sarcoidosis or hypersensitivity pneumonitis. Clubbing is a useful sign because it points strongly to IPF or asbestosis; clubbing is rare in sarcoidosis, hypersensitivity pneumonitis, and pulmonary fibrosis associated with connective tissue disease (with the exception of rheumatoid arthritis). However, no diagnostic conclusions can be drawn from the absence of clubbing. Mid to late inspiratory squawks, an under-recognized sign, are strongly indicative of an underlying bronchiolitic disorder, including hypersensitivity pneumonitis (in which the bronchiolitic component may be prominent). Central cyanosis, tachypnea, and pulmonary hypertension are nonspecific findings in end-stage DLD; however, when pulmonary hypertension is associated with limited DLD, underlying connective tissue disease (especially systemic sclerosis and systemic lupus erythematosus) should be suspected.

BLOOD TESTS

In most cases, specific diagnostic tests for DLD are confined to autoimmune serology and precipitins against organic antigens. Serologic evidence of rheumatoid arthritis and the other major connective tissue diseases should be sought in any patient with apparently idiopathic DLD, in whom the diagnosis is uncertain. This is particularly important when the diagnosis appears to be cryptogenic organizing pneumonia because underlying connective disease is frequent and, when present, the prognosis is not always good and prolonged treatment may be necessary. The antisynthetase syndrome is characterized by Jo1 antibody positivity, polymyositis, and progressive pulmonary fibrosis, and lung disease often precedes systemic manifestations. However, although antibodies to extractable nuclear antigens tend to be disease specific, antinuclear antibodies and rheumatoid factor levels are often moderately increased in IPF and are less useful diagnostically unless titers are markedly elevated. The presence of precipitins to organic antigens increases the likelihood of hypersensitivity pneumonitis but should never be considered in isolation. Positive precipitins denote exposure to an antigen, with immune recognition, but are not in themselves indicative

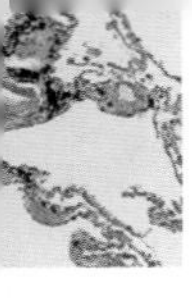

of clinically significant DLD; bird breeders often have avian precipitin positivity without overt lung disease. Moreover, in many patients with convincing exposure histories and a histologic diagnosis of hypersensitivity pneumonitis, the appropriate precipitins are not present; avian antigens, for example, vary between bird species and, to a lesser extent, between individual birds.

PULMONARY FUNCTION TESTS

Most DLDs are characterized by a restrictive ventilatory defect, a reduction in gas transfer, and variable hypoxia at rest or exercise. A pure obstructive defect is often present in Langerhans cell histiocytosis and lymphangioleiomyomatosis, and is sometimes a feature of fibrotic pulmonary sarcoidosis. A mixed ventilatory defect, which usually denotes an airway-centered component, is often present in hypersensitivity pneumonitis, sarcoidosis, and connective tissue disease (in which bronchiolitis or bronchiectasis may coexist with pulmonary fibrosis). Paradoxically normal lung volumes in association with severe reduction in gas transfer levels are the hallmark of the combination of emphysema and pulmonary fibrosis. The often-cited phenomenon of a marked increase in gas transfer (measured using single-breath techniques) due to diffuse alveolar hemorrhage is rarely clinically useful because this abnormality persists for only 36 hours after hemorrhage. The most diagnostically useful pulmonary function pattern is preservation of gas transfer in association with irreversible airflow obstruction, a combination that points strongly toward intrinsic airways disease (i.e., bronchiolitis) rather than emphysema. However, the delineation of the pattern of pulmonary function impairment seldom makes a major contribution to refining the differential diagnosis.

CHEST RADIOGRAPHY

With recent attention focused on the diagnostic value of HRCT, it is often forgotten that the plain chest radiograph provides invaluable information in DLD. Sometimes the chest radiograph points strongly toward a specific diagnosis. Sarcoidosis, the most prevalent DLD encountered in clinical practice, can be diagnosed with confidence in many cases from the clinical and chest radiographic features at presentation; HRCT seldom adds useful diagnostic information in this context.

Several chest radiographic features have useful positive predictive values for individual diseases. The presence of hilar lymphadenopathy on chest radiography is particularly strongly predictive of sarcoidosis in the correct clinical context, although the radiographic differential diagnosis includes tuberculosis and malignancy, especially when hilar lymphadenopathy is asymmetrical. Pleural effusions are a feature of connective tissue disease, lymphangioleiomyomatosis, and asbestos-related disease (as well as disease processes that sometimes mimic DLD, including heart failure, infection, and malignancy). The distribution of disease on chest radiography is also diagnostically useful; granulomatous diseases (tuberculosis, sarcoidosis, hypersensitivity pneumonitis) tend to be more prominent in the middle to upper zones, whereas fibrotic diseases (IPF, fibròtic NSIP, asbestosis) have a predominantly lower zone distribution.

However, apart from a large subgroup of patients with sarcoidosis, diagnoses based on chest radiography are seldom confident. Chest radiography is sometimes insensitive; in the often-quoted series of Epler and colleagues, 10% of patients with biopsy-proven DLD had normal chest radiographic appearances. The superior diagnostic accuracy of HRCT, compared with chest radiography, has been well documented, and the increased confidence associated with an HRCT diagnosis is a considerable aid to management. Moreover, although there is a long tradition of characterizing chest radiographic abnormalities as nodular, reticulonodular, or reticular, this provides relatively little diagnostic information. Predominantly basal honeycombing on chest radiography (which is invariably associated with honeycombing on HRCT) may be diagnostically useful in increasing the likelihood of IPF, but is radiographically obvious in surprisingly few patients with that disease. It is now generally accepted that, except in patients with obvious sarcoidosis, routine HRCT is almost always warranted in DLD, although occasional exceptions exist (e.g., elderly patients with obvious lower zone honeycombing on chest radiography, indicative of IPF; patients with long-standing pulmonary fibrosis on serial chest radiography and an obvious underlying cause, such as coal mining).

Two chest radiographic appearances pose particular diagnostic difficulties. *Persistent unexplained multifocal consolidation* has usually been treated unsuccessfully as for community-acquired pneumonia and has a wide differential diagnosis. Serial chest radiography tends to be more useful than HRCT in refining further investigation because the crucial diagnostic distinction lies between fixed infiltrates (nonbacterial infection including tuberculosis, alveolar cell carcinoma, and other malignant processes) and changing infiltrates in which these diagnoses are effectively excluded. However, immunologically mediated diseases (including eosinophilic pneumonia, cryptogenic organizing pneumonia, and vasculitic disorders) may give rise to either fixed or evanescent radiographic abnormalities, and a histologic diagnosis is often warranted. *Diffuse alveolar filling processes* giving rise to widespread airspace consolidation are usually indicative of life-threatening disease. Although this picture may represent DLD (e.g., acute interstitial pneumonitis, acute eosinophilic syndromes, drug-induced pulmonary infiltration), it is essential to broaden the differential diagnosis beyond DLD to include diffuse pulmonary infection, toxic inhalation, severe aspiration, opportunistic infection (especially *Pneumocystis* pneumonia), diffuse alveolar hemorrhage syndromes, mitral stenosis, and, above all, heart failure. In both of these radiographic presentations, successful management often depends on consideration of a wide differential diagnosis from the outset.

HIGH-RESOLUTION COMPUTED TOMOGRAPHY

HRCT has been the most important diagnostic advance in DLD in the last two decades. Numerous studies have confirmed the overall diagnostic accuracy of HRCT against findings at surgical biopsy, with a striking increase in sensitivity and specificity for individual diseases, compared with chest radiography. However, academic series understate the impact of HRCT, for the most important benefit has been to increase clinician confidence in noninvasive diagnosis, with a corresponding reduction in the numbers of patients needing to undergo surgical biopsy. Before HRCT, diagnoses based on clinical data and chest radiographic findings were seldom confident and management was necessarily tentative in many cases. The combination of clinical and

HRCT information now provides a confident first-choice diagnosis in most patients, and in many other cases the realistic differential diagnosis is shortened to two or three disorders. This allows surgical biopsy to be reserved for cases in which the distinction between a small group of possible disorders has important management implications, and for occasional cases in which HRCT appearances are not suggestive of any single disorder. Thus, routine surgical biopsy, as a diagnostic gold standard, can no longer be justified in the HRCT era.

The question of histospecific diagnosis aside, HRCT plays an important role in identifying DLD in some contexts. The superior sensitivity of HRCT against chest radiography has been an invariable finding in a wide range of disorders. This feature of HRCT is particularly useful when symptoms or lung function impairment are associated with normal chest radiographic appearances and the indications for surgical biopsy are marginal. In connective tissue disease, pulmonary involvement is a leading source of mortality and early treatment of progressive lung disease is desirable; by identifying limited pulmonary fibrosis, HRCT allows clinicians to select patients in whom more intensive monitoring is required, even when immediate treatment is not warranted. In workers previously exposed to asbestos, HRCT often discloses pulmonary fibrosis, which is obscured on chest radiography by concurrent pleural disease. However, the sensitivity of HRCT occasionally creates its own difficulties. When interstitial abnormalities are limited, their clinical significance is sometimes difficult to rationalize; disease that is evident only on HRCT should not be extrapolated, in terms of natural history and management, to the more extensive disease described in historical clinical series. It is essential that HRCT findings be integrated with other clinical and investigative features and not interpreted in isolation.

The distinction between predominantly inflammatory and predominantly fibrotic disease can usually be made with reasonable confidence from HRCT. Anatomic distortion and reticular abnormalities are strongly indicative of irreversible fibrotic disease and this is invariably true of honeycomb change (Fig. 42.1). Consolidation is usually reversible, although it may occasionally represent dense fibrosis, especially in sarcoidosis. Ground-glass attenuation is often more difficult to interpret. In early work, this HRCT sign was shown to identify a substantial increase in the likelihood of significant inflammation, especially in the absence of concurrent reticular abnormalities. However, it is now clear that ground-glass attenuation denotes fine fibrosis in many cases, and this is especially the case in NSIP, in which ground-glass attenuation is the cardinal HRCT feature (Fig. 42.2), and in sarcoidosis. Traction bronchiectasis is a key HRCT discriminator because it is invariably indicative of underlying fibrosis. Thus, reversible inflammatory disease is likely only when ground-glass attenuation is not associated with traction bronchiectasis or admixed with reticular abnormalities.

A wide range of HRCT profiles, encompassing the distribution and pattern of disease, is strongly suggestive of individual DLDs. The cardinal findings in the more commonly encountered DLDs are summarized in Table 42.3. As with all other applications of HRCT, it is essential that HRCT findings are integrated with the pretest diagnostic probability, distilled from the history, clinical signs, previous natural history or treated course, and investigative findings (especially chest radiography, pulmonary function tests, and serology for autoimmune disease and environmental antigens). In particular, the diagnostic interpretation of HRCT can usefully be considered separately for cases in which the likely etiology is apparent and for idiopathic disease. In patients with appropriate environmental antigen or drug exposures (hypersensitivity pneumonitis, pneumoconioses, drug-induced lung disease), malignant disease (lymphangitis carcinomatosis), clinical or serologic evidence of connective tissue disease, or a heavy smoking history (Langerhans cell histiocytosis, RBILD), the diagnostic weighting required from HRCT can be reduced. In these clinical contexts, compatible but not classic HRCT appearances often allow a sufficiently confident diagnosis to obviate diagnostic surgical biopsy. By contrast, HRCT is more frequently pivotal to diagnosis when disease is idiopathic, but in the absence of a high pretest clinical probability the diagnosis is seldom confident unless HRCT findings are typical.

In the diagnosis of idiopathic DLD, the use of HRCT can be summarized in a simple algorithm. The first step is to determine whether HRCT abnormalities are fibrotic or inflammatory, as discussed previously. If disease is fibrotic, as in a large majority of cases, the next important question is whether HRCT findings are typical of IPF. As stated in the recent American Thoracic Society/European Respiratory Society (ATS/ERS) recommendations, IPF can be diagnosed confidently on HRCT when there is honeycombing with little ground-glass attenuation in a predominantly basal and subpleural distribution. It is logical to focus on IPF because it is the most prevalent idiopathic fibrotic disease among cases in which the diagnosis is not obvious from clinical and chest radiographic findings. Most cases of sarcoidosis are diagnosed without recourse to HRCT (Fig. 42.3).

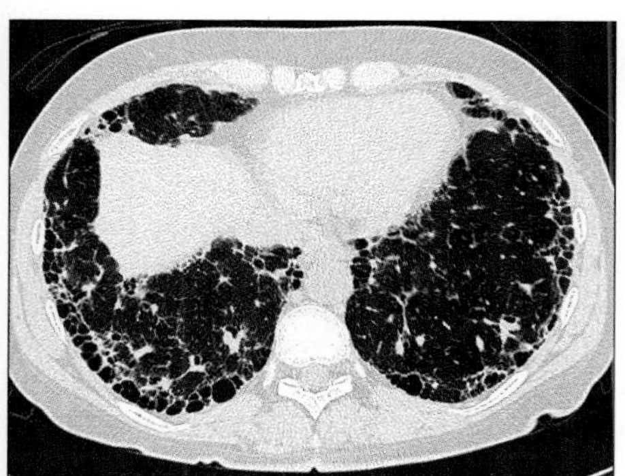

Figure 42.1 High-resolution computed tomography appearances in a patient with idiopathic pulmonary fibrosis (IPF). There is prominent subpleural honeycombing with no ground-glass attenuation. In the correct clinical context, this picture is virtually pathognomonic of IPF.

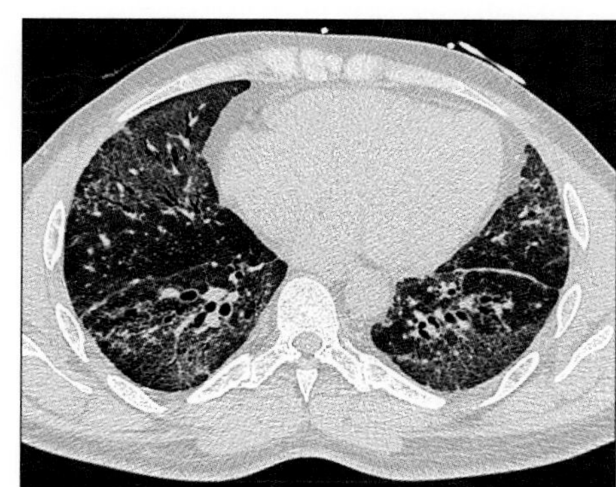

Figure 42.2 In a patient with nonspecific interstitial pneumonia, the predominant abnormalities on high-resolution computed tomography are ground-glass attenuation, with variable admixed fine reticular abnormalities, and traction bronchiectasis. Notably, there is no honeycomb change.

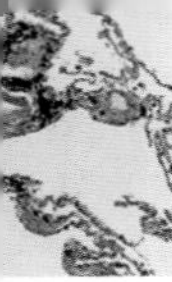

Table 42.3
High-Resolution Computed Tomography Features Recognized as Typical of Selected Diffuse Lung Diseases

Idiopathic pulmonary fibrosis: Lower zone, subpleural predominance, maximal posterobasally, predominantly reticular pattern with associated honeycombing.
Nonspecific interstitial pneumonia: Two frequent appearances. The variant that overlaps with idiopathic pulmonary fibrosis in disease distribution: ground-glass attenuation predominates, with a variable fine reticular component and traction bronchiectasis, but no honeycombing. The variant that overlaps with cryptogenic organizing pneumonia: consolidation with surrounding ground-glass attenuation and a variable fine reticular pattern.
Desquamative interstitial pneumonia: Ground-glass attenuation, sometimes diffuse, sometimes basal and peripheral centered, frequent associated fibrotic cysts with anatomic distortion and traction bronchiectasis.
Acute interstitial pneumonia: Widespread ground-glass attenuation admixed with features of fibrosis, usually with airspace consolidation, and occasional emphysema.
Respiratory bronchiolitis—interstitial lung disease: Patchy ground-glass attenuation, poorly defined centrilobular nodules, occasional mosaic attenuation, prominent bronchial wall thickening.
Sarcoidosis: Highly variable. Nodules distributed along bronchovascular bundles, interlobular septa, and subpleurally including the fissure; ground-glass attenuation that may represent either inflammation or fine fibrosis; reticular abnormalities, representing fibrosis; distortion most commonly occurring in upper zones with posterior displacement of the upper lobe bronchus; air trapping; associated hilar and mediastinal lymphadenopathy.
Subacute hypersensitivity pneumonitis: Widespread ground-glass attenuation, often containing poorly defined centrilobular nodules, admixed with areas of black lung (mosaic attenuation), representing air trapping and enhanced on expiratory high-resolution computed tomography.
Cryptogenic organizing pneumonia: Bilateral patchy consolidation, subpleural and predominantly basal in the majority, occasional peribronchial distribution, associated often sparse nodules up to 1 cm in diameter.
Constrictive bronchiolitis: Patchy areas of hyperlucency enhanced on expiration, which may not change in cross-sectional diameter on full expiration; associated bronchiectasis and bronchial wall thickening.
Langerhans cell histiocytosis: Bizarre cyst shapes and associated nodules throughout the lung fields but sparing the costophrenic angles and tips of the lingula and middle lobes. Associated emphysema common.
Pulmonary lymphangioleiomyomatosis: Homogeneously distributed, thin-walled parenchymal cysts, varying from a few millimeters to several centimeters in diameter; associated with retrocrural adenopathy, pleural effusion, thoracic duct dilatation, pericardial effusion, and pneumothorax.

Furthermore, IPF has a much worse prognosis than other fibrosing processes and is, therefore, the most important diagnosis to confirm or exclude from the outset. It is now known that HRCT appearances considered typical of IPF by experienced thoracic radiologists have a positive predictive value of over 95%. Based on their prevalence in clinical practice, the five most important differential diagnoses are IPF with atypical HRCT appearances, sarcoidosis, NSIP, hypersensitivity pneumonitis (with the antigen unknown), and the fibrotic sequelae of cryptogenic organizing pneumonia. Amongst these, IPF with atypical HRCT appearances is the most prevalent disorder in most populations: up to 30% of IPF cases have atypical HRCT features.

The weighting given to HRCT in the diagnosis of DLD varies from case to case but can usefully be considered in three categories. In some patients, HRCT appearances are virtually pathognomonic: This includes many cases of IPF, Langerhans cell histiocytosis, sarcoidosis, and lymphangitis carcinomatosis. Often, HRCT findings are diagnostic when combined with clinical information. A good example is the combination of widespread ground-glass attenuation (often with poorly defined

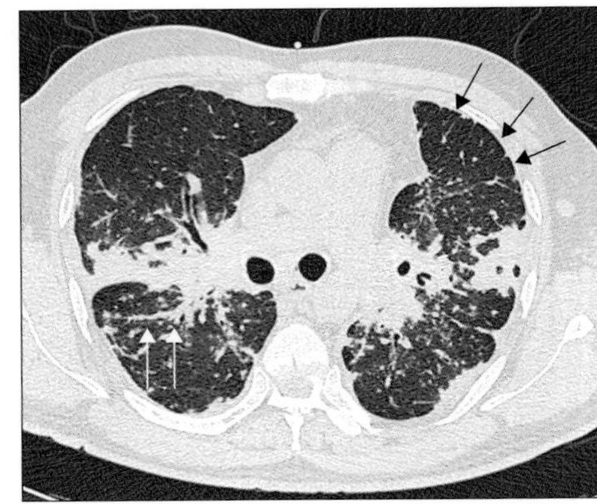

Figure 42.3 In this high-resolution computed tomography scan from a patient with sarcoidosis, abnormalities suggesting the diagnosis include multiple, well-defined nodules, surrounding bronchovascular beading (*white arrows*), micronodules (especially in the left anterior lung, indicated by *black arrows*), septal thickening (by granulomatous infiltration), and areas of dense consolidation which may be reversible (coalescence of granulomata) or irreversible (fibrosis). This combination of abnormalities is virtually pathognomonic of sarcoidosis.

centrilobular nodules) with mosaic attenuation, which may be strongly indicative of hypersensitivity pneumonitis in nonsmokers with a compatible exposure history, or of RBILD in current smokers (Fig. 42.4). Finally, even when not conclusive in its own right, HRCT may also be invaluable when considered in conjunction with diagnostic surgical biopsy. The histologic entity of NSIP is found in a variety of clinicoradiologic contexts, including an entity overlapping clinically with IPF, fibrosing organizing pneumonia, and hypersensitivity pneumonitis; HRCT evaluation is central to the distinction between these variants.

BRONCHOSCOPIC PROCEDURES

Although endobronchial and transbronchial biopsies are straightforward and relatively noninvasive procedures, the volume of tissue taken is small and only bronchial and peribronchial tissue is sampled. Thus, both procedures have a high yield in diseases that have a peribronchial distribution, especially sarcoidosis and lymphangitis carcinomatosis. Occasionally, transbronchial biopsy findings can help to cement a diagnosis of hypersensitivity pneumonitis, although bronchoalveolar lavage (BAL) tends to be more rewarding in this regard. Bronchoscopic biopsy procedures have little or no diagnostic value in the idiopathic interstitial pneumonias. Hemorrhage and pneumothorax (with transbronchial biopsy) are the important risks associated with bronchoscopic procedures. Major hemorrhage is rare, but pneumothoraces complicate transbronchial biopsies in 1% to 2% of procedures, although intercostal tube drainage is not always required.

In the 1980s, BAL was regarded by many as an important part of the diagnostic algorithm in DLD. The distinction between a BAL neutrophilia and a BAL lymphocytosis was considered to be particularly useful, with the former being strongly indicative of IPF, rather than hypersensitivity pneumonitis or sarcoidosis. However, as experience accumulated, it became apparent that conclusions drawn from BAL findings were robust when groups of patients with different diseases were compared, but that many exceptions occurred in individual cases. The

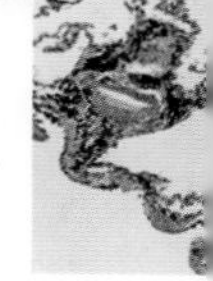

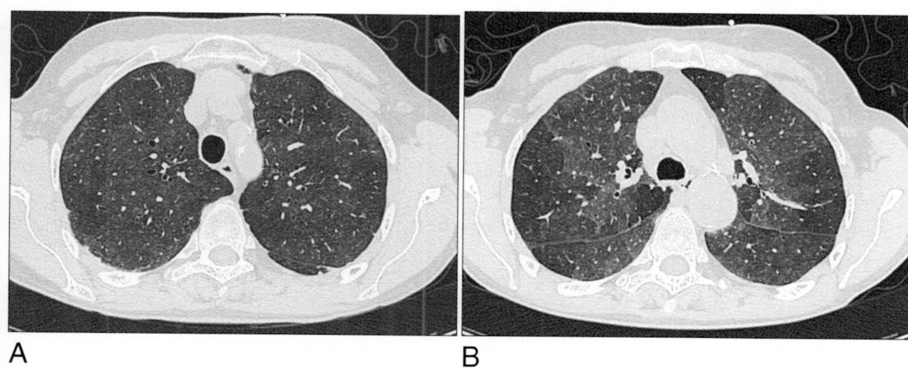

Figure 42.4 In hypersensitivity pneumonitis, abnormalities on inspiratory high-resolution computed tomography (HRCT), consisting of widespread ground-glass attenuation, often with poorly formed centrilobular nodules, are often extremely subtle and HRCT appearances may be virtually normal **(A)**. However, on expiratory HRCT **(B)**, striking regional variation in lung attenuation is often apparent, with areas of darker lung representing gas trapping (due to the bronchiolitic component of the disease).

advent of HRCT, with the wealth of additional diagnostic information that it provided, also limited the role of BAL, which had been more influential in the pre-HRCT era, when most noninvasive diagnoses were tentative.

There are currently no published evaluations of the diagnostic value added by BAL, once HRCT findings are taken into account. However, in the last 5 years, BAL has enjoyed a renaissance in some centers. In recent ATS/ERS recommendations, compatible BAL findings (i.e., no lymphocytosis) are a requirement for the noninvasive diagnosis of IPF; this criterion reflects the diagnostic value of BAL findings when HRCT appearances are suggestive of IPF but are not definitive. However, a BAL lymphocytosis has an even greater diagnostic impact in some patients with sarcoidosis or hypersensitivity pneumonitis; when significant fibrosis supervenes in these disorders, HRCT appearances often becomes atypical and IPF is frequently the preferred diagnosis before the performance of BAL. A BAL lymphocytosis in the setting of fibrotic DLD is sometimes an important justification for diagnostic surgical biopsy. Thus, BAL continues to play a useful diagnostic role in a significant subset of patients when clinical and HRCT features are inconclusive, although adding little to diagnosis in most DLD cases.

SURGICAL BIOPSY

Surgical biopsy, formerly performed as an open procedure but now obtained using video-assisted thoracoscopic surgery (VATS), was once regarded as the diagnostic gold standard and, until recently, its routine performance in DLD has been advocated by some authorities. However, routine surgical biopsy is impracticable outside referral centers, and in the 1980s, even before HRCT had a significant diagnostic impact, it was performed in less than 15% of patients with IPF in the United Kingdom. Even in referral centers, the performance of diagnostic surgical biopsies has been radically reduced with the application of HRCT. In one U.K. referral center (the Royal Brompton Hospital), biopsy was performed in over 50% of IPF cases in the 1980s but in less than 15% of IPF cases in the mid-1990s. Moreover, it is increasingly clear that open or VATS biopsy is not a true diagnostic gold standard. Variation between 10 thoracic pathologists in assigning a histologic diagnosis in DLD was recently found to be considerable, with agreement only moderate (kappa coefficient of agreement of 0.38). In over 20% of biopsies, the first-choice diagnosis was assigned with low confidence. Thus, although biopsy procedures add invaluable information in selected cases, there is never an absolute guarantee of a secure histologic diagnosis in an individual patient.

Sometimes, the histologic diagnosis appears to be at odds with clinical and HRCT information. In this situation, it is essential that histologic findings are not considered as a gold standard but are integrated with other information. In some patients with fibrotic hypersensitivity pneumonitis, a histologic pattern of usual interstitial pneumonia (which is normally indicative of IPF) is disclosed at biopsy, despite clinical, HRCT, and BAL features of hypersensitivity pneumonitis and an indolent course during follow-up. Similarly, in a cohort of over 100 patients with either IPF or fibrotic NSIP recently reported by Flaherty and colleagues, a combination of histologic and HRCT findings provided more accurate prognostic information than either modality in isolation. Thus, surgical biopsy is now best viewed, like HRCT, as a diagnostic "silver standard," and can often be avoided when HRCT and clinical features are typical of an individual DLD.

The morbidity and mortality associated with surgical biopsy in DLD are low in patients with an adequate pulmonary reserve but increase significantly in severe disease. In the series of Utz et al., patients with advanced IPF (with a mean gas transfer level of <35% of predicted) had a mortality rate ascribable to biopsy of 15%. Although this figure is usually regarded as an overstatement of the risk of the procedure, based on widespread anecdotal experience, a surgical biopsy should not be performed unless central to management if the gas transfer is less than 30% of predicted. Moreover, in advanced idiopathic fibrotic disease, the prognostic value of a histospecific diagnosis diminishes. In the recent series of Latsi and coworkers, mortality rates were identical in IPF and fibrotic NSIP when the gas transfer was less than 35%, despite major differences in survival in less severe disease.

Thus, in younger patients (<60 years) presenting with a typical clinical picture of severe IPF and HRCT features suggestive of fibrotic NSIP, immediate referral for consideration of lung transplantation is warranted without a histologic diagnosis. The exception is the patient presenting with overwhelmingly severe acute DLD, in whom the diagnosis is unclear and realistic differential diagnoses include acute interstitial pneumonia, severe infection (including opportunistic infection), and malignancy. Bronchoalveolar lavage may be required to exclude infection and occasionally a histologic diagnosis is required to rationalize management. Both procedures can be performed in ventilated patients, and if disease is slightly less severe, elective mechanical ventilation may be warranted to investigate appropriately.

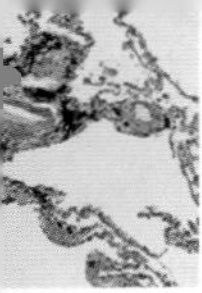

INTEGRATED DIAGNOSIS IN DIFFUSE LUNG DISEASE

The central diagnostic challenge for the clinician is to integrate the information discussed previously into a final diagnosis, without overemphasizing any single clinical or investigative feature in isolation. Indeed, only the clinician is able to play this role, for both histologic and HRCT diagnoses made without reference to other information are seriously flawed in a significant proportion of cases. The most difficult dilemma, when noninvasive evaluation discloses two or more realistic diagnoses, is whether to accept diagnostic uncertainty without investigating further or to resort to invasive (surgical biopsy) or semi-invasive (BAL, transbronchial biopsy) procedures.

This decision should be made pragmatically and not by protocol. The value of a specific diagnosis in DLD is that the clinician is informed of the probable natural history and the likelihood that treatment will play a useful role; from these considerations, the optimal approach to monitoring disease during follow-up will usually be apparent. Thus, the essential purpose of pursuing a diagnosis is to identify probable disease behavior with and without treatment. Broadly, with occasional exceptions, longitudinal disease behavior in DLD can be subdivided into the five patterns listed in Table 42.4. When an individual patient can be subclassified confidently into one of these groups, invasive investigation often adds little to short- and long-term management. Three strands of information are of particular value in making these distinctions: the underlying cause (if any), a morphologic assessment using HRCT (and histologic evaluation in selected cases), and observed longitudinal disease behavior.

The identification of an underlying cause is vital because it may, when considered in conjunction with HRCT appearances, allow disease to be classified confidently as self-limited inflammation (e.g., acute drug-induced lung disease, hypersensitivity pneumonitis, RBILD in smokers), with a good outcome provided that the offending agent is removed. In long-standing disease, knowledge of a cause often allows the clinician to classify fibrotic abnormalities on HRCT as stable fibrotic disease (e.g., the fibrotic sequelae of nitrofurantoin lung, silicosis, and other pneumoconioses); the confidence of this conclusion is increased by the documentation of stable longitudinal disease behavior based on previous chest radiographs, symptoms, and, occasionally, pulmonary function tests. In both self-limited inflammation and stable fibrotic disease, invasive diagnostic investigations are seldom warranted and potentially toxic treatments can usually be minimized.

A histologic diagnosis is required more frequently in apparently idiopathic disease to draw two essential distinctions: between inherently stable and potentially progressive fibrotic disease, and between major inflammation (with a high risk of evolution to fibrosis with undertreatment) and inexorably progressive fibrotic disease. In both scenarios, therapeutic intervention may be the key to a substantially better outcome. Knowledge of likely intrinsic disease behavior is invaluable because it allows decisive management and increases patient confidence considerably. A confident diagnosis of hypersensitivity pneumonitis, NSIP, or cryptogenic organizing pneumonia associated with significant fibrosis justifies aggressive intervention with a higher risk of drug toxicity because the treated outcome is often good. By contrast, in IPF, in which the benefits of treatment may be marginal, a more cautious therapeutic approach is often warranted, and in younger patients, the timing of consideration of transplantation can be rationalized. As a general principle, BAL or surgical biopsy should always be pursued in patients fit for these procedures (as judged by age, disease severity, and comorbidity) if a confident management

Table 42.4
The Most Frequent Patterns of Longitudinal Disease Behavior in Diffuse Lung Disease with Selected Examples of Underlying Diagnoses that May Appear in Several Categories*

Self-limited inflammation	Drug-induced lung disease (acute onset) Hypersensitivity pneumonitis (usually short-term exposure) Sarcoidosis (distinct subset with, usually, acute onset)
Stable fibrotic disease	Drug-induced lung disease (residual fibrosis after cessation) Hypersensitivity pneumonitis (after prolonged exposure) Sarcoidosis (residuum of burnt-out disease) Nonprogressive pneumoconioses after exposure (e.g., silicosis)
Major inflammation, risk of fibrotic progression	Drug-induced lung disease (unusually florid reactions) Hypersensitivity pneumonitis (usually continuing exposure) Sarcoidosis (prolonged severe inflammation)
Inexorably progressive fibrosis	Drug-induced lung disease (continuing exposure) Hypersensitivity pneumonitis (antigen usually unknown) Sarcoidosis (small subset of patients) Progressive pneumoconioses after exposure (e.g., asbestosis)
Explosive acute diffuse lung disease	Drug-induced lung disease

*Excluding the idiopathic interstitial pneumonias, covered in Table 42-5.

Table 42.5
ATS/ERS Consensus Classification of the Idiopathic Interstitial Pneumonias, and the Most Frequent Patterns of Longitudinal Behavior Associated with Individual Diagnoses

Clinicopathologic Diagnosis	Likely Longitudinal Behavior
Idiopathic pulmonary fibrosis/ cryptogenic fibrosing alveolitis	Inexorably progressive fibrosis
NSIP	Cellular NSIP: self-limited or major inflammation Fibrotic NSIP: stable or progressive fibrosis
Cryptogenic organizing pneumonia	Self-limited or major inflammation
Acute interstitial pneumonia	Explosive acute disease
Desquamative interstitial pneumonia	Self-limited or major inflammation
Respiratory bronchiolitis–associated interstitial lung disease	Self-limited inflammation
Lymphocytic interstitial pneumonia	Self-limited or major inflammation

NSIP, nonspecific interstitial pneumonia.

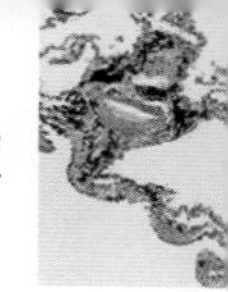

strategy, based on disease behavior, cannot be constructed from noninvasive evaluation.

These principles apply especially to the most common presentation of nongranulomatous idiopathic DLD: the clinical entity of IPF/cryptogenic fibrosing alveolitis. In previous decades, underlying histologic appearances have tended to be lumped together, but the recent ATS/ERS reclassification of the idiopathic interstitial pneumonias (Table 42.5) has provided a framework for the separation of a number of disease entities with strikingly diverse natural histories and treated outcomes. In an evaluation by Nicholson et al. of biopsy diagnoses of "cryptogenic fibrosing alveolitis" made in the 1980s, in patients presenting with the clinical features of IPF, an alternative histologic diagnosis was evident on review (associated with a much better observed outcome) in over 50% of cases. The ATS/ERS classification system is logical and pragmatic because, as shown in Table 42.5, each individual entity tends to fall into a particular category of longitudinal disease behavior (although a certain amount of overlap is inevitable). Thus, when a confident noninvasive diagnosis is unattainable in patients with idiopathic interstitial pneumonia, surgical biopsy should always be considered.

SUGGESTED READINGS

American Thoracic Society: Idiopathic pulmonary fibrosis: Diagnosis and treatment. International consensus statement. Am J Respir Crit Care Med 161:646-664, 2000.

American Thoracic Society/European Respiratory Society: American Thoracic Society/European Respiratory Society international multidisciplinary consensus classification of the idiopathic interstitial pneumonias. Am J Respir Crit Care Med 165:277-304, 2002.

Bertorelli G, Bocchino V, Olivieri D: Hypersensitivity pneumonitis. Eur Respir Monogr 14:120-136, 2000.

Coultas DB, Zumwalt RE, Black WC, Sobonya RE: The epidemiology of interstitial lung diseases. Am J Respir Crit Care Med 150:967-972, 1994.

Epler GR, McLoud TC, Gaensler EA, et al: Normal chest radiographs in chronic diffuse infiltrative lung disease. N Engl J Med 298:934-939, 1978.

Flaherty KR, Thwaite EL, Kazerooni EA, et al: Radiological versus histological diagnosis in UIP and NSIP: Survival implications. Thorax 58:143-148, 2003.

Hunninghake GW, Zimmerman MB, Schwartz DA, et al: Utility of a lung biopsy for the diagnosis of idiopathic pulmonary fibrosis. Am J Respir Crit Care Med 164:193-196, 2001.

Latsi PI, Du Bois RM, Nicholson AG, et al: Fibrotic idiopathic interstitial pneumonia: The prognostic value of longitudinal functional trends. Am J Respir Crit Care Med 168:531-537, 2003.

Nicholson AG, Colby TV, du Bois RM, et al: The prognostic significance of the histologic pattern of interstitial pneumonia in patients presenting with the clinical entity of cryptogenic fibrosing alveolitis. Am J Respir Crit Care Med 162:2213-2217, 2000.

Utz JP, Ryu JH, Douglas WW, et al: High short-term mortality following lung biopsy for usual interstitial pneumonia. Eur Respir J 17:175-179, 2001.

Wells AU: High resolution computed tomography in the diagnosis of diffuse lung disease: A clinical perspective. Semin Respir Crit Care Med 24:347-356, 2003.

CHAPTER 43 Idiopathic Pulmonary Fibrosis and Other Idiopathic Interstitial Pneumonias

Ulrich Costabel and John R. Britton

Our understanding of idiopathic pulmonary fibrosis (IPF), or, more generally speaking, of the idiopathic interstitial pneumonias, has undergone major changes in recent years. The term (which is synonymous with *cryptogenic fibrosing alveolitis* in the United Kingdom) has been used as an umbrella label to describe all patients with pulmonary fibrosis of unknown cause, regardless of differences in histologic patterns. Today IPF is defined more rigorously and is limited to the histologic pattern of usual interstitial pneumonia (UIP) as presented in the International Consensus Statement on IPF of 2000 and the American Thoracic Society and European Respiratory Society (ATS/ERS) Consensus Classification of 2002. Under these systems, IPF with UIP is just one of seven subsets of the idiopathic interstitial pneumonias (Table 43.1). IPF remains the most common diagnosis, accounting for 50% to 60% of all cases, followed by nonspecific interstitial pneumonitis (NSIP), which represents 20% to 40% of the idiopathic interstitial pneumonias; the remaining conditions are much more rare. IPF with UIP has the worst prognosis after acute interstitial pneumonia (AIP), with a median survival of only 2.8 years, compared with 5 years in previous studies. However, the older studies included patients with other histologic patterns that are associated with a better prognosis. Cryptogenic organizing pneumonia (COP) (which is synonymous with idiopathic), bronchiolitis obliterans organizing pneumonia (BOOP), and lymphoid interstitial pneumonia (LIP), which is rarely idiopathic, are covered elsewhere (see Chapters 46 and 47).

Historically, Hamman and Rich were the first to describe pulmonary fibrosis of unknown cause. In 1944 they reported on four patients with acute diffuse interstitial fibrosis who died within 1 to 6 months. It is now clear that these patients had AIP, and not IPF with UIP.

DEFINITION OF IDIOPATHIC PULMONARY FIBROSIS

The new definition, as written in the ATS/ERS classification of 2000, reads as follows:

> IPF is a specific form of chronic fibrosing interstitial pneumonia of unknown etiology, limited to the lung and with the histopathologic appearance of UIP on surgical lung biopsy with:
>
> - Exclusion of known causes of interstitial lung disease such as drug toxicities, environmental exposures, and connective tissue diseases
> - Abnormal pulmonary function tests with evidence of restriction and/or impaired gas exchange
> - Characteristic abnormalities on chest radiography or high-resolution computed tomography (HRCT) scans
>
> In the absence of a surgical lung biopsy, the diagnosis of IPF is less secure. However, in the immunocompetent adult, the presence of all of the following major diagnostic criteria, as well as at least three of the four minor criteria, increases the likelihood of a correct clinical diagnosis.

Major Criteria

- Exclusion of known causes (see preceding section)
- Abnormal pulmonary function tests with evidence of restriction and impaired gas exchange
- Bibasilar reticular abnormalities with minimal or no ground-glass opacities on HRCT scans
- Transbronchial biopsy or bronchoalveolar lavage showing no features to support an alternative diagnosis

Minor Criteria

- Age over 50 years
- Insidious onset of otherwise unexplained dyspnea on exertion
- Duration of illness more than 3 months
- Bibasilar inspiratory crackles on chest auscultation

EPIDEMIOLOGY

Patients with IPF are usually between age 50 and 70 years, with a mean age at diagnosis of 67 years, and about two thirds of patients are over the age of 60. Patients with the other forms of idiopathic interstitial lung disease, such as desquamative interstitial pneumonitis (DIP), NSIP, or AIP, usually are younger at presentation (Table 43.2). Males are affected slightly more frequently than females.

Data on the incidence and prevalence of IPF are scant and variable. Most are based on older studies that did not distinguish between IPF and UIP and the other subsets of the idiopathic interstitial pneumonias. There is evidence that the incidence is increasing, based on the mortality statistics for England and Wales. The incidence has been estimated at 10.7 per 100,000 per year for males and 7.4 per 100,000 for females, and a prevalence of 20.2 per 100,000 for males and 13.2 per 100,000 for females was seen in the early 1990s in New Mexico in the

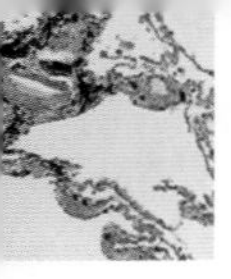

United States. The nationwide prevalence of IPF in Finland as defined by the new ATS/ERS criteria was recently estimated to be 16 to 18 per 100,000. The incidence and prevalence of IPF increases markedly with age (e.g., prevalence among persons aged 35 to 44 years is 2.7 per 100,000, and prevalence among persons over 75 years of age is 250 per 100,000).

Routine mortality statistics for IPF did not become available until 1979, when the introduction of the ninth revision of the International Classification of Diseases first provided a specific code for this disease. Registered mortality from IPF has since risen substantially in many countries (Fig. 43.1) to a degree that seems unlikely to result purely from increased recognition or a change in diagnostic labeling. Annual mortality in the United Kingdom in the early 1990s amounted to approximately 15 per million, which has been estimated to represent approximately one half of those who die with (but not necessarily from) clinically recognized IPF. Death from IPF is approximately 1.5 to 2 times more common in men than in women, and is much more common in older age groups. Registered mortality in the United States and in Germany is much lower than that in the United Kingdom and most other developed countries, to a degree incompatible with contemporary estimates of prevalence in the United States. This suggests that reporting or labeling artifacts are problematic in these countries.

RISK FACTORS

Several risk factors for IPF have now been identified, in particular, occupational exposure to metal or wood dust. Occupational exposure to organic solvents, mycotoxins, hydrogen peroxide,

Table 43.1
American Thoracic Society and European Respiratory Society Classification of Idiopathic Interstitial Pneumonias

Histologic Pattern	Clinical-Radiologic-Pathologic Diagnosis
Usual interstitial pneumonia	Idiopathic pulmonary fibrosis or cryptogenic fibrosing alveolitis
Nonspecific interstitial pneumonia	Nonspecific interstitial pneumonia (provisional)
Organizing pneumonia	Cryptogenic organizing pneumonia (synonymous with idiopathic bronchiolitis obliterans organizing pneumonia)
Diffuse alveolar damage	Acute interstitial pneumonia
Respiratory bronchiolitis	Respiratory bronchiolitis interstitial lung disease
Desquamative interstitial pneumonia	Desquamative interstitial pneumonia
Lymphocytic interstitial pneumonia	Lymphocytic interstitial pneumonia

Unclassifiable Interstitial pneumonias: Some cases of interstitial pneumonia are unclassifiable for a variety of reasons. Such cases constitute a heterogeneous group with poorly characterized clinical and radiologic features.

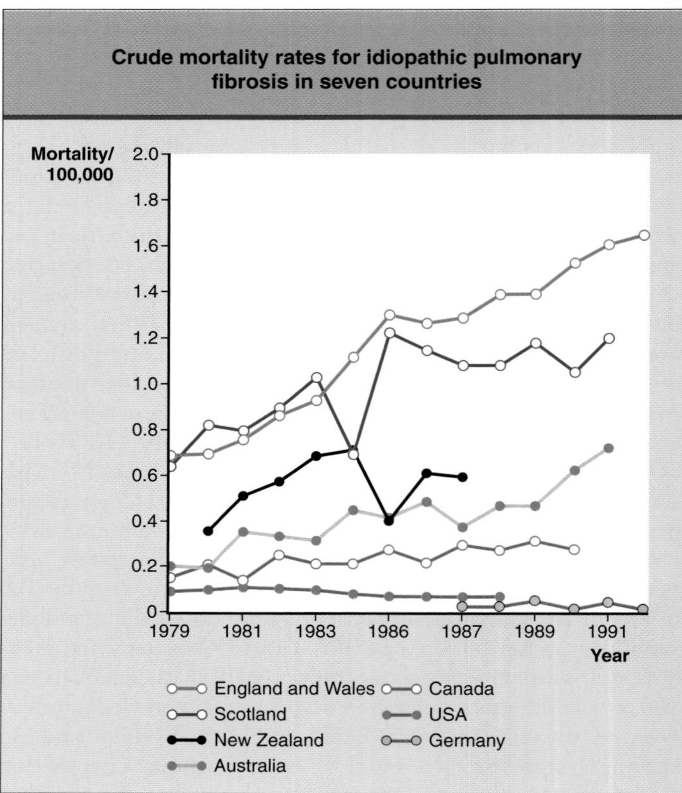

Figure 43.1 Crude mortality rates for idiopathic pulmonary fibrosis (IPF) in seven countries. (Adapted with permission from Coultas DB, Zumwalt RE, Black WC, Sobonya RE: The epidemiology of interstitial lung diseases. Am J Respir Crit Care Med 150:967-972, 1994.)

Table 43.2
Contrasting clinical features of idiopathic interstitial pneumonias

	IPF	DIP	RB-ILD	AIP	COP	NSIP*
Age (years)	65	40	35	50	55	55
Occurrence in children	No	Rare	No	Rare	No	Occasional
Onset	Chronic	Chronic	Chronic	Acute	Acute or subacute	Subacute or chronic
Clubbing	Frequent	Frequent	No	No	No	Occasional
Fever	Rare	No	No	50%	70%	10%-30%
Mortality (%)	70-90	0-27	0	80	13	11-60
Mean survival	2.8 years	12 years	Not reduced	1.5 months	>10 years	4-13 years
Response to corticosteroids	Poor	Good	Good	Poor	Good	Good

AIP, acute interstitial pneumonia; COP, chronic organizing pneumonia; DIP, desquamative interstitial pneumonia; IPF, idiopathic pulmonary fibrosis; NSIP, nonspecific interstitial pneumonia; RBILD, respiratory bronchiolitis interstitial lung disease.
*NSIP has a variable prognosis: favorable for cellular type, intermediate for fibrotic type.

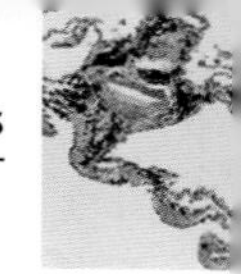

and various other occupational substances has also been implicated. Epstein-Barr virus, cytomegalovirus, and hepatitis C virus infections have been suggested to have a role in the etiology of IPF, although the evidence is not yet conclusive. IPF is probably more common among cigarette smokers than nonsmokers, and it has recently been suggested that IPF may be related to use of some antidepressant drugs. The prevalence of chronic aspiration secondary to gastroesophageal reflux is increased in patients with IPF.

Some evidence suggests that genetic factors may contribute to the risk of developing IPF. Reported associations with the human leukocyte antigen (HLA) phenotype have not proved consistent, but the increased prevalence of autoantibodies in individuals with IPF is well recognized. The significance of this association, either in etiologic or pathogenetic terms, is not yet established. Familial IPF is also a well-documented condition but in practice is extremely rare, accounting for only 0.5% to 3.5% of all IPF cases in studies from the United Kingdom and Finland.

CLINICAL FEATURES

Typically, IPF is seen in older patients and usually has an insidious onset and slow disease progression. In a nationally representative sample of nearly 600 new cases of IPF that occurred over a 2-year period in the United Kingdom, the mean age at presentation was the late sixties, with a male-female ratio of 1.7:1. The most common presenting symptoms are breathlessness and dry cough of gradual onset, with the breathlessness having been present for a median of 9 months before presentation. Hemoptysis is uncommon and, if present, should raise the suspicion of an underlying lung cancer, the relative risk of which increases 7- to 14-fold with IPF. On physical examination, the most frequent signs are bilateral fine crackles on auscultation (in 96% of patients in one series). They are typically end inspiratory and most prevalent in the lung bases but tend to extend to the upper zones with progression of the disease. Finger clubbing is present in approximately 50% of patients, and arthralgia or arthritis, in the absence of more overt clinical evidence of connective tissue disease, in about 20% (Table 43.3). Constitutional signs and symptoms, including malaise and weight loss, are recognized but uncommon. Fever is rare, and its presence suggests an alternative diagnosis. In more advanced disease, cyanosis and cor pulmonale may also be present.

Table 43.3
Clinical features at presentation in patients who have idiopathic pulmonary fibrosis

Features		Males	Females	Total
Age (mean in years)		67	68	67
Symptoms (%)	Breathlessnes	87	92	89
	Cough	73	77	75
	Arthritis/arthralgia	17	24	19
	Asymptomatic	5	4	5
	Finger clubbing	54	40	49
Lung function (% predicted)	Forced expiratory volume in 1s	78	79	78
	Forced vital capacity	78	79	78
	Residual volume	70	74	71
	Diffusing factor for carbon monoxide (DLCO)	48	53	50
	Diffusion coefficient (DLCO/accessible alveolar volume)	58	65	60
Smoking history	Current	22	13	19
	Ex-smoker	70	36	58
	Never	8	51	24

Data from Johnston IDA, Prescott RJ, Chalmers JC, Rudd RM: British Thoracic Society study of cryptogenic fibrosing alveolitis: Current presentation and initial management. Thorax 52:38-44, 1997.

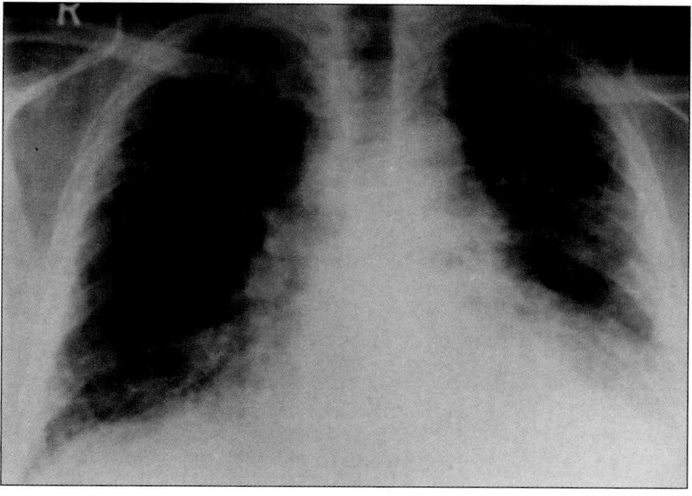

Figure 43.2 Typical chest radiograph appearance in idiopathic pulmonary fibrosis (IPF), with reticular and some nodular shadowing at both bases and some reduction of lung volume. (Radiograph courtesy of Dr. Andrew Evans, Nottingham City Hospital, UK.)

The chest radiograph is abnormal at presentation in virtually all patients with IPF. Typical chest radiographic appearances are of bilateral linear (reticular) shadowing, often also with fine nodules, predominantly at the periphery and at the lung bases, and usually with associated evidence of reduced lung volume (Fig. 43.2). In most cases, the shadowing leads to a loss of definition of the cardiac and diaphragmatic outline. In more advanced disease the reticular shadowing becomes more prominent and combines with multiple cystic translucencies to produce the appearance of honeycomb lung. The soft, ground-glass appearance of alveolar shadowing is also sometimes seen, but not usually in isolation from more marked reticulonodular shadowing.

HRCT now has a central role in the diagnostic approach to diffuse lung diseases. It can reveal disease before the chest radiograph becomes abnormal, helps to narrow the differential diagnosis based on the CT pattern, and allows the identification of associated emphysema. The primary role of HRCT in suspected idiopathic interstitial pneumonia is to separate patients with the typical findings of IPF and UIP from those with the less-specific findings associated with other idiopathic interstitial pneumonias. The typical HRCT changes associated with IPF and UIP consist of a reticular pattern in a subpleural and peripheral distribution, usually patchy and bilateral (Fig. 43.3). A variable amount of ground-glass opacification may be present; such opacification is usually minor and limited in extent to the areas of involvement

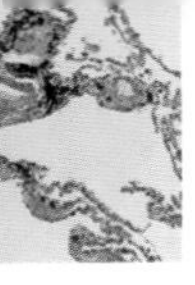

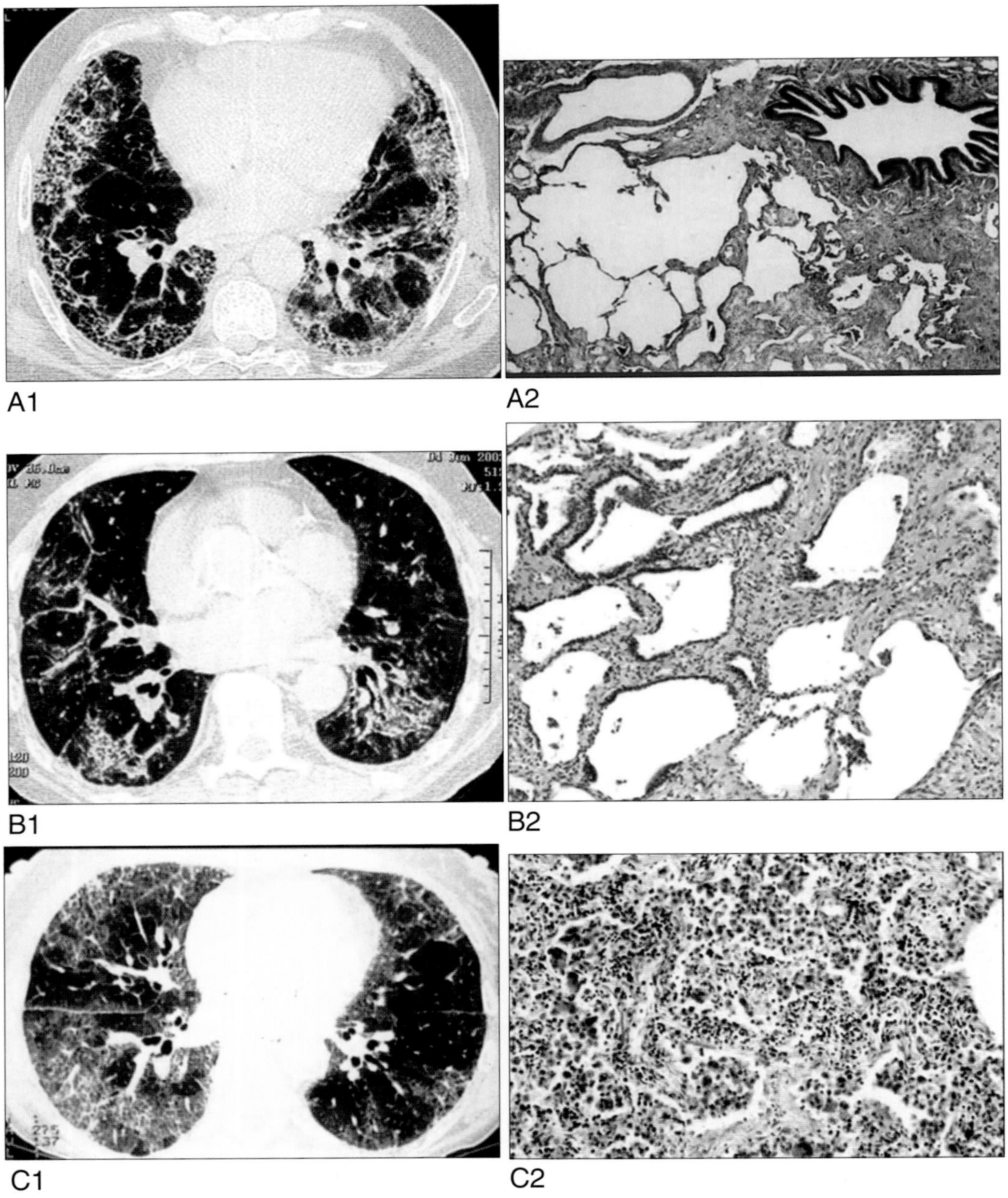

Figure 43.3 Typical HRCT scans and histopathologic patterns. **A,** IPF and UIP. **B,** NSIP. **C,** DIP. The patterns are described in detail in Table 43.4. (Histology courtesy of Dr. Dirk Theegasten, Department of Pathology, Ruhr University, Bochum, Germany.)

by the reticular pattern. The distribution is predominantly in the posterior part of the bases, but it affects the anterior regions with progression of disease before spreading centrally and to the upper zones. In areas of more severe involvement, traction bronchiectasis and subpleural cysts (honeycombing) are seen. Consolidation and nodules are absent. When all these radiologic features are present (characteristic IPF/UIP pattern), then the changes are virtually pathognomonic, and the clinical diagnosis of IPF is correct in more than 90% of cases (specificity ranging between 90% and 97% in various studies). In a recent study, honeycombing on HRCT indicated the presence of UIP with a sensitivity of 90% and a specificity of 86%, confirming that this feature is an important diagnostic criterion. Extensive ground-glass opacity on CT should prompt consideration of a diagnosis other than IPF, particularly DIP, but also respiratory bronchiolitis interstitial lung disease (RBILD), NSIP, or COP (Table 43.4). The role of HRCT in prognosis and response to treatment is discussed under "Clinical Course and Prevention."

The characteristic lung function abnormalities in IPF are restrictive, with reduction of vital capacity, forced expiratory volume in 1 second (FEV_1), and residual volume. Often at presentation the impairment of FEV_1 and forced vital capacity (FVC) is relatively minor, but measures of gas transfer show a more marked reduction. However, in practice a high proportion of patients with IPF are or have been active smokers, and this has led to some degree of airflow obstruction. In these individuals lung function tests may reveal a mixed restrictive and obstructive pattern. Arterial blood gas tensions may be normal in early disease but more commonly demonstrate hypoxemia and, in later stages of disease, hypercapnia.

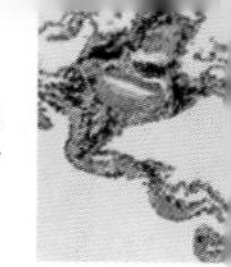

Table 43.4
Contrasting histopathologic and HRCT characteristics of idiopathic interstitial pneumonias

Histological pattern	Histopathological findings	Usual CT findings
Usual interstitial pneumonia	Architectural destruction, fibrosis with honey-combing, fibroblastic foci. Non-uniformity of these changes within biopsy specimen (temporal heterogeneity)	Peripheral, sub-pleural and basal distribution. Irregular reticular changes with honey-combing, traction bronchiectasis and architectural distortion. Focal, but minimal, ground glass change.
Non-specific interstitial pneumonia	Variable interstitial inflammation and fibrosis. Uniformity of changes within biopsy specimen. Fibroblastic foci inconspicuous/absent	Peripleural, peribronchial, basal; subpleural sparing possible. More ground glass attenuation. Reticular changes and traction bronchiectasis seen, but honeycombing is not prominent. Little consolidation may be present.
Lymphocytic interstitial pneumonia	Extensive lymphocytic infiltration in the inter-stitium often associated with peribronchiolar lymphoid follicles (follicular bronchiolitis)	Centrilobular nodules, ground glass attenuation, septal and bronchovascular thickening, thin walled cysts.
Diffuse alveolar damage	Diffuse. Alveolar septal thickening, airspace organization, hyaline membranes	Gravity-dependent consolidation, ground glass opacification – often with lobular sparing. Traction bronchiectasis occurs later
Organising pneumonia	Lung architecture preserved. Patchy distri-bution of intraluminal organizing fibrosis in distal air spaces	Patchy consolidation and/or nodules. May have a ground glass component.
Desquamative interstitial pneumonia	Uniform involvement of parenchyma. Alveolar macrophages filling the alveoli with little interstitial disease	Peripheral, subpleural, basal distribution. Ground glass attenuation, minor reticular changes, "geographic pattern."
Respiratory-bronchiolitis associated interstitial lung disease	Bronchiolocentric alveolar macrophage accumulation, Minor inflammation and fibrosis	Patchy ground glass. Bronchial wall thickening with centrilobular nodules.

Bronchoalveolar lavage differential cell counts in a patient with typical IPF usually shows elevated neutrophils and eosinophils. This pattern may be helpful in narrowing the differential diagnosis but is not diagnostic of IPF, because it is also observed in other fibrosing lung conditions. A neutrophilia is noted in 70% to 90% of patients, an associated increase in eosinophils in 40% to 60%, and a mild additional lymphocytosis in 10% to 20%. Higher percentages of lymphocytes (greater than 30%) are uncommon in IPF, and, when they are present, other disorders should be excluded (e.g., granulomatous infectious disease, sarcoidosis, hypersensitivity pneumonitis, COP, NSIP, or LIP).

Transbronchial biopsy is not very useful in the diagnosis of UIP but may suggest an alternative specific diagnosis (e.g., malignancy, infections, sarcoidosis, hypersensitivity pneumonitis, COP, eosinophilic pneumonia, or Langerhans-cell histiocytosis).

Up to one third of patients have antinuclear antibodies or rheumatoid factor in their serum at presentation, despite the conventional exclusion of patients who show overt clinical evidence of connective tissue disease from the diagnosis of IPF.

DIAGNOSIS

The diagnostic process in a patient suspected of having an idiopathic interstitial pneumonia is dynamic (Fig. 43.4). The first question is whether the disease is idiopathic or associated with known causes of interstitial fibrosis, or whether it represents another form of interstitial lung disease of unknown cause such as Langerhans-cell histiocytosis, eosinophilic pneumonia, and others. The next question is whether the disease is IPF or one of the other interstitial pneumonias.

The clinical diagnosis of IPF depends primarily on the identification of symptoms and signs of breathlessness, basal crackles, and finger clubbing (often seen on examination); the finding of characteristic radiographic appearances; and the demonstration of restrictive lung function. The clinical history must, however, also explore and exclude other possible causes of interstitial fibrosis, such as occupational exposure or exposure to drugs, allergens, and other substances as outlined in Chapter 42. It is therefore especially important to establish details of occupations in which the patient has worked, as well as to elicit a history of recreational activities, to establish whether the patient has been exposed to birds, hay, or other known causes of extrinsic allergic alveolitis. It is also important to obtain a drug history to identify potentially relevant current or previous drug exposures. While taking the history and conducting the examination, the examiner should also seek evidence of skin rashes, arthritis, or arthralgia as markers of connective tissue disease and general markers of other contributors to breathlessness, such as chronic obstructive pulmonary disease, respiratory infections, cardiac disease, primary or metastatic lung cancer, pulmonary embolus or hemorrhage, sarcoid, and so on. A full smoking history is also important, because smoking is a risk factor for IPF and because lung function test data in these patients may show a mixed obstructive and restrictive defect.

HRCT has a central role in the evaluation of a patient with idiopathic interstitial pneumonia (see Fig. 43.4). If, on the basis

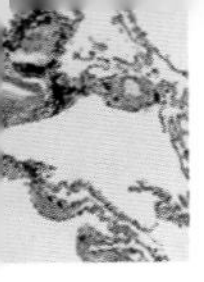

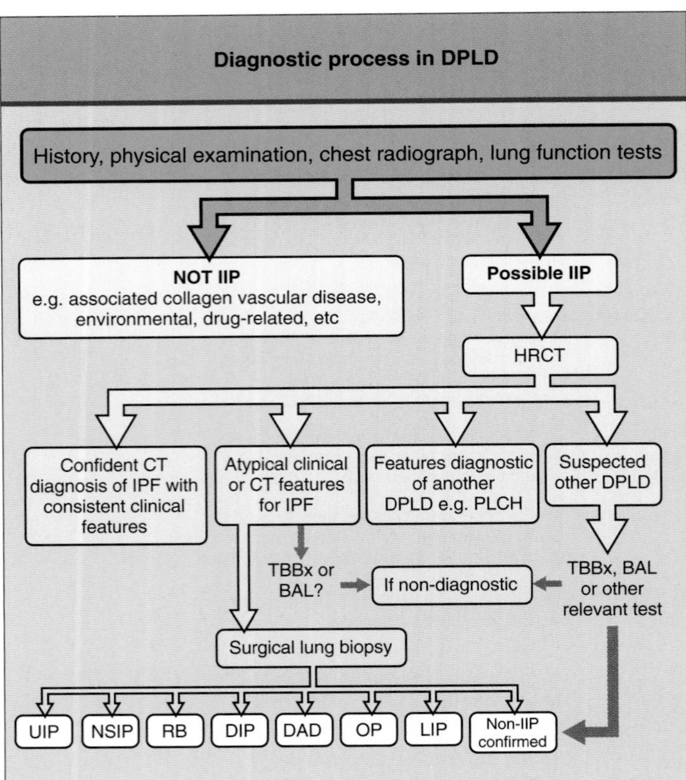

Figure 43.4 Suggested diagnostic algorithm for the evaluation of patients with diffuse parenchymal lung disease (DPLD). The importance of the HRCT is highlighted. BAL, bronchoalveolar lavage; DAD, diffuse alveolar damage; DIP, desquamative interstitial pneumonia; IIP, idiopathic interstitial pneumonia; LIP, lymphocytic interstitial pneumonia; NSIP, nonspecific interstitial pneumonia; OP, organizing pneumonia; PLCH, pulmonary Langerhans cell histiocytosis; RB, respiratory bronchiolitis; TBBx, transbronchial biopsy; UIP, usual interstitial pneumonia. (Adapted with permission from Travis WD, King TE, Bateman ED, et al: ATS/ERS international multidisciplinary consensus classification of idiopathic interstitial pneumonias. General principles and recommendations. Am J Respir Crit Care Med 165:277-304, 2002.)

of the history, physical examination, chest radiograph, and lung function tests, a patient possibly has idiopathic interstitial pneumonia, the next and obligatory step is to perform HRCT. This may also provide clues to the presence of nonidiopathic interstitial pneumonias such as sarcoidosis, extrinsic allergic alveolitis, lymphangioleiomyomatosis, Langerhans-cell histiocytosis, and alveolar proteinosis. After CT, if the clinician is confident of a diagnosis of IPF and the clinical features are consistent (see the major and minor ATS/ERS criteria), a surgical lung biopsy is not necessary. A transbronchial biopsy is usually not helpful in diagnosing IPF, as the biopsy does not usually yield a sufficiently substantial sample to make a confident diagnosis of UIP or any other idiopathic interstitial pneumonia, but it may provide a specific histopathology of other diseases as described previously. Most of these diagnoses would be evident, however, if not obvious, from the history, HRCT scan, or results of other clinical investigations.

In summary the diagnosis of IPF requires combined clinical, radiologic, and pathologic efforts. A surgical biopsy can no longer be considered the gold standard in making the diagnosis of IPF. The histopathologic pattern of UIP (Table 43.5) is not specific for IPF and may also be associated with collagen vascular disease, drug toxicity, chronic hypersensitivity pneumonitis, and asbestosis. Along the same lines, the NSIP pattern may be associated with no detectable cause (idiopathic NSIP) or may be associated with collagen vascular disease, hypersensitivity pneumonitis, drug-induced pneumonitis, infections, and immunodeficiency including that related to human immunodeficiency virus (HIV) infection. The same is true for the organizing pneumonia pattern (see Chapter 46) and the diffuse alveolar damage pattern in AIP, which is also associated with infection, collagen vascular disease, drug toxicity, and inhalation of toxic entities. Given the importance of a confident diagnosis in determining possible treatment and defining the prognosis, a clear diagnosis should be obtained early in the course of illness or before commencement of therapy.

TREATMENT

There is no established optimal treatment for IPF. The usual treatment strategy is anti-inflammatory, but anti-inflammatory therapy is unsuccessful in preventing the progression of IPF in most patients. For decades the leading hypothesis with regard to the pathogenesis of IPF was that the initial event is an inflammatory process (alveolitis characterized by infiltration of inflammatory cells such as macrophages, lymphocytes, and neutrophils). Inflammation was believed to lead to recruitment of fibroblasts and myofibroblasts and finally to collagen formation and irreversible fibrosis. The new theory is that IPF is a primary epithelial and fibroblastic disease, and not a primary inflammatory disorder. Inflammation is considered to be the secondary and not the primary event. This new hypothesis is the basis for understanding the disappointing results with an isolated anti-inflammatory treatment. New strategies are targeted at developing truly antifibrotic drugs.

Despite the widespread use of corticosteroids to treat IPF, no definitive evidence shows that these drugs improve either

Table 43.5
Key Differences among the Histopathological Features of Usual Interstitial Pneumonia, Nonspecific Interstitial Pneumonia, and Desquamative Interstitial Pneumonia

Usual Interstitial Pneumonia	Nonspecific Interstitial Pneumonia	Desquamative Interstitial Pneumonia
Dense fibrosis and honeycombing	Preserved architecture, variable fibrosis and cellularity	Intra-alveolar macrophage accumulation
Fibroblastic foci prominent	Few fibroblastic foci	No fibroblastic foci
Patchy, heterogeneous pattern	Temporally homogenous	Uniform involvement
Subpleural, paraseptal distribution	Inconsistent distribution	Diffuse distribution

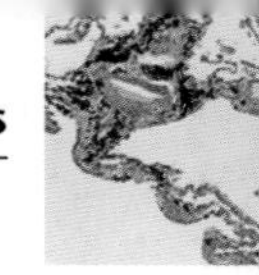

survival or quality of life. The available evidence on corticosteroid effects is based entirely on observational or retrospective comparative studies, none of which has involved a randomized, placebo-controlled, double-blind design. In addition, many of these studies included patients with other idiopathic interstitial pneumonias. Corticosteroid therapy is associated with significant morbidity, with adverse effects reported in a quarter of those treated.

Typical corticosteroid doses are 40 to 60 mg of prednisolone per day, or the equivalent, for at least 1 month, tapering down after stabilization of the disease to around 20 mg every other day. Of other proposed therapies for IPF, some have been assessed in randomized controlled trials. All are based on small numbers of subjects. Improved survival relative to prednisone therapy, albeit only to a borderline level of statistical significance, has been reported for treatment with a combination of azathioprine and modest doses of corticosteroids. A similar study in a small number of patients found no significant benefit from the addition of cyclophosphamide to prednisolone. Evidence of benefit from treatment with colchicine, penicillamine, and cyclosporin is limited to small, uncontrolled trials.

The ATS/ERS consensus statement recommends that treatment offered to a patient with IPF be combined therapy, including corticosteroids and either azathioprine or cyclophosphamide (Table 43.6). If therapy is offered to a patient, it should be started early, at the first identification of clinical or physiologic evidence of impairment or documentation of decline in lung function. Response rates may be better in patients in whom irreversible fibrosis has not yet developed. Treatment should be limited to those patients who have been given adequate information regarding the advantages and risks of treatment. The combined therapy should be continued for at least 6 months, and close monitoring every 3 to 6 months is recommended. If the patient's condition is found to be improved or stable, which occurs transiently in 10% to 30% of patients, this improvement or stabilization can be regarded as a beneficial effect of treatment, and the combined therapy should be continued using the same doses of medication. In patients in whom the disease progresses, treatment can be modified by switching to a different cytotoxic agent, or an alternative therapy or lung transplantation may be considered.

As disease progresses, patients with IPF can derive some benefit from more general methods of management of dyspnea and respiratory failure, such as supplemental oxygen, help with mobility outside and inside the home, opiates for respiratory distress, and other general social and nursing supportive measures. Radical therapy of IPF by lung transplantation is also an option for some patients and provides improved quality of life and survival for those who have advanced disease, but the availability of this procedure is obviously limited.

Potential opportunities for therapeutic intervention in the future include the use of antifibrotic agents, such as interferon-γ and pirfenidone; antagonists to cytokines such as TNF-α; to growth factors; and to endothelin receptors, thought to be involved in the pathogenesis of pulmonary fibrosis. Antioxidant drugs currently under development and the existing antioxidant *N*-acetylcysteine, which is currently being tested in a multinational clinical trial, may also have a role. For the present, however, the drug therapy of IPF remains an area of substantial controversy, and some physicians still elect not to intervene with drugs in this disease.

There are no prospective trials on treatment of the other idiopathic interstitial pneumonias. Therapy for fibrotic NSIP is the same as that for IPF. The suggested treatment for the other chronic idiopathic entities is administration of prednisone with the addition of other immunosuppressive agents later if necessary. AIP requires intravenous administration of high-dose corticosteroids and/or cyclophosphamide. Patients with DIP and RBILD should also stop smoking.

Table 43.6
American Thoracic Society and European Respiratory Society Recommendations for Treatment of Idiopathic Pulmonary Fibrosis

Corticosteroid (prednisone or equivalent)
0.5 mg per kilogram of body weight per day orally for 4 weeks
0.25 mg/kg/day for 8 weeks
Taper to 0.125 mg/kg/day or 0.25 mg/kg/day on alternate days

PLUS

Azathioprine
2-3 mg/kg/day
Maximum dose 150 mg daily
Begin dosing at 25-50 mg/day; increase in 25-mg increments every 1-2 weeks until the maximum dose is achieved

OR

Cyclophosphamide
2 mg/kg/day
Maximum dose 150 mg daily
Begin dosing at 25-50 mg/day; increase in 25-mg increments every 1-2 weeks until the maximum dose is achieved

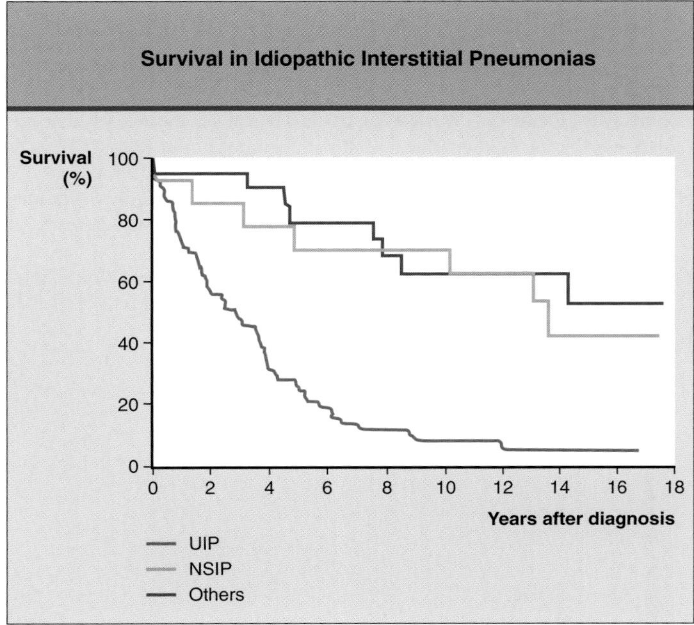

Figure 43.5 Survival in idiopathic interstitial pneumonias according to histopathological subgroups. Patients with UIP had a significantly worse survival compared with the other subgroups. Median survival for UIP patients was 2.8 years. NSIP, nonspecific interstitial pneumonia; UIP, usual interstitial pneumonia. (Adapted with permission from Bjoraker JA, Ryu JH, Edwin MK, et al: Prognostic significance of histopathologic subsets in idiopathic pulmonary fibrosis. Am J Respir Crit Care Med 157:199-203, 1998.)

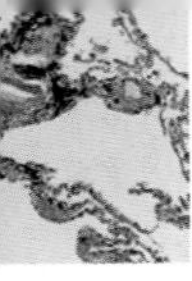

CLINICAL COURSE AND PREVENTION

The clinical course of IPF is variable but in most cases involves a progressive deterioration to death from respiratory failure. Life expectancy as estimated from follow-up of patients with IPF who attended specialist clinics has usually been approximately 5 years, but these figures can be substantially biased by the inclusion of other idiopathic interstitial pneumonias and by the tendency for longer-term survivors to be overrepresented in such populations. Most survival data come from specialist centers, and these may be unrepresentative of the disease spectrum. Typical survival in new cases of IPF is probably closer to 3 years, which, when compared with individuals of similar age and sex, represents a reduction in normal life expectancy of approximately 7 years. Most of the excess mortality in these patients is directly or indirectly attributable to IPF, but there may also be an increased risk of death from cardiovascular conditions or lung cancer.

The histologic diagnosis of UIP is the most important factor in determining survival in patients with suspected idiopathic interstitial pneumonia. All other histologic entities except AIP have a significantly better prognosis (Fig. 43.5). According to a recent study, the presence of honeycombing on HRCT is a good surrogate for UIP and could be useful in diagnosing patients unable to undergo surgical lung biopsy or in those in whom the recent ATS/ERS criteria for making a confident clinical diagnosis are fulfilled. Patients with NSIP are more likely to respond to or remain stable after a course of therapy with prednisone. Patients whose condition remains stable after steroid therapy have the best prognosis.

Markers of a poor prognosis of IPF include a relatively low FVC, diffusing factor for carbon monoxide, and arterial oxygen level at presentation; male sex; older age; lack of lymphocytosis in bronchoalveolar lavage fluid; and high counts of fibroblastic foci on biopsy. Evidence of improvement after a trial of corticosteroid therapy is associated with a favorable prognosis and may in turn be more likely in those with a relatively cellular histologic pattern on lung biopsy or a predominantly ground-glass pattern on HRCT of the lung. Extensive ground-glass shadowing is, however, atypical for IPF and UIP and suggests an alternative diagnosis. Current cigarette smoking at the time of diagnosis has been associated with improved survival—a finding that remains unexplained.

Because the cause of IPF is not clearly understood, prevention is not feasible. A number of potentially avoidable risk factors, such as occupational exposure to metal and wood dust and the use of common drugs, have now been identified, but none has yet been established with sufficient confidence to justify attempts at primary prevention. Secondary prevention is also not currently a practical option for IPF, though the implication of viral infections in the pathogenesis of IPF presents potential opportunities for future investigation.

SUGGESTED READINGS

Bjoraker JA, Ryu JH, Edwin MK, et al: Prognostic significance of histopathologic subsets in idiopathic pulmonary fibrosis. Am J Respir Crit Care Med 157:199-203, 1998.

Coultas DB, Zumwalt RE, Black WC, Sobonya RE: The epidemiology of interstitial lung diseases. Am J Respir Crit Care Med 150:967-972, 1994.

Flaherty KR, Toews GB, Travis WD, et al: Clinical significance of histological classification of idiopathic interstitial pneumonia. Eur Respir J 19:275-283, 2002.

Hunninghake GW, Zimmermann MB, Schwartz DA, et al: Utility of a lung biopsy for the diagnosis of idiopathic pulmonary fibrosis. Am J Respir Crit Care Med 164:193-196, 2001.

Katzenstein ALA, Myers JL: Idiopathic pulmonary fibrosis. Clinical relevance of pathologic classification. Am J Respir Crit Care Med 157:1301-1315, 1998.

King TE, Costabel U, Cordier JF, et al: ATS/ERS International Consensus Statement. Idiopathic pulmonary fibrosis: Diagnosis and treatment. Am J Respir Crit Care Med 161:646-664, 2000.

King TE: Idiopathic interstitial pneumonias. In Schwarz MI, King TE (eds): Interstitial Lung Disease. Hamilton-London, BC Decker, 2003, pp 701-786.

Nicholson AG, Fulford LG, Colby TV, et al: The relationship between individual histologic features and disease progression in idiopathic pulmonary fibrosis. Am J Respir Crit Care Med 166:173-177, 2002.

Selman M, King TE Jr, Pardo A: Idiopathic pulmonary fibrosis: Prevailing and evolving hypotheses about its pathogenesis and implication for therapy. Ann Intern Med 134:136-151, 2001.

Travis WD, King TE, Bateman ED, et al: ATS/ERS international multidisciplinary consensus classification of idiopathic interstitial pneumonias. General principles and recommendations. Am J Respir Crit Care Med 165:277-304, 2002.

CHAPTER 44 Extrinsic Allergic Alveolitis

C. J. Corrigan and A. J. Newman-Taylor

EPIDEMIOLOGY, RISK FACTORS, AND PATHOPHYSIOLOGY

Extrinsic allergic alveolitis (EAA) is a disease that arises from hypersensitivity to inhaled organic dust. The resulting inflammatory response is confined to the lungs, but not the alveoli, as the name suggests; hence, some prefer the term *hypersensitivity pneumonitis.* The prototype disease, farmer's lung, was described in 1932, and Pepys and colleagues associated it with development of serum precipitins to antigens derived from moldy hay contaminated with the spores of the thermophilic actinomycetes *Micropolyspora faeni* and *Thermoactinomyces vulgaris.* Since then, many microbial spores have been recognized as potential causes, along with other antigens derived from plants, animals, and chemicals (the last probably acting as haptens, antigenically modifying intrinsic or extrinsic proteins). A list of these agents, with their typical sources and associated "common parlance" diseases, is given in Table 44.1; most of these microorganisms may contaminate vegetable and cereal produce. The contamination is not present when the produce is harvested, but only after storage, particularly under warm, damp conditions.

In the United Kingdom, new cases of EAA occur primarily from occupational exposure, particularly in farmers, and from the keeping of domestic birds (budgerigars and pigeons). Nevertheless, EAA accounts for only about 2% of the incidence of all reported occupational lung diseases reported to Surveillance of Work and Occupational Respiratory Disease (SWORD) (compared with occupational asthma, the most common, which accounts for 26%). Corresponding with the "at-risk" groups, allergy to microorganisms is responsible for 50% of new cases of occupational EAA, although in over 25% of cases a causal antigen is not immediately identifiable. Individual risk is difficult to assess, because individual exposure varies widely within a given at-risk occupation or environment. Among farmers the mean incidence in the United Kingdom is 40 per million per year, with wide geographic variability. Apart from relevant exposure, no individual risk factors have been identified. Sporadic cases are familial.

Rough estimates of the prevalence of the more common forms of EAA in the United Kingdom are given in Table 44.2. Again, "spot" prevalences, both within and among countries, vary markedly. For example, the prevalence of EAA within the at-risk population exposed to contaminated air conditioners within single-office complexes in the United States has been reported to be as high as 70%, whereas in Japan the summer growth of *Trichosporon cutaneum* within unsanitary houses accounts for about 75% of all cases of EAA, which is 10 times more prevalent than farmer's lung in the United Kingdom.

EAA has been reported as being caused by molds and also recently by nontuberculous bacteria growing in hot tubs and saunas. The responsible molds include *Cladosporium cladosporides* and *Pullularia* species; these have been cultured from the water, and precipitins and inhalation-provoked symptoms have been identified in affected subjects. *Mycobacterium avium* complex may also grow in hot tubs and cause diffuse, granulomatous pulmonary disease. It is still not clear whether this should be considered an infection or a hypersensitivity reaction; some reported cases have resolved after treatment with oral steroids, others after antimycobacterial therapy. Therefore, although the majority of cases of EAA occur in the workplace, these cases highlight the importance of considering domestic allergens other than birds as potential causes of the disease.

Pathophysiology

Limited data are available on the histology of the lung after acute exposure, because tissue is rarely available. Acutely, nonspecific, diffuse pneumonitis with inflammatory cell (mononuclear cell, neutrophil) infiltration of the bronchioles, alveoli, and interstitium is accompanied by edema and luminal exudation. With ongoing continuous or intermittent exposure, a lymphocytic alveolitis centered on the bronchioles develops. Noncaseating epithelioid granulomata may also form quite rapidly (within 3 weeks), but these are often not a prominent feature of the pathology and furthermore are evanescent and usually resolve on cessation of exposure. Cellular infiltration (monocytes, lymphocytes, and plasma cells) with continued exposure is accompanied by progressive fibrosis in the interstitium and alveolar spaces, with obliteration of the bronchioles. Peribronchial and foreign body granulomata may reflect reactions to particulate matter. Finally, fibrosis (collagen deposition) becomes extensive, with loss of lung architecture and "honeycombing" typical of any cause of this process, except that upper lobe involvement may be more prominent. Vasculitis is not a feature at any stage.

The discovery of circulating precipitins (usually immunoglobulin [Ig] G, and also IgA and IgM) to relevant sensitizing agents in patients who have EAA led to the original concept that this disease is caused by deposition of antigen-antibody complexes within the alveolar wall (type III hypersensitivity). Subsequent investigation, however, has revealed many anomalies that do not support this hypothesis. In many patients with EAA, precipitin formation is not prominent and may wane with time although disease persists. On the other hand, many exposed subjects develop precipitins but no disease. Histologically, in chronic EAA many of the features of the prototype type III Arthus reaction (local immunocomplex deposition and complement fixa-

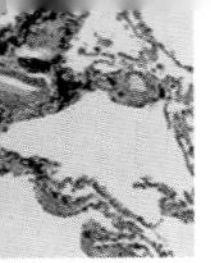

Table 44.1
Agents reported to cause extrinsic allergic alveolitis

Agent	Source	Disease
Microorganisms		
Alternaria spp.	Wood, wood pulp	Wood pulp and woodworker's lung
Aspergillus spp.	Whisky maltings	Malt worker's lung
	Vegetable compost	Farmer's lung
	Animal bedding	Dog house disease
Aureobasidium pullulans	Redwood	Sequoiosis
Penicillium chrysogenum *Merulius lacrymans* *Saccharomonospora viridis*	Wood	Woodworker's lung
Cephalosporium	Sewage	Sewage worker's lung
Cryptostroma corticale	Maple	Maple bark stripper's lung
Lycoperdon spp.	Puffballs	Lycoperdonosis
Mucor stolonifer	Paprika	Paprika splitter's lung
Penicillium casei	Cheese	Cheese washer's lung
Penicillium frequentens	Cork	Suberosis
Streptomyces albus	Soil, peat	Farmer's lung
Micropolyspora faeni	Hay, straw, grain	Farmer's lung
Thermoactinomyces spp.	Mushroom compost	Mushroom worker's lung
	Bagasse	Bagassosis
Trichosporon cutaneum	Japanese houses in summer	Summer-type extrinsic allergic alveolitis
Naegleria gruberi *Acanthamoeba castellani* *Other bacterial/ fungal/debris*	Water in air conditioners and humidifiers	Ventilation pneumonitis and humidifier lung
Botrytis cinera	Wine grapes	Spaetlese lung
Animals		
Wheat weevil (*Sitophilus granarius*)	Grain dust	Wheat weevil disease
Birds (budgerigars, pigeons, ducks)	Bloom? Excreta?	Bird fancier's lung
Fish	Meal	Fish-meal worker's lung
Pituitary extracts (bovine, porcine)	Pituitary snuff	Snuff taker's lung
Animal furs	Hair	Furrier's lung
Plants		
Coffee	Coffee bean dust	Coffee worker's lung
Trees (*e.g. Gonystylus bacanus*)	Wood dust	Woodworker's lung
Cotton	Bract of cotton flower	Byssinosis
Chemicals and drugs		
Drugs	Amiodarone, gold, procarbazine	Drug-induced extrinsic allergic alveolitis
Bordeaux mixture (fungicide)	Vineyards	Vineyard sprayer's lung
Diisocyanates	Plastics industry	–
Trimellitic anhydride	–	–
Pyrethrum	Insecticide sprays	–

Table 44.2
More common causes of extrinsic allergic alveolitis in the UK

Disease	'At-risk' population (%)	Prevalence in 'at-risk' population (%)
Farmer's lung	1–2	2–3
Budgerigar (parakeet)-induced extrinsic allergic alveolitis	10–12	0.5–7.5
Pigeon fancier's lung	0.25–0.3	Up to 21

tion, vasculitis, neutrophil infiltration) are characteristically absent, although neutrophil infiltration is a feature of acute exposure, and some organic dusts can activate complement directly through the alternative pathway. Thus, despite the presence of precipitating antibodies in most patients affected by EAA, the histology is one of a lymphocytic alveolitis with granuloma formation more consistent with cell-mediated (type IV) hypersensitivity. It is unclear why the disease develops in only a minority of exposed individuals, although it is known that cigarette smoking is associated with a reduced risk of the disease in such individuals. It has been postulated that the disease may be triggered in certain individuals by concurrent acute inflammation, such as that associated with viral infections or other unidentified stimuli.

CLINICAL FEATURES

The spectrum of clinical illness associated with EAA varies, which probably reflects factors specific to the individual as well as the frequency and degree of exposure to the relevant sensitizing antigen.

The acute form is most characteristic and specific and most probably reflects repeated, high-level exposure. Following a period of exposure and sensitization (which may last weeks to years) in an at-risk environment, the patient suffers repeated episodes of an influenza-like illness (malaise, fever, anorexia, headache, and fatigue) associated with dry cough, breathlessness, and occasionally wheeze 3 to 9 hours after the onset of exposure. Systemic symptoms are generally more prominent than respiratory symptoms, particularly because they may occur at night once the patient has gone to bed. Most patients, especially well-informed, high-risk groups such as farmers and pigeon fanciers, are able to associate these symptoms with exposure to an at-risk environment. However, patients may suppress symptoms, for example, if they fear loss of employment. The ease of association of symptoms with the environment also depends on the degree of exposure; mild symptoms may occur the same day and be missed, whereas heavy exposure may cause symptoms that last days to weeks. Clinical examination during an acute attack of EAA following exposure typically reveals respiratory distress with fast, shallow breathing, fever, and symmetrical basal crackles in the chest. Finger clubbing is very unusual. Blood gas analysis typically shows type I respiratory failure with hypoxia and hypocapnia. A peripheral blood lymphopenia is characteristic. The chest radiograph may show diffuse alveolitis with a "ground-glass" appearance, especially in the lower and middle zones (Fig. 44.1), but early changes may be evanescent so that the appearance may be normal between attacks. High-

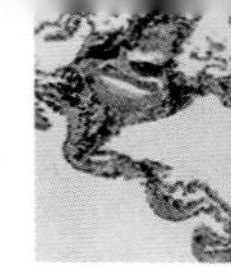

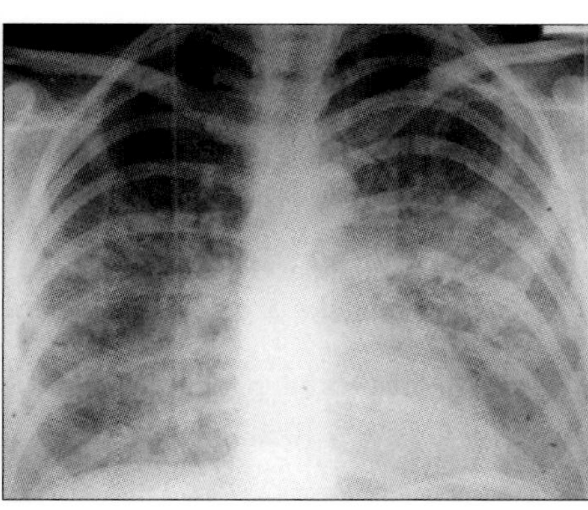

Figure 44.1 Chest radiograph of extrinsic allergic alveolitis (EAA) in the acute form showing alveolitis with basal ground-glass opacification.

resolution computed tomographic (CT) scanning during the acute episode characteristically shows ground-glass shadowing with discrete ("geographic") variation, which may be associated with nodular and reticular opacities. Characteristically the radiographic changes wax and wane with time, which is a helpful diagnostic pointer. Spontaneous resolution of clinical symptoms within days and radiographic changes within weeks are the general rules.

Presenting signs of the chronic form include an insidious loss of exercise tolerance and increasing breathlessness. No history of systemic symptoms may be found, although weight loss is often marked because of progressive pulmonary fibrosis with hypoxemia, which may progress to pulmonary hypertension and right-sided cardiac failure. Finger clubbing and chest crackles are uncommon. The chest radiograph shows signs of diffuse fibrosis with honeycombing, which, in contrast to the changes seen in the acute disease, usually affects the upper zones (Fig. 44.2). This type of disease is often, but not exclusively, seen in patients who keep one or a few birds at home and is caused by chronic, low levels of exposure to relevant antigens. The situation is probably more complicated, however, than this simple scenario suggests, and a spectrum of host responses to the antigen probably also influences the course of the disease.

Between these extreme ends of the spectrum of clinical disease, acute episodes with systemic symptoms may be superimposed on a background of more chronic, progressive disease. The clinical and radiographic changes accordingly show a mixed picture.

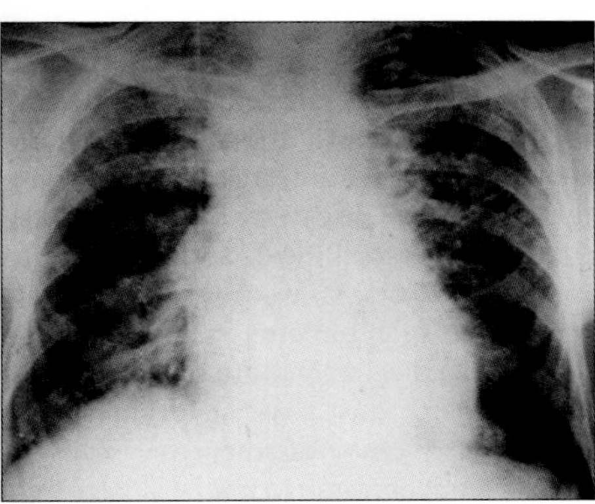

Figure 44.2 Chest radiograph of extrinsic allergic alveolitis (EAA) in the chronic, insidious form showing apical pulmonary fibrosis.

DIAGNOSIS

The diagnosis of EAA rests upon the demonstration of the following:

- Periodic or continuous exposure to a relevant sensitizing antigen
- Appropriate changes in lung physiology and pathology
- Evidence of immunologic sensitization to the suspected provoking agent

Periodic or Continuous Exposure to a Relevant Sensitizing Antigen

Periodic or continuous exposure to a relevant sensitizing antigen may be obvious from the history and the temporal pattern of symptoms in relation to exposure to an at-risk environment. In more chronic disease, a high index of suspicion may uncover chronic exposure to a recognized sensitizing antigen.

Appropriate Changes in Lung Physiology and Pathology

High-resolution CT scans demonstrate more clearly the changes seen on the chest radiography, but no single feature of these scans is pathognomonic of EAA. Acutely, discrete parenchymal reticular or nodular infiltration with ground-glass shadowing is seen. More chronically, diffuse fibrosis with honeycombing is more widespread and less confined to the upper lobes than suggested by chest radiography (Fig. 44.3).

Lung function varies with exposure and disease activity and may range from normal to a pattern of progressive restrictive lung disease. Total lung capacity is typically reduced, but the chronic bronchiolitis may cause gas trapping with elevated residual volume. Carbon monoxide transfer is eventually impaired with hypoxia, particularly on exercise. Airway obstruction is unusual. In addition to the clinical history, corresponding changes in lung function on alternative exposure to, and isolation from, the suspected environment may help to establish the diagnosis. Bronchoalveolar lavage typically shows markedly elevated percentages of bronchial, luminal T lymphocytes (typically

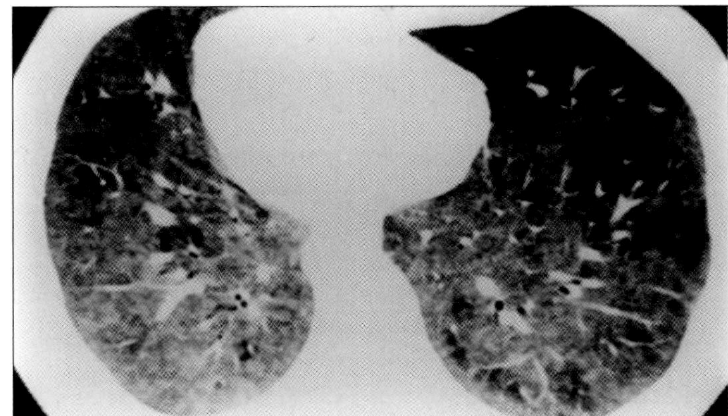

Figure 44.3 Thin-layer computed tomographic (CT) scan of extrinsic allergic alveolitis (EAA) showing reticular and nodular shadowing, interstitial fibrosis, and ground-glass opacification. Note the discrete (geographic) distribution of the changes.

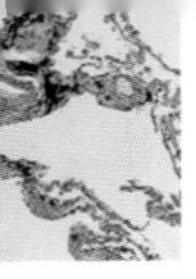

60% or more of the total cells) and, acutely, neutrophils. Elevated mast-cell numbers are also characteristic. The CD4/CD8 T-cell ratio is typically abnormal (<1). Although these changes are not specific and are quite variable among individuals, in practice few diseases cause such a characteristic cellular profile (the principal alternative being sarcoidosis). Transbronchial or open lung biopsy may be necessary to establish a definitive diagnosis in cases in which it is not evident from the history.

Evidence of Immunologic Sensitization to the Suspected Provoking Agent

Immunologic sensitization to the suspected provoking agent is demonstrated by the presence of IgG precipitins to the inducing organic agent in the serum of the affected patient. This has classically been assessed by radial diffusion (Ouchterlony) analysis (Fig. 44.4), although enzyme-linked immunosorbent assay (ELISA), which is more sensitive, is increasingly being used. These tests are very sensitive, especially for the diagnosis of farmer's or pigeon fancier's lung. Sensitivity may be further improved by concentrating the serum. Unfortunately, however, the tests are not very specific, because they are also positive in many exposed, nondiseased patients and, at the population level, reflect exposure rather than disease development. Nevertheless, it is true to say that nearly all diseased patients have detectable precipitins to the relevant sensitizing agent (although the concentration of these precipitins may wane with disease progression and they may be further depressed by concurrent smoking), so that their absence makes the diagnosis of EAA very unlikely. In contrast to type I hypersensitivity to allergens, skin-prick testing has no place in the detection of precipitins.

TREATMENT

Acute exacerbations of disease are generally manageable conservatively with bed rest, nonsteroidal anti-inflammatory agents, and supplementary oxygen therapy. In severe cases, mechanical ventilatory support may be required. Spontaneous recovery (over days or weeks, depending on the level of exposure) is the general rule.

The cornerstone of management is to remove the patient from further exposure. Although this may be straightforward in some cases, it can be extremely difficult if the patient fears loss of employment or refuses to discontinue a beloved hobby. Furthermore, it is difficult for the physician to insist on complete cessation of exposure because continued exposure does not inevitably result in progressive disease. In an industrial setting it is often possible to reduce exposure significantly by moving the employee to a lower exposure environment, and on farms, simple precautions, such as the thorough drying of hay prior to storage, are often beneficial. Industrial respirators, which filter up to 99% of respirable dust from inhaled air, are helpful but cumbersome to wear for long periods and are not suitable for heavy manual labor.

Once these measures are in place the patient should be assessed periodically to monitor disease progression or regression. If no evidence of progression is found, the patient may reasonably tolerate existing exposure conditions. However, with evidence of progression, the patient must be advised to cease further exposure. Further management includes investigation of the at-risk environment, with identification of others who have the disease or are at risk.

The role of systemic glucocorticoid therapy at any stage of the disease is unclear. Although such therapy accelerates recovery from acute illness following relevant exposure, it does not provide any long-term benefit, and it does carry its own added risks. Nevertheless, many patients are given glucocorticoids acutely to hasten improvement. There is also a risk that continual treatment of patients in this fashion may encourage carelessness about avoiding further exposure.

CLINICAL COURSE AND PREVENTION

If the diagnosis of EAA is made early and further relevant exposure is avoided, little risk of permanent lung damage exists, and most changes resolve. It is not always safe to assume, however, that patients will continue to avoid exposure in the future, so follow-up is desirable. Permanent pulmonary impairment is relatively uncommon but is most likely to occur in those patients who experience continuous, symptomatic exposure, although even at this stage the majority of such patients do improve if exposure is eliminated and pulmonary fibrosis is not advanced. A minority, however, show relentless progression even if exposure is stopped. Unfortunately, patients may not present with EAA until pulmonary fibrosis is well established and respiratory failure advanced.

PITFALLS AND CONTROVERSIES

The diagnosis of EAA is easy to miss. It is facilitated by maintaining a high index of suspicion and paying close attention to the patient's occupational and environmental history. In patients with an acute, influenza-like illness and impairment of lung function, the differential diagnosis is obviously wide, and the diagnosis of EAA should be considered in patients being investigated for possible viral, bacterial, and fungal pneumonias (especially atypical pneumonias such as psittacosis), tuberculosis, aspiration pneumonia, transient pulmonary infiltrates (such as those associated with collagen vascular diseases, drug reactions, eosinophilic vasculitis, and other vasculitides), and exposure to poisons or nonorganic industrial dusts. Coexisting asthma, particularly occupational asthma, in such patients may be a source of confusion. Specific differential diagnoses more relevant to the at-risk environment include organic dust toxic syndrome (transient, usually harmless respiratory embarrassment on exposure to very heavy, physically toxic concentrations of microbial spores

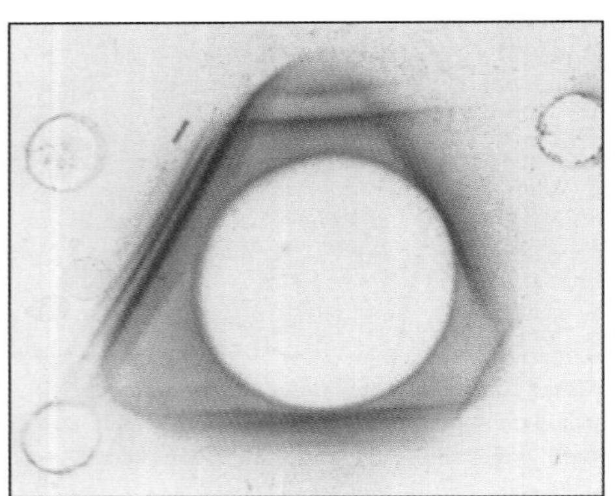

Figure 44.4 Radial precipitin (Ouchterlony) analysis of extrinsic allergic alveolitis (EAA) showing precipitin lines formed by interaction of the patient's serum and relevant antigen.

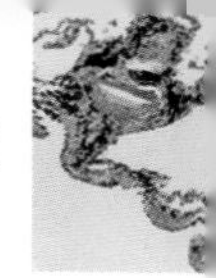

in contaminated vegetable and cereal produce) and nitrogen dioxide toxicity.

Current controversies in EAA concern the precise pathogenesis of the disease, especially the role of type III, as opposed to type IV, hypersensitivity; the spectrum of the host response in sensitized individuals; and the merits or otherwise of systemic glucocorticoid therapy.

SUGGESTED READINGS

Braun SR, doPico GA, Tsiatis A, et al: Farmer's lung disease: Long-term clinical and physiologic outcome. Am Rev Respir Dis 119:185-191, 1979.

Cormier Y, Lacasse Y: Keys to the diagnosis of hypersensitivity pneumonitis: The role of precipitins, lung biopsy and high-resolution computed tomography. Clin Pulm Med 3:72-77, 1996.

Fan LL: Hypersensitivity pneumonitis in children. Curr Opin Pediatr 14:323-326, 2002.

Fink JN: Hypersensitivity pneumonitis. Chest 13:303-309, 1992.

Hansell DM, Wells AU, Padley SPG, Muller NL: Hypersensitivity pneumonitis: Correlation of individual CT patterns with functional abnormalities. Radiology 199:123-128, 1996.

Jacobs RL, Thorner RE, Holcomb J, et al: Hypersensitivity pneumonitis caused by *Cladosporium* in an enclosed hot tub area. Ann Intern Med 105:204-206, 1986.

Khom A, Leslie KO, Tazelaer HD, et al: Diffuse pulmonary disease caused by non-tuberculous mycobacteria in immunocompetent people (hot tub lung). Am J Clin Pathol 115:755-762, 2001.

McSharry C, Anderson K, Bourke SJ, Boyd G: Takes your breath away—the immunology of allergic alveolitis. Clin Exp Immunol 128:3-9, 2002.

Meredith SK, Taylor VM, McDonald JC: Occupational respiratory disease in the United Kingdom, 1989: A report to the British Thoracic Society and the Society of Occupational Medicine by the SWORD project group. Br J Ind Med 48:292-298, 1991.

Reynolds HY: Hypersensitivity pneumonitis: Correlation of cellular and immunologic changes with clinical phases of disease. Lung 169(suppl.): S109-S128, 1991.

Richerson HB, Bernstein IL, Fink JN, et al: Guidelines for the clinical evaluation of hypersensitivity pneumonitis. J Allergy Clin Immunol 84:839-844, 1989.

CHAPTER 45 Sarcoidosis

David Moller

Sarcoidosis is a multisystem disorder of unknown cause characterized by noncaseating, epithelioid granulomas in affected organs. Although the disease most commonly affects the lungs and intrathoracic lymph nodes, granulomatous inflammation may be present in any organ system. Eye and skin involvement is seen in as many as 25% of patients, and symptomatic involvement of other organs occurs less frequently. Although the cause of sarcoidosis is unknown, clinical, epidemiologic, family, and laboratory-based studies support the hypothesis that sarcoidosis is triggered by exposure to microbial agent(s) in individuals who have genetic susceptibility to the disease. The pathogenesis of the granulomatous inflammation involves cytokine-producing $CD4^+$ T-helper-1 (TH1) lymphocytes and mononuclear phagocytes. A diagnosis of sarcoidosis is most securely established by a compatible clinical history together with a biopsy that demonstrates noncaseating granulomas in affected organs and the absence of competing diagnoses such as tuberculosis, fungal disease, or malignancy. The clinical course is highly variable, with a disease-related mortality of 1% to 6%. Corticosteroids remain the mainstay of treatment when sarcoidosis needs to be treated because of organ-threatening or chronic progressive disease.

EPIDEMIOLOGY

Sarcoidosis is found worldwide, although the prevalence is strikingly different in different geographic areas and racial groups. The prevalence of sarcoidosis ranges from 10 to 40 per 100,000 population in North America, Britain, and southern Europe, but less than 10 in 100,000 in Japan. Higher prevalence rates have been noted in Scandinavian countries and among African Americans in the United States. The age-adjusted incidence rate in the United States is estimated at 35.5 per 100,00 in the black population and 10.9 per 100,000 in the white population. In underdeveloped countries where tuberculosis is common, no reliable epidemiologic data are available because of the difficulty in distinguishing these diseases. Worldwide, a slight female predominance is found. Although all ages can be affected, over 80% of affected patients are between the ages of 20 to 50 years.

The frequencies of different clinical presentations of sarcoidosis vary among different groups. Erythema nodosum, which carries a good prognosis in sarcoidosis, has a particularly high frequency among Scandinavians, Irish female immigrants in Britain, and Puerto Rican women in New York City. In contrast, this presentation is less common in African Americans and Japanese patients. Lupus pernio, a disfiguring, nodular facial condition associated with chronic sarcoidosis, is more frequent in patients of African descent. Cardiac sarcoidosis and ocular sarcoidosis are more common in Japan than in Europe and the United States. Hospital statistics and anecdotal experience suggest that race is an important prognostic indicator, with African-American patients more likely to have chronic persistent disease and to suffer from increased morbidity and mortality than white patients who have sarcoidosis.

Retrospective studies suggest that sarcoidosis is the direct cause of death in 1% to 6% of patients. A recent analysis of mortality data from hospitals in the United States from 1979 to 1991 found that 0.02% of deaths were caused by sarcoidosis. Age-adjusted mortality was consistently higher among African Americans than among whites and among women compared with men. In the United States, autopsy studies and hospital data suggest that 40% to 80% of sarcoidosis deaths are the result of respiratory insufficiency, cor pulmonale, or massive hemoptysis. In Sweden and Japan, in contrast, most of the deaths from sarcoidosis are the result of cardiac involvement. Uremia from chronic renal failure and hepatic failure are less common causes of death related to sarcoidosis. These statistics are likely to underestimate the problem, given the potential for underdiagnosis of this disease.

ETIOLOGY AND RISK FACTORS

Infection

The cause of sarcoidosis remains unknown. Since sarcoidosis was first described, investigators have postulated an infectious cause of the disease based on the clinical similarities to tuberculosis. Environmental, presumably microbial, exposures have been linked to sarcoidosis because of seasonal variation and time-space clustering. However, despite considerable efforts to link specific infectious agents to sarcoidosis, conclusive evidence for a role for infectious agents remains elusive.

Early reports of acid-fast organisms, cultivable mycobacterial, cell-wall deficient organisms, and other bacterial, fungal, and viral agents have not been confirmed. Recently, polymerase chain reaction methods have been used to search for traces of genetic elements from microbial organisms. Different studies have found mycobacterial DNA in 0% to 80% of biopsy specimens, but also in 0% to 30% of control tissues. Propionibacterial DNA has also been found to be present more frequently and in greater quantities in sarcoidosis than in control tissues. Other microbial agents such as *Borrelia burgdorferi*, *Chlamydia pneumoniae*, and *Rickettsia helvetica* have been implicated in sarcoidosis by biopsy or serologic studies. Although no consensus has been reached, many investigators favor the hypothesis that certain microbial agents such as mycobacterial or propionibacterial

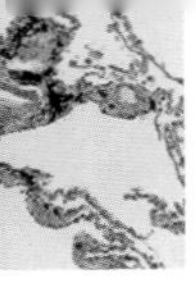

organisms may trigger sarcoidosis in susceptible individuals, but that sarcoidosis is not caused by an active, ongoing infection.

Noninfectious environmental triggers of sarcoidosis have also been hypothesized to cause the disease. Chronic beryllium disease results in a granulomatous pneumonitis that is histologically identical to sarcoidosis and results from immunologic sensitization to beryllium in less than 5% of exposed workers. However, the clinical overlap with multisystem sarcoidosis is small—restricted to those with interstitial lung disease without extrapulmonary involvement. Results from a large case-control study in the United States called ACCESS (A Case Controlled Etiologic Study of Sarcoidosis) showed no environmental or occupational associations positively linked to sarcoidosis risk with an odds ratio greater than 2.0 and an exposure prevalence of greater than 5%. The study found positive associations with insecticides, mold and mildew, and musty odors with odds ratios approximating 1.5, suggesting possible links to microbe-rich environments. Sarcoidosis was not associated with exposure to heavy metals or wood dusts or with rural residence as previously hypothesized. The ACCESS study found a robust negative association between smoking and sarcoidosis risk, confirming previous, more limited studies. Overall, the ACCESS study provided few data to support an environmental (noninfectious) cause for sarcoidosis.

Autoimmunity

Some investigators suggest that sarcoidosis is a result of autoimmunity, perhaps from molecular mimicry of autoantigens to proteins from infectious agents. The presence of antinuclear antibodies, rheumatoid factor, hypergammaglobulinemia, and immune complexes in sarcoidosis supports a possible autoimmune origin of sarcoidosis.

Kveim-Siltzbach reaction

In the 1860s, Ansgar Kveim found that the intradermal inoculation of a suspension of sarcoidosis lymph-node tissue resulted in a nodular skin reaction that contained sarcoid-like granulomas in patients who had suspected sarcoidosis, but not in control individuals. Subsequent investigators found that this reaction (using validated spleen tissue) occurs in 70% to 80% of patients early in the disease, with a less than 1% false-positive rate. In this reaction, well-formed granulomas take 2 to 4 weeks to develop. Attempts have been made to identify the granuloma-inducing factor contained in the Kveim reagent, but precise characterization has yet to be accomplished. Given the concerns of injecting allogeneic material into patients, clinical use of this reagent is restricted to a few specialized centers with archived tissue.

Genetic Factors

Substantial evidence exists for a genetic predisposition to sarcoidosis. Familial clustering of sarcoidosis occurs in 3% to 14% of patients, with a greater frequency among African-American compared with white populations. The U.S. ACCESS study found sarcoidosis cases were almost five times as likely as controls to report a sibling or parent with a history of sarcoidosis. Siblings had a higher relative risk (odds ratio 5.8) than parents (odds ratio 3.8), whereas spouses of cases were less likely to report a family history of sarcoidosis than controls (odds ratio 0.2). Significantly higher adjusted familial relative risk estimates were reported for whites in both the U.S. ACCESS study (RR = 20) and in a U.K. study involving mostly whites (RR = 36 to 73) than in African Americans (RR = 3) in ACCESS, suggesting familial factors may have a greater influence in susceptibility to sarcoidosis in whites than African Americans. Monozygotic twins appear two to four times more likely to develop sarcoidosis than dizygotic twins, which strongly suggests a genetic component to the disease. The lack of a clear genetic pattern indicates that susceptibility to sarcoidosis is polygenic and interacts with environmental factors.

Table 45.1
Genetic basis for sarcoidosis

Antigen subtype	Sarcoidosis risk
Class 1 HLA-B8	Associated with disease susceptibility in several populations
Class 2 HLA-DR1 HLA-DR4	Associated with disease protection in several populations
HLA-DR17 (DR3) HLA-DRB1 HLA-DQB1	Associated with presentations of sarcoidosis with favorable outcomes in European and Japanese populations. Favorable outcomes: Löfgren's syndrome, acute arthritis. Stage 1 radiograph, or remission in 2 years.
HLA-DRB1 HLA-DQB1	Associated with more severe or chronic sarcoidosis
Tumor necrosis factor-α gene in MHC locus	Associated with sarcoidosis subgroups
CCR2	
CCR5	
Angiotensin converting enzyme	Only one of several studies showed sarcoidosis risk association

Recent studies using a candidate gene approach or family linkage data have begun to elucidate the genetic basis of sarcoidosis. A recent genome-wide microsatellite analysis of 63 German families demonstrated strongest linkage to the *MHC* locus on chromosome 6. This finding is consistent with multiple prior studies that found certain Human Leukocyte Antigen (HLA) class I or II alleles were associated with susceptibility to sarcoidosis or its different clinical presentations. Table 45.1 presents the correlation of HLA subtypes and chemokine receptors to sarcoidosis outcomes.

PATHOPHYSIOLOGY

The histologic hallmark of sarcoidosis is the presence of discrete, noncaseating granulomas (Fig. 45.1). The dominant cell in the central core is the epithelioid cell, thought to be a differentiated form of a mononuclear phagocyte. Mature macrophages and $CD4^+$ lymphocytes are interspersed throughout the epithelioid core, whereas both $CD4^+$ and $CD8^+$ lymphocytes are seen around the periphery of the granuloma. Multinucleated giant cells, which often contain cytoplasmic inclusions such as Schaumann bodies or asteroid bodies, are scattered throughout the inflammatory locus. In the lung, granulomas tend to form along bronchovascular, bronchial submucosal, subpleural, and

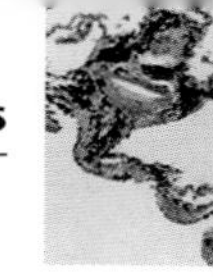

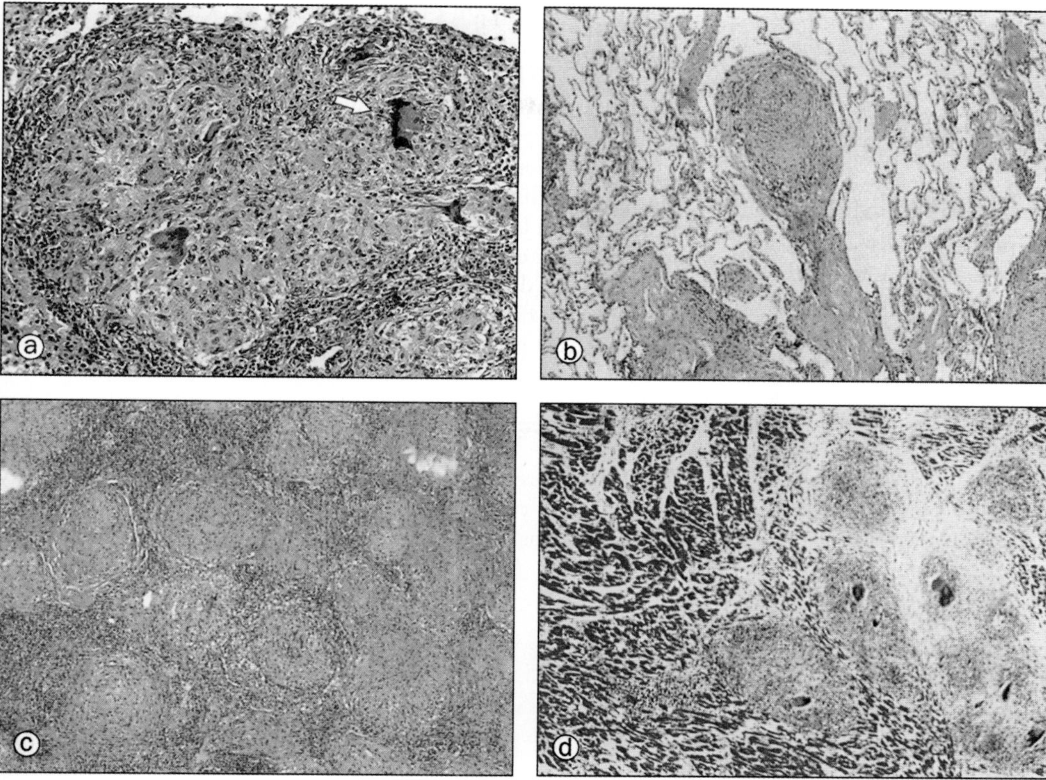

Figure 45.1 Noncaseating granulomatous inflammation in sarcoidosis. A, Close-up of epithelioid granuloma with giant cells and mononuclear cell infiltration. **B,** Open lung biopsy showing granulomas, giant cells, and lymphocytic infiltrates in lung parenchyma and within interlobular septal and subpleural regions. **C,** Lymph node biopsy showing extensive replacement with typical sarcoid-type epithelioid granulomas. Fibrinoid necrosis, but not overt caseation, may be seen in the center of granulomas. **D,** Myocardial biopsy showing patchy granulomatous inflammation with giant cells.

interlobular septal regions, areas rich in lymphatic vessels (see Fig. 45.1B). Hyalinized, relatively acellular ghosts of granulomas are thought to be a later development in granulomatous inflammation.

Current concepts of the immunopathogenesis of sarcoidosis have been derived in large part from studies of lung cells and fluid recovered from the alveolar surface by bronchoalveolar lavage (BAL). Samples of BAL fluid from patients who have sarcoidosis are characterized by an increased proportion of lymphocytes (Fig. 45.2). These lung T cells are predominantly of the $CD4^+$ phenotype, typically with a CD4/CD8 ratio between 3:1 and 10:1, compared with a ratio of 2:1 in healthy individuals. Greater than normal numbers of these lung T cells express the activation markers, VLA-1 (very late activation antigen–1, CD49a) and HLA-DR molecules. Sarcoidosis lung T cells demonstrate reduced surface density of the CD3/T-cell receptor complex, a hallmark of T cells activated through the T-cell antigen receptor (TCR) pathway. BAL lung T-cell populations in sarcoidosis are characterized by expanded oligoclonal T cells that express specific gene segments from the variable regions of the TCR β-, α-, γ-, or δ-chains. These studies provide direct evidence that granulomatous inflammation in sarcoidosis is driven by an immune response to conventional antigens.

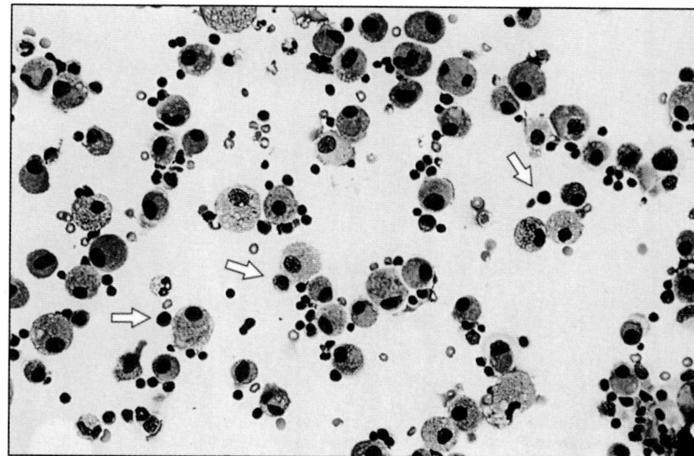

Figure 45.2 Cytospin of bronchoalveolar lavage (BAL) cells from a patient with sarcoidosis. Image shows a higher than normal proportion of lung lymphocytes (small, dark staining cells with unilobular nuclei and scant cytoplasm). Larger cells are alveolar macrophages that normally constitute 90% or more of recovered cells from BAL fluid of healthy individuals.

Alveolar macrophages are thought to play a central role in the development of granulomatous inflammation in pulmonary sarcoidosis. Sarcoidosis alveolar macrophages spontaneously produce tumor necrosis factor (TNF)-α, interleukin (IL)-6, IL-12, and IL-18, cytokines that are known to regulate granuloma formation. These cells also produce increased amounts of lysozyme, angiotensin-converting enzyme (ACE), and reactive oxygen species. Lung macrophages release increased amounts of transforming growth factor (TGF)-β, fibronectin, and insulin-like growth factor (IGF)-1, which are important in fibroblast recruitment and replication, as occurs in fibrotic wound healing. Osteopontin, a glycoprotein cytokine important in granuloma formation, is expressed by alveolar macrophages, T cells, epithelioid histiocytes, and multinucleated giant cells and likely plays a role in granuloma formation.

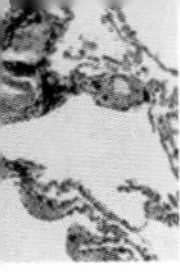

Sarcoidosis as a TH1-driven Disorder

Recent evidence supports the concept that sarcoidosis is a polarized TH1 disorder with spontaneous production of the TH1 cytokines, interferon (IFN)-γ, and IL-2 by lung T cells and the IFN-γ costimulatory factors, IL-12 and IL-18, by lung macrophages (Fig. 45.3A and B). In contrast, low or undetectable levels of the TH2 cytokines IL-4 and IL-5 occur in most patients who have sarcoidosis. One hypothesis suggests that successful removal of the inciting antigens by the immune response results in resolution of the disease (Fig. 45.3C). In a subgroup of patients, enhanced in vitro production of TGF-β from lung macrophages has been associated with remission of active disease, suggesting this cytokine may be critical to downregulating the TH1 inflammatory process in sarcoidosis. If the immune response ineffectively removes the stimulating antigens or autoimmunity develops, dysregulated cytokine production driven by a positive feedback loop between IFN-γ and IL-12 and IL-18 results in maintenance of granulomatous inflammation (see Fig. 45.3B). TNF is a major effector cytokine of granuloma formation in sarcoidosis, as evidenced by the fact that enhanced release of TNF by BAL cells is associated with persistent disease. A fibrotic outcome may occur in response to unremitting inflammation, with tissue injury from the local release of reactive oxygen species, proteases, and lysosomal products from phagocytic cells in the presence of profibrotic cytokines such as TGF-β and IGF-1 (Fig. 45.3D). Theoretically, fibrosis can be prevented by suppressing the inflammatory response early in the course of the disease. Consistent with this scenario, drugs able to suppress TH1 cytokines and TNF production (e.g., corticosteroids, pentoxifylline, thalidomide, anti-TNF biologics) may be beneficial in the treatment of sarcoidosis.

CLINICAL FEATURES

The clinical presentation and natural course of sarcoidosis vary greatly. Up to two thirds of patients are asymptomatic but have sarcoidosis diagnosed on the basis of an incidental radiographic

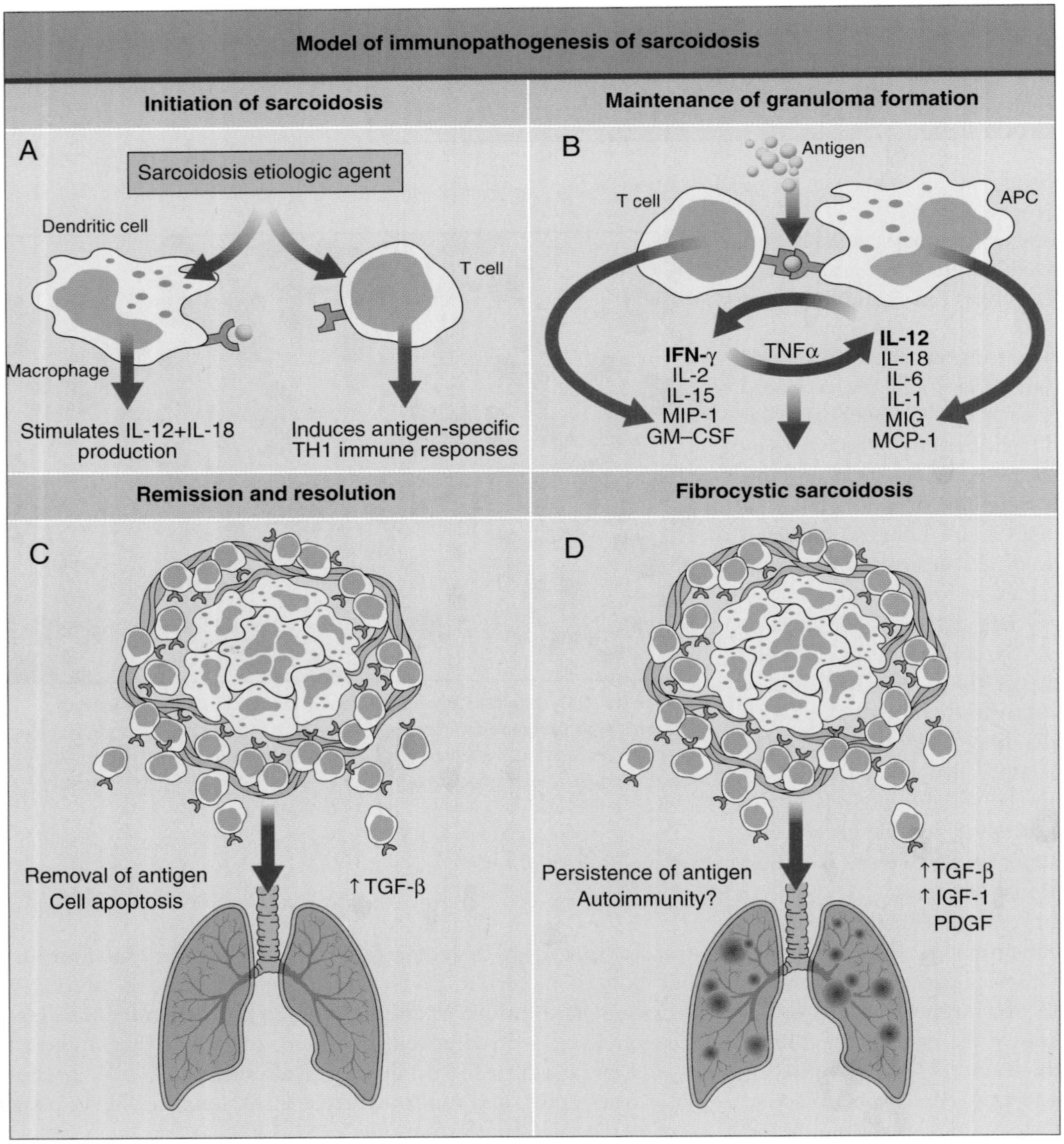

Figure 45.3 Model of the immunopathogenesis of sarcoidosis. Initiation of sarcoidosis involves stimulation of IL-12+IL-18 production from mononuclear phagocytes and dendritic cells and adaptive T-cell immunity to an inciting agent. Maintenance of granuloma formation by a TH1 immune response driven by IFN-γ and IL-12+IL-18. Resolution of sarcoidosis after removal of stimulating antigen, suppression of T-cell responses by TGF-β and other mediators, and granuloma resorption by cell apoptosis. Fibrotic outcome from persistent, possibly autoimmune, antigenic stimulation in the presence of TGF-β and other profibrotic mediators.

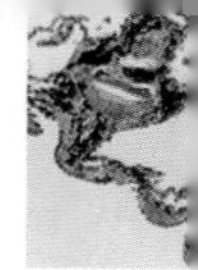

finding of bilateral hilar adenopathy or, occasionally, of an abnormal liver profile. Symptomatic presentations of sarcoidosis most frequently involve the respiratory system. Systemic constitutional symptoms, such as fever, malaise, and weight loss, may be prominent features, particularly in those patients who have Löfgren's syndrome or hepatic sarcoidosis. One possible presenting sign of sarcoidosis is fever of unknown origin.

Asymptomatic Sarcoidosis

Based on population screening with chest radiographs, it is estimated that 30% to 60% of patients who have sarcoidosis are asymptomatic. Patients in this subgroup usually have bilateral hilar adenopathy on the chest radiograph. Occasionally, interstitial infiltrates are also seen in association, more commonly in white individuals.

Löfgren Syndrome

Löfgren syndrome is a well-defined presentation of sarcoidosis that consists of erythema nodosum, polyarthritis, and (in over 90% of cases) bilateral hilar adenopathy. The polyarthritis, which may be severe, commonly involves the ankles, knees, and wrists, sometimes with heel pain and Achilles tendinitis. Fever and lassitude are often prominent manifestations, and uveitis is found in 50% or more cases. The onset of symptoms is usually abrupt. In most cases, spontaneous remission occurs within several weeks to months. This presentation is common in European and white populations but occurs in less than 5% of African-American patients who have sarcoidosis.

Pulmonary Sarcoidosis

The most common symptoms of pulmonary sarcoidosis are shortness of breath, cough, and chest discomfort (Table 45.2). Dyspnea is most marked on exertion and typically progresses in active, untreated disease. Cough is usually nonproductive early in the course of sarcoidosis and can vary greatly in severity. Dyspnea and cough may reflect parenchymal (interstitial) involvement, endobronchial disease, or both. Chronic sputum production and hemoptysis are more frequent in advanced fibrocystic disease. Chest pain is common, is often difficult to describe, and varies in location and severity. Chest tightness and wheezing are frequent in patients who have chronic fibrocystic sarcoidosis or bronchial hyper-reactivity. Typically, the physical findings of pulmonary sarcoidosis are few. Lung crackles are heard in less than 20% of patients, even in those who have advanced disease. Clubbing is rare, but when present it is usually associated with advanced bronchiectasis.

Symptomatic bronchial or tracheal stenosis is rare, but may be associated with dyspnea, stridor, wheezing, or cough. Lobar atelectasis, usually of the upper or right middle lobes, may be seen. Mechanisms include compression by nearby lymph nodes, fibrotic distortion of major airways, endobronchial disease, and mediastinal fibrosis.

Chronic pulmonary hypertension and cor pulmonale are seen in 1% to 4% of patients and usually arise from severe fibrocystic sarcoidosis. Rarely, dyspnea from pulmonary hypertension is seen without severe interstitial lung disease. Causes include extrinsic compression of pulmonary vessels by enlarged lymph nodes or fibrosing mediastinitis, or a granulomatous vasculitis of pulmonary vessels. Superior vena cava syndrome rarely occurs from extensive mediastinal lymphadenopathy and fibrosis as a result of sarcoidosis; more commonly, histoplasmosis or malignancy is the cause.

Table 45.2
Major clinical features of pulmonary and upper respiratory tract sarcoidosis

Symptoms	Signs	Tests
Dyspnea	Wheezes (occasional)	Lung function
Cough	Crackles (uncommon)	Restrictive impairment
Chest pain	Clubbing (rare)	Obstructive impairment
Sputum production	Stridor	Hypoxemia
	Sinus tenderness	Hypercapnia (late)
Hemoptysis	Cobblestoning, edema, erythema of nasal mucosa, laryngeal structures	Bilateral hilar and mediastinal adenopathy
Hoarseness		Diffuse infiltrates
Nasal congestion	Saddle nose deformity	Upper lobe fibrosis
Sinus pain		Bronchiectasis
		Mycetomas

Chest Radiology

Chest radiographs are abnormal in more than 90% of patients who have sarcoidosis. By international convention, the chest radiograph is divided into the following stages or types (Fig. 45.4):

- Stage 0—normal chest radiograph
- Stage I—bilateral hilar adenopathy
- Stage II—bilateral hilar adenopathy plus interstitial infiltrates
- Stage III—interstitial infiltrates only (nonfibrotic)
- Stage IV—fibrotic interstitial lung disease

A normal chest radiograph is found in 5% to 10% of patients who have sarcoidosis, frequently in those who show extrathoracic manifestations of sarcoidosis. Stage I is seen in 40% to 50% of cases on initial presentation (Fig. 45.4A). Typically, the hilar adenopathy is discrete and symmetrical and stands away from the right heart border to give the appearance of "potato nodes"; paratracheal adenopathy, particularly on the right side, is a common accompaniment. A stage II chest radiograph is seen in 20% to 30% of cases on initial presentation (Fig. 45.4B). Typically the infiltrates demonstrate fine, linear markings, reticulonodules, or confluent shadows. A mid- or upper-zone predominance is frequently seen and may mimic tuberculosis or histoplasmosis. A stage III chest radiograph has interstitial infiltrates and no discernable hilar adenopathy and is seen in 10% to 20% of cases on initial presentation (Fig. 45.4C). Chest radiographs that have extensive fibrocystic changes and scarring are frequently placed under a separate subgroup, stage IV, in recognition of the poor outcome of this group of patients (Fig. 45.4D). Destruction of lung tissue, fibrous traction on airways with upward hilar retraction, and multiple bullous and cystic changes are typically seen.

More unusual patterns of lung infiltrates may occur in some patients. Larger, more well-defined nodular infiltrates may mimic granulomatous infections, Wegener's granulomatosis, or

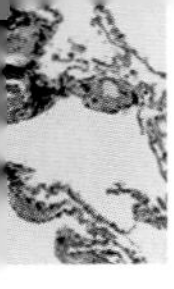

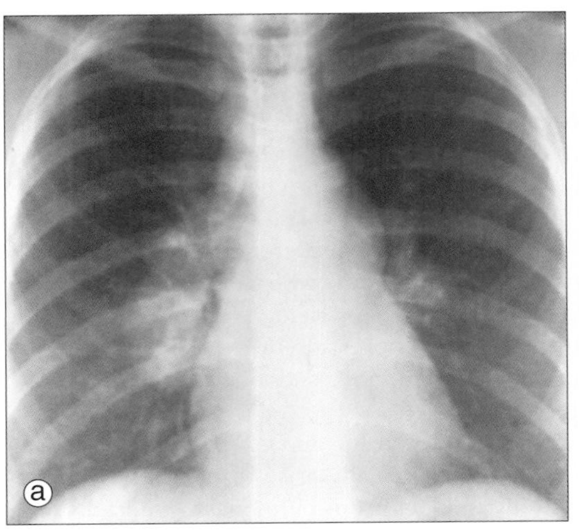

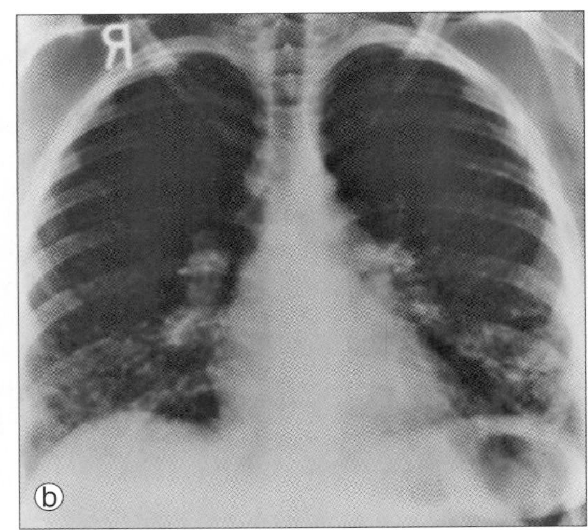

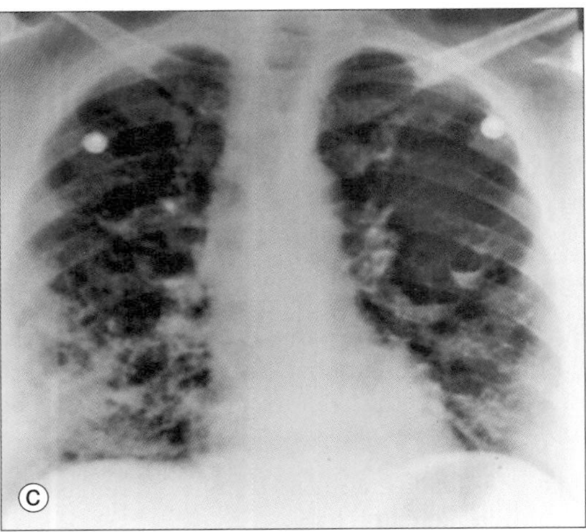

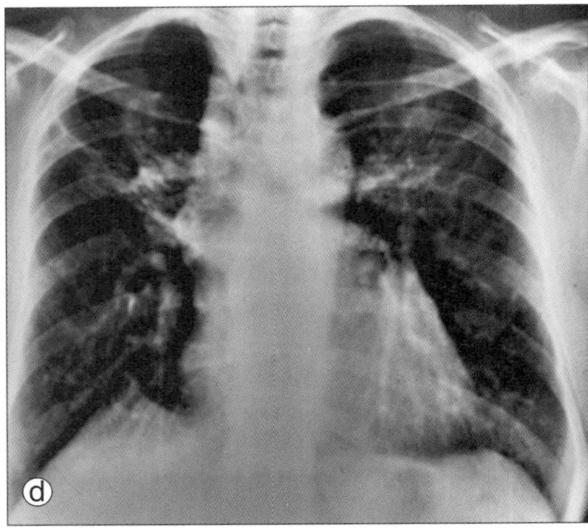

Figure 45.4 Chest radiograph stages of sarcoidosis. A, Stage I sarcoidosis with bilateral hilar and right paratracheal adenopathy. **B,** Stage II sarcoidosis with bilateral hilar adenopathy and reticulonodular infiltrates. **C,** Stage III sarcoidosis with bilateral infiltrates without adenopathy. Multiple cystic areas are also seen, which could lead to a classification of stage IV disease. **D,** Stage IV fibrocystic sarcoidosis with typical upward hilar retraction and large cystic and bullous changes.

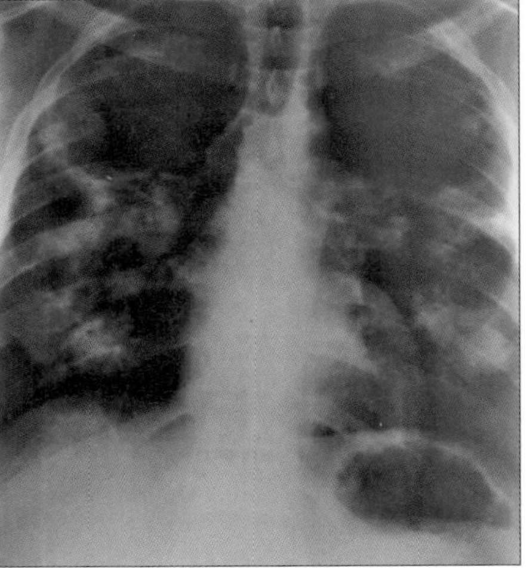

Figure 45.5 Nodular sarcoidosis with multiple bilateral pulmonary nodules.

malignancy (Fig. 45.5). Less commonly a miliary pattern is seen, suggestive of tuberculosis. Occasionally, a pattern with patchy areas of air-space consolidation and air bronchograms, termed *alveolar sarcoidosis*, is seen and may simulate infection, malignancy, eosinophilic pneumonia, or Wegener's granulomatosis (Fig. 45.6). Mycetomas are mobile fungus balls that colonize preexisting cystic spaces in fibrocystic sarcoidosis (Fig. 45.7).

Although pleural effusions have been reported in less than 1% to 3% of chest radiographs, evidence that sarcoidosis involvement is the direct cause is usually not present. Rigorous exclusion of more common causes of pleural effusions (heart failure, infection, pulmonary embolism) is mandatory. Pleural fluid from sarcoidosis has been reported to be either transudative or exudative, and the latter effusions usually contain predominantly lymphocytes on cell differential. Pneumothorax is rare and usually occurs in the context of fibrocystic disease. Pleural thickening occurs in fibrocystic sarcoidosis, often prior to the development of mycetomas (Fig. 45.8).

Pulmonary Function Tests

Pulmonary function tests have only a modest correlation with the chest radiograph. Such tests are normal in about 80% of patients who have stage I chest radiographs; others may have only an isolated reduction in diffusing capacity for carbon monoxide (DLCO). When pulmonary infiltrates are present on the chest radiograph, restrictive impairment with reduction in lung volumes, forced vital capacity (FVC), and forced expiratory volume in 1 second (FEV_1) is found in 40% to 70% of cases. The DLCO is also frequently reduced in conjunction with restrictive impairment but can occur as an isolated deficit. However, FVC, FEV_1, and DLCO may be normal in patients who have pulmonary infiltrates.

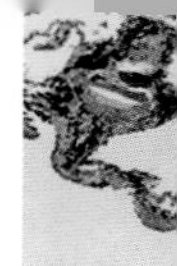

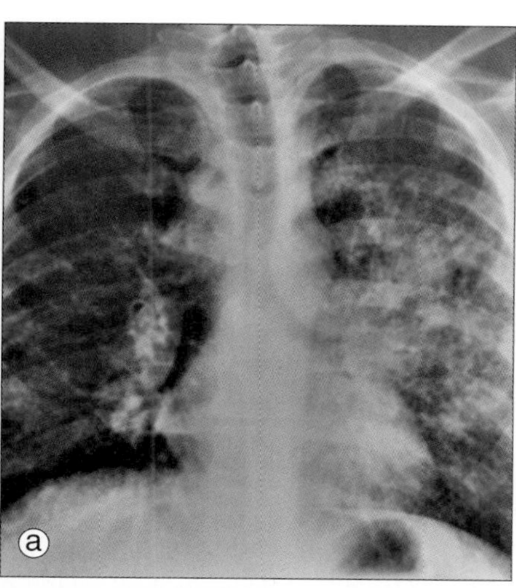

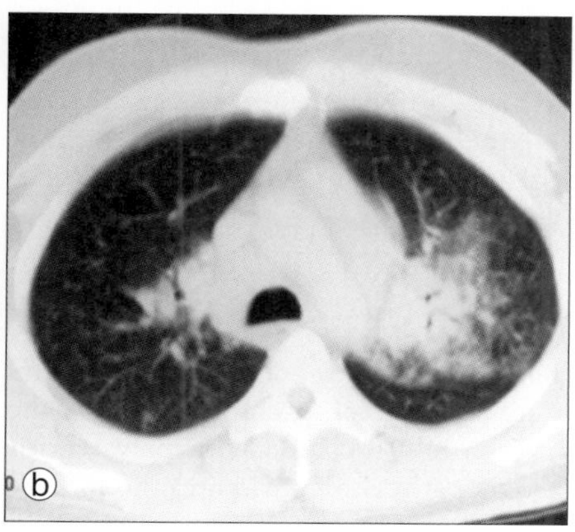

Figure 45.6 Stage II sarcoidosis. A, Chest x-ray film showing extensive alveolar and interstitial infiltrates, predominantly on the left side. Air bronchograms and extensive hilar and right paratracheal adenopathy are seen. **B,** Chest CT demonstrates a consolidated, nodular appearance of the infiltrates, which involve the central portion of the lung along bronchovascular bundles. Air bronchograms and extensive adenopathy are also clearly seen. Because this patient had prominent fevers, weight loss, and respiratory symptoms for less than 2 months, mediastinoscopy was performed to rule out malignancy or infection. Lymph node biopsy was consistent with sarcoidosis.

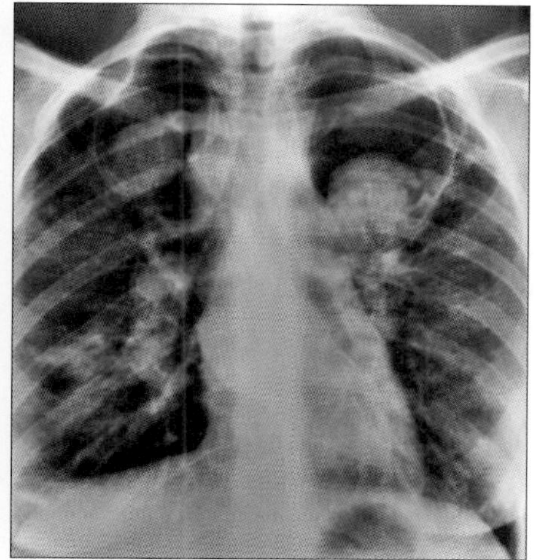

Figure 45.7 Fibrocystic sarcoidosis demonstrating bilateral upper lobe mycetomas (aspergillomas) in pre-existing cystic lesions.

Obstructive impairment is present in greater than 30% to 50% of patients. Reduced FEV_1/FVC ratios, increased upstream airway resistance (Raw), and positive tests for small-airway obstruction may be found in patients with any stage of chest radiograph. Tests for bronchial hyper-reactivity are positive in 0% to 30% of patients. Obstructive impairment is most often severe in advanced fibrocystic sarcoidosis. Gas exchange is usually preserved until extensive fibrocystic changes are evident, in contrast to idiopathic pulmonary fibrosis, in which hypoxemia tends to be found early in the disease. With severe parenchymal involvement (stages III and IV), reduced FEV_1 from both restrictive and obstructive impairment, reduced diffusing capacity, and abnormal gas exchange are typical. Carbon dioxide retention is rare, except in advanced fibrocystic disease and cor pulmonale.

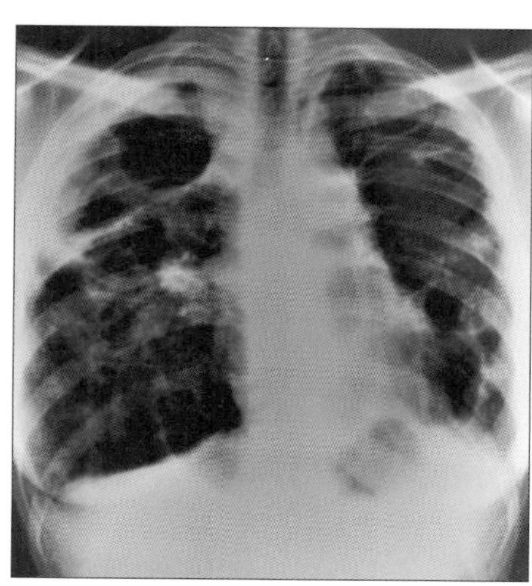

Figure 45.8 Fibrocystic sarcoidosis with marked pleural thickening of the right upper lobe that presaged development of an aspergilloma.

Computed Tomography of the Chest

Computed tomography (CT) scans of the chest demonstrate enlarged lymph nodes and pulmonary infiltrates with more sensitivity than plain chest radiographs. Pretracheal, paratracheal, para-aortic, and subcarinal adenopathy (in addition to bilateral hilar adenopathy) may be seen even when not apparent on plain chest radiographs. High-resolution, thin-section CT typically demonstrates nodular infiltrates that follow central bronchovascular structures (see Fig. 45.6B). Lymphangitic carcinomatosis also follows a bronchovascular distribution and must be considered in the differential diagnosis. Occasionally, alveolar infiltrates (with or without air bronchograms), miliary infiltrates, ground-glass opacities, or distinct, larger-sized nodules are clearly visualized on CT scan. Similar to plain chest radiography, CT scans correlate poorly with functional impairment.

Necrotizing Sarcoid Granulomatosis

Often considered a variant of sarcoidosis, this disease is characterized by large, confluent, noncaseating granulomas associated with a granulomatous vasculitis that involves both arteries and veins. Systemic vasculitis is not present. Patients may be asymptomatic or have cough, dyspnea, fever, chest pain, or constitutional symptoms. Chest radiographs typically demonstrate multiple, usually noncavitating, nodules (Fig. 45.9). Surprisingly, the prognosis is good, with spontaneous remission or a rapid response to corticosteroid therapy occurring in most cases.

Extrapulmonary Sarcoidosis

Although pulmonary symptoms are the most common initial complaint, many patients have clinically important involvement of one or more organ systems, either with or without pulmonary sarcoidosis (Table 45.3). The recent ACCESS study found that African Americans more frequently demonstrated extrathoracic lymphadenopathy and eye, liver, skin (other than

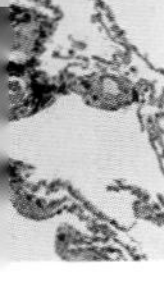

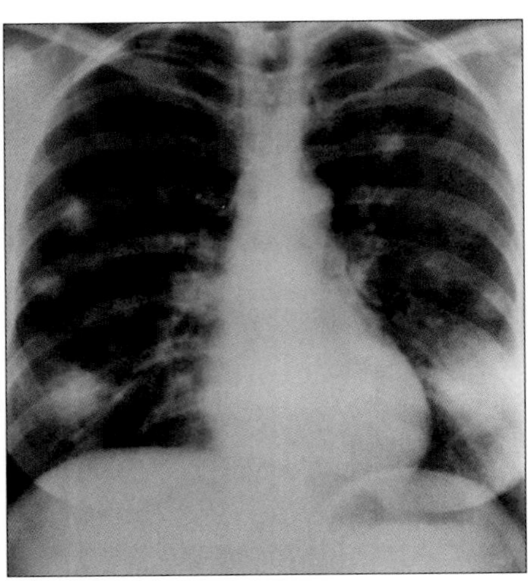

Figure 45.9 Necrotizing sarcoid granulomatosis in a patient with pleuritic chest pain, fevers, and mild dyspnea. Nodular infiltrates may simulate malignancy, classic sarcoidosis, Wegener's granulomatosis, or infections. The diagnosis was confirmed by open lung biopsy.

Table 45.3
Recommended tests for an initial evaluation of sarcoidosis

Chest radiograph	**Liver function tests**
Pulmonary function tests	Alkaline phosphatase Aspartate aminotransferase Alanine aminotransferase Total and indirect bilirubin
Spirometry Diffusing capacity of lung for carbon monoxide Lung volumes	**Calcium level**
Renal function tests	**Extrapulmonary organ-specific tests (for symptomatic organ involvement)**
Blood urea nitrogen Creatinine Urinalysis	Neurosarcoidosis – magnetic resonance imaging with gadolinium enhancement, cerebral spinal fluid examination, nerve conduction studies
Ophthalmologic (slit lamp) examination	
Electrocardiogram	Cardiac sarcoidosis – Holter monitor, 2D-echocardiogram, Thallium-201 myocardial imaging
Purified protein derivative skin test	

erythema nodosum), and bone marrow involvement than whites, whereas calcium metabolism abnormalities were more frequent in the latter group.

Sarcoidosis of the Upper Respiratory Tract

Sarcoidosis of the upper respiratory tract occurs in approximately 10% of patients, usually in those with long-standing disease. The mucosa of the nasal septum and inferior turbinates, overlying skin, nasal bone, nasopharyngeal mucosa, and laryngeal structures may be involved. Typical presenting signs and symptoms include nasal congestion, dizziness, crusting, epistaxis, anosmia, or rhinorrhea. Nasal congestion may be severe and unresponsive to decongestants and topical corticosteroids. Nasal septal perforation, a "saddle-nose" deformity, or palatal perforation may occur, particularly in patients who have had previous submucous resections. Sarcoidosis may affect the maxillary, ethmoid, and sphenoid sinuses, which may lead to obstruction and sinusitis. Direct invasion into contiguous bone may be seen on CT scan or magnetic resonance imaging (MRI).

Laryngeal Sarcoidosis

Laryngeal sarcoidosis is an uncommon manifestation of sarcoidosis, occurring in less than 1% to 5% of patients, and rarely as the sole manifestation of disease. Presenting signs usually include hoarseness or dysphonia, dysphagia, or dyspnea. Less frequently, stridor and acute respiratory failure secondary to upper airway obstruction may occur, requiring urgent tracheostomy. Physical signs of laryngeal sarcoidosis include edema, diffuse thickening, and nodules of laryngeal structures. Frequently, laryngeal sarcoidosis and nasal sarcoidosis are associated with chronic skin lesions, particularly lupus pernio.

Ocular Sarcoidosis

Anterior uveitis is the most common presenting eye lesion, may be unilateral or bilateral, and is usually associated with bilateral hilar adenopathy. Chronic uveitis occurs in as many as 20% of patients who have chronic sarcoidosis, more frequently in African-American populations. Other manifestations include posterior uveitis, granulomatous conjunctivitis, and severe chorioretinitis or optic neuritis; the latter conditions may occur acutely with blindness.

Cutaneous Sarcoidosis

Erythema nodosum is characterized by tender, reddish nodules that are several centimeters in diameter, usually located on the lower extremities. When seen in association with polyarthritis and bilateral hilar lymphadenopathy, Löfgren syndrome may be diagnosed. Chronic skin sarcoidosis usually manifests as plaques and subcutaneous nodules that have a propensity to involve the skin around the hairline, eyelids, ears, nose, mouth, and extensor surfaces of the arms and legs. Lesions in the scalp are sometimes associated with alopecia. Skin lesions may be either hyperpigmented or hypopigmented and are usually nontender and nonpruritic. Lupus pernio is a particularly disfiguring form of cutaneous sarcoid of the face, with violaceous plaques and nodules that cover the nose, nasal alae, malar areas, and areas around the eyes. Chronic skin lesions appear more common and severe in the African-American population.

Cardiac Sarcoidosis

Cardiac sarcoidosis appears to be more common in Japan than in other parts of the world; one autopsy series from Japan demonstrated cardiac sarcoidosis in almost 50% of cases, whereas 27% of cases were found to have cardiac involvement in a series from Baltimore. In North America and Europe, cardiac sarcoidosis is clinically apparent in approximately 5% patients who have sarcoidosis. Most patients present with either cardiomyopathy or conduction abnormalities with heart block or ventricular arrhythmias. Valvular dysfunction, pericardial disease, or a process that mimics myocardial infarction are less frequently seen. Sudden death from cardiac sarcoidosis is a major cause of mortality in young adults with sarcoidosis, primarily from heart block or arrhythmias. Extensive involvement of the myocardium can lead to progressive congestive heart failure and is responsible for most of the other deaths related to cardiac sarcoidosis.

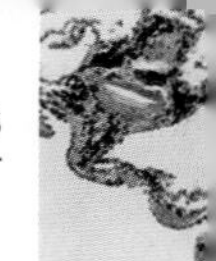

Hepatic Sarcoidosis

Noncaseating granulomas are found by percutaneous biopsy in 40% to 70% of patients, but clinical manifestations are seen in less than 10% of cases. Symptomatic hepatic sarcoidosis often manifests with fever and tender hepatomegaly. Pruritus can be severe and disabling in a small number of patients. Characteristically, the serum alkaline phosphatase and γ-glutamyl transferase are elevated proportionately higher than aspartate aminotransferase, alanine aminotransferase, and bilirubin, although all patterns can be seen. Hepatic sarcoidosis may mimic primary biliary cirrhosis, except that antimitochondrial antibodies are absent.

Joints and Bones

Arthralgias are common in active multisystem sarcoidosis. Acute, often incapacitating, migratory polyarthritis is seen in Löfgren syndrome. In such instances, joint radiographs are negative, and the arthritis usually regresses within weeks to several months with or without therapy. Persistent joint disease is found in less than 5% of patients who have chronic sarcoidosis. Pain, swelling, and tenderness of the phalanges of the hands and feet are most common. Joint radiographs may demonstrate "punched-out" lesions with cystic changes and marked loss of trabeculae, but with no evidence of erosive chondritis. Cystic lesions of the long bones, pelvis, sternum, skull, and vertebrae rarely occur.

Neurosarcoidosis

Neurosarcoidosis occurs in 5% to 10% of patients who have sarcoidosis. The most common manifestation is cranial neuropathy, with bilateral or unilateral seventh nerve (Bell's) palsy seen in 50% to 70% of cases. Cranial neuropathies may resolve spontaneously or with corticosteroids and rarely recur years later. Optic neuritis, the second most common cranial neuropathy in sarcoidosis, can result in blurred vision, field defects, and blindness. Less commonly, involvement of the glossopharyngeal, auditory, oculomotor, trigeminal, or other cranial nerves occurs. Manifestations of central nervous system (CNS) involvement include mass lesions, aseptic meningitis, obstructive hydrocephalus, and hypothalamic and/or pituitary dysfunction. Seizures, headache, change in mental status, confusion, and diabetes insipidus may be presenting symptoms. Spinal cord involvement is rare, but quadriparesis, paraparesis, hemiparesis, back and leg pains, and dysesthesias have been described. Peripheral neuropathies account for about 15% of cases of neurosarcoidosis, and often manifest as mononeuritis multiplex or a primary sensory neuropathy. One recent study suggested small-fiber neuropathy is frequent in sarcoidosis and a potential cause of diffuse pain and dysesthesias.

Salivary, Parotid, and Lacrimal Gland Sarcoidosis

Heerfordt syndrome, also called *uveoparotid fever,* manifests as fever, parotid and lacrimal gland enlargement, uveitis, and bilateral hilar adenopathy. This uncommon presentation of acute sarcoidosis may be associated with cranial neuropathies, usually facial palsy.

Hematologic Sarcoidosis

Peripheral lymph-node enlargement occurs in 20% to 30% of patients as an early manifestation of sarcoidosis, but this typically undergoes spontaneous remission. Chronic bulky lymphadenopathy occurs less than 10% of the time. Splenomegaly, occasionally massive, occurs in less than 5% of cases. Hypersplenism with anemia and thrombocytopenia are rare and should be investigated for alternative causes. Peripheral leukopenia in sarcoidosis is common, usually as a result of $CD4^+$ lymphopenia from altered trafficking of lymphocytes rather than splenic trapping. Splenomegaly is often associated with hepatomegaly and, less frequently, with hypercalcemia in a characteristic triad that may present without pulmonary involvement. Nonclonal hypergammaglobulinemia is present in 25% or more of patients. Occasionally, common-variable immunodeficiency is found in association with sarcoidosis and should be suspected in the presence of recurrent pulmonary or sinus infections and splenomegaly. Cutaneous anergy to recall antigens for tuberculin, mumps, and *Candida* species is characteristic of patients who have sarcoidosis; the mechanisms underlying this phenomena are unknown.

Sarcoidosis Myopathy

Although random muscle biopsies in autopsy series demonstrate muscle granulomas in a majority of patients who have sarcoidosis, symptomatic myopathy with weakness and tenderness is uncommon. Rarely, sarcoidosis can manifest as a polymyositis with profound weakness and elevated serum creatine kinase and aldolase. Fibromyalgia may be associated with sarcoidosis; this condition is not thought to result from direct granulomatous inflammation of the muscle, because it does not respond to anti-inflammatory therapy.

Hypercalcemia, Hypercalciuria, and Renal Disease

Hypercalcemia is present in 2% to 5% of patients; hypercalciuria is more common. Abnormal calcium regulation is thought to result from an increased conversion of 1-hydroxyvitamin D_3 to the active 1,25-dihydroxyvitamin D_3 by macrophages and epithelioid cells from the granulomas. Chronic hypercalcemia or hypercalciuria most commonly manifests as kidney stones. Renal failure from chronic, often asymptomatic, nephrocalcinosis may result if left undetected. Granulomatous involvement of the kidneys is uncommon and usually not a cause of renal failure. Nephrotic syndrome and chronic membranous glomerulonephritis are also associated with sarcoidosis.

Psychosocial Aspects

A Dutch study found the prevalence of depression was 4% in asymptomatic patients and 30% in symptomatic patients with sarcoidosis. The prevalence of depression was found to be 60% in a U.S. study of both white and African-American patients with sarcoidosis and was associated with female sex, lower socioeconomic status, poor access to care, and increased disease severity, but not race. Although the data are limited, there is increasing recognition of the need to treat depression to improve the overall health of patients with sarcoidosis.

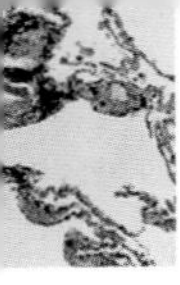

DIAGNOSIS

An initial diagnostic evaluation of a patient who possibly has sarcoidosis consists of tests to evaluate the presence and extent of pulmonary involvement and to screen for extrathoracic disease (Table 45.3). The chest radiograph is an important starting point, because it is abnormal in over 90% to 95% of known cases of sarcoidosis and carries prognostic implications. Spirometry, diffusing capacity, and lung volume testing are used to detect the presence and extent of parenchymal lung involvement. Flow-volume curves are indicated when laryngeal or upper airway obstruction is possible. Arterial blood gas measurement is not routinely needed unless evidence of moderate or severe pulmonary impairment is found. Oxygen saturation and exercise studies (e.g., 6-minute walk) may help to determine subtle changes in pulmonary involvement in response to treatment or the need for supplemental oxygen, but are not needed for most patients initially. An initial slit-lamp examination is recommended in all cases to exclude uveitis, which may be clinically silent. Blood testing is performed to exclude significant hepatic, renal, or hematologic involvement. An electrocardiogram is indicated to detect evidence of arrhythmias or heart block from possible cardiac sarcoidosis. A purified protein derivative skin test should be performed to help exclude tuberculosis.

Chest CT is not routinely needed in the evaluation of patients who are suspected to have pulmonary sarcoidosis. Occasionally, CT is useful to define the pattern of hilar or mediastinal adenopathy to assist the bronchoscopic needle biopsy of mediastinal lymph nodes. Chest CT may also help to define the extent of fibrocystic disease or unusual radiographic features, such as masses, bronchial or tracheal stenosis, atelectasis, or bronchiectasis.

Diagnostic Approach

A diagnosis of sarcoidosis is based on a compatible clinical picture, histologic evidence of noncaseating granulomas, and the absence of other known causes of this pathologic response. There is no pathognomonic histology that enables a definitive diagnosis of sarcoidosis. The presence of compatible multiorgan involvement increases the likelihood of sarcoidosis. The need to exclude alternate diagnoses increases as the clinical manifestations deviate from those usual for sarcoidosis. Tuberculosis, fungal diseases, and lymphoma are usually the most important diseases to be excluded in patients who have chest disease. Chronic beryllium disease, hypersensitivity pneumonitis, and drug reactions must be excluded when the history suggests these possibilities. In the absence of defined multiorgan disease, a diagnosis of sarcoidosis is presumed, because local "sarcoid" reactions may occur in response to infection, tumor, or foreign material.

In general, the easiest accessible biopsy site is used for biopsy confirmation. Biopsy of a skin nodule, superficial lymph node, lacrimal gland, nasal mucosae, conjunctivae, or salivary gland (lip biopsy) can often be used to establish a diagnosis. Biopsy of these sites is generally performed only if the tissue is abnormal, because blind biopsies are usually unhelpful. Biopsy of the liver or bone marrow is nonspecific and is used to support a diagnosis of sarcoidosis only after malignancy and infectious granulomatous diseases or other competing diagnoses have been excluded. When superficial abnormalities are not apparent or when infectious or malignant chest disease should be excluded, bronchoscopic biopsy is usually performed.

Biopsy confirmation of sarcoidosis is usually not necessary in Löfgren syndrome. An exception to this recommendation may exist in regions in which histoplasmosis is endemic, such as the Mississippi Valley, where some authorities recommend routine bronchoscopy to exclude infection, particularly before corticosteroid therapy is initiated.

The need for tissue confirmation of asymptomatic bilateral hilar adenopathy is unclear. In one classic study, over 95% of asymptomatic individuals who had bilateral hilar adenopathy and a normal physical examination and laboratory tests had sarcoidosis. Those patients with erythema nodosum or uveitis also were diagnosed with sarcoidosis. Patients with bilateral hilar adenopathy from malignant disease were all symptomatic or had an abnormal physical examination. Based on this study, many authorities suggest that histologic confirmation is not needed for asymptomatic patients who have bilateral hilar adenopathy and normal physical examinations and laboratory tests. However, some authorities favor biopsy in all cases of bilateral hilar adenopathy to exclude with certainty the possibility of lymphoma, particularly if the adenopathy is asymmetrical, massive, or associated with symptoms.

Bronchoscopy

Biopsy by fiberoptic bronchoscopy is now the most frequent procedure used to diagnose pulmonary sarcoidosis because of its relative safety and high yield. The yield of transbronchial biopsy approaches 90% when pulmonary infiltrates are seen radiographically and at least 4 to 6 transbronchial biopsy specimens are taken (Fig. 45.10). Studies suggest the yield may approach 50% with stage I chest radiographs, although the absence of infiltrates on chest CT significantly reduces this yield. Recently, several studies emphasized the utility of an endobronchial biopsy, which is safer than a transbronchial biopsy. Endobronchial biopsy directed to abnormal airways (nodularity, mucosal edema, hypervascularity) has a greater than 50% positive yield (Fig. 45.11). In the absence of visual abnormalities, the yield of endobronchial biopsy may approach 30% to 50%. When endobronchial biopsy is used together with transbronchial biopsy, the yield increases beyond that of either technique alone. Extensive fibrocystic sarcoidosis has a low yield because of extensive parenchyma fibrosis and distorted airways.

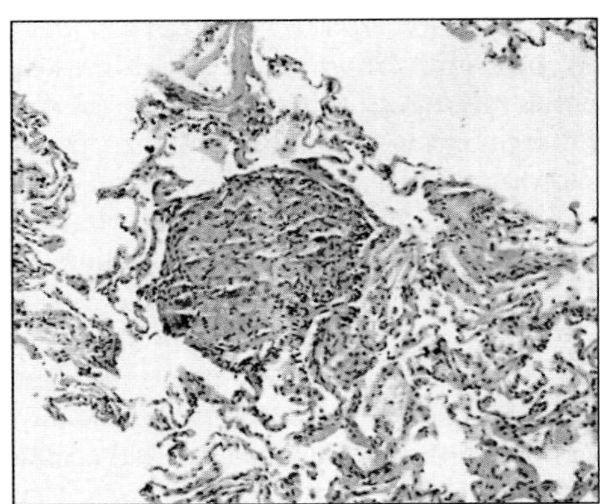

Figure 45.10 Epithelioid granuloma in a transbronchial biopsy from a patient with sarcoidosis.

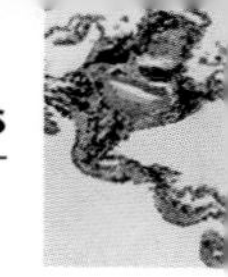

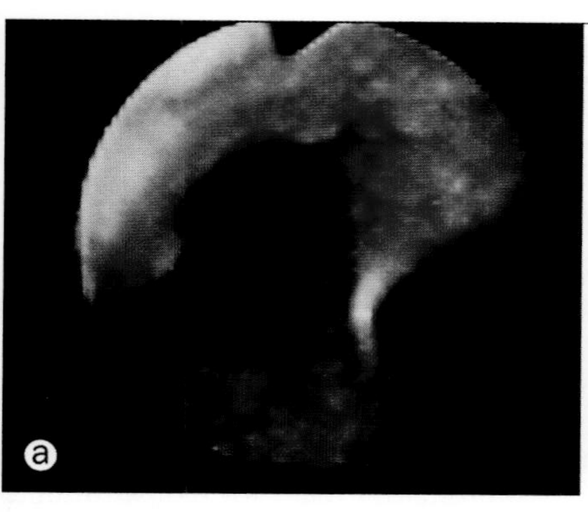

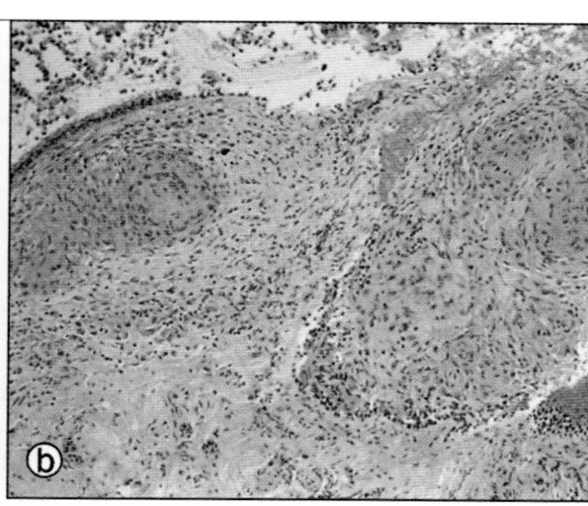

Figure 45.11 Endobronchial sarcoidosis.
A, Bronchoscopic view shows extensive nodularity of bronchial mucosa, that is, "cobblestoning" of the airway. Rarely, Wegener's granulomatosis, tuberculosis, or fungal disease demonstrates similar airway abnormalities.
B, Endobronchial biopsy demonstrating several granulomas and giant cells beneath bronchiolar epithelium.

Transbronchial needle aspiration (TBNA) increases the yield of bronchoscopy by sampling enlarged mediastinal lymph nodes. In expert hands, the yield of TBNA may exceed 80% in patients with stage I chest radiographs and slightly increases the overall 90% yield of bronchoscopy in stage II disease (when used together with transbronchial biopsy). Advantages of this procedure include a lower incidence of bleeding and pneumothorax than in transbronchial biopsy, although expertise in the technique is required.

Mediastinoscopy

Mediastinoscopy is rarely required to establish a diagnosis of sarcoidosis, but it is considered for cases in which lymphoma or other intrathoracic malignancy cannot be reasonably excluded. For example, mediastinoscopy may be indicated when there is an unusual radiographic pattern or asymmetrical or marked enlargement of hilar or mediastinal adenopathy, even with a positive bronchoscopic biopsy (see Fig. 45.6A). Given the yield of bronchoscopy and mediastinoscopy, thoracoscopic or open lung biopsy is usually not needed to establish a diagnosis of sarcoidosis.

Specialized Testing

Specialized testing is indicated when symptoms or signs suggest extrapulmonary involvement.

CARDIAC SARCOIDOSIS

In the presence of cardiac symptoms, a two-dimensional (2D) echocardiogram, Holter monitor, and often a gated thallium-201 mycocardial scan are used to evaluate for the presence of cardiac sarcoidosis. In cardiac sarcoidosis, a 2D echocardiogram may demonstrate abnormal myocardial wall motion, reduced left ventricular ejection fraction, valvular abnormalities, or evidence of pulmonary hypertension. Radionuclide imaging with gated thallium-201 scanning may show segmental areas of decreased uptake that correspond to areas involved with granulomatous inflammation or fibrosis. During exercise, the magnitude of these defects tends to decrease or remain fixed if related to sarcoidosis, but worsen with ischemic disease. A Holter monitor is used to detect serious conduction system abnormalities. Even in the absence of serious arrhythmias on Holter monitoring, electrophysiologic testing may be indicated to detect the presence of serious, inducible arrhythmias if suspicion remains that sarcoidosis-related cardiac arrhythmias are present. Other tests that have been used to detect myocardial abnormalities in sarcoidosis include gallium scanning, cardiac MRI, and positron emission tomography (PET) scanning. These tests are nonspecific, and their sensitivity remains uncertain. A diagnosis of cardiac sarcoidosis is usually made within the context of a compatible clinical picture in a patient with sarcoidosis confirmed by biopsy of a site other than the heart. Endomyocardial biopsy is an established diagnostic tool but is positive in less than 20% of cases because of inhomogeneities of the granulomatous inflammation and sampling inefficiencies (see Fig. 45.1D); thus, a negative biopsy never excludes the diagnosis.

NEUROSARCOIDOSIS

When CNS or spinal cord sarcoidosis is considered, MRI with gadolinium enhancement is now considered the optimal test to detect characteristic inflammatory lesions that have a propensity for periventricular and leptomeningeal areas. CT of the head with contrast enhancement is a less sensitive test in those who cannot undergo MRI. The images from both MRI and CT are nonspecific and can be produced by infectious disease (tuberculosis, fungal disease), malignant disease (lymphoma, carcinomatosis), or demyelinating disease. A normal scan does not exclude neurosarcoidosis, particularly for cranial neuropathies or if corticosteroid therapy is being used. Cerebral spinal fluid (CSF) examination provides useful data in neurosarcoidosis; characteristic findings include lymphocytic pleocytosis, elevated protein levels, and, in less than 50% of cases, elevated ACE concentration. Most patients who have neurosarcoidosis provide an abnormal chest radiograph that leads to consideration of this diagnosis. A diagnosis is usually confirmed by biopsy of a non-CNS site, generally a bronchoscopic or lymph node biopsy. In some patients there is no clinical evidence of sarcoidosis involvement outside the CNS. In this situation, MRI, PET, or gallium scanning may be used to search for an appropriate biopsy site to confirm a diagnosis. Rarely, brain biopsy is needed to exclude infectious or malignant disease. In cases of peripheral neuropathy, nerve conduction studies and peripheral nerve biopsy may be indicated.

Other Diagnostic Studies

BRONCHOALVEOLAR LAVAGE

Landmark studies in the early 1980s established that active pulmonary sarcoidosis in nonsmokers is usually characterized by a marked increase in the proportion of lymphocytes recovered by

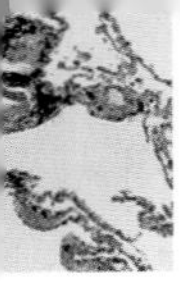

BAL (20% to 50%, compared with less than 10% lymphocytes in healthy controls; see Fig. 45-2). In more than 90% of cases, BAL lymphocytosis is typified by a dominance of $CD4^+$ T cells in contrast to the $CD8^+$ BAL lymphocytosis seen in patients who have hypersensitivity pneumonitis, viral infections, and many drug reactions. Studies show that elevated $CD4^+$ BAL lymphocytosis or an elevated CD4/CD8 BAL ratio is not sufficiently specific to establish a diagnosis of sarcoidosis, however.

SERUM ANGIOTENSIN-CONVERTING ENZYME

Levels of serum ACE (SACE) are elevated in 40% to 90% of patients with clinically active disease. This protein has been detected in sarcoid granulomas, BAL fluid, tears, and CSF. The likely source is activated epithelioid cells and macrophages at sites of inflammation. Elevated SACE levels are found in other granulomatous diseases, however (e.g., chronic beryllium disease, fungal and mycobacterial disease, silicosis, leprosy, extrinsic allergic alveolitis, Hodgkin's disease), and in some non-granulomatous conditions (e.g., Gaucher's disease, hyperthyroidism, hepatic cirrhosis, and diabetes mellitus). The lack of specificity for sarcoidosis limits its utility for diagnosis.

SPECIAL IMAGING STUDIES

Gallium-67 scans often demonstrate enhanced uptake in the lungs and mediastinal lymph node area in patients who have active pulmonary sarcoidosis, but the pattern is nonspecific and can persist for years after regression of active pulmonary disease. One study suggests that the combination of a lambda sign (highlighting of bilateral hilar and right paratracheal adenopathy) and panda sign (uptake in the parotid, lacrimal, and salivary glands) is highly specific for sarcoidosis. Occasionally, a gallium scan may be used to search a potential biopsy site of an inflammatory focus. With this possible exception, the lack of specificity, the cost, and the considerable radiation exposure with this test have led most clinicians to abandon its use in sarcoidosis.

More recently, MRI with gadolinium enhancement (to improve sensitivity) has been used to detect organ involvement, particularly of the CNS, spinal cord, heart, muscle, and bones. PET scanning frequently demonstrates increased activity at sites of granulomatous inflammation. Both of these techniques are non-specific and may reveal clinically inapparent inflammation. These imaging techniques may, however, be used to localize a potential biopsy site for diagnosis. Both procedures may also help assess response to therapy, although further studies are needed to better define their utility in the management of sarcoidosis.

TREATMENT

Corticosteroids are the cornerstone of therapy for serious or progressive pulmonary or extrapulmonary sarcoidosis (Table 45.4). Guidelines for when to initiate therapy are formulated on the basis of different patterns of organ involvement and disease progression. A decision to treat is tempered and complicated by the fact that a majority of patients undergo spontaneous remission. Early treatment is indicated for serious pulmonary or extrapulmonary disease. Although the overall effectiveness of corticosteroids in altering the long-term course of the disease is not proven (see later discussion), it is clear that corticosteroids acutely provide symptomatic relief and reverse organ dysfunction in more than 90% of patients who have symptomatic pulmonary disease. The optimal doses and duration of corticosteroid treatment have not been established by rigorous clinical studies. Corticosteroid-sparing agents are used when corticosteroid therapy is not tolerated or is ineffective; their benefit has also not been established by controlled clinical trials. Nonetheless, there is widespread agreement on the basic treatment principles outlined in the following sections.

Löfgren Syndrome

Bed rest and nonsteroidal anti-inflammatory drugs (NSAIDs) are recommended for symptomatic relief of constitutional symptoms and joint pains. Corticosteroids are almost immediately effective but are recommended only in cases in which symptoms are disabling and unresponsive to NSAIDs. Generally, the corticosteroids can be tapered over a few weeks to months without recrudescence of symptoms.

Pulmonary Sarcoidosis

Indications for observation are as follows:

- Asymptomatic patients who have normal lung function
- Patients who have minimal symptoms and mild functional abnormalities until disease progression

Indications for treatment are as follows:

- Moderate or severe symptomatic pulmonary disease
- Progressive symptomatic pulmonary disease
- Persistent pulmonary infiltrates or abnormal lung function for 1 to 2 years with mild symptoms (to assess reversibility)

CORTICOSTEROIDS

Initial treatment of pulmonary sarcoidosis with corticosteroids usually does not require more than prednisone 30 to 40 mg/day. Higher doses are rarely needed. A recommended regimen for treating pulmonary sarcoidosis with corticosteroids is outlined in Table 45.4. Treatment should ordinarily be continued for a minimum of 8 to 12 months, because premature tapering is likely to result in relapse of disease. A maintenance dose of prednisone 5 to 15 mg/day is usually sufficient to suppress persistent pulmonary disease. Alternate-day therapy (e.g., 10 to 30 mg every other day) is suggested by some investigators, although such a regimen may not be effective in a subgroup of patients who respond to daily dosing, and compliance may be more difficult. Intermittent attempts to taper corticosteroids are appropriate in the first several years of treatment, but those patients who have repetitive relapses usually require indefinite suppressive therapy. Patients with advanced fibrocystic disease often have only a modest or no improvement in lung function because of the presence of irreversible fibrosis. A maintenance dose (e.g., prednisone 10 to 20 mg/day) is usually indicated, however, to prevent or slow further progression of respiratory insufficiency, because open lung biopsies or "explants" from lung transplant patients usually show active granulomatous inflammation in patients with fibrocystic disease.

Low-dose corticosteroid therapy is usually well tolerated. The most common complaint is weight gain. Patients are instructed early in the treatment about caloric and salt restriction to minimize this effect. Insomnia and euphoria may also

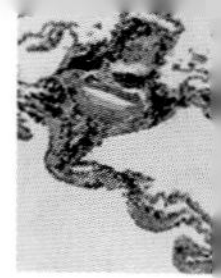

Table 45.4
Treatment of sarcoidosis

Drug group and indications	Specific drug	Dosage and duration	Side effects
Corticosteroids for pulmonary or systemic sarcoidosis	Prednisone	Initial regimen: 40 mg q24h for 2 weeks 30 mg q24h for 2 weeks 25 mg q24h for 2 weeks 20 mg q24h for 2 weeks 10-15 mg q24h for 6–8 months Taper to 2.5 mg every 2–4 weeks; if relapse, reinstitute lowest prior effective dose	Increased appetite, weight gain Cushingoid habitus Hyperglycemia Adrenal axis suppression Emotional lability, depression Psychosis, pseudotumor cerebri Hypertension Sodium, fluid retention Glaucoma, cataracts Osteoporosis, osteonecrosis Compression fractures Myopathy Pancreatitis Striae, easy bruisability, acne
Antimalarials for mucocutaneous sarcoidosis	Chloroquine phosphate	500 mg q24h for 2 weeks then 500 mg q48h for 6 months followed by 6-month drug-free period	Retinopathy Gastrointestinal upset Headache Discoloration of nailbeds Reversible dermatitis
	Hydroxychloroquine sulfate	200 mg q12h or q24h, may be given indefinitely	Retinopathy (rare) Gastrointestinal symptoms Dermatitis
Alternative therapies for			
Mild disease or as corticosteroid-sparing agent	Pentoxifylline	400 mg q6h or q8h, may be given indefinitely	Gastrointestinal upset Headache
Severe, refractory sarcoidosis and as corticosteroid-sparing agent	Azathioprine	50 mg q24h for 2 weeks Increase by 50mg every 2–4 weeks Maximum suggested: 150–200 mg q24h	Bone marrow suppression Hepatic toxicity Gastrointestinal toxicity Carcinogenicity Opportunistic infections
	Methotrexate	10–20 mg once a week plus folic acid 1 mg/day	Hepatic toxicity Gastrointestinal toxicity Pulmonary toxicity (hypersensitivity pneumonitis) Bone marrow suppression Opportunistic infections
Experimental	Doxycycline Minocycline	200 mg/day 200 mg/day	Photosensitivity Gastrointestinal upset
	Thalidomide	100-150 qhs	Teratogenicity Peripheral neuropathy Sedation Skin reactions
	Infliximab	Infusion	Infusion reactions Opportunistic infections Tuberculosis/fungal infections, serious infections, sepsis Hypersensitivity reactions
	Etanercept	Injection	Injection site reactions serious infections, sepsis, death Gastrointestinal upset CNS demyelination disorders

occur; psychosis is rare but can occur with higher doses. Glaucoma is a potential complication of long-term corticosteroid therapy (or chronic ocular sarcoidosis). Osteoporosis and osteonecrosis are potential complications in patients treated with chronic corticosteroid therapy. Use of supplemental calcium to delay these complications should be carefully monitored; vitamin D supplementation is generally not recommended to avoid the potential for hypercalcemia and hypercalciuria. Bisphosphonate therapy is often used in patients receiving maintenance corticosteroid therapy, particularly when bone density scanning demonstrates reduced bone density. Although clinical experience suggests these drugs are beneficial,

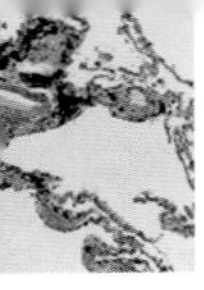

clinical trials with sarcoidosis are lacking. Although reports of *Pneumocystis pneumonia* are rare in sarcoidosis, with doses exceeding 20 mg/day, prophylaxis against *Pneumocystis* is reasonable.

INHALED CORTICOSTEROIDS

Inhaled corticosteroids may help to reduce the cough and airway irritability seen with endobronchial sarcoidosis. A role for inhaled corticosteroids in the treatment of parenchymal pulmonary sarcoidosis is uncertain, as most studies have failed to demonstrate significant improvement in lung function or chest radiographs in patients with stage II or III disease. Whether potent inhaled corticosteroids will find a place as systemic corticosteroid-sparing agents, particularly in mild disease, remains uncertain.

OTHER TREATMENTS

Supportive management of patients who have advanced fibrocystic sarcoidosis and cor pulmonale includes supplemental oxygen, diuretics, and bronchodilators for obstructive impairment. Aggressive antibiotic treatment of bronchitis and bronchiectasis is indicated, often employed on a rotating monthly regimen, to reduce the frequency of infectious episodes.

Extrapulmonary Sarcoidosis

Indications for treatment are as follows:

- Threatened organ failure (e.g., severe ocular, cardiac, or CNS disease)
- Posterior uveitis or anterior uveitis that does not respond to local corticosteroids
- Persistent hypercalcemia
- Persistent renal or hepatic dysfunction
- Pituitary disease
- Myopathy
- Palpable splenomegaly or evidence of hypersplenism
- Severe fatigue and weight loss
- Painful lymphadenopathy
- Disfiguring skin disease

OCULAR SARCOIDOSIS

Topical corticosteroids are usually sufficient in anterior uveitis, but oral corticosteroids are necessary in posterior uveitis, chorioretinitis, and optic neuritis. These last two disorders may present as ocular emergencies that require high doses of intravenous corticosteroids initially. Close ophthalmologic follow-up is necessary in all patients who have ocular sarcoidosis. Methotrexate and azathioprine have been used as steroid-sparing drugs with anecdotal effectiveness in serious ocular sarcoidosis.

CARDIAC SARCOIDOSIS

Treatment of cardiac sarcoidosis consists of anti-inflammatory therapy along with appropriate antiarrhythmic, diuretic, and afterload-reducing agents, depending on the cardiac abnormalities. Automatic implantable defibrillators and/or pacemakers can prevent sudden death in individuals who have serious arrhythmias or heart block and are indicated in patients at risk for sudden death. A standard approach is to use corticosteroids in moderate doses (prednisone 40 to 60 mg/day followed by a slow taper to a maintenance dose of 10 to 20 mg/day), as clinical experience indicates that corticosteroid therapy can reverse heart block, reduce arrhythmias, and improve ejection fraction. Methotrexate and azathioprine have most often been used as steroid-sparing agents in patients who do not maintain stable cardiac function on maintenance doses, but experience remains limited. Extensive myocardial fibrosis may result in dilated cardiomyopathy resistant to corticosteroids and immunosuppressive drugs.

NEUROSARCOIDOSIS

High doses of oral corticosteroids (60 to 80 mg/day) or high-dose pulse intravenous therapy are often employed for serious CNS involvement. Tapering to more modest doses is performed over several months, following evidence of persistent suppression of disease by objective criteria (e.g., serial MRI scans). Neurosarcoidosis that is severe in its presentation tends to be chronic and requires long-term therapy. Methotrexate, azathioprine, and hydroxychloroquine have been used effectively in anecdotal cases as corticosteroid-sparing drugs.

HEPATIC SARCOIDOSIS

Patients with persistently elevated liver function tests (e.g., alkaline phosphatase greater than 2 to 3 times normal) should generally be treated, even if asymptomatic, to prevent progressive hepatic dysfunction and cirrhosis. Low-dose corticosteroids (e.g., prednisone 10 to 15 mg/day) are usually sufficient to suppress the hepatic inflammation and prevent progressive organ dysfunction. Patients should be monitored for hyperglycemia, as it is a frequent complication of corticosteroid therapy in the setting of hepatic sarcoidosis.

HYPERCALCEMIA

Persistent hypercalcemia is an indication for treatment because of the risk of nephrocalcinosis or (rarely) of acute hypercalcemic crisis. Prednisone in small to moderate doses is generally effective. If it is not, primary hyperparathyroidism should be considered. Case reports also document that chloroquine, hydroxychloroquine (see the following discussion), and ketoconazole may effectively treat hypercalcemic sarcoidosis.

BONE AND JOINT SARCOIDOSIS

Corticosteroids usually result in marked improvement in symptoms. Over months, new bone formation can occur with a return to a normal radiographic bone appearance. Chloroquine, hydroxychloroquine, and methotrexate may also be effective.

HEMATOLOGIC SARCOIDOSIS

Corticosteroids usually effectively shrink an enlarged spleen, though some splenic enlargement may persist. Hypersplenism also frequently responds, at least in part, to low or moderate doses of corticosteroids.

MUCOCUTANEOUS SARCOIDOSIS

The antimalarial drugs chloroquine and hydroxychloroquine have been used as first-line drugs for lupus pernio, other disfiguring sarcoid skin disease, and nasal and sinus sarcoidosis. Response rates approximate 50% and are higher with chloroquine than with hydroxychloroquine. Beneficial effects may not be evident for 2 to 3 months. Chloroquine may be useful

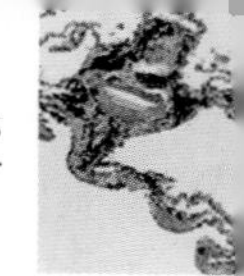

in chronic laryngeal sarcoidosis, although corticosteroids are usually used initially to prevent acute airway obstruction.

Immunosuppressive and Other Alternative Therapies

HYDROXYCHLOROQUINE AND CHLOROQUINE

Hydroxychloroquine, because of its overall relative safety, is frequently used in treatment of mucocutaneous sarcoidosis and also as a steroid-sparing drug in conjunction with low doses of corticosteroids for pulmonary and systemic sarcoidosis. Occasionally the drug has been reported to be beneficial in neurologic sarcoidosis. Chloroquine is less frequently used because of a concern for ocular toxicity (which occurs more frequently than with hydroxychloroquine). This complication is rare, however, when low doses are used with drug-free periods and ophthalmologic exams are conducted every 3 to 4 months during therapy (see Table 45.4). One study found chloroquine effective in pulmonary sarcoidosis, but wider clinical experience has not found these drugs to be useful alone in many patients with pulmonary or systemic disease.

METHOTREXATE

Methotrexate has found increasing use in the treatment of chronic sarcoidosis when corticosteroid therapy is poorly tolerated. Initially the drug was used to treat severe sarcoidosis of the skin with anecdotal success. More recently, methotrexate in low, weekly doses (10 to 20 mg/week) has been used to treat pulmonary, ocular, and other systemic involvement. Response rates range from 50% to 70% as a corticosteroid-sparing drug; response rates as a corticosteroid-replacing drug are lower. Beneficial responses are often not noted until at least 6 months of therapy, which diminishes the utility of the drug in the acute treatment of sarcoidosis. Methotrexate has known potential to cause hepatic toxicity (which limits its use in hepatic sarcoidosis), opportunistic infections, hypersensitivity pneumonitis, and bone marrow suppression. Because methotrexate is cleared by the kidneys, renal insufficiency also limits its use. A complete blood count and liver and renal function tests should be performed at least monthly during therapy. The need for routine liver biopsy to monitor for hepatic fibrosis is not clear, although it is recommended by some authorities after patients have received a total of 1 to 1.5 g of the drug. One study found hepatic toxicity by liver biopsy in more than 10% of patients with sarcoidosis treated for more than 2 years with methotrexate, and this finding was not predicted by changes in liver function tests.

AZATHIOPRINE

Anecdotal experience suggests that azathioprine in a dose of 100 to 200 mg/day may be useful in corticosteroid-resistant sarcoidosis. Low doses of corticosteroids (e.g., 10 mg of prednisone per day) are often prescribed concomitantly; beneficial effects may require 3 months or more of therapy. Bone marrow suppression, gastrointestinal symptoms, hepatotoxicity, skin rashes, and arthralgias are serious drawbacks, and the drug may be associated with a slightly increased risk of malignancy. Nonetheless, because it is often well tolerated for prolonged periods of treatment, azathioprine remains a useful corticosteroid-sparing drug for serious pulmonary, neurologic, cardiac, and other forms of extrapulmonary sarcoidosis.

OTHER CYTOTOXIC AND IMMUNOSUPPRESSIVE AGENTS

Cyclophosphamide has been used with anecdotal success in some forms of severe sarcoidosis including sinus sarcoidosis and neurosarcoidosis that are resistant to corticosteroid and other therapies. Chlorambucil also been reported to be beneficial in some cases of steroid-resistant sarcoidosis. The oncogenic potential of both of these drugs suggests that their use should be extremely limited. Most experts favor cyclophosphamide over chlorambucil. Cyclosporin A, a drug known to inhibit T-cell activation, is ineffective in pulmonary sarcoidosis and systemic sarcoidosis except for possibly a few cases of steroid-resistant neurosarcoidosis. Cyclosporin A and other immunophilins used for transplant rejection therapy also do not prevent recurrent granulomas in organ transplantation in sarcoidosis. Given the overall toxicities in these drugs, there is little clinical basis for their use in sarcoidosis.

PENTOXIFYLLINE

A recent clinical study found that pentoxifylline was beneficial when used alone or with corticosteroids in the initial treatment of sarcoidosis, although it was not clear how many of the patients studied actually required treatment. Wider clinical experience suggests that the drug has limited effectiveness but may be helpful in some cases of mild pulmonary or hepatic disease or as a corticosteroid-sparing agent. Gastrointestinal side effects and headache may limit dosing, but given the relative safety of the drug, further studies seem merited.

THALIDOMIDE

Small clinical series or case reports have found that thalidomide maybe beneficial in steroid-recalcitrant cutaneous sarcoidosis, including lupus pernio. One study found that the drug was not beneficial for pulmonary sarcoidosis. Peripheral neurotoxicity and the well-known teratogenicity of the drug limit its usefulness as a therapeutic agent.

TETRACYCLINES

Doxycycline and minocycline have been reported to be beneficial in a few cases of cutaneous sarcoidosis but have not been shown to be effective in pulmonary or other organ involvement.

ANTI–TUMOR NECROSIS FACTOR THERAPY

The premise that TNF inhibition may be beneficial in sarcoidosis is based on the concept that TNF plays a critical role in granuloma formation. Although drugs such as pentoxifylline and thalidomide inhibit production of TNF in vitro, the effective mechanism of these drugs in sarcoidosis is not clear, because these drugs have other immunomodulatory effects. Newer anti-TNF biologic response modifiers include immunoglobulin-derived agents against TNF (infliximab, adalimumab) or soluble TNF receptor fusion protein (etanercept). Although case reports suggest that infliximab may be beneficial in some patients with corticosteroid-resistant sarcoidosis, experience remains extremely limited. Because these anti-TNF biologics are associated with increased risk for tuberculosis reactivation and serious infections including sepsis, clinical trials are needed to define their role in sarcoidosis.

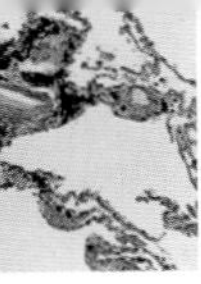

Role of Transplantation in Sarcoidosis

Successful lung, heart, kidney, and liver transplantations have been performed in small numbers of patients with sarcoidosis. Several reports document the recurrence of noncaseating granulomas in the lungs of transplanted patients, however. The recurrence of granulomas generally is transient, self-limited, and responsive to an increase in immunosuppression. Overall, the survival rate for lung transplantation for end-stage pulmonary sarcoidosis appears to be similar to that for other pulmonary diseases. One study found that evidence of pulmonary hypertension was associated with reduced survival in patients with advanced pulmonary sarcoidosis awaiting lung transplant. Experience with heart transplantation for advanced sarcoid cardiomyopathy is limited. Recurrence of heart granulomas has been documented in a few cases but has not seemed to alter overall outcome.

CLINICAL COURSE AND PREVENTION

The clinical course is highly variable in sarcoidosis. Overall, 50% to 65% of patients undergo spontaneous remission, usually (greater than 85%) within the first 2 years. From 80% to 95% of patients with Löfgren syndrome experience spontaneous remissions. Patients who have lupus pernio, bony involvement, nephrocalcinosis, hepatomegaly, and fibrocystic lung disease rarely undergo spontaneous remission. Initial severity of symptoms and type of organ involvement may provide important prognostic information. Extrathoracic disease that is asymptomatic and detected as part of an initial evaluation may not indicate a poor prognosis, as it likely reflects incidental granulomatous inflammatory disease. When extrathoracic disease is symptomatic and severe on presentation, the disease tends to be persistent and requires treatment. It is interesting to note that the pattern of organ involvement typically declares itself during the first year of clinical disease and usually does not change with time. Peripheral adenopathy, salivary gland enlargement, and Bell's palsy generally subside spontaneously or with treatment and do not recur. Neurologic deficits may remain following involvement of cranial nerves. Elevated serum liver function tests also may revert to normal spontaneously.

Studies from both the United States and the United Kingdom show that the chest radiograph stage provides useful prognostic information in pulmonary sarcoidosis.

The rates of spontaneous remission for the different stages are as follows:

- Stage I—greater than 50% to 80%
- Stage II—30% to 60%
- Stage III—20% to 30%
- Stage IV—less than 5% to 10%

The prognosis associated with cardiac sarcoidosis is uncertain. Early case series or autopsy reports emphasized that median survival is limited to about 2 years. At least one large series suggested that a 10- to 20-year survival is not unusual. In my experience, a treatment approach employing maintenance therapy with moderate doses of corticosteroids, with or without steroid-sparing drugs, together with appropriate cardiac management of arrhythmias, heart block, and congestive heart failure is associated with a longer than 5-year survival in over 90% of patients with cardiac sarcoidosis.

Clinical Follow-up

Direct serial measurement of organ function provides the most important data for following the course of the disease and response to treatment. For patients who have pulmonary sarcoidosis, serial spirometry, in particular the FVC, is considered the most reliable indicator of pulmonary status. Diffusing capacity is more variable but may reveal early progressive disease, and correlates best with exercise responses. Other organ-specific tests (e.g., echocardiogram, Holter monitor in cardiac sarcoidosis, MRI in neurosarcoidosis, liver function tests in hepatic sarcoidosis) are indicated to follow response to therapy.

Biomarkers of Disease Activity

BRONCHOALVEOLAR LAVAGE STUDIES

Early research suggested that the extent of $CD4^+$ lymphocytosis or the CD4/CD8 ratio of BAL cells in pulmonary sarcoidosis correlates with disease activity. More recent data from studies around the world, however, have led to the generally accepted conclusion that these measurements (or other BAL findings) are not sufficiently predictive to assist in clinical decision making.

SERUM ANGIOTENSIN-CONVERTING ENZYME AND OTHER BIOCHEMICAL TESTS

Several studies have shown that initial SACE levels do not predict those patients who will improve or deteriorate. Although elevated SACE levels usually decrease as the disease regresses or responds to starting corticosteroids, these changes do not correlate with response to therapy and may lead to overtreatment. Many other serum and urine biochemical tests (e.g., soluble IL-2 receptor, b_2-microglobulin, urinary neopterin) have been proposed for following disease activity, but most reflect only a measure of immunologic activation. Although these tests provide important insights into the pathogenesis of granulomatous inflammation in sarcoidosis, none of them has been proved to be useful in clinical management.

Management Problems

RESPIRATORY DECOMPENSATION

Respiratory infection is the most common cause of pulmonary decompensation in pulmonary sarcoidosis. Progressive granulomatous lung disease is an unlikely cause if the patient is on a previously effective maintenance dose of corticosteroids unless poor compliance is occurring. Other causes of respiratory decompensation include congestive heart failure and pulmonary embolism. Opportunistic lung infection is a consideration in patients on immunosuppressive therapy, but appears to be rare in sarcoidosis. A temporary, modest increase in corticosteroid therapy may be indicated, but return to a previously successful maintenance dose must be planned following treatment of the primary cause.

MYCETOMAS AND HEMOPTYSIS

Fibrocystic sarcoidosis may be complicated by mycetomas, bronchiectasis, and hemoptysis (see Figs. 45.9 and 45.10). *Aspergillus* species are the usual organisms to form mycetomas and can often be cultured from sputum or biopsy. Aspergillomas may be asymptomatic or may cause hemoptysis. Hemoptysis i

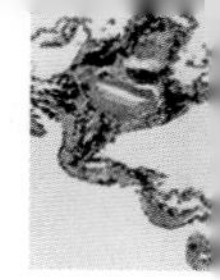

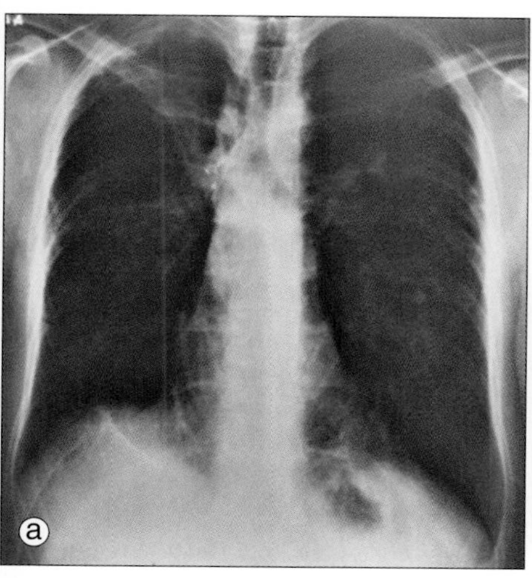

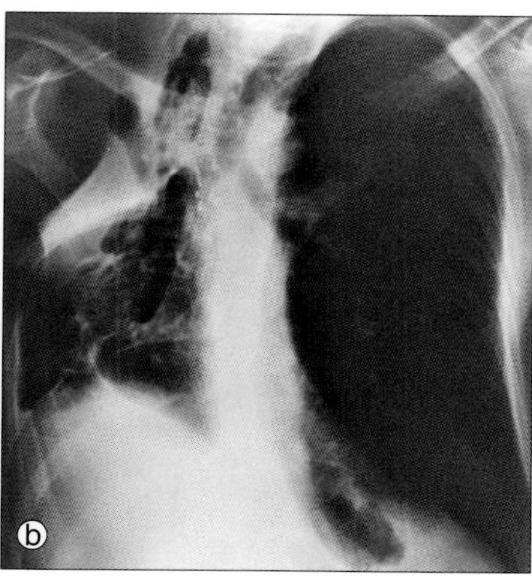

Figure 45.12 Chronic fibrocystic sarcoidosis. **A,** Marked bullous changes in a patient with chronic fibrocystic sarcoidosis with chronic recurrent hemoptysis. **B,** After an episode of massive hemoptysis, patient underwent right upper lobe resection and thoracoplasty that was complicated by empyema and bronchopleural cutaneous fistulae. (Courtesy of C. Johns, Johns Hopkins University.)

almost always the result of associated bronchiectasis and/or bronchitis (and not caused by angioinvasion by *Aspergillus* species), because most episodes respond to conservative therapy with bed rest, cough suppression, moderate corticosteroid doses, and parenteral or oral antibiotics. Rotation of monthly antibiotics and low-dose maintenance corticosteroids often effectively minimize repeated episodes. Amphotericin therapy has not been recommended in the past, because the drug did not appear to be effective and toxic side effects were common. A role for newer oral antifungal agents with activity against *Aspergillus* species to reduce episodes of hemoptysis is unknown. Occasionally, mycetomas are associated with massive hemoptysis, with mortality ranging from less than 10% to 50%. Significant recurrent or submassive hemoptysis may be treated with embolotherapy of the appropriate bronchial or collateral artery following bronchoscopic localization of the bleeding segment. External beam irradiation may also be effective. Surgical resection is usually not feasible or desirable because of the risk of significant morbidity and mortality in patients who usually have severe respiratory insufficiency (Fig. 45.12).

PREGNANCY

In general, pregnancy has little effect on the long-term course of sarcoidosis. Sometimes, spontaneous improvement in chronic sarcoidosis occurs during pregnancy, which allows a temporary reduction in corticosteroid dosage. However, in these patients, an exacerbation typically follows pregnancy and requires a return to a maintenance corticosteroid dose.

PITFALLS AND CONTROVERSIES

The overall effectiveness of corticosteroid therapy in sarcoidosis is controversial. It is agreed that corticosteroids are effective in initially reversing pulmonary and extrapulmonary organ dysfunction in most patients. Long-term benefits of corticosteroid therapy in sarcoidosis are less clear, in large part because of the difficulties engendered by a disease with a highly variable course, a high rate of spontaneous remission, and variable degrees of inflammation and fibrosis, both of which impair organ function. Several prospective studies failed to find any long-term benefit of corticosteroid therapy in altering outcomes in pulmonary sarcoidosis, although the patient groups had a high likelihood of spontaneous remission. In contrast, retrospective studies from centers that treat patients at high risk for chronic disease provide data in support of the clinical impression that corticosteroids have a favorable impact on the course of chronic sarcoidosis. Two recent prospective studies of patients with stage II or III disease in the United Kingdom and Finland found that corticosteroids significantly improved long-term pulmonary function compared with comparison groups. Further studies are needed to corroborate these results, but most authorities favor the view that corticosteroid therapy improves outcome in most patients who have chronic disease by preventing or delaying progressive pulmonary fibrosis and organ dysfunction.

The role of corticosteroid-sparing medications in sarcoidosis continues to evolve. Hydroxychloroquine is often tried first as a corticosteroid-sparing drug, given its overall relative safety, but frequently it has little impact on more severe disease. Methotrexate and, less commonly, azathioprine are used as second-line drugs in corticosteroid-recalcitrant sarcoidosis or when corticosteroid therapy is not tolerated in serious disease. None of these practices has been established by controlled clinical trials. Newer anti-TNF therapies are promising options for patients who do not tolerate "standard" therapies, but all have serious potential adverse effects, and experience in the use of these drugs remains limited. The need for clinical trials to evaluate the benefits of these agents is agreed. Furthermore, agreement is universal on the need for safer and more effective therapies for those patients who have chronic, sometimes devastating, sarcoidosis. Recent advances in our understanding of the pathogenesis of sarcoidosis and the rapid pace of biotechnologic innovation encourage optimism that such therapies will continue to be developed.

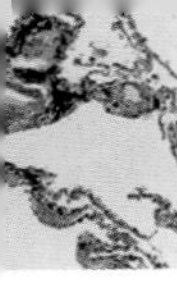

SUGGESTED READINGS

American Thoracic Society, European Respiratory Society, World Association of Sarcoidosis and Other Granulomatous Disorders: Statement on sarcoidosis. Joint Statement of the American Thoracic Society (ATS), the European Respiratory Society (ERS) and the World Association of Sarcoidosis and Other Granulomatous Disorders (WASOG) adopted by the ATS Board of Directors and by the ERS Executive Committee, February 1999. Am J Respir Crit Care Med 160:736-755, 1999.

Baughman RP, Lynch JP: Difficult treatment issues in sarcoidosis. J Intern Med 253:41-45, 2003.

Baughman RP, Tierstein AS, Judson MA, et al: Clinical characteristics of patients in a case control study of sarcoidosis. Am J Respir Crit Care Med 164:1885-1889, 2001.

du Bois RM, Goh N, McGrath D, Cullinan P: Is there a role for microorganisms in the pathogenesis of sarcoidosis? J Intern Med 253:4-17, 2003.

Johns CJ, Michele TM: The clinical management of sarcoidosis. A 50-year experience at the Johns Hopkins Hospital. Medicine (Baltimore) 78:65-111, 1999.

Moller DR: Treatment of sarcoidosis: From a basic science point of view. J Intern Med 253:31-40, 2003.

Muller-Quernheim J: Sarcoidosis: Immunopathogenetic concepts and their clinical application. Eur Respir J 12:716-738, 1998.

Rybicki BA, Iannuzzi MC, Frederick MM, et al: Familial aggregation of sarcoidosis: A case control etiologic study of sarcoidosis (ACCESS). Am J Respir Crit Care Med 164:2085-2091, 2001.

Sharma OP: Cardiac and neurologic dysfunction in sarcoidosis. Clin Chest Med 18:813-825, 1997.

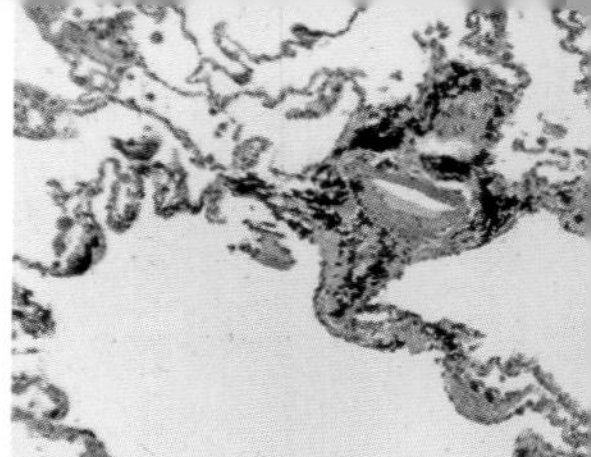

CHAPTER 46 Eosinophilic Lung Disease and Bronchiolitis Obliterans Organizing Pneumonia

Sanjay Kalra, Jeffrey L. Myers, and Jay H. Ryu

The term *eosinophilic lung disease* encompasses diverse pulmonary disorders associated with peripheral blood eosinophilia, bronchoalveolar lavage (BAL) eosinophilia, or eosinophilic infiltrates in the lung tissue. These disorders may manifest as acute or chronic illnesses or may cause no symptoms. Some manifest features of airways obstruction, while others are predominantly parenchymal with a restrictive type of physiologic impairment. Although most of the symptoms of eosinophilic lung diseases are confined to the respiratory tract, in some, such as Churg-Strauss syndrome (CSS, also called *allergic angiitis and granulomatosis*) and idiopathic hypereosinophilic syndrome (HES), a wide variety of extrapulmonary involvement occurs.

Bronchiolitis obliterans organizing pneumonia (BOOP) refers to a nonspecific tissue reaction in the lung and is characterized by the presence of intraluminal plugs of connective tissue in the bronchioles that extend distally into alveolar ducts and alveolar spaces. This pattern has been termed *proliferative bronchiolitis* and may be seen in a variety of clinical contexts. Its presence does not constitute a discrete clinicopathologic entity on its own. However, an idiopathic form of BOOP is recognized and is synonymous with cryptogenic organizing pneumonia (COP).

EOSINOPHILIC LUNG DISEASE

Many pulmonary disorders have been associated with eosinophilia (defined as >6% eosinophils) in the peripheral blood, BAL fluid (normal is <1% eosinophils), or lung tissue (Table 46.1). However, other pulmonary disorders in which peripheral blood, BAL fluid, or tissue eosinophilia occurs include asthma, idiopathic pulmonary fibrosis, Langerhans cell histiocytosis, and hypersensitivity pneumonitis, as well as various infectious and neoplastic disorders. These disorders have their own distinctive features and are generally not included under the category of eosinophilic lung diseases.

Epidemiology, Risk Factors, and Pathophysiology

Eosinophilic lung diseases occur worldwide. Parasites are probably the most common cause of eosinophilic lung disease, and the prevalence of individual infections varies from one geographic location to another. In the United States, *Strongyloides stercoralis*, *Ascaris lumbricoides*, *Toxocara canis*, and *Ancylostoma duodenale* are the most frequent parasitic infections associated with eosinophilic lung disease. Parasites gain entry into the human body by being ingested (*Ascaris*, *Toxocara*) or by penetration through the skin (*Strongyloides*, *Ancylostoma*). Tropical eosinophilia is caused by the filarial worms *Wuchereria bancrofti* and *Brugia malayi*. These parasites are widely distributed in the tropics and are transmitted to humans by mosquitoes. Eosinophilic pulmonary reaction occurs when parasites migrate to the lungs.

Eosinophilic lung diseases are uncommon or rare in developed countries. They occur in subjects of all ages and have no particular gender predominance, although some exceptions to this are found. For example, chronic eosinophilic pneumonia (CEP) occurs mostly in adults, with peak incidence in the fourth decade, and women are affected more than twice as frequently as men. Idiopathic HES occurs mostly in adults in the age range 20 to 50 years, with a 9:1 male predominance, and CSS develops mainly in older adults, with no sex predominance. In contrast, children are at high risk of certain parasitic infections such as *Toxocara canis* (the dog roundworm), which is associated with pica, close contact with pets, and outside play.

In about two thirds of patients who have Löffler's syndrome, a parasitic infestation or drug reaction is the underlying cause. An atopic history, in particular of asthma, is often present in patients who develop CEP and CSS. Asthma is also present in about one third of patients who have bronchocentric granulomatosis (BG). No cause or risk factor is known for acute eosinophilic pneumonia (AEP) or HES although an acute hypersensitivity phenomenon to unknown inhaled antigens has been suggested as the possible cause of the former, which has also been reported in the setting of the acquired immunodeficiency syndrome (AIDS).

The list of drugs that cause eosinophilic pulmonary disorders is growing, typified by the acute reaction to nitrofurantoin. Most of these drug reactions appear to be idiosyncratic, but eosinophilic disorders of epidemic proportions have occurred with ingestion of contaminated L-tryptophan (eosinophilia-myalgia syndrome) and contaminated rapeseed oil (toxic oil syndrome).

Clinical Features

LÖFFLER'S SYNDROME (SIMPLE PULMONARY EOSINOPHILIA)

Löffler's syndrome is characterized by migratory pulmonary infiltrates that are often peripheral in location. These transient infiltrates may be unilateral or bilateral, and of mixed alveolar and interstitial pattern. Peripheral blood eosinophilia is present with minimal or no pulmonary symptoms.

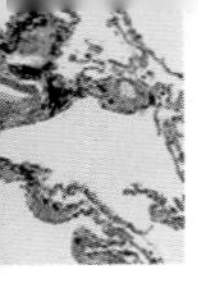

Table 46.1
Eosinophilic lung diseases

Löffler's syndrome	Bronchocentric granulomatosis
Acute eosinophilic pneumonia	Idiopathic hypereosinophilic syndrome
Chronic eosinophilic pneumonia	Parasitic infections
Allergic bronchopulmonary aspergillosis	Drug reactions
Churg–Strauss syndrome	

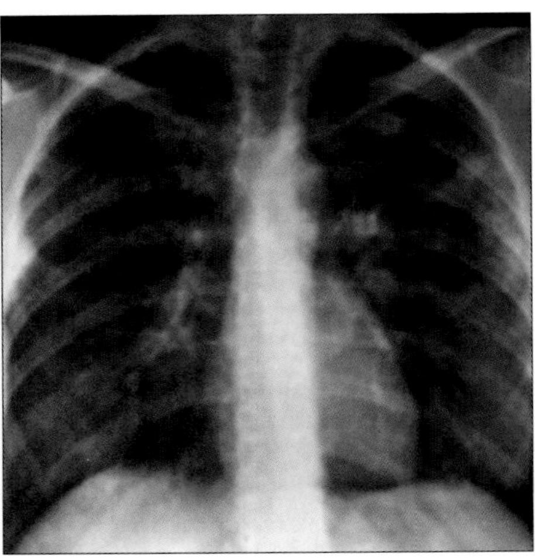

Figure 46.1 Chronic eosinophilic pneumonia (CEP). Chest radiograph of a 42-year-old woman who has CEP, which shows peripheral alveolar infiltrates bilaterally. Patient had cough and dyspnea of 3 months' duration.

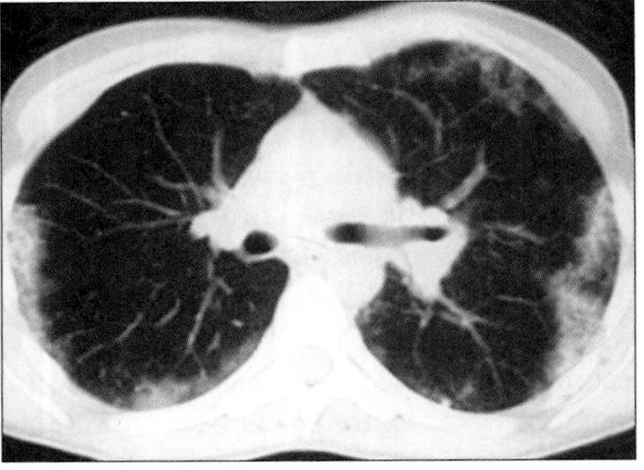

Figure 46.2 Chronic eosinophilic pneumonia (CEP). Computed tomogram of the chest on the same patient as in Figure 46.1 demonstrates the peripheral nature of the infiltrates.

CHRONIC EOSINOPHILIC PNEUMONIA

CEP is associated with respiratory and/or constitutional symptoms that have been progressing over several months. Respiratory symptoms commonly include cough and dyspnea, which may be accompanied by fever, weight loss, and malaise. Less common symptoms include wheezing, night sweats, hemoptysis, chest pain, and myalgias. Peripheral blood eosinophilia is usually present, but may be absent in up to 30% of patients. Erythrocyte sedimentation rates and serum immunoglobulin E (IgE) levels are usually elevated. Peripheral alveolar infiltrates are seen in about two thirds of affected patients, but the so-called "photographic negative" of pulmonary edema pattern (extensive, dense, peripheral alveolar infiltrates) is seen in only 25% of cases (Fig. 46.1). In other cases, unilateral and nonperipheral opacities are observed. Chest computed tomography (CT) generally confirms the peripheral nature of the alveolar infiltrates (Fig. 46.2), and mediastinal adenopathy may be seen.

ACUTE EOSINOPHILIC PNEUMONIA

AEP is an acute illness of 1 to 5 days' duration and rapid progression. Presenting symptoms include myalgias, pleuritic chest pain, and dyspnea. Fever and crackles on auscultation are notable findings on physical examination. The chest radiograph reveals interstitial infiltrates that may be subtle in the early phases but progresses to diffuse alveolar infiltrates that are not peripherally based. Small to moderate-sized, usually bilateral pleural effusions are common. Pleural and BAL fluids contain a high percentage of eosinophils, but peripheral blood eosinophilia is uncommon.

ALLERGIC BRONCHOPULMONARY ASPERGILLOSIS

Allergic bronchopulmonary aspergillosis (ABPA) generally is seen in asthmatic patients who have recurrent or persistent lung infiltrates. It can also occur in association with cystic fibrosis. The clinical features include those of asthma, as well as peripheral blood eosinophilia, elevated total serum IgE level (>1000 ng/mL), and an immediate skin reaction to *Aspergillus* antigen. ABPA is discussed in more detail in Chapter 39.

CHURG-STRAUSS SYNDROME

Asthma, peripheral blood eosinophilia, and systemic vasculitis characterize CSS (or allergic angiitis and granulomatosis). Manifestations develop several years after the onset of asthma symptoms. CSS primarily affects the lungs, upper respiratory tract, skin, and peripheral nerves, but other organs, which include kidneys, gastrointestinal tract, and heart, may also be involved. Several cases have been reported in patients treated with leukotriene antagonists for asthma, where it is likely the accompanying reduction in maintenance corticosteroids led to an unmasking of CSS. Serum IgE level is usually elevated and appears to correlate with disease activity. Perinuclear-staining antineutrophil cytoplasmic autoantibody (p-ANCA) may be detected in the serum in more than 50% of affected patients. The chest radiograph may show various abnormalities, which include patchy, transient infiltrates, nodules of varying sizes, diffuse interstitial infiltrates, and pleural effusions.

BRONCHOCENTRIC GRANULOMATOSIS

The diagnosis of BG is made on the basis of histologic features. Although initially regarded as a distinct category of pulmonary angiitis and granulomatosis, it is now considered a nonspecific reaction of the lung that occurs in a variety of clinical settings, which include infections and other inflammatory disorders, including ABPA. About one third of affected patients manifest asthma symptoms and peripheral eosinophilia, and in these patients BG is a manifestation of ABPA. Findings on chest radiographs include nodular or mass lesion(s) and focal consolidation.

IDIOPATHIC HYPEREOSINOPHILIC SYNDROME

Idiopathic HES is defined by the presence of peripheral blood eosinophilia of greater than 1500/mL for more than 6 months in the absence of both an identifiable cause and evidence of end-organ damage related to increased eosinophils. Recent data suggest that underlying genetic deletions may lead to a gain-of-function fusion tyrosine kinase that may not only produce HES but also be a target for future treatments. Large numbers of eosinophils are present in the bone marrow and account for

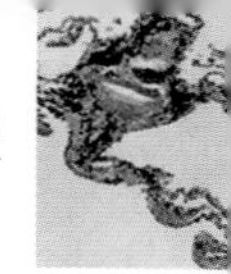

about 30% to 70% of peripheral white blood cells. Night sweats, weight loss, anorexia, pruritus, cough, and fever are common presenting symptoms that tend to be insidious. Cardiac involvement is the major cause of morbidity and mortality and includes endocardial fibrosis, restrictive cardiomyopathy, valvular insufficiency, mural thrombus formation, and embolization. Pulmonary manifestations occur in about 40% of affected patients and reflect eosinophilic infiltration of the lungs, congestion caused by heart failure, and pulmonary embolism from right ventricular thrombi. Focal or diffuse lung infiltrates are seen in 14% to 28% of patients who have HES. Pleural effusions are seen in about one half of those affected by pulmonary involvement. Arterial thromboembolism and eosinophilic infiltration of other organs cause a variety of extrapulmonary symptoms. Serum levels of soluble interleukin-5 receptor are increased and correlate with disease activity.

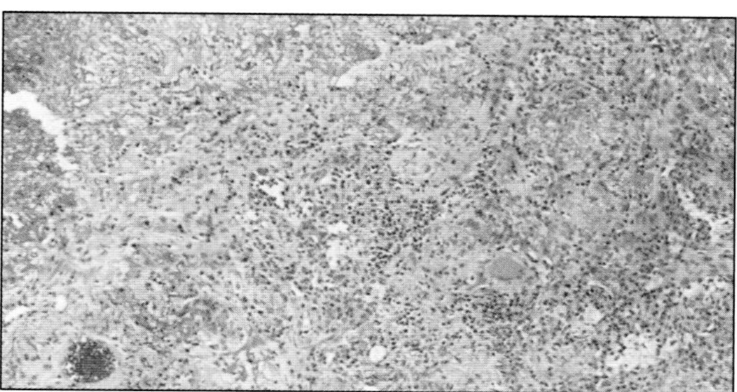

Figure 46.3 Histopathology of Churg-Strauss syndrome (CSS). This photomicrograph shows a combination of parenchymal necrosis and focally marked tissue eosinophilia in CSS. The inflammatory infiltrate includes a combination of eosinophils and variable numbers of epithelioid histiocytes in a vaguely granulomatous appearance.

PARASITIC INFECTIONS

Parasitic infections that cause lung involvement generally are associated with cough, lung infiltrates, and peripheral blood eosinophilia. Skin rashes may be seen with certain parasitic infestations, such as strongyloidiasis, ascariasis, and ancylostomiasis. Other respiratory symptoms may include dyspnea, wheezing (especially nocturnal), and hemoptysis. Systemic manifestations, which include, malaise, fever, fatigue, and weight loss, may be prominent in the earlier stages of tropical eosinophilia. Pulmonary auscultation may reveal crackles and wheezes. Chest radiographs can show transient, migratory infiltrates to diffuse, alveolar, or interstitial infiltrates. Pleural effusions and hilar adenopathy are uncommon.

DRUG-INDUCED EOSINOPHILIC PNEUMONIAS

Drug-induced eosinophilic pneumonias generally begin within days of drug intake. Typical symptoms include dry cough, dyspnea, fever, and chills. Patchy or diffuse infiltrates may be seen on the chest radiograph, sometimes accompanied by pleural effusions.

Diagnosis

Most of the eosinophilic lung diseases can be tentatively diagnosed on the basis of the clinical picture, laboratory tests, and chest radiographic findings. Bronchoalveolar lavage and/or lung biopsy may be useful for diagnosing AEP, CEP, and CSS. Open (or thoracoscopic) lung biopsy remains the diagnostic “gold standard” for identifying cases of CSS and BG. The histopathologic lesions of CSS include necrotizing vasculitis (which primarily affects small to medium vessels), eosinophilic infiltration, and extravascular granulomas (Fig. 46.3). Transbronchial biopsy generally provides inadequate tissue samples. Similarly, it is difficult to diagnose BG without a surgical biopsy. Characteristic histologic features include necrosis and a mixed inflammatory cell infiltrate, with granulomatous features that involve small bronchi and bronchioles. Chronic inflammatory changes and eosinophilic infiltrates may be seen in the surrounding lung parenchyma, but vasculitis is absent. Because infections and a wide variety of inflammatory conditions may cause a similar histologic picture, BG is a diagnosis of exclusion.

Current diagnostic criteria for AEP include acute onset (onset of any symptoms within 7 days of presentation); fever (37.2°C [≥99°F]); bilateral infiltrates on chest film; severe hypoxemia; lung eosinophilia (BAL differential with ≥25% eosinophils or predominance of eosinophils on open lung biopsy); and exclusion of other known causes of eosinophilic lung disease, including drug hypersensitivity and infection. Histopathologic findings include a combination of diffuse alveolar damage and eosinophilia.

Diagnostic criteria for ABPA include asthma, peripheral blood eosinophilia (>1000/mm^3 or μL), elevated total serum IgE level (generally exceeding 1000 ng/mL), the presence of serum-precipitating antibodies against *Aspergillus* antigens, immediate cutaneous reactivity to *Aspergillus* antigens, current or previous chest radiographic infiltrates, and central bronchiectasis. Although central bronchiectasis is present in most patients who have ABPA at the time of the diagnosis, it may be absent in early disease. Surgical specimens typically show a combination of BG, mucoid impaction of bronchi, and eosinophilic pneumonia.

The diagnosis of HES requires the presence of peripheral blood eosinophilia greater than 1500/mm^3 or μL for longer than 6 months, signs and symptoms of end-organ damage related to eosinophilia, and exclusion of other known causes for eosinophilia.

Although some parasitic infections may be diagnosed by stool examination for ova, others cannot be diagnosed in this fashion because pulmonary manifestations occur before the mature worms develop. This is true of strongyloidiasis and visceral larva migrans (toxocariasis), which are diagnosed by enzyme-linked immunosorbent assays in patients who have compatible epidemiologic and clinical features. This is also true of ascariasis, in which the ova may not be seen in the stool for up to 8 weeks after the onset of respiratory symptoms. The larvae of *Ascaris* may occasionally be detected in the sputum. The diagnosis of *Ancylostoma* infection and tropical eosinophilia is usually made on the basis of clinical presentation and exposure history. This is also true of most drug reactions that cause eosinophilic lung disease, which are usually diagnosed without lung biopsy. Resolution of pulmonary manifestations after withdrawal of the offending drug provides further evidence for the causal relationship.

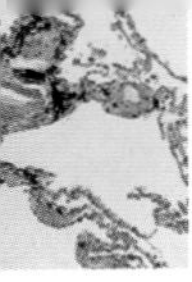

Treatment

Because some of the eosinophilic lung diseases have specific causes such as parasitic infections and drug reactions, treatment issues can be addressed only after an adequate search has been conducted to identify an underlying cause. Parasitic infections and Löffler's syndrome caused by parasitic infestations are treated with appropriate antihelminthic or antifilarial drugs. Thiabendazole 25 mg/kg q12h is used for uncomplicated strongyloidiasis and *Ancylostoma* infection. Visceral larva migrans is generally self-limited, and the role of antihelminthic drugs is unclear. Mebendazole 100 mg q12h for 3 days is appropriate for ascariasis. Tropical eosinophilia responds promptly to treatment with diethylcarbamazine (a piperazine derivative) 6 to 12 mg/kg/day given in three divided doses for 1 to 3 weeks. Drug reactions usually resolve after discontinuation of the offending drug. A brief course of corticosteroid therapy may help in severe or persistent cases of drug reactions, as well as for certain severe, acute parasitic infections such as visceral larva migrans.

Corticosteroid therapy is commonly used for ABPA as well as for various idiopathic eosinophilic lung diseases, which include AEP, CEP, CSS, BG, and HES. An initial prednisone dose of 0.5 mg/kg is generally sufficient to treat ABPA, with the dose tapered after 2 weeks and over the following months, while asthma symptoms, lung infiltrates, and total serum IgE levels are monitored. Concurrent use of the antifungal agent itraconazole has also been shown to be useful. Patients who have AEP respond within 24 to 48 hours to administration of high doses of corticosteroids, for example 60 to 125 mg of methylprednisolone every 6 hours. As the patient improves, oral prednisone at 40 to 60 mg/day is given for 2 to 4 weeks and gradually tapered over the subsequent weeks. Patients who have CEP are treated with moderate doses of prednisone (e.g., 30 to 40 mg/day), which produces dramatic relief of symptoms within the first few days. However, symptomatic relapses are frequent if corticosteroids are discontinued within the first 6 months. Maintenance therapy on a low, alternate-day dose of prednisone for a year or more is frequently necessary, and some patients require even more prolonged treatment. Inhaled corticosteroid therapy has occasionally been reported to be useful in patients who have CEP. Rare instances of spontaneous disease resolution have been reported with AEP and CEP.

Prednisone dosage of 40 to 60 mg/day for several weeks is usually required to treat Churg-Strauss syndrome. Subsequently, lower doses are continued for several months to 1 year. In patients who do not respond adequately to corticosteroid therapy, other immunosuppressive agents, such as cyclophosphamide and azathioprine, may be useful. Similarly, patients who suffer BG generally respond to corticosteroid therapy, but cyclophosphamide may be useful in some cases; however, some patients undergo surgical resection for mass lesions.

Treatment with prednisone 60 mg/day for 1 week, followed by 60 mg every other day for 3 months, is recommended for patients who have demonstrable end-organ damage because of HES. About one half of these patients experience a good response to corticosteroid therapy. Other useful therapeutic agents include interferon-α, hydroxyurea, azathioprine, cyclophosphamide, busulfan, cyclosporin-A, etoposide, and vincristine, as well as leukapheresis and bone marrow transplantation. Successful treatment of HES has recently been described using imatinib, a tyrosine kinase inhibitor. This represents a significant advance in the treatment of this disease as well as in the understanding of the underlying pathogenetic mechanism.

Clinical Course and Prevention

Löffler's syndrome is generally a benign disorder with an excellent prognosis. Although patients affected by AEP may be severely ill at presentation, they also have an excellent prognosis if the underlying disorder is promptly recognized and treated with corticosteroids. After the initial improvement, corticosteroids can be gradually tapered with full recovery in most cases and no relapse. Despite recurrent relapses, most patients who have CEP also have an excellent prognosis with corticosteroids; residual pulmonary dysfunction is unusual.

Although relapses can usually be prevented with corticosteroid therapy, patients who suffer ABPA may develop long-term complications of central bronchiectasis, irreversible airway obstruction, aspergilloma, pulmonary fibrosis, and eventual respiratory failure. This progressive course of ABPA has been described in five stages: acute, remission, exacerbation, corticosteroid-dependent asthma, and fibrosis. Early diagnosis and treatment may slow or prevent progression.

Although the untreated course of Churg-Strauss syndrome can be devastating, a mean survival of 9 years has been reported for patients treated with corticosteroids. Death occurs when various organs are affected by complications, particularly coronary arteritis and myocarditis, as well as from respiratory failure. The outcome of patients who have BG is favorable with surgical resection or corticosteroid therapy.

Pitfalls and Controversies

A potential pitfall in the diagnosis of eosinophilic lung diseases is an inadequate search for an underlying cause. Thus, a patient may be treated inappropriately with corticosteroids for presumed AEP or BG when a fungal infection may be responsible for the clinical picture. A serious hyperinfection syndrome with *Strongyloides stercoralis* may be precipitated by corticosteroid or other immunosuppressive treatment. It is important to note that the idiopathic eosinophilic diseases such as AEP, CEP, and HES are diagnoses of exclusion.

BRONCHIOLITIS OBLITERANS ORGANIZING PNEUMONIA

Bronchiolitis is a generic term used to describe various inflammatory disorders of bronchioles. The category of bronchiolar diseases remains a confusing one for the clinician, and no classification for subsets of bronchiolitis is universally accepted. The term *bronchiolitis obliterans* has been used to refer to diverse conditions, which include a rare syndrome of progressive airflow limitation caused by bronchial and peribronchial fibrosis (often referred to as "constrictive" or "obliterative" bronchiolitis) and the distinctive histologic lesion in which intraluminal polyps of organizing connective tissue are seen (BOOP). It is crucial that both of these lesions be recognized as nonspecific reactions that may occur in a variety of clinical contexts. The focus of this section is BOOP.

Synonyms for BOOP in current terminology include *organizing pneumonia* and *proliferative bronchiolitis*. As a

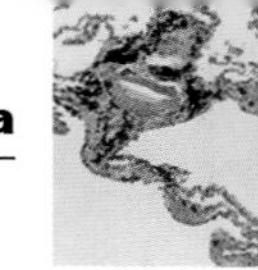

histopathologic lesion, BOOP is characterized by the presence of intraluminal plugs of connective tissue in the bronchioles that extend distally into adjacent alveolar ducts and alveoli (Fig. 46.4). The lesion appears temporally uniform with a patchy distribution and general preservation of the background architecture. Idiopathic BOOP is considered a discrete clinicopathologic entity and is increasingly also referred to as COP.

Epidemiology, Risk Factors, and Pathophysiology

As already mentioned, BOOP or proliferative bronchiolitis can be seen in various clinical settings. The term *BOOP* was popularized by Epler in 1985, who described 57 cases of BOOP, of which 50 were idiopathic. However, BOOP may be associated with connective tissue disorders (which include rheumatoid arthritis, systemic lupus erythematosus, polymyositis and/or dermatomyositis, mixed-connective tissue disease), and other conditions listed in Table 46.2. It may also occur in a focal form on its own or around other processes such as an infarct or abscess, including those associated with necrotizing vasculitides such as Wegener's granulomatosis. Most patients affected by idiopathic or secondary forms of BOOP are in their fifth to seventh decades, and no sex predominance exists.

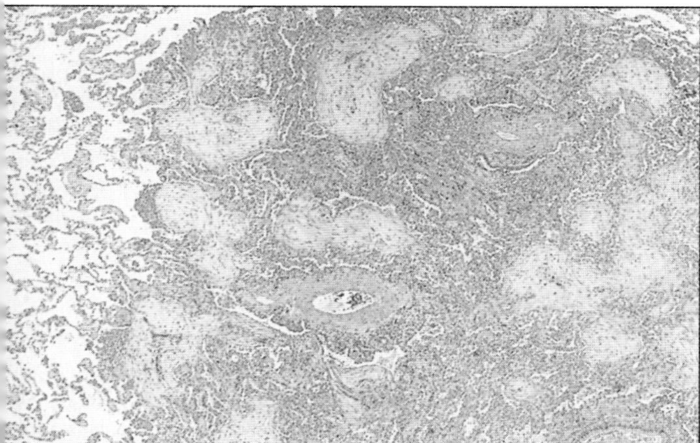

Figure 46.4 Histopathology of bronchiolitis obliterans organizing pneumonia (BOOP). This low-magnification photomicrograph shows BOOP in a patient who has the syndrome of idiopathic BOOP. The main change is the presence of intraluminal plugs of pale-staining, fibroblastic tissue. The configuration of the plugs betrays their distribution within distal bronchioles and alveolar ducts.

Clinical Features

Patients with BOOP usually have new cough and dyspnea of several weeks' duration. Constitutional symptoms are common and include malaise, fever, and weight loss. In idiopathic cases a preceding upper respiratory infection may occur. On physical examination, crackles and tachypnea are observed in most patients, but clubbing of the digits is rarely seen. The chest radiograph shows bilateral, patchy alveolar infiltrates (Fig. 46.5). A peripheral distribution, which resembles that of CEP, may be seen. At times the infiltrates may appear to be "migratory," with resolution of infiltrates in one region of the lung followed by appearance of new infiltrates in another region. Less commonly, linear and nodular opacities or diffuse interstitial infiltrates may be seen. Pleural effusions are uncommon but are reported in 30% of patients affected by secondary forms of BOOP. High-resolution CT of the chest also demonstrates patchy areas of consolidation and/or ground-glass density with a subpleural predominance. Bronchial wall thickening and dilatation are seen in those who have severe disease. Honeycombing is not seen in idiopathic BOOP. Pulmonary function tends to reveal a restrictive defect with a reduced diffusing capacity and resting and/or exercise-induced hypoxemia. Pulmonary function may be normal in up to one fifth of patients. Typically, BAL fluid shows an increased percentage of lymphocytes, but this is a nonspecific finding.

Diagnosis

A tentative diagnosis of BOOP may be made by recognizing the characteristic patchy, peripheral, alveolar infiltrates on a chest radiograph in an appropriate clinical setting. However, other disorders such as CEP, lymphoproliferative disorders, bronchoalveolar cell carcinoma, infections, and drug reactions may have a similar appearance. Thus, histopathologic confirmation by lung biopsy should be pursued before corticosteroid therapy is initiated. Although open (or thoracoscopic) lung biopsy is generally preferred, the diagnosis of BOOP can be made on transbronchial

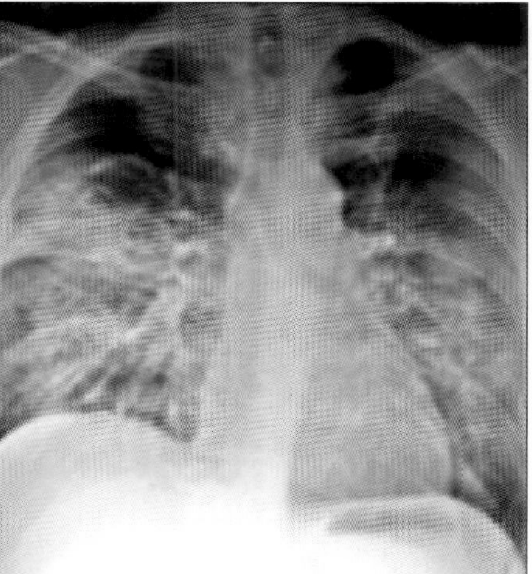

Figure 46.5 Bronchiolitis obliterans organizing pneumonia (BOOP). This radiograph of a 51-year-old man shows bilateral alveolar infiltrates. The patient had exertional dyspnea, malaise, and low-grade fever of 2 months' duration. Transbronchial lung biopsy showed BOOP, but no underlying cause or associated disorder was identified (idiopathic BOOP).

Table 46.2 Clinical classification of bronchiolitis obliterans organizing pneumonia

Type	Cause
Idiopathic	–
Secondary	Connective tissue disorders or vasculitides Inhaled or systemic toxins or drugs Infections Hypersensitivity pneumonitis Obstructive pneumonia Aspiration Chronic eosinophilic pneumonia Diffuse alveolar damage Myelodysplastic syndrome or hematologic malignancies Radiation therapy Allograft transplant (bone marrow, heart, lung)

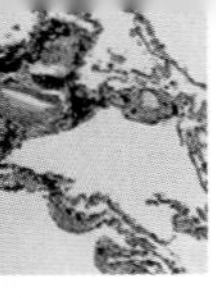

biopsy if the specimen is adequate in size to reveal the characteristic lesion. The histologic features of BOOP may be confused with those of usual interstitial pneumonia (UIP) or organizing diffuse alveolar damage. Clinically, BOOP is generally not difficult to differentiate from UIP, given the differences in clinical and radiographic features.

After biopsy confirmation of BOOP, the clinician needs to search for an underlying cause or associated disorder. The diagnosis of idiopathic BOOP or COP is reached if this search reveals no possible cause or association.

Treatment

Appropriate treatment for BOOP is determined by the underlying cause or associated condition. Specific therapy is employed when possible—for example, BOOP caused by infections is treated using effective antimicrobial therapy. If the cause is drugs or toxins, management may involve withdrawal of the offending agent and initiation of supportive measures. For BOOP resulting from many other causes, which include idiopathic cases and those associated with connective tissue disorders, corticosteroid therapy remains the treatment of choice. However, occasional cases of spontaneous recovery occur.

Corticosteroid therapy is generally begun with prednisone 1 mg/kg/day given for 1 to 3 months and slowly tapered over several months. Clinical and radiographic improvement is seen within days to weeks. The duration of corticosteroid therapy is usually 6 months or more because relapses are frequent if the corticosteroid is administered for less than 3 months. In contrast to UIP, most patients respond to corticosteroid therapy. Idiopathic cases appear to respond better than secondary forms of BOOP, which include those with associated connective tissue disorders. About two thirds of patients who have idiopathic BOOP experience complete resolution of symptoms, physiologic dysfunction, and radiographic abnormalities.

Clinical Course and Prevention

For the majority of patients affected by BOOP, and in particular those who have the idiopathic form, prognosis is excellent and recovery is complete. Some patients may require maintenance, low-dose corticosteroid therapy for several years to prevent relapse. Death from BOOP has been observed in 5% of cases. In particular, a small subset of patients has a fulminant course that resembles adult respiratory distress syndrome, which may result in death or severe residual fibrosis.

Pitfalls and Controversies

The classification and terminology of bronchiolar diseases remain unclear. In particular, the term *bronchiolitis obliterans* is used in reference to diverse bronchiolar conditions that have differing clinical, physiologic, and radiographic features. We prefer the pathologic classification that separates bronchiolitis obliterans into two major forms—constrictive bronchiolitis and proliferative bronchiolitis (BOOP). It is emphasized, however, that both of these lesions are nonspecific reaction patterns, and the clinician needs to correlate the histologic lesion with the clinical setting to assess its diagnostic, therapeutic, and prognostic significance.

SUGGESTED READINGS

Allen JN, Davis WB: State of the art: Eosinophilic lung diseases. Am J Respir Crit Care Med 150:1423-1438, 1994.

American Thoracic Society: American Thoracic Society/European Respiratory Society International Multidisciplinary Consensus Classification of the Idiopathic Interstitial Pneumonias. Am J Respir Crit Care Med 165:277-304, 2002.

Brito-Babapulle F: The eosinophilias, including the idiopathic hypereosinophilic syndrome. Br J Haematol 121:203-223, 2003.

Epler GR, Colby TV, McCloud TC, et al: Bronchiolitis obliterans organizing pneumonia. N Engl J Med 312:152-158, 1985.

Greenberger PA: Allergic bronchopulmonary aspergillosis. J Allergy Clin Immunol 110:685-692, 2002.

Katzenstein AL: Diagnostic features and differential diagnosis of Churg-Strauss syndrome in the lung. A review. Am J Clin Pathol 114:767-772, 2000.

Marchand E, Reynaud-Gaubert M, Lauque D, et al: Idiopathic chronic eosinophilic pneumonia. A clinical and follow-up study of 62 cases. The Groupe d'Etudes et de Recherche sur les Maladies "Orphelines" Pulmonaires 77:299-312, 1998.

Myers JL, Colby TV: Pathologic manifestations of bronchiolitis, constrictive bronchiolitis, cryptogenic organizing pneumonia, and diffuse panbronchiolitis. Clin Chest Med 14:611-622, 1993.

Philit F, Etienne-Mastroianni B, Parrot A, et al: Idiopathic acute eosinophilic pneumonia: a study of 22 patients. Am J Respir Crit Care Med 166:1235-1239, 2002.

Savani DM, Sharma OP: Eosinophilic lung disease in the tropics. Clin Chest Med 23:377-396, 2002.

CHAPTER 47 Other Diffuse Lung Diseases

Eric J. Olson, Jeffrey L. Myers, and Jay H. Ryu

The term *diffuse lung diseases* encompasses a broad array of disorders, many of which are covered in other chapters. This chapter focuses primarily on four distinct diffuse lung diseases: pulmonary lymphangiomyomatosis (LAM), pulmonary Langerhans cell histiocytosis (LCH), lymphoid interstitial pneumonia (LIP), and alveolar proteinosis. The unique epidemiologic, pathophysiologic, clinical, radiographic, management-related, and prognostic features will be described. In addition, this chapter briefly reviews several other rare forms of diffuse lung disease.

The terms *lymphangiomyomatosis*, *lymphangioleiomyomatosis*, and *pulmonary lymphangiomyomatosis* are used interchangeably. This process may involve pulmonary and/or extrapulmonary sites, including the mediastinal or retroperitoneal lymphatic system and abdominal or pelvic organs such as the uterus. The discussion will concentrate on pulmonary LAM, which is the most common presentation. LAM is characterized by atypical smooth muscle proliferation in the lung that results in diffuse cystic changes and airway obstruction, recurrent pneumothoraces, and chylous pleural effusions. *Pulmonary LCH* is the preferred term for the disease characterized by the proliferation and infiltration of the lung by Langerhans cells, with or without involvement of other organs, superseding other terms such as *primary pulmonary histiocytosis X*, *pulmonary eosinophilic granuloma*, *Langerhans cell granulomatosis*, *Letterer-Siwe disease*, and *Hand-Schüller-Christian* disease. Diffuse cystic changes in the lungs, airways obstruction, and recurrent pneumothoraces may also be seen with pulmonary LCH, and the condition is strongly associated with smoking. LIP, initially described by Liebow and Carrington as a subtype of the idiopathic interstitial pneumonias, is marked by diffuse interstitial infiltration of the lung with lymphocytic and plasma cell components. It may be associated with a variety of underlying disorders, and most authors consider it to be a type of lymphoproliferative disease. Pulmonary alveolar proteinosis (PAP), also called *alveolar phospholipidosis*, *alveolar lipoproteinosis*, and *pulmonary alveolar phospholipoproteinosis*, is either a primary (idiopathic) or secondary (associated with underlying disorders) process characterized by accumulation of lipoproteinaceous material in the alveolar spaces (Fig. 47.1).

EPIDEMIOLOGY, RISK FACTORS, AND PATHOPHYSIOLOGY

LAM is almost exclusively a disease of women of childbearing age, with an average age of onset of approximately 35 years. However, several cases have been reported in postmenopausal women, sometimes in association with postmenopausal hormone replacement, and biopsy-confirmed disease has also been documented in a man. The cause of LAM is unknown, but its predilection for women, association with postmenopausal hormonal therapy, and occasional acceleration during pregnancy suggests a pathogenic role for estrogenic hormones. LAM can occur sporadically or in women with tuberous sclerosis complex (TSC). TSC is an autosomal-dominant form of congenital hamartomatosis. Up to 30% to 40% of women with TSC may have radiographic changes consistent with LAM. The pathophysiologic basis of sporadic LAM (Fig. 47.2) and TSC-LAM, namely, atypical smooth muscle cell proliferation, is believed to be similar. TSC results from mutations of either the hamartin *(TSC1)* gene on chromosome 9 or the tuberin *(TSC2)* gene on chromosome 16, both tumor suppressor genes. Mutations in *TSC1* and *TSC2* genes have been found in sporadic LAM cells, supporting a role for *TSC* genes in LAM pathogenesis. In TSC-LAM, it remains unclear how *TSC1* or *TSC2* mutations correlate with the expression of the LAM features.

Langerhans cells are present in the normal lung, almost exclusively intercalated between epithelial cells of the airways, and they have potent antigen-presenting capabilities. Langerhans cells are distinguished by their characteristic pentalaminar, plate-like cytoplasmic organelles (Birbeck granule or X-body) seen on electron microscopy, and their strong expression of the CD1a antigen on the cell surface. They also stain with S-100 and CD45 antibodies. The cause of the excessive proliferation of Langerhans cells in pulmonary LCH is not known, although the strong association with cigarette smoking suggests a causal link. Most studies have shown that more than 90% of patients who have LCH are current or previous cigarette smokers who are typically in their third to fifth decade of life. It is postulated that cigarette smoking leads to recruitment and proliferation of Langerhans cells in the lung parenchyma. In extrapulmonary sites, the Langerhans cell proliferation may be monoclonal; however, pulmonary LCH is believed to represent a reactive, not neoplastic, process. Morphologic studies show proliferating Langerhans cells involved in a bronchocentric process accompanied by mixed cellular infiltrates (Fig. 47.3). Adjacent blood vessels and lung parenchyma are also involved. As this granulomatous-like reaction evolves, collagen fibrosis and scarring occur, with associated paracicatricial air-space enlargement that accounts for the concomitant cystic changes. The incidence and prevalence of pulmonary LCH are not known. Most cases occur sporadically, usually in whites, and there are no known predisposing genetic factors.

Although LIP was initially described in 1969 as a distinct form of idiopathic interstitial pneumonia, it appears that this disorder is rarely idiopathic and more commonly is associated

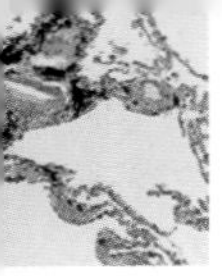

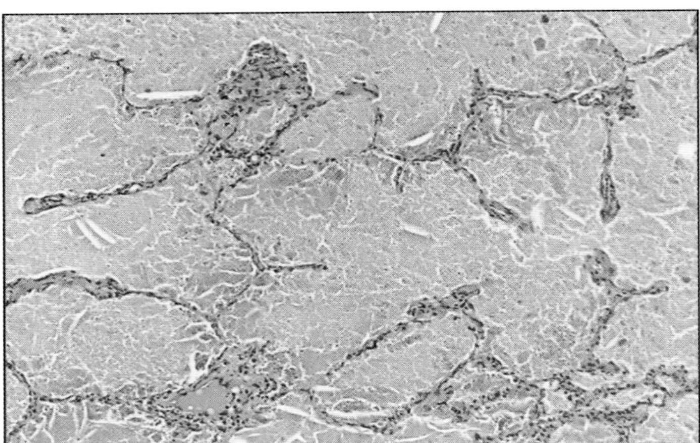

Figure 47.1 Histopathology of pulmonary alveolar proteinosis (PAP). Photomicrograph of PAP showing alveolar spaces filled with amorphous granular eosinophilic debris. The proteinaceous exudate includes scattered cell "ghosts." Alveolar septa are only minimally thickened in this predominantly air-space lesion.

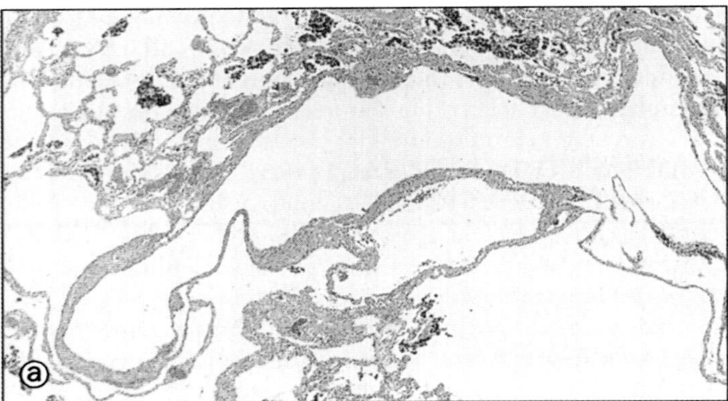

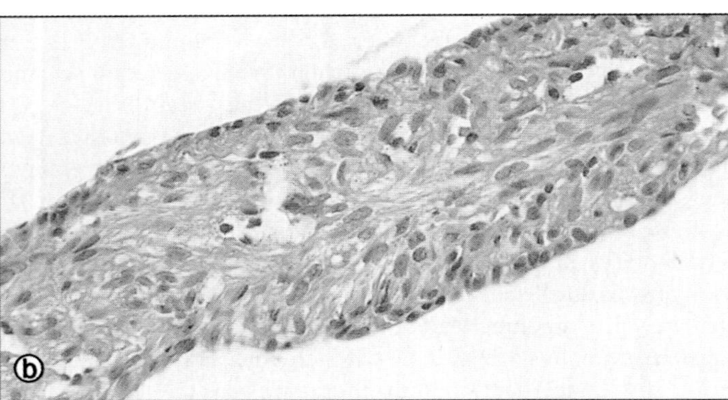

Figure 47.2 Histopathology of lymphangiomyomatosis (LAM). **A,** Low-magnification photomicrograph of LAM showing cystic spaces surrounded by a variably thick wall containing proliferating spindle cells. Hemosiderin pigment is present in adjacent air spaces, which attests to the presence of alveolar hemorrhage. **B,** Higher-magnification photomicrograph showing smooth muscle cells within thickened peribronchiolar interstitium in LAM.

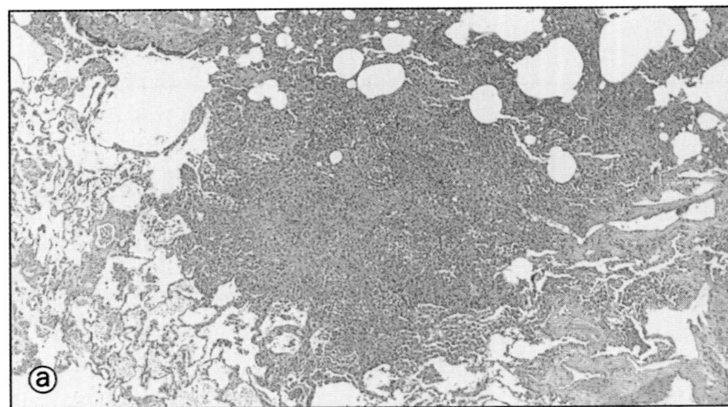

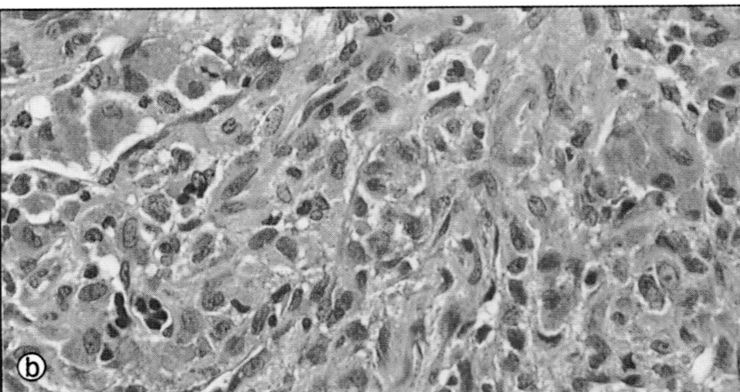

Figure 47.3 Histopathology of Langerhans cell histiocytosis (LCH). **A,** Low-magnification photomicrograph showing stellate, bronchiolocentric nodule in LCH. **B,** High-magnification photomicrograph showing a polymorphic, interstitial infiltrate in LCH. The cellular infiltrate includes a mixture of mononuclear cells and eosinophils. Langerhans cells predominate and are differentiated by highly convoluted nuclei with nuclear grooves, which result in nuclear configurations that resemble crumpled paper or coffee beans.

with a variety of underlying conditions, including human immunodeficiency virus (HIV) infection, Sjögren's syndrome, Hashimoto's thyroiditis, chronic active hepatitis, primary biliary cirrhosis, myasthenia gravis, rheumatoid arthritis, pernicious anemia, and autoimmune hypogammaglobulinemia. In a small number of cases, LIP is thought to transform into lymphoma or represent lymphoma de novo. The Epstein-Barr virus genome has been identified in some patients who have LIP. The majority of HIV-negative patients who have LIP are adults in their fourth to seventh decades. Women are more commonly affected than men. However, those who have LIP in association with HIV infection tend to be younger, with a male predominance.

PAP is an uncommon disorder that occurs in patients over a wide age range, with most cases occurring in people 30 to 50 years old. Few familial cases have been reported, men are affected about twice as often as women, and the disorder has been encountered in virtually all industrialized countries. PAP is restricted to the lungs and is characterized by accumulation of Periodic Acid Schiff (PAS)–positive, acellular, lipoproteinaceous surfactant component material in the alveolar spaces with negligible interstitial inflammation. PAP can occur as a congenital disorder, a primary (idiopathic) acquired form, or as a secondary form in association with pulmonary infections, exposure to inhaled chemicals (insecticides) and minerals (silica, aluminum dust, titanium), immunodeficiency disorders (severe combined immunodeficiency disorder, immunoglobulin A deficiency, HIV), and hematologic disorders (lymphoma, leukemia). Pathogenesis appears to primarily involve disrupted clearance of surfactant-like material by alveolar macrophages, and in some situations this may be related to impaired action of granulocyte-macrophage colony-stimulating factor (GM-CSF). Some acquired cases may result from GM-CSF blocking autoantibodies demonstrable in bronchoalveolar lavage (BAL) fluid, whereas congenital cases may be linked to GM-CSF receptor defects.

CLINICAL FEATURES

The characteristic presentation of LAM includes progressive breathlessness and recurrent pneumothoraces. Less common symptoms include chest pain, cough, hemoptysis, pleural effusions (usually chylous), chylous ascites, and (rarely) chyloptysis. Physical examination is usually unremarkable except for signs of a pleural effusion (if present) or occasional wheezes or basal crackles. Those patients who have TSC-LAM usually show pathognomonic findings of TSC, which include facial angiofibromas, periungual or ungual fibromas, and retinal astrocytomas.

The clinical presentation of pulmonary LCH most commonly includes dyspnea and nonproductive cough in a current or former smoker. A history of pneumothorax is obtained in about 15% to 25% of patients, with a similar percentage of patients having no symptoms or only mild, nonspecific symptoms in the early stages of disease. Other symptoms may include wheezing, fever, fatigue, weight loss, and chest pain. Hemoptysis is uncommon (less than 5% of patients). Examination sometimes reveals crackles, wheeze, and digital clubbing. Approximately 15% of patients have extrapulmonary manifestations, including diabetes insipidus from hypothalamic involvement, pain from bone involvement, adenopathy from lymph node infiltration, rash from cutaneous involvement, and abdominal discomfort from hepatosplenic involvement.

LIP patients are usually symptomatic at presentation, most commonly reporting gradually progressive dyspnea and cough. Less common symptoms include weight loss, fever, chest pain, and arthralgias. On examination, bibasilar crackles are heard in most patients, but digital clubbing and pneumothorax are unusual. Physical signs of associated conditions, such as connective tissue disorders, should be sought, because idiopathic LIP is considered a rare entity. Dysproteinemia, most commonly polyclonal hypergammaglobulinemia, is found in the majority of patients. Rheumatoid factor and antinuclear antibody titers may be elevated in those who have Sjögren's syndrome in association with LIP.

Clinical presentation of PAP is nonspecific, with dyspnea and a dry cough in most patients. Less common symptoms include chest pain, hemoptysis, weight loss, chills, fatigue, and arthralgias. Fever is also unusual and should raise suspicion for a superimposed process, such as infection. Crackles occur over the involved areas of lung in about 20% of patients. Digital clubbing occurs in about 20% of patients and cyanosis is seen with severe disease. Mildly elevated serum lactate dehydrogenase level is common, and increased levels of lung surfactant A and D (SP-A and SP-D) and mucin-like glycoprotein (KL-6) in the serum have also been found in PAP; however, these findings are not specific. Patients affected by PAP may have PAS-positive material or elevated SP-A levels in their sputum, but these findings are also nonspecific.

Chest radiographs of LAM patients are usually abnormal and show diffuse reticular and nodular densities, without sparing of the costophrenic angles (Fig. 47.4). As the disease progresses, cystic changes may become apparent, together with signs of hyperinflation. Pneumothorax and/or pleural effusions may accompany infiltrates. However, in early disease the chest radiograph may be entirely normal. High-resolution computed tomography (HRCT) of the chest reveals well-defined cystic spaces throughout both lungs, even in those patients with normal chest radiographs (Fig. 47.5). Cystic changes are diffuse, with no sparing of the costophrenic angles. The cysts have uniformly thin walls and measure a few millimeters to several centimeters in diameter. Most are round, but they can coalesce into bizarre shapes as the disease progresses. Pleural effusions, pneumothoraces, and mediastinal adenopathy, which sometimes are not apparent on the chest radiograph, may also be seen. Most of the lung parenchyma between the cystic spaces appears normal. No difference is found in the appearance of the lungs of patients who have sporadic LAM versus those who have TSC-LAM. When CT of the chest is performed in a woman suspected of having LAM, it is useful to extend the scanning to include the kidneys, as one third or more of patients have renal angiomyolipomas (AMLs). Also, CT of the abdomen may reveal unsuspected retroperitoneal lymphangiomyomas or adenopathy.

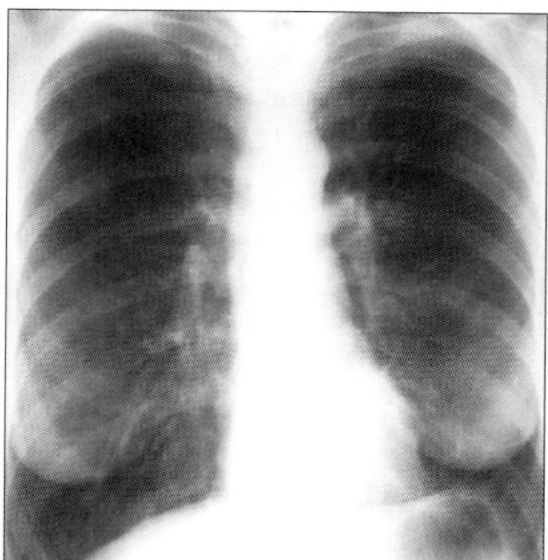

Figure 47.4 Lymphangiomyomatosis (LAM). This posteroanterior chest radiograph of a 37-year-old woman with LAM shows hyperinflation and diffuse reticular infiltrates.

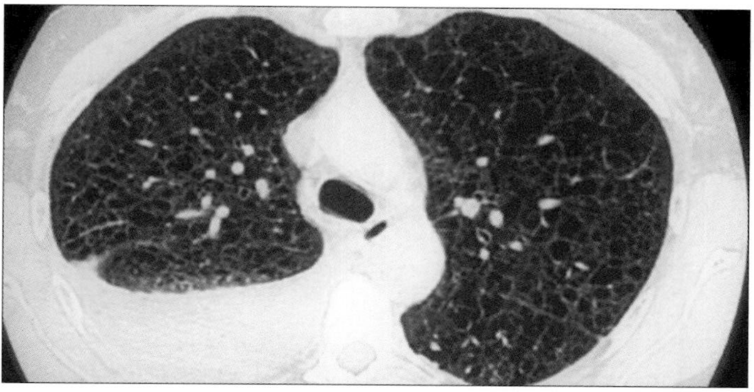

Figure 47.5 Lymphangiomyomatosis (LAM). High-resolution computed tomogram of a 42-year-old woman with tuberous sclerosis complex (TSC) with lung involvement (lymphangiomyomatosis) showing diffuse cystic changes and a right pleural effusion (chylothorax).

The typical chest radiographic finding in pulmonary LCH is reticulonodular infiltrates, most prominent in the middle and upper zones (Fig. 47.6). Often the costophrenic angles are spared and the lung volume appears normal or increased. As the disease advances, cystic changes and bullae appear. Pleural disease (except for pneumothorax) or adenopathy is unusual.

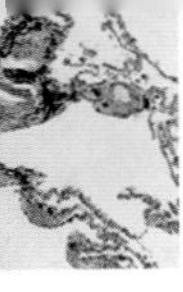

Predilection for the middle and upper lung zones is confirmed by HRCT of the chest, which also shows thin-walled cysts and nodules (with or without cavitation), reticular densities, and some areas of ground-glass opacity (Fig. 47.7). The cysts are irregularly shaped and more complex than those seen in LAM.

Chest radiography reveals basilar-predominant reticulonodular opacities in patients with LIP. Superimposed, patchy alveolar (Fig. 47.8) or nodular infiltrates are present in about half of the patients. HRCT of the chest patterns shows ground-glass opacities, reticular infiltrates, nodules, diffuse consolidation, and, in advanced cases, honeycombing. Mediastinal or hilar adenopathy and pleural effusions are infrequent in HIV-negative patients. However, intrathoracic adenopathy may be seen in up to one third of HIV-infected patients with LIP.

The intra-alveolar buildup of surfactant-like material in patients with PAP results in bilateral, patchy air-space infiltrates on chest radiographs (Fig. 47.9). Less commonly, an interstitial pattern may be seen. Infiltrates are often more prominent in the perihilar regions, and this "bat-wing" pattern may be mistaken for pulmonary edema. The radiographic differential diagnosis can include sarcoidosis, infections, bronchoalveolar cell carcinoma, pneumoconiosis, and other diffuses diseases. About one third of patients have asymmetrical or unilateral infiltrates. HRCT of the chest demonstrates ground-glass and/or consolidative infiltrates in patchy or diffuse distributions. Distinct central or peripheral distribution is usually not seen, but sharp demarcation of the infiltrates from surrounding normal lung tissue is commonly observed. Reticular opacities or interlobular septal thickening are present within the air-space infiltrates, creating a "crazy-paving" pattern.

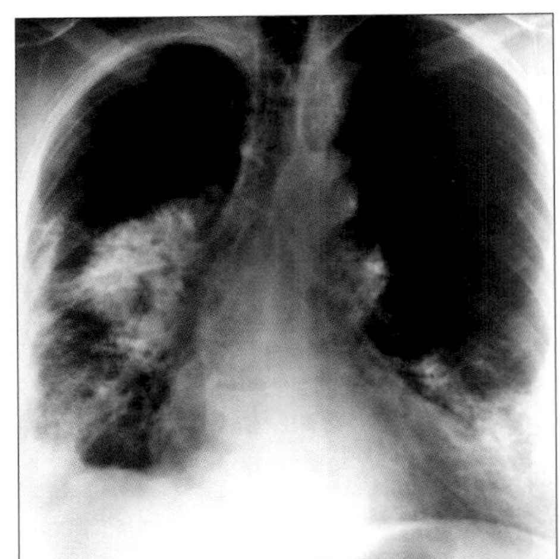

Figure 47.8 Lymphoid intersitial pneumonia (LIP). Posteroanterior chest radiograph of a 73-year-old woman with LIP showing consolidative infiltrates in the right midlung and lung base as well as the left lung base.

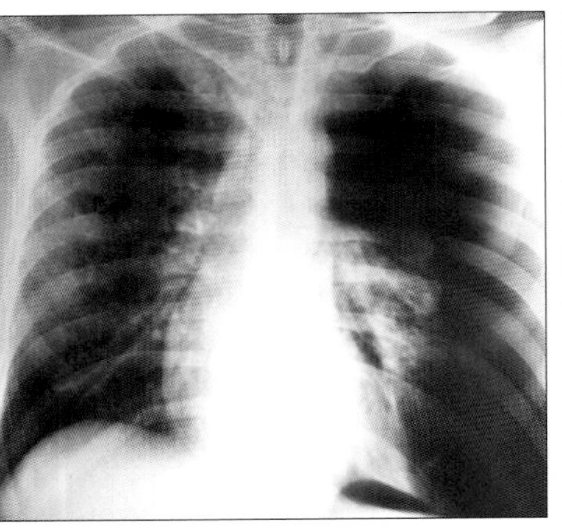

Figure 47.6 Langerhans cell histiocytosis (LCH). Posteroanterior chest radiograph of a 25-year-old male smoker with dyspnea. Massive left pneumothorax and interstitial infiltrates are seen in the right lung.

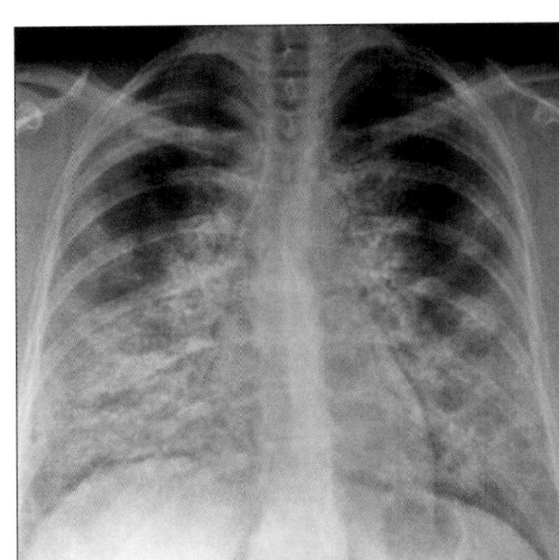

Figure 47.9 Pulmonary alveolar proteinosis (PAP). Posteroanterior chest radiograph of a 53-year-old woman with PAP shows diffuse alveolar infiltrates. She presented with progressive exertional dyspnea of 1.5 years' duration.

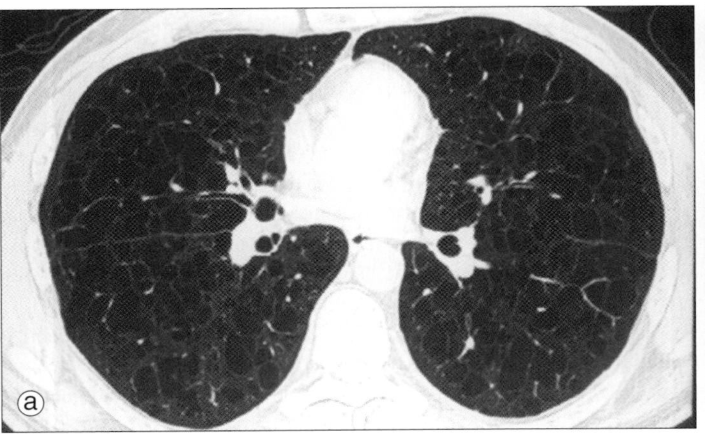

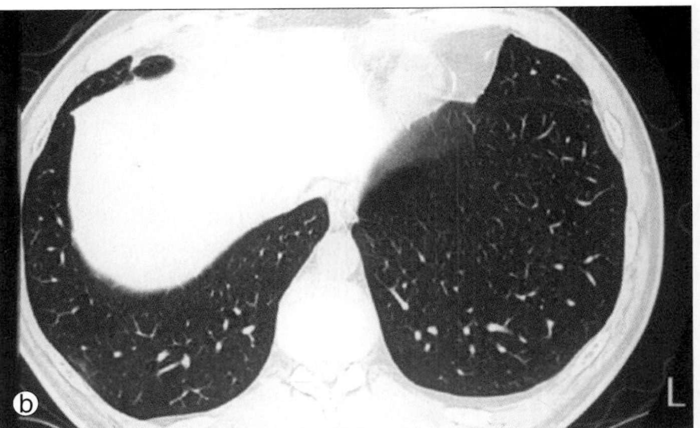

Figure 47.7 Langerhans cell histiocytosis (LCH). High-resolution computed tomograms of the same patient shown in Figure 47.6 taken 6 years after presentation. **A,** Diffuse cystic changes are seen with **(B)** relative sparing of bibasilar regions.

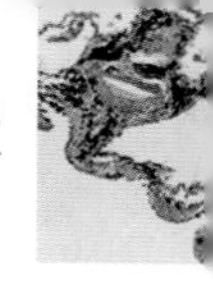

Pulmonary function testing in LAM patients usually reveals airflow obstruction, increased lung volumes, air trapping, and a decreased diffusing capacity. Hypoxemia is seen in late stages of the disease. Obstructive and/or restrictive changes may occur in patients with pulmonary LCH. The relative contributions of cigarette smoking and the disease itself may be difficult to define. Diffusing capacity is usually abnormal and correlates with impairment in exercise performance. Restrictive changes with diffusion capacity reduction are found in patients with LIP and PAP. Hypoxemia is common in PAP patients, resulting from shunt physiology.

DIAGNOSIS

LAM, LCH, LIP, and PAP may be strongly suspected on the basis of epidemiologic, clinical, radiographic, and physiologic features. For example, diffuse interstitial infiltrates in a nonsmoking woman of childbearing age who has a history of recurrent pneumothoraces and/or chylous pleural effusions strongly suggests LAM. Similarly, diffuse interstitial infiltrates predominantly in the middle and upper lung fields and sparing the costophrenic angles with normal or increased lung volume in a young adult smoker suggests the diagnosis of pulmonary LCH. A history of never having smoked makes the diagnosis of pulmonary LCH very unlikely. Predominantly bibasilar reticulonodular infiltrates with superimposed patchy alveolar opacities in a middle-aged individual with dysproteinemia suggest LIP. The diagnosis of PAP should be considered in a patient who has persistent perihilar alveolar infiltrates without evidence of congestive heart failure or infection.

The diagnosis of these four disorders generally requires histologic confirmation, but the use of HRCT and bronchoscopy provides some exceptions to this rule; the HRCT finding of diffuse cystic changes with no sparing of the costophrenic angles in the lungs of a young woman can be nearly pathognomonic for LAM, especially if renal AMLs coexist. Nonetheless, biopsy confirmation of LAM is generally recommended, as occasional cases of pulmonary LCH or metastatic sarcoma may be difficult to differentiate from LAM on HRCT. Transbronchial lung biopsy may suffice for this purpose, especially if the lung biopsy specimen stains positively for HMB-45, a highly sensitive and specific marker for LAM cells.

PAP and pulmonary LCH may be confirmed by BAL. Although Langerhans cells can be found in other disorders, which include idiopathic pulmonary fibrosis, the presence of 5% CD1a-positive cells in the BAL fluid is highly specific for LCH. If this criterion is not met, histologic confirmation of LCH is pursued by lung biopsy. Transbronchial biopsy may provide adequate tissue but requires a high index of suspicion and an experienced pathologist for proper interpretation. If transbronchial lung biopsy or BAL does not confirm the diagnosis, surgical lung biopsy or biopsy of bone lesions, if present, may provide diagnostic material.

In an appropriate clinical setting, the diagnosis of PAP may be made by BAL, which typically yields a milky effluent (Fig. 47.10). Under light microscopy, this fluid shows large amounts of PAS-positive lipoproteinaceous material. Transbronchial biopsy also provides the diagnosis in most cases and demonstrates accumulation of granular, PAS-positive, lipoproteinaceous material within the alveolar spaces with alveolar architecture usually preserved, although thickening of the alveolar septa and interstitial fibrosis may occur in some cases. In the absence of a superimposed infection, very few inflammatory cells are seen in the lung tissue. Surgical biopsy is now being used less frequently to confirm a PAP diagnosis. Although a transbronchial biopsy may occasionally suffice, the diagnosis of LIP usually requires a lung biopsy. An open or thoracoscopic lung biopsy (Fig. 47.11A and B) is frequently needed. Infectious processes should be excluded. Immunohistochemical stains are valuable in the dense interstitial lymphoid infiltrate of LIP from other lymphoproliferative disorders, such as lymphoma, diffuse lymphoid hyperplasia, nodular lymphoid hyperplasia, chronic lymphocytic leukemia, and multiple myeloma. BAL typically shows a nonspecific lymphocytosis in LIP.

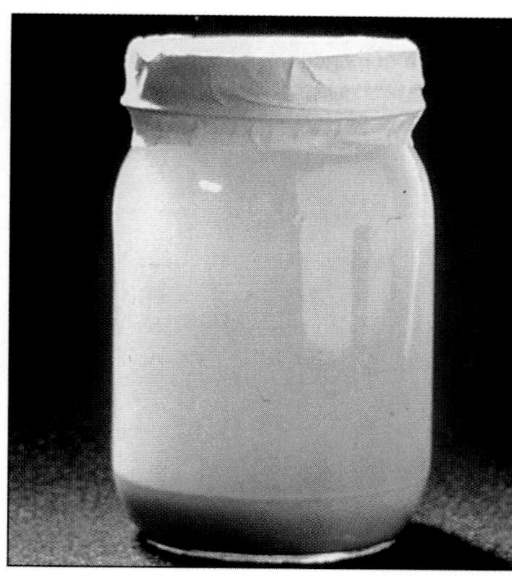

Figure 47.10 Lung lavage fluid in pulmonary alveolar proteinosis (PAP). A sample of lung lavage fluid in PAP showing the typical cloudy appearance and sediment that forms over 30 minutes.

TREATMENT

The traditional treatment for LAM is hormonal manipulation, typically intramuscular medroxyprogesterone injections at a dose of 400 mg/month; however, the evidence supporting the use of hormonal therapy in this disease is relatively weak. Gonadotropin-releasing hormone analogs, such as leuprolide, have also been used. Tamoxifen and oophorectomy are less frequently employed. Patients who suffer recurrent pneumothoraces or chylothorax may require pleurodesis. Lung transplantation is an option for patients affected by advanced LAM. Corticosteroids are not helpful in LAM. Smoking cessation should be the initial intervention in all cases of pulmonary LCH and may be all that is required. Corticosteroids are initiated for progressive or systemic disease despite smoking cessation, although data are insufficient to definitively support their role. Radiation therapy for bone lesions provides symptomatic relief. In those patients who suffer progressive disease despite smoking cessation and corticosteroids, options include cytotoxic drugs, which generally are of limited benefit, and lung transplantation.

Most patients affected by LIP are treated with corticosteroids with or without chlorambucil. The response is variable, and optimal dosing of corticosteroids has not been defined. Chlorambucil and other cytotoxic agents probably provide no significant benefit. Vigilance for and prompt treatment of superimposed pulmonary infections are important.

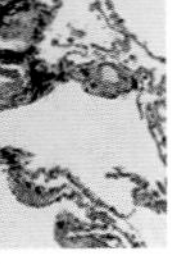

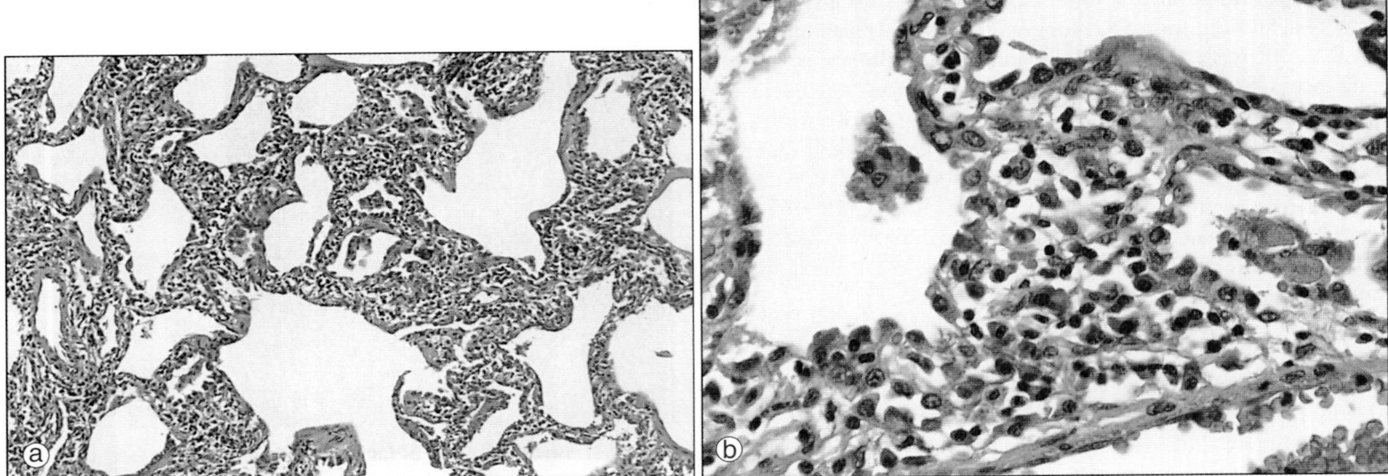

Figure 47.11 Histopathology of lymphoid interstitial pneumonia (LIP). A, Low magnification photomicrograph demonstrating features of LIP. Alveolar septa are diffusely expanded by a cellular infiltrate characterized by a combination of lymphocytes and plasma cells. **B,** High-magnification photomicrograph showing LIP. The expanded alveolar septum contains an infiltrate of mononuclear cells that, in this example, includes mainly mature plasma cells.

The treatment mainstay for PAP is whole lung lavage. This is performed with the patient under general anesthetic via a bronchoscope passed through a double-lumen endotracheal tube. The procedure typically lasts 1 to 2 hours, during which repeated instillation and drainage of the lung with up to 20 to 30 L of isotonic saline is performed until the run-off is clear. Only one lung is usually lavaged at a session, with the other lung treated similarly 2 to 3 days later if necessary, although single-session, sequential, bilateral whole lung lavage has been performed. Chest percussion during the lavage may help. More than 80% of patients show improvement after lung lavage. The median duration of clinical benefit is approximately 15 months. Eventually, 60% to 70% of patients require repeat lavage, and the median total number of procedures is two. Consistent with its proposed importance in surfactant clearance, preliminary experience with GM-CSF administration in PAP has shown potential. Corticosteroids have no beneficial effect.

CLINICAL COURSE AND PREVENTION

The clinical course varies greatly among these four diffuse lung diseases. Most LAM patients experience slow progression of their disease. However, recent studies report survival rates of 38% to 78% 8.5 years after the onset of symptoms, figures better than initially reported. Our experience suggests that the rate of progression varies among LAM patients. Postmenopausal women tend to have a more benign course. Exogenous estrogens may exacerbate the disorder and should be avoided. Properly designed clinical trials of progesterone therapy have not been performed, but clinical experience in the United States and Europe suggests intramuscular progesterone slows the rate of decline in the forced expiratory volume in 1 second (FEV_1). A review of 34 LAM patients who underwent lung transplantation revealed survival rates of 69% and 58% at 1 and 2 years after transplantation, respectively—values similar to transplant experience with other chronic pulmonary conditions. About half the patients had substantial pleural adhesions that caused intraoperative difficulties. Recurrent pneumothorax in the remaining native lung and chylothorax were the main postoperative problems. Recurrent LAM has occurred in allografts and was found in 1 patient in this series.

Substantial variation is also found in the natural history of pulmonary LCH. A recent retrospective review from Mayo Clinic of 102 patients with histopathologically confirmed pulmonary LCH and with median follow-up of 4 years reported 33 deaths (15 due to respiratory failure) and overall median survival of 12.5 years. Univariate analysis revealed poorer prognosis with older age and greater impairment of pulmonary function (lower FEV_1, higher residual volume, lower ratio of FEV_1 to forced vital capacity, and lower diffusing capacity). Patients affected by only pulmonary involvement follow a more benign course. Cigarette smoking must be discouraged. Pulmonary LCH has recurred in transplanted lungs, with or without smoking cessation.

The clinical course of LIP includes progression to diffuse pulmonary fibrosis in one third of cases. Some patients diagnosed with LIP probably have lymphoma from the outset, but cases in which LIP has transformed to lymphoma have occurred. Death may result from progressive lung involvement with cor pulmonale, malignant lymphoma, or complications of treatment. Those individuals with LIP in the setting of HIV usually die from complications of the HIV infection. Spontaneous improvement of LIP may occur.

Spontaneous resolution occurs in about one third of patients with PAP. Death from progressive disease, pulmonary fibrosis, and respiratory failure is rare. Superimposed infection, such as nocardiosis, may occur. Lung transplantation is an option in those individuals affected by progressive disease. Recurrent PAP following double lung transplantation has been reported.

PITFALLS AND CONTROVERSIES

Several lines of evidence have led to the hypothesis that pulmonary LAM represents metastatic disease. Renal AML cells and pulmonary LAM cells in sporadic LAM have been shown to contain the identical *TSC2* mutation not present in other, normal cells. LAM cells from recurrent disease in an engrafted lung have been shown to contain the same *TSC2* mutation

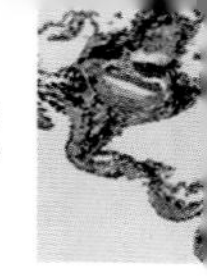

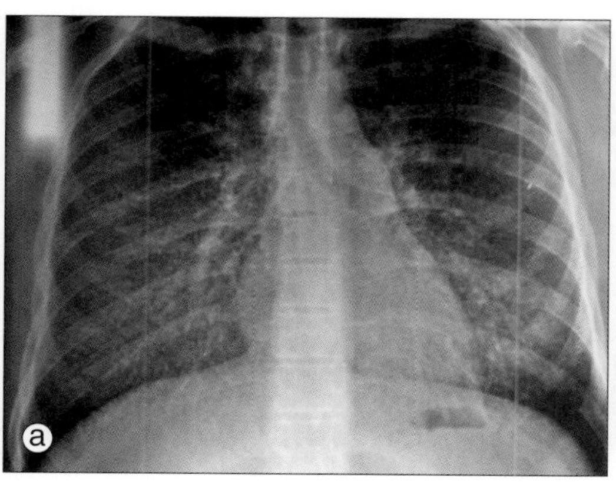

Figure 47.12 Pulmonary alveolar microlithiasis. A, Posteroanterior chest radiograph of an 18-year-old asymptomatic man who has pulmonary alveolar microlithiasis showing numerous tiny opacities present throughout both lungs. **B,** Magnified view of the right lower lung showing numerous opacities that measure less than 1 mm.

present in native LAM cells before transplant. This patient, however, did not have renal AMLs, but the *TSC2* mutation was also found in four separate mediastinal lymph nodes. The risks of pregnancy and air travel are not fully defined, and counseling must be handled on a patient-by-patient basis. The optimal timing for initiation of progesterone therapy remains unclear. Eight women in a cohort of 250 sporadic LAM patients were found to have brain lesions compatible with meningiomas, a finding of concern because progesterone is a putative growth factor for meningiomas. Whether all LAM patients require screening for meningiomas and how this information should influence treatment decisions remain unclear.

There may be an increased risk for neoplasms in pulmonary LCH. In the Mayo Clinic series, six hematologic cancers were diagnosed, so clinicians are advised to be mindful of malignancy in these patients, especially those with hemoptysis. The diagnosis of LIP should not be made without immunohistochemical staining to exclude lymphoma. It is likely that some cases diagnosed as the transformation of LIP to lymphoma represented lymphoma de novo.

OTHER RARE DIFFUSE LUNG DISEASES

The remaining disorders described in this section are a diverse group of diseases the pulmonary manifestations of which stem from excessive accumulation of various types of material in the respiratory system.

Neurofibromatosis

Neurofibromatosis is a variably expressed autosomal dominant disorder characterized by café-au-lait spots, subcutaneous neurofibromas, axillary freckling, and iris hamartomas (Lisch nodules). Thoracic involvement is estimated to occur in 10% to 15% of patients who show manifestations, which include a predominantly bibasilar interstitial fibrosis in middle-aged patients, apical bullous disease alone or in conjunction with interstitial fibrosis, kyphoscoliosis, and meningoceles. Intrathoracic neurofibromas may occur in the pulmonary parenchyma, either as primary or as metastatic lesions, in the posterior mediastinum, and on the chest wall.

Pulmonary Alveolar Microlithiasis

Pulmonary alveolar microlithiasis results from the unexplained and extensive intra-alveolar deposition of concentrically lamellated calcium phosphate spheres, which produces a distinctive calcific, micronodular infiltrate on the chest radiograph. Most patients are asymptomatic, but dyspnea, cough, and right-sided cardiac failure may occur in later stages with interstitial fibrosis. Microlith expectoration is uncommon. A familial incidence occurs in approximately 50% of cases, and diagnosis is usually made on the unique "sandstorm" chest radiographic appearance (Fig. 47.12). Supporting evidence can be obtained by transbronchial lung biopsy or by the demonstration of extensive pulmonary uptake during technetium-99m diphosphonate scanning. No consistently effective therapy is known, although lung transplant has been attempted and regression of the calcific infiltrates has been reported in pediatric patients treated with disodium editronate.

Amyloid

Amyloid, a fibrillar, homogeneous, proteinaceous material usually derived from immunoglobulin light chains, can deposit in the tracheobronchial tree or pulmonary parenchyma in either localized or diffuse patterns. This accumulation can be part of a systemic process (primary systemic amyloidosis, secondary amyloidosis, familial amyloidosis) or can be isolated to the lung (localized pulmonary amyloidosis). The incidence of pulmonary amyloid deposition with secondary and familial amyloidosis is low, whereas pulmonary involvement by primary systemic amyloidosis is common and usually takes the form of diffuse, alveolar, septal amyloid accumulation that manifests radiographically as reticular or reticulonodular infiltrates. Pleural effusions may also occur because of simultaneous pleural involvement or from heart failure caused by cardiac amyloid deposition. Prognosis is poor for patients with primary systemic amyloidosis who have pulmonary involvement.

A diffuse interstitial pattern is rare with localized pulmonary amyloidosis. Instead, pulmonary parenchymal involvement manifests as single or multiple nodules that are often detected incidentally on the chest radiograph. These nodules may grow slowly, cavitate, or calcify. Localized amyloid masses or multifocal, submucosal plaques characterize the tracheobronchial forms of localized pulmonary amyloidosis. Diffuse endobronchial involvement is recognizable bronchoscopically as shiny, pale plaques with scattered focal stenoses. Symptoms depend on the extent of luminal compromise and include dyspnea, cough, hemoptysis, wheeze, atelectasis, and recurrent pneumonia. Severe localized stenosis can be treated with repeated bron-

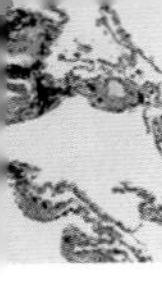

choscopic resection, perhaps incorporating laser ablation, or surgery. Other pulmonary manifestations of amyloid deposition, whether caused by a systemic or localized process, are mediastinal and/or hilar adenopathy, mediastinal masses, and macroglossia that results in obstructive sleep apnea.

Tracheobronchial and diffuse parenchymal forms of pulmonary amyloidosis can be safely diagnosed at bronchoscopy, although the endoscopist must be prepared for potential bleeding. Lung nodules are diagnosed by needle aspiration or resection. Biopsy material reveals the characteristic apple-green birefringence with polarized microscopy after staining with Congo red.

Hermansky-Pudlak Syndrome

The Hermansky-Pudlak syndrome is a triad of oculocutaneous albinism, platelet aggregation dysfunction, and visceral ceroid deposition. It is an autosomal recessive disorder with a high frequency among Puerto Ricans. At least four different genes may cause HPS. Mutations in the *HSP1* gene are associated with a progressive interstitial fibrosis that may develop during the second and fourth decades and for which there is no reliable treatment. The interstitial lung disease is felt to be related to the interaction of alveolar macrophages with ceroid, a material derived from incompletely processed lysosomal membranes. Such ceroid-laden macrophages have been demonstrated by Fontana-Masson staining of BAL fluid.

Lipoid Storage Disorders

Several autosomal-recessive, inborn errors of sphingolipid metabolism may have pulmonary manifestations that result from the intracellular accumulation of metabolic products induced by enzymatic defects. Gaucher's disease is caused by a deficiency of β-glucosidase, which leads to the formation of the characteristic Gaucher cell, a reticuloendothelial cell packed with glucose-1-ceramide. With Niemann-Pick disease, deficiencies in sphingomyelinase or cholesterol esterification lead to the development of foamy-appearing cells. Reticular or reticulonodular infiltrates can occur in Gaucher's and Niemann-Pick disease, as alveolar macrophages filled with material accumulate in the interstitium and alveolar spaces. Patients who have Fabry's disease, an X-linked sphingolipidosis caused by the absence of α-galactosidase A, may exhibit airflow obstruction and reduced diffusing capacities. In general, the pulmonary manifestations in these metabolic disorders are incompletely described, have a variable course, may occur in childhood, and are often overshadowed by the extrapulmonary manifestations.

SUGGESTED READINGS

American Thoracic Society/European Respiratory Society International Multidisciplinary Consensus Conference of the Idiopathic Interstitial Pneumonias: Am J Respir Crit Care Med 165:277-304, 2002.

Garay SM, Gardella JE, Fazzini EP, Goldring RM: Hermansky-Pudlak syndrome: pulmonary manifestations of a ceroid storage disorder. Am J Med 66:737-747, 1979.

Kelly J, Moss J: Lymphangioleiomyomatosis. Am J Med Sci 321:17-25, 2001.

Long RG, Lake BD, Pettit JE, et al: Adult Niemann-Pick disease. Am J Med 62:627-635, 1977.

Riccardi VM: Von Recklinghausen's neurofibromatosis. N Engl J Med 305:1616-1627, 1981.

Rosenberg DM, Ferrans VJ, Fulmer JD, et al: Chronic airflow obstruction in Fabry's disease. Am J Med 68:898-904, 1980.

Seymour JF, Presneill JJ: Pulmonary alveolar proteinosis: progress in the first 44 years. Am J Respir Crit Care Med 166:215-235, 2002.

Utz JP, Swensen SJ, Gertz MA: Pulmonary amyloidosis: The Mayo Clinic experience from 1980 to 1993. Ann Intern Med 124:407-413, 1996.

Vassallo R, Ryu JH, Colby TV, et al: Pulmonary Langerhans'-cell histiocytosis. N Engl J Med 342:1969-1978, 2000.

Vassallo R, Ryu JH, Schroeder DR, et al: Clinical outcomes of pulmonary Langerhans'-cell histiocytosis in adults. N Engl J Med 346:484-490, 2002.

Wolsen AH: Pulmonary findings in Gaucher's disease. AJR Am J Roentgenol 123:712-715, 1975.

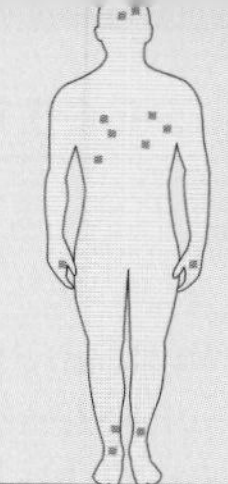

CHAPTER 48 Connective Tissue Disorders

A. G. Bradbeer, R. G. Stirling, and R. M. du Bois

EPIDEMIOLOGY AND RISK FACTORS

Although the lung can be affected in many ways in connective tissue disease (CTD), the prevalence and incidence of lung disease in CTD, along with the associated risk factors, are largely unknown. Reasons for this include the following:

- Variable reporting of prevalence and incidence rates depending on how closely lung disease is sought
- Past tendency for all lung diseases associated with CTD to be grouped as a single entity; it is now well understood that focus of disease can be in different compartments of the lung (e.g., alveolus, small airway, large airway, interstitium, vasculature)
- The great functional reserve of the lung; considerable function may be lost before symptoms prompt investigation
- Reduction or worsening of the expression of lung disease in CTD by medications, as a result of immunosuppression, direct toxicity, and/or opportunistic infection
- The fact that pulmonary manifestations of CTD may precede extrapulmonary evidence of disease by several years
- Increased sensitivity of high-resolution computed tomography (HRCT), which results in diagnosis of disease that previously would not have been recognized

PATHOGENESIS

In CTD, lung disease generally results from chronic inflammation affecting the airways and/or the lung parenchyma. This occurs as a result of an inflammatory and subsequently a fibrotic response to an insult, the nature of which is unknown but which may result from immunologic responses to an initiating agent. For example, in progressive systemic sclerosis (PSS), presentation of epitopes of the Scl-70 antibody is thought to be one of the early initiating events in the immune response. Similarly, viral epitopes have been incriminated in Sjögren's syndrome, and other infective agents are thought to function as inciting agents in the immune response in rheumatoid arthritis (RA). Regardless of the specific trigger factor(s) there is no doubt that in all of the CTDs, there is evidence of immune activation in the form of activated T-cells, usually bearing the CD45 RO phenotype, at whichever pulmonary site(s) are affected. Prominent lymphoid follicles are seen with true germinal centers, indicating local antibody production, and high levels of immunoglobulin are seen in lung lavage fluid, tissue, and serum; often, circulating immune complexes are seen in peripheral blood and lavage fluid.

The immune response is followed by an influx of other inflammatory cells, most notably granulocytes and mononuclear phagocytes. These cells elaborate injurious enzymes including proteases and elastases, together with oxidant radicals that promote tissue injury. In response to, but ultimately in parallel with, the cellular infiltration is an ongoing connective tissue matrix response consisting of an influx of connective tissue matrix cells such as myofibroblasts, myocytes, and fibroblasts that produce a wide range of connective tissue matrix proteins. As part of the regulatory process, there is often an upregulation of connective tissue matrix protein breakdown enzymes, such as collagenase, and other metalloproteinases and serine proteases, such as elastase. The result is chronic inflammation with damage to the original architecture and scarring.

Unanswered questions pertaining to the pathogenesis of CTD-related lung disease include the following:

- Why are individual lung compartments affected more in one disease than in another?
- Why is there so much individual variation in disease expression?
- Is the specific lung disease in one CTD driven by the same etiopathologic process as that seen in another?

In this regard, evidence is now emerging that the pathogenesis of the fibrosing lung disease in idiopathic interstitial pneumonias might be quite different from that in CTD. In particular, the differentiation of nonspecific interstitial pneumonia (NSIP) as a histopathologic entity distinct from usual interstitial pneumonia (UIP) is having a great impact on our understanding of fibrosing lung disease in CTD. This issue will be addressed in greater detail in the next section.

CLINICAL FEATURES

Respiratory Disease Patterns

DIFFUSE INTERSTITIAL LUNG DISEASE

The range of histopathologic and radiologic subtypes of diffuse interstitial lung disease (DLD) encountered in patients with CTD mirrors the idiopathic interstitial pneumonias, although the clinical course and prognosis are different and often less aggressive. NSIP is probably the most common form of diffuse lung disease encountered in CTD. It is clinically, radiologically, and histopathologically indistinguishable from idiopathic NSIP, but the clues that suggest CTD include the presence of pleural disease (not seen in idiopathic disease); a disproportionate distribution of upper lung zone involvement (as seen in RA); concomitant airway disease, particularly bronchiectasis (a combination that suggests RA or Sjögren's syndrome); and, of course, clinical evidence of systemic disease elsewhere. Chest radiographs are markedly less sensitive than HRCT. Biopsy and postmortem figures put the prevalence of DLD at approximately

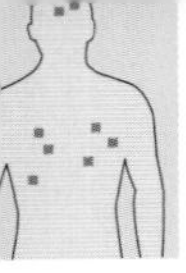

80% in PSS (e.g., scleroderma) and 40% in Japanese patients with dermatomyositis and polymyositis (DM/PM). The mortality of DLD in patients with various types of CTDs is generally lower than that found with idiopathic pulmonary fibrosis.

Typical clinical features are a dry cough, progressive shortness of breath, digital clubbing (the prevalence of which varies considerably in different CTDs), and bibasal fine inspiratory crepitations. Lung function tests show a restrictive ventilatory defect with reduced gas transfer but relatively well preserved PaO_2 until late in the disease.

Chest radiographs reveal peripheral reticulonodular shadowing, most prominent in the lower lung zones, that obscures the right and left heart borders and the diaphragms and is quite indistinguishable from that seen in idiopathic pulmonary fibrosis. HRCT identifies more disease than chest radiographs, is more specific, and has a greater ability to demonstrate coexistent pleural disease, small airway disease, bronchiectasis, and pulmonary nodules. HRCT can also be useful in choosing the best sites for open or thoracoscopic lung biopsy, or for demonstrating the extent of the irreversible "honeycomb" component of the fibrosing alveolitis. See Figure 48.1.

Until recently, the most common histopathologic pattern has been thought to be UIP (Table 48.1). With the definition of NSIP as a subgroup of fibrosing lung disease distinct from UIP, it has become apparent that many CTD patients previously thought to have a UIP histopathologic pattern of DLD actually fit the definition of NSIP much more closely. Whereas in idio-

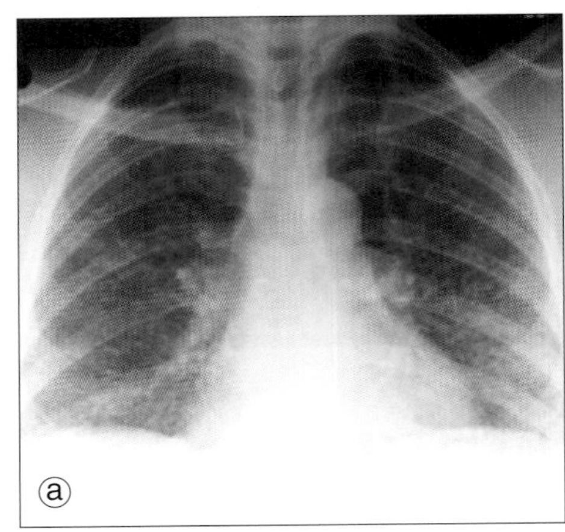

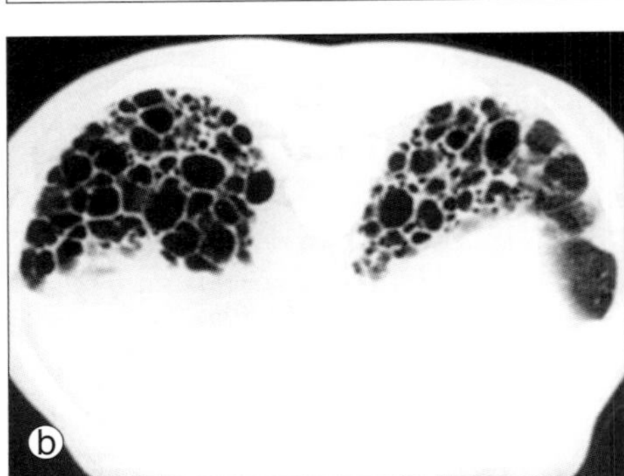

Figure 48.1 Fibrosing alveolitis (FA). **A,** Diffuse fibrosing lung disease of nonspecific interstitial pneumonia (NSIP) or usual interstitial pneumonia (UIP) pattern has a characteristic chest radiographic appearance with fine reticular shadowing that progressively obliterates heart borders and diaphragm. **B,** Honeycombing and cystic change appear in late fibrosis in this case of FA with systemic sclerosis (SSc).

Table 48.1
Diffuse lung disease - summary of histological and high-resolution computed tomography appearance

Histological pattern	Histopathological findings	Usual CT findings
Usual interstitial pneumonia	Architectural destruction, fibrosis with honeycombing, fibroblastic foci. Non-uniformity of these changes within biopsy specimen (temporal heterogeneity)	Peripheral, sub-pleural, and basal distribution. Irregular reticular changes with honeycombing, traction bronchiectasis, and architectural distortion. Focal, but minimal, ground-glass change.
Non-specific interstitial pneumonia	Variable interstitial inflammation and fibrosis. Uniformity of changes within biopsy specimen. Fibroblastic foci inconspicuous/absent	Symmetric, peripheral, basal, sub-pleural. More ground-glass attenuation. Reticular changes and traction bronchiectasis seen, but honeycombing is not prominent.
Lymphocytic interstitial pneumonia	Extensive lymphocytic infiltration in the interstitium often associated with peribronchiolar lymphoid follicles (follicular bronchiolitis)	Centrilobular nodules, ground-glass attenuation, septal and bronchovascular thickening, thin walled cysts.
Diffuse alveolar damage	Diffuse. Alveolar septal thickening, airspace organization, hyaline membranes	Gravity-dependent consolidation, ground-glass opacification – often with lobular sparing. Traction bronchiectasis occurs later.
Organizing pneumonia	Lung architecture preserved. Patchy distribution of intraluminal organizing fibrosis in distal air spaces	Patchy consolidation and/or nodules. May have a ground-glass component.
Desquamative interstitial pneumonia	Uniform involvement of parenchyma. Alveolar macrophages filling the alveoli with little interstitial disease	Ground-glass attenuation, "geographic distribution"
Respiratory—bronchiolitis associated interstitial lung disease	Bronchiolocentric alveolar macrophage accumulation, minor inflammation, and fibrosis	Patchy ground-glass. Bronchial wall thickening with centrilobular nodules.

pathic disease the distinction between NSIP and UIP serves to distinguish a group of patients (those with NSIP) who may have a better response to treatment, this is not necessarily the case in patients with CTD. In CTD even those with a UIP pattern on biopsy have a better chance of response to treatment than their counterparts with idiopathic disease. Other patterns seen in the context of connective tissue disease include the following:

- Lymphocytic interstitial pneumonia (LIP). LIP is seen particularly in Sjögren's syndrome and RA.
- Desquamative interstitial pneumonia (DIP), which is thought to overlap with the pattern of respiratory bronchiolitis–associated interstitial lung disease (RB-ILD). Each of these is regarded as a complication of cigarette smoking in the "idiopathic" classification system, and the same may be true in patients with CTD.
- Diffuse alveolar damage, manifesting as acute respiratory failure and described in association with systemic lupus erythematosus (SLE), polymyositis, and RA.
- Organizing pneumonia, which is listed alongside diffuse lung diseases in the consensus classification of idiopathic interstitial pneumonias, although the focus of the inflammation is the lumen of the small airways as well as the alveoli. Most common in patients with RA, and some patients with polymyositis, this entity is rare in SLE, systemic sclerosis (SSc), and Sjögren's syndrome. (In those conditions the presence of consolidation should prompt consideration of more sinister diagnoses such as bronchoalveolar cell carcinoma or lymphoma—Fig. 48.2). Onset is generally acute, with systemic features including fever and high sedimentation rate and white cell count. Chest radiographs show patchy consolidation that may fluctuate and that is usually peripheral, often bilateral, and often in the lower zones. CT confirms more graphically the consolidating nature of the lesions. The response to corticosteroids is usually excellent. Organizing pneumonia has often been confused with obliterative bronchiolitis (OB)—a condition affecting the small airways in patients with CTD and discussed in some detail later in this chapter. This confusion is compounded by use of the term *bronchiolitis obliterans organizing pneumonia* (BOOP). The two conditions differ from each other in many respects, as summarized in Figure 48.3.

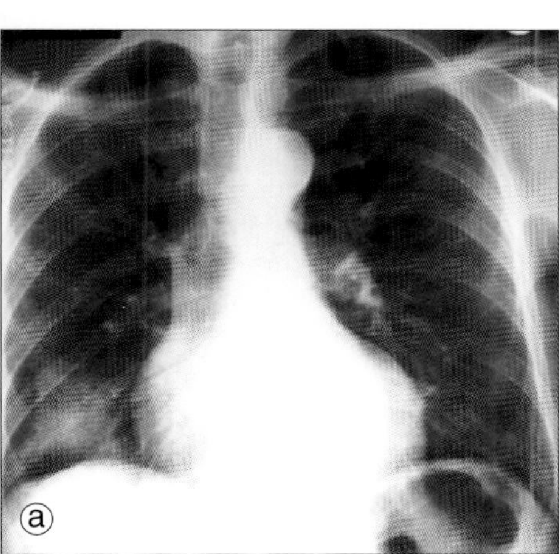

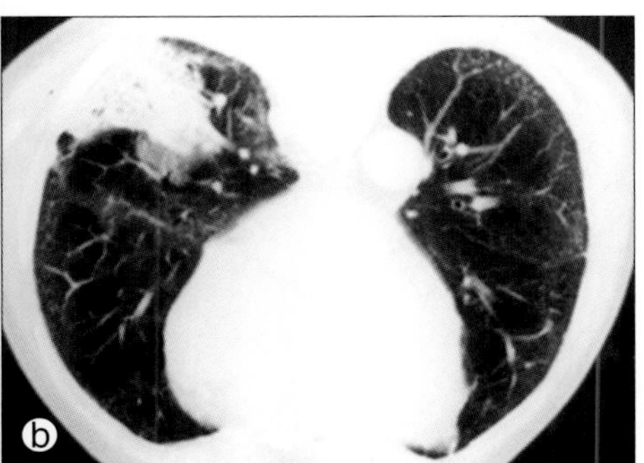

Figure 48.2 Bronchoalveolar cell carcinoma. This complication of fibrosing alveolitis or diffuse fibrosing lung disease is associated radiologically with patchy alveolar infiltrate **(A)** on chest radiography. **B,** An air bronchogram is seen more clearly on the computed tomogram.

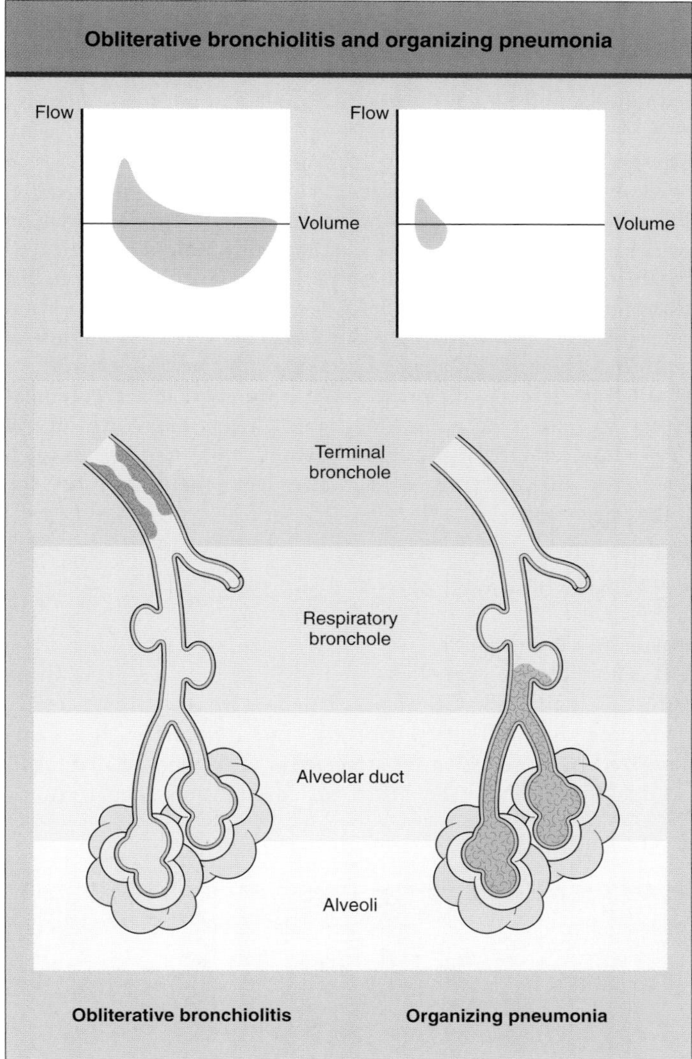

Figure 48.3 Obliterative bronchiolitis organizing pneumonia (BOOP). Obliterative bronchiolitis (OB) and organizing pneumonia (OP) have distinctive pathology and lung function features. In OB hyperinflation and fixed airflow obstruction result from fibrous obliteration of terminal bronchioles with gross reduction of flow particularly in the small airways (left flow volume curve). Restrictive pulmonary function defects in OP reflects loose connective tissue in terminal bronchioles, respiratory ducts, and alveoli, with less impact on flow rates, but huge impact on lung volume (right flow volume curve).

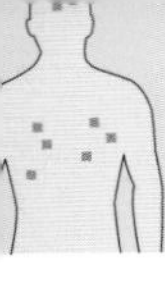

Chronic DLD increases the risk of lymphoma and carcinoma, and focal change in disease pattern should be viewed with suspicion (see Fig. 48.2).

ASPIRATION PNEUMONIA

Pharyngeal muscle weakness involving the tongue, soft palate, and upper esophageal muscles affects 15% of patients with DM/PM and is closely linked to aspiration, nasal regurgitation, and dysphagia. It may also be a complication of PSS because of regurgitation of pooled contents from a fibrotic, ectatic esophagus (Fig. 48.4). Aspiration-related infection can be worsened by therapeutic immunosuppression, respiratory muscle weakness, and structural interstitial lung disease, which broaden the array of infectious agents observed and hinder normal protective clearance mechanisms.

AIRWAY DISEASE

Airway disease is a common finding in some of the CTDs, most notably RA and Sjögren's disease. Small airway disease has also been reported in SLE and, more rarely, in PSS. Airway disease can usually be differentiated from parenchymal disease by the predominance of cough, with or without sputum production. Furthermore, wheezing may be a presenting feature and may be evident on examination. Chest radiography, unless complicated by diffuse lung disease, will show hyperexpanded lung fields; this finding is confirmed on HRCT scan, which may in addition reveal evidence of frank bronchiectasis, as well as small airway wall thickening. Pulmonary physiology will show an obstructive ventilatory defect with preserved gas transfer. It is rarely necessary to undertake open lung biopsy in patients with airway disease unless OB is suspected but not confirmed on imaging. The two major types of airway involvement include the following:

- OB
- Follicular bronchiolitis

Obliterative Bronchiolitis

OB occurs chiefly in patients with RA but is also seen in those with SLE and PSS. OB associated with RA has a particularly poor prognosis, and death within 3 years is common. It is characterized by progressive breathlessness with wheeze. An inspiratory "squeak" may be heard on auscultation. The terminal bronchioles are obliterated by dense fibrous tissue, with sparing of the respiratory bronchioles and alveoli. Response to treatment is poor, but occasionally disease may be held stable with corticosteroids and immunosuppression. The entity was initially thought to be caused by d-penicillamine, a medication used to treat RA, but is now considered to be a complication of RA per se.

Follicular Bronchiolitis

This term *follicular bronchiolitis* refers to the appearance of numerous lymphoid follicles around small airways. This pattern is rarely seen as an isolated entity and is more usually found in association with DLD. It is a particular feature of RA and Sjögren's syndrome.

VASCULAR DISEASE AND ALVEOLAR HEMORRHAGE

Pulmonary vessels may be involved by inflammation (vasculitis) or by concentric fibrosis. Vasculitis affects all levels of the pulmonary circulation, and pulmonary capillaritis manifests as diffuse alveolar hemorrhage. This unusual condition occurs in association with a number of systemic conditions including microscopic polyarteritis, SLE, PSS, Wegener's granulomatosis, Behçet's syndrome, Henoch-Schönlein purpura, the antiphospholipid antibody syndromes, Goodpasture's syndrome, idiopathic pulmonary-renal syndrome, and IgA nephropathy.

Shortness of breath, hemoptysis, and fever are the principal symptoms. Physical examination may reveal diffuse crackles but often is normal. Chest radiographs show diffuse bilateral alveolar infiltrates that clear within 2 or 3 days. Lung function tests are characterized by increased diffusion in the first 24 hours following a bleeding episode (as a result of intra-alveolar hemoglobin) and hypoxemia. In less acute, lower volume bleeds, chronic hemorrhage provokes a fibrotic response, and diffusion is reduced. Subsequent acute bleeds may increase diffusion to more normal values. Normochromic, normocytic anemia is seen with acute disease, and iron deficiency with more chronic bleeding. Bronchoalveolar lavage (BAL) can confirm alveolar hemorrhage by revealing red blood cells in the acute stages or iron-laden macrophages in patients with chronic disease. A specific diagnosis, particularly pulmonary capillaritis, may be made only after histologic examination of lung tissue obtained via an open or thoracoscopic procedure.

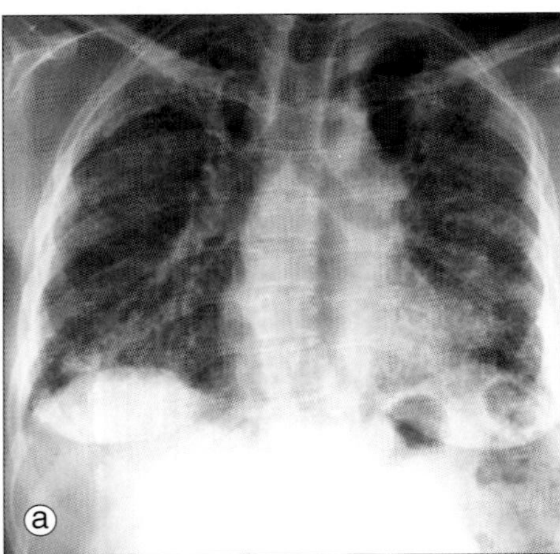

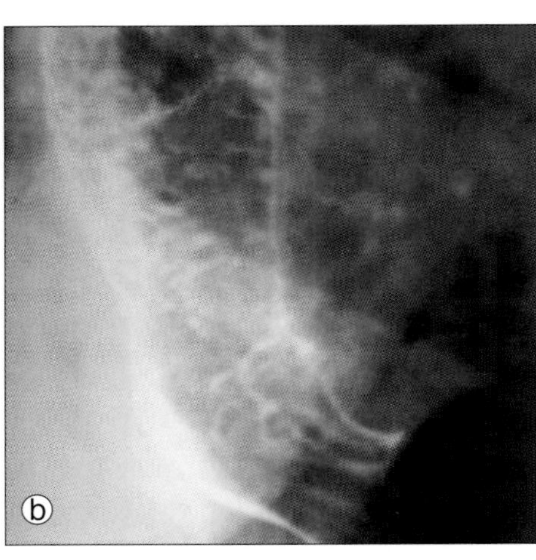

Figure 48.4 Systemic sclerosis (SSc). Pulmonary disease in SSc can be exacerbated by gastrointestinal dysmotility. Here a widely patent esophagus appears on chest radiography.

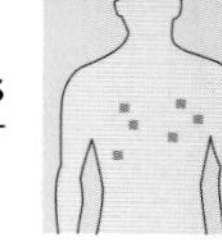

Pleural Disease

Pleural disease is the most common manifestation of connective tissue disorder, being particularly common in patients with SLE and RA. Manifestations include pleurisy, pleural thickening, and/or pleural effusion. Differentiation of effusions due to different CTDs is not possible except for the classical low glucose in RA and the presence of lupus erythematosus cells in patients with SLE.

RESPIRATORY MUSCLE WEAKNESS

Respiratory muscle weakness may occur in DM/PM and SLE, although it is uncommon. Presenting symptoms include breathlessness, and chest roentgenograms may show small lung fields. Although lung volumes will show a restrictive pattern, diffusion is normal, and maximum inspiratory and expiratory flows and pressures may be reduced. Hypercapnic respiratory failure is usual when the vital capacity falls below 55% predicted.

Ventilatory failure may develop rapidly in patients with DM/PM, and patients with proximal weakness or oropharyngeal weakness need to be closely monitored for this complication. Nocturnal noninvasive ventilation is being used with some success, although daytime hypercapnia may persist.

Specific Diseases

RHEUMATOID ARTHRITIS

RA is more common in women (2-3 : 1), but lung involvement and other extra-articular features are more common in men. The peak prevalence is in the fifth and sixth decades, and risk factors appear to include smoking and the class II MHC HLA-DR4 phenotype. Joint manifestations precede interstitial lung disease in 90% of cases. When lung disease precedes joint disease it is usually associated with a positive rheumatoid factor. Rheumatoid factor, specifically the IgM directed against the Fc portion of IgG, is found in 75% to 80% of patients at some stage during the course of the disease.

RA can involve any part of the respiratory tract, including the cricoarytenoid joint, the airways, the parenchyma, and the pleura (Table 48.2). Usually only one of these disorders is predominant in a single individual, although the parenchymal interstitial processes are often associated with subtle-change, HRCT evidence of airway disease. In one study of 77 patients, bronchiectasis was seen in 30%, pulmonary nodules in 22%, subpleural micronodules and/or pseudoplaques in 17%, ground-glass attenuation in 14%, honeycombing in 10%, and pleural effusions in 5%. Abnormal CT findings were found in 29% of asymptomatic and 69% of symptomatic patients. Lung biopsy in unselected patients with RA shows interstitial inflammation and fibrosis in up to 60%, the majority of whom are asymptomatic.

Table 48.2
Lung involvement in rheumatoid arthritis

Diffuse fibrosing lung disease of NSIP or UIP pattern
Lymphocytic interstitial pneumonia
Organizing pneumonia
Obliterative bronchiolitis
Bronchiectasis
Vasculitis
Alveolar hemorrhage
Pulmonary nodules
Pleural disease

Obliterative Bronchiolitis

OB is an uncommon but severe complication of RA and typically occurs in a rapidly progressive form in HLA-DR4–positive patients who have severe, nodular deforming disease. Death commonly occurs within 3 years of onset, reflecting the fact that the condition responds poorly to steroids.

Pulmonary Vasculitis

RA-associated pulmonary vasculitis is uncommon but may coexist with systemic vasculitis (e.g., cutaneous infarcts, mononeuritis multiplex, and visceral involvement).

Pulmonary Nodules

Pulmonary nodules are uncommon, may be multiple, can mimic malignancy, and may spontaneously resolve and recur. Nodules may vary in size from millimeters to several centimeters and may occur in any lung zone. Histopathologically they have necrotic centers surrounded by palisades of histiocytic epithelioid cells rimmed by fibroblasts and occasional chronic inflammatory cells. Nodules occurring in miners (Caplan's syndrome) show scattered dust particles at microscopy. Rarely, a large nodule may cavitate and manifest as hemoptysis or pneumothorax. Cavitation requires further investigation, as these lesions may mimic bronchogenic scar carcinoma, tuberculosis, granulomatous vasculitis, and aspergilloma. Previous chest radiography and rate of change in the size of the nodules may help in differentiation. If the lesion is solitary, excision may be needed to exclude malignancy.

Pleural Disease

RA-associated pleural disease is seen in up to 50% of patients at postmortem examination and is asymptomatic in the majority, although presenting signs and symptoms can include fever, pleuritic chest pain, and shortness of breath. The effusions are generally small and unilateral and associated with chronic disease, but rarely occur acutely, in large volume, or bilaterally. The fluid is exudative and frequently cloudy (protein >30 g/L) and characteristically has a low glucose (<1.4 mmol/L; < 25 mg/dL), an elevated lactate dehydrogenase (LDH; greater than 200 IU/mL), a low pH, and a high cholesterol. Effusions are usually paucicellular (<5,000/mm^3) with lymphocyte predominance, but neutrophilic and frank pus exudates are also seen. Intercurrent infection, especially tuberculosis and bacterial empyemas, must be excluded. Pleural biopsy is infrequently helpful, but thoracoscopy may reveal a fine granular appearance to the pleural wall. Histopathologic examination of these micronodules shows the same palisading of histiocytes and chronic inflammatory cells described above, with the exception that central fibrinoid necrosis is rare. The usual course of pleural effusion is that of spontaneous resolution.

SYSTEMIC SCLEROSIS

The prevalence of PSS is 30 to 120 per 10^6 with a 4 : 1 to 9 : 1 female preponderance. The incidence is approximately 2 to 20

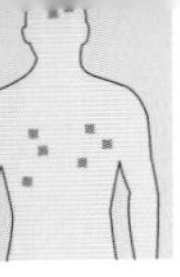

per 10^6 per year, peaking in the fourth to sixth decades. HLA-DRB1*11 and HLA-DPB1*1301 are associated with the development of diffuse lung disease in PSS, and a number of agents have been associated with development of SSc-like lung abnormalities, including d-penicillamine, tryptophan, bleomycin, pentazocine, vinyl chloride, benzene, toluene, and trichloroethylene. Silica exposure increases the odds ratio of PSS, and silicosis increases the rate even further. A toxic oil syndrome occurred in Madrid in 1981 in patients who ingested cooking oil that contained rapeseed oil denatured with aniline. This substance provoked a scleroderma-like syndrome with pulmonary involvement. Some researchers have hypothesized an association with silicone breast implants, but this has not been established.

PSS is a heterogeneous condition affecting skin and viscera to a variable degree. Distinct patterns of disease are discernible, defined by the extent of skin involvement and autoantibody status. There are fewer patterns of lung disease seen in patients with PSS than in those with RA (Table 48.3).

Pulmonary involvement has emerged as the major cause of excess morbidity and mortality in SSc since the emergence of angiotensin-converting enzyme inhibitors to prevent renal crisis and omeprazole and other gastrointestinal motility agents to treat upper gastrointestinal symptoms. Autopsy studies indicate that at least some degree of DLD is present in up to 79% of patients, and pulmonary vascular disease occurs in 29%.

Table 48.3 Lung involvement in progressive systemic sclerosis
Diffuse fibrosing lung disease
Organizing pneumonia
Isolated pulmonary vascular disease
Aspiration pneumonia
Chest wall restriction

Antinuclear antibodies are found in 90% to 100% of patients with PSS, but in 30% the specific antigen is unidentified. Three major autoantibodies include anticentromere, occurring in 70% to 80% of patients with limited disease; antitopoisomerase (Scl-70), occurring in 30% of patients with DLD; and polymyositis-Scl, occurring in a small fraction of patients who have an overlap syndrome with polymyositis (Table 48.4). DLD is rare in the presence of the anticentromere antibody, and a protective role for this autoantibody has been suggested but not substantiated. Diffuse cutaneous PSS is more strongly associated with DLD and the Scl-70 antibody; limited cutaneous disease is associated with the vascular disease and with the anticentromere antibody. Both forms of lung disease may progress to pulmonary hypertension.

DIFFUSE FIBROSING LUNG DISEASE

The fibrosing lung disease seen in PSS is indistinguishable from idiopathic NSIP radiographically, physiologically, and histopathologically in 80% of cases. Patients with PSS may, however, also have evidence of pulmonary vascular disease.

Vascular Involvement

Unlike the other CTDs, vascular involvement in PSS is caused by concentric fibrosis of small arterioles. Plexiform lesions and fibrinoid necrosis of primary pulmonary hypertension are not seen (Fig. 48.5). Pulmonary vascular disease occurs in the limited form of PSS (defined as skin disease not extending proximal to the elbow, except for the face and serologic evidence of the anticentromere antibody in approximately 70% to 80% of patients). Associated features include those of the CREST syndrome (i.e., calcinosis cutis, Raynaud's phenomenon, esophageal disease, sclerodactyly, and telangiectasia). Chest radiography and CT scan are normal. BAL fluid is normal. Lung function studies show an isolated reduction in diffusion. When damage to the pulmonary vascular bed is extensive (gas transfer less than 50% predicted) the risk of pulmonary hypertension increases. Echocardiography indicates indirect evidence of pulmonary hypertension, which should be confirmed by right heart catheterization in a specialized center.

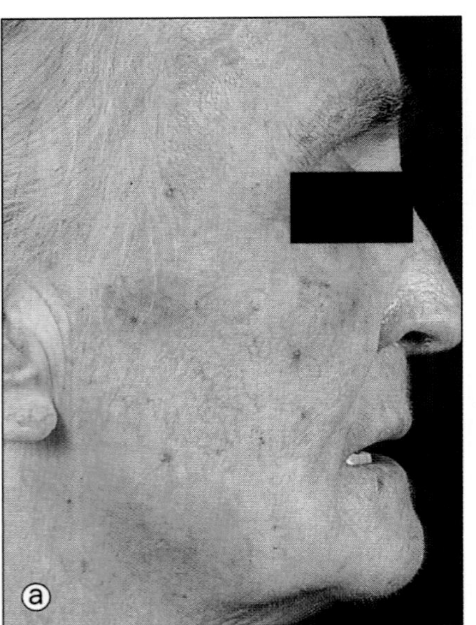

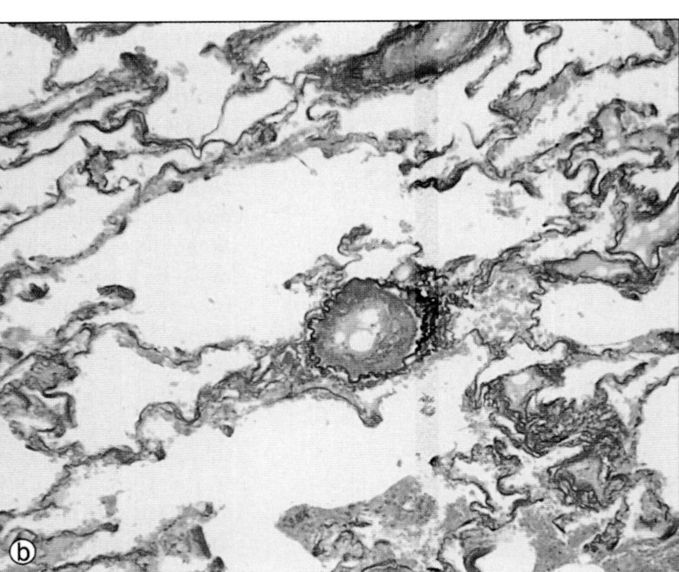

Figure 48.5 Systemic sclerosis (SSc). Lone pulmonary vascular disease in SSc is more common in limited cutaneous disease and is associated with the presence of anticentromere antibodies. **A,** Facial telangiectasia are more prominent. **B,** Intralobular vessels show collagenous thickening of the intima and luminal narrowing. (**A,** courtesy of Dr. H. Beynon, Royal Free Hospital, London; Elastin von Gieson stain in [**B**] reproduced by permission of Prof. B. Corrin, National Heart and Lung Institute, London.)

Table 48.4
Autoantibody specificity in connective tissue disease

Connective tissue disease	Autoantibody	Target	Comments
Rheumatoid arthritis	Rheumatoid factor	IgG	Seropositive disease more frequent with pulmonary nodules
	Antinuclear antibody	–	–
	Histone	Histone proteins	5% rheumatoid vasculitis
Systemic sclerosis	**Anticentromere**	Centromere proteins (CENP A–F)	20–40% total systemic sclerosis, wide racial variation; 70–80% limited cutaneous variant with pulmonary hypertension
	Scl-70	DNA topoisomerase-1	28–70% total systemic sclerosis, wide racial variation; >30% diffuse cutaneous disease with interstitial lung disease
	PM-Scl	–	Scleroderma–myositis overlap syndromes
	Antinucleolar	RNA polymerase-1	8–20% systemic sclerosis suggests poorest 10-year survival, renal crisis
	Ku	DNA binding proteins	Scleroderma–myositis overlap syndromes
Systemic lupus erythematosus	**dsDNA**	Double-stranded DNA	50–75%, strong association with nephritis
	Antinuclear antibody	–	90–95%
	Ro/La	RNA transcription factors	60%/20%
	Histone	Histone proteins	>90% drug-induced lupus, 20–30% primary systemic lupus erythematosus
	Sm	–	10% Caucasians, 30% African Americans and Chinese
	Lupus anticoagulant	Phospholipid	20–30%
Mixed connective tissue diseases	**U1-RNP**	Small nuclear proteins	Myositis overlap syndromes (10% systemic sclerosis)
	U2-RNP	–	Myositis, systemic lupus erythematosus, systemic sclerosis
Dermatomyositis/polymyositis	**Jo-1**	Histidyl tRNA synthetase	20–30% inflammatory myopathy but 50–100% when associated with diffuse interstitial lung disease
	PL-7	Threonyl tRNA synthetase	<3% antisynthetase syndrome
	PL-12	Alanyl tRNA synthetase	<3% antisynthetase syndrome
	EJ	Glycyl tRNA synthetase	<2% antisynthetase syndrome
	OJ	Isoleucyl tRNA synthetase	<2% antisynthetase syndrome
			Antisynthetase antibodies 25–30% dermatomyositis/polymyositis (Jo-1 most prevalent)
	Mi-2	Nuclear proteins	<8% dermatomyositis
Antiphospholipid syndrome	**Anticardiolipin**	Membrane phospholipids	Disease diagnosis depends on presence of clinical features
	Lupus anticoagulant	–	–
Relapsing polychondritis	**Anticartilage**	Cartilage	Unknown sensitivity
	Anticollagen	Collagen	–
Sjögren's syndrome	**Ro (SS-A)**	RNA transcription factors	40–50% primary Sjögren's syndrome (25–30% systemic lupus erythematosus)
	La (SS-B)	–	50% Sjögren's (10% systemic lupus erythematosus)

POLYMYOSITIS AND DERMATOMYOSITIS

The inflammatory myopathies dermatomyositis and polymyositis present a characteristic clinical picture of proximal muscle weakness associated with other features of CTD. Dermatomyositis is distinguished by the presence of scaly cutaneous eruptions affecting the extensor surfaces of the finger joints (Gottron's tubercles) or the characteristic edema and violaceous or purplish, heliotrope rash that surrounds the eyelids (Fig. 48.6). Diagnostic criteria include progressive, symmetrical proximal muscle weakness, elevated muscle enzymes, compatible electromyographic abnormalities, muscle biopsy evidence of noninfective myopathy, and typical cutaneous changes. Diagnosis is considered "definite" if four and "probable" if three criteria are present. Proximal muscle weakness tends to be insidious, progressive, and painless, affecting head, neck, and limb girdles, eventually involving the muscles of tongue, pharynx, and thorax. Pulmonary complications occur in approximately 45% of patients and are the most frequent cause of death.

The inflammatory myopathies are relatively rare, affecting 2 to 10 per 1,000,000 people, with a female-to-male predominance of 2.5:1 and a bimodal age distribution peaking in childhood and in the fourth to fifth decades. DM appears to have a higher expression of HLA-B8 and HLA-DR3, B14, and B40, whereas PM associates with HLA-B8 and HLA-DR3 and in blacks with B7 and DRw6.

Pulmonary manifestations are listed in Table 48.5. The most common problems are infection and DLD. Aspiration pneumonia should be differentiated from organizing pneumonia. The most distinctive features of DM/PM-associated DLD are the presence of highly specific autoantibodies and the occasional very rapid onset as an acute pneumonitis. Digital clubbing is uncommon. There is an associated risk of both pulmonary and extrapulmonary cancer (DM relative risk, 3.8; PM relative risk, 1.7, but DM and PM are well-recognized paraneoplastic phenomena, so it is sometimes difficult to determine which condition manifested first).

Autoantibodies occur in 80% to 90% of patients with DM/PM. Antibodies directed against the aminoacyl tRNA synthetases are most specific for the inflammatory myopathies and diffuse lung disease. Anti-Jo-1 (antihistidyl tRNA synthetase) is

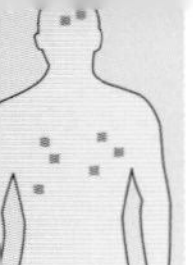

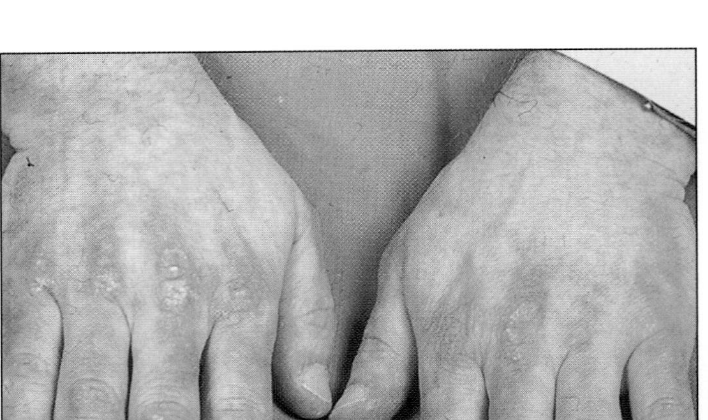

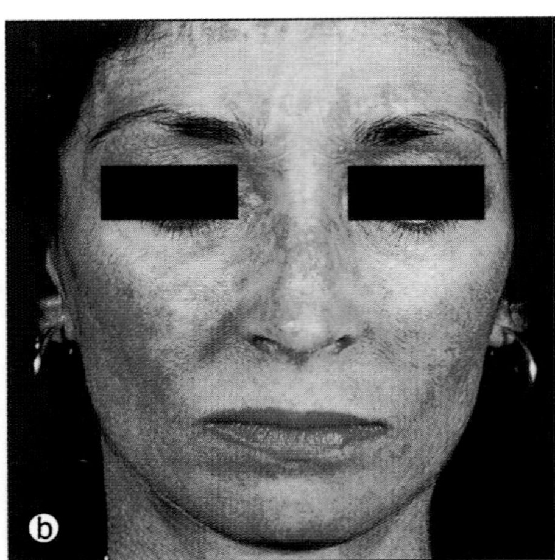

Figure 48.6 Dermatomyositis (DM). A, Gottron's plaques are seen over the metacarpophalangeal joints. Facial rash may be periorbital, malar, or more widespread **(B)**. (Courtesy of Dr. H. Beynon, Royal Free Hospital, London.)

Table 48.5 Lung involvement in dermatomyositis/polymyositis
Diffuse fibrosing lung disease
Aspiration pneumonia
Respiratory muscle weakness
Organizing pneumonia
Pulmonary vasculitis
Alveolar hemorrhage

the most common autoantibody, occurring in 20% to 30% of patients with inflammatory myopathy but in 50% to 100% of cases of inflammatory myopathy and DLD, in contrast to less than 5% patients without diffuse lung disease. Anti-PM/Scl-70 often signifies a dermatomyositis-polymyositis-scleroderma overlap syndrome and is also associated with pulmonary hypertension. A variety of other autoantibodies have been described with affinity for other tRNA synthetase molecules—PL12, PL7, EJ, Mi-2, and OJ (see Table 48.4). These molecules help define the antisynthetase syndrome that includes features of myositis, DLD, and arthritis.

SYSTEMIC LUPUS ERYTHEMATOSUS

SLE is a multisystem immunologic disorder that occurs in up to 1 in 2000 individuals, with a marked female preponderance (10:1) and a peak age of onset in the third decade. Evidence of B- and T-cell dysfunction with prominent autoantibody expression, hypergammaglobulinemia, circulating immune complexes, and complement activation confirms the immune basis to the disorder. Diagnosis requires that at least four of the findings summarized in Table 48.6 be present at some stage. The patterns of pulmonary disease are quite unlike those seen in other CTDs (Table 48.7), and good responses to treatment are less frequent.

Acute Lupus Pneumonitis

Acute lupus pneumonitis can occur in a number of CTDs and is the counterpart of idiopathic "acute interstitial pneumonitis," or AIP. (This presentation is likely to be more common in RA and DM/PM than in SLE). Presentation is with acute respiratory failure in patients with no other previous evidence of respiratory disease. Chest radiography and HRCT may show a more widespread alveolar filling pattern than in diffuses lung disease. The incidence of this complication is not known, but it may occur in as many as 15% of patients with SLE. The associated fever raises concerns for infection, and the sudden onset of breathlessness and cyanosis would be compatible with alveolar

Table 48.6 Diagnostic features of systemic lupus erythematosus
Malar (i.e., butterfly) rash
Discoid skin lesions
Photosensitivity
Oral ulcers
Nonerosive arthritis
Serositis
Nephritis
Hematologic involvement
Central nervous system involvement
Immunologic abnormalities (i.e., double-stranded DNA, anti-Sm antibodies)
Positive antinuclear antibody

Table 48.7 Lung involvement with systemic lupus erythematosus
Acute lupus pneumonitis
Pulmonary vasculitis
Alveolar hemorrhage
Shrinking lung syndrome
Antiphospholipid antibody syndrome
Organizing pneumonia
Atelectasis
Pleural disease
Diffuse fibrosing lung disease

hemorrhage and cardiogenic edema. BAL is frequently performed to exclude these concerns. Open lung biopsy may be necessary if doubt remains.

Shrinking Lung Syndrome

The term *shrinking lung syndrome* refers to a constellation of findings including dyspnea and orthopnea, a restrictive ventilatory defect, elevation of one or both hemidiaphragms, clear lung fields, and reduced diaphragmatic excursion. The cause of this syndrome is unclear. Diaphragmatic dysfunction has been suggested as a possible cause, but this is disputed because diaphragm function seems to be normal when direct phrenic nerve stimulation is used. Impairment of chest wall excursion has also been proposed. Diaphragm function generally remains stable for protracted periods. Theophyllines and $\beta 2$ agonists have been reported to be beneficial.

Antiphospholipid Antibodies

Antiphospholipid antibodies are antibodies that bind to negatively charged phospholipids and include the anticardiolipin antibody, the lupus anticoagulant, and an antibody causing a false-positive venereal disease research laboratory (VDRL) test result. These antibodies are associated with in situ arterial and venous thrombosis at multiple sites, including the lung, and thromboembolic disease. Independent arterial and venous thromboses occur in up to half of patients, and arterial thrombosis together with venous thrombosis occurs in up to 14%.

Presentation may be subacute, with features suggesting pulmonary hypertension, or it may involve acute-onset dyspnea, tachypnea, fever, and hypoxemia. Prominent bilateral pulmonary infiltrates are also seen, as is vasculitis.

Treatment is supportive, and a good response is seen in general with prednisolone, although a number of immunosuppressive regimens have also been employed, including intravenous immunoglobulin and cyclophosphamide, when the syndrome occurs with a CTD such as SLE. Long-term anticoagulation is needed in patients with thrombosis.

Pleural Involvement

Pleural involvement is by far the most common pulmonary manifestation of SLE and is identified in up to 100% of patients postmortem. As many as 56% of patients will develop pleural effusions. Pleural fluid is exudative with excess neutrophils and lymphocytes and a normal glucose concentration. It does not generally require specific treatment.

Diffuse Fibrosing Lung Disease

Diffuse fibrosing lung disease and organizing pneumonia are rare in SLE, but linear atelectasis is a common finding on chest radiography. Vasculitis is a common systemic manifestation of SLE and may be the presenting pulmonary feature.

SJÖGREN'S SYNDROME

Sjögren's syndrome is an autoimmune inflammatory disease principally affecting the exocrine glands and may be primary or secondary. A predominantly lymphocytic infiltrate destroys glandular tissue and reduces glandular secretion. Clinical features include mucosal dryness affecting the eyes (keratoconjunctivitis sicca), mouth, trachea (xerostomia, xerotrachea), and vagina.

The incidence of primary Sjögren's syndrome in the general population is unknown but approaches 30% in patients with RA, PSS, and SLE. Female predominance is 9:1, and the condition affects all age groups, including children.

Hypergammaglobulinemia is a common feature, and a variety of autoantibodies are found, particularly in secondary disease. The most specific autoantibodies are the extractable nuclear antigens SSA (Ro) in 40% to 50% of patients and SSB (La) in 50%.

Both the airways and the lung parenchyma may be affected. The airway manifestations are most common and include dryness, cough, wheeze, and airflow limitation. Treatment is symptomatic, and patients improve with inhaled corticosteroids and/or inhaled β_2-agonists. Pulmonary parenchymal involvement is less common, affecting 10% to 20% of cases, with LIP with high level $CD8^+$ expression, other diffuse fibrosing lung disease, pseudolymphoma, or malignant lymphoma. Radiographic and physiologic features are nonspecific. Lymphoma and pseudolymphoma, which some argue may be a low-grade lymphoma, are of major concern, as B-cell lymphoma was seen in 9% of patients in one series, with the lung as the most common site of involvement. Biopsy is necessary for confirmation, as the treatment of pseudolymphoma involves chemotherapy as would be given for primary lymphoma.

MIXED CONNECTIVE TISSUE DISEASE

Mixed connective tissue disease (MCTD) is defined by the presence of more than one CTD in association with high titers (greater than 1 : 1600) of an autoantibody directed against the extractable nuclear antigen U1-RNP. The difference between MCTD and the CTD overlap syndromes may be semantic, but the former often manifests more acutely and with greater specificity for U1-RNP. Some patients have only one symptom, or a few symptoms that defy categorization into a recognizable CTD syndrome, but progress to exhibit typical findings of PSS, SLE, DM/PM, or Sjögren's syndrome over time.

Mixed CTD affects approximately 1 per 10,000 people, with a 9 : 1 female preponderance. Pulmonary involvement, investigations, and treatment are as for the individual CTD.

RELAPSING POLYCHONDRITIS

Relapsing polychondritis is a very rare disorder that is characterized by episodic, painful, and destructive cartilaginous inflammation. The condition affects men and women equally and has a peak incidence between ages 40 to 60 years. Relapsing polychondritis is considered an autoimmune process, and autoantibodies directed against cartilage and type II collagen have been found. Diagnosis is made on the basis of the clinical presentation but can be confirmed at biopsy. The condition is usually multifocal, affecting the cartilage of the ear in 88% of patients, the nose in 82%, the upper respiratory tract in 56% to 70%, and the thyroid and ribs less commonly. Additionally, patients frequently suffer ocular inflammation, nonerosive arthropathy (80%), and vestibulocochlear dysfunction that may occur as part of a CTD (Fig. 48.7).

Respiratory involvement probably accounts for approximately 10% of deaths in this condition. Pulmonary parenchymal disease is rare, but vasculitis may occur. Destruction and obstruction of the glottis, trachea, and/or bronchi leads to airway stricture and collapse followed by distal infection. Lung

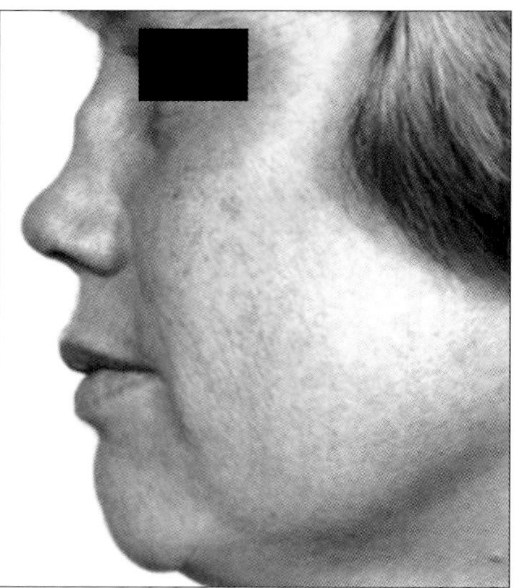

Figure 48.7 Relapsing polychondritis. This process affects the cartilage of the nose, ears, and airways, and cartilaginous nasal collapse may be characteristic.

function testing may show inspiratory and/or expiratory airflow limitation, and flow-volume curves may target the site of airflow limitation to the upper airway.

Treatment depends on disease severity. Mild cases may be controlled with nonsteroidal anti-inflammatory agents, whereas relapses may require short-term, high-dose corticosteroids. Steroid-resistant lesions have been treated with immunosuppressive agents such as cyclophosphamide. Tracheostomy and stenting are occasionally indicated, but other surgical treatment is difficult because of the extent of involvement.

ANKYLOSING SPONDYLITIS

Ankylosing spondylitis is a seronegative spondyloarthropathy that is characterized by its predilection for the sites of ligamentous attachment to bone and joint capsules. Its prevalence is 1.5 per 10,000 white men (lower prevalence in Afro-Caribbean men), and there is a 10:1 male predominance (although the prevalence in women may be underestimated, as they seem to be affected by a milder form of disease). There is a high familial inheritance, and subsequently a strong correlation has been noted with the major histocompatibility antigen HLA-B27. HLA-B27 is present in 7% of whites and 95% of patients with ankylosing spondylitis, and 2% to 20% of HLA-B27–positive patients develop the condition.

Sacroiliac pain is frequently the initial manifestation, and involvement spreads through the axial spine. Uveitis and iridocyclitis may affect 25% of patients, and asymptomatic cardiac involvement occurs in 20% to 30%. Some 10% of cases progress to symptomatic aortic incompetence. Pleuropulmonary involvement is uncommon, affecting only 1% of cases. It usually occurs late in the disease course.

Apical Fibrobullous Disease

Apical fibrobullous disease is a late complication of ankylosing spondylitis that usually first appears as unilateral fibrotic, upper lobe stranding that becomes bilateral and more extensive with time. Cystic spaces may develop that may mimic tuberculosis may develop. Mycetoma may also develop. Surgical treatment is occasionally required for debilitating infection or for persistent, or life-threatening hemoptysis.

Chest Wall Disease

Chest wall disease results from inflammation of costovertebral and costosternal joints, along with kyphoscoliosis, which can result in restriction of the chest wall. Despite the reduction in total lung capacity, the residual volume may be elevated because exhalation is limited by the inability of thorax to become smaller.

MARFAN SYNDROME

Marfan syndrome is a rare, autosomal dominant CTD attributed to abnormalities of type I procollagen gene regulation. The condition affects 4 to 6 per 100,000 people with variable penetrance and a relatively high spontaneous mutation rate.

Affected individuals have long limbs, arachnodactyly, joint laxity, and a high frequency of ocular (50% to 80%) and cardiovascular (60%) abnormalities. Diagnosis is established by finding at least two of the following:

1. Consistent family history
2. Ocular system involvement
3. Cardiovascular system involvement
4. Skeletal system involvement

Pulmonary involvement occurs in 10% to 16% of patients and may occur at any age.

Structural lung changes are well described and include patchy emphysema, cysts, and bullous degeneration. Aberrant lobulation and anomalous development, particularly of the right middle lobe, have been described. Pneumothorax affects 4% to 11% of patients, and 10% of these suffer bilateral or recurrent disease. Upper lobe fibrosis is seen in 4% of reported series.

BEHÇET'S DISEASE

This rare vasculitis is seen most frequently in Turkey, Japan, and the Mediterranean vicinity. Prevalence approaches 80 to 300 per 100,000 in Turkey, but the disease is rarer elsewhere. Male and female patients are affected equally, and a strong association has been noted with the HLA-B51 allele.

Mucocutaneous ulceration is the clinical hallmark, with apthous oral and genital ulceration seen in almost all patients. Other cutaneous features include erythema nodosum, an acneiform rash, and papular lesions of cutaneous vasculitis. Uveitis is the major cause of morbidity, but systemic vasculitis may affect all systems.

Pulmonary involvement is seen in 1% to 7% of patients and tends to affect HLA-B51–positive males who are younger than age 25 years more severely. Symptoms include dyspnea, chest pain, and recurrent hemoptysis that can be massive and fatal. Pathology reveals pulmonary arterial aneurysms, arterial and venous thrombosis, pulmonary infarcts, and occasional pleural effusions. Radiography is nonspecific but may demonstrate the features of pulmonary hemorrhage, vascular occlusion, or mass lesions representing arterial aneurysm(s).

Treatment is complex and depends on presentation. Steroids and immunosuppressive agents are used to control vasculitis, and colchicine has been helpful in some patients. Anticoagulants may be required for thrombosis, but the risk of hemorrhage is significant. Pulmonary embolization and surgical resection have been reported, but aneurysms at the anastomosis site may occur.

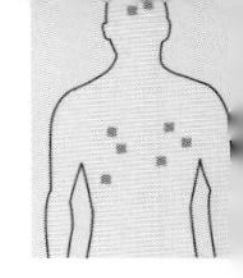

DIAGNOSIS

Although the evaluation of patients for CTD-associated lung involvement may follow a common algorithm (Fig. 48.8), the approach is critically dependent on the findings of a thorough history and physical examination.

Chest Radiography

Chest radiography should be performed in every patient with CTD, regardless of whether they have any pulmonary complaints or findings. The pattern of abnormalities may distinguish among some of the CTDs, although the extent of disease is often underestimated. If any abnormality is seen, no matter how trivial it may appear, HRCT should be performed.

High-resolution Computed Tomography

The value of HRCT scanning is established in the evaluation of patients suspected of having CTD-related pulmonary disease. This study offers particular benefit in detection and assessment of the severity of DLD and airways diseases. Standard chest radiographs may contribute to a diagnosis in up to 50% of patients with DLD, but in the remainder they may be either normal or nonspecific. HRCT is a more sensitive test for DLD, and the pattern of abnormality may frequently be informative. A ground-glass pattern denotes predominantly inflammatory disease, whereas a reticular pattern correlates well with the presence of fibrosis. These patterns are also relatively accurate with regard to predicting the likelihood of response to treatment: patients with the ground-glass pattern generally improve, and those with the reticular pattern, particularly honeycombing, do not. In certain situations (see Biopsy later in this chapter) the constellation of typical clinical and radiographic features precludes the need for lung biopsy. If there is any doubt about the nature of the problem, however, CT can indicate the most appropriate site for biopsy.

Technetium-labeled Diethylenetriaminepentacetate Clearance

Enhanced clearance of diethylenetriaminepentacetate (DTPA), a 500-Da molecule, is an early index of the lung inflammation accompanying PSS, RA, and SLE. Persistently normal DTPA clearance suggests that patients with SSc-associated fibrosing alveolitis will maintain stable lung function.

Pulmonary Function Tests

Any clinical suspicion of lung disease should be investigated with full lung function tests, including a cardiopulmonary exercise test (or, at the least, exercise oximetry). Restrictive and obstructive disease can be readily distinguished by spirometry. DLD is associated with a rightward shift of the static lung pressure-volume curve on its volume axis, indicating that compliance is reduced. Increases in the alveolar-to-arterial O_2 difference at rest are largely explained by ventilation-perfusion heterogeneity. Abnormalities in diffusion play a greater role during exercise. Decreases in diffusion indicate abnormalities in the pulmonary vascular bed. Increases suggest alveolar hemorrhage. Coexistent impairment of inspiratory and expiratory flow suggests respiratory muscle weakness.

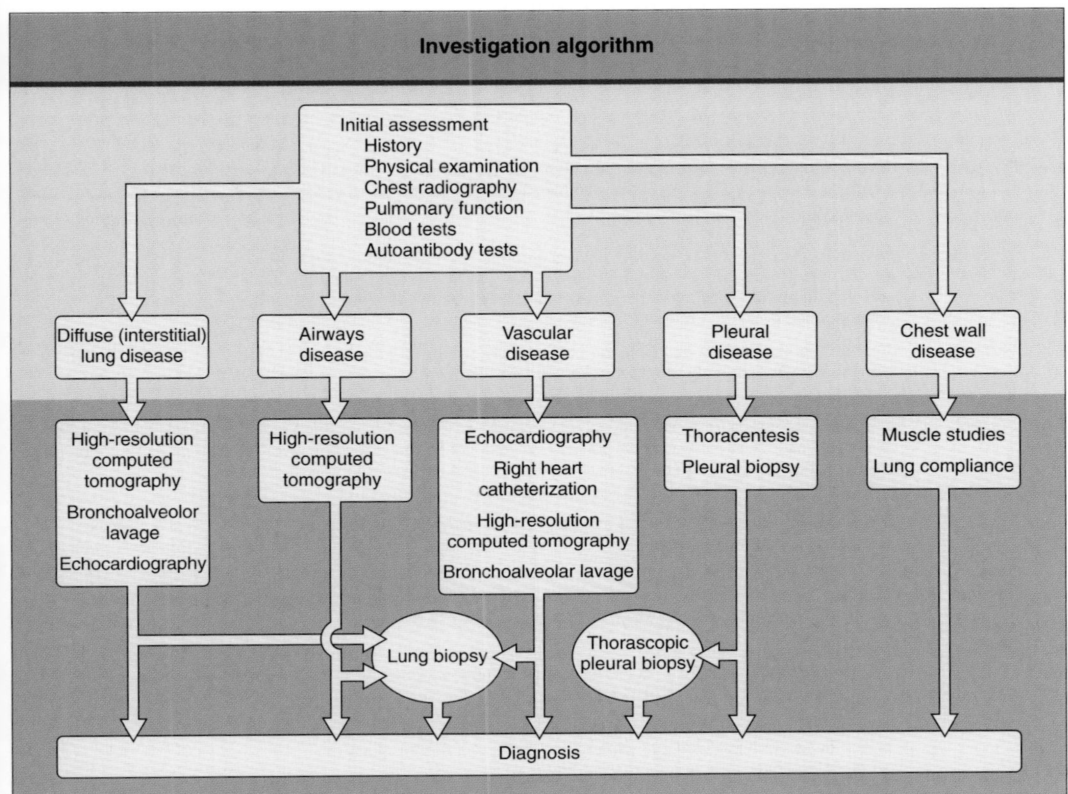

Figure 48.8 Investigation algorithm. Clinical history and examination are crucial in guiding appropriate investigation in connective tissue diseases (CTDs). Two key decisions are needed to establish diagnosis. First, the lung compartment predominantly affected must be identified and appropriate investigations pursued. Second, if the boxed investigations do not allow a diagnosis, or if the findings are atypical, inconsistent, or unconvincing then an open lung biopsy may need to be considered.

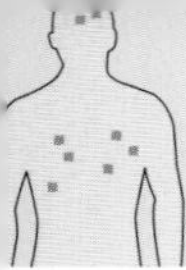

Exercise Testing

Exercise testing allows early detection and quantification of subclinical pulmonary disease and also quantifies the respective contributions of the heart, lung, and peripheral vascular system in causing exercise limitation.

Echocardiography

In any of the CTDs in which cardiac disease or pulmonary hypertension occurs, echocardiography should be performed. The test can demonstrate cardiac muscle infiltration as seen in PSS, poor ventricular function if small vessel vasculitis is present, pericardial disease in patients with SLE or PSS, and evidence of pulmonary hypertension (e.g., right ventricular hypertrophy or dilatation and, if tricuspid regurgitation is present, a measure of pulmonary arterial systolic pressure).

Bronchoalveolar Lavage

BAL is commonly included in the evaluation of diffuse lung disease in patients with CTD. It is of no clinical value in patients with suspected airway disease. The predominant cell type is usually the neutrophil, but excess numbers of eosinophils and lymphocytes may be seen. BAL may be abnormal before patients have clinical evidence of CTD. In patients with PSS the predominant cell type seems to relate to the extent of the disease, and therefore to the prognosis (e.g., neutrophil predominance is thought to predict deterioration), but the independence of this relationship has not yet been established.

BAL is the best method for detecting chronic alveolar hemorrhage, as iron-laden macrophages can be found; infection can be diagnosed using quantitative culturing, special stains, and viral cultures; drug-induced lung diseases can be supported (e.g., an excess percentage of $CD8^+$ lymphocytes); and supervening malignancy such as alveolar cell carcinoma, bronchogenic carcinoma, and, occasionally, lymphoma, can be discovered.

Autoantibodies

Eosinophils may be seen in some variants of PSS and can help discriminate Churg-Strauss vasculitis from other forms of vessel disease. Autoantibodies occur in the majority of patients with CTD and can point to a specific CTD when the lung disease precedes other manifestations. The type of autoantibody is highly specific (see Table 48.4).

Biopsy

Biopsy should be performed if there is any doubt about the diagnosis and in cases with unusual clinical or radiologic features. In general a thoracoscopic approach should be used for diffuse lung disease because transbronchial samples do not provide sufficient material to assess the pattern of disease. If the process is thought to be bronchocentric, however (e.g., as with Sjögren's syndrome), then bronchial and/or transbronchial biopsies can be helpful. If other comorbid conditions such as tuberculosis or sarcoidosis are suspected, then transbronchial biopsy is the more appropriate procedure. Transbronchial biopsies should *not* be used for suspected vascular disease because of the risk of uncontrolled bleeding.

TREATMENT

In general, the approach to treatment is focused on the specific type of lung disease and is independent of the specific type of CTD. In most instance there is a paucity of large scale, properly controlled trials of any treatment, and the following guidelines represent what is thought, at present, to be the best approach (Table 48.8).

Table 48.8
Immunosuppressive therapy for the major pulmonary complications of connective tissue diseases

Drug	Dose	Duration	Comments	Monitoring
Azathioprine	2.5mg/kg per day; max 200mg/day	Continuous	Maximal effect may not be evident for 6–9 months, but has better adverse-effect profile than cyclophosphamide; may be used long term; starting dose 50mg daily with monitoring full blood count in case of thiopurine methyltransferase deficiency, maintenance dose for 1 month	Full blood count Liver function tests
Cyclophosphamide, p.o.	2mg/kg per day	Variable	Oral cyclophosphamide may be used continuously or substituted at 3 months for azathioprine because of more favorable adverse-effect profile in diffuse interstitial lung disease	Full blood count
Cyclophosphamide, i.v.	15mg/kg monthly for 1–6 months	Variable	Intravenous therapy for rapid induction of remission at 2–4mg/kg per day for 3–4 days, especially for vasculitis; pulsed i.v. cyclophosphamide may be given at 1–3 monthly intervals, with better adverse-effect profile and lower long-term cumulative dose, particularly in nonvasculitic disease	Liver function tests Urinalysis for blood
Cyclosporin A	5mg/kg per day	Continuous	Bioavailability variable, thus blood monitoring necessary; may be used in combination with prednisolone	Blood pressure Urea and creatinine Cyclosporin level
Methotrexate	7.5–25mg/week	Continuous	Little information to support use except as second-line therapy after first-line treatment; pulmonary toxicity may be limiting	Full blood count Liver function tests
Prednisolone	1mg/kg per day or 20mg alternate days	Continuous	Prednisolone used alone in high dose for cellular diffuse interstitial lung disease and then titrated to control; in conjunction with immunosuppressants, the low-dose regimen is used	Blood pressure Blood glucose Weight
Methylprednisolone, i.v.	500–1000mg daily	3–5 days	Used for aggressive induction of remission, particularly for vasculitis or acute pneumonitis, then followed by maintenance therapy of prednisolone or prednisolone plus immunosuppressive agent	

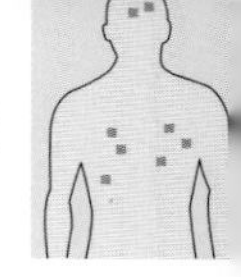

Diffuse Lung Disease

Treatment is with low-dose corticosteroids and either azathioprine or cyclophosphamide. Azathioprine is preferred, although historically, cyclophosphamide has been used in PSS-associated DLD, with anecdotal evidence of benefit. Mycophenolate is increasingly used in patients who have not tolerated azathioprine. Cyclosporin A is occasionally successful.

Airway Disease

Treatment is with inhaled corticosteroids and bronchodilators for milder disease. Corticosteroids alone or in combination with immunosuppression may be used in some situations, but this should not be expected to do more than stabilize obliterating bronchiolitis at best.

High-dose intravenous corticosteroids given intravenously at the inception of treatment is the mainstay of treatment for organizing pneumonia. Response is usually rapid and complete (Fig. 48.9) but the condition may have a relapsing, remitting course once steroids are tapered. Occasionally immunosuppression is required as a steroid sparing strategy.

Vessel Disease

Vasculitis must be treated aggressively. The most accepted regimen is high-dose corticosteroids, together with oral or pulsed cyclophosphamide. Other medications and approaches include azathioprine (often after 3 months of cyclophosphamide), methotrexate, plasmapheresis, and intravenous immunoglobulin.

Vessel disease in SSc is treated differently because it is *not* a vasculitis. Vasodilators such as captopril and nifedipine are effective in studies of acute disease, and more modestly so in longer term trials, but the high doses required for meaningful improvements in pulmonary vascular resistance often produce unacceptable side effects such as systemic hypotension and peripheral edema.

A variety of options are now available for treatment of pulmonary hypertension, although the relative clinical benefit of each still requires closer definition. For this reason, treatment of pulmonary hypertension should be undertaken in a highly specialized setting in which patients can participate in clinical trials where appropriate. Current options include stable prostacyclin analogues—either by regular infusion or very frequent nebulization—and/or the oral endothelin-receptor antagonist bosentan. Oral sildenafil has been demonstrated to reduce pulmonary artery pressure in pulmonary hypertension, but its role, if any, in this group of patients requires further study.

Anticoagulation is indicated when pulmonary hypertension is documented.

Pleural Disease

Large, persistent, or symptomatic effusions may rarely require treatment with systemic corticosteroids or other immunosuppressive agents. Occasionally, intercostal catheter drainage and pleurodesis have been used.

CLINICAL COURSE AND PREVENTION

The treatment of lung disease in CTD can give rise to two pulmonary complications: opportunistic infection and idiosyncratic drug-induced lung disease (Table 48.9). Infection is relatively easy to exclude. Differentiating drug-induced from disease-induced lung problems is more difficult because of the wide

Table 48.9
Toxicity of drugs commonly used to treat connective tissue diseases and patterns of lung disease

Pulmonary effect	Drug				
	Penicillamine	Methotrexate	Gold	Cyclophosphamide	Sulfasalazine
Hypersensitivity pneumonitis		+	+		
Pulmonary infiltrate with eosinophilia	++	++	+	+	+
Fibrosing alveolitis	++	++	+	+	+
Obliterative bronchiolitis	+		+		
Organizing pneumonia	+		+		+
Pleural effusion/ thickening	+	+		+	+
Alveolar hemorrhage/ vasculitis	++				+
Anaphylaxis/ bronchospasm	+	+		+	
Acute pulmonary edema		+		+	+

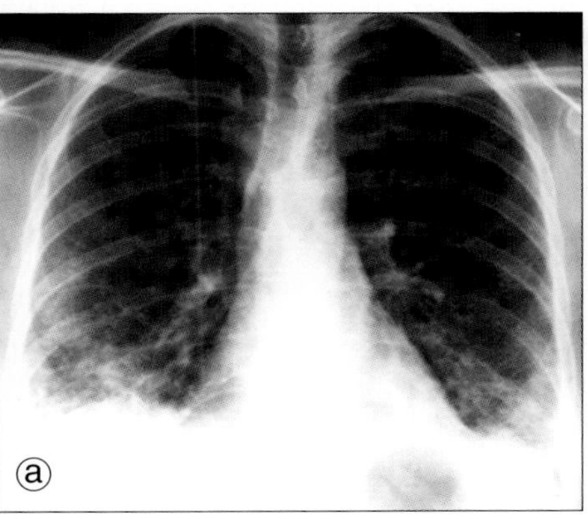

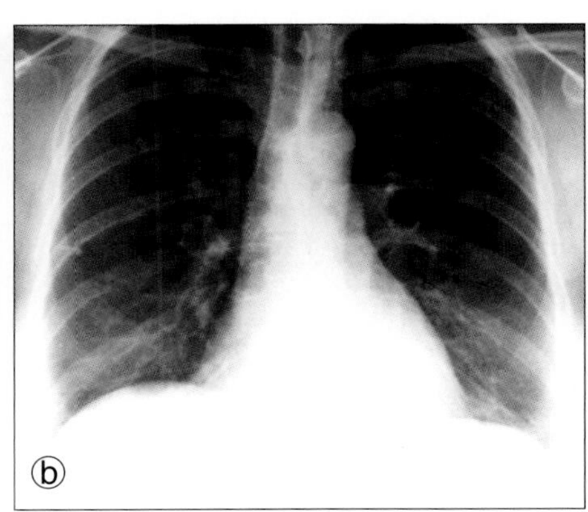

Figure 48.9 Organizing pneumonia.
A, Radiographically, organizing pneumonia is characterized by diffuse patchy bilateral consolidation. Lung biopsy is required to confirm the diagnosis as there are multiple causes of bilateral consolidation. **B,** Radiograph (see biopsy clip, right mid zone) revealing marked radiologic clearance after treatment with corticosteroids.

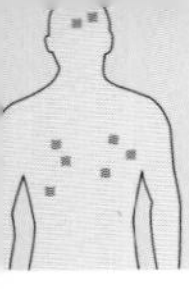

range of drug effects that can also affect all compartments. Symptoms are usually subacute. Clinical signs and the results of lung function tests are dependent on the specific compartment(s) involved. Peripheral blood eosinophilia may be seen with methotrexate, but in general, blood tests are not helpful. BAL characteristically returns an excess of lymphocytes that are predominantly $CD8^+$. Eosinophilic parenchymal infiltration will be reflected in the BAL. Occasionally, biopsy is needed to confirm the pattern of disease. As a general rule, if a patient is receiving any therapy at or before the time of presentation with pulmonary complaints or findings, drug-induced disease must always be considered. Treatment is drug withdrawal. Occasionally, in severe cases, treatment with corticosteroids is required.

Supportive therapy should include assistance with cessation of smoking and the early treatment of infection and heart failure. Influenza and pneumococcal vaccinations are recommended. Long-term oxygen therapy should be considered if hypoxia is chronic, as this provides general systemic support, especially of renal function.

Transplantation, either single lung or heart and lung, should be considered if the systemic aspects of the CTD are not severe and are under satisfactory control. Adequate renal function is essential.

Smoking cessation is critical in patients with RA, as lung involvement in this condition seems to be more common in smokers. Patients with PSS, DM/PM, or MCTD should have maximal prophylaxis against esophageal reflux and aspiration.

PITFALLS AND CONTROVERSIES

Lung Transplantation

There are few case series of lung transplantation in patients with CTD who also have progressive pulmonary disease. Some have reported reasonable survival outcomes, and consideration of the possibility of future lung transplantation is appropriate in this group of patients. Whether transplantation eventually occurs is, of course, dependent on many variables, which are often idiosyncratic to the transplant service.

Diffuse Fibrosing Lung Disease

Diffuse fibrosing lung disease in CTD is not the same as idiopathic pulmonary fibrosis. Fibrosing lung diseases in patients with connective diseases will have histopathologic and radiologic features in common with idiopathic interstitial pneumonias (usually NSIP, but often UIP). The poor prognosis of idiopathic pulmonary fibrosis and UIP must not, however, be transferred on to this group. Judicious use of corticosteroids and immunosuppressive medication is more likely to be effective in stalling disease progression and even improving lung function in the CTD group.

Pulmonary Vascular Disease

A fall in gas transfer on lung function testing does not always signify worsening parenchymal lung disease. One must always be alert to the possible diagnosis of independent pulmonary vascular disease, particularly in patients with PSS. Pulmonary embolism should also be considered.

Interventions Not Targeted at Disease

Continued careful attention must be given to the appropriate use of oxygen therapy as well as the treatment and prevention of osteoporosis and other drug side effects. These measures are often of the greatest benefit to the patient's quality of life.

SUGGESTED READINGS

American Thoracic Society/European Respiratory Society: International Multidisciplinary Consensus Classification of the Idiopathic Interstitial Pneumonias. Am J Respir Crit Care Med 165:277-304, 2002.

Bouros D, Wells AU, Nicholson AG, et al: Histopathologic subsets of fibrosing alveolitis in patients with systemic sclerosis and their relationship to outcome. Am J Respir Crit Care Med 165:1581-1586, 2002.

Davidson BK, Kelly CA, Griffiths ID: Ten year follow up of pulmonary function in patients with primary Sjögren's syndrome. Ann Rheum Dis 59:709-712, 2000.

Dawson JK, Fewins HE, Desmond J, et al: Fibrosing alveolitis in patients with rheumatoid arthritis as assessed by high resolution computed tomography, chest radiography, and pulmonary function tests. Thorax 56:622-627, 2001.

Douglas WW, Tazelaar HD, Hartman TE, et al: Polymyositis-dermatomyositis-associated interstitial lung disease. Am J Respir Crit Care Med 164:1182-1185, 2001.

Kim EA, Lee KS, Johkoh T, et al: Interstitial lung diseases associated with collagen vascular diseases: radiologic and histopathologic findings. Radiographics 22:S151-S165, 2002.

Lynch JP III, McCune WJ: Immunosuppressive and cytotoxic pharmacotherapy for pulmonary disorders. Am J Respir Crit Care Med 155:395-420, 1997.

Veeraraghavan S, Nicholson AG, Wells AU: Lung fibrosis: new classifications and therapy. Curr Opin Rheumatol 13:500-504, 2001.

Wells AU: Lung disease in association with connective tissue disease In du Bois RM, Olivieri D (eds): Interstitial Lung Diseases. European Respiratory Monograph 14. Vol 5, European Respiratory Society Journals, 2000, pp 137-164.

Wells AU, Hansell DM, Rubens MB, et al: Functional impairment in lone cryptogenic fibrosing alveolitis and fibrosing alveolitis associated with systemic sclerosis: A comparison. Am J Respir Crit Care Med 155:1657-1664, 1997.

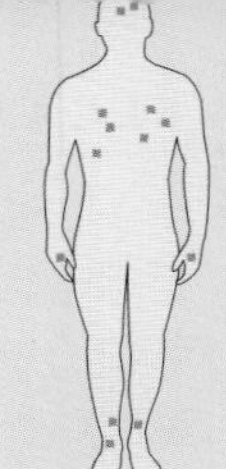

CHAPTER 49 Pregnancy

Stephen E. Lapinsky and Arthur S. Slutsky

The pregnant patient who has pulmonary disease presents a unique challenge to the physician with regard to altered maternal physiology, the occurrence of diseases specific to pregnancy, and the need to consider two patients in all therapeutic decisions. In this chapter, the focus is on the changes in pulmonary physiology associated with pregnancy, certain pregnancy-specific disorders, and other pulmonary diseases encountered in the pregnant patient.

PULMONARY PHYSIOLOGY

Physiologic Changes in Pregnancy

Hormonal changes in pregnancy affect the upper respiratory tract and cause airway hyperemia, edema, and increased friability. Estrogens are likely responsible for many of these effects by producing capillary congestion and hyperplasia of mucus glands. Changes to the thoracic cage result from both the enlarging uterus and from hormonal effects that produce ligamentous laxity. The diaphragm is displaced cephalad by up to 4 cm, but the potential loss of lung capacity is partially offset by an increase in the anteroposterior and transverse diameters, and by widening of the subcostal angle (Fig. 49.1). Despite these anatomic changes, diaphragmatic function remains normal and diaphragmatic excursion is not reduced. The maximum transdiaphragmatic inspiratory pressures that can be generated near term are similar to values generated by patients who are not pregnant. The changes in the chest wall return to normal within 6 months of delivery, although the costal angle may remain widened. The aforementioned changes in the thorax produce a progressive decrease in functional residual capacity (FRC), to 10% to 25% of normal by term (Fig. 49.2). Residual volume decreases slightly, but the major change is in expiratory reserve volume. These alterations are measurable at 16 to 24 weeks' gestation, and progress to term. The increased diameter of the thoracic cage and the preserved respiratory muscle function allow the vital capacity to remain unchanged, and total lung capacity decreases only minimally. Measurements of airflow and lung compliance are not affected, but chest wall and total respiratory compliance are reduced in the third trimester because of the chest wall changes and increased abdominal pressure. Inconsistencies in results reported in studies of diffusing capacity during pregnancy likely arise from the effects of anemia, variable changes in intravascular volume, and the increase in cardiac output. A small increase may be noted in early pregnancy with a subsequent decrease to normal values by term.

Minute ventilation increases markedly in pregnancy, beginning in the first trimester and reaching 20% to 40% above baseline at term (see Fig. 49.2), produced mainly by an increase in tidal volume of approximately 30% to 35%. These changes are mediated by the increase in respiratory drive that results from elevated serum progesterone levels. A respiratory alkalosis with compensatory renal excretion of bicarbonate results, with $PaCO_2$ falling to 4.5 to 4.9 kPa (28 to 32 mm Hg) and plasma bicarbonate falling to 18 to 21 mEq/L. Alveolar-to-arterial oxygen tension differences (PAO_2–PaO_2) are similar to nonpregnant values, and mean PaO_2 usually exceeds 21 kPa (100 mm Hg) at sea level throughout pregnancy. Mild hypoxemia and an increased PAO_2–PaO_2 may develop in the supine position because of airway closure as FRC diminishes near term. A recent study suggests that shunt is normally increased in the third trimester to approximately 15%, and is not changed significantly by posture. Oxygen consumption increases, beginning in the first trimester, and reaches 20% to 33% above baseline by the third trimester because of fetal demands and maternal metabolic processes. The combination of a reduced FRC and increased oxygen consumption lowers oxygen reserve, which renders the pregnant patient susceptible to the rapid development of hypoxia in response to hypoventilation or apnea.

During labor, hyperventilation increases and tachypnea (caused by pain or anxiety) may result in marked respiratory alkalosis. Superimposed metabolic alkalosis can be produced by volume depletion and vomiting. Alkalosis adversely affects fetal oxygenation by reducing uterine blood flow. In some patients, severe pain and anxiety may lead to rapid, shallow breathing with alveolar hypoventilation, atelectasis, and mild hypoxemia. Achieving adequate pain relief with narcotics or epidural analgesia blunts the ventilatory response, and can correct the gas exchange abnormalities associated with active labor. The pregnancy-associated changes in lung function reverse significantly in the first 72 hours postpartum, and return to baseline within a few weeks.

Dyspnea in Pregnancy

Dyspnea is a common complaint in women who have otherwise normal pregnancies, and often is an isolated symptom that results from the normal physiologic changes in the respiratory system. Although a number of mechanisms have been proposed, the symptom most likely arises from a normal perception of the increased minute ventilation that accompanies pregnancy. Diagnosis of this benign condition is based on the presence of isolated dyspnea not usually affecting daily activities, the absence of associated symptoms, and the exclusion of other pathologic conditions.

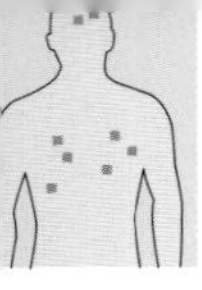

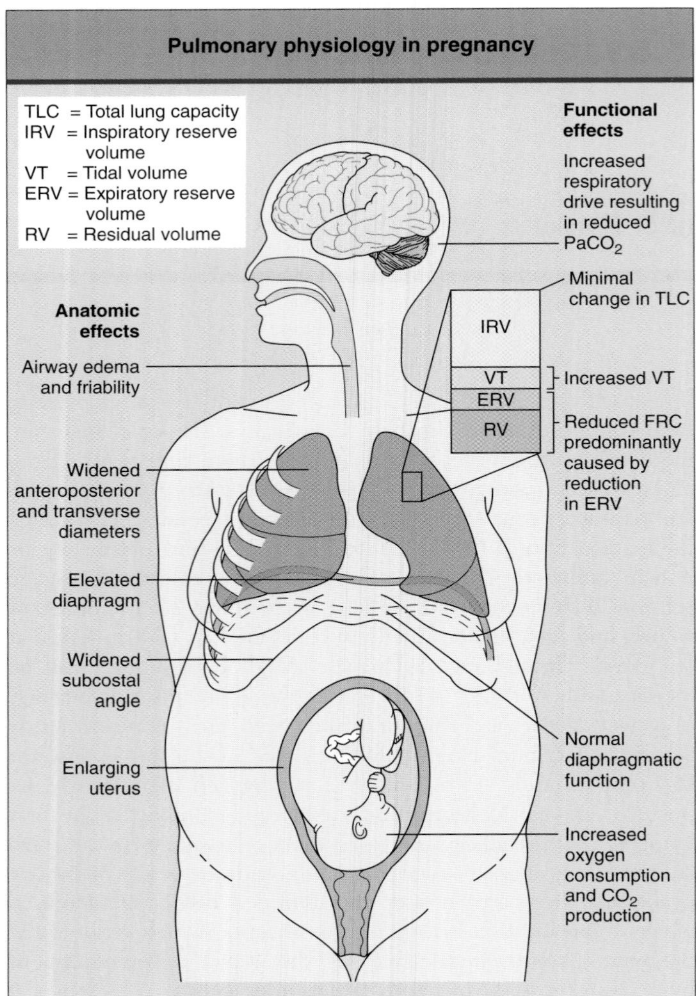

Figure 49.1 Pulmonary physiology in pregnancy: anatomic and functional effects of pregnancy that influence pulmonary physiology.

Physiologic changes in pregnancy

Change from prepregnancy level (%)

Functional residual capacity

Minute ventilation

Cardiac output

Blood volume

Glomerular filtration rate

Weeks of pregnancy

Weeks postpartum

Delivery

Figure 49.2 Physiologic changes in pregnancy. Shown are some of the physiologic changes that occur during pregnancy and the postpartum period. (Reproduced with permission from Lapinsky SE, Kruczynski K, Slutsky AS: Critical Care in the Pregnant Patient. Am J Respir Crit Care Med 152:427-490, 1995.)

PREGNANCY-SPECIFIC DISORDERS

Amniotic Fluid Embolism

EPIDEMIOLOGY AND PATHOPHYSIOLOGY

Amniotic fluid embolism is a rare (between 1/8000 and 1/80,000 live births) but potentially catastrophic obstetric complication (mortality rate of 10% to 86%) that may account for 10% of maternal deaths. Amniotic fluid embolism is usually associated with labor and delivery, but it may also occur with uterine manipulations or uterine trauma, or in the early postpartum period. The mechanism appears to involve amniotic fluid that enters the vascular circulation through endocervical veins or uterine tears. Particulate cellular contents or humoral factors in the amniotic fluid produce acute pulmonary hypertension, both by obstructing the pulmonary vessels and by causing vascular spasm (Fig. 49.3). Acute left ventricular dysfunction may also occur, either secondary to the initial pulmonary embolic event or in response to humoral events mediated by cytokines. The cardiovascular changes of amniotic fluid embolism closely resemble those of anaphylaxis, and sensitivity to amniotic fluid contents may be responsible.

CLINICAL FEATURES

The clinical presentation usually involves the sudden onset of severe dyspnea, hypoxemia, and cardiovascular collapse, often accompanied by seizures. Less common presentations are with hemorrhage caused by disseminated intravascular coagulation, or with fetal distress. Up to one half of the patients may die within the first hour, and cardiac arrest during this period is common.

DIAGNOSIS

The diagnosis of amniotic fluid embolism is usually based on observing the typical clinical picture. Fetal squames in a wedged pulmonary capillary aspirate have been used to confirm the diagnosis, but this does not appear to be a specific finding. Newer, less invasive diagnostic tests may soon be available (e.g., monoclonal antibodies to fetal mucin, measurement of maternal serum zinc coproporphyrin).

The differential diagnosis includes septic shock, pulmonary thromboembolism, abruptio placentae, tension pneumothorax, or a myocardial ischemic event.

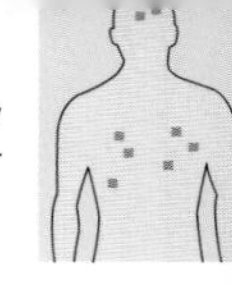

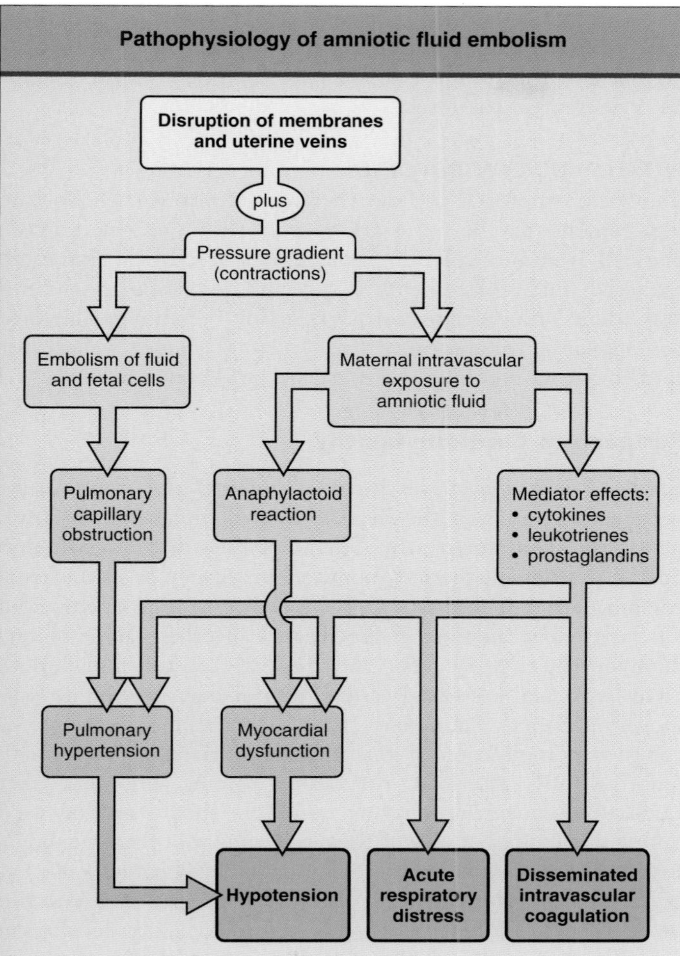

Figure 49.3 Pathophysiology of amniotic fluid embolism: proposed pathophysiologic mechanisms for the development of circulatory shock caused by amniotic fluid embolism.

TREATMENT

Treatment involves routine resuscitative and supportive measures, with prompt attention to adequate oxygenation, mechanical ventilation, and inotropic support. No specific therapy has been shown to be effective, but some suggest a role for corticosteroids. In view of the inconsistent hemodynamic findings, invasive monitoring may be of value.

CLINICAL COURSE AND PREVENTION

Survivors of the initial resuscitation are likely to experience the complications of disseminated intravascular coagulation or acute respiratory distress syndrome (ARDS). Neurologic damage caused by hypotension and hypoxemia is common.

PITFALLS AND CONTROVERSIES

Predisposing factors, pathophysiology, and therapy of this condition are poorly understood. Accordingly, given that only supportive therapy can be undertaken, little can be done to prevent the condition or to reduce its morbidity or mortality. Concerns regarding use of Swan-Ganz catheters, oxygen toxicity, or ventilator-induced acute lung injury apply to the resuscitative measures used in this setting.

Table 49.1
Acute respiratory distress in pregnancy

Disorder	Distinguishing features
Amniotic fluid embolism	Cardiorespiratory collapse, seizures, disseminated intravascular coagulopathy
Pulmonary edema secondary to preeclampsia	Hypertension, proteinuria
Tocolytic pulmonary edema	Tocolytic administration, rapid improvement
Aspiration pneumonitis	Vomiting, aspiration
Peripartum cardiomyopathy	Gradual onset, cardiac gallop
Venous thromboembolism	Evidence of deep venous thrombosis; positive ventilation–perfusion scan, venous Doppler, computed tomography angiogram
Pneumomediastinum	Occurs during delivery, subcutaneous emphysema
Air embolism	Sudden hypotension, cardiac murmur

Tocolytic Pulmonary Edema (Drug-Induced, During Labor)

EPIDEMIOLOGY AND PATHOPHYSIOLOGY

β-Adrenergic agonists, particularly ritodrine and terbutaline, are used to inhibit uterine contractions in preterm labor. A complication of β-agonists that is unique to pregnancy is the development of pulmonary edema. The frequency of tocolytic-induced pulmonary edema varies in published series, from 0.3% to 9%. Postulated mechanisms include prolonged exposure to catecholamines, which causes myocardial dysfunction; increased capillary permeability; large volumes of intravenous fluid administration, often in response to maternal tachycardia; reduced osmotic pressure; or hypotension induced by β-stimulation. Glucocorticoids are often administered in preterm labor to enhance fetal lung maturity and may compound fluid retention.

CLINICAL FEATURES

The clinical presentation is of acute respiratory distress with features of pulmonary edema. No specific features characterize this condition.

DIAGNOSIS

The diagnosis is a clinical one, made in the presence of acute pulmonary edema occurring in the appropriate clinical situation. The differential diagnosis includes cardiogenic pulmonary edema, amniotic fluid embolism, and other conditions (Table 49.1). Failure of the pulmonary edema to resolve in 12 to 24 hours prompts a search for alternative causes.

TREATMENT AND CLINICAL COURSE

The β-agonist must be discontinued, whereupon pulmonary edema should resolve rapidly; additional treatment is supportive and includes diuresis. Early recognition and management should reduce the need for invasive hemodynamic monitoring and mechanical ventilation.

PITFALLS AND CONTROVERSIES

Recent studies suggest that tocolytics do not improve the outcome in preterm labor. Accordingly, prolonged use of these agents may become less common. The condition remains of

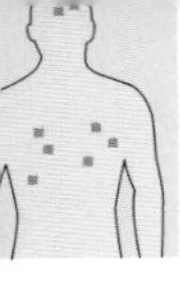

physiologic interest because the pathophysiologic process has not yet been clarified.

Preeclampsia and Pulmonary Edema

EPIDEMIOLOGY AND PATHOPHYSIOLOGY

Pulmonary edema may rarely occur in association with preeclampsia (i.e., perhaps 3% of preeclamptic patients). The preeclamptic patient is usually volume depleted, and pulmonary edema most commonly occurs in the early postpartum period and is often associated with aggressive, intrapartum fluid replacement. Other factors that may contribute to the pathogenesis include reduced serum albumin, elevated left ventricular afterload, and systolic and diastolic myocardial dysfunction (Fig. 49.4). Increased capillary permeability may also occur, aggravated by concomitant conditions such as sepsis, abruptio placentae, or massive hemorrhage.

Pulmonary edema has been described in chronically hypertensive, obese, pregnant patients in whom preeclampsia develops. Diastolic left ventricular dysfunction results from both the hypertension and the obesity, and pulmonary edema is precipitated by volume overload of pregnancy and hemodynamic stresses of preeclampsia.

CLINICAL FEATURES

The presentation is of acute respiratory distress in the preeclamptic patient, often in the early postpartum period.

DIAGNOSIS

Preeclampsia is characterized by hypertension, proteinuria, and peripheral edema, usually in the third trimester.

TREATMENT AND CLINICAL COURSE

The standard approach is to restrict fluid and to administer supplemental proteins and diuresis. Invasive monitoring may be useful if inotropic or vasodilator therapy becomes necessary, particularly in the presence of renal dysfunction. Aggressive diuresis must be avoided because filling pressures should not be reduced to the point of compromising cardiac output and reducing placental perfusion. The ultimate treatment of preeclampsia is delivery of the fetus.

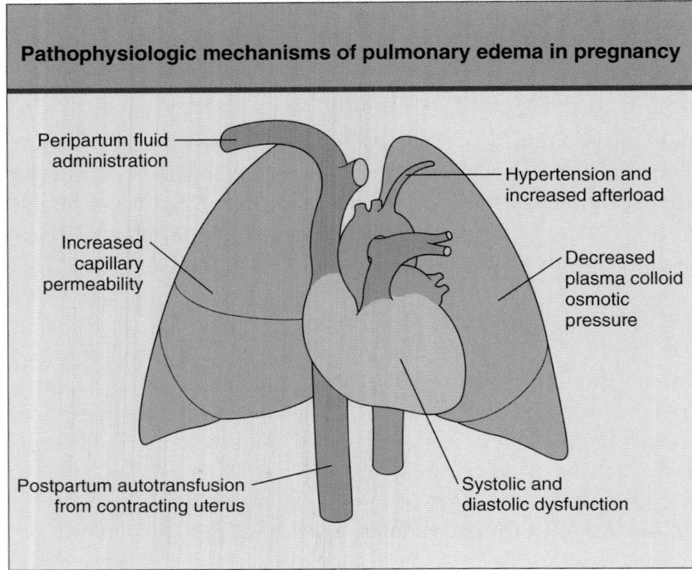

Figure 49.4 Pathophysiologic mechanisms responsible for the development of pulmonary edema in preeclampsia.

PITFALLS AND CONTROVERSIES

The "best" approach to fluid therapy is controversial. Volume replacement may be necessary because these patients may be markedly volume depleted, particularly if vasodilators are used. Excessive fluid replacement may precipitate pulmonary or cerebral edema, however. Accordingly, many recommend invasive hemodynamic monitoring. The "correct" target values for cardiac output and filling pressure are not known, however.

Peripartum Cardiomyopathy

Cardiac failure may occur in the absence of preexisting heart disease as a result of the hypertension of pregnancy, or from peripartum cardiomyopathy. This idiopathic dilated cardiomyopathy presents in the last month of pregnancy or in the postpartum period. The diagnosis is by demonstration of impaired left ventricular function in the absence of other causes of cardiomyopathy. During labor and the early postpartum period, tachycardia and increased cardiac output may precipitate pulmonary edema. Pulmonary thromboembolic events are a common complication of this condition. Management is with diuretics and afterload reduction, bearing in mind that angiotensin-converting enzyme inhibitors should not be used during pregnancy because of the development of fetal renal dysfunction. Anticoagulation is recommended in all patients. Recovery occurs in approximately 50% to 60% of patients within 6 months, but persistent or progressive cardiac failure develops in a significant proportion, with a mortality rate in the range of 12% to 18%.

Gestational Trophoblastic Disease

Pulmonary hypertension and pulmonary edema may complicate benign hydatidiform mole, caused by trophoblastic pulmonary embolism. This most commonly occurs during evacuation of the uterus, and the incidence of pulmonary complications is higher in later gestations. Molar pregnancy may be associated with choriocarcinoma, which can produce multiple, discrete pulmonary metastases, and occasionally pleural effusions.

OTHER PULMONARY DISORDERS IN PREGNANCY

Asthma

EPIDEMIOLOGY AND PATHOPHYSIOLOGY

Asthma affects 5% to 10% of the population and can, accordingly, be expected to affect a similar proportion of pregnant women; during pregnancy, asthma may improve, worsen, or remain unchanged. Although pregnancy does not affect airflow in normal subjects, airway hyperreactivity in asthmatic subjects can be altered. Asthma severity usual returns to prepregnancy levels within 3 months postpartum.

CLINICAL FEATURES

The clinical features of asthma during pregnancy are the same as those in patients who are not pregnant.

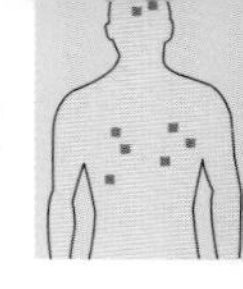

DIAGNOSIS

Objective assessment using pulmonary function tests is essential to assess the presence of airflow obstruction. Gastroesophageal reflux is increased in both frequency and severity during pregnancy, and the symptoms of this condition should be sought as a contributing factor.

TREATMENT

Management is similar to that in patients who are not pregnant (Table 49.2), and includes adequate monitoring, avoidance of precipitating factors, and adequate education. Although physicians may be reluctant to prescribe medications during pregnancy, poorly controlled asthma is potentially more dangerous for the fetus. Inhaled corticosteroids remain the mainstay of therapy. The use of a spacer device is encouraged to reduce local side effects and systemic absorption. Although animal data suggest a small risk of cleft palate with systemic corticosteroid use, this has not been demonstrated in humans. Short courses of prednisone should be used to manage poorly controlled asthma where clinically indicated. Inhaled β-agonists appear safe and should be used as required for symptomatic relief. Acute attacks are treated by ensuring adequate oxygenation, closely monitoring the fetus, and administering appropriate medications. Antireflux measures may markedly reduce asthmatic symptoms.

CLINICAL COURSE AND PREVENTION

Poor asthma control has been reported to cause an increased incidence of preterm births and low birth weight, as well as increased prenatal mortality. Acute exacerbations may be associated with hypoxemia, which may, in turn, compromise the fetus.

PITFALLS AND CONTROVERSIES

Concerns over fetal effects of drugs should not cause physicians and patients inappropriately to avoid the use of effective pharmacologic therapy. Gastroesophageal reflux, a potentially preventable cause of worsening asthma, is frequently overlooked.

Table 49.2
Asthma therapy in pregnancy

Drug	Clinical use	US Food and Drug Administration Classification
Inhaled bronchodilators		
Albuterol (salbutamol)	Common	C
Terbutaline	Common	B
Ipratropium	Occasional	B
Salmeterol	Occasional	C
Formoterol	Occasional	C
Inhaled corticosteroids		
Beclomethasone	Common	C
Budesonide	Common	B
Fluticasone	Common	C
Leukotriene antagonists		
Zafirlukast	Little information available	B
Montelukast	Little information available	B
Theophylline	Uncommon	C
Cromolyn (cromoglycate)	Occasional	B
Systemic corticosteroids	If necessary	B

Pulmonary Thromboembolic Disease

EPIDEMIOLOGY AND PATHOPHYSIOLOGY

Pulmonary thromboembolism occurs in up to 1.3% of pregnancies, both during pregnancy and in the postpartum period; it is an important cause of maternal mortality. The increased incidence results from a hypercoagulable state that occurs with pregnancy, from hormonally mediated venous stasis, and from local pressure effects of the uterus on the inferior vena cava. Pulmonary embolism occurs more frequently in the early postpartum period than during pregnancy, particularly after cesarean section. Deep venous thrombosis occurs with almost equal frequency in all trimesters.

CLINICAL FEATURES

The presentation is similar to that in the patient who is not pregnant. However, the clinical diagnosis of deep venous thrombosis and pulmonary embolism is notoriously inaccurate. The overwhelming predilection for left leg deep venous thrombosis in pregnancy is likely to be the result of anatomic factors.

DIAGNOSIS

Investigation of suspected pulmonary embolism follows a similar approach to that in the patient who is not pregnant, and the diagnosis must be pursued aggressively. Duplex ultrasonography is useful for the diagnosis of deep venous thrombosis, although venous Doppler can give false-positive results because of venous obstruction by the gravid uterus. Ventilation–perfusion scanning can be performed with less than 0.5 mGy (<50 mrad) exposure to the fetus and, if necessary, a computed tomography pulmonary angiogram may be carried out with similarly low fetal exposure (Table 49.3). Such levels of exposure are not believed to cause teratogenicity, which is associated with exposure of greater than 50 to 100 mGy (5 to 10 rad). However, an increased incidence of childhood leukemia has been documented with lower fetal radiation exposure, in the range of 20 to 50 mGy (2 to 5 rad).

Table 49.3
Management of thromboembolic disease in pregnancy – fetal risk of diagnostic procedures

Investigation	Fetal radiation exposure (mGy)	Comments
Duplex ultrasound	Nil	Initial procedure of choice, false positives from ultrasound alone
Chest radiograph (abdomen shielded)	0.01–0.08	Minimal risk
Ventilation–perfusion scan		
Perfusion	0.1–1.0	Low risk, begin with perfusion scan
Ventilation	0.1–0.4	
Computed tomography angiogram	0.1–0.5	Low risk
Pulmonary angiogram		
Brachial route	c. 0.5	Perform if indicated
Femoral route	2.2–4.0	

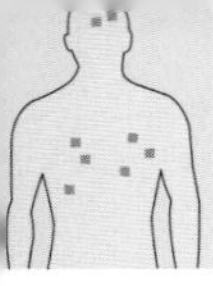

TREATMENT

Warfarin therapy during the first trimester has been associated with development of an embryopathy, and central nervous system abnormalities have been described with second- and third-trimester exposure. Accordingly, warfarin should be avoided (Table 49.4). The anticoagulant of choice is heparin, which does not cross the placenta, is not associated with adverse fetal outcome, and can be readily reversed. Low–molecular-weight heparins do not appear to cross the placenta, and increasing clinical evidence suggests that they are both safe and effective in pregnancy.

When administered with adequate precautions, streptokinase, urokinase, and tissue plasminogen activator have been used successfully without major hemorrhagic complications or significant adverse effects on the fetus or placenta. Use of these agents should nevertheless be limited to life-threatening situations. Where clinically indicated, transvenous placement of an inferior vena cava filter can be performed, although there is some risk of dislodgment because of the dilated venous system and pressure effects during labor.

CLINICAL COURSE AND PREVENTION

Women who have a known hypercoagulable state and those who have had a previous thromboembolism are at increased risk and should receive prophylaxis with anticoagulation throughout pregnancy.

PITFALLS AND CONTROVERSIES

The use of radiologic investigations during pregnancy remains a concern for the fetus. It is nevertheless important to establish a diagnosis of pulmonary embolism because of the major implications if such a diagnosis is missed, and the effects of unnecessary therapy on the health of mother and fetus.

Lower Respiratory Tract Infections

EPIDEMIOLOGY AND PATHOPHYSIOLOGY

Lower respiratory tract infections are an infrequent occurrence, but an important cause of indirect obstetric death. The pregnant patient is susceptible to the usual bacterial pathogens such as *Streptococcus pneumoniae*, *Haemophilus influenzae*, and *Mycoplasma pneumoniae*; less common diseases include varicella pneumonia (Fig. 49.5) and coccidioidomycosis (with dissemination). *Pneumocystic carinii* pneumonia is seen in human immunodeficiency virus–positive patients. Pregnancy does not appear to affect the course or incidence of reactivation of tuberculosis.

CLINICAL FEATURES

The clinical features are similar to those in patients who are not pregnant. Although dyspnea and an increased minute ventilation are common in pregnancy, the respiratory rate is not elevated by the pregnant state.

DIAGNOSIS

A chest radiograph is essential for the diagnosis of lower respiratory tract infections, and must be considered in any pregnant woman who has a clinical presentation suggestive of pneumonia. Further diagnostic investigations include the usual microbiologic cultures, sputum microscopy, and serologic tests.

TREATMENT

Tetracyclines should be avoided in pregnancy. Treatment of varicella pneumonitis is with acyclovir, which decreases mortality and has not been associated with fetal anomalies. Coccidioidomycosis is associated with an extremely high mortality rate and disseminated disease should be treated with antifungal agents. *P. carinii* pneumonia requires treatment with trimethoprim-sulfamethoxazole (Cotrim) with folate supplementation, as well as with corticosteroids if indicated clinically. Although folic acid antagonists and sulfa drugs carry risks for the fetus, pentamidine is associated with higher risks for mother and fetus. Tuberculosis treatment is with isoniazid and rifampin (rifampicin), which have a low risk of adverse fetal effects, as well as ethambutol initially, until sensitivities are available. Pyrazinamide has been used in pregnancy and is recommended by some authorities.

Table 49.4
Management of thromboembolic disease in pregnancy – treatment of pulmonary thromboembolism

Therapy	US Food and Drug Administration classification	Comments
Heparin	C	Treatment of choice
Low–molecular-mass heparin	B/C	Increasing evidence of safety
Warfarin	X	Embryopathy and central nervous system abnormalities
Thrombolytics	C	Consider in acute, life-threatening situations

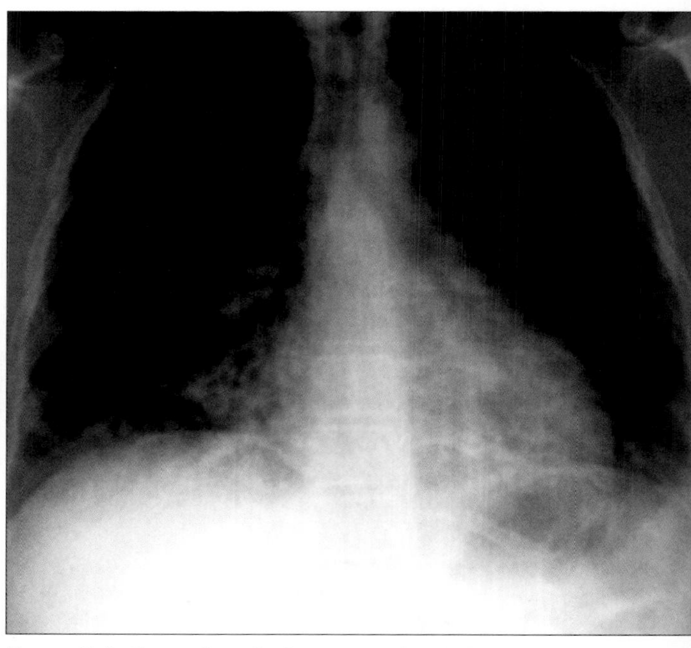

Figure 49.5 Chest radiograph of a woman with varicella pneumonitis that developed at 29 weeks' gestation. Note the diffuse, bilateral, fluffy nodular infiltrate. (Courtesy of Dr. M. Steinhardt, Mount Sinai Hospital, Toronto.)

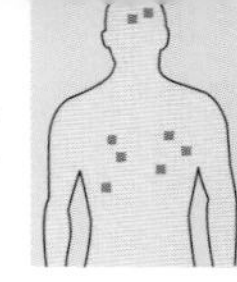

:LINICAL COURSE AND PREVENTION

Although pneumonia is associated with an increased risk of mor-ality, this is probably attributable to underlying diseases rather han to the pneumonia per se. Fetal complications may occur, s may preterm labor. Transplacental transmission of varicella-oster virus occurs uncommonly (<5%), but can produce limb leformities and neurologic involvement. The nonimmune preg-ant woman exposed to varicella-zoster should receive prophy-axis with varicella-zoster immunoglobulin within 96 hours of xposure, and acyclovir if clinical disease develops. Unlike the reatment of active disease, tuberculosis prophylaxis can usually e deferred until after pregnancy, except in the case of recent xposure or skin test conversion.

ITFALLS AND CONTROVERSIES

Vhen investigating and managing lower respiratory tract infec-ions it is important to consider effects on the fetus (i.e., radi-tion exposure, drug toxicities), but necessary evaluations and nterventions should not be avoided inappropriately.

Acute Respiratory Distress Syndrome in Pregnancy

PIDEMIOLOGY AND PATHOPHYSIOLOGY

'he pregnant patient is at risk for development of ARDS from number of pregnancy-associated problems (Table 49.5). Iatro-enic factors such as excessive fluid administration and tocolytic herapy may contribute, as may a reduced albumin level.

:LINICAL FEATURES

'he clinical features are similar to those in the patient who is ot pregnant.

)IAGNOSIS

'he diagnosis is by the usual criteria of hypoxemia in the pres-nce of diffuse pulmonary infiltrates and in the absence of left entricular failure. A detailed history is critical to identification f the underlying problem.

'REATMENT

'here are no major differences in the management of pregnant atients who have ARDS compared with those who are not regnant, other than the need for continuous assessment of the fetus. When administering pharmacologic therapy, it is critical to assess the effects on both the fetus and the mother. Ventilatory management includes consideration of the normal physiologic changes of pregnancy. Adequate maternal oxygen saturation is essential for fetal well-being. Alkalosis has an adverse effect on placental perfusion and should be limited. Acidosis appears to be reasonably well tolerated by the fetus. Fetal delivery may benefit both the mother and the fetus. Epidural anesthetic may reduce the increased oxygen demand produced by uterine contractions.

Table 49.5
Acute lung injury in pregnancy

Relationship to pregnancy	Injury
Pregnancy specific	Preeclampsia Amniotic fluid embolism Chorioamnionitis Trophoblastic embolism
Risk increased by pregnancy	Gastric acid aspiration Pyelonephritis Sepsis Air embolism Massive hemorrhage
Nonspecific	Trauma Drugs/toxins Pancreatitis

CLINICAL COURSE AND PREVENTION

Survival appears to be similar or better than that in the general population, possibly because of the young age of the patients and the reversibility of many of the predisposing conditions.

PITFALLS AND CONTROVERSIES

Specific causes of ARDS that pertain to pregnancy should be sought when assessing patients who have this syndrome. When women of childbearing age present with ARDS, they should be checked for pregnancy.

Pleural Disease

Although pleural effusions may accompany obstetric complications, such as preeclampsia and choriocarcinoma, small, asymptomatic pleural effusions develop in a significant proportion of women in the postpartum period. These result from the increased blood volume and reduced colloid osmotic pressure that occur in pregnancy, as well as from impaired lymphatic drainage caused by Valsalva maneuvers during labor. Moderate-size effusions or the presence of symptoms should prompt a full clinical evaluation. The repeated Valsalva maneuvers of labor may also cause spontaneous pneumothorax and pneumomediastinum, particularly in patients affected by predisposing conditions such as asthma. This diagnosis should be considered in the patient who experiences chest discomfort and dyspnea during or immediately after delivery.

Interstitial Lung Disease

Interstitial lung disease is uncommon in pregnant women, with most cases occurring in women who are older than their childbearing years. When it exists in pregnant women, however, certain physiologic aspects must be considered. A reduced diffusing capacity may lead to difficulty in meeting the increased oxygen consumption requirements of pregnancy. Pulmonary hypertension carries increased risks because cardiac output must increase during pregnancy. Little data exist on the management and outcome in these patients, but restrictive lung disease appears reasonably well tolerated in pregnancy. Patients who have a vital capacity less than 1 L and those who have pulmonary hypertension should consider avoiding pregnancy. Lymphangioleiomyomatosis and systemic lupus erythematosus may worsen as a result of pregnancy.

Management involves careful assessment and monitoring of respiratory and cardiovascular status. Exercise intolerance is common, and patients may require supplemental oxygen therapy early in pregnancy to avoid hypoxemic episodes, which may be dangerous for the fetus. During labor, maternal effort should be limited and oxygen saturation must be monitored.

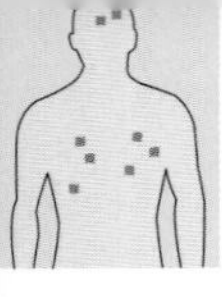

Invasive hemodynamic monitoring may be indicated in the presence of pulmonary hypertension.

Obstructive Sleep Apnea

Pregnancy may be complicated by obstructive sleep apnea (OSA), with potential adverse effects for both the mother and fetus. In general, apnea and hypopnea are uncommon in pregnancy because of the respiratory stimulatory effect of progesterone. Usually OSA is confined to obese patients, perhaps being precipitated by the pregnancy-associated airway mucosal edema and vascular congestion. There is an association between OSA and preeclampsia, probably because of the generalized edema that occurs. Nocturnal hypoxemia may adversely affect the fetus, and poor fetal growth has been documented in these patients. Treatment with nasal continuous positive airway pressure is safe and effective. Snoring is not associated with fetal risk and is not a good marker for OSA in pregnant women.

Cystic Fibrosis

Advances in the management of patients who have cystic fibrosis have extended life expectancy into the childbearing age. Although fertility is impaired, contraception and planned pregnancy should be considered in the management of these patients. Available data indicate that pregnancy does not increase mortality in patients who have stable disease, but poor outcomes can occur in those affected by advanced disease. Those who have both a forced vital capacity less than 50% of predicted and pulmonary hypertension before pregnancy are at greatest risk. Perinatal mortality is increased, related largely to preterm delivery that occurs spontaneously or to maternal complications of cystic fibrosis. Management requires a multidisciplinary approach, with careful attention to nutrition, glucose monitoring, and genetic counseling. Respiratory exacerbations require early aggressive therapy, with due consideration of the potential fetal toxicity of antibiotics such as aminoglycosides and quinolones, and the altered maternal pharmacokinetics.

Gastric Aspiration

Gastric acid aspiration may occur during labor because of delayed gastric emptying, reduced lower esophageal sphincter tone, and the effects of increased intra-abdominal pressure. The presentation is with cough, bronchospasm, and dyspnea, which can progress to ARDS. Prophylaxis with antacids, histamine-2 receptor antagonists, or proton pump inhibitors is often given before cesarean section.

Pulmonary Vascular Disease

Pregnancy in the patient with pulmonary hypertension is associated with an extremely high mortality rate. The increased blood volume and cardiac output during pregnancy may precipitate right ventricular failure. Left ventricular filling may also be impaired as a result of ventricular interdependence. Hospitalization is recommended early in the third trimester, with close monitoring and anticoagulation and oxygen therapy. The cardiovascular effects of labor pose a particular risk, and hemorrhage is poorly tolerated. Invasive hemodynamic monitoring may be of value. Successful pregnancy in these patients requires a multidisciplinary team approach in a referral center.

Pulmonary arteriovenous malformations expand during pregnancy because of the increase in blood volume and venous distensibility, which increases the likelihood of bleeding. Embolization and surgical management have been described in pregnancy.

SUGGESTED READINGS

Clark SL, Hankins GDV, Dudley DA, et al: Amniotic fluid embolism: Analysis of the national registry. Am J Obstet Gynecol 172:1158-1167, 1995.

Elkus R, Popovich J: Respiratory physiology in pregnancy. Clin Chest Med 13:555-565, 1992.

Frangolias DD, Nakielna EM, Wilcox PG: Pregnancy and cystic fibrosis: A case-controlled study. Chest 111:963-969, 1997.

Greer IA: Prevention and management of venous thromboembolism in pregnancy. Clin Chest Med 24:123-137, 2003.

Lapinsky SE, Kruczynski K, Slutsky AS: State of the art: Critical care in the pregnant patient. Am J Respir Crit Care Med 152:427-455, 1995.

Lim WS, Macfarlane JT, Colthorpe CL: Pneumonia and pregnancy. Thorax 56:398-405, 2001.

Miller KS, Miller JM: Tuberculosis in pregnancy: Interactions, diagnosis and management. Clin Obstet Gynecol 39:120-142, 1996.

Nelson-Piercy C: Asthma in pregnancy. Thorax 56:325-328, 2001.

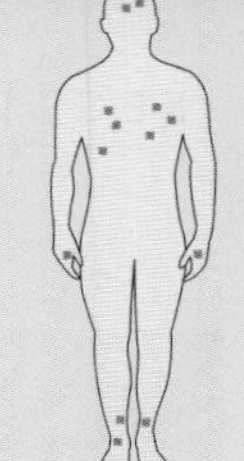

CHAPTER 50 Hematopoietic Stem Cell Transplantation

Stephen W. Crawford

EPIDEMIOLOGY

The procedure of transplanting a marrow graft is now called *hematopoietic stem cell transplantation* (HSCT), in place of the previously used term *bone marrow transplantation*. This reflects the broader range of donor stem cells sources available. These sources include bone marrow, fetal cord blood, and growth-factor–stimulated peripheral blood.

Historically, 40% to 60% of patients experience pulmonary problems some time after HSCT. Up to one third of these patients require intensive care. The incidence of complications increases with the age of the patient, the intensity of the cytoreductive regimen, transplantation for malignant disease, and allogeneic (as opposed to autologous or syngeneic) HSCT. The incidence of these complications appears to be lower after nonmyeloablative HSCT, but the absolute degree of reduction is unclear.

Pneumonia is the leading infectious cause of death. The incidence of some pulmonary infections, such as *Pneumocystis carinii* pneumonia, has decreased because of the routine use of prophylactic antimicrobial agents. Diffuse "idiopathic" pulmonary injury continues to be a problem and has a mortality rate that exceeds 60%. Newer understanding of idiopathic lung injury has led to the delineation of the idiopathic pneumonia syndrome.

Defects in airflow obstruction occur in at least 10% of patients with chronic graft-versus-host disease (GvHD) and have been seen, albeit rarely, in recipients of autologous HSCT. Obliterative bronchiolitis is the most commonly identified obstructing lesion and may progress to profound respiratory insufficiency and death.

Bacteremia or serious bacterial infection is noted in up to 50% of HSCT recipients. Central venous access lines, neutropenia, and immunosuppression to prevent GvHD pose risks for bacterial and fungal infections. Colonization and infection with *Aspergillus* species and *Candida* species are emerging as increasingly frequent problems.

The principles and approaches to the care of HSCT recipients are similar to those for other immunosuppressed patients. The chief distinctive features of HSCT recipients are the high prevalence of graft rejection, GvHD, and chemotherapy and radiation therapy regimen–related toxicities. The HSCT recipient may present a less confusing clinical diagnostic picture than other immunosuppressed patients because specific complications tend to occur within well-defined time periods.

Complications that predispose to, or are associated with, critical illness are listed in Table 50.1. Most notable among these are relapse, rejection, GvHD, and hepatic veno-occlusive disease (VOD).

Temporal Sequence of Pulmonary Disease Syndromes

Specific complications tend to occur within well-defined periods that correspond to the state of immune reconstitution. These complications may be grouped according to the time of presentation relative to the day of HSCT transplantation. The groupings are based in part on the fact that chronic GvHD occurs approximately at or beyond day 100 after allogeneic transplantation, delimiting a "late" from an "early" period.

Complications within the first 30 days are dominated by regimen-related toxicities (Table 50.2). Pancytopenia is common, although administration of hematopoietic colony-stimulating factors may shorten its duration. Pulmonary edema syndromes caused by excess fluid administration have been reported in up to one half of HSCT transplant recipients but should be expected less frequently with appropriate attention to fluid management. In addition, congestive heart failure due to cardiotoxic chemotherapy, adult respiratory distress syndrome due to chemoradiation therapy injury or sepsis, and pulmonary hemorrhage in the presence of thrombocytopenia all contribute to the diffuse infiltrates. The patients frequently have multiorgan disease with regimen-related toxicities or, among allogeneic HSCT recipients, grade 2 to 4 (moderate to severe) acute GvHD. Severe oral mucositis is common and may result in recurrent aspiration of oral secretions. Secondary infection of the denuded oral mucosa with herpes simplex virus or gram-negative bacilli may delay healing and increase the risk of pneumonia. During this period, diffuse pulmonary infiltrates are rarely infectious, and opportunistic infections are not common.

During days 30 to 150, granulocyte number and function have usually returned to normal, but defects in humoral and cell-mediated immunity persist. Both opportunistic and idiopathic pneumonias occur in this period (see Table 50-2). Historically, viral pneumonias, especially cytomegalovirus (CMV) pneumonia, used to be the most frequent cause of diffuse pulmonary infiltrates. More recently, the advent of effective prophylaxis and early treatment strategies has markedly decreased the incidence of CMV and herpes simplex virus pneumonia.

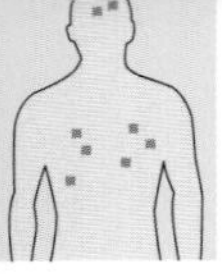

Table 50.1
Complications of hematopoietic stem cell transplantation

Graft failure	**Respiratory disease**
Relapse of malignancy	Pneumonia
Secondary malignancy	Aspiration
Reactions to marrow infusion	Infection
Bronchospasm	Idiopathic
Anaphylaxis	Acute respiratory distress syndrome
Hypotension	Interstitial idiopathic
Pulmonary fat emboli	Chronic fibrosis
Graft-versus-host disease	Airflow obstruction
Acute	Asthma
Chronic	Bronchiolitis
Gastrointestinal disease	Pleural effusion
Oral mucositis	Diaphragmatic paralysis
Esophagitis or gastritis	**Neuromuscular**
Hemorrhage	Metabolic encephalopathy
Diarrheal syndromes	Leukoencephalopathy
Pancreatitis	Seizures
Hepatic insufficiency	Polyneuropathy
Veno-occlusive disease	**Infection**
Drug toxicity	Bacterial
Infection	Viral
Cardiac disease	Herpes group
Tachyarrhythmias	Respiratory viruses
Myocarditis	Respiratory syncytial virus
Pericarditis	Adenovirus
Pericardial effusion	Influenza virus
Renal insufficiency	Parainfluenza virus
Hepatorenal syndrome	Fungal
Nephrotoxicity	*Candida* spp.
	Filamentous fungi
	Pneumocystis carinii
	Protozoal

Table 50.2
Timing and incidence of pulmonary complications

Complications		Approximate incidence (%)
Early complications (<100 days)	Pulmonary edema syndromes	0–50
	Infectious pneumonia	30–40
	Bacterial	2–30
	Fungal	10–20
	Viral	20–30
	Protozoal	<5
	Idiopathic pneumonia (including alveolar hemorrhage)	7–12
	Oral mucositis	50–70
	Pulmonary veno-occlusive disease	rare
Late complications (>100 days)	Bronchopneumonia	20–30
	Idiopathic pneumonia	10–20
	Viral pneumonia	0–10
	Obstructive air flow	10–20

Influence of Transplantation Techniques

Hematopoietic stem cells are the precursors for the three lines of blood cells, red cells, white cells, and platelets. They are recognized and sorted by their CD34-positive surface markers. The stem cells that serve as a marrow graft may come from autologous (same patient), syngeneic (identical twin), or allogeneic (nonself—sibling or unrelated) donor sources. Cells from the former two sources are immunologically identical to the recipient and avoid most reactions between graft and host. Fewer than 30% of patients who require an allogeneic HSCT have a suitable sibling donor. The disparity in match between the donor graft and the recipient for the human leukocyte antigens (HLA) mediates GvHD and graft rejection (host-versus-graft reactions). However, it is now clear that some differences are responsible for favorable results in allogeneic HSCT. A graft-versus-malignancy effect is thought to improve antileukemic responses to allogeneic HSCT.

HSCT usually entails preparing the recipient with marrow-ablative doses of chemotherapy (and, often, radiation therapy) and infusing the donor cells intravenously. Donor cells may be processed by stem cell enrichment techniques, and may be cryopreserved before administration. Refinements in the technique of HSCT include eradicating malignant cells before transplantation with biologic response modifiers (e.g., interleukins) or targeted monoclonal antibodies, treatment of autologous marrow after harvest to destroy malignant cells, accelerating engraftment of the transplanted marrow with growth factors (e.g., granulocyte–macrophage colony-stimulating factor), and positive selection of the hematopoietic stem cells from the marrow or peripheral blood. The period of immune and hematopoietic reconstitution requires intensive blood support and infection precautions. In most myeloablative transplantations, there is an inevitable period of neutropenia and profound immunosuppression.

Recently, nonmyeloablative HSCT has been performed. These procedures use less intensive chemotherapy regimens along with infusion of allogeneic stem cells. The beneficial effects of these "mini-allotransplants" take advantage of the graft-versus-malignancy effect in eradicating malignancy, while not inducing an ablation of the host defenses and marrow. These less chemotherapy- and radiation-intensive techniques may have greater application among older patients and those with multiple medical problems.

The incidence of infections and late airflow obstructive defects is less after autologous transplantation than after allogeneic transplantation. Viral pneumonia is markedly less common among autologous HSCT recipients, presumably owing to the lower level of suppression of cytotoxic T lymphocytes from GvHD and its treatment and prophylaxis. CMV pneumonia occurs in 4% or less of autologous stem cell recipients, and invasive fungal disease after the initial period of neutropenia appears to be less common. Idiopathic lung injury, associated with chemoirradiation or sepsis syndrome, occurs after both allogeneic and autologous HSCT with similar frequency (5% to 7%).

The use of alternative hematopoietic precursor sources (e.g., mobilized peripheral blood stem cells) and cytokines (e.g., hematopoietic cell colony-stimulating factors) have shortened the time to engraftment. The shorter period of neutropenia should decrease the incidence of pulmonary complications. Improved granulocyte numbers and shorted duration of hospitalization reduce the risk of opportunistic infections, and improved platelet counts decrease the hemorrhage associated with lung injury (Table 50.3). Decreased toxicity and improved survival associated with the use of peripheral blood stem cells in allogeneic transplantation are largely related to modifications in GvHD prophylaxis rather than the stem cell source (Table 50.4).

CLINICAL FEATURES

Pulmonary Function Testing

BEFORE TRANSPLANTATION

Pulmonary function testing (PFT) is a standard part of the pretransplantation evaluation. The results form baseline data for comparison with later testing and have been used as a contraindication to transplantation. Abnormalities in the measures of airflow, lung volume, and diffusing capacity have been associated with increased risk of pulmonary complications after transplantation.

Abnormal PFT results before transplantation are predictive of mortality. After accounting for other clinical characteristics associated with death after transplantation (e.g., age, relapsed malignancy, HLA-mismatched graft), restrictive lung defects, hypoxemia, and reduced diffusing capacity are associated with statistically increased risk of death, especially within the first few months after transplantation.

Pretransplantation PFT results are statistically associated with complications and death; however, there are no values for these tests that predict these outcomes with certainty. On average, a total lung capacity (TLC) or diffusing capacity value (corrected for hemoglobin content) below the lower limits of normal is associated with a 20% decreased probability of survival. Such information should not used as an absolute contraindication to transplantation, but rather used in combination with other known risks for transplant-related mortality to assess the risks fully.

Table 50.3
Variables influencing outcome of critical care complications of hematopoietic stem cell transplantation

Stem cell source	Graft-versus-host disease prophylaxis
Bone marrow	Methotrexate
Peripheral blood	Corticosteroids
Growth factors	Underlying disease
Granulocyte colony-stimulating factor	Previous treatments
Granulocyte–macrophage colony-stimulating factor	

Table 50.4
Advantages of peripheral blood stem cells over bone marrow cells in allogeneic transplantation

Peripheral blood stem cells offer
- Decreased regimen-related toxicity
- Improved survival, secondary to the use of FK-506 plus corticosteroids
- Improved platelet and neutrophil recovery, secondary to the use of corticosteroids instead of methotrexate

AFTER TRANSPLANTATION

There are both acute and long-term decrements in pulmonary function after intensive chemotherapy and irradiation as used in HSCT transplantation. Reductions in lung volumes, diffusing capacity, and exercise tolerance have been documented after treatment for leukemia in children as well, and they are thought to be a complication of chemotherapy. Abnormalities in PFTs in HSCT recipients include decreases in lung volume, gas diffusion, and airflow. Reductions in lung volume and diffusing capacity are common early (i.e., within months) after HSCT transplantation. The declines in lung volumes may be at least partially reversible within the first 2 years of transplantation, whereas the low diffusing capacity reportedly persists for several years. Development of airflow obstruction has been seen in approximately 10% of allogeneic HSCT recipients in the presence of chronic GvHD and is most often related to obliterative bronchiolitis.

A few reports have examined abnormalities in other PFTs for association with increased mortality. Both relapses of malignancy and overall mortality correlated with falls in lung volumes and diffusion 1 year after HSCT transplantation. At 3 months after transplantation, the mean values for TLC and diffusing capacity are decreased, and restrictive ventilatory defects (TLC <80% of predicted value) are noted in 34% of the recipients. Airflow rates (forced expiratory capacity in 1 second/forced vital capacity) remain largely unchanged. A restrictive lung defect at 3 months after transplantation or a significant decline (>15%) in TLC from baseline despite remaining within the normal range is associated with a twofold increased risk for nonrelapse mortality. Neither airflow obstruction nor impairment in diffusing capacity is associated with an increased risk. Abnormalities of the TLC at 3 months after transplantation are associated with death with respiratory failure but not with an increased risk of chronic GvHD.

Radiography

Attention to radiographic abnormalities of the chest is crucial for avoiding unnecessary complications. Focal abnormalities represent opportunistic infection in over 80% of cases in neutropenic hosts and those with malignancy, even in the absence of symptoms. Focal lung lesions among patients with non-Hodgkin's lymphoma and Hodgkin's lymphoma are most often parenchymal lymphoma. However, fungal pneumonia may present after chemotherapy and be indistinguishable on radiographs from malignancy. In addition, tuberculosis after transplantation most often occurs in patients with evidence of prior parenchymal lung disease.

Presence of focal lesions on chest radiography should prompt aggressive diagnostic evaluation before transplantation. Computed tomography (CT) scans may help to localize the lesion and define it anatomically. Depending on the number, size, and location of the lesions, diagnostic procedures are warranted for

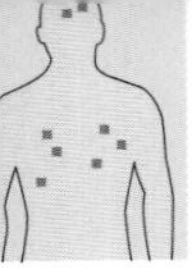

planning treatment. Bronchoscopy, percutaneous needle aspiration, or lung resection should usually follow radiographic identification of lesions.

Predicting Respiratory Failure

Respiratory failure is the most common cause of critical illness after HSCT (Table 50.5). The risk factors for respiratory failure that are present at the time of transplantation are

- Receipt of an HLA-nonidentical donor marrow
- Active phase of malignancy
- Older age (>21 years)

The incidence of respiratory failure is between 10% and 13% in patients with no risk factors, increasing to over 50% when all three risk factors are present.

DIFFUSE INFILTRATES

Idiopathic Pneumonia Syndrome

INCIDENCE AND EPIDEMIOLOGY

Although pneumonia develops in 40% to 60% of patients after allogeneic marrow transplantation, no infectious etiology is identified in 30% to 45% of cases. These episodes are referred to as *idiopathic pneumonias* (or *idiopathic interstitial pneumonias*) to indicate the lack of documented infection and the uncertainty regarding the precise etiologies. Several studies have reported the incidence of idiopathic pneumonia to be 11% to 17% after allogeneic marrow transplantation, with a median onset of 39 to 52 days and an associated mortality rate of 60% to 70%.

The risk factors associated with idiopathic pneumonia in most studies were transplantation for malignancy and age greater than 20 years. Suggested etiologies for the apparently noninfectious lung injury after marrow transplantation have included chemoirradiation damage, occult CMV infection, and a graft-versus-host reaction.

DEFINITION

A National Institutes of Health workshop addressed the issues of definitions and diagnostic criteria for idiopathic pneumonia after marrow transplantation and recommended that the process be referred to as *idiopathic pneumonia syndrome* (IPS) to reflect the diversity of clinical presentations and probable multifactorial etiologies of the apparently noninfectious diffuse lung injuries. IPS was defined as "evidence of widespread alveolar injury in the absence of active lower respiratory tract infection" after marrow transplantation (Table 50.6). Bronchoalveolar lavage (BAL), rather that lung biopsy, was recommended as the primary diagnostic approach.

CLINICAL PRESENTATION AND COURSE

The usual clinical presentation of "interstitial pneumonia" is described as diffuse radiographic infiltrates, fever, dyspnea, and hypoxemia. However, this presentation is also consistent with viral pneumonia, and there is no apparent distinction in presentation for the idiopathic processes. The diagnosis of idiopathic pneumonia requires the exclusion of infection. Large studies of pneumonia after marrow transplantation have therefore required examination of lung tissue either from lung biopsy or autopsy for the diagnosis. The histology of IPS is usually found to be either idiopathic interstitial pneumonia or diffuse alveolar damage when lung biopsy is performed (Table 50.7).

The incidence of IPS appears lower, the onset earlier, and the risk factors changed from those previously reported for idiopathic pneumonia. The major risks appear to be regimen-related toxicity and multiple-organ dysfunction associated with alloreactive processes. Among 1165 consecutive marrow recipients in Seattle in the United States, the estimate of the incidence of IPS within 120 days of transplantation was 7.7%. The median time to onset was 21 days (mean 34 ± 30). The in-hospital mortality rate was 79%, a similar result to that of previous studies.

Table 50.5
Reasons for admissions to critical care units after hematopoietic stem cell transplantation

Reasons for admissions	Percentage of patients
Respiratory failure	46
Shock	17
Arrhythmias	9
Neurologic complications	7
Postoperative care	7
Bleeding	3
Multiple organ dysfunction syndrome	3
Procedures	
Ventilation	58
Insertion of arterial line	61
Insertion of Swan–Ganz catheter	26
Hemodialysis	15

Table 50.6
Criteria for diagnosis of idiopathic pneumonia syndrome after hematopoietic stem cell transplantation

Evidence of widespread alveolar injury
Multilobar infiltrates on chest radiograph or computed tomography; and
Symptoms and signs of pneumonia; and
Evidence of abnormal physiology; and
Absence of active lower respiratory tract infection documented by
Negative bronchoalveolar lavage, lung biopsy, or autopsy with examination of stains and cultures for bacteria, fungi and viruses, including cytomegalovirus centrifugation culture; and
Cytology for viral inclusions and *Pneumocystis carinii*; and
Immunofluorescence monoclonal antibody staining for cytomegalovirus, respiratory syncytial virus, influenza virus, parainfluenza virus, and adenovirus

Table 50.7
Histology of idiopathic pneumonia syndrome

Histologic pattern	Number of cases (%)
Interstitial pneumonia	25 (59%)
Diffuse alveolar damage	15 (37%)
Bronchopneumonia	2 (5%)
Bronchiolitis obliterans	1 (2%)

Fifty-three transplant recipients (62%) died with progressive respiratory failure. IPS resolved in 22 patients (26%), and 18 patients (21%) survived to discharge (Fig. 50.1). Mechanical ventilation was required for 59 marrow recipients (69%) within a median of 2 days of onset of infiltrates, and 2 of these (3%) survived to discharge. Pulmonary infection (predominantly fungal) was noted in 7 of 25 (28%) marrow recipients who had an autopsy.

Although there was no significant difference in the incidence of IPS between autologous (5.7%) and allogeneic marrow recipients (7.6%), risks were identified only for the latter: malignancy other than leukemia and grade 4 GvHD. No factors were associated with recovery.

An "engraftment syndrome" has been described among autologous HSCT recipients (Fig. 50.2). A combination of fever, diffuse pulmonary infiltrates, and generalized capillary leak occurred in most of the patients approximately 1 week after transplantation. The syndrome appeared related, in part, to administration of a growth factor, granulocyte colony-stimulating factor. A prompt response to corticosteroids was reported.

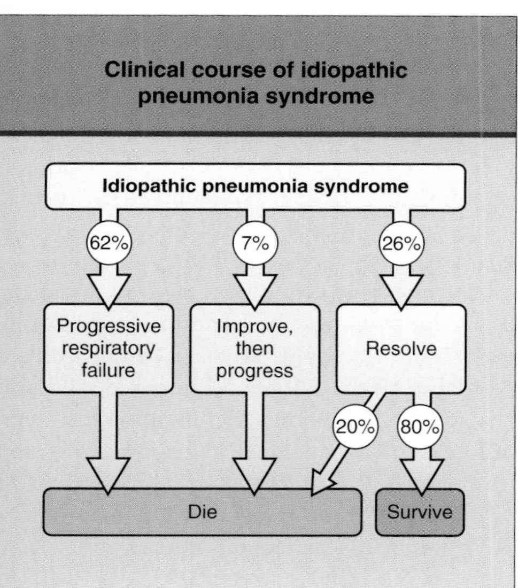

Figure 50.1 Clinical course of idiopathic pneumonia syndrome.

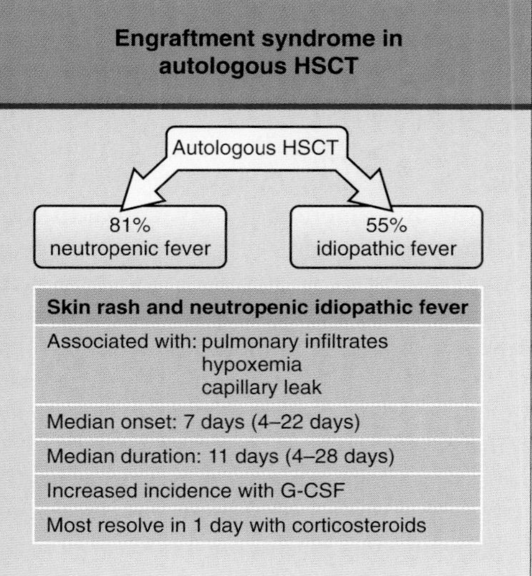

Figure 50.2 Engraftment syndrome in autologous hematopoietic stem cell transplantation (HSCT). G-CSF, granulocyte colony-stimulating factor.

TREATMENT

There are no proven effective treatments for IPS. High-dose corticosteroids are the conventional therapy on the basis of anecdotal successes. Prednisone has been associated with improvement in reduced lung diffusing capacity for carbon monoxide (DLCO) after autologous HCST for breast cancer. Similarly, the noninfectious lung complications associated with acute GvHD reportedly respond well to corticosteroids after allogeneic HCST. The optimal dosing and duration of treatment are unknown.

Other therapeutic options have been investigated. The administration of etanercept, a soluble, dimeric tumor necrosis factor-α (TNF-α)–binding protein, in combination with standard immunosuppressive therapy, was well tolerated by three consecutive pediatric allogeneic BMT recipients with IPS and associated with significant improvements in pulmonary dysfunction within the first week of therapy.

Pulmonary Hemorrhage

EPIDEMIOLOGY, CLINICAL PRESENTATION, AND COURSE

A syndrome of diffuse pulmonary infiltrates, fever, hypoxemia, thrombocytopenia, and renal insufficiency occurring within the first few weeks after autologous marrow transplantation for solid tumor has been described. The hallmark of the syndrome was progressively bloodier return from BAL and the absence of infection in the lungs. This diffuse alveolar hemorrhage syndrome was associated with a greater than 90% mortality rate. Diffuse alveolar hemorrhage appeared to be unrelated to the platelet count, but it correlated with increased requirements for platelet transfusion.

Initially seen in 29% of the patients at the University of Nebraska in the United States, the incidence of this syndrome has declined markedly, to less than 7%, presumably owing to alterations in either patient selection or transplantation conditioning regimens. Among marrow recipients with lymphoma at the Memorial Sloan-Kettering Cancer Center in the United States, the reported incidence is 8%. All centers reporting the syndrome note mortality rates over 67%.

Studies of alveolar hemorrhage suggest that the finding of blood in BAL fluid may not represent a specific syndrome. Among a cohort of 194 immunosuppressed patients undergoing BAL, detection of alveolar bleeding by the presence of alveolar siderophages did not correlate with specific lung disease, presence of infection, or clinical outcome. Siderophages did correlate with uremia, thrombocytopenia, coagulopathies, and a long history of tobacco smoking. This quantitative measure of alveolar bleeding circumvents the subjective nature of recognizing "progressively bloodier" BAL. The correlations support a contention that alveolar blood is a sign of disease and not a specific diagnostic category. Spanish investigators noted that there was poor correlation between the presence of blood in the lungs at autopsy and the results of BAL during life among patients after allogeneic marrow transplantation or hematologic malignancy, thereby further questioning the specificity of the BAL findings as representing a specific syndrome.

PATHOGENESIS AND PATHOLOGY

All cases of diffuse alveolar hemorrhage that have come to autopsy have demonstrated diffuse alveolar damage, alveolar desquamation, and hyaline membrane formation, typical findings of the acute respiratory distress syndrome. Because the incidence of the syndrome correlates with the recovery of circulating granulocytes in affected patients, investigators have proposed that neutrophilic inflammation plays a pathogenetic role. Supporting this contention, visual evidence of airway inflammation (ascertained by a bronchitis index) before transplantation was associated with the syndrome.

The timing and pathologic features of the syndrome suggest that chemoirradiation injury to multiple organs is central to its etiology. It remains unclear whether the hemorrhage is an essential element to the pathogenesis and outcome or merely an expected consequence of diffuse lung injury in the presence of a coagulopathy.

TREATMENT

There are no controlled studies of the treatment of diffuse alveolar hemorrhage. Retrospective data and anecdotal reports suggest that high-dose corticosteroids may improve the survival rates. Doses of methylprednisolone ranging from 30 mg/day to 1 g/day have been associated with a decrease in mortality rates from over 90% to 67%. Clouding the interpretation of this finding was the simultaneous declining incidence of the syndrome at the center where this finding occurred, suggesting that influences on the course and severity of the disease may have been altered as well.

Late-Onset Noninfectious Pulmonary Complications

Approximately 5% to 15% of patients surviving for more than 3 months after HSCT experience late-onset noninfectious pulmonary complications (LONIPC). These diverse processes include obliterative bronchiolitis, bronchiolitis obliterans with organizing pneumonia, diffuse alveolar damage, lymphocytic interstitial pneumonia, and nonclassifiable interstitial pneumonia. These diagnoses were based on clinical investigation, radiologic imaging, lung function tests, BAL, and biopsies. Chronic GvHD appeared to be the only significant risk factor for the development of these "late" complications. The frequency of LONIPC is low in autologous (5%) compared with allogeneic transplants (14.7%), but this difference was not statistically significant. Various methods of enhanced immunosuppressive therapy (most often with corticosteroids) results in marked durable remission in half of the case. The response rates for obliterative bronchiolitis are lower. Overall, the development of these late pulmonary complications had no adverse effect on survival. With the exception of obliterative bronchiolitis, the data do not support that diffuse lung diseases are significantly different in pathogenesis or response to treatment than those that occur earlier.

Similarly, at Duke University, close follow-up of women undergoing high-dose chemotherapy (cyclophosphamide/cisplatin/BCNU) and autologous HSCT for primary breast cancer with pulmonary function testing and CT at regular intervals revealed a high incidence of interstitial pneumonia requiring steroids (64%), but no deaths due to pulmonary toxicity. The DLCO reached a nadir of 58% of baseline at 15 to 18 weeks. Spirometry suggested mild restrictive changes without significant obstruction. Patients in whom pulmonary symptoms of cough or dyspnea developed had a corresponding significantly greater and earlier decline in DLCO. Chest CT was neither sensitive nor specific for diagnosing pulmonary toxicity. For patients who received steroids for pulmonary toxicity, there was a subsequent improvement in DLCO of 17% ($p = .0001$). Such changes may represent a form of delayed pulmonary toxicity. The role of and necessity for corticosteroids are unclear in these conditions.

Diagnosis

DIFFUSE INFILTRATES

HSCT recipients with diffuse pulmonary infiltrates after transplantation require a thorough clinical evaluation. Empirical treatment with broad-spectrum antibiotics, diuresis, and sodium restriction should usually be instituted. A trial of diuretics may help differentiate the presentation of diffuse infiltrates due to IPS from pulmonary edema due to volume excess or left ventricular failure. Occasionally, pulmonary artery wedge pressure measurement (or cardiac echocardiography) to exclude pulmonary edema and guide therapy is recommended if renal insufficiency or respiratory compromise exist. Bleeding disorders should be corrected and adequate platelet support provided to prevent further pulmonary hemorrhage. If the response to these emprical treatments is not rapid, or if edema is not considered a component of the infiltrates, HSCT recipients with diffuse infiltrates after transplantation usually should undergo fiberoptic bronchoscopy with BAL (Fig. 50.3). Pulmonary infection is confirmed with cytology, histology, or culture by demonstrating infection from BAL or lung biopsy. In addition to bacterial, fungal, and cytologic stains, a quantitative bacterial culture should be performed (Table 50.8). These specimens should also be processed with rapid detection techniques for viral pathogens. Direct fluorescent monoclonal antibody stains and centrifugation culture (shell vial) are indicated if the patient or donor is seropositive for CMV. Outbreaks of viral pneumonias due to respiratory syncytial virus and parainfluenza virus have recently been recognized in HSCT units. BAL, as well as nasopharyngeal and throat swabs for virologic studies, should be performed to exclude treatable pulmonary infection, especially during autumn and winter.

FOCAL INFILTRATES

Focal, multifocal, or patchy infiltrates after HSCT frequently represent bacterial or fungal infection. Bacteria are an unusual cause of diffuse infiltrates. The proportion of focal infiltrates that resolve spontaneously or with empiric antibacterial therapy is unknown. Focal radiographic lesions with a masslike appearance that develop or persist despite antibiotics at any time after HSCT are, in most cases, due to pulmonary fungal infection. The incidence of invasive fungal infections after HSCT has increasing to more than than 11%. Occasionally, *Legionella* species and *Pseudomonas* species, and, rarely, *Nocardia* species are identified in localized lesions.

Noninfectious causes of focal lung lesions after HSCT include resolving (sterile) abscess, lymphoma or Hodgkin's disease, and organizing pneumonia with bronchiolitis obliterans. A clinical history of recent bacteremia, previous solid tumor, and

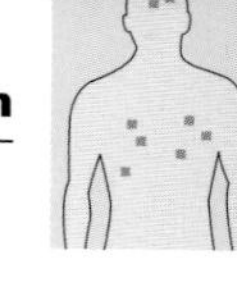

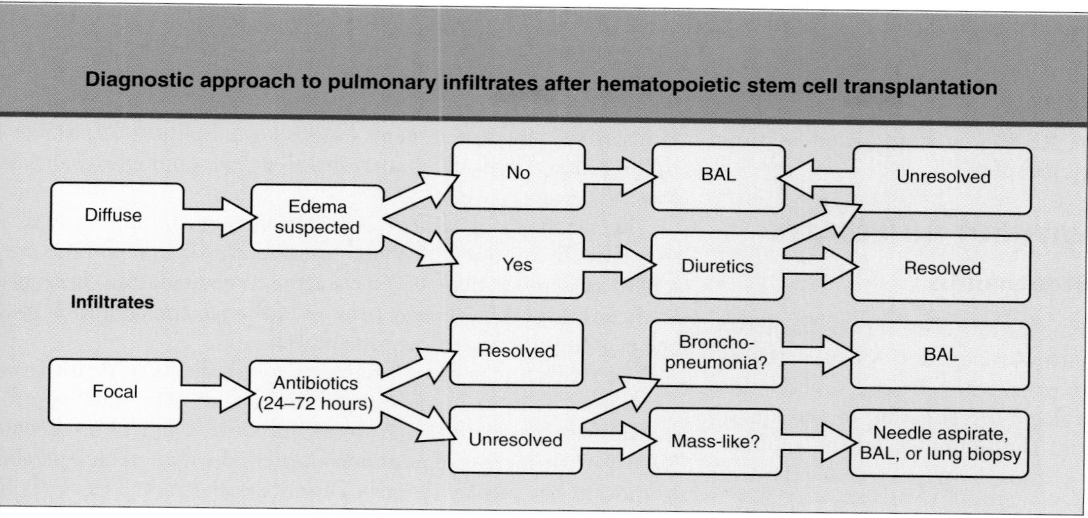

Figure 50.3 Diagnostic approach to pulmonary infiltrates after hematopoietic stem cell transplantation. BAL, bronchoalveolar lavage.

Table 50.8
Routine laboratory evaluation of bronchoalveolar lavage specimens after hematopoietic stem cell transplantation

Pathology	Stains
	Wright–Giemsa stain
	Papanicolaou stain
	Silver stain
	Modified Jimenez stain (or other stain suitable for detecting *Legionella* spp.)
	Monoclonal fluorescent antibody stain for *Pneumocystis carinii* (consider in exceptional setting)
Microbiology	Stains
	Gram stain
	Wet mount potassium hydroxide stain or calcofluor white stain
	Modified acid-fast stain
	Fluorescent antibody stain for *Legionella* spp.
	Culture
	Bacterial (aerobic), semiquantitative method
	Fungal
	Legionella spp. (chocolate yeast extract)
	Acid-fast
Virology	Fluorescent antibody stains
	Cytomegalovirus
	Herpes simplex virus
	Respiratory syncytial virus, parainfluenza and influenza viruses pooled antibodies
	Culture (rapid centrifugation technique preferred)
	Cytomegalovirus
	Herpes simplex virus
	Adenovirus
	Respiratory syncytial virus, parainfluenza, and influenza viruses (in appropriate clinical setting)

Table 50.9
Invasive pulmonary aspergillosis after hematopoietic stem cell transplantation: the bronchogenic carcinoma equivalent

- Presentation most often focal
- Patients have identified risk factors
- Chemotherapy alone of limited value
- Cause of death
  - Spread to brain or heart
  - Erosion into vessels (causing hemoptysis)
- Consider surgical resection
  - Potentially curative
  - "Debulking" of devascularized tissue

clinical acute pneumonia that is resolving are important clues to the differential diagnosis. Unfortunately, the absence of fever and clinical symptoms does not exclude the diagnosis of filamentous fungal infection.

HSCT recipients with focal pulmonary lesions should be evaluated aggressively because there is a high probability of infection. CT scanning of the chest should usually be included in the diagnostic evaluation. A fungal infection often has a masslike appearance with a zone of attenuation that is highly suggestive of tissue invasion. Additional lesions that are not appreciated on plain chest radiographs may also be seen.

The diagnostic approach to localized lesions is dictated by their radiographic appearance and locations. Areas of apparent bronchopneumonia are approached with fiberoptic bronchoscopy and BAL, whereas peripheral, consolidated lesions are amenable to percutaneous needle aspiration for diagnosis (see Fig. 50.3). A nondiagnostic result by any technique should be repeated, or alternative measures for diagnosis should be attempted. If bronchoscopy or needle aspirations are not diagnostic, the most definitive study is biopsy at thoracotomy. Surgical resection should be considered when the pulmonary lesions can be removed completely because this may be both diagnostic and curative in patients with a localized fungal infection (Table 50.9).

The presentation of basilar infiltrates without masslike consolidation that occur within the first several weeks after marrow infusion in the setting of oral mucositis should prompt evaluation for recurrent aspiration. A history of recurrent cough induced by attempts at swallowing or nocturnal paroxysms of cough in the setting of severe mucositis is common. The appropriate approach to such patients is conservative—moderating

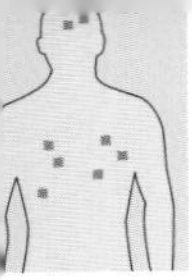

the administration of sedatives, encouraging pulmonary toilet, and avoiding mucosal bleeding by adequate platelet support. Most patients receive broad-spectrum antibiotics. Rarely, tracheal intubation is required to avoid massive aspiration in a profoundly obtunded patient or acute airway obstruction in the presence of severe upper airway bleeding.

RESPIRATORY FAILURE WITHOUT INFILTRATES

Airflow Obstruction and Bronchiolitis

Several centers report that chronic airflow obstruction develops in 6% to 10% of allogeneic marrow recipients. Most of these cases are among long-term survivors with chronic GvHD. In 70% of the reported cases, histologic investigation of the lungs showed obliterative bronchiolitis. The obliterative bronchiolitis lesions in the lungs of marrow transplantation recipients are occasionally, but not always, accompanied by interstitial infiltrates of mononuclear cells. However, interstitial fibrosis and bronchitis without obliteration have also been noted among patients with airflow obstructive physiology. Airflow obstruction with obliterative bronchiolitis has been reported after autologous marrow transplantation. Based on these findings, new-onset airflow obstruction, not the presence of obliterative bronchiolitic lesions, is the hallmark of this problem.

The etiology of obliterative bronchiolitis after marrow transplantation is unknown. Those causes recognized in otherwise normal hosts (e.g., recurrent aspiration, viral infection with influenza, adenovirus, or measles, and bacterial or mycoplasma infection) have not been found consistently in HSCT recipients with obliterative bronchiolitis. Immunologic mechanisms inducing bronchial epithelial injury are suggested by the strong association between chronic GvHD and the development of obliterative bronchiolitis. Factors associated with the increased risk of GvHD, such as increasing age and HLA-nonidentical marrow grafts, are not independent risk factors for the development of obliterative bronchiolitis. The lung epithelium may be the target of immune-mediated injury in chronic GvHD through the expression of Ia antigens and subsequent activation of donor cytotoxic T lymphocytes. The reported association with the administration of methotrexate also raises the possibility of direct drug-related injury to the pulmonary bronchial epithelium. Furthermore, there is a higher incidence of decreased levels of immunoglobulin G among patients with obliterative bronchiolitis than that seen in other marrow recipients. This hypogammaglobulinemia may be a manifestation of the immunologic lesion responsible for the airway disease, or it may merely be related to the presence of chronic GvHD.

Airflow obstruction is occasionally seen within 100 days of transplantation. Histologic results are available for fewer of these cases, and the defect is possibly related to airway infection. This early presentation is often associated with acute GvHD.

CLINICAL PRESENTATION AND COURSE

Typical manifestations of airflow obstruction due to obliterative bronchiolitis after marrow transplantation are

- Insidious progression of tachypnea
- Dyspnea on exertion
- Dry, nonproductive cough

Fever is not common. Physical findings may be minimal. Scattered expiratory wheezing and occasionally diffuse inspiratory crackles may be heard, but results of chest auscultation sometimes are normal. The chest radiograph is commonly interpreted as negative; however, recent studies reveal almost all affected children have typical abnormalities noted on high-resolution chest CT scans.

The diagnosis of airflow obstruction is made among HSCT recipients by routine pulmonary function testing. When the presentation is more than 150 days after transplantation, evidence of chronic GvHD is usually present, although the condition may occur at any time after transplantation.

The syndrome is often progressive and results in death from respiratory failure. A more rapid onset and faster rate of progression are associated with worse outcome. Control of chronic GvHD with increased immunosuppression may achieve stabilization of the airway disease. Patients with gradual declines in airflow tend to have courses that are more benign. Patients who have the onset of airflow obstruction beyond 150 days after transplantation tend to have a more gradual decline in lung function. Airflow may stabilize in 50% of these. Reversal of the obstruction is reported in only 8% of cases.

TREATMENT

There are no prospective studies of the treatment of new-onset airflow obstruction after HSCT. Airflow obstruction in the presence of chronic GvHD is managed primarily by controlling the GvHD with increased immunosuppression (Table 50.10). Airflow obstruction has improved in some patients with increased immunosuppression. Experience with obliterative bronchiolitis among the recipients of heart-lung transplants suggests the addition of azathioprine (1 to 1.5 mg/kg/day) to cyclosporine may be effective in arresting the decline in airflow in these patients. In addition, aerosolized bronchodilator treatment for symptomatic patients is appropriate. Early and aggressive antibiotic treatment for any potential lower respiratory infection should be initiated. Prophylactic trimethoprim-sulfamethoxazole (co-trimoxazole; or another form of prevention of *P. carinii* infection) should be continued for the duration of

Table 50.10
Approach to treatment of airflow limitation after hematopoietic stem cell transplantation

1.	Control associated chronic graft-versus-host disease (cyclosporin-A, FK-506)
2.	Prophylaxis for *Pneumocystis carinii* pneumonia
3.	Treat any intercurrent respiratory infection
4.	Augment low serum immunoglobulin levels
5.	Administer aerosolized adrenergic agonists to symptomatic patients
6.	Prednisone (or its equivalent) 1–1.5 mg/kg/day (up to 100 mg/day) for 4–6 weeks
7.	Repeat pulmonary function testing monthly
8.	If there is no improvement or if there is deterioration after 1 mon of corticosteroid therapy, begin azathioprine (up to 3 mg/kg/day, 200 mg/day maximum)
9.	If there is no response, add mycophenolate mofetil or thalidomide

immune suppression. Routine intravenous replacement of immunoglobulin for those with low class or subclass levels is usual.

Similar immunosuppressive management is recommended for airflow obstruction that develops early in the transplant course in the absence of chronic GvHD. Evaluation for possible airway infection by respiratory viruses or fungus should be undertaken in rapidly developing obstruction, especially in the presence of acute GvHD.

Early recognition and treatment may improve outcome. Therefore, routine spirometry after marrow transplantation among patients with chronic GvHD is encouraged to detect the insidious onset of this process.

Pulmonary Veno-occlusive Disease

Pulmonary VOD is a rare complication of HSCT. Cases of pulmonary VOD are most common in children with acute lymphocytic leukemia and are usually associated with bis-chloroethyl-1 nitrosourea therapy; it is a very rare a complication after cytoreductive conditioning for HSCT with cyclophosphamide and total-body irradiation.

Pulmonary VOD presents with the insidious onset of dyspnea on exertion, hypoxemia, and resting tachypnea within 3 to 4 months after HSCT. Chest radiography has been reported as negative. Clinical examination, electrocardiography, and ultrasound studies are consistent with pulmonary hypertension. Perfusion–ventilation radionuclide scans have been negative, excluding the diagnosis of pulmonary embolism, which may present similarly. Pulmonary function studies have failed to demonstrate airflow obstruction consistent with bronchiolitis. The diagnostic procedure of choice is right heart catheterization with a pulmonary angiogram or possibly a spiral CT angiogram. Right heart catheterization reveals elevated pulmonary artery pressure with normal pulmonary artery wedge pressures. Angiography excludes the presence of thrombi as a cause for the pulmonary hypertension.

Pulmonary VOD has been recognized most often at autopsy after conventional chemotherapy treatment for malignancy. These patients had an insidious course with progressive hypoxemia and dyspnea on exertion due to pulmonary hypertension. Prompt recognition and diagnosis may be important because response to high-dose corticosteroid therapy (methylprednisolone 2 mg/kg/day) has been reported.

Clinical Approach to Respiratory Failure without Pulmonary Infiltrates

The patient who presents with marked tachypnea or hypoxemia after HSCT in the absence of radiographic infiltrates should be evaluated for the presence of obstructive airway disease, pulmonary VOD, and pulmonary vascular disease. Diagnostic evaluation should include complete pulmonary function testing and arterial blood gas analysis. The absence of airflow obstruction rules out bronchiolitis. If restrictive ventilatory defects are noted, a CT scan of the chest should be performed to look for subtle interstitial disease suggestive of idiopathic pneumonia not otherwise noted on routine radiographs. The evaluation would then proceed as for diffuse infiltrates.

Patients with hypoxemia but no obstructive or restrictive lung defects should proceed to echocardiography to look for the right ventricular failure and pulmonary arterial hypertension that is typical of pulmonary VOD. If these signs are present, right heart catheterization should be performed to confirm the diagnosis of pulmonary VOD. In the rare patient with dyspnea despite normal pulmonary function testing and echocardiographic results, a cardiopulmonary exercise test is indicated to detect pulmonary vascular disease or myocardial limitations.

PLEURAL DISEASE

Pleural effusions are common during the first weeks after HSCT, but they are rarely related to an identifiable infectious source. Pleural effusions may be associated with fluid retention of any cause and especially with ascites secondary to hepatic VOD or vascular leak due to GvHD. Bilateral pleural effusions in the presence of weight gain can be approached conservatively without diagnostic thoracentesis. Cautious diuresis often produces satisfactory results.

Bacterial empyema is rare after HSCT, probably because of the frequent administration of broad-spectrum antibiotics during the neutropenic period. However, a large unilateral or rapidly accumulating effusion in the presence of fever or ipsilateral chest pain should be evaluated promptly by thoracentesis. Unusual causes of pleural effusion include chylothorax, candidal empyema, toxoplasmosis, and *Legionella* (non-*pneumophila* species) empyema.

BRONCHOSCOPY

BAL is safe in marrow transplantation recipients and it may be carried out in profoundly thrombocytopenic patients with little risk of bleeding or infection, even when performed by the transnasal route. Although BAL can document the presence of viral and bacterial infection, negative results do not exclude the presence of fungal infection, nor do they confirm the diagnosis of idiopathic pneumonia. The use of additional invasive procedures must be individualized according to the likelihood of undiagnosed, treatable infection. The yield in *P. carinii* infection is unclear; however, we have never confirmed the presence of this organism by any other means after BAL failed to detect an infection. Transbronchial lung biopsy does not appear to improve the diagnostic yield in marrow recipients with diffuse infiltrate; furthermore, it is not specific for an idiopathic process and it may be unsafe in thrombocytopenic patients.

VIDEO-ASSISTED THORACOSCOPIC SURGERY

Most reports note that thoracotomy may be undertaken with acceptable morbidity and mortality, even in severely immunosuppressed patients, as long as the platelet count is adequate (usually >50,000/mm^3). Among the available procedures, open lung biopsy has the highest probability of rendering a specific diagnosis, and it was the mainstay of diagnosis for diffuse pulmonary infiltrates before the advent of rapid and sensitive virologic diagnostic techniques applied to bronchoscopy specimens.

The morbidity of lung biopsy may be diminished in the hands of a surgeon who is skilled in the use of a thoracoscope. Thoracoscopically directed biopsy permits diagnostic tissue to be obtained without a formal thoracotomy incision. In most patients, the postoperative recovery is faster and there is less incision pain. Access to thoracoscopic lung biopsy has increased our willingness to subject marrow transplant recipients to surgery. One limitation of the procedure is the requirement for bilateral bronchial intubation to permit deflation of the involved lung. Patients with little pulmonary reserve or severe bilateral disease may tolerate this procedure poorly.

Thoracoscopic lung biopsy also has a role in the diagnosis and management of focal lung lesions, especially those close to the pleural surface. Surgical resection of a focal fungal lesion may be curative while also being diagnostic. Caution must be exercised, however, in discounting fungal disease because of a negative open lung biopsy. Despite the relatively large tissue specimen that can be sampled, the diagnoses may not be evident in the pathologic examination. Invasive filamentous fungi, by their focal nature and accompanying large degree of tissue infarction and hemorrhage, may not be seen in as many as 20% of cases in which they are present. Therefore, it is difficult to withdraw or withhold empirical antifungal therapy in the neutropenic patient despite "negative" results.

PITFALLS AND CONTROVERSIES

Mortality Predictions

The number of transplantation procedures being performed continues to increase as the indications expand and the sources of donor stem cells enlarge. More patients are at risk of complications and require supportive care.

The precision with which we can predict those patients who are at risk of complications is increasing such that we are better able to predict those who are less likely to survive. This both improves and complicates the decision regarding whether to advise and accept transplantation.

It is important that transplantation units and patients have adequate information to assess the associated risks. Such information is crucial to discussions of advanced care directives and cost containment. Given the difficulty in assessing medical futility in patients with HSCT with respiratory failure, autonomous decisions by the patient should be followed. Advanced care directives should be obtained before transplantation from all recipients, but particularly from those who are at risk of respiratory failure, and the estimated risk of complications should be used in counseling before marrow transplantation.

Predicting Outcome

Studies of intensive care for respiratory failure of patients with cancer, hematologic malignancy, and marrow transplantation have reported low survival rates. In reports from Seattle, the University of Minnesota, and others, approximately 3% of marrow recipients receiving mechanical ventilation survived to 6 months after transplantation. Studies of pediatric marrow transplant recipients find the same poor prognosis as noted among adults. Improvement in survival may be seen with increased use of noninvasive ventilation and earlier intervention, as well as with less intensive radiochemotherapy regimens ("mini-allotransplantation").

Investigators at the Fred Hutchinson Cancer Research Center in the United States have identified specific predictors of nonsurvival in mechanically ventilated marrow transplant recipients. Survival was statistically associated with younger age, lower score in the Acute Physiology and Chronic Health Evaluation III (APACHE III), and a shorter time from transplantation to intubation, but these associations lacked sensitivity for clinical use. There were, however, no survivors among an estimated 398 patients who had severe lung injury (as evidenced by fraction of inspired oxygen >0.6 or positve end-expiratory pressure >5 cm H_2O) who also required more than 4 hours of vasopressor support or who sustained combined hepatic and renal insufficiency (Table 50.11). Using these factors, an accurate prediction of death could be made within 4 days of mechanical ventilation in 90% of nonsurvivors. Over the last 5 years of the review, there was a statistically significant improvement in survival rates (from 5% to 16%; $p = .008$), which was not explained by a change in patient age, the rate or timing of intubation, or the percentage of HLA-nonidentical allogeneic transplants.

These data appear to conflict with those presented by others, who found that, among 191 marrow recipients requiring mechanical ventilation, age over 40 years and respiratory failure within 90 days of transplantation were usually associated with fatality. The bases for the differences in the data are unclear. The data from the Fred Hutchinson Cancer Research Center were largely confined to several months after transplantation, whereas the University of Minnesota experiences included patients several years after transplantation. Regional differences in patient care may also contribute. Regardless, the two reports agree that severe multiple-organ failure with mechanical ventilation after marrow transplantation is fatal.

Pulmonary dysfunction, central nervous system dysfunction, and hepatic dysfunction are all associated with significant decreases in the levels of antithrombin III and protein C and an increase in the platelet transfusion requirement. Patients with these organ dysfunctions have higher levels of interleukin-6, interleukin-10, and TNF-α than patients who never experience these complications. Mortality rates for patients with these organ dysfunctions vary from 15% in patients with only one organ dysfunction to 100% in patients who have progressed to all three. Patients in whom none of these organ dysfunctions develop have a mortality rate that approaches zero.

Table 50.11
Probability of survival after mechanical ventilation following hematopoietic stem cell transplantation

Risk factors for in-hospital mortality for patients receiving mechanical ventilation

Severe lung injury (FIO_2 >0.6 or PEEP >5 cm H_2O [0.5 kPa] after the first 24 hr)
Hypotension requiring vasopressor support for more than 4 hours
Combined hepatic and renal dysfunction (bilirubin >4 mg/dL and creatinine >2 mg/dL)

Risk factor(s) present	Probability of survival
None	27%
Hepatic and renal dysfunction only	16%
Lung injury only	8%
Hypotension only	1.5%
Any two risk factors	0.2%
All three risk factors	0%

Severe lung injury combined with hemodynamic instability or hepatorenal insufficiency is a sensitive and highly specific predictor of nonsurvival in mechanically ventilated HSCT recipients. These overwhelmingly negative results justify restricting prolonged care of mechanically ventilated HSCT recipients. We use such information to counsel patients and families on the expected outcomes of such situations, and will withdraw life support based on these data.

SUGGESTED READINGS

Baron F, Beguin Y: Nonmyeloablative allogeneic hematopoietic stem cell transplantation. J Hematother Stem Cell Res. 11:243-263, 2002.

Bhalla KS, Wilczynski SW, Abushamaa AM, et al: Pulmonary toxicity of induction chemotherapy prior to standard or high-dose chemotherapy with autologous hematopoietic support. Am J Respir Crit Care Med 161:17-25, 2000.

Duncker C, Dohr D, Harsdorf S, et al: Non-infectious lung complications are closely associated with chronic graft-versus-host disease: A single center study of incidence, risk factors and outcome. Bone Marrow Transplant 25:1263-1268, 2000.

Haire WD: Multiple organ dysfunction syndrome in hematopoietic stem cell transplantation. Criti Care Med 30:S257-S262, 2002.

Wilczynski SW, Erasmus JJ, Petros WP, et al: Delayed pulmonary toxicity syndrome following high-dose chemotherapy and bone marrow transplantation for breast cancer. Am J Respir Crit Care Med 157:565-573, 1998.

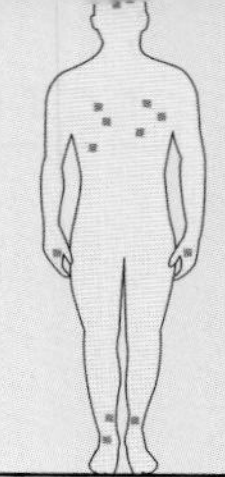

SECTION 12
Pulmonary Manifestations of Systemic Conditions

CHAPTER 51 Hepatic and Biliary Disease

Michael J. Krowka

EPIDEMIOLOGY, RISK FACTORS, AND PATHOPHYSIOLOGY

The pulmonary consequences of liver disorders can be classified according to whether they predominantly affect the pleural space, the lung parenchyma, or the pulmonary circulation (Table 51.1). Unique pulmonary abnormalities occur in the setting of severe alpha$_1$-antitrypsin deficiency, primary biliary cirrhosis (PBC), and primary sclerosing cholangitis (PSC).

Hepatopulmonary syndrome (HPS) and portopulmonary hypertension (PortoPH) are the major pulmonary vascular problems that complicate portal hypertension from any cause. HPS, a pulmonary vascular dilatation problem leading to arterial hypoxemia, occurs in 5% to 15% of patients with portal hypertension. PortoPH, resulting from pulmonary vascular obstruction or obliteration, has been reported in 4% to 8.5% of patients with advanced liver disease. Pleural effusions related to the formation of ascites develops in 5% to 10% of cirrhotic patients.

Pulmonary function abnormalities can be demonstrated in approximately 50% of patients with advanced liver disease. The most common abnormality is a reduced diffusing capacity. Abnormal oxygenation (measured by an increased alveolar-arterial oxygen gradient or reduced PaO_2) is frequent (20% to 40%). Specific reasons for such abnormalities are usually multifactorial, resulting from problems listed in Table 51.1 as well as the effects of smoking and abdominal ascites.

Risk Factors

Portal hypertension appears to be a prerequisite for the development of either HPS or PortoPH. Previous portosystemic surgical shunts have been reported in up to 30% of patients with PortoPH. Conditions leading to abdominal ascites usually precede the development of pleural effusions ("hepatic hydrothorax"). Smoking in the setting of ZZ or SZ antitrypsin deficiency phenotypes leads to the greatest risk of emphysema. The Child-Pugh classification for the severity of liver diseases correlates poorly with most pulmonary consequences, with the exception of hepatic hydrothorax. The epidemic of hepatitis C disease does not appear to be related to any unique pulmonary abnormality.

Pathophysiology

Intuitively, circulating mediators associated with the appropriate genetic predisposition would appear to be the cause of HPS or PortoPH. Such mediators (causing vasodilatation or vasoconstriction, respectively) should arise because of the abnormal metabolism of the dysfunctional liver. In humans, such specific circulating mediators have yet to be identified. HPS is characterized by arterial hypoxemia caused by precapillary-capillary dilatations or direct arteriovenous communications. Excess perfusion for a given area of ventilation, diffusion limitation, and true anatomic shunting contribute to the degree of abnormal arterial oxygenation (Fig. 51.1). Increased amounts of exhaled nitric oxide have been demonstrated in HPS.

PortoPH results from vasoproliferation (endothelium and smooth muscle), along with in situ thrombosis, which results in increased pulmonary vascular resistance (PVR). It is important to note the various pulmonary hemodynamic patterns that may exist in the setting of advanced liver disease (Table 51.2). Lung biopsies have confirmed the pulmonary vascular consequences of portal hypertension (Fig. 51.2).

Hepatic hydrothorax is a transudative pleural effusion caused by the formation of ascitic fluid. A combination of negative pleural pressure and positive abdominal pressures force ascitic fluid into the pleural spaces via diaphragmatic defects and lymphatics. Rarely, the fluid may be chylous.

PBC has systemic manifestations presumably because of autoimmune phenomena. Pulmonary granulomas, lymphocytic infiltrates, and bronchiolitis obliterans organizing pneumonia (BOOP) can result. Rarely, PSC may be associated with airway inflammation and hilar and mediastinal adenopathy for reasons that are unclear.

CLINICAL FEATURES

Exertional dyspnea is the most common, nonspecific presentation of any pulmonary consequence of liver dysfunction.

Hepatopulmonary Syndrome

Clubbing, cyanosis of the digits, and spider angiomas suggest the arterial hypoxemia of HPS. The chest examination is usually unremarkable. Worsening dyspnea (platypnea) and oxygenation (orthodeoxia) as one moves from the supine to the standing position is frequently noted in HPS.

Portopulmonary Hypertension

Chest pressure, syncope, and palpitations suggest later manifestations of PortoPH. An accentuated second heart sound (increased P2) is frequent when PortoPH is advanced.

Primary Biliary Cirrhosis/Primary Sclerosing Cholangitis

Inspiratory crackles may be associated with the interstitial lung problems that complicate PBC or chronic aspiration in patients

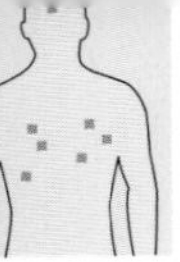

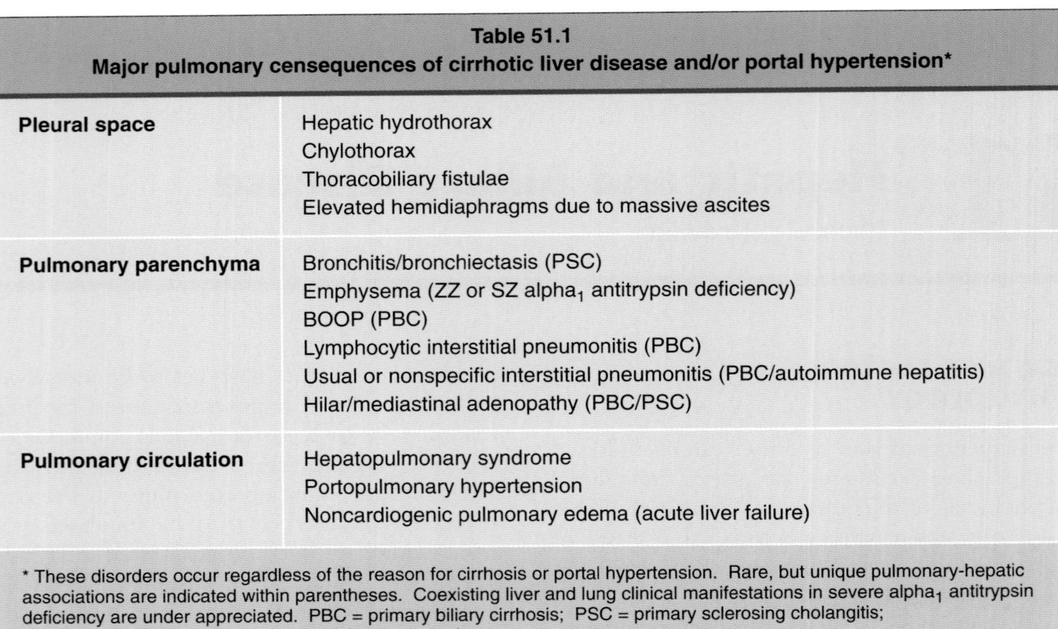

Table 51.1
Major pulmonary censequences of cirrhotic liver disease and/or portal hypertension*

Pleural space	Hepatic hydrothorax Chylothorax Thoracobiliary fistulae Elevated hemidiaphragms due to massive ascites
Pulmonary parenchyma	Bronchitis/bronchiectasis (PSC) Emphysema (ZZ or SZ alpha$_1$ antitrypsin deficiency) BOOP (PBC) Lymphocytic interstitial pneumonitis (PBC) Usual or nonspecific interstitial pneumonitis (PBC/autoimmune hepatitis) Hilar/mediastinal adenopathy (PBC/PSC)
Pulmonary circulation	Hepatopulmonary syndrome Portopulmonary hypertension Noncardiogenic pulmonary edema (acute liver failure)

* These disorders occur regardless of the reason for cirrhosis or portal hypertension. Rare, but unique pulmonary-hepatic associations are indicated within parentheses. Coexisting liver and lung clinical manifestations in severe alpha$_1$ antitrypsin deficiency are under appreciated. PBC = primary biliary cirrhosis; PSC = primary sclerosing cholangitis; BOOP = bronchiolitis obliterans organizing pneumonia

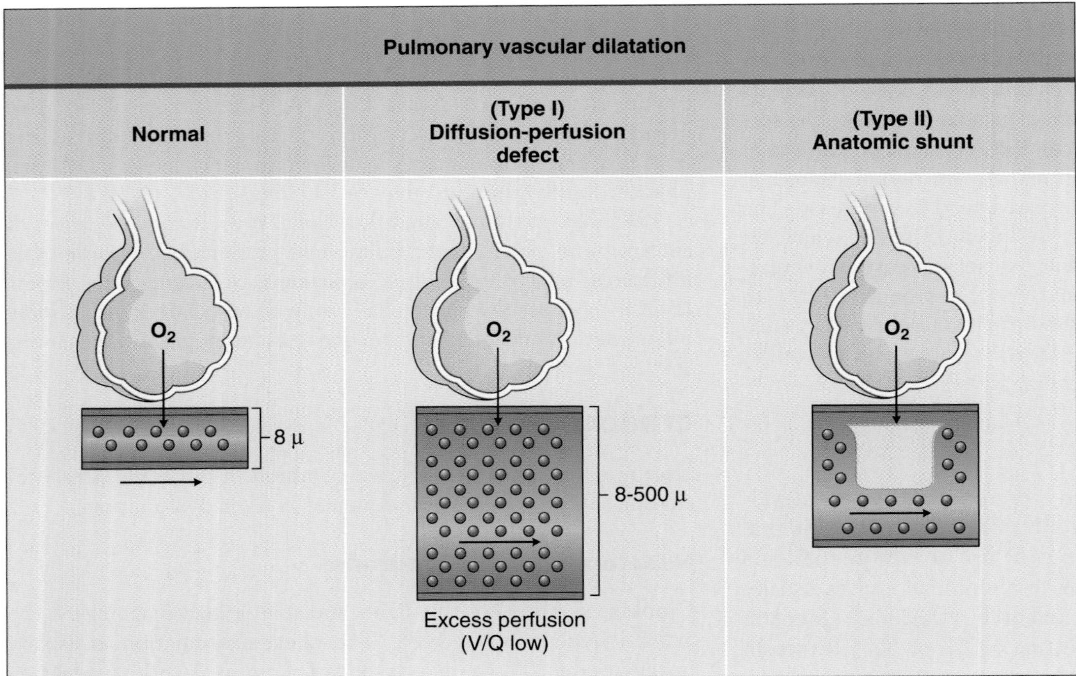

Figure 51.1 Schematic showing the two types of pulmonary vascular dilatation that result in the arterial hypoxemia of hepatopulmonary syndrome (HPS).

with hepatic encephalopathy. Productive sputum may be related to the airway abnormalities (bronchiectasis) associated with antitrypsin deficiency or PSC (bronchitis).

Hepatic Hydrothorax

Pleural effusion caused by liver dysfunction will be associated with diminished breath sounds depending on the location and extent of the pleural effusion. Egophony suggests atelectatic lung caused by compressive pleural effusions; affected patients may have significant hypoxemia. Pleuritic or chest wall pain is not a symptom of hepatic hydrothorax and suggests another diagnosis.

Antitrypsin Deficiency

Signs and symptoms are similar to advanced chronic obstructive lung disease. Chest radiography and computed tomographic imaging, however, suggest predominantly lower lung field distribution of emphysematous or bullous abnormality. Such

Table 51.2
Pulmonary hemodynamics and chronic liver disease

	MPAP	CO	PVR	PCWP
High flow, hyperdynamic circulatory state*	↑	↑↑↑	↓	↓
Excess central volume	↑	↑	↑	↑
PortoPH (arterial vasculopathy; vaso-proliferation and obstruction to flow)**	↑↑↑	↑↔↓	↑↑↑	↓

MPAP = mean pulmonary artery pressure (mm Hg)
CO = cardiac output (L/min)
PVR = pulmonary vascular resistance (dynes/sec/cm^{-5})
PCWP = pulmonary capillary wedge pressure (mm Hg)

* This is the usual hemodynamic pattern documented in HPS
** Initially CO increases, but as MPAP amd PVR markedly increase, the right heart fails and CO decreases

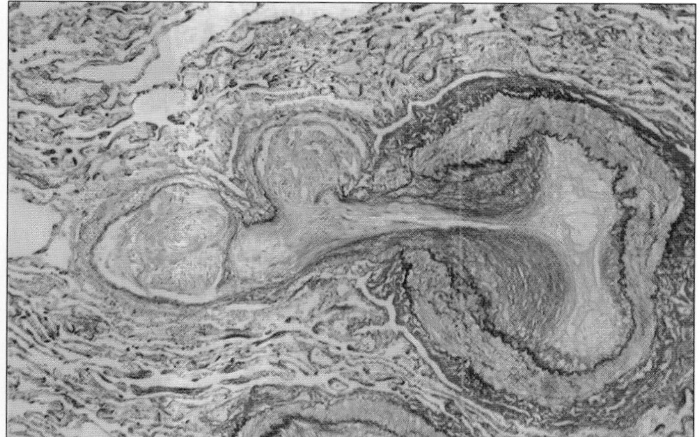

Figure 51.2 Plexogenic arteriopathy documented in the setting of primary biliary cirrhosis (PBC) complicated by severe portopulmonary hypertension. Specimen was obtained from the lung explant. Combined heart-lung-liver transplant was accomplished. (Reprinted with permission from Krowka MJ, Plevak DJ, Findlay J, et al: Pulmonary hemodynamics and perioperative cardiopulmonary mortality in patients with portopulmonary hypertension undergoing liver transplantation. Liver Transpl 6:443–450, 2000.)

changes are seen only in the severely deficient ZZ or SZ phenotypes. Approximately 50% of cirrhotic patients with ZZ or SZ phenotypes have abnormal pulmonary function tests, such as increased residual volume, and/or reduced forced expiratory volume in 1 second.

DIAGNOSIS

Hepatopulmonary Syndrome

This diagnosis is established by demonstrating pulmonary vascular dilatation as the cause for hypoxemia. Hypoxemia is usually defined as PaO_2 less than 70 mm Hg or alveolar-arterial oxygen gradient greater than 15 to 20 mm Hg. Two noninvasive methods are available to document abnormal pulmonary vascular dilatation. Qualitatively, a positive contrast enhanced transthoracic echocardiogram reflects the passage of microbubbles (usually absorbed during a first pass through normal lungs) through dilated pulmonary vessels, with subsequent detection in the left atrium. Quantitatively, an abnormal brain uptake of technetium (^{99m}Tc)–macroaggregated albumin (^{99m}Tc MAA) (uptake >6%) following lung perfusion reflects the passage of radiolabeled albumin aggregates through the lungs and subsequent uptake in the brain (Fig. 51.3). Contrast echocardiography is more sensitive than ^{99m}Tc lung scanning to detect pulmonary vascular dilatation. A lung biopsy is not necessary. A practical clinical algorithm for the evaluation of suspected HPS is shown in Figure 51.4.

Portopulmonary Hypertension

Screening for pulmonary hypertension is accomplished by Doppler echocardiography. Increased right ventricular systolic pressures greater than 50 mm Hg suggest clinically significant PortoPH. A right heart catheterization must be accomplished to establish the diagnosis. Most centers adhere to the triad of mean pulmonary artery pressure (MPAP) greater than 25 mm Hg, pulmonary capillary wedge pressure (PCWP) less than 15 mm Hg, and PVR greater than 120 dynes/sec/cm^{-5} as definitive criteria for PortoPH. A lung biopsy is not advised. Chronic pulmonary emboli should be excluded.

Hepatic Hydrothorax

This is a clinical diagnosis based on the chest radiograph showing a pleural effusion that can be right sided (70%), left sided (15%), or bilateral (15%). Thoracentesis is usually performed only when atypical symptoms (e.g., pain) exist or there are suspicions of another process such as empyema. Hepatic hydrothorax may occur in the absence of clinical ascites.

Antitrypsin Deficiency

Pulmonary dysfunction in the setting of severe alpha$_1$-antitrypsin deficiency should be established by standard pulmonary testing (assess degree of expiratory airflow limitation and hyperinflation) and high-resolution computed tomography of the chest (assess for subclinical emphysema, bullae, and bronchiectasis). Serum phenotypes and levels should be obtained.

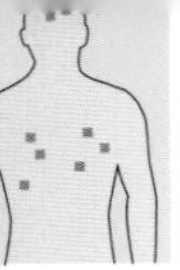

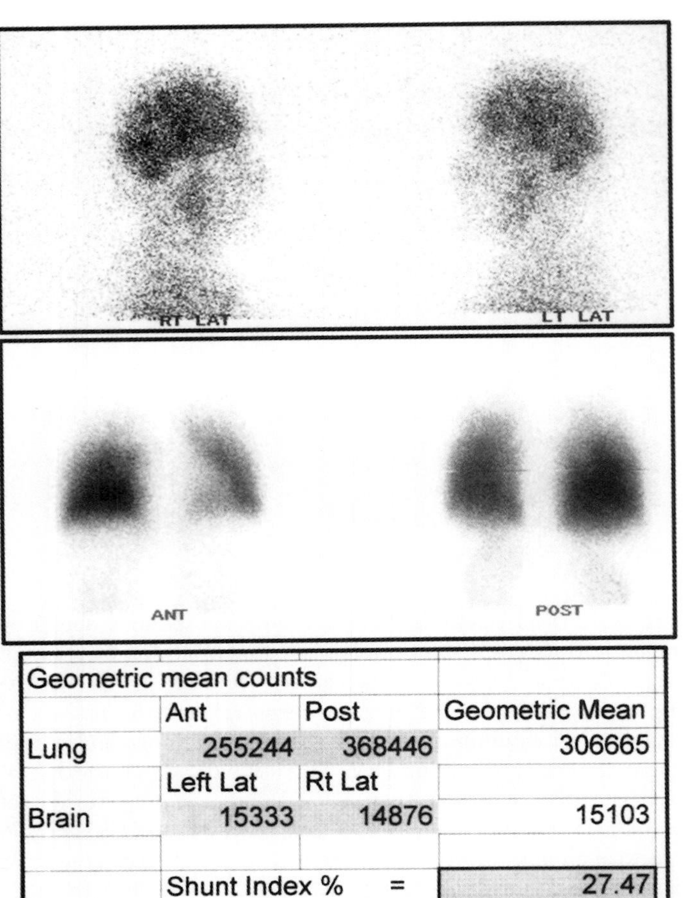

Geometric mean counts			
	Ant	Post	Geometric Mean
Lung	255244	368446	306665
	Left Lat	Rt Lat	
Brain	15333	14876	15103
	Shunt Index % =		27.47
	Normal shunt index < 5%		

Figure 51.3 Lung perfusion scan with quantified technetium 99 macroaggregated albumin (MAA) abnormal uptake over the brain in a patient with hepatopulmonary syndrome (HPS). (From Krowka MJ, Wiseman GA, Burnett OL, et al: Hepatopulmonary syndrome: a prospective study of relationships between severity of liver disease, PaO_2 response to 100% oxygen, and brain uptake after ^{99m}Tc MAA lung scanning. Chest 118:615-624, 2000.)

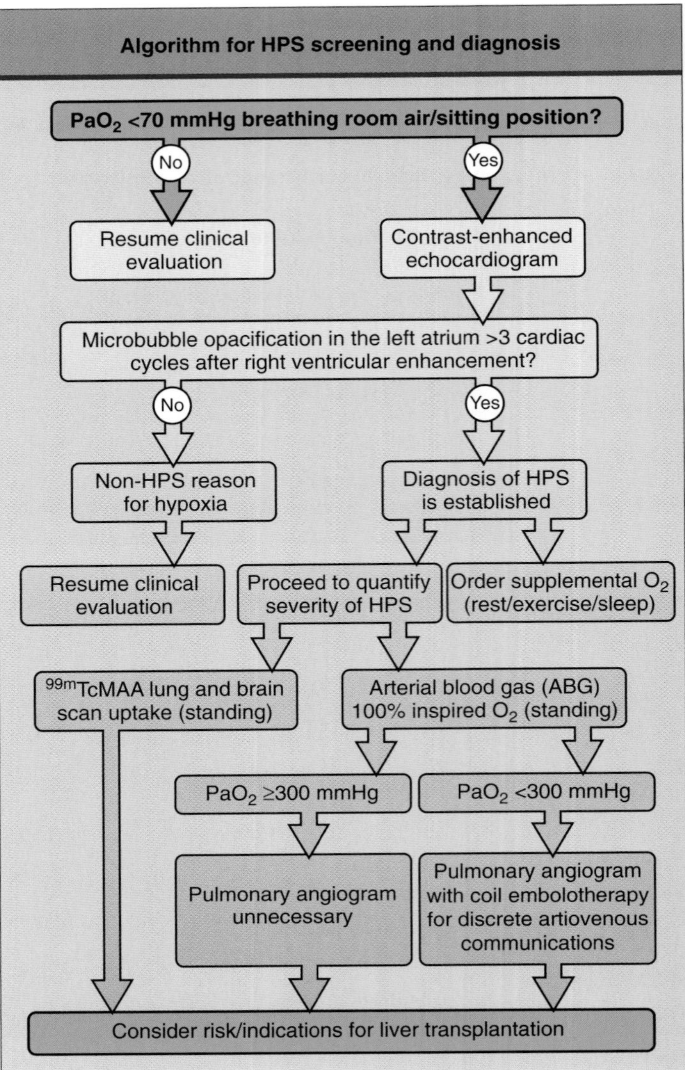

Figure 51.4 Current screening and diagnostic algorithm followed at the Mayo Clinic for patients with suspected hepatopulmonary syndrome (HPS).

TREATMENT

Hepatopulmonary Syndrome

No pharmacologic treatments have proved efficacious in improving arterial hypoxemia due to HPS. Liver transplantation (cadaveric or living donor) is the treatment of choice. Rarely, coil embolization of discrete arteriovenous communications that occur in HPS can result in improvement in oxygenation.

Portopulmonary Hypertension

Significant improvement in pulmonary hemodynamics has been reported with the long-term use of continuous 24-hour intravenous infusion of the prostacyclin epoprostenol (Flolan). However, unless liver transplantation can be accomplished, there has been no proved survival benefit to date with long-term epoprostenol use in PortoPH (Fig. 51.5). Liver transplantation is a high-risk procedure in the setting of PortoPH.

Hepatic Hydrothorax

Repeated thoracentesis is not advised. Chest tube drainage with pleurodesis and video-assisted thoracoscopy rarely provide long-term improvement, by obliterating the pleural space and repairing diaphragmatic defects, respectively. Transjugular intrahepatic portosystemic shunting (TIPS) is appropriate treatment for refractory hepatic hydrothorax, as is liver transplantation.

Severe Antitrypsin Deficiency and Abnormal Pulmonary Function

In the setting of clinically significant liver disease and severe serum $alpha_1$-protein deficiency (less than 80 mg/dL), therapy to replace the $alpha_1$-protein is appropriate and safe. The goal is to minimize lung function deterioration. Liver transplantation results in the phenotype of the donor liver and usually normalizes the serum $alpha_1$ level. Lung transplantation in the setting of serious liver dysfunction due to ZZ or SZ phenotype may be problematic and must be considered on a case-by-case basis.

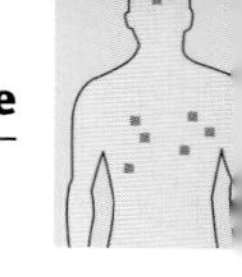

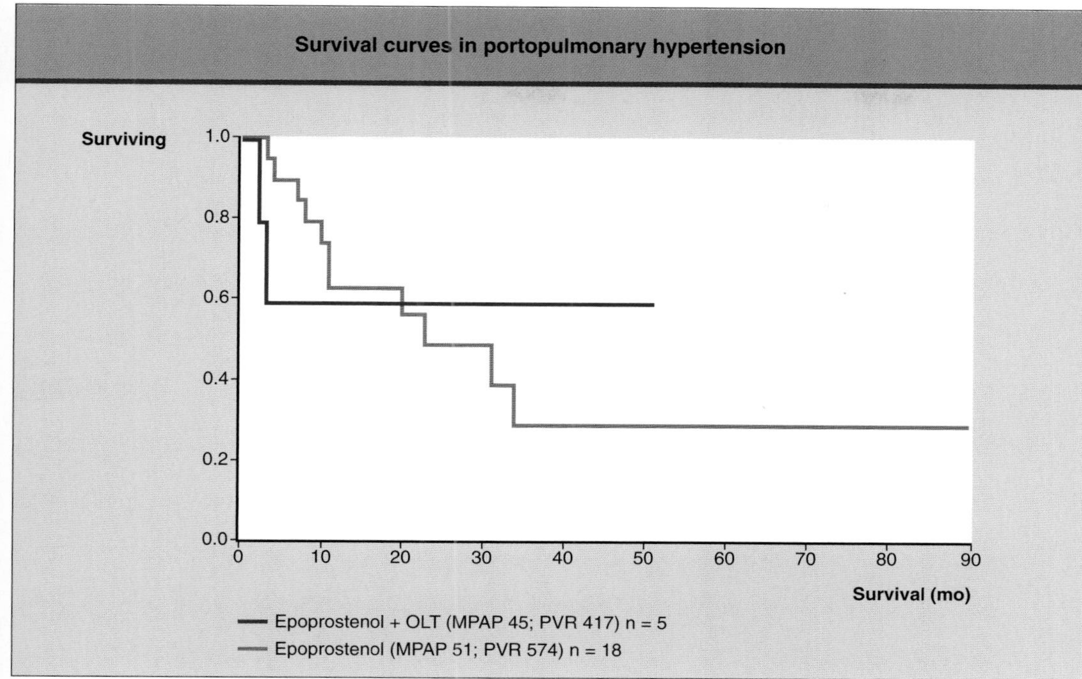

Figure 51.5 Survival curves in portopulmonary hypertension (PortoPH); nonrandomized results of standard treatment versus continuous intravenous epoprostenol with and without orthotopic liver transplantation (OLT). (Swanson KL, Wiesner RH, McGoon MD, Krowka MJ: Survival in portopulmonary hypertension with the use of intravenous epoprostenol. Am J Respir Crit Care Med 167:A693, 2003.)

CLINICAL COURSE

Hepatopulmonary Syndrome

Few data exist to accurately characterize the clinical course in HPS. Retrospective data from before the liver transplant era suggest that the 2.5-year survival rate was 41%. Current data suggest long-term survival if liver transplantation can be successfully accomplished. Deterioration in PaO_2 while the patient is awaiting liver transplantation is approximately 5 mm Hg per year. Mortality is rarely a direct consequence of hypoxemia.

Portopulmonary Hypertension

The 5-year survival ranges from 30% to 50%. Mortality is frequently due to progressive right-sided heart failure, as well as the complications directly related to liver disease.

Antitrypsin Deficiency

In those with the ZZ phenotype, long-term survival is significantly reduced in smokers. There are no data that describe the long-term outcomes in patients with ZZ phenotype, cirrhosis, and pulmonary function abnormalities.

CAVEATS AND CONTROVERSIES

Transjugular intrahepatic portosystemic shunting may or may not have a therapeutic role in the treatment of HPS. TIPS may acutely worsen pulmonary hemodynamics because of increased preload and therefore may be contraindicated in the setting of PortoPH.

The optimal treatment of PortoPH is unclear. Guidelines regarding which patients can safely undergo liver transplantation are empiric and evolving. The highest risk for perioperative mortality appears to be associated with MPAP greater than 35 mm Hg and PVR greater than 250 dyne/sec/cm^{-5}.

SUGGESTED READINGS

Budhiraja R, Hassoun PM: Portopulmonary hypertension: a tale of two circulations. Chest 123:562-576, 2003.

Fallon MB, Abrams GA: Pulmonary dysfunction in chronic liver disease. Hepatology 32:859-865, 2000.

Krowka MJ: Pulmonary manifestations of liver disease. In Schiff ER, Sorrell MF, Maddrey WC (eds): Schiff's Diseases of the Liver, 9th ed. Philadelphia, Lippincott Williams & Wilkins, 2003, pp 543-558.

Krowka MJ, Plevak DJ, Findlay J, et al: Pulmonary hemodynamics and perioperative cardiopulmonary mortality in patients with portopulmonary hypertension undergoing liver transplantation. Liver Transpl 6:443-450, 2000.

Lazidaris KN, Frank JM, Krowka MJ, Kamath PS: Hepatic hydrothorax: pathogenesis and management. Am J Med 107:262-267, 1999.

Mahadeva R, Lomas DA: $Alpha_1$ antitrypsin deficiency, cirrhosis and emphysema. Thorax 53:501-505, 1998.

Swanson KL, Wiesner RH, McGoon MD, Krowka MJ: Survival in portopulmonary hypertension with the use of intravenous epoprostenol. Am J Respir Crit Care Med 167:A693, 2003.

Taille C, Cadranel J, Bellocq A, et al: Liver transplantation for hepatopulmonary syndrome: a ten-year experience in Paris, France. Transplantation 75:1482-1489, 2003.

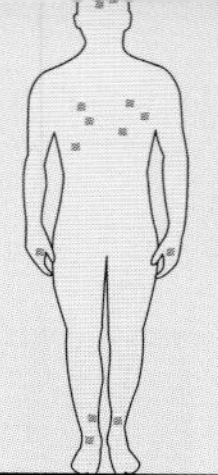

CHAPTER 52 Inflammatory Bowel Disease

Philippe Camus and Thomas Colby

Several intrathoracic complications can develop in patients with inflammatory bowel diseases (IBDs), including both ulcerative colitis (UC) and Crohn's disease (CD). This supports the view that IBDs are systemic diseases.

The most distinctive form of respiratory involvement in IBD is chronic airway inflammation, often with suppuration, a pattern typically seen in patients with UC, as opposed to patients with CD, who more often develop infiltrative lung disease (ILD) corresponding to several distinct histopathologic patterns. Less common thoracic manifestations in IBD include pleurisy or pericarditis and, rarely, sterile, neutrophil-rich masses that may cavitate and correspond to visceral (pulmonary) pyoderma gangrenosum. The latter pattern has been reported only in patients with UC. Severe pulmonary embolism or hypoproteinemia-related pulmonary edema develops in a minority of patients.

Medications used to treat IBD, such as sulfasalazine, mesalazine, methotrexate, and anti–tumor necrosis factor-α (TNF-α) antibodies, can also affect the lung in the form of diffuse ILD (not in the form of large airway disease), with histologic patterns corresponding to nonspecific interstitial, eosinophilic, or organizing pneumonia. In addition, methotrexate and anti–TNF-α drugs predispose patients to the development of opportunistic pulmonary infections, which need to be carefully excluded. Iatrogenic (especially drug-induced) lung or, rarely, pleural involvement is often difficult to distinguish clinically, pathologically, and on imaging from the respiratory involvement associated with IBD, and drug withdrawal or rechallenge of patients with the drug may be needed to solve this issue.

EPIDEMIOLOGY

Thoracic manifestations affect approximately 0.1% to 0.2% of patients with IBD. Therefore, there are few large series of patients with the association. The thoracic manifestations of IBD may develop on a background of quiescent or active IBD, or even after colectomy. Consequently, the causal association may be difficult to recognize, and patients may be diagnosed late after prolonged periods of disabling respiratory symptoms that may have been controllable earlier by appropriate treatment with corticosteroids. Had the association been recognized at the initial time of presentation with thoracic symptoms and treated earlier, the outcome might have been better. Temporally, the respiratory involvement in IBD can develop at any time during the course of the bowel disease: before the clinical onset, at the time of diagnosis, concomitant with a flare-up or relapse of the disease, in patients with quiescent disease, or days to many years after colectomy. Statistically, however, thoracic involvement follows the clinical onset of the IBD (by months to years) in approximately 80% of patients. Among the whole group of patients, airway disease preferentially develops in those who have had colectomy, whereas ILD more often develops in the others.

CLINICAL MANIFESTATIONS

The inflammatory respiratory involvement in IBD can involve the bronchial tree, lung parenchyma, or serosal surfaces, with variable combinations of dyspnea, fever, cough, expectoration, or chest pain.

Involvement of the bronchial tree is the most common pattern of involvement, and develops preferentially in patients with UC compared with CD. The inflammatory process can localize in the glottic/subglottic area, where it produces stenosis with the corresponding symptoms of cough, stridor, and sometimes asphyxia. Involvement of the large airways manifests with otherwise unexplained chronic cough productive of variable, sometimes large amounts of mucopurulent sputum. This corresponds to bronchial inflammation and suppuration, and evolves into basilar bronchiectasis in some patients. Involvement of the small airways (bronchiolitis) is unusual, and manifests as chronic airflow obstruction with or without chronic sputum production.

ILD manifests with roughly symmetrical parenchymal involvement, with mild or moderate symptoms of dyspnea and fever. Acute respiratory failure is encountered in some patients. Cryptogenic organizing pneumonia or bronchiolitis obliterans organizing pneumonia (BOOP) usually manifests with bilateral subpleural opacities or masses containing air bronchograms; less often, it is diffuse. In addition to organizing pneumonia/BOOP, other histopathologic patterns of ILD include granulomatous interstitial pneumonia, nonspecific interstitial pneumonia, eosinophilic pneumonia, and acute bronchiolitis. Patients may present with a lymphocytic or, less often, eosinophilic bronchoalveolar lavage (BAL) pattern. Clinical, BAL, or imaging data usually do not permit one to forecast the histologic pattern of ILD, except in patients with dense, patchy infiltrates, which suggest organizing pneumonia/BOOP, or if the BAL contains high numbers of eosinophils, which suggests the diagnosis of eosinophilic pneumonia.

Necrobiotic nodules is a characteristic but unusual UC-associated pattern of lung involvement. Patients with necrobiotic nodules usually present with fever and multiple parenchymal lung nodules, which tend to cavitate rapidly. Associated dermatologic lesions with the same histopathologic appearance of neutrophilic infiltration are present in some patients.

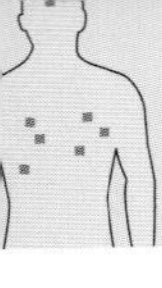

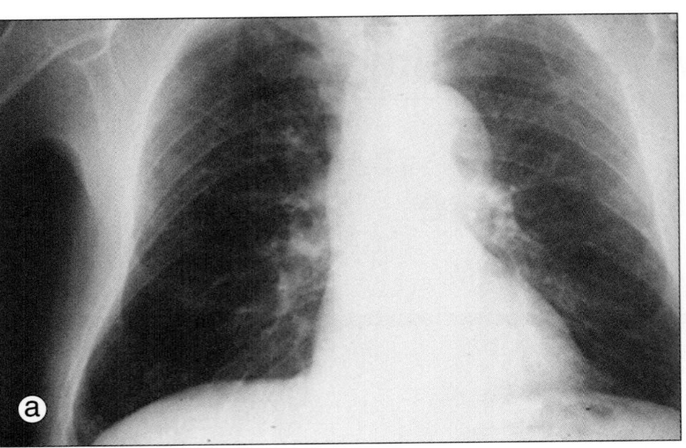

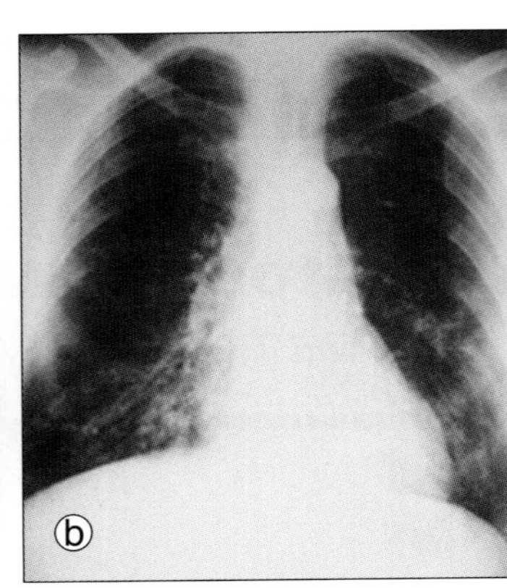

Figure 52.1 Chest radiographs in patients with large airway involvement associated with chronic ulcerative colitis. Slight basilar volume loss, increased density, small, irregular opacities, and tram lines reflecting increased bronchial thickness are seen in the bases bilaterally **(A)**. With time, especially if untreated, patients with bronchial suppuration tend to develop basilar bronchiectatic changes, which are irreversible and less amenable to treatment with corticosteroids **(B)**. Early recognition and treatment are recommended. Treatment often brings definite improvement.

Patients with serositis usually present with chest pain and sometimes fever. The presence of arrhythmia, heart block, or left ventricular failure suggests myocarditis. Rarely, pleural thickening has been found.

Rarely, pneumomediastinum has been observed in patients with active IBD.

ESTABLISHING THE DIAGNOSIS OF INFLAMMATORY BOWEL DISEASE–RELATED THORACIC INVOLVEMENT

Bronchoscopy

Bronchoscopy is the key step to the diagnosis of upper and large airway involvement. The degree of inflammation seen at endoscopy ranges from simple redness of the bronchial walls to exuberant pseudotumoral and hemorrhagic granulation tissue that restricts the airway lumen. The tracheal or bronchial narrowing may impair the progression of the fiberoptic bronchoscope through and beyond the inflammatory area. The bronchoscopic appearance is normal in patients with involvement restricted to the small airways, or in those with ILD. BAL typically yields large numbers of neutrophils in patients with airway involvement, and lymphocytosis, eosinophilia, or a mixed pattern in those with ILD.

Imaging

Radiographs and computed tomography (CT) in patients with upper airway obstruction may show airway stenosis. The chest radiographic appearance in patients with large airway involvement ranges from near normal to a pattern of increased bronchial markings (Fig. 52.1) or, in advanced or rapidly progressive disease, bibasilar bronchiectasis (Fig. 52.2). Mucoid impaction is a relatively common finding on CT distal to bronchiectasis; rarely, it occurs as an isolated finding. In a few patients, simple bronchial distention has been visualized on CT.

Pulmonary Function Testing

Patients with airway involvement usually demonstrate an obstructive or mixed obstructive/restrictive functional pattern that is little influenced by bronchodilators but often improves if corticosteroids are given. The changes in pulmonary function roughly correlate with the extent and severity of involvement seen at endoscopy or imaging. Although minor changes in pulmonary function can be found in patients free from respiratory involvement, these changes do not predict the development of overt respiratory disease.

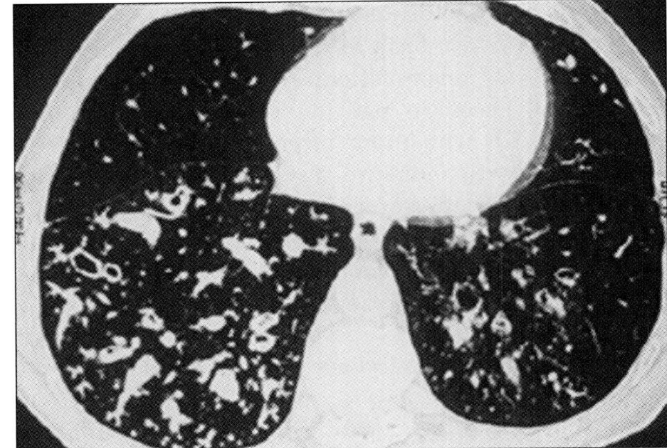

Figure 52.2 Computed tomography scan corresponding to bronchiectasis in chronic ulcerative colitis. More-or-less symmetrical bronchiectatic changes develop bilaterally with time. Mucoid/mucopurulent impaction is a common finding distal to bronchiectasis, and is clearly visible here in the right lower lobe, peripherally.

Histopathology

Histopathologic evaluation of airway or lung tissue may be required to confirm the diagnosis of IBD-related respiratory involvement, to rule out other causes, and to guide or follow treatment. In patients with airway involvement, bronchial biopsies demonstrate luminal exudate with neutrophils, mucosal epithelial metaplasia, and a submucosal inflammatory infiltrate composed of mononuclear cells. The inflammation is responsible for airway narrowing, and is often amenable to treatment with corticosteroids. Involvement of the small airways can be seen in association with involvement of larger airways, or is the sole site of involvement in the form of an active suppurative or fibrosing bronchiolitis. In some cases, the appearance is indistinguishable from diffuse panbronchiolitis, with prominent interstitial foamy histiocytes around the respiratory bronchioles. Late changes include constrictive bronchiolitis obliterans, which correlates with severe airflow obstruction.

Lung biopsy may be required in patients with diffuse lung disease in whom the diagnosis was not established by noninva-

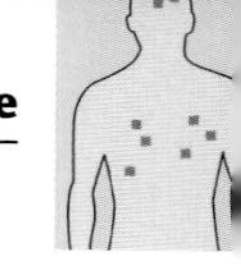

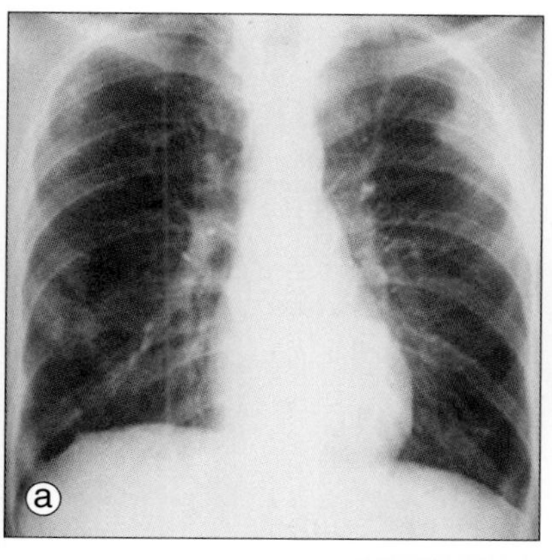

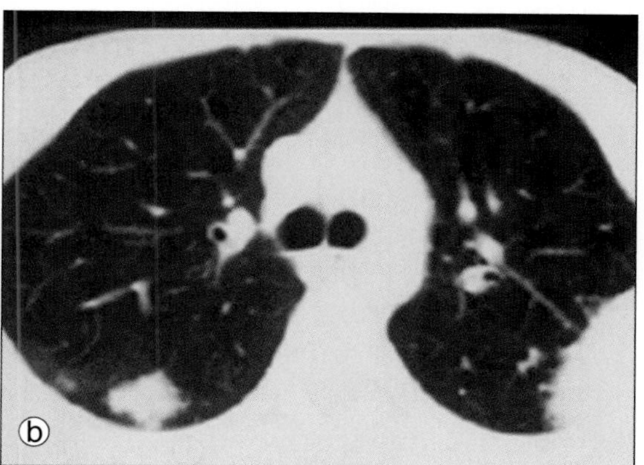

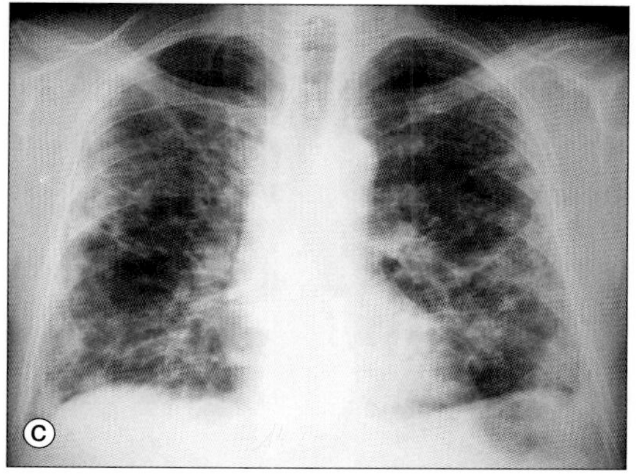

Figure 52.3 Organizing pneumonia (bronchiolitis obliterans organizing pneumonia) associated with inflammatory bowel diseases. In a typical chest radiograph, the extent of involvement ranges from dense peripheral subpleural infiltrates **(A, B)**, to a pattern of diffuse infiltrative lung disease **(C)**. Diffuse infiltrative lung disease corresponds to several other patterns of involvement (see Table 52.1).

sive methods. The patterns of ILD include nonspecific interstitial pneumonia (cellular), cryptogenic organizing pneumonia (BOOP) (Fig. 52.3), granulomatous interstitial pneumonia, eosinophilic pneumonia, and desquamative interstitial pneumonia. Although some of these patterns may simulate sarcoidosis or hypersensitivity pneumonitis, subtle histopathologic differences usually allow segregation of these entities. The pattern of diffuse lung disease on imaging may also result from lesions in the distal airways, such as chronic bronchiolitis (with or without non-necrotizing granulomatous inflammation) or acute bronchiolitis associated with a neutrophil-rich sterile bronchopneumonia.

Necrobiotic nodules (Fig. 52.4) are sterile and resemble abscesses with central fibrinous exudate with neutrophils, necrosis of lung tissue (which explains the cavitation seen radiologically), and a rim of histiocytes and chronic inflammation without giant cells or non-necrotizing granulomas, as seen in granulomatous infections and Wegener's granulomatosis. The lesion resembles pyoderma gangrenosum in the skin. The main differential diagnosis is pyogenic abscesses, and special stains and cultures are required to rule out an infection. Anti-neutrophil cytoplasmic antibodies with a perinuclear, not a cytoplasmic staining pattern are found in a fraction of patients with IBD.

The possibility that disease-modifying drugs play a role in patients with ILD should always be considered. Drugs are extremely unlikely to play a causative role in patients with involvement of the airways or necrobiotic nodules because these are not recognized patterns of involvement due to drugs. Moreover, severe airway involvement can develop in patients with IBD with a history of colectomy who are no longer receiving drugs. The issue is more complex in patients with IBD treated with drugs in whom diffuse ILD develops; in these patients, a drug reaction and opportunistic infections (including tuberculosis) should be considered, especially in those on chronic treatment with corticosteroids, immunosuppressive drugs, or anti–TNF-α agents. Accordingly, special stains and cultures of BAL fluid or lung tissue should be routinely performed, and an infection should be searched for aggressively. In some patients, the issue remains unclear even though lung tissue is available for review. Drug withdrawal or prudent rechallenge with the drug may be helpful to establish or rule out the drug etiology. Should drug withdrawal be considered, care must be taken to avoid a relapse of the IBD.

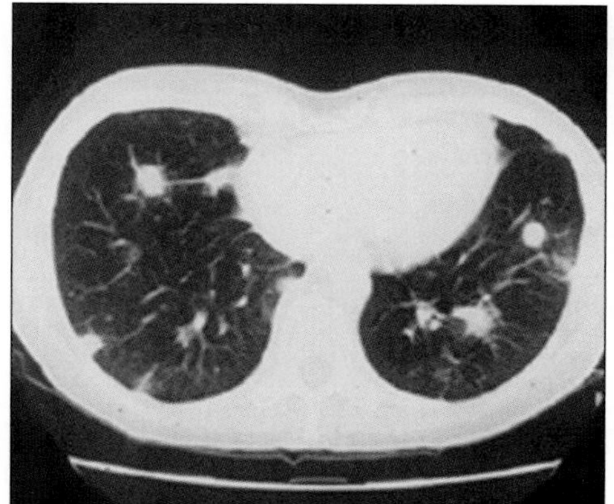

Figure 52.4 Necrotic lung nodules in a patient with ulcerative colitis and pyoderma of the skin. The nodules correspond to neutrophilic aggregates and tend to cavitate within a few days.

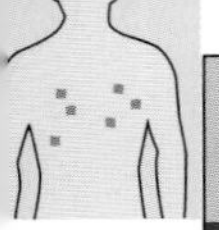

Table 52.1
Thoracic involvement in inflammatory bowel disease

Site of Predominant Involvement	Pattern	UC	CD	Presenting Symptoms	Imaging	Bronchoscopy	BAL	Recommended Treatment	Outcome
Large airways									
Larynx/glottis	Glottic/subglottic stenosis	++	+	Cough, dyspnea, hoarseness, stridor, asphyxia	Narrowing	Glottic/subglottic edema and inflammation (granulomatous in CD)	ND	IV steroids with or without laser ablation	Favorable
Trachea	Tracheal inflammation/stenosis	++	+	Cough, dyspnea, hemoptysis, chronic expectoration	Narrowing	Tracheal stenosis/inflammation	ND	IV/oral steroids (laser ablation?)	Favorable
Major bronchi	Simple chronic bronchitis	++	±	Slightly productive cough, wheeze	Normal	Mild/moderate inflammation of large airways	PMN	Inhaled steroids	Favorable
	Bronchial distention*†	+	–	Cough, asymptomatic	Distention on CT	ND	ND	Inhaled steroids?	Favorable
	Mucoid impaction†	++	–	Asymptomatic	Branched shadow on CT	ND	ND	Inhaled steroids, follow-up	Favorable
	Spotted bronchial granulomas	–	+	Cough, hoarseness	Normal	Spotted granulomas	ND	Oral steroids with or without inhaled steroids	Favorable
	Chronic bronchial suppuration	++	±	Cough, wheeze, copious sputum	Thickened bronchial walls	Large airways inflammation, often severe	PMN	Inhaled/oral/nebulized steroids	Variable; residual impairment common
	Bronchiectasis	++	+	Cough, wheeze, abundant sputum	Thickened /dilated bronchi	Extensive airway inflammation/narrowing	PMN	Inhaled/nebulized/oral steroids serial bronchial lavages with steroids. Rarely surgery	Variable; residual impairment or progression common
Small airways‡	Granulomatous bronchiolitis†	–	+	Nonproductive cough	Mosaic at CT, ILD	Normal	Ly	Oral steroids	Favorable
	Acute purulent bronchiolitis*	+	+	Dyspnea		ND	ND	ND	Favorable
	Diffuse panbronchiolitis pattern‡	+	–	Dyspnea with or without sputum	Tree-in-bud or mosaic on CT	Normal/mild inflammation	ND	Inhaled/oral steroids	Usually severe
	Bronchiolitis obliterans	+	–	Dyspnea, chronic airflow obstruction	ND	Normal	ND	Inhaled/oral steroids	Usually severe
Lung parenchyma	Bronchiolitis obliterans and organizing pneumonia	++	+	Dyspnea/fever/ acute respiratory failure	Bilateral infiltrates or diffuse	Normal	Variable	Oral/IV steroids	Favorable (possibly caused by drugs)
	Nonspecific interstitial pneumonia, cellular	+	+	Dyspnea	Basilar opacities	Normal	Ly	Oral/IV steroids	Favorable (possibly caused by drugs)
	ILD, granulomatous	±	++	Dyspnea	Diffuse shadows	Normal	Ly	Oral/IV steroids	Favorable
	Desquamative interstitial pneumonia	+	–	Dyspnea	Bilateral opacities	Normal	ND	Oral/IV steroids	Favorable
	Pulmonary infiltrates and eosinophilia§	+	±	Dyspnea ± fever	Bilateral opacities	Normal	Eo	Oral/IV steroids	Favorable (possibly caused by drugs)
	Sterile necrobiotic nodules	+	+	Dyspnea, chest pain; sometimes pyoderma present in the skin	Multiple lung nodules/ cavitation	Normal	ND	Oral/IV steroids	Favorable
Pleura	Pleural effusion	+	+	Chest discomfort, chest pain	Effusion	–	–	Drainage, NSAIDs/steroids	Favorable
Pericardium	Pericardial effusion	+	+	Chest pain, tamponade, arrhythmias, heart block, heart failure	Enlarged heart	–	–	Drainage, NSAIDs/steroids	Favorable; constriction unusual

*Some patterns have been seen in patients submitted to our International Registry for Bowel and Lung Disease but have not yet been validated by peer review and publication.

†Very few cases/data available for review.

‡May be associated with pneumothorax or pneumomediastinum.

§Some of these patterns of ILD may be induced by the bowel disease-modifying drugs sulfasalazine and mesalazine.

BAL, bronchoalveolar lavage; CD, Crohn's disease; CT, computed tomography; Eo, eosinophils; ILD, infiltrative lung disease; IV, intravenous; Ly, lymphocytes; ND, no data; NSAIDs, nonsteroidal anti-inflammatory drugs; PMN, neutrophils; UC, ulcerative colitis; ++, typical/common; +, occasional; ±, unusual; –, not described, does not apply.

TREATMENT

Among various drugs, only corticosteroids have demonstrated convincing clinical efficacy in the management of thoracic complications in IBD. There is usually no response to immunosuppressive agents, and only anecdotal responses to anti–TNF-α drugs.

In patients with airway disease, the site, extent, and degree of involvement influence treatment options and the route of administration of corticosteroids (Table 52.1). It is important to achieve clinical remission as early as possible and to control subsequent flare-ups of airway symptoms carefully.

Involvement of the large airways (trachea excepted) represents the most common type of involvement and is often amenable to topical corticosteroids. A fairly high initial dosage is recommended (e.g., 2000 to 2500 μg of beclomethasone or budesonide, or equivalent) until symptom relief is obtained, to be prudently decreased after 2 to 4 weeks to 800 to 1000 μg. Tapering must be slow, and is guided by symptoms and pulmonary function. Initially, oral corticosteroids may be given in association with inhaled corticosteroids (e.g., 40 to 50 mg prednisolone for 4 weeks, to be tapered over a further 4 to 8 weeks), in the hope of accelerating recovery. In some patients with severe involvement, higher corticosteroid dosages may be needed initially. If this treatment option fails, 500 to 1000 μg nebulized budesonide three to four times daily can be tried, in conjunction with inhaled and oral corticosteroids. Involvement of the airways in some patients is so severe and refractory to treatment that endoscopic administration of corticosteroids has been proposed in an attempt to enhance drug delivery. Twice- or thrice-weekly instillations or bronchial lavages with methylprednisolone (40 to 80 mg dissolved in 50 to 125 mL saline) are given through the fiberoptic bronchoscope, whereas oral and inhaled corticosteroids are continued as described previously. This may provide at least transient improvement. Corticosteroid tapering is not possible in all patients with severe involvement.

Follow-up includes symptom reporting, imaging, endoscopy, pulmonary function testing, and monitoring for adverse effects of corticosteroids. Patients with airway involvement should be treated early and aggressively to minimize the symptoms of cough and expectoration and to avoid the development of irreversible bronchiectatic changes. There is clinical evidence that corticosteroids are less effective in patients with advanced disease, which encourages early recognition and treatment of airway involvement.

Acute upper airway stenosis requires expeditious laser or surgical treatment, in addition to high-dose intravenous corticosteroids.

Patients with ILD usually respond to high(er) doses of systemic or oral corticosteroids, and the prognosis is good.

Pleural drainage, pericardiocentesis, and surgical pericardial drainage are needed in some patients.

CLINICAL COURSE AND PREVENTION

It is important that physicians caring for patients with IBD are cognizant of the many possible patterns of respiratory involvement in this setting.

Airway involvement should be recognized as early as possible, which may help avoid long periods of disabling or debilitating symptoms and the development of irreversible bronchiectatic changes, which are more difficult to control than early stages of the disease. However, progression of airway disease varies among patients and is sometimes refractory to any form or dosage of corticosteroids. A few patients die from uncontrollable airway inflammation.

Patients in whom ILD develops may simply be observed if they present with patchy infiltrates suggesting cryptogenic organizing pneumonia (BOOP; see Fig. 52.3), if features of eosinophilic pneumonia are present, or if drug withdrawal translates into definite improvement of symptoms and imaging. Otherwise, accurate labeling of the ILD is advisable and a lung biopsy (preferably a wedge biopsy) should be discussed to rule out an infection, establish the diagnosis, and guide treatment. A trial of corticosteroids without documentation of the nature of the ILD usually is not recommended.

Note: A Registry of Cases is kept by the authors, who are happy to discuss clinical or histopathological data (philippe.camus@chu-dijon.fr or colby.thomas@mayo.edu). Inquiries about the possibility of drug-induced involvement are also welcome on Pneumotox.com.

SUGGESTED READINGS

Alrashid AI, Brown RD, Mihalov ML, et al: Crohn's disease involving the lung: Resolution with infliximab. Dig Dis Sci 46:1736-1739, 2001.

Camus P, Piard F, Ashcroft T, et al: The lung in inflammatory bowel disease. Medicine (Baltimore) 72:151-183, 1993.

Camus P, Colby TV: The lung in inflammatory bowel disease. Eur Respir J 15:5-10, 2000.

Casey MB, Tazelaar HD, Myers JL, et al: Noninfectious lung pathology in patients with Crohn's disease. Am J Surg Pathol 27:213-219, 2003.

Eaton TE, Lambie N, Wells AU: Bronchiectasis following colectomy for Crohn's disease. Thorax 53:529-531, 1998.

Foucher P, Camus P: Pneumotox web site. Available at http://www.pneumotox.com. 1997; last update, December, 2003.

Higenbottam T, Cochrane GM, Clark TJH, et al: Bronchial disease in ulcerative colitis. Thorax 35:581-585, 1980.

Hotermans G, Benard A, Guenanen H, et al: Nongranulomatous interstitial lung disease in Crohn's disease. Eur Respir J 9:380-382, 1996.

Mahadeva R, Walsh G, Flower CD, et al: Clinical and radiological characteristics of lung disease in inflammatory bowel disease. Eur Respir J. Jan; 15(1):41-48, 2000.

Spira A, Grossman R, Balter M: Large airway disease associated with inflammatory bowel disease. Chest 113:1723-1726, 1998.

Ward H, Fisher KL, Waghray R, et al: Constrictive bronchiolitis and ulcerative colitis. Can Respir J 6:197-200, 1999.

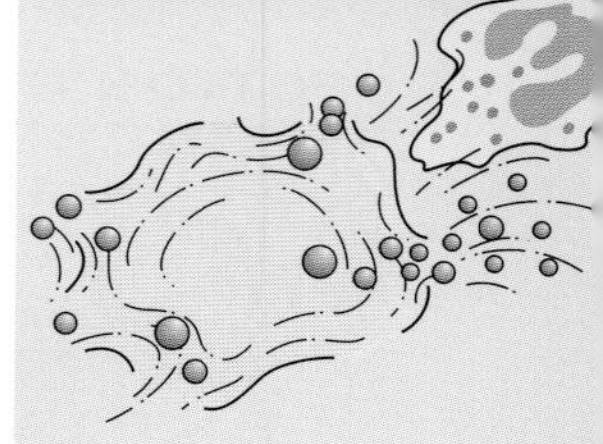

CHAPTER 53

Pulmonary Embolism

Alexander Bankier, Otto Burghuber, Christian Herold, Erich Minar, and Herbert Watzke

Pulmonary embolism (PE) is caused by the obstruction of the pulmonary artery(ies) by clots from the veins of the systemic circulation that embolize to the lungs. Although obstructive material other than blood can cause PE in certain situations (e.g., fat embolism after severe trauma, postpartum amniotic fluid), venous thromboembolism (VTE) is by far the most common cause. However, the differential diagnosis of PE is broad and can present significant difficulties in accurate diagnosis (Table 53.1). In addition, accurate diagnosis is complicated by the fact that a PE can present in a variety of ways, depending on the size, location, number of emboli, and the underlying condition of the patient (Table 53.2). For clinical purposes, PE and deep venous thrombosis (DVT) represent variations of the common clinical entity VTE. Significant morbidity and mortality can result from PE, particularly when it is unrecognized or undertreated. Research has focused on the prevention, diagnosis, and treatment of this condition and has led to a reduction in mortality from PE.

EPIDEMIOLOGY, RISK FACTORS, AND PRIMARY PREVENTION

Epidemiology

In the United States, PE is common—at least 50,000 people die annually of PE, and 300,000 to 600,000 hospital admissions each year are associated with PE or DVT. Similar statistical data are available from several European countries. Age-adjusted hospital diagnosis rates and mortality rates from PE are higher in men than in women and are higher in African Americans than in Caucasians. The incidence rate of PE is also age-dependent, with rates of 130 per 100,000 in those ages 65 to 69 years, and 280 per 100,000 in those ages 85 to 89 years. Mortality rates from PE have changed in the past few decades—they doubled from 1962 to 1974 and then declined by 25% between 1974 and 1979, with a further small decline thereafter. This pattern is paralleled by the decline in incidence rates of PE, which were 92 per 100,000 population in 1975 and 51 per 100,000 in 1995, which suggests that the decline in incidence is the primary reason for the decline in death rates from PE. This is further supported by primary prevention trials of postoperative VTE, which show consistent rates of mortality for patients who have suffered PE in the past two decades. Consequently, the identification and avoidance of clinical situations that carry a high risk for PE or the development of strategies to prevent high-risk states may be the best strategies to combat mortality.

Risk Factors

The clinical significance of a risk factor is determined by its prevalence in the population and by the relative risk it confers to the carrier. These two key features are important for both genetic (inherited thrombophilia) and acquired risk factors (acquired thrombophilia).

INHERITED THROMBOPHILIA

A family history of VTE (inherited thrombophilia) is a strong positive predictor for PE because of the inherited defects in proteins, many of which are involved in the regulation of the coagulation cascade (Fig. 53.1).

However, such defects do not explain all cases of familial thrombosis, and other genetic defects must exist. Testing for genetic risk factors is considered in patients who have established PE and one or more of the following typical features of hereditary thrombophilia: VTE at a young age; family history of VTE; no evidence for acquired risk factors for VTE; and PE that originates from a spontaneous venous thrombosis other than leg vein thrombosis.

Antithrombin Deficiency

Antithrombin (AT), initially designated antithrombin III, is an important inhibitor of coagulation. It binds and inactivates predominantly thrombin (and hence is designated *antithrombin*) but also coagulation factors IXa, XIa, and XIIa. The inhibitory activity of AT itself is low, but is enormously enhanced by heparin. AT deficiency is inherited in an autosomal-dominant manner with incomplete penetrance and is found in 1% of unselected patients with VTE. The prevalence of AT deficiency (including acquired AT deficiency) in the general population is 1 in 2000 to 5000. It increases the lifetime relative risk of VTE to 8.1 in families with AT deficiency but only to 2.2 in unselected patients with VTE.

Protein C (PC) Deficiency

Protein C (PC) is a vitamin K–dependent zymogen that, after being converted into the active enzyme APC (activated protein C), exerts its antithrombotic function by inactivating factors Va and VIIIa. The activation of PC to APC is mediated by thrombin, predominantly by thrombomodulin-bound thrombin. The prevalence of PC deficiency in the general population is 1 in 200 to 500. It can be found in 2% to 9% of individuals with a history of venous thrombosis. It increases the lifetime relative risk of

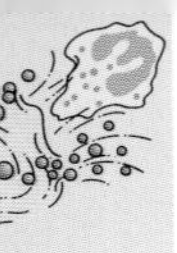

Table 53.1
Differential diagnosis of acute pulmonary embolism

Myocardial infarction
Pneumonia
Congestive heart failure
Asthma and chronic obstructive pulmonary disease
Intrathoracic cancer
Pleuritis/pericarditis
Rib fracture
Pneumothorax
Musculoskeletal pain

Table 53.2
Incidence of symptoms and signs in angiographically proven pulmonary embolism. (Data from Bell WR, Simon TL, DeMets DL: The clinical features of submassive and massive pulmonary emboli. Am J Med 62:355-360,1977.)

	Symptom/sign	Percentage
Symptoms	Chest pain	88
	Pleuritic chest pain	74
	Dyspnea	84
	Cough	53
	Hemoptysis	30
	Syncope	13
Signs	Tachypnea	92
	Crackles	58
	Rales	48
	Tachycardia (>100/min)	44
	Fever (>37.8°C)	43
	Gallop	34
	Phlebitis	32
	Edema	24

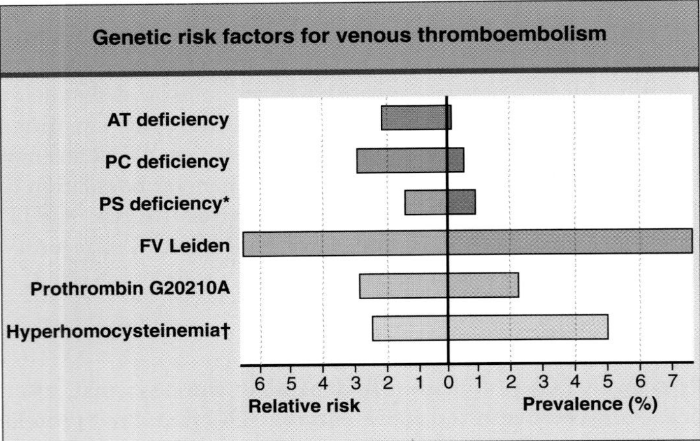

Figure 53.1 Genetic risk factors for venous thromboembolism. (Data from the Leiden Thrombophilia study for heterozygous defects. Van er Meer FJM, Koster T, Vandenbroucke JP, et al: The Leiden thrombophilia study. Thromb Haemost 78: 631-635, 1997.)
*The prevalence of PS deficiency is unknown.
†Includes acquired defects.

VTE to 7.3 in families with PC deficiency but only to 3.1 in unselected patients with VTE.

Protein S Deficiency

Protein S (PS), as with PC, is a vitamin K–dependent protein. It acts as a cofactor for APC in the inactivation process of factors Va and VIIIa. Much of PS is bound to C4b-binding protein in plasma and is without cofactor activity. Only unbound PS ("free PS"), which constitutes 40% of the total PS, has cofactor activity.

It enhances the inactivation of FVa (and FVIIIa) approximately 20-fold. The prevalence of PS deficiency in the general population is unknown. It can be found in around 1% of consecutive patients with VTE and in approximately 10% of patients with a family history of thrombophilia. It increases the lifetime relative risk of VTE to 8.6 in families with PS deficiency but only to 1.6 in unselected patients with VTE. Familial PS deficiency is inherited in an autosomal manner. However, there are numerous causes of acquired PS deficiency, such as acute and chronic inflammatory disease, disseminated intravascular coagulopathy, human immunodeficiency virus infection pregnancy, or the use of oral contraceptives. In addition, PS levels decrease with increasing age and are generally lower in females compared with males. This makes a clear distinction between genetic and acquired cause of PS deficiency occasionally difficult.

The antithrombotic properties of PC and PS are related to inactivation of the activated factors Va and VIIIa by the serin protease APC; PS is the cofactor in this reaction. Both PC and PS deficiencies are inherited in an autosomal-dominant manner. A sixfold risk of VTE is conferred by PC deficiency. The prevalence of PS deficiency is unknown and is associated with only a slightly increased risk of DVT. The cumulative incidence of VTE at age 40 years is 10%.

Factor V Leiden

A single point mutation in the gene coding for FV results in a FV protein that is relatively resistant to the inactivation by activated PC. The mutation leads to a substitution of an arginine by glutamine at amino acid 506, which is part of the cleavage site for APC. The mutation arose about 20,000 years ago from a single founder and occurs today predominantly in Caucasians, with a frequency of the heterozygous state of 1 in 20 to 30 in the general population. It is present in 20% to 30% of consecutive patients with VTE. It increases the lifetime risk of thrombosis by a factor of 6.6. Individuals who are homozygous for the mutation carry a much higher risk (odds ratio of 80). The high prevalence of FV Leiden in the general population increases the likelihood of a coincidence with other genetic or acquired risk factors for thrombophilia. The combination of FV Leiden with hyperhomocysteinemia increases the risk for a thrombotic event between 10- and 20-fold. The incidence of thrombotic events is doubled by the presence of FV Leiden in individuals with PC, PS, or AT deficiency. The thrombotic risk is increased by FV Leiden in women taking the oral contraceptive pill from 7-fold in women without the mutation to 30-fold in the presence of FV Leiden.

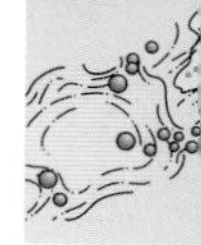

Prothrombin G20210A

A single nucleotide change in the 3′-untranslated region of prothrombin (guanosine to adenosine at nucleotide 20210 of the prothrombin gene) results in elevated prothrombin levels and is associated with a fivefold increase in risk for DVT. It is found in 2.3% of the general population and in 6.2% of consecutive patients with thrombosis. It increases the risk for VTE 2.8-fold.

Hyperhomocysteinemia

Hyperhomocysteinemia can be acquired through diminished intakes of folic acid or vitamins B_{12} and B_6 or it can be genetic through defects in enzymes that affect homocysteine disposal. Individuals with a plasma homocysteine level above 18.5 μmol/L have a 2.5-fold risk of developing VTE. Among the genetic causes, cystathionine b-synthetase deficiency is the most common entity. In the homozygous state, it is associated with the early onset of VTE and a high relative risk of arterial thrombosis. Mutations have also been described in the MTHFR gene that increase plasma levels of homocysteine. However, the corresponding phenotype is not independently associated with VTE.

Factor VIII

An increased level of factor VIII is an independent risk factor for VTE, with a relative risk of 4.8.

Blood Group

Carriers of blood groups other than group O have a twofold increased risk of DVT compared with those who have blood group O.

Acquired Risk Factors

Acquired risk factors in hospitalized patients are given in Table 53.3.

Surgery and Trauma

Surgery, whether elective or posttraumatic, is the most significant acquired risk factor for VTE. Surgery is performed on an ever-increasing number of patients (high prevalence) and, at the same time, confers a substantial risk of VTE (high relative risk); several thrombogenic factors account for this:

- Blood stasis in the lower extremities is caused by preoperative, intraoperative, and postoperative immobilization, or by cast immobilization after trauma
- General anesthetic itself disturbs the delicate balance between the level of coagulation factors and their inhibitors and thereby generates a prothrombotic state
- Local tissue trauma and vessel damage releases tissue factors that cause a hypercoagulable state

Thus, the risk of PE after surgery or trauma is related, on the one hand, to specific surgical factors such as the site and extent of the trauma, the actual surgical procedure, and the time of perioperative immobilization. On the other hand, it is also related to patient-specific factors such as age, underlying disease, and other medical conditions. The interplay of these factors determines the actual risk of VTE for an individual surgical patient.

Table 53.3
Frequency of acquired risk factors in hospitalized patients. Conditions with a particularly high relative risk are highlighted in bold. (Adapted from Anderson FA, Wheeler HB, Goldberg RJ, Hosmer DW, Forcier A: The prevalence of risk factors for venous thromboembolism among hospital patients. Arch Intern Med 152:1660-1664, 1992.)

Age 40 years or more	**Stroke**
Obesity	Oral contraceptives
Surgery/trauma	Hormone replacement therapy
Prolonged immobilization	**Pregnancy**
Malignancy	**Nephrotic syndrome**
Left ventricular failure	**Lupus anticoagulant**
Myocardial infarction	Myeloproliferative disorders
Previous venous thromboembolism	Paroxysmal nocturnal hemoglobinuria
Heparin-induced thrombocytopenia	Waldenström's macroglobulinemia

Medical Conditions

Autopsy studies show that the vast majority of patients who die from PE in hospital had underlying medical illnesses. The most frequent medical conditions associated with an increased risk for DVT can occur singly or in combination (e.g., left ventricular failure and immobilization). In addition, increasing age contributes to the risk of VTE and must be accounted for when thrombotic risk is estimated in a given individual.

Gynecology

During pregnancy and in the month after delivery, PE is a major risk factor and is still the most prevalent cause of maternal mortality.

Oral Contraceptives

The estrogen content of oral contraceptives increases the risk of VTE sevenfold, which is particularly important in women who undergo elective surgery. The risk is further increased if the patient is also heterozygous for FV Leiden—30-fold compared with women who do not take the contraceptive pill and have a normal FV genotype.

Heparin-induced Thrombocytopenia

Heparin-induced thrombocytopenia (HIT) is an immune-mediated condition. It is precipitated by the use of heparin and is characterized by a sudden onset of moderately severe thrombocytopenia in association with life-threatening venous or arterial thromboembolism. The main pathologic event in HIT is formation of heparin-dependent immunoglobulin-G antibodies that activate platelets, bind to platelet factor 4, and increase thrombin generation. This leads to formation of platelet clots that consume platelets and provide the basis for thromboembolic events. It typically begins after 5 to 10 days of heparin use but can occur several weeks after initiating heparin therapy. The incidence of HIT (defined as a reduction in platelet count to 50,000/μL or less than 50% of initial count in the presence of anti-PF4 antibodies) is approximately 3% in surgical patients on unfractionated heparin but is much less in patients receiving low molecular-weight heparin (LMWH). Approximately 50% of all patients with HIT develop clinically overt DVT, and about half

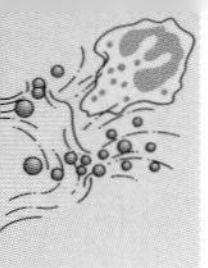

of these have PE. Patients with DVT can develop severe limb ischemia including phlegmasia cerulea dolens.

Primary Prevention

The need for primary prevention is determined by the nature of the individual patient's risk (e.g., surgery, stroke, delivery) in conjunction with the patient's profile of thromboembolic risk factors (genetic or acquired). Areas that carry a high risk for VTE, such as orthopedic surgery, demand maximum prophylactic measures for patients who have no predisposing thromboembolic risk factors. Conditions that carry a low risk for VTE, such as pneumonia, need prophylactic measures only when additional acquired risk factors (e.g., immobilization, left ventricular failure, advanced age) or genetic risk factors (e.g., ATIII deficiency) are present.

Posttraumatic and elective orthopedic surgery carry the highest risk for postoperative PE. Because orthopedic procedures are standardized, the efficacy of various prophylactic measures for PE has been extensively tested in this setting (Fig. 53.2). It is evident that medical prophylaxis with heparin is the treatment of choice for the primary prevention of VTE; aspirin is of no value in such cases.

For patients who undergo orthopedic surgery, LMWHs are superior to unfractionated heparins (UFHs). The incidence of postoperative PE was reduced from 4.1% in patients who received UFH to 1.7% in patients who received LMWH (relative risk 0.43), with a concomitant reduction in fatal PEs and no increased risk of perioperative bleeding (Table 53.4). The same is true for patients who have severe trauma and those who suffer spinal cord injuries. Hirudin may be superior to LMWHs in the primary prophylaxis of VTE in orthopedic patients.

For preventive postoperative VTE, LMWHs are not superior to UFHs in general surgery, obstetrics, or gynecology. However, several other advantages of LMWHs make them the drug of choice in such cases. Their excellent bioavailability leads to a highly predictive anticoagulant response and makes laboratory tests unnecessary. Their long half-life provides protection from VTE for 24 hours after a single subcutaneous dose. In addition, the risks of osteoporosis and heparin-associated thrombocytopenia are much less than with UFHs.

Also, LMWHs can be administered safely preoperatively. Preliminary data suggest even greater protection from VTE without increased perioperative bleeding when LMWHs are given before surgery. The optimum duration of prophylaxis after surgery has been addressed in many studies. Discontinuation of prophylactic treatments after discharge from the hospital leads to a peak of occasionally fatal thromboembolic complications within 2 weeks. These events can be significantly reduced by prolonging prophylactic treatment with LMWHs for 4 weeks postoperatively. Nonmedical prophylaxis, such as graduated compression stockings, intermittent pneumatic compression, or foot impulse pumps, is valuable in various postoperative risk categories, particularly for patients who have contraindications to anticoagulants.

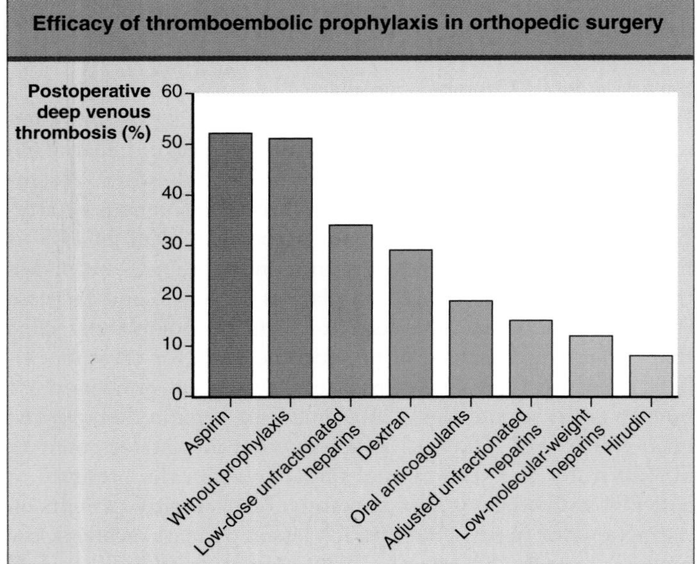

Figure 53.2 Efficacy of thromboembolic prophylaxis in orthopedic surgery.

CLINICAL FEATURES

Pathophysiology

To suspect and subsequently diagnose PE, it is crucial to understand the respiratory and hemodynamic consequences of partial obstruction of the pulmonary vascular bed.

The initial phase is primarily dependent upon the extent of occlusion of the pulmonary bed. Anatomic obstruction of pulmonary arteries by the emboli and pulmonary arterial constriction leads to an increased pulmonary vascular resistance. This places a greater workload on the right ventricle, which is unprepared for high-pressure loads. In the absence of preexisting cardiopulmonary disease, acute elevation of mean pulmonary artery pressure greater than 5.3 kPa (greater than 40 mmHg) leads to right ventricular failure. Even smaller increases can lead to marked right ventricular dilatation and a decrease in cardiac output, which increases the arteriovenous oxygen content difference. To lower the mixed venous oxygen content seems to be the major mechanism of arterial hypoxemia in the initial phase of massive PE. A right-to-left shunt through an already patent or newly patent foramen ovale can also contribute to arterial hypoxemia. At the same time, tachycardia and hyperventilation occur, although the mechanisms responsible for these are uncertain. Both arterial hypoxemia and hypocapnia cause a widening

Table 53.4
The perioperative frequency of pulmonary embolism and fatal pulmonary embolism without and with low–molecular-weight heparin prophylaxis

Type of surgery	Without prophylaxis		Prophylaxis with low–molecular-weight heparin	
	Incidence of pulmonary embolism (%)	Incidence of fatal pulmonary embolism (%)	Incidence of pulmonary embolism (%)	Incidence of fatal pulmonary embolism (%)
Post-traumatic orthopedic	6.9	4	–	–
Elective orthopedic	4	1.65	1.7	<1
General	1.6	0.87	0.23	<0.1

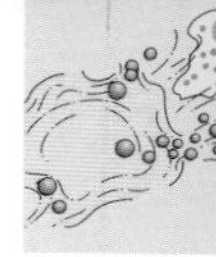

of the alveolar-arterial oxygen difference, but in submassive PE with no pulmonary hypertension the alveolar-arterial oxygen difference remains normal.

In the adaptation phase, partial lysis of the thrombus allows the right ventricle to recover and the cardiac output to increase. Perfusion is enhanced to poorly ventilated lung zones. Normally, perfusion to hypoventilated zones is decreased by hypoxic pulmonary vasoconstriction. However, if PE causes pulmonary hypertension, this vasoconstriction can be overcome; increased perfusion therefore occurs in poorly ventilated areas, which results in hypoxemia. This is accompanied by a decrease in minute ventilation to high ventilation/perfusion ($\dot{V}/\dot{Q}$) areas, which lowers mixed venous oxygen partial pressure. Again, in submassive PE, $\dot{V}/\dot{Q}$ mismatch may not occur.

Approximately 24 hours after the acute event, structural changes develop (the compensation phase). Surfactant is depleted in the obstructed alveolar zones, and atelectasis and edema develop, which (together with necrosis in the case of infarction) increases shunt, which keeps PaO_2 low, even when the acute phase of pain, hyperventilation, and decreased cardiac output has settled.

The influence of the preexisting cardiopulmonary status of the patient is often overlooked, but significant cardiopulmonary disease plus a relatively small embolic event may have severe hemodynamic consequences, whereas in a previously normal individual, substantial embolic occlusion may be tolerated with limited cardiopulmonary dysfunction.

DIAGNOSIS

Diagnosis of Acute Pulmonary Embolism

Clinical suspicion is of crucial importance to guide diagnostic testing. In autopsy studies, rates of 62% and 84% were reported for over- and underdiagnosis, respectively. Furthermore, the Prospective Investigation of Pulmonary Embolism Diagnosis (PIOPED) study showed that to combine clinical probability with lung scan probability establishes the likelihood of PE more accurately. Therefore, to suspect PE in the initial examination is essential for an early diagnosis, with confirmation given by subsequent examinations (e.g., lung scan, pulmonary angiography [PA], spiral CT pulmonary angiography [CTPA]).

The preliminary procedures employed in suspected PE include a good medical history (to identify patients at risk), recognition of common symptoms, physical findings, standard laboratory tests including D-dimer testing, chest radiography, electrocardiography (ECG), arterial blood gas analysis, echocardiography, and examination of the lower extremities (compression ultrasound and venography).

MEDICAL HISTORY

Congenital, prothrombotic coagulopathies (see previous section) need to be suspected if a family history is apparent, particularly in a young person who carries no acquired risk factor.

Acquired major risk factors for VTE include pelvic and lower extremity fracture or surgery (especially hip and knee replacement), surgical procedures that required more than 30 minutes of general anesthetic, and any cause of prolonged immobility or venous stasis. More modest risk is imposed during the third trimester of pregnancy, the postpartum period, and by cancer, obesity, and the use of estrogen-containing medications.

SYMPTOMATOLOGY

The most common symptoms (see Table 53-2) are unexplained acute dyspnea, tachypnea (more than 20 breaths/minute), or substernal chest discomfort—97% of symptomatic patients who have PE show one of or more of these. Shock or syncope is rare and is associated with massive PE. Hemoptysis, often found with an infiltrate localized in the periphery of the lung, is associated with smaller emboli that involve segmental or subsegmental vessels. In fact, pleurisy and hemoptysis are uncommon manifestations of pulmonary infarction, which occurs in a minority of patients who have embolism. In addition, a significant proportion of patients affected by PE may be asymptomatic.

FINDINGS AT PHYSICAL EXAMINATION

The physical findings in PE are also nonspecific. They include tachycardia, a pleural rub and rales, a right-sided gallop, and an increased pulmonary component of the second heart sound, with perhaps a right ventricular "tap" palpable on the right sternal border in massive PE associated with pulmonary hypertension. With right ventricular failure, fixed splitting of the second sound, a right ventricular S3, an elevated jugular venous pulse, and a tender liver may occur. Fever is uncommon if no complicating infection or infarction is present.

STANDARD LABORATORY TESTS

Standard laboratory tests contribute little specificity. Leukocytosis and elevation of the erythrocyte sedimentation rate are rarely present without infarction. Plasma D-dimer measurement (a degradation product of cross-linked fibrin) has been used in suspected PE because its level is highly sensitive for acute VTE. Hence, a normal D-dimer level (less than 500 mg/L) probably excludes VTE. In contrast, a high D-dimer level is not helpful because so many other diseases exhibit high levels.

ELECTROCARDIOGRAPHY

Abnormalities of ECG are also nonspecific. The classic electrocardiographic findings of acute right ventricular strain are observed in some patients who have massive PE. However, ECG is useful to exclude competing diagnoses—myocardial infarction or a rapid atrial arrhythmia, with the caveat that T-wave inversion may suggest an early myocardial infarct, and embolism may induce atrial flutter or fibrillation. Characteristic ECG findings in acute PE include (Fig. 53.3) right ventricular strain pattern with a negative T-wave or ST segment depression in leads V1-V3, or incomplete or complete right bundle branch block. In the limb leads, P pulmonale, rotation of the QRS axis to the right with a deep S wave in lead I, or the development of the so-called SI-QIII-TIII pattern are found. This pattern comprises a deep S wave in lead I, a deep Q wave in lead III, and an inverted T wave in lead III, and can be very similar to that in posterior myocardial infarction. Ultimately, PE often is accompanied by sinus tachycardia, and sometimes by paroxysms of atrial flutter or fibrillation.

CHEST RADIOGRAPHY

Chest radiography may demonstrate radiologic signs compatible with PE (and raise the level of clinical suspicion), may demonstrate or exclude other diseases potentially responsible for a patient's symptoms, and is needed to adequately evaluate a V/Q scan.

A chest radiograph from a patient who is suspected to have PE is neither sensitive nor specific. Notably, a negative chest radiograph is one of the most common presentations of PE, because changes only occur when a fairly large segmental or even more proximal vessel is occluded or when obstruction of many small vessels impairs pulmonary hemodynamics. Up to 80% of patients who have confirmed PE have an abnormal chest radiograph. Findings include loss of lung volume with platelike atelectasis or diaphragmatic elevation, and pleural effusion. Less often, a prominent pulmonary hilus (which represents a large central pulmonary artery) with inadequate tapering of vessels (Fleischner sign) can be seen and may or may not be associated with peripheral regional oligemia (Westermark sign). Infarcts are rare and, if present, appear as peripheral, wedge-shaped densities (Hampton hump). Most commonly, radiographic abnormalities in PE are located in the lower portion of the chest, because approximately 90% of all emboli are lodged in lower lobe vessels.

Unfortunately, none of these signs have a high enough specificity to allow a straightforward diagnosis of PE. Radiographic abnormalities, including pleural effusion or platelike atelectasis, may also be found in other thoracic or even abdominal disorders. Nevertheless, the chest radiograph fulfills a very distinct role in the evaluation of patients suspected to have PE, and provides potentially important information on a patient's pulmonary and cardiovascular state (Fig. 53.4).

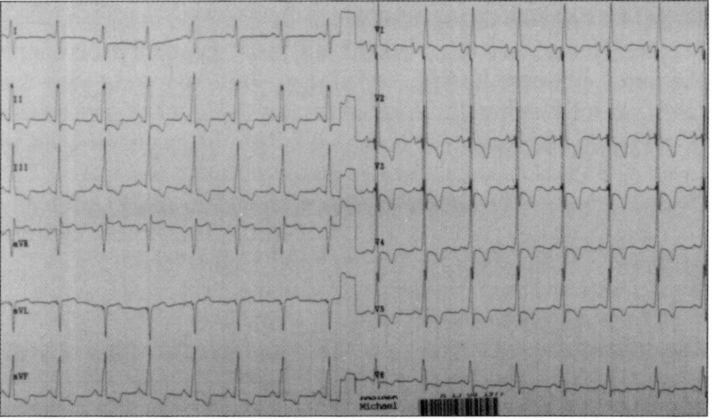

Figure 53.3 Characteristic electrocardiographic findings in acute pulmonary embolism. Right ventricular strain is seen in the precordial leads, and P pulmonale in limb leads II and III, and right axis deviation.

ARTERIAL BLOOD GAS ANALYSIS

In the vast majority of patients who have acute PE, the partial pressures of arterial blood gases demonstrate hypocapnia and respiratory alkalosis. The PaO_2 when breathing room air drops with massive PE, but in submassive embolism it may be normal or near normal if no underlying pulmonary disease is present. Hypoxemia is very common in cardiopulmonary disease, but it is not specific and should be interpreted with caution in the assessment of PE.

DOPPLER ECHOCARDIOGRAPHY

Echocardiography, both transthoracic and, in particular, transesophageal, may identify thrombi in the central pulmonary arteries; it does not reliably identify emboli in the lobar and segmental arteries. Echocardiography may prove useful in massive PE associated with pulmonary hypertension. It can be performed rapidly at the bedside and may reveal significant disease. Doppler echocardiographic features that suggest acute massive PE include a dilated, hypokinetic right ventricle, absence of right ventricular hypertrophy, distortion of the interventricular septum toward the left ventricle (mainly in diastole), the presence of tricuspid regurgitation with increased flow velocity (3 to 3.5 m/sec) compatible with mild-to-moderate elevation of pulmonary artery systolic pressure, and the absence of significant pathologic left ventricular conditions.

Diagnosis of Deep Venous Thrombosis

More than 90% of all emboli arise from DVT, which is a progressive process that usually begins in the deep veins of the calf and propagates through the popliteal and into the iliofemoral system. Thrombosis of the popliteal or more proximal veins is more likely to cause PE. Consequently, the approach to the diagnosis of PE must also include a search for DVT of the lower extremities.

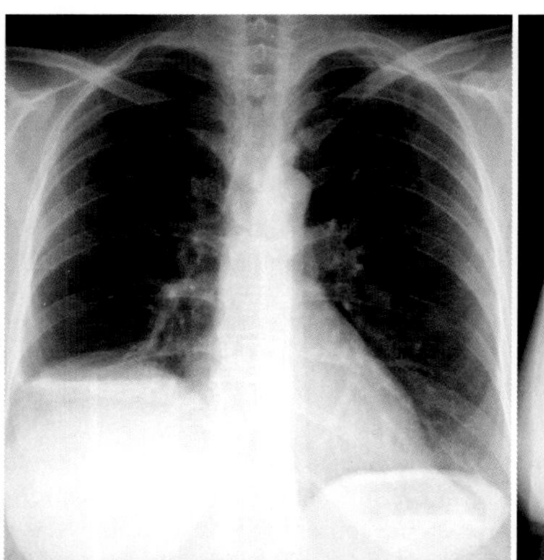
A

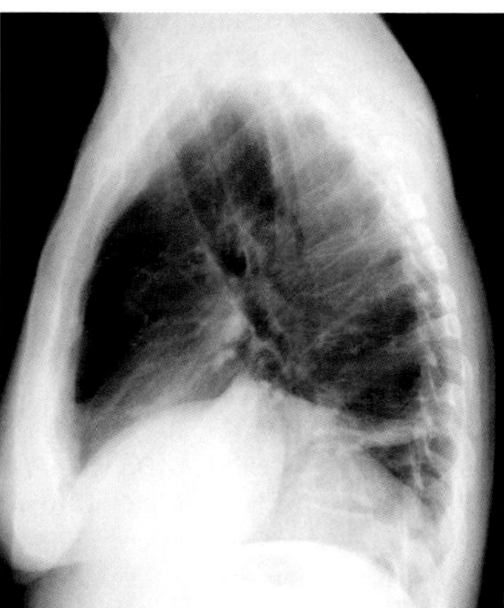
B

Figure 53.4 Multiple atelectatic lines in the right lower zone of the chest X-ray of a patient with acute pulmonary embolism seen **(A)** on PA film, and **(B)** in the lateral projection.

Although DVT can be silent, symptoms include leg pain, tenderness, and swelling, while the major signs are edema, discomfort in the calf upon forced dorsiflexion of the foot (Homan sign), venous distension of subcutaneous vessels, discoloration, and a palpable cord (Fig. 53.5). Clinical evaluation is by B-mode compression ultrasonography (CUS), which not only establishes the diagnosis, but also (when it is repeatedly negative), identifies a low-risk group for subsequent PE or proximal DVT. Consequently, the test can be used to stratify the risk of individuals suspected to have PE for subsequent morbid events over a 3-month period. B-mode compression ultrasonography is so reliable, inexpensive, and safe that it has rapidly supplanted leg phlebography as the gold standard. Phlebography, therefore, is reserved for those situations in which the ultrasound examination is normal despite high clinical suspicion for DVT.

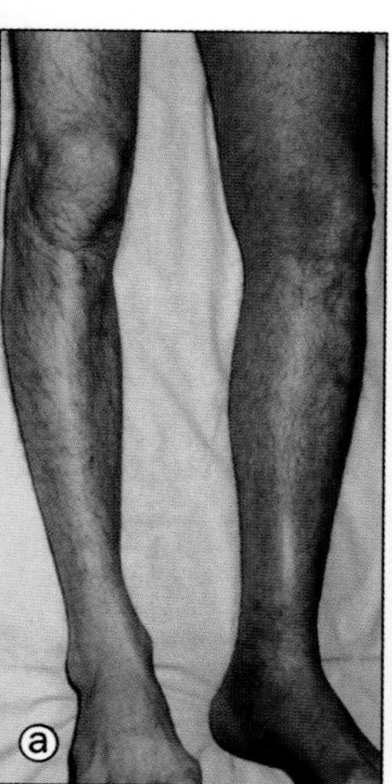

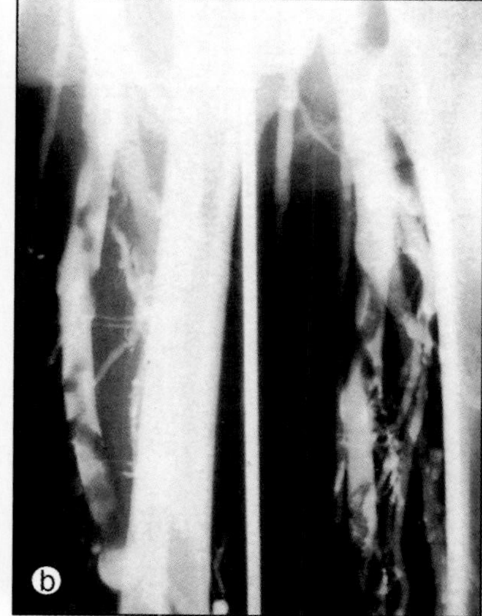

Figure 53.5 Deep venous thrombosis. A, Leg edema, venous distension of subcutaneous vessels and skin discoloration are seen. **B,** Phlebography of the same patient. Multiple filling defects are seen in the femoral vein. These defects correspond to thrombi.

Common Clinical Syndromes of Acute Pulmonary Embolism

The clinical features of acute PE can be divided into several syndromes, but they have considerable overlap (Table 53.5).

MASSIVE PULMONARY EMBOLISM

Massive pulmonary embolism is defined as right-sided ventricular failure with or without cardiovascular collapse, hypotension, and shock. When encountered in its classic form in a predisposed patient, acute massive PE that obstructs more than 60% to 70% of the pulmonary circulation is rarely a diagnostic problem. The common features are profound dyspnea, tachypnea, tachycardia, and, occasionally, hypotension. Syncope, cardiogenic shock, and cardiac arrest (particularly with electromechanical dissociation) are life-threatening events, which lead to death in most cases. Signs of acute right ventricular failure are usually present. The differential diagnosis includes acute myocardial infarction, superior vena cava syndrome, pericardial tamponade, hypovolemia, and sepsis. The classic electrocardiographic finding in patients who have massive PE may be present (see the previous section). The chest radiograph is not often helpful, whereas the diagnosis may be established by two-dimensional echocardiography, which shows a thrombus in the central part of a pulmonary artery. Indirect echocardiographic features include a dilated, hypokinetic right ventricle, absence of right ventricular hypertrophy, distortion of the interventricular septum toward the left ventricle, and the presence of tricuspid regurgitation.

SUBMASSIVE PULMONARY EMBOLISM

Submassive pulmonary embolism is an acute, transient unexplained dyspnea and tachycardia. The most difficult diagnostic challenge is posed by transient, mild, or moderate pulmonary hypertension caused by submassive PE. If PE obstructs less than 60% of the pulmonary circulation, acute right ventricular failure does not occur, which makes the diagnosis of submassive PE difficult. No clinical signs of right ventricular failure are found, and ECG remains normal. If pulmonary infarction has not occurred, pleuritic chest pain is absent and no abnormalities are found on chest radiography or ECG. In such cases, the clinician must rely

Table 53.5
Common clinical syndromes of acute pulmonary embolism

	Massive pulmonary embolism		Submassive pulmonary embolism	
	With/without hypotension and shock	**With transient dyspnea and tachycardia**	**With pulmonary hemorrhage or infarction**	**Without any symptoms**
Symptoms	Dyspnea, tachypnea, syncope, +/- shock, cardiac arrest	Dyspnea, anxiety, tachypnea	Pleuritic chest pain, hemoptysis	None
Clinical signs	Tachycardia, splitting 2nd heart sound, right ventricular–S3, elevates jugular venous pulse, tender liver	Tachycardia	Rales, wheezes, pleural friction rub	None
Differential diagnosis	Myocardial infarction, pericardial tamponade, hypovolemia, superior vena caval syndrome	Left ventricular failure, pneumonia, hyperventilation syndrome	Pneumonia	None
Electrocardiogram	Negative T wave in V1–V3, S1–Q3 type, P-pulmonale, incomplete or complete right bundle branch block	Normal	Normal	Normal
Chest radiograph	May be "knuckle" or Westermark sign	Normal	Pulmonary infiltrate	Normal
Arterial blood gas tension	Often hypoxemia despite hypocapnia, Aa-oxygen gradient↑	Hypoxemia, often Aa-oxygen gradient↑	Hypocapnia, respiratory alkalosis	Normal
Echo	Dilated, hypokinetic right ventricule, no right ventricular hypertrophy, distortion of interventricular septum, TI	Normal	Normal	Normal

on the clinical symptoms of sudden onset of dyspnea, tachypnea, and possibly tachycardia and anxiety. The differential diagnosis includes left ventricular failure, pneumonia, and the hyperventilation syndrome. Patients who present with dyspnea caused by acute PE may also be hypoxic.

PULMONARY HEMORRHAGE OR INFARCTION

Pulmonary infarction occurs with pleuritic chest pain, with or without dyspnea, and occasionally hemoptysis. The clinical diagnosis of infarction caused by PE cannot be confirmed unless an infiltrate is present on the chest radiograph. Signs of right ventricular failure are absent. Examination of the lungs may reveal rales, wheezes, or evidence of pleural effusion or a friction rub. The most useful laboratory tests include arterial blood gases, differential white blood cell count, and chest radiography. The arterial blood gas partial pressures usually demonstrate hypocapnia and respiratory alkalosis, whereas PaO_2 may be normal. The white blood cell count and differential help to diagnose bacterial pneumonia, although a high white blood cell count does not rule out PE.

NO SYMPTOMS (SILENT PULMONARY EMBOLISM)

It has been argued that approximately 10% of patients who have submassive PE may show no symptoms at all; thus, it is crucial to periodically reevaluate these patients.

CHRONIC THROMBOEMBOLIC PULMONARY HYPERTENSION

Recurrent PE causes chronic pulmonary hypertension associated with a clinical syndrome of progressive right ventricular failure and cor pulmonale. This develops insidiously and diagnosis is often made only when the disease is far advanced.

Definition of Clinical Probability

INTEGRATED APPROACH TO DIAGNOSIS

Although no algorithms to estimate the clinical probability of PE are validated, it has been suggested that a high-probability patient (80% to 100%) shows a plausible risk factor, one or more of the common screening findings, and a radiographic or gas-exchange abnormality. A low-probability patient (1% to 19%) shows no risk factor, clinical symptoms or findings that are explainable by another disease, or radiographic or gas-exchange abnormalities that are also explainable by another condition. Intermediate category patients (20% to 79% probability) are those who do not meet the criteria for either of the above categories (Table 53.6). Consequently, the integrated approach to the diagnosis of VTE relies both on the clinical estimation of probability and on the use of the two major screening tests—that is, CTPA and B-mode compression ultrasonography of the lower extremities (Fig. 53.6).

Table 53.6 Estimation of clinical probability in acute pulmonary embolism. Data from Hyers. TH: Diagnosis of pulmonary embolism. Thorax 50:930-932, 1995.

Category	Finding
High probability (80–100%)	Risk factor present Otherwise unexplained dyspnea, tachypnea, or pleuritic chest pain Otherwise unexplained radiographic or blood-gas abnormality
Intermediate probability (20–79%)	Neither high nor low clinical probability
Low probability (1–19%)	Risk factor not present Dyspnea, tachypnea, or pleuritic chest pain may be present, but explainable by another condition Radiograph or blood-gas abnormality may be present, but explainable by another condition

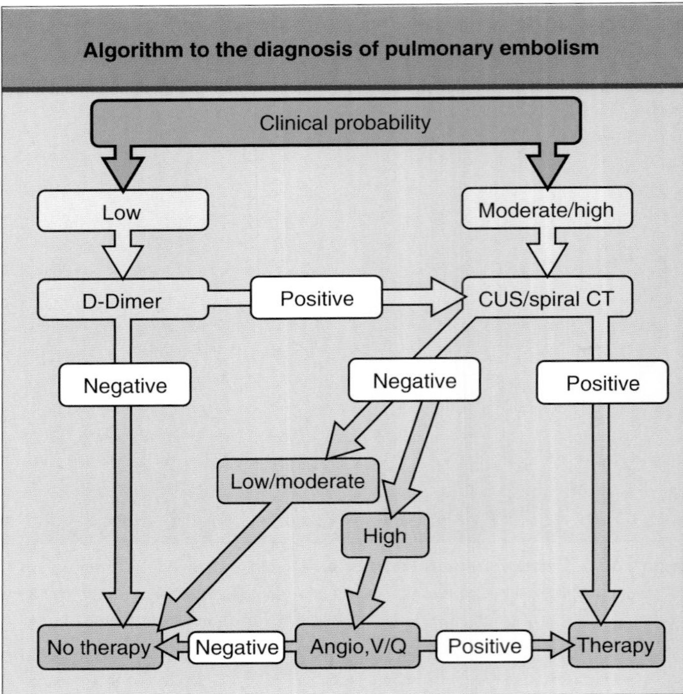

Figure 53.6 Algorithm to the diagnosis of pulmonary embolism.

Imaging in Venous Thromboembolism

GENERAL PRINCIPLES

In patients who have suspected VTE, it is of paramount importance to identify those patients in whom PE or DVT is present and who therefore receive anticoagulant treatment. In principle, the diagnosis of either PE or DVT alone suffices to institute therapy. Nevertheless, an examination of the complementary portion of the vascular bed (i.e., the lower extremity veins in PE or the pulmonary arteries in DVT) may provide important information for the treatment plan, duration of anticoagulation therapy, and use of alternative treatment options in cases of treatment failure. For example, in patients who have PE, it may be important to know whether a thrombus load is present in the lower extremity veins with the potential to cause recurrent (and potentially fatal) PE. Likewise, the diagnosis of PE in a patient who has DVT may have significant therapeutic implications in the case of a recurrent event, which represents treatment failure (and is an indication for a vena cava filter).

Of equal importance is the selection of cases in which the exclusion of PE and DVT obviates the need for treatment, because long-term anticoagulation carries significant risks, such as hemorrhage. Thus, for management, a multimodality approach is required in many cases to achieve a coherent

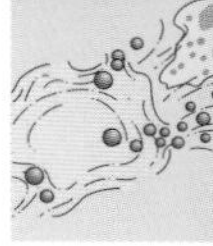

diagnosis based on the findings in the pulmonary arterial bed and the lower extremity veins.

Because few clinical signs that suggest PE or DVT are reliable enough to confirm or exclude the disease, imaging modalities play a major role in patients suspected to have these disorders. Requirements of the "ideal" imaging modality are multiple—availability, high sensitivity and specificity, good positive and negative predictive values, cost-effectiveness, low invasiveness, and patient acceptance. In addition, the imaging modality should help to depict other diseases that may be the cause the patient's complaints. Unfortunately, none of the imaging modalities available to date fulfills all these criteria.

IMAGING PULMONARY EMBOLISM

Chest Radiograph

For a discussion of the use of chest radiography in PE, see the section on clinical diagnosis.

Scintigraphy

In patients who have suspected PE, the first-line imaging evaluation usually includes a chest radiograph and V/Q scintigraphy. The latter couples the scintigraphic assessment of lung perfusion (in which the diagnosis of PE is not based on the direct visualization of the embolus, but rather on the detection of perfusion abnormalities subsequent to the embolic event) with the pattern of lung ventilation. The two studies are analyzed together and, in cases of PE, classically display a mismatch between perfusion and ventilation, that is a lung segment distal to an obstructing embolus is not perfused, but is still ventilated (Fig. 53.7).

Although V/Q scans do not confirm or exclude PE, they give an estimate of its likelihood. In most classifications, the results of V/Q scanning are reported to show high (more than 90%), intermediate, or low (less than 10%) probability, or to be normal. In clinical practice, the results of V/Q scintigraphy are most usefully interpreted together with the clinical estimate of the likelihood of acute PE (pretest probability). It has been shown that a normal perfusion scan virtually excludes clinically relevant PE. The PIOPED study has shown that PE may be confidently excluded in patients whose scan shows a low probability and who have a low clinical suspicion of acute PE. Conversely, a high-probability scan (together with a high clinical suspicion of acute PE) is sufficiently reliable to initiate anticoagulant treatment. The PIOPED study also showed that to combine clinical probability with lung scan probability establishes the likelihood of PE more accurately.

The clinical relevance of V/Q scintigraphy is limited because only 25% to 40% of patients referred with acute PE fall into the previously named categories. The remaining cases (the majority) either show intermediate probability results or a clinical assessment that suggests a probability of PE discordant with the probability indicated by the V/Q scan. In these patients, the average risk for PE is high (approximately 34%) and a diagnosis must be

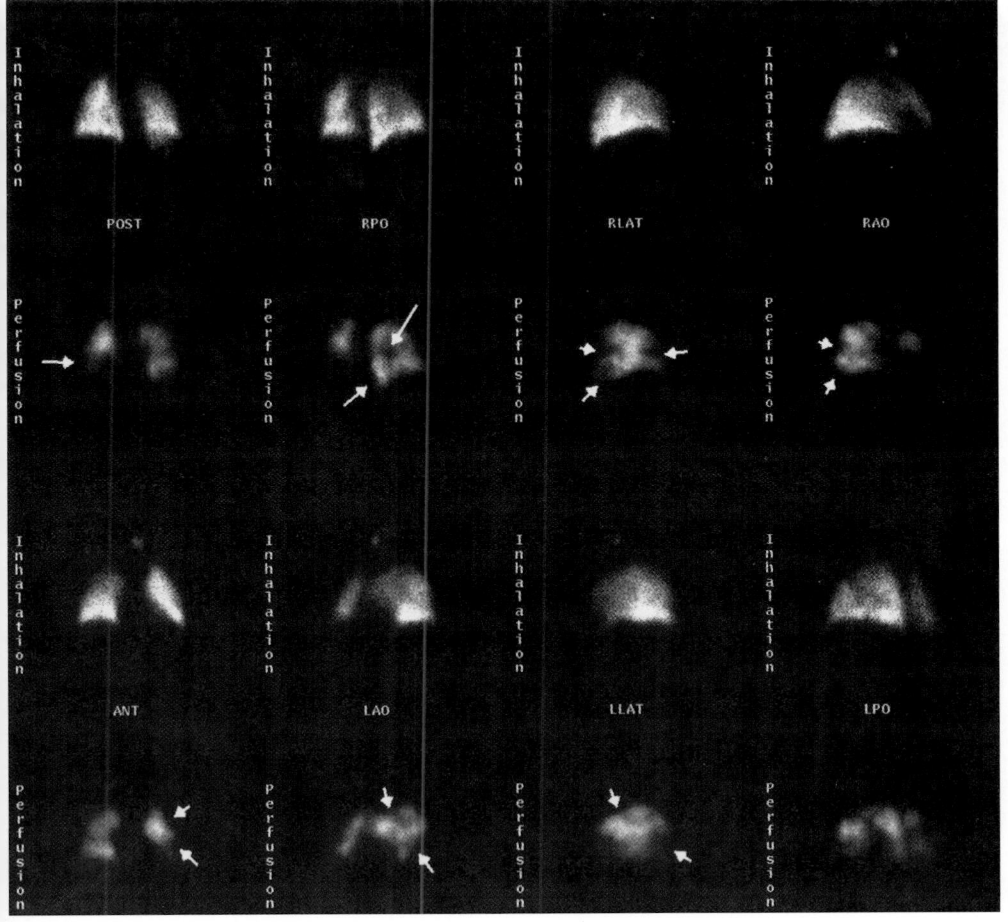

Figure 53.7 Ventilation and perfusion scans in a patient who has multiple pulmonary emboli. Ventilation inhalation scan is normal. Perfusion shows large segmental defect caused by an embolus in a segmental pulmonary artery.

13

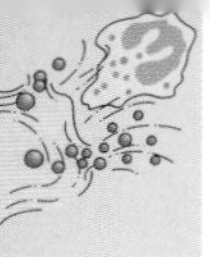

made using another modality. The major limitation of V/Q scintigraphy, therefore, is that clinical decisions can be based on this method only in a minority of patients. The majority of cases suspected to have PE require further testing.

Pulmonary Angiography

The gold standard in the diagnosis of acute PE is PA. Compared with all other imaging methods, PA has a superior ability to depict embolic filling defects in the central vessels (Fig. 53.8 A). In addition, it also detects emboli in the subsegmental or even more peripheral arteries, although the accuracy is limited but reasonable. A negative PA is an excellent indicator of a good prognosis.

Unfortunately, PA also has disadvantages, mainly its non-availability as an urgent investigation, if at all, and it is invasive. Thus, it suffers from a low level of use, and most cases are treated on the basis of the best clinical guess. With the advent of spiral CT and the ever-increasing use of this technique in the work-up of patients with PE, angiography is less and less performed, which also leads to a decrease in number of radiologic investigators experienced with this technique.

Spiral Computed Tomography Pulmonary Angiography

Spiral (helical) CTPA allows rapid and contiguous data acquisition and enables investigation of the pulmonary vasculature at peak contrast opacification within a single breath-hold. The result is a truly two-dimensional angiographic visualization of the pulmonary arteries that enables the viewer to depict directly or to exclude emboli in the pulmonary arterial system (see Fig. 53.8 B).

The sensitivity and specificity of CTPA for pulmonary embolism is approximately 90%. In addition to the diagnosis or exclusion of PE, spiral CTPA may demonstrate or exclude other abnormalities in the lung or the mediastinum that may be responsible for the patient's symptoms. It may also quantify the severity of the embolic event. Limitations of CTPA include potentially suboptimal contrast opacification of pulmonary arteries in certain groups of patients (notably in those who have cardiac insufficiency, elevated pulmonary arterial pressure, and congenital cardiac abnormalities) and decreased sensitivity in the analysis of subsegmental and peripheral arteries. However, the clinical relevance of isolated subsegmental PE is still unclear.

In most centers where it is available, CTPA is already incorporated into the diagnostic algorithms used to investigate patients who suspected to have PE. A key factor that increases acceptance is the cost-effectiveness. Diagnostic issues such as the visualization of subsegmental thrombi have been resolved with technical improvements, refinements of examination protocols, and with the introduction of multislice, rapid sequence CT machines. These last-generation CT scanners allow for improved intravascular contrast and faster examination times. This will often result in increased image quality, given that many patients with PE are breathless and cannot easily breath-hold for long.

Although the role of CT in the diagnosis of PE has been intensively discussed during the past decade, CT has now found its role in virtually all widely accepted diagnostic algorithms (see Fig. 53.6). Although the position of CT in these algorithms depends on patient selection, pretest probability, availability, and local factors, the role of CT per se is now beyond doubt. Spiral CT angiography particularly benefits from its high negative predictive value (i.e., patients with a negative CTPA examination have a high likelihood of not having a pulmonary embolism). In cases negative for PE, spiral CTPA also has the ability to depict other abnormalities that may explain the patient's symptoms. In this light, the acceptance of CT by clinicians has substantially increased as the method provides an integral assessment of the individual patient and does not remain focused on confirming or excluding PE. Although not yet confirmed by large multicenter trials, and encouraged by the decrease in use of PA, the general trend indicates that CTPA might become the reference imaging technique in the diagnosis of PE.

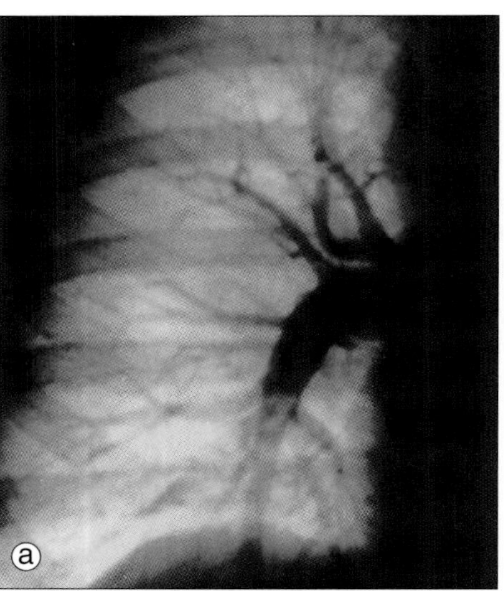

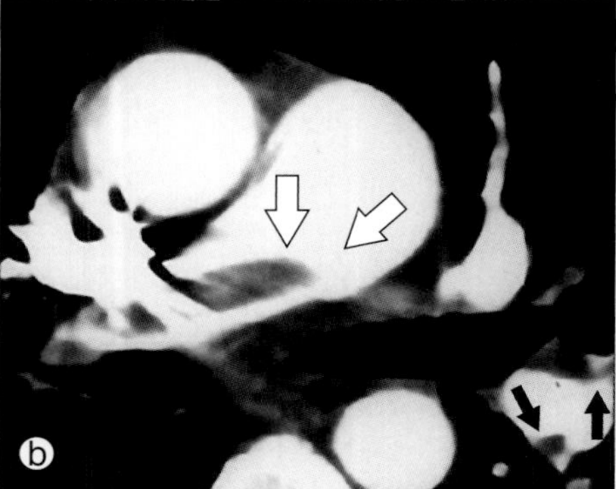

Figure 53.8 Pulmonary imaging for embolism. **A,** Pulmonary angiogram showing a filling defect in the right lower lobe pulmonary artery. **B,** A spiral computed tomography angiogram in another patient showing multiple filling defects (arrows).

Magnetic Resonance Angiography

Technical improvements and the use of contrast material have expanded the role of magnetic resonance angiography (MRA) in patients who have suspected PE. Imaging of the pulmonary arteries beyond the segmental level is possible using MRA, and in the detection of emboli in the central arteries sensitivities of 70% to 90%, and specificities of 77% to 100% have been reported (see Chapter 1). A potential advantage of MRA is that it allows the study of the pulmonary arteries and the deep veins of the lower extremities within a single examination.

Conversely, MRA clearly suffers from limited availability and, because MRA examinations usually require more time than CT, MRA is not an ideal imaging modality in the emergency setting. Finally, MRA is highly sensitive to motion, which results in

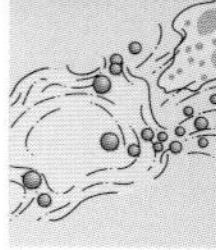

substantially poor image quality in patients unable to hold their breath. In the clinical work-up of PE, the use of MRA is therefore generally restricted to occasional patients in whom either irradiation or ionic contrast material might pose a problem. These include pregnant women or patients with severe renal disorders.

IMAGING OF DEEP VENOUS THROMBOSIS

Venography is still the gold standard for DVT. After compression of superficial veins, contrast material is injected into the deep venous system. The advantages of this method include high sensitivity and specificity, direct visualization of thrombi depicted as filling defects in the contrasted veins, and visualization of other venous pathologies such as venous insufficiency. Potential drawbacks may arise from the administration of contrast material and from patient irradiation.

In most centers, sonography has superseded venography as the first-line imaging of DVT. Suitable sonographic techniques include:

- Compression ultrasound, which is sonography combined with an operator-induced compression of the ultrasonographically visible veins via the transducer
- Duplex Doppler sonography, which combines the analysis of the sonographic picture of the veins with the analysis of venous flow
- Color-encoded duplex sonography, the most modern approach to venous imaging, which offers a colored picture of venous flow

Sonography offers a high level of sensitivity and specificity in symptomatic patients, but suffers from a lack of sensitivity in asymptomatic patients. Also it has limitations for the calf veins. Finally, sonography is (as are other imaging techniques) operator-dependent.

IMAGING STRATEGIES

In patients suspected to have PE, the choice of imaging strategy depends not only on the accuracy of methods, but particularly on local equipment availability and acceptance of the tools at hand. The goal must be to maximize the number of patients who are given a definite diagnosis—PE or no PE. When this is provided using the first-line imaging method, treatment is instituted or withheld based on the findings of the imaging test. An inconclusive result must be clarified using an angiographic method, such as PA or CTPA. Traditional concepts favor V/Q scintigraphy as a first-line imaging tool, whereas more recent views suggest that CTPA could be used as a first, or even only, method to confirm or to exclude PE, and only those patients who show inconclusive results be referred for PA. However, recent developments clearly show an increasing use of CTPA and, simultaneously, a decreasing use of both V/Q scanning and PA as first-line imaging tools in the work-up of patients with PE. Given the potential limitations of CTPA in the diagnosis of subsegmental and peripheral PE (although less of a problem with the modern multislice, rapid-sequence CT scanners), it appears to be advantageous to combine it with venous imaging using sonography and clinical tests, such as D-dimer, to evaluate the risk of underlying venous thrombosis. Cases that have a high clinical suspicion of PE and a negative imaging work-up should be treated whenever possible (see the following section) and could be brought back for a follow-up examination of the veins after 2 to 3 weeks. A further difficulty with V/Q scans is their unavailability outside working hours. Performing a scan 1 to 2 days after anticoagulation has begun makes the normal or low probability scan hard to interpret because the PE may have been lysed.

TREATMENT AND SECONDARY PREVENTION OF PULMONARY EMBOLISM

The objectives for treatment of patients who have pulmonary embolism are to prevent death, to reduce morbidity from the acute event, and to prevent thromboembolic pulmonary hypertension. Treatment regimens for DVT and PE are similar because the two conditions are manifestations of the same disease process.

Treatment in the Acute Phase

GENERAL MEASURES

For patients who have massive embolism, management must be a coordinated effort, because survival may hinge on a matter of minutes. Careful monitoring is mandatory. General therapeutic measures include the administration of oxygen, intravenous fluids, vasopressor agents, and other resuscitory measures depending on the clinical status of the patient. Specific therapeutic measures include anticoagulants and thrombolytic agents.

ANTICOAGULANT THERAPY

The anticoagulant agents commonly used for treatment of PE are UFH and, more recently, LMWH, and oral anticoagulants.

Unfractionated Heparin

The mainstay of treatment for PE has been UFH, based on the results of a single study that involved only a few patients. Until recently, UFH was the treatment of choice for most patients who had PE, except those affected by hemodynamic instability. Although UFH is highly effective and safe for the initial treatment of patients who suffer VTE, it is not an ideal antithrombotic agent because of its pharmacologic and biophysical limitations. It binds to endothelial cells and plasma proteins, such as fibrinogen and fibronectin, or to platelet factor IV, which limits its bioavailability and anticoagulant effects in an unpredictable manner.

Administration of UFH is by continuous intravenous infusion or by subcutaneous injection. A bolus application of 5000 IU is followed by continuous infusion of about 30,000 to 35,000 IU per day. Because its antithrombotic efficacy is related to an adequate level of anticoagulation, the dose of UFH must be titrated on the basis of a coagulation test sensitive to heparin, usually the activated partial thromboplastin time (APTT) test. An APTT 1.5 to 2.5 times the control level is regarded as therapeutic. The risk of hemorrhagic complications does not correlate well with APTT, and such complications appear to be related more to other patient-dependent factors such as significant coexisting diseases.

Heparin-induced Thrombocytopenia

Heparin can cause thrombocytopenia, either as a relatively mild form or as a delayed form. The mild occurs early and is caused

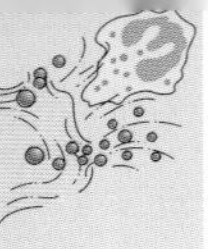

by platelet aggregation induced by heparin itself. It is reversible and improves during continued heparin therapy with no clinical sequelae. A delayed form (type II) is an antibody-mediated adverse reaction to heparin, the antigen being a multimolecular complex of heparin and PF4 (a platelet granule protein). There are different laboratory assays (activation and antigen assays) to detect heparin-induced thrombocytopenia (HIT) antibodies. However, the results have to be interpreted cautiously in clinical context. The HIT type II is associated with thromboembolic complications in the arterial and venous system with high morbidity and mortality. Recent studies indicate that the frequency of this complication is less than 1% when heparin is given for no more than 5 to 7 days. Heparin therapy must be stopped and replaced by an alternative rapidly acting anticoagulant (hirudin, lepirudin [a recombinant hirudin derivative], or danaparoid [a heparinoid]). In the near future newer classes of antithrombotic agents such as ximelagatran (a direct thrombin inhibitor) or fondaparinux (a selective Xa inhibitor) will become available.

The most significant risk associated with long-term heparin use is osteopenia.

Low Molecular-weight Heparins

During the past several years, LMWHs have become available for prophylaxis and also treatment of VTE, at least in Europe. Their elimination half-life is longer than that of UFH, and they are not specifically bound by plasma proteins, which improves the predictability of their anticoagulant effect. This enables weight-adjusted, fixed-dose subcutaneous applications of LMWHs without laboratory monitoring in the initial treatment of VTE. Furthermore, LMWH is less likely to cause HIT antibody formation.

Randomized trials in patients who have proximal DVT showed that LMWH given once or twice daily subcutaneously in a weight-adjusted dosage is at least as effective and safe as unfractionated heparin. However, these trials did not include patients who had symptomatic PE. In 1997, two large, randomized studies demonstrated that fixed-dose, unmonitored subcutaneous LMWH is as effective and safe as adjusted-dose intravenous UFH for the initial management of VTE, regardless of whether the patient has PE, symptomatic DVT, or both (Table 53.7).

Furthermore, LMWH regimens offer the potential for treating most patients with DVT and selected patients with stable PE on an early discharge outpatient basis. Recent trials have demonstrated the feasibility and safety of such an outpatient management in selected patients. Besides the previously mentioned advantages of LMWH compared with unfractionated heparin, potential cost savings associated with home therapy or early hospital discharge are also in favor of LMWH.

THROMBOLYSIS

Thrombolysis was introduced for acute PE more than 30 years ago. However, contrary to the general acceptance and frequency of use of thrombolytic therapy for acute myocardial infarction, the situation is different for pulmonary embolism. Because most hospitals have only a few patients each year who present with recognized massive PE, most physicians have limited experience of thrombolysis for acute PE.

Randomized controlled studies of hemodynamically stable patients who had PE showed that thrombolysis causes more rapid resolution of the pulmonary angiographic, perfusion lung scan, and hemodynamic abnormalities than does anticoagulant therapy alone. However, these benefits are short-lived and results are similar a few days after treatment. Thrombolysis may have lifesaving potential in patients affected by hemodynamic instability caused by massive PE, but the impact of the rapid hemodynamic improvement on the clinical outcome—with mortality being the most important endpoint—of patients who have major PE has not yet been investigated in large, randomized trials.

The major problem of thrombolytic treatment is the risk of severe bleeding—intracranial hemorrhage occurs in approximately 1% of patients. Therefore, in most centers thrombolysis is reserved for massive PE and hemodynamic instability.

Thrombolytic regimens approved by the US Food and Drug Administration for the treatment of PE are listed in Table 53.8.

Table 53.7

Randomized trials comparing low–molecular-weight heparin (LMWH) subcutaneously with unfractionated heparin (UFH) intravenously in patients with venous thromboembolism (VTE) and pulmonary embolism (PE)

Study	End points	Drug	Recurrent thromboembolism	Major bleeding	Death
Columbus Study (patients who had venous thromboembolism)	After 12 weeks	Low–molecular-weight heparin (reviparin), twice daily subcutaneously (n = 510)	27 (5.3%)	16 (3.1%)	36 (7.1%)
	After 12 weeks	Unfractionated heparin, intravenously (n = 511)	25 (4.9%)	12 (2.3%)	39 (7.6%)
THÉSÉE Study Group (patients who had pulmonary embolism)	Combined after 8 days	Low–molecular-weight heparin (tinzaparin) once daily subcutaneously (n = 304)	9 (3%)	–	–
		Unfractionated heparin, intravenously (n = 308)	9 (2.9%)	–	–
	Combined after 90 days	Low–molecular-weight heparin (tinzaparin) once daily subcutaneously (n = 304)	–	–	18 (5.9%)
		Unfractionated heparin, intravenously (n = 308)	–	–	22 (7.1%)

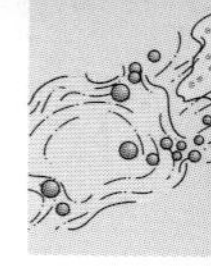

Table 53.8
Thrombolytic regimens approved by the US Food and Drug Administration for the treatment of pulmonary embolism

Drug	Regimen
Streptokinase (approved in 1977)	Loading dose: 250,000IU/30 minutes 100,000IU/h for 24h
Urokinase (approved in 1978)	Loading dose: 4400IU/kg per 10 minutes 4400IU/kg per h for 12–24h
Recombinant tissue plasminogen activator (approved in 1990)	100mg/2h (continuous infusion)

Because all regimens use fixed or weight-adjusted doses with no further dose adjustments, coagulation laboratory tests are not needed during thrombolysis.

It probably does not matter which thrombolytic agent is used. It is much more important that patients receive one treatment quickly. Several trials of thrombolytic therapy in acute PE showed that the administration of recombinant tissue plasminogen activator or urokinase over a short period of time produced faster improvement than the earlier regimens of thrombolytic therapy administered over 12 to 24 hours. Favorable results have been reported with urokinase at a dose of 3 million units over 2 hours, and with streptokinase at a dose of 1.5 million units over 1 hour. As most recent trials were conducted using recombinant tissue plasminogen activator, this thrombolytic agent is increasingly used despite its higher cost.

Thrombolytic therapy has also been administered successfully in patients after recent surgery and in pregnancy complicated by major PE. However, in such cases thrombolytic therapy is employed only in the most life-threatening situations because of major hemorrhagic problems.

Thrombolysis can also reduce the risk of recurrence by dissolving the thrombus in the deep leg and pelvic veins. In a German multicenter trial, the patients who received thrombolytic agents had a reduced rate of recurrent PE (7.7%) compared with those treated with anticoagulants (18.7%).

It is reasonable to use thrombolytic therapy in patients who have major PE if the clinician judges the patient to be at risk of dying from the consequences of the pulmonary artery obstruction. However, a potentially life-threatening disorder may be masked by apparent hemodynamic stability at presentation. It is most important to identify those patients with PE who, despite being initially hemodynamically stable, have an increased risk of deterioration. Echocardiography should be used for risk stratification in these patients to detect right ventricular dysfunction. A recent randomized trial comparing heparin plus alteplase with heparin alone in 256 hemodynamically stable patients with submassive pulmonary embolism and echocardiographically detected right ventricular dysfunction (defined as right ventricular enlargement combined with loss of inspiratory collapse of the inferior vena cava) has been reported. Patients with echocardiographically detected pulmonary artery hypertension—defined as tricuspid regurgitant jet velocity greater than 2.8 m per second—were also included. The incidence of the primary endpoint (in-hospital death or clinical deterioration requiring an escalation of treatment, which was defined as catecholamine infusion, secondary thrombolysis, endotracheal intubation, cardiopulmonary resuscitation or emergency surgical embolectomy or thrombus fragmentation by catheter) was significantly higher in the heparin only compared with the heparin plus alteplase group. This difference was mainly the result of the higher incidence of treatment escalation in the heparin group (24.6% versus 10.2%) because the mortality rate was low in both groups (2.2% in the heparin and 3.4% in the thrombolysis group). Interestingly, no fatal bleeding or cerebral bleeding occurred in patients receiving heparin plus alteplase (a dose of 100 mg of alteplase was given as a 10-mg bolus followed by a 90-mg intravenous infusion over 2 hours).

In conclusion, the most important points to consider when thrombolysis is indicated are risk stratification (e.g., by determining whether right ventricular dysfunction exists) and risk assessment for intracranial hemorrhage (e.g., in patients who have uncontrolled hypertension, prior stroke, and seizure disorder). For patients with contraindications to thrombolysis who nevertheless require more intensive therapy than anticoagulation alone, alternative strategies such as catheter-based or surgical embolectomy should be considered.

PULMONARY EMBOLECTOMY

In patients who have hemodynamic instability, both surgical embolectomy and percutaneous transvenous removal or fragmentation of emboli can replace thrombolytic therapy, depending on local hospital facilities and experience. Surgical intervention for massive PE is now restricted to patients whose circulation is severely compromised and who do not improve rapidly after thrombolytic treatment has commenced or who have an absolute contraindication to thrombolysis. In emergency situations, the decision to operate may be based only on clinical factors with no time available for imaging diagnostic procedures. In experienced teams the mortality of surgical embolectomy is confined to the most severe cases, often with of preoperative cardiac arrest. In small series excellent early and late results have been reported.

Recently, percutaneous catheter techniques were introduced for the treatment of acute severe PE as an alternative to surgical embolectomy. Removal of emboli by suction via a catheter or successful mechanical fragmentation of massive PE that obstructs the main pulmonary arteries using conventional angiographic catheters or special devices has been reported in small series. Mechanical fragmentation can be combined with intrapulmonary thrombolysis. If these strategies fail, acute surgical pulmonary embolectomy can be undertaken.

Long-term Treatment (Secondary Prevention)

The need for long-term treatment using anticoagulants in patients who have VTE is demonstrated by a high incidence of recurrence in patients treated using short-term heparin alone. Therefore, the initial treatment is followed by secondary prophylaxis with heparin or oral anticoagulants such as coumarins. Patients with VTE who receive adequate anticoagulation have a low risk for dying of recurrent disease. However, this risk is four times higher during the first year in patients who are treated for PE compared with patients who are treated for DVT (1.7% versus 0.4%).

ORAL ANTICOAGULANTS

The coumarin dosage is adjusted according to the prothrombin time, International Normalized Ratio (INR). Heparin treatment

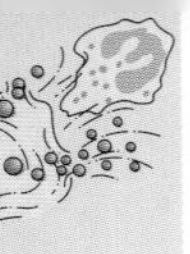

is continued until the INR has been in the therapeutic range (2 to 3 INR) for more than 24 hours. Higher values are associated with more bleeding, but no greater efficacy. The traditional therapeutic concept that heparin should be administered for 7 to 10 days before treatment using oral anticoagulants is initiated has been superseded to rapid initiation of therapy using oral anticoagulant.

Long-term subcutaneous heparin therapy instead of oral anticoagulants for secondary prophylaxis is used only in special cases, such as pregnancy, because coumarin has been linked with fetal abnormalities.

No data are available for the optimal duration of anticoagulant treatment. The risk of bleeding should be balanced against the risk of recurrence when therapy is discontinued. Furthermore, patients who have cardiorespiratory disease might tolerate recurrent PE poorly. Generally, 6 months of anticoagulation can be recommended after the first episode of VTE. However, anticoagulant therapy is given for longer periods—probably indefinitely—in patients who suffer two or more recurrent documented episodes of VTE and in patients whose risk factors are persistent. Recently it could be demonstrated that long-term, low-intensity oral anticoagulant therapy (target INR is 1.5 to 2.0) is an effective method of preventing recurrent VTE with an acceptably low bleeding risk.

VENA CAVA FILTERS

The placement of a vena cava filter must be considered to prevent recurrent episodes of PE. The two major indications are VTE in the setting of absolute contraindication to anticoagulant therapy (e.g., active, clinically important bleeding) and in recurrent PE despite adequate anticoagulant therapy. A rare indication for mechanical protection against recurrent PE is a patient who has sustained massive PE that requires surgical embolectomy.

Many different devices or filters are available and in clinical use. These filters are inserted into the inferior vena cava via the femoral or jugular veins and are lodged below the renal veins.

CLINICAL COURSE OF PULMONARY EMBOLISM

The prognosis for patients who have PE depends on the underlying or concomitant diseases and on the appropriate diagnosis and treatment being carried out. The majority of patients who are treated using anticoagulants survive and have no long-term sequelae. Because the endogenous thrombolytic system is a potent one, resolution of emboli within a few days or weeks is the rule. With heparin therapy alone, embolic resolution proceeds rapidly during the first 2 weeks after the embolic event; at 5 days of therapy, 36% of the scan defects are resolved; at 2 weeks, this is 52%, and at 3 months, 73%.

Significant long-term residual disease after PE is uncommon, particularly pulmonary hypertension. Only a small (unknown) percentage of patients who survive the initial event develop chronic thromboembolic pulmonary hypertension. Many who suffer major residual disease are not treated during the acute event because no definitive diagnosis is made, and pulmonary hypertension seems primarily a complication of chronic recurrent PE. Furthermore, pulmonary emboli may accumulate gradually over a prolonged period if they are small enough to produce microemboli.

Death usually occurs soon after the acute event. The mortality rate in patients who have undiagnosed PE is about 30%, often because of recurrence in those who survived the initial episode and remained untreated. Thus, it is imperative that treatment is initiated as soon as possible as the evidence suggests strongly that PE tends to recur if left untreated. Patients who have major PE frequently exhibit evidence of prior minor embolism. Residual thrombus can be detected in the leg veins of most patients who have PE, and the risk of recurrent PE is related to the presence of proximal venous thrombosis. In a German multicenter trial, 17.2% of patients affected by proximal DVT had recurrent PE, compared with 11.4% of patients who showed negative vein studies or thrombosis restricted to the calf veins. Factors also associated with a high risk of death include syncope, arterial hypotension, history of congestive heart disease, and chronic pulmonary disease.

The PIOPED study reported on the clinical course of 399 patients who had angiographically proved PE. The 1-year mortality rate was 24%, primarily because of cardiac disease, recurrent PE, infection, and cancer. Clinically apparent recurrences of PE developed in 33 patients (8.3%). Fatal recurrences of PE were usually identified during the first 2 weeks of follow-up. However, because patient population was highly selected, these data cannot be considered representative for all patients who present with PE.

CONTROVERSIES

The role of therapeutic thrombolysis in patients whose hemodynamic condition is stable remains uncertain, because no trial has been large enough to demonstrate clinically important differences in mortality in these patients. In most of these studies, angiographic, scintigraphic, and hemodynamic results have been used as surrogate measures. However, a recent multicenter randomized trial of 256 patients suggests that thrombolysis may favorably affect the clinical outcome of hemodynamically stable patients who have submassive PE according to clinical, echocardiographic, and cardiac catheterization criteria. The data from this study provide the first link between the hemodynamic benefits of thrombolysis and clinically relevant endpoints.

Treatment with LMWH enables outpatient treatment. However, criteria for selecting patients for therapeutic management on an early discharge outpatient basis have to be defined. No randomized studies deal with the question of immediate mobilization of patients who have submassive PE and a stable hemodynamic condition. Studies in patients who have massive DVT suggest that the risk of further embolization is very low in mobilized patients on adequate anticoagulation.

The idea that traditional imaging algorithms, which combine V/Q scintigraphy and PA for the diagnosis of acute PE, are suboptimal or underused and the perception that CTPA could provide a minimally invasive, fast, and accurate diagnosis of pulmonary emboli has intensified the search for an "ideal" diagnostic algorithm and discussion of the role of different imaging methods. As the debate continues, the diversification of diagnostic approaches and the heterogeneity of imaging strategies increases. Traditionalists still favor the combination of V/Q scanning and PA for the diagnosis of acute PE. In contrast, others argue for the use of CTPA as a primary or secondary tool, in combination with examination of the lower extremity veins.

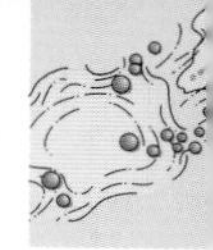

Researchers increasingly stress the future role of magnetic resonance imaging, because this method may also provide a unifying method that provides information on the pulmonary arteries and the leg veins in one single examination using blood pool contrast agents. Although no single diagnostic strategy can be clearly identified as being superior to another, the trend indicates that CTPA will carry the role of leading imaging modality in the diagnostic evaluation of patients with suspected PE. For practical purposes, a number of factors must be considered in addition to the accuracy of the various diagnostic tests to shape the best possible imaging strategy. Factors that play a role in decision making include local equipment availability, acceptance of the various diagnostic tests by clinicians and radiologists, cost-effectiveness analyses, and stratification of patients according to different parameters. An algorithm is summarized in Fig. 53.6.

SUGGESTED READINGS

Agnelli G: Anticoagulation in the prevention and treatment of pulmonary embolism. Chest 107(Suppl.):39-44, 1995.

Bell WR, Simon TL, DeMets DL: The clinical features of submassive and massive pulmonary emboli. Am J Med 62:355-360, 1977.

Erdman WA, Peshok RM, Redman HL, et al: Pulmonary embolism: Comparison of MR images with radionuclide and angiographic studies. Radiology 190:499-508, 1994.

Goodman LR, Curtin JR, Mewissen MW, et al: Detection of pulmonary embolism in patients with unresolved clinical and scintigraphic diagnosis: Helical CT versus angiography. Am J Roentgenol 164:1369-1374, 1995.

Konstantinides ST, Geibel A, Heusel G et al: Heparin plus alteplase compared with heparin alone in patients with submassive pulmonary embolism. New Engl J Med 347:1143-1150, 2002.

Lane D, Manucci PM, Bauer KA et al: Inherited thrombophilia: Part 1. Thromb Haemost 76:651-662 ,1996.

PIOPED Investigators: Value of ventilation/perfusion scan in acute pulmonary embolism: Results of the prospective investigation of pulmonary embolism diagnosis. JAMA 263:2753-2759, 1990.

Ridker PM, Goldhaber SZ, Danielson E et al: Long-term, low-intensity warfarin therapy for the prevention of recurrent venous thromboembolism. New Engl J Med 348:1425-1434, 2003.

Simonneau G, Sors H, Charbonnier B et al: A comparison of low-molecular-weight heparin with unfractionated heparin for acute pulmonary embolism. New Engl J Med 337:663-669, 1997.

The Columbus Investigators: Low-molecular-weight heparin in the treatment of patients with venous thromboembolism. New Engl J Med 337:657-662, 1997.

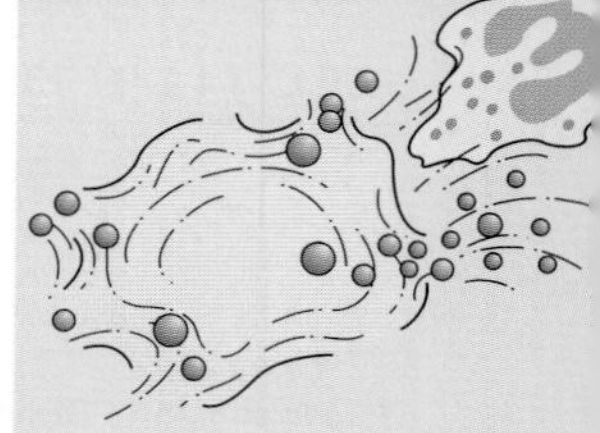

CHAPTER 54 Pulmonary Hypertension

Andrew Jones and Timothy W. Evans

EPIDEMIOLOGY, RISK FACTORS, AND PATHOPHYSIOLOGY

Pulmonary hypertension is defined as a mean pulmonary artery pressure greater than 3.3 kPa (>25 mm Hg) at rest, or greater then 4 kPa (>30 mm Hg) on exercise. Historically, pulmonary hypertension has been classified as primary (idiopathic) or as developing in association with another disease (secondary). Using this approach, conditions that are pathologically and physiologically distinct were classified together merely because their etiologies were unknown. Realization that both the pathologic abnormalities and the response to treatment could be similar in patients with pulmonary hypertension attributable to different etiologies promoted the development of a new World Health Organization (WHO) classification in 1998 (Table 54.1), which also identified known risk factors for the development of the disease (Table 54.2). This chapter reviews pulmonary vascular hypertension, with primary pulmonary hypertension (PPH) being the sine qua non of this condition. Other conditions associated with pulmonary hypertension are mentioned where they are relevant to establishing a diagnosis, but are otherwise discussed in detail elsewhere.

Primary Pulmonary Hypertension

The incidence of PPH is approximately 1 to 2 cases per million population. It can present at any age, but the peak incidence is in the third and fourth decades. In childhood, the sex distribution is almost equal, but in adults the female-to-male ratio is approximately 2 : 1. The pathogenesis of PPH remains a matter of speculation. Current concepts propose that a triggering stimulus in a susceptible individual leads to pulmonary vascular endothelial injury, vasoconstriction, and subsequent repair with vascular remodeling (Fig. 54.1). Genetic susceptibility has long been recognized in familial disease, but accounts for only 6% of the 187 cases in the National Institutes of Health (NIH) registry. More recently, the first PPH gene (*PPH1*)—encoding type II bone morphogenic protein receptor (BMPR2)—has been localized to chromosome 2q31-32. More than 70% of familial cases analyzed show either BMPR2 mutations or linkage to the BMPR2 locus. Moreover, 26% of apparently sporadic cases of PPH also demonstrate germline BMPR2 mutations. Inheritance is believed to occur in an incomplete dominant fashion. The exact role of BMP proteins in the development of PPH remains unknown, but they are known to regulate growth, differentiation, and apoptosis of diverse cell lines, including mesenchymal and epithelial cells. Potassium channel abnormalities have also been described. The resulting membrane depolarization can lead to increased calcium influx, which, in turn, causes vasoconstriction and possibly stimulates vascular smooth muscle proliferation and inhibits apoptosis. Finally, vascular smooth muscle proliferation may be the result of increased expression of a serotonin transport protein resulting from a polymorphism in the promoter region.

Histopathologically, PPH is characterized by intimal fibrosis, in situ thrombosis, and hypertrophy of the smooth muscle cells of the media. Three distinct pathologic patterns have been described:

Plexogenic arteriopathy (30% to 60%) has the worst prognosis and is associated with the plexiform lesion, a mass of disorganized vessels associated with endothelial cells, smooth muscle cells, and myofibroblasts, believed to represent an angiogenic response to vascular injury.

Thrombotic arteriopathy (40% to 50%) is characterized by a vascular histologic appearance similar to that of plexiform arteriopathy, but multiple thrombi are prominent, possibly developing owing to endothelial injury. This entity may explain the benefits of anticoagulation in patients with PPH.

Veno-occlusive disease (<10%) appears to be a separate condition in which the predominant histopathologic changes are occlusive intimal lesions that occur in the pulmonary veins, with arterialization of these vessels. Although rare, it is important to diagnose because the use of intravenous vasodilators can be fatal.

The endothelium is thought to play a central role in the development of PPH, perhaps through its ability to elaborate a number of vasoactive mediators. An imbalance between the production of vasoconstrictor and vasodilator substances could result in vasoconstriction. The endothelium is also intimately involved in the control of platelet function and coagulation, and endothelial cell damage may lead to a prothrombotic state in the pulmonary vasculature and in situ thrombosis. In addition, endothelial cell products may modulate vascular remodeling—for example, endothelin-1 is known to promote smooth muscle cell proliferation, and nitric oxide (NO) and epoprostenol may have opposing effects. Other factors are also likely to be involved in the pathobiology, including chemokines such as interleukin-1 and growth factors such as transforming growth factor-β and fibroblast growth factor.

Other Conditions Associated with Pulmonary Arterial Hypertension

CONNECTIVE TISSUE DISORDERS

Pulmonary arteriopathy may develop in association with many connective tissue disorders, including systemic sclerosis (particularly the "CREST" variant of calcinosis cutis, Raynaud's

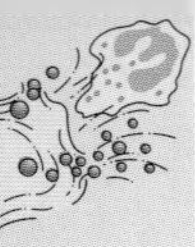

Table 54.1
World Health Organization classification of pulmonary hypertension

1. **Pulmonary arterial hypertension**
   1.1 Primary pulmonary hypertension
   a) Sporadic
   b) Familial
   1.2 Related to:
   a) Collagen vascular disease
   b) Congenital systemic–pulmonary shunts
   c) Portal hypertension
   d) Human immunodeficiency virus infection
   e) Drugs/toxins
   1) Anorexigenics
   2) Other
   f) Persistent pulmonary hypertension of the newborn
   g) Other
2. **Pulmonary venous hypertension**
   2.1 Left-sided atrial or ventricular heart disease
   2.2 Left-sided valvular heart disease
   2.3 Extrinsic compression of central pulmonary veins
   a) Fibrosing mediastinitis
   b) Adenopathy/tumors
   2.4 Pulmonary veno-occlusive disease
   2.5 Other
3. **Pulmonary hypertension associated with disorders of the respiratory system and/or hypoxemia**
   3.1 Chronic obstructive pulmonary disease
   3.2 Interstitial lung disease
   3.3 Sleep-disordered breathing
   3.4 Alveolar hypoventilation disorders
   3.5 Chronic exposure to high altitude
   3.6 Neonatal lung disease
   3.7 Alveolar-capillary dysplasia
   3.8 Other
4. **Pulmonary hypertension due to chronic thrombotic and/or embolic disease**
   4.1 Thromboembolic obstruction of proximal pulmonary arteries
   4.2 Obstruction of distal pulmonary arteries
   a) Pulmonary embolus (thrombus, tumor, ova and/or parasites, foreign material)
   b) In situ thrombosis
   c) Sickle cell disease
5. **Pulmonary hypertension due to disorders directly affecting the pulmonary circulation**
   5.1 Inflammatory
   a) Schistosomiasis
   b) Sarcoidosis
   c) Other
   5.2 Pulmonary capillary hemangiomatosis

Table 54.2
World Health Organization classification of risk factors for pulmonary hypertension

A. Drugs and toxins
   1. Definite
   Aminorex
   Fenfluramine
   Toxic rapeseed
   2. Very likely
   Amphetamines
   L-Tryptophan
   3. Possible
   Methamphetamines
   Cocaine
   Chemotherapeutic agents
   4. Unlikely
   Antidepressants
   Oral contraceptives
   Estrogen therapy
   Cigarette smoking
B. Demographic and medical conditions
   1. Definite
   Sex
   2. Possible
   Pregnancy
   Systemic hypertension
   3. Unlikely
   Obesity
C. Diseases
   1. Definite
   Human immunodeficiency virus infection
   2. Very likely
   Portal hypertension/liver disease
   Collagen vascular disease
   Congenital systemic–pulmonary cardiac shunts
   3. Possible
   Thyroid disorders

disease, esophageal dysmotility, sclerodactyly, and telangiectasis), systemic lupus erythematosus, mixed connective tissue disease, and, to a lesser extent, rheumatoid arthritis, polymyositis, and dermatomyositis. The strongest association seems to be with disorders associated with Raynaud's disease, which occurs exclusively in women and often predates the development of pulmonary hypertension. Histologic findings may be indistinguishable from those seen in PPH. In view of the high incidence of pulmonary hypertension in this patient group, and the difficulty in making an early diagnosis, the WHO recommends that echocardiography be performed annually in all patients with limited systemic sclerosis, regardless of symptoms.

PORTAL HYPERTENSION

Pulmonary hypertension has been reported in 2% to 10% of patients admitted with hepatic cirrhosis. The etiology is unknown, but cirrhosis without the presence of portal hypertension does not seem to be related to the development of pulmonary hypertension. An endogenous or exogenous vasoconstrictor in the splanchnic circulation may bypass the liver, thereby affecting the pulmonary vasculature. It has not been possible to produce pulmonary hypertension by surgically creating portal hypertension in animal models, however.

HUMAN IMMUNODEFICIENCY VIRUS

Severe pulmonary hypertension, clinically indistinguishable from PPH, can develop in human immunodeficiency virus–infected individuals (estimated incidence, 0.5%). Although pulmonary hypertension develops more frequently in those infected through intravenous drug abuse, no clear etiologic link has been established with either foreign body embolus or portal hypertension related to cirrhosis from hepatitis C and B infection.

DRUG- OR TOXIN-INDUCED PULMONARY HYPERTENSION

In the late 1960s, a 20-fold increase in the incidence of unexplained pulmonary hypertension was seen after the introduction of the appetite suppressant aminorex fumarate in Switzerland, Austria, and West Germany. Histologically, the condition was indistinguishable from the plexogenic arteriopathy of PPH. Aminorex resembles ephedrine and amphetamine in structure, and the release of catecholamines from endogenous stores was suggested as a cause, although attempts to reproduce chronic

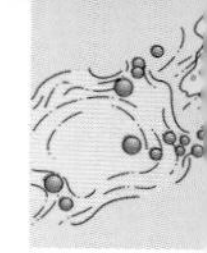

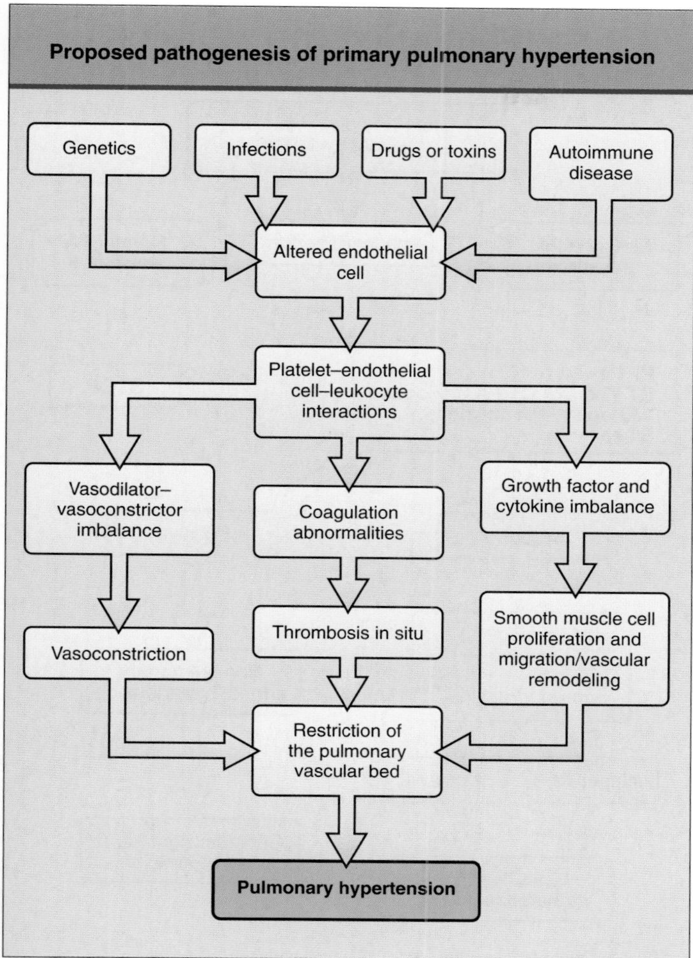

Figure 54.1 Proposed pathogenesis of primary pulmonary hypertension.

pulmonary hypertension with prolonged administration of aminorex to animals failed. Moreover, pulmonary hypertension developed in only 2% of all patients who took aminorex. Pulmonary hypertension has also been reported in association with use of the anorexic agents fenfluramine and dexfenfluramine. These agents are now either used within strict guidelines or, in certain countries, have been withdrawn from clinical use.

An epidemic of a previously unrecognized multisystem disorder that occurred in Spain in 1981 was related subsequently to the ingestion of illegally marketed rapeseed oil. The syndrome presented initially as pneumonia, but patients failed to respond to conventional therapy. A second stage of fever, myalgia, and neurologic deficits followed, and a later stage resembled scleroderma. Follow-up studies found that pulmonary hypertension developed in 8% of patients thus afflicted, although in most cases it regressed with time, and a malignant or progressive form developed in only 2%. Pathologically, the condition most closely resembled pulmonary venous occlusive disease. The toxin responsible was not identified, although oleoanilides or their metabolites were implicated.

L-Tryptophan is a food supplement used for ailments such as premenstrual syndrome, insomnia, and depression. After an epidemic in New Mexico in 1989, it has been linked with a syndrome characterized by diffuse myalgia, fatigue, and blood eosinophilia, with the later development of polyneuropathy, scleroderma-like skin changes, and pulmonary complications. The latter include eosinophilic infiltrates and effusions, vasculitis, interstitial disease, and chronic pulmonary hypertension with a frequency of 5% to 7%. Tryptophan is produced by the action of bacteria on several nutrients, including anthranilic acid, a compound similar to aniline, which was strongly implicated in the pathogenesis of the syndrome seen with rapeseed oil.

Solvent abuse and inhalation of crack cocaine have been associated with the development of pulmonary hypertension.

The role of genetic susceptibility in the development of pulmonary arterial hypertension (PAH) is strengthened by the fact that not all of those who are exposed to the aforementioned triggers acquire the condition.

PATHOPHYSIOLOGY

The normal pulmonary circulation is a high-flow, low-resistance system, and blood flow can increase threefold to fivefold with minimal changes in pulmonary artery pressures because of recruitment and distention of the pulmonary vasculature. Under normal conditions, the right ventricle is a thin-walled cavity that can accommodate large changes in venous return with little change in filling pressures, but is poorly equipped to generate significant systolic pressures. Prolonged pulmonary hypertension reduces the cross-sectional area and the distensibility of the pulmonary vasculature, resulting in increased pulmonary vascular resistance and right ventricular afterload. Initially, cardiac output may remain normal at rest through a compensatory tachycardia and right ventricular hypertrophy, but fails to increase appropriately with exercise. Increased heart rate and systolic pressures may compromise right ventricular myocardial blood flow, which results in right ventricular ischemia. Eventually, cardiac output falls, even at rest, as right ventricular afterload increases further. Increased right ventricular pressures can, in addition, cause septal shift and impair left ventricular filling and performance. Fluid retention occurs secondary to the low output state, which results in peripheral edema, hepatic congestion, and ascites. Most patients die from right ventricular failure, but sudden death is seen in approximately 7%. Common precipitating events are believed to be arrhythmias and pulmonary emboli.

CLINICAL FEATURES

History

Early diagnosis of pulmonary hypertension is difficult and requires a high index of suspicion because of the nonspecific nature of the symptoms and the subtle findings on physical examination. Patients are therefore frequently misdiagnosed, and are identified only when the later and more severe stages of the condition have been reached. In the NIH registry of PPH, the mean length of time from onset of first symptoms to diagnosis was more than 2 years. Dyspnea is the presenting complaint in 60% of patients, and is eventually reported by virtually all as the disease progresses. It may be graded I to IV according to the New York Heart Association (NYHA) criteria, which reflect both the severity of the pulmonary hypertension and the prognosis. Fatigue is common. Angina occurs in 47% of patients, and is usually caused by right ventricular ischemia. Coronary

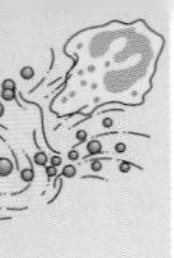

angiography usually is negative. Syncope or presyncope, especially on exertion, is an ominous complaint, and indicates severe limitation of cardiac output.

Physical Examination

Careful examination may alert the physician to other causes of "non–pulmonary arterial" pulmonary hypertension (see Table 54.1) or may establish the presence of PAH associated with other systemic disease processes. Establishing an accurate diagnosis has important implications for therapy. Physical findings due to pulmonary hypertension may be few and subtle in the earliest stages of the condition. With progression, tachycardia occurs, with a low-volume pulse. Poor peripheral perfusion results in cold extremities, with peripheral cyanosis. Central cyanosis is common, but finger clubbing is not a feature of PPH, and its presence should alert the examiner to consider other conditions that result in pulmonary hypertension. The jugular venous pressure is often raised, frequently with cannon v waves resulting from tricuspid regurgitation. A parasternal heave may be found on palpation, along with a palpable pulmonary component of the second heart sound (P_2). Auscultation reveals a loud P_2, and right ventricular gallops (i.e., S_3 or S_4) are present in more severe cases. Tricuspid regurgitation is very common, and evidence may also be found for pulmonary valvular insufficiency (i.e., Graham Steell's murmur, resulting from dilatation of the pulmonary valve ring). Peripheral edema and ascites may be present in severe disease.

DIAGNOSIS

Once the suspicion of pulmonary hypertension has been raised, subsequent investigation has three specific aims:

1. *To identify* or exclude all known causes of the condition because different therapeutic strategies may apply depending on etiology
2. *To confirm* and document the severity of the pulmonary hypertension
3. *To assess* the response to vasodilator therapy

An appropriate approach is presented in Figure 54.2.

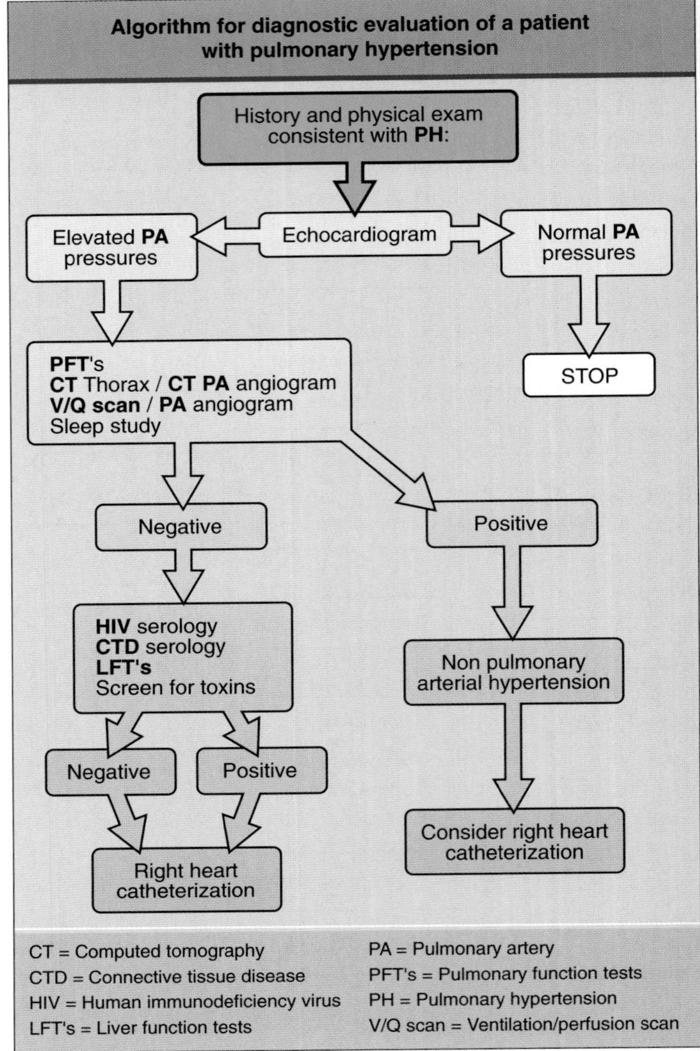

Figure 54.2 Algorithm for diagnostic evaluation of patients with pulmonary hypertension.

Electrocardiogram

The electrocardiogram typically shows right-axis deviation with evidence of right ventricular hypertrophy and strain, although the degree of these changes does not always reflect the severity of the pulmonary hypertension.

Echocardiography

Transthoracic echocardiography is important to exclude cardiac causes of pulmonary hypertension, as well as to provide a noninvasive estimation of right ventricular function and pulmonary artery pressure. Typically, right ventricular and right atrial enlargement are apparent, with a normal left ventricular cavity size. In severe cases, intraventricular septal curvature may be reversed and the left ventricular cavity compromised. Pulmonary and tricuspid regurgitation are identified and quantified using Doppler techniques, the latter of which permits the noninvasive estimation of pulmonary artery pressures (pulmonary arterial pressure $\approx 4v^2 +$ right atrial pressure, where v is velocity). Such studies also provide an index of disease progression, removing the need for repeated right heart catheterizations. Although more invasive and more expensive, transesophageal echocardiography provides a superior assessment of structural cardiac defects, and may be used to exclude proximal (large) pulmonary thromboembolism.

Chest Radiography

The chest radiograph may reveal abnormalities suggestive of an alternative diagnosis as the cause of the pulmonary hypertension (e.g., emphysema, interstitial lung disease). Chest radiography shows abnormalities in over 90% of cases of PPH. Prominence of the main pulmonary arteries (90%), enlargement of the hilar vessels (80%), and peripheral pruning (51%) are the most common abnormalities (Fig. 54.3). Of patients enrolled in the NIH registry, only 6% had a negative chest radiograph.

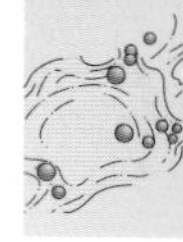

Pulmonary Function Tests

Mild restrictive defects and evidence of small airways dysfunction can be seen in PPH, but the main role of pulmonary function testing is to exclude parenchymal lung disease as an underlying cause of the pulmonary hypertension. Significant impairment of gas exchange may occur in PPH, with reduced transfer capacity of the lung for carbon monoxide, hypoxemia, hypocapnia secondary to alveolar hyperventilation, and an increased alveolar–arterial oxygen (P_{AO_2}–Pa_{O_2}) gradient. Severe hypoxemia in PPH may result from intracardiac shunting caused by a patent foramen ovale, or may be a consequence of severely depressed cardiac output with resultant mixed venous hypoxemia.

Cardiopulmonary Exercise Test

Cardiopulmonary exercise studies show reduced maximal oxygen consumption, increased minute ventilation, low anaerobic threshold, a large amount of dead space that fails to decrease with progressive exercise, and increased P_{AO_2}–Pa_{O_2} that widens with progressive exercise. The specificity and sensitivity of such findings for pulmonary hypertension remain to be determined, however.

Lung Scanning

Ventilation–perfusion scintigraphy is essential to exclude chronic thromboembolic disease. The scan is typically negative in PAH or displays only minor, patchy perfusion defects. In patients who have pulmonary hypertension as a result of thromboembolic disease, at least one, but often several, major segmental or subsegmental mismatches in ventilation–perfusion relationships are seen (Figs. 54.4 and 54.5). A negative or low-probability scan effectively excludes thromboembolic disease. In uncertain cases, pulmonary angiography or, increasingly, contrast-enhanced spiral computed tomography (CT) may be obtained.

If the lung scan shows one or more segmental ventilation–perfusion mismatches, pulmonary angiography should be performed to exclude chronic thromboembolic disease (Fig. 54.6). In experienced hands the procedure is quite

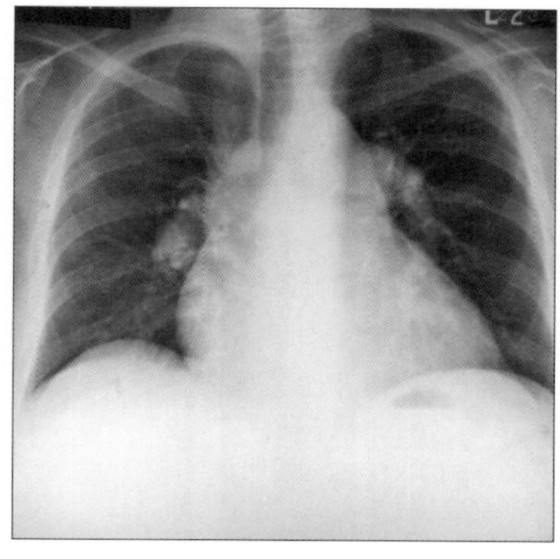

Figure 54.3 Chest radiograph in primary pulmonary hypertension. Note enlargement of the proximal pulmonary arteries (spurious cardiomegaly caused by poor inspiration).

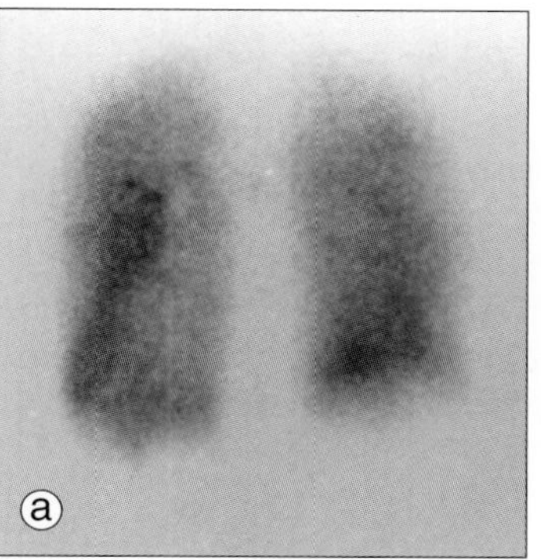

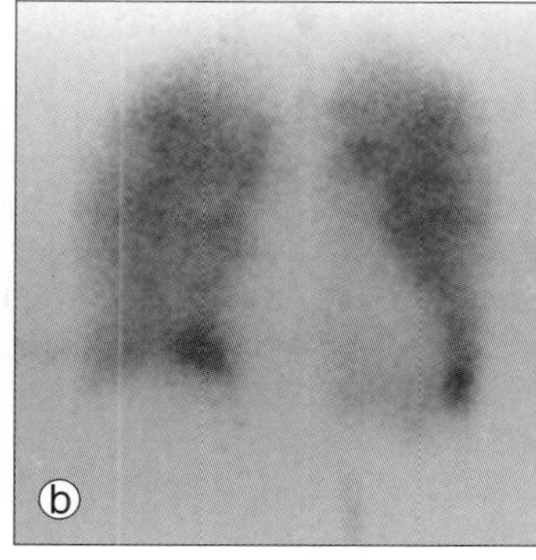

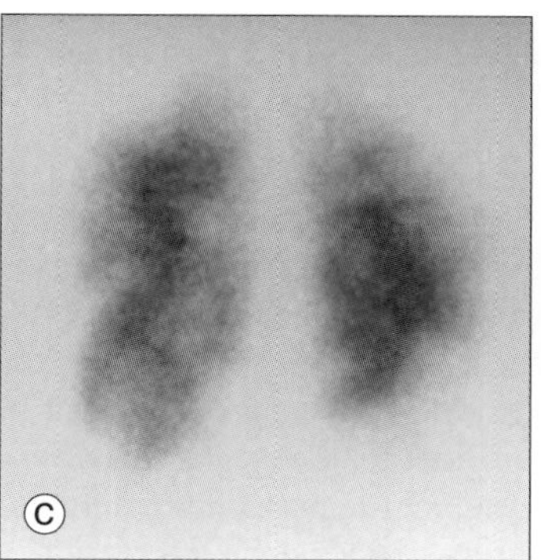

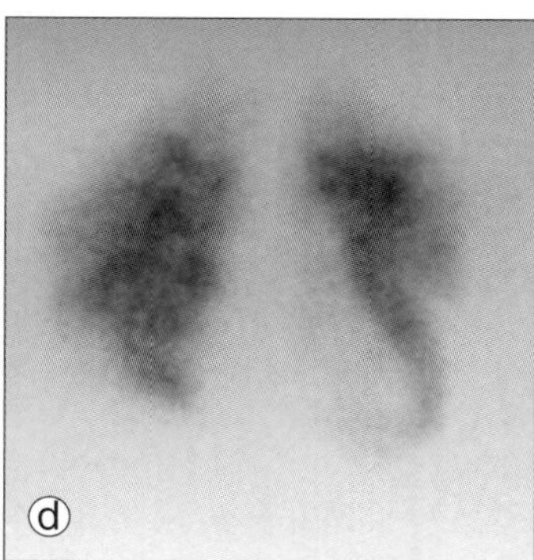

Figure 54.4 Typical ventilation–perfusion scan in primary pulmonary hypertension. Ventilation scan **(A)**, perfusion scan **(B)**, and patchy subsegmental perfusion defects **(C)**.

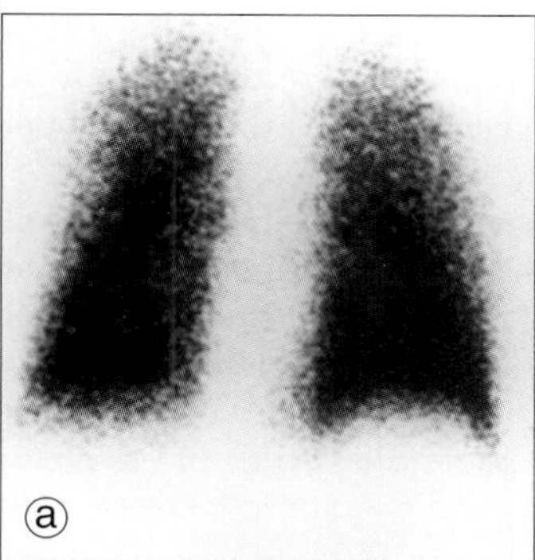

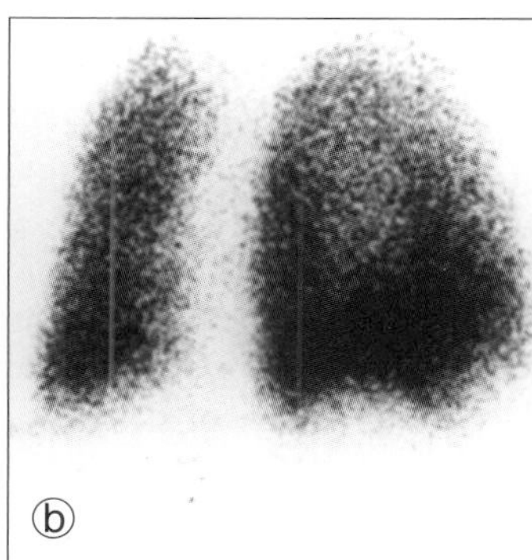

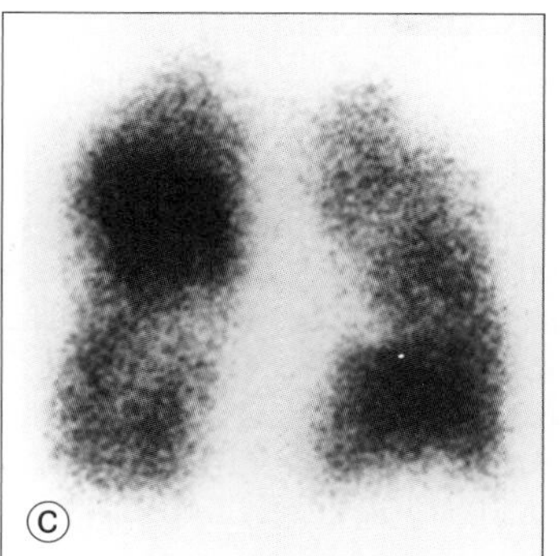

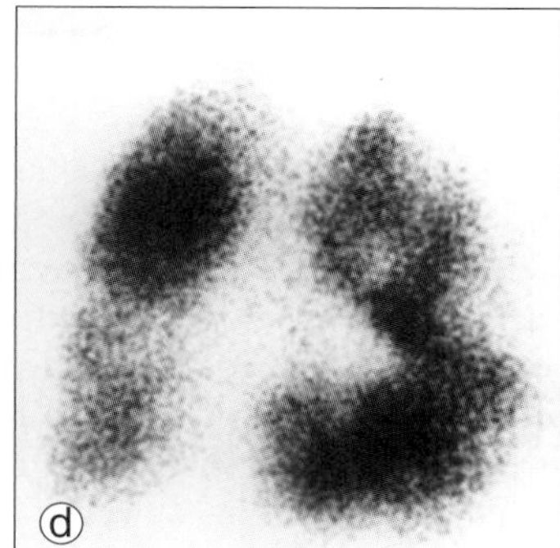

Figure 54.5 Chronic thromboembolic hypertension. Multiple **(A)**, segmental **(B)**, and larger perfusion defects **(C** and **D)**.

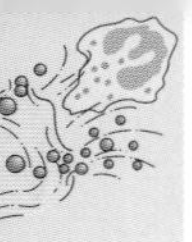

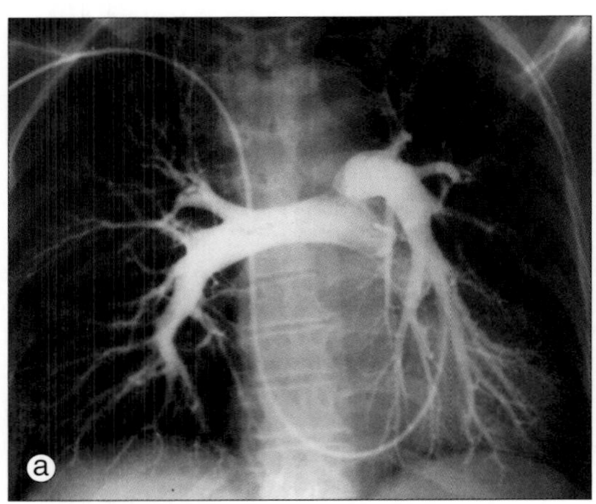

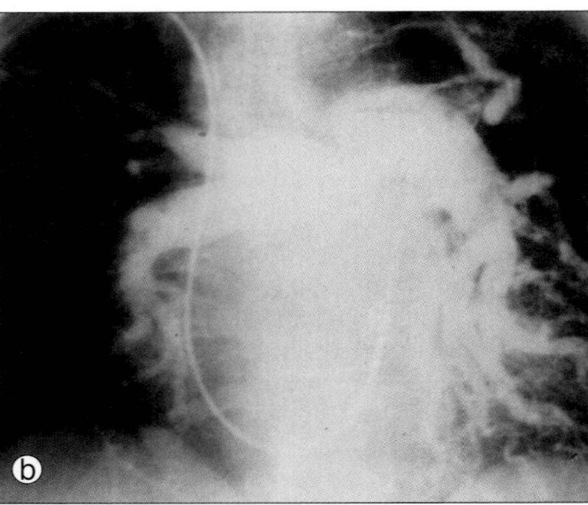

Figure 54.6 Pulmonary angiograms. **A**, Normal, **B**, in primary pulmonary hypertension with marked peripheral pruning of pulmonary vasculature.

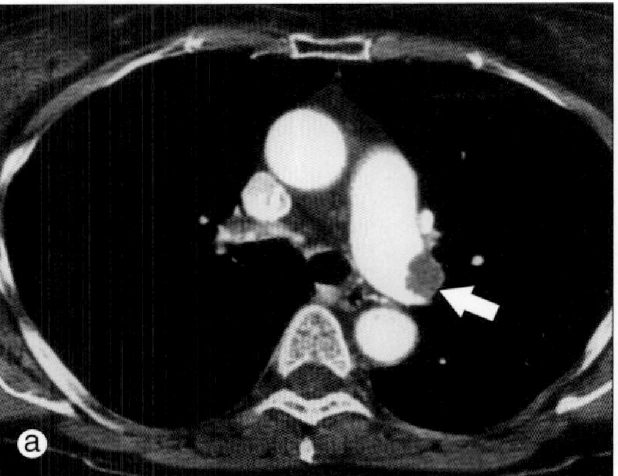

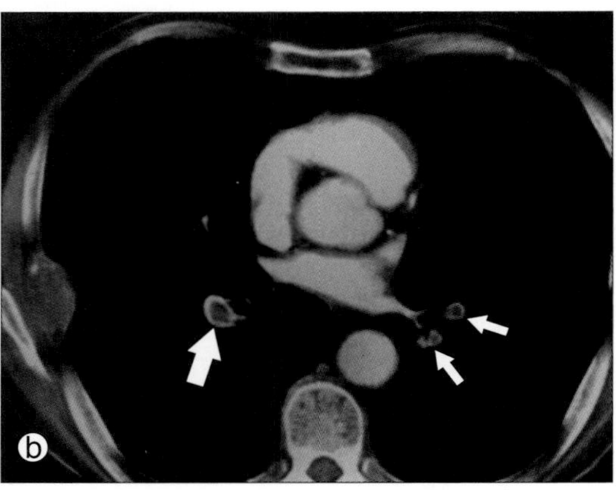

Figure 54.7 Spiral computed tomography. A, Massive filling defect in the main pulmonary artery (*arrow*). **B,** Filling defects in lobar (*large arrow*) and segmental (*small arrows*) pulmonary arteries.

safe, even in patients who have high pulmonary pressures and low cardiac outputs.

Computed Tomography

Recent experience indicates that contrast-enhanced, continuous-volume (i.e., spiral) CT scanning provides a less invasive alternative to lung scans for investigating suspected pulmonary thromboembolic disease because thrombi in the proximal pulmonary arteries can be readily identified. This test can also be combined with high-resolution CT to exclude parenchymal lung disease as the cause of the pulmonary hypertension. Interpretation of spiral CT images may be highly observer dependent, however, and only sixth- or seventh-generation pulmonary arteries can be visualized with confidence (Fig. 54.7).

Heart Catheterization

Pulmonary arterial catheterization is an essential procedure, not only to confirm the presence and degree of pulmonary hypertension but to guide therapy and estimate prognosis. Pulmonary arterial pressures are often increased to three times normal, right atrial pressure is elevated, and cardiac output is reduced. Pulmonary capillary occlusion pressure is usually normal in PAH, and may not be elevated even in pulmonary venous obstructive disease because of the patchy nature of this condition. In the setting of severe right ventricular dilatation, left ventricular filling can be reduced and left ventricular end-diastolic pressure and left atrial pressure may be elevated.

Serology

Antinuclear antibody testing is frequently positive in patients with PPH (29% in the NIH registry), despite the absence of connective tissue disease. These are usually of a nonspecific pattern, and are present in low titers. Strongly positive serology should lead to further, more specific serologic testing to exclude PAH related to connective tissue disease because in such cases, therapeutic strategies for other systemic conditions may need to be considered.

TREATMENT

General

Treatment of pulmonary hypertension centers around therapy for any associated condition, and for the pulmonary hypertension itself. Here we describe therapies directed specifically at the treatment of significant PAH, using PPH as the main model because of its prominence in clinical studies (Fig. 54.8).

The rarity and life-threatening nature of severe PAH, as well as the complexities of therapy suggest that patients are more likely to be optimally managed if they are referred to regional centers that have greater experience with the condition. Education is a critical aspect of care because patients must live as active a life as possible but at the same time avoid excess physical exertion, which can abruptly and markedly increase pulmonary artery pressure and precipitate arrhythmias. Altitude, with its associated hypoxia, must be avoided. Commercial air

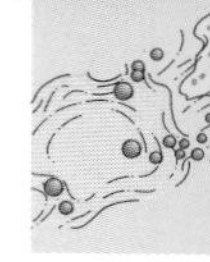

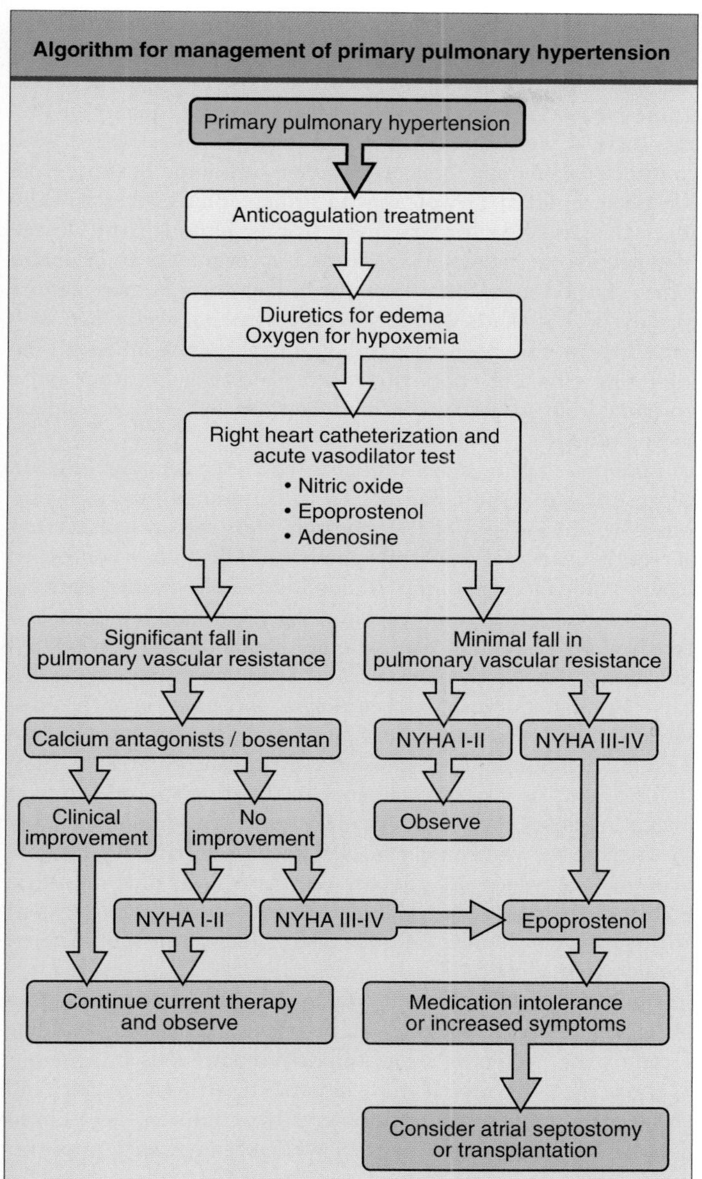

Figure 54.8 Algorithm for management of primary pulmonary hypertension.

travel is usually safe for those with mild or moderate disease, although supplementary oxygen should be available, and a fitness-to-fly test before the trip should be considered. Pregnancy, in particular the postpartum period, is poorly tolerated and effective birth control is therefore essential. Oral contraceptives are now thought unlikely to be implicated in the development of PAH. Women who do become pregnant, however, should be referred to centers with high-risk obstetrical expertise.

If right ventricular failure develops, with the resultant hepatic congestion and peripheral edema, diuretics are warranted, but these must be prescribed with caution because right ventricular performance is highly dependent on preload and overaggressive diuresis may markedly reduce cardiac output. If diuresis cannot be accomplished without diminishing cardiac output, the discomfort and problems that result from edema may be controlled with compressive stockings extended at least to the midthigh.

The use of cardiac glycosides in PAH is controversial. Some investigators recommend their use to improve right ventricular performance, whereas others use them to counteract the negative inotropic effects of calcium channel blocking agents when the latter are used as pulmonary vasodilators. The risk of digitalis toxicity may be aggravated by the concomitant use of diuretics in this group of patients.

There is no role for routine long-term oxygen administration unless patients are hypoxemic. Supplemental oxygen may, however, reduce dyspnea and improve exercise tolerance and is recommended for symptom control in more severely affected patients.

Anticoagulation

Extensive thrombosis is a common histopathologic finding in patients with PPH. Patients with severe PAH are also at increased risk of thromboembolic events because of diminished venous return, high right-sided filling pressures, a dilated and poorly contracting right ventricle, reduced pulmonary blood flow, and reduced activity. Even a small embolic event may have serious consequences because of the lack of pulmonary vascular reserve. Although evidence is limited to the results of a large, retrospective study, and a recent small, nonrandomized, prospective study, both found that patients treated with oral anticoagulants had an improved survival compared with those who were not. Warfarin is the anticoagulant of choice, with doses adjusted to achieve an international normalized ratio of 2 to 3. In patients who experience adverse effects from warfarin or in those with an increased risk of bleeding, twice-daily subcutaneous heparin may be an alternative. Initial studies suggest that low–molecular-weight heparins cause fewer long-term side effects (e.g., osteoporosis, thrombocytopenia).

Vasodilator Therapy

Vasodilators are used on the premise that vasoconstriction is an important contributor to the pathophysiologic process of the condition. Unfortunately, there is no way noninvasively to predict which patients are likely to respond to treatment, and the agents used are all associated with considerable morbidity and mortality. The standard approach is to administer a potent, short-acting, titratable vasodilator during pulmonary artery catheterization and monitor the result. The effects of such a drug should be confined to the pulmonary circulation. Because these acute pharmacologic tests are not without risk, they must be performed by experienced clinicians in an appropriate setting. Repeated measurements of pulmonary artery and right atrial pressures, systemic blood pressure, arterial oxygenation, and cardiac output are made in response to increasing doses of the test drug. In theory, the short half-lives and relative pulmonary selectivity of the agents used enable any adverse effects to be reversed quickly by discontinuing the drug. Several vasodilators have been used in this way, including inhaled NO, intravenous epoprostenol, and intravenous adenosine (Table 54.3). In general, the acute response is useful in predicting the response to longer-acting, orally administered compounds (see later). The use of empirical oral vasodilator therapy,

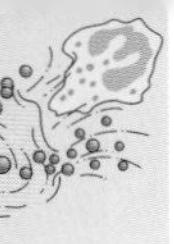

Table 54.3
Vasodilators frequently used in the investigation and management of primary pulmonary hypertension

Drug	Route	Dose range	Half-life
Epoprostenol[a]	Intravenous	2–20 ng/kg of body weight/minute	3–5 min
Adenosine	Intravenous	50–200 mg/kg of body weight/minute	5–10 sec
Nitric oxide	Inhaled	5–80 parts per million	15–30 sec
Nifedipine[b]	Oral	30–240 mg/day	2–5 hr
Diltiazem[b]	Oral	120–900 mg/day	2–4.5 hr
Bosentan	Oral	125–500 mg/day	4–5 hr

[a]The dose range shown is for a short-term infusion; the dose range for long-term infusions often exceeds 100–150 ng/kg per minute.
[b]The half-life shown refers to conventional preparations; sustained-release preparations may be administered once daily.

without prior acute vasoreactivity testing, is strongly to be discouraged.

CALCIUM CHANNEL BLOCKERS

The calcium channel antagonists nifedipine and diltiazem have been the most commonly used agents for long-term vasodilator therapy. The dose required to produce a beneficial response tends to greater than that usually used to treat systemic hypertension or coronary artery disease (see Table 54.3), although a wide variation exists in requirement and tolerance between individual patients. Verapamil has marked negative inotropic effects and should be avoided. The main limitations to therapy are systemic hypotension, peripheral edema, and hypoxia due to increased ventilation–perfusion mismatch. More severe adverse effects, including arrhythmias, cardiogenic shock, and death, have been reported.

ENDOTHELIN-1 RECEPTOR ANTAGONISTS

More encouraging has been the use of the dual endothelin receptor antagonist bosentan. When given orally in doses up to 250 mg/day in divided doses, bosentan improves cardiopulmonary hemodynamics, exercise tolerance, dyspnea score, and WHO functional class. The therapy is well tolerated, with asymptomatic elevation of liver function test results noted in a small number of patients. The use of an endothelin antagonist has theoretical advantages in addition to initial vasodilatory effect because endothelin-1 is also believed to play an important role in inflammation, proliferation, fibrosis, and bronchoconstriction in the lung, and it is likely that some, if not all, of these processes are involved in the pathobiology of PAH. At present, bosentan is indicated for the treatment of patients with stable functional class III or IV disease. A study is under way to assess possible synergy with epoprostenol.

PROSTACYCLIN ANALOGS

Epoprostenol, the synthetic analog of prostaglandin I_2, has selective vasodilatory effects on the pulmonary circulation when given intravenously. In a 3-month, randomized, open-label trial, patients with NYHA grade III or IV dyspnea were treated with a continuous infusion of epoprostenol (in addition to standard therapy, which included oral vasodilators). Improved hemodynamic parameters and better exercise tolerance, quality of life, and survival were found compared with patients treated with conventional therapy. Longer-term hemodynamic benefits have also been reported, as well as echocardiographic evidence of the reversal of right ventricular hypertrophy, although the dosage may need to be increased for these improvements to be maintained. Importantly, improvements in long-term hemodynamics may occur in patients who receive epoprostenol even when they have little or no vasodilatory response to the acute infusion. The inhibiting effect of epoprostenol on platelet aggregation and a potential role in vascular remodeling are believed to explain these findings.

Epoprostenol must be administered by continuous infusion because it has a short half-life (3 to 5 minutes) and is inactivated by the low pH of the stomach. This requires placement and maintenance of a central venous catheter that is connected to a portable infusion pump. Minor adverse effects are relatively common, including flushing, skin rashes, joint and jaw pain, and diarrhea. More serious adverse effects include catheter-related infections, venous thrombosis, and pump malfunction, which can result in underdosing or overdosing. Interruption of the infusion because of pump failure or line occlusion may lead to rebound pulmonary hypertension, which can be fatal. In addition, patients do develop tolerance to the drug and may require increasing doses over time. As a result of these difficulties, only those patients who remain in NYHA classes III or IV, despite maximal "conventional" therapy (i.e., anticoagulants, diuretics, oral vasodilators, cardiac glycosides, and supplemental oxygen) are usually considered candidates for long-term epoprostenol therapy (see Table 54.3).

Iloprost is a stable prostacyclin analog with a longer duration of vasodilatation. It can be given by inhalation, thereby avoiding some of the problems associated with continuous intravenous epoprostenol. In a recent study in patients with severe PAH and chronic thromboembolic pulmonary hypertension, aerosolized iloprost (six to nine times a day) was associated with improvements in pulmonary hemodynamics, NYHA class, exercise capacity, dyspnea, and quality of life. No direct comparison between iloprost and intravenous epoprostenol has been performed. At the time of writing, iloprost is not available in the United States.

Treprostinil, a second prostacyclin analog administered by continuous subcutaneous infusion, has been shown to improve 6-minute walking distance, dyspnea, and hemodynamics in patients with PAH, benefits that have been sustained for up to 18 months. Unfortunately, pain at the site of injection is common and may be severe. Moreover, pump disconnection may have catastrophic consequences and gastrointestinal bleeding has been reported.

The only oral prostacyclin analog so far developed, beraprost, improves hemodynamics in short-term pilot studies and, in a retrospective analysis, it also improved exercise tolerance, hemodynamics, and survival up to 3 years after the initiation of therapy compared with control subjects. No controlled trials have been performed using these analogs and no firm recommendations can yet be made regarding their use.

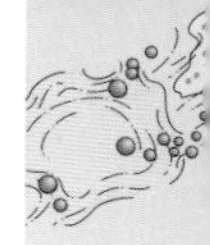

Surgical Treatment

ATRIAL SEPTOSTOMY

In patients who do not respond to maximal medical therapy, creation of an artificial atrial septal defect may be considered. In theory, creating a right-to-left shunt to improve left-sided filling should increase cardiac output. Although the oxygen content of arterial blood falls, the improvement in cardiac output may be sufficient to increase oxygen delivery—the more important parameter. The procedure can be performed by either balloon or blade septostomy. To date, however, a survival benefit has not been demonstrated. As such, this procedure should be performed only in experienced centers and in patients with severe symptoms (e.g., recurrent syncope, intractable right heart failure) despite maximal therapy, in whom transplantation is the only other therapeutic option.

TRANSPLANTATION

Before the emergence of epoprostenol, heart-lung or lung transplantation was the only treatment option for severe, intractable pulmonary hypertension. Interestingly, there seems to be little difference in efficacy between single-lung, double-lung, and heart-lung transplantation, with survival rates of 70% to 80% at 1 year and 50% to 60% at 3 years with all. Right ventricular remodeling occurs within 3 to 6 months after single-lung transplantation for PAH, suggesting that heart-lung transplantation may not be required. This is an important consideration when the main limitation to transplantation in Western countries is organ availability. This shortage of organs has prompted some centers to undertake live donation from relatives, but the associated ethical and moral dilemmas are considerable.

The main complication after transplantation is obliterative bronchiolitis. To date, no recurrence of PPH in the transplanted lung has been reported. With transplantation comes the onerous requirement for continuous immunosuppression and its risks. The decision of when to perform transplantation is difficult, especially in light of the improved survival seen with recently introduced medical therapies. This, in addition to the relative shortage of suitable organs, has led to the general recommendation that transplantation should be considered only in those patients who are unable to tolerate epoprostenol, or in whom progressive right ventricular failure develops despite its use.

CLINICAL COURSE AND PREVENTION

Historically, the course of PPH was one of unrelenting, progressive deterioration, with a median survival of 2.5 years. After the introduction of newer therapies, however, survival has improved. Long-term anticoagulation seems to double the predicted 3-year survival, and patients who respond to calcium channel blockers have a 5-year survival rate approaching 95%. Continuous intravenous infusion of epoprostenol in patients with NYHA class III and IV disease doubled their 5-year survival rate compared with historical control subjects (54% versus 27%).

Several factors identifiable at presentation predict shorter survival, including:

- Higher pulmonary vascular resistance and pressures
- Absence of a favorable response to vasodilator therapy
- Worse NYHA classification
- Elevated right atrial pressure
- Decreased cardiac output (<2 L/min/m)
- Pulmonary arterial oxygen saturation less than 63%
- Shorter distance walked in the 6-minute walking test

PITFALLS AND CONTROVERSIES

Classification

Misclassification of pulmonary hypertension remains the greatest pitfall. It is essential that all associated conditions be vigorously sought and excluded because the distinction between PAH and other causes of pulmonary hypertension has important implications regarding management and prognosis.

Screening

Because of its nonspecific presentation, the diagnosis of PPH is often delayed. Prognosis, however, probably depends on making a diagnosis early when the pulmonary circulation is compliant and responsive to vasodilator therapy. Until recently, full assessment of the pulmonary circulation required right heart catheterization, which is not without risk. However, the advent of widely available echocardiography has transformed our ability to screen patients at risk for development of pulmonary hypertension. The recent WHO classification provides a useful stratification of risk that can be used as a basis for screening patients in whom pulmonary hypertension may develop (see Table 54.2).

Angiography

Misinterpretation of pulmonary angiograms is another important pitfall because of the possibility that central thrombi caused by the low cardiac output state can be seen in PPH. Accordingly, angiography should be performed and interpreted only by physicians experienced in the study of patients who have PPH.

Anticoagulation

With progressive disease, right-sided heart failure may lead to hepatic congestion, which can impair hepatic function and alter the extent of anticoagulation observed with warfarin therapy. Accordingly, more frequent monitoring of prothrombin times is warranted.

SUGGESTED READINGS

Eddahibi S, Humbert M, Fadel E, et al: Serotonin transporter overexpression is responsible for pulmonary artery smooth muscle hyperplasia in primary pulmonary hypertension. J Clin Invest 108:1141-1150, 2001.

Jeffery TK, Morrell NW: Molecular and cellular basis of pulmonary vascular remodeling in pulmonary hypertension. Prog Cardiovasc Dis 45:173-202, 2002.

Olschewski H, Rose F, Grunig E, et al: Cellular pathophysiology and therapy of pulmonary hypertension. J Lab Clin Med 138:367-377, 2001.

Paramothayan NS, Lasserson TJ, Wells AU, Walters EH: Prostacyclin for pulmonary hypertension. Cochrane Database Syst Rev CD002994, 2002.

Peacock AJ. Primary pulmonary hypertension. Thorax 54:1107-1118, 1999.

Rich S (ed): Primary Pulmonary Hypertension. Executive Summary from the World Symposium. Primary Pulmonary Hypertension. Geneva, World Health Organization, 1998.

Runo JR, Loyd JE: Primary pulmonary hypertension. Lancet 361:1533-1544, 2003.

Sitbon O, Humbert M, Simonneau G: Primary pulmonary hypertension: Current therapy. Prog Cardiovasc Dis 45:115-128, 2002.

Strange JW, Wharton J, Phillips PG, Wilkins MR: Recent insights into the pathogenesis and therapeutics of pulmonary hypertension. Clin Sci (Lond) 102:253-268, 2002.

Trulock EP: Lung transplantation for primary pulmonary hypertension. Clin Chest Med 22:583-593, 2001.

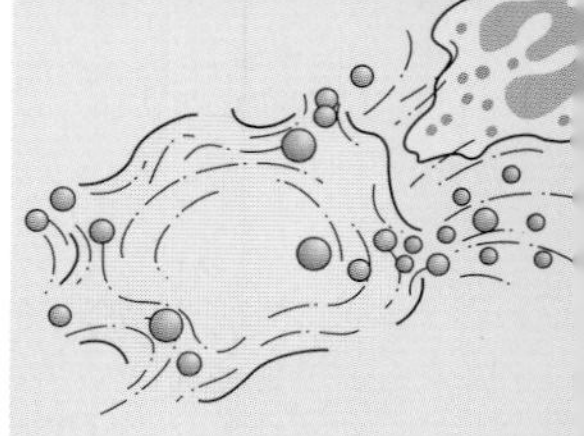

CHAPTER 55 Pulmonary Vasculitis and Hemorrhage

Marvin Schwarz

PULMONARY VASCULITIDES

Epidemiology, Risk Factors, Pathophysiology

The pulmonary vasculitides are one component of a group of systemic disorders (Table 55.1) that are characterized by vascular inflammation, which in turn leads to tissue necrosis and eventual end-organ dysfunction. Although pulmonary vasculitis can complicate an established autoimmune disorder (the connective tissue or collagen vascular diseases) the others conditions listed in Table 55.1 for the most part occur without a definable, underlying precipitating cause. Although this disease category has been recognized for more than 60 years, specific etiologies, or even identifiable risk factors, have not been elucidated. In general, the vasculitides are uncommon conditions and involve the lung with a variable frequency (see Table 55.1). It does appear, however, that the incidence of systemic vasculitis is increasing. This most likely relates to the widespread availability of antineutrophil cytoplasmic antibody (ANCA) testing. These antibodies are found in the serum of four of these disorders (i.e., Wegener's granulomatosis, microscopic polyangiitis, polyarteritis nodosa, and Churg-Strauss syndrome). The projected annual incidence for most of the disorders ranges from 2 to 13 cases per million population.

Vasculitis implies inflammation which can progress to necrosis of the vascular walls. If medium or large sized vessels are involved, infarction, necrosis and end-organ dysfunction will result. When smaller vessels are affected (i.e., capillaries, arterioles, and venules), there is a loss of vascular integrity and leakage of blood into the tissue. When this small-vessel vasculitis occurs in the lung, it is referred to as pulmonary (or alveolar) capillaritis, and results in the clinical syndrome of diffuse alveolar hemorrhage (DAH). When it occurs in the skin it is described as a leukocytoclastic vasculitis and manifests as visible, raised palpable purpura, and sometimes as petechiae. In the kidney, small vessel involvement results in a focal, segmental necrotizing glomerulonephritis, which can be either subclinical (manifesting only as hematuria, red blood cell casts, and proteinuria) or present as renal insufficiency, which can lead to chronic renal insufficiency, sometimes requires dialysis. Any organ system may, however, be affected by the vasculitic process.

A granulomatous vasculitis involving small and medium sized vessels is the characteristic histologic feature of Wegener's granulomatosis. Here, in addition to vascular inflammation and tissue necrosis, there is a necrotizing granulomatous process in the tissue adjacent to, and within the wall of, the affected blood vessel. An area of central necrosis is seen, surrounded by mixed acute and chronic inflammatory cells, palisading histiocytes, and giant cells (Fig. 55.1) is characteristic and most readily apparent in tissue obtained from the lung, which is involved in 75% to 90% of cases. Renal tissue may only show a small-vessel vasculitis (capillaritis) appearing as focal segmental necrotizing glomerulonephritis, often with crescent formation (Fig. 55.2). These renal findings are nonspecific and common to many of the systemic vasculitides.

Another form of systemic vasculitis that often affects the lung and causes granulomatous inflammation is the Churg-Strauss syndrome. Here, the medium- and small-vessel inflammation includes numerous eosinophils and is associated with eosinophilic pneumonia. Giant-cell arteritis, the most common type of vasculitis, is also granulomatous in character; however, it rarely involves the lungs. Necrotizing sarcoidal granulomatosis is another example of a granulomatous vasculitis involving medium sized vessels and has been considered to be a variant of sarcoidosis. Necrotizing sarcoidal granulomatosis only involves the lung. Takayasu arteritis is a large and medium sized vessel vasculitis of a granulomatous nature that infrequently can lead to major pulmonary artery occlusion.

The causes of this group of diseases remain unknown. There is some evidence to suggest that exacerbations in Wegener's granulomatosis are more likely to occur in those patients whose upper respiratory tract is chronically colonized by staphylococci. Similarly, some cases of polyarteritis nodosa, cryoglobulinemia, and microscopic polyangiitis are associated with chronic hepatitis B and C viral infections. Takayasu arteritis is most often seen in young women of Asian descent. Churg-Strauss syndrome follows a several-year prodrome of allergic rhinitis and asthma.

At present, two pathogenetic pathways for the development of systemic vasculitis have been suggested. The first involves development of antibodies to various neutrophil cytoplasmic components or ANCA. In Wegener's granulomatosis more than 85% of patients demonstrate a serum antibody to a serine proteinase (i.e., proteinase 3 or c-ANCA), which is found in neutrophils and macrophages. In microscopic polyangiitis and the Churg-Strauss syndrome, 85% and 45% of patients, respectively, develop antibodies directed against the neutrophil cytoplasmic myeloperoxidase (p-ANCA). Approximately 10% to 20% of cases of polyarteritis nodosa also demonstrate serum p-ANCA; however, lung involvement is rare in this disorder. The c and p prefixes refer to the pattern of immunofluorescent staining, cytoplasmic or perinuclear.

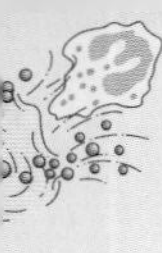

Table 55.1 The systemic vasculitides and relative frequencies of lung involvement

Entity	Serum antineutrophil cytoplasmic antibody	Vessels involved	Cases/million per year	Lung involvement
Takayasu's arteritis	No	L and M	?	Common
Giant cell arteritis	No	L and M	13	Rare
Behçet's syndrome	No	L, M, and S	?	Uncommon
Wegener's granulomatosis	Yes	M and S	3–9	Common
Churg–Strauss syndrome	Yes	M and S	2–3	Common
Polyarteritis nodosa	Yes	M and S	3–4	Rare
Collagen vascular disease	No	M and S	12	Common
Kawasaki's disease	No	M	?	Rare
Necrotizing sarcoid granulomatosis	No	M	?	Common
Microscopic polyangiitis	Yes	S	3	Common
Isolated pauci-immune pulmonary capillaritis	Yes/no	S	?	Common
Henoch–Schönlein purpura	No	S	?	Uncommon
Cryoglobulinemia	No	S	2–3	Rare
Goodpasture's syndrome	Yes/no	S	?	Common

The systemic vasculitidies and their relative frequency of lung involvement. L, large pulmonary arteries (major branches); M, medium sized muscular pulmonary arteries; S, small pulmonary vessels (arterioles, venules, and capillaries); ANCA, antineutrophil cytoplasmic antibody.

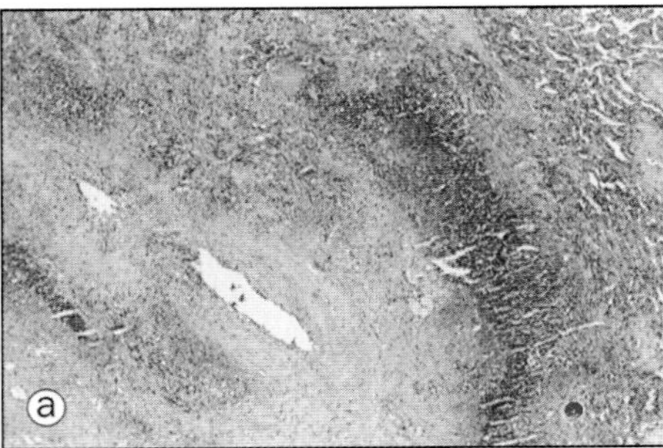

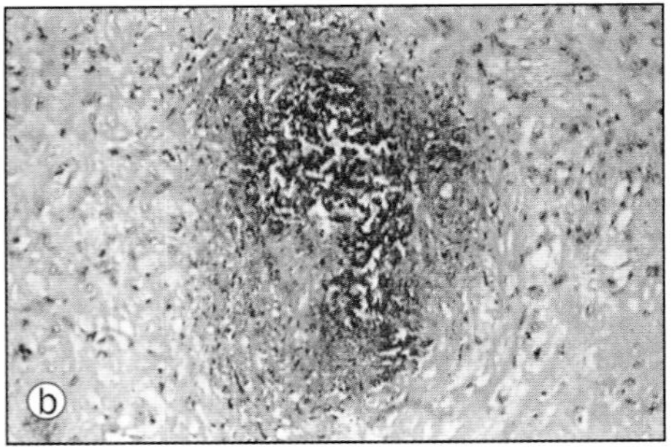

Figure 55.1 Wegener's granulomatosis. **A,** Pulmonary artery demonstrating broadening of the vessel wall resulting from acute and chronic inflammation, cell infiltration, and an area of geographic necrosis outside the vessel, which stains dark blue. **B,** Total destruction of an arteriole with a giant cell visible in the lower right-hand corner.

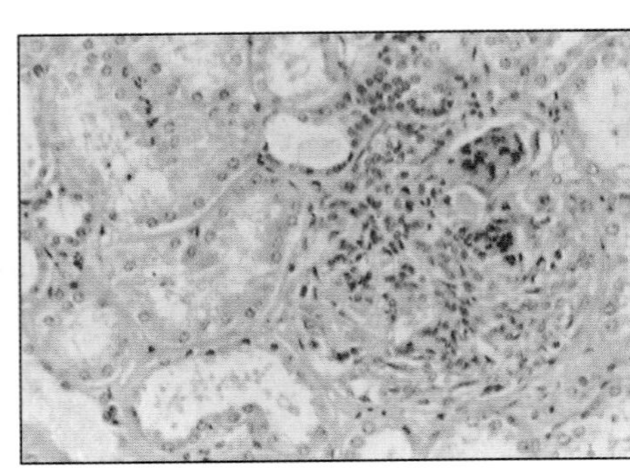

Figure 55.2 Renal biopsy. Focal segmental necrotizing glomerulonephritis with crescent formation.

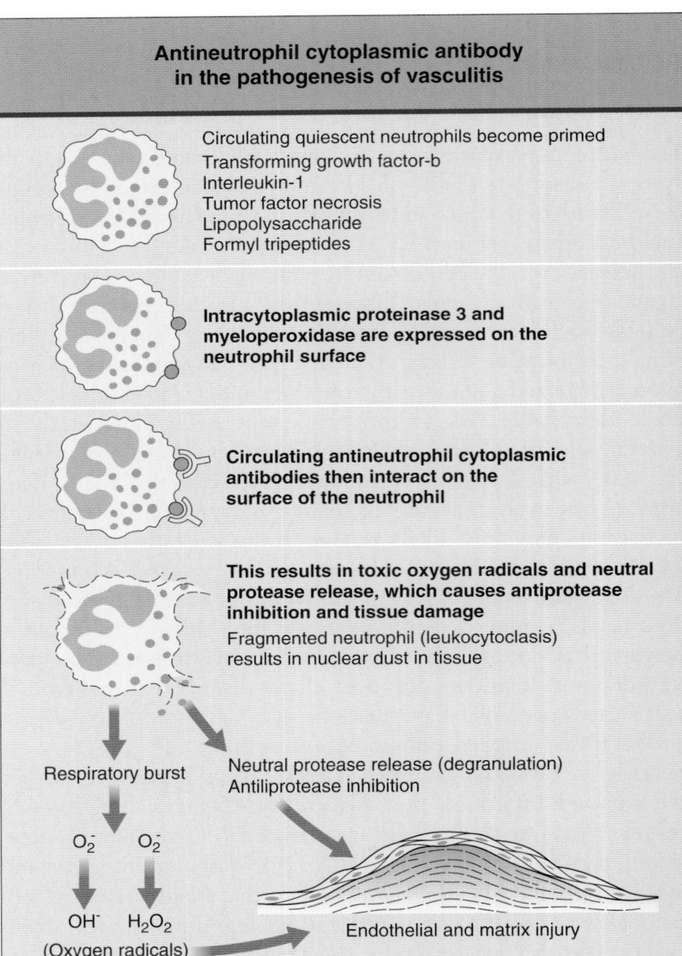

Figure 55.3 Antineutrophil cytoplasmic antibody in the pathogenesis of vasculitis.

Figure 55.3 outlines the potential role for ANCA in the pathogenesis of vasculitis. Circulating neutrophils become primed by either inflammatory cytokines or bacterial products. It is proposed that the primed neutrophils express proteinase 3 or myeloperoxidase on their cell surfaces, thereby allowing ANCA to bind to the target sites on the neutrophil cell membrane. The neutrophil then undergoes a respiratory burst and degranulates as it fragments and undergoes apoptosis (cell death). This results in the release of toxic oxygen radicals and cytoplasmic proteolytic enzymes into the surrounding tissue

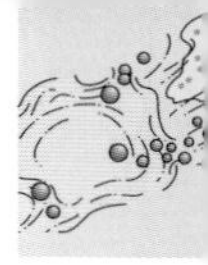

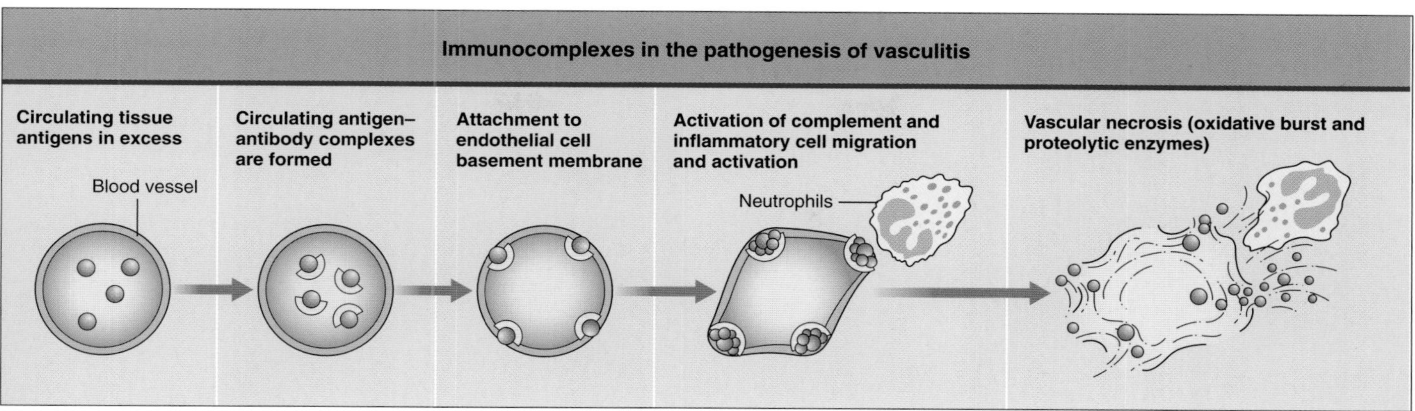

Figure 55.4 Immune complexes in the pathogenesis of vasculitis.

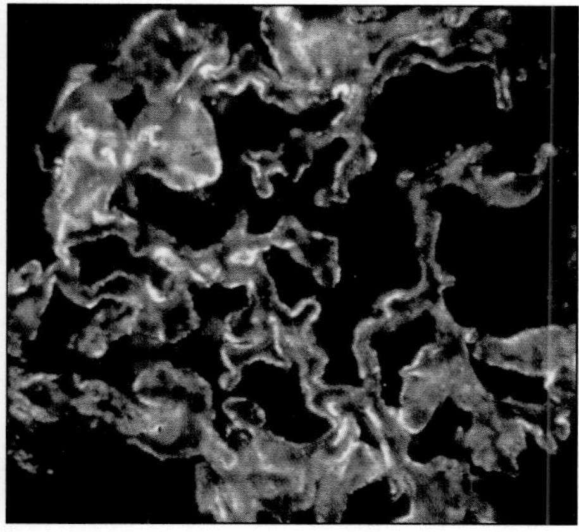

Figure 55.5 Goodpasture's syndrome. Linear immunofluorescence (antibody to immunoglobulin-G) in a lung biopsy.

that, in turns, causes endothelial and eventually tissue matrix injury. Antineutrophil cytoplasmic antibodies also inhibit the naturally occurring anti-inflammatory α-1 antiprotease inhibitor, thereby enhancing the enzymatic injury caused by the serine proteases. There is also evidence to support a role for ANCA in direct endothelial cell cytotoxicity and in the release of chemokines that are capable of attracting inflammatory cell populations. Although this pathogenetic potential role for ANCA is appealing, similar vasculitic changes can occur in patients without circulating ANCA. Moreover, ANCA levels do not necessarily correlate with clinical activity.

The second proposed pathogenetic mechanism involves immune complexes (Fig. 55.4). Immune complex deposition has been found in the kidney and lungs of patients with systemic lupus erythematosus, mixed connective tissue disease, rheumatoid arthritis, Henoch-Schönlein purpura, and Goodpasture's syndrome. All of these conditions can have underlying pulmonary capillaritis and focal segmental necrotizing glomerulonephritis. Figure 55.5 shows that antigens that are either acquired or derived from a tissue component form circulating antigen-antibody complexes, particularly when there is antigen excess. These complexes attach to the vascular endothelium and activate complement that, in turn, results in the chemotaxis and adhesion of inflammatory cells and subsequent vascular necrosis. In Goodpasture's syndrome a specific antibody, the antibasement membrane antibody, is found in both the lung and the kidney. This antibody is directed against an antigen found in type 4 collagen, the major component of basement membranes. The antibody is present in the serum of the majority of cases of Goodpasture's, and stains as a linear, continuous immunofluorescence along the basement membranes in renal and lung tissue (Fig. 55.5). Immune complexes in the other aforementioned entities produce a granular, interrupted pattern of immunofluorescence, indicating immune complex formation in the circulation and subsequent attachment to the tissue. In contrast to this, despite being ANCA-positive, Wegener's granulomatosis, microscopic polyangiitis, and Churg-Strauss syndrome are not associated with tissue immune complex deposition, and are referred to as pauci-immune.

Clinical Features

In general, patients with systemic vasculitis have musculoskeletal complaints such as myalgias and arthralgias. Fever, malaise, and anorexia and weight loss of varying durations are also common. With respiratory tract involvement cough, dyspnea, and hemoptysis are reported.

WEGENER'S GRANULOMATOSIS

Wegener's granulomatosis affects the upper and lower respiratory tract early in the course of the disease and may represent the only manifestation (i.e., limited Wegener's granulomatosis). These patients may present with chronic pansinusitis. Involvement of the nose with crusting, nose bleeds, and septal perforation leading to saddle nose deformity is also seen. Sinus and nasal manifestations are often the first signs of the disease. Chronic otitis media and mastoiditis are occasional complications as well. Eye involvement appears in up to 70% of patients and includes conjunctivitis, episcleritis, uveitis, and retinal artery occlusion resulting from the vasculitis.

Acute involvement of the trachea or the major bronchi can result in tracheobronchial inflammation, ulceration, and malacia, which can ultimately lead to stenosis, causing upper airway obstruction. Airway involvement may result in permanent air flow limitation. In the lung parenchyma the most typical lesions are single or multiple nodules that undergo cavitation (Fig. 55.6). These heal by forming scars. Other lung manifestations include atelectasis and postobstructive pneumonias resulting from primary endobronchial obstruction. Another, often dramatic presentation is hemoptysis with widespread infiltration

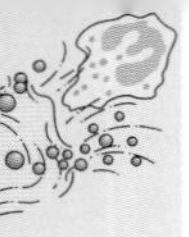

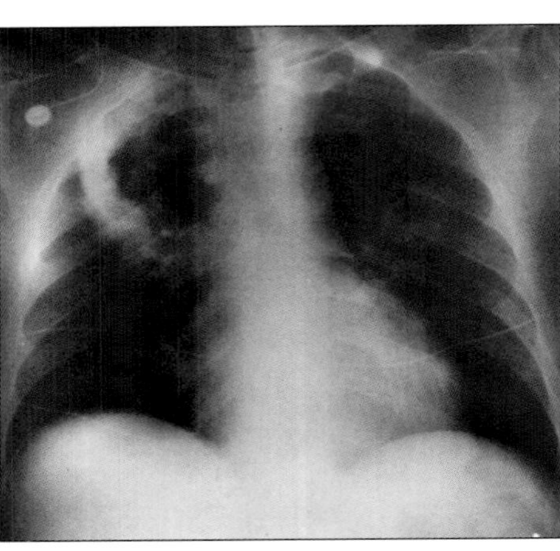

Figure 55.6 Wegener's granulomatosis. Two cavitating lesions.

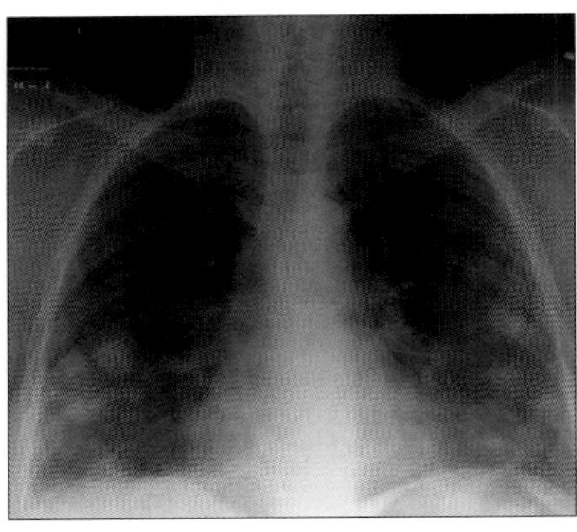

Figure 55.7 Necrotizing sarcoid granulomatosis. A young woman with a slight cough. Chest radiograph indicates multiple lower zone nodules. Diagnosis was proven by biopsy.

resulting from DAH from pulmonary capillaritis. Pulmonary capillaritis and DAH may appear in conjunction with typical cavitating lesions, may be the sole presenting manifestation, or may represent an exacerbation in a previously established case. In a small percentage of patients, pleural effusions or hilar lymphadenopathy may be seen.

Other systemic manifestations, which can appear initially or at a later date, include palpable purpura (leukocytoclastic vasculitis), peripheral neuropathy (mononeuritis multiplex), cranial neuropathies, and pituitary gland involvement causing diabetes insipidus. Glomerulonephritis (focal segmental necrotizing glomerulonephritis) is a common manifestation of the generalized forms of Wegener's granulomatosis and often causes substantial renal impairment that sometimes requires chronic dialysis and, eventually, renal transplantation. The glomerular lesion is not specific for Wegener's granulomatosis because it is also seen in the glomerulonephritis associated with other systemic vasculitidies, Goodpasture's syndrome, and the collagen vascular diseases.

CHURG-STRAUSS SYNDROME

The vasculitis component of the Churg-Strauss syndrome follows a several-year history of atopy (i.e., rhinitis, nasal polyps, asthma, peripheral eosinophilia, and sometimes chronic eosinophilic pneumonia). The vasculitis, when it appears, is characterized by tissue eosinophil infiltration, extravascular granulomas, and necrotizing vasculitis of small and medium sized vessels. Sinus involvement in the form of an allergic rhinitis, and asthma are present in all affected individuals. Parenchymal infiltration, with or without a pleural effusion, is present in 66% to 75% of cases. Differentiating Churg-Strauss from chronic eosinophilic pneumonia is sometimes difficult, because 50% of patients with the latter also have an allergic prodrome, and chronic eosinophilic pneumonia may also lead to the development of the Churg-Strauss syndrome. Subcutaneous skin nodules occur in 66% of patients, mononeuritis multiplex is seen in 65% to 75%, and cardiac disease manifesting as congestive heart failure, pericardial effusion, or a restrictive cardiomyopathy is present in 50%. When present, cardiac involvement results in considerable morbidity and increases the mortality. Abdominal pain, gastrointestinal bleeding, and diarrhea occur in up to 66% of affected individuals. Glomerulonephritis is less likely to be present in the Churg-Strauss syndrome than in Wegener's granulomatosis.

POLYARTERITIS NODOSA

Up to one third of patients with polyarteritis nodosa have evidence of hepatitis B infection. Other viruses implicated in the pathogenesis include the human immunodeficiency virus, cytomegalovirus, parvovirus B19, and hepatitis C virus. The clinical manifestations of polyarteritis nodosa are similar to the vasculitic phase of the Churg-Strauss syndrome, except that:

1. There is no atopic prodromal phase in polyarteritis nodosa
2. There is a higher incidence of glomerulonephritis that often results in hypertension
3. Lung parenchymal involvement is almost never seen

Microscopic polyangiitis, thought by some to represent a small-vessel variant of polyarteritis nodosa, is discussed with the diffuse alveolar hemorrhage syndromes in the next section.

NECROTIZING SARCOIDAL GRANULOMATOSIS

Necrotizing sarcoidal granulomatosis occurs in young individuals, only affects the lung, and the pulmonary nodules are often only discovered after routine chest radiography (Fig. 55.7). Although this rare entity is thought to represent a variant of sarcoidosis by some, the localization to the lung and the distinct vasculitic features are distinguishing features.

Diagnosis

All the aforementioned vasculitic syndromes cause increases in the peripheral blood sedimentation rate, often to levels exceeding 75 mm/hr, increases in serum c-reactive proteins and nonspecific elevations of serum rheumatoid factors and antinuclear antibody titers. Leukocytosis is common, but peripheral eosinophilia should suggest the Churg-Strauss syndrome. Nonspecific elevations of serum immunoglobulins can be expected, but an elevated serum immunoglobulin (Ig)E also supports the diagnosis of the Churg-Strauss syndrome. A urinalysis indicating red blood cells, red blood cell casts, and protein indicates the presence of active glomerulonephritis, a complication common to many of the syndromes. Ordering a microscopic examination of the urine cannot be overemphasized.

A positive serum c-ANCA level confirmed by an enzyme-linked immunosorbent assay (ELISA), which demonstrates antibodies to proteinase 3, is highly specific for Wegener's granulomatosis; however, the sensitivity of this test is lower in patients with disease that is limited to the respiratory tract. In these, tissue biopsy, preferably via a thoracoscopic approach, is indicated. Nasal, sinus, or even endobronchial biopsies often only shows inflammation or necrosis, but not granulomatous vasculitis. Although a positive serum p-ANCA representing antibodies to neutrophil cytoplasmic myeloperoxidase supports the diagnosis of either the Churg-Strauss syndrome, polyarteritis nodosa, or microscopic polyarteritis, it can also be positive in up to 15% of patients with Wegener's granulomatosis. Lung tissue is required to definitely establish the diagnosis of necrotizing sarcoidal granulomatosis.

Treatment and Outcome

The primary therapy for systemic vasculitis is a corticosteroid preparation, usually in combination with cyclophosphamide. In the majority of cases oral preparations (e.g., prednisone 1 mg/kg ideal body weight/day and cyclophosphamide 2 mg/kg ideal body weight/day) are all that is required. The prednisone is tapered and discontinued over a several-month period. Full doses of cyclophosphamide are continued for 6 to 12 months, and then gradually tapered over the next 2 to 6 months. Intravenous therapy with methylprednisolone, up to 1 g daily in divided doses, is recommended for vasculitic syndromes which cause DAH leading to acute respiratory failure or to rapidly progressive renal failure. Intravenous cyclophosphamide 2 to 4 mg/kg ideal body weight should also be administered for several days. Cyclophosphamide occasionally seems to be necessary in the treatment of the Churg-Strauss syndrome, although its role not been well-established. Necrotizing sarcoid granulomatosis resolves in essentially all patients after treatment with corticosteroids alone and, as opposed to what is seen with the other vasculitic syndromes, recurrences are rare.

Although adding cyclophosphamide to the treatment regimen of the vasculitidies has significantly improved survival (particularly in patients with Wegener's granulomatosis, microscopic polyarteritis, and polyarteritis nodosa), the medication has a number of important complications including sterility, alopecia, bone marrow suppression, and an increased incidence of opportunistic infections. Moreover, the development of transitional cell carcinoma of the bladder and non-Hodgkin's lymphoma are long-term complications of cyclophosphamide treatment. For this reason, after induction of remission with prednisone and cyclophosphamide oral weekly, weekly oral methotrexate is applied for long-term immunosuppression in some treatment protocols. New therapies, such as tumor necrosis factor blockade, are currently being evaluated.

Trimethoprim-sulfamethoxazole prophylaxis is recommended to reduce the incidence of *Pneumocystis jiroveci* pneumonia when treating patients with corticosteroids, cyclophosphamide, or other immunosuppressive agents.

Clinical Course and Prevention

More than 90% of patients with Wegener's granulomatosis achieve complete remission with the currently available therapeutic options summarized previously, and up to 80% survive at least 8 years. Patients with more limited forms of the disease (i.e., no renal or central nervous system involvement) have an even better prognosis. Relapses are not uncommon, however, and monitoring of the urine, sedimentation rate, and possibly the serum c-ANCA levels is advised. There are limited data regarding the survival of patients with the Churg-Strauss syndrome. There is no known method to prevent any of these disorders.

Pitfalls and Controversies

A potentially fatal complication of cyclophosphamide therapy, particularly in older individuals, is hemorrhagic cystitis. Accordingly, monitoring of the urine sediment is important. Azathioprine or methotrexate can be substituted in those who develop hemorrhagic cystitis. A late complication is transitional cell cancer of the bladder, particularly in those with persistent microscopic hematuria after cessation of treatment.

There is disagreement in the literature about whether an asymptomatic rise in c-ANCA necessarily portends an impending exacerbation of Wegener's granulomatosis. Accordingly, some suggest that the c-ANCA should not be routinely monitored but only measured in conjunction with clinical findings that may represent an exacerbation of the disease. In patients with Wegener's granulomatosis that is limited to the respiratory tract, trimethoprim-sulfamethoxazole alone can induce remissions. Adding trimethoprim-sulfamethoxazole to the standard therapeutic regimen of patients with systemic forms of Wegener's granulomatosis reduces relapse rates by 50%. Accordingly, there is debate about whether and when to include trimethoprim-sulfamethoxazole with corticosteroids and cyclophosphamide.

DIFFUSE ALVEOLAR HEMORRHAGE

Pathophysiology

A clinical syndrome, DAH is caused by diffuse intraalveolar bleeding from the small vessels of the lungs, particularly the alveolar capillaries, but also the arterioles and venules. It is recognized by finding intraalveolar collections of red blood cells and fibrin, as well as hemosiderin-bearing macrophages and free hemosiderin, in the lung parenchyma. The causes of DAH represent a broad spectrum of etiologies with dissimilar underlying histologies (Table 55.2).

Pulmonary (alveolar) capillaritis defines a small-vessel vasculitis of the lungs, which may be isolated to the lung, but may also appear as a component of a number of systemic disorders. The distinct histologic finding is neutrophilic infiltration of the alveolar wall, with many of the cells being fragmented and appearing pyknotic. Because these cells are undergoing apoptosis (cell death), nuclear dust collects in the tissue. The alveolar interstitium becomes thickened by the neutrophilic infiltration, edema, and fibrinoid necrosis. It is hypothesized that the fragmented, dying neutrophils cause fibrinoid necrosis of the alveolar walls and disruption of the alveolar capillaries via their oxidative burst and the release of cytoplasmic enzymes. This leads to leakage of red blood cells, fibrin, and the fragmented neutrophils into the alveolar spaces, producing the histologic picture of DAH (Fig. 55.8). Pulmonary capillaritis is primarily associated with a number of systemic vasculitidies, as well as with the collagen vascular diseases (see Table 55.2). There are also newly defined associations, such as with isolated pauciimmune pulmonary capillaritis, lung allograft rejection, and some of the collagen vascular diseases. Lung allograft rejection and the

Table 55.2
Histologic and clinical classification of diffuse alveolar hemorrhage

Histology	Frequency	Disease
Pulmonary capillaritis and glomerulonephritis (pulmonary–renal syndrome)	More common	Wegener's granulomatosis Microscopic polyangiitis **Systemic lupus erythematosus** **Goodpasture's syndrome**
	Less common	**Rheumatoid arthritis** **Mixed connective tissue disease** **Scleroderma** Henoch–Schönlein purpura IgA nephropathy Pauci-immune glomerulonephritis Drug-induced (propylthiouracil, penicillamine, diphenylhydantoin) Cryoglobulinemia Behçet's syndrome
Pulmonary capillaritis without glomerulonephritis	More common	Isolated pauci-immune/pulmonary capillaritis Acute lung transplant rejection
	Less common	Polymyositis Rheumatoid arthritis Mixed connective tissue disease Retinoic acid toxicity Goodpasture's syndrome Primary acute phospholipid antibody syndrome
Bland pulmonary hemorrhage	More common	Idiopathic pulmonary hemosiderosis **Goodpasture's syndrome** **Systemic lupus erythematosus**
	Less common	Coagulopathies Trimellitic anhydride exposure Mitral stenosis Drugs (amiodarone, nitrofurantoin) Subacute bacterial endocarditis
Diffuse alveolar damage(acute lung injury)	More common	Idiopathic pneumonia syndrome (bone marrow transplantation) Crack cocaine inhalation Cytotoxic drug injury Acute respiratory distress syndrome
	Less common	Acute radiation pneumonitis **Systemic lupus erythematosus**
Other histologies	More common	Lymphangioleiomyomatosis Pulmonary veno-occlusive disease
	Less common	Pulmonary capillary hemangiomatosis Fibrillary glomerulonephritis Malignancy (renal cell carcinoma, hemangioepithelioma, angiosarcoma choriocarcinoma, Kaposi's sarcoma)

Entities with more than one underlying histology. Adapted from Schwarz MI: Diffuse alveolar hemorrhage. In Schwarz MI, King TE (eds): Interstitial lung disease, ed. 3. Hamilton, Canada, BC Decker, 1998, pp 535-558.

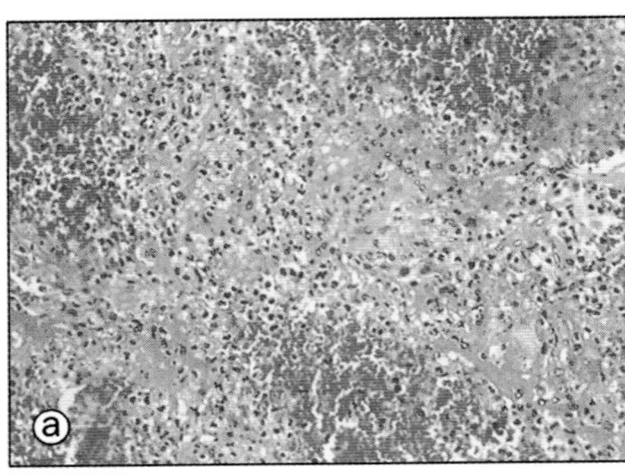

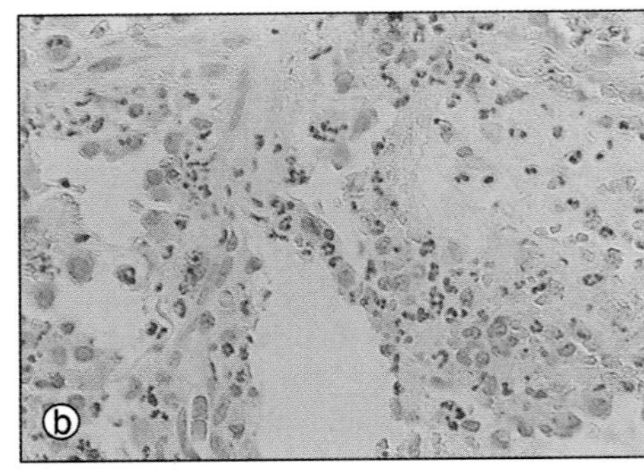

Figure 55.8 Pulmonary capillaritis and diffuse alveolar hemorrhage. A, The alveolar spaces are filled with blood in the biopsy of this patient with microscopic polyangiitis. Note the marked broadening and destruction of the intervening alveolar walls. An area of fibrinoid necrosis is visible in the lower left-hand corner. **B,** Note the neutrophilic infiltration of the alveolar walls (interstitium) in this earlier stage. Some of these cells appear pyknotic and fragmented.

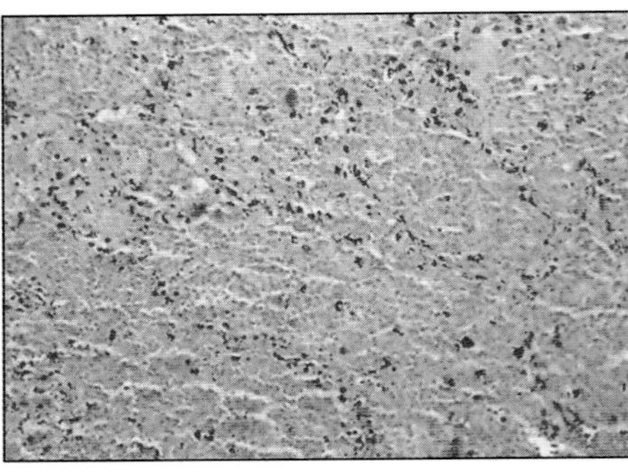

Figure 55.9 Goodpasture's syndrome. Bland pulmonary hemorrhage. The alveoli are filled with blood, and the alveolar walls are intact.

isolated forms of pulmonary capillaritis are examples of lung limited disease and represent an isolated lesion in the lung and is not a component of a systemic disease process.

The term *bland alveolar hemorrhage*, on the other hand, refers to a form of DAH in which there is no evidence of alveolar wall inflammation or necrosis and the histologic appearance is that of DAH alone (Fig. 55.9). This implies a type of capillary endothelial injury occurring without inflammation. In idiopathic pulmonary hemosiderosis and Goodpasture's syndrome, for example, disruptions in the alveolar-capillary basement membrane have been identified by electron microscopy.

Diffuse alveolar damage, the underlying histology associated with the acute respiratory distress syndrome, and other conditions listed in Table 55.2, can result in DAH, particularly if the insult is acute and extensive. In addition to DAH, other features of diffuse alveolar damage include alveolar wall and intraalveolar edema and fibrin deposition, as well as capillary congestion, capillary microthrombi, and the characteristic intraalveolar hyaline membrane formation. There are also a number of rare miscellaneous, but characteristic, histologies that present with DAH (see Table 55.2).

Clinical Features

Hemoptysis is the hallmark of DAH. It may be present in variable amounts ranging from intermittent to continuous, lasting from several weeks to several days before presentation. In some instances (e.g., crack cocaine inhalation) hemoptysis only occurs for a few hours before presentation. Cough, progressive dyspnea, fatigue, and low-grade fever may accompany the

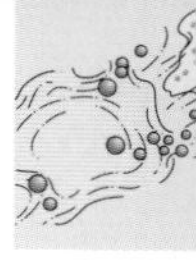

hemoptysis. With extensive DAH, blood gas abnormalities can be so severe that mechanical ventilation for respiratory failure may be necessary. Other systemic symptoms, such as skin rash, visual disturbances, myalgias, and arthralgias may also be reported depending on the underlying etiology. Considerable intraalveolar bleeding may occur, as manifested by a falling hematocrit and a hemorrhagic bronchoalveolar lavage, without the patient experiencing hemoptysis. In fact, as many as 33% of patients with DAH present without hemoptysis.

A prior history of hemoptysis should be sought as DAH, particularly one that occurs with the vasculitic syndromes—the collagen vascular diseases, mitral stenosis, idiopathic pulmonary hemosiderosis, and pulmonary venoocclusive disease—is often recurrent. Conversely, DAH is frequently the first and only apparent manifestation of these disorders. It is important to obtain a medication history because penicillamine, crack cocaine, diphenylhydantoin, amiodarone, propylthiouracil, nitrofurantoin, and various cytotoxic drugs have all been associated with DAH. Penicillamine, propylthiouracil, and diphenylhydantoin can produce hypersensitivity vasculitis with skin and renal involvement as well. Spontaneous DAH may occur in patients receiving anticoagulant and thrombolytic agents. A history of prior cardiac problems may be found in patients with mitral stenosis; however, DAH may also be the first manifestation of this disorder.

Extrapulmonary physical findings are often helpful. The presence conjunctivitis, iridocyclitis, or episcleritis points to a systemic disease, as does palpable purpura and active synovitis. Cardiac examination may disclose a heart murmur. The pulmonary examination is nonspecific.

The chest radiograph demonstrates diffuse or scattered, patchy alveolar infiltrates (Fig. 55.10). Occasionally, DAH has a more localized radiograph distribution early in its course. The heart should be examined for mitral stenosis. In pulmonary venoocclusive disease or mitral valve disease, Kerley B lines may be seen. High-resolution computed tomographic scans of the lung offer no advantage over conventional radiograph. The urine is tested for proteinuria, microscopic hematuria, and red blood cell casts, all of which are indicative of focal segmental necrotizing glomerulonephritis, a lesion common to the systemic vasculitidies, the collage vascular diseases, and Goodpasture's syndrome. The hemoglobin level is decreased and often continues to fall, and the white blood cell count may be elevated. The platelet count is either normal or increased except in those patients with DAH secondary to bone marrow suppression occurring as a result of the primary disease process (e.g., leukemia) or the ensuing cytotoxic therapy. DAH can also complicate thrombotic thrombocytopenic purpura, idiopathic thrombocytopenic purpura, and the primary antiphospholipid antibody syndrome—conditions associated with thrombocytopenia.

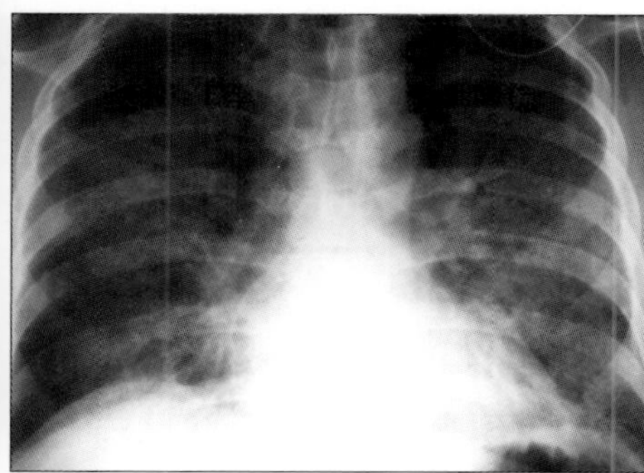

Figure 55.10 Diffuse alveolar hemorrhage. The biopsy shows nonspecific diffuse alveolar infiltration.

Clinical Features of Selected Entities

WEGENER'S GRANULOMATOSIS

DAH with underlying pulmonary capillaritis is the initial manifestation of 5% to 10% of patients with Wegener's granulomatosis. All reported cases are also associated with a focal segmental necrotizing glomerulonephritis. DAH and capillaritis may be seen in lung biopsies in addition to the more typical granulomatous vasculitis. In patients whose initial manifestation is DAH, the more characteristic clinicohistologic picture may evolve months to years after the initial episode. Moreover, in patients with more classic disease, exacerbations may appear in the form of acute DAH. Because of the association with glomerulonephritis, the DAH presentation in Wegener's granulomatosis mimics microscopic polyangiitis. A positive serum c-ANCA establishes the diagnosis of Wegener's granulomatosis.

MICROSCOPIC POLYANGIITIS

Microscopic polyangiitis possibly represents the small vessel variant of polyarteritis nodosa. The lack of medium vessel involvement, the relatively high incidence of lung involvement in the form of DAH because of capillaritis (33% of cases), and the absence of hypertension characterize and differentiate microscopic polyangiitis from polyarteritis nodosa. All patients with microscopic polyangiitis have focal segmental necrotizing glomerulonephritis. Additional clinical features that are similar to other systemic vasculitides include a dermatologic vasculitis, arthritis, myositis, gastrointestinal bleeding resulting from mucosal vasculitis, and a peripheral neuropathy. Nonspecific laboratory findings include an elevated sedimentation rate and increases in both serum rheumatoid factors and antinuclear antibodies. More specifically, antibodies to either hepatitis B or C virus are present in 33% and serum p-ANCA is found in more than 90% of patients.

Two related entities deserve comment. The first is pauci-immune idiopathic glomerulonephritis. This histologic pattern is associated with serum p-ANCA positivity and is considered to be a localized form of renal vasculitis. In 50% of these subjects, however, DAH and other systemic manifestations are found. It is likely that this entity initially is a localized form of microscopic polyangiitis. There is also a recently reported localized form of alveolar capillaritis and DAH associated with p-ANCA positivity. It is not known whether these patients develop a more generalized form of vasculitis because follow-up data are not available.

CONNECTIVE TISSUE OR COLLAGEN VASCULAR DISEASES

Of patients who suffer systemic lupus erythematosus, DAH develops in 3% to 4% of patients. In a study of 15 patients, the underlying histology in the majority was capillaritis, but bland pulmonary hemorrhage and diffuse alveolar damage were also found. Although 80% to 90% of the time DAH occurs in patients with established disease, up to 20% of the time it may be the initial manifestation. Most also have lupus nephritis.

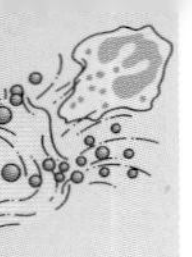

DAH infrequently complicates the other collagen vascular diseases. In polymyositis, rheumatoid arthritis, and mixed connective tissue disease, DAH resulting from pulmonary capillaritis has been described, but without evidence of generalized systemic vasculitis. In these patients, and in those with systemic lupus erythematosus, granular deposition of immune complexes is often, but not always seen. There is also a report of p-ANCA–positive DAH and glomerulonephritis in rheumatoid arthritis, but this may represent a complicating microscopic polyangiitis. Isolated DAH has also been reported to occur in the primary antiphospholipid antibody syndrome.

GOODPASTURE'S SYNDROME

Goodpasture's syndrome (antibasement membrane antibody disease) is a distinct pulmonary-renal syndrome that causes DAH and glomerulonephritis, but without other systemic findings. Both pulmonary capillaritis and bland pulmonary hemorrhage may be responsible for the DAH. It is thought to be caused by the development of an antibody that is specific to an antigen found in the type 4 collagen of alveolar and glomerular basement membranes. This antibasement membrane antibody is also present in the serum of affected patients and is expressed in tissue as noninterrupted linear immunofluorescence with antibody to IgG and complement (see Fig. 55.5). Most cases occur in the second or third decade of life, the condition is more frequent in men, and it may develop after a viral upper respiratory tract infection. In 60% to 80% of patients the lung and kidney disease appear simultaneously, in 10% to 30% glomerulonephritis is the only manifestation, and in 5% to 10% DAH occurs without renal disease. Older affected individuals are more apt to have isolated renal disease, and active smokers in all age groups are more likely to develop DAH alone or in combination with renal disease.

ISOLATED PAUCI-IMMUNE PULMONARY CAPILLARITIS

Isolated pauci-immune pulmonary capillaritis is a newly described, small-vessel vasculitis that is confined to the lungs without serologic or clinical evidence of an accompanying collagen vascular disease or one of the systemic vasculitides that are listed in Table 55.2. Immunofluorescent examination of lung tissue does not reveal evidence of granular or linear immune complex deposition, and an extended follow-up of these patients failed to demonstrate the development of a systemic disease.

HENOCH-SCHÖNLEIN PURPURA

Henoch-Schönlein purpura is a systemic vasculitis typified by circulating and tissue immune complexes consisting of IgA antibodies. Although the condition is most common in children, adults can sometimes be affected, and, in several of these, pulmonary capillaritis causing DAH has been described. Although immunoglobulin A nephropathy is a common form of glomerulonephritis in adults and includes the presence of serum and renal IgA immune complexes, DAH is a rare complication.

IDIOPATHIC PULMONARY HEMOSIDEROSIS AND MISCELLANEOUS DISORDERS

A bland, recurrent form of DAH is idiopathic pulmonary hemosiderosis (IPH), which has a poorly understood pathogenesis. More than 75% of patients develop the condition in childhood. A review of some adult cases indicates that they represented isolated pauci-immune pulmonary capillaritis. Moreover, several cases of IPH have developed a full-blown systemic vasculitis (microscopic polyangiitis) or a collagen vascular disease (systemic lupus erythematosus and rheumatoid arthritis) years after initial diagnosis. However, there are unexplained cases of recurrent bland pulmonary hemorrhage in adults that are considered to be recurrent IPH. In addition to familial and geographic clustering of cases, there is an association of IPH with celiac disease.

Pulmonary venoocclusive disease, another usual cause of DAH, is caused by fibrous obliteration of the postcapillary venules, leading to severe progressive pulmonary hypertension that is complicated by episodes of DAH. It has recently been found that, in some cases, there is a mutation in the bone morphogenesis protein receptor gene that also occurs in some cases of familial primary pulmonary hypertension. Although most cases are idiopathic, pulmonary venoocclusive disease has been reported as a complication of both bleomycin and carmustine therapy, thoracic radiation, human immunodeficiency virus infection, and collagen vascular disease.

Diagnosis

Establishing a diagnosis of DAH is not difficult in patients who present with hemoptysis, radiographic diffuse pulmonary infiltrates, a falling hematocrit, and a sequential hemorrhagic bronchoalveolar lavage. In those without hemoptysis, however, the bronchoalveolar lavage differentiates DAH from other acute infectious and noninfectious pulmonary processes. Table 55.3 outlines the expected findings for the more common causes of DAH.

Treatment

Treatment for the systemic vasculitides and the collagen vascular disease associated DAH is identical to that already described for vasculitis in the previous section of this chapter. One major addition is the use of plasmapheresis in patients with Goodpasture's syndrome. In patients with collagen vascular disease and Wegener's granulomatosis–induced DAH, plasmapheresis is ineffective. For the treatment of diffuse alveolar damage-induced DAH, high-dose intravenous methylprednisolone is recommended (see previous section). Mitral stenosis causing DAH requires surgical intervention. Patients with Goodpasture's syndrome must stop smoking.

Clinical Course and Prevention

DAH occurring in the setting of a systemic vasculitis or collagen vascular disease adversely affects the outcome. More than half of these patients require mechanical ventilation, and death frequently occurs as a result of respiratory and renal failure or of superimposed infection resulting from the immunosuppressive therapies. Only 50% of patients with systemic lupus erythematosus survive the initial episode of DAH. In Wegener's granulomatosis and microscopic polyangiitis, the initial mortality is 25% to 30%. Furthermore, 5-year survival rates are also reduced (65%). The mortality and survival data are more encouraging in isolated pauci-immune pulmonary capillaritis. In

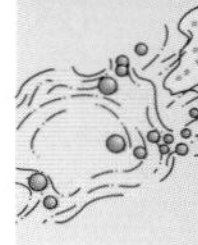

Table 55.3
Diagnosis of diffuse alveolar hemorrhage

Disease	Glomerulo-nephritis	Arthritis	Dermat-ologic vasculitis	Anti-nuclear antibody	Rheuma-atoid factor	Serum complement	Antibasement antibody syndrome	Cytoplasmic antineutrophil cytoplasmic antibody	Perinuclear antineutrophil cytoplasmic antibody	Antideoxy-ribonucleic acid antibody	Tissue immuno-complex antibody
Wegener's granulomatosis	+	+	+	±	±	Within normal limits	–	+	±	–	–
Microscopic polyangiitis	+	+	+	±	±	Within normal limits	–	–	+	–	–
Systemic lupus erythematosus	+	+	±	+	±	Low	–	–	±	+	+ (granular)
Goodpasture's syndrome	+	–	–	–	–	Within normal limits	+	±	±	–	+ (linear)
Henoch–Schönlein purpura	+	±	+	–	–	Within normal limits	–	–	–	–	+ (IgA)
Idiopathic pauci-immune pulmonary capillaritis	–	–	–	–	–	Within normal limits	–	–	–	–	–
Idiopathic pulmonary hemosiderosis	–	–	–	–	–	Within normal limits	–	–	–	–	–
Pulmonary veno-occlusive disease	–	–	–	±	±	Within normal limits	–	–	–	–	Occasional

(Adapted from Schwarz MI, Cherniack RM, King TE: Diffuse alveolar hemorrhage and other rare pulmonary infiltrative disorders. In Murray J, Nadel J (eds): Textbook of Respiratory Medicine, ed 2. WB Saunders, Philadelphia, 1993, pp 1889-1912.)

Goodpasture's syndrome, the 2-year survival rate is 50%. Lower survival rates in Goodpasture's syndrome are to be expected in patients with severe renal failure and persistent DAH. An early mortality (25%) can be expected in IPH; however, 50% survive for 5 years.

The only known preventive approach that can be suggested for patients with this group of disorders is smoking cessation in patients with Goodpasture's syndrome.

Pitfalls and Controversies

In adults with isolated DAH who do not have evidence of a drug exposure, mitral stenosis, or a coagulopathy, a lung biopsy to differentiate between IPH, isolated pauci-immune pulmonary capillaritis, and Goodpasture's syndrome without renal involvement should be performed. In fact, in those patients who present with isolated DAH, open or thoracoscopic lung biopsy should be performed after mitral valve disease, a coagulopathy, a potential drug exposure, or conditions that can lead to diffuse alveolar damage are excluded. The clinical and radiographic features of pulmonary veno-occlusive disease can be confused with mitral stenosis.

There are two potential pulmonary complications related to recurrent DAH. One is pulmonary fibrosis causing a progressive restrictive lung disease; the other is a progressive obstructive lung disease in patients with recurrent DAH resulting from pulmonary capillaritis. It is unclear why recurrent bleeding in the lung causes interstitial fibrosis. In iron-overload states such as transfusion hemosiderosis or primary hemochromatosis, pulmonary fibrosis does not occur. Obstructive lung disease is thought to be due to the development of emphysema in patients with pulmonary capillaritis because of the release of neutral proteases from destroyed neutrophils and ANCA inhibition of antiproteases.

The use of plasmapheresis in patients with microscopic polyangiitis is debated.

SUGGESTED READINGS

D'Agati V: Antineutrophil cytoplasmic antibody and vasculitis: Much more than a disease marker. J Clin Invest 110:919-921, 2002.

Fauci AS, Haynes BF, Katz P, Wolff SM: Wegener's granulomatosis: Prospective clinical and therapeutic experience with 85 patients for 21 years. Ann Intern Med 98:76-85, 1983.

Jennette JC, Falk RJ, Andrassy K, et al: Nomenclature of systemic vasculitides: A proposal of an international consensus conference. Arthritis Rheum 37:187-192, 1994.

Jennings CA, King TE, Tuder R, et al: Diffuse alveolar hemorrhage with underlying isolated, pauciimmune pulmonary capillaritis. Am J Respir Crit Care Med 155:1101-1109, 1997.

Kelly PT, Haponik EF: Goodpasture's syndrome: Molecular and clinical advances. Medicine 73:171-185, 1994.

Schwarz MI, Brown KK: Small vessel vasculitis of the lung. Thorax 55:502-510, 2000.

Schwarz MI, Cherniack RM, King TE: Diffuse alveolar hemorrhage and

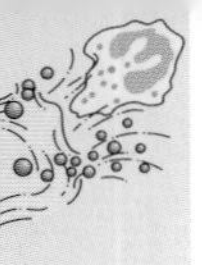

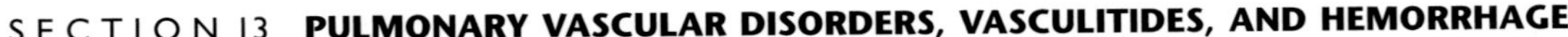

other rare pulmonary infiltrative disorders. In Murray J, Nadel J (eds). Textbook of respiratory medicine, 3rd ed. WB Saunders, Philadelphia, 2000, pp 1733-1756.

Specks U: Diffuse alveolar hemorrhage syndromes. Curr Opin Rheumatol 13:12-17, 2001.

Specks U: Pulmonary vasculitis. In Schwarz MI, King TE (eds). Interstitial Lung Disease, 3rd ed. BC Decker, Hamilton, Canada, 1998, pp 507-534.

Travis WD, Hoffman GS, Leavitt RY, et al: Surgical pathology of the lung in Wegener's granulomatosis. Am J Surg Pathol 15:315-333, 1991.

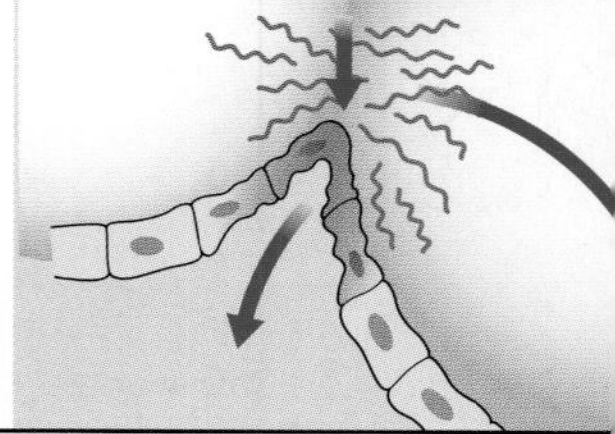

CHAPTER 56

Disability Evaluation

Robin Rudd

In patients with occupational respiratory disease, it is often necessary to assess disability for purposes of determining compensation and fitness for work. In considering respiratory disability it is important to distinguish between impairment of respiratory function and disability that results from the impairment. Respiratory disability has been defined by the World Health Organization as a reduction in exercise capacity secondary to impaired lung function and the resulting social and occupational disadvantage is designated handicap. The assessment of respiratory disability requires information about impairment of respiratory function and its effect on exercise performance. The former is easily obtained by standard tests of static lung function. The latter is most easily obtained by interviewing the subject, but much effort has been expended on trying to devise more objective methods.

ASSESSMENT OF IMPAIRMENT OF LUNG FUNCTION

Impairment of respiratory function is assessed by a range of lung function tests, the results of which are commonly interpreted by comparison with reference values. These are values determined in subjects without known respiratory disease or respiratory symptoms. In some, but not all, series used to determine reference values, smokers have been excluded. It is important to appreciate that reference values represent only the mean of a population of similar age, sex, and height so that, by definition, some healthy individuals will have values well above or below the reference value.

Rating scales for impairment of respiratory function have been formulated by working groups of the American Thoracic Society and European Society for Clinical Respiratory Physiology. The proposals differed in their definitions of the lower limit of normal, respectively 20% and 1.64 standard deviations below the reference value. The latter has more statistical validity because it defines the lowest 5% of the population at any age, whereas a criterion based upon percentage predicted will define more patients as abnormal with increasing age. The categories of impairment defined by the two scales are shown in Table 56.1. As well as being statistically questionable, these grades are arbitrary and their descriptions were not accompanied by evidence that validated their selection as reflecting loss of exercise capacity. There is only a weak correlation between loss of lung function and the resultant loss of exercise capacity. These guidelines relate to persons with chronic stable respiratory disease and are inappropriate for patients with asthma, the impairment that is, by definition, variable. The American Thoracic Society has proposed a scoring system for the evaluation of disability in patients with asthma.

ASSESSMENT OF EXERCISE ABILITY

Questionnaires

Assessment of disability therefore should include an assessment of the extent to which exercise capacity is impaired. The simplest structured method of assessing limitation of exercise capacity is by means of a validated questionnaire. One of the earliest and most widely used is that devised by the Medical Research Council in the United Kingdom. The questions regarding breathlessness are shown in Table 56.2. A more detailed questionnaire assessing grades of breathlessness was devised by McGavin and colleagues, who found the grades correlated with measured walking distance. A system for assessing respiratory disability in percentage terms was devised for dealing with compensation claims by coal miners in the United Kingdom. It relates symptom descriptions to lung function impairment as categorized by the American Thoracic Society impairment scale (Table 56.3). When there is conflict between reported symptoms and objective measurements, more weight is accorded to the latter.

Exercise Tests

For healthy subjects, the level of energy expenditure that can be sustained during exercise is determined mainly by the ability of the circulation to deliver blood to the muscles. For the subject with impaired lung function, the limiting factor is usually the ventilatory capacity. The energy cost of activity may be related to ventilatory capacity or gas exchange. Figure 56.1 shows approximate relations between a range of everyday activities, energy expenditure, and minute ventilation. The relations are loose and there is considerable variation in the ventilation required for a given degree of energy expenditure. In general, people who are physically unfit and overweight have higher ventilatory requirements for a given energy expenditure.

Ability to exercise may be assessed directly by means of an exercise test. One of the simplest tests is the timed walk in which the subject is asked to walk as far as he or she can along a level corridor in the specified time, with stopping allowed within that period. The 6-minute period has been found to be as reproducible as the 12-minute and is therefore more convenient. The usefulness of the test can be improved by assessing breathlessness after the walk in addition to measuring the distance walked. The shuttle walk requires that patients walk back and forth between two markers set 10 meters apart. The walking speed is paced by an audio signal and the walking speed is increased each minute in a graded fashion. The end of the test occurs when the patient is too breathless to maintain the

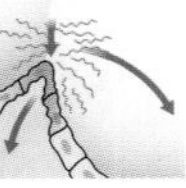

Table 56.1
Impairment of lung function as defined by the American Thoracic Society and European Society for Clinical Respiratory Physiology. The rating is based upon the index that deviates most from normality

Impairment	American Thoracic Society	European Society for Clinical Respiratory Physiology
None	FEV_1, FVC, and DLCO ≥80%; FEV_1% ≥75%	> Reference value – 1.64 standard deviations
Mild	FEV_1, FVC, or DLCO 60–79%; FEV_1% 60–74%	Not normal, but ≥60% reference value
Moderate	FEV_1, FEV_1%, or DLCO 41–59%; or FVC 51–59%	40–59% reference value
Severe	FEV_1, FEV_1%, or DLCO <40%; or FVC <50%	<40% reference value or FVC <50%

FEV_1, forced expiratory volume in 1s; FVC, forced vital capacity; DLCO, diffusing capacity of lung for carbon monoxide; FEV_1%, FEV_1/FVC%.

required speed. In one study, inability to complete 25 shuttles on two occasions suggested a maximal oxygen uptake (VO_2max) of less than 10 mL/kg/min. Walking tests are dependent on good motivation, which may be lacking in the context of assessment of disability for compensation and do not provide information as to the cause of impaired exercise capacity.

A more detailed approach employs measurement of maximal oxygen uptake during a progressive exercise test on a treadmill or cycle ergometer (Fig. 56.2). On a cycle ergometer the work rate is increased progressively while the subject is asked to exercise until symptoms oblige him or her to cease and he or she is asked to report the reasons for stopping. For the result to be considered evidence of respiratory disability, exercise must be terminated because of breathlessness rather than, for example, by chest pain, leg pain, or fatigue. During exercise, successive measurements of ventilation and consumption of oxygen are

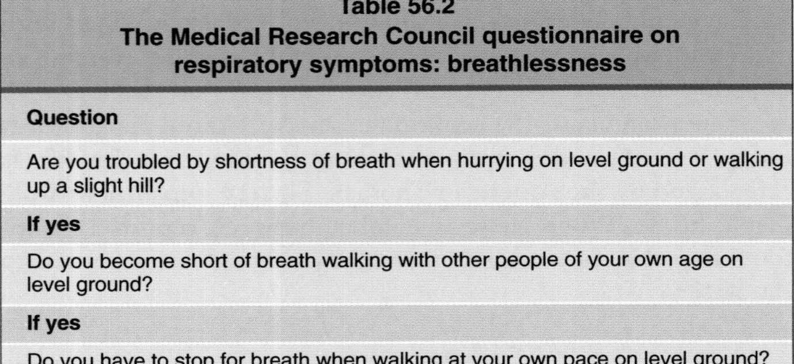

Table 56.2
The Medical Research Council questionnaire on respiratory symptoms: breathlessness

Question
Are you troubled by shortness of breath when hurrying on level ground or walking up a slight hill?
If yes
Do you become short of breath walking with other people of your own age on level ground?
If yes
Do you have to stop for breath when walking at your own pace on level ground?

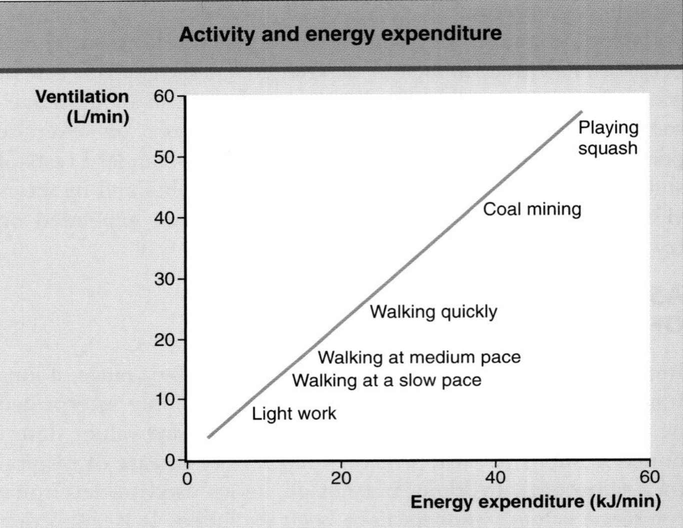

Figure 56.1 The relationship between levels of energy expenditure during everyday tasks and ventilation.

Table 56.3
UK coal miner's respiratory disability rating scale. Lung function impairment based on American Thoracic Society criteria (see Fig. 56.1)

Disability score	Symptoms	Lung function impairment
0%	Not breathless on exercise	None
10%	Breathless on prolonged or heavy exertion	Mild
20%	Breathless on walking uphill or climbing stairs or on hurrying on level ground	Mild
30%	Breathless at normal pace for age walking on level ground	Moderate
40%	Breathless on walking 100 yards or climbing one flight of stairs at a slow pace	Moderate
50%	Breathless on walking 100 yards at a slow pace or climbing one flight of stairs at a slow pace	Moderate
60%	Breathlessness prevents walking 100 yards at a slow pace without stopping or climbing one flight of stairs without stopping	Severe
70%	Breathlessness prevents activity outside the home without assistance or supervision	Severe
80%	Breathlessness limits activities to within home	Severe
90%	Able to walk only a few steps because of breathlessness	Severe
100%	Bed and chair bound, totally dependent on caregivers because of breathlessness	Severe

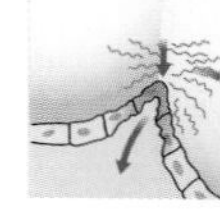

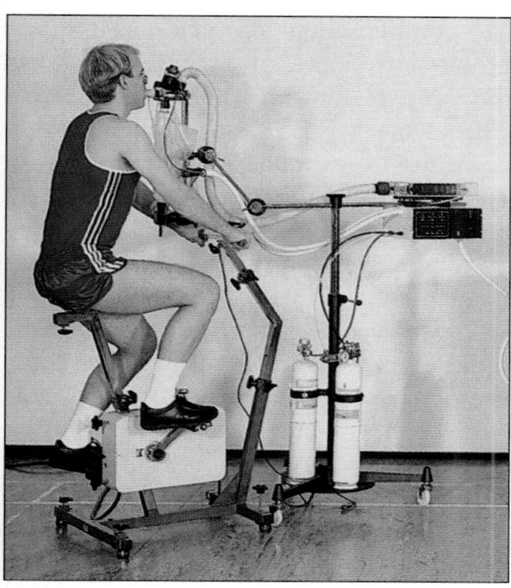

Figure 56.2 A progressive exercise test using a cycle ergometer. Measurements are made each minute of heart rate, ventilation, oxygen uptake, carbon dioxide output, and work rate.

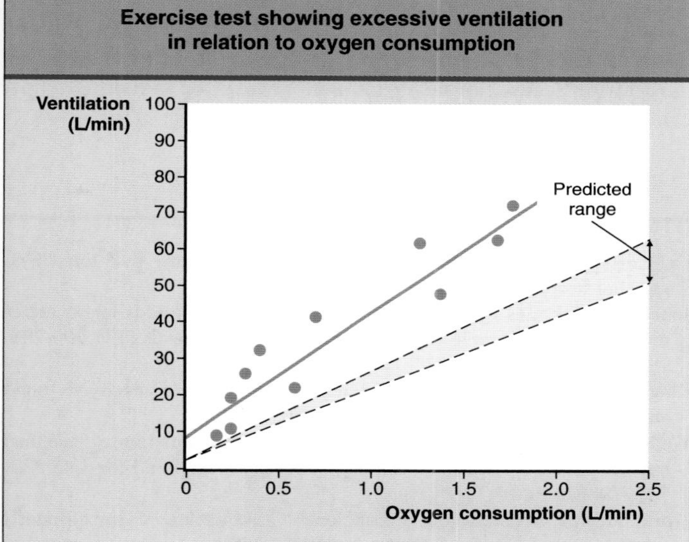

Figure 56.3 Exercise test showing ventilation in relation to oxygen consumption. The maximum ventilation is 72 L/min; the FEV_1 is 2.0 L. Maximum exercise ventilation is approximately $FEV_1 \times 35$. Thus the test was maximal, with ventilation levels above the normal range indicating respiratory impairment.

made. Traces must be inspected to ensure that these measurements lie along a reasonably smooth curve and that tidal volume is appropriate for the vital capacity. At the point of stopping the ventilation should be around the maximum value predicted by the subject's forced expiratory volume in 1 second (FEV_1) (Fig. 56.3). The electrocardiogram is also monitored and exercise terminated if the electrocardiogram becomes abnormal. Two sets of reference values that yield similar results are available.

Many untrained subjects do not perform a maximal exercise test satisfactorily. Some decline to try hard enough whereas other, particularly older, subjects develop nonrespiratory symptoms or electrocardiogram changes that necessitate cessation of exercise. Many more people are capable of completing a submaximal exercise test, and this can be used to measure ventilation at a given oxygen uptake, commonly 45 $mmol/min^{-1}$ (VE_{45}) (to convert from $mmol/min^{-1}$ to L/min^{-1}, divide by 44.6), a reflection of the increased ventilatory cost of exercise resulting from respiratory impairment. Maximal oxygen uptake can then be estimated from an equation relating it to VE_{45}, FEV_1, age, and fat-free mass (FFM):

$$VO_2 \text{ max (L/min)} = 1.49 + 0.3\ FEV_1 \text{ (L)} - 0.021\ VE_{45}\ VE_{45} \text{ (L/min)} + 0.45\ FFM \text{ (kg)} - 0.007 \text{ age (years)}$$

A disability rating scale based upon the results of maximal exercise testing has been devised by the European Society for Clinical Respiratory Physiology. Zero disability was defined as a maximal oxygen uptake at or above the lower limit of the normal range, defined as reference value 1.64 residual standard deviations, and 100% disability was defined as inability to achieve during exercise an oxygen uptake more than twice that used as rest. Between these limits, disability was assessed on a linear scale. However, the correlation between the grade of disability assessed by this means and breathlessness grade was poor.

The disability rating scale was later systematically evaluated in a comparison with assessments of disability made by the Medical Boarding Centre (Respiratory Diseases), a panel of doctors that determines awards of state compensation for occupational respiratory disease in the United Kingdom. There was a significant correlation between the percentage disability assessed by exercise test and the board's assessment of total cardiorespiratory disability ($r = .51$) but a poor correlation between the exercise test and breathlessness grade. The disability scores assessed from directly measured maximal oxygen uptake and estimated from VE_{45} were moderately well correlated ($r = .72$), but the two disability scores differed by more than 25% in 18% of subjects. The authors suggested that the directly measured maximal oxygen uptake is more likely to be reduced by negative attitudes and that the estimated maximal uptake may be more representative of respiratory disability.

A study that assessed anxiety, depression, and attitudes and beliefs about health and personal disability in welders and other tradesmen found that these factors were significantly associated with clinical grade of breathlessness, lung function, and the physiologic response to exercise. The general attitude score accounted for more than half the explained variance in the clinical grade of breathlessness and contributed more to the variance in maximal oxygen uptake than FEV_1. Thus attitude to disability reflected the subject's assessment of his or her exercise capacity and was closely related to the clinical grade of breathlessness that is an index of performance with a large subjective component.

In routine practice detailed assessment of psychologic factors as well as full lung function testing and exercise testing is not a practical proposition. The clinician faced with the task of assessing the disability of a patient with occupational respiratory disease will usually have to proceed on the basis of a clinical assessment, including structured questions about breathlessness on exertion and the ways in which it impairs everyday life and working capacity and lung function tests. For most patients this is adequate, and evidence that more complex tests increase the validity of the assessment is lacking. A progressive exercise test may be helpful, particularly in cases in which the claimed disability is not in keeping with the results of clinical assessment and lung function tests. In the United States the Social Security Administration requires a measure of exercise capacity in assessing disability.

OVERALL ASSESSMENT OF DISABILITY

In assessing the effect of respiratory impairment on disability, it is often necessary to take into account the combined effects of the occupational disease and other conditions. Many subjects with occupational lung disease also have smoking-induced respiratory disease. A given decrement in lung function caused by occupational disease will give rise to a greater increment in disability in a subject who has already lost a substantial amount of lung function because of smoking than in a subject with otherwise healthy lungs. Respiratory impairment may also interact with other disease processes. For example, symptoms of ischemic heart disease or peripheral arterial disease may be worsened by hypoxemia on exercise caused by respiratory disease. Impaired cardiac function and obesity may contribute to breathlessness.

In assessing patients with occupational respiratory disease in the context of compensation, it is important to take into account psychologic factors. The compensation claimant has obvious reasons for maximizing the reported level of disability, and it has been shown that, for the same level of breathlessness, subjects claiming compensation had a mean FEV_1 that was significantly higher than those who consulted doctors because of respiratory symptoms. However, apparent overstatement of disability may not necessarily reflect deliberate exaggeration. Patients may have a psychologic adverse reaction to the diagnosis of an occupational respiratory disease, for example, excessive anxiety about future risks of malignant disease in a patient with asbestosis, which may make respiratory symptoms subjectively worse. Such an effect is properly regarded as a consequence of the occupational disease and should be taken into account in assessing overall disability.

It is also important to bear in mind the subject's way of life. A subject accustomed to a sedentary job and leisure activities may not be at all disabled by a degree of respiratory impairment that causes substantial disability to another subject employed in work involving heavy exertion or enjoying strenuous sporting activities. An adequate assessment of disability should take into account the effect of the physical impairment upon the individual subject; this requirement ensures that standard rating scales can never be a substitute for individual clinical assessment.

SUGGESTED READINGS

American Thoracic Society, Medical Section of the American Lung Association: Evaluation of impairment/disability secondary to respiratory disease. Am Rev Respir Dis 133:1205-1209, 1986.

American Thoracic Society, Medical Section of the American Lung Association: Guidelines for the evaluation of impairment/disability in patients with asthma. Am Rev Respir Dis 147:1056-1061, 1993.

Cotes JE, Chinn DJ, Reed JW, Hutchinson JE: Experience of a standardised method for assessing respiratory disability. Eur Respir J 7:875-880, 1994.

Cotes JE, Zejda J, King B: Lung function impairment as a guide to exercise limitation in work-related lung disorders. Am Rev Respir Dis 137:1089-1093, 1988.

Cotes JE: Rating respiratory disability: A report on behalf of a working group of the European Society for Clinical Respiratory Physiology. Eur Respir J 3:1074-1077, 1990.

De Coster A. Respiratory impairment and disablement. Bull Eur Physiopathol Respir 19:1-3P, 1983.

Jones NL, Makrides L, Hitchcock C, et al: Normal standards for an incremental progressive cycle ergometer test. Am Rev Respir Dis 131:700-708, 1985.

King B, Cotes JE: Relation of lung function and exercise capacity to mood and attitudes to health. Thorax 44:402-409, 1989.

Weller JJ, el-Gamal FM, Parker L, et al: Indirect estimation of maximal oxygen uptake for study of working populations. Br J Ind Med 45:532-537, 1988.

World Health Organization: International Classification of Impairments, Disabilities and Handicaps. Geneva, WHO, 1980.

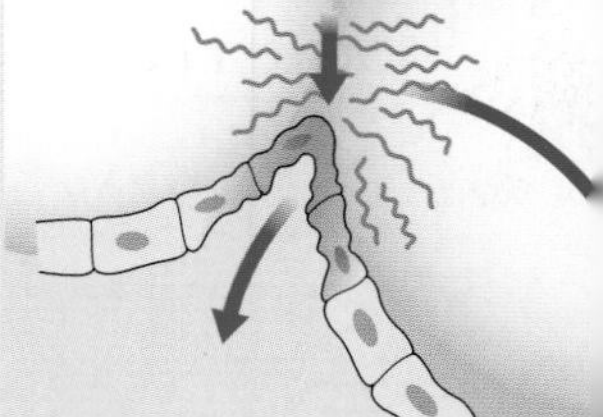

CHAPTER 57 Silicosis and Coal Worker's Pneumoconiosis

Benoit Wallaert and Sylvie Leroy

Pneumoconiosis has been defined as the non-neoplastic reaction of the lung to inhaled mineral or organic dust. The prolonged inhalation of coal mine dust may result in the development of coal worker's pneumoconiosis (CWP), silicosis, and industrial chronic bronchitis and emphysema, either singly or in various combinations. CWP is the term generally applied to interstitial disease of the lung resulting from chronic exposure to coal dust, its inhalation and deposition, and the tissue reaction of the host to its presence, whereas silicosis is due to inhalation of dust containing silica. The pneumoconioses differ in a number of ways from the acute allergic and toxic interstitial diseases, which are associated with exposure to organic dusts, principally because of their long latency periods (usually 10 to 20 years or more) between exposure onset and disease recognition.

SOURCES OF EXPOSURE

Coal is not a mineral of fixed composition. Coal is graded by rank, reflecting its carbon content and thus combustibility: anthracite is the highest ranked coal, with a carbon content around 98%. Lower ranked coals, bituminous and sub-bituminous, have carbon contents around 90% to 95% carbon. The rank of coal has an influence on the risk of disease: higher rank coals entail higher risk than lower rank coals. However, exposure to coal dust with a quartz concentration greater than 15% is associated with a high risk of a rapidly progressive form of pneumoconiosis that has the characteristics of silicosis. In open mines, dust levels rarely approach those of underground mines.

The most common form of crystalline silica is quartz. Quartz is almost pure silicone dioxide but often contains traces of other elements. Other crystalline forms of silica are cristobalite and tridymite. The importance of silica as a health hazard is due to its ubiquity (Table 57.1). Diatomite is a siliceous sedimentary rock used for filtration; for heat and sound insulation; as an adsorbent; as a filter for plastics, paper, and insecticides; and for floor coverings.

It appears that development and progression of silicosis depend on the total amount of quartz to which workers are exposed, the time over which that exposure occurs, and the presence of others minerals that may interfere with the toxicity of the quartz.

Epidemiology

CWP was first recognized in Scottish miners in 1830. In recent decades the incidence of CWP has been declining in industrial countries because of improved dust controls, though increased mechanization in the mid-1960s led to a temporary increase in dust levels. In parallel, through the period 1950-1980, the annual United Kingdom rate for the recognition of CWP for state compensation in current and retired miners decreased from about 7% to 1%-2%. The overall prevalence of CWP, which reflects more distant exposure and earlier incidence, declined from about 13% to 5%, but there were substantial regional differences. Similar regional differences and similar declines have been noted in the United States and other countries.

PATHOPHYSIOLOGY

There are three groups of factors known to influence the character and severity of lung tissue reaction to the mineral dusts. The risk of pneumoconiosis is related to the intensity and years of exposure. However, among a group of workers exposed to the same dust, only a fraction develops pneumoconiosis because of an individual susceptibility. The nature and properties of each specific dust constitute the third factor under consideration. For each mineral, geometric and aerodynamic properties, chemistry, and surface properties have to be considered. The particles that can cause pneumoconiosis are those aerodynamically and geometrically small enough to reach the respiratory bronchioles and be deposited there—this generally means spherical particles between 0.5 and 5 μm.

The pathogenesis of pneumoconiosis is similar to that of all interstitial lung diseases. There is a chronic inflammatory state (alveolitis) in which inflammatory cells are activated and damage the pulmonary architecture. Inorganic particles are phagocytosed by alveolar macrophages, causing activation and the release inflammatory mediators such as cytokines and arachidonic acid metabolites. The mediators in turn induce the recruitment of other inflammatory cells within the alveolar wall and on the alveolar epithelial surface. The alveolitis is dominated by alveolar macrophages. Toxic oxygen derivatives and proteolytic enzymes are released by the inflammatory cells, which cause cellular damage and disruption of the extracellular matrix.

The inflammatory phase is followed by a reparative phase in which growth factors stimulate the recruitment and proliferation of mesenchymal cells and regulate neovascularization and reepithelialization of injured tissues. During this phase, abnormal, or uncontrolled, reparative mechanisms may result in the development of fibrosis. Fibrogenic particles activate proinflammatory cytokine production within the respiratory tract. Tumor

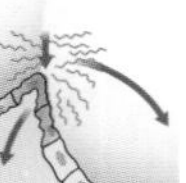

Table 57.1 Major industries with silica exposure	
Occupation	**Exposure**
Sand blaster	Ship building, oil rig maintenance, preparing steel for painting
Miner	Surface coal mining, roof bolting, shot firing, drilling, tunneling
Miller	Silica flour
Glass maker	Polishing with sand and enamel work
Potter	Crushing flint and fettling, foundry work, mold making and cleaning, vitreous enameling, manufacture of cultured quartz crystal
Quarry and stone worker	Cutting of slate, sandstone, and granite
Abrasive worker	Inhalation of fine particles during grinding

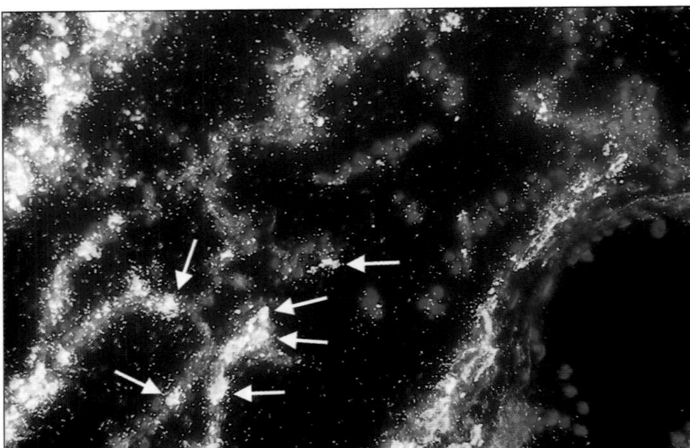

Figure 57.1 Expression of tumor necrosis factor-α messenger RNA. Tumor necrosis factor-α messenger RNA (by in situ hybridization) is expressed in alveolar macrophages in lung section from a patient with coal worker's pneumoconiosis.

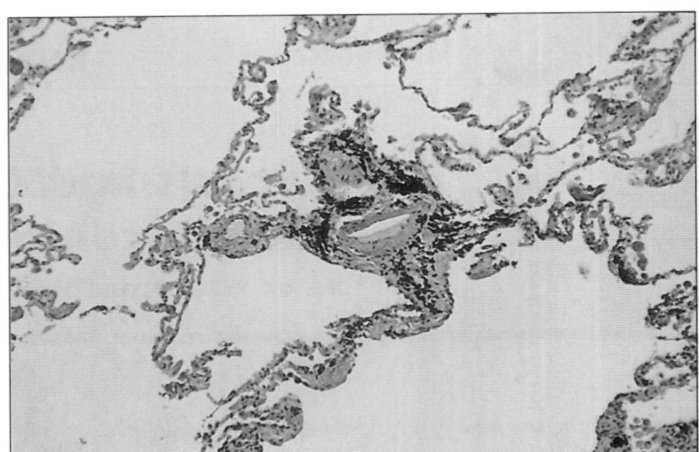

Figure 57.2 Macular lesion of coal worker's pneumoconiosis. This coal macule consists of collections of macrophages that are laded with coal dust and extend into the connective tissue surrounding the respiratory bronchioles.

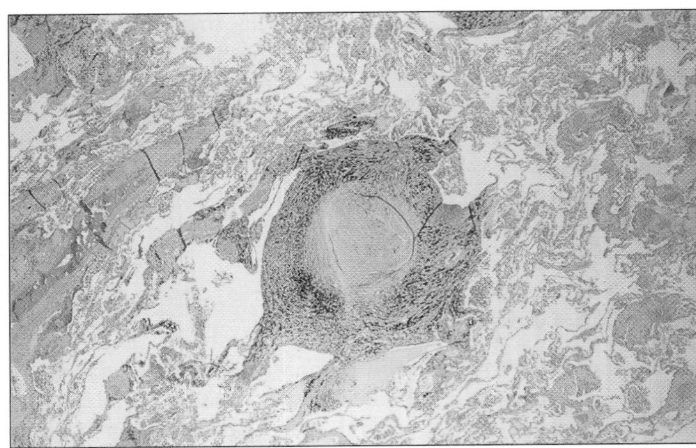

Figure 57.3 Coal nodule. Coal nodule is a rounded lesion with a collagenous center and a peripheral anthracotic pigmented area. This nodule shows a smooth, sharp border, dust-laden macrophages, and laminated collagen deposition within the interstitium of the lung. The small central area is pale and rich in collagen, and the periphery contains a varying amount of fibrogenic dust.

necrosis factor-α seems to play a key role in the recruitment of inflammatory cells induced by toxic dusts (Fig. 57.1). In addition, neutrophils recruited in the area of inflammation may contribute to the alveolitis, and respiratory and endothelial cells may play a further role by releasing various chemokines such as interleukin-8. Last, growth factors such as platelet-derived growth factor, insulin-like growth factor, fibroblast growth factor, and transforming growth factor-β are involved in the pathogenesis of lung fibrosis and in the proliferative response of type II epithelial cells, which occurs in progressive massive fibrosis.

PATHOLOGY

The lesions of CWP are focal. Simple CWP is associated with the macular and nodular lesions, whereas complicated CWP is associated with progressive massive fibrosis (PMF) and the lesions of rheumatoid pneumoconiosis (Caplan syndrome).

The initial lesions in the lung are the coal dust macules, which correspond macroscopically to focal areas of black pigmentation. Microscopically, the macule is composed of coal-dust-laden macrophages within the walls of the respiratory bronchioles and adjacent alveoli (Fig. 57.2). Focal emphysema around the coal dust macule is common and is considered an integral part of the lesion of simple CWP.

The histologic hallmark of simple CWP is the nodule. The nodules are rounded lesions with collagenous centers. Microscopically, the nodule can be divided into three zones: a central zone composed of whorls of dense, hyalinized fibrous tissue; a middle zone made up of concentrically arranged collagen fibers (onion skinning); and a peripheral zone of more randomly oriented collagen fibers, mixed with dust-laden macrophages and lymphoid cells (Fig. 57.3). "Old" inactive nodules are often relatively acellular. Particles of silica may be demonstrated in the nodules as birefringent particles under polarized light. Nodules represent a form of mixed dust fibrosis (i.e., coal dust plus silica exposure), are usually found in association with macules, and in some instances may develop from preexisting macules. They are not confined to the respiratory bronchioles, but are also seen in the subpleural and peribronchial connective tissues. There is a tendency for nodules to cluster and eventually coalesce to produce PMF. Degenerative changes are commonly observed in

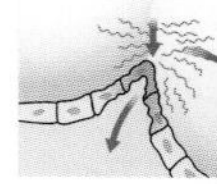

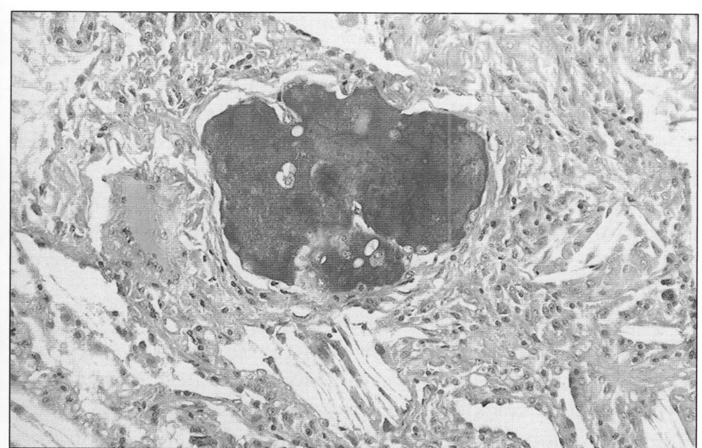

Figure 57.4 Acute silicosis. Infiltration of the alveolar walls by plasma cells and lymphocytes. Note the alveoli filled with an eosinophilic coagulum.

Table 57.2
International Labour Organization radiographic classification of pneumoconioses.

Small opacities*		
	Regular	**Irregular**
< 1.5 mm in diameter	p	s
> 1.5 mm but < 3 mm in diameter	q	t
> 3 mm but < 10 mm in diameter	r	u
Profusion: 0-3**		
Large opacities (PMF or complicated CWP)***		
> 10 mm in diameter		

Category
A - sum of diameters of lesions is not more than 50 mm
B - total area occupied by lesions is not greater than the area of the right upper lobe
C - total area occupied by lesions is greater than the area of the right upper lobe
*Small opacities are defined by their average size and profusion
**Profusion categories (0–3) are the number of small opacities apparent on the radiograph: category 0, small opacities are absent or less profuse than category 1; 1, few in number; 2, numerous; 3, opacities are very numerous and obscure the normal radiographic markings.
***Complicated pneumoconiosis or progressive massive fibrosis is divided into categories based on the size of the large opacities. To be classified as progressive massive fibrosis, at least one nodule should be 1cm or greater.

the nodular lesions, including calcification, cholesterol clefts, and cavitation. In severe silicosis, there may be structural alterations of the pulmonary vasculature resulting from the accumulation of dust in the adventitia of large vessels and involvement of the smaller blood vessels by silicotic nodules.

PMF is defined as an opacity or fibrotic pneumoconiotic lesion of 1 cm in diameter or greater. PMF lesions appear as black fibrotic masses that may be round, oval or irregular in shape. The lung and bronchovascular rays become markedly distorted. Microscopically, the lesions are composed of bundles of haphazardly arranged hyalinized collagen fibers and/or reticulin fibers and coal dust. Dust particles near the periphery of the lesion are mainly found within macrophages, whereas in the center, the dust tends to lie free in clefts and cavities. Areas of liquefactive necrosis containing fragments of degenerating collagen and cholesterol crystals are frequently observed.

The pathology of acute silicosis is quite different from the chronic form. There is infiltration of the alveolar walls with plasma cells, lymphocytes and fibroblasts with some collagenation. The alveoli are filled with an eosinophilic coagulum (Fig. 57.4). Electron microscopy shows widening of alveolar walls with some collagen and clusters of type II cells; the alveolar spaces contain degenerating cells that are probably type II alveolar cells and macrophages. Silica particles may be demonstrated in the lungs and lymph nodes; silicotic nodules are few or absent.

CLINICAL FEATURES AND DIAGNOSIS

Coal worker's pneumoconiosis and silicosis are generally first recognized from the plain chest radiograph, which is critical also in evaluating disease progression. Requirements for the diagnosis include a history of significant exposure, radiographic features consistent with these illnesses and the absence of illnesses that may mimic these diseases (primarily infections with a predominantly miliary radiographic pattern, such as tuberculosis, fungal infections, or sarcoidosis). The radiographic appearances are most usefully described by the coding system devised for standard films of pneumoconiosis under the auspices of the International Labour Office (ILO) (Table 57.2). In clinical practice simple CWP is characterized by small rounded opacities (nodules) rather than small irregular opacities, though the latter may be seen in much lesser profusion (profusion categories [0-3] are the number of small opacities apparent on the chest radiograph). When large opacities occurred, the term progressive massive fibrosis (PMF) or complicated CWP is in common use.

Clinical Features

Simple CWP and category A complicated CWP are not associated with respiratory symptoms. As in most populations engaged in manual work, breathlessness and cough in coal miners are usually a consequence of cigarette smoking. However, coal mine dust may itself cause chronic bronchitis and chronic obstructive pulmonary disease, which together are known as industrial bronchitis. The evidence that coal dust exposure is associated with the development of significant respiratory impairment has led to it becoming a compensable disease despite the absence of CWP.

By contrast, complicated pneumoconiosis (PMF) at categories B and C may present with undue breathlessness and productive cough. Melanoptysis is the result of necrosis within the conglomerate, coal-containing lesions that characterize PMF. Progressive, undue exertional dyspnea is usually the dominant symptom, but rarely there may be breathlessness at rest.

There are no specific abnormal physical signs in CWP. Finger clubbing and fine inspiratory crackles are not features of the disease and, if these are present, another explanation should be sought. Only in a small proportion of severe cases of complicated disease does CWP evolve to produce chronic respiratory failure and cor pulmonale.

Irrespective of PMF, there are a number of other disorders with which CWP may be associated—most notably the autoim-

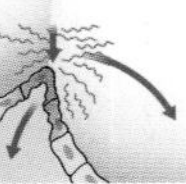

mune disorders of rheumatoid disease and progressive systemic sclerosis. The association of rheumatoid disease with CWP is known as Caplan syndrome. The diagnosis is suggested by the association of coal dust exposure, rheumatoid arthritis, and multiple well-defined large, rounded opacities (nodules with diameter greater than 10 mm) on the chest radiograph (Fig. 57.5). Spontaneous disappearance is common, with or without initial cavitation, and new nodules commonly emerge in different locations. The Caplan nodule is also more likely to cavitate, thereby producing a concentric ring pattern, and so is also known as a necrobiotic nodule. Central necrosis is rare in nodules of CWP, though it may occur in conglomerate lesions.

CWP has also been linked with a number of specific infections, the most prominent of which has been tuberculosis. In contrast to silicosis, however, CWP does not increase significantly the risk for infection with *Mycobacterium tuberculosis*. Nontuberculous mycobacteria, on the other hand, may infect lungs damaged by CWP and other types of pneumoconiosis with greater than usual frequency, and so CWP does appear to increase the risk for infection with opportunistic organisms. *Mycobacterium avium* is probably the most important of these and is poorly sensitive to antibiotic agents. *Mycobacterium kansasii* and *Mycobacterium malmoense* may also be pathogenic in this setting. It may similarly be difficult to attribute change in the radiographic appearances to advancing infection or progressive PMF. Experimental studies additionally suggest that mycobacterial infection is a factor that helps explain the progression from simple to complicated pneumoconiosis.

Other opportunistic infections reported in association with CWP have included nocardiosis, sporotrichosis, and cryptococcosis; and *Aspergillus* spp have been noted to colonize cavities in conglomerate lesions of complicated CWP.

A further association with complicated CWP, if manifested by bullous emphysema, is spontaneous pneumothorax. The advanced stages of complicated CWP are additionally associated with recurrent episodes of acute and subacute bronchitis.

Figure 57.5 Caplan syndrome. High-resolution computed tomography scan obtained at the level of the upper lobes showing bilateral parenchymal micronodules and coalescence in the right upper lobe. Note the cavitation of the nodule in the left upper lobe.

Persistent productive cough is common in coal miners in the absence of CWP. There is no evidence of a causal relationship between CWP and carcinoma of the lung, though there is strengthening evidence linking silica exposure with lung cancer. Thus, CWP and silicosis should be considered conditions that predispose workers to an increased risk of lung cancer.

Accelerated silicosis is rare and is clinically identical to the classic forms of silicosis, except that the time from initial exposure to the onset of disease is shorter and the rate of progression of disease is dramatically faster.

Acute silicosis is rare. Symptoms begin with cough, weight loss, and fatigue; there may be rapid progression to fulminant respiratory failure over several months. Chest auscultation reveals diffuse crackles, and workers with this clinical picture rapidly develop cor pulmonale and progress to a respiratory death. Survival after the onset of symptoms is often less than 2 years. Diffuse alveolar filling, most apparent at the bases, is the most prominent finding on the chest X-ray (Fig. 57.6). Although serial chest X-rays from workers with this illness have been infrequently reported, it appears that the bibasilar filling pattern progresses into large opacities located in the middle zones rather than the upper zones.

CHEST RADIOLOGY

The radiographic pattern of simple CWP is typically one of small rounded opacities that appear first in the upper zones (Fig. 57.7). The middle and lower zones become involved as the number of opacities increases. The nodules increase in profusion with increasing dust exposure; a change in profusion after dust exposure has ceased is very unusual. Calcification of the nodules may occur (10% to 20% of cases).

Complicated pneumoconiosis is defined as a lesion of 1 cm or greater in longest diameter. The large opacities are usually predominant in the upper lobes, may be unilateral or bilateral, and are symmetrically or asymmetrically distributed. The pattern of change in size is variable and unpredictable. Most PMF occurs on a background of simple pneumoconiosis, but this is not invariably so, and it may occur after dust exposure has ceased. Cavitation can develop within a PMF lesion, and occasionally there is a dense peripheral arc or rim at its lower pole that represents calcification. Dense calcification with the lesion is also sometimes seen. PMF is often associated with bullous

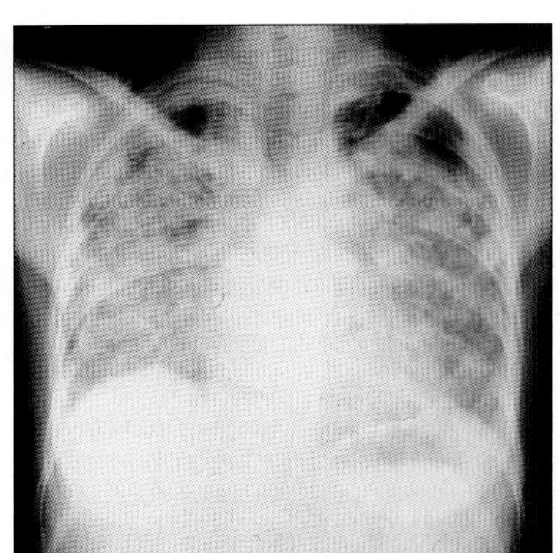

Figure 57.6 Chest X-ray showing alveolar filling in acute silicosis. A 28-year-old woman inhaled fine particles of silica from abrasive powder. The disease that has developed was rapidly progressive silicosis, which was typically fatal over the next several years.

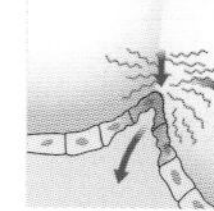

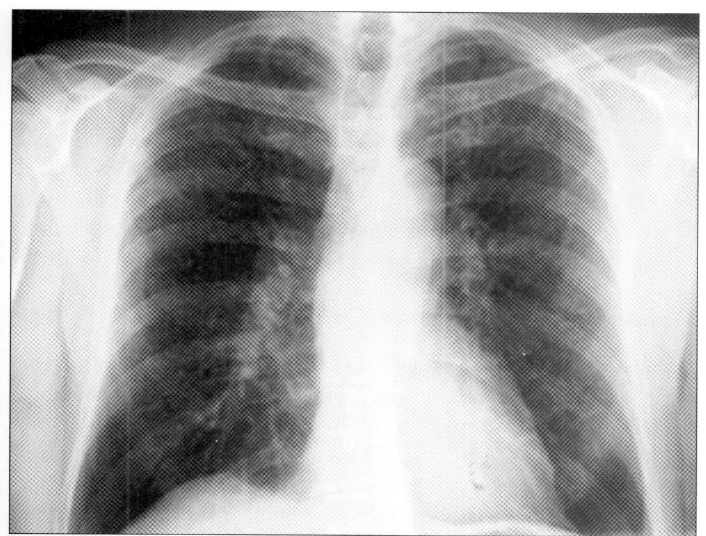

Figure 57.7 Chest X-ray of simple coal worker's pneumoconiosis. Simple coal worker's pneumoconiosis in a 55-year-old man who had worked for 18 years in an underground coal mine. He was a nonsmoker with a chronic cough and normal lung function. The X-ray shows a diffuse distribution of small rounded opacities, more prominent in the upper zones than the lower zones.

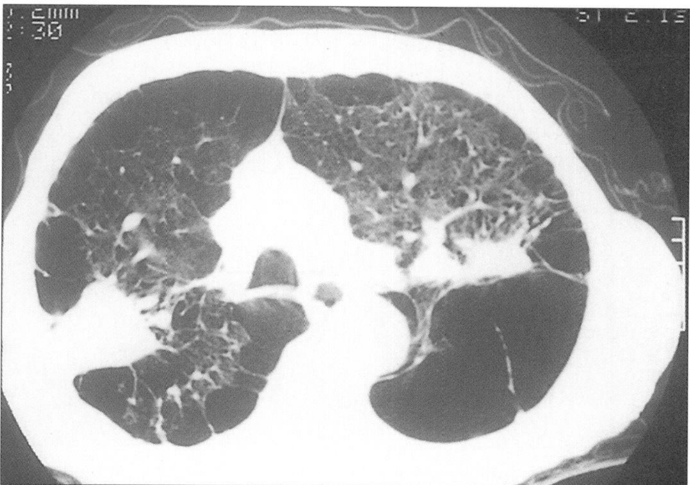

Figure 57.8 Progressive massive fibrosis. High-resolution computed tomography scan showing bilateral masses consistent with progressive massive fibrosis. There is a background of nodules associated with bullous changes around progressive massive fibrosis lesions referred to as paracicatricial emphysema.

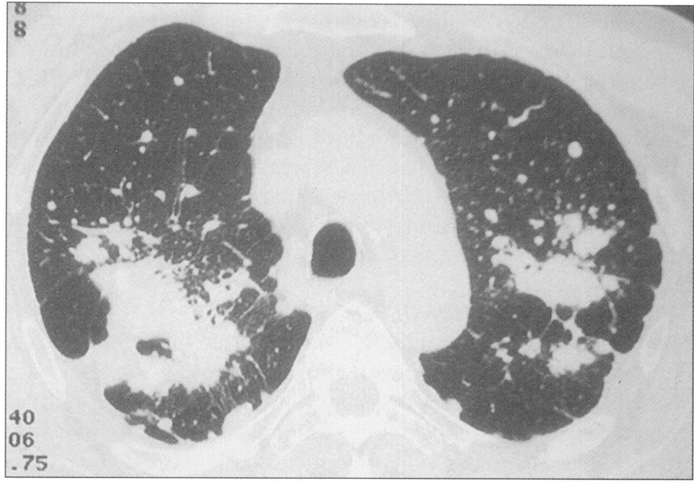

Figure 57.9 Aseptic necrosis. Computed tomography scan showing bilateral masses with necrosis of the right upper lobe mass and bilateral emphysema.

emphysema and fibrotic scarring, leading to distortion of the lung and shift of the trachea and mediastinum to the affected side. Irregular, mainly basal, opacities may also be seen on standard radiographs. Eggshell calcification is uncommon in CWP but may occur in intrapulmonary, hilar, or mediastinal lymph nodes, possibly because of concomitant exposure to silica. Pleural effusion is uncommon in CWP. Its presence may be related to an associated infection or an interaction with a systemic collagen vascular disease.

In simple CWP, computed tomography (CT) shows parenchymal lesions that can be detected in miners with normal chest radiographs. There is thus greater sensitivity compared with plain radiographs in detecting simple CWP, but less obvious benefit for complicated pneumoconiosis. There is a posterior and right-sided predominance in the upper zones. Detection is dramatically influenced by CT technique, and a 10-mm collimation is considered the best technique.

Nodules are usually observed against a background of parenchymal micronodules and are generally associated with subpleural micronodules. Two categories of lesions can be observed in PMF: lesions with irregular borders that are associated with disruption of the pulmonary parenchyma and lead to typical scar emphysema (Fig. 57.8), and lesions with regular borders that are unassociated with scar emphysema. When the lesions are larger than 4 cm in diameter, irregular areas of aseptic necrosis can be observed with or without cavitation (Fig. 57.9).

Two major forms of emphysema occurring in coal workers can be detected on CT: bullous changes around PMF lesions, referred to as paracicatricial or scar emphysema, whereas nonbullous emphysematous lesions are defined as irregular emphysema (Fig. 57.10). Lesions of diffuse pulmonary fibrosis can be detected on high-resolution CT as honeycombing or areas of ground-glass attenuation. Two specific etiologies of fibrosis of coal miners should be considered: a direct effect of deposited coal or silica particles and an indirect effect resulting from an association with scleroderma.

LUNG FUNCTION

In all studies about lung function of pneumoconiotic patients, account should be taken of a number of different and confounding influences; the effects of smoking need to be considered. It can be stated that simple CWP has no important effect on spirometric measures when prior dust exposure is taken into account and when smoking habits are also considered. Similarly, simple silicosis has no appreciable effect on lung function. In more advanced disease, slight reduction in volumes, compliance, and gas transfer can be present; there is a predominantly restrictive pattern. Slight reduction in arterial oxygen tension on effort may be observed in advanced disease. Oxygen desaturation is not present at rest or on moderate effort in the nonconglomerate stages of disease. As in the case of radiographic progression, the changes in pulmonary function are more likely to occur in

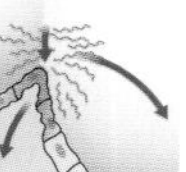

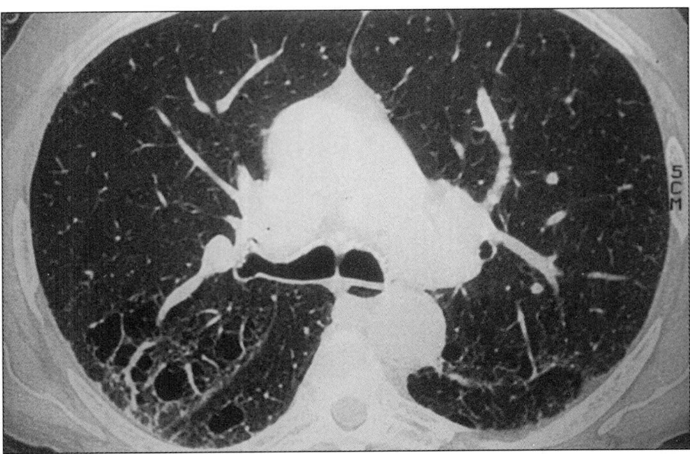

Figure 57.10 Nonbullous emphysema. High-resolution computed tomography scan showing small bullae and low attenuation, without progressive massive fibrosis lesions, defined as centrilobular or non-paracicatricial emphysema.

workers who have had intense exposure to dust. In addition, it must be pointed out that miners who did not have CWP on chest radiography exhibited lower forced expiratory volume in 1 second than controls, suggesting the frequent presence of coal dust–induced chronic obstructive pulmonary disease. In PMF, lung function depends on the extent of the lesions and of associated emphysema. Studies of lung function in the more advanced stages of PMF have shown an obstructive and restrictive pattern; therefore, diffusing capacity is usually reduced. Compliance is usually somewhat decreased. Ultimately, hypoxemic respiratory failure may occur.

SEROLOGIC AND IMMUNOLOGIC FEATURES

There are no specific biologic features of pneumoconiosis. However, immunologic abnormalities are now well described: positive circulating antinuclear antibodies or rheumatoid factor. Serum immunoglobulins A and G have significantly raised levels in miners with pneumoconiosis. Finally, increased serum angiotensin-converting enzyme level was observed in 45% of pneumoconiotic coal miners, whatever the radiologic classification of pneumoconiosis.

BRONCHOALVEOLAR LAVAGE

There was no change in differential cell count, in contrast to a number of other interstitial disorders of the lung. Alveolar inflammatory cells from patients with CWP, especially those with PMF, released spontaneously more superoxide anions, proinflammatory cytokines, and profibrotic mediators than did those from control subjects.

CLINICAL COURSE, TREATMENT AND PREVENTION

Prognosis

Simple CWP is not associated with premature mortality, but approximately 4% of deaths in coal miners are due directly to complicated pneumoconiosis. In categories 1, 2, and 3 of simple CWP and category A of complicated CWP, life expectancy is the same as that among the general population without pneumoconiosis.

The rate of progression to PMF appears to be influenced chiefly by the age at which the miner begins to show radiographic changes of CWP; the earlier the diagnosis, the more likely there is to be progression reflecting individual susceptibility and the level of cumulative exposure.

Management

No specific treatment affects the course of CWP, though treatment options are available for complications such as tuberculosis, pneumothorax, and chronic hypoxemia.

When a miner is found to have CWP, further dust exposure should be excluded. Simple pneumoconiosis does not necessarily imply complete exclusion from mining, whereas when PMF is detected, all further dusty works should be prevented. Additional information is given from pulmonary function tests because the development of an obstructive ventilatory defect (resulting from dust exposure) may occur in the absence of CWP. In all smoking patients, advice and support of smoking cessation should be given. If a physician concludes there is disability from CWP, he or she should be able to direct the patient toward whatever mechanism exists for compensation.

Prevention

The prevention of pneumoconiosis depends on controlling exposure concentrations of ambient dust to levels known to be associated with minimal and acceptable risk. Dust control is affected primarily by ventilation, though water sprayed at points of dust generation is a useful measure of dust suppression. The effectiveness of such measures should be monitored by regular measurement of dust concentrations, and by regular clinical and radiologic surveillance of the workforce. Surveillance allows early recognition of workers with simple pneumoconiosis, who are likely to be those with greatest susceptibility, so that ongoing exposure can be restricted (perhaps by transfer to jobs with lower exposure) and the risk of future disablement from PMF reduced.

Variability of individual susceptibility is likely to be an important determinant for CWP, as it is for most occupational disorders, and a number of predictive factors may be useful in identifying miners with higher than average risk: initially presence of expiratory wheezes, obstructive pattern of lung function, and more micronodules on CT scan. An alternative approach for the future might involve genetic screening evaluating polymorphism in the promoter of various mediators. In any event, control of exposure levels alone is likely to prevent most cases of disabling PMF, and it has been predicted that an exposure concentration over 35 working years that does not exceed an average of 4.3 mg/m^3 is associated with a probability for the development of category 2 or more CWP of no more than 3.4%. This represents a dramatic reduction in risk over the last 50 years.

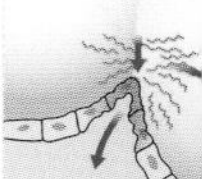

SUGGESTED READINGS

Attfield MD, Seixas NS: Prevalence of pneumoconiosis and its relationship to dust exposure in a cohort of U.S. bituminous coal miners and ex-miners. Am J Ind Med 27:137-151, 1995.

Begin R, Cantin A, Massé S: Recent advances in the pathogenesis and clinical assessment of mineral dust pneumoconioses: Asbestosis, silicosis and coal pneumoconiosis. Eur Respir J 2:988-1001, 1989.

Piguet PF, Collart MA, Grau GE, Sappino AP, Vassalli P: Requirement of tumour necrosis factor for development of silica-induced pulmonary fibrosis. Nature 344:245-247, 1990.

Remy-Jardin M, Remy J, Farre I, Marquette CH: Computed tomography evaluation of silicosis and coal worker's pneumoconiosis. Radiol Clin N Am 30:1155-1176, 1992.

Rom WN, Bitterman PB, Rennard SI, Cantin A, Crystal RG: Characterization of the lower respiratory tract inflammation of nonsmoking individuals with interstitial lung disease associated with chronic inhalation of inorganic dust. Am Rev Respir Dis 136:1429-1434, 1987.

Seaton A: Coal mining, emphysema, and compensation. Editorial. Br J Ind Med 47:433-435, 1990.

Vanhee D, Gosset P, Boitelle A, Wallaert B, Tonnel AB: Cytokines and cytokine network in silicosis and coal workers' pneumoconiosis. Eur Respir J 8:1-9, 1995.

Wouters EFM, Jorna THJM, Westenend M: Respiratory effects of coal dust exposure: Clinical effects and diagnosis. Exp Lung Res 20:385-394, 1994.

Zhai R, Jetten M, Schins RP, Franssen H, Borm J: Polymorphisms in the promoter of the tumor necrosis factor alpha in coal miners. Ann J Ind Med 34:318-324, 1998.

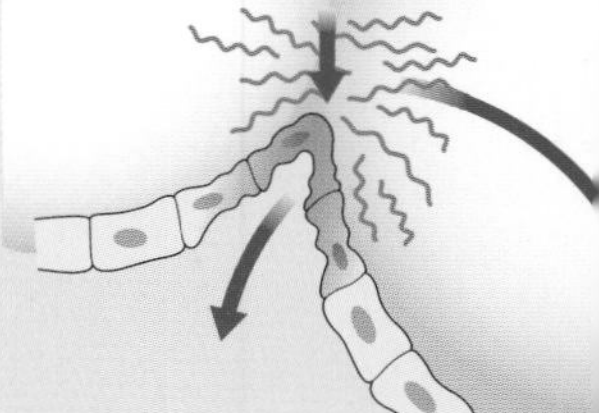

CHAPTER 58 Asbestosis

Lee S. Newman and E. Brigitte Gottschall

Inhalational exposure to asbestos produces both malignant and nonmalignant diseases of the chest. In this chapter, the focus is on the two major categories of nonmalignant disease—asbestosis and asbestos-related pleural disorders, presented in Table 58.1. These conditions have received a great deal of attention from the scientific and medical communities because of the ubiquitous use of asbestos in modern society and its diverse and pernicious toxicities. Despite major progress in the awareness and control of exposure, a large burden of asbestos-related disease will continue because of ongoing exposure and because of disease latency.

EPIDEMIOLOGY, RISK FACTORS, AND PATHOLOGY

Epidemiology

The first well-documented cases of asbestosis were reported in 1906 among asbestos textile workers. Through the 1920s and 1930s, reports emerged of asbestosis, pleural thickening, pleural calcification, and right ventricular failure in asbestos-exposed workers. Radiographic studies that began in the 1930s documented an asbestosis prevalence of 25% to 55% in these workers, especially among those who have greater cumulative exposure. With thousands of commercial applications and the mineral's resistance to degradation, asbestos remains ubiquitous. Between 1940 and 1979, more than 20 million people had potential exposure in the United States alone. Given the long latency required before asbestosis becomes clinically apparent, past and current asbestos workers must all be considered to be at risk of this fibrosing lung disorder. Disability and mortality from asbestosis will continue well into the 21st century.

Etiology and Risk Factors

The minerals referred to herein as asbestos are a family of naturally occurring, flexible, fibrous hydrous silicates found in soil worldwide. Mined asbestos fibers are categorized as either long and curly (serpentine) or straight and rodlike (amphibole). The serpentine fiber, chrysotile, accounts for most of the commercially used asbestos, favored for its properties of heat resistance, flexibility, and ease of spinning for textiles. There are five categories of amphiboles—crocidolite, amosite, anthophyllite, tremolite, and actinolite. These more rigid fibers are less commonly used, but still pathogenic. All major commercial forms have been associated with nonmalignant respiratory disorders and with lung cancer and mesothelioma, as discussed in Chapters 41 and 64.

Asbestosis is the result of either direct or bystander exposure to asbestos-containing materials. Major sources of exposure are summarized in Table 58.2. During the first half of the 20th century, high exposures to asbestos dust occurred in the manufacturing of asbestos textiles and construction materials and in the construction and shipbuilding trades. Potential exposures still occur in the construction trades and in the process of asbestos abatement. Although the use of asbestos has been curtailed in many developed nations since the 1970s, in less-developed countries this inexpensive but hazardous material continues to be used widely. High cumulative, occupational exposures in these settings are still commonplace.

A clear dose-response relationship exists between asbestos exposure and asbestosis, although controversy remains concerning risks at low-level exposure. Risk for asbestosis varies widely among industries, with more disease seen in textile and construction workers compared with those in mining. Development of the disease is associated with factors such as how respirable the fiber type is, the cumulative dose of exposure, the capacity of the lung to clear the fibers, and the biopersistence of the asbestos. In general, the relative risk of developing asbestosis for asbestos workers increases in proportion to the asbestos exposure levels in the workplace. More severe disease has been associated with higher retention of asbestos fiber in the lungs. Typical asbestos fibers found in the lungs are 20 to 50 μm long, and are initially deposited at the bifurcations of conducting airways. Thin fibers, of diameters less than 3 μm, translocate readily into the alveolar space, interstitium, and pleural space. Thicker fibers tend to be incompletely phagocytosed by alveolar macrophages and are retained in the lung, where they can trigger the inflammatory events that lead to fibrosis, as discussed in the following section.

Pathology

Asbestosis is defined pathologically as bilateral, diffuse interstitial fibrosis of the lungs caused by the inhalation of asbestos fibers (Fig. 58.1). Gray streaks of fibrosis can be seen in the parenchyma along interlobar and interlobular septa. Later, the pleural surface becomes more nodular in appearance, and the parenchyma loses volume and elasticity and forms more fibrotic scars and honeycombing. The gross pathologic appearance is most obvious in the lower lung zones bilaterally, with the worst disease nearest to the pleura. The pathology definition remains unclear. The College of American Pathologists has defined four grades of severity:

- Grade 1—fibrosis that involves the wall of a respiratory bronchiole

Table 58.1
Nonmalignant asbestos-related diseases

Condition	Pathologic effect	Description
Asbestosis	Parenchymal effect	Interstitial pulmonary fibrosis
Benign nodules	Parenchymal effect	Lymphoid or fibrotic nodular scars
Benign pleural effusion	Pleural effect	Exudative, transient effusion
Pleural plaques	Pleural effect	Collagenous, hyalinized masses; circumscribed, avascular, usually affecting the parietal pleura
Diffuse pleural thickening	Pleural effect	Collagenous, hyalinized masses; diffuse, avascular, affecting the parietal and visceral pleura, and interlobular space
Rounded atelectasis	Combined pleural and parenchymal effects	Scarring of pleura and adjacent lung tissue, resulting in retraction, entrapment, and local partial collapse of lung

The nonmalignant diseases caused by asbestos. Categorization is based on the effects on the lung parenchyma and pleura.

- Grade 2—Grade 1 plus involvement of alveolar ducts and adjacent alveoli, but with some nonfibrotic adjacent alveolar septae
- Grade 3—Grade 2 fibrosis, but with coalescence, such that all alveoli between two adjacent bronchi show fibrotic septa, with some complete obliteration
- Grade 4—Grade 3 fibrosis plus honeycombing

A supplementary scoring system has been developed to describe the degree of airway involvement.

Although histologic evidence of pulmonary fibrosis may occasionally be obtained in the course of clinical evaluation, routine lung biopsy and lavage are not recommended, and microscopic evidence is rarely required to diagnose asbestosis.

Occasionally, the determination of asbestos fibers in lung tissue, bronchoalveolar lavage, or sputum may be used to document past exposure, although these measurements are neither usually relied upon nor required for the clinical diagnosis of asbestosis. Under light microscopy or using transmission electron microscopy, uncoated fibers or fibers coated with proteinaceous material may be detected. These latter so-called asbestos bodies or ferruginous bodies are nonspecific, because they can be found in occupationally unexposed individuals, in occupationally exposed individuals who have no asbestos-related lung disease, and in workers who suffer asbestosis. Generally, the most exposed and most severely affected individuals have higher asbestos fiber counts, but a significant interlaboratory variability is found in these measures.

Table 58.2
Major asbestos uses and sources of exposure

Environment	Type of exposure	Source of exposure
Occupational	Asbestos–cement products	Construction industry (sheeting used in roofing and cladding of structural materials, molded into roof tiles, pipes, gutters; filler for wall cracks, cement, joint compound, adhesive, caulking putty)
	Floor tiling	Filler and reinforcing agent in asphalt flooring, vinyl tile, adhesive
	Insulation, fireproofing	Insulators, pipefitters Construction industry (pipes, boiler covers, ship bulkheads, sprayed on walls and ceilings as fireproofing, soundproofing)
	Textiles	Fireproof textiles used in clothing, blankets
	Paper products	Roofing felt, wall coverings, mill board, insulating paper
	Friction materials	Brake linings
	Rubber, plastic manufacture	Filler in rubber and plastics
	Building trades, secondhand exposure	Building maintenance activities, pipefitting, electrical repair, boiler tending and repair, power station maintenance Carpenters, plumbers, welders
Domestic	'Fouling the nest'	Carrying home asbestos in hair and clothes of exposed workers results in exposure to family members
	Secondhand exposure	Residential remodeling, removal, handling of frayed, friable asbestos in homes can cause environmental exposure
General	Contaminated buildings	Found in low levels in buildings under normal use Elevated exposures from remodeling, renovation, asbestos removal, disturbance of contaminated materials such as acoustic ceiling tiles, vinyl floor tiles, paints, plaster, pipes, boilers, steel beams
	Geologic exposure	Living near asbestos mines or cement factories, or in geographic areas in which naturally occurring asbestos is found in ambient air
	Urban environment	Ambient air levels slightly higher in cities, perhaps because of automotive brakes, and high concentration of industry and construction

The major environmental and occupational sources of asbestos exposure. Categorization is based on exposures in the workplace, home, or general environment.

Pathogenesis

Some of the major events thought to be involved in the pathogenesis of asbestosis are summarized in Fig. 58.2. Within minutes after asbestos fibers having been inhaled, a local tissue response is initiated at the bifurcations of terminal bronchioles and alveolar ducts. The first changes occur in epithelial cells and then in alveolar macrophages as they attempt to engulf and are pierced by the fibers. In addition to cell death, which leads to the release of macrophage contents, asbestos-activated macrophages release reactive oxygen species that directly damage the tissue through peroxidation and direct cytotoxicity. Asbestos can also induce toxicity by mechanisms independent of its ability to promote reactive oxygen species.

Increasing numbers of alveolar macrophages accumulate within 48 hours of first exposure. With chronic inhalation, a localized fibrosing alveolitis in the peribronchiolar region develops, followed by diffuse fibrotic scarring. Increasing the dose of asbestos increases the cellular response. A cascade of events ensues, in which the macrophages and neutrophils release various cytokines (such as interleukin-8 and gamma-interferon), chemokines, oxidants, and growth factors (such as fibronectin, platelet-derived growth factor, insulin-like growth factor, transforming growth factor-β, tumor necrosis factor-α, and fibroblast growth factor). These attract and alter the function of other inflammatory cells and resident cells, and thus promote inflam-

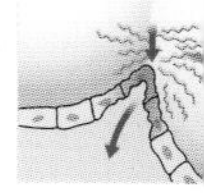

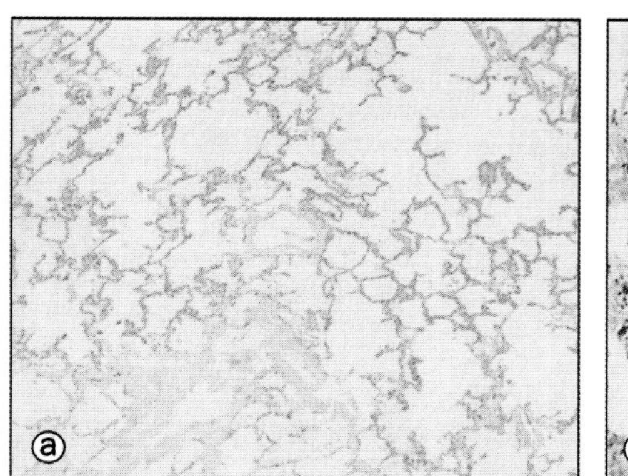

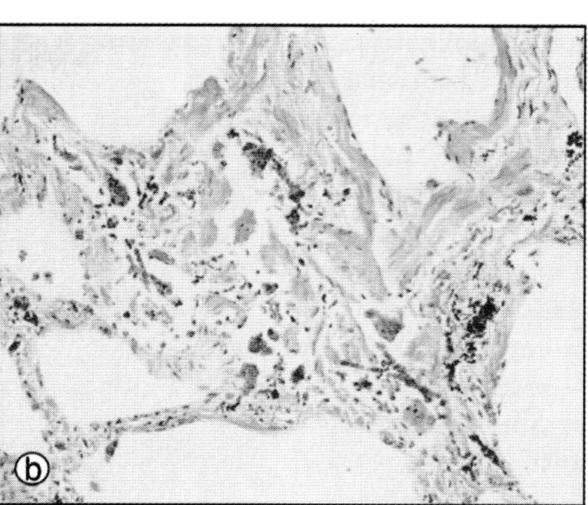

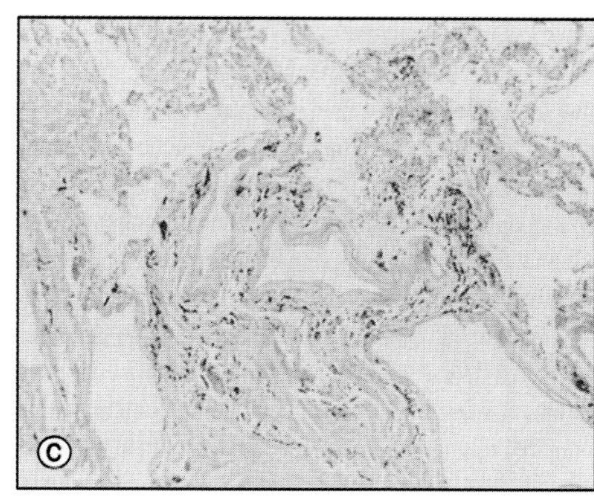

Figure 58.1 Histology of asbestosis. A, In this grade 1 lesion, fibrosis is limited to the peribronchiolar tissue and the walls of the respiratory bronchioles (hematoxylin and eosin). **B,** Enlargement of a grade 1 lesion illustrates presence of asbestos bodies (hematoxylin and eosin). **C,** In this grade 3 lesion, fibrosis extends into the interstitial space between the respiratory units and into the alveolar ducts (hematoxylin and eosin). (Courtesy of Dr. Val Vallythan, National Institute for Occupational Safety and Health, Morgantown, West Virginia).

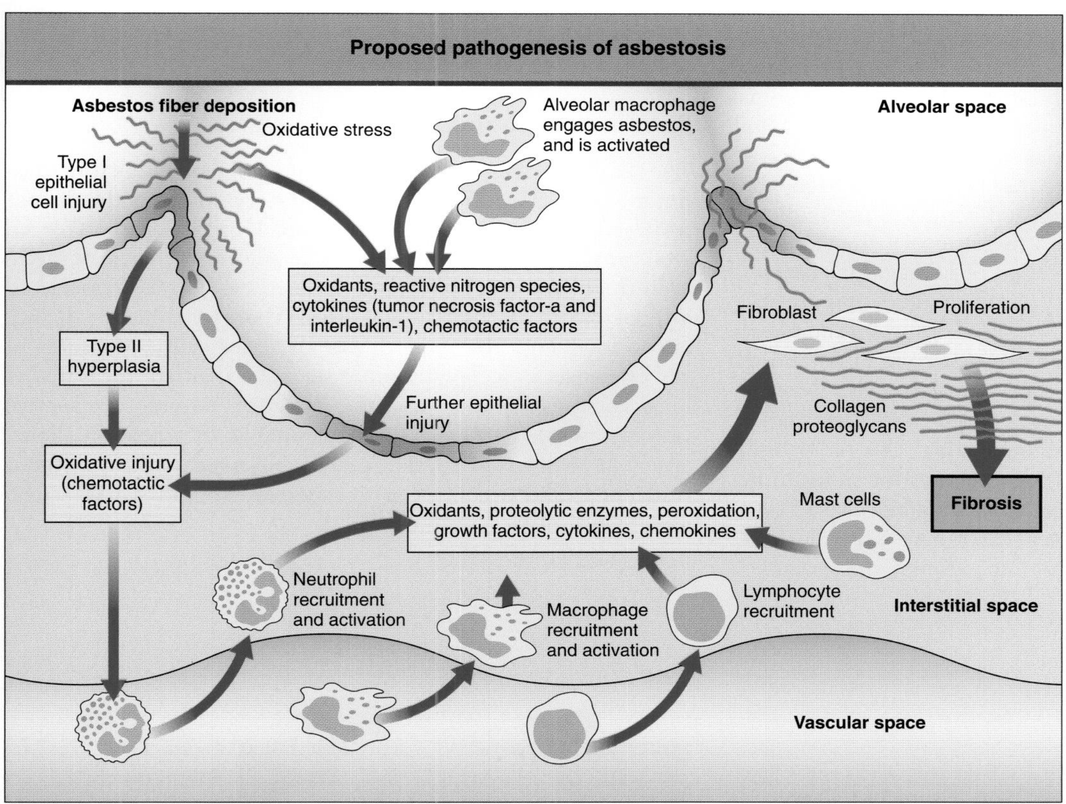

Figure 58.2 Proposed pathogenesis of asbestosis. Asbestos fibers deposit at branch points in the distal airways and alveolar ducts, which prompts an inflammatory cascade characterized by cellular activation, recruitment, and injury. The result is fibroblast proliferation and extracellular matrix deposition in the interstitial space.

mation and fibrosis. The response of fibroblasts to these signals is to proliferate and produce the constituents of extracellular matrix (e.g., collagen, proteoglycans) in the pulmonary interstitium. Resident cells themselves are both targets and perpetrators of the fibrotic response. The pathogenesis of the chronic fibrotic response remains sketchy. However, it is clear that this chronic response is progressive and that, apart from macrophage, neutrophil, and epithelial cells, a number of other cell types, such as lymphocytes and mast cells, contribute to the cycle of lung remodeling and fibrosis. Multiple, functionally overlapping, redundant inflammatory events occur in the lung simultaneously during the period of fibrogenesis. The consequence is an irreversible alteration in the structure and function of the lung.

CLINICAL FEATURES

Asbestosis is the pulmonary fibrotic disease that results from asbestos exposure. It affects the lungs symmetrically and is typically diagnosed on the basis of a consistent occupational or environmental history of asbestos exposure plus evidence of pulmonary fibrosis, usually by chest radiography. The latency period from first exposure to clinical disease is 10 to 20 years, but can be up to 40 years or more, with shorter latency and more severe disease seen in those workers who have the highest inhalational exposures. In some situations the exposure history may be difficult to document. If needed, further evidence of occupational exposure can be verified by identifying high

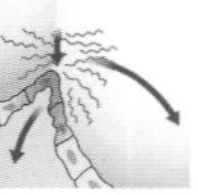

numbers of asbestos bodies in bronchoalveolar lavage fluid, sputum, or lung tissue, as discussed previously. Evidence of bilateral pleural plaques is pathognomonic for previous asbestos exposure. The radiographic finding of bilateral interstitial markings in the lower lung zone is sufficient radiographic evidence of asbestosis, although (as discussed in the following section) other tools such as computed tomography and measures of lung physiology also aid diagnosis.

The most common symptoms of asbestosis are the insidious onset of dyspnea on exertion (and eventually at rest), dry cough that can be paroxysmal, and fatigue. Hemoptysis, chest pain, and weight loss are not common and should raise suspicion of asbestos-related malignancy. Although physical abnormalities are uncommon at the early stages of asbestosis, over time these patients may develop dry, bilateral basilar rales at end inspiration, digital clubbing cyanosis, and signs of cor pulmonale.

Radiologic Findings

Radiographically, asbestosis typically presents in the lower lobes with irregular "reticular" markings toward the lung periphery and costophrenic angles (Fig. 58.3). Linear opacities that resemble extensions of vascular markings may assume a netlike appearance. In early or less severe disease, the middle and upper lung zones may appear relatively spared. With progression, the linear and irregular opacities thicken and spread to the midlung zones, but rarely to the apex. The International Labor Organization (ILO) International Classification of Radiographs characterizes each type of irregular opacity based on increasing size and thickness as either *s*, *t*, or *u*, and on a scale of profusion (number) of opacities from normal profusion (0/–, 0/0, 0/1) to severe (3/2, 3/3, 3/+; see Chapter 57, Table 57.2 for classification details). When irregular opacities are seen on the chest radiograph in conjunction with pleural thickening, the radiograph can be considered virtually pathognomonic for asbestosis. However, the chest radiograph lacks sensitivity, because 15% to 20% of symptomatic, biopsy-proved cases have normal chest radiographs. Focal masses are uncommon except those caused by rounded atelectasis.

Computed Tomography

As a result of the limited sensitivity of the radiograph, computed tomography has been thoroughly investigated. High-resolution computed tomography (HRCT), obtaining 1-to 3-mm slices, has sensitivity superior to the plain chest radiograph in detection of the fine reticular opacities in this disease. Of asbestos-exposed workers who have normal chest radiographs, 10% to 30% have HRCT scans that suggest underlying interstitial disease. Thus, the HRCT can prove useful when the clinical index of suspicion for asbestosis is high, but the chest radiograph appears normal. The most common HRCT findings in asbestosis are short, peripheral septal lines, subpleural curvilinear lines, peripheral cystic lesions (honeycombing), parenchymal bands adjacent to areas of pleural thickening, and bronchiolar thickening (Fig. 58.4). The density of interstitial abnormalities found on HRCT has been shown to correlate with the symptoms, and with physiologic and inflammatory indicators of asbestosis, although in general both the chest radiograph and the HRCT show only a limited correlation with disease severity measured physiologically.

Pulmonary Physiology

The earliest physiologic changes include small airway dysfunction (e.g., decreased forced expiratory flow). As the disease progresses, restriction (diminished total lung capacity and forced vital capacity) is observed, as is worsening gas exchange as measured by diffusing capacity, and by exercise- and rest-associated arterial blood gas partial pressures. These parameters do not necessarily show the same degree of abnormality. Measures of gas exchange are generally more sensitive than are measures of lung volumes in this disorder. Isolated, severe, obstructive airway disease is usually not attributable to asbestosis alone, although airflow obstruction can be observed with or without restriction, and occurs even in asbestos-exposed workers who were nonsmokers.

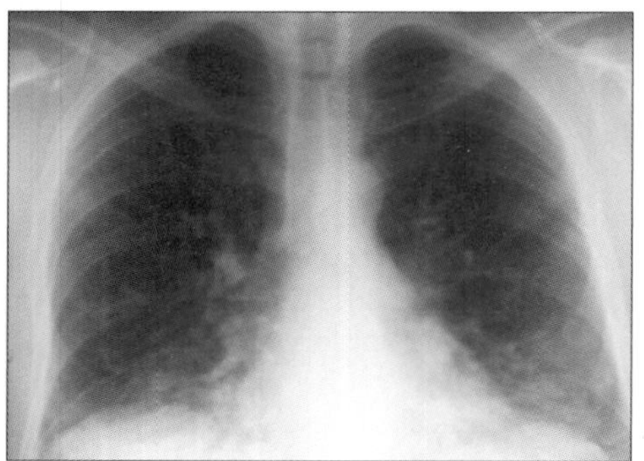

Figure 58.3 Chest radiograph illustrating parenchymal abnormalities in asbestosis. Descriptive terms from the International Labor Organization's classification for the radiographic appearance of pneumoconioses are used here (see Chapter 57, Table 57. 2). Coarse "u" and "t" reticular opacities can be seen in the lower lung zones. In this advanced case, the profusion of small opacities is 3/3.

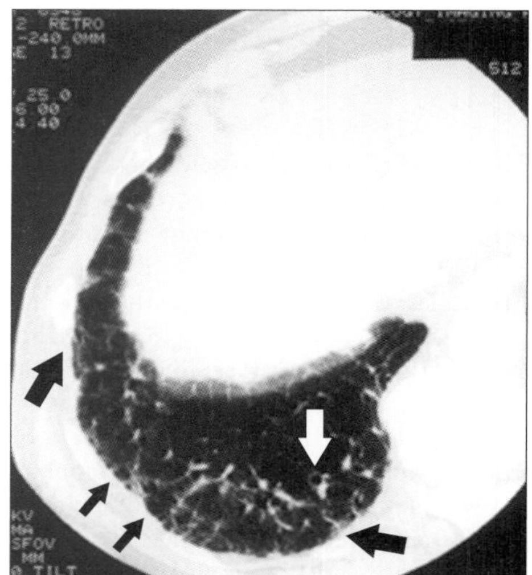

Figure 58.4 Asbestosis. High-resolution computed tomography of an asbestos-exposed worker who has asbestosis and mild pleural thickening. Patchy subpleural accentuation of interstitial markings (thick arrows) with honeycombing (thin arrows) and traction bronchiectasis (white arrow) are classic for the computed tomography appearance of advanced asbestosis.

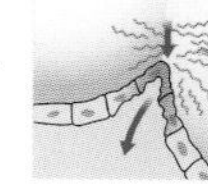

DIAGNOSIS

The long latency between asbestos exposure and development of asbestosis and the gradually progressive nature of the symptoms mean that this disease has a tendency to remain undetected until fairly late in its course. Efforts to conduct workplace surveillance using the chest radiograph and ILO readings of these films have improved disease detection. The diagnosis is based on a consistent history of exposure to asbestos, with sufficient latency, and evidence of interstitial fibrosis. A careful work and environmental history holds the key to determining that past exposure has occurred. As discussed previously, the presence of bilateral pleural plaques or demonstration of asbestos bodies in lavage or on biopsy can also aid in the assessment of exposure. Although most algorithms for diagnosis of asbestosis suggest that the combination of histologic material plus mineralogic assessment is the most sensitive and specific method of diagnosis, frequently such biopsy material is unavailable and unnecessary in making a probable determination of disease. Even the lung pathology should be considered in context with clinical data. The main considerations in the histologic differential diagnosis include the other pneumoconioses and other causes of pulmonary fibrosis such as pharmaceutic drugs, metal dusts, infectious agents, autoimmune disorders, and idiopathic pulmonary fibrosis.

In the absence of lung histology and mineralogic analysis, the clinical diagnosis of asbestosis can be made with reasonable confidence based on:

- History of significant asbestos exposure
- Appropriate time interval between exposure and disease detection (latency)
- Radiographic evidence of bilateral lung fibrosis by chest radiograph or HRCT (especially with coexisting pleural plaques).

Helpful, but less essential, criteria include evidence of restrictive lung function, abnormalities of gas exchange, bilateral inspiratory crackles (rales), and digital clubbing.

TREATMENT

Presently, no cure exists for asbestosis and no benefit from the use of corticosteroids or other immunosuppressive therapy has been documented. After exposure and early disease have occurred, no prophylactic measures are available.

Medical management in cases of asbestosis focuses on:

- Supplemental oxygen therapy in the face of hypoxemia or pulmonary hypertension
- Treatment of intercurrent infections
- Treatment of right ventricular failure in advanced disease
- Immunization for influenza and pneumococcal infections
- Appropriate medical documentation of the degree of physical impairment and appropriate advice to the patient to apply for workers' compensation benefits if exposure was occupational
- Education on the signs and symptoms of lung cancer and mesothelioma
- Assistance in smoking cessation among current smokers who have asbestosis to help reduce the risk of lung cancer
- Cessation of ongoing asbestos exposure is advisable, because it may slow disease progression, based on experimental evidence

CLINICAL COURSE

The prognosis for patients with asbestosis varies widely. It is dependent, in part, on the magnitude of exposure. In 1906, the disease was almost uniformly fatal by the third decade of life. However, with fewer exposures and lower exposure times, and with superior detection and supportive care, few patients demonstrate such severe progression of their disease. After removal from exposure, progression is usually slow, and occurs in 5% to 40% of patients over approximately a decade of follow-up. Thus, if clinical deterioration occurs over a period of days or weeks, the clinician must look first for other explanations, such as infection or malignancy. Many patients may remain mildly symptomatic for many years, and show little or no objective signs of disease progression, whereas others show steady, inexorable decline in lung function, gas exchange, worsening symptoms, development of end-stage respiratory insufficiency, and cor pulmonale with right ventricular failure.

Patients who suffer asbestosis are at increased risk of intercurrent lung infections and lung cancer. The best prognosis is found in those workers who have the lowest ILO profusion scores (i.e., chest radiographs that show the fewest irregular opacities) at time of termination of exposure. Tobacco smoking contributes to radiographic evidence of disease severity. Greater age at time of diagnosis is a strong predictor of progression; both smoking and duration of exposure contribute relatively smaller, yet significant, effects also. Multiple studies demonstrate that those with the greatest average and cumulative dust exposures tend to have the higher initial profusions of small opacities on chest radiographs and more rapid disease progression.

Based on National Center for Health Statistics data through 1992, for US residents the age-adjusted mortality rate attributable to asbestosis began to plateau in the 1990s, but only after having risen from an age-adjusted mortality rate of 0.44 per 1,000,000 population in 1968 to 3.01 per 1,000,000 in 1990. Mortality rates are much higher among men than among women, and the age at which people die of asbestosis has risen from a median of 60 years in 1968 to approximately 74 years in 1992. In 1992, asbestosis resulted in nearly 12,000 years of potential life lost to life expectancy. Lung cancer is a significant contributing cause of increased mortality in asbestosis patients.

ASBESTOS-RELATED, NONMALIGNANT PLEURAL DISORDERS

The most common pleural changes caused by asbestos are pleural plaques, with or without pleural calcification and diffuse pleural thickening. Presence of pleural thickening is a marker of exposure. Pleural changes are now known to contribute to the lung function abnormalities seen in asbestos-exposed workers. Both types of pleural alteration contribute independently to restrictive lung physiology (reduced vital capacity), reduced lung compliance, and diminished diffusing capacity. Of asbestos-exposed construction workers, 20% to 60% demonstrate chest radiographic evidence of pleural disease, which is remarkable in light of the insensitivity of the radiograph.

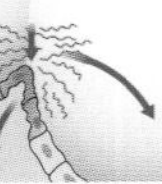

Circumscribed pleural plaques that involve the parietal pleura are usually symmetrical and bilateral, most commonly between the fifth and eighth ribs toward the posterolateral aspects of the thorax (Fig. 58.5); they also frequently involve the diaphragmatic pleura (Fig. 58.6). These lesions remain discrete. Thus, if radiographic evidence of more diffuse thickening is found, either mesothelioma or diffuse pleural thickening must be considered. Histologically, pleural plaques are hyalinized, acellular, avascular masses, and rarely contain asbestos bodies. They have a tendency to calcify, which can be mistaken for nodular infiltrates on the chest radiograph. Although the ILO classification system has an elaborate section devoted to characterization of pleural abnormalities on the chest radiograph, interreader agreement is relatively low. Because HRCT is more sensitive than chest radiography in the detection of pleural plaques, it helps to determine past asbestos inhalation, because these plaques are pathognomonic for that exposure. Also, HRCT helps to differentiate plaques from extrapleural fat pads. Asbestosis can occur in the absence of pleural disease and, inversely, pleural disease can occur without underlying pulmonary fibrosis, although autopsy studies suggest that when pleural changes are seen there is often histologic evidence of asbestosis even if the radiograph is normal. Pleural plaques rarely, if ever, undergo malignant transformation.

Diffuse pleural thickening involves both parietal and visceral pleura and is strongly associated with prior, benign asbestos pleural effusions. It may also develop when subpleural parenchymal fibrosis extends to the visceral pleura. Diffuse pleural thickening is most commonly located in the lower thorax, can blunt the costophrenic angles, and may be either unilateral or bilateral. Because it is so diffuse, this form of pleural thickening can produce dyspnea on exertion and dry cough as well as loss of lung function. Other conditions that can induce similar diffuse thickening include past tuberculosis, thoracic surgery, chest trauma with hemorrhage, adverse drug reactions, and infection.

After direct contact of asbestos fibers and the pleural space, an inflammatory, exudative, and often hemorrhagic effusion can develop. It is asymptomatic in two thirds of cases, but can be associated with acute chest pain with or without fever. It can occur in the presence or absence of asbestosis. Its incidence in asbestos-exposed workers has been estimated to be less than 5%. Although it can be the first manifestation of asbestos-related disease, the mean latency for benign, asbestos-related pleural effusions is 30 years. These effusions often resolve spontaneously, but recur in approximately one third of cases. The regression may be associated with pain. The consequences include not only diffuse pleural thickening, but also the formation of adhesive fibrothorax. Benign pleural effusion is considered a diagnosis of exclusion.

Rounded atelectasis, while uncommon, is important to recognize because of its tendency to mimic lung tumors. It is thought to occur when visceral pleural thickening invaginates and folds upon the lung parenchyma, resulting in atelectasis—computed tomography is the preferred method of detecting its typical cicatricial pattern. Malignancy has only rarely been described in areas of rounded atelectasis. A positron emission tomography scan is usually negative in rounded atelectasis and may help differentiate the lesion from a lung cancer.

PITFALLS AND CONTROVERSIES

The threshold of asbestos exposure below which asbestosis will not occur is unclear, and so any asbestos exposure carries some potential risk of asbestos-related disease. Prevention is superior to treatment of disease because there is no cure. The best preventive measure is to eliminate inhalational exposure by:

- Not working with asbestos
- Not disturbing asbestos in buildings or other locations where it has been used in the past
- Encapsulating exposed areas of friable asbestos
- Having asbestos removed by those experienced in asbestos abatement technologies

Substitute materials that have less toxicity must be considered in industrial applications. When asbestos substitutes are not available, appropriately designed and maintained engineering controls must be used, such as local exhaust ventilation systems. Personal respiratory protection is appropriate for short periods of exposure or when other controls are not feasible. Such respirators must be appropriately fitted to the individual and tested for the degree of protection they afford the worker by quantitative fit-testing. Showering and changing of work clothes at the end of work shifts help to eliminate take-home exposures.

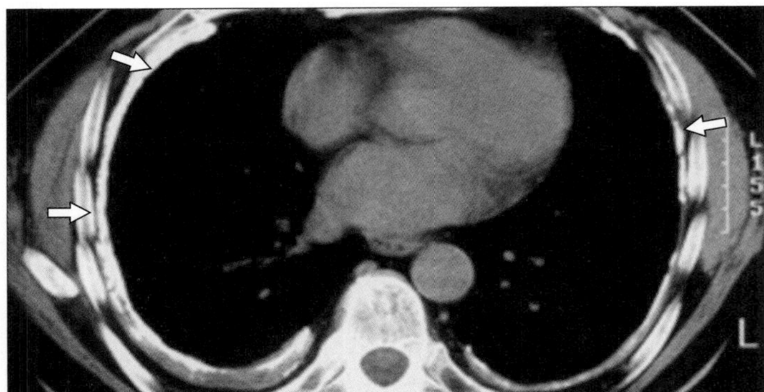

Figure 58.5 Pleural plaque. A conventional computed tomography scan of an asbestos worker shows extensive bilateral pleural calcifications (arrows).

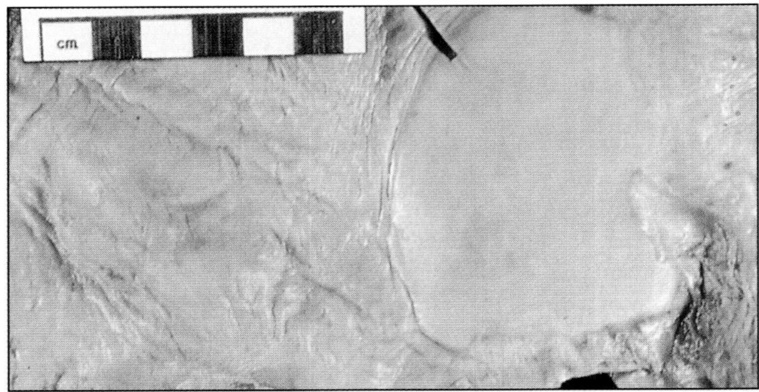

Figure 58.6 The gross pathologic appearance of a pleural plaque adjacent to the diaphragm of a construction worker. The benign pleural plaques that form as a consequence of asbestos inhalation have a smooth, shiny appearance and are usually well circumscribed.

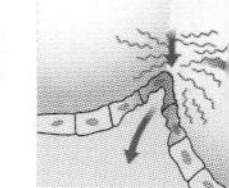

Workers must be educated about the combined risks of asbestos exposure and smoking for lung cancer, and must be counseled to avoid future asbestos exposure. Companies that use asbestos must strictly comply with government regulations as to the permissible exposure limits and appropriate medical surveillance of workers.

SUGGESTED READINGS

Asbestos, asbestosis, and cancer: The Helsinki criteria for diagnosis and attribution. Scand J Work Environ Health 23:311-316, 1997.

Burgess WA: Asbestos products. In Burgess WA (ed): Recognition of health hazards in industry. New York, John Wiley & Sons, 1995, pp 443-451.

Craighead JE, Abraham JL, Churg A, et al: The pathology of asbestos-associated disease of the lung and pleural cavities: Diagnostic criteria and proposed grading scheme. Arch Pathol Lab Invest 106:544-595, 1982.

Division of Respiratory Disease Studies, National Institute for Occupational Safety and Health (NIOSH): Work-related Lung Disease Surveillance Report 2002 (DHHS [NIOSH] Publication No. 2003-2111). Washington, DC: U.S. Government Printing Office.

Hillerdal G: Rounded atelectasis: clinical experience with 74 patients. Chest 9:836-841, 1989.

International Labor Office (ILO)/University of Cincinnati: International classification of radiographs of pneumoconiosis 1980, No. 22 revised, Occupational safety and health series. Geneva, International Labor Office, 1980.

Kamp DW, Weitzman SA: The molecular basis of asbestos induced lung injury. Thorax 54:638-652, 1999.

Rudd RM: New developments in asbestos-related pleural disease. Thorax 51:210-216, 1996.

Sluis-Cremer GK, Hnizdo E: Progression of irregular small opacities in asbestos miners. Br J Ind Med 46:846-852, 1989.

Tossavainen A: International expert meeting on new advances in the radiology and screening of asbestos-related diseases. Scand J Work Environ Health 26:449-454, 2000.

Yamamoto S: Histopathological features of pulmonary asbestosis with particular emphasis on the comparison with those of usual interstitial pneumonia. Osaka City Med J 43:225-242, 1997.

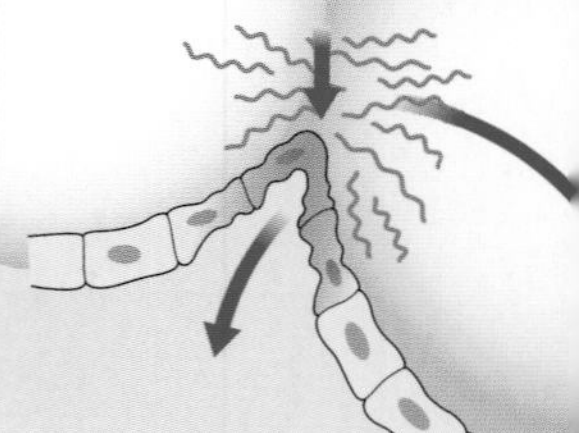

CHAPTER 59

Beryllliosis, Byssinosis, and Occupational Chronic Obstructive Pulmonary Disease

Anthony C. Pickering

Beryllium is a rare element used in industry for its properties of lightness, strength, and resistance to high temperatures and corrosion. It is the lightest of all chemically stable substances. Beryllium alloys have a wide and increasing use in modern technology, including the aerospace and nuclear industries and telecommunications and computer industries. Other industries involving potential exposure to beryllium include ceramics, dentistry (dental alloys), scrap metal reclamation, and metal machining.

The majority of cases of beryllium disease occur in workers directly exposed through handling beryllium alloys. It has also been described in vicinity workers including a secretary, a security guard, a cleaner in the reclamation of nonferrous alloys, and in the families of workers returning home wearing contaminated overalls.

EPIDEMIOLOGY, RISK FACTORS, AND PATHOPHYSIOLOGY

Epidemiology

Chronic beryllium disease is rare in the United Kingdom, with only seven new cases diagnosed by the medical respiratory boards under the Industrial Injuries Scheme between 1982 and 1996, and no claims for injury or disablement benefits since 1996. Epidemiologic studies in the ceramic and nuclear industries have revealed sensitization and disease rates varying between 2.9% and 15.8% in differing exposure categories. Prospective studies have shown that, despite a decline in exposures to beryllium, there has not been a matched decline in sensitization and disease.

Pathophysiology

The histopathology is characterized by the development of noncaseating granulomas in the lung parenchyma and hilar lymph nodes (Fig. 59.1). The granulomas consist of epithelioid cells, multinucleate giant cells, macrophages, and numerous lymphocytes. An alveolar wall infiltration by lymphocytes and histiocytes is a constant finding. The disease may progress to end-stage interstitial lung fibrosis with honeycomb changes. Granulomas may also be present in the skin; cervical, hilar and abdominal lymph nodes; liver; spleen; kidneys; adrenals; and the central nervous system. The disease process is one of the development of a cell-mediated immune response to the beryllium antigen leading to the development of noncaseating granulomata. Helper T lymphocytes (CD4+) are the major lymphocyte population involved in the response to beryllium. Usually 80% to 90% of the T lymphocytes from bronchoalveolar lavage in patients with beryllium disease are CD4+. The T-cell response is interleukin-2 dependent.

Clinical Features

Two forms of pulmonary disease are recognized: acute and chronic berylliosis.

ACUTE BERYLLIOSIS

Acute berylliosis follows an intense exposure to beryllium and is now rarely seen. The clinical features are those of a chemical pneumonitis associated with conjunctivitis, rhinitis, and tracheitis. Lower respiratory symptoms include a paroxysmal cough with occasionally blood-stained sputum and breathlessness on exertion. There may be a fever, tachycardia, and inspiratory crackles throughout the lung fields. The symptoms usually occur within 72 hours of exposure.

CHRONIC BERYLLIOSIS

The disease is a chronic granulomatous disorder predominantly affecting the lungs. Involvement of other organs can occur but is rare. Beryllium sensitization and evidence of chronic disease may be rapid and can occur within 50 days of first exposure. The clinical symptoms are those of a nonproductive cough with the insidious onset of exertional dyspnea and fatigue. These may be associated with nonspecific symptoms including fever, anorexia, weight loss, lassitude, and malaise. In early, mild disease physical signs may be absent. As the disease progresses, bilateral basal inspiratory crackles develop, finger clubbing may be present (10% to 20%) and signs of cor pulmonale ensue.

DIAGNOSIS

The diagnosis of berylliosis is based on a history of exposure to beryllium salts, the clinical features and the immunologic, radiologic, and physiologic findings.

Serology and Bronchoalveolar Lavage

This lymphocytic response in beryllium disease is specific to beryllium salts and has led to the development of the beryllium lymphocyte proliferation assay (BeLT). The test is now reliable, reproducible, and is elevated on bronchoalveolar lavage lym-

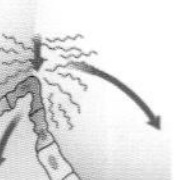

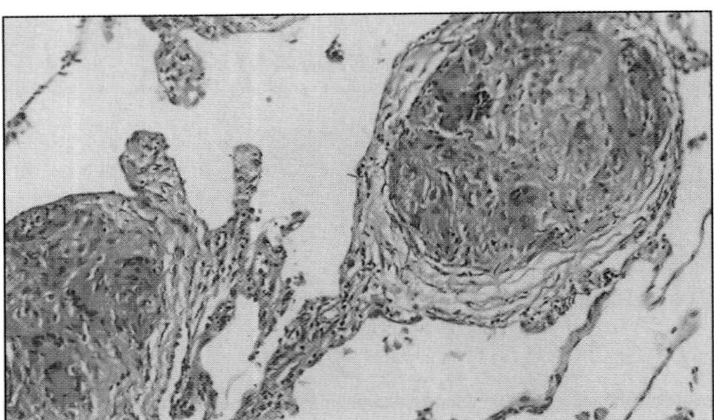

Figure 59.1 A lung biopsy from a case of berylliosis, with two areas of confluent granulomas surrounded by a rim of loose connective tissue. (Courtesy of Dr. Alan Gibbs.)

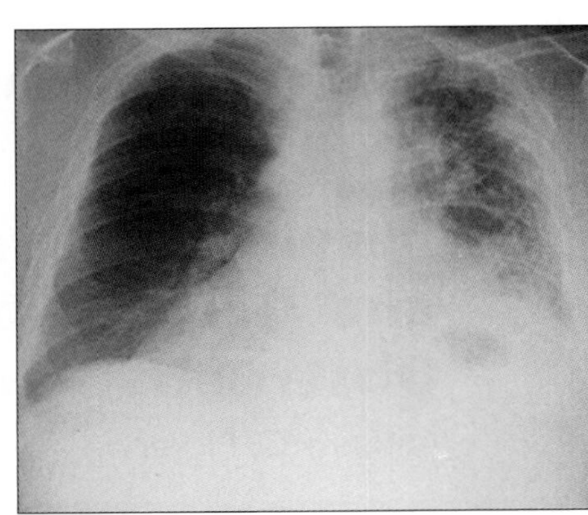

Figure 59.2 Chronic beryllium disease in a beryllium-cooper alloy worker treated by single lung transplantation. (Courtesy of Professor A.J. Newman Taylor.)

phocytes in individuals with beryllium disease and normal in unexposed subjects and in beryllium-exposed normal subjects. Bronchoalveolar lavage BeLT and bronchoalveolar lavage lymphocytosis correlate with disease severity in berylliosis. The picture may be obscured by cigarette smoking habits that partially normalize the bronchoalveolar lavage differential cell count. In some individuals the blood BeLT may be abnormal in the face of negative lavage lymphocyte reactivity to beryllium. Follow-up studies of such individuals suggest a significant number (even in those who have left the industry) go on to develop pulmonary disease. Nevertheless, blood BeLT has a high positive predictive value in determining the presence or absence of chronic beryllium disease.

Radiology

The radiographic abnormalities of berylliosis may precede the onset of symptoms by a number of years. Characteristically there are bilateral widespread opacities, initially predominantly round opacities, with disease progression becoming more irregular, accompanying hilar gland enlargement is uncommon and when present modest in degree. High-resolution computed tomography scanning identifies the earliest radiographic changes when the plain chest radiograph is normal. The most frequent abnormalities described on computed tomography scanning are nodules, septal lines, areas of ground glass attenuation, and bronchial wall thickening.

Lung Function

In the earliest stages of the disease (before the development of symptoms or radiologic changes), abnormalities in exercise physiology may be demonstrable, with reduced exercise tolerance, a rise in dead space to tidal volume ratio, and an increased alveolar-arterial oxygen tension difference. In more advanced disease a mixed picture may be present of obstructive and restrictive lung defects with impaired gas transfer.

The differential diagnosis of chronic beryllium disease includes all those conditions characterized by the formation of multiorgan noncaseating granulomas, especially sarcoidosis, and to a lesser extent extrinsic allergic alveolitis. The features that may help to distinguish berylliosis from sarcoidosis are the absence of ocular, bone and neurologic manifestations; normal tuberculin skin reactivity; and elevated levels of blood and bronchoalveolar lavage BeLT.

Treatment

Acute disease is treated immediately with high-dose steroids and, if indicated, oxygen. The majority of cases make a full recovery within 1 to 6 months; however, a small proportion—17% in one series—progress to chronic disease.

The management of chronic beryllium disease is based on the concept that the suppression of granulomas will prevent the development of fibrosis. It involves the early introduction of corticosteroids before there is significant established fibrosis and, because beryllium is only slowly cleared from the lung, the treatment period is likely to be prolonged. In chronic disease initial treatment is with prednisolone 40 mg on alternate days for 6 months; it should then be reduced by 10 mg per month until there is evidence of renewed disease activity. It is not known whether the introduction of steroids would be beneficial at a stage when evidence of lymphocyte sensitization is present, but no clinical evidence of disease. In the presence of end-stage disease, lung transplantation has been performed (Fig. 59.2).

Course and Prognosis

The prognosis of chronic beryllium disease is poorly documented. The longitudinal studies recently initiated in the nuclear and ceramic industries in the United States will provide this information. Preliminary results have shown sensitization in the absence of chronic beryllium disease, the progression of sensitization to clinical disease in a significant proportion of a small number of individuals followed for 5 years and, in some cases, progression of disease producing increasing disability and death.

Pitfalls and Controversies

The most important aspect of diagnosing berylliosis is to consider it as a possible diagnosis, and subsequently take an adequate occupational history (bearing in mind the possibility of a vicinity exposure).

BYSSINOSIS AND ALLIED RESPIRATORY DISEASES

The early description of respiratory symptoms in cotton workers reported "work-related cough associated with a sensation of uneasiness beneath the sternum." It was 14 years later, in 1845,

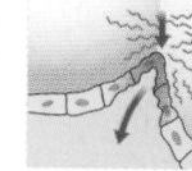

when the specific periodicity of these symptoms, which characterize byssinosis, was described: "All the workers have told us that the dust bothered them much less on the last days of the week than on Monday or Tuesday." The diagnosis remains based on a clinical history of work-related respiratory symptoms most severe on the first day returning to work after a period away from the workplace such as a weekend or holiday. In the last decade new terminology has been introduced in the literature, and byssinosis has been divided into "acute" and "chronic" forms. Acute byssinosis refers to the acute airway response to both cotton and flax dust seen in subjects exposed to these dusts for the first time. This type of response may account for the substantial labor turnover observed during the first year of employment in cotton-spinning mills. Chronic byssinosis is applied to the symptoms and disability that develop after many years of exposure to cotton dust reported in the early epidemiologic studies.

Epidemiology, Risk Factors, and Pathophysiology

EPIDEMIOLOGY

Epidemiologic studies in the United Kingdom have documented a progressive fall in the prevalence of byssinosis over the past 30 years. For example, a 50% prevalence of byssinosis in the highest dust exposure areas of cotton spinning, such as the Lancashire cotton-spinning mills, which has fallen progressively to a current level of 3%. However, in the Middle and Far East, the prevalence rates of byssinosis in cotton mills remain high, including 40% in Ethiopia, up to 50% in India, 30% in Indonesia, and 37% in the Sudan.

PATHOGENESIS

Both the mechanisms and the causative agents of byssinosis remain a matter of speculation. The etiologic factor is likely to be water soluble because washed cotton loses its ability to induce symptoms in affected individuals. Various mechanisms have been proposed including antigen-antibody reactions (immunoglobulin E– and non–immunoglobulin E–mediated responses are not supported either by the pattern of disease development or by challenge testing); nonimmunologic release of histamine; bacterial endotoxin; fungal enzymes and nonspecific pharmacologic release of mediators. None of these factors individually fully explain all the clinical features of byssinosis.

PATHOLOGY

The pathologic features of byssinosis have been poorly defined in published studies that have included small numbers of workers and a few nonsmokers. The main abnormalities include mucous gland hypertrophy and basement membrane thickening, features that do not differentiate byssinosis from chronic bronchitis or asthma. These studies have not shown an association between byssinosis and pulmonary emphysema or interstitial lung fibrosis.

Clinical Features

ACUTE BYSSINOSIS

The artificial card room experiments demonstrating acute airway responses to cotton dust on first exposure to that dust have been attributed to the individual's inherent airway reactivity. This is supported by a study of normal, cotton-naive subjects in whom their response to cotton dust was significantly associated with their prechallenge airway reactivity, using a methacholine challenge system.

The card room experiments have shown a spectrum of responses in naive subjects, varying between small asymptomatic falls in lung function to large changes, exceeding 30%, with associated symptoms after exposure to cotton dust. Because there have been no longitudinal studies of workers from the time of their first employment in the industry, the fate of low-level responders is unknown. Longitudinal studies of cohorts of cotton workers have suggested that cross-shift changes in lung function are associated with accelerated lung function decline (see chronic obstructive pulmonary disease). It is possible that this population of asymptomatic cotton dust responders, identified by card room experiments, forms a susceptible group of textile workers.

CHRONIC BYSSINOSIS

The classic form of byssinosis (chronic byssinosis) is characterized by a feeling of chest tightness and difficulty in breathing that the worker experiences on his first day back at work after a period of absence from work. Additional symptoms that may be present include a cough, which is initially nonproductive, and wheezing. Two patterns of symptomatology are seen in the workplace. Approximately one half the workers experience their most severe symptoms during the first half of the working shift, developing symptoms shortly after starting work. The remainder are most affected over the second half of the shift. Most symptomatic workers experience a further exacerbation of their symptoms on leaving work in the evening; these may last through the evening and keep the individual awake during the night. There is a subjective improvement in symptoms over subsequent days of the working week, with a further exacerbation of symptoms when cleaning procedures are undertaken at the end of the working week.

The frequency of the symptoms formed the basis of Schilling's original classification of byssinosis that has been widely used in epidemiological studies of the textile industry. This grading system, however, does not take account of the irritant effects of cotton dust or the pulmonary function changes that may occur in the absence of symptoms. As a result of these deficiencies, a new grading system has been proposed by the World Health Organization (Table 59.1), which addresses these problems and includes the symptoms of byssinosis, chronic bronchitis, and physiological measurement of cross-shift and permanent reductions in lung function.

In addition to the classic symptoms of byssinosis, studies of cotton workers report a number of work-related symptoms that do not have the characteristic periodicity of byssinosis; these include ocular and nasal irritation, cough, chest tightness and wheeze.

Chronic bronchitis, defined as cough and sputum production, was first described in association with byssinosis in 1970. Subsequently the prevalence of bronchitis was found to be greater in cotton than in manmade fiber mills, being in males, 44.9% in cotton and 26% in manmade fiber mills. By 1997 the prevalence of bronchitis in the Lancashire cotton mills had fallen to 7.15%. Differentiating the relative contributions of cotton dust exposure and cigarette smoking to the development of bronchitis in

Table 59.1
World Health Organization grading system for byssinosis

Classification		Symptoms
	Grade 0	No symptoms
Byssinosis	Grade B1	Chest tightness and/or SOB on most of first days back at work
	Grade B2	Chest tightness and/or SOB on the first and other days of the working week
Respiratory tract irritation	Grade RTI 1	Cough associated with dust exposure
	Grade RTI 2	Persistent phlegm (i.e., on most days during 3 months of the year) initiated or exacerbated by dust exposure
	Grade RTI 3	Persistent phlegm initiated or made worse by dust exposure either with exacerbations of chest illness or that persists for 2 years or more
Lung function	***Acute changes***	
	No effect	A consistent decline in FEV_1 of less than 5% or an increase in FEV_1 during the work shift
	Mild effect	A consistent decline of between 5% and 10% in FEV_1 during the work shift
	Moderate effect	A consistent decline of between 10% and 20% in FEV_1 during the work shift
	Severe effect	A decline of 20% or more in FEV_1 during the work shift
	Chronic changes	
	No effect	FEV_1 - 80% of predicted value
	Mild to moderate effect	FEV_1 - 60% - 80% of predicted value
	Severe effect	FEV_1 - less than 60% of predicted value

[a] A decline occurring in at least the last three consecutive tests made after an absence from dust exposure of two days or more.

[b] By a preshift test after an absence from dust exposure of two days or more. Predicted values should be based on data obtained from local populations or similar ethnic and social class groups.

mill workers has been difficult, due to the small numbers of nonsmokers in the cotton industry. However, in a large study of 3000 textile workers the role of cotton dust exposure in the development of chronic bronchitis has been clearly defined. Chronic bronchitis was more prevalent in cotton workers than in those working with manmade fiber, and exposure was additive to the effect of smoking. Effectively, the risk of developing chronic bronchitis for a nonsmoking cotton worker is the same as that of a smoking manmade fiber worker. The diagnosis of chronic bronchitis was associated with a small but significant decrement in lung function.

Diagnosis

The diagnosis of byssinosis is based on a history of work-related respiratory symptoms (chest tightness or breathing difficulty), which are most severe on the first day back at work after a break away from work. The diagnosis may be supported by measurement of lung function.

Acute cross-shift changes in lung function have frequently been demonstrated in byssinotic workers. The magnitude of change determines the grade of byssinosis. Serial measurements of lung function in the industry have demonstrated varying patterns of lung function change. The clinical history of byssinosis is one of respiratory symptoms most severe on the first day on returning to work. This, to some extent, is reflected in changes in lung function, in that the largest fall in lung function is seen to occur across the first working shift. Subsequent cross-shift falls over the remainder of the week are less marked, although the overall level of airway obstruction may in fact increase, the lowest measurement of lung function being recorded at the end of the working shift on the final working day. In other individuals there is a progressive improvement in lung function over the working week consistent with the clinical history. Whatever the pattern of pulmonary change that is recorded the diurnal variation in lung function appears to be greatest on the first working day on returning to work after a break.

In addition to abnormalities in spirometry, cotton workers have changes in airway reactivity. The highest level of airway reactivity is found in byssinotics; workers with nonspecific work-related symptoms form an intermediate group and asymptomatic workers have the lowest levels of airway reactivity. In one study of cotton textile workers, increased airway reactivity occurs in about 80% of byssinotics, 35% of those with nonspecific symptoms and 20% of asymptomatic workers.

No changes in gas transfer in workers exposed to cotton, hemp, or flax have been reported. A study of smoking and nonsmoking byssinotic workers found changes in gas transfer only in the smoking workers and showed a dose-response relationship between the number of cigarettes smoked and the impairment of gas transfer. This finding, combined with pathologic studies of cotton workers, indicate that the development of emphysema in byssinotic workers is attributable to their cigarette smoking habits rather than their exposure to cotton dust. There are no specific changes on the chest radiograph in byssinotic workers.

Treatment

As with all forms of occupational lung disease, treatment should consist of the early identification of disease and removal of the individual from exposure to the causative agent. In the textile industry this involves either moving the individual to an area of lower dust exposure or transferring him or her from cotton spinning to manmade fiber production.

Course and Prevention

It has always been assumed that with continued exposure to cotton dust the disease progresses from one grade to the next. However, two longitudinal studies have suggested that this is not the case in all individuals. In both studies cotton workers were recorded as initiating their disease at grade 2 or 3 without passing through the earlier grades. In addition, individuals have been reported in whom symptoms have remitted despite remaining exposed to cotton dust. This may reflect reducing levels of exposure to cotton dust or its contaminants. The end stage of byssinosis is one of fixed airway obstruction with associated disability.

The ultimate aim should be to reduce dust exposure to a level that prevents disease development. This has been achieved by investment in modern, enclosed machinery. The automation of the opening room and the enclosure of the blowing and carding processes are of particular importance in reducing dust exposure

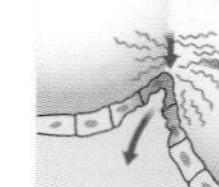

levels in the areas most frequently associated with lung disease (Figs. 59.3 and 59.4).

Pitfalls and Controversies

The steady reduction in cotton dust exposure levels in Western countries has lead to the virtual disappearance of chronic byssinosis and to changes in the patterns of disease. The diagnosis of byssinosis remains a difficult area. Epidemiologic studies have identified a full range of symptoms associated with exposure to cotton dust, including chest tightness, breathlessness, cough, and wheeze. These symptoms may occur in combination or singly and may or may not be most severe on the first day of the working week. The World Health Organization grading system, based on the Schilling questionnaire, establishes a diagnosis of byssinosis on symptoms of chest tightness or shortness of breath present on the first day back at work after a break. Other symptoms are not included and there is no reference to the variation in severity that is characteristically described in this disease. Recent epidemiologic studies have varied in both the symptoms and periodicities they have used to define this condition. This makes comparisons between studies difficult and raises the issue of how byssinosis should be defined. It was believed that individuals progressed through the various stages of the Schilling classification; however, longitudinal studies have not confirmed this. In some individuals, symptoms of byssinosis may resolve despite continued exposure to cotton dust. Questions regarding the relationship between acute and chronic byssinosis, such as whether these are separate diseases or one is a continuation of the other, remain unresolved.

OCCUPATIONAL CHRONIC BRONCHITIS AND CHRONIC OBSTRUCTIVE PULMONARY DISEASE

Chronic bronchitis, defined by the presence of regular cough and sputum, is well established as an occupational disease that is independent of cigarette smoking habits. The relationship between industrial exposures to dust or fume and the development of obstructive airway disease in exposed workers is a source of considerable controversy. The methodology of many studies has been criticized on the basis of small cohort numbers, inappropriate case controls, confounding of smoking habits, and lack of lung function data and of exposure data. Recent epidemiologic studies have addressed these criticisms and provide a clearer picture of the effects on the lung of chronic exposures to certain dusts and fumes, including coal dust (see Chapter 57), cadmium, welding fume, cotton dust, and farming exposures.

There is now a considerable weight of evidence that exposure to dust and fume in the workplace contributes to the development of both chronic bronchitis and chronic obstructive pulmonary disease in a proportion of the exposed population. The overall cost of occupational chronic obstructive pulmonary disease in 1996 in the United States was estimated to be $5 billion.

Two approaches to identifying the prevalence of these diseases and their relationship to occupational exposures have been adopted: community respiratory health surveys and studies in specific industries.

Community Health Respiratory Health Surveys

Large cross-sectional population surveys have been carried out in Europe and the United States. Comparisons between these and other studies are difficult because of the different age groups and diagnostic criteria used in the various studies. In a European study of an age group of 20 to 45 years, an increased risk of chronic bronchitis was found in agricultural, textile, paper, wood, chemical, and food processing workers, but this was not associated with abnormalities in lung function. The effect was more pronounced in smokers. In an older, North American population group, ages 30 to 75 years, after taking into account confounding variables, industries associated with increased odds ratios for chronic obstructive pulmonary disease in never-smokers were rubber, plastics, and leather manufacturing; utilities; textile mill products manufacturing; armed forces; food products manufacturing; chemicals; petroleum; coal manufacturing; sales; construction; transportation and trucking; personal services (hairdressers, cosmetics experts); and health care. This study concluded that 19% of chronic obstructive pulmonary disease in the United States' working population, as a whole, ages 30 to 75 years, is attributable to occupational exposures, and in never-smokers the attributable fraction is 31%.

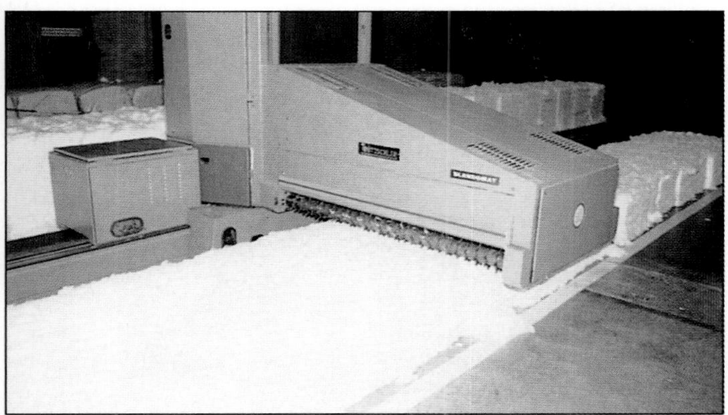

Figure 59.3 Automated opening and blending process previously conducted by manual feeding.

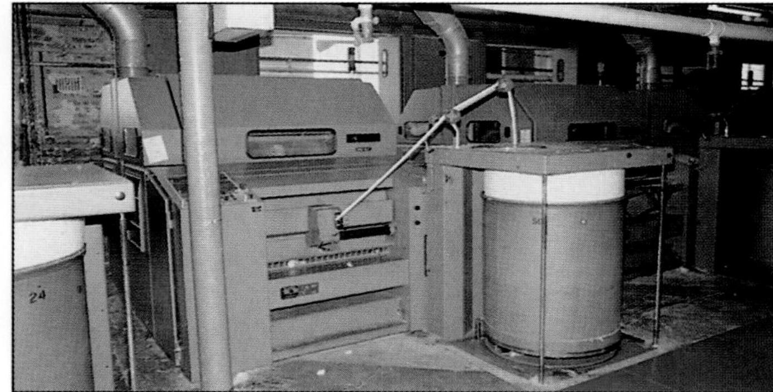

Figure 59.4 Totally enclosed cotton carding machine.

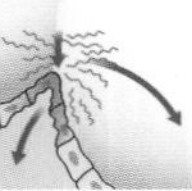

Specific Industries

CADMIUM

The inhalation of cadmium fume at high concentrations may cause a chemical pneumonia. For many years it has been suggested that there is an association between fume exposure and the development of emphysema. In a case-control study of cadmium workers, a dose response was demonstrated between cumulative exposures to cadmium and impairment of forced expiratory volume in 1 second (FEV_1) and diffusion coefficient. This decrement was independent of smoking habit and was consistent with the functional and radiologic changes of emphysema present in the studied workers.

WELDING FUME

Many studies of welders have demonstrated an increased prevalence of chronic cough and sputum. A cross-sectional study of shipyard workers exposed to welding fume has shown a small but significant impairment in FEV_1 of 250 mL compared with nonexposed workers. A 7-year follow-up study of these workers demonstrated an annual decline in FEV_1 of 16 mL in nonsmoking nonexposed workers, with declines attributable to smoking of 18 mL and to welding fume of 16 mL per year. An interaction was noted between smoking and welding fume exposure, with a disproportionate effect of fume on smokers compared with nonsmokers.

COTTON DUST

Although chronic bronchitis associated with cotton dust exposure was described 40 years ago, it is only in recent years that accelerated lung function decline associated with cotton dust exposure has been definitely identified. A longitudinal study of cotton workers in the United States has shown that the annual decline in FEV_1 in cotton workers is related to dust exposure category. In this lowest exposure category (150 mcg/m^3) the annual decline in FEV_1 in nonsmokers is 18 mL and in smokers 41.2 mL. In the highest exposure category (250 mcg/m^3) the decline in nonsmokers is 35 mL and in smokers 57 mL. The excess decline in lung function was identifiable at mean annual cotton dust exposures of only 200 mcg/m^3 and by cross-shift changes in FEV_1 of 200 mL. This study suggests that to prevent dust-related declines in lung function, exposures should be reduced to 100 mcg/m^3 and smokers should be excluded from the high dust exposure areas. The current UK maximum exposure limit for cotton, using a personal sampling device, is 2.5 mg/m^3. Dust measurements in the United States are made using a different measuring device: a vertical elutriator. The level equivalent, to the US measurement of 100 μg/m^3 of cotton dust, using the UK sampling device, is unknown.

DAIRY FARMING

An increased risk of chronic bronchitis is well established among dairy farmers in Europe, with a strong positive relationship with clinical farmer's lung and an increasing prevalence with altitude. Over the age of 50, chronic bronchitis is a risk factor for airway obstruction.

Pitfalls and Controversies

Epidemiologic studies in industry of rates of decline in lung function are expensive and difficult to conduct and analyze. Cigarette smoking, where a pollutant is inhaled in high concentrations far exceeding occupational exposures, remains a major confounding factor. Adequate information on the effects of many industrial exposures on the airway is not available; there is an urgent need for further research in this area.

SUGGESTED READINGS

Chinn DJ, Stevenson IC, Cotes JE: Longitudinal respiratory survey of shipyard workers—effects of trade and atopic status. Br J Ind Med 47:83-90, 1990.

Fishwick D, Pickering CAC: Byssinosis—a form of occupational asthma? Thorax 47:401-403, 1992.

Glindmeyer HW, Lefante JJ, Jones RN et al: Cotton dust and across-shift change in FEV_1 as predictors of annual change in FEV_1. Am J Respir Crit Care Med 149:584-590, 1994.

Glindmeyer HW, Lefante JJ, Jones RN, et al: Exposure-related declines in lung function of cotton textile workers. Am Rev Respir Med 144:675-683, 1991.

Henneberger PK, Cumro D, Deuber DD, et al: Beryllium sensitization and disease among long-term and short-term workers in a beryllium ceramics plant. Int Arch Occup Health 74:167-176, 2001.

Newman LS: Beryllium disease and sarcoidosis: Clinical and laboratory links. Sarcoidosis 12:7-19, 1995.

Newman LS, Bobka C, Schumacher B: Compartmentalized immune response reflects clinical severity of beryllium disease. Am J Respir Crit Care Med 150:135-142, 1994.

Niven RMcL, Pickering CAC: Byssinosis: A review. Thorax 51:632-637, 1996.

Niven RMcL, Fletcher AM, Pickering CAC, et al: Chronic bronchitis in textile workers. Thorax 52:22-27, 1997.

Schilling RSF: Byssinosis in cotton and other textile workers. Lancet 1:319-324, 1956.

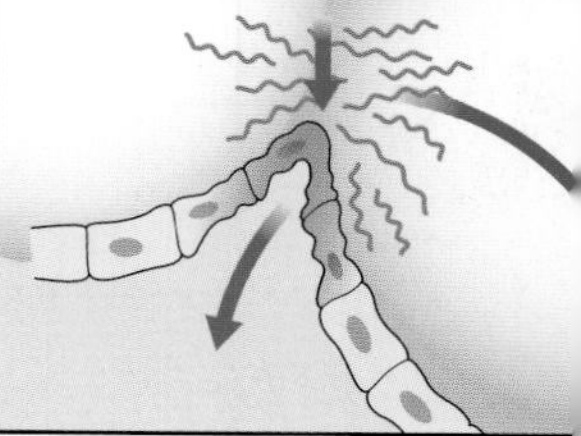

CHAPTER 60 Occupational Asthma

Moira Chan-Yeung and Jean-Luc Malo

There has been a growing interest in occupational asthma (OA) recently for several reasons:

- The frequency of asthma has increased progressively during the last two decades and occupational exposure may be a contributing factor.
- The list of agents that can cause OA is steadily lengthening (www.asmanet.com; www.asthme.csst.qc.ca).
- Occupational asthma has become the most prevalent occupational lung disease in many developed countries, resulting in an increased burden to society.
- Moreover, OA is an excellent model to study the epidemiology, pathophysiology, genetics, and other aspects of asthma in humans.

OA is defined as a disease characterized by variable airflow limitation or bronchial hyperresponsiveness resulting from causes and conditions attributable to a particular working environment and not to stimuli encountered outside the workplace. OA can be classified according to the pathogenic mechanisms: immunologically or nonimmunologically mediated. Immunologically mediated OA is characterized by a latency period that is necessary for acquiring sensitization, whereas nonimmunologically mediated OA has no latency period.

EPIDEMIOLOGY AND RISK FACTORS

It has been estimated that 5% to 15% of adult-onset asthmatic subjects relate that their workplace makes their asthma worse, though it can be suspected that the workplace causes asthma in only a portion of them. Several types of studies have been used to estimate the frequency of immunologic OA: population-based surveys, cross-sectional surveys in high-risk workplaces, registry based on physician reporting, and medicolegal statistics. Some results of these approaches are summarized in Table 60.1. In general, the prevalence of OA resulting from high-molecular-weight agents is less than 5% and from 5% to 10% from low-molecular-weight agents. Reactive airway dysfunction syndrome (RADS) or irritant-induced asthma accounted for 17% of 154 consecutive cases of OA in one series. This is the most common form of nonimmunologically induced asthma.

The degree of exposure is the most important determinant of OA. Exposure-response relationships may also be affected by individual susceptibility and timing of exposure. Levels of exposure at critical points may be more relevant to the development of occupational asthma than cumulative doses of exposure or current levels of exposure. It is now possible to measure levels of exposure by personal sampling using direct chemical analytic methods or, in the case of protein-derived allergens, by immunologic methods. Some agents appear to be more potent in inducing sensitization than others. Gautrin and coworkers found that laboratory animals caused the onset of sensitization more often than latex and flour.

PATHOPHYSIOLOGY

The development of occupational asthma results from a complex interaction between environmental factors and individual susceptibility. Asthma is a multifactorial disease and appears to be genetically heterogeneous. Most reported genetic studies of occupational asthma have investigated the importance of human leukocyte antigen class II polymorphism in increasing or decreasing the risk of developing sensitization and OA. Glutathione-S-transferase is an important protector of cells from oxidative stress products. The polymorphic glutathione-S-transferase seems to play an important role in occupational asthma because of isocyanates.

There is now overwhelming evidence of a dose-response relationship between the level of exposure to occupational agents and the development of sensitization or work-related symptoms.

Occupational asthma induced by immunologic mechanisms is characterized by a latency period. Only a small proportion of the exposed subjects are affected, and exposure to a minute quantity of the offending agent can lead to a severe asthmatic reaction. Although some agents induce asthma through the production of specific immunoglobulin (Ig)E antibodies in others, the immunologic mechanism responsible has not yet been identified.

Immunologic, Immunoglobulin E–Mediated

High-molecular-weight occupational agents act as complete antigens and induce specific IgE antibody production. The best examples are laboratory animals and flour. Some low-molecular-weight occupational agents, including platinum salts, trimellitic anhydride, and other acid anhydrides, also induce specific IgE antibodies and some others induce specific IgG antibodies. They probably act as haptens and bind with proteins to form complete antigens. Quantitative structure-activity relationship models have recently contributed to characterize further the structural and physicochemical properties that determine the potential for inducing respiratory sensitization.

Reactions between specific IgE and IgG antibodies and antigens lead to a cascade of events that results in the release of inflammatory mediators and influx of cells in the airway resulting in airway inflammation and development of airway hyperresponsiveness as in asthma resulting from common allergens. There are no apparent differences in the pathogenetic

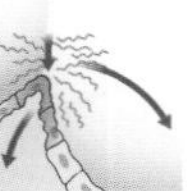

Table 60.1 Frequency of occupational asthma				
Survey type	**Population**	**Number of subjects**	**Participation (%)**	**Prevalence**
Population-based	Spain	2646	61	5.0–7.7%
	New Zealand	1609	64	1.9–3.1%
Registry based on voluntary reporting	United Kingdom	554	Not relevant	22/million per year
	Quebec	287	Not relevant	60/million per year
	British Columbia	124	Not relevant	92/million per year
	Sweden	1010	Not relevant	80/million per year
Survey in high-risk workplaces	Agents of high molecular weight			
	Snow-crab processors	303	97	15%
	Clam/shrimp	57	93	4%
	Psyllium (pharmacists)	130	93	4%
	Psyllium (nurses)	194	91	4%
	Guar gum	151	96	3%
	Agents of low molecular weight			
	Isocyanates	51	100	12%
	Spiramycin	51	100	8%
	White cedar	31	94	10%
Medicolegal	Quebec	c. 60/year	Not relevant	c. 20/million per year
	Finland	352	Not relevant	c. 156/million per year

mechanisms between OA induced by high-molecular-weight occupational agents and those of allergic nonoccupational asthma.

Immunologic, Non–Immunoglobulin E–Mediated

Many low-molecular-weight agents, including isocyanates and plicatic acid (responsible for red cedar asthma), have been shown to cause OA, and yet specific IgE antibodies cannot be found or are found in only a small percentage of the affected subjects. Specific IgG antibodies are also found and have been found to be significantly associated with the development of OA. The significance of IgE and IgG antibodies in the pathogenesis of asthma is not clear.

Bronchial biopsies of subjects with OA have shown activation of T lymphocytes, suggesting that T lymphocytes may play a direct role mediating airway inflammation. This hypothesis has been substantiated by the finding of proliferation of peripheral blood lymphocytes when stimulated with the appropriate antigen in a proportion of affected subjects with nickel-induced asthma and Western red cedar asthma. In isocyanate-induced asthma, an increase of CD8+ cells and eosinophils were found in the peripheral blood of subjects during a late asthmatic reaction induced by exposure testing. Cloning of T cells from bronchial biopsies of these subjects showed that the majority of the clones exhibited CD-8 phenotype that produced interferon-γ (IFN-γ) and interleukin-5, with very few clones producing interleukin-4. This finding provides supportive evidence that CD-8 cells may play a direct role in OA without the necessity of producing IgE antibodies.

Although asthma and OA have both been identified as diseases in which eosinophilic inflammation plays a key role, the role of neutrophils has recently been examined. Induced sputum is a noninvasive means to assess cell profiles and is more often used as an interesting investigative tool. Eosinophilic and neutrophilic variants of OA have been found in the case of OA resulting from low-molecular-weight agents, especially isocyanates.

Some low-molecular-weight agents have pharmacologic properties that cause bronchoconstriction. For example, isocyanates may block the β_2-adrenergic receptor. Isocyanates and other occupational agents may also stimulate sensory nerves to release substance P and other peptides that have been shown to inhibit neutral endopeptidases necessary for the inactivation of neuropeptides. Neuropeptides affect many cells in the airways, causing cough, smooth muscle contraction, and mucous production in subjects with asthma. Thus, low-molecular-weight occupational agents such as isocyanates may have a variety of proinflammatory effects and induce asthma through more than one mechanism.

An autopsy study of the lung of a subject with isocyanate-induced asthma who died after re-exposure showed denudation of airway epithelium, subepithelial fibrosis, infiltration of the lamina propria by leukocytes, mainly eosinophils, and diffuse mucous plugging of the bronchioles, similar to those who died from nonoccupational asthma. Bronchial biopsies of 18 subjects with proven OA have also shown extensive epithelial desquamation, ciliary abnormalities of the epithelial cells, smooth muscle hyperplasia, and subepithelial fibrosis (Fig. 60.1). The total cell count, eosinophils, and lymphocytes were increased compared with healthy controls.

Nonimmunologic

Occupational asthma resulting from nonimmunologic mechanisms is characterized by the absence of latency. The underlying mechanism of reactive airway dysfunction syndrome is not known. It has been postulated that the extensive denudation of the epithelium in these conditions leads to airway inflammation and airway hyperresponsiveness for several reasons, including loss of the epithelium-derived relaxing factors, exposure of the

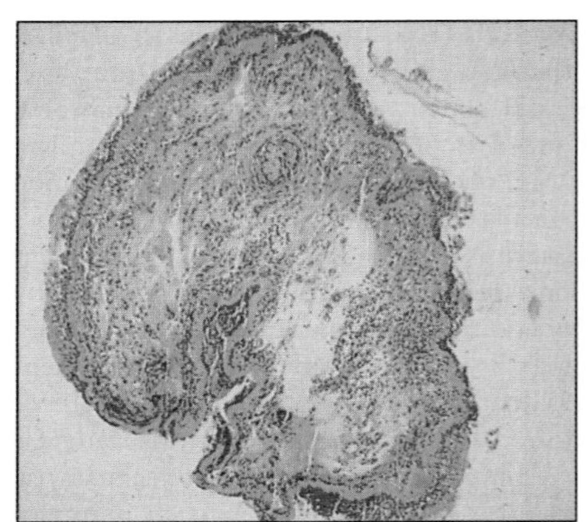

Figure 60.1 Bronchial biopsy of patient who had occupational asthma caused by toluene di-isocyanates. After removal from exposure, partial desquamation of the epithelium, thickened basement membrane, and some cellular infiltration were found.

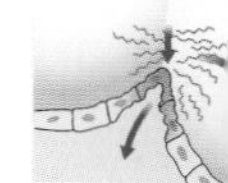

nerve endings leading to neurogenic inflammation, and nonspecific activation of mast cells with release of mediators and cytokines (Fig. 60.2).

Sequential changes in the airways of a subject with reactive airway dysfunction syndrome or irritant-induced asthma have been described. In the acute phase of RADS, there is rapid denudation of the mucosa with fibrinohemorrhagic exudate in the submucosa; this was followed by regeneration of the epithelium with proliferation of basal and parabasal cells and subepithelial edema (Fig. 60.3). In the chronic phase of RADS, there is marked thickening of the airway wall (Fig. 60.4). In a study of irritant-induced asthma resulting from multiple exposures to an irritant, inflammatory infiltrate with eosinophils and lymphocytes as well as diffuse deposition with collagen fibers were found.

CLINICAL FEATURES

There are many agents that can cause occupational asthma. Agents that cause immunologically mediated OA include a broad spectrum of protein-derived and natural and synthetic chemicals used in various workplaces. Extensive lists of causative agents and workplaces have been published and databases on computer diskettes and web sites (www.asmanet.com/asmapro/, www.asthme.csst.qc.ca) have been made available by professional agencies. The most common workplaces and agents causing immunologically mediated OA are listed in Table 60.2. These agents can be classified according to their molecular weight: high (greater than 5000 daltons) and low (less than 5000 daltons).

Table 60.3 shows some of the agents reported to have given rise to reactive airway dysfunction syndrome. All agents in exceedingly high concentrations can theoretically cause OA through nonimmunologic mechanisms, especially for agents occurring in vapor or gaseous form such as chlorine and ammonia.

The clinical signs and symptoms of occupational asthma are similar to those of other types of asthma. However, it is not uncommon for rhinitis to occur several months before the onset of asthma. At the onset of the illness, many patients present with cough, wheeze, and shortness of breath after working hours, with improvement during the evening. Their symptoms improve whenever they are away from work and recur when they return to work. As they continue to be exposed, symptoms tend to occur earlier during the shift. In some individuals, symptoms may develop immediately on exposure to the causative agent. At this stage, there is no remission of symptoms during weekends; a much longer period is necessary for improvement to take place.

Proposed pathophysiology of reactive airway dysfunction syndrome

Irritant agent
Eosinophil
Macrophage
O_2^-
Major basic protein
Platelet-activating factor
Mast cell
Hypersecretion
Bronchial epithelium
Neutral endopeptidase
Sensitive afferent nerve
Increase in vascular permeability
Nonadrenergic, noncholinergic pathways
Efferent nerve
Neuro-kinin A
Acetylcholine
Substance P
Neurokinin A
Bronchoconstriction
Prostaglandin-2
Lymphotoxin
Prostaglandin-4
Histamine

Figure 60.2 Proposed pathophysiology of reactive airways dysfunction syndrome.

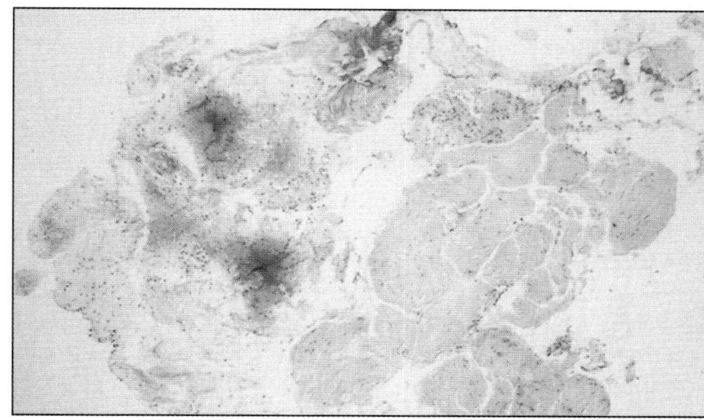

Figure 60.3 Bronchial biopsy taken 3 days after an acute accidental inhalation of a high concentration of chlorine. This shows almost complete desquamation of bronchial mucosa with fibrinohemorrhagic deposit (Weigert-Masson stain).

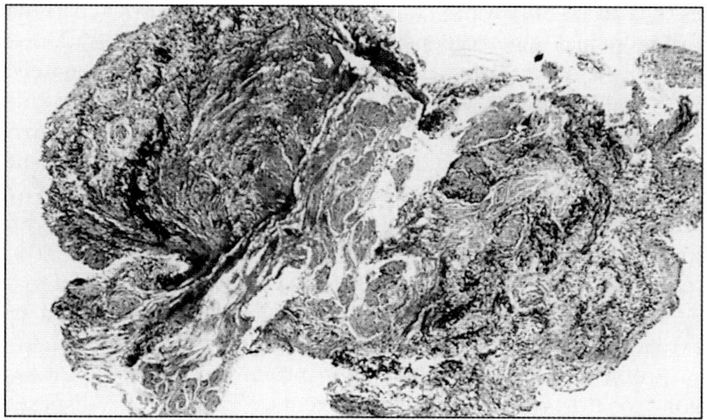

Figure 60.4 Bronchial biopsy taken 2 years after an acute accidental inhalation of chlorine showing severe desquamation of epithelial cells. Smooth muscle cells are surrounded by reticulocollagenic fibrous tissue (Weigert-Masson stain).

Table 60.2
Common agents that cause immunologically mediated occupational asthma and at-risk occupations

Agent	Agent
High molecular weight	
Cereals	Bakers, millers
Animal-derived allergens	Animal handlers
	Detergent users, pharmaceutical workers
Enzymes	Bakers
Gums	Carpet makers, pharmaceutical workers
Latex	Health professionals
Seafoods	Seafood processors
Low molecular weight	
Isocyanates	Spray painters, insulation installers, manufactures of plastics, rubbers, foam
Wood dusts	Forest workers, carpenters, cabinetmakers
Anhydrides	Users of plastics, epoxy resins
Amines	Shellac and lacquer handlers, solderers
Fluxes	Electronics workers
Chloramine-T	Janitors, cleaners
Dyes	Textile workers
Persulfate	Hairdressers
Formaldehyde, glutaraldehyde	Hospital staff
Acrylate	Adhesive handlers
Drugs	Pharmaceutical workers, health professionals
Metals	Solderers, refiners

Common agents that cause immunologically mediated occupational asthma and at-risk occupations. (Reproduced from Chan-Yeung M, Malo J-L: Occupational asthma. N Engl J Med 333:107-112, 1995. ©1995 Massachusetts Medical Society. All rights reserved.)

Table 60.3
Agents responsible for reactive airway dysfunction syndrome

Acetic acid	Diesel exhaust	Spray paint
Sulfuric acid	Diethylaminoethanol	Sulfur dioxide
Chloridric acid	Epichlorohydrin	Gas (chlorine, mustard, phosgene, etc.)
Heated acid	Ethylene oxide	Fire/smoke
Ammonia	Isocyanates	Floor sealant
Bleaching agent	Metal remover	Formol–Zenker
Chlorine	Oxide (calcium)	Cleaning mist
Chloropicrin	Paints (heated)	Hydrazine
Cleaning agents	Phthalic anhydride	

Agents responsible for reactive airway dysfunction syndrome. (Reproduced with permission from Lemiere C, Malo JL, Gautrin D: Nonsensitizing causes of occupational asthma. Med Clin North Am 80:749-774, 1996.)

There are differences in the clinical presentation of subjects with occupational asthma resulting from IgE- and non–IgE-mediated causes. The latency period is longer for high molecular-weight than for low molecular-weight agents. The temporal pattern of bronchial reactions on specific inhalation challenges in the laboratory is different. Immediate or dual reactions occur more frequently for high-molecular-weight agents, whereas isolated late or atypical reactions develop for low-molecular-weight agents.

The presence of sensitization to occupational agents can be detected either by skin tests or by RAST or ELISA tests. In subjects with a compatible clinical history of occupational asthma and bronchial hyperresponsiveness, a positive skin or RAST test probably has a diagnostic accuracy close to 80%. Unfortunately, there are very few standardized commercially available materials for skin tests or for RAST tests in occupational asthma. Recently, stimulation production of monocyte chemoattractant protein-1 in vitro from peripheral blood mononuclear cells by diisocyanates conjugated with human serum albumin has been shown to have sensitivity and specificity of 79% and 91%, respectively, in the diagnosis of isocyanate-induced asthma. Further studies are necessary to confirm the findings and to extend this test to other low-molecular-weight agents.

Atopic subjects are much more prone to develop sensitization to high-molecular-weight agents. Smoking predisposes workers to sensitization to some agents, including platinum salts. On the other hand, nonatopic subjects and nonsmokers are more often affected in OA caused by agents that induce asthma through non–IgE-mediated mechanisms. Certain HLA class II antigens have been reported to confer susceptibility to, whereas others provide protection from, OA because of low-molecular-weight compounds.

The reactive airway dysfunction syndrome originally described by Brooks and colleagues is due to acute airway injury from accidental exposure to high doses of irritants. The typical clinical presentation is the development of symptoms of asthma within a few hours of acute exposure in a subject without history of any respiratory symptoms. The symptoms of asthma usually last for more than 3 months and are associated with nonallergic bronchial hyperresponsiveness.

DIAGNOSIS

It is necessary to confirm the diagnosis of OA with objective means for several reasons. The diagnosis of OA has considerable socioeconomic implications for the worker and his or her family; it usually means a change of job in most instances with its financial consequences. In Quebec, each accepted claim of OA costs the compensation board USD$55,000 (amount in 2003); thus, it is costly to the society. Asthma is a common disease, affecting 6% to 8% of the adult population in Canada and is higher in other parts of the world. Having asthma and working in an environment with an agent known to give rise to OA do not make the diagnosis of OA.

An occupational cause should be suspected for all new cases of adult-onset asthma, especially those subjects who report worsening of their asthma symptoms at work (see Epidemiology and Risk Factors). A detailed occupational history on past and current exposure to possible causal agents in the workplace, work processes, and specific job duties should be obtained. In addition, the intensity, frequency, and peak concentrations of exposure in the workplace should be assessed qualitatively. Information can be requested from the work site, including material safety data sheets, although in some instances, the information is incomplete on all constituents of the product, especially those with concentrations of less than 1%. Computerized databases and published lists of agents and workplaces are very useful. Walk-through visits of the workplace may be necessary. Industrial hygiene data and employee health records can be obtained.

Open medical questionnaires should be regarded as fairly sensitive, but not specific, tools for diagnostic purposes. Temporal

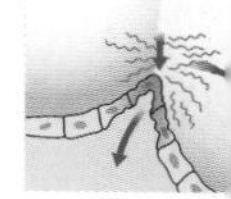

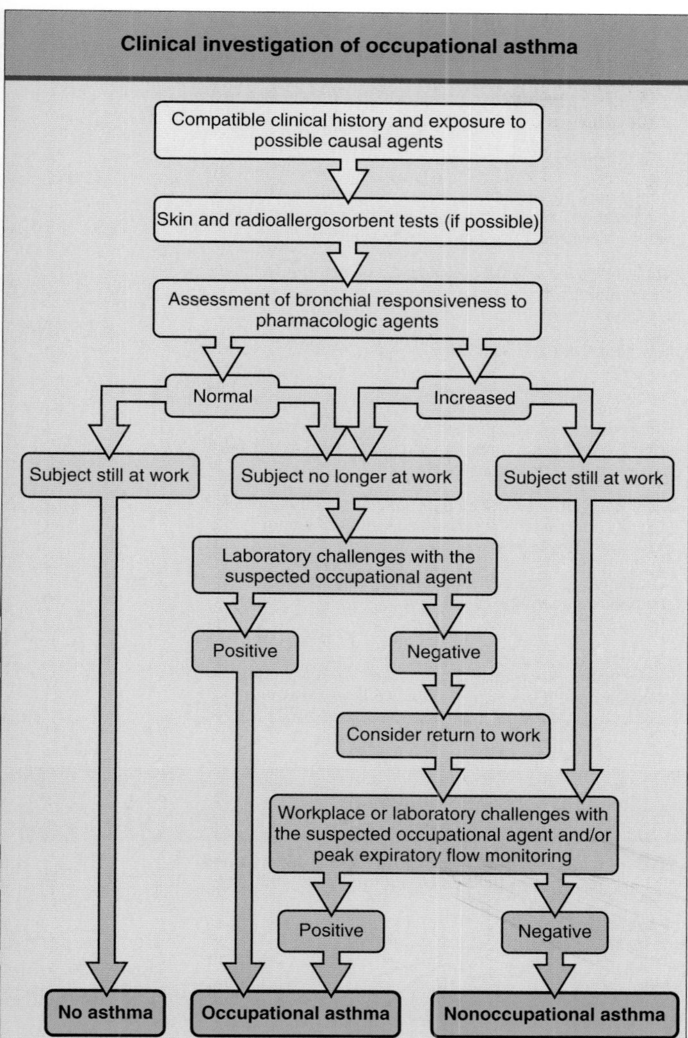

Figure 60.5 Clinical investigation of occupational asthma. (Reproduced from Chan-Yeung M, Malo J-L: Occupational asthma. N Engl J Med 333:107-112, 1995. ©1995 Massachusetts Medical Society. All rights reserved.)

associations are not sufficient to diagnose work-related asthma. Ocular and nasal symptoms often accompany respiratory symptoms. They are more frequent in OA because of high-molecular-weight than low-molecular-weight agents and usually precede the onset of asthma symptoms.

An individual with suspected OA should be best assessed by a specialist in this area. The role of this specialist is to confirm the diagnosis of OA by objective means if possible and to assess impairment or disability. A delay in referral may jeopardize the chance of confirming the diagnosis with objective measurements because the subject may have left the workplace and recovered or the working conditions may have changed. However, in cases of OA, inhalation challenges with a specific agent generally remain positive even 2 years or more after cessation of exposure.

An algorithm for the clinical investigation of occupational asthma is shown in Figure 60.5. The advantages and pitfalls of the various tools in confirming the diagnosis of OA are listed in Table 60.4. For high-molecular-weight agents, skin tests to detect immediate reactivity or measurements of specific IgE antibodies are important tools. Although having immediate skin reactivity to an inhalant only reflects immunologic "sensitization" and not necessarily the disease, it has been shown that having both immediate skin reactivity and increased bronchial hyperresponsiveness results in an 80% likelihood of developing an asthmatic attack on laboratory exposure to this agent. Unfortunately, reagents used for skin and in vitro testing are not standardized and are generally prepared from occupational agents in individual laboratories.

The absence of nonallergic bronchial hyperresponsiveness in a subject at the end of 2 weeks of working under the usual conditions virtually excludes the diagnosis of asthma and OA. If there is nonallergic bronchial hyperresponsiveness, further testing is required. Measuring spirometry before and after a work shift has not been found to be sensitive or specific. Two options can be considered for objective confirmation depending on availability. First, exposure to the suspected agent under control conditions in a hospital laboratory can be done as originally described by Pepys and Hutchcroft. Attempts have been made to improve specific challenge tests by exposing subjects in the laboratory to low and stable levels of dry or wet aerosols and vapors to avoid nonspecific reactions. However, these tests can be falsely negative if the wrong agent is used for testing or if the subject has been away from work for too long, although such occurrences are rare. If this is the case, the subject should be instructed to return to the workplace if feasible, and specific laboratory or work site challenges should be repeated at a later time.

Burge and coworkers were the first to propose the use of serial measurement of peak expiratory flow (PEF) using portable devices in the diagnosis of OA. An example of serial PEF recording is shown in Figure 60.6. Although there is relatively good correlation between results of serial PEF monitoring and OA as confirmed by specific inhalation challenges in the laboratory, there are several limitations and pitfalls in PEF monitoring. When PEF monitoring is suggestive of occupational asthma, and specific inhalation challenges in the laboratory are not possible or negative, it is advisable to confirm OA by sending a technician to the workplace to record spirometry serially throughout a work shift. The use of computerized peak flow meters is very helpful in overcoming some of the problems of PEF monitoring. Computerized programs to assess changes in PEF are currently available. Combining PEF monitoring with serial assessments of nonallergic bronchial responsiveness can provide further objective evidence, although this does not add to the sensitivity and specificity of PEF monitoring alone. Finally, assessment of airway inflammation (% eosinophils) in induced sputum has recently been found to be sensitive and specific in the diagnosis of OA.

TREATMENT

The ideal treatment for patients with occupational asthma is removal from the causal exposure permanently, retraining for alternative employment if necessary. Larger companies may be able to relocate the affected worker to another job in the same plant or another plant with no exposure; they may also be able to improve ventilation or change work practices to eliminate or reduce exposure. This is usually not possible for smaller companies. Any subject with OA who remains in the same job

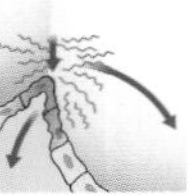

Table 60.4
Advantages and disadvantages of diagnostic methods in occupational asthma

Method	Advantages	Disadvantages
Questionnaire	Simple, sensitive	Low specificity
Immunologic testing	Simple, sensitive	Only for agents of high molecular weight and for some of low molecular weight; identifies sensitization, not disease; no 'standardized' and commercially available agents
Bronchial responsiveness to methacholine/histamine	Simple, sensitive	Not specific for asthma or occupational asthma; occupational asthma not ruled out by a negative test if workers are no longer exposed
Measurement of forced expiratory volume in 1s (FEV_1) before and after a work shift	Simple, inexpensive	Low sensitivity and specificity
Peak expiratory flow monitoring	Relatively simple, inexpensive	Requires patient's cooperation and honesty; not as sensitive as FEV_1 or a computerized method to assess airway caliber to interpret changes
Specific inhalation challenges in a hospital laboratory	If positive, confirmatory	Diagnosis not ruled out by a negative confirmatory test; (e.g., if wrong agent or subject no longer at work); expensive; few referral centers
Serial FEV_1 measurement at work under supervision	If negative, rules out diagnosis when patient tested under usual work	A positive test may be result from conditions of irritation; requires collaboration of employer

Advantages and disadvantages of diagnostic methods in occupational asthma. (Reproduced from Chan-Yeung M, Malo J-L: Occupational asthma. N Engl J Med 333:107-112, 1995. ©1995 Massachusetts Medical Society. All rights reserved.)

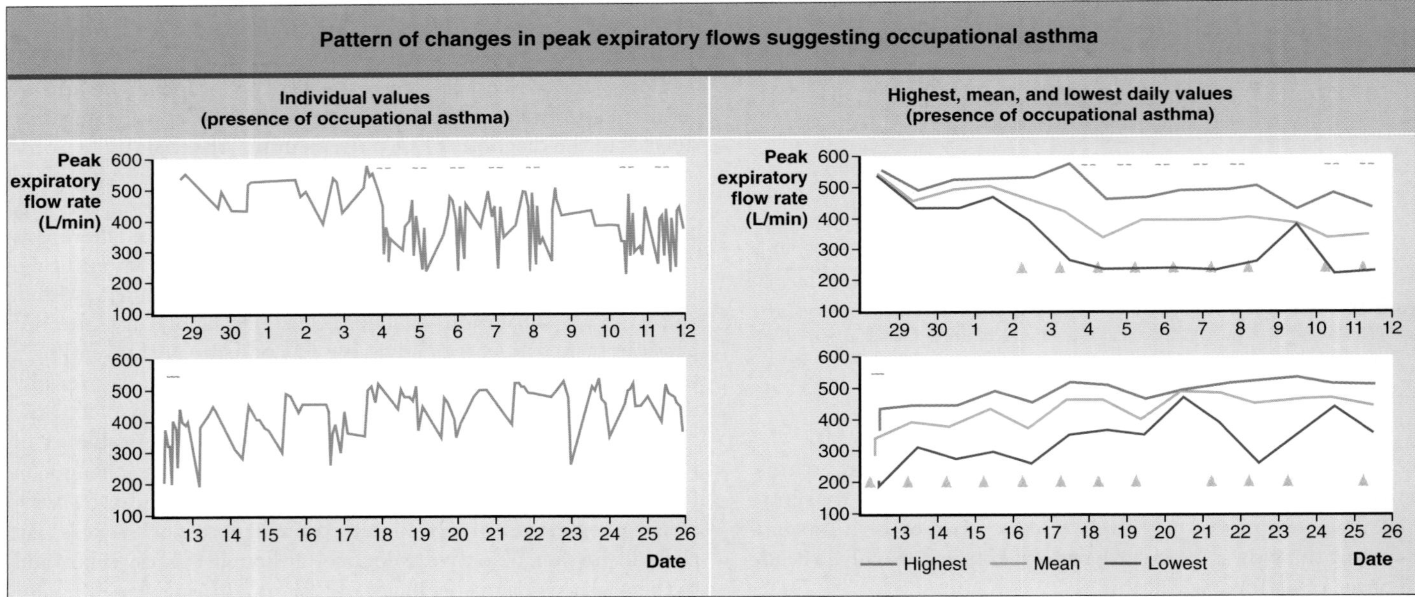

Figure 60.6 Pattern of changes in peak expiratory flows that suggest occupational asthma. The horizontal lines show the periods at work; the triangles illustrate the need for an inhaled bronchodilator. (Reproduced from Malo JL, Cote J, Cartier A, Boulet LP, L'Archeveque J, Chan-Yeung M: How many times per day should peak expiratory flow rates be assessed when investigating occupational asthma? Thorax 48:1211-1217, 1993.)

should have respiratory protection and have close medical follow-up. Worsening of asthma should lead to immediate removal from exposure. Pharmacologic treatment of patients with OA is similar to other types of asthma. Although removal from exposure generally results in improvement, patients generally (approximately 75% of the time) continue to require medication and have airflow limitation or nonallergic bronchial hyperresponsiveness.

After the diagnosis is made, physicians should counsel patients concerning compensation; the specifics vary from country to country. The appropriate public health authority should be notified. Such agencies should initiate surveillance programs when sentinel cases have been identified. Patients should also be referred to compensation boards or similar agencies when appropriate. Patients should be evaluated for temporary impairment when their asthma is under control. Evaluation for permanent impairment and disability should take place when improvement is maximal, which may take 1 to 2 years. The guidelines for assessment of impairment and disability for patients with chronic irreversible lung diseases are

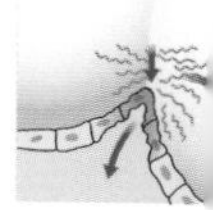

inappropriate for patients with asthma. The American Thoracic Society guidelines attempt to take into account all the special features of asthma. In addition to measurements of lung function, assessment of impairment includes the degree of nonallergic bronchial hyperresponsiveness or airway reversibility, the minimum amount of medication required for maintaining control of asthma and the effects of asthma on the quality of life. When there is a change in clinical status, reassessment is recommended.

CLINICAL COURSE

Subjects with OA deteriorate if they continue in the same job without protection. Fatalities in workers who continue to be exposed have been reported. A scheme of the progressive natural history of OA is shown in Fig. 60.7.

The majority of patients with occupational asthma improve but do not recover completely, even several years after removal from exposure. Table 60.5 shows some of the studies indicating this. The proportion of subjects followed up in these studies is high, suggesting that the high rate of persistence of asthma is not due to bias (i.e., "sick" ones came for the follow-up examination). Follow-up studies of patients with various types of OA have shown that subjects who became asymptomatic after leaving exposure had higher lung function and a lower degree of nonallergic bronchial hyperresponsiveness at the time of diagnosis and a shorter duration of exposure after the onset of symptoms. These findings suggest that they were diagnosed at an earlier stage of the disease. Early diagnosis and removal from exposure are essential in ensuring recovery.

Although symptoms and lung function improve within 1 year of leaving exposure, improvement in nonallergic bronchial hyperresponsiveness depends on the length of interval from cessation of exposure. Specific IgE antibodies decrease even more slowly with no plateau after 5 years, as shown in subjects with snow crab–induced asthma. It has been recommended that assessment of permanent respiratory impairment or disability take place after at least 2 years of cessation of exposure.

The rate of decline in lung function of subjects with OA with continuous exposure is greater than subjects without asthma. Moreover, specific bronchial reactivity to the offending occupational agents often persists after the subject has left exposure for 2 or more years. Thus, it is not advisable for these patients to return to the same job after they become asymptomatic.

Table 60.5
Retrospective evidence for the persistence of symptoms and bronchial hyperresponsiveness after removal from the offending agent

Agent	Number of cases	Duration of follow-up (years)	Persistence of symptoms (%)	Nonspecific bronchial hyperreactivity	
				Number	Percentage
Red cedar	38	0.5–4	29	38/38	100
	75	1–9	49	25/33	76
Colophony	20	1.3–3.8	90	7/20	35
Snow-crab	31	0.5–2	61	28/31	90
	31	4.8–6	100	26/31	84
Various	32	0.5–4	93	31/32	97
Isocyanates	12	1–3	66	7/12	58
	50	>4	82	12/19	63
	20	0.5–4	50	9/12	75
	22	1	77	17/22	77
Various	28	4–11	100	25/26	96

Retrospective evidence for the persistence of symptoms and bronchial hyperresponsiveness after removal of the offending agent. (Reproduced from Chan-Yeung and Malo by courtesy of Marcel Dekker Inc. Chan-Yeung M, Malo JL: Natural history of occupational asthma. In Bernstein IL, Chan-Yeung M, Malo JL, Bernstein D (eds): Asthma in the workplace. New York, Marcel Dekker, 1993, pp 299-322.)

There is a histologic basis to the persistence of symptoms and nonallergic bronchial hyperresponsiveness in patients with OA. Higher total cell count and eosinophils in bronchoalveolar lavage fluid were found in subjects with Western red cedar asthma who did not recover compared with those who recovered completely after removal from exposure. Saetta and coworkers have documented improvement in airway wall remodeling (thickness of subepithelial fibrosis and number of subepithelial fibroblasts) in patients with toluene diisocyanate (TDI)-induced asthma 6 months after the cessation of exposure, but there was no improvement in bronchial inflammation and in the degree of nonallergic bronchial hyperresponsiveness. The reasons for the

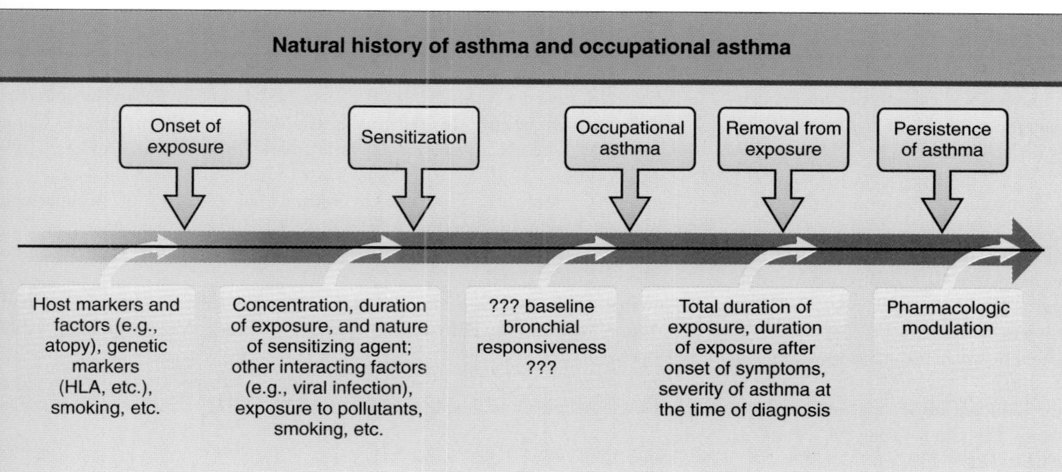

Figure 60.7 Natural history of asthma and occupational asthma. The boxes illustrate the steps, whereas the modifying factors before each step are listed under the horizontal line. (Reproduced from Malo JL, Ghezzo H, D'Aguino C, L'Archeveque J, Cartier A, Chan-Yeung M: Natural history of occupational asthma: Relevance of type of agent and other factors in the rate of development of symptoms in affected subjects. J Allergy Clin Immunol 90:937-943, 1992.)

persistence of symptoms, nonallergic bronchial hyperresponsiveness, and airway inflammation after removal from exposure are not known.

Some researchers have explored the possibility of "curing" subjects with OA with inhaled steroids to reduce the degree of airway inflammation after the patients have been removed from the workplace. Although some improvement in various clinical and functional parameters was found, no case of cure from asthma was documented.

Because most cases of reactive airway dysfunction syndrome occur in isolation, it is difficult to study the natural history involving a series of such patients. However, improvement and cure in the first 2 to 3 years after the inhalational accident have been described in approximately 25% of subjects.

PREVENTION

Primary prevention programs should be implemented for OA in high-risk industries. The most important measure is to reduce the level of exposure. For example, with the introduction of powder-free gloves with reduced protein levels, education about natural rubber latex allergies in health care facilities led to a decline in the number of suspected cases of occupational allergies and asthma caused by enzymes and to natural latex allergies. Other measures may include the use of alternative nonsensitizing agents, improved ventilation, and the use of appropriate ventilators. Permissible exposure limits should be established for all high-risk agents for OA as they have for flour. It should be noted that after a person is sensitized, he or she may react to a much lower level of exposure. Another method is to identify susceptible subjects at the time of preemployment examination and exclude them from employment. Unfortunately, there are no reliable markers of susceptibility. Atopy is one of the predisposing factors for sensitization in OA resulting from high-molecular-weight compounds; however, atopy has a low predictive value for the development of asthma. Moreover, 40% to 50% of young adults are atopic; thus, atopic subjects should not be excluded from high-risk workplaces. Genetic studies are, for the moment, at a very early stage, and genetic markers should not be used in surveillance programs.

Secondary prevention by early detection of workers with OA and removal from exposure before development of irreversible airflow obstruction have been found to be effective in isocyanate workers and platinum refinery workers. Secondary prevention requires the institution of a medical surveillance program that includes a preemployment medical questionnaire followed by a periodic questionnaire every 6 to 12 months in high-risk industries. Some surveillance programs include periodic skin tests if the sensitizing agent is a high-molecular-weight compound or for some chemical sensitizers such as platinum salts or measurement of specific IgE, whereas others include periodic spirometry.

PITFALLS AND CONTROVERSIES

It is important to have objective evidence that the patient's asthma is due to occupational exposure. There are many pitfalls in confirming the diagnosis of OA. Although lists of agents causing OA found in published articles and databases are useful to alert the physician, the absence of an agent on such lists does not exclude the possibility of OA, because new chemicals are constantly being introduced into the market. Patients are often asked to leave the job when the diagnosis is suspected. However, one of the objective tests is to ask the patient to do serial monitoring of PEF for a period at work and a period away from work. Unless the patient has severe symptoms, it is best to obtain objective evidence first before asking the patient to resign from his or her job. PEF monitoring also has limitations, as discussed previously. It should be done properly according to a protocol and using a logged device or together with serial measurement of nonallergic bronchial hyperresponsiveness. Specific challenge tests have been said to be the "gold standard" in diagnosing OA. It is not without pitfalls because there are both false-positive and false-negative results. When a new agent is suspected, investigators often use several methods to confirm the diagnosis.

Although most people include RADS as a form of occupational asthma, others think that it is an entirely different condition because of differences in pathologic features. There is still considerable controversy as to whether exposure to low levels of irritant gases or fumes in the workplace or in the environment can actually induce asthma de novo. The long-term outcome of RADS has yet to be studied.

Despite the great deal that has been learned about OA over the last few years, there are still many gaps in our knowledge. Future research priorities should include further improvement in diagnosis, screening methods, and control of exposures to prevent the development of the disease.

SUGGESTED READINGS

Becklake MR, Malo JL, Chan-Yeung M: Epidemiological approaches in occupational asthma. In: Bernstein IL, Chan-Yeung M, Malo JL, Bernstein DI (eds): Asthma in the workplace. New York, Marcel Dekker, 1999, pp 27-65.

Bernstein IL, Chan-Yeung M, Malo JL, Bernstein D: Asthma in the workplace, 2nd ed. New York, Marcel Dekker, 1999.

Burge PS, Moscato G: Physiologic assessment: Serial measurements of lung function. In: Asthma in the workplace. Bernstein IL, Chan-Yeung M, Malo JL, Bernstein DI (eds): New York, Marcel Dekker, 1999, pp 193-210.

Chan-Yeung M, Malo JL, Tarlo SM, Bernstein L, Gautrin D, Mapp C, et al: Proceedings of the first Jack Pepys Occupational Asthma Symposium. Am J Respir Crit Care Med 167:450-471, 2003.

Chan-Yeung M, Malo JL: Tables of major inducers of occupational asthma. In: Asthma in the workplace. Bernstein IL, Chan-Yeung M, Malo JL, Bernstein DI (eds): New York, Marcel Dekker, 1999, pp 683-720.

Fabbri LM, Ciaccia A, Maestrelli P, Saetta M, Mapp CE: Pathophysiology of occupational asthma. In: Asthma in the workplace. Bernstein IL, Chan-Yeung M, Malo JL, Bernstein DI (eds): New York, Marcel Dekker, 1999, pp 81-110.

Lemière C, Malo JL, Gautrin D: Nonsensitizing causes of occupational asthma. Med Clin North Am 80:749-774, 1996.

Malo JL, Chan-Yeung M: Occupational asthma. J Allergy Clin Immunol 108:317-328, 2001.

Newman-Taylor AJ: Genetics and occupational asthma. Bernstein IL, Chan-Yeung M, Malo JL, Bernstein DI (eds): New York, Marcel Dekker, 1999, pp 67-80.

Vandenplas O, Malo JL: Inhalation challenges with agents causing occupational asthma. Eur Respir J 10:2612-2629, 1997.

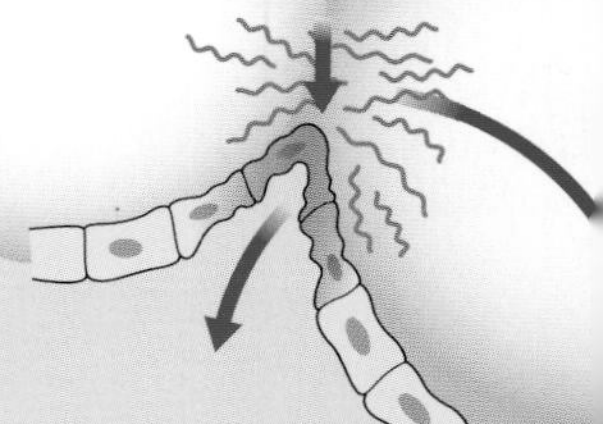

CHAPTER 61

Air Pollution

Helgo Magnussen and Rudolf A. Jörres

The risk of air pollution for human health has been extensively studied over the last several decades. Classically, sulfur dioxide and particles are important components of winter smog episodes ("London type"), whereas ozone and nitrogen dioxide are major constituents of photochemical smog in summertime ("Los Angeles type"). In recent years, the focus has shifted to components of air pollution that are less dependent on seasonal variations, because many of them are directly or indirectly generated by traffic, such as fine and ultrafine particles. These are a major concern regarding morbidity and mortality in the elderly and in patients with cardiovascular disease. This chapter presents a brief overview of the effects of different components of air pollution and provides a few selected readings from a great number of papers published on these issues.

PARTICULATE MATTER

Particle Fractions

Within the last several years the interest in the health effects of particulate matter has gained much attention. Acute and chronic exposure to inhalable particles were found to be associated with adverse health effects, with mortality closely related to particle exposure, especially small size particles (Fig. 61.1). The harmful effects also seem to be related to chemical properties of particles—for example, acidity. Clearly, their deposition within the respiratory tract depends on aerodynamic diameter—larger particles being deposited in extrathoracic airways and smaller ones entering the lower airways and alveoli. The particle fractions that are most often considered are those smaller than 2.5 or 10 μm ($PM_{2.5}$ and PM_{10}, respectively). Although much evidence points toward major effects of smaller particles, the larger ones are still considered important, and not only because they represent the size fraction that is more amenable to individual monitoring. As with gaseous air pollutants, there can be major differences between personal exposure levels and ambient air levels as determined in outdoor measurements.

Fine and Ultrafine Particles

There is considerable evidence that fine (0.1 to 2.5 μm) and ultrafine (0.01 to 0.1 μm) particles are even more strongly related to morbidity and mortality, in particular from cardiovascular diseases, than are larger particles. Owing to their great number compared with their minor mass, these particles can induce acute and chronic effects within the lung, which may be exaggerated through oxidative mechanisms, such as the catalytic activity of transition metals that are found on the surface of small particles.

Ultrafine particles can also cross the alveolocapillary barrier and move through the circulation—for example, into the heart. Besides other mechanisms, their effects may ultimately lead to changes in blood viscosity, causing alterations in systolic pressure or arrhythmias and thereby increasing the health risk in subjects with preexisting cardiovascular disease. Most of the evidence stems from animal experiments and from epidemiologic studies. Only few experimental data in humans are available, and the current research is trying to derive adequate estimates of the impact of fine particles on human health. As an additional effect on lung function, symptom scores and lung function deterioration in subjects with asthma may be more closely related to fine and ultrafine particles than to total particle mass or larger particles.

OZONE

Formation and Exposure Levels

Ozone (O_3) is mainly generated from hydrocarbons and NO_2 under the presence of ultraviolet radiation. Average levels are lowest during the winter and highest in the summer, and concentrations normally peak in the afternoon. In most areas of industrialized countries, annual average levels range from 20 to 40 ppb (parts per billion, v/v). Annual and daily cycles can lead to peak concentrations reaching or exceeding 100 ppb. It has been estimated that, for example, about half of the US population lives in areas with maximal concentrations exceeding 120 ppb. The situation in many other parts of the world is probably similar.

Epidemiologic Studies

There is no doubt that epidemiologic studies have consistently demonstrated the onset of symptoms and a decline in spirometric volumes even after short-term ozone exposure. In addition, there is mounting evidence for an association between short-term ozone levels and hospital admissions for respiratory disorders in subjects with preexisting airway diseases, and possibly even the prevalence of atopic asthma. Furthermore, long-term exposure to ozone has been found to be associated with symptoms of chronic respiratory disease and an accelerated rate of decline of forced expiratory volume in 1 second (FEV_1).

Exposure Studies

According to experimental exposure studies, ozone causes pain on deep inspiration and a transient reduction in inspiratory capacity as reflected in FEV_1 or forced vital capacity. Parameters indicative of small airway narrowing can show longer-lasting

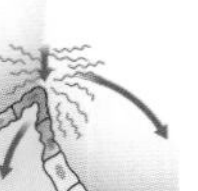

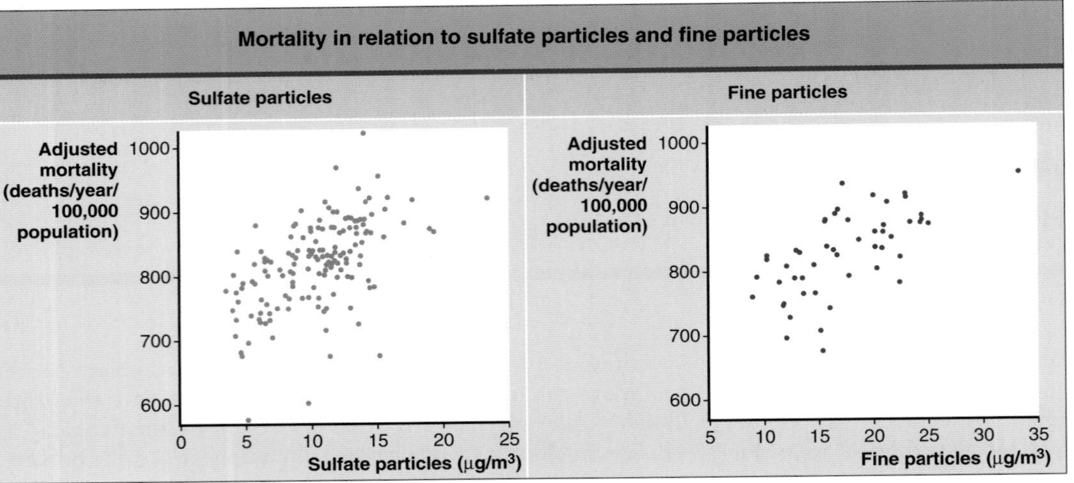

Figure 61.1 Mortality in relation to sulfate particles and fine particles. Relationship between mortality per year per 100,000 inhabitants adjusted for age, sex, and ethnic origin versus concentrations of **A,** sulfate particles and **B,** fine particles. The analysis is based on a comparison of 151 urban areas in 1980. (Data from Pope CA III, Thun MJ, Namboodiri MM, et al: Particulate air pollution as a predictor of mortality in a prospective study of US adults. Am J Respir Crit Care Med 151:669-674, 1995.)

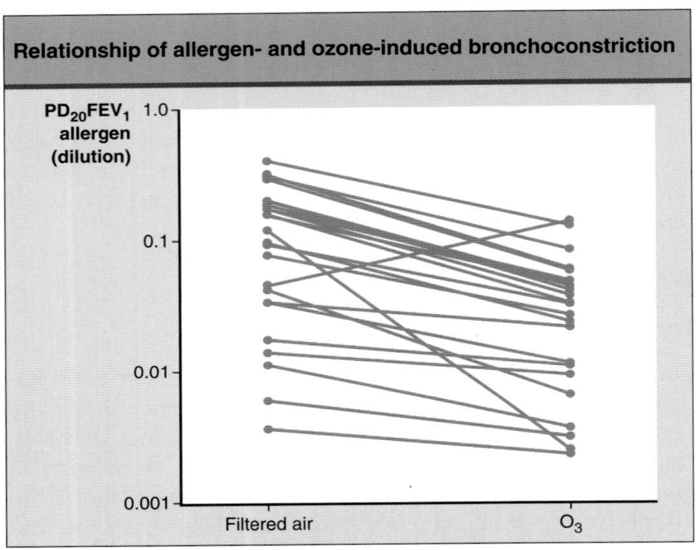

Figure 61.2 Interrelationship of allergen- and ozone-induced bronchoconstriction. Individual values of cumulative doses of allergen ($PD_{20}FEV_1$) in subjects with mild asthma (n = 24) that were needed to elicit a 20% fall in FEV_1, after previous exposure to filtered air or 250 ppb O_3 for 3 hours of intermittent exercise. O_3,ozone; FEV_1, forced expiratory volume in 1 second; ppb, parts per billion. (Data from Jörres R, Nowak D, Magnussen H: The effect of ozone exposure on allergen responsiveness in subjects with asthma or rhinitis. Am J Respir Crit Care Med 153:56-64, 1996.)

or more exaggerated effects. Compared with spirometric (volume) responses, changes in airway resistance (obstruction) seem to be minor. Responses are a function of concentration, minute ventilation, and time, with considerable individual variability. Studies involving prolonged exposures over 6.6 hours with nearly continuous exercise demonstrated that 80 ppb of ozone is sufficient to elicit a measurable effect. When ozone exposures are repeated, a reduction of lung function responses occurs, which is called adaptation or tolerance. The underlying mechanism is unknown. It should be noted that, on average, subjects with mild asthma experience lung function responses to ozone that are equal to or not much greater than those of normal subjects.

Ozone induces a transient increase in airway responsiveness to methacholine that is not related to the changes in lung function. Whereas exercise-induced asthma is not exaggerated, allergen responses are enhanced by ozone. For example, a 3-hour exposure to 250 ppb ozone including intermittent moderate exercise led to a significant increase in bronchial allergen responsiveness (Fig. 61.2). There was even a slight bronchial allergen response after ozone in subjects with allergic rhinitis. Furthermore, four-times repeated exposure to a concentration as low as 125 ppb was capable of increasing the magnitude of early and late phase responses to allergen, as well as the associated airway inflammation, even in subjects with allergic rhinitis. In addition, nasal allergen responses, in terms of the concentrations of eosinophils and eosinophil cationic protein, can be enhanced by ozone. Whether the amplification of allergen responses by ozone is a major factor under ambient air exposure conditions has, however, not yet been established.

Mechanisms of Action

Ozone elicits a number of cellular and biochemical changes that are detectable in the bronchoalveolar lavage (BAL) fluid or in induced sputum. The most prominent feature is the neutrophil influx. Inflammation occurs in the upper and lower airways and seems to be stronger in subjects with asthma compared with controls. Responses are indicated by elevated levels of prostanoids such as prostaglandins $(PG)E_2$, $PGF_{2\text{-alpha}}$, and thromboxane B_2 (but not leukotrienes) in BAL fluid, and of cytokines and chemokines such as interleukin-6, interleukin-8, and granulocyte-monocyte colony-stimulating factor. Possibly, stimulation of nonmyelinated C-fibers and release of neuropeptides are also involved, because substance P and bradykinin levels in BAL fluid are elevated after exposure.

Additionally, ozone causes cellular damage and an increase in epithelial permeability as indicated by the levels of lactate dehydrogenase, total protein, fibronectin, fibrinogen, IgG, albumin, and other markers. Interestingly, lung function responses to ozone in terms of FEV_1 do not correlate with airway inflammation, although both of them are individually reproducible. However, a relationship between indices of small airway function and fibrinogen, as a tentative marker of vascular permeability, has been reported.

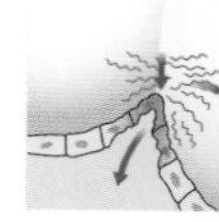

As major effects, ozone causes lipid peroxidation, loss of functional groups of biomolecules, and cellular activation, which leads to the release of inflammatory mediators. Owing to its low solubility in water, it can penetrate into the lung periphery. Pharmacologic trials suggest that β_2-agonists and atropine only partially prevent the ozone-induced airway response, if at all, and that indomethacin can reduce this response, but without attenuating the increase in methacholine responsiveness. Similarly, when dogs were treated with budesonide, the increase in pulmonary resistance and the neutrophil influx were reduced, but airway hyperresponsiveness was not prevented. There are also animal and human data indicating a role of antioxidants in attenuating the response to ozone, but it is not clear whether these compounds markedly reduce the individual susceptibility to ozone under ambient air exposure conditions.

NITROGEN DIOXIDE

Formation and Exposure Levels

Nitrogen dioxide (NO_2) is predominantly generated by motor vehicles, power stations, and industrial processes. It also occurs in the workplace and can be a part of indoor air pollution. NO_2 concentrations in urban areas are, on average, below 50 ppb, but may show peak values of 100 to 400 ppb. Indoor concentrations may exceed these values especially when poorly ventilated high-temperature combustion occurs.

Epidemiologic Studies

Outdoor and indoor levels of NO_2 have been found to be correlated with the frequency or duration of respiratory illness and functional impairment in children, even at low levels. Results in adults and patients with respiratory diseases are less consistent. Some investigators found an association between NO_2 levels and respiratory symptoms or peak flow rates in patients with asthma, whereas others did not. Most of these studies are hampered by the strong associations between different air pollutants.

Exposure Studies

Experimental studies have demonstrated that NO_2 does not affect lung function to a major extent in healthy subjects or patients with mild asthma. Patients with chronic obstructive pulmonary disease might show deteriorations after inhalation of 300 ppb NO_2 but data are not consistent. Subjects with asthma can show enhanced airway responsiveness to histamine or methacholine after inhalation of NO_2. In this respect, they seem to be more sensitive than healthy subjects, but, again, such findings, particularly in asthmatic subjects, are not consistent. The same is true for the enhancement of exercise-induced bronchoconstriction and the airway response to hyperventilation of cold air by NO_2. Although the bronchoconstrictor response to hyperventilation of air containing SO_2 was increased by NO_2, it is likely that this effect is not specific for SO_2. Similar to ozone, NO_2 can facilitate bronchial allergen responses in subjects with asthma, in terms of both early and late phase responses (Fig. 61.3), but it appears that the effects of NO_2 in experimental studies are strongly influenced by the choice of subjects and the study protocol.

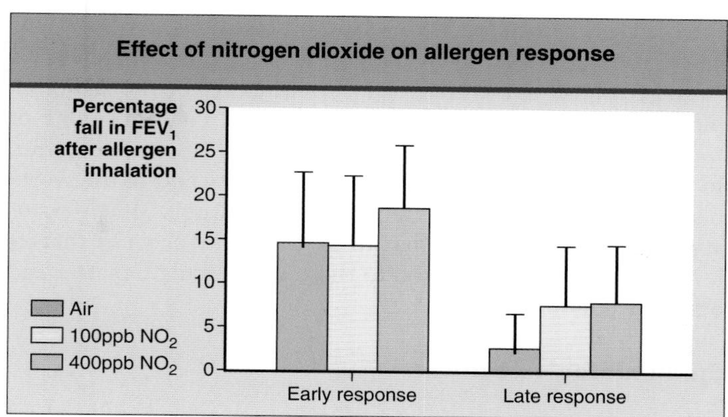

Figure 61.3 Interrelationship of NO_2 and bronchial reactivity to allergen. Mean values (± standard deviation) of the percent fall in FEV_1 after allergen inhalation after exposure to clean air, 100 ppb, or 400 ppb NO_2 for 1 hour at rest. The study included eight subjects with mild allergic asthma. NO_2, nitrogen dioxide; FEV_1, forced expiratory volume in 1 second; ppb, parts per billion. (Data from Tunnicliffe WS, Burge PS, Ayres JG: Effect of domestic concentrations of nitrogen dioxide on airway responses to inhaled allergen in asthmatic patients. Lancet 344:1733-1736, 1994.)

Mechanisms of Action

According to BAL studies, healthy subjects exposed to 3000 to 4000 ppb of NO_2 can show a reduction in the inhibitory capacity of the alpha-1-proteinase inhibitor, in contrast to continuous exposure to a lower concentration or discontinuous exposure with intermittent peaks. Cell numbers in BAL fluid are altered in a concentration-dependent manner, and numbers of mast cells and lymphocytes are increased, with slight differences in cellular response pattern between smokers and nonsmokers. In subjects with mild asthma, exposure to 1000 ppb NO_2 led to an increase in the concentration of thromboxane B_2 and PG D_2 and a decrease in the concentration of 6-keto $PGF_{1\text{-alpha}}$, without significant changes in cell counts. Although in most studies concentrations of total protein, albumin, and lactate dehydrogenase in BAL fluid were not altered by NO_2, changes in alveolar permeability have been shown to occur with a delay of several hours. There are also time-dependent effects on the antioxidant status within the airways.

Owing to its oxidative properties, NO_2 leads to lipid peroxidation and generates reaction products with constituents of airway surfaces. Therefore, one way to achieve protection against NO_2 could be given by antioxidants. Indeed, pretreatment with vitamins C and E diminished the degree of lipid peroxidation in BAL fluid, and pretreatment with vitamin C inhibited the increase in methacholine responsiveness induced by NO_2. Interestingly, the NO_2-induced bronchoconstriction in subjects with chronic bronchitis could be attenuated by antihistamines, whereas atropine or β_2-adrenoceptor agonists were not effective.

SULFUR DIOXIDE

Formation and Exposure Levels

Sulfur dioxide (SO_2) is mainly produced by combustion of fossil fuels. Owing to the reduction of coal burning in individual households and the increased number of large emission sources such as power plants, the distribution of sources changed over

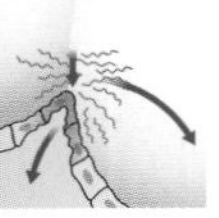

time. SO_2 is associated with weather conditions, whereby low air exchange can lead to elevated levels over prolonged periods. Average annual ambient air concentrations are below 20 ppb in most areas. During air pollution episodes, concentrations of more than 100 ppb, with peaks exceeding 200 ppb, may occur. In some places, particularly in Eastern Europe and in the workplace, SO_2 concentrations can still reach 500 ppb. When evaluating the effects of SO_2 it has to be taken into account that its levels are often closely linked to those of particulate matter and other air pollutants.

Epidemiologic Studies

Epidemiologic data have suggested that extremely high levels of SO_2 are associated with daily mortality, with a delay over days, and with respiratory morbidity resulting from asthma and bronchitis. Such observations are in accordance with those made during the London smog episode in December 1952; the pollutant mixture encountered there contained high levels of SO_2 plus suspended particles. At lower concentrations, subjects with preexisting respiratory and cardiovascular diseases appear to be at partial risk from SO_2. The Six Cities Study, however, which analyzed the effects of lower levels of SO_2 and particles as compared with the London smog episode, found that mortality was less closely related to SO_2 than to particulate matter. Despite this, there seem to be independent effects of SO_2, even with regard to the triggering of ischemic cardiac events.

Long-term exposure to SO_2 (plus particles) can be associated with increased prevalence of cough and phlegm but relationships seem to be complex and difficult to disentangle. Data from reunified Germany, for example, indicated that the higher levels of SO_2 and particles in Eastern compared with Western Germany were not associated with an increased prevalence of atopy, hay fever, or asthma in children and adults.

Exposure Studies

Inhalation of SO_2 induces symptoms such as cough, chest tightness, and wheezing that are closely related to airflow obstruction. SO_2 is a potent bronchoconstrictor in subjects with asthma. Approximately 20% to 25% of subjects with nonspecific airway hyperresponsiveness show airway hyperresponsiveness to SO_2 (Fig. 61.4). The degree of bronchoconstriction depends on minute ventilation and the route of inhalation. In dry or dry cold air, SO_2 responses are stronger than in humidified air. Although airway hyperresponsiveness to methacholine or histamine appears to be a prerequisite for hyperresponsiveness to SO_2, its magnitude does not correlate with the magnitude of SO_2 responsiveness. SO_2 itself does not exert major effects on nonspecific airway responsiveness or allergen responsiveness in human subjects. When exposures are repeated within short intervals of time, bronchoconstrictor responses are attenuated.

Mechanisms of Action

As SO_2 readily dissolves in the fluid layer of airway epithelium, it undergoes a variety of chemical reactions yielding sulfuric acid, sulfites, bisulfites and sulfates, all of which can induce harmful effects. SO_2 and its reaction products interfere with disulfide bonds in biologic macromolecules. Several other mechanisms causing cell damage seem to be possible. The subsequent release of inflammatory mediators can induce mucus hypersecretion and stimulation of sensory nerve endings.

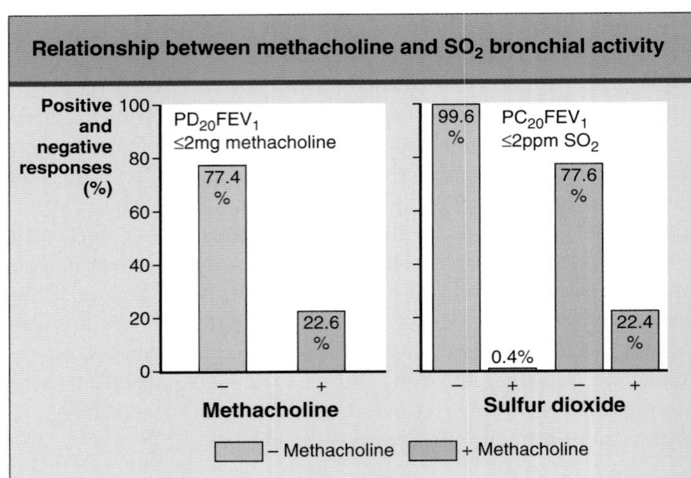

Figure 61.4 Relationship between methacholine and SO_2 bronchial reactivity. Percentages of positive response to inhalation of SO_2 within a population-based sample (n = 780) ages 20 to 44 years (lower panel) in relation to airway responsiveness to methacholine (upper panel). Positive responses were defined as a 20% fall in FEV_1 after inhalation of concentrations of at maximum 2 ppm SO_2 and 2 mg methacholine. SO_2, sulfur dioxide; ppm, parts per million. (Data from Nowak D, Jörres R, Berger J, Claussen M, Magnussen H: Airway responsiveness to sulfur dioxide in an adult population sample. Am J Respir Crit Care Med 156:1151-1156, 1997.)

The hypothesis that relaxation of bronchial smooth muscle or blocking of C-fibers and irritant receptors are means to attenuate the SO_2 response is suggested by the findings of pharmacologic interventions. β_2-adrenoceptor agonists, disodium cromoglycate, nedocromil sodium, and theophylline are capable of either attenuating or completely blocking the bronchoconstrictor response to SO_2. In contrast, inhaled corticosteroids seem to exert only weak protection, and ipratropium bromide had no effect. The data on protective effects of drugs may also help when estimating the potential risk for patients, particularly those with asthma. Prolonged exposure to extremely high concentrations of SO_2 causes structural and functional alterations similar to those observed in chronic bronchitis. Such conditions, however, are not met in human exposures.

MIXTURES OF AIR POLLUTANTS

In daily life, air pollution is mostly the result of a complex mixture of components whose harmful effects may also be modified by factors such as temperature and humidity. In epidemiologic settings, the separation and combination of effects might be achieved by multivariate analyses. Experimental studies of mixtures of air pollutants demonstrated that, for example, preexposure to NO_2 exerts a delayed effect on ozone response and that, in patients with asthma, SO_2-induced bronchoconstriction is facilitated by preexposure to ozone. The available data suggest that the time pattern of exposures and concentrations, as well as the characteristics of the subjects, are key determinants of responses.

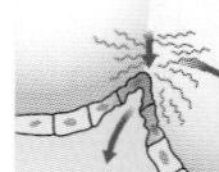

SUGGESTED READINGS

Dockery DW, Pope CA, Xiping X, et al: An association between air pollution and mortality in six U.S. cities. N Engl J Med 329:1753-1759, 1993.

Jörres R, Nowak D, Magnussen H: The effect of ozone exposure on allergen responsiveness in subjects with asthma or rhinitis. Am J Respir Crit Care Med 153:56-64, 1996.

Nowak D, Jörres R, Berger J, Claussen M, Magnussen H: Airway responsiveness to sulfur dioxide in an adult population sample. Am J Respir Crit Care Med 156:1151-1156, 1997.

Peters A, Liu E, Verrier RL, et al: Air pollution and incidence of cardiac arrhythmia. Epidemiology 11:2-4, 2000.

Pope CA III, Thun MJ, Namboodiri MM, et al: Particulate air pollution as a predictor of mortality in a prospective study of US adults. Am J Respir Crit Care Med 151:669-674, 1995.

Sunyer J, Ballester F, Tertre AL, et al: The association of daily sulfur dioxide air pollution levels with hospital admissions for cardiovascular diseases in Europe (The Aphea-II study). Eur Heart J 24:752-760, 2003.

Sunyer J, Basagana X: Particles, and not gases, are associated with the risk of death in patients with chronic obstructive pulmonary disease. Int J Epidemiol 30:1138-1140, 2001.

Tunnicliffe WS, Burge PS, Ayres JG: Effect of domestic concentrations of nitrogen dioxide on airway responses to inhaled allergen in asthmatic patients. Lancet 344:1733-1736, 1994.

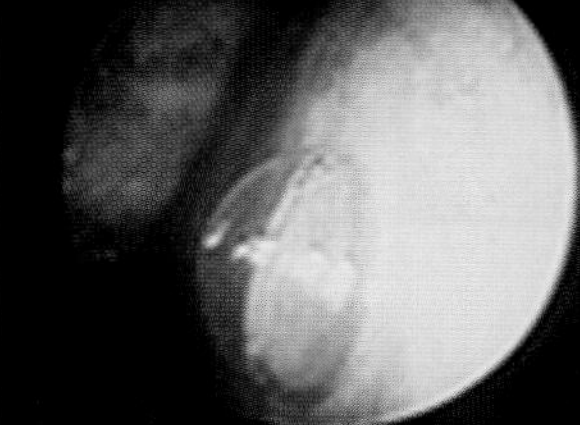

CHAPTER 62 Pneumothorax

Roland Vanderschueren

The term pneumothorax refers to the presence of free air between the visceral pleura and the parietal pleura. Pneumothoraces are either spontaneous or iatrogenic; spontaneous pneumothorax has an unknown cause or occurs as a consequence of the natural course of a disease process.

Primary spontaneous pneumothoraces usually occur in apparently healthy people, whereas secondary spontaneous pneumothoraces are associated with underlying pulmonary pathology, usually chronic obstructive pulmonary disease (COPD), although acquired immunodeficiency syndrome (AIDS) and *Pneumocystis jiroveci* infection appear to play an increasing role in the etiology of primary spontaneous pneumothoraces.

Iatrogenic pneumothoraces occur as the result of diagnostic or therapeutic medical procedures. These pneumothoraces can be intentional or a complication associated with pleural puncture.

Traumatic pneumothoraces can follow any penetrating or nonpenetrating chest trauma, with or without bronchial rupture (Table 62.1).

PRIMARY SPONTANEOUS PNEUMOTHORAX

Spontaneous pneumothorax usually occurs in young male smokers between 20 and 40 years of age. The male-female ratio is about 5:1. Cigarette smoking is probably one of the most important risk factors.

Pathophysiology

Affected patients have no obvious underlying pulmonary disease. Thoracoscopic studies show that blebs and bullae play a role in pathogenesis and are frequently seen in patients with spontaneous pneumothorax. Pulmonary blebs (Fig. 62.1) are air-filled spaces between the lung parenchyma and the visceral pleura; in contrast, pulmonary bullae (Fig. 62.2) are air-filled spaces within the lung parenchyma itself. Blebs and bullae are also known as *emphysema-like changes*. The probable cause of the pneumothorax is rupture of an apical bleb or bulla, because the compliance of blebs and bullae in the apices is low compared with that of similar lesions situated in the lower parts of the lungs. It is often hard to assess whether bullae are the sites of leakage and where the site of rupture of the visceral pleura is. Smoking causes a ninefold increase in the relative risk of a pneumothorax in females and a 22-fold increase in males, with a dose-response relationship between the number of cigarettes smoked per day and the occurrence of primary spontaneous pneumothorax.

Clinical Features

Symptoms are not always present, and sometimes a small apical pneumothorax is found on routine chest x-ray. In the majority of cases, however, the patient develops sudden unilateral chest pain and dyspnea, which is related to the size of the pneumothorax. Physical examination reveals hyper-resonant percussion and reduced breath sounds. In left-sided pneumothorax, Hamman's sign may be heard, i.e., a clicking sound synchronous with the heartbeat. Another symptom is dry cough. In rare cases subcutaneous emphysema may be obvious on inspection of the neck, face, or chest. In a tension pneumothorax, breathlessness can be severe, and there may be hypotension with cardiac tamponade.

Diagnosis

Spontaneous pneumothorax is usually suggested by the history and physical examination. A chest x-ray is needed to establish the diagnosis. If a small pneumothorax is suspected but not apparent on the chest x-ray, another film taken with the patient in complete expiration often reveals the lesion, because during expiration air is expelled into the pleural cavity, making the pneumothorax more obvious. When there are adhesions between the pleurae and the lung cannot collapse completely, a partial pneumothorax is seen (Fig. 62.3). Often some displacement of the mediastinum toward the normal side is evident. Mediastinal emphysema and subcutaneous emphysema are rare.

Treatment

The choice of the best treatment method is still somewhat controversial. Several choices are available:

- Rest and oxygen therapy
- Needle aspiration
- Simple intercostal drainage
- Medical thoracoscopy with talc poudrage
- Video-assisted thoracic surgery (VATS) with pleural abrasion or partial pleurectomy and bullectomy
- Full thoracotomy

The choice of initial treatment depends on the presentation (Fig. 62.4). The size of the pneumothorax and the presence and extent of bullae are important. In a fit young person who is not distressed, management is conservative and includes weekly chest x-rays taken on an outpatient basis. If the patient is breathless, then needle aspiration through the second intercostal space anteriorly should be performed. Up to 2.5 L of air can be aspi-

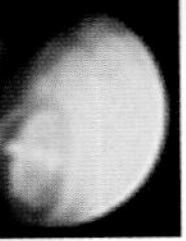

Table 62.1
Classification of pneumothoraces

Spontaneous pneumothoraces	Iatrogenic pneumothoraces
Primary idiopathic spontaneous pneumothorax Secondary spontaneous pneumothorax	Traumatic pneumothorax Diagnostic (intentional) pneumothorax Inadvertent pneumothorax

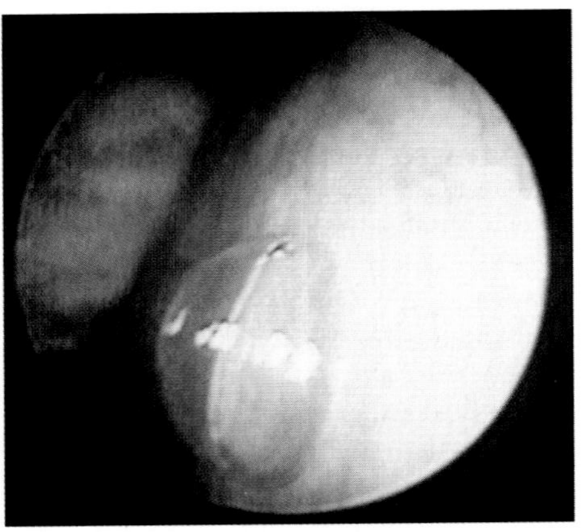

Figure 62.1 Thoracoscopic view of a bleb.

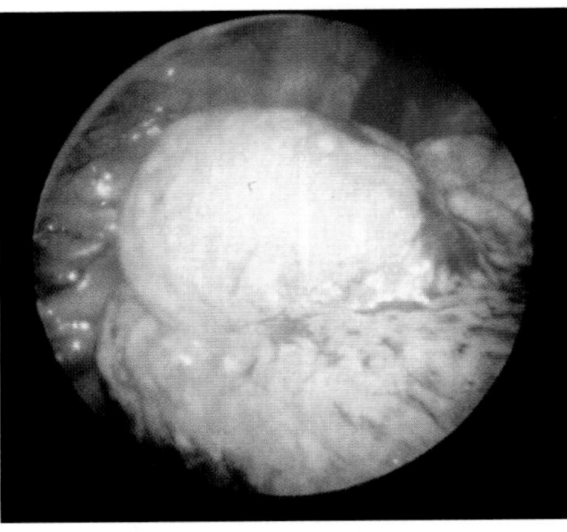

Figure 62.2 Thoracoscopic view of a bulla.

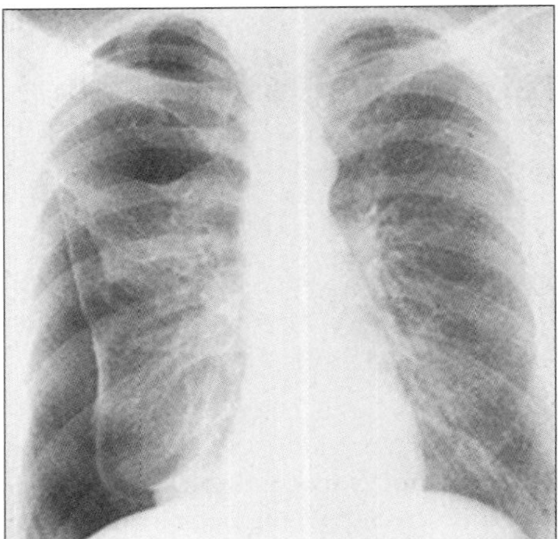

Figure 62.3 Partial pneumothorax with adhesions.

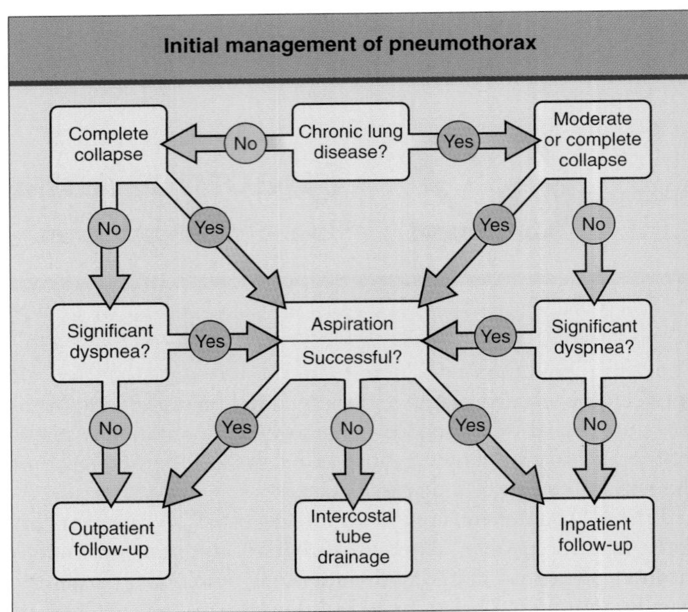

Figure 62.4 Initial management of a pneumothorax. (Adapted from Miller AC, Harvey JE: Guidelines for the management of spontaneous pneumothorax. Br Med J 307:114-116, 1993.)

rated with a 50-mL syringe and a three-way tap. If the lung re-expands and the patient is comfortable, overnight observation is advised, with a goal of discharge and weekly follow-up. However, if the pneumothorax does not respond to aspiration, an intercostal tube should be inserted. If the lung is totally collapsed at presentation, aspiration should still be the first choice of treatment. If an intercostal tube is inserted, high concentrations of inspired oxygen may encourage re-expansion by the washout of nitrogen in the pleural cavity.

A recurrence of a spontaneous pneumothorax is an indication for more invasive therapy, such as pleural drainage with a chemical pleurodesis or surgical intervention.

CHEMICAL PLEURODESIS

Needle aspiration, intercostal tube drainage, and the use of a Heimlich flutter valve have proved to be safe procedures in the treatment of primary spontaneous pneumothorax, with few side effects, but most studies report a recurrence rate of 30% to 50%. On recurrence, talc or 3 g of tetracycline have proved to be effective sclerosing agents and can be instilled via an intercostal tube. In the case of talc poudrage, 4 to 6 g of talc are insufflated by means of a talc atomizer or disposable single-use spray canister (Fig. 62.5); for best results this procedure should be performed under direct vision at VATS or thoracotomy. Chemical pleurodesis with talc slurry or tetracycline is very painful, and 100 to 200 mg of lidocaine should be added to the sclerosing solution. Sedation or parenteral analgesia is also recommended. In general, pleurodesis via an intercostal drain is not as effective as pleurodesis performed under direct vision, and reviews report a recurrence rate of 8% in 1030 patients.

Concerns have been raised regarding the safety of pleurodesis with talc, particularly the possibility that talc slurry may cause acute pneumonitis and adult respiratory distress syndrome. However, this seems to occur only if more than 10 g of talc are administered or if vascular injury is present. No evidence

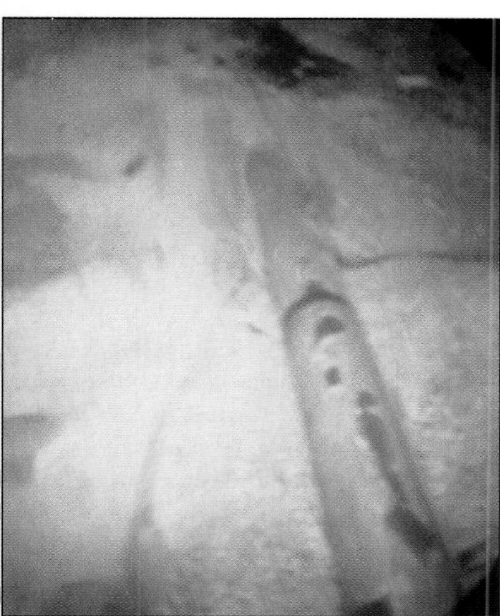

Figure 62.5
Thoracoscopic view after pleural talc poudrage.

of mesothelioma was found in two studies that followed patients for up to 35 years after talc pleurodesis, although some pleural thickening and calcification were seen.

SURGICAL TREATMENT

Minimally invasive surgical procedures, particularly VATS, have developed rapidly, and a recent review of 805 patients with spontaneous pneumothorax treated with VATS had a mean recurrence rate of 4%, which was higher than that after conventional surgical therapy (the recurrence rate of which was 1.5%). During VATS, bullae can be stapled with endostaplers or resected by a neodymium:yttrium-aluminium-garnet (Nd:YAG) laser. In addition, tetracycline or talc is usually instilled or a pleural abrasion performed. Thoracotomy is now indicated only if thoracoscopy and VATS are not available or in cases of failure or recurrence after treatment with sclerosing agents, VATS, or both.

SECONDARY SPONTANEOUS PNEUMOTHORAX

Patients with secondary pneumothorax have an underlying pulmonary disease, often with diminished lung function, making the symptoms worse than those associated with primary spontaneous pneumothorax and sometimes life threatening.

A summary of the most frequent underlying diseases is given in Table 62.2. The most common underlying association is COPD; infection with *P. jiroveci* in patients with AIDS is becoming more common.

Clinical Features

The symptoms of secondary spontaneous pneumothorax are identical to those of primary spontaneous pneumothorax but are frequently disproportionate to the size of the pneumothorax. In some patients clinical deterioration occurs suddenly and rapidly, and fatal episodes have been documented. Patients with COPD already have hyperexpanded lungs, so physical examination is less helpful in these patients than in patients with primary spontaneous pneumothorax, because a contralateral difference may not be so apparent.

Table 62.2
Causes of pneumothorax

Iatrogenic	Spontaneous
Penetrating chest wounds	Primary (most common in young men)
Iatrogenic – including chest aspiration, intercostal nerve block, subclavian cannulation, transbronchial biopsy, needle aspiration lung biopsy, positive pressure ventilation	Secondary Chronic obstructive pulmonary disease Asthma Congenital cysts and bullae Pleural malignancy Interstitial lung fibrosing diseases Bacterial pneumonia Tuberculosis Whooping cough
Chest compression injury – including external cardiac massage	Cystic fibrosis Histiocytosis X Tuberous sclerosis Lymphangiomyomatosis Endometriosis of the pleura Marfan syndrome Sarcoidosis Esophageal rupture *Pneumocystis jiroveci* pneumonia

Diagnosis

The diagnosis is established by examining the chest x-ray. In patients with COPD, emphysematous changes are present in both lungs, and often hyperlucent or bullous areas can be seen that could be confused with or mistaken for the appearance of a pneumothorax. The recognition of a visceral pleural line on the radiograph is essential. In uncertain cases computed tomography may be helpful, although it is not useful for differentiating a large bulla from a pneumothorax unless there are strands of tissue seen running within the bulla.

Treatment

Treatment options in primary and secondary spontaneous pneumothorax are similar, but because of the more severe symptoms and the impaired lung function associated with secondary spontaneous pneumothorax, more patients with the latter condition require treatment with intercostal tube thoracostomy. In the event of a recurrence of the pneumothorax, pleurodesis should be performed. Because many of these patients have underlying lung disease and are not fit for surgery (even VATS), the pleurodesis is likely to be "medical" (i.e., talc or tetracycline administered via an intercostal tube). However, if the patient is a potential candidate for lung transplantation, thoracoscopy with Nd:YAG treatment of blebs and stapling of bullae are preferable.

In patients with AIDS and *P. jiroveci* infection, the occurrence of pneumothorax is an ominous prognostic sign. Pneumothorax in these patients is most often caused by a rupture of a subpleural necrotic cavity. Simple tube thoracostomy is seldom successful, and the simplest alternative seems to be the use of a Heimlich valve, which allows the patient to be discharged from the hospital. If the fistula does not close, then talc slurry should be used before invasive treatment such as VATS or thoracotomy is undertaken.

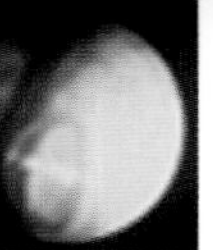

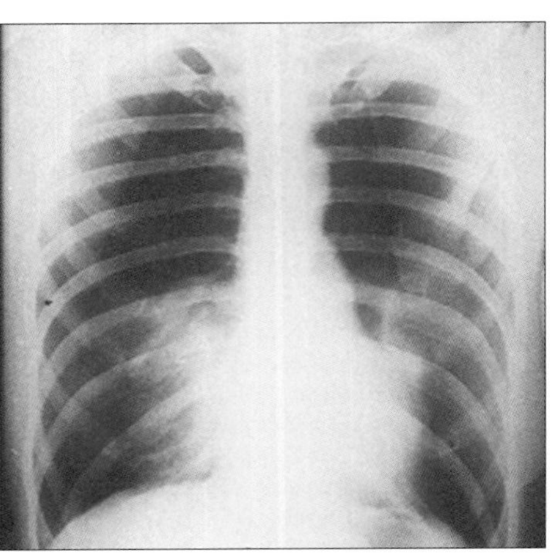

Figure 62.6 Catamenial pneumothorax (bilateral).

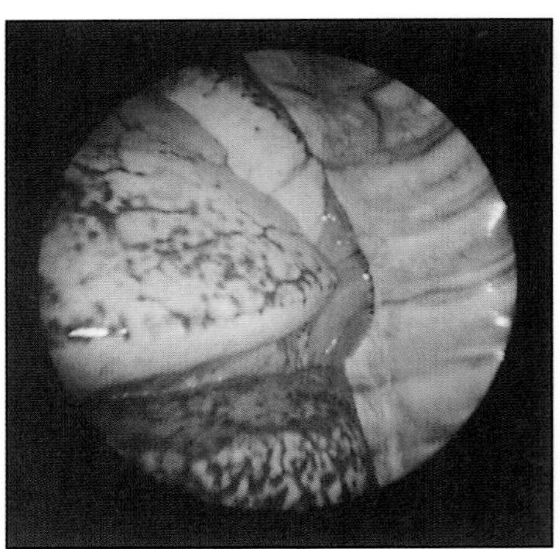

Figure 62.7 Idiopathic spontaneous pneumothorax. Thoracoscopic image of a normal lung in a patient with idiopathic spontaneous pneumothorax.

CATAMENIAL PNEUMOTHORAX

Catamenial pneumothorax occurs in conjunction with menstruation and is for the most part recurrent (Fig. 62.6). The pathogenesis is still unclear. One of the hypotheses is that during menstruation air enters the peritoneal cavity and also the pleural cavity through a defect in the diaphragm. However, these defects are not always seen in patients treated for catamenial pneumothorax. Pleural or diaphragmatic endometriosis could also be of importance. The diagnosis of catamenial pneumothorax is obvious, and, if the pneumothorax is recurrent, treatment should be the administration of ovulation-suppressing drugs. In cases in which this treatment is not wanted or tolerated, thoracoscopy and pleurodesis are advised.

PITFALLS AND CONTROVERSIES

Optimal treatment of pneumothorax is still controversial. The ideal treatment should aim at expanding the lung rapidly and completely, with restoration (or improvement) of pulmonary function. It should also be associated with minimal morbidity and mortality, a low cost, and a short hospital stay. After conservative treatment (i.e., rest, simple aspiration, or drainage) of a first pneumothorax the recurrence rate is as high as 30% to 50%.

Thoracoscopy is now performed more routinely for first pneumothoraces (in some cases) and for recurrent pneumothoraces (in most cases). At thoracoscopy, radiologically occult anomalies (e.g., blebs or cysts) can be identified, and a more effective subsequent surgical repair is possible. If the pleura and lung are normal at thoracoscopy (Fig. 62.7) in a young patient, pleurodesis is the best method of treatment, with a recurrence rate of 6% to 8%. Other patients need surgical treatment, either by VATS or thoracotomy, in which the usual procedure is pleurodesis by abrasion after repair of any lung abnormality. Pleurectomy should be performed in patients with secondary pneumothorax if pleurodesis fails.

In cases of life-threatening pneumothorax, the findings at physical examination are usually sufficient for the diagnosis to be made. The most important step is to insert a large-bore needle to evacuate the pneumothorax. The definitive treatment procedure can then be performed later. In a young patient with severe underlying disease who may be a candidate for lung transplantation, pleurodesis and thoracotomy should be avoided. The profession of the patient can also be of importance in choosing the type of treatment (e.g., pilots, construction workers).

SUGGESTED READINGS

Gerlinzani S, Tos M, Poliziani D: Catamenial pneumothorax. Surg Endosc 16:870-871, 2002.

Light RW: Pneumothorax. In Light RW (ed): Pleural Diseases, 3rd ed. Baltimore, Williams and Wilkins, 1995, pp 242-277.

Research Committee of the British Thoracic Association and the Medical Research Council Pneumoconiosis Unit: A survey of long-term effects of talc and kaolin pleurodesis. Br J Dis Chest 73:285-288, 1997.

Schramel FMNH, Postmus PE, Vanderschueren RGJRA: Current aspects of spontaneous pneumothorax. Eur Respir J 10:1372-1379, 1997.

Tschopp JM, Bolliger CT, Boutin C: Treatment of spontaneous pneumothorax: Why not simple talc pleurodesis by medical thoracoscopy? Respiration 67:108-111, 2000.

Tschopp JM, Boutin C, Astoul P: Talcage by medical thoracoscopy for primary spontaneous pneumothorax is more cost-effective than drainage: A randomised study. Eur Respir J 20:1003-1009, 2002.

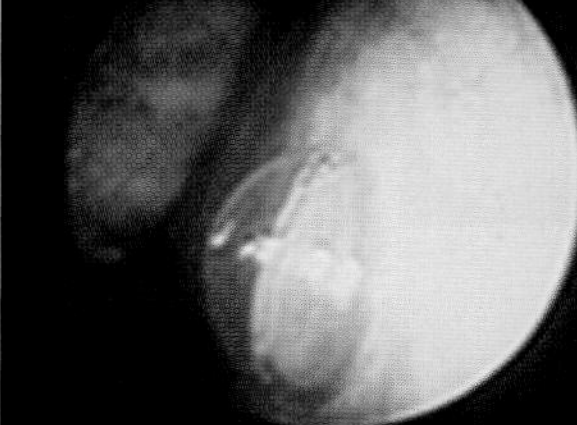

CHAPTER 63 Pleural Effusion

Robert Loddenkemper

Pleural effusion is defined as accumulation of fluid in the pleural space that exceeds the physiologic amounts of 10 to 20 mL. Pleural effusion develops either when the formation of pleural fluid is excessive or when fluid resorption is disturbed. Pleural effusions may represent a primary manifestation of many diseases, but most often they are observed as secondary manifestations or complications of other diseases.

EPIDEMIOLOGY AND PATHOPHYSIOLOGY

Epidemiology

Pleural effusion is found in almost 10% of patients who have internal diseases, and the main cause in 30% to 40% of these is cardiac failure (Table 63.1). Among the noncardiac effusions, parapneumonic effusions are the most common at 48%, of which approximately 75% are of bacterial and 25% of viral origin. Malignant pleural effusions follow with 24% of cases, more than half of which are caused by lung or breast cancer. Pleural effusion is secondary to pulmonary embolism in 18% of cases, to liver cirrhosis in 6%, and to gastrointestinal diseases—mainly pancreatitis—in 3% of cases. Many other possible causes, albeit extremely rare, play an important role in differential diagnosis. The discrepancy between these estimated incidences and the frequency distribution in the respiratory literature, in which malignant causes are the most common at 42%—followed by infectious causes at 29% and idiopathic effusions at 15%—most probably results from patient selection (Table 63.2). Conversely, it may be concluded that, apart from cardiac effusions, effusions as sequelae of pneumonia, pulmonary embolism, and gastrointestinal diseases are easy to diagnose and, therefore, less frequently referred to the pulmonary specialist.

Pathophysiology

Pleural effusion may result from a number of pathophysiologic mechanisms, all of which disturb the physiologic balance between the formation and removal of pleural fluid (normal production estimated at 15 mL/day in a 60-kg person). Most effusions develop from both an increase in the entry rate of liquid into the pleural space and a decrease in the maximal exit rate of liquid from the pleural space. Transudative effusions are either caused by increased hydrostatic pressure (e.g., in cardiac failure) or by reduced plasma oncotic pressure because of protein deficiency (e.g., liver cirrhosis, nephrotic syndrome). The pleura itself remains intact. Rarely, transudates may arise from the entry of liquids with low protein concentrations (e.g., urine [ipsilateral obstructive uropathy], cerebrospinal fluid [duropleural fistula], or iatrogenic intrapleural infusion of fluids). In contrast, pathologic changes in the pleura result in exudation caused by a diffuse increase of capillary permeability, to localized ruptures (e.g., blood vessels, lymphatic vessels, lung abscess, esophagus) or to disturbed absorption (e.g., lymphatic blockage).

A wide spectrum of diseases may be associated with pleural effusion. Table 63.3 shows the relevant etiologic groups together with their most important characteristics, such as appearance, protein and cell content, and other possible features. In some diseases, the pleural effusion may either be an exudate or a transudate.

CLINICAL FEATURES

Pleural effusion may present at all ages, but is mainly found in adults. Malignant pleural effusions are observed mainly in patients older than age 60 years. The most common presentations are dyspnea and chest pain, and those of the individual underlying diseases. Physical examination reveals dullness on percussion, usually at the base of the thorax, and decreased breath sounds.

Imaging Techniques

Pleural effusion may be demonstrated by a number of techniques with different sensitivities. The demonstration by percussion requires at least 300 to 400 mL of fluid, whereas at least 200 to 300 mL is necessary for standard chest radiography. Smaller amounts can be recognized by lateral decubitus radiography, which also demonstrates whether the fluid is moving freely (Fig. 63.1). Ultrasound is able to demonstrate small effusions, and the sensitivity is almost 100% for volumes of 100 mL and above. Computed tomography and magnetic resonance imaging have very similar sensitivities, but require a more advanced technology and are therefore much more expensive.

DIAGNOSIS

In the majority of cases, the etiology is based on the case history, clinical presentation, imaging techniques, and examination of the pleural fluid.

Diagnostic Approach

The presence of a pleural effusion is established only by thoracentesis. The site should be selected according to the results of the diagnostic procedures. If the effusion is small, thoracentesis can be performed under ultrasound guidance. Thoracentesis is indicated in all cases of pleural effusion of unknown origin, and in effusions that do not resolve after appropriate treatment. If

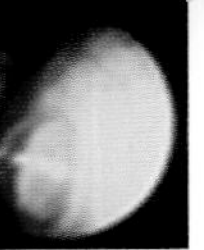

Table 63.1
Approximate annual incidence of various types of pleural effusions in the United States

Etiology	Number	Percentage	Percentage of noncardiac effusions
Congestive heart failure	500,000	37.5	
Other causes		63.5	
Pneumonia	400,000		48.0
Malignant disease	200,000		24.0
Pulmonary embolism	150,000		18.0
Cirrhosis with ascites	50,000		6.0
Gastrointestinal disease	25,000		3.0
Collagen vascular disease	6,000		0.7
Tuberculosis	2,500		0.3
Asbestos pleuritis	2,000		0.25
Mesothelioma	1,500		0.2
Total	1,337,000	100.0	100.0

(Adapted with permission from Light RW (ed): Pleural Diseases (4th ed). Philadelphia, Lippincott Williams & Wilkins, 2001.)

Table 63.2
Frequency distribution of noncardiac effusions

Authors	Number	Neoplastic (%)	Infectious (%)	Various (%)	Idiopathic (%)
Storey et al. JAMA/1976	115	56	6	16	22
Hirsch et al. Thorax/1979	295	39	31	9	21
Lamy et al. Poumon-Coeur/1979	194	46	33.5	12	20
Engel Nordd Ges Lungen-u Bronchialheilkunde/1980	646	34.5	26.5	15	12.5
Loddenkemper Poumon-Coeur/1981	250	34	39	18	9
Total	1500	42	29	14	15

the results of pleural fluid examination are not conclusive, thoracentesis may be repeated. However, additional biopsy procedures, such as closed pleural needle biopsy (see Chapter 10) or medical thoracoscopy (see the following section), may become necessary to confirm or exclude malignant or tuberculous causes. These are performed in a stepwise diagnostic approach (Fig. 63.2). Careful thoracentesis is generally safe. Complications include pneumothorax and bleeding; a less common event is reexpansion pulmonary edema attributed to changes in transpulmonary pressure gradients and endothelial disruption from rapid removal of large volumes of fluid. Edema is usually seen in the ipsilateral lung, although both contralateral and bilateral involvement have been described.

Evaluation of the Pleural Fluid

In many cases, evaluation of the pleural fluid yields valuable diagnostic information or even permits a clear diagnosis. The most important criteria are appearance, protein content, and cellular components. In cases of more specific diagnostic questions, routine measurement of the glucose content is supplemented by determination of further laboratory parameters and bacterial culture (Table 63.4).

The appearance may be serous (light to dark, clear to turbid), serosanguineous (blood-tinged, in some cases because of thoracentesis), hemorrhagic (bloody), purulent (fetid odor in anaerobic effusions), or chylous (milky). Bilious (cholohemothorax), brown (perforated amebic abscess), black (aspergillar infection), or yellowish green (rheumatoid pleuritis, pancreatic effusion) appearances are extremely rare. Blood-tinged effusions that occur with no trauma are mainly caused by tumors (hemorrhagic in 50%) or pulmonary infarction. Hemothorax is characterized by purely bloody effusions and hematocrit values that exceed those in peripheral blood by more than 50%. Increased triglycerides distinguish chylous from pseudochylous effusions. Viscous effusions are rare and may indicate increased hyaluronic acid in malignant pleural mesothelioma, whereas ammonia odor may indicate urinothorax and food particles indicate esophageal perforation. Purulent effusions must be analyzed for infecting organisms (aerobic and anaerobic, tuberculous, and fungal).

The most important laboratory parameter is total protein content in the effusion, for which a threshold value of 30 g/L separates a transudate from an exudate effusion. However, this value is not exclusive, and additional parameters such as lactate dehydrogenase (LDH greater than 200 U/L) or cholesterol (greater than 1.55 mmol/L [60 mg/dL]) may be helpful (Table 63.5). The simultaneous determination of serum values is important, because these may strongly influence the values in the pleura. Thus, the quotient of total pleural protein and total serum protein (higher than 0.5), pleural LDH and serum LDH (higher than 0.6), pleural cholesterol (higher than 60 mg/dL), or pleural versus serum bilirubin (less than 0.6) permits a safer classification as exudate, although recent meta-analysis suggests that the three-test combination of pleural fluid protein, pleural fluid LDH, and pleural fluid cholesterol has high diagnostic accuracy.

Low glucose values under 3.33 mmol/L (60 mg/dL) or an effusion:serum quotient less than 0.5 (alternatively, a pH value lower than 7.3 with normal serum pH or LDH [greater than 1000 U/L]) may indicate rheumatoid pleuritis, lupus pleuritis, empyema, tuberculous or malignant effusion, or esophageal perforation. However, these entities differ in the frequency of decreased glucose values (Table 63.6).

The lowest glucose values (less than 0.56 mmol/L [10 mg/dL]) are found in rheumatoid effusions and empyema. Parapneumonic effusions with values less than 2.22 mmol/L (40 mg/dL) are frequently associated with bacterial infection. In tuberculous effusions, the chance of a positive culture improves markedly with decreased glucose concentrations. Low glucose content in malignant effusions indicates more extensive involvement and a poorer prognosis. A low pH reflects intensive, anaerobic metabolism of leukocytes, bacteria, or tumor cells.

Markedly elevated amylase values—higher and more persistently increased than in serum—are observed in acute pancreatitis and pancreatic pseudocysts (often greater than 1000 U/L), esophageal perforation (salivary amylase, pH markedly decreased to 6.0), and occasionally in malignant effusions.

Table 63.3
Etiology and characteristics of pleural effusions

Etiologic disease groups	Disease	Results of pleural fluid examination; those in brackets to be clarified			
		Appearance	Protein content (exudate >30g/L; transudate <30g/L)	Cells (if relatively typical)	Other features
Oncotic and hydrostatic disturbances	Cardiac insufficiency	Serous	Transudate	–	Pseudoexudate possible
	Superior vena cava obstruction	Serous	Transudate	–	–
	Constrictive pericarditis	Serous	Transudate	–	–
	Liver cirrhosis with ascites	Serous	Transudate	–	–
	Hypoalbuminemia	Serous	Transudate	–	–
	Salt retention syndrome	Serous	Transudate	–	–
	Peritoneal dialysis	Serous	Transudate	–	–
	Hydronephrosis	Serous	Transudate	–	–
	Nephrotic syndrome	Serous	Transudate	–	–
Infectious	Tuberculosis	Serous, hemorrhagic, purulent, chylous	Exudate	Lymphocytes (neutrophilic granulocytes)	Rarely, microscopic detection of bacteria, elevated adenosine deaminase, glucose decrease possible
	Viruses and mycoplasmas	Serous, (hemorrhagic)	Exudate	Lymphocytes	Giant cells possible
	Parapneumonic	Serous, (hemorrhagic)	Exudate	Neutrophilic granulocytes +	Bacteria +
	Nonspecific empyema	Purulent, (serous)	Exudate	Neutrophilic granulocytes ++	Bacteria +, glucose and pH decreased
	Fungi and parasites	Serous, (hemorrhagic)	Exudate	–	Infecting organisms microscopically or in culture
Neoplastic	Diffuse malignant mesothelioma	Serous, hemorrhagic	Exudate, (transudate)	Tumor cells	–
	Metastatic extrathoracic tumor	Serous, hemorrhagic, chylous	Exudate, (transudate)	Tumor cells	(Tumor markers) (Chromosome analysis)
	Bronchial carcinoma	Serous, hemorrhagic, chylous	Exudate, (transudate)	Tumor cells	Low glucose possible
	Lymphomas and leukemia	Serous, hemorrhagic, chylous	Exudate, transudate	Tumor cells	–
	Localized pleural tumors	Serous, (hemorrhagic)	Exudate, transudate	–	–
	Kaposi's sarcoma (AIDS)	Hemorrhagic	Exudate	–	–
	Chest wall tumors	Serous, hemorrhagic	Exudate	Tumor cells	–
	Accompanying effusion in tumors	Serous	Exudate, transudate	–	–
Vascular	Pulmonary infarction	Hemorrhagic, serous	Exudate, transudate	–	–
	Collaterals in liver cirrhosis	Hemorrhagic, serous	Exudate, transudate	–	Markedly decreased
Autoimmune	Rheumatoid arthritis	Serous, chylous	Exudate	Lupus erythematosus cells	Glucose and C3/C4
	Systemic lupus erythematosus	Serous, (hemorrhagic)	Exudate	–	–
	Sjögren's syndrome	Serous	Exudate, (transudate)	–	–
	Mixed connective tissue disease	Serous	Exudate	–	–
Originating from the abdomen	Pancreatitis, pseudocyst	Serous, (hemorrhagic)	Exudate, (transudate)	–	Elevated amylase
	Subdiaphragmatic abscess	Serous, purulent	Exudate	Neutrophilic granulocytes	–
	Liver cirrhosis with ascites	Serous, (purulent)	Transudate, (exudate)	–	–
	Abdominal tumor with ascites	Serous	Transudate	–	–
	Meigs' syndrome	Serous	Transudate, (exudate)	–	–
	Cholohemothorax (biliary fistula)	Bilious	Exudate	–	Bilirubin
	Endometriosis	Hemorrhagic	Exudate	–	–
Traumatic	Hemothorax	Hemorrhagic	Exudate	Erythrocytes	High hemoglobin
	Chylothorax	Chylous	Transudate, (exudate)	–	Chylomicrons, elevated triglycerides
	Esophageal perforation	Purulent	Exudate	Neutrophilic granulocytes	Elevated amylase, low pH
	Surgery (thorax, abdomen)	Serous, hemorrhagic	Exudate, transudate	–	–
	Seropneumothorax	Serous, (hemorrhagic)	Exudate	–	–
Miscellaneous	Uremic pleuritis	Serous, (hemorrhagic)	Exudate	–	–
	Myxedema	Serous	Transudate	–	–
	Yellow nail syndrome	Serous, (chylous)	Exudate	–	–
	Postmyocardial infarction syndrome	Serous, (hemorrhagic)	Exudate	–	–
	Periarteritis nodosa	Serous	Exudate	–	–
	Sarcoidosis	Serous, (hemorrhagic)	Transudate, (exudate)	–	–
	Familial Mediterranean fever	Serous	Exudate	–	–
	Benign asbestos effusion	Serous, (hemorrhagic)	Exudate	–	–
	Drug-induced	Serous	Exudate	–	–
	Radiation pneumonia	Serous, (hemorrhagic)	Exudate	–	–
	Lymphangioleiomyomatosis	Chylous	Transudate, (exudate)	–	–
	Tuberous sclerosis	Chylous	Transudate, (exudate)	–	–
	Cholesterol pleuritis (pseudochylothorax)	Chylous	Transudate, exudate	–	Cholesterol (crystals), low triglycerides
	Intrapleural infusion	Serous, (hemorrhagic)	Exudate, transudate	–	–
	Idiopathic	Serous, (hemorrhagic)	Exudate, transudate	Eosinophils	–

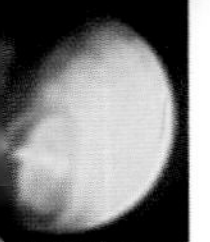

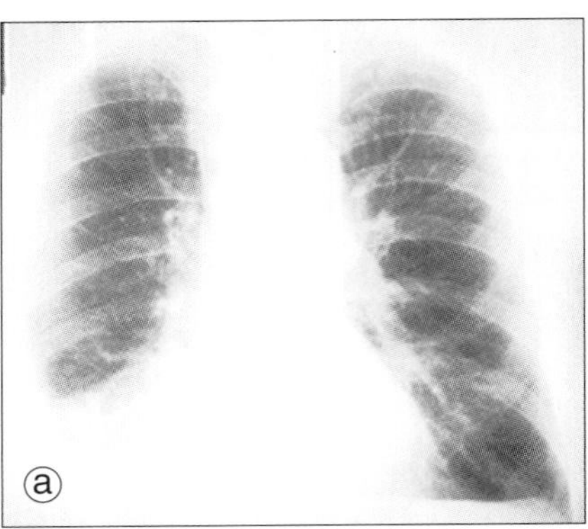

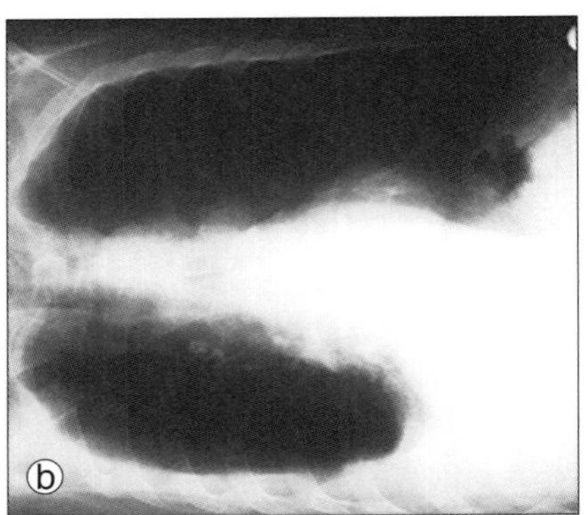

Figure 63.1 Right-sided basal pleural effusion. **A,** Posteroanterior view. **B,** Lateral decubitus view.

Table 63.4
Investigative parameters of pleural effusion

Obligatory	Optional
Appearance	Glucose (pH)
Total protein	Lactate dehydrogenase
Cell differentiation (cytology)	Cholesterol
	Triglycerides
	Amylase
	Bilirubin
	Creatinine
	Hematocrit
	Immunocytology
	Tumor markers
	Adenosine deaminase
	Lysozymes
	Antinuclear factor, rheumatoid factors, etc.
	Search for infecting organisms
	Tubercle bacilli
	Gram staining
	Anaerobic, aerobic bacteria
	Fungi, parasites

Triglyceride content greater than 1.24 mmol/L (110 mg/dL) strongly suggests a chylous effusion (intermediate values are further assessed by lipoprotein electrophoresis). Because chylous effusions are not necessarily milky in appearance, triglycerides are determined in all effusions of uncertain etiology. Chylothorax is a rare cause of increased bilirubin in pleural effusions, whereas increased creatinine may be caused by urinothorax.

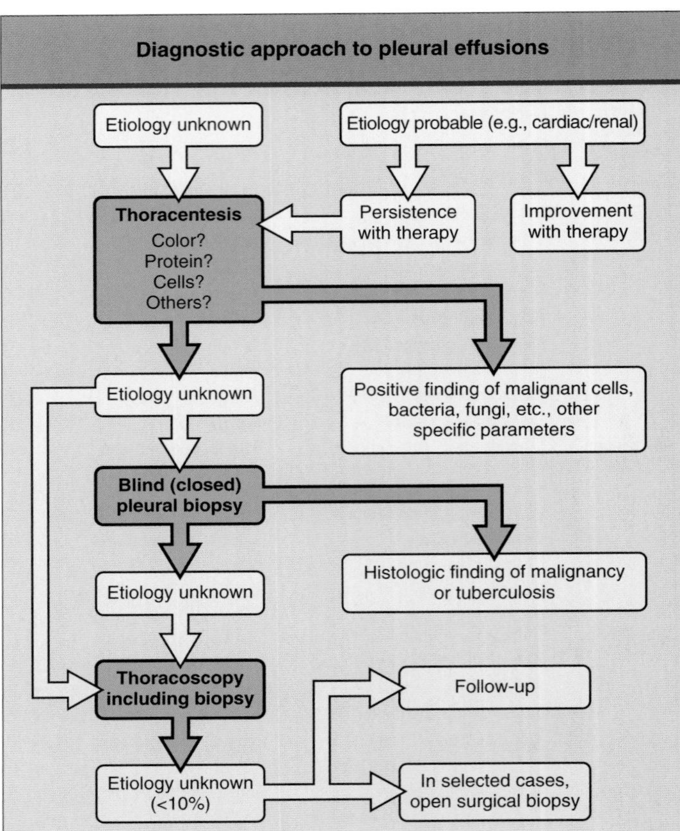

Figure 63.2 Diagnostic approach to pleural effusions.

Table 63.5
Differentiation between transudate and exudate

Parameter	Transudate	Exudate
Total protein (TP)	<3 g/dL	>3 g/dL
Ratio of TP pleura to TP serum	<0.5	>0.5
Lactate dehydrogenase (LDH)	<200 U/L	>200 U/L
Ratio of LDH pleura to LDH serum	<0.6	>0.6
Cholesterol	<1.55 mmol/L (<60 mg/dL)	>1.55 mmol/L (>60 mg/dL)
Bilirubin pleura:serum ratio	<0.6	>0.6

When pleural effusion is associated with rheumatoid arthritis or systemic lupus erythematosus, immunologic parameters (rheumatoid factor, antinuclear antibodies, lupus erythematosus cells, and complement values) are assessed in addition to the glucose levels.

Although nonspecific, adenosine deaminase and lysozymes are frequently increased in tuberculous effusions.

The search for tumor cells focuses on analysis of the cellular components. In an analysis of 4000 cases of malignant effusions, the mean sensitivity of cytologic diagnostic procedures was 58% (range 41% to 88%, standard deviation ±14%). The results were partly improved by repeat analysis. The sensitivity was also

Table 63.6
Frequency of low glucose values in pleural effusions

Entity	Frequency (%)
Rheumatoid pleuritis	85
Empyema	80
Malignant effusion	30
Tuberculous effusion	20
Lupus pleuritis	20

(Adapted with permission from Sahn SA: The diagnostic value of pleural fluid analysis. Semin Respir Crit Care Med 16: 269–278, 1995.)

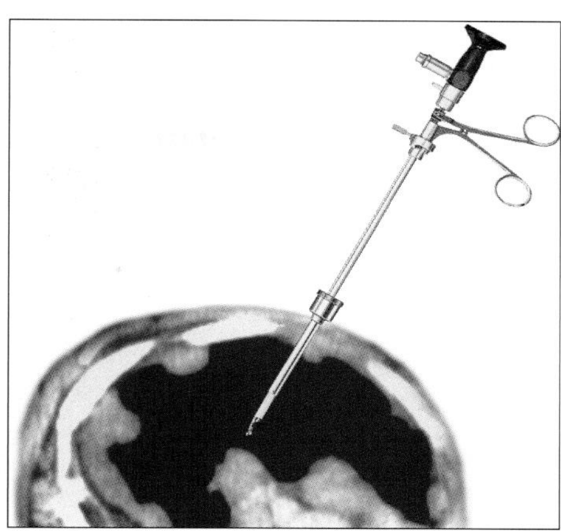

Figure 63.3 Technique of thoracoscopy. Computed tomography scan of a patient with malignant pleural effusion with large nodules on the chest wall and the mediastinum, onto whose hemithorax the thoracoscope with the biopsy forceps is projected.

dependent on the tumor type and the primary tumor. Differences in the accuracy of cytologic tests were found in lung carcinomas, extrathoracic primary tumors, and primary pleural mesotheliomas.

The red cell count, the relative and absolute numbers of lymphocytes, and neutrophilic and eosinophilic granulocytes are rarely important in the differential diagnosis. Although usually rich in lymphocytes, tuberculous effusions in the early stages may contain a preponderance of granulocytes, which is also typical of nonspecific bacterial effusions. Increased eosinophils are of no great diagnostic value, but are very frequently observed in effusions of uncertain etiology and in chronic effusions.

Diagnostic testing for the infecting organisms that cause pleural effusion is indicated in empyemas with aerobic and anaerobic cultures and in suspected tuberculous, fungal, or parasitic effusions.

Medical Thoracoscopy

Medical thoracoscopy (pleuroscopy) is an invasive technique that may be used when other simpler methods fail. The technique is similar to chest tube insertion by means of a trocar, the difference being that, in addition, the pleural cavity can be visualized, and biopsies can be taken from all areas of the pleural cavity, including the chest wall, diaphragm, mediastinum, and lung (Fig. 63.3). The main advantage of medical thoracoscopy compared with surgical thoracoscopy, which is video-assisted thoracic surgery, is that the examination can be performed under local anesthetic and sedation after adequate premedication, and thus an anesthesiologist is not required. Furthermore, medical thoracoscopy is less expensive, because it may be safely performed with nondisposable instruments and in an appropriate endoscopy room. One technique favors a single entry using a 9-mm thoracoscope with a working channel for accessory instruments and optical biopsy forceps, and local anesthetic. Another technique favors two entry sites using a 7-mm trocar for the examination telescope and a 5-mm trocar for accessory instruments, including the biopsy forceps, under sedative or (general) anesthetic.

Medical thoracoscopy is safe if the contraindications are observed and if certain standard criteria are fulfilled. An obliterated pleural space is an absolute contraindication. Relative contraindications include bleeding disorders, hypoxemia, an unstable cardiovascular state, and persistent, uncontrollable cough. Complications, such as benign cardiac arrhythmias, low-grade hypertension, or hypoxemia, can be minimized by oxygen administration. The most serious, but rare, complication is severe hemorrhage caused by blood vessel trauma during the procedure. However, this, and lung perforation, can be avoided by using safe points of entry and a cautious biopsy technique. A serious complication of pneumothorax induction is air or gas embolism, which occurs very rarely (less than 0.1%). Several liters of fluid can be removed during thoracoscopy with little risk of pulmonary edema, because immediate equilibration of pressures is provided by direct entrance of air through the cannula into the pleural space.

Medical thoracoscopy is primarily a diagnostic procedure, but it can also be applied for therapeutic purposes. Pleural effusions are the leading indication for medical thoracoscopy, both for diagnosis and staging of diffuse malignant mesothelioma or lung cancer and for treatment by talc pleurodesis in malignant or other recurrent effusions, or occasionally in empyema. If the facilities are available, medical thoracoscopy is performed in pleural effusions when the etiology remains undetermined after thoracentesis and closed pleural biopsy. This applies to at least 20% to 25% of effusions. Medical thoracoscopy has a sensitivity of about 95% in malignant pleural effusions and of almost 100% in tuberculous pleurisy (Table 63.7). In addition, it allows a fast and more definite biopsy diagnosis, including a higher yield in tuberculosis cultures, and the determination of hormone receptors in some malignancies. Underlying malignancy or tuberculosis is excluded with high probability. Surgery, including surgical thoracoscopy, is not only much more invasive and expensive, but it also does not produce better results than medical thoracoscopy and is therefore reserved for carefully selected cases. In cases with effusions that are neither malignant nor tuberculous, thoracoscopy may give macroscopic clues to their etiology (e.g., in rheumatoid effusions, or effusions after pancreatitis, liver cirrhosis, extension from the abdominal cavity, or trauma, although in these entities the history, pleural fluid analysis, and other examinations are usually sufficient for diagnosis). When pleural effusion is secondary to the underlying primary lung diseases, such as pulmonary infarction or pneumonia, the diagnosis can frequently be made on macroscopic examination and be confirmed microscopically from lung biopsy specimens. Medical thoracoscopy is well suited to the diagnosis of benign, asbestos-related pleural effusions, which, by definition, are a diagnosis of exclusion. After thoracoscopy, the

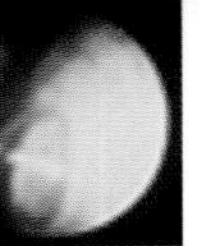

Table 63.7
Sensitivity of medical thoracoscopy in malignant and tuberculous pleural effusions: Intrapatient comparison with pleural fluid examination and closed needle biopsy

Biopsy procedure	Malignant; n = 208 (%)	Tuberculous; n = 100 (%)
Pleural effusion	62 (cytology)	28 (culture)
Closed needle biopsy	44	51
Effusion plus needle	74	61
Medical thoracoscopy	95	99
Effusion plus thoracoscopy	96	100
All materials	97	100

Table 63.8
Complete success rates of commonly used pleurodesis agents

Chemical agent	Total patients (n)	Successful (%)	Dose
Talc	165	93	2.5–10g
Corynebacterium parvum	169	76	3.5–14mg
Doxycycline	60	72	500mg (often multiple doses)
Tetracycline	359	67	500mg, up to 20mg/kg
Bleomycin	199	54	15–240 units

(Adapted with permission from Walker-Renard PB, Vaughn LM, Sahn SA: Chemical pleurodesis for malignant pleural effusions. Ann Intern Med 120:56–64, 1994.)

proportion of idiopathic pleural effusions usually falls below 10%.

Medical thoracoscopy can also be useful in the management of early empyema. In cases with multiple loculations, it is possible to open these spaces to remove the fibrinopurulent membranes by forceps and to create one single cavity, which can be drained and irrigated much more successfully. This treatment is carried out early in the course of empyema before the adhesions become too fibrous and adherent. Thus, if an indication for placement of a chest tube is present and if the facilities are available, medical thoracoscopy is performed at the time of chest tube insertion. In general, the technique of medical thoracoscopy is similar to that of chest tube placement, but allows the potential restoration of a single pleural cavity, and thus better local treatment. Thoracotomy or pleurectomy remains an option if these measures fail.

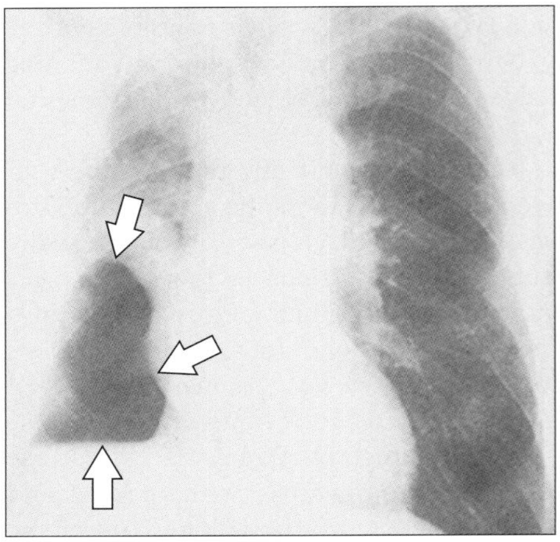

Figure 63.4 Radiograph of a patient with a trapped lung on the right side. The patient had an epidermoid bronchial carcinoma with massive pleural effusion on the right. Thoracoscopically, a trapped lower lobe was present, and the lung was unable to expand.

TREATMENT

Therapeutic aims in patients with pleural effusion are palliation of symptoms (pain, dyspnea), treatment of underlying diseases, prevention of pleural fibrosis with reduction of pulmonary function, and prevention of recurrences. The therapeutic approach depends on the availability of options for causal or only symptomatic treatment. Details are given in the descriptions of the specific disease entities.

Pleurodesis

The aim of pleurodesis is to achieve fusion between visceral and parietal pleural layers to prevent reaccumulation of fluid (or air) in the pleural space. Its main indications are malignant pleural effusions or, rarely, benign, recurrent pleural effusions when other treatments have failed (e.g., for liver cirrhosis, nephrotic syndrome, chylothorax, cardiac failure).

To achieve a complete pleural symphysis, several conditions need to be fulfilled. In particular, the fluid must be removed completely from the pleural space to keep the visceral and parietal pleural layers in close contact. This is achieved with application of suction through appropriate drainage, provided a trapped lung (Fig. 63.4) and bronchial obstruction have been ruled out. Furthermore, to achieve complete fusion, the pleural surface needs to be irritated, either mechanically with pleural abrasion or through application of a sclerosing agent. Various chemicals have been used in attempts to induce pleurodesis (Table 63.8). The most effective and also least expensive agent is talc, which has been used in most series via medical thoracoscopy. For thoracoscopic talc poudrage, general anesthetic or tracheal intubation is not necessary, but careful local anesthetic with parenteral analgesia is mandatory. If thoracoscopy is not available, many groups use a talc slurry (talcum powder suspended in variable amounts of saline), with a reported overall success rate of 91%, which is comparable to that of talc insufflation, but fewer studies have been carried out using talc slurry than talc poudrage. The advantage of thoracoscopic talc poudrage compared with slurry is probably the more even distribution over the whole pleural surface, which can be achieved under visual control. A randomized trial is currently underway in North America to evaluate these two methods. Complications related to talc are rare, provided a sterile and asbestos-free form is used. Severe pain is usually less frequent than with tetracycline, and mild fever (probably related to the inflammatory process) can be observed for 2 to 3 days after the procedure. A few major complications (acute respiratory distress syndrome, acute pneumonitis, and respiratory failure) have been reported, but these may be related to particle size or dosage (doses of talc larger than 5 g) or other factors related to its instillation. It is remarkable that several large series from Europe and from Israel did not observe these complications after thoracoscopic talc insufflation.

Tetracycline hydrochloride has a reportedly wide range of efficacy (45% to 77%). It requires heavy analgesia, but production of the parenteral form has been discontinued in the United States. Moreover, a relatively high rate of late recurrences has been reported. An alternative is doxycycline, but repeated dosages are frequently necessary. Minocycline has also been proposed as a replacement for tetracycline, but it may provoke vestibular symptoms when the dosages required for pleurodesis are used. Bleomycin is more effective in clinical practice than in experimental animal studies, but its main drawbacks are cost and systemic absorption, with the risk of significant toxicity. Quinacrine (mepacrine) is frequently used in Scandinavia. It may provoke serious toxicity of the central nervous system, probably because of the high dosages required. *Corynebacterium parvum* is almost exclusively used in some European centers, and the average effectiveness of this procedure has been reported to be 76%. However, in a randomized study with bleomycin, it was effective in only 32% of cases. The use of fibrin glue is controversial because of the cost and lack of evidence of experimental effectiveness. Moreover, it has been demonstrated that failure of pleurodesis in malignant effusions is associated with increased pleural fibrinolysis, which could lead to rapid destruction of the fibrin glue. Silver nitrate (20 mL, 0.5%) has been shown to be an effective agent for pleurodesis and is also inexpensive, widely available, and associated with tolerable side effects. More sophisticated agents, such as transforming growth factor-β, which may produce pleurodesis without inducing pleural inflammation, are not yet available (and would be quite expensive).

In conclusion, if the facilities for medical thoracoscopy are available, talc poudrage is performed. This technique has many advantages, not only for diagnostic purposes, but also because large amounts of fluid can be removed immediately and completely during medical thoracoscopy with little risk of pulmonary edema because of the immediate equilibration of pressures by direct entrance of air into the pleural space. Furthermore, the reexpansion potential of the lung can be evaluated directly. In addition, the extent of intrapleural tumor spread can be identified. Talc poudrage is the best conservative option for pleurodesis, possibly because of even distribution of the talc to all parts of the pleura. Surgical pleurectomy is indicated rarely for pleurodesis, although it is the procedure of choice in units that do not have thoracoscopy if the patient is fit and, in the case of a malignant effusion, likely to survive months or years (e.g., breast cancer). The insertion of a pleuroperitoneal shunt is another important alternative if reexpansion of a trapped lung is impossible because of tumor and the effusion reaccumulates rapidly. The fluid drains into the abdominal cavity with remarkably few complications.

SPECIFIC ENTITIES ASSOCIATED WITH PLEURAL EFFUSION

Oncotic and Hydrostatic Effusions

CARDIAC EFFUSIONS

Cardiac effusions are predominantly caused by left ventricular failure, which leads to increased formation of pleural fluid through the visceral pleura because of elevated pulmonary capillary pressure. Right ventricular failure, which interferes in particular with lymphatic drainage through the parietal pleura because of increased venous pressure, is rarely the sole cause. Dyspnea predominates and, on auscultation, additional rales are often present because of left ventricular failure; furthermore, signs of right ventricular failure can be found. More than half of effusions are bilateral, and 27% are right sided only and 15% left sided only. Usually, the heart is enlarged. Chest radiography may reveal so-called pseudotumor, predominantly in the right horizontal or the oblique fissure, which disappears with diuretic treatment (Fig. 63.5).

Diagnostic thoracentesis is indicated only if cardiac treatment is not successful. Pleural effusions caused by heart failure are usually transudates; however, the protein content may be increased as a result of diuretic treatment (so-called pseudoexudate). In the differential diagnosis, constrictive pericarditis, pulmonary infarction, and pneumonia must also be considered.

The treatment of these effusions is that for heart failure, and therapeutic thoracentesis to relieve dyspnea is rarely necessary.

Hepatic and Other Abdominal Effusions

Pleural effusions secondary to liver cirrhosis are usually caused by the passage of ascitic fluid into the pleural cavity or (less frequently) by decreased oncotic pressure caused by hypoalbuminemia. Hemorrhage from congested collateral veins is another, extremely rare, cause. The clinical picture is of cirrhosis and ascites, and the diagnosis is based on thoracentesis and paracentesis with demonstration of transudates.

Differential diagnosis must exclude all other diseases that may be associated with simultaneous ascites and pleural effu-

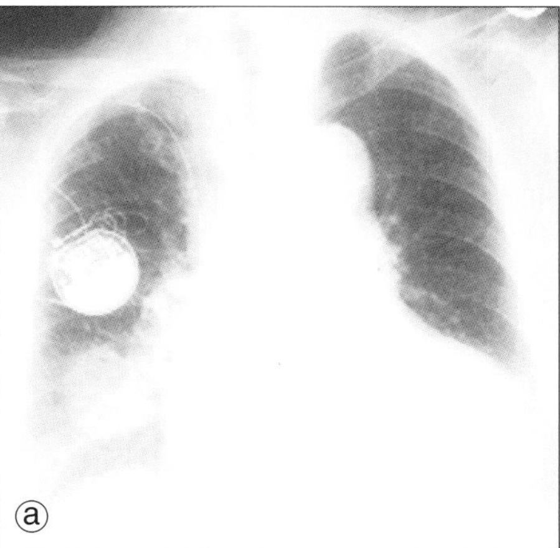

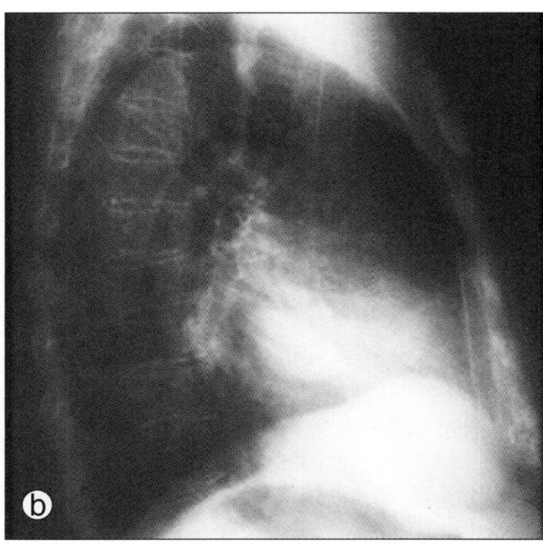

Figure 63.5 Pseudotumor of the lung. A, Posteroanterior and **B,** lateral chest radiographs showing a mass caused by fluid trapped in a fissure.

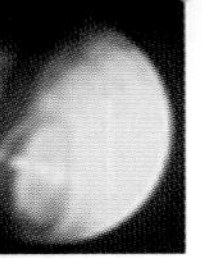

sion. In women, Meigs syndrome, tuberculosis, and pleural carcinomatosis secondary to cirrhosis-induced hepatic carcinoma must be ruled out. Other rare causes of pleural effusion are viral hepatitis and intrahepatic abscess. Pleural effusion may rarely occur during peritoneal dialysis or abdominal surgery. Subphrenic abscess is associated with pleural effusion in more than 50% of cases.

Approximately 20% of cases of acute pancreatitis develop pleural effusions, of which two thirds are left-sided, whereas one third is right-sided or bilateral. Crucial diagnostic factors are amylase values in the effusion persistently above those in serum. The effusion may be serosanguineous or bloody. In cases of persistent effusion, a pancreatic abscess or pseudocyst must be excluded. In the case of high amylase values, esophagus perforation must be excluded (salivary amylase).

Gallstone perforation into the pleura is extremely rare and results in a bilious effusion (cholohemothorax). Diaphragmatic hernia occurs most frequently on the left side after trauma and may resemble or, in cases of incarceration, even result in an effusion.

In the treatment of cirrhosis the goal is to remove ascites. Occasionally, therapeutic thoracentesis is indicated to relieve dyspnea. Pleurodesis may be attempted in therapy-resistant cases. In effusions from other abdominal causes, therapy is directed at the underlying disease.

Renal Effusions

Renal causes of pleural effusions are nephrotic syndrome, acute glomerulonephritis, uremia, and (rarely) hydronephrosis, which may result in retroperitoneal fluid collecting and causing a so-called urinothorax with increased creatinine values in the pleural fluid. The increased values are caused by retroperitoneal urinary leakage from trauma, retroperitoneal inflammatory or malignant processes, failed nephrostomy, or even kidney biopsy. The usually right-sided effusion observed in peritoneal dialysis corresponds chemically closely to dialysis fluid. Hemorrhagic effusion may develop during hemodialysis as a complication of anticoagulant treatment.

Infectious Pleurisy, Empyema

Infections of the pleura usually result in an effusion. However, initially only an inflammatory process that has no associated pleural fluid is possible (pleuritis sicca; dry pleurisy).

Pleuritis sicca is characterized by acute chest pain, in particular when breathing and coughing, which may radiate to the abdominal region or shoulder if the diaphragmatic pleura is involved, and thus make differential diagnosis more difficult. Clinical examination often reveals a circumscribed sensitivity to pressure or pain on percussion in the area of the diseased pleura. On auscultation, inspiratory and expiratory pleural rub of different intensity may be present. The affected side of the chest may be less active in breathing, whereas further symptoms depend on the underlying disease. Chest radiography often reveals an elevation of the hemidiaphragm and rib crowding because of efforts to limit respiratory movement and pain.

In the exudative stage, the pleuritic pain disappears and dyspnea may develop. The effusion may be parapneumonic without infection (uncomplicated) or culture positive (complicated). Empyema is apparent by the macroscopic appearance of thick and turbid fluid (pus). The differentiation is important because a complicated parapneumonic empyema usually requires tube thoracotomy.

Bacterial pneumonia is associated with an effusion in approximately 40% of cases, and is thus one of the main causes, although the frequency has been reduced by early antibiotic treatment. The spectrum of infecting organisms has also changed. In adults, anaerobic bacteria or a mixture of aerobic and anaerobic bacteria are found frequently. Among the aerobic bacteria, pneumococci predominate by more than 50%, and usually cause an uncomplicated effusion. Depending on the etiology of pneumonia, gram-negative bacteria may play a role, in particular *Klebsiella pneumoniae* and *Pseudomonas aeruginosa*. In *Legionella* spp. pneumonia, small pleural effusions occur in approximately 25% of patients. In children, pleurisy is mainly caused by staphylococci, pneumococci, or *Haemophilus influenzae*, whereas anaerobes are extremely rare.

The development of pleural effusion is correlated with the length of time the pneumonia remains untreated, but has little influence on symptoms. If fever persists for more than 48 hours after initiation of antibiotic treatment, a complicating effusion (empyema) is likely. In contrast, patients who suffer anaerobic infections tend to have subacute symptoms over several days and can develop an effusion at any time.

Depending on the clinical picture and size of the effusion (more than a 10-mm thickness on the decubitus radiograph), a diagnostic thoracentesis is performed to ascertain bacterial contamination before the start of antibiotic treatment. The appearance (turbid, thick, and putrid) and odor (foul in anaerobic infection) signal pleural empyema. Important parameters are Gram stain, protein content, glucose, LDH, amylase pH, and leukocyte count. An uncharacteristic appearance, glucose values lower than 2.22 mmol/L (40 mg/dL), and pH values less than 7.2 suggest bacterial infection.

The antibiotic treatment of pneumonia with and without accompanying effusion is the same. However, empyema, which occurs in approximately 10% of pneumonias, may require additional pleural drainage. Resolution may be further facilitated by the instillation of a fibrinolytic agent. In the American College of Chest Physician guidelines, a risk categorization for poor outcome in parapneumonic pleural effusions has been proposed, which is based on pleural anatomy, pleural fluid bacteriology and chemistry. For category 3, which is defined as an effusion occupying more than half the hemithorax, which may be loculated and in which the parietal pleura may be thickened, with a positive culture or Gram stain and a pleural pH less than 7.2, and for category 4, which is characterized by the additional finding of pus in the pleural cavity, it is proposed to use, besides drainage, either percutaneous intrapleural fibrinolytics or a surgical approach (video-assisted thoracic surgery [VATS] or thoracotomy).

Tuberculous Pleurisy

Tuberculous pleurisy mainly affects younger patients and is twice as frequent in males as in females. However, the trend is toward the development of tuberculous pleural effusions in older age groups. Tuberculous pleuritis usually occurs soon after the primary tuberculosis infection.

The onset of symptoms may be acute (severe pleuritic chest pain, nonproductive cough, high temperature, and dyspnea) or subacute (loss of appetite, weight loss, and night sweats). In many cases of acute onset, auscultation reveals only dry pleurisy, with the symptoms of effusion following later. Tuberculin skin tests are usually positive. The involvement of the lung parenchyma and lymph nodes found in 37% to 83% of patients is frequently not detected by radiography before the effusion disappears. The transition to an empyema may be insidious.

The old rule that any exudative pleural effusion of uncertain etiology and a positive tuberculin skin test must be considered and treated as tuberculous is no longer valid. Tuberculosis can be proved by granulomata in a pleural biopsy specimen and from biopsy specimen culture. The effusion is usually clear and serous and seldom turbid and serous. Predominantly, lymphocytes are present, but in the very early stages, neutrophils may be prominent. Low glucose values are found in only 20% to 50% of cases; however, the chances of a positive *Mycobacterium tuberculosis* culture from the exudate are higher in these cases. Molecular methods such as polymerase chain reaction (PCR) and others have in general—up to now—not achieved higher sensitivities, but may allow, if positive, a more rapid diagnosis. The most promising laboratory test is adenosine deaminase, which has a sensitivity of 73% to 100% and a specificity of 81% to 97%. High levels of adenosine deaminase can also be found in other diseases, such as empyema, malignant lymphoma, and collagen-vascular diseases. Its use is highly recommended in countries with a high prevalence of tuberculosis, but may not be very distinctive in low-prevalence countries. The most important diagnostic tools, closed pleural biopsy and thoracoscopy, permit a fast diagnosis based on histologic findings and also increase the chances of bacteriologic proof.

The treatment of tuberculosis is covered in Chapter 27.

Pleurisy Caused by Other Organisms

Small pleural effusions are found in approximately 20% of infections by viruses, *Mycoplasma* spp or *Rickettsia* spp, but do not necessarily affect the lungs. The diagnosis is based mainly on the clinical picture, and on serum titers, virus culture, or virus antibodies in the pleural fluid. The exudate is characterized by lymphocytes and initially also by neutrophils. Thoracoscopy can be a valuable tool to exclude tuberculosis. Virus infections are frequently accompanied by pericarditis. Differential diagnosis must exclude pleurodynia (Bornholm disease caused by coxsackievirus B_6).

Although unusual, pleural effusion may occur in all mycotic lung diseases. The effusion is usually lymphocytic, but may also be eosinophilic. *Aspergillus fumigatus* infection is occasionally found after artificial pneumothorax treatment for tuberculosis or postoperatively after lobectomy or pneumonectomy, especially in the presence of a bronchopleural fistula. Pleural effusion is observed in approximately 4% of blastomycoses and 20% of coccidioidomycosis. Cryptococci or other fungi are very rare causes of pleural effusion, but occur mainly in immunocompromised patients.

Parasitic pleural diseases are extremely rare and include amebiasis (perforation of a liver abscess into the pleural cavity), echinococcosis, paragonimosis, and the *Pneumocystis carinii* infection related to acquired immunodeficiency syndrome.

Malignant Pleural Effusions Other Than Mesothelioma

Malignant pleural diseases are mainly caused by hematogenic or lymphogenic metastases from extrathoracic primary tumors or by direct tumor spread from adjacent organs. However, increased asbestos exposure has also led to more cases of primary, diffuse, pleural mesothelioma. Tumor-related pleural effusions may have direct and indirect causes. Direct causes are increased capillary permeability caused by pleural metastases, obstruction of mesothelial capillaries, or disturbed reabsorption through insufficient lymphatic drainage caused by pleural metastases, involvement of mediastinal lymph nodes, or blockage of the thoracic duct. Indirect, paramalignant causes may be postobstructive pneumonia with pleuritis, atelectasis with decreased intrapleural pressure, pericardial involvement, vena cava syndrome, late effects of radiotherapy-induced pleuritis, pulmonary infarction, or hypoproteinemia. The distinction between these paramalignant and true malignant effusions is important when deciding on possible resection of bronchial carcinoma.

The majority of pleural tumors are not primary, but represent metastases or direct spread from adjacent organs. The most frequent primary tumors are bronchial (10% to 50%) and breast (20% to 50%) carcinoma, followed by lymphomas, ovarian cancer, and others. Any malignant tumor, except for primary brain tumors, may metastasize into the pleura. In 20% to 50% of cases, the primary tumor cannot be localized. Pleural effusion develops in 8% to 15% of all patients who have bronchial carcinoma, with a rate of up to 27% in small-cell carcinomas and up to 50% in metastasizing carcinomas. Malignant pleural effusion is found in approximately 7% of breast cancer patients at some point during their disease and is a first symptom of metastasis in 43% of these. Between 5% and 33% of malignant lymphomas are associated with pleural effusion. Malignant effusions can be huge, filling the entire hemithorax, and shift the mediastinum to the unaffected side. Lung involvement and mediastinal lymph node enlargement are best detected by computed tomography. Cytologic investigation of the effusion and closed pleural biopsy yield success rates between 20% and 84%, depending on the primary tumor. Carcinoembryonic antigen is characteristically elevated with adenocarcinoma, but is not diagnostic of cancer. The safest diagnostic procedure, with a sensitivity of 90% to 98%, is medical thoracoscopy, in which biopsy specimens may also be taken from the lung. Histologic evaluation of large biopsy specimens additionally provides information on undetected primary tumors. Cytologic evaluation of the effusion is more successful for breast cancer than for other tumors. Histologic specimens for hormone-receptor determination may be taken during thoracoscopy. Malignant lymphomas are frequently accompanied by chylous effusions, for which cytologic evaluation and blind needle biopsy have low diagnostic sensitivities. Chromosome analysis and thoracoscopy are clearly superior in this respect. Benign ovarian tumors (Meigs syndrome) and fibromyomas of the uterus are occasionally accompanied by pleural effusions. Pleural endometriosis is extremely rare.

With the diagnosis of a malignant pleural effusion, palliative therapy should be considered, necessitating evaluation of the patient's symptoms, general health and functional status, and expected survival. The major indication for treatment is relief

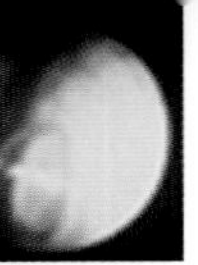

of dyspnea. Therapeutic thoracentesis or chest tube drainage combined with chemical pleurodesis or medical thoracoscopy with talc poudrage are the preferred options for local treatment. Rarely, major surgical procedures, such as pleurectomy or decortication, or insertion of a pleuroperitoneal shunt, are indicated.

In malignant pleural effusions resulting from tumors likely to respond to chemotherapy (e.g., small-cell lung cancer, breast cancer, lymphoma, and others), systemic treatment should be started and may be combined with therapeutic thoracentesis or pleurodesis, if necessary. In hormone-sensitive tumors (e.g., breast and prostate cancer), hormonal treatment may often be applied successfully. Intrapleural treatment with cytotoxic drugs and cytokines such as interleukin-2, interferon (IFN)-β, and IFN-γ, as well as gene therapy, may offer new therapeutic approaches, but are currently unproven.

Pleural Effusions of Other Etiologies

Effusions may be observed in connection with autoimmune diseases, especially rheumatoid arthritis and systemic lupus erythematosus. Sjögren's syndrome, dermatomyositis, scleroderma, mixed connective tissue disease, polyarteritis nodosa, and Wegener's granulomatosis are rarely associated with pleural effusion.

Pleural effusion is the most frequent thoracic manifestation of rheumatoid arthritis and occurs in 3% to 5% of cases, usually several years after the onset of arthritic symptoms. The effusion is characterized by very low glucose (less than 1.67 mmol/L [30 mg/dL]), low pH (less than 7.2), increased LDH (greater than 700 U/L), elevated rheumatoid factor, and low complement levels. The course of rheumatoid pleurisy may vary, and spontaneous resorption is frequently observed. Recurrences are rare, but systemic corticosteroid therapy may be necessary. A chronic, sterile, therapy-resistant, pleural empyema may develop.

In systemic lupus erythematosus, the pleura is affected in approximately 50% of patients who have pleuritic symptoms and in 20% to 30% of cases by a pleural effusion, and is bilateral in more than half the cases. The frequent cardiac involvement is reflected by cardiomegaly. Antinuclear antibodies are typically increased in the pleural effusion; lupus erythematosus cells are characteristic if present. The changes of glucose, pH, and LDH values are less pronounced than in rheumatoid pleurisy. Corticosteroid treatment results in a rapid, satisfactory response.

Effusions caused by pulmonary infarction are nonspecific and may be exudative or transudative. More than 70% are blood tinged, and approximately 20% are bloody.

Asbestos exposure may cause a bilateral, benign effusion that often recurs after spontaneous resorption. The exudate is sanguineous in over 30% of cases. The diagnosis must be based on at least 2 years of observation after exclusion of other causes.

Exudative effusions may also be associated with familial Mediterranean fever, yellow-nail syndrome, sarcoidosis, radiation pneumonia, long-term medication (especially with nitrofurantoin, bromocriptine, procarbazine, methotrexate, mitomycin, amiodarone, methysergide, or practolol [now withdrawn]), drug-induced lupus erythematosus, Dressler syndrome after myocardial infarction, cardiac surgery, and other diseases.

Approximately 15% of pleural effusions remain undiagnosed, particularly in young males, and eosinophils are frequently increased in these effusions, possibly because of virus infection. However, eosinophilia is also observed in other types of pleurisy.

Hemothorax

Hemothorax is mainly caused by trauma, pulmonary infarction, or tumors, and is characterized by hematocrit values more than 50% above those in serum.

Traumatic hemothorax usually results from penetrating or contused thoracic injuries that lead to rib fracture and damage of intercostal or pulmonary vessels. The treatment depends on the clinical picture and on the severity of hemorrhage, which is monitored by intrapleural drainage. Thoracotomy is indicated if blood volumes exceed 100 to 200 mL/h. The prognosis depends largely on the patient's other injuries.

Chylothorax

Chylothorax is characterized by the direct passage of chyle from the thoracic duct into the pleural cavity. The pleural fluid is usually milky. The triglyceride content needs to be determined because not all chylous effusions are milky in appearance and because some milky effusions may be pseudochylous. Triglyceride values greater than 1.24 mmol/L (110 mg/dL) indicate chylothorax, which may be excluded if the content is less than 0.56 mmol/L (50 mg/dL). Results between these values need to be tested further for chylomicrons. Pseudochylothorax, which must be excluded in differential diagnosis, is characterized by high cholesterol values and by the absence of chylomicrons.

The cause in more than 50% of cases is tumor, predominantly lymphomas. Approximately 25% are secondary to trauma to the thoracic duct, especially during surgery. Further rare causes are congenital defects, lymphangioleiomyomatosis, and others. The etiology remains unclear in 15% of patients.

The treatment of chylothorax depends on the cause. Irradiation of the mediastinum or systemic chemotherapy is indicated in cases of lymphoma or metastasizing tumor. Chylothorax after trauma is treated by pleural drainage. Pleurodesis may be successful in some patients. In individual cases, surgical ligature of the thoracic duct or pleurectomy may be indicated. A pleuroperitoneal shunt may be indicated if the effusions continue despite parenteral feeding followed by a fat-reduced diet with medium-chain fatty acids and surgery is not feasible. Surgical ligation of the thoracic duct as it enters the chest through the esophageal hiatus is usually accomplished via video-assisted thoracic surgery.

Pleural Thickening

The main cause of pleural thickening is fibrothorax, which may be secondary to empyema, tuberculous pleuritis, or hemothorax. It can cause dyspnea and the affected side of the chest may shrink and become distorted. The only possible treatment is decortication, which should be performed early whenever possible.

Asbestos exposure may lead to the formation of hyaline, sometimes sclerotic, pleural thickening (pleural plaques). This must be distinguished from other localized pleural thickenings, such as tumors, lipomas, lymphoma, and inflammatory changes.

The much less frequent diffuse pleural fibrosis after asbestos exposure is often preceded by an asbestos effusion.

PITFALLS AND CONTROVERSIES

The indication for thoracentesis in pleural effusions is sometimes arbitrary—its main purpose is to differentiate between transudate and exudate effusions and to rule out empyema. Cardiac effusions may become "exudative" after treatment. Another pitfall is the so-called pseudotumor (fluid in a fissure), which vanishes after cardiac failure treatment. In infectious pleural effusions, it is important to differentiate between uncomplicated and complicated parapneumonic effusions. The role of pH and glucose is helpful in this respect. In tuberculous pleurisy, the diagnosis may be made by biopsy of the pleura.

In malignant pleural effusions, the differentiation between true malignant and paramalignant effusions is essential, especially in lung cancer, where it changes the stage of the disease. Mesothelioma and adenocarcinoma of the pleura are often difficult to distinguish (see Chapter 64). Medical thoracoscopy plays an important role in the diagnostic approach to the evaluation of pleural effusions when the initial thoracocentesis is not diagnostic.

In the treatment of pleural effusions, the indications for drainage and fibrinolytic treatment in parapneumonic effusions are now better defined. A good option for pleurodesis is talc poudrage, which can only be applied adequately by medical thoracoscopy. The alternatives are talc slurry and other sclerosing substances. A pleuroperitoneal shunt or surgery is indicated in selected cases in which the lung fails to reexpand. The best timing for surgical decortication in empyema and fibrothorax is still unclear.

SUGGESTED READINGS

Antony VB, Loddenkemper R, Astoul P, Boutin C, Goldstraw P, Hott J, et al: Management of malignant pleural effusions (ATS/ERS statement). Am J Respir Crit Care Med 162:1987-2001, 2000.

Colice GL, Curtis A, Deslauriers J, Heffner J, Light R, Littenberg B et al (for the American College of Chest Physicians Parapneumonic Effusions Panel): Medical and surgical treatment of parapneumonic effusions: An evidence-based guideline (ACCP consensus statement). Chest 18:1158-1171, 2000.

Heffner JE, Sahn SA, Brown LK: Multilevel likelihood ratios for identifying exudative pleural effusions. Chest 121:1916-1920, 2002.

Light RW, Lee YCG (eds): Textbook of Pleural Diseases. London, Arnold, 2003.

Loddenkemper R: Thoracoscopy—state of the art. Eur Respir J 11:213-221, 1998.

Loddenkemper R, Antony VB (eds): Pleural diseases (European Respiratory Monograph 22). Sheffield, England, ERS Journals, 2002.

Rodriguez-Panadero F, Antony VB: Pleurodesis: State of the art. Eur Respir J 10:1648-1654, 1997.

CHAPTER 64 Malignant Pleural Mesothelioma

James R. Jett and Marie Christine Aubry

Malignant mesothelioma originates from the lining cells (mesothelium) of the pleural and peritoneal cavities as well as the pericardium and the tunica vaginalis. The tumor may be restricted to a small area or involve the lining cells in a multifocal or continuous manner. One of the first epidemiologic studies to link malignant mesothelioma and asbestos was reported by Wagner and colleagues using data collected in 1960 among South African mine workers. This association has been confirmed by subsequent studies. The delay between exposure and development of disease is generally 20 to 40 years.

EPIDEMIOLOGY, RISK FACTORS, AND PATHOLOGY

Epidemiology

There are an estimated 2000 to 3000 cases per year in the United States, and the annual deaths from mesothelioma peaked at 3060 cases in 2002 and will begin to diminish. The estimates for mesothelioma mortality in Britain are similar, with a peak in about the year 2020 of 2700 to 3300 deaths. A report estimating current trends was based on data from the Surveillance Epidemiology and End Results program for 1973-1992 in the United States. There was a virtually constant rate of mesothelioma for females and a consistently higher rate for males that increased during the study period. The growth rate for disease incidence among males was 14% for 1973-1974, which dropped to 0.4% for 1991-1992. There was no growth rate for females. The lifetime risk of mesothelioma peaks at 200 per 100,000 for men in the birth cohort for 1925-1929 and then decreases. The lifetime risk for females is essentially constant at 25 per 100,000. These data estimate the annual number of male mesothelioma cases will peak at 2300 and are consistent with other estimates. After the peak of mesothelioma rates in the United Sates and Western Europe, the numbers of cases will drop because of legislation that has decreased the exposure to asbestos in the workplace and ambient environment. That has not been the case in most developing countries.

Etiology and Risk Factors

Asbestos is naturally occurring fibrous silicate that is present in the soil. The main asbestos mineral groups are serpentine fibers (long and curly) or amphibole fibers (straight and rodlike). Chrysotile, the only serpentine fiber, accounts for 95% of the asbestos used commercially. The distinction between the serpentine group and amphibole group is important because the serpentine fiber shape is more easily cleared from the respiratory tract. Fibers with the greatest length-to-diameter ratios have been shown to be the most carcinogenic. Epidemiologic data suggest that the amphibole, crocidolite, is associated with the highest risk of malignant mesothelioma and that chrysotile has the lowest risk. Another amphibole, amosite, carries an immediate risk. Roggli and colleagues quantified the number of asbestos bodies in the lung tissue of:

1. Patients who died with asbestosis (fibrosis of the lung resulting from asbestos) without malignant pleural mesothelioma (MPM),
2. A group of patients with MPM without asbestosis, and
3. Fifty patients who died of other causes.

The lungs of patients with asbestosis without MPM had the highest fiber counts and those with MPM, but without asbestosis, had an intermediate number of fibers. Some of the MPM patients had fiber counts that overlapped with the 50 patients who died of other causes. It is, therefore, uncertain if there is a threshold of exposure to asbestos below which there is no risk of MPM, or if some individuals are predisposed to the disease because of inherited or acquired genetic mutations.

Asbestos, especially the amphiboles, is the main cause of MPM but does not account for all cases. Asbestos exposure is documented in only 50% to 70% of cases in most series. In asbestos-related cases, the disease is diagnosed 20 to 40 years after the first exposure, and the incidence of MPM increases with greater exposure. Among a population of asbestos insulation workers from North America, 8% of deaths were due to mesothelioma. There is also an increased incidence of MPM among the wives of asbestos workers. Presumably, this was due to asbestos that was brought home on the hair or clothing of the spouse exposed to asbestos. To avoid this risk, work practices have been put in place since 1972 that state that asbestos workers must shower and change their clothing before leaving work. Cases of MPM with no history of asbestos exposure are common. The most notable other causal factor is radiation exposure. In one series of five cases of MPM in patients with a prior history of treated Hodgkin's disease, the average interval from radiotherapy to diagnosis of MPM was 15 years. The role of simian virus (SV40) in the etiology of MPM is controversial. SV40 has been shown to cause malignant mesotheliomas in 100% of hamsters when it is injected intrapleurally. Using polymerase chain reaction analysis, SV40 DNA sequences have been documented in 60% to 80% of human MPM samples, except those from Finland, which have consistently tested negative. Some scientists believe that viral products of SV40 infection help to promote the genetic damage caused by asbestos by interference with tumor suppressor genes such as p53. Others have

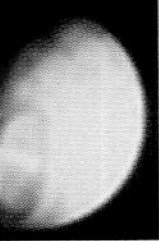

countered that technical factors produce false positive results that suggest SV40 infection is present when it is not. Further information is needed to resolve this debate.

Multiple genetic alterations are involved in the development of most malignancies. In one series of 20 malignant mesotheliomas that were karyotyped, more than 10 clonal chromosomal alterations were noted in all but one case. Although a specific chromosomal change is not shared by all MPM, the most common changes are losses or structural rearrangements of 1p, 3p, 6p, 9p, and 22q. Homozygous deletions of the tumor suppressor gene p16 on chromosome 9p 21-23 have been identified in 34 of 42 (85%) of malignant mesothelioma cell lines and in 5 of 23 (22%) of primary tumors. Losses involving 22q were documented in 14 of 24 mesothelioma cell lines in one study and 7 of 7 in another, whereas loss of 22q has been described less frequently in primary tumors (20%). Many of the chromosomal abnormalities in Finnish and US cases have been identical, but there are some distinct differences. It is uncertain if these discrepancies are related to the presence of SV40 in MPM cases from the United States and absence in Finnish cases. Several proteins are overexpressed in MPM including vascular endothelial growth factor and its receptors (VEGFR-1, -2, -3), which are potential targets for novel therapies.

Pathology

According to the World Health Organization classification of 1999, MPM are classified as epithelioid, sarcomatoid—which includes desmoplastic mesothelioma—biphasic, and others. Epithelioid MPM comprise tubules, acini, papillae, or solid sheets of atypical polygonal cells, whereas sarcomatoid MPM consist of a pure spindled pattern. Biphasic MPM represent a combination of epithelioid and sarcomatoid patterns, with at least 10% of each pattern. A large number of less common patterns have been described, including deciduoid, lymphohistiocytoid, small cell, clear cell, poorly differentiated, and MPM containing heterologous elements such as chondrosarcoma, osteosarcoma, and rhabdomyosarcoma.

This variety of patterns raises a wide differential diagnosis, which more commonly includes metastatic adenocarcinoma and sarcoma. Histochemistry and immunohistochemistry, using polyclonal or monoclonal antibodies, can be helpful in this distinction (Table 64.1). MPM often produce intracellular and extracellular hyaluronic acid (Alcian blue positive removed by hyaluronidase). Only very rarely have focal intracellular neutral mucin (diastase-resistant periodic acid Schiff [PAS-d] and mucicarmine [hyaluronidase-resistant]) been identified. In contrast, adenocarcinomas usually show intracellular neutral mucin. MPM should stain for cytokeratin (intermediate filament present in epithelial neoplasms) and are nearly always negative for glycoproteins such as polyclonal carcinoembryonic antigen (pCEA), Leu-M1 (CD15), B72.3, MOC-31, and Ber-EP4. Adenocarcinomas also stain positive for cytokeratin; however, they will usually immunoreact with at least one of the glycoproteins. The search for a specific MPM marker has been frustrating, and several markers have been studied, including cytokeratin 5/6, calretinin, thrombomodulin, and WT-1. Because the expression of the glycoproteins varies with the degree of differentiation and the site of origin of the adenocarcinoma, and no entirely specific and sensitive mesothelioma marker exists, a panel approach is therefore recommended to increase the sensitivity of the testing procedure. The most specific and sensitive markers for mesothe-

Table 64.1
Immunohistochemistry staining results for malignant pleural mesothelioma histologic types and adenocarcinomas

	MPM, epithelioid	MPM, sarcomatoid	Adenocarcinoma, pulmonary	Adenocarcinoma, NOS
Keratin (AE1/AE3/CAM5.2)	100%	95%	100%	100%
Keratin 5/6	92-100%	26%	0-19%	15%
pCEA	4%	0%	>80%	78%
Leu-M1	0-6%	10%	73-85%	70-75%
B72.3	2-14%	6%	35-84%	82%
Ber-EP4	0-26%	0%	93-100%	81-99%
MOC-31	0-9%	0%	97-100%	89-98%
TTF-1	0%	ND	76%	0%
Calretinin	83%	50%	18%	0-33%
Thrombomodulin	59-100%	31%	31-58%	21%
WT-1	72-95%	34%	0-31%	0-83%*

* Serous carcinomas of the ovary or peritoneum commonly express WT-1; however, nonpulmonary and nonovarian adenocarcinomas are rarely positive.

lioma are calretinin and cytokeratin 5/6 (sensitivity 90% and specificity 80% to 90%). However, calretinin is positive in 10% of lung adenocarcinoma, whereas cytokeratin 5/6 is expressed in squamous cell carcinomas of the lung and in 15% of nonpulmonary adenocarcinomas. Although less sensitive, calretinin has the advantage of not being expressed in squamous cell carcinoma; however, it is not as useful in the differential diagnosis of peritoneal malignant mesothelioma. The best negative markers, both sensitive and specific for MPM, are pCEA, B72.3, and MOC-31. Usually a panel of four markers (two positive and two negative) will be sufficient to make the diagnosis. These stains do not help to differentiate sarcomatoid mesothelioma from sarcoma. The most useful marker to help differentiate sarcomatoid mesothelioma from sarcoma is cytokeratin, positive in MPM and negative in most sarcomas. Calretinin is not valuable because it is not expressed in more than half of sarcomatoid MPM and has been described in sarcomas. Electron microscopic evidence of long, thin, bush surface microvilli has been found in epithelioid mesothelioma, whereas short blunt microvilli are seen in adenocarcinomas. A length-to-diameter ratio of microvilli greater than 15 should be considered strongly supportive of the diagnosis of epithelioid MPM. Electron microscopy is less effective in diagnosing poorly differentiated epithelioid mesothelioma or in distinguishing sarcomatous mesothelioma from sarcoma.

MPM also needs to be distinguished from benign mesothelial epithelial, and spindled (fibrous pleurisy/fibrosing pleuritis) proliferation. MPM shows complex growth pattern, dense cellularity in stroma, stromal invasion, absence of zonation, storiform pattern, increased cytologic atypia, lack of capillaries, and necrosis. Immunohistochemical studies play a small role in this differential diagnosis except keratin to demonstrate invasion.

Partly because of its rarity, the histologic diagnosis of MPM is difficult, and there is considerable variation in the diagnosis arrived at by different observers, which is as high as 50% in some studies. Pathology panels have been formed in a number of countries to address this problem and for purposes of referral. The members of the North American mesothelioma panel reached a consensus of 75% or more on 70% of the referral material sent to them. It is obvious, therefore, that even the experts do not always agree.

CLINICAL FEATURES

MPM is primarily a disease of adults and presents when the patient is in the fifth to seventh decade (median age 60 years). Those diagnosed between ages 20 to 40 years usually have a history of childhood exposure. Children have rarely been reported to develop this disease. Men account for 70% to 80% of cases. The most common presentations are dyspnea, nonpleuritic chest pain, or both. Table 64.2 outlines the initial presentation of 90 cases of MPM in our previously reported series and does not differ substantially from the results that have appeared in other publications. The physical examination is usually unremarkable except for dullness to percussion at the base of one lung caused by pleural effusion and tumor infiltrating the pleura. Palpable metastatic lymph nodes may occasionally be present, and digital clubbing is observed in less than 10% of cases.

Table 64.2
Initial symptoms in 90 cases of malignant pleural mesothelioma

Symptom	Number of cases	%
Pain	62	69
Nonpleuritic	56	–
Pleuritic	6	–
Shortness of breath	53	59
Fever, chills, or sweats	30	33
Weakness, fatigue, or malaise	30	33
Cough	24	27
Weight loss	22	24
Anorexia	10	11
Sensation of heaviness or fullness in chest	6	7
Hoarseness	3	3

Symptoms at initial presentation in 90 evaluable cases of malignant pleural mesothelioma. Modified with permission from Adams et al: Cancer 58:1540-1551, 1986.

The tumor originates mainly on the parietal pleura and progressively spreads to encase the lung surfaces and individual lobes by tracking along fissures. The tumor may reach several centimeters in thickness. It can penetrate into the chest wall, along needle tracts, infiltrate the diaphragm, invade mediastinal structures, and encase the heart and pericardium. Peritoneal involvement is found in about one third of cases at autopsy. Localized malignant mesotheliomas, sessile or pedunculated, can occur.

RADIOLOGIC FINDINGS

At the time of diagnosis, approximately 75% of patients will have a pleural effusion. In one series of 37 patients with pleural effusion, the effusion was greater than one third of the hemithorax in 19 (51%). The next most frequent abnormality on the chest radiograph is nodular thickening of the pleura and irregular thickening of the interlobar fissure (Fig. 64.1, A and B). A localized mass may be the only radiologic abnormality in 5% to 10% of individuals. Spontaneous pneumothorax has been reported occasionally. When the disease is more advanced, diffuse thickening of the pleura can produce decreased volume of the affected hemithorax (see Fig. 64.2). Calcified or noncalcified plaques may also be identified. A prospective series followed more than 1500 Swedish men with pleural plaques for 16,000 plus person-years and observed a risk of MPM of 1 in 1700 per year.

Computed Tomography

Computed tomography (CT) provides more information on the extent of disease. CT examination of 50 patients with MPM showed pleural thickening that varied in extent and nodularity in 92% of patients (Figs. 64.2 and 64.3). Thickening of the interlobar fissure was observed in 86% of cases and pleural effusion in 74%. Calcified pleural plaques were seen in 10 patients (20%) and were assimilated into the mesothelioma in six cases. There was contraction of the involved hemithorax in 42% of patients,

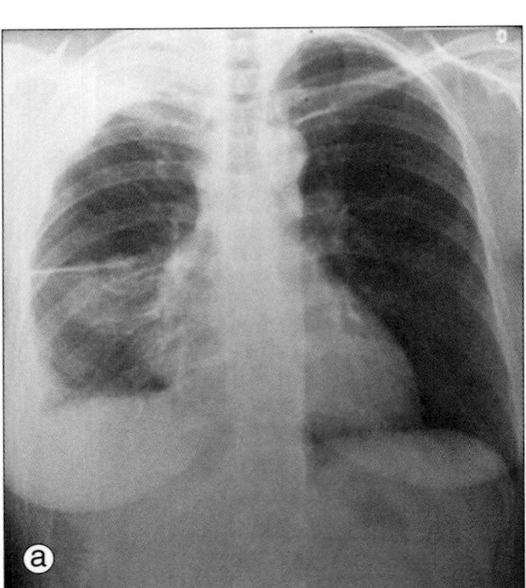

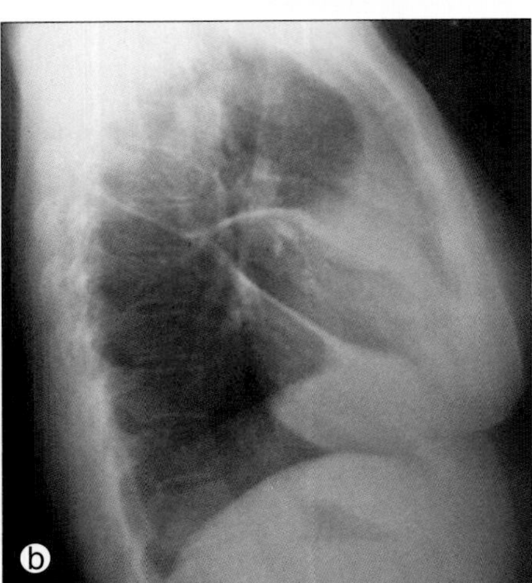

Figure 64.1 **A,** Posteroanterior and **B,** lateral chest radiographs of a patient with malignant pleural mesothelioma. Thickening of the pleura of the major fissure is most clearly visible in the lateral view.

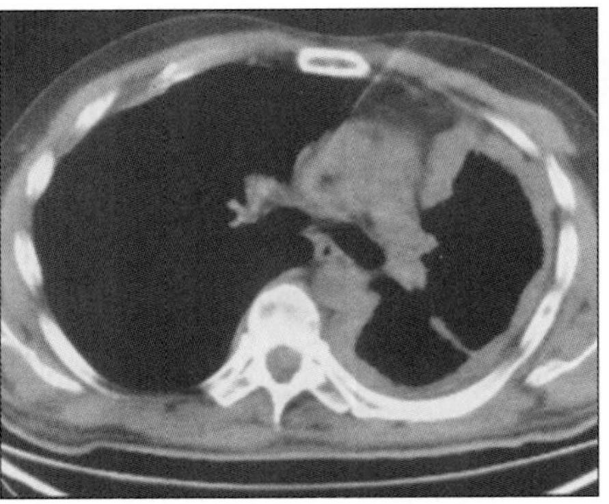

Figure 64.2 Computed tomography scan of chest of patient with malignant pleural mesothelioma. Thickening of the entire circumferential pleura and invasion of the fissure can be seen on this cut. Note the associated loss of volume of the involved hemithorax.

but a mediastinal shift was present in only seven (14%). Extension of the tumor into the chest wall and abdomen, as well as involvement of the mediastinal pleura, pericardium, and lymph nodes, was documented in some cases. Magnetic resonance imaging of the thorax with the use of multidimensional planes is superior to CT scans for evaluating the relationship of the tumor to the great vessels if surgery is being considered. In one large, prospective study of 65 patients comparing CT and magnetic resonance imaging, the latter was significantly better at demonstrating invasion of the diaphragm and chest wall.

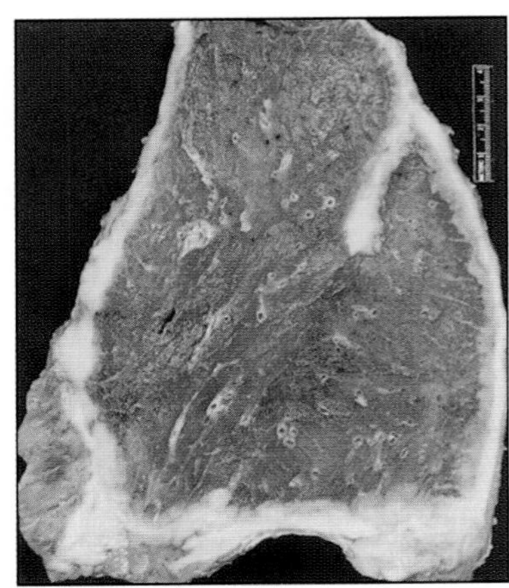

Figure 64.3 Pleural thickening. A cross section of a lung removed at surgery by pleuropneumonectomy. This specimen was taken from the patient whose computed tomography scan is shown in

Staging

The literature contains at least six different staging systems for MPM. The lack of a universal system has hindered comparison of reports. The International Mesothelioma Interest Group proposed a modified staging system (Tables 64.3 and 64.4) that reconciles and updates previous systems. In 2002, this system was adopted by the International Union Against Cancer and the American Joint Committee on Cancer. These staging categories have been validated on a series of 131 patients from Memorial Sloan-Kettering Cancer Center, and 48 patients from a National Cancer Institute series. Most patients have an advanced stage at diagnosis. In the National Cancer Institute series, 4 patients had stage I, 4 had stage II, 38 had stage III, and 2 had stage IV disease. In the surgical staging series of 131 patients from Memorial Sloan-Kettering, 12% were stage I, 15% stage II, 44% stage III, and 29% stage IV. In most reported series, very few patients have stage IA or IB disease at diagnosis.

DIAGNOSIS

The initial diagnosis can be difficult and is frequently delayed. Pleural fluid cytology is positive for malignant cells in one third of cases, but it is uncommon for the pathologist to make a definitive diagnosis of MPM on cytology alone. Percutaneous or closed needle biopsy of the pleura yields adequate tissue for diagnosis in approximately one third of cases. Thoracoscopy with direct visualization of the pleura yields diagnostic tissue in more than 90% of samples. Before thoracoscopy, open pleural biopsy had been the gold standard for diagnosis, but even this method is not absolutely definitive in all cases because of problems encountered both with sampling and with pathologic interpretations. The typical visual appearance at thoracoscopy or open biopsy is that of multiple pleural nodules or masses. The nodules are usually larger and more numerous on the parietal pleura, but frequently involve the visceral pleura. A dominant mass surrounded by numerous scattered smaller nodules may occur. Pleural effusion with pleural thickening may be the only finding, and pleural symphysis with obliteration of the pleural space is encountered occasionally.

Because initial pleural fluid examination is often inconclusive, cytology, in general, is an unsatisfactory technique for diagnosing this type of tumor. Some physicians may accept a diagnosis on the basis of clinical presentation, exposure history, and typical chest radiographs and CT scans, but a tissue diagnosis is strongly

Table 64.3
Tumor - nodes - metastasis (TNM) staging system for malignant pleural mesothelioma

Primary tumor (T)	
TX	Primary tumor cannot be assessed
T0	No evidence of primary tumor
T1	Tumor involves ipsilateral parietal pleura, with or without focal involvement of visceral pleura
T1a	Tumor involves ipsilateral parietal (mediastinal, diaphragmatic) pleura. No involvement of visceral pleura
T2	Tumor involves any of the ipsilateral pleural surfaces with at least one of the following: • confluent visceral pleural tumor (including fissure) • invasion of diaphragmatic muscle • invasion of lung parenchyma
T3*	Tumor involves any of the ipsilateral pleural surfaces with at least one of the following: • invasion of the endothoracic fascia • invasion into mediastinal fat • solitary focus of tumor invading the soft tissues of the chest wall • non-transmural involvement of the pericardium
T4**	Tumor involves any of the ipsilateral pleural surfaces with at least one of the following: • diffuse or multifocal invasion of soft tissues of the chest wall • any involvement of the rib • invasion through the diphragm to the peritoneum • invasion of any mediastinal organ(s) • direct extension to the contralateral pleura • invasion into the spine • extension to the internal surface of the pericardium • pericardial effusion with positive cytology • invasion of the myocardium • invasion of the brachial plexus
Regional lymph nodes (N)	
NX	Regional lymph nodes cannot be assessed
N0	No regional lymph node metastases
N1	Metastases in the ipsilateral bronchopulmonary and/or hilar nodes
N2	Metastases in the subcarinal lymph node(s) and/or the ipsilateral internal mammary or mediastinal nodes
N3	Metastases in the contralateral mediastinal, internal mammary, or hilar lymph node(s) and/or the ipsilateral or contralateral supra-clavicular or scale lymph node(s)
Distant metastases (M)	
MX	Distant metastases cannot be assessed
M0	No distant metastases
M1	Distant metastases

* Describes locally advanced, but potentially resectable tumor.
** Describes locally advanced, technically unresectable tumor.

Tumor-nodes-metastasis staging system for malignant pleural mesothelioma. This system was developed by the International Mesothelioma Interest Group to reconcile and update previous systems. In 2002, it was accepted by the International Union Against Cancer and the American Joint Committee on Cancer.

advised for almost all cases. Closed pleural biopsy with an Abrams needle is technically difficult because the pleura is often very thick and fibrous. In general, a core of tissue is required. Physicians may be reluctant to insert a large needle through the chest wall because of the high risk of tumor growing out along the tract formed, thus producing a painful mass. This can be prevented by prophylactic radiotherapy (see the following section). CT-guided core biopsies give a fair diagnostic yield, and thoracoscopy is the procedure of choice when a tissue diagnosis is in doubt.

Table 64.4
Stage grouping for diffuse MPM

Stage I	T1	N0	M0
Stage IA	T1a	N0	M0
Stage IB	T1b	N0	M0
Stage II	T2	N0	M0
Stage III	T1,T2	N1	M0
	T1,T2	N2	M0
	T3	N0, N1, N2	M0
Stage IV	T4	Any N	M0
	Any T	N3	M0
	Any T	Any N	M1

Staging system for diffuse malignant pleural mesothelioma. Stage groupings are based on tumor-nodes-metastasis categories as defined in Table 64.3.

TREATMENT

The beneficial effects of treatment for MPM of the pleura are controversial. Perhaps the major area of debate about treatment is the role of surgery. It is estimated that 50% or fewer of all patients with MPM are potentially resectable. Two large retrospective series concluded that patients undergoing either decortication/pleurectomy or extrapleuropneumonectomy did not show improved survival compared with other treatments or with simply the best supportive care. However, a number of recent reports have suggested that surgery may have an effect on survival. Sugarbaker and associates performed pleuropneumonectomy in 183 selected patients who were then treated with adjuvant chemotherapy and ipsilateral hemithoracic irradiation. The overall median survival was 19 months with 38% alive at 2 years and 15% at 5 years. Epithelioid histology was associated with a better survival (median 26 months, 21% 5-year survival). In those patients with mixed or sarcomatoid histology, only 2 of 72 patients were alive at 3 years. Additionally, none of the patients with N2 or N3 lymph node involvement survived for 3 years. In another surgical series from Memorial Sloan-Kettering Cancer Center, 88 patients were operated with extrapleuropneumonectomies (n=62), pleurectomy/decortications (n=5), or exploration only (n=21). Adjuvant hemithoracic radiotherapy of 54 Gy was given to those undergoing resection. The median survival was 17 months with a 27% 3-year survival. In both of these series, the patients with stage I/II disease had a much better survival (median 24 to 33 months) than did patients with stage III disease (median 10 months). The promising results may reflect the treating physician's ability to select the best patients for operation. Some surgeons advise only pleurectomy/decortication or talc pleurodesis to control the malignant effusions. Ideally, when surgery is part of the treatment, it should be performed in the setting of a controlled clinical trial. This would be the most effective way of advancing our knowledge on the usefulness of surgery as part of the therapeutic approach.

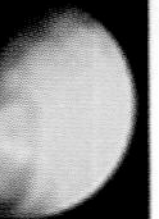

Radiotherapy

Radiotherapy causes occasional regression of disease, but does not alter survival compared with supportive care alone. If radiotherapy is to be used as a cure, treatment of the entire hemithorax and ipsilateral pleura is necessary. Treating such a large tumor volume carries with it a significant risk to underlying normal structures. However, short courses of 20 Gy in 5 fractions or 30 Gy in 10 fractions are effective for palliating symptoms. As mentioned previously, radiation can prevent seeding of biopsy tracts and surgical wounds. Boutin and colleagues gave 7 Gy/fraction for 3 consecutive days to 20 patients and observed no local recurrences after needle biopsy, chest tube, or thoracoscopy. In contrast, 8 of 20 patients not treated developed entry tract metastasis. Radiotherapy may be more effective when treating microscopic diseases compared with gross disease. In a recent series from Memorial Sloan-Kettering Cancer Center, 57 patients received hemithoracic radiotherapy (54 Gy) after extrapleuropneumonectomy. Locoregional recurrences occurred in 7 patients and distant metastases only occurred in 30 patients. This suggests that hemithoracic radiation after extrapleural pneumonectomy decreases the rate of local recurrences.

Chemotherapy

There is no single drug or combination chemotherapy regimen that would be considered standard therapy for MPM. No drug has consistently produced a partial response (50% or greater shrinkage in tumor mass) in more than 20% of cases and complete clinical remissions are rare. Agents that produce partial response rates in 10% to 20% of patients include:

- Doxorubicin
- Epirubicin
- Mitomycin
- Cyclophosphamide
- Ifosfamide
- Cisplatin
- Carboplatin
- Vinorelbine
- Pemetrexed

Combination chemotherapy has not demonstrated consistently greater response rate than single agents. In one trial of single-agent intrapleural recombinant gamma-interferon, twice a week for 8 weeks, a response rate of 20% was observed. This, however, included eight complete responses. The response rate for stage I patients was 45%, but no other group has been able to reproduce these encouraging results. Very few centers see patients presenting with the early-stage disease (stage IA) identified in this particular trial. A recent phase III international trial randomized patients with unresectable MPM to chemotherapy with cisplatin and pemetrexed versus cisplatin alone. The response rate was twice as high with the combination treatment (41% versus 17%) and survival was significantly better (median survival time 12.1 versus 9.3 months). This is only the second prospective phase III trial conducted with MPM, but we can anticipate more. Whenever possible, patients with MPM should be enrolled in prospective clinical trials. Currently, there is a Phase III trial in The United Kingdom comparing chemotherapy with best supportive care only.

Control of Pleural Effusion

In many patients, no specific therapy to reduce the tumor mass will be offered. Patients frequently present with large pleural effusions causing troublesome breathlessness. Although pleural effusions can be aspirated repeatedly, this may fail to relieve symptoms for long. With repeated thoracentesis, the pleural fluid may undergo loculation and be difficult to drain. If a clinically significant pleural effusion is present, it may be most effective to treat the patient initially with either thoracoscopy and talc pleurodesis or chest tube drainage and talc pleurodesis.

One risk of thoracoscopy or tube drainage is that on emptying the pleural cavity, the lung may be encased by tumor and not fully expand to obliterate the pleural space, thus making pleurodesis impossible. Should the space obliterate, then intrapleural talc may be instilled. However, when the space persists, drainage of pleural fluid into the peritoneal cavity via a pleuroperitoneal (i.e., Denver) shunt or an indwelling pleural catheter with external drainage can be extremely effective for many months. Control of the pleural fluid, if effective, is likely to bring significant symptom relief. The primary tumor does not usually metastasize outside the involved hemithorax until later in the clinical course and local symptoms are the immediate priority.

Prognosis and Survival

The enumeration of prognostic factors has varied in different series. Histologic type has been identified as important in numerous reports, with epithelioid histology patients surviving longer than others. The Cancer and Leukemia Group B and the European Organization for Research and Treatment of Cancer each performed multivariate analyses of large numbers of patients enrolled in treatment trials for MPM through their cooperative groups. The following are the poor prognostic factors identified in one or both of these reports:

- Nonepithelioid histology
- Poor performance score
- Chest pain
- Age older than 75 years
- Male gender
- White blood cell count 8.3×10^9/L or greater
- Platelets greater than 400,000 μL
- LDH greater than 500 IU/L

The median survival time varies from 8 to 12 months and less than 20% of patients survive beyond 2 years. The majority of those who survive for 2 years have epithelioid histology. Patients

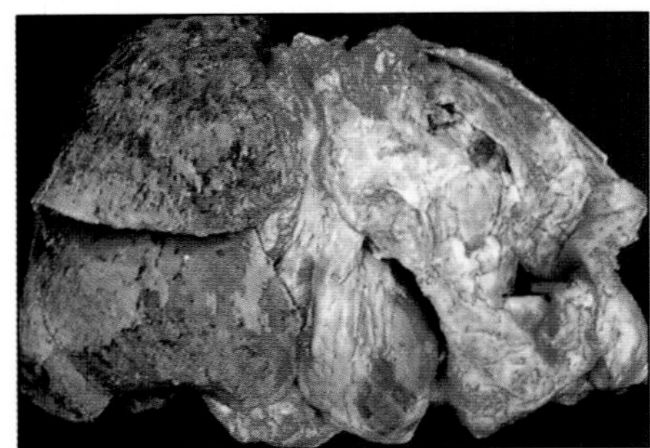

Fig. 64.2.
Figure 64.4 An intact heart and lung block from necropsy. This demonstrates encasement of one lung and heart by tumor. This 68-year-old male garage worker's noninvolved lung appears black secondary to inhaled

Table 64.5
Necropsy findings in 92 patients with malignant pleural mesothelioma

Site	Number of patients	%
Local extension		
Mediastinum	58	63
Pericardium	45	49
Diaphragm	60	65
Lung	51	55
Opposite pleura	34	37
Chest wall	32	35
Peritoneum	36	39
Lymph node involvement		
Mediastinum	37	40
Retroperitoneum	19	21
Metastases	45	49
Liver	28	30
Contralateral lung	15	
Adrenal(s)	11	
Kidney(s)	12	
Bone	9	
Pancreas	5	
Brain	3	
Spleen	4	
Skin	4	
Thyroid	4	

Necropsy findings in 92 patients with malignant pleural mesothelioma. Other sites of metastasis occurred in two or fewer cases. Modified with permission from Ruffie et al: J Clin Oncol 7:1157-1168, 1989.

generally die of respiratory failure because of local extension of the disease. Some deaths are caused by pericardial constriction, congestive heart failure or cardiac arrhythmias (Fig. 64.4). Ascites and small-bowel obstruction can occur because of intraabdominal extension of the tumor. The sites of tumor involvement in a necropsy series of 92 patients are listed in Table 64.5.

PITFALLS AND CONTROVERSIES

It is important that MPM be considered part of the differential diagnosis of any new pleural effusion, especially in males, and more particularly, in those with a significant history of occupational exposure to asbestos. To determine exposure, a careful occupational history is required, including information about occupations and exposures that date back 30 to 40 years to the individual's initial employment or hobbies. Exposure history should include questions about occupations during military service. In 30% to 50% of cases, there may be no significant history of asbestos exposure.

Cytologic evaluation of pleural effusion is notoriously insensitive. A negative cytology or closed pleural biopsy should not, therefore, dissuade the physician from pursuing a definitive diagnosis. If the etiology of the pleural effusion is still uncertain after adequate attempts at closed biopsy, then thoracoscopy should be considered as a further means of investigation to obtain a definitive histologic diagnosis.

Occasionally, the pleural fluid cytology will yield malignant cells without further definition. In such cases, additional tissue should be obtained by closed biopsy or thoracoscopy. If the physician is obviously dealing with a malignancy at the time of thoracoscopy, then it may be beneficial to proceed with talc pleurodesis after obtaining the appropriate biopsies. The difficulties with definitive histologic diagnosis of MPM were described previously. It is important to distinguish metastatic disease to the pleura from MPM. It is especially important to rule out cancers of other sites that have a good chance of responding to therapy, such as carcinoma of the breast, ovary, or prostate or a germ cell tumor.

Treatment of MPM is controversial. No single modality or combination of therapies promises prolonged survival. Some recent reports suggest that surgery may benefit patients with an early stage of disease, especially if they have epithelioid histology and if lymph node metastases (N2 or N3) are absent. Chemotherapy has not been shown to be superior to supportive care alone, although some agents offer a 10% to 20% chance of partial response. New agents or modalities of therapy are needed to combat this recalcitrant disease. Progress in discovering these new agents or modalities will be made only if we treat MPM patients in controlled clinical trials. Investigators have recently demonstrated the ability to conduct randomized phase III trials with national or international cooperation to answer important treatment questions.

SUGGESTED READINGS

American Joint Committee on Cancer: Cancer Staging Manual, 6th ed. New York, Springer-Verlag, 2002.

Heelan RT, Rusch VW, Begg CB et al: Staging of malignant pleural mesothelioma: Comparison of CT and MR imaging. Am J Roentgenol 172:1039-1046, 1999.

Herndon II JE, Green MR, Chahinian AP et al: Factors predictive of survival among 337 patients with mesothelioma treated between 1984 and 1994 by the cancer and leukemia group B. Chest 113:723-731, 1998.

Ordonez NG: Immunohistochemical diagnosis of epithelioid mesothelioma: A critical review of old markers and new markers. Human Pathol 33:953-967, 2002.

Peto J, Hodgson J, Matthews F et al: Continuing increase in mesothelioma mortality in Britain. Lancet 345:535-539, 1995.

Price B: Analysis of current trends in United States mesothelioma incidence. Am J Epidemiol 145:211-218, 1997.

Rusch VW, Rosenzweig K, Venkatraman E et al: A phase II trial of surgical resection and adjuvant high-dose hemithoracic radiation for malignant pleural mesothelioma. J Thorac Cardiovasc Surg 122:788-795, 2001.

British Thoracic Society Standards of Care Committee: Statement on malignant mesothelioma in the United Kingdom. Thorax 56:250-265, 2001.

Sugarbaker DJ, Flores RM, Jaklitsch MT et al: Resection margins, extrapleural node status, and cell type determine postoperative long-term survival in trimodality therapy of malignant pleural mesothelioma: Results in 183 patients. J Thorac Caradiovasc Surg 117:54-65, 1999.

Vogelzang NJ: Emerging insights into the biology and treatment of malignant mesothelioma. Semin Oncol 29(6 Suppl 18):35-42, 2002.

World Health Organization: International Histological Classification of Tumors. In Travis WD, Colby TB, Corrin B, Shimosah Y, Brambella E (eds): Histological Typing of Lung and Pleural Tumors, 3rd ed. Berlin, Springer-Verlag, 1999, pp 51-54.

CHAPTER 65 Acute Respiratory Distress Syndrome

Luciano Gattinoni, Paolo Pelosi, Luca Brazzi, and Franco Valenza

Since its first description more than 25 years ago, the acute respiratory distress syndrome (ARDS; originally known as *adult respiratory distress syndrome*) has received more attention than any single entity in critical care medicine. The syndrome consists of an acute, severe alteration in lung structure and function characterized by hypoxemia, low respiratory system compliance, low functional residual capacity, and diffuse radiographic infiltrates, along with increased lung endothelial and alveolar epithelial permeability.

EPIDEMIOLOGY, RISK FACTORS, AND PATHOPHYSIOLOGY

Epidemiology

As a consequence of the different definitions of ARDS (see later), it has always been difficult to estimate the true incidence of this condition. The 1972 report of the National Heart, Lung, and Blood Institute of the National Institutes of Health (NIH) suggested that approximately 150,000 cases of ARDS occurred per year in the United States, which represents an incidence of 60/100,000 population per year. This figure has been challenged in a number of reports (Table 65.1), all of which give an incidence that is an order of magnitude lower than the NIH estimates. Two points must be stressed, however. First, different ARDS definitions play an obvious role when its incidence is estimated. Not surprisingly, defining ARDS according to more or less strict criteria results in incidence estimates that differ by more than 100%. Second, some studies suffer from substantial methodologic problems. Moreover, it has been recently reported that more or less selective criteria to recruit the intensive care units in which the incidence is measured may greatly affect the results.

RISK FACTORS

The results of a systematic overview of the incidence and risk factors for ARDS (Table 65.1) found that the strongest evidence to support a cause-and-effect relationship between ARDS and a risk factor was identified for sepsis, trauma, multiple transfusions, aspiration of gastric contents, pulmonary contusion, pneumonia, and smoke inhalation. The weakest evidence was identified for disseminated intravascular coagulation, fat embolism, and cardiopulmonary bypass.

Pathophysiology

Whenever an insult is applied to the lung, a host response is triggered that is characterized by a close interplay of cells and humoral factors and results in lung inflammation (Fig. 65.1). Epithelium and endothelium are both involved, although injury to one or the other barrier may predominate. It is useful to consider two pathways—the effect of the insult directly on the lung (direct insult), and pulmonary lesions that result from an acute systemic inflammatory response (indirect insult). This distinction may be important because the pathway affected may govern the expression of the pulmonary abnormalities.

DIRECT INSULT

Lung injury has been reproduced in animal models by direct application of the insult to the alveoli (as with intratracheal instillation of endotoxin or live bacteria, complement, tumor necrosis factor, and the like). Pulmonary epithelium was thus subjected to the initial injury, with activation of alveolar macrophages. These, in turn, activate the inflammatory network, which leads to the pulmonary inflammation. The prevalent damage after the direct insult is intra-alveolar, with alveolar filling by edema, fibrin, collagen, neutrophilic aggregates, or blood, and often described as *pulmonary consolidation*.

INDIRECT INSULT

Pulmonary lesions may originate indirectly through mediators released from extrapulmonary foci into the blood, as during peritonitis, pancreatitis, and various abdominal diseases. The primary target in such cases is the pulmonary endothelial cell. The activation of the inflammatory network results in increased permeability of the endothelial barrier and recruitment of monocytes, polymorphonuclear neutrophil leukocytes, platelets, and other cells. Consequently, the prevalent damage is represented by microvessel congestion and interstitial edema, whereas intra-alveolar spaces are relatively spared.

It is likely that direct and indirect insults can coexist. This may occur, for example, in patients who have pneumonia when one lung is initially directly affected, and the other is indirectly injured hours or days later as the inflammation spreads by means of loss of compartmentalization (indirect insult).

It is important to differentiate between direct and indirect pathophysiologic pathways because the underlying pathologic process (i.e., predominantly consolidation versus interstitial edema and collapse) seems different in the two conditions, at least during the early phases, as recently confirmed in both pathologic and imaging studies. This may have an important effect on the approach to treatment. Figure 65.2, taken from the first report of the effect of positive end-expiratory pressure (PEEP) in ARDS studied using computed tomography (CT) scans, clearly emphasizes the point. Application of PEEP overdistended previously inflated lung regions in one patient,

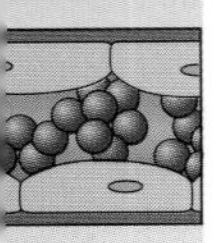

and resulted in a remarkable recruitment in the second. Intuitively, the different responses of the respiratory system to the same perturbation suggest different underlying conditions.

MODELS OF ACUTE RESPIRATORY DISTRESS SYNDROME

Before the introduction of CT scan technology, imaging of ARDS was limited to chest radiographs, which showed (and this was part of the ARDS definition) a widespread and bilateral appearance of "pulmonary infiltrates." Thus, ARDS was considered to be a homogeneous alteration of the lung parenchyma, with reduced gas content, characterized by an abnormal stiffness. The CT scan completely changed this model because it has been consistently observed that the densities, which reflect the

Table 65.1
Incidence and mortality of acute respiratory distress syndrome

Author	Patient number	Incidence (100,000 population/year)	Mortality rate (%)
National Heart, Lung, and Blood Institute	–	60	–
Fowler	88	5.2	65
Webster	139	4.5	38
Evans	62	25	60
Villar	30/74	1.5/3.5	70/50
Thomsen	110/83	8.3/4.8	–
Lewandowski	17	3	58.8

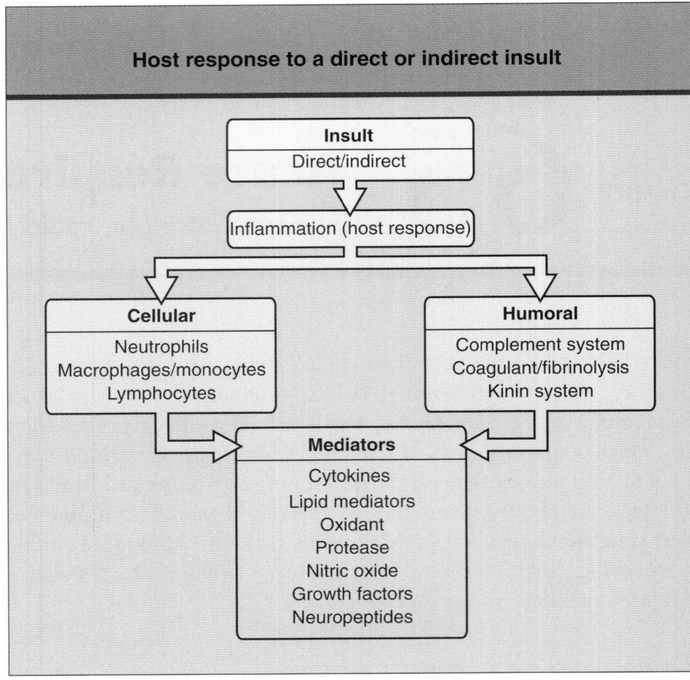

Figure 65.1 Host response to a direct or indirect insult.

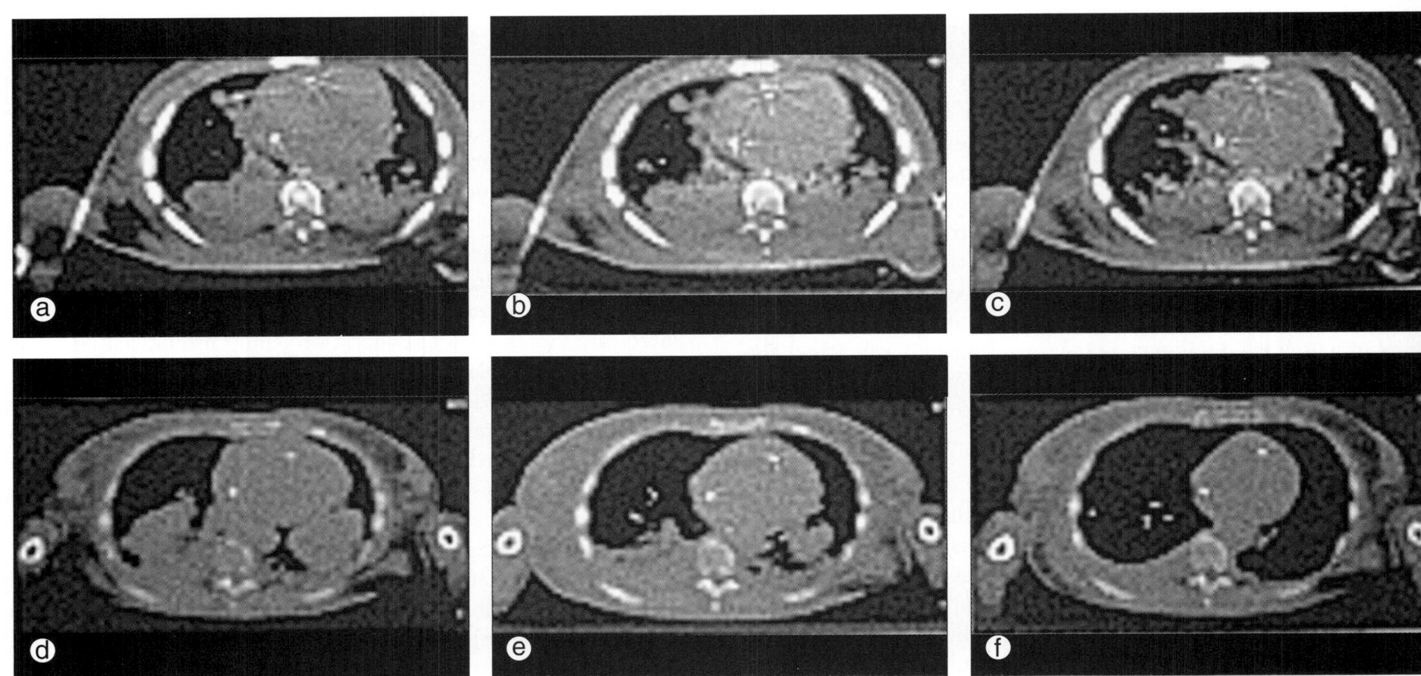

Figure 65.2 Computed tomography scans of the caudal lung at various positive end-expiratory pressures (PEEP). **A–C,** Acute respiratory distress syndrome (ARDS) from bacterial pneumonia (direct insult). No changes in density (i.e., air space collapse or parenchymal consolidation) and arterial partial pressure of oxygen (PaO_2) are observed with increasing levels of PEEP. **A,** At 5 cm H_2O, PaO_2 is 12.9 kPa (97 mm Hg), density 59%. **B,** At 10 cm H_2O, PaO_2 is 13.7 kPa (103 mm Hg), density 56%. **C,** At 15 cm H_2O, PaO_2 is 13.8 kPa (104 mm Hg), density 53%. **D–F,** ARDS from sepsis caused by peritonitis (indirect insult). There is substantial clearing of the densities (which, in this instance, seem to represent air space collapse) with changes in PEEP. **D,** At 5 cm H_2O, PaO_2 is 4.5 kPa (34 mm Hg), density 70%. **E,** At 10 cm H_2O, PaO_2 is 6.5 kPa (49 mm Hg), density 52%. **F,** At 15 cm H_2O, PaO_2 is 16.1 kPa (121 mm Hg), density 32%. (10 cm H_2O = 1 kPa.)

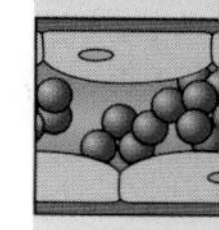

ratio of gas volume to the total lung volume, are primarily distributed in dependent lung regions such that nondependent lung regions are relatively normally inflated, whereas the intermediate regions are poorly inflated (Fig. 65.3). Typically, the normally inflated volume of lung tissue approximates 200 to 400g in a lung that weighs as much as 2000 to 4000g (compared with 1000 to 1200g for a normal lung).

These observations led to the model of the so-called "baby lung" because the amount of residual, normally inflated lung had the volume of a lung of a 5- or 6-year-old child. The baby lung presents with the following characteristics:

- Small and a normal or near-normal compliance
- Located in the nondependent lung regions
- Associated with a variable amount of abnormal lung, in part poorly inflated and in part collapsed or consolidated

Accordingly, the ARDS lung could be modeled as a mixture of three zones:

1. Normally inflated (the baby lung, nondependent);
2. Recruitable (i.e., collapsed lung that could be opened with adequate inflation pressure)
3. Consolidated lung (i.e., lung consists of alveolar filling such that it cannot be opened by increased alveolar pressure)

This model, however, implies that the lung in the nondependent regions is spared by the disease process. However, when patients are studied in the prone position, a partial redistribution of densities from the dorsal to the ventral region can occur (Fig. 65.4). Accordingly, the original baby lung model does not hold true because although the inflated tissue (the baby lung) is nondependent, the anatomic regions affected change.

The most important finding of regional chest CT analysis is that the excess tissue mass, which likely derives from edema, is not distributed according to gravity, but is evenly distributed throughout the parenchyma, from ventral to dorsal in the supine position. Thus, the acute lung injury (ALI)/ARDS lung is characterized by diffuse, increased permeability (the whole lung is diseased), and its edema increases at each level, as a sponge soaks up water. The increased lung mass in a gravitational field, however, means increased lung weight, and the most dependent levels are compressed by the increased weight of the levels above. In other words, if it is assumed that the lung behaves as a fluid, each lung level from sternum to vertebra in the supine

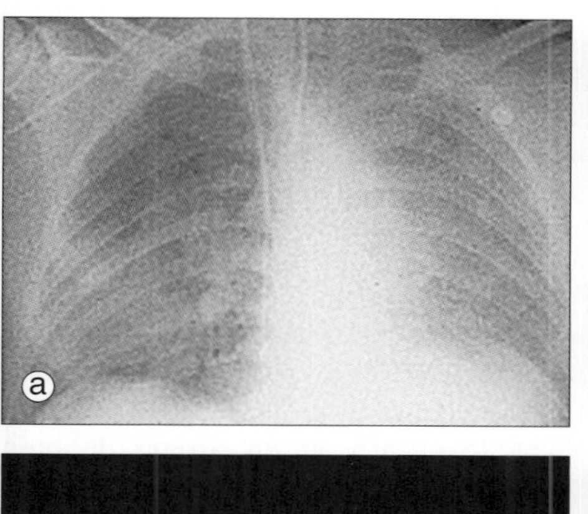

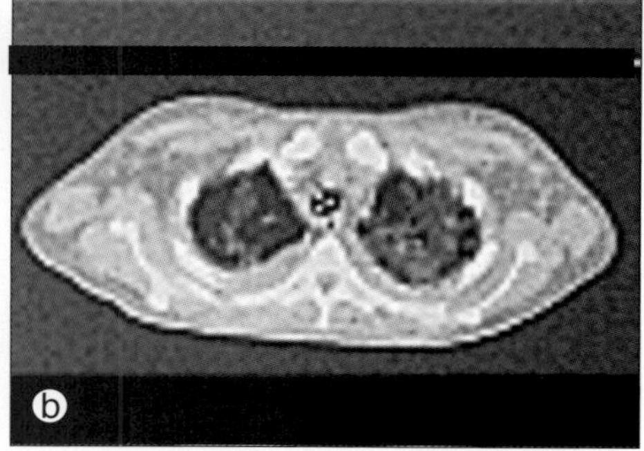

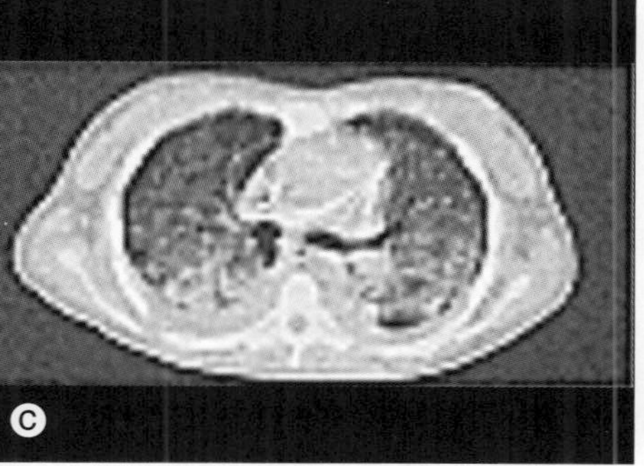

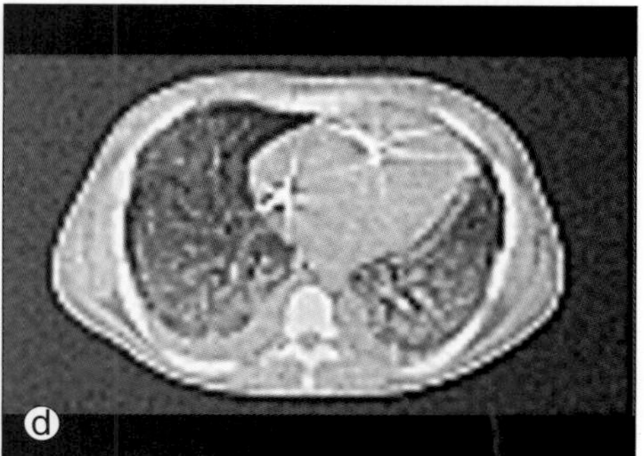

Figure 65.3 Acute respiratory distress syndrome in the early phase. Chest radiograph **(A)**, computed tomography (CT) scan in the apical lung region **(B)**, CT scan at hilum **(C)**, and CT scan in the basilar lung region **(D)**. All the images are at 10cm H_2O positive end-expiratory pressure. Although the chest radiograph shows mainly a diffuse involvement, the CT scans clearly demonstrate a predominantly dependent distribution of the densities.

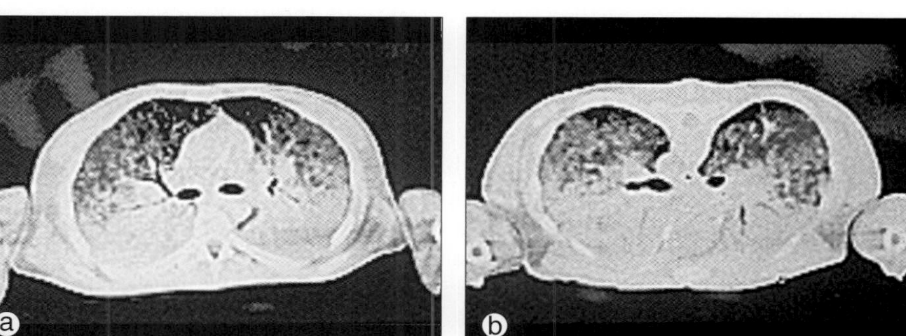

Figure 65.4 Redistribution of the lung densities shown in a patient lying supine (A), and in the same patient turned prone **(B)**.

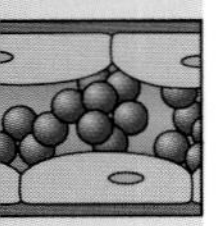

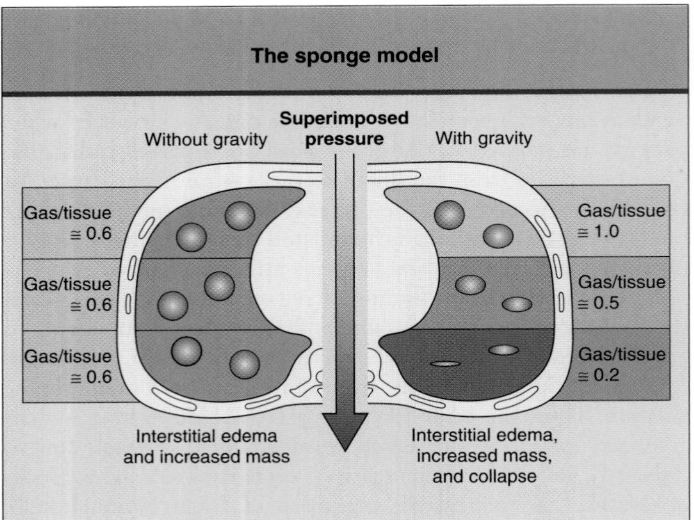

Figure 65.5 The sponge model. The edema is homogeneously distributed throughout the lung. In the absence of gravity, the lung would have pulmonary units of equal size (i.e., same gas/tissue ratio). In the presence of gravity, the superimposed pressure causes a size reduction and collapse of the dependent lung regions.

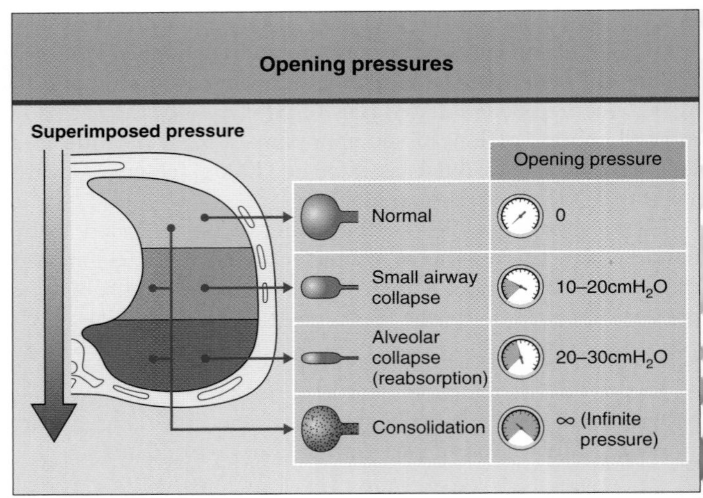

Figure 65.6 Opening pressures. The lung with acute respiratory distress syndrome is composed of normally inflated lung regions, consolidated lung regions, and collapsed (atelectatic) lung regions. Atelectasis may be caused by both compression atelectasis (needing up to 10 to 20 cm H_2O of transpulmonary pressure to reopen) and reabsorption atelectasis (which needs up to 20 to 30 cm H_2O of transpulmonary pressure to reopen. (10 cm H_2O = 1 kPa.)

position is compressed by the pressure exerted by the levels above. This pressure, called *superimposed pressure*, equals, as in a fluid model, the density times the height of the superimposed lung. As shown in Figure 65.5, in the absence of gravity a lung outside the thorax would have pulmonary units of equal size, and each level would have the same gas/tissue ratio. In a gravitational field, on the contrary, and with the addition of the condition that when it is placed in the thorax the lung must fit within the thoracic cage, the superimposed pressure causes size reduction (poorly inflated) and collapse (noninflated) of the pulmonary units of the dependent lung regions. This model accounts for the density redistribution seen in the prone position, as the gravitational forces compress the previously open ventral regions, while the dorsal regions become decollapsed. Therefore, the "sponge model" indicates the following:

- Whole lung is altered
- Normally inflated tissue (baby lung) still occurs in the nondependent regions
- Baby lung is not an anatomic reality, but a functional concept

The sponge model seems most appropriate when ARDS results from an indirect insult to the lung, such that the diffuse increase in permeability leads to widespread interstitial edema and collapse. This model, however, is less applicable to ARDS that results from a direct insult, in which the primary problem is consolidation with alveolar filling and the amount of recruitable lung (i.e., previously collapsed) is scarce.

The sponge model is also limited because many patients have little or no reversal of lung density on turning prone, which implies that other factors (i.e., the effects of the lung having to fit into the thorax) contribute to the positional differences in the extent of lung collapse. Possibilities include the generally triangular shape of the lung, the effect of the weight of the heart on the dorsal lung units, the effect of differences in ventral and dorsal aspects of the diaphragm with regard to the transmission of abdominal pressure to the lung, or regional differences in chest wall compliance.

The lung sponge model theory has been recently challenged on the basis of previous experimental work in which regional volumes were measured by intraparenchymal markers. The newly proposed model is that in the edematous lung, increasing air space pressure first causes the air–fluid interface to penetrate into the mouth of the alveolus (airway pressure approximately 20 cm H_2O), after which the air–fluid interface is inside the alveoli and the lung becomes compliant. The basic difference between the two views is that in the sponge model the edema is believed to be predominantly in the interstitium (causing alveolar collapse by compression), whereas in the air–fluid interface model, the edema is predominantly in the alveoli. In both models, the total lung volume is near normal.

MECHANISMS OF POSITIVE PRESSURE

Mechanisms of Lung Opening (Inspiration)

When a tidal volume (VT) is delivered in ARDS, two phenomena may occur—inflation and recruitment. Recruitment is defined as the inflation of previously noninflated regions, and the pressures required to open the lung are known to be greater than those required to keep the lung open. Two kinds of collapse may coexist: one is collapse of the small airways, and the other is alveolar collapse from complete reabsorption of gases.

When the small airways collapse, some gas remains trapped behind the region of closure. If the small-airway collapse persists, it evolves into alveolar collapse. The distinction between small airway and alveolar collapse is important because the pressures required for opening may be greatly different—10 to 20 cm H_2O to open small airways, and 30 to 35 cm H_2O to re-expand alveoli that have collapsed because of gas reabsorption. Consequently, as shown in Figure 65.6, a complete range of opening pressures is found in ARDS, from 0 to 1 cm H_2O to inflate open units (not exactly an opening pressure), to 10 to 20 cm H_2O to counteract the small-airway collapse (a pressure normally reached during normal tidal ventilation), and up to 30 to 35 cm H_2O transmural pressure to open areas of alveolar collapse (pressures not normally generated during normal tidal

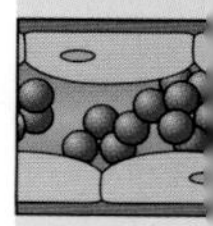

ventilation). At the end of the spectrum is the area of consolidation in which opening is impossible because the air spaces are occupied with inflammatory exudate and cells.

Indeed, it has been shown both in experimental animals and in humans with ARDS that lung opening (i.e., recruitment) is an inspiratory phenomenon that occurs, to a different extent, along a wide airway pressure range.

Keeping the Lung Open (Exhalation)

The primary role of PEEP in ARDS is to keep pulmonary units open at end exhalation when they would otherwise collapse. For years, the "best PEEP" has been sought on the assumption that for each ARDS lung there is an ideal level of PEEP. That such a level does not exist is clearly shown by CT scans, and PEEP is always a compromise between lung stretching and lung recruitment (at least when patients are supine). Indeed, in a study of a series of supine patients using PEEP levels from 0 to 20 cm H_2O, regional quantitative analysis of the gas/tissue ratio showed, as expected from the sponge model, that the various levels of the same lung, from sternum to vertebra, require different levels of PEEP to stay open.

According to the sponge model, the superimposed pressure over a given lung level is a function of density of the levels above times their height. It follows that the level of PEEP required to keep ventral regions open (in the supine position) is 0 cm H_2O (no compression, no atelectasis). In the middle of the lung, the PEEP needed to counteract the superimposed pressure is higher, and it is highest in the most dependent lung regions. It follows that to keep the most dorsal regions open, the most ventral regions must be overexpanded, and consequently the PEEP used is not "best," but always a compromise (Fig. 65.7).

In the sponge model, the superimposed pressure causes compression atelectasis as a function of density and lung height, and accordingly:

- Body size (the larger body has a larger lung) is an important variable to consider when deciding what PEEP level is appropriate to counteract superimposed pressure.
- Baseline lung density decreases with age, such that in neonates the baseline density is almost twice that of adults (thus, high levels of PEEP are sometimes required to keep the lung open in a small child who has ALI/ARDS).

Redistribution of Ventilation–Perfusion

Although explaining the effect of PEEP on lung inflation is quite straightforward using the sponge model, to explain its beneficial effects on oxygenation is more difficult. Compression atelectasis is much less prevalent in late-phase ARDS and in ARDS that results from primary lung injury. Accordingly, the ability to obtain recruitment with PEEP is limited. Although not proved, the authors believe that the mechanism of PEEP in this setting is not the prevention of air space closure and end exhalation, but possibly involves redistributing ventilation from ventral to dorsal regions. In fact, overstretching the nondependent regions using PEEP decreases the compliance of these regions such that ventilation may be diverted toward the middle and dependent regions, and increases the ventilation–perfusion ($\dot{V}/\dot{Q}$) ratio of the poorly inflated regions. Unfortunately, no data are available on regional distribution of blood flow in humans, and thus a real understanding of the ventilation and perfusion redistribution phenomena is not possible.

MECHANISMS OF DISTRIBUTION OF TIDAL VOLUME

Distribution of the insufflated volume is a function of two factors—airway resistance and regional respiratory system compliance. The CT scan, taken in static conditions, enables inferences to be made regarding variations in regional compliance. The authors found that, in ARDS, the distribution of insufflated VT is a function of PEEP. In fact, on increasing PEEP from 0 to 20 cm H_2O, the fraction of VT that was distributed to nondependent lung compared with that which was distributed to dependent lung decreased from 2.5 : 1 to approximately 1 : 1 (i.e., the ventilation became more homogeneous). This phenomenon has always been associated with better oxygenation. The mechanism by which the VT is redistributed with PEEP is as follows: In the most ventral regions, which are already open, increasing PEEP causes a progressive stretching of the lung with a decrease of the regional compliance. In the most dorsal regions, PEEP maintains recruitment of otherwise collapsing lung, and thereby increases the compliance of this region as more pulmonary units become available for inflation. The final effect depends on the balance between the overstretching and recruitment phenomena (Fig. 65.8).

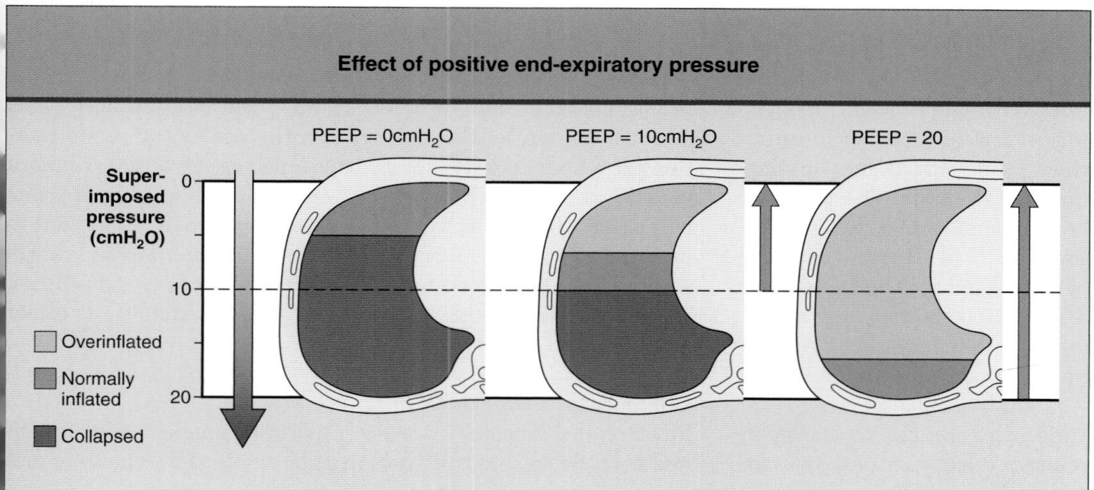

Figure 65.7 Effect of positive end-expiratory pressure (PEEP). Because PEEP acts as a counterforce to the superimposed pressure over a given lung level (indicated by *arrows*), at zero end-expiratory pressure the superimposed pressure is 0 in the ventral regions and 20 cm H_2O in the dorsal ones. To counterbalance 20 cm H_2O of superimposed pressure (dependent lung regions), a PEEP of 20 cm H_2O is necessary. However, while dependent lung regions are kept open, the nondependent ones become overinflated. (10 cm H_2O = 1 kPa.)

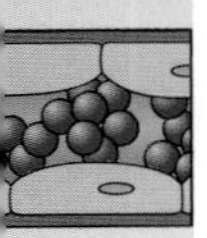

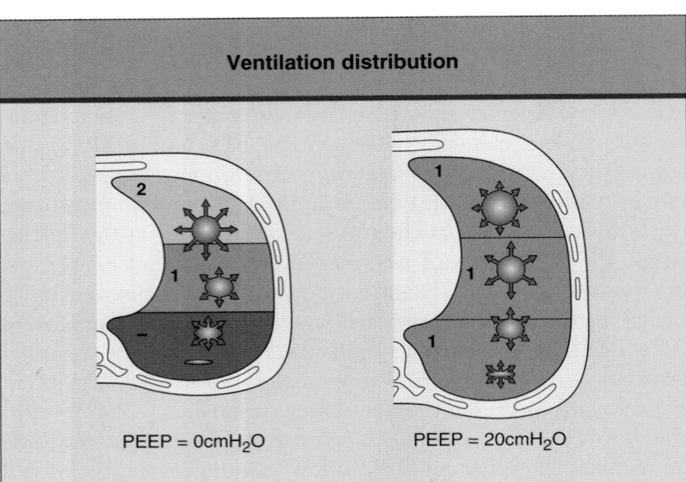

Figure 65.8 Effects of positive end-expiratory pressure (PEEP) on distribution of ventilation. At zero end-expiratory pressure, ventilation is preferentially distributed to the nondependent lung region (2 : 1 : 0) because the dependent regions are partially collapsed at end expiration. At high PEEP, the distribution of ventilation is more homogeneous (1 : 1 : 1) because of overstretching of nondependent units and recruitment of the dependent ones. (10 cm H_2O = 1 kPa.)

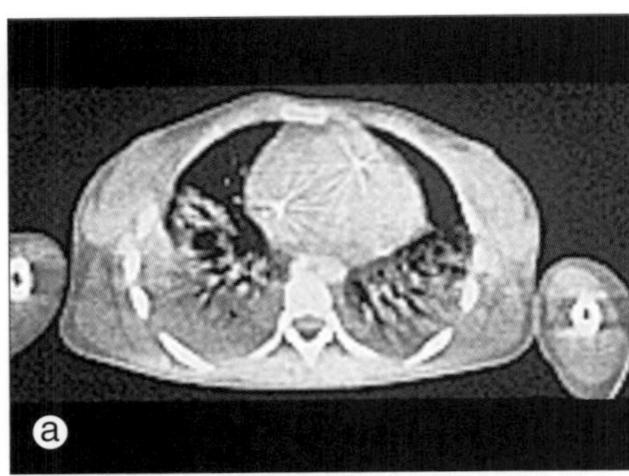

Figure 65.9 Distribution of lung densities that arise from consolidation, not collapse. Change of position from supine **(a)** to prone **(b)** does not affect the distribution of lung densities. Compare with Figure 65-4.

POSITIONING

An important maneuver that is increasingly being used in ARDS is to place the patients in the prone position. In Figure 65-4, the effects on density redistribution from dorsal to ventral are shown. This effect does not arise from a variable distribution of edema. In ARDS, the interstitial edema, rich in proteins, is not "free" to move throughout the lung parenchyma. Instead, the density redistribution, according to the sponge model, results from "squeezing out" the gas from the dependent lung regions because of the superimposed pressure. According to the mandate that the lung fit within the thorax, density redistribution on turning indicates that the lung fits better within the thorax when patients are prone compared with when they are supine.

The redistribution of lung density induced by the prone position may be more pronounced in ARDS that results from extrapulmonary disease. In ARDS caused by pulmonary disease, densities change much less on going from the supine to the prone position (Fig. 65.9). The prone position, in approximately 60% to 70% of patients with ARDS, is associated with increased oxygenation. Several mechanisms are likely to be involved, and important differences may arise when ARDS occurs as a result of pulmonary versus extrapulmonary disease. In the latter, because atelectasis depends on lung density and height, a larger volume of lung opens in the prone position. In ARDS that results from pulmonary disease, the authors found that changes in thoracic compliance play a substantial role. In the prone position, for anatomic reasons, the dorsal component of the chest wall is stiffer than the anterior wall, and the VT is distributed more toward the ventral and abdominal regions, where the higher lung densities predominate (Fig. 65.10). Indeed, human and animal studies conclude that more homogeneous inflation or ventilation is the main mechanism of oxygenation improvement in the prone position.

Although prone positioning improves the gas exchange in most patients with ARDS, its positive effects on outcome are

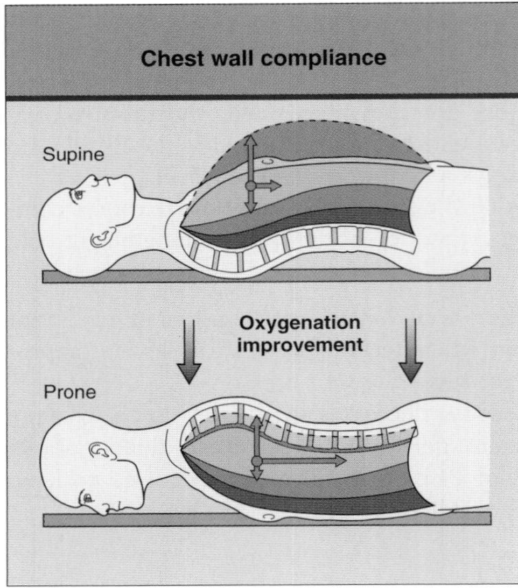

Figure 65.10 Effect of prone position on ventilation distribution. In the supine position, the distribution of ventilation is preferentially distributed to the ventral regions. When the patient is prone, the stiffness of the dorsal chest wall favors the distribution of ventilation to the dorsal regions, facilitating reinflation in this area.

unproved. Although experimental work has shown that the prone position may protect against ventilator-induced lung injury, a randomized clinical trial on the use of the prone position for 6 hours per day for 10 days failed to show improvement in survival. The study, however, was criticized because of treatment rules, limited hours in the prone position, and late enrollment of part of the patients. Indeed, the prone position is still widely used and recommended for gas exchange problems, whereas further studies are recommended to establish its effect on outcome.

CHEST WALL COMPLIANCE

Most of the available data on respiratory mechanics in ARDS relate to the respiratory system as a whole (i.e., the lung and

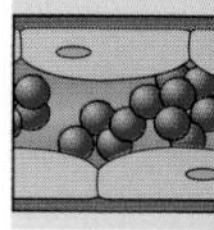

the chest wall). The mechanical alterations observed were mainly attributed to the lung because chest wall compliance was considered to be normal. The few studies that investigated chest wall compliance per se found it to be decreased. More recently, it has become clear that in ARDS caused by pulmonary disease, chest wall compliance is normal, whereas in that from extrapulmonary disease it is greatly decreased. It is more convenient to use the elastance (the reciprocal of compliance) to discuss the partitioning of compliance between chest and lung because the elastance of the respiratory system is the sum of chest wall and lung elastances.

Elastance is the pressure required to keep the respiratory system inflated. Part of this pressure is spent to keep the lung inflated, and part to keep the thoracic cage (which includes the abdominal wall) expanded. Normally, lung and chest wall elastances are similar, such that half of the applied pressure keeps the lung inflated and half expands the thoracic cage when inflated. In ARDS caused by extrapulmonary disease, however, more pressure is required to expand the thorax. The reverse is true for ARDS that results from pulmonary disease. Thus, although the total respiratory system elastance is similar in ARDS from pulmonary and that from extrapulmonary disease, its partitioning is different. This explains, for instance, why in ARDS from pulmonary disease, heart size tends to remain normal when PEEP is increased (i.e., low pleural pressure around the heart), whereas it decreases in ARDS caused by extrapulmonary disease (i.e., progressively higher pleural pressure because of the relative stiffness of the thorax; see Fig. 65.10). Accordingly, PEEP may have different hemodynamic consequences in ARDS that results from direct or indirect insults.

In this context, the issue of intra-abdominal pressure must be discussed. Normally, intra-abdominal pressure measured through the bladder is in the range 5 to 10 cm H_2O. In ARDS caused by extrapulmonary diseases (most of which occur mainly in the abdominal compartment) intra-abdominal pressure is greatly increased. The authors found a strict correlation between abdominal pressure and chest wall elastance (i.e., increasing the abdominal pressure increases chest wall elastance, which reflects an increased stiffness of the thoracic cage). Because the importance of chest wall elastance is becoming increasingly clear, the authors believe that the measurement of intra-abdominal pressure must be part of the assessment of patients with ARDS (both for respiratory treatment and hemodynamic consequences). In fact, many patients admitted to the intensive care unit present with an abdominal pressure greater than 12 mm Hg, a condition that is not detectable on a clinical basis and requires objective measurement (bladder pressure).

PULMONARY CIRCULATION

The ARDS lung is usually characterized by increased pulmonary artery pressure and increased pulmonary vascular resistances. A mean pulmonary artery pressure of 4 kPa (30 mm Hg) or greater is a universal hallmark of ARDS, regardless of etiology. A single mechanism is unlikely to explain the increased resistances. Moreover, the causes of the pulmonary hypertension may change over time. Indirect evidence suggests that a generalized vasoconstriction exists in ARDS and that this can be modulated with vasodilatation. Moreover, inhaled nitric oxide may selectively dilate vessels in ventilated areas, which suggests that hypoxemia (arterial and mixed venous) is not the cause of the observed functional vasoconstriction. Eicosanoids and other mediators are likely to be responsible. A second possible mechanism is vessel compression by the increased lung weight and superimposed perivascular pressure. The authors found, in vivo, that every increase of 0.13 kPa (1 mm Hg) of pulmonary artery pressure is associated with a 14% increase in the original lung weight. Unfortunately, it is not possible to determine an independent variable because, if it is possible that edema causes vessel compression, it is also possible that increased pulmonary artery pressure increases the interstitial edema through increased microfiltration. Anatomic alterations in the vascular wall have also been described, such as swelling of the endothelial cells and, with time, a medial hypertrophy. Finally, evidence of fibrin clot and cellular obstruction in the capillaries is found in 20% to 30% of patients with ARDS. With time, the collapsed or obstructed vessels undergo remodeling or become completely obliterated by fibrotic processes, which leads to microvascular destruction. A summary of pulmonary circulation alterations is presented in Figure 65.11.

In considering the overall circulatory function, however, it is noteworthy that in ARDS, despite the generalized vasoconstriction, collapsed lung regions are appropriately underperfused compared with the inflated regions. Indeed, it is not rare to find 50% to 60% of collapsed lung associated with a shunt fraction (i.e., the flow through the collapsed regions) of 20% to 30% of the cardiac output, which suggests that a somewhat appropriate flow diversion is still occurring.

The pathophysiologic consequences of elevated pulmonary vascular resistances depend on the cardiac reserve of each patient. If the right ventricle is able to increase its work, the hemodynamic consequences are nil. If right ventricular dysfunction is present, numerous systemic consequences arise.

GAS EXCHANGE ALTERATIONS

The main alteration of gas exchange in ARDS is hypoxemia because of shunt, and is usually associated with normocapnia or hypocapnia. However, although the hypoxemia persists, a progressive rise in the arterial partial pressure of carbon dioxide (Pa_{CO_2}) occurs if the minute ventilation is maintained constant. Gas exchange is the final result of the match between ventilation and perfusion, which in turn depends on the anatomic structure of the lung (which changes with time and with the prevalent underlying pathologic process). An attempt to correlate lung structure with gas exchange alterations is given in Table 65.2.

Early Acute Lung Injury/Acute Respiratory Distress Syndrome, Indirect Insult

In early ALI/ARDS caused by an indirect insult, the lung architecture is preserved and the primary pathophysiologic abnormality is edema with consequent collapse of dependent regions. The pulmonary blood flow through these regions is the main cause of shunt. The midlung regions are poorly inflated and, if perfused, could contribute to hypoxemia because of low $\dot{V}/\dot{Q}$. The nondependent regions are open and likely to be hyperventilated because of the preferential distribution of VT to these regions. Thus, carbon dioxide elimination is not a problem. The application of PEEP may keep open the otherwise collapsing regions and increase ventilation of the poorly inflated

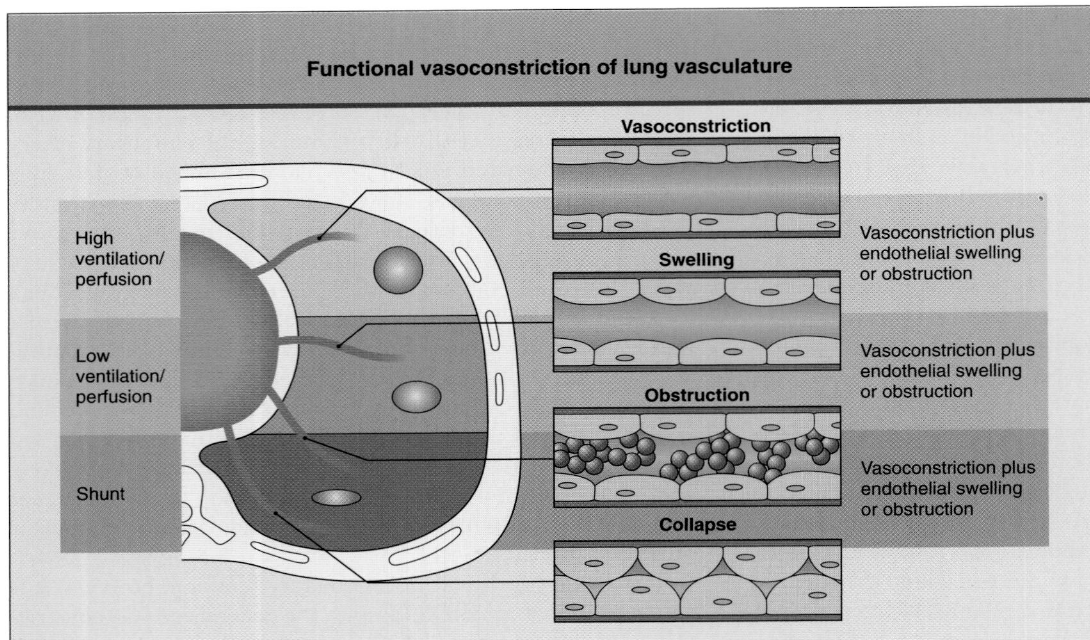

Figure 65.11 All the lung vasculature is functionally vasoconstricted. Moreover, endothelial swelling and obliteration may further increase pulmonary vascular resistance. In the dependent lung regions, vessel compression may also be present.

Table 65.2
Gas exchange

Acute respiratory distress syndrome	Lung injury	Lung structure	Pulmonary circulation	Mechanism of gas exchange	Corrections (other than fraction of inspired oxygen)
Early	Direct	Collapse in the dependent regions	Vasoconstriction and partial collapse	Shunt	Positive end-expiratory pressure (PEEP; re-expansion)
		Poorly inflated in middle regions	Vasoconstriction	Low ventilation/ perfusion ($\dot{V}/\dot{Q}$)?	PEEP (normalizing inflation)
		Inflated in upper regions	Vasoconstriction	High $\dot{V}/\dot{Q}$	Nitric oxide (increasing perfusion) Inhaled prostaglandin
		Consolidation and collapse in dependent regions	Vasoconstriction plus possible collapse	Shunt	PEEP (re-expansion)
	Indirect	Possible consolidation foci in middle regions	Vasoconstriction and low $\dot{V}/\dot{Q}$?	Shunt in consolidated area and low $\dot{V}/\dot{Q}$?	PEEP (?)
		Possible consolidation foci in nondependent regions	Vasoconstriction and high $\dot{V}/\dot{Q}$	Shunt in consolidated area	PEEP [ventilation redistribution to lower regions (?) by stretching upper regions?] plus nitric oxide – prostaglandins
		Consolidation	Vasoconstriction	Shunt	PEEP (ventilation redistribution to lower regions?)
Late	Widespread lesions	Fibrosis	Microvessel destruction and obliteration	Diffusion impairment?	No recruitment evident
		Bullae and emphysema-like alterations	–	Increased dead space	Nitric oxide?

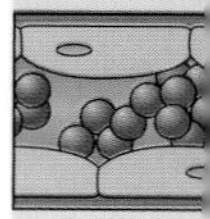

regions to the extent that shunt decreases and low $\dot{V}/\dot{Q}$ is possibly corrected. If the PEEP level is excessive, however, the upper regions are kept open but are overstretched, with less capability of ventilation. Oxygen may be exchanged (a kind of "regional apneic oxygenation"), but the carbon dioxide clearance is impaired. This is one possible explanation why, with excessive PEEP, shunt decreases but the $PaCO_2$ may increase.

Early Acute Respiratory Distress Syndrome, Direct Insult

In early ARDS caused by a direct insult, the overall lung architecture is preserved but the prevalent damage is intra-alveolar, with edema and collapse being secondary phenomena and quantitatively less important than in ARDS that results from indirect insult. The consolidated regions, if perfused, cause shunt just as if they were collapsed. It is likely that PEEP works by keeping the otherwise collapsing regions open. It is possible, however, that PEEP also works by redistributing V_T from nondependent to dependent regions, thus improving the ventilation of low $\dot{V}/\dot{Q}$ regions. The shunt decrease may also be associated with a $PaCO_2$ increase in this instance, which suggests a ventilation diversion with PEEP.

Late-Phase Acute Lung Injury/Acute Respiratory Distress Syndrome

The situation is likely to be different in the late stage of ALI/ARDS, in which the lung architecture is markedly altered because of fibrosis, capillary destruction, and emphysema-like lesions. In such conditions, PEEP is still required to maintain oxygenation, but it does not work by "keeping open" the recruited units because collapse is scarce, if it occurs at all. Redistribution of ventilation or perfusion is a possible mechanism. Moreover, the structural changes of the lung may contribute to hypoxemia by some impairment of oxygen diffusion (fibrosis and interstitial thickening), whereas the emphysema-like lesions are likely to be the anatomic basis for carbon dioxide retention.

CLINICAL FEATURES

Originally, ARDS was defined as the presence of severe dyspnea, tachypnea, hypoxemia refractory to oxygen therapy, reduced lung compliance, and diffuse alveolar infiltration seen on chest radiographs. Subsequent authors used a PaO_2/fraction of inspired oxygen (FIO_2) ratio of less than 150 to characterize ARDS. In 1979, the National Heart, Lung, and Blood Institute introduced criteria based on time (fast and slow) and threshold oxygenation values at defined levels of FIO_2 and positive expiratory pressure. The explicit exclusion of cardiogenic pulmonary edema was introduced next with suggestions for a quantitative threshold for pulmonary wedge capillary pressure, and this was followed by the introduction of a quantitative measurement of respiratory system compliance. In 1988, a new approach was proposed that involved a "lung injury score" to quantify, albeit roughly, the presence, severity, and evolution of acute and chronic damage involving lung parenchyma.

Recently, the American-European Consensus Conference on ARDS recommended that ARDS be described as a particularly severe subset of ALI, the latter of which was defined as a "syndrome of inflammation and increased permeability that is associated with a constellation of clinical, radiologic and physiologic abnormalities that cannot be explained by, but may coexist with, left arterial or pulmonary capillary hypertension." A summary of ALI/ARDS definitions is presented in Table 65.3.

Table 65.3
Acute respiratory distress syndrome definitions

Reference	Clinical	Oxygenation threshold	Bilateral infiltrates	Respiratory system compliance	Threshold wedge pressure
Ashbaugh et al.	1	None	Yes	None	Clinical judgment
Bone et al.	1	Partial pressure of arterial oxygen (PaO_2)/fraction of inspired oxygen (FIO_2) ≤21 kPa (≤150 mmHg)	Yes	None	Clinical judgment
Zapol et al.	1	PaO_2 <6.6 kPa (<50 mmHg) 100% FIO_2 after 2 h 60% FIO_2 after 24 h Positive end-expiratory pressure (PEEP) 5 cmH_2O	Yes	None	Clinical judgment
Pepe et al.	1	PaO_2 <10.0 kPa (<75 mmHg) FIO_2 ≥50%	Yes	None	>2.4 kPa (>18 mmHg)
Bell et al. and Fein et al.	1	PaO_2 ≥6.6 kPa (50 mmHg) FIO_2 ≥50%	Yes	None	>2.0 kPa (>15 mmHg)
Fowler et al.	1	PaO_2/alveolar PO_2 <0.2	Yes	>50 mL/cmH_2O	>1.6 kPa (>12 mmHg)
Murray et al.	1	PaO_2/FIO_2 score 0–4 PEEP score 0–4	Chest radiograph score 0–4	Compliance score 0–4	Clinical judgment
Bernard et al.	1	PaO_2/FIO_2 <26.6 kPa (<200 mmHg), acute respiratory distress syndrome PaO_2/FIO_2 <40 kPa (<300 mmHg), acute lung injury	Yes	None	Clinical judgment

The definitions of ALI/ARDS are not of merely academic interest because testing new treatments requires trials in which the homogeneity of the study population plays a substantial role. Interestingly, considering the evolution of ARDS definitions, it is clear that more extensive and quantitative criteria were added over the years to define a more homogeneous population, but the recent American-European Conference almost represents a return to the original, very simple definition. The dilemma is still unsolved—simple criteria mean that a large trial with a very inhomogeneous population is feasible; strict criteria result in a homogeneous population and a large trial becomes unfeasible. In the authors' opinion, work is still required to find the best compromise between these opposing needs.

DIAGNOSIS

The diagnosis of ALI/ARDS is simple, according to its current definition, because it requires only a known predisposing factor, bilateral pulmonary infiltrates on the chest radiograph, and a threshold PaO_2 value normalized for the FIO_2 in use.

An accurate patient history is of paramount importance to infer the etiology and pathogenesis of ALI/ARDS, and assessment of traditional signs must be carried out despite the availability of newer technology. Respiratory frequency, dyspnea, symmetry or asymmetry of thoracic movements, percussion, and auscultation may provide insights into the etiology, prevalent underlying pathologic process, and the patient's ability to deal with the respiratory distress (e.g., signs of muscle fatigue must be carefully investigated so as not to delay initiating mechanical ventilatory support).

Etiologic Diagnosis

In most instances, the etiology that leads to ALI/ARDS is clear, as in aspiration or lung contusion. In some patients, however, the etiology is not apparent. In patients who have ALI/ARDS and signs of sepsis, a systematic search for all possible infection foci must be carried out, using all the available facilities.

Pathogenic Diagnosis

The authors suggest that ALI/ARDS be distinguished according to pulmonary and extrapulmonary causes. In most circumstances, this is an easy distinction based on an accurate history and clinical assessment. Such a distinction is more useful in the early phases of ALI/ARDS. With time, and with the structural changes that occur in the lung, the two processes are likely to overlap.

Pathophysiologic Characterization

Together with etiologic and pathogenic screening, the authors believe that every patient who has ALI/ARDS must be carefully investigated to define specific pathophysiologic characteristics because this enables treatment to be tailored more precisely.

GAS EXCHANGE

Characterization of the degree of gas exchange impairment is the most common way of defining the severity of ALI/ARDS. To infer the underlying pathophysiologic process, it is always useful to observe the oxygenation response at different FIO_2 values (the authors believe a brief test with an FIO_2 of 1.0 is useful) and to conduct a formal PEEP trial (e.g., 5, 10, and 15 cm H_2O). Changes in FIO_2 may markedly affect the PaO_2/FIO_2 ratio, and the response may help to estimate a possible $\dot{V}/\dot{Q}$ mismatch. The PEEP trial (in which hemodynamic status is controlled) may enable effective recruitment maneuvers to be inferred. The $PaCO_2$ response during the PEEP trial (in which minute ventilation is kept constant) may also be informative. An increase in PaO_2 with a decrease in the $PaCO_2$ indicates effective recruitment. An increase in PaO_2 with an increase in $PaCO_2$ could indicate overstretching of the nondependent lung (in addition to recruitment).

In some circumstances, it may be necessary to measure mixed venous (or central venous) blood gases. This is particularly true when cardiac output is low because the fraction of shunt flow is directly related to the cardiac output. In some cases, an increase in PaO_2 occurs simply because of a decrease in cardiac output, with no improvement in lung function.

IMAGING

Although not proven to alter outcomes, we believe that chest CT scans should be obtained in all patients with ALI/ARDS. In a series of 74 patients with ALI/ARDS, 24 had pneumothoraces, and in 37% of these the pneumothorax was ventral in location and detected only by CT scan. Although this has not been well studied, cross-table lateral films may have discovered many of these. Moreover, in 60% of the cases the CT scan provided additional clinical information compared with conventional radiology, and in 22% the findings resulted in a change in the clinical management. These and other data emphasize the importance of this technology in routine clinical management. Also, CT scans are the best tool with which to discriminate between recruitment and consolidation, and the authors routinely perform a PEEP trial during the CT scan, taking images at different pressures. This may be of great help when tailoring the respiratory support because the potential for recruitment in a given patient is assessed precisely. Unfortunately, the pathology and physiology of ALI/ARDS evolve over time, which renders the findings less useful the longer the patient requires support.

RESPIRATORY MECHANICS

Lung Volume

The authors believe that measurements of respiratory mechanics may be better interpreted if the starting lung volume is known. Accordingly, a simplified helium method is routinely used to determine the lung gas volume.

Pressure–Volume Relationship

Another way to characterize the underlying pathologic process is the pressure–volume (PV) curve of the total respiratory system, from which several inferences may be derived (Fig. 65.12). The initial slope of the PV curve (also called the *starting compliance*) was thought to give an idea of the dimensions of the "baby lung" at atmospheric pressure. In adult men, starting compliances of 20, 30, and 40 cm H_2O roughly correspond to baby lung volumes of 20%, 30%, and 40%, respectively, of the original healthy lung. The inflection point (or, more precisely, the inflection zone) has been thought to suggest a potential for recruitment and indicates the pressures over which most

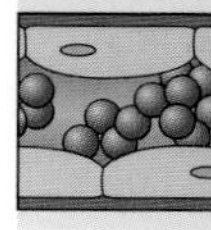

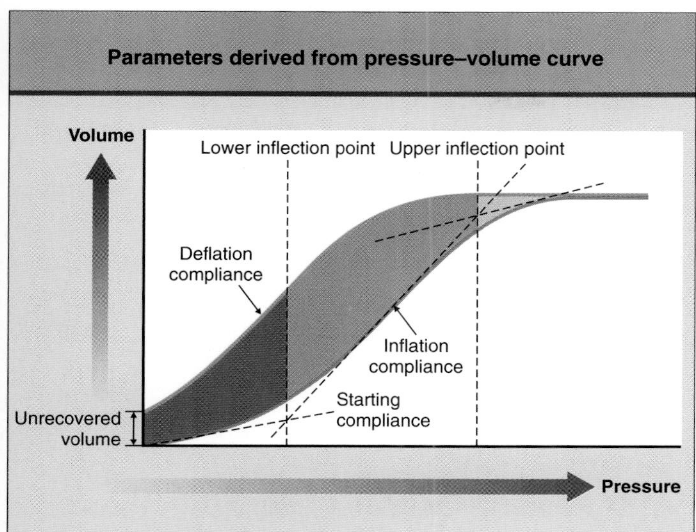

Figure 65.12 Parameters derived from the pressure–volume curve of the total respiratory system. (For explanation, see text.)

of the recruitment may occur. The slope of the PV curve after the inflection point (inflation compliance) was thought to give some estimate of the amount of recruitment (the steeper the PV curve, the greater the recruitment). Finally, the upper inflection point indicates the pressure at which the stretching of pulmonary units becomes the prevalent phenomenon.

Recent theoretical and experimental data have challenged these views, however, because it has been shown that recruitment occurs along the entire PV curve.

Indeed, to date, we know that the lower inflection point, more than the recruitment zone, may indicate the "start" of recruitment, that recruitment occurs along the entire PV curve, that it may occur even above the upper inflection point, and that the PV curve is also a "recruitment curve." Unfortunately, it gives the fraction of the recruitment occurring at different pressures, but not the absolute amount of total recruitment actually occurring.

Partitioning; Respiratory System Mechanics

The authors believe that this measurement should also be included in the routine assessment of patients with ALI/ARDS because the same applied pressure may result in completely different transmural pressure depending on the relative elastance of the lung and chest wall, and because these may be considerably different in ALI/ARDS that results from pulmonary and extrapulmonary diseases. Although the utility of this information has not yet been determined with regard to outcomes, the authors feel that this information is of great importance for the prevention of barotrauma and hemodynamic impairment. In this context, the intra-abdominal pressure, because of its profound effect on the elastance of the thoracic cage, should also be measured.

Hemodynamics

In addition to a clinical assessment of cardiac output (e.g., skin perfusion, pulse volume, skin and mucous membrane color, extremity temperature, urine output), invasive monitoring, including central venous pressure and arterial lines, is usually routine and safe in these patients. The utility of pulmonary artery catheters and other invasive means of monitoring the cardiac output is unclear. Quantitative assessment of hemodynamics has been deleted from the definition of ALI/ARDS. In some circumstances, however, measurement of cardiac output or pulmonary vascular pressures may still be necessary.

TREATMENT

Etiologic Treatment

A summary of most of the risk factors that lead to ALI/ARDS is given in Table 65.4. The search for etiology is as urgent and important as selecting the type of ventilatory support. The results of treatment strongly depend on the specific problem that leads to the episode of ALI/ARDS, whereas the type of ventilatory support may only "buy time" for the correct treatment to work.

In some instances, the etiology of the injury occurred in the past (e.g., trauma with lung contusion, an episode of smoke inhalation, or near drowning). In these, only symptomatic, and possibly pathogenic, treatments are possible. In other instances, however, ARDS results from etiologic factors present while patients are treated (e.g., pneumonia sepsis). Two rules must be followed:

1. Any etiologic factor found must be treated aggressively (be it surgical or medical treatment).
2. If a microorganism is suspected, no antibiotic, antifungal, or antiviral agent should be given until the appropriate sampling (e.g., bronchoalveolar lavage, blood, urine) has been carried out.

Pathogenic Treatment

One animal model commonly chosen to study lung injury that resembles ALI/ARDS is lipopolysaccharide (LPS) administration, which can cause a direct injury when instilled into the trachea or an indirect injury when given intravenously. Both the complement system and alveolar macrophages can be activated by LPS. Both events trigger a complex cytokine network that recruits cells and releases numerous humoral mediators. A simplified sequence of events is outlined in Figure 65.13. Although incomplete, it indicates the pathogenic targets of a number of clinical trials that have been conducted on patients who have ALI/ARDS or sepsis. Some strategies were based on blocking the trigger of the inflammatory response (e.g., anti-LPS antibodies), or focused on single elements of the inflammatory network (e.g., anti–tumor necrosis factor antibodies, soluble tumor necrosis factor receptors, interleukin-1 receptor antagonist), or modified neutrophil function (liposomal prostaglandin E_1, antioxidants); yet others addressed the consequences of inflammation such as hemodynamic imbalances (e.g., inhibitors of nitric oxide synthase, prostaglandin E_1). A summary of these is given in Table 65.5. Almost all the studies found either no major benefit or that the intervention was actually harmful. Given the complexity of the network, perhaps multiple sites should be blocked or potentiated simultaneously as opposed to selectively blocking single events or mediators of the overall process.

In recent years, it has been shown in septic patients (most of whom present with ALI/ARDS) that 4 days of treatment with

Table 65.4
Distribution of risk factors for acute respiratory distress syndrome (ARDS)

	Pepe et al.	Fowler et al.	Mancebo and Artigas	Villar and Slutsky	Suchyta et al.	Hudson et al.	Milberg et al.	Heffner et al.
Total patients who had ARDS/ total patients in study (%)	46/136 (34)	68/936 (7)	35/35 (100)	74/1997 (4)	215/215 (100)	179/695 (26)	918/918 (100)	50/50 (100)
Cardiopulmonary bypass	–	4/237 (2)	–	–	–	–	–	–
Burn	–	2/87 (2)	–	–	–	–	–	–
Bacteremia	–	9/239 (4)	–	–	–	–	–	–
Massive blood transfusion	19/42 (45)	9/197 (5)	–	–	–	28/77 (36)	48/918 (5)	4/50 (8)
Bone fractures	15/34 (44)	2/38 (5)	–	–	–	7/63 (11)	–	–
Pneumonia	–	10/84 (12)	9/35 (25)	5/74 (7)	76/215 (35)	–	–	20/50 (40)
Disseminated intravascular coagulation	–	2/9 (22)	–	–	–	–	–	–
Pulmonary aspiration	10/32 (31)	16/45 (36)	–	9/74 (12)	25/215 (11)	13/59 (22)	85/918 (9)	5/50 (10)
Sepsis	9/19 (47)	–	6/35 (17)	30/74 (41)	31/215 (14)	56/136 (41)	340/918 (37)	9/50 (18)
Major trauma	–	–	4/35 (11)	14/74 (19)	20/215 (9)	–	230/918 (25)	6/50 (12)
Drug overdose	–	–	1/35 (2)	3/74 (4)	–	14/164 (8)	54/918 (6)	–
Near drowning	3/4 (75)	–	–	1/74 (1)	–	2/6 (33)	–	1/50 (2)
Pulmonary contusion	19/50 (38)	–	–	–	–	12/55 (22)	–	–
Abdominal surgery	–	–	–	4/74 (5)	–	–	–	–
Thoracic surgery	–	–	–	2/74 (3)	–	–	–	–
Postanoxic coma	–	–	–	2/74 (3)	–	–	–	–
Cerebral hemorrhage	–	–	–	2/74 (3)	–	–	–	–
Pancreatitis	1/1 (100)	–	5/35 (14)	–	–	–	–	–
Prolonged hypotension	2/4 (50)	–	–	–	–	–	–	–
Shock	–	–	2/35 (5)	–	–	–	–	3/50 (6)
Fat embolism	–	–	–	–	–	–	–	1/50 (2)
Smoke inhalation	–	–	–	–	–	–	–	1/50 (2)
Peritonitis	–	–	7/35 (20)	–	43/215 (20)	–	–	–
Systemic lupus	–	–	1/35 (2)	–	–	–	–	–
Others	–	–	–	–	20/215 (9)	–	–	–

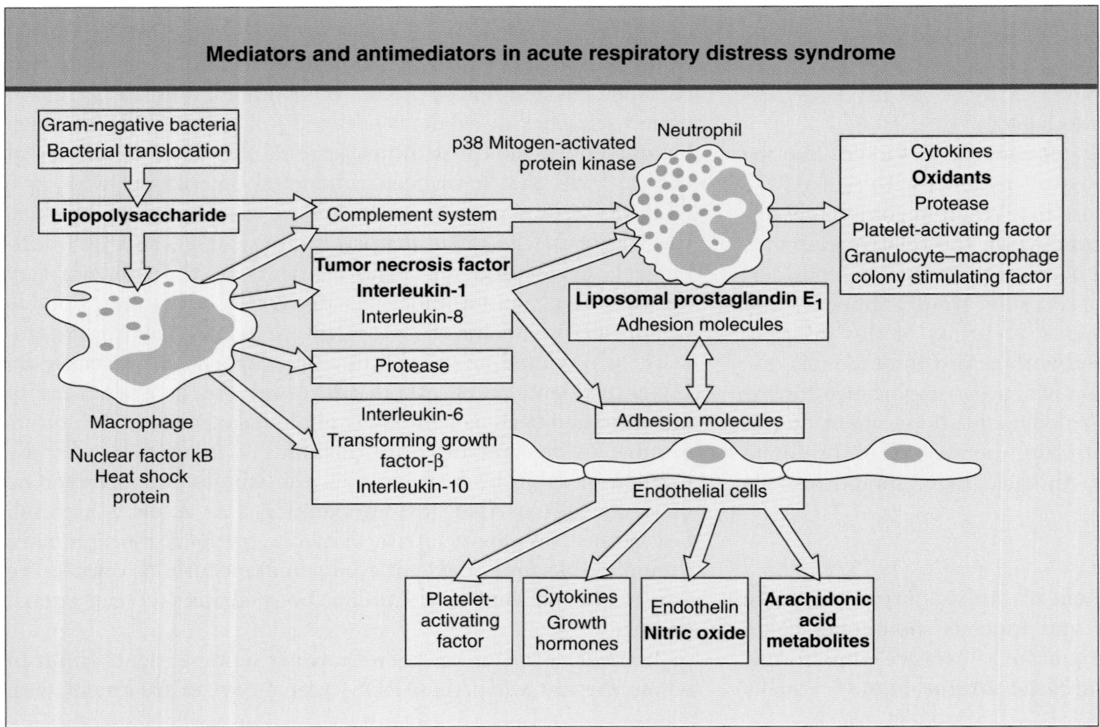

Figure 65.13 Mediators and antimediators involved in the inflammatory response in acute respiratory distress syndrome. The mediators against which pathogenic therapy has been tested in clinical trials are indicated in bold.

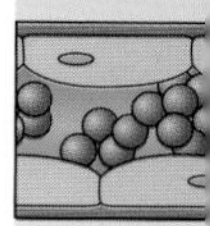

Table 65.5
Clinical trials directed at the pathogenesis

Strategy	Author	Study characteristics present						Number of patients	Diagnosis	Results	
		p	r	d1	d2	c	n			Overall	Stratified
Antilipopolysaccharide	McCloskey et al.	No	Yes	Yes	No	Yes	No	2199	Sepsis	=	na
	Ziegler et al.	No	Yes	Yes	No	No	No	543	Sepsis	=	+
Interleukin-1 receptor antagonist	Fisher et al.	Yes	No	No	Yes	Yes	No	99	Sepsis/shock	+	na
	Fisher et al.	No	No	Yes	No	No	No	893	Sepsis	=	+
	Opal et al.	Yes	Yes	Yes	No	Yes	No	696	Sepsis stratified	=	na
Antibodies against tumor necrosis factor (TNF)-α	Abraham et al.	No	No	No	Yes	No	No	994	>50% acute lung injury	=	+
	Cohen and Carlet	Yes	Yes	No	Yes	Yes	Yes	553	Sepsis/shock	=	+
	Reinhart et al.	Yes	Yes	No	Yes	Yes	Yes	122	Sepsis/shock	=	+
Antibodies against soluble TNF receptor	Abraham et al.	Yes	Yes	Yes	Yes	Yes	Yes	498	Sepsis/shock	=	+
Cortisone	Bernard et al.	Yes	Yes	Yes	No	No	No	99	Acute respiratory distress syndrome (ARDS)	=	na
	Bone et al.	Yes	Yes	Yes	No	Yes	No	382	ARDS	=	na
	Luce et al.	Yes	Yes	Yes	No	No	No	87	ARDS	=	na
	Meduri et al.	Yes	Yes	Yes	No	Yes	No	24	ARDS (late)	+	na
Liposomal prostaglandin E_1	Abraham et al.	Yes	Yes	Yes	No	Yes	No	25	ARDS	=	na
Prostaglandin E_1	Bone et al.	Yes	Yes	Yes	No	No	No	100	ARDS	=	na
	Holcroft et al.	Yes	Yes	Yes	No	No	No	41	ARDS	+	na
Antioxidants	Jepsen et al.	Yes	Yes	Yes	No	No	No	66	ARDS	=	na
	Suter et al.	No	No	No	Yes	No	No	61	ARDS	=	na
	Bernard et al.	Yes	Yes	Yes	No	Yes	No	48	ARDS	=	na
Inducible nitric oxide synthase	Petros et al.	No	Yes	Yes	No	No	No	12	Sepsis	=	na
Anticyclo-oxygenase	Haupt et al.	No	Yes	Yes	No	Yes	No	29	Sepsis	=	na
	Yu and Tomasa	Yes	Yes	Yes	No	No	No	54	Sepsis	+	na

p, prospective; r, randomized; d1, double-blind; d2, dose ranging (more than one dose tested); c, multicenter; n, multinational; =, no positive result; +, positive result; na, not available.

activated protein C results in a significant improvement in survival. Activated protein C, compared with other molecules tested in sepsis treatment, presents the widest range of actions on the complex network of coagulation/inflammation. In fact, it has anticoagulant, anti-inflammatory, and profibrinolytic effects.

Other positive results have been reported in septic patients given low-dose corticosteroid replacement. It is important to emphasize, however, that the positive effects are present when patients are characterized by relative adrenal insufficiency.

Symptomatic Treatment

Symptomatic (i.e., supportive) treatment is currently the cornerstone of ARDS therapy. The possible changes in mortality of ALI/ARDS over time that have been reported by some groups may result from differences in supportive treatment, or from differences in the iatrogenic nature of the treatments themselves.

BLOOD GAS TARGETS

In the past few years, the "lung rest" philosophy (i.e., permissive hypercapnia) has become more accepted, which has led to the acceptance of arterial blood gases that may be markedly abnormal with respect to $PaCO_2$. Although it may be reasonable to accept a high $PaCO_2$, the authors believe that PaO_2 should be maintained at approximately 10.6 kPa (80 mm Hg) instead of 8.0 kPa (60 mm Hg), as suggested by other investigators, to avoid the risk of sudden deterioration of oxygen saturation.

LUNG OPENING

Regardless of the prevalent damage that underlies ALI/ARDS, some degree of lung collapse is always present when the patient is referred to the intensive care unit. For hours or days before admission to the intensive care unit, most patients are likely to have secretions, high respiratory frequency, or low VT, which are all risk factors for atelectasis. To reach the goal of an open, expanded lung, airway patency must be ensured (consider bronchoscopy) and atelectasis reversed if possible. Although formal rules to recruit the lung are not established, transmural pressure and respiratory system compliance must be considered.

Transmural Pressure

The air space opening pressure is the transmural pressure (i.e., the difference between intra-alveolar and pleural pressures). Transmural pressure is a function of the pressure applied to the airways and of the elastances of the lung and chest wall, according to the following equation, in which PAW is the applied airway pressure, EL is the elastance of the lung, and EW is the elastance of the chest wall.

EQUATION 65.1

$$\text{Transpulmonary pressure} = \text{P}_{\text{AW}} \times [\text{E}_{\text{L}}/(\text{E}_{\text{L}} + \text{E}_{\text{W}})]$$

Normally, EL equals EW, and the transmural pressure, as an average, would be approximately half of the pressure applied to the airways. However, as previously discussed, in ALI/ARDS caused by direct or indirect insult, the EL/(EL + EW) value may be very different. For example, in ARDS that results from direct insult, the ratio is less than 1 for patients who have extrapulmonary disease. It follows that to achieve the same opening transmural pressure, a higher PAW is required in ARDS that arises from extrapulmonary problems than in ARDS that results from pulmonary conditions.

Respiratory System Compliance

The recruitment maneuver may be difficult when respiratory system compliance is relatively good (as in moderate ALI), or when one lung has a good compliance compared with the other. In such conditions, it is difficult to achieve the adequate transmural pressure unless volumes up to 2 L or more are insufflated. Artificially reducing the total respiratory system compliance (by applying external compression or turning prone) may help to reach the required transmural pressure without insufflating excessive volumes.

Once opened, the lung must be kept open, and PEEP is the leading strategy used to prevent lung collapse. The level of PEEP is a compromise between that required to keep the lung open and that which results in overstretching, as noted earlier.

IATROGENIC COST OF MECHANICAL VENTILATION

Inspired Oxygen Fraction

The suggestion that a high FIO_2 (i.e., >0.6) causes lung damage is based on experimental studies carried out on normal animals, in which, in most cases, the inspired air was not appropriately humidified. In the authors' opinion, no consistent evidence shows that high FIO_2 is dangerous in ALI/ARDS because there is worldwide experience with patients treated for days or weeks with 100% oxygen who ultimately survive.

Plateau Pressures and Pressure Swings

It has been suggested that 35 cm H_2O of plateau airway pressure is the safe upper threshold for mechanical ventilation. However, pressure per se is not dangerous (e.g., a diver may have an alveolar pressure of several atmospheres!). What is important is the transmural pressure, and possibly the difference in pressure between end expiration and end inhalation. A plateau pressure of 35 cm H_2O may be associated with a wide range of transmural pressures, depending on the relationship between the lung and chest wall elastances and, in nonparalyzed patients, on the action of respiratory muscles.

The effect of high inflation pressures differs markedly depending on the starting inflation pressure or, more specifically, the lung volume present at end exhalation.

Intratidal Collapse and Decollapse

Intratidal collapse and decollapse are forms of barotrauma that may be most likely when compression atelectasis is the primary type of lung damage. In fact, during inspiration even low plateau pressures (20 to 25 cm H_2O) are sufficient to open the dependent lung regions in which "loose" compression atelectases, probably caused by small airway collapse, are recruited. However, if the PEEP level is not adequate, at end expiration the dependent lung regions collapse again. To avoid this phenomenon, a PEEP level sufficient to counteract the lung weight is required.

VENTILATION STRATEGIES

The authors believe that a single "best" pattern of ventilatory support does not exist for all patients who have ALI/ARDS. To clarify and understand the differences between the various strategies, it is useful to start from the equation of motion for the respiratory system:

EQUATION 65.2

$$\text{Muscle pressure} + \text{ventilator pressure} = (\text{V}_{\text{T}} \times \text{E}) + (\text{resistance} \times \text{flow})$$

Respiratory support may thus be applied in three ways:

1. Driving pressure needed to overcome the elastic and resistive load of the respiratory system is furnished by the ventilator (i.e., the muscle pressure equals zero).
2. Driving pressure is furnished by a combination of muscle pressure and ventilator pressure.
3. Driving pressure is totally furnished by the respiratory muscles (i.e., the ventilator pressure equals zero).

Driving Pressure Provided by the Ventilator Only (Controlled Mechanical Ventilation)

The mode chosen to deliver the ventilation may be volume or pressure targeted. In the volume preset modes, VT is delivered with a predefined inspiratory flow–time profile. As seen from the equation for motion for the respiratory system, the pressure that the ventilator must generate depends on the mechanics of the respiratory system: the higher the elastance, the higher the ventilation pressure. During pressure preset ventilation, the ventilator applies a predefined pressure to the airways. In this case, the higher the elastance, the lower the VT.

Driving Pressure Furnished by Both Respiratory Muscles and Ventilator

In general, ventilators deliver a positive-pressure breath at a preset T (assisted ventilation) or a preset pressure (pressure support), and the muscles of respiration activate the ventilator-delivered breath. A combination of pressure–volume targets is synchronized with intermittent mandatory ventilation, usually given along with pressure support, in which a low-rate, volume-targeted VT is associated with pressure-supported spontaneous ventilation. Some types of combined-modality support may be delivered without intubation (i.e., noninvasive positive-pressure ventilation).

Driving Pressure Furnished Exclusively by Respiratory Muscles

Driving pressure furnished exclusively by respiratory muscles is more a respiratory support than a ventilatory support because the respiratory muscles are sufficiently strong to overcome the impedance of the respiratory system.

Choice of Ventilation Strategy

Over the last few years, a number of studies have been performed to investigate the effects on outcome of low VT versus high VT ventilation for patients with ARDS. These studies, although based on the same rationale (gentle lung treatment),

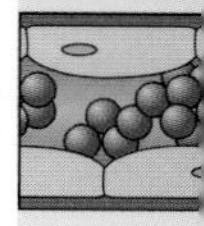

had different powers and different designs. Three studies compared 7 mL VT/kg with 10 to 10.5 mL VT/kg ideal body weight and were not able to show any difference in outcome. One compared two ventilatory strategies, high PEEP/low VT versus low PEEP/high VT, and found impressive differences in mortality. The study was criticized, however, because of reporting an extremely high mortality rate (70%) in the high VT/low PEEP group. The last study of this series is the NIH Network trial, which was the only study adequately powered and found a 9% reduction in mortality rate in patients treated with 6 mL VT/kg as opposed to 12 mL VT/kg. In most of these studies, a "safety limit" for plateau pressure was set at 35 cm H_2O. The contradictory results generated considerable controversy, to the point that a recent review suggested that the 6 mL VT/kg ventilation was unsafe because the relationship between VT and outcome was U shaped, with greater mortalities being associated with both low and high VTs.

However, the "lung protective strategy" (i.e., high PEEP to maintain an open lung and plateau pressures <35 cm H_2O, excepting hypercapnia) is a well accepted form of treatment.

When patients begin to improve, we begin weaning by lowering the FIO_2. Once the FIO_2 reaches 0.4, we slowly start to wean mean airway pressure (1 to 2 cm H_2O/hour lower). At this point, we switch to a mixed form of ventilatory support (e.g., synchronized intermittent mandatory ventilation and pressure support). Spontaneous breathing is tested using continuous positive airway pressure when the patient maintains target blood gases with 5 to 10 cm H_2O PEEP and 5 to 10 cm H_2O pressure support. In less severe ALI/ARDS, noninvasive ventilation or continuous positive airway pressure may be the first approach. Whichever approach is selected, the first principle is *primum non nocere* with regard to the iatrogenic factors discussed previously.

With regard to fluids, the authors believe that the risks of fluid restriction to hemodynamics and kidney function outweigh any limited potential advantage relative to reducing lung edema. The edema in ALI/ARDS has a high protein concentration and, as such, is not easily removed unless the permeability defects are solved. Similarly, "normal" hemodynamic values are sought because studies have not shown any advantages in achieving supranormal values. Finally, enteral nutrition is instituted as soon as possible. If parenteral nutrition is used, the authors limit the caloric intake to 20 to 25 kcal/kg to avoid increasing the carbon dioxide load in a respiratory system that is already compromised, particularly during the weaning process. All of these approaches, however, are a matter of personal opinion, and none can be supported by randomized, controlled trials.

OTHER EXPERIMENTAL STRATEGIES

Strategies able regionally to redistribute VT may allow recruitment while preserving pressures within a safe range. Prone ventilation seems to redistribute VT more homogeneously. Other strategies include extracorporeal membrane oxygenation, high-frequency ventilation, and (more recently) ventilation with perfluorocarbons (i.e., liquid ventilation) and extracorporeal carbon dioxide removal along with low frequency, positive-pressure ventilation. Intratracheal ventilation has been used to facilitate decreasing dead space while using low VT ventilation. Aside from prone positioning, only centers with the required experience and equipment should attempt these more complicated interventions, and then perhaps only in selected patients with ARDS using prospectively designed research protocols, because all these interventions remain experimental and, again with the exception of prone ventilation, carry high risks of complication.

Lung inflammation and epithelial cell injury result in a quantitative and qualitative surfactant deficiency in ALI/ARDS. Unfortunately, inhalation of synthetic surfactant has not yet been shown to be beneficial. Inhaled pulmonary vasodilators have also been tested, but a recent controlled trial of nitric oxide indicated that its beneficial effect on oxygenation is small and is limited to the first 24 hours of treatment.

CLINICAL COURSE AND PREVENTION

Independent of the initial etiology, other insults may occur during the course of the basic disease (i.e., nosocomial pneumonia, iatrogenic barotrauma, appearance of new foci of infection on heart valves or liver). Accordingly, a systematic daily consideration of the etiologic factors and their control, persistence, or development is mandatory.

Pathophysiologic characterization must also be repeated intermittently during the course of the syndrome because lung lesions evolve and the pathophysiologic process, and therefore the approach to treatment, changes.

Intra-alveolar (direct insult) or interstitial (indirect insult) edema characterizes the "early" phases of ARDS, with neutrophilic exudate at first, followed by monocytic and lymphocytic cell recruitment, which further contributes to the epithelial and endothelial injury. Although several proinflammatory and anti-inflammatory mediators and neutrophil markers have been found in patients with ARDS, the complexity of the defense mechanism is such that its efficacy is difficult to evaluate. The response may be homeostatic, which allows recovery to occur, or overwhelming, which perpetuates the lung injury and limits the repair process.

After approximately 1 week, during the so-called "intermediate" phase of ARDS, death of type I cells together with dysfunction of the remaining type II cells, which are unable to produce sufficient surfactant and actively transport sodium, contribute to maintaining lung edema, and thus further distort lung mechanical properties. Endothelial dysfunction and death contribute to plasma and cell transfer from the vascular compartment to the lung, whereas basement membrane collagen exposed to platelets leads to intravascular coagulation, which further compromises lung function.

Meanwhile, under the influence of a set of newly synthesized growth factors, interstitial fibroblasts differentiate into myofibroblasts and migrate into alveolar clots, thus initiating a fibroproliferative response that progressively leads to a fibrous, noncompliant lung. Thus, so-called "late" phase ARDS (>2 weeks) develops, in which several functional and structural modifications occur, such as resorption of the edema, widespread development of fibrosis, microvascular destruction, and development of emphysema-like lesions in the parenchyma (Fig. 65.14). The sponge lung model is not applicable in these conditions because the transmission of superimposed pressures is prevented by fibrosis. These differences in pathologic process imply that the approach to treatment of late-phase ARDS must also differ.

The value of $PaCO_2$ has not been used in classifying ALI/ARDS severity. The authors believe, however, that change in $PaCO_2$ (at a constant minute ventilation) is more informative

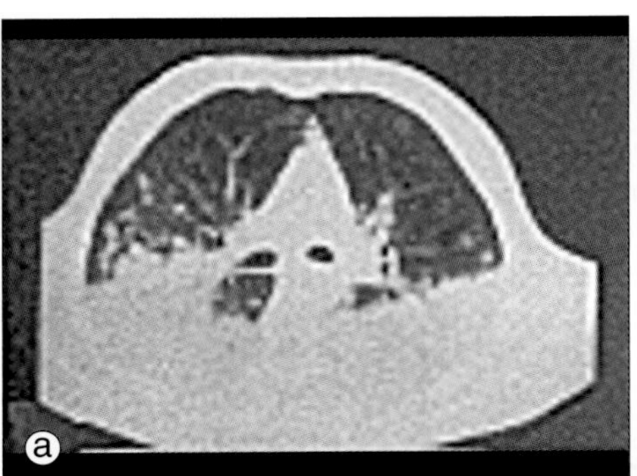

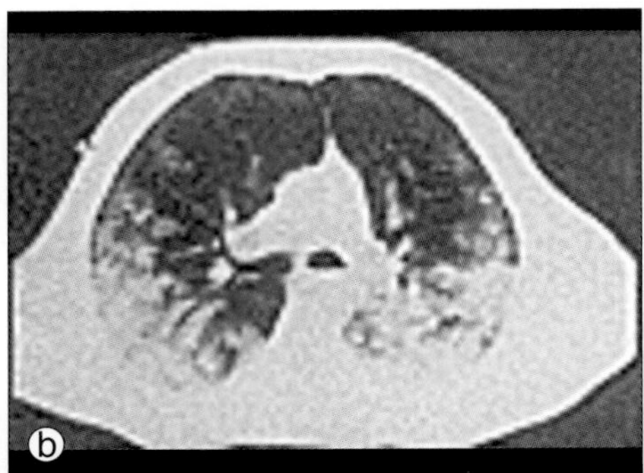

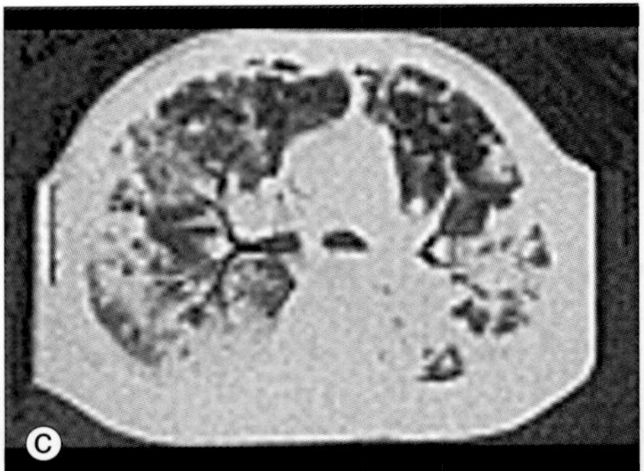

Figure 65.14 Evolution of the acute respiratory distress syndrome (ARDS) lung with time. **a,** Early ARDS (acute phase, week 1). **b,** Intermediate ARDS (week 2). **c,** Late ARDS (week >3). Note the presence of dependent lung densities in the acute phase. In the late phase, lung densities disappeared while emphysema-like lesions appeared throughout the lung.

than changes in oxygenation during the course of ALI/ARDS because this may predict the development of emphysema-like lesions that result from ongoing injury or repair.

The mortality rate of ALI/ARDS in its first description was 7 of 12 patients. Despite nearly three decades of progress in the supportive care of patients who have ARDS, recent studies and reviews continue to report mortality rates that range between 40% and 70%. A recent study that evaluated changes in outcome and severity of ALI/ARDS (as indicated by PaO_2/FIO_2 ratio or lung injury scores) over the past three decades showed that the mortality rate of patients with ARDS remained constant throughout the period studied. Different conclusions were reached in another review, which concluded that in the past 10 years the mortality rate decreased by approximately 20%. In the authors' opinion, a discussion on differences of outcome over the years is academic only. Differences in technology, patient populations, and overall treatments make comparisons extremely difficult.

Although the ability to prevent the development of ALI/ARDS is limited if aspiration pneumonia, pulmonary emboli, or indwelling catheters are considered as a source of sepsis in hospitalized patients, it is clear that careful attention to risk factors that may predispose to ALI/ARDS may be useful. In this context, for example, the efficacy of selective digestive decontamination to prevent secondary lung infection may be useful. In addition, if ventilatory-induced lung injury is a substantial cause of ALI/ARDS, minimization of those factors thought to contribute to this phenomenon (e.g., overstretching, repetitive air space opening and closing, surfactant inactivation) may be helpful.

SUGGESTED READINGS

ARDS Network: Ventilation with lower tidal volumes as compared with traditional tidal volumes for acute lung injury and the acute respiratory distress syndrome. The Acute Respiratory Distress Syndrome Network. N Engl J Med 342:1301-1308, 2000.

Bernard GR, Vincent JL, Laterre PF, et al: The Recombinant Human Protein C Worldwide Evaluation in Severe Sepsis (PROWESS) Study Group. Efficacy and safety of recombinant human activated protein C for severe sepsis. N Engl J Med 344:699-709, 2001.

Gattinoni L, Caironi P, Pelosi P, Goodman LR: What has computed tomography taught us about the acute respiratory distress syndrome? Am J Respir Crit Care Med 164:1701-1711, 2001.

Gattinoni L, Tognoni G, Pesenti A, et al: The Prone-Supine Study Group: Effect of prone positioning on the survival of patients with acute respiratory failure. N Engl J Med 345:568-573, 2001.

Gattinoni L, Vagginelli F, Chiumello D, et al: Physiologic rationale for ventilator setting in acute lung injury/acute respiratory distress syndrome patients. Crit Care Med 31(4 Suppl):S300-S304, 2003.

Goss CH, Brower RG, Hudson LD, et al: Incidence of acute lung injury in the United States. Crit Care Med 31:1607-1611, 2003.

Vincent JL, Sakr Y, Ranieri VM: Epidemiology and outcome of acute respiratory failure in intensive care unit patients. Crit Care Med 31(4 Suppl):S296-S299, 2003.

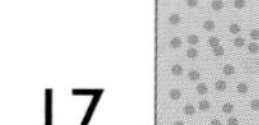
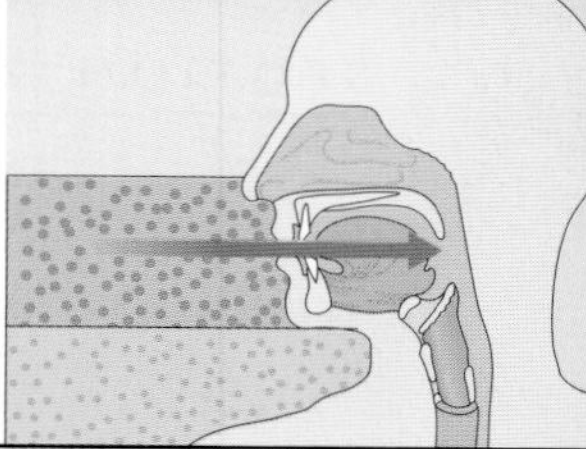

CHAPTER 66 Toxic Inhalational Lung Injury

Lee S. Newman and E. Brigitte Gottschall

A variety of chemicals when liberated into the atmosphere as gases, fumes, or mist can cause irritant lung injury or asphyxiation. As summarized in Table 66.1, any level of the respiratory tract can be the target for toxins, which produce a wide range of disorders from tracheitis and bronchitis to pulmonary edema.

EPIDEMIOLOGY, RISK FACTORS, AND PATHOLOGY

Epidemiology

Smoke inhalation is common among the general population. The use of potentially toxic chemicals in industry continues to rise, and accidental spills, explosions, and fires can result in complex exposures for which little is known of the health consequences. It is challenging to estimate the potential magnitude of the health effects produced by inhaled toxins. For example, in the United States alone, more than 500,000 workers are at risk of exposure to ammonia (NH_3) and other gases such as sulfur dioxide (SO_2). More than 100,000 individuals have potential exposure to hydrogen sulfide (H_2S). Tens of thousands risk smoke inhalation from household fires. The number of people environmentally exposed to potentially hazardous levels of air pollutants such as ozone can be estimated in the tens of millions.

Etiology and Risk Factors

Major risk factors for inhalational exposure and injury are related to the environment and not to the host. Exposures occur randomly in the general environment, such as when a chemical spill occurs on a highway or railroad, carbon monoxide (CO) leaks in a home, or a person incorrectly mixes household chemicals together and releases a gas or aerosol. Smoke that comprises the pyrolysis products of synthetic materials is a common cause of injury to the respiratory tract, as well as a cause of pulmonary insufficiency and death from fires.

Occupational injuries are more common, and occur especially when workers handle chemicals, work in areas that are inadequately ventilated, or enter exposed areas with improper protective equipment. Sources of occupational exposure to major chemical causes of irritant lung injury and asphyxiation are given in Table 66.2.

Factors that influence the acute effects of toxic chemicals include solubility, particle size, concentration, duration of exposure, chemical properties, and host factors such as minute ventilation of the exposed individual. The more water-soluble compounds dissolve in the upper respiratory tract and airways, whereas the less water-soluble agents tend to bypass the upper airway and affect peripheral airways and pulmonary parenchyma, as summarized in Figure 66.1.

Pathology

In general, the upper airway can be affected by most inhaled toxins, which result in edema of the nasal passage, posterior oropharynx, and larynx. In severe cases, mucous membrane ulceration and hemorrhage can ensue. Toxins of low water solubility may reach the lung parenchyma without necessarily producing upper airway lesions. If breath holding, laryngospasm, and normal "scrubbing" activities of the nasopharynx fail to contain the exposure, lesions develop in the trachea and bronchi (e.g., paralysis of cilia, increased mucus production, goblet cell hyperplasia, injury to airway epithelium, epithelial denudation, exudation, submucosal hemorrhage, and edema). Pseudomembranes may form along the trachea and bronchi. The consequences may include various degrees of bronchiolitis, bronchiolitis obliterans (Fig. 66.2), and organizing pneumonia (Fig. 66.3). Bronchiolitis has been associated with exposures to nitrogen oxides (nitric oxide [NO], nitrogen dioxide [NO_2], and nitrogen peroxide [N_2O_4]), sulfur dioxide, ammonia, chlorine (Cl_2), phosgene, fly ash that contains trichloroethylene (C_2HCl_3), ozone (O_3), hydrogen sulfide, hydrogen fluoride (HF), metal oxide fumes, dusts (e.g., asbestos, silica, talc, and grain dust), free-base cocaine, tobacco smoke, and fire smoke.

Parenchymal injury is less common than airway damage. When alveolar or interstitial injury occurs, both epithelial and endothelial damage is observed. Injury typically results in alveolar–capillary leak, and the pathologic changes of acute respiratory distress syndrome (ARDS). Diffuse alveolar damage is a common histologic pattern in acute interstitial lung disease caused by inhaled toxins. It is characterized by widespread, diffuse edema, epithelial necrosis and cell sloughing (with exudates that fill the alveolar spaces), and formation of hyaline membranes (Fig. 66.4). Later, diffuse alveolar damage may organize, which leads to proliferation of type II pneumonocytes, resorption of the hyaline membranes and exudates, and fibroblast proliferation. Long-term survivors of such parenchymal injury may fully recover or be left with various degrees of permanent interstitial fibrosis.

Pathogenesis

Asphyxiants, such as methane (CH_4) and carbon dioxide (CO_2), displace oxygen (O_2) from the air or, in the case of carbon monoxide, interfere with normal oxidative metabolism and oxygen transport. Typically, the more soluble gases produce greater injury in the upper airway, whereas less soluble gases

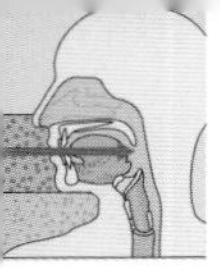

Table 66.1 Range of toxicity produced by inhaled agents	
Example of toxins	**Effect**
Carbon monoxide, cyanide, hydrogen sulfide	Asphyxiation
Ammonia	Mucous membrane irritation and sloughing
Ammonia, phosgene, hydrogen sulfide	Laryngeal edema and obstruction
Hydrogen chloride, chlorine	Tracheobronchitis
Ammonia	Bronchiectasis
Sulfur dioxide, hydrogen chloride, oxides of nitrogen, ozone	Bronchoconstriction, airway edema, asthma
Oxides of nitrogen, sulfur oxides	Bronchiolitis obliterans
Hydrogen fluoride, mustard gas	Chemical pneumonitis
Chlorine, phosgene	Acute respiratory distress syndrome
Hydrogen sulfide	Bacterial pneumonia
Ammonia	Pulmonary interstitial fibrosis
Hydrofluoric acid	Systemic effects, hypocalcemia, hypomagnesemia
Nitric oxide	Systemic effects, methemoglobinemia

Table 66.2 Sources of exposure to inhalational toxins	
Toxin	**Sources of exposure**
Ammonia	Agriculture, explosives, plastics
Hydrogen chloride	Fertilizers, textiles, dyes, rubber manufacture
Hydrofluoric acid	Fertilizers, insecticides, glass and ceramic etching, masonry, metal working, pharmaceuticals, chemical manufacture
Sulfur dioxide	Air pollution, smelting, power plants, chemical manufacture, paper manufacture, food preparation
Chlorine	Household cleaners, paper, textiles, sewage treatment, swimming pools
Oxides of nitrogen	Air pollution, welding, hockey rinks, chemical and dye manufacture, agriculture
Phosgene	Firefighters; paint strippers; chemical, pharmaceutical, and dye manufacturing; and chemical warfare
Mustard gas	Chemical warfare
Ozone	Welding, air pollution, high altitude, chemical manufacture
Carbon monoxide	Firefighters, smoke inhalation, smelters, miners, transportation, home furnaces
Hydrogen cyanide	Metallurgy, electroplating, plastics, polyurethane manufacture
Hydrogen sulfide	Metallurgy, chemical manufacture, wastewater treatment, natural gas and oil drilling, paper mills, coke ovens, rayon manufacture, rubber vulcanization

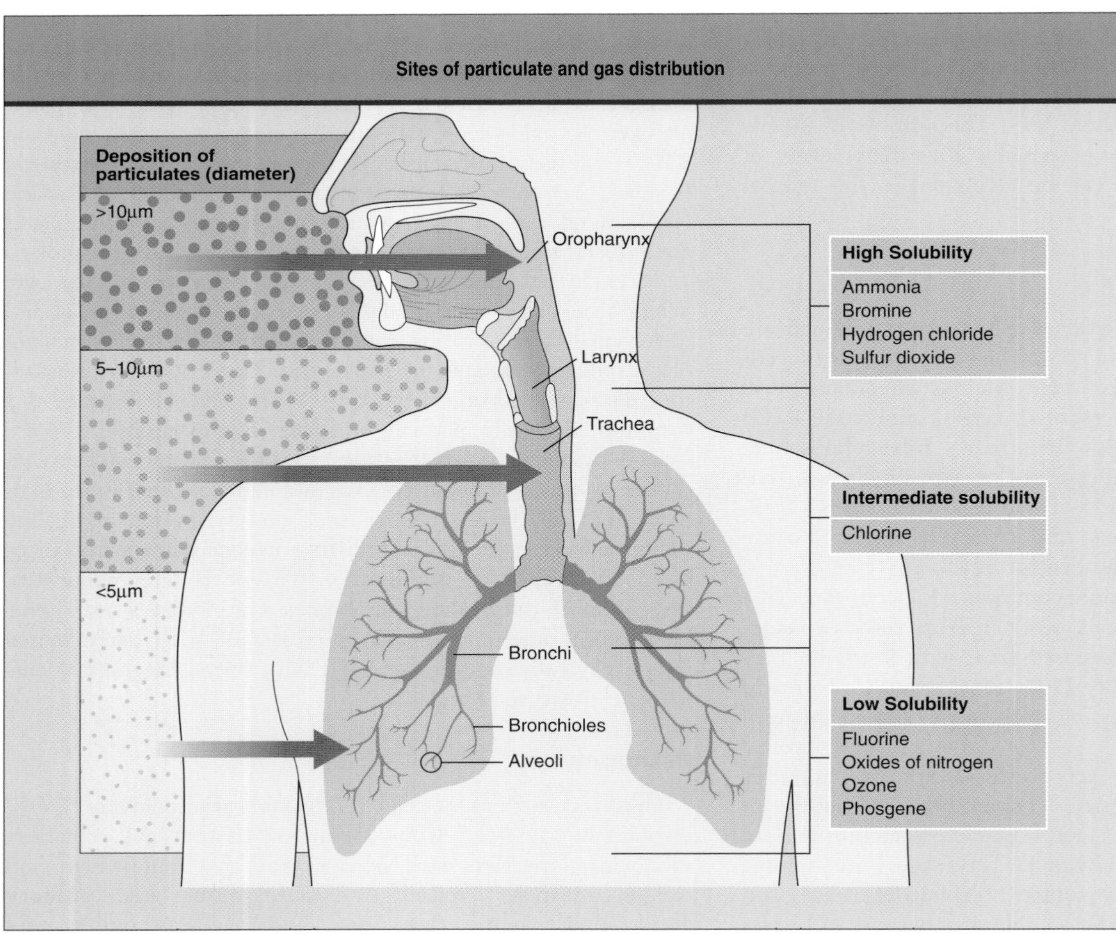

Figure 66.1 Distribution of gases and particulate matter in the respiratory tract influences the site of toxic injury.

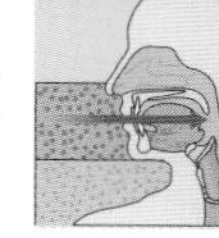

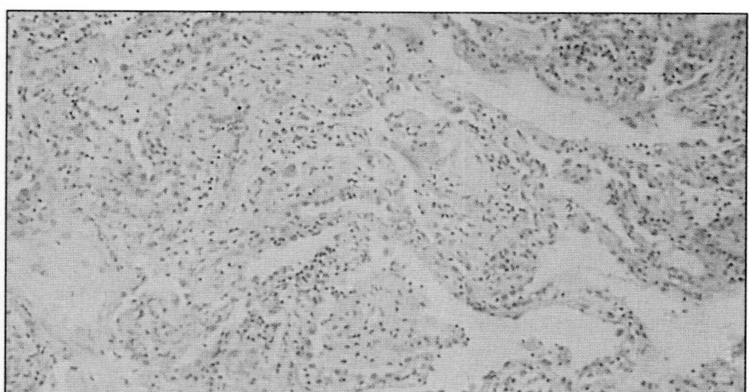

Figure 66.2 Bronchiolitis obliterans organizing pneumonia caused by inhalation of oxides of nitrogen in a silo filler.

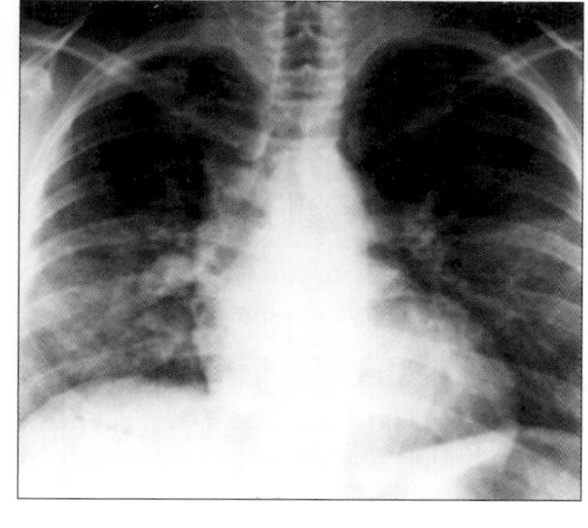

Figure 66.5 Radiographic changes produced by diffuse alveolar damage. Chest radiograph of the same patient as in Figure 66-4 shows acute, diffuse alveolar and interstitial infiltrates.

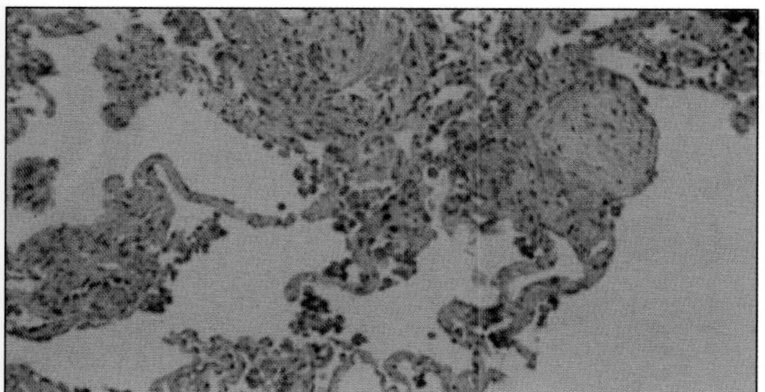

Figure 66.3 Organizing pneumonia after sulfur dioxide intoxication.

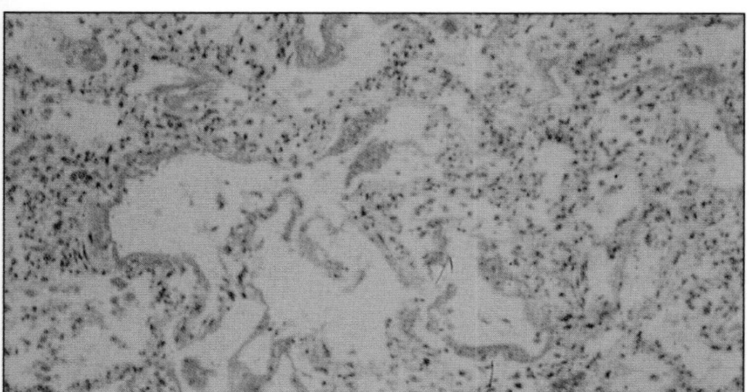

Figure 66.4 Diffuse alveolar damage caused by anhydrous ammonia inhalation. An agricultural worker inhaled the gas when a hose broke during the transfer of this fertilizing agent.

injure distal airways and parenchyma. Some of the irritant gases produce direct cellular injury because they are alkalis (e.g., ammonia) or acids (e.g., phosgene). Others, such as ozone and oxides of nitrogen, form oxygen free radicals that cause respiratory tract injury. These gases may also produce smooth muscle bronchoconstriction and stimulate afferent parasympathetic receptors, which explain some of their ability to induce airway hyperreactivity and bronchoconstriction. Chronic lower-level exposures to various toxic gases, such as sulfur dioxide and chlorine, can induce copious mucus secretion, cough, bronchoconstriction, and bronchitis as a physiologic response to the inhalational exposure. Chronic bronchitis is common among workers exposed to relatively low levels of irritants and may increase their risk for development of chronic airflow obstruction and accelerated longitudinal decline in forced expiratory volume in 1 second (FEV_1). In some instances, nonspecific airway hyperreactivity is induced by persistent, nonspecific irritant exposures.

CLINICAL FEATURES AND DIAGNOSIS

Initial efforts at diagnosis focus on the nature of the compound inhaled, approximating the probable circumstances of exposure (including the magnitude and duration of exposure), determining the water solubility of the inhaled agent, and determining whether the individual was exposed to multiple irritants and asphyxiants simultaneously, as occurs in firefighters or others subjected to smoke inhalation. Inhalational injury is suspected in those who have facial burns or inflamed nares. Headache and dizziness, along with chest pains and emesis, suggest systemic poisons, such as cyanide or hydrogen sulfide. Unconscious victims found in confined spaces are assumed to have received longer inhalational exposures than conscious ones because of the unprotected airways and concentrated exposures. Evidence of hoarseness, upper airway stridor, wheezing or rales, cough, and sputum production is assessed. Chest radiographs may show pulmonary edema, atelectasis, or infiltrates (Fig. 66.5), although they are often negative early after exposure. Flow–volume loops are the most sensitive noninvasive indicators of upper and lower airway obstruction. Hypoxemia in the face of a normal arterial partial pressure of oxygen suggests carbon monoxide toxicity. Carboxyhemoglobin levels are obtained for all fire and explosion victims. Metabolic acidosis may indicate cyanide or hydrogen sulfide intoxication.

In individuals who have persistent symptoms months after exposure, bronchial provocation tests with methacholine may help assess whether the individual has reactive airway dysfunction syndrome. Computed tomography may help determine if permanent fibrotic changes have developed.

Chemical Irritants

AMMONIA

Ammonia is a colorless, water-soluble, alkaline gas with a pungent odor. Because it is usually transported as a liquid, many accidents occur when it is being transferred from tanks to farm

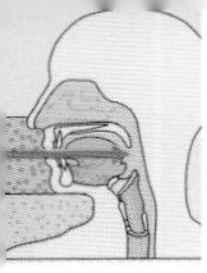

equipment. When it comes in contact with the mucosa, ammonia reacts with water to form a strong alkali, ammonium hydroxide (NH_4OH). Acute irritation of mucous membranes can be followed within hours by sloughing of the upper airway mucosa, edema, and obstruction. Laryngeal edema can present without other obvious clinical signs of burns, but if skin burns are present, inhalational injury is likely. Unusual complications include pneumonia and ARDS, which occur within hours to a few days of exposure. Long-term consequences include persistent bronchitis, bronchiectasis, airflow obstruction, interstitial fibrosis, and impaired gas exchange. Treatment is supportive—bronchodilators, oxygen therapy, and observation for need for airway protection. Early intubation may be required to defend the airway from acute laryngeal obstruction.

HYDROGEN CHLORIDE

Hydrogen chloride (HCl) is highly water soluble, and injures the mucosa of the upper airways because of its acidity. Typically encountered in the manufacture of fertilizers, textiles, rubber, and dyes, acute exposure causes mucous membrane irritation of the eyes and airways at levels as low at 5 to 10 parts per million (ppm). Acute higher levels of exposure can cause acute airflow obstruction and gas exchange abnormalities. Meat wrappers become exposed to hydrogen chloride when they heat polyvinyl chloride film.

HYDROFLUORIC ACID

Hydrofluoric acid (HF) is highly corrosive, and most of the health effects from hydrofluoric acid involve dermal injury to the hands. Hydrofluoric acid releases free hydrogen ions that penetrate and corrode the skin, potentially down to bone, and even produce bone demineralization and necrosis. The respiratory effects parallel those of the skin, except that in the lungs the effects have a very rapid onset and patients present with acute respiratory distress. Hydrofluoric acid is water soluble and thus exerts its predominant effects on the upper airways, which results in the rapid onset of tissue damage and bronchoconstriction, and sometimes even leads to chemical pneumonitis, delayed-onset pulmonary edema, and death.

SULFUR DIOXIDE

Sulfur dioxide and sulfuric acid (H_2SO_4) aerosols are produced by fossil fuel combustion. They are encountered in power plants and in various industrial processes such as smelting, chemical manufacture, paper manufacture, food preservation, metal and ore refining, and refrigeration. Past sulfur dioxide air pollution catastrophes have been associated with increased death rates for patients with chronic lung disease and the elderly.

As little as 0.5 ppm of sulfur dioxide can be detected in air from its characteristic odor. At levels of 6 to 10 ppm, immediate irritation of eyes and nasopharynx are reported. High exposures ($\geq$50 ppm) injure the larynx, trachea, bronchi, and alveoli. A wide range of individual variability in the response to this substance is found, but atopic and asthmatic subjects show the most susceptibility. Prior exposure to ozone may potentiate the effect of sulfur dioxide in asthmatic subjects. Classically, patients first experience a burning of the eyes, nose, and throat (with associated cough, chest pain, chest tightness, and dyspnea), along with conjunctivitis, corneal burns, and pharyngeal edema, followed hours later by pulmonary edema. Bronchiolitis obliterans can develop 2 to 3 weeks after exposure. Persistent airflow obstruction has been observed in smelter workers up to 4 years after overexposure, probably because of bronchiolitis obliterans.

Treatment is symptomatic. Systemic corticosteroids may be beneficial in acute toxicity. Bronchospasm in asthmatic patients may reverse spontaneously after removal from exposure, or may require administration of bronchodilators and inhaled corticosteroids.

CHLORINE

Chlorine is of intermediate solubility, and liberates hydrogen chloride and oxygen free radicals when it contacts water. The result is dose-dependent epithelial cell injury. At low levels of exposure, the upper airways and eyes are irritated. Increasing levels of exposure injure the nasopharynx and larynx. Higher exposures result in pulmonary edema within 6 to 24 hours. Pulmonary function tests typically show airflow obstruction and air trapping. Long-term consequences include persistent airflow obstruction in some survivors. Clinical management is supportive. Even symptomatic individuals who have negative physical examinations and laboratory tests must be observed for at least 6 hours because of the potential for a delay in the onset of significant airway toxicity. If symptoms persist, corticosteroids may improve outcome.

OXIDES OF NITROGEN

The oxides of nitrogen (NO, NO_2, N_2O_4) can produce fatal respiratory injury for some of the millions of workers who come into contact with these gases. Occupations at risk include coal miners after firing of explosives, welders who work with acetylene torches in confined spaces, hockey rink workers, and chemical workers who may be exposed to byproduct fumes in the manufacture of dyes, lacquers, and nitric acid (HNO_3). "Silo-filler's disease" is caused by inhalation of nitrogen dioxide that forms when corn or alfalfa stored in a silo ferments. The risk is greatest in the first few weeks after the silo is filled. Because the oxides of nitrogen have low water solubility, the lower respiratory tract can be exposed to these potent oxidizers with little warning. Nitrogen dioxide reacts with water in the lung to form nitric and nitrous (HNO_2) acids. The oxides dissociate into oxygen free radicals, nitrates, and nitrites, which cause tissue inflammation, lipid peroxidation, and impairment of surfactant activity (among other cellular changes). Notably, nitric oxide has a high affinity for hemoglobin, and so causes methemoglobinemia.

With exposures of 15 to 25 ppm, acute mucous membrane irritation affects the eyes and throat. At exposure levels of 25 to 100 ppm, toxic pneumonitis and bronchiolitis can develop, often with a smothering sensation and dyspnea. Exposures above 150 ppm are often fatal, and are associated with bronchiolitis obliterans, chemical pneumonitis, and pulmonary edema. Nitrogen oxide and nitrogen dioxide produce the greatest degree of toxicity, which includes pulmonary edema and subsequent bronchiolitis obliterans. Symptom onset may be delayed and patients are also cautioned that relapses can occur 3 to 6 weeks after initial exposure, with symptoms of cough, chills, fever, and shortness of breath. In some individuals, persistent obstructive lung disease and chronic bronchitis develop. Case reports suggest improvement after corticosteroids in those who manifest bronchiolar inflammation.

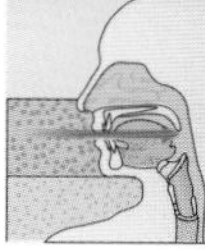

PHOSGENE

Also called carbonyl chloride, phosgene replaced chlorine as the preferred chemical weapon of World War I, and resulted in the majority of gas attack fatalities. Phosgene is an intermediate product in the manufacture of isocyanates, pesticides, dyes, and pharmaceuticals. It has a low odor threshold at 1 ppm, and produces a characteristic smell of musty hay. As a result of its poor water solubility, phosgene causes only mild upper airway and eye irritant symptoms, and deposits distally in the lung where it hydrolyzes to form hydrochloric acid (aqueous HCl) and carbon dioxide. At high levels of exposure, dyspnea, chest tightness, and cough occur. Acute exposure produces necrosis and sloughing of tracheal, bronchial, and bronchiolar mucosa with associated edema, hemorrhage, and atelectasis. Progressive respiratory failure and ARDS may follow.

MUSTARD GAS

Sulfur mustard gas was first used as a chemical warfare agent in Europe in 1917. Mustard agents are not gases, but liquids at environmental temperatures. They are volatile, enter vapor phase at ambient temperatures, and have low water solubility. Exposure to sulfur mustard produces eye irritation and swelling within 2 to 3 hours. With higher exposure, blurred vision, conjunctival edema, and iritis can occur, with potential for corneal ulceration. The skin itches, becomes pruritic and erythematous, and, 4 to 16 hours later, forms blisters. Acute respiratory damage in this setting may be evident within a few hours or, more commonly, several days later. Chemical pneumonitis and pulmonary edema can also occur, with upper airway irritation, sneezing, hoarseness, epistaxis, cough, and dyspnea. Acute injury includes edema, inflammation, and destruction of the airway epithelium, with pseudomembranes developing that are similar to those seen with diphtheria. Secondary complications include infection and airway stenosis. The long-term effects include death caused by respiratory infections, chronic bronchitis, and accelerated longitudinal decline in airflow.

OZONE

Ozone is a light blue gas with an acrid "electric" odor. It occurs naturally in the stratosphere, where it is produced by the interaction between oxygen and ultraviolet light. In the troposphere, it is produced as a result of photochemical reactions between oxides of nitrogen and volatile organic compounds. Ozone is a major component of environmental air pollution and remains a serious pollutant for urban populations worldwide. Its low water solubility means that ozone principally affects the lower respiratory tract. In healthy individuals exposed to low concentrations of ozone, acute increases in airway resistance and decreases in FEV_1 and forced vital capacity have been reported, probably through a neural reflex mechanism. With acute exposures to low concentrations, patients can experience chest pain, dyspnea, and cough. Exposure to concentrations as low as 0.08 ppm for 6 hours with intermittent exercise has been shown to cause lung function and inflammatory changes. Exposure to 0.12 ppm for 1 hour is the U.S. Environmental Protection Agency Air Quality Standard.

Chemical Asphyxiants

Nitrous oxide, carbon monoxide, hydrogen cyanide (HCN), and hydrogen sulfide interfere with oxygen delivery, which results in asphyxiation. Others, such as methane, ethane (C_2H_6), argon (Ar), and helium (He_2), are more innocuous at low concentrations, but at high exposure levels can displace oxygen or block the reaction of cytochrome oxidase or hemoglobin, impairing cellular respiratory and oxygen transport. Several important asphyxiants are discussed in the following sections.

CARBON MONOXIDE

Carbon monoxide is colorless, tasteless, and odorless, and is the major cause of death by poisoning in the United States and most industrialized countries. Exposure results from incomplete combustion of carbon-containing materials such as gasoline, coal, and wood. Home exposures occur from furnace gas leaks or fire smoke inhalation. Methylene chloride (CH_2Cl_2), which is used in paint strippers and as a household solvent, metabolizes into carbon monoxide and can be deadly if handled in poorly ventilated areas.

Severe forms of carbon monoxide poisoning are characterized by unconsciousness, seizures, syncope, coma, neurologic deficits, pulmonary edema, myocardial ischemia, and metabolic acidosis. Lower exposures produce symptoms of headache, nausea, weakness, giddiness, and tinnitus. Confusion typically occurs at carboxyhemoglobin levels greater than 30%, with coma ensuing at 35% to 45%, and death at 50%. In addition to acute toxic effects, victims are at risk for delayed neuropsychological effects. Carboxyhemoglobin levels correlate poorly with the clinical severity of neurologic sequelae. Carbon monoxide half-life in individuals at rest is approximately 4 hours and can be reduced to 60 to 90 minutes by breathing 100% oxygen by face mask or to less than 60 minutes with oxygen administered by manual bag-assisted ventilation.

Nonrandomized studies have found that hyperbaric oxygen reverses the acute effects of carbon monoxide poisoning and is the most rapid means of reversing acute poisoning. Additional treatments may improve acute neurologic defects. Results of controlled trials are unclear as to the efficacy of hyperbaric oxygen as a treatment for the delayed neuropsychological symptoms. Cardiac monitoring is warranted for individuals who have carboxyhemoglobin levels greater than 25% because of the risk of arrhythmias and myocardial infarction.

HYDROGEN CYANIDE

Individuals exposed to smoke generated by the combustion or pyrolysis of plastics and polyurethanes are at particular risk of hydrogen cyanide toxicity. The fumes are absorbed through the skin and respiratory tract. By binding to the cytochrome A–cytochrome A_3 subcomplex, hydrogen cyanide blocks oxidative phosphorylation and mitochondrial oxygen utilization, which results in lactic acidosis.

Symptoms produced by exposures to 50 ppm of cyanide gas include headache, tachycardia, tachypnea, and dizziness. Exposures greater than 100 ppm can cause confusion, apnea, and seizures. The patient may emit a bitter almond odor, but this is not a reliable or consistent marker of exposure. The key to diagnosis rests with the occupational and environmental history. Venous blood appears hyperoxygenated and the patient may have a distinctive red appearance before respiratory insufficiency, although, as in carbon monoxide poisoning, this is not a reliable clinical sign. Carboxyhemoglobin levels are measured to help separate cyanide intoxication from carbon monoxide poisoning. Treatment focuses on life support measures and detoxification. Early mechanical ventilation, hyperoxygenation, and treatment of metabolic acidosis are critical. Both amyl nitrate and sodium nitrite are recommended. Amyl nitrate and sodium nitrite form methemoglobin.

HYDROGEN SULFIDE

Hydrogen sulfide is both a respiratory irritant and asphyxiant. As a colorless, naturally occurring gas, it is found in marshes and sulfur springs, and as a decay product of organic matter. It is known for its typical "rotten egg" odor. Occupational exposure occurs in the manufacture of chemicals and metals, and in petroleum refineries, natural gas plants, coke ovens, paper mills, rubber vulcanization, rayon manufacture, and tanneries. Heavier than air, hydrogen sulfide accumulates in low-lying areas; it causes poisoning during oil drilling and wastewater treatment and as a result of natural gas field leaks. The hydrogen sulfide reaction with metalloenzymes, such as cytochrome oxidase, accounts for much of its toxicity in humans.

The odor threshold for this gas is low (0.13 ppm). At concentrations of 50 ppm, hydrogen sulfide is a mucous membrane irritant. Above 100 ppm, the gas fatigues the sense of olfaction, which makes individuals insensitive to its continued presence. When inhaled, it preferentially affects the lower respiratory tract. At concentrations of 250 ppm, pulmonary edema can occur. At 500 ppm, systemic and neurologic effects develop, with sudden loss of consciousness seen above 700 ppm. Above 1000 ppm, the gas produces hyperpnea and apnea, which paralyze respiratory drive centers. Thus, death caused by asphyxia can result at 1000 ppm or above.

Prolonged low-level (50 ppm) exposures can cause respiratory tract inflammation and drying; typical symptoms of cough, sore throat, hoarseness, rhinitis, and chest tightness occur between 50 and 250 ppm. At higher acute exposure levels, such symptoms may not manifest because of the rapid absorption of the gas through the lung into the bloodstream.

Management is generally supportive, with prompt endotracheal intubation and mechanical ventilation for severe cases of intoxication. Oxygen enhances sulfide metabolism and benefits hypoxic tissue. Because the mechanism of toxicity is similar to that of cyanide, induction of methemoglobinemia with infusion of 3% sodium nitrite or inhalation of amyl nitrate is recommended. Hyperbaric oxygen therapy may be beneficial.

Complex Exposures

In practice, individuals who suffer inhalational injuries are frequently exposed to complex mixtures of toxic compounds, rather than a single agent. Such mixtures may be poorly characterized, but can contain admixtures of combustion products, pyrolysis products, metals, particulates, and gas. Recent studies illustrate the ability of such mixtures to produce a range of airway and diffuse interstitial lung lesions. For example, as a consequence of exposures immediately after the World Trade Center attack, rescue workers experienced acute, and often prolonged, cough and airway hyperreactivity consistent with reactive airway dysfunction syndrome. Factors such as dust alkalinity may have contributed to this condition, although, as is often the case in acute situations, detailed information about the inhalational exposures in those workers is limited.

PITFALLS AND CONTROVERSIES

Many of the uncertainties in this arena of pulmonary medicine pertain to the management and treatment of inhalational injury, for which a few general comments apply. In cases of severe inhalational injury, intubation may be required for airway protection. Careful observation, preferably in an intensive care setting, is recommended for suspected cases of significant inhalational injury. Direct laryngoscopy or fiber-optic bronchoscopy is advocated by some investigators to assess for laryngeal edema. However, no clear guidelines are available to direct clinicians as to when intubation, laryngoscopy, or bronchoscopy is warranted. Although many clinicians may empirically prescribe corticosteroids, such medications have not been proved efficacious. We depend on case reports and small case series to justify the use of corticosteroids.

A common clinical pitfall is to dismiss patients prematurely who may be at risk for delayed-onset respiratory disorders such as asthma, bronchiolitis obliterans, chemical pneumonitis, or pulmonary edema. Given sufficient dose and solubility, most acutely inhaled substances pose a risk for immediate or delayed-onset pulmonary edema, which warrants careful observation. Even those toxin victims who are thought to be stable and ready for discharge from the emergency department must be given detailed instructions about the warning signs of delayed-onset respiratory tract injury.

SUGGESTED READINGS

Amshel CE, Fealk MH, Phillips BJ, Caruso DM: Anhydrous ammonia burns: Case report and review of the literature. Burns 26:493-497, 2000.

Das R, Blanc PD: Chlorine gas exposure and the lung: A review. Toxicol Ind Health 9:439-455, 1993.

Dorevitch S, Forst L, Conroy L, Levy P: Toxic inhalation fatalities of US construction workers, 1990 to 1999. J Occup Environ Med 44:657-662, 2002.

Douglas WW, Hepper NGG, Colby TV: Silo-filler's disease. Mayo Clin Proc 64:291-304, 1989.

Hnizdo E, Sullivan PA, Moon Bang K, Wagner G: Association between chronic obstructive pulmonary disease and employment by industry and occupation in the US population: A study of data from the Third National Health and Nutrition Examination Survey. Am J Epidemiol 156:738-746, 2002.

Kennedy SM: Acquired airway hyperresponsiveness from nonimmunogenic irritant exposure. In Beckett WS, Bascome R (eds): Occupational Medicine: State of the Art Reviews. Philadelphia, Hanley and Belfus, 1992, pp 287-300.

Malo JL, Chan-Yeung M: Occupational asthma [review]. J Allergy Clin Immunol 108:317-328, 2001.

Martyny J, Glazer CS, Newman LS: Respiratory protection. N Engl J Med 347:824-830, 2002.

Miller K, Chang A: Acute inhalation injury. Emerg Med Clin North Am 21:533-557, 2003.

Newman LS: Current concepts: Occupational illness. N Engl J Med 333:1128-1134, 1995.

Perkner JJ, Fennelly KP, Balkissoon R, et al: Irritant-associated vocal cord dysfunction. J Occup Environ Med 40:136-143, 1998.

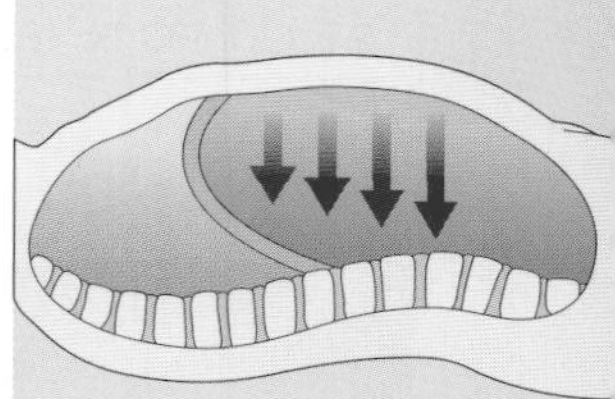

CHAPTER 67 Scoliosis and Kyphoscoliosis

Anita K. Simonds

Spinal curvature is the most common cause of chest wall deformity. The term *scoliosis* refers to lateral curvature of the spine (Fig. 67.1) and was described by Hippocrates as early as 500 BC. Kyphosis indicates backward curvature in an anteroposterior (median) plane, and lordosis forward curvature. Many patients who have a thoracic scoliosis are mistakenly described as having a kyphoscoliosis, because the rib angle prominence is misinterpreted as a kyphotic component. In fact, most idiopathic thoracic scolioses incorporate a lordotic and rotatory element. The degree of lateral curvature is expressed by the Cobb angle, which is calculated from a radiograph as shown in Figure 67.2.

EPIDEMIOLOGY, RISK FACTORS, AND PATHOPHYSIOLOGY

The causes of chest wall deformity due to spinal deformity are shown in Table 67.1. By far the most common form of scoliosis is the idiopathic variety, which accounts for approximately 80% of cases. Scoliotic curves of more than 35 degrees affect 1 in 1000 people, and those that exceed 70 degrees are estimated to occur at a rate of 0.1 per 1000; females are at greater risk of severe curves than are males. About 3 or 4 children per 1000 require supervision by a specialist for their spinal curvature, and a third of these will require intervention, such as corrective surgery or bracing. Idiopathic scoliosis occurs more often with increasing maternal age and in higher socioeconomic groups, but there is no association between the incidence of scoliosis and birth order or season of birth.

Marfan syndrome affects 1 in 5000 people, and around 63% of affected individuals develop a spinal deformity. Diagnosis can be confirmed by linkage to the Marfan syndrome gene *MFS1*, which produces fibrillin. Related syndromes may result from mutations in microfibrils that interact with fibrillin in the extracellular matrix. Congenital contractual arachnodactyly (Beals syndrome), in which scoliosis is common, has also been shown to be caused by fibrillin deficiency. The genetic basis of idiopathic scoliosis remains unclear, and causation may be multifactorial in that particular growth patterns may exacerbate a genetic predisposition. Approximately 30% of individuals with an idiopathic scoliosis have an affected first-degree relative. A mouse model for idiopathic scoliosis has recently been identified.

Spinal curvature is acquired in neuromuscular disorders that involve the chest wall and thoracic musculature before skeletal maturity occurs. More than 50% of boys who have Duchenne muscular dystrophy develop scoliosis, and spinal curvature is common in many of the other congenital muscular dystrophies, myopathies, and conditions such as types I and II spinal muscular atrophy. Scoliosis often develops in children and young adults who undergo thoracotomy.

Kyphosis

Idiopathic kyphosis is rare (see Table 67.1). An increase in thoracic kyphosis occurs with age and is exacerbated by factors that increase a tendency to osteoporosis such as oral corticosteroid therapy. Pott's tuberculosis (TB) of the spine is still a common cause of acquired kyphosis.

Effects of Chest Wall Deformity on Respiratory and Cardiac Function

Chest wall disorders affect respiratory function and cause a restrictive ventilatory defect. Any significant scoliosis or kyphosis results in a loss of height, so that arm span is used to predict normal lung volumes. As a rule of thumb, patients who have a thoracic curve greater than 70 degrees are subject to significant ventilatory limitation.

LUNG VOLUMES

Although both scoliosis and kyphosis diminish lung volumes, which results in a restrictive ventilatory defect, lateral curvature has a more profound effect on chest wall mechanics. Total lung capacity is reduced in all chest wall disorders. In a pure scoliosis, both vital capacity (VC) and expiratory reserve volume are decreased with relative preservation of residual volume (Table 67.2). An obstructive ventilatory defect is rare in scoliosis and kyphosis, unless the individual is a smoker or has coexistent asthma or the scoliosis results in bronchial torsion.

The relationship between pulmonary impairment and the deformity is complex and cannot be predicted accurately from the Cobb angle alone. The four major determinants of a reduced VC are the number of vertebrae involved in the curve, the cephalad position of the curve, the Cobb angle, and the degree of loss of normal thoracic kyphosis.

In paralytic scoliosis, lung volumes are reduced not only by chest wall restriction, but also by inspiratory muscle weakness.

CHEST WALL MECHANICS

Chest wall compliance is an important determinant of lung volumes and the work of breathing. Individuals with a Cobb angle of less than 50 degrees experience a minimal reduction in chest wall compliance, whereas the compliance is likely to be significantly reduced if the Cobb angle is greater than 100 degrees. A direct relationship between Cobb angle and chest wall compliance is not seen in patients who have neuromuscular disorders, as respiratory muscle weakness contributes independently to chest wall stiffness. Alteration in chest wall properties cannot solely be attributed to the mechanical deformity of scoliosis, as a decrease in chest wall compliance has been

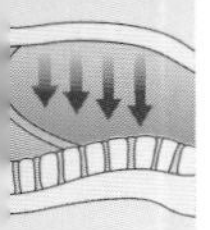

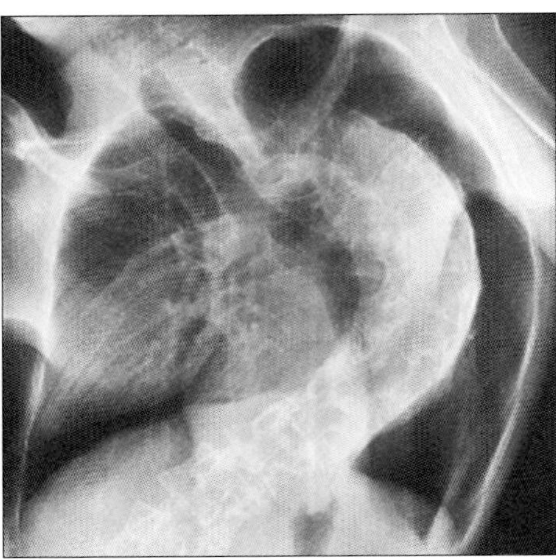

Figure 67.1 Early-onset thoracic scoliosis caused by arthrogryposis.

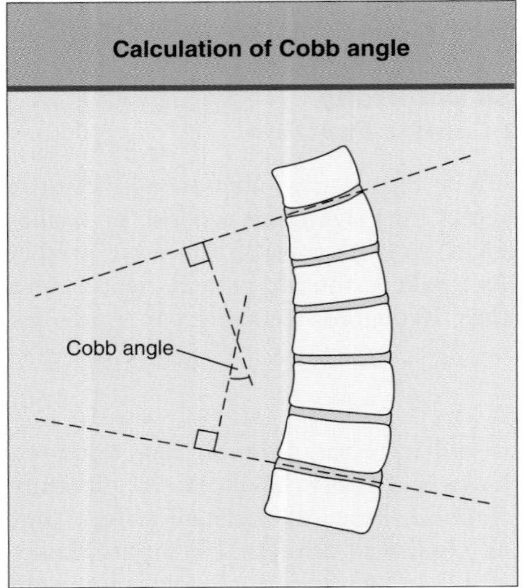

Figure 67.2 Method of calculation of Cobb angle. From the vertebral bodies at the top and bottom of the curve, lines are drawn parallel to the planes of the vertebral bodies. Lines perpendicular to these are then drawn, and the Cobb angle is found at the intersection.

Table 67.1
Classification of spinal deformity

Idiopathic deformities	Associated with neuromuscular disease
Idiopathic scoliosis	Cerebral palsy
Idiopathic kyphosis	Poliomyelitis
Congenital deformities	Muscular dystrophies
Bone	Myopathies
Scoliosis	Hereditary sensory motor neuropathies
Kyphosis	Friedreich's ataxia
Cord	Syringomyelia
Myelodysplasia	**Acquired deformity caused by**
Syndromes in which scoliosis is common	Surgery/trauma
Neurofibromatosis	Infection
Marfan syndrome	Pyogenic
Osteogenesis imperfecta	Tuberculosis (Pott's kyphosis)
Klippel–Feil syndrome	Radiotherapy
Mucopolysaccharidoses	Tumor
Treacher Collins syndrome	Neuroblastoma
Goldenhar's syndrome	Osteoma
Apert's syndrome	Hemangioma
Ehlers-Danlos syndrome	Chordoma
Vertebral and epiphyseal dysplasias	Eosinophilic granuloma
Arthrogryposis	

Table 67.2
Typical pulmonary function results in idiopathic thoracic scoliosis

Parameter	Effect
Forced expiratory volume in 1 s (FEV_1)	Reduced
Forced vital capacity (FVC)	Reduced
FEV_1/FVC	Normal
Residual volume	Normal
Total lung capacity	Reduced
Transfer factor for carbon monoxide (DLCO)	Reduced
Transfer coefficient (DLCO /accessible alveolar volume; KCO)	Supranormal

Diffusion coefficient is usually supranormal, but it is reduced in the presence of pulmonary hypertension.

found in patients affected by chronic respiratory muscle weakness in the absence of a scoliosis.

LUNG COMPLIANCE

Although lung expansion is compromised by chest wall properties, primary pulmonary pathology is unusual in patients who have idiopathic scoliosis. However, lung compliance is reduced because of a shift in the pressure-volume curve to the right. These changes in pulmonary characteristics largely arise from an alteration in alveolar forces caused by chronic hypoventilation. In neuromuscular patients, microatelectasis and macroatelectasis may complicate the picture. Microatelectasis seems relatively rare, however, as fine-section computed tomographic (CT) scans have shown areas of atelectasis in only a minority of patients affected by respiratory muscle weakness. Recurrent pneumonia may occur in neuromuscular patients who have bulbar weakness or an ineffectual cough. Pulmonary fibrosis is also seen in patients who have old TB, and these individuals may have areas of bronchiectasis. Cystic lung changes affect some individuals with neurofibromatosis.

The gas transfer coefficient (KCO) tends to be raised in scoliotic patients in the presence of a low transfer factor (see Table 67.2), because extrathoracic compression squeezes more air than blood out of the lungs, and thereby decreases accessible alveolar volume.

RESPIRATORY MUSCLES AND THORACIC PUMP DURING SLEEP

Impaired respiratory muscle function might be expected in idiopathic scoliosis, as the respiratory muscles work at a mechanical disadvantage when chest wall shape is altered. Reductions in transdiaphragmatic pressure and static respiratory mouth pressures have been demonstrated in patients who have scoliosis or a thoracoplasty. These findings tend to support the contention that the efficiency of the respiratory muscles may be affected by relatively small degrees of chest wall deformity. Respiratory muscle action is further reduced by the loss of intercostal muscle tone during rapid eye movement (REM) sleep and a reduced ability to compensate for added respiratory load. This explains why early features of ventilatory failure during sleep predate the development of daytime ventilatory failure.

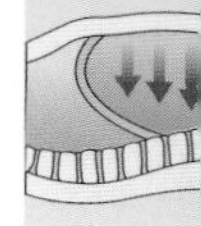

CONTROL OF BREATHING

Impaired hypercapnic ventilatory drive is usually secondary to chronic CO_2 retention in scoliotic patients. However, primary drive disorders may complicate some neuromuscular conditions (e.g., myotonic dystrophy) and may be acquired in patients who have poliomyelitis that affects brainstem control mechanisms. Generally, however, ventilatory drive is increased in neuromuscular patients to compensate for respiratory muscle insufficiency.

PULMONARY AND CARDIAC HEMODYNAMICS

Cor pulmonale is the end-stage result of severe, untreated chest wall deformity. Pulmonary artery pressure becomes elevated at rest with an inverse correlation between pulmonary artery pressure and arterial oxygen tension. In some patients with severe scoliosis a disproportionate rise in pulmonary artery pressure on exercise can be seen in the absence of hypoxemia, as the restricted thorax is unable to accommodate the increase in cardiac output on exertion.

An additional stress on hemodynamics is the effect of nocturnal hypoventilation on pulmonary artery pressure. The exact level of nocturnal hypoxemia that generates pulmonary hypertension is unknown, but severe, nocturnal arterial blood gas disturbances inevitably lead to daytime problems if untreated.

CLINICAL FEATURES

Spinal abnormalities are best understood by describing the age of onset, cause, and location of the curve (e.g., adolescent onset, idiopathic thoracic scoliosis). During physical examination, accompanying features should be sought, such as café-au-lait spots and neurofibromata. Marfan syndrome is a clinical diagnosis that requires the involvement of two of the three main systems (ocular, cardiac, and skeletal). A careful search for cardiac lesions is mandatory in early-onset scoliosis, which is associated with an increased incidence of congenital heart disease. Lesions demonstrated radiologically, such as hemivertebrae and rib fusion, suggest the presence of a congenital scoliosis.

Patients are observed while they are standing and while they are bending forward, so that an indication of the degree of lateral rib hump deformity can be determined. The lower back is examined for hairy tufts and other cutaneous stigmata of spinal dysraphism.

Progression of Curvature

Only one in five curves that is less than 20 degrees progresses. Detailed studies of the natural history of untreated idiopathic scoliosis are rare, but the younger the age at presentation, the greater the potential for progression as more of the growth spurt needs to be accommodated, and spinal growth continues until at least the age of 25 years. High and low thoracic curves together with thoracolumbar curves seem to be more unstable than lumbar deformities. Curves most likely to progress include those caused by congenital failure of segmentation, infantile idiopathic scoliosis, the angular curve of neurofibromatosis, pronounced paralytic curves, and scoliosis associated with progressive childhood neuromuscular conditions.

DIAGNOSIS

Cardiopulmonary Decompensation—Identification of High-Risk Cases

The vast majority of patients who have a thoracic spinal curvature do not develop cardiorespiratory problems and therefore do not require long-term respiratory follow-up. However, it is important to be able to identify the minority of patients at risk for problems so that appropriate monitoring and therapeutic intervention can be carried out.

Cor pulmonale was the primary cause of death in a series of 102 untreated idiopathic thoracic scoliosis patients. Age at onset of the scoliosis is crucial. Branthwaite showed that in patients who developed cardiorespiratory problems attributable to their scoliosis, 90% had an early-onset curvature (i.e., onset before the age of 5 years).

A VC of 50% of that predicted is an important cut-off figure, as those with a VC less than 50% predicted at presentation are much more likely to develop respiratory decompensation than those who have higher lung volumes.

In a study at the Royal Brompton Hospital, the mean age of patients in respiratory failure who required ventilatory support was 49 years in idiopathic scoliosis patients, 51 years in patients who had previous poliomyelitis, and 62 years in those who suffered sequelae of pulmonary TB. Pehrsson and colleagues followed lung function over a period of 20 years in idiopathic scoliosis patients. Respiratory failure occurred in 25%, all of whom had a VC less than 45% predicted and a thoracic Cobb angle greater than 110 degrees.

Monitoring High-Risk Patients

Pulmonary function, arterial blood gas tensions, and assessment of respiratory muscle strength using mouth pressures is helpful, particularly in patients who have neuromuscular disease. A fall in VC greater than 15% predicted on assumption of the supine position indicates significant diaphragm weakness. Daytime hypercapnia is associated with an inspiratory mouth pressure less than 30% predicted.

In addition to inquiries about breathlessness and exercise tolerance, patients should be asked about symptoms of nocturnal hypoventilation (morning headache, poor sleep quality, frequent arousals, nocturnal confusion, and morning anorexia), and if any are present the patient should undergo monitoring of respiration during sleep. A characteristic picture of nocturnal hypoventilation is usually found with episodes of desaturation and CO_2 retention, most pronounced in rapid eye movement (REM) sleep (Fig. 67.3).

TREATMENT

Management of Spinal Deformity

CONSERVATIVE MANAGEMENT

The success of a conservative approach depends on the age of the patient, the curve size at presentation, and the propensity of the curve to progress.

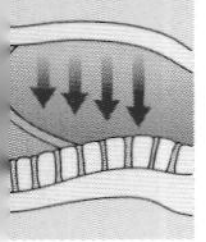

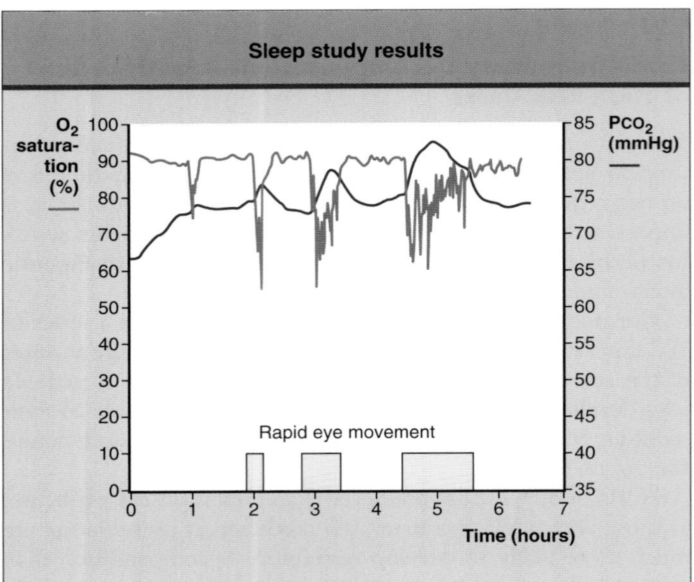

Figure 67.3 Sleep study results. Overnight monitoring of arterial oxygen saturation and transcutaneous CO_2 in an individual with congenital scoliosis who had morning headaches. Note the marked desaturation and CO_2 retention during episodes of rapid eye movement (REM) sleep.

BRACING

Devices such as the Milwaukee and Cotrell braces have been used extensively. The mechanical aim of the brace is to recreate a normal thoracic kyphosis, hyperextend the spine, and limit forward flexion, all of which will act to derotate the scoliosis. Bracing probably works more effectively in kyphosis than scoliosis. In paralytic disorders, a circumferential brace can support the trunk and make sitting more comfortable. VC should always be measured with and without the brace in place.

Surgery for Scoliosis

In general, surgery is performed to correct unacceptable deformity and prevent progression. It is not carried out to improve ventilatory function.

Thoracic scolioses greater than 45 degrees are usually judged unacceptable. However, a lesser curve associated with a greater degree of rotation may create a rib hump, which is just as concerning to the patient. It is a surgical maxim that even the best operative technique does not completely straighten a spine. About a 50% correction of the Cobb angle in smaller curves can be expected from a Harrington rod procedure. The best guide to a successful result is the initial amount of spinal flexibility. Also, the greater the degree of rotation, the greater the inflexibility of the curve.

Spinal fusion followed by casting has now been superseded in many situations by Harrington rod instrumentation. The system provides distraction to the concave side of the spine and compression to the convex side, which enhances stabilization and reduces any rotational tendency.

Ventilatory Impairment

OPTIMIZATION OF RESPIRATORY FUNCTION

Patients must be advised about the adverse effects of smoking and obesity. The influenza and pneumococcal vaccines are recom-mended for those who have ventilatory limitations.

Osteoporosis should be actively sought and treated. Care should be taken not to miss the reactivation of TB in patients with a thoracoplasty. Patients with Marfan syndrome may require β-adrenergic blocker therapy to reduce the risk of aortic dissection.

Exercise should be encouraged, except in patients with pulmonary hypertension and those who have Marfan syndrome. Pulmonary rehabilitation programs suggest that exercise and a reduction in deconditioning are just as valuable in restrictive disorders as in chronic obstructive pulmonary disease.

Ventilatory Failure

The evidence now clearly shows that ventilatory failure in patients who have chest wall disease can be successfully treated using noninvasive ventilation at night. Negative-pressure devices are effective but have been largely supplanted by nasal positive-pressure ventilation (NIPPV). In scoliotic patients who receive NIPPV, 5-year survival is around 80%, with 100% in patients with previous poliomyelitis and over 90% in those with post-tuberculous conditions. It seems increasingly likely that individuals who have nonprogressive disorders may have a normal or near-normal life span, provided NIPPV is introduced before the development of intractable pulmonary hypertension. Patients report good quality of life using NIPPV, and many are able to return to work.

Also, NIPPV can be used to palliate symptoms of breathlessness and cor pulmonale in patients who have progressive disorders and will alter the natural history of these conditions. A 5-year survival as high as 73% can be achieved in Duchenne muscular dystrophy.

PITFALLS AND CONTROVERSIES

Clinical Signs in Scoliosis

In patients who have severe scoliosis and who develop asthma, a characteristic wheeze may not be heard because of low airflow. Measurement of spirometry and home peak-flow monitoring is useful in these cases.

Pregnancy and Scoliosis

A successful outcome after pregnancy is usual in most patients who have adolescent-onset idiopathic scoliosis. In a survey of 118 pregnancies in 64 women who had thoracic scoliosis, no serious medical problems were encountered, with a cesarean rate of 17% for obstetric reasons. However, cardiorespiratory complications can be expected in those with a VC less than 1.25 L. Pregnancy is contraindicated in the presence of pulmonary hypertension and hypoxemia. If ventilatory problems arise in pregnancy, the situation may be successfully managed using noninvasive ventilation.

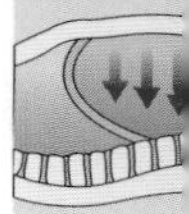

SUGGESTED READINGS

Bergofsky EH: Thoracic deformities. In Roussos C (ed): The Thorax. Part C. Disease. New York, Marcel Dekker, 1995, pp 1915-1949.

Branthwaite MA: Cardiorespiratory consequences of unfused idiopathic scoliosis. Br J Dis Chest 80:360-369, 1986.

Dubowitz V: The muscular dystrophies. In Dubowitz V (ed): Muscle Disorders in Childhood. London, WB Saunders, 1995, pp 34-133.

Giampietro PF, Raggio C, Davis JG: Marfan syndrome: orthopedic and genetic review. Curr Opin Pediatr 14:35-41, 2002.

Kearon C, Guillermo RV, Kirkly A, Killian KJ: Factors determining pulmonary function in adolescent idiopathic thoracic scoliosis. Am Rev Respir Dis 148:288-294, 1993.

Leatherman KD, Dickson RA: Basic principles. In Leatherman KD, Dickson RA (eds): The Management of Spinal Deformities. London, J Wright (Butterworth & Co Ltd), 1988, pp 1-27.

Leger P, Bedicam JM, Cornette A, et al: Nasal intermittent positive pressure ventilation: Long term follow-up in patients with severe chronic respiratory insufficiency. Chest 105:100-105, 1994.

Lowe TG, Edgar M, Margulies JY, et al: Etiology of idiopathic scoliosis: Current trends in research. J Bone Joint Surg 82-A:1157-1168, 2000.

Pehrsson K, Bake B, Larsson S, Nachemson A: Lung function in adult idiopathic scoliosis: a 20 year follow up. Thorax 46:474-478, 1991.

Simonds AK: Domiciliary non-invasive ventilation in restrictive disorders and stable neuromuscular disease. In Simonds AK (ed): Non-Invasive Respiratory Support: A Practical Handbook. London, Arnold, 2001, pp 133-145.

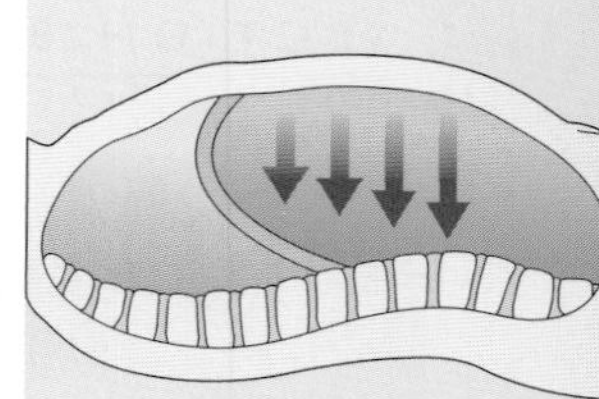

CHAPTER 68 Acute and Chronic Neuromuscular Disorders

Jean-William Fitting

PATHOPHYSIOLOGY

The exchange of carbon dioxide and oxygen between the blood and the atmosphere results from an integrated process that involves the ventilatory pump and the lungs. The ventilatory pump is complex and extends from the central nervous system to the chest wall; its engines are the respiratory muscles. A variety of neuromuscular disorders may affect the ventilatory pump at different sites (Fig. 68.1). When severe, acute neuromuscular disorders result in respiratory failure. Chronic neuromuscular disorders manifest with progressive respiratory insufficiency, but they may also have acute respiratory failure as the initial manifestation, an intercurrent complication, or the terminal event. With few exceptions, these disorders induce respiratory muscle weakness, which itself results in alveolar hypoventilation and impaired cough.

Lung Volumes

Inspiratory and expiratory muscle weakness reduces the vital capacity (VC) and its components. The end-expiratory lung volume, or functional residual capacity (FRC), is decreased, whereas residual volume (RV) may be normal or increased (Fig. 68.2). As a consequence of the sigmoidal shape of the pressure-volume relationship of the respiratory system, large changes in inspiratory pressure exerted near total lung capacity (TLC), or large changes in expiratory pressure exerted near RV, produce only small changes in lung volume (Fig. 68.3). Nevertheless, the actual loss of lung volume is always higher than expected for a given loss of muscle strength in neuromuscular disorders because of alterations of lung and chest wall mechanics, which occur even in the absence of associated scoliosis.

Lung and Chest Wall Mechanics

Acute respiratory muscle weakness results in loss of lung volume without change in compliance. In contrast, long-standing respiratory muscle weakness is associated with a number of modifications of the lung pressure-volume relationship, including the following:

1. Lung elastic recoil pressure is lower than normal at TLC (which is itself reduced).
2. Lung elastic recoil is higher than normal at any absolute lung volume.
3. Lung compliance is reduced.
4. Chest wall compliance is lower than normal.

The likely causes of these alterations in lung mechanics are a reduced number of alveoli in patients suffering from neuromuscular disorders from early childhood and a stiffening of lung elastic fibers induced by shallow breathing. Areas of microatelectasis are an additional contributing factor, but are present in only a minority of patients. The reduction in chest wall compliance occurs because of stiffening of the costosternal and costovertebral joints, tendons, and ligaments. The stiffening of the lung and chest wall is responsible for the lower level of the equilibrium position of the respiratory system (i.e., FRC) and contribute with respiratory muscle weakness to the drop in TLC and VC.

Forced Expiration and Cough

Expiratory muscle weakness modifies the contour of the flow-volume curve during a forced expiration, with a slower rise of flow, a lower peak expiratory flow, and an abrupt cessation of flow at end expiration. Because maximum expiratory flow requires only a low driving pressure over most of VC, however, the ratio of forced expiratory volume in 1 second to forced VC (FEV_1/FVC) is usually normal (or may be supranormal) despite expiratory muscle weakness. In contrast, cough is generally inefficient because expiratory muscles are unable to produce the high positive pleural pressure that normally induces dynamic compression of the central airways and transient acceleration of flow. This problem leads to frequent pulmonary infections.

Dyspnea

Patients with neuromuscular disorders often complain of dyspnea despite having reduced physical activity. The cause of the dyspnea may be the increased respiratory effort required when the ratio between tidal inspiratory pressure and maximal inspiratory pressure increases (PI/PI_{max}). In neuromuscular disorders, PI may increase because of lower lung and chest wall compliances, and PImax is reduced because of inspiratory muscle weakness. When muscle weakness is reversible, the sensation of dyspnea may fluctuate markedly (Fig. 68.4).

Respiratory Failure

With progressive respiratory muscle weakness, breathing becomes rapid and shallow. As tidal volume decreases, the ratio of dead space to tidal volume increases, causing hypercapnia and ultimately hypoxemia as alveolar ventilation falls. The

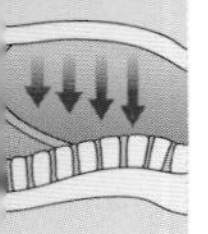

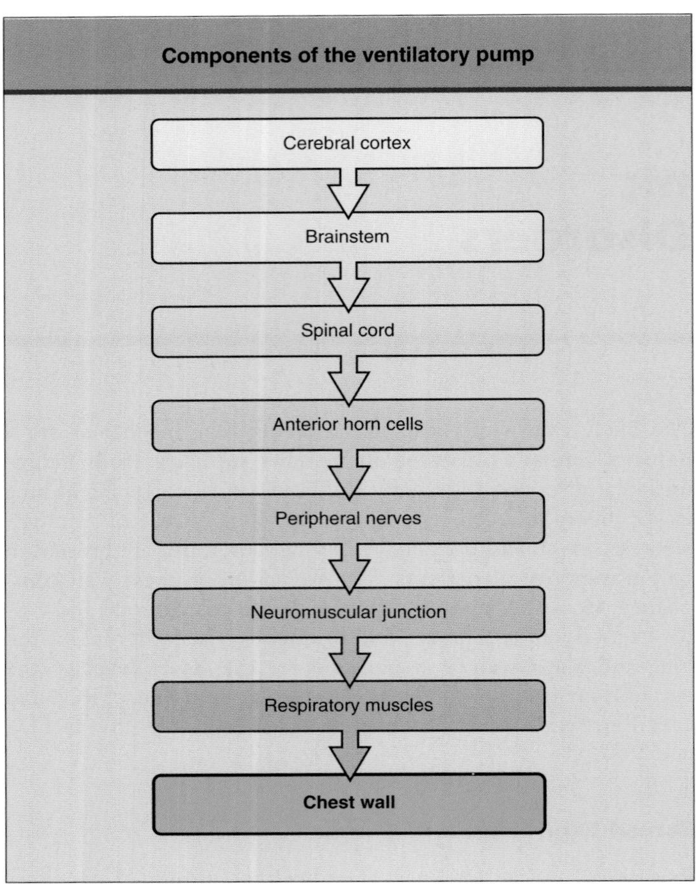

Figure 68.1 Components of the ventilatory pump.

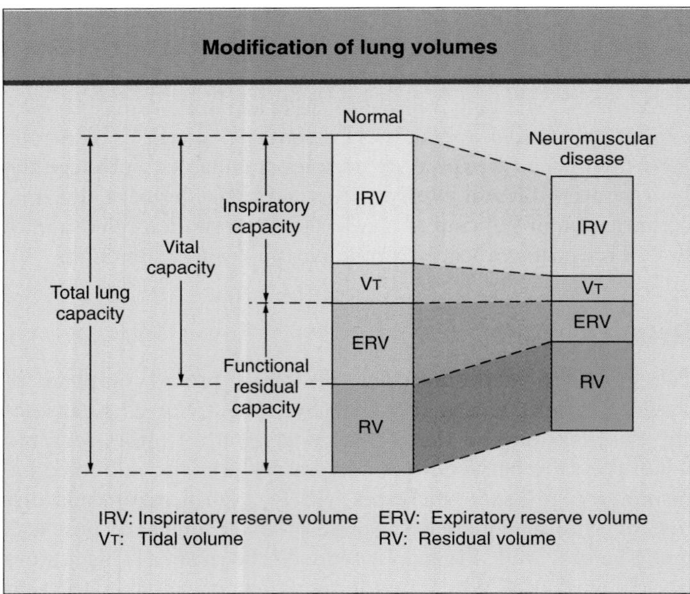

Figure 68.2 Modification of lung volumes in neuromuscular diseases.

prevalence of hypercapnic respiratory failure increases with the degree of respiratory muscle weakness, being more common when respiratory muscle strength is less than 30% of normal. Considerable individual variability occurs, however, and the risk of respiratory failure cannot be predicted with certainty from measurement of VC or PImax.

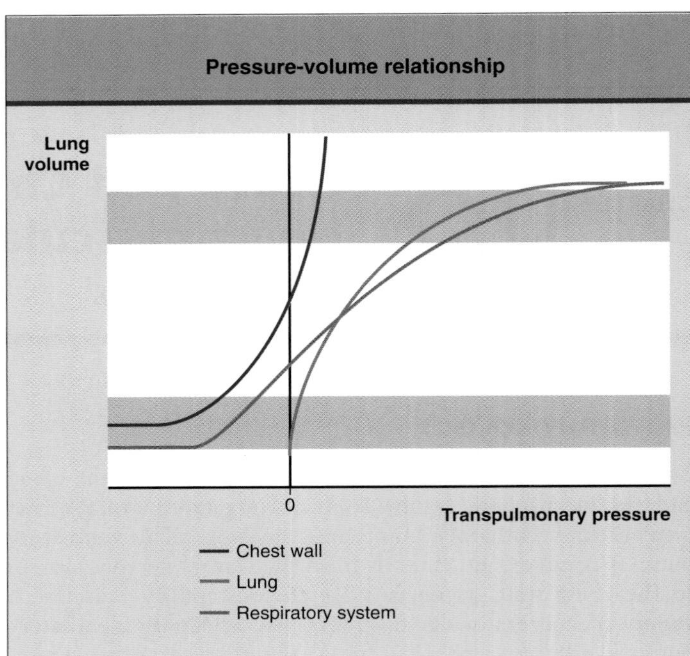

Figure 68.3 Minimal changes in lung volume occur with marked changes in transpulmonary pressure near total lung capacity or residual volume (shaded areas).

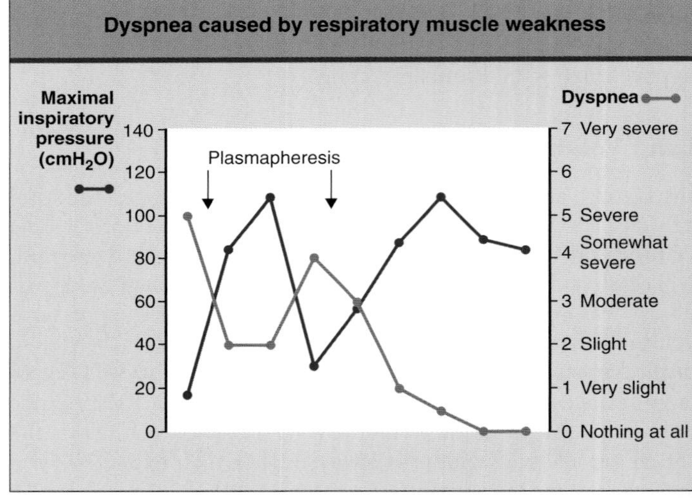

Figure 68.4 Dyspnea caused by respiratory muscle weakness in a patient who has myasthenia gravis.

Part of this variability can be explained by the respiratory problems that occur during sleep. Nocturnal studies show that alveolar hypoventilation develops initially at night, particularly during rapid eye movement (REM) sleep. This sleep stage is normally characterized by shallow breathing and inhibition of the intercostal muscles. In patients with neuromuscular disorders, REM sleep is often associated with transient hypercapnia and profound desaturation. These nocturnal anomalies precede and predispose to diurnal respiratory failure.

EPIDEMIOLOGY AND CLINICAL FEATURES

A variety of neurologic disorders can affect respiration. The most important are presented here according to the anatomic level of the lesion. They are classified as acute or chronic, but

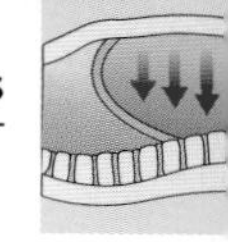

some acute disorders have permanent consequences, and some chronic disorders may manifest with acute respiratory failure (Table 68.1).

Central Nervous System

ACUTE DISORDERS

Head and Spinal Cord Injury

Traumatic injury to the brain and the spinal cord may result in total or subtotal loss of respiratory muscle function and a number of resulting acute complications. Patients with brain injury develop early arterial hypoxemia related to ventilation-perfusion inequality. Neurogenic pulmonary edema is frequent and is believed to result from massive α-adrenergic discharge, pulmonary vasoconstriction, systemic hypertension, and capillary disruption. Other early complications include pulmonary embolism, hypersecretion of tenacious bronchial mucus, and pneumonia. Tetraplegia results from cervical spinal cord trauma, spinal artery infarction, or compression by tumor. In all instances, the function of intercostal and abdominal muscles is lost, and the only remaining expiratory muscle is the clavicular portion of the pectoralis major. This results in a profound impairment in expiratory force and cough efficacy. The degree of inspiratory muscle impairment depends on the level of the lesion with respect to the phrenic nerve roots, which originate from C3 to C5. Diaphragmatic function is intact in patients with lower cervical lesions. Their inspiratory function is, however, impaired by a paradoxical movement of the upper rib cage that occurs because of the intercostal muscle paralysis. Lesions at C3 to C5 induce a variable loss of diaphragmatic function. Ventilatory autonomy often improves after the initial phase of spinal shock in these patients. Higher cord injuries result in a nearly complete loss of respiratory muscle function, which necessitates immediate and long-term ventilatory assistance.

Table 68.1
Acute and chronic neuromuscular disorders that cause respiratory failure

Level of lesion	Acute disorders	Chronic disorders
Central nervous system	Head and spinal cord injury Stroke Tetanus	Multiple sclerosis Parkinson's disease Shy–Drager syndrome
Anterior horn cells	Paralytic poliomyelitis Rabies Flavivirus encephalomyelitis	Amyotrophic lateral sclerosis Spinal muscular atrophies Postpoliomyelitis atrophy
Peripheral nerves	Guillain–Barré syndrome Critical illness polyneuropathy Diphtheria Herpes zoster Neuralgic amyotrophy Phrenic nerve injury Metabolic and toxic causes	Hereditary neuropathies
Neuromuscular junction	Botulism Organophosphate poisoning Snake bite, tick paralysis	Myasthenia gravis Lambert–Eaton syndrome
Muscles	Acute corticosteroid myopathy Electrolyte disorders	Duchenne's muscular dystrophy Myotonic dystrophy Facioscapulohumeral disease Limb girdle dystrophy Congenital myopathies Acid maltase deficiency Mitochondrial myopathies Inflammatory myopathies

Stroke

Hemispheric strokes affect the voluntary pathway of respiration, with elevation and decreased voluntary activation of the contralateral hemidiaphragm. Cheyne-Stokes breathing may develop, particularly in patients with bilateral hemispheric lesions. These alterations have only modest clinical consequences, however, because the automatic pathway is preserved. Brainstem strokes may affect respiratory rhythm in various ways. Lesions of the dorsolateral medulla result in fatal apnea. In contrast, injuries that spare the dorsolateral medulla do not impair automatic respiratory rhythm, even when the strokes are extensive and patients are left with the locked-in syndrome. Lateral medullary strokes that result from occlusion of a distal vertebral artery induce the loss of automatic breathing, or Ondine's curse. While breathing is maintained during wakefulness, potentially fatal hypoventilation and central apnea develop during sleep. This must be differentiated from obstructive apnea, which may also be associated with lateral medullary strokes and which results from paralysis of pharyngeal muscles.

Tetanus

Tetanus toxin produced by *Clostridium tetani* reaches the central nervous system via retrograde axonal transport and blocks the synaptic release of inhibitory transmitters. Localized or generalized spasms develop through loss of central inhibition, and death results from respiratory failure due to laryngospasm or generalized spasms of the respiratory muscles. Specific therapy includes antibiotics, human tetanus immune globulin, muscle relaxants or neuromuscular blockade, and intubation and mechanical ventilation.

CHRONIC DISORDERS

Multiple Sclerosis

Multiple sclerosis is an inflammatory, demyelinating disease that can affect almost any area of the central nervous system. Different types of respiratory anomalies may develop depending on the location of the lesion, and occasionally these abnormalities can be life threatening. Respiratory control can be affected by loss of automatic breathing, loss of voluntary breathing, or both. Bulbar dysfunction increases the risk of respiratory failure from aspiration and pneumonia. Respiratory muscle weakness is usually moderate in degree, but may become severe and include diaphragmatic paralysis during relapses of the disease. Patients are particularly at risk of acute respiratory failure when infection and fever accompany an exacerbation. In these circumstances, severe respiratory muscle weakness can occur acutely because of a conduction block of demyelinated fibers.

Extrapyramidal Diseases

Parkinson's disease is associated with frequent respiratory complications, including pneumonia, which is the most common cause of death in these patients. Abnormal control of breathing is

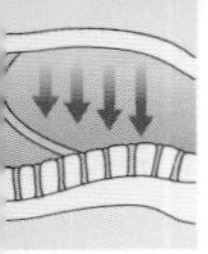

frequently present, with tachypnea accompanied by dyspnea. Respiratory muscle weakness manifests by reduced lung volumes, impaired ability to clear secretions, and a delay in achieving peak expiratory flow. Finally, some patients with Parkinson's disease have dynamic instability of upper airway patency, which can be recognized as manifesting a sawtooth pattern on both the inspiratory and expiratory loops of a flow-volume curve. Respiratory dysfunction can also be induced by L-dopa therapy in patients with Parkinson's disease. Some patients develop dyskinesias associated with tachypnea and dyspnea within 1 hour of drug administration as a result of choreiform movements and rigidity-akinesis of the respiratory muscles.

The Shy-Drager syndrome is a multiple system atrophy that manifests by parkinsonism and autonomic failure. It is often associated with abnormal control of breathing, including irregular respiratory rate and tidal volume, central apneas, Cheyne-Stokes breathing, apneustic breathing, or central hypoventilation. The most dangerous anomaly is bilateral vocal cord abductor paralysis, which can result in obstructive sleep apnea and death.

Anterior Horn Cells

ACUTE DISORDERS

Paralytic Poliomyelitis

Before the advent of poliovirus vaccines, poliomyelitis was the most frequent neuromuscular disorder causing respiratory failure. It is now rare, and usually attributed to live, attenuated polio vaccines. The acute infection has few symptoms, with fever and myalgia occurring in adults and upper airway infection in children. Only a minority of infected persons develop paralysis, which is widely and asymmetrically distributed. Respiratory complications include irregular breathing and apneas, upper airway obstruction, aspiration, and respiratory muscle weakness or paralysis. About 25% of patients require ventilatory assistance during the acute infection, but ventilatory autonomy is often recovered within months through reinnervation of denervated fibers.

Rabies

Rabies is an almost universally fatal disorder. The virus is transported along the peripheral nerves and enters the central nervous system, where it induces inflammation. In 20% of cases, the inflammation predominates in the spinal cord and manifests as paralytic rabies with progressive, ascending paralysis that may lead to respiratory muscle weakness and eventual respiratory arrest in a fashion that may be indistinguishable from the Guillain-Barré syndrome (GBS). Immediate prophylaxis is mandatory for subjects likely to be exposed to rabies and consists of human rabies immune globulin and rabies vaccine.

Flavivirus Encephalomyelitis

Tick-born encephalitis is caused by a flavivirus and is endemic in Central Europe. In a minority of patients, acute myelitis develops in which paralysis and areflexia predominate in upper limbs. Severe weakness of respiratory muscles may develop, requiring prolonged mechanical ventilation.

CHRONIC DISORDERS

Amyotrophic Lateral Sclerosis

Amyotrophic lateral sclerosis (ALS) is a progressive degenerative disorder characterized by loss of both upper and lower motor neurons. With an incidence of 1 to 2 per 100,000 persons, ALS is the most frequently occurring motor neuron disorder in developed countries. It affects predominantly middle-aged to older subjects, with a male-to-female ratio of 2:1. The cause is unknown, but 5% to 10% of cases are familial, usually with autosomal dominant transmission, caused by a defect localized in chromosome 21. ALS has a very poor prognosis, with 50% of patients dying within 3 years and 80% within 5 years, usually of respiratory failure.

The clinical features are not uniform, however. Loss of lower motor neurons often predominates, resulting in fasciculations, amyotrophy, and weakness, whereas loss of upper motor neurons manifests with spasticity and hyperreflexia. In the majority of cases, weakness initially develops in the extremities; in a minority the bulbar lesions are most prominent. Similarly, respiratory muscle dysfunction is quite variable during the course of ALS. In some patients, respiratory muscle strength and lung volumes are relatively preserved even when peripheral muscle weakness has progressed to the point where the patients are wheelchair bound. Abdominal muscle dysfunction usually occurs before diaphragmatic dysfunction, leading to expiratory muscle weakness. In rare cases, however, the initial manifestation may be severe respiratory weakness from phrenic motor neuron lesions. Ultimately, most patients develop alveolar hypoventilation unless ventilatory support is initiated. Death most commonly occurs as a result of acute respiratory failure that develops as a result of aspiration pneumonia.

Spinal Muscular Atrophies

The spinal muscular atrophies (SMAs) have an autosomal recessive inheritance pattern and arise from an anomaly of chromosome 5. All are characterized by weakness and amyotrophy, which predominates in the proximal muscles and begins in the lower limbs. Respiratory muscle weakness is caused by paralysis of intercostal muscles, whereas the diaphragm is preserved. The SMAs are classified into three types according to the age of onset; types I and II are also termed *Werdnig-Hoffmann disease*, and type III is *Kugelberg-Welander disease*. Type I SMA begins before the age of 6 months and results in death from respiratory failure before the age of 2 years. Type II begins before the age of 18 months, progresses more slowly, and leads to death in late childhood as a result of both respiratory muscle weakness and scoliosis. Type III begins after 18 months and is associated with late respiratory complications resulting mainly from kyphoscoliosis.

Postpoliomyelitis Muscular Atrophy

Approximately 25% of patients with previous poliomyelitis have further muscular weakness as a result of degeneration of reinnervated motor units 20 to 40 years after the initial episode. In patients with respiratory muscle sequelae and kyphoscoliosis, further dysfunction of respiratory muscles may induce alveolar hypoventilation. The loss of muscle strength is gradual, however, and can be detected by appropriate tests before respiratory failure develops.

Peripheral Nerves

ACUTE DISORDERS

Guillain-Barré Syndrome

An acute, multifocal, demyelinating polyradiculoneuropathy, GBS is of uncertain pathogenesis. *Campylobacter* infection is

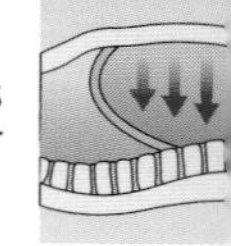

the most common predisposing factor, although some patients have exposures to a variety of viral illnesses, as well (e.g., varicella-zoster virus, cytomegalovirus, Epstein-Barr virus, human immunodeficiency virus). The condition has also been reported to occur after *Mycoplasma pneumoniae* infection, receipt of the influenza vaccine, surgery, and in the setting of concurrent malignancy. Cerebrospinal fluid is characterized by elevated proteins and a cell count of 10 or fewer mononuclear leukocytes per cubic millimeter. Muscle weakness and paralysis commonly begin in the lower extremities and progress in an ascending pattern to include the respiratory muscles. Maximum weakness is attained within 2 weeks in 50% of cases, and within 4 weeks in 90%. Respiratory failure develops as a result of both respiratory muscle weakness and pulmonary infections caused by aspiration and requires mechanical ventilation in 15% to 30% of patients. Sensory impairment is minor, but autonomic dysfunction may be severe and include arrhythmias and hypertension or hypotension. Presently, specific therapy is limited to plasmapheresis, which may limit progression of the disease and accelerate recovery when given early. Corticosteroids are ineffective and may be harmful. Most patients recover fully from GBS, but 15% manifest residual weakness and 5% develop a chronic form with relapsing episodes of demyelination.

Critical Illness Polyneuropathy

Patients who stay for longer than 5 days in the intensive care unit and who suffer from sepsis and failure of two or more organs are at high risk for developing critical illness polyneuropathy. This is an acute, reversible axonal neuropathy manifested by symmetrical and predominantly distal weakness or paralysis. Cerebrospinal fluid is unremarkable, in contrast to GBS. Electrophysiologic examination shows normal nerve conduction velocities but low or absent action potential amplitudes. Neural biopsies show no inflammation. The resulting respiratory muscle weakness is a frequent cause of prolonged and difficult weaning from mechanical ventilation. Electrophysiologic and clinical recovery occurs within 6 to 12 months.

Diphtheria

Diphtheria, caused by *Corynebacterium diphtheriae*, is characterized by a pharyngeal and tracheal inflammatory membrane. In 20% of cases, an exotoxin provokes cardiac and neurologic complications, beginning with palatal paralysis. A demyelinating polyneuropathy develops 6 weeks after the initial infection and can result in respiratory failure if the respiratory muscles are involved. Neurologic symptoms progress over 1 to 2 weeks, then stabilize and regress over several months. Antitoxin is the only specific therapy and must be administered as early as possible.

Herpes Zoster

Herpes zoster is caused by reactivation of varicella-zoster infections and generally affects sensory nerves, causing a unilateral vesicular eruption involving a single dermatome. Motor neurons may occasionally be affected, with resultant flaccid paralysis. The phrenic nerve may be involved in midcervical lesions and this can result in complete and permanent hemidiaphragmatic paralysis—a cause of dyspnea, but not of respiratory failure. Since herpes zoster is not invariably accompanied by a cutaneous eruption, it may remain undetected in cases of unexplained, usually unilateral, diaphragmatic paralysis.

Neuralgic Amyotrophy

Neuralgic amyotrophy (Parsonage-Turner syndrome) is an acute neuritis that affects cervical roots and is manifested by sudden onset of neck and shoulder pain, followed by sensory and motor impairment with prominent weakness and amyotrophy of the shoulder and arm muscles. A recent history of viral infection or immunization is present in a minority of patients. Diaphragmatic paralysis, commonly bilateral, may ensue and induce dyspnea and orthopnea (see Table 68-1). Diaphragmatic function appears to recover slowly but only in a minority of patients.

Phrenic Nerve Injury

Damage to or compression of the phrenic nerves induces unilateral or bilateral diaphragmatic paralysis. Such injury can be caused by trauma, surgery, mediastinal tumors, pleural space infections, or forceful manipulation of the neck. Diaphragmatic paralysis is a common complication of open-heart surgery and results from cold- or stretch-induced injury to the nerve. This dysfunction is reversible, with recovery of 80% of cases within 6 months, and 90% within 1 year.

Metabolic and Toxic Causes

Acute intermittent porphyria causes an axonal neuropathy, which may be severe enough to induce respiratory failure. Acute hyperkalemic paralysis, commonly triggered by drugs in patients with acute or chronic renal failure or, less commonly, with adrenal insufficiency, may be complicated by respiratory failure. Other causes of acute neuropathy that result in respiratory muscle paralysis include poisoning with ciguatoxin (produced by protozoan algae and transmitted by fish), saxitoxin (transmitted by shellfish), tetrodotoxin (elaborated by the pufferfish), and thallium.

CHRONIC DISORDERS

Hereditary Neuropathies

Hereditary motor and sensory neuropathies represent a group of inherited, autosomal dominant or recessive disorders that are characterized by chronic degeneration of the peripheral nerves and roots. Muscle weakness affects the extremities but may also progress to diaphragmatic paralysis after a long evolution.

Neuromuscular Junction

ACUTE DISORDERS

Botulism

Botulism is caused by an exotoxin elaborated by *Clostridium botulinum*, a gram-positive, spore-forming anaerobe widely present in soil. The disease can be acquired three ways: food-borne organisms can be acquired from the consumption of improperly cooked food that contains the spores and toxin; infantile botulism can be acquired by colonization of the gastrointestinal tract in the first 6 months of life; and wound botulism can be acquired from entry of the organism through breaks in the skin or from injectable drugs, given either intravenously or subcutaneously. The toxin is hematogenously disseminated, enters the neurons via endocytosis, binds irreversibly to calcium channels, and blocks acetylcholine release at the neuromuscular junction and at postganglionic parasympathetic nerve terminals. The incubation period lasts hours to days in food-borne disease, and days to 2 weeks in wound botulism. Gastrointestinal symp-

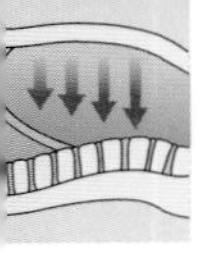

toms appear first, with nausea and vomiting, followed by blurred vision, diplopia, and a descending paralysis, which includes the respiratory muscles. Mortality is less than 10% with the use of mechanical ventilation, but support may be required for up to 3 months in severe cases. Respiratory muscles appear to recover more slowly than other muscle groups. The diagnosis is made by isolating the toxin or the organism in food remnants or from gastric aspirate, stools, or serum in food-borne botulism, and in serum and wound tissue in wound botulism. Specific therapy includes enemas and gastric lavage, surgical débridement of wounds, high-dose penicillin, and antitoxin within the first days.

Organophosphate Poisoning

Poisoning occurs with ingestion, inhalation, or absorption via mucous membranes of organophosphate insecticides. These compounds are anticholinesterases, which induce a cholinergic crisis and skeletal muscle weakness from dysfunction of postsynaptic neuromuscular junctions. The acute intoxication presents as a potentially fatal cholinergic crisis. An intermediate form may develop 1 to 4 days after intoxication, and manifest with cranial and proximal muscle weakness and respiratory failure. Specific therapy includes atropine and the cholinesterase reactivator pralidoxime.

Snake Bite and Tick Paralysis

Snake neurotoxins act by preventing the release of acetylcholine at the neuromuscular junction. Paralysis develops 6 to 12 hours after the bite, with ptosis, diplopia, blurred vision, dysphagia, proximal muscle paralysis, and respiratory failure. After mechanical ventilation is initiated, paralysis usually regresses in 2 to 3 days. Specific therapy includes monovalent or polyvalent antivenin.

Tick paralysis is also caused by a neurotoxin that blocks the release of acetylcholine. After a 5-day latent period, a rapidly ascending paralysis develops and leads to respiratory failure. Removal of the tick rapidly reverses the process.

CHRONIC DISORDERS

Myasthenia Gravis

Myasthenia gravis is the most common disorder of the neuromuscular junction and is mediated by antibodies against acetylcholine receptors. Muscle weakness, which is exacerbated by exercise, is due to a reduction of available acetylcholine receptors. The onset of the disease is usually insidious but may be abrupt. Weakness most commonly affects the extraocular muscles (causing ptosis and/or diplopia), but also affects facial muscles (causing weakness or paralysis), bulbar muscles (causing aspiration), laryngeal muscles (causing stridor), and truncal and limb muscles. Exacerbations may occur with exertion, infection, surgery, or a variety of drugs (most commonly the neuromuscular blocking agents, aminoglycosides, clindamycin, tetracycline, propranolol, quinidine, procainamide, lidocaine, corticosteroids, chlorpromazine, and phenytoin). Treatment includes cholinesterase inhibitors, immunosuppression, thymectomy, and plasmapheresis.

Acute respiratory failure may develop during a myasthenic crisis, defined as a rapid worsening of symptoms caused by a triggering factor, like surgery, infection, stress, or drugs. A cholinergic crisis results from an excess of anticholinesterase agents. Weakness worsens because of a cholinergic blockade and is associated with muscarinic symptoms, which include hypersalivation, increased bronchial secretions, bradycardia, nausea, and vomiting. A mixed or brittle crisis causes both myasthenic and cholinergic symptoms. Because the respiratory muscles are usually affected less severely, they may suffer cholinergic block when other muscles require more anticholinesterase agents. Apart from mechanical ventilation, the treatment of acute respiratory failure includes corticosteroids and plasmapheresis, and temporary discontinuation of anticholinesterase medication. An insidious form of respiratory failure may develop in those who have long-standing, generalized muscle weakness.

Of patients with the Lambert-Eaton myasthenic syndrome, 50% have small-cell carcinoma of the lung. Weakness is caused by a reduction of acetylcholine release and predominates in the pelvic girdle and thigh muscles. Some respiratory muscle weakness is frequent, but respiratory failure is rare. It can precede the presentation of the tumor by several months.

Diseases of Muscle

ACUTE DISORDERS

Acute Corticosteroid Myopathy

Severe generalized weakness may develop in critically ill patients treated with high-dose corticosteroids and neuromuscular blocking agents. Rhabdomyolysis can be detected by increased serum creatine kinase levels and myoglobinuria. Histologic changes are found, with widespread muscle necrosis and atrophy and loss of myosin filaments. This syndrome is often observed in patients treated by mechanical ventilation, and severe respiratory muscle weakness may prolong weaning, or even necessitate long-term ventilatory support.

Electrolyte Disorders

Hypophosphatemia is common in chronic alcoholism, diabetic ketoacidosis, and gram-negative infections and induces generalized weakness, hypotonia, and areflexia. Acute respiratory failure can occur in patients with hypophosphatemia as a result of respiratory muscle weakness, but this is rapidly reversed by phosphate administration. Severe hypokalemia is another cause of respiratory muscle weakness. Respiratory failure can result from acute hypokalemic paralysis (as a complication of treatment for diabetic ketoacidosis), barium sulfide poisoning, or ureterosigmoidostomy.

CHRONIC DISORDERS

Duchenne's Muscular Dystrophy

Duchenne's muscular dystrophy (DMD) is an X-linked recessive disorder that is caused by a variety of mutations of the gene for the protein dystrophin. Weakness, clumsiness, and waddling gait are observed in early childhood. With progressive muscle weakness, most patients are wheelchair dependent by the age of 12 years. Absolute values of VC increase until age 10 to 12 years, then plateau, and inexorably diminish. From age 10 to 12 on, the ventilatory decline is further aggravated by the development of scoliosis. Patients with DMD may remain clinically stable despite considerable loss of lung volume. Eventually, they develop nocturnal hypoxemia and hypercapnia and commonly die of acute respiratory failure secondary to pulmonary infection at 20 to 25 years of age. Congestive heart failure may also occur as a result of left ventricular fibrosis. Surgical correction of the scoliosis improves comfort but not the lung volumes. Noninvasive or invasive home mechanical ventilation should be considered before the stage of terminal respiratory failure.

Myotonic Dystrophy

Myotonic dystrophy is the most common muscle dystrophy in adults, with an incidence of 1 in 8000. It is inherited in an autosomal dominant pattern and is characterized by myotonia (delayed muscular relaxation), progressive muscle weakness, cardiac conduction defects, endocrine abnormalities, cataracts, ptosis, frontal baldness, and temporal wasting. Respiratory failure is frequent because of respiratory muscle weakness. Aggravating factors include central or obstructive sleep apnea and pharyngeal and laryngeal dysfunction that predisposes to aspiration. Rarely, severe dyspnea may result from myotonia of the respiratory muscles; this can be alleviated by antimyotonic therapy. Patients affected by myotonic dystrophy have an increased sensitivity to anesthetic agents and respiratory depressants. When surgery is needed, close postoperative monitoring is mandatory for at least 24 hours. Congenital myotonic dystrophy occurs in the offspring of 15% of affected mothers. It is manifested by hypotonia, severe facial weakness, and frequent respiratory failure that necessitates mechanical ventilation. The prognosis is good for those who survive the respiratory complications of the neonatal period.

Other Adult Muscular Dystrophies

Facioscapulohumeral muscular dystrophy is an autosomal dominant condition that affects the face and arm muscles. The trunk muscles are involved in 20% of patients, and in these patients respiratory failure may ensue. The limb girdle dystrophies are a group of autosomal and recessive conditions that can lead to respiratory failure.

Congenital Myopathies

Congenital myopathies are characterized by definitive abnormalities on muscle biopsy. The form most often associated with respiratory failure is nemaline myopathy, which can appear in neonates, children, or adults and is characterized by accumulation of rodlike bodies in muscle fibers. Centronuclear myopathy affects mainly slow-twitch oxidative fibers (type I). An X-linked recessive form often requires mechanical ventilation at birth. Autosomal dominant forms develop in childhood and adulthood but rarely lead to respiratory failure.

Metabolic Myopathies

Acid maltase deficiency is a glycogen storage disease. In the infantile form, all organs accumulate glycogen, and death ensues from cardiorespiratory failure by the age of 2 years. In the childhood form, organomegaly is variable and respiratory failure is common because of severe muscle weakness. In the adult form, organomegaly is rare, and nocturnal hypoxemia and respiratory failure are frequent and caused by predominant dysfunction of the diaphragm.

Mitochondrial myopathies represent a group of systemic diseases in which mitochondrial disorders are recognized in muscle biopsies by the presence of "ragged, red fibers." The following three mitochondrial myopathies are associated with respiratory failure, either initial or precipitated by anesthesia or respiratory depressants:

- Kearns-Sayre syndrome
- Myoclonic epilepsy and ragged-red fibers (MERRF)
- Mitochondrial myopathy, encephalopathy, lactic acidosis, and stroke-like episodes (MELAS)

Depressed ventilatory response to hypoxia and hypercapnia may occur independently of respiratory muscle weakness.

Inflammatory Myopathies

Polymyositis, dermatomyositis, and inclusion body myositis are characterized by lymphocytic infiltration of the muscles. Respiratory muscle weakness is frequent, but ventilatory failure is relatively rare. Interstitial lung disease is present in up to 30% of patients and is often associated with antibodies to histidyl-transfer RNA synthetase (Jo-1 antigen). Systemic lupus erythematosus (SLE) is frequently associated with respiratory muscle weakness without signs of generalized muscle involvement. The "shrinking lung syndrome" observed in patients who have SLE results from dysfunction and elevation of the diaphragm, caused by both muscle atrophy and fibrosis.

DIAGNOSIS

History

The cause of respiratory failure is often a previously diagnosed, long-standing neuromuscular disorder. If no such disorder is present, evidence of trauma, wounds, infection, exposure to insects, drugs, or toxic agents is sought. Clues to an underlying neuromuscular disorder may include a history of fatigability on repetitive tasks, difficulty standing up from a chair or in performing tasks with the arms elevated, difficulty with speech or swallowing liquids, tracheal aspiration, or impaired cough.

Dyspnea is a common symptom of respiratory insufficiency, although obviously not specific. Typically, dyspnea occurs on exertion, but may be masked in patients whose exercise capacity is severely restricted by limb weakness. Dyspnea at rest is an alarm signal for imminent acute respiratory failure. Bilateral diaphragmatic paralysis causes orthopnea, and this problem can be severe enough to prevent normal sleep and necessitate nocturnal ventilatory support. Nocturnal hypoventilation commonly develops before the onset of diurnal hypercapnia and may be recognized by the presence of early morning headache and daytime sleepiness.

Physical Examination

Patients who complain of dyspnea of unexplained origin, or those for whom a neuromuscular disorder is suspected, are given a detailed neurologic examination. This includes assessment of the presence and distribution of muscle atrophy and weakness, fasciculation, spasticity, and abnormal tendon reflexes.

The clinical examination is often unremarkable when weakness is mild or even moderate. Rapid, shallow breathing typically accompanies more severe involvement. Signs of diaphragmatic paralysis are sought with the patient in the supine position—elevation of respiratory rate, prominent contraction of the sternocleidomastoid and scalene muscles, and abdominal paradox (i.e., an indrawing of abdominal wall during inspiration, instead of the normal synchronized outward movement of both rib cage and abdomen [Fig. 68.5]). The signs of spinal cord injury vary according to the level of lesion. Patients injured above the

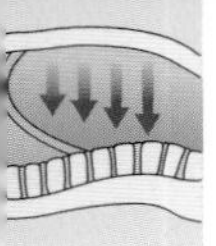

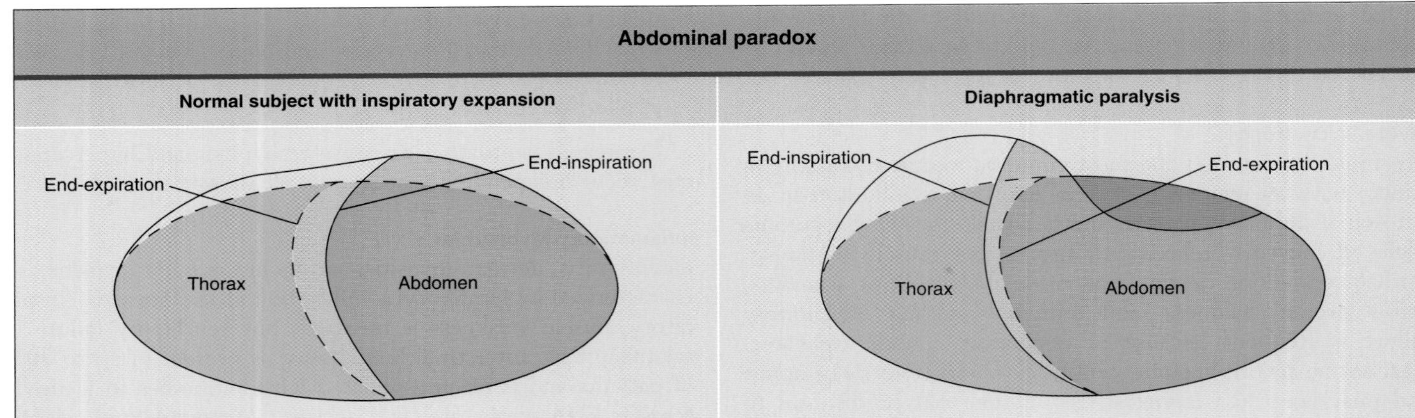

Figure 68.5 Abdominal paradox caused by severe dysfunction or paralysis of the diaphragm. A, Normal subject with inspiratory expansion of both the thorax and abdomen. **B,** Diaphragmatic paralysis with marked expansion of the thorax and paradoxical motion of the diaphragm and abdomen. Abdominal paradox should be looked for in the supine position.

C3 to C5 level are extremely dyspneic and tachypneic, have clear use of the inspiratory neck muscles, and show abdominal paradox. Diaphragmatic function is preserved in lesions below C5. During inspiration, these patients show a normal expansion of the abdomen but often a paradoxical inward movement of the upper rib cage because of paralysis of the inspiratory rib cage muscles.

Imaging

Chest radiographs showing elevation of one hemidiaphragm suggest paralysis on that side, but other causes, such as atelectasis and subpulmonary pleural effusion, must be eliminated. Elevation of both hemidiaphragms is compatible with diaphragmatic paralysis but can also result from inadequate inspiration or diffuse interstitial lung disease. Comparison with previous radiographs is most helpful (Fig. 68.6). Examination of diaphragmatic movements under fluoroscopy with the patient in the supine position may be useful. During sniffing, both hemidiaphragms normally show a brisk caudad displacement. In hemidiaphragmatic paralysis, the corresponding side shows a paradoxical cephalad movement. In bilateral paralysis, both hemidiaphragms show this paradoxical shift. The hemidiaphragmatic movement can also be seen with ultrasound.

Arterial Blood Gases

The hallmarks of severe respiratory muscle weakness are hypercapnia and hypoxemia. Diaphragmatic paralysis does not cause hypercapnia, unless it is associated with an increased load caused by a lung or chest wall problem. When caused by respiratory muscle weakness, hypercapnia is a late sign and usually develops only when respiratory muscle strength is markedly reduced. In chronic disorders, global respiratory muscle weakness results in progressive hypercapnia with markedly elevated bicarbonates and a normal pH. Initially, alveolar hypoventilation develops only during the night, in particular during REM sleep. Such episodes can be detected by falls in arterial oxygen saturation during nocturnal pulse oximetry.

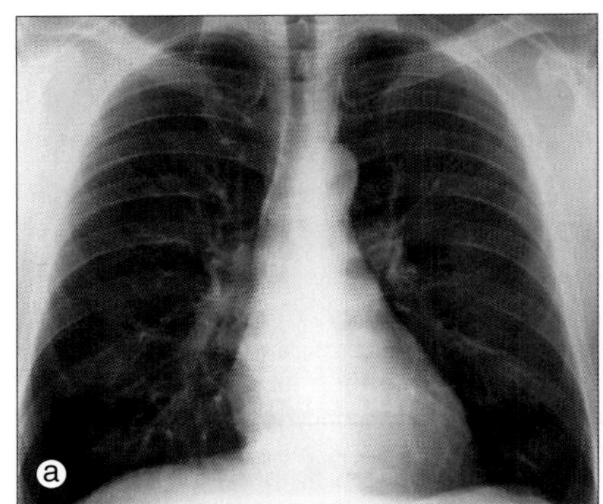

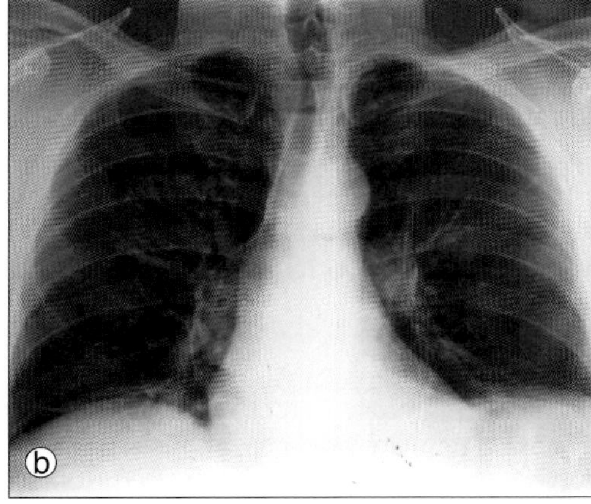

Figure 68.6 Bilateral diaphragmatic paralysis. A, Normal diaphragmatic location. **B,** Chest radiograph during acute neuralgic amyotrophy with elevation of both hemidiaphragms.

Pulmonary Function Tests

In the absence of associated lung or skeletal disease, a reduction of VC suggests respiratory muscle weakness. However, this simple test is not sensitive in mild neuromuscular disorders because the VC falls significantly only when respiratory muscle strength is reduced by 50% or more. Normally, VC decreases by 5% to 10% when moving from an upright to a supine position,

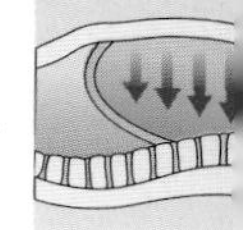

whereas a 30% to 50% fall strongly suggests diaphragmatic weakness or paralysis. In neuromuscular disorders, FRC is normal or decreased, RV is normal or increased, and TLC is decreased. The RV/TLC ratio is increased but does not reflect obstructive lung disease in this setting.

The flow-volume loop may show several anomalies: a delay in reaching peak expiratory flow, a truncation of peak expiratory and peak inspiratory flow, and/or an abrupt drop of expiratory flow at the end of expiration. In contrast to normal subjects, the forced *inspiratory* volume in 1 second is often smaller than FEV_1 because of muscle weakness and/or bulbar involvement with upper airway obstruction.

Gas transfer (DLCO) is reduced with respiratory muscle weakness, but less so than the lung volumes. The gas transfer coefficient (KCO, or DLCO/VA) is typically raised, as would be seen during a voluntary, incomplete inspiration in a normal subject.

Respiratory Muscle Function

Because loss of lung volume is neither a sensitive nor a specific test for respiratory muscle weakness, the direct measurement of respiratory muscle strength is often needed in patients who have neuromuscular disorders. Measurement of respiratory muscle function is discussed in Chapter 6. The decline of inspiratory and expiratory muscle strength may not be synchronous, and separate consequences may ensue. Inspiratory muscle weakness is a major determinant of dyspnea and hypercapnia. Expiratory muscle weakness leads to impaired cough and pulmonary infection. Hence, it is important to test *both* inspiratory and expiratory muscles in these patients.

INSPIRATORY MUSCLES

Maximal Inspiratory Pressure

The maximal inspiratory pressure (PImax) developed during a volitional effort from FRC or RV is the test most commonly used to assess inspiratory muscle strength. A PImax lower than 30% of normal value is a predictor of hypercapnia in patients with neuromuscular disorders. The main limitation of PImax is its difficulty for the subject. As a consequence, low values are difficult to interpret, because, although they reflect true muscle weakness, they can also be found in normal subjects. Moreover, PImax often cannot be interpreted in neuromuscular disorders because of air leaks around the mouthpiece caused by orofacial muscle weakness.

Sniff Nasal Inspiratory Pressure

The nasal sniff test is not hampered by orofacial muscle weakness, and it is therefore particularly useful for patients with neuromuscular disorders (Fig. 68.7). Normal values are similar or slightly higher than for PImax (Table 68.2). The sniff nasal inspiratory pressure (SNIP) declines linearly in patients with ALS and is a good predictor of hypercapnia when it falls below 32% of normal value (Fig. 68.8).

Sniff Transdiaphragmatic Pressure

The formal evaluation of diaphragmatic strength requires specialized equipment (see Chapter 6). A maximum transdiaphragmatic pressure generated during a sniff less that 30 cm H_2O accurately predicts hypercapnia in patients with ALS.

EXPIRATORY MUSCLES

Maximal Expiratory Pressure

A normal value of maximal expiratory pressure (PEmax) is useful to exclude expiratory muscle weakness in neuromuscular disorders. Low values are more difficult to interpret because of

Table 68.2
Sniff nasal inspiratory pressure (SNIP)

Gender	Age (years)	SNIP (cm H_2O)
Male	6-17	110 (60-160)
	20-65	110 (70-150)
	66-80	90 (50-130)
Female	6-17	95 (50-140)
	20-65	85 (50-120)
	66-80	75 (50-100)

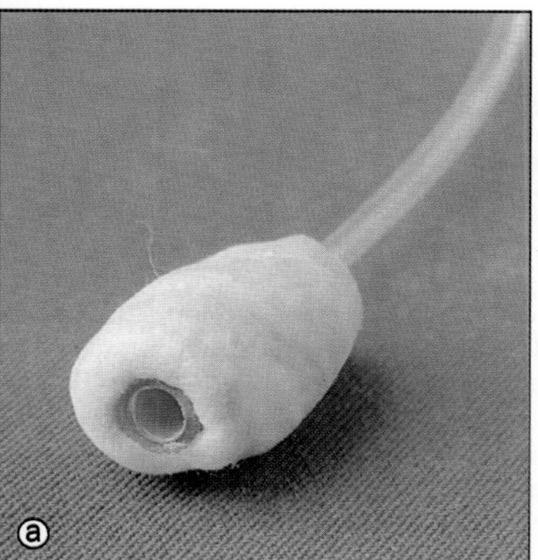

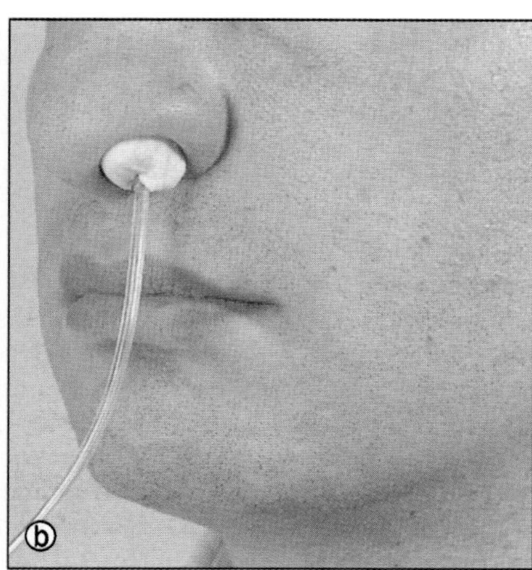

Figure 68.7 Method for performing sniff nasal inspiratory pressure. A, A plug made of two to three waxed ear plugs is hand fitted around the tip of a catheter. **B,** The plug and catheter are inserted into one nostril, which enables the measurement of sniff nasal inspiratory pressure while the subject performs a maximal sniff through the contralateral nostril.

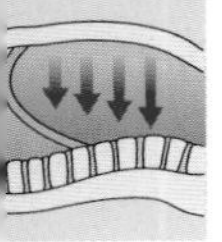

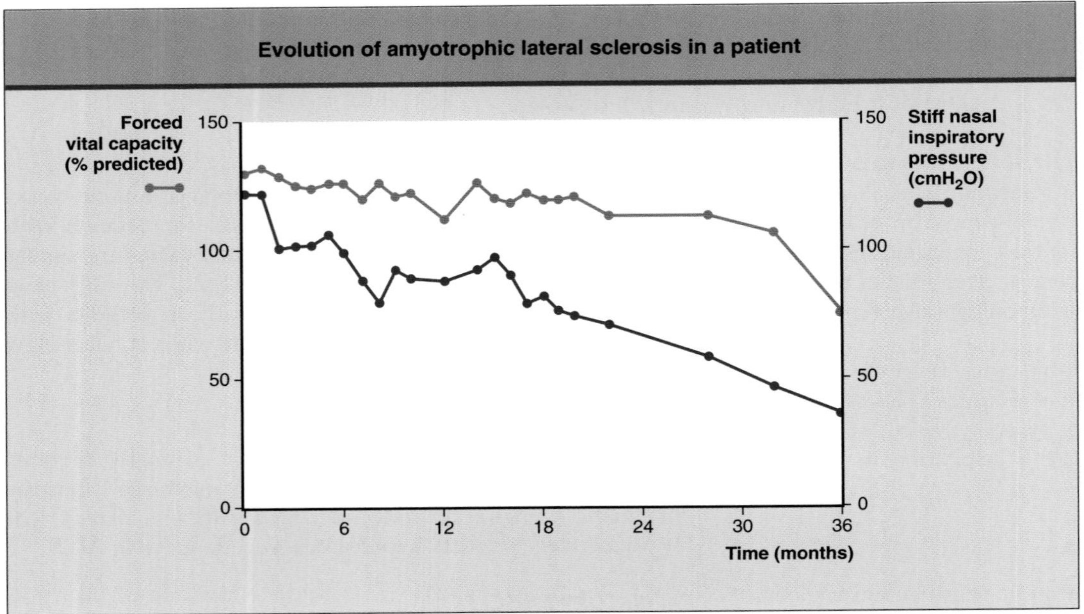

Figure 68.8 Evolution of a patient with amyotrophic lateral sclerosis (ALS). In this case, forced vital capacity (VC) remains initially stable and drops after 30 months. In contrast, sniff nasal inspiratory pressure falls early, heralding progression of the disease.

possible air leaks with orofacial weakness. Unfortunately, the loss of cough function cannot be reliably predicted from PEmax alone.

Cough Tests

The measurement of cough gastric pressure (cough Pga) is more invasive but is also more relevant than PEmax in neuromuscular disorders. Values of cough Pga below 50 cm H_2O are associated with an impaired cough function. A simple and noninvasive test consists of measuring peak expiratory flow during a maximal cough effort (cough peak flow). Whereas the normal cough peak flow ranges between 360 and 1200 L/min, values below 160 L/min are associated with the inability to clear secretions from central airways.

If the diaphragmatic function is to be specifically assessed because of concern about a suspected neuromuscular disease, often the patient should be referred to a specialized laboratory for testing (Table 68.3). Simple and noninvasive tests of lung function and respiratory muscle strength are preferred to monitor the evolution over time, however.

Table 68.3
Respiratory assessment in neuromuscular disorders

Type	Notes
Clinical assessment	History – dyspnea, orthopnea, difficulty in coughing or swallowing, early morning headache, daytime somnolence Examination – tachypnea, cyanosis, abdominal or rib cage paradox, contraction of abdominal or neck muscles, amyotrophy
Imaging	Static – chest radiography Dynamic – fluoroscopy, ultrasound
Functional assessment	Simple tests Sitting and supine vital capacities Lung volumes Flow–volume loop Arterial blood gases Nocturnal oximetry Maximal inspiratory and expiratory pressures Sniff nasal inspiratory pressure Cough peak flow
	Specialized tests Sniff transdiaphragmatic pressure Cough gastric pressure Phrenic nerve stimulation Twitch transdiaphragmatic pressure Twitch mouth pressure Conduction time

TREATMENT

Indications for Mechanical Ventilation

Whenever possible, specific treatment of the causal neurologic process is applied. This is not possible for some of the neuromuscular disorders and is often not adequate to prevent respiratory failure in many of the others. In many cases, the primary therapeutic option is ventilatory support. The methods of invasive and noninvasive mechanical ventilation are described in Chapters 14 and 15.

Mechanical ventilation may be indicated when patients develop severe dyspnea, tachypnea, and acute CO_2 retention from acute pulmonary infections. Endotracheal intubation is mandatory if the patient cannot protect the airway, if retention of secretions occurs, or if any associated acute dysfunction is present. Otherwise, noninvasive mechanical ventilation may be tried if the patient is cooperative. In other patients, chronic respiratory failure develops with no or only few symptoms. The time at which ventilatory assistance must be initiated in this setting is not clear, and many patients may not accept this therapy without subjective benefit. Nocturnal ventilatory assistance should be initiated when there are symptoms of chronic hypoventilation or when the daytime $PaCO_2$ exceeds 6.6 kPa (50 mm Hg). Noninvasive positive-pressure ventilation is the ventilatory mode of choice in these circumstances, but patients

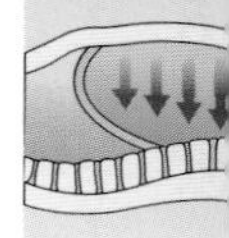

with severe respiratory muscle weakness that necessitates more than 16 hours of ventilatory assistance per day generally require invasive mechanical ventilation via a tracheostomy.

Mechanical Ventilation in Specific Disorders

ACUTE RESPIRATORY FAILURE

In spinal cord injury, the degree of ventilator dependence is mainly determined by the level of the lesion with respect to phrenic nerve roots. Endotracheal mechanical ventilation is initiated after the acute injury, but weaning or transfer to noninvasive mechanical ventilation is often possible later because of partial neurologic recovery, conditioning of the diaphragm, and/or decreased flaccidity of the chest wall.

Patients with GBS are intubated when their VC falls below 15 to 20 mL/kg, and they can be weaned when this value is exceeded during recovery. Intubation may be necessary earlier to protect the airway. Prolonged mechanical ventilation is common, and tracheostomy should be considered early, but virtually all patients eventually can be weaned from the ventilator. Myasthenia gravis can lead to acute respiratory failure. Intubation is often indicated, especially because of pharyngeal muscle dysfunction, but the duration of mechanical ventilation is usually short and tracheostomy is often not necessary.

CHRONIC RESPIRATORY FAILURE

Patients with muscular dystrophies or progressive myopathies develop chronic respiratory insufficiency at some point, starting with nocturnal hypoventilation and hypoxemia. Noninvasive positive-pressure ventilation is the preferred mode of treatment and is initially used only during the night. Support is extended to the daytime when mandated by progressive weakness. Ultimately, survival can be prolonged only by positive-pressure ventilation via a tracheostomy.

In selected cases, ALS may be an indication for mechanical ventilation. Noninvasive positive-pressure ventilation can relieve dyspnea or symptoms of nocturnal hypoventilation in patients who do not have significant bulbar involvement. Tracheostomy is the only way of providing mechanical ventilation in this setting when the respiratory and bulbar muscle weakness progresses. Although ventilation will prolong survival while the disease progresses to complete paralysis, this option must be discussed in advance to allow the patient to make a considered choice. Under these circumstances, only about 10% of patients opt for tracheostomy.

DIAPHRAGMATIC PACING

Patients who are ventilator dependent because of a high cervical-cord lesion or central alveolar hypoventilation are potential candidates for diaphragmatic pacing. This technique consists of stimulation of the phrenic nerves via intrathoracic implanted electrodes, the receiver being activated by radiofrequency waves generated by an external power source. Diaphragmatic pacing is an effective method of supporting ventilation in patients who have good phrenic nerve and diaphragmatic function, but its use is limited by high costs and the required specialized skills.

Assisted Cough

The most common cause of acute respiratory failure in patients with chronic neuromuscular disorders is ineffective cough during airway infections. Assisted cough techniques must be introduced to prevent this potentially lethal complication. If bulbar function is preserved, patients can be taught air stacking. The patient receives consecutive volumes of air delivered via a volume-cycled ventilator or a manual resuscitator and holds the air in with a closed glottis until maximal lung expansion has occurred. Coughing is then manually assisted by a chest squeeze or an abdominal thrust timed to glottic opening. Alternatively, mechanical insufflation-exsufflation can be used: a positive-pressure deep insufflation is provided through a face mask, followed by an abrupt negative pressure. When combined with a manually assisted cough, this technique is highly efficient for the clearing of airway secretions in patients with severe respiratory muscle weakness (Fig. 68.9).

Respiratory Muscle Training

The potential benefits and adverse effects of muscle training are controversial in neuromuscular disorders. Recent data suggest that inspiratory muscle training can improve respiratory muscle strength and endurance in Duchenne's muscular dystrophy and in spinal muscular atrophy. This benefit is limited to patients with a VC greater than 25% of predicted value.

PITFALLS AND CONTROVERSIES

In the presence of a neuromuscular disorder, the main omission is to miss the diagnosis and fail to appreciate the likelihood of impending respiratory failure. This frequently occurs as a result of mistakenly attributing symptoms to other, more common conditions. Accordingly, in the absence of evidence of cardiac or pulmonary disease, dyspnea should not automatically be attributed to a psychogenic cause. Orthopnea is a frequent symptom of left-sided heart failure, but it may also herald diaphragmatic paralysis. Unexplained fatigue and lack of concentration should not be attributed simply to age, but should raise the suspicion of alveolar hypoventilation.

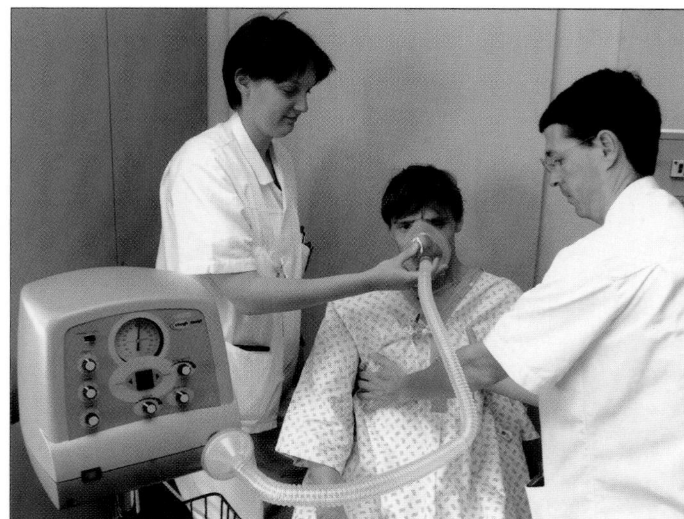

Figure 68.9 Mechanical insufflation-exsufflation. A manual chest squeeze is applied during the exsufflation phase of mechanical insufflation-exsufflation.

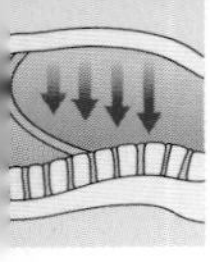

The physical examination of the respiratory system should not be performed with the patient only in the sitting position; abdominal paradox, which accompanies diaphragmatic paresis or paralysis, can be recognized only when the patient is supine. On the chest radiograph, small but normal lungs may not reflect poor inspiratory effort, but true inspiratory muscle weakness. Hypercapnia should not always be ascribed to chronic obstructive pulmonary disease, even with a positive smoking history or a mild degree of airflow limitation.

In summary, the main danger is failure to consider respiratory muscle dysfunction and to take the appropriate measurements. Respiratory muscle weakness can be diagnosed only if it is measured. The second danger is to minimize or ignore the risk of acute respiratory failure. In a patient who has a neuromuscular disorder, hypercapnia should be sought and must be considered as a sign of imminent ventilatory failure. Techniques of assisted cough must also be introduced early enough to prevent dangerous consequences of minor airway infections.

SUGGESTED READINGS

American Thoracic Society/European Respiratory Society: ATS/ERS Statement on respiratory muscle testing. Am J Respir Crit Care Med 166:518-624, 2002.

Chatwin M, Ross E, Hart N, et al: Cough augmentation with mechanical insufflation/exsufflation in patients with neuromuscular weakness. Eur Respir J 21:502-508, 2003.

Fromageot C, Lofaso F, Annane D, et al: Supine fall in lung volumes in the assessment of diaphragmatic weakness in neuromuscular disorders. Arch Phys Med Rehabil 82:123-128, 2001.

Lyall RA, Donaldson N, Polkey MI, et al: Respiratory muscle strength and ventilatory failure in amyotrophic lateral sclerosis. Brain 124:2000-2013, 2001.

Similowski T, Attali V, Bensimon G, et al: Diaphragmatic dysfunction and dyspnoea in amyotrophic lateral sclerosis. Eur Respir J 15:332-337, 2000.

Stefanutti D, Benoist MR, Scheinmann P, et al: Usefulness of sniff nasal pressure in patients with neuromuscular or skeletal disorders. Am J Respir Crit Care Med 162:1507-1511, 2000.

Suarez AA, Pessolano FA, Monteiro SG, et al: Peak flow and peak cough flow in the evaluation of expiratory muscle weakness and bulbar impairment in patients with neuromuscular disease. Am J Phys Med Rehabil 81:506-511, 2002.

Tzeng AC, Bach JR: Prevention of pulmonary morbidity for patients with neuromuscular disease. Chest 118:1390-1396, 2000.

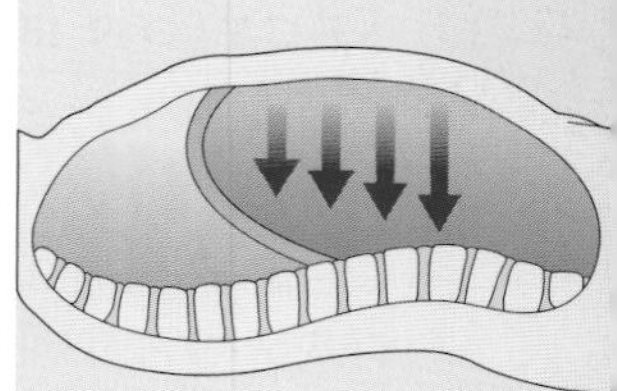

CHAPTER 69 Obesity

Richard K. Albert

Obesity increases the risk of heart disease, diabetes, hypertension, and cancer and has a number of adverse effects on the respiratory system (Table 69.1). Sleep apnea is discussed in Chapter 7 and is not considered here.

EPIDEMIOLOGY

The prevalence of obesity continues to increase. As of the year 2001, 21% of Americans and 15% of Canadians were overweight (defined as a body mass index greater than 30), and 2.3% were severely obese (i.e., a body mass index greater than 40). Similar prevalence rates have been observed in Eastern Mediterranean and Eastern European countries, North Africa, and Latin America, and recent reports document an increasing prevalence in Egypt, Australia, and China.

RISK FACTORS

Obesity

Previously, obesity was attributed to the result of an imbalance between the number of calories ingested versus those expended, with the idea that obese patients either eat excessively, do not undertake sufficient exercise, or both. Recent studies of the genetics of obesity have considerably altered this simplistic approach. Both caloric intake and energy expenditure are now known to be carefully autoregulated by a variety of mediators that act both centrally and peripherally (Table 69.2). In an average adult, body weight increases only slightly over any 10-year period, but the total caloric intake during this period approximates 10 million kilocalories. To account for the only modest weight gain that occurs, energy output must match caloric input within 0.17% per decade. Over 70 genetic loci predicting obesity have been identified in mice and a number of chromosomal abnormalities have been described in patients with rare genetic syndromes that have obesity as one of the distinguishing features (e.g., Prader-Willi syndrome). Mutations in a melanocyte-stimulating hormone receptor (MC4R), which causes leptin resistance, has been found in 3% to 5% of extremely obese subjects. Patients with cachexia in association with chronic obstructive pulmonary disease have lower levels of leptin than healthy controls.

Blunted Hypoxic and Hypercarbic Drives

A number of investigators have documented that the ventilatory responses to carbon dioxide and oxygen have a wide range in the general population. Accordingly, it may be that only patients with inherently low drives who also become obese are affected by the adverse clinical consequences. If this pathophysiologic scenario is correct, having a low ventilatory drive would represent a risk factor for many obesity-related pulmonary problems. Alternatively, reduced ventilatory drives may be the result of the mechanical limitations associated with obesity, coupled with a failure to increase inspiratory muscle activity, rather than abnormalities in the neural drive to breathe.

PATHOPHYSIOLOGY

The increase in rest and work-associated ventilation seen in obesity results from an increase in body mass without a commensurate increase in the size of the heart or lungs. Chest wall restriction is caused by the increased weight of the thoracic and abdominal walls that must be displaced by the respiratory muscles (Fig. 69.1). In some patients, obesity puts the abdomen on the flat portion of its pressure-volume curve. This, in turn, increases the work of breathing, reduces the functional residual capacity (FRC), and causes small airway closure. Chest wall restriction limits the inspiratory capacity such that the increase in tidal volume that accompanies the increased ventilatory demands associated with exercise is reduced. The reduction in FRC is magnified when patients lie supine, as large areas of the dorsal lung are exposed to abdominal pressure (Fig. 69.2), which can be considered equivalent to a fluid pressure that is equal to the ventral-dorsal span of the abdominal cavity. It is interesting to note that in contrast to normal subjects, in obese patients sitting versus supine FRCs are similar, perhaps because of the adverse effects of the sitting position on abdominal compliance in the setting of obesity. Pulmonary vascular resistance may also be increased as a result of pulmonary vascular kinking associated with the low lung volumes (Fig. 69.3). Breathing at low lung volumes redistributes ventilation to nondependent lung regions (a situation that is the opposite of normal). Because regional perfusion is not similarly affected, dependent lung regions become overperfused relative to their ventilation, resulting in hypoxemia.

DIAGNOSIS

Although obese patients may be dyspneic, the symptom is commonly attributed to the obesity per se, by both the physician and the patient, such that the link to a specific pulmonary problem may be overlooked. This is an important oversight, because some of the obesity-related pulmonary abnormalities can be treated successfully. Therefore, the pulmonary complications of obesity must be sought in every obese patient, regardless of whether pulmonary symptoms are present or clinical manifestations of pulmonary disease are apparent. Screening should seek historical evidence supporting sleep apnea and include a hematocrit (for detection of erythrocythemia from chronic hypoxemia) and measurement of lung volumes, the maximum voluntary ventilation, and resting, supine oximetry.

Obesity reduces the FRC with little or no effect on the residual volume (RV). Accordingly, the expiratory reserve volume (ERV) is markedly reduced (see Fig. 69.1). The reduction in ERV directly correlates with the increase in body weight, whereas reductions in the total lung capacity (TLC), FRC, and vital capacity (VC) are not seen until the ratio of the weight (in kilograms) to height (in centimeters) exceeds 1. The reduction in FRC (and in ERV) is most striking when patients lie supine (see Fig. 69.2). The maximum voluntary ventilation is frequently reduced in obese patients as a result of the mechanical effects of the increased body mass on chest wall movement and on the work required of the inspiratory muscles. Diffusion may be increased in obese patients, presumably because of an increased pulmonary blood volume, but this has not been a uniform finding in all studies.

Although not routinely performed, the single-breath oxygen test is abnormal in obese patients and vividly illustrates the adverse effects of obesity on airway closure. The test is carried out by having patients perform a slow inhalation of 100% oxygen, starting at RV and ending at TLC, followed by a slow exhalation back to RV while the exhaled nitrogen concentration is continuously monitored (Fig. 69.4). The initial approximately 150 mL of gas exhaled (i.e., the anatomic dead space) contains only oxygen. Subsequently, the exhaled gas contains a mixture of oxygen and nitrogen, with the nitrogen concentration being inversely related to the degree of alveolar expansion that occurred during the inhalation of oxygen from RV. The more constant the exhaled nitrogen concentration over a range of lung volumes (i.e., the slope of phase III), the more uniform the alve-

Table 69.1
Effects of obesity on the respiratory system

- Increases oxygen consumption and carbon dioxide production at rest and during exercise
- Chest wall restriction, which increases work of breathing and reduces maximum voluntary ventilation
- Reduces functional residual capacity, which causes premature closure of small airways and can cause hypoxemia
- Reduces the ventilatory response to hypoxia and hypercarbia
- Causes upper airway constriction

Table 69.2
Molecules involved with regulation of energy balance and body weight

Molecule	Effect on food intake	Effect on central nervous system activity
Corticotropin-releasing hormone	↓↓	↑↑
Bombesin	↓	↑
Somatostatin	↓	?
Cholecystokinin	↓	↑
Thyrotropin-releasing hormone	↓	?
Calcitonin gene-related peptide	↓	↑
α-melanocyte-stimulating hormone	↓	↑
Cocaine/amphetamine-related transcript	↓	↑
Neurotensin	↓	↑
Serotonin	↓	↑
Leptin	↓	↑
Glucagon-like peptide-1	↓	?
Neuropeptide Y	↑↑	↓↓
Galanin	↑	?
β-Endorphin	↑	↓
Dynorphin	↑	?
Growth hormone-releasing hormone	↑	↓
Norepinephrine	↑	↓
Agouti-related protein	↑	↓
Ghrelin	↑↑	↓

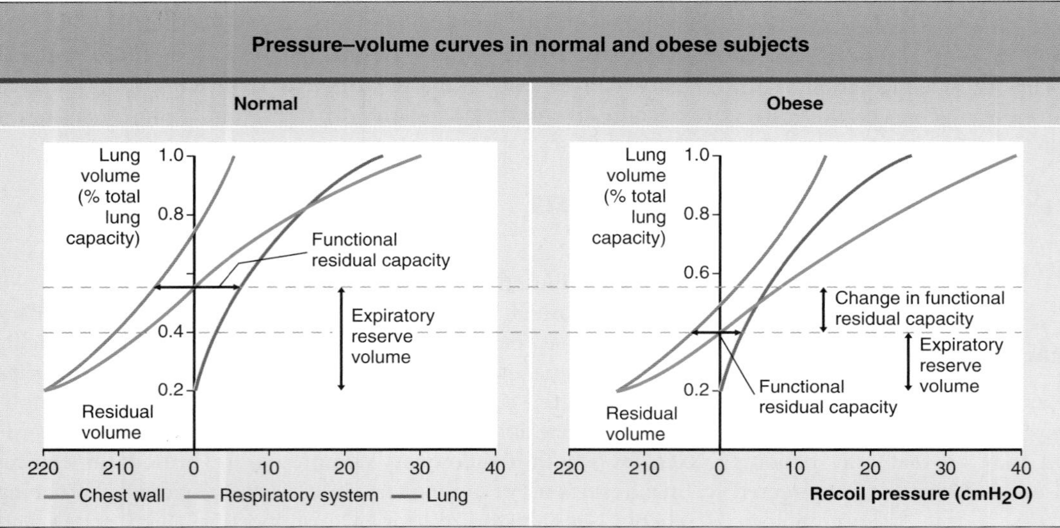

Figure 69.1 Lung, chest wall, and respiratory system pressure-volume curves in normal and obese subjects. Note the effect of the rightward shift in the chest wall curve on the respiratory system pressure-volume curve and on the functional residual capacity and the expiratory reserve volume (as the residual volume is unchanged).

olar ventilation. Near the end of exhalation the exhaled nitrogen concentration increases rather abruptly. Extrapolation of this point to the volume axis identifies the closing volume (CV), that is, the lung volume at which airway closure in the dependent lung regions begins. When this occurs, the exhaled gas starts to come from nondependent regions preferentially. These areas have higher nitrogen concentrations because they were more distended at RV as a result of the gravitational difference in pleural (and therefore in transpulmonary) pressure. Accordingly, these areas received less volume per alveolus of 100% oxygen during the inhalation. In normal subjects, CV occurs at a lung volume that is well below FRC, so that tidal breathing is occurring at a lung volume well above the volume at which airway closure occurs. In obese subjects, however, the FRC may be reduced below CV, particularly when patients lie supine. This abnormality explains the increased small airway closure, the regional alveolar hypoventilation, and the resultant hypoxemia that occur.

Hypoxemia and hypercarbia are the cardinal manifestations of the obesity-hypoventilation syndrome. Accordingly, all obese patients should have oximetry performed in both the upright and supine positions. In some patients the hypoxemia is manifested only when they are supine. In patients who have more

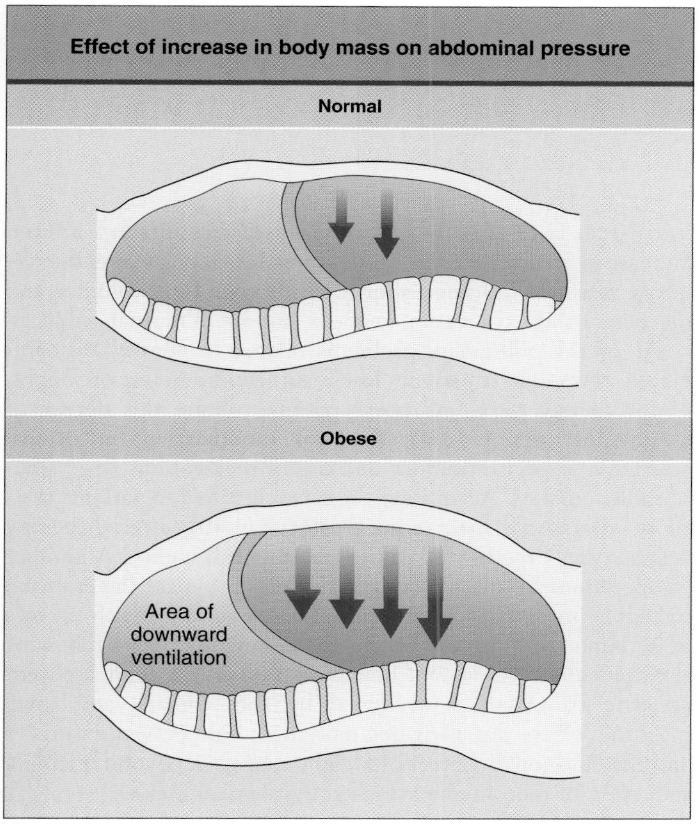

Figure 69.2 Effect of the increase in body mass on abdominal (liquid) pressure. In turn, this effect adversely affects the dorsal lung regions, which causes a reduction in ventilation.

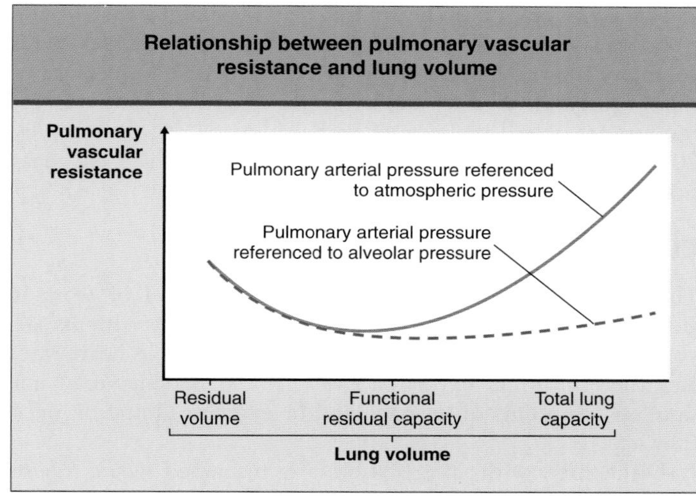

Figure 69.3 Relationship between pulmonary vascular resistance and lung volume. The solid line represents the relationship when pulmonary arterial pressure is referenced to atmospheric pressure, and the dashed line is the relationship when pulmonary arterial pressure is referenced to alveolar pressure. Note the increase in resistance that occurs with the reduction in lung volume, which is attributed to kinking of the larger pulmonary arteries and veins.

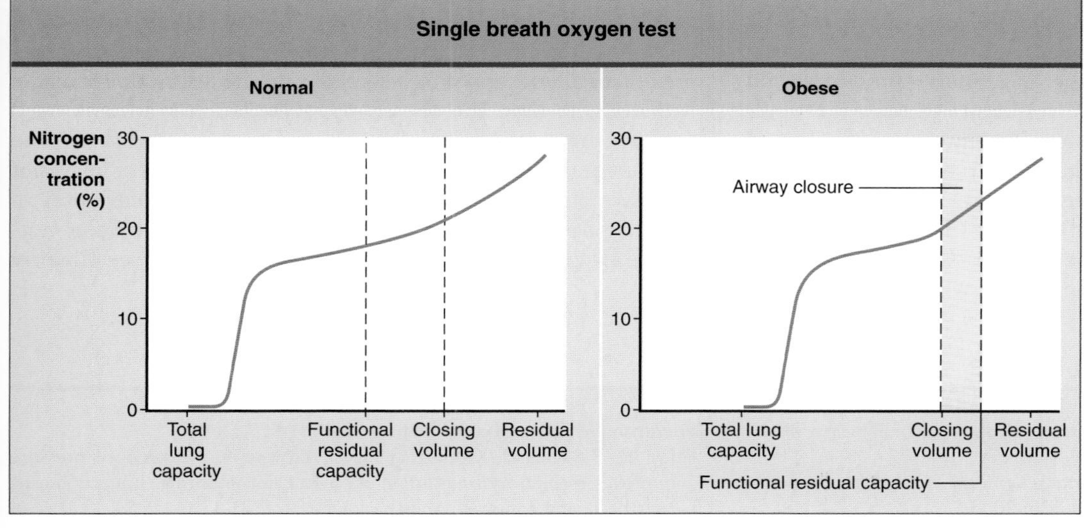

Figure 69.4 Single-breath oxygen test in a normal versus an obese subject. The reduction in functional residual capacity below the closing volume in the obese patient accounts for the reduction in dorsal lung ventilation depicted in Figure 69.2.

18

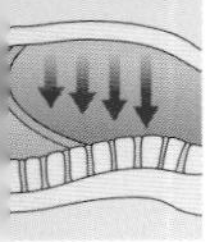

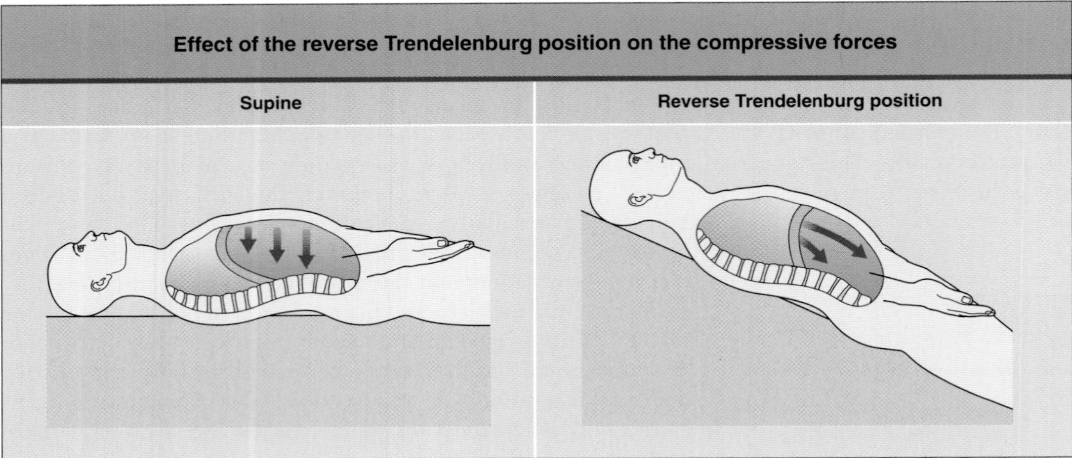

Figure 69.5 Effect of the reverse Trendelenburg position on the compressive forces. This results from the increase in body mass and abdominal pressure seen in obese patients and depicted in Figure 69.2.

advanced disease, hypoxemia is observed when they are sitting and worsens when they lie supine. The hypoxemia that results from the obesity-hypoventilation syndrome improves with voluntary, slow, deep breathing, as well as with the increase in tidal volume that may occur during exercise. On average, the arterial partial pressure of carbon dioxide can decrease by 20% to 30%. Obesity is the only condition in which oxygenation improves during exercise.

CLINICAL COURSE AND PREVENTION

The increased oxygen consumption for any level of work is generally tolerated with no symptoms when obese patients are young. Because aging limits the maximal attainable heart rate, and thereby limits oxygen delivery, obese patients may not develop symptoms of dyspnea and/or exercise limitation until they age.

Difficulties with oxygenation are magnified when obese patients lie supine (e.g., during sleep, during surgery, or when in the hospital). Because the hypoxemia is a function of the posture-associated reductions in FRC, limitation of the reduction in FRC that occurs on lying supine reduces the degree of hypoxemia. This can be accomplished to some extent by positioning patients in steep reverse Trendelenburg position so that the vector of the gravitational gradient of abdominal pressure is directed caudally, away from the diaphragm (Fig. 69.5).

Another way to limit the fall in FRC is to have patients breathe through a mask that provides continuous positive airway pressure (CPAP), which causes the lung volume present at end exhalation to increase by the resultant increase in end-expiratory transpulmonary pressure. Patients generally find it uncomfortable to wear CPAP masks that provide more than 10 cm H_2O of pressure, and the pressure that the CPAP is trying to counter (i.e., abdominal pressure) frequently exceeds 40 cm H_2O. Accordingly, the effect of CPAP is probably restricted to a small zone in the mid-lung where the additional 5 to 10 cm H_2O of end-expiratory pressure results in a limited increase in airway patency. During anesthesia, positive end-expiratory pressure has been shown to improve lung volumes and mechanics and oxygenation in obese, but not in normal, subjects.

All of the pulmonary problems related to obesity are completely reversible if patients lose a sufficient amount of weight. Unfortunately, very few obese patients obtain this degree of weight loss despite diet, behavior modification, nutritional education, exercise training, and use of medications (e.g., sibutramine, orlistat). Accordingly, in severely affected patients (i.e., those with a body mass index greater than 40), surgical therapy is increasingly recognized as the treatment of choice. A number of operations have been designed to either bypass the stomach or reduce its size, and these have been associated with up to a 50% reduction in excess weight for as long as 9 years following the procedure. The recent demonstration that ghrelin, a potent appetite stimulant, is produced by the stomach and small intestine offers an intriguing potential link between surgery and the hormonal control of weight that goes beyond a simple reduction in food intake achieved by physical means.

PITFALLS AND CONTROVERSIES

It is important to determine whether the hypoxemia encountered in obese patients is the result of the obesity-hypoventilation syndrome and/or of blunted ventilatory drives (with or without obstructive sleep apnea). Either or both of these problems may contribute to the hypoxemia, and an appropriate treatment cannot be selected until the distinction is made. Patients who have the obesity-hypoventilation syndrome need not have any type of sleep-disordered breathing, and those who have central and/or obstructive sleep apnea may or may not also have obesity-hypoventilation syndrome that contributes to their hypoxemia. Sleep oximetry and even formal sleep testing are frequently needed to make the distinction (see Chapter 72).

SUGGESTED READINGS

Brolin RE: Bariatric surgery and long-term control of morbid obesity. JAMA 288:2793-2796, 2002.

Cummings DE, Shannon MH: Roles for ghrelin in the regulation of appetite and body weight. Arch Surg 138:389-396, 2003.

Friedman JM (ed): Obesity. Nature 404:631-677, 2000.

Pelosi R, Ravagnan I, Guirati G, et al: Positive end-expiratory pressure improves respiratory function in obese but not in normal subjects during anesthesia and paralysis. Anesthesiology 91:1221-1231, 1959.

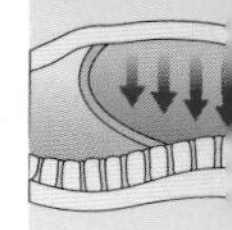

Perilli V, Sollazzi L, Bozza P, et al: The effects of the reverse Trendelenburg position on respiratory mechanics and blood gases in morbidly obese patients during bariatric surgery. Anesth Analg 91:1520-1525, 2000.

Ray CS, Sue DY, Bray G, et al: Effects of obesity on respiratory function. Am Rev Respir Dis 128:501-506, 1983.

Rotsztain A, Haddad R, Canter HG: Blood gas changes during voluntary hyperventilation in normal and disease states. Am Rev Respir Dis 102:205-212, 1979.

World Health Organization: Obesity: preventing and managing the global epidemic. Technical report series no. 894. Geneva, World Health Organization, 2000.

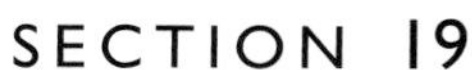
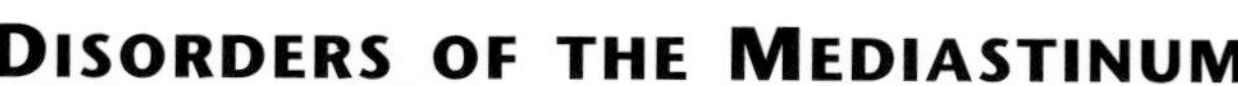
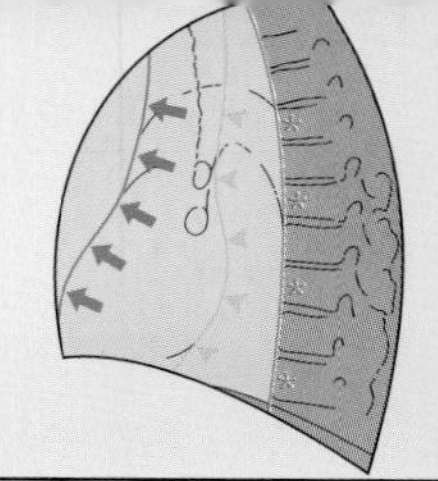

CHAPTER 70 Disorders of the Mediastinum

Diane C. Strollo, Melissa L. Rosado-de-Christenson, and Selim M. Arcasoy

ANATOMY OF THE MEDIASTINUM AND GENERAL CONSIDERATIONS

The mediastinum is the central space within the thoracic cavity, bounded by the sternum anteriorly, the parietal pleura and lungs laterally, the vertebral column posteriorly, the thoracic inlet superiorly, and the diaphragm inferiorly. Although the mediastinum may be arbitrarily divided into three or four compartments, true anatomic planes do not exist, and a mediastinal lesion can occupy more than one compartment. Anatomists and surgeons traditionally divide the mediastinum into four compartments: superior, anterior, middle, and posterior. Because the initial evaluation of mediastinal disease usually begins with chest radiography, radiologists employ the location of a mass on the lateral chest radiograph to place it into an anterior, middle, or posterior compartment. Radiologists usually do not employ the superior mediastinal compartment, as masses of the mediastinum may occur anywhere from the thoracic inlet to the diaphragm. This chapter divides the mediastinum into three compartments (Fig. 70.1). The anterior mediastinum is the space anterior to the heart and great vessels and posterior to the sternum and contains the thymus gland, lymph nodes, and connective tissue. The middle mediastinum is located between the anterior and posterior compartments and contains the heart, pericardium, ascending aorta and aortic arch, brachiocephalic vessels, vena cava, main pulmonary vessels, trachea, main bronchi, phrenic and upper aspects of the vagus nerves, and lymph nodes.

In adults, 65% of primary mediastinal lesions are located in the anterior mediastinum, 10% in the middle, and 25% in the posterior compartment. In contrast, 38% of childhood mediastinal lesions are located in the anterior, 10% in the middle, and 52% in the posterior mediastinum (Table 70.1). The most common mediastinal masses are neurogenic neoplasms, thymic lesions, cysts, lymphomas, and germ-cell neoplasms. Thymic and neurogenic neoplasms and foregut cysts are the most frequent lesions in adults, and neurogenic neoplasms, foregut cysts, and lymphoma are the predominant lesions in children. Less frequent mediastinal lesions include goiter, lymphangioma, intrathoracic hernia, pancreatic pseudocyst, extramedullary hematopoiesis, and meningocele.

The nature of mediastinal diseases varies significantly with the patient's age and the clinical presentation. Overall, approximately one third of mediastinal neoplasms are malignant. The mediastinal neoplasms that affect children (40% to 50%) are more likely to be malignant when compared with those affecting adults (25%). The majority (80% to 90%) of masses in asymptomatic individuals are benign, whereas approximately 50% of the lesions that produce symptoms are malignant. Conversely, approximately 75% of patients who have malignant neoplasms also have symptoms, in comparison with less than 50% of patients with benign lesions. Patients with mediastinal masses may experience constitutional symptoms, paraneoplastic syndromes, and symptoms related to compression or invasion of adjacent mediastinal structures. The latter may herald a large, aggressive, or malignant lesion.

The initial evaluation of patients with mediastinal abnormalities includes a detailed history and physical examination targeted for specific symptoms and signs of various mediastinal disorders and associated diseases (Table 70.2). Posteroanterior (PA) and lateral chest radiographs, computed tomography (CT), and occasionally magnetic resonance imaging (MRI) are used for lesion detection and characterization, usually followed by an invasive procedure for tissue diagnosis. However, some mediastinal lesions have a characteristic radiologic appearance, and biopsy may be unwarranted or contraindicated, as in pericardial cysts and vascular lesions, respectively. In addition, laboratory evaluation to include a complete blood count, electrolytes, renal and liver function tests, and serologic tests for various autoantibodies and tumor markers may be useful in the initial evaluation and in posttherapy follow-up.

DISEASES OF THE ANTERIOR MEDIASTINUM

Neoplasms of the Thymus Gland

THYMOMA

Thymoma is the most common primary mediastinal neoplasm in adults and the most frequent tumor of the anterior mediastinum. It usually affects adults over age 40 years, with no gender predilection, and is rarely found in children. Approximately 30% of patients with thymoma have thoracic symptoms of cough, dyspnea, and/or chest pain; 40% to 70% have symptoms related to one or more of the parathymic syndromes, typically myasthenia gravis (MG), hypogammaglobulinemia, pure red-cell aplasia, and nonthymic malignancies. Some patients are asymptomatic and are diagnosed incidentally on radiography. Although the association of thymoma and MG is well recognized, approximately 85% of patients with MG have thymic lymphoid hyperplasia, and only 15% are found to have thymoma. In contrast, up to 30% to 50% of patients with thymoma develop MG. Hypogammaglobulinemia and pure red-cell aplasia occur in 10% and 5% of patients who have thymoma, respectively. Nonthymic malignancies occur in 12% to 20% of patients with thymoma and include thyroid carcinoma, bronchogenic carcinoma, and lymphoma.

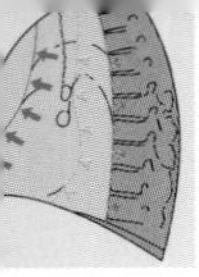

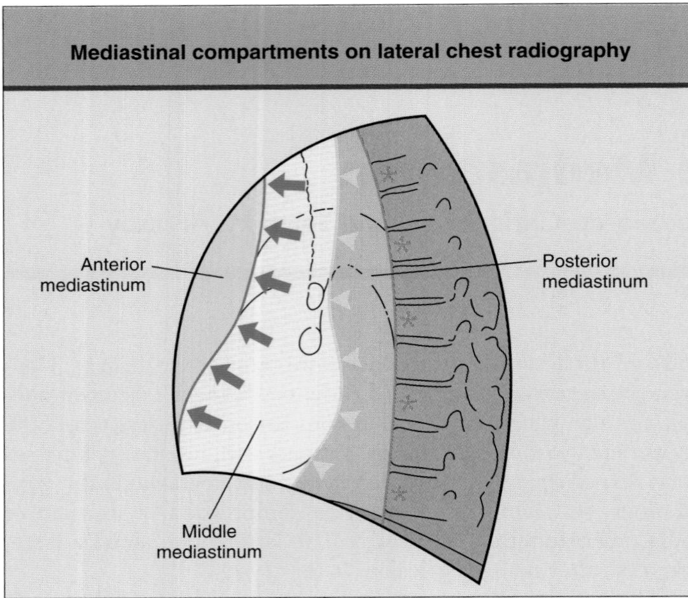

Figure 70.1 Mediastinal compartments on lateral chest radiography. The anterior mediastinum is the area between the sternum anteriorly and the heart and great vessels *(arrows)* posteriorly. A line placed along the posterior aspect of the trachea and heart *(arrowheads)* divides the middle from the posterior mediastinum, which is defined posteriorly by the vertebrae *(asterisks)*.

Table 70.1
Compartmental classification of mediastinal disorders

Location	Source of abnormality	Disorder
Anterior mediastinum	Disorders of the thymus gland	Thymoma Thymic carcinoma Thymic carcinoid Thymolipoma Thymic cyst Thymic hyperplasia
	Lymphoma	Hodgkin disease Non-Hodgkin lymphoma
	Germ cell neoplasms	Benign Mature teratoma
		Malignant Seminoma Non-seminomatous germ cell neoplasms
	Thyroid	Intrathoracic goiter
	Parathyroid	Parathyroid adenoma
	Miscellaneous	Mesenchymal neoplasms (lipoma, liposarcoma, angiosarcoma, leiomyoma) Cystic hygroma (mediastinal lymphangioma)
Middle mediastinum	Lymph node enlargement	Lymphoma
		Benign mediastinal lymphadenopathy Granulomatous disease Infectious (tuberculosis, fungal infections) Noninfectious (sarcoidosis, silicosis) Miscellaneous causes Castleman disease Amyloidosis
		Metastatic mediastinal lymphadenopathy Lung, renal cell, gastrointestinal carcinoma, breast
	Cysts	Foregut cysts Bronchogenic and enteric cysts
		Pericardial cysts
	Vascular lesions	Aneurysms, hemangioma
	Miscellaneous lesions	Diaphragmatic hernias Pancreatic pseudocyst
Posterior mediastinum	Neurogenic neoplasms	Peripheral nerve neoplasms Schwannoma, neurofibroma, malignant peripheral nerve sheath neoplasm
		Sympathetic ganglia neoplasms Ganglioneuroma, ganglioneuroblastoma, neuroblastoma
		Paraganglionic neoplasms Pheochromocytoma, paraganglioma
	Esophageal disorders	Achalasia Benign tumors Esophageal carcinoma Esophageal diverticulum
	Spinal	Lateral thoracic meningocele Paraspinal abscess (Pott's disease)
	Miscellaneous	Extramedullary hematopoiesis Thoracic duct cysts

Table 70.2
Constitutional and paraneoplastic findings of mediastinal disorders

Diseases	Clinical findings
Lymphoma	Fever, weight loss, night sweats, pruritus, hypercalcemia
Thymoma	Myasthenia gravis, hypogammaglobulinemia, pure red-cell aplasia
Thymic carcinoid	Cushing's syndrome, syndrome of inappropriate antidiuretic hormone secretion
Germ cell neoplasms	Gynecomastia, Klinefelter syndrome, hematologic neoplasms
Intrathoracic goiter	Hyper/hypothyroidism
Pheochromocytoma	Hypertension, hypercalcemia, polycythemia, Cushing syndrome
Autonomic ganglia neoplasms	Opsomyoclonus, hypertension, watery diarrhea, Horner syndrome
Sarcoidosis	Hypercalcemia

Thymomas manifest on radiography as rounded, well-circumscribed, unilateral, anterior mediastinal masses (Fig. 70.2). They are typically located anterior to the aortic root, but may be found anywhere from the thoracic inlet to the diaphragm, and rarely in the neck. On cross-sectional imaging, thymomas are typically homogeneous, soft-tissue masses (Fig. 70.3), but may exhibit heterogeneity because of cystic change, hemorrhage, or necrosis, especially in large neoplasms. "Drop metastases" to the ipsilateral pleura, pericardium, or upper abdomen via a diaphragmatic hiatus are well documented and represent invasive disease. Pleural drop metastases may encase the lung and mimic diffuse malignant mesothelioma, although

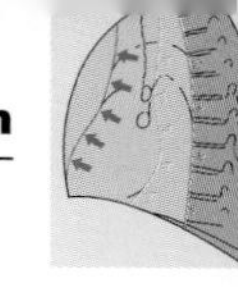

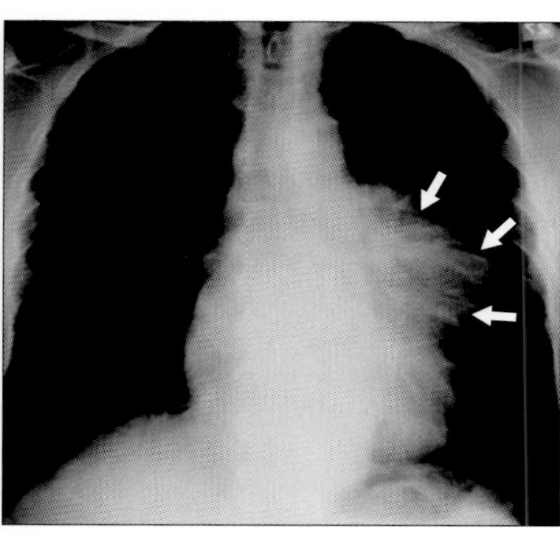

Figure 70.2 Posteroanterior (PA) chest radiograph of a patient with thymoma. A large, lobular, left anterior mediastinal thymoma ***(arrows)*** extends into the inferior mediastinum. Thymomas occur anywhere between the thoracic inlet and the diaphragm.

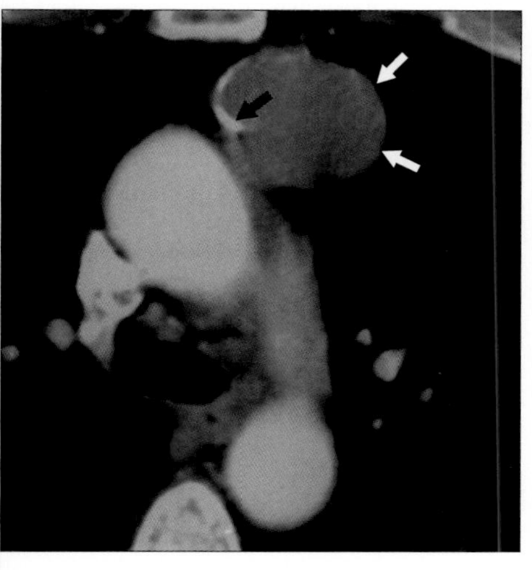

Figure 70.3 Contrast-enhanced chest computed tomographic (CT) scan (mediastinal window) of a patient with thymoma. A sharply marginated thymoma ***(white arrows)*** arises from the left thymic lobe and exhibits capsular calcification ***(black arrow)***.

associated pleural effusion is infrequent. Lymph node and hematogenous metastases are rare. Mediastinal invasion may be detected with CT and may manifest as an irregular tumoral surface, contralateral extension of thymoma across the midline, and obvious invasion of mediastinal fat and structures. Imaging evidence of local invasion must be correlated with microscopic evidence of capsular transgression and tissue invasion, as encapsulated thymomas may produce fibrous adhesions to adjacent structures. MRI is more sensitive than CT in the detection of vascular invasion. CT-guided needle biopsy, mediastinotomy, mediastinoscopy, and/or video-assisted thoracoscopy may establish the diagnosis. However, histologic diagnosis prior to excisional surgery may not be required in classic cases of thymoma.

Thymomas represent neoplastic proliferation of thymic epithelial cells, intermixed with mature lymphocytes. The Revised 1999 World Health Organization (WHO) classification divides thymic epithelial neoplasms into three types (A, B, and C) based on epithelial cell morphology, the ratio of lymphocytes to epithelial cells, and prognosis. Type A corresponds to neoplastic "atrophic" changes that resemble the adult thymus, type B reflects "bioreactive" changes characteristic of thymic activity of fetuses and infants, and type C denotes "carcinoma." Types A and B are "organotypic" and correlate with the traditional four major histologic subtypes of thymoma—epithelial, lymphocytic, mixed lymphoepithelial, and spindle cell. Anatomic staging is based on the presence or absence of capsular invasion determined macroscopically during surgery and confirmed microscopically. The majority of thymomas are completely encapsulated; however, approximately 30% are invasive and grow through the capsule into surrounding adipose tissue, pleura, pericardium, great vessels, and/or heart. Encapsulated and invasive thymomas are microscopically identical and lack histologic features of malignancy, and thus the term "invasive" rather than "malignant" thymoma is used to denote capsular invasion.

The treatment of choice for encapsulated and invasive thymomas confined to the mediastinum is surgical resection. Postoperative radiation therapy is included in the treatment of invasive thymoma, but the role of preoperative irradiation is controversial. Chemotherapy with cisplatin-based regimens is generally recommended for metastatic or unresectable recurrent disease, with an overall response rate of 50% to 70% in small studies.

The prognosis of patients with thymoma varies with the stage and extent of surgical resection. Patients with completely resected, encapsulated lesions have the best prognosis. The overall 5- and 10-year survival rates in patients who have encapsulated thymomas are 75% and 63%, respectively, whereas patients with invasive thymoma have survival rates of 50% and 30%, respectively. Delayed recurrence of thymomas may occur, even in patients with completely resected encapsulated lesions, which emphasizes the importance of long-term follow-up.

The role of thymectomy in the treatment of parathymic syndromes is controversial. Thymectomy is more effective in patients with MG in the absence of a thymoma, with a clinical remission rate of approximately 35% and improvement in another 50%. Neurologic improvement is less likely when MG is associated with thymoma. Thymectomy in patients with pure red-cell aplasia results in a 40% to 50% remission rate, in contrast to those with hypogammaglobulinemia, who do not benefit from thymic resection.

THYMIC CARCINOMA

Thymic carcinomas are a heterogeneous group of aggressive, epithelial malignancies with a tendency for early local invasion and distant metastases. Men are more commonly affected (mean age, 46 years). The Revised 1999 WHO classification of thymic epithelial neoplasms describes thymic carcinomas as "non-organotypic" malignancies (type C) that resemble carcinomas of extrathymic origin, such as lung carcinomas. By traditional histopathologic classification, the two most common cell types are squamous cell and lymphoepithelial-like carcinoma. Unlike thymoma, thymic carcinoma has malignant histologic features and typically manifests as a large, poorly defined, infiltrative, anterior mediastinal mass, frequently with regional lymph node and pulmonary metastases, and pleural and/or pericardial effusions.

The histologic grade and neoplastic staging determine the therapy and prognosis. Surgical resection, when feasible, is the preferred treatment. Adjuvant cisplatin-based chemotherapy and concurrent radiotherapy may be employed. Response rates are generally poor, with 5-year survival rates of approximately 30%.

THYMIC CARCINOID

Thymic carcinoid is a rare, aggressive neuroendocrine neoplasm that typically affects men in the fourth and fifth decades. These

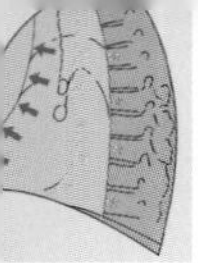

are large, symptomatic, locally invasive neoplasms with frequent distant metastases. Approximately 35% of affected patients develop endocrine abnormalities caused by ectopic hormone production, most commonly Cushing syndrome. Multiple endocrine neoplasia syndrome type I may also occur. However, the syndrome of inappropriate antidiuretic hormone secretion and the carcinoid syndrome are rare. Radiologically, thymic carcinoid is a large, lobular, heterogeneous, and usually invasive anterior mediastinal mass indistinguishable from thymic carcinoma or thymoma. Surgical resection, when feasible, is the treatment of choice, and response to chemotherapy and radiotherapy is poor.

THYMOLIPOMA

Thymolipoma is a rare, benign thymic neoplasm, composed of mature adipose and thymic tissues. It usually affects young adults and has no gender predilection. Thymolipomas grow slowly, frequently reaching a large size before diagnosis, and nearly half of the patients are asymptomatic. Thymolipomas manifest as large, anterior, inferior mediastinal masses that conform to adjacent thoracic structures and may mimic diaphragmatic elevation and cardiac enlargement. CT and MRI demonstrate soft-tissue and adipose tissue components and may show positional change in lesion shape (Fig. 70.4). The treatment of choice is surgical resection. The prognosis is excellent.

THYMIC CYST

Thymic cysts are rare, anterior mediastinal masses that may be congenital or acquired. Congenital thymic cysts are usually found in the first two decades of life, whereas acquired thymic cysts are seen in adults in association with the acquired immunodeficiency syndrome or thymic inflammation or malignancy, such as thymic carcinoma or Hodgkin's disease (HD). Radiologically, thymic cysts are well-defined anterior mediastinal masses with cystic unilocular or multilocular appearances on cross-sectional imaging. Surgical excision is the recommended treatment. The diagnosis of cystic neoplasm should be considered and excluded, and inflammatory cysts must be carefully examined to exclude associated malignancy.

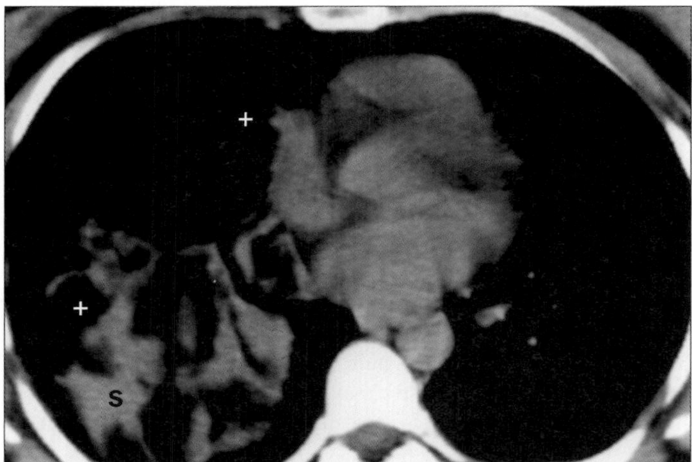

Figure 70.4 Unenhanced chest CT (mediastinal window) of a patient with thymolipoma. A large anterior mediastinal mass preferentially occupies the right inferior hemithorax. Note the anatomic connection with the thymus and an admixture of fat (+) and soft-tissue (S) elements.

THYMIC HYPERPLASIA

Thymic hyperplasia is most commonly seen as a rebound phenomenon in patients who have received chemotherapy for treatment of lymphoma or germ-cell neoplasms. Diffuse hyperplasia occurs within 2 weeks to 12 months after chemotherapy and may manifest with mediastinal enlargement on radiography or may mimic thymic neoplasia on cross-sectional imaging. Differentiation from recurrent neoplasia is difficult, and close follow-up or biopsy is required.

Mediastinal Lymphoma

Lymphoma represents 10% to 20% of all mediastinal neoplasms in adults. Approximately two thirds of all lymphomas are non-Hodgkin's lymphoma (NHL). Mediastinal involvement typically denotes systemic lymphoma, but may also represent primary disease. Although both HD and NHL may affect the mediastinum, mediastinal involvement from systemic lymphoma is much more common in HD than in NHL. Nodular sclerosis is the most common subtype of HD to affect the mediastinum. Diffuse, large B-cell and lymphoblastic lymphomas represent the most common primary mediastinal subtypes of NHL. Patients affected by NHL have a higher incidence of systemic symptoms and concomitant involvement of extrathoracic and extranodal lymphoid tissue.

HODGKIN'S DISEASE

HD is most commonly seen in adults age 20 to 30 years and in those over the age of 50 years. Even though the nodular sclerosis subtype is more common in women, HD in general does not exhibit a gender predilection in young patients. Patients who have mediastinal lymphoma tend to be younger. The usual presenting finding is cervical and supraclavicular lymphadenopathy. In less than 25% of patients HD is limited to the thorax. Approximately one third of patients have systemic symptoms. Patients with mediastinal involvement are generally asymptomatic, although bulky lymphadenopathy may induce symptoms related to mediastinal compression.

Radiologically, the majority of patients with HD have bilateral, asymmetrical, mediastinal lymphadenopathy, which frequently involves the prevascular and paratracheal lymph nodes and rarely the posterior mediastinal or paracardiac lymph nodes. Nodular sclerosis HD can manifest as large, lobular, coalescent lymphadenopathy in the anterior mediastinum or as a discrete mass (Fig. 70.5). Invasion, compression, and displacement of mediastinal structures, lung, pleura, and/or chest wall may occur. Affected lymph nodes usually exhibit homogeneous attenuation but may be heterogeneous because of hemorrhage, necrosis, or cystic change. De novo lymph node calcification rarely occurs but may develop 1 to 5 years after radiation therapy. Direct invasion of the lung occurs in 8% to 14% of untreated patients and is usually associated with hilar lymphadenopathy. The diagnosis is established with either core biopsy or surgical excision of affected palpable lymph nodes or masses found on imaging.

HD spreads via contiguous nodal chains and is staged anatomically according to the modified Ann Arbor Classification,

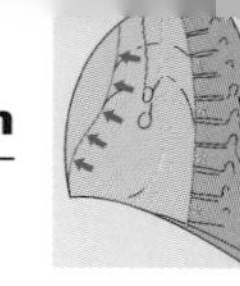

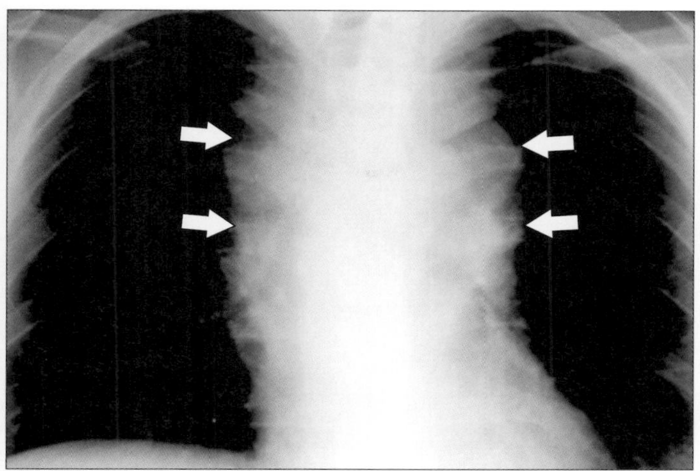

Figure 70.5 Posteroanterior (PA) chest radiograph of a patient with Hodgkin's disease (HD). A large predominantly anterior mediastinal mass ***(arrows)*** extends to both sides of midline.

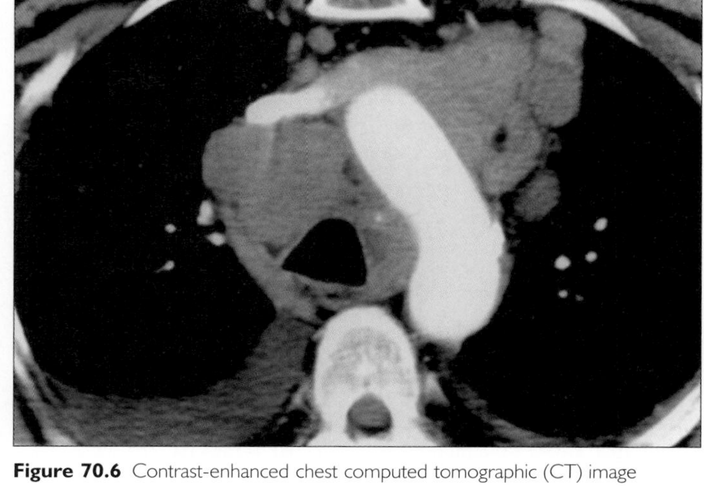

Figure 70.6 Contrast-enhanced chest computed tomographic (CT) image (mediastinal window) of a patient with large B-cell non-Hodgkin's lymphoma (NHL). There is bulky, conglomerate anterior and middle mediastinal lymphadenopathy and bilateral pleural effusions.

combined with histologic staging (nodular sclerosis, mixed cellularity, lymphocyte predominant, lymphocyte depletion, and unclassified). Stages IA and IIA HD (asymptomatic disease on the same side of the diaphragm, without bulky lymphadenopathy) have historically been treated with radiation therapy alone. At this time limited chemotherapy and limited radiotherapy are being evaluated for early stage disease. More advanced stages are treated with systemic chemotherapy. Bulky mediastinal lymphoma or HD is treated with chemotherapy followed by radiation therapy. Prognosis depends on the stage of the disease, with cure rates of over 90% achieved in stage IA and IIA disease; even with diffuse or disseminated involvement of one or more extranodal tissues (stage IV), 50% to 60% of patients can be cured with combination chemotherapy. Recurrences may be cured with salvage chemotherapy.

NON-HODGKIN'S LYMPHOMA

NHL typically affects older patients (when compared with those affected by HD) and exhibits a slight male predilection. Diffuse, large B-cell and lymphoblastic lymphomas, the most commonly diagnosed subtype in the mediastinum, occur in younger patients. Diffuse large B-cell lymphoma is more common in females, and lymphoblastic lymphoma is more common in males and is frequently associated with acute lymphoblastic leukemia (Fig. 70.6). Both may produce symptoms related to rapid growth and mediastinal invasion, including the superior vena cava syndrome. The majority of patients with NHL present with advanced disease and systemic symptoms, and approximately half have intrathoracic lymph node enlargement. Thoracic lymphadenopathy is typically isolated or noncontiguous and tends to occur in unusual sites, such as the posterior mediastinal, paracardiac, and retrocrural lymph node groups. Anterior mediastinal involvement is less common than in HD, but imaging features are similar to those of HD.

NHL is usually systemic upon presentation and spreads unpredictably; thus, histologic classification has a better prognostic value than anatomic staging. According to the Revised European-American Classification of Lymphoid Neoplasms, NHL can be classified as indolent, aggressive, or highly aggressive. Indolent NHLs are associated with a more favorable histology and a higher likelihood of nodal disease, but a more advanced clinical stage than the aggressive variety, with a propensity to transform into higher grade lymphomas. Aggressive NHLs have a less favorable histology, with a tendency for extranodal involvement. Although their prognosis is poor if untreated, they are potentially more curable than indolent lymphomas. The treatment of indolent NHLs is palliative, and use of radiotherapy and/or chemotherapy depends on disease stage.

Mediastinal Germ-Cell Neoplasms

The most common primary extragonadal site of germ-cell neoplasms is the anterior mediastinum. These lesions account for 10% to 15% of anterior mediastinal neoplasms in adults. Mediastinal germ-cell neoplasms are a diverse group of benign and malignant neoplasms, which may originate from ectopic primitive germ cells "misplaced" in the mediastinum during embryogenesis. The majority of neoplasms that occur in adulthood are benign, but childhood neoplasms are more commonly malignant. Adults in the third decade of life are most commonly affected. Benign, mature teratomas affect males and females equally, but the majority of malignant mediastinal germ-cell neoplasms affect males. Although malignant germ-cell neoplasms that manifest as mediastinal masses are typically primary lesions, secondary neoplasia from a primary gonadal germ-cell neoplasm should be excluded. Elevation of serum levels of tumor markers, such as α-fetoprotein (AFP) and β-subunit of human chorionic gonadotropin (B-HCG), in a male with an anterior mediastinal mass strongly suggests the diagnosis of a malignant, nonseminomatous germ-cell neoplasm.

TERATOMAS

Teratomas represent the most common mediastinal germ-cell neoplasms, accounting for 60% to 70% of cases, and consist of tissues that may be derived from more than one of the embryonic germ-cell layers (Fig. 70.7). The overwhelming majority of

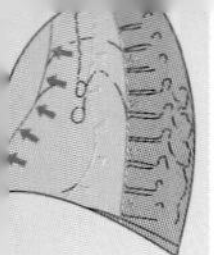

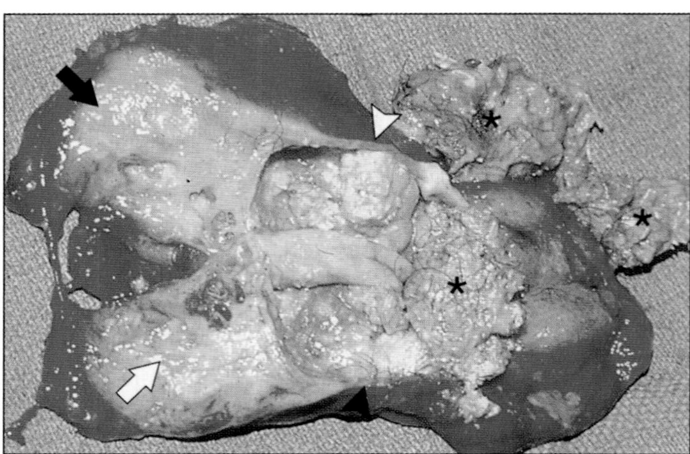

Figure 70.7 Gross specimen of mature cystic teratoma. The cut section demonstrates an encapsulated cystic mass with fat ***(arrow)***, calcification ***(arrowhead)***, and debris ***(asterisk)***.

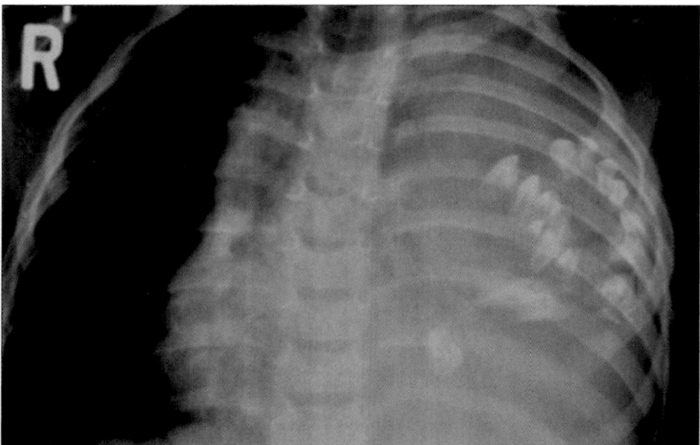

Figure 70.8 Posteroanterior (PA) chest radiograph of a patient with mediastinal mature teratoma. A large mass occupies the entire left hemithorax with mass effect on the mediastinum. Well-formed teeth within the mass, although highly specific for the diagnosis, are an extremely unusual finding.

teratomas are well differentiated and benign, hence the term *mature teratoma*. Uncommon categories include immature teratoma and malignant teratoma or teratocarcinoma.

Mature teratoma typically affects children and young adults. Whereas large tumors may result in symptoms related to local compression, patients with mature teratoma are frequently asymptomatic. Characteristic but uncommon symptoms include expectoration of hair (trichoptysis), sebum, or fluid as a result of communication between the tumor and the airways.

Radiologically, teratomas are spherical, lobular, well-circumscribed, anterior mediastinal masses that may exhibit calcification on radiography (Fig. 70.8). CT typically demonstrates a multilocular cystic mass, and 75% of lesions contain fat attenuation. The treatment of choice is surgical excision, and the prognosis is excellent.

SEMINOMAS

Mediastinal seminomas typically affect men in the third and fourth decades of life and represent 40% to 50% of mediastinal malignant germ-cell neoplasms of a pure histology. Most patients are symptomatic. B-HCG levels are elevated in 10% of the patients, but AFP level is normal in pure seminomas. The tumor manifests as a large, lobular, well-defined, anterior mediastinal mass. Invasion of mediastinal structures is uncommon, but lymph node, lung, and skeletal metastases may occur.

Cisplatin-based chemotherapy for four cycles has largely replaced previously employed radiotherapy alone and results in cure rates of approximately 80%. Radiotherapy is still employed in combination with chemotherapy to treat bulky disease and residual neoplasm after chemotherapy.

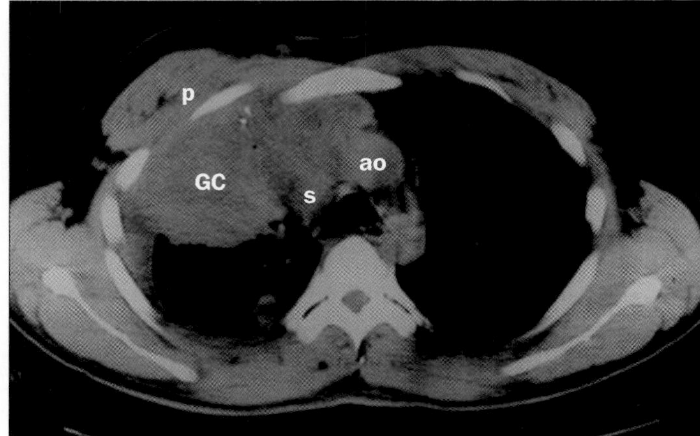

Figure 70.9 Unenhanced chest computed tomographic (CT) image (mediastinal window) of a patient with nonseminomatous, malignant germ-cell neoplasm. A large, predominantly right-sided, anterior mediastinal neoplasm (GC) is intimately associated with the superior vena cava (s) and aorta (ao) and invades the chest wall and pectoral muscles (p). A small right-sided pleural effusion is present.

NONSEMINOMATOUS, MALIGNANT GERM-CELL NEOPLASMS

Nonseminomatous, malignant germ-cell neoplasms affect young, symptomatic men and include choriocarcinoma, embryonal carcinoma, endodermal sinus (yolk sac) tumor, and mixed germ-cell neoplasms. Tumor markers (AFP and HCG) are elevated in the majority of patients. A significantly elevated AFP level is usually found in endodermal sinus tumor and embryonal carcinoma, whereas HCG is typically elevated in choriocarcinoma. Nonseminomatous, malignant germ-cell neoplasms may be associated with various hematologic neoplasms, such as acute leukemia or myelodysplastic syndrome, and up to 20% of affected patients have Klinefelter's syndrome. These tumors manifest radiologically as large heterogeneous masses with internal low attenuation areas corresponding to central necrosis surrounded by enhancing nodular irregular soft tissue. Invasion of adjacent structures, pleural and pericardial effusions, and lymph node and distant metastases are common (Fig. 70.9).

Standard treatment involves systemic chemotherapy with cisplatin-containing regimens, followed by surgical resection of residual neoplasm if a positive response is achieved. Patients who respond to therapy are followed with serum tumor markers, which are expected to normalize after treatment. Compared with seminoma, the prognosis is less favorable; however, complete remission rates of 50% to 70% and 5-year survival rates of approximately 50% can be achieved.

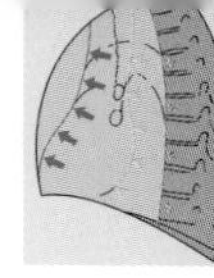

Intrathoracic Goiter

Most intrathoracic goiters result from extension of cervical thyroid goiters into the mediastinum, and typically affect women. Although patients are usually asymptomatic, compression of the trachea or esophagus rarely causes symptoms such as dyspnea or dysphagia. The risk of malignant degeneration is small. The majority of intrathoracic goiters are located in the anterior-superior mediastinum, usually on the right side, but other compartments may be affected. Ectopic intrathoracic goiter without a cervical component rarely occurs. Chest radiography often reveals a cervicothoracic mass that produces a mass effect on the trachea. CT demonstrates a lobular, well-defined mass with heterogeneous attenuation resulting from hemorrhage, cystic change, and calcification (Fig. 70.10). Intense and sustained contrast enhancement is common. In functioning goiters, uptake of radioactive iodine (iodine 123 [^{123}I] or iodine 131 [^{131}I]) and technetium 99m (^{99m}Tc) pertechnetate is diagnostic. Symptomatic or large goiters may be surgically excised.

Parathyroid Adenoma

Ectopic parathyroid glands in the mediastinum are usually located within or near the thymus gland. The majority are encapsulated, functioning, benign adenomas, most commonly seen in older women who have persistent hyperparathyroidism after surgical parathyroidectomy. Because of their small size, they are rarely detected on chest radiography and frequently mimic lymph nodes on CT. Localization may be achieved by ^{99m}Tc sestamibi scintigraphy or dual isotope digital subtraction imaging using ^{99m}Tc pertechnetate and thallium-201 chloride. Scintigraphic (functional) localization is correlated with CT or MRI (anatomic) visualization of a mediastinal soft-tissue nodule or mass. Selective venous sampling for parathyroid hormone levels may be necessary. Surgical excision is the treatment of choice.

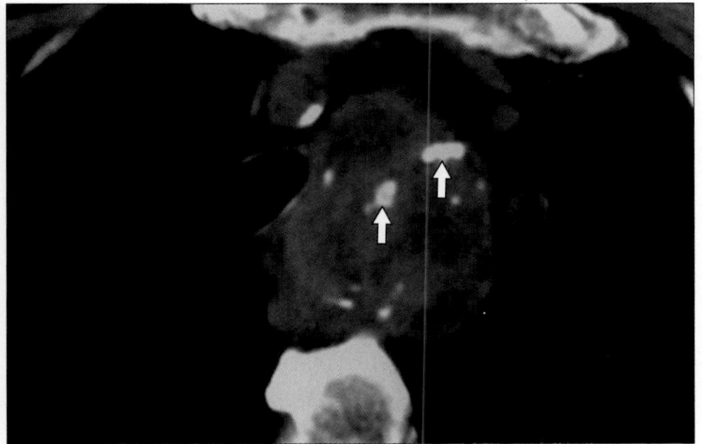

Figure 70.10 Unenhanced chest computed tomographic (CT) image (mediastinal window) of a patient with intrathoracic goiter. A heterogeneous soft-tissue mass has large flocculent calcification *(arrows)* and produces mass effect on the trachea.

DISEASES OF THE MIDDLE MEDIASTINUM

Benign Mediastinal Lymphadenopathy

Infectious and noninfectious granulomatous diseases may involve the mediastinal lymph nodes. Infectious granulomatous diseases include tuberculosis and fungal infections, such as histoplasmosis and coccidioidomycosis. The most important noninfectious granulomatous diseases include sarcoidosis and silicosis. Lymphadenopathy associated with granulomatous infection is usually unilateral and asymmetrical, in contrast to bilateral and symmetrical lymph-node enlargement with sarcoidosis and silicosis. Many of these disorders cause lymph node calcification, which may exhibit an "eggshell" configuration, characteristic of silicosis and, less commonly, sarcoidosis. Although calcified lymph nodes generally represent a benign process, definitive exclusion of malignant lymphadenopathy is frequently impossible by CT alone, and histologic examination may be required.

Other benign causes of lymph node enlargement include reactive hyperplasia from bacterial or viral lung infections, amyloidosis, drugs such as phenytoin, and Castleman's disease (angiofollicular lymphoid hyperplasia or giant lymph node hyperplasia). Castleman's disease usually manifests in young, asymptomatic adults as incidental, large, well-circumscribed, middle mediastinal lymph nodes. Nodal hypervascularity results in intense, homogeneous enhancement following intravenous contrast administration on cross-sectional imaging. The hyaline vascular histologic type accounts for 80% to 90% of cases, whereas the plasma cell and multicentric types represent only 10%. Patients with the hyaline vascular type are typically asymptomatic, although symptoms of compression may occur. The plasma cell variety may be associated with constitutional symptoms and signs of fever, weight loss, fatigue, anemia, and hypergammaglobulinemia, which may improve following surgical excision. The multicentric type is rare and is associated with severe systemic symptoms in older patients, generalized lymphadenopathy, and hepatosplenomegaly, with eventual development of NHL.

Metastatic Middle Mediastinum and Hilar Lymphadenopathy

Primary lung, breast, renal cell, gastrointestinal, and prostate carcinomas and malignant melanoma may metastasize to mediastinal and/or hilar lymph nodes and may manifest as a solitary mass, a dominant mass with lymphadenopathy, or multifocal enlarged lymph nodes. Ipsilateral mediastinal metastases from lung carcinoma represent N2 disease and may be operable. The diagnosis of metastases is established by a history of a known primary malignancy confirmed by biopsy. The treatment depends on the underlying neoplasm and its stage.

Mediastinal Cysts

FOREGUT CYSTS

Congenital foregut cysts represent 20% of mediastinal masses, and 50% to 60% of these are bronchogenic cysts. Enteric cysts, which include esophageal duplication and neurenteric cysts, account for approximately 10% to 15%. Up to 20% of foregut cysts cannot be histologically classified and hence are termed *nonspecific* or *indeterminate* cysts.

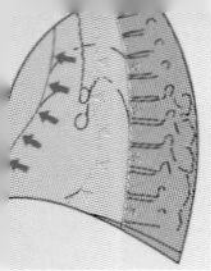

BRONCHOGENIC CYSTS

Bronchogenic cysts are thought to originate from abnormal budding of the ventral foregut. The majority are located in the mediastinum, most commonly in subcarinal or paratracheal locations. Up to 15% are reported to arise in the lung; other locations (pleura, diaphragm, pericardium) are rare. These cysts are lined by a pseudostratified, columnar, ciliated (respiratory) epithelium and may contain serous fluid, mucus, milk of calcium, blood, or purulent material (Fig. 70.11).

Bronchogenic cysts typically occur in adult males and females but may affect all age groups. Patients are commonly asymptomatic, but infection or bleeding eventually produces symptoms in up to two thirds of cases. Radiography usually reveals a well-circumscribed, spherical, middle mediastinal mass. On CT, these cysts are homogeneous, nonenhancing masses of variable attenuation depending on the composition of the fluid (Fig. 70.12). The cyst wall may contain calcification or enhance. A gas-fluid level within the cyst is exceptionally rare in mediastinal cysts but commonly occurs in pulmonary cysts and indicates communication with the airways or infection. Large cysts in children may compress the airways, with resultant atelectasis, bronchopneumonia, or air trapping. The treatment of choice is surgical resection (even in the absence of symptoms), although incidental cysts in asymptomatic adults have been followed clinically and radiologically. Bronchoscopic or thoracoscopic needle drainage of cyst fluid typically reveals mucus and bronchial epithelial cells and is reserved for patients with a high risk of surgical complications.

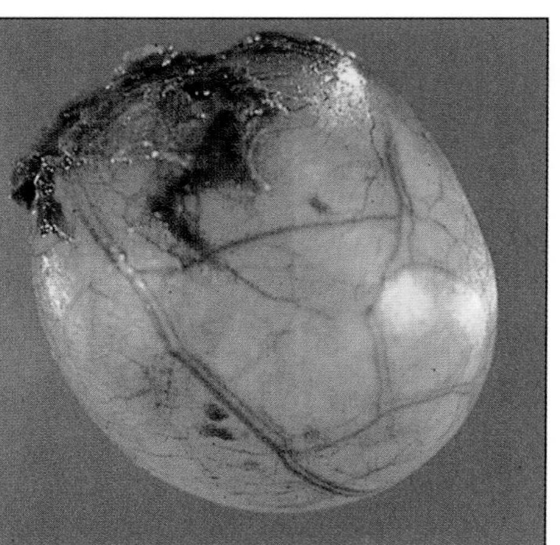

Figure 70.11
Gross specimen of bronchogenic cyst. The cyst has a spherical morphology and a thin wall with numerous vascular structures.

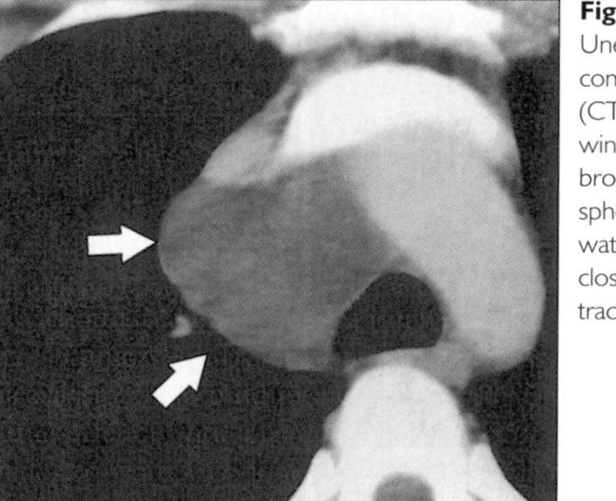

Figure 70.12
Unenhanced chest computed tomographic (CT) scan (mediastinal window) of a patient with bronchogenic cyst. A spherical mass ***(arrows)*** of water attenuation is closely related to the tracheal carina.

ENTERIC CYSTS

Enteric (esophageal duplication and neurenteric) cysts originate from the dorsal foregut, are usually located in the middle or posterior mediastinum, and typically manifest in childhood. Enteric cysts are lined by squamous or enteric epithelium and may contain gastric mucosa and/or pancreatic and neural tissue. The cyst walls have two well-defined, smooth muscle layers with a myenteric plexus. Esophageal duplication cysts almost always adhere to the esophagus or are located within its wall and can be associated with gastrointestinal malformations. Similarly, neurenteric cysts may be associated with gastrointestinal and/or cervical or upper thoracic vertebral anomalies, occasionally with a fibrous attachment to the spine or intraspinal extension.

Most enteric cysts are diagnosed during childhood. Hemorrhage or rupture may occur, especially when gastric epithelium or pancreatic tissue is present. The radiologic features of enteric cysts are similar to those of bronchogenic cysts. Esophageal duplication cysts are usually located close to the distal esophagus on the right side. Most neurenteric cysts are located in the posterior mediastinum, above the level of the carina on the right side, and approximately one half are associated with scoliosis, anterior spina bifida, vertebral fusion, hemivertebrae, and other vertebral anomalies. MRI is indicated to exclude intraspinal extension. Surgical excision is the treatment of choice. Prognosis following complete resection is excellent.

PERICARDIAL CYSTS

Pericardial cysts, also termed *spring water cysts* or *clear water cysts* because of their clear fluid contents, are uncommon developmental lesions of the anatomic middle mediastinum. The vast majority are discovered incidentally in asymptomatic middle-aged adults. These cysts are well circumscribed and usually abut the heart, the diaphragm, and the anterior chest wall, typically in the right cardiophrenic angle. CT typically demonstrates a nonenhancing cystic mass of water attenuation and an imperceptible wall (Fig. 70.13). Unless significant symptoms or atypical imaging features are found, pericardial cysts are followed clinically and radiologically.

Vascular Lesions

Vascular lesions constitute approximately 10% of all mediastinal masses and may originate from the arterial or venous portions of the systemic or pulmonary circulation. They may mimic neoplasms on chest radiographs and should be considered in the differential diagnosis before biopsy is performed. The diagnosis is usually established with contrast-enhanced CT, MRI, and/or angiography.

Diaphragmatic Hernias

Hiatal hernias are common and result when an abdominal structure, usually the stomach, extends through the esophageal hiatus into the thorax and manifests as a retrocardiac mass. Congenital defects in the diaphragm, with omental herniation or herniation of other abdominal contents into the thorax, include Morgagni hernias, which manifest as right cardiophrenic angle

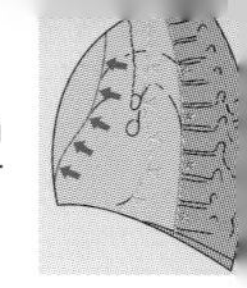

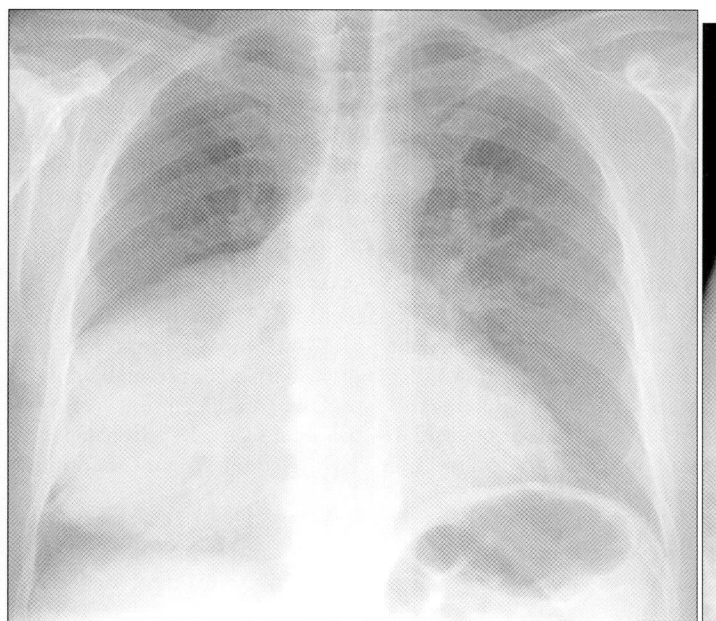

A

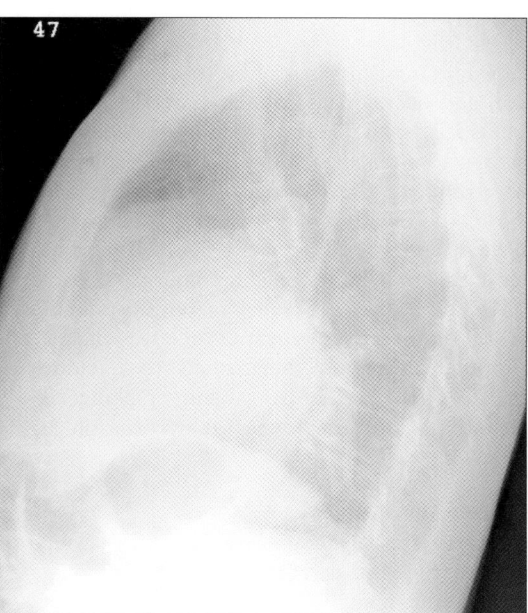

B

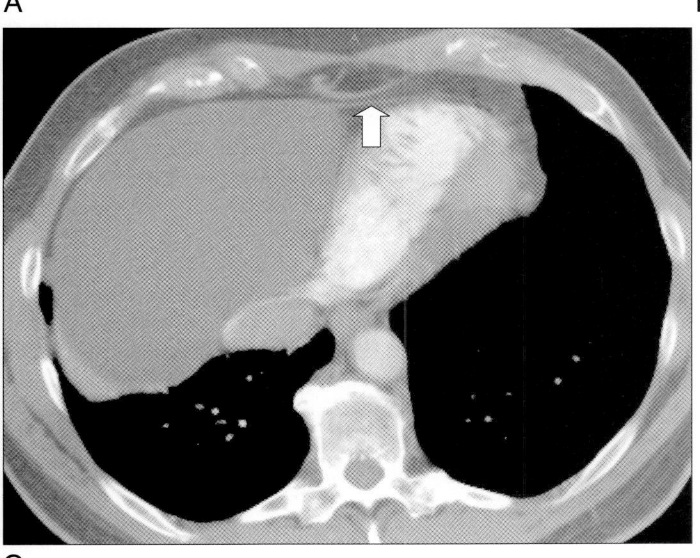

C

Figure 70.13 A, Posteroanterior; **B,** lateral chest radiograph; and **C,** unenhanced chest computed tomographic (CT) image (mediastinal window) of an asymptomatic patient with a giant pericardial cyst. A sharply marginated, predominantly middle mediastinal mass exhibits water attenuation contents and an imperceptible wall and abuts the anterior chest wall, pericardium ***(arrow)***, and diaphragm.

masses. Diagnosis can be established by a gastrointestinal barium study or cross-sectional imaging. Treatment of symptomatic cases is surgical.

DISEASES OF THE POSTERIOR MEDIASTINUM

Neurogenic Neoplasms

Neurogenic neoplasms constitute 15% to 20% of adult and 40% of pediatric mediastinal tumors. Approximately 90% occur in the posterior mediastinum. A neurogenic neoplasm is the most common cause of a posterior mediastinal mass and accounts for 75% of primary posterior mediastinal neoplasms. Approximately 50% of neurogenic neoplasms in children are malignant, whereas in adults the majority are benign. Half of the patients are asymptomatic. Neurogenic neoplasms are generally grouped into three categories according to their structure of origin: peripheral nerve, sympathetic ganglia, and paraganglionic neoplasms.

PERIPHERAL NERVE NEOPLASMS

Schwannoma and Neurofibroma

Schwannoma (also termed *neurilemmoma*) and neurofibroma are the most common mediastinal neurogenic neoplasms. Over 90% are benign, and 10% are multiple. They are slow-growing neoplasms and usually arise from a posterior spinal nerve root, but can involve any nerve in the thorax. Schwannoma and solitary neurofibroma affect men and women equally in the third and fourth decades. Although these neoplasms may attain large sizes, most patients are asymptomatic. Approximately 30% to 45% of neurofibromas occur in individuals who have neurofibromatosis (von Recklinghausen disease). The presence of multiple neurofibromas or a single plexiform neurofibroma is pathognomonic of this disorder. Malignant transformation of a solitary schwannoma is extremely rare. Patients with neurofibromatosis and neurogenic neoplasms are at increased risk for malignant transformation of one or more lesions.

Patients with neurofibromatosis may also develop ganglion cell neoplasms.

Radiologically, schwannomas and neurofibromas are sharply marginated, spherical, and occasionally lobular posterior mediastinal masses, which usually span one to two rib interspaces but can attain large sizes. Up to one half of the cases cause splaying and benign pressure erosion of the ribs, vertebral bodies, and neural foramina. Approximately 10% of schwannomas and neurofibromas grow through and widen adjacent neural foramina and expand on either end with a "dumbbell" or "hourglass" configuration (Fig. 70.14). Typically, CT reveals a heterogeneous mass, which may contain punctate calcification or areas of low attenuation. MRI should always be performed to exclude intraspinal extension (Fig. 70.15). The treatment of choice is surgery. Recurrences are uncommon, even when excision is incomplete.

Malignant Peripheral Nerve Sheath Neoplasms

Malignant peripheral nerve sheath neoplasms are a rare group of spindle cell sarcomas thought to represent the malignant counterparts of schwannomas and neurofibromas. They occur equally in men and women in the third to fifth decades, and approximately half occur in individuals who have neurofibromatosis. The incidence of sarcomatous degeneration of a neurogenic neoplasm in patients with neurofibromatosis is approximately 5%. Malignant peripheral nerve sheath neoplasms may also occur sporadically or be induced by radiation. Pain and an enlarging mass are common presenting manifestations. Radiologically, mediastinal malignant peripheral nerve sheath neoplasms manifest as sharply marginated, spherical, heterogeneous masses on cross-sectional imaging and may exhibit explosive growth.

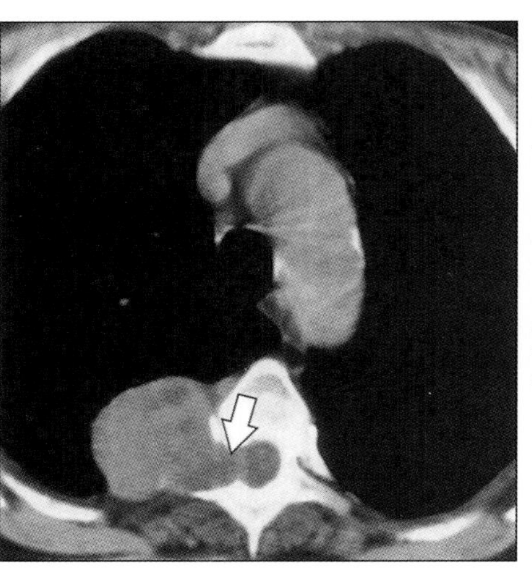

Figure 70.14 Unenhanced chest computed tomographic (CT) image (mediastinal window) of a patient with neurofibroma. A spherical mass of heterogeneous attenuation exhibits intraspinal extension ***(arrow)*** with enlargement and pressure erosion of the adjacent neural foramen.

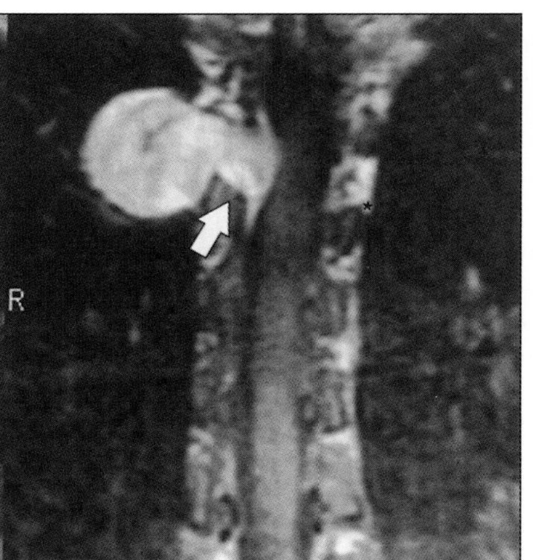

Figure 70.15 Gadolinium-enhanced coronal T1-weighted MRI of a patient with neurofibroma. There is a spherical heterogeneously enhancing mass that exhibits intraspinal extension ***(arrow)*** and mass effect on the spinal cord.

SYMPATHETIC GANGLIA NEOPLASMS

Neoplasms of sympathetic ganglia affect both children and young adults, but malignant lesions are most common in children. Ganglioneuroma and ganglioneuroblastoma usually arise in sympathetic ganglia in the posterior mediastinum. Approximately one half of neuroblastomas arise from the adrenal glands, and one third are located in the mediastinum, the most common extra-abdominal location.

Ganglioneuromas

Ganglioneuromas are benign neoplasms that affect males and females equally. Patients are older children (over age 3 years) and young adults. One half of the patients are symptomatic from local effects of the tumor or intraspinal extension. Radiologically, they are well circumscribed, oblong, paraspinal masses that usually span three to five vertebrae and may exhibit skeletal displacement or pressure erosion. MRI is indicated to exclude intraspinal extension. Surgical excision is the treatment of choice and may necessitate a combined thoracic and neurosurgical approach.

Ganglioneuroblastomas

Ganglioneuroblastomas are malignant neoplasms that usually affect children under the age of 10 years, with no gender predilection. They demonstrate composite histologic, biologic, and radiologic features of ganglioneuromas and neuroblastomas and are not usually distinguishable on imaging. Symptoms, when present, are caused by local mass effect, invasion of adjacent structures, or metastases. Staging and treatment are the same as for neuroblastomas.

Neuroblastomas

Neuroblastomas are highly malignant neoplasms that affect children under age 5 years, typically boys. Neuroblastomas in children older than 5 years have no gender predilection. Two thirds of patients have constitutional symptoms, pain, cough, dyspnea, paraplegia, opsomyoclonus, and Horner's syndrome. Systemic effects, such as hypertension, tachycardia, perspiration, flushing, and severe watery diarrhea, may result from elevation of catecholamine and vasoactive intestinal peptide levels. Radiologically, the masses are paraspinous, occasionally with local invasion, contralateral extension, and/or skeletal erosion. Approximately one third exhibit extensive calcification on radiography. On CT, the tumors are heterogeneous because of hemorrhage and necrosis, and calcification may be detected in 80% of cases. MRI should always be used to exclude intraspinal extension and vascular or skeletal involvement. Metaiodobenzylguanidine scintigraphy (^{123}I or ^{131}I) may demonstrate uptake in both primary and metastatic sites.

Neuroblastomas and ganglioneuroblastomas are treated with surgical resection. Adjuvant chemotherapy and irradiation may

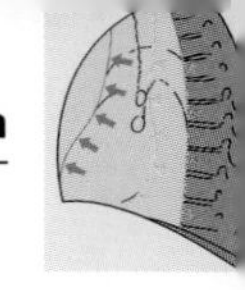

be used for residual disease or as a primary treatment modality in advanced cases. Radiotherapy in children can lead to delayed complications such as myelitis and scoliosis. The prognosis is generally poor and depends on the age at diagnosis, the size, the degree of histologic differentiation, and the neoplastic stage. Patients with congenital and thoracic lesions have the best prognosis.

PARAGANGLIONIC NEOPLASMS

Pheochromocytoma

Pheochromocytomas are functioning paragangliomas that most commonly arise from the adrenal glands and occur more frequently in men in the third to fourth decades of life. Approximately 10% of pheochromocytomas are extra-adrenal, and less than 2% are intrathoracic; the latter tend to be more aggressive and multicentric. Symptoms relate to excessive systemic catecholamines or local mass effect. Pheochromocytomas may be part of a multisystem endocrine syndrome, such as type 2a or 2b multiple endocrine neoplasia syndrome. Diagnosis can be established by measurement of urine catecholamines and their metabolites (vanillyl mandelic acid, homovanillic acid, metanephrine, and normetanephrine). Typically, CT and MRI reveal a well-delineated, enhancing, posterior mediastinal mass. The neoplasm is typically ^{123}I and ^{123}I metaiodobenzylguanidine avid. Treatment includes sympathetic alpha- and beta-blockade for 1 to 2 weeks, followed by surgical excision. Chemotherapy and/or radiotherapy can be used to treat metastatic disease.

Paraganglioma

Paragangliomas are rare neoplasms of paraganglionic tissue. Most are benign, asymptomatic, and nonfunctioning. Radiologically, they typically manifest as a sharply marginated, middle or posterior mediastinal nodule or mass, usually located adjacent to the aorta, pulmonary arteries, heart, or costovertebral sulci or within the left atrial wall. They are hypervascular lesions and demonstrate marked contrast enhancement. The treatment is surgical excision.

Lateral Thoracic Meningocele

Lateral thoracic meningoceles are rare tumors that consist of redundant meninges that protrude through the neural foramen and contain cerebrospinal fluid. They do not exhibit a gender predilection and may occur in neurofibromatosis. Patients are usually asymptomatic adults in the fourth to fifth decades of life. Radiologic studies demonstrate a well-circumscribed, paraspinous, cystic lesion, frequently associated with vertebral erosion, kyphoscoliosis, and/or widening of adjacent neural foramina. Cross-sectional imaging may demonstrate continuity with the thecal sac. CT demonstrates a homogeneous nonenhancing mass of water attenuation, and MRI shows signal intensity equal to that of adjacent cerebral spinal fluid. Symptomatic lesions are treated with surgical excision.

MISCELLANEOUS DISORDERS OF THE MEDIASTINUM

Mediastinitis

The term *mediastinitis* is used to refer to a variety of infectious and inflammatory conditions. Acute mediastinitis is more common than the chronic form and may be caused by esophageal or tracheobronchial perforation, penetrating chest trauma, postoperative sternal wound infection, extension of an oropharyngeal infection, a paravertebral or vertebral abscess, radiation therapy, malignancy, and rarely anthrax.

Patients with acute mediastinitis usually have had sudden onset of high fever, chills, chest pain, dyspnea, and dysphagia. Physical examination may reveal systemic toxicity, respiratory distress, Hamman sign, subcutaneous emphysema, chest-wall tenderness, and edema. Chest radiography and CT show mediastinal widening, pneumomediastinum, mediastinal air-fluid levels or fluid collections, and pleural effusions. An esophagram may reveal perforation. Acute mediastinitis is generally diffuse but may be localized when secondary to sternal wound infection. The treatment includes surgical drainage, débridement, repair of the traumatic injury, and broad-spectrum antibiotics. The mortality rate is high, especially when the diagnosis is delayed.

Chronic mediastinitis, also termed *fibrosing mediastinitis* or *granulomatous mediastinitis*, is caused by various infectious and inflammatory processes. Histoplasmosis and tuberculosis account for most cases. Noninfectious causes include mediastinal hematoma, radiation therapy, and drugs such as methysergide and hydralazine. Chronic mediastinitis can be associated with various idiopathic and autoimmune diseases, such as retroperitoneal fibrosis, Riedel's thyroiditis, pseudotumor of the orbit, sclerosing cholangitis, systemic lupus erythematosus, and rheumatoid arthritis. Dense fibrous tissue, most commonly located in the paratracheal, carinal, and hilar regions, compresses and obstructs mediastinal structures such as the superior vena cava, pulmonary vessels, airways, and esophagus. Superior vena cava syndrome is the most common clinical manifestation. Chest radiographs, CT, MRI, and perfusion scintigraphy, in addition to endoscopy, help to suggest the diagnosis. The typical CT finding is an infiltrative mediastinal soft-tissue mass with calcification and coexistent pulmonary or hepatosplenic calcified granulomas. Histologic examination of mediastinal tissue may be necessary to exclude a neoplastic process or active infection. Treatment is ineffective and mostly palliative; the benefit of corticosteroids is controversial. In the presence of viable fungal organisms or rising serum antibody titers, antifungal agents can be administered. With superior vena cava syndrome, long-term anticoagulation and vascular stents may be very effective.

Pneumomediastinum

Pneumomediastinum is typically caused by overdistention and rupture of alveoli due to increased intrathoracic volume or pressure that results from mechanical ventilation, blunt trauma, asthma, or spontaneous rupture. Air dissects along the pulmonary interstitium into the peribronchovascular tissues and mediastinum and frequently decompresses into the soft tissues of the neck. Less commonly, pneumomediastinum can be secondary to tracheobronchial or esophageal perforation, a gas-forming infection, traumatic direct entry of air, or cervical emphysema or pneumoperitoneum that tracks into the mediastinum.

Mediastinal Hemorrhage

Mediastinal hemorrhage can be spontaneous from rupture of a thoracic or other vascular aneurysm or dissection or secondary to blunt or penetrating trauma or invasive medical procedures. Chest radiography typically reveals mediastinal widening. Unenhanced chest CT may show hyperdense areas within the mediastinum or aortic wall, and contrast-enhanced chest CT may reveal an intimal flap or dissection, a contained pseudoaneurysm, or frank extravasation of blood into the mediastinum, pericardium, and/or pleural space. The treatment depends on the cause and typically involves surgical repair.

Differential Diagnosis

Many mediastinal masses are benign and are found incidentally in asymptomatic patients. Large lesions may manifest with symptoms related to compression of adjacent structures. Aggressive or malignant neoplasms may produce constitutional symptoms, paraneoplastic syndromes, invasion of adjacent structures, or metastases. The radiologic evaluation of these patients begins with chest radiography and is followed by cross-sectional imaging with CT and occasionally MRI. CT is useful in excluding vascular lesions and some benign causes of mediastinal widening such as lipomatosis. In addition, confident diagnosis of some lesions such as mature teratoma, mediastinal goiter, pericardial cyst, foregut duplication cyst, and lateral thoracic meningocele can be established. Adjacent structures may also be evaluated for mass effect or invasion. Patients with primary mediastinal masses and cysts usually undergo surgical resection. The presence of lymphadenopathy (in cases of lymphoma and metastatic disease) or certain positive tumor markers may prompt limited biopsy sampling of the lesion followed by oncologic consultation and chemotherapy and/or radiation therapy when appropriate. Resection of residual neoplasm will follow in some cases.

The most common primary anterior mediastinal neoplasms are thymoma, teratoma, substernal goiter, and lymphoma. All other lesions are extremely rare. In the correct clinical setting, patients with an anterior mediastinal mass should have serologic evaluation for detection of antibodies to acetylcholine receptors or elevation of AFP and B-HCG to exclude MG and nonseminomatous malignant germ-cell neoplasm, respectively. Most primary thymic neoplasms arise in one lobe of the thymus and exhibit unilateral growth; thus, an anterior mediastinal mass that extends across the midline is likely an aggressive neoplasm or diffuse malignant lymphadenopathy. Whereas thymoma typically manifests as a homogeneous unilateral thymic mass, invasive thymoma may exhibit irregular margins, invasion of mediastinal tissue planes and structures, and/or drop metastases. Mature teratoma typically manifests as a large unilateral multilocular cystic mass that often exhibits intrinsic fat and/or calcification. Intrathoracic goiter almost always results from contiguous extension of a cervical goiter. Lymphoma may affect any mediastinal compartment and classically manifests as lymph node enlargement. The diagnosis is frequently made by biopsy of a palpable peripheral lymph node, and mediastinal involvement is determined by cross-sectional imaging studies. Diagnostic problems may arise when lymphoma manifests with primary mediastinal lymphadenopathy or focal mass.

Middle mediastinal masses include lesions from many causes. Mediastinal lymphadenopathy is common and may be of benign or malignant etiology to include lymphoma. Mediastinal cysts are typically congenital, classically affect predominantly the middle mediastinal compartment, and are often surgically excised because of the high incidence of symptoms and complications. Radiologic characteristics can establish the diagnosis of congenital cysts in most cases. Pericardial cysts and lateral thoracic meningoceles are often followed clinically and on imaging.

Neurogenic neoplasms are common posterior mediastinal masses. Based on morphology, patient age, and presence or absence of symptoms or associated conditions, a prospective diagnosis can usually be established. Lesions of peripheral nerve origin typically affect asymptomatic adults, have a spherical morphology, and are cured by excision. Multiple lesions suggest the diagnosis of neurofibromatosis. Neoplasms of sympathetic ganglial origin usually affect children and young adults, have an elongate morphology, and have a variable prognosis due to higher frequency of malignant histologic types. Preoperative assessment usually includes MRI to exclude intraspinal extension and exclusion of elevated levels of serum and urine catecholamines in some cases to exclude malignancy or clinically active neoplasms.

SUGGESTED READINGS

Chalabreysse L, Roy P, Cordier JF, et al: Correlation of the WHO schema for the classification of thymic epithelial neoplasms with prognosis: A retrospective study of 90 tumors. Am J Surg Pathol 26:1605-1611, 2002.

Fraser RS, Müller NL, Colman N, Paré PD: The normal chest. In Fraser RS, Müller NL, Colman N, Paré PD (eds): Diagnosis of Diseases of the Chest, 4th ed. Philadelphia, WB Saunders, 1999, pp 2875-2937.

Lonergan GJ, Schwab CM, Suarez ES, Carlson CL: Neuroblastoma, ganglioneuroblastoma, and ganglioneuroma: Radiologic-pathologic correlation. Radiographics 22:911-934, 2002.

Moeller KH, Rosado-de-Christenson ML, Templeton PA: Mediastinal mature teratoma: Imaging features. AJR Am J Roentgenol 169:985-990, 1997.

St-Georges R, Deslauriers J, Duranceau A, et al: Clinical spectrum of bronchogenic cysts of the mediastinum and lung in the adult. Ann Thorac Surg 52:6-13, 1991.

Strollo DC, Rosado-de-Christenson ML: Tumors of the thymus. J Thorac Imaging 14:152-171, 1999.

Strollo DC, Rosado-de-Christenson ML: Primary mediastinal malignant germ cell neoplasms: Imaging features. Chest Surg Clin N Am 12:645-658, 2002.

Strollo DC, Rosado-de-Christenson ML, Jett JR: Primary mediastinal tumors. Part I. Tumors of the anterior mediastinum. Chest 112:511-522, 1997.

Strollo DC, Rosado-de-Christenson ML, Jett JR: Primary mediastinal tumors. Part II. Tumors of the middle and posterior mediastinum. Chest 112:1344-1357, 1997.

Wychulis AR, Payne WS, Clagett OT, Woolner LB: Surgical treatment of mediastinal tumors. J Thorac Cardiovasc Surg 62:379-391, 1971.

CHAPTER 71 Obstructive Sleep Apnea

Charles W. Atwood, Jr. and Patrick J. Strollo, Jr.

Obstructive sleep apnea (OSA) is a disorder characterized by collapse of the pharyngeal airway during sleep. A sleep apnea event is defined as a 10-second cessation of airflow. The presence of continued ventilatory effort characterizes it as an obstructive apnea rather than a central apnea, in which airflow and ventilatory effort are both absent. Sleep hypopnea, a related condition, is a reduction in airflow by a defined amount, accompanied by a desaturation of 3% to 4%. *Sleep-disordered breathing* (SDB) is a more general term used to encompass both sleep apneas and hypopneas. Sleep apnea–hypopnea syndrome (SAHS) is used to define patients who have a sleep-study–based diagnosis of sleep apneas and hypopneas associated with clinical symptoms of the disorder. Examples of sleep apneas and hypopneas are shown in Figure 71.1.

EPIDEMIOLOGY

SAHS is a common disorder. A large epidemiologic study of the prevalence of SDB in middle-aged Americans found that 4% of men and 2% of women have SAHS, defined as a positive sleep study with appropriate clinical symptoms. Abnormal sleep-study results without the presence of symptoms were found in 24% of men and 9% of women. Other epidemiologic studies have found similar degrees of prevalence.

RISK FACTORS

Several conditions predispose an individual to sleep apnea. These include age, male gender, obesity, increased neck circumference, use of alcohol or sedative or hypnotic medications, and craniofacial abnormalities, such as retrognathia. A recent study demonstrated that certain craniofacial abnormalities, such as retrognathia and a decreased intermolar distance (resulting in a high, arched palate), when combined with the body mass index (kg/m^2), were strongly predictive of SDB.

Weight gain is an important risk factor for sleep apnea. One recent study found that a 10% weight gain predicted a 32% increase in the number of apneas and hypopneas during sleep. Similarly, weight loss was associated with a corresponding decrease in sleep apnea activity.

Alcohol use close to the sleep period appears to predispose to SDB. This is thought to be due to a greater relaxation effect on the upper airway dilator muscles, such as the genioglossus, compared with the effect on the diaphragm, resulting in a more negative upper airway pressure generated during inspiration than can be defended against by activation of pharyngeal dilator muscles.

PATHOPHYSIOLOGY

The pathophysiology of OSA is complex and incompletely understood. Anatomic features of the upper airway such as pharyngeal diameter, the presence of tonsils, hyoid bone position, and relative upper and lower jaw structure interact with "neuromuscular factors," such as resting muscle tone of the pharyngeal dilator muscle group and the effects of state (sleep versus wakefulness) to determine upper airway caliber. Upper airway tone and patency involve a dynamic process.

Upper airway size is an important determinant of OSA. A smaller airway is more prone to closure for a given degree of upper airway tone than a larger airway, because the amount of narrowing until closure is complete will be less than for a larger airway. Tonsils or other intraluminal soft-tissue obstruction can contribute to pharyngeal narrowing at specific airway sites.

Upper airway muscle tone is dynamic and is important in the pathophysiology of OSAs. In normal persons without sleep apnea, muscle tone of the genioglossus, the chief pharyngeal dilator muscle, increases during inspiration and decreases during exhalation. This pattern is maintained during non-REM sleep. Furthermore, in normal persons, during wakefulness the genioglossus contracts in response to sudden negative intrapharyngeal pressure. This airway reflex is normally decreased during non-REM sleep (Fig. 71.2), a finding that may predispose to upper airway collapse. In patients with OSA, resting genioglossal tone is generally increased during wakefulness, which may be due to the need for greater neuromuscular compensation for the smaller pharyngeal airway present in OSA patients. Obstructive apneas occur when the smaller-than-normal airway narrows further during sleep as the genioglossal tone present during wakefulness is significantly decreased.

In addition to differences in genioglossal tone during sleep, anatomic factors such as neck soft-tissue mass, parapharyngeal fat, upper airway vascular engorgement, and intraluminal adhesive surface forces, all of which favor pharyngeal narrowing, are likely to play a role in the development of OSA. As airflow through the narrowed pharynx becomes turbulent, vibrations occur in the soft tissues of the pharynx. As pharyngeal intraluminal pressure becomes negative with each inspiratory effort, the likelihood of airway collapse increases, with apneas and hypopneas occurring as a result (Fig. 71.3).

A common feature of sleep apnea is the lack of awareness of it by the patient. Frequently, patients with moderate or even severe SAHS deny having a problem with sleep or daytime functioning and make excuses for actions or behaviors ultimately attributable to sleep apnea. A concerned spouse or bedpartner may be the motivating force bringing the patient to clinical

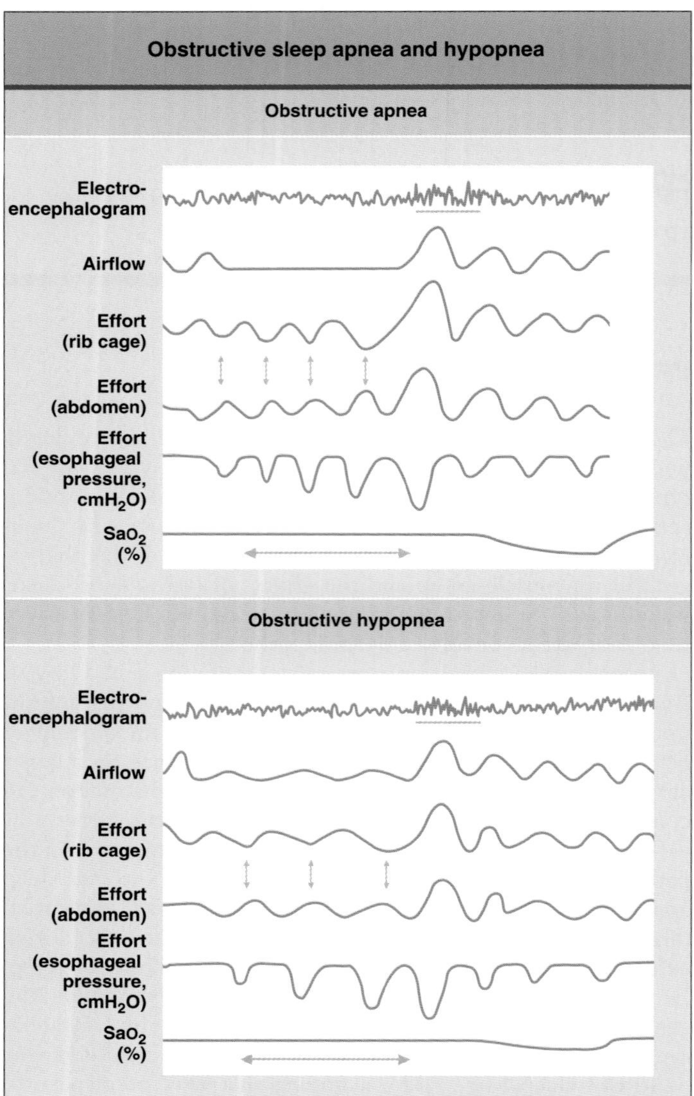

Figure 71.1 Obstructive sleep apnea (OSA) and hypopnea. *Top*, Example of key elements of OSA. Note cessation of airflow for at least 10 seconds, out-of-phase (paradoxic) movement of thoracic and abdominal respiratory effort signal, increasingly negative deflections of esophageal pressure (which indicates increasing airway resistance), oxygen desaturation, and arousal from sleep. *Bottom*, Example of key elements of obstructive sleep hypopnea. Note reduction (but not cessation) in airflow for at least 10 seconds, out-of-phase (paradoxic) movement of thoracic and abdominal respiratory effort signals, increasingly negative esophageal pressure deflections (which indicates increased airway resistance), oxygen desaturation, and arousal from sleep.

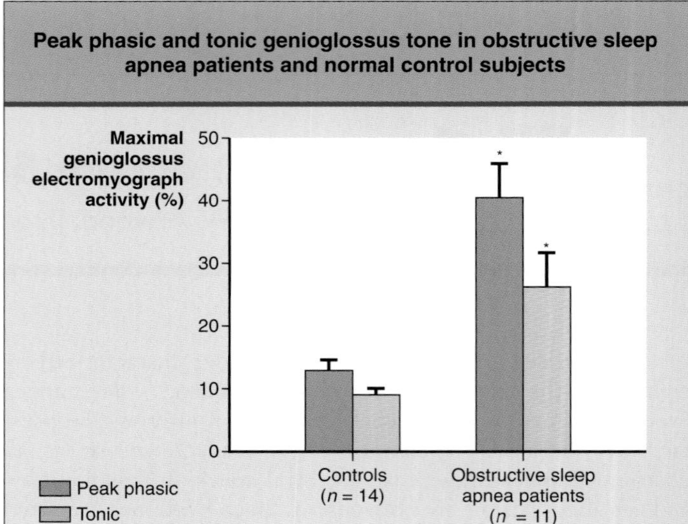

Figure 71.2 Peak phasic and tonic genioglossal tone in patients with obstructive sleep apnea (OSA) and normal control subjects. Mean data from all subjects demonstrate that both peak phasic and tonic genioglossal electromyogram activities are higher in patients with OSA than in normal subjects. Asterisks denote $P < 0.005$ versus controls. (Adapted from Mezzanote WS, Tangel DJ, White DP: Waking genioglossal electromyogram in sleep apnea patients versus normal controls (a neuromuscular compensatory mechanism). J Clin Invest 89:1571-1579, 1992. Copyright American Society for Clinical Investigation. Used with permission.)

attention. It may not be until the OSA has been treated and the symptoms unmasked that the patient realizes how impaired he or she was. Not surprisingly, the time from onset of symptoms to clinical diagnosis and treatment is frequently many years.

CLINICAL FEATURES

Important clinical features of sleep-disordered breathing are shown in Table 71.1. Snoring is frequently associated with sleep apnea but may occur independently. Many patients are unaware of the effects of sleep apnea on their sleep and awaken feeling unrefreshed without realizing why. This leads to daytime sleepiness and measurable effects on cognitive functioning. Sleep fragmentation from repetitive arousals from sleep contributes to the symptom of daytime hypersomnolence, although influences from oxyhemoglobin desaturation may also be important.

Hypersomnolence

When a sleep history is taken, it is important to ask about the daytime somnolence and to recognize its significance. That excessive sleepiness contributes to reduction in work performance, concentration lapses, inattention, and decreased reaction times has been well documented. Depending on the patient's occupation, this may lead to unacceptable risks to the patient and the general public. For example, in truck or school bus drivers, untreated sleep apnea with excessive daytime sleepiness may cause catastrophic accidents. Disabling daytime sleepiness may lead to disciplinary actions against employees who fall asleep on the job. Productivity is decreased due to errors and loss of time from work due to sleepiness.

Hypoxemia

Nocturnal hypoxemia is another important feature of sleep apnea. Depth and frequency of oxygen desaturation are commonly used methods of classifying severity of sleep apnea; the deeper and more frequent the desaturation, the greater the severity of the disorder.

The physiologic impact of desaturation in sleep apnea is not completely understood. In severe cases, it is associated with erythrocythemia and the possible development of pulmonary hypertension. It may also contribute to the development of neu-

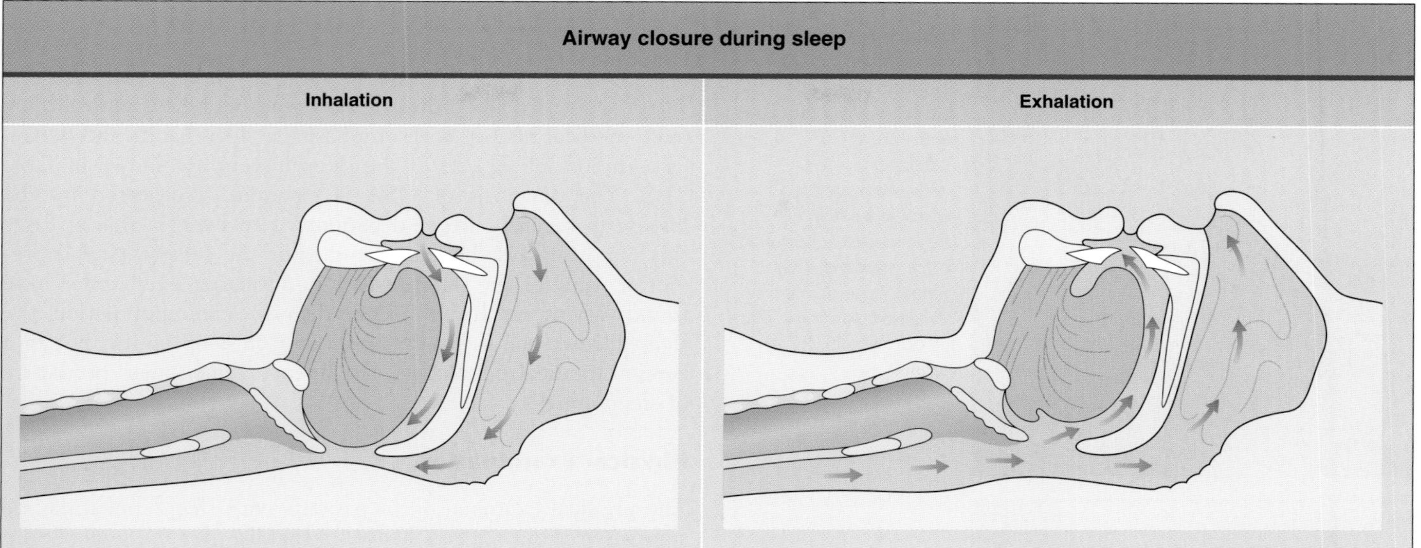

Figure 71.3 Airway closure during sleep demonstrates an upper airway segment that is narrowed and susceptible to airway closure during inhalation, when pharyngeal intraluminal pressure is negative. During exhalation, the segment remains narrowed and unstable, which sets up the upper airway segment for a repeat cycle of closure with the next inhalation.

Table 71.1
Clinical features of obstructive sleep apnea

Symptoms	Signs
Excessive daytime sleepiness	Snoring
Unrefreshing sleep	Nocturnal choking
Restless sleep	Nocturnal cardiac arrhythmia
Morning dry mouth	Sleeping at inappropriate times
Morning headache	Cor pulmonale
Difficulty concentrating	Erythrocythemia
Irritability, mood changes	

rocognitive deficits and to vascular disease through release of inflammatory mediators. However, isolating the effect of desaturation from other aspects of sleep apnea, such as sleep fragmentation and changes in activation of the sympathetic nervous system, is difficult. Clinically, patients with sleep apnea have a mix of clinical symptoms and physiologic perturbations, which are generally treated simultaneously.

Obesity

Patients with sleep apnea are frequently obese, although severe forms of the disorder can occur in individuals of normal body weight. Severity of sleep apnea tends to increase with increasing weight. The typical male obesity pattern of central or truncal weight distribution is more common than the more typical female pattern of obesity, which has a more peripheral distribution. Neck circumference is strongly predictive of sleep apnea, even more so than the body mass index in some studies.

Craniofacial and Airway Abnormalities

In patients who are not obese, craniofacial structural abnormalities may contribute to sleep apnea. A retrognathic mandible and an inferiorly displaced hyoid bone have been associated with sleep apnea. Because these abnormalities tend to occur over time, it is not known whether they are causative of sleep apnea or reflect changes in facial structure that are the result of having sleep apnea. These and other craniofacial structural features can be assessed with a lateral cephalometric radiograph (Fig. 71.4). These x-ray films may be helpful in management of sleep apnea, especially if reconstructive upper airway surgery is contemplated. In selected cases, other forms of upper airway imaging, such as computed tomography (CT) or magnetic resonance imaging (MRI), may be helpful.

Some patients with sleep apnea have large palatine tonsils that may partially obstruct the pharyngeal lumen (Fig. 71.5). These tend to be seen in younger patients but may be seen in older patients occasionally. Sleep apnea due to large palatine tonsils has been reported in patients with AIDS and is a result of HIV-related tonsillar hypertrophy. Surgical removal of palatine tonsils is not uniformly successful in treating sleep apnea. Caution is recommended before proceeding with this surgery alone for treating OSA.

Other medical conditions that can affect upper airway function can contribute to OSA, including hypothyroidism (especially myxedema), acromegaly, macroglossia (from any cause), and Down syndrome.

Overlap Syndrome

The overlap syndrome is the concurrent presence of OSA and another form of serious lung disease, usually chronic obstructive pulmonary disease (COPD) or severe obesity with consequent diurnal and nocturnal hypoxemia. Patients with both COPD and obesity have an increased risk of developing pulmonary hypertension and tend to have more symptoms and a worse clinical course. Overlap syndrome is frequently seen in chest clinics; one study at a European chest clinic found that 11% of patients with an apnea-hypopnea index (AHI) higher than 20 also had a forced expiratory volume in 1 second (FEV_1) of less than 60%, indi-

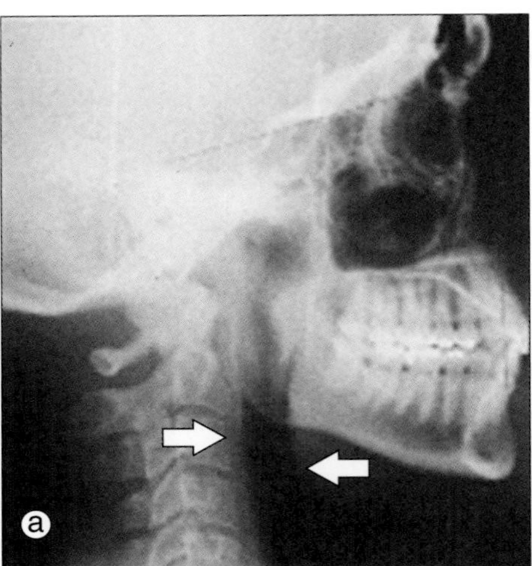

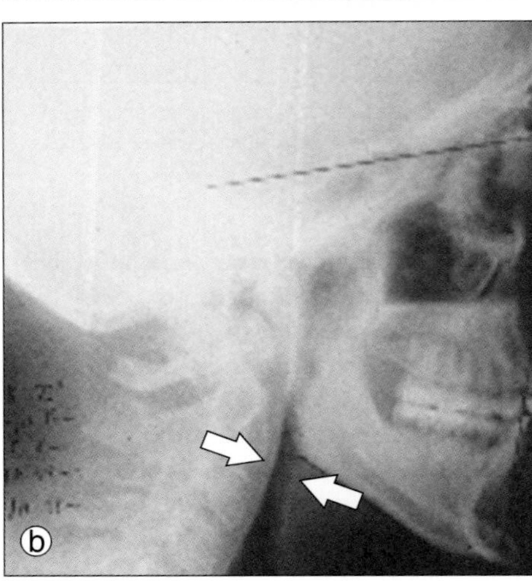

Figure 71.4 Lateral cephalometric radiographs.
A, Normal subject.
B, Patient with obstructive sleep apnea (OSA). Radiograph shows a narrowed posterior airway space (thin dark line immediately posterior to the mandible) and steeper plane of mandible compared with those of the normal subject *(arrows)*.

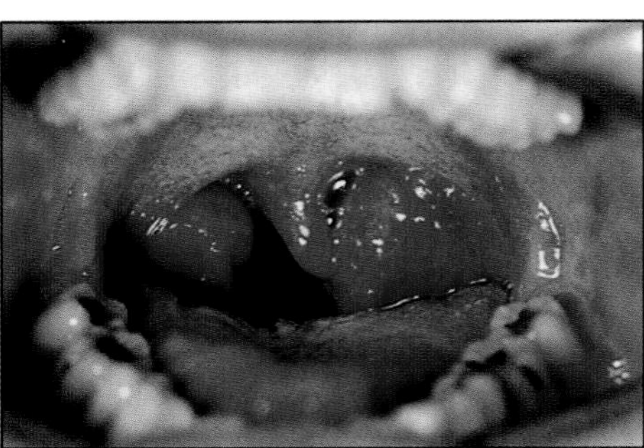

Figure 71.5 Obstructing palatine tonsils. Example of palatine tonsils that nearly obstruct the posterior oropharyngeal airway. Surgical removal of tonsils is not always curative of obstructive sleep apnea (OSA).

cating moderate to severe COPD. Commonly, these patients have been untreated for many years and have developed right-sided heart failure as a complication of their two conditions. It is not uncommon for patients with the overlap syndrome to come to medical attention with acute respiratory failure requiring orotracheal intubation and mechanical ventilation. Pulmonary hypertension is common in these patients, although its severity is usually moderate at worst. Its response to oxygen for the diurnal hypoxemia and treatment of sleep apnea is variable, but some improvements usually occur.

DIAGNOSIS

History

The diagnosis of sleep-disordered breathing begins with a thorough medical history with emphasis on sleep habits and behaviors. Important aspects of the sleep history are shown in Table 71.2. The diagnosis of OSA is frequently suggested by the history in severely affected patients. However, in milder cases this is not always the case. Studies of the sensitivity and predictive value of the sleep history in detecting sleep apnea have found varying results. In a sleep disorder clinic population, the sleep history can be quite predictive of sleep apnea, but in a general medical population, the history alone is less predictive of sleep apnea.

Physical Examination

The physical examination of patients with sleep apnea may be suggestive of but not conclusive for the disorder. General obesity and body mass index should be noted; they are strongly predictive of sleep apnea. If the circumference of the neck is more than 42 cm for a male patient and 40 cm for a female patient, it is considered enlarged; this is also strongly associated with sleep apnea.

Other aspects of the general medical examination in patients with suspected sleep apnea should be emphasized. The oral cavity, the size of the tongue, the presence of tonsils, and the position of the posterior portion of the soft palate should be noted. Obstructing tonsils similarly may contribute to upper airway narrowing.

General craniofacial structure and the degree of retrognathia should be noted. Deviation of the nasal septum should be assessed, because this may contribute to snoring and cause positive airway pressure therapy for OSA to be less comfortable. An examination of the soft and hard palates and oral cavity may reveal a narrowed intermolar distance and a high-arched hard palate. These are suggestive of abnormal craniofacial features that are associated with increased risk for sleep apnea.

Table 71.2
What to assess in a sleep history

General problem area	Particular difficulties
Daytime sleepiness	Sleep at work or other inappropriate times or places Difficulty driving a car because of sleepiness Daytime napping
Bed habits and behaviors	Bedtime – restlessness throughout night Out-of-bed time – can be substantial Number of awakenings Insomnia
Snoring and apneas	Patient history of snoring and apneas given by partner Patient awakenings with choking, gasping, or dyspnea
Habits	Alcohol, Cigarettes, Caffeine – all worsen obstructive sleep apnea
Other medical history	Hypertension, Cardiopulmonary disorders, Cerebrovascular disease – may be made worse by obstructive sleep apnea

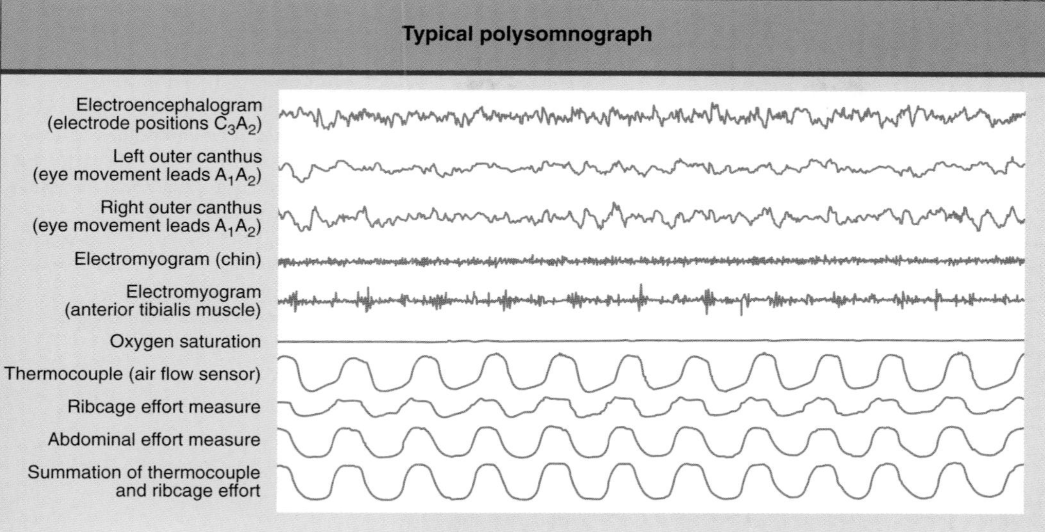

Figure 71.6 A typical polysomnogram.

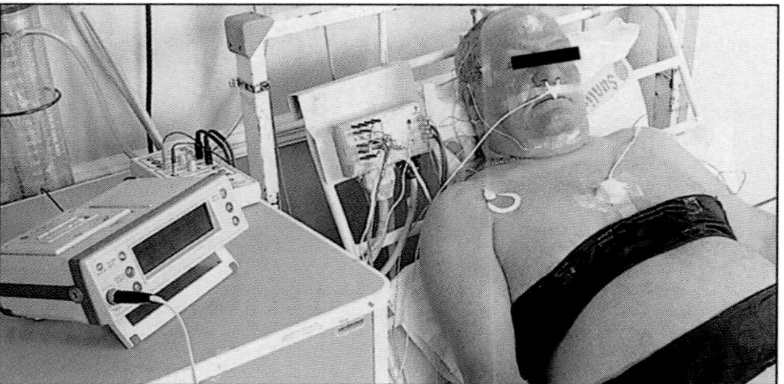

Figure 71.7 Polysomnography. Example of a patient set up to undergo polysomnography.

During the cardiopulmonary examination, evidence of heart failure should be sought. Chronic peripheral edema may be a clue to severe right-sided heart failure associated with significant and untreated sleep apnea. Left-sided heart failure and congestive heart failure have been associated with an increased likelihood of sleep-disordered breathing. The presence of concomitant pulmonary disease should be determined because of the likelihood of more serious desaturation during sleep apneas and hypopneas.

Sleep Laboratory Diagnosis

The diagnosis of sleep apnea requires measurement of the abnormal breathing patterns and associated abnormalities that define the syndrome. Traditionally, this entails a full polysomnogram that measures a large number of physiologic signals during sleep (Figs. 71.6 and 71.7). Polysomnograms are typically performed in sleep disorder laboratories and are monitored by trained technicians. They are therefore labor intensive and costly. However, they do provide the clinician with an enormous amount of useful information about the sleep of the patient, including whether sleep-disordered breathing is present and its severity, as well as other physiologic data. A variety of non–breathing-related sleep disorders also have characteristic findings on polysomnography.

The indications for polysomnography include the following:

- Evaluation of patients with snoring, excessive daytime sleepiness, and other features of OSA; the diagnosis can be confirmed and treatment confidently started
- Evaluation of patients with snoring but a lower likelihood of OSA based on clinical features; OSA can be excluded and the snoring treated by other means, possibly surgery; evaluation of SDB in patients with neuromuscular or chest wall disorders in whom nocturnal hypoventilation is being evaluated
- Exclusion of other sleep disorders that may be in the differential diagnosis of patients with excessive daytime sleepiness (e.g., periodic limb movement disorder, narcolepsy)
- Assessment of response to therapy after a treatment intervention for SDB (or other disorders)

Another diagnostic approach that has been adopted in some centers is to record a fewer number of variables overall but to focus on the key respiratory variables that define OSA. These include oronasal airflow, respiratory effort, pulse oximetry, and heart rate. Studies such as the electroencephalogram (EEG) and electromyogram (EMG) are omitted, and sleep stages are not recorded. Sleep apnea disease burden is measured in terms of apnea and hypopnea frequency and desaturations, and without reference to its effect on sleep. These sleep apnea diagnostic systems are easily portable and relatively simple to operate and provide information about sleep-disordered breathing that is minimal but frequently sufficient to diagnose sleep apnea. Their role in routine diagnosis remains controversial, primarily because of the limited degree to which they have been validated against traditional studies in sleep laboratories. Nonetheless, they play a growing role in OSA diagnosis. Frequently, simple continuous oximetry alone may strongly suggest sleep apnea (Fig. 71.8).

TREATMENT

Positive Airway Pressure

A variety of medical and surgical treatments for SAHS have been described. The mainstay of treatment, however, is positive airway pressure therapy. The most widely used of the positive

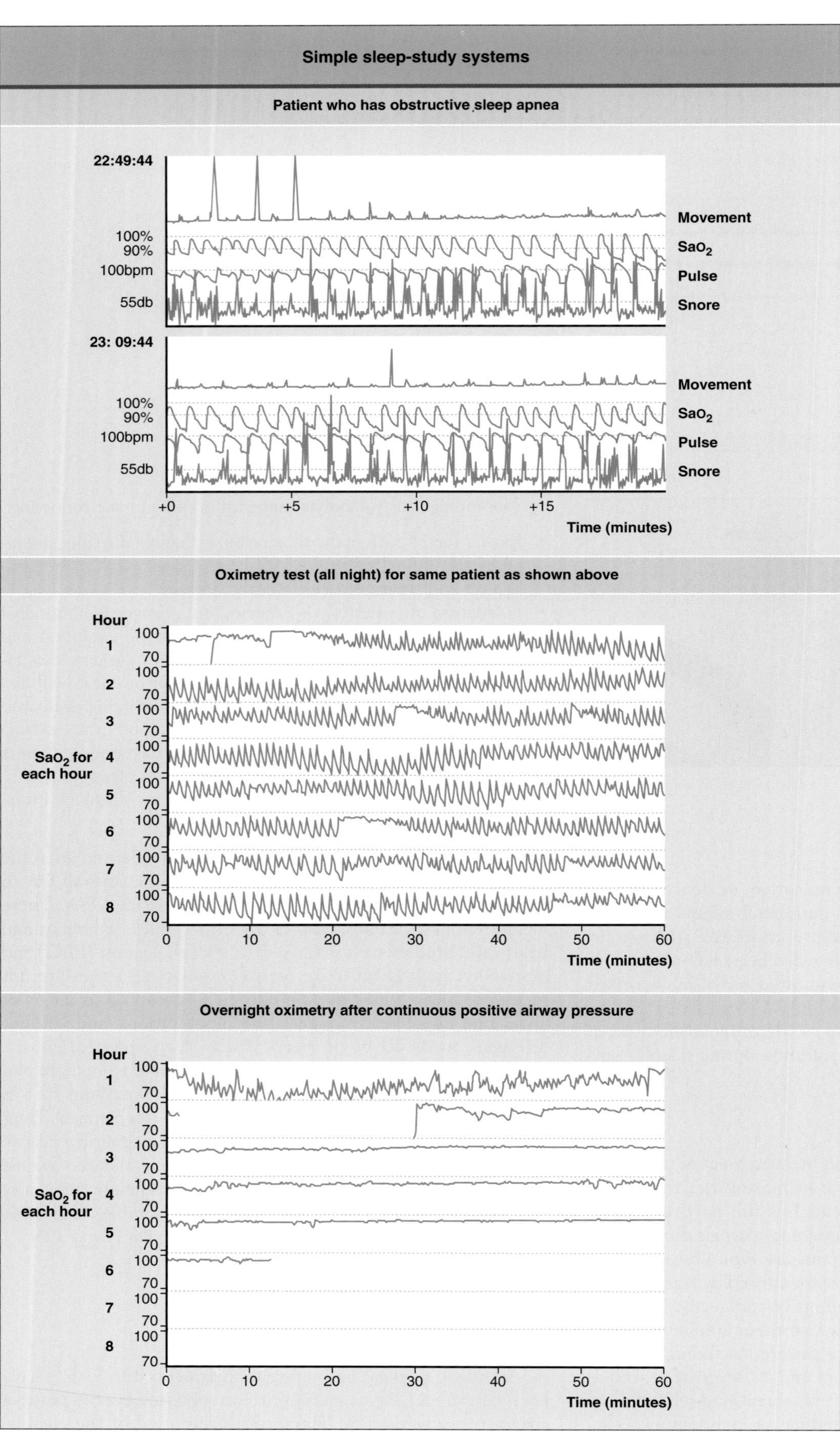

Figure 71.8 Simpler sleep-study systems. Top, Recording of body movement (Movement), oximetry (Sao_2), heart rate (Pulse), and snoring (Snore, in decibels) that clearly shows obstructive sleep apnea (OSA). **Middle,** The same patient's oximetry trace is shown for the whole night with desaturation throughout the night (i.e., severe OSA). **Bottom,** Oximetry for 4 hours after commencement of continuous positive airway pressure (CPAP) (following a 1-hour period of observation), with complete control of the OSA.

airway pressure therapies is nasal continuous positive airway pressure (CPAP). The main way in which nasal CPAP, and all other positive pressure therapies, function in the treatment of OSA is to pneumatically dilate the upper airway, preventing its closure (Fig. 71.9).

Bilevel positive airway pressure (BPAP) is an alternative to CPAP for OSA treatment. It operates on the principle that a higher level of positive airway pressure is required to open the obstructed pharyngeal airway segment than is required to maintain its patency. Therefore, during BPAP therapy, the inspiratory pressure is higher than the expiratory pressure. Some patients who complain about exhaling against an elevated pressure during CPAP therapy find bilevel PAP more comfortable to use.

Self-adjusting CPAP (or autoCPAP) machines are increasingly being used in the treatment of OSA. The function of these devices is based on the idea that the upper airway closure is a dynamic process and that the same amount of pressure is not needed at all times. AutoCPAP machines adjust pressure on the basis of changes in upper airway physiology. Manufacturers of these devices have proprietary algorithms that monitor aspects of upper airway physiology and control pressure adjustments. AutoCPAP therapy seems to be equivalent to standard fixed pressure CPAP therapy, but how these units fit into treatment plans is still a matter of controversy.

In order for treatment with positive pressure therapy (PAP) to be successful, the patients must be willing to use the prescribed therapy on a nightly basis. As with any type of therapy, attention must be paid to the patient's experience with therapy and its inevitable side effects.

PAP has frequent side effects, but they are usually correctable. Common problems include mask leaks (sometimes directed to the eyes), air leaks from the mouth, dry mouth, nasal congestion and/or rhinitis, skin irritation, aerophagia, and claustrophobia. Instructing the patient to work with a knowledgeable sleep laboratory technologist or home equipment specialist can help the patient overcome these side effects. Patients should be reassured at every opportunity that PAP therapy is helpful and that the side effects can be successfully managed. For nasal problems, nasal decongestants are frequently helpful; in some cases, an otolaryngologist may need to be consulted. Comfortable PAP masks are available and have steadily improved in design and comfort over the past decade.

Patients on PAP therapy should be offered follow-up care, just as any patient with a chronic disease would be. The location and frequency of follow-up care are best left up to local agreements between primary care and specialist physicians. In some locations, nurse-managed programs may be successful in accomplishing this.

Follow-up sleep studies are not routinely needed in all patients. However, in regular follow-up with patients, changes in therapy will be required. Significant weight gain or loss is a common reason for adjustments in PAP prescriptions. Others include changes in other medical conditions, especially cardiopulmonary problems, and reports by the patient that once-effective therapy is no longer effective.

Dental Appliances

Dental appliances are an alternative therapy to PAP for OSA. These devices come in two types: tongue retainers and mandibular advancement splints (MAS). The latter type has predominated in the past 5 years. The splints work by causing mandible protrusion, which results in an increased opening in the posterior airway space (Fig. 71.10). These splints are made by a dentist and individually fitted to the patient. Advancement of the mandible is done slowly (usually over weeks); the time is based on patient comfort and reduction in snoring and OSA symptoms. The maximum protrusion is usually 4 to 5 mm. Randomized clinical studies have found MAS to be effective, although not as effective as PAP, in reversing OSA symptoms.

Surgical Therapy

Surgical treatments for OSA seek to alter the upper airway anatomy in order to eliminate sites of obstruction. Recent studies have shown than the upper airway tends to be diffusely affected in the majority of cases, as opposed to having segments of discrete obstruction. This finding has important implications for planning surgical therapy, because the most commonly performed OSA surgeries have mostly been focused on a single part, or site, of the upper airway: the soft palate.

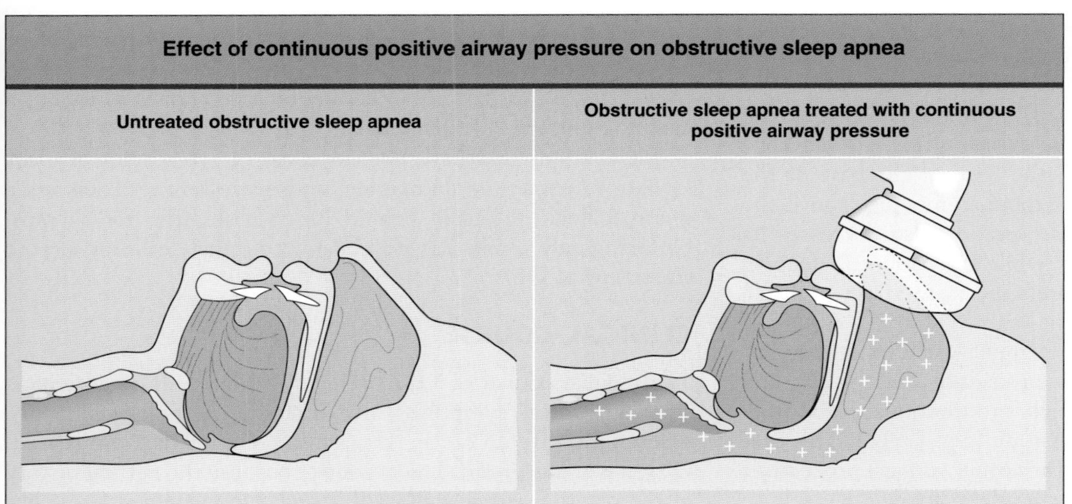

Figure 71.9 Effect of continuous positive airway pressure (CPAP) on obstructive sleep apnea (OSA). The chief mechanism of CPAP in the treatment of OSA is airway splinting and dilatation of obstructed pharyngeal segments. Both untreated OSA and OSA treated using CPAP are shown.

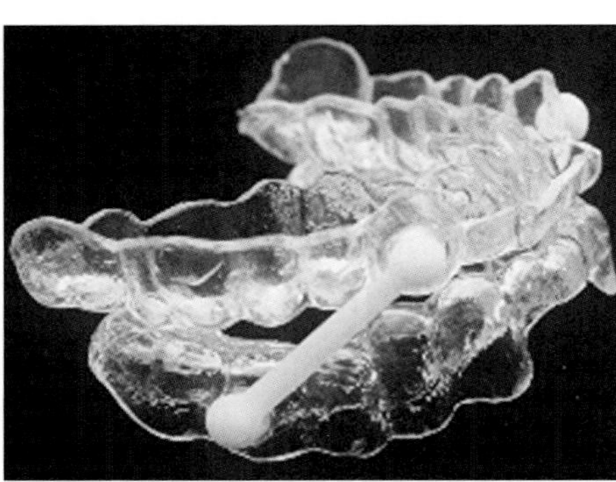

Figure 71.10 A mandibular advancement splint—inserted before sleep.

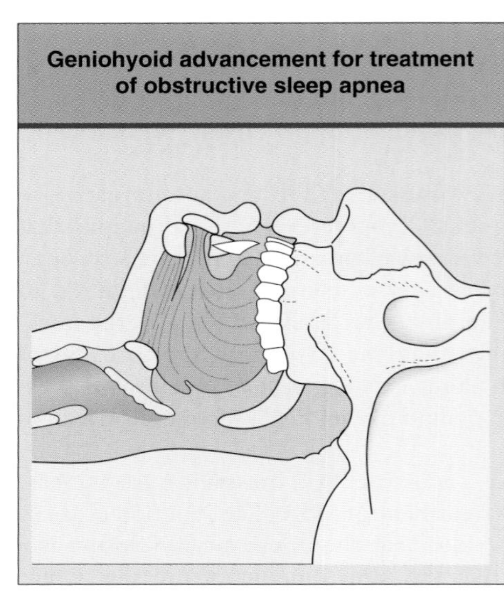

Figure 71.11 Geniohyoid advancement to treat obstructive sleep apnea (OSA). The geniotubercle (insertion site of the genioglossus) is advanced after a small mandibular osteotomy. The hyoid bone is resuspended in a more superior and anterior position, which results in advancement of the anterior pharyngeal wall and an increase in the posterior pharyngeal airway diameter.

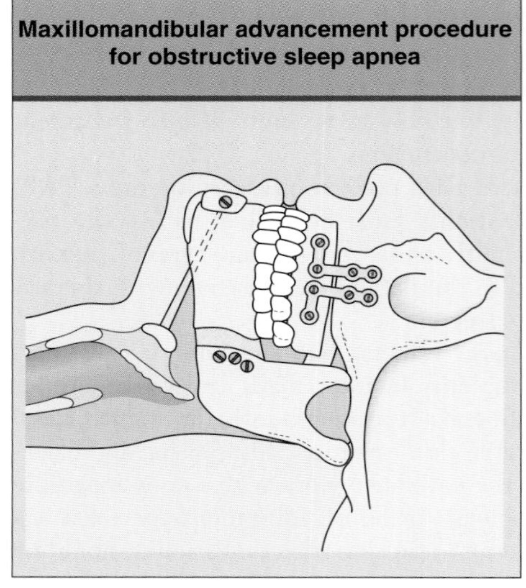

Figure 71.12 Maxillomandibular advancement procedure for obstructive sleep apnea (OSA). A maxillary and mandibular LeFort I osteotomy is performed. Both maxilla and mandible are advanced by 6 to 8 mm and refixed in a forward position. In this example, note the prior geniotubercle advancement and hyoid suspension.

Tracheostomy is an effective treatment for SAHS but is disfiguring and is unacceptable to many patients. Uvulopalatopharyngoplasty (UPPP), which is a soft palate–specific therapy developed as a less disfiguring alternative to tracheostomy in the early 1980s, has been the most commonly performed operation for OSA since the mid 1980s. Despite initial enthusiasm for the procedure, subsequent studies have shown a response rate of less than 50% in unselected patients. The diffuse nature of pharyngeal involvement in OSA probably accounts for the poor success rate of UPPP. Even when patients are selected on the basis of having obstruction at the level of the soft palate, which should be correctable with UPPP, cure rates are still lower than ideal. Furthermore, no clear consensus exists among surgeons about the best way to evaluate and select candidates for UPPP.

Laser-assisted uvuloplasty (LAUP) was developed in Europe for treatment of snoring. It is very successful in treating uncomplicated snoring. Over time, LAUP has been used for treatment of OSA. Unfortunately, results in treating OSA with LAUP have not been as successful.

Considering the observations that OSA usually occurs because of upper airway obstruction at multiple sites, the approach favored by surgeons expert in sleep apnea therapy involves procedures that can be used in the treatment of multiple segments of the upper airway obstruction.

A geniohyoid advancement procedure with or without a traditional UPPP may be curative of SAHS in approximately 70% of patients. In this procedure, the genioglossus is advanced through a mandibular osteotomy at the geniotubercle, the site of genioglossus insertion on the anterior mandible. This “plug” of bone and tongue-muscle insertion is advanced several millimeters and resecured to the mandible. The hyoid bone is then resuspended in a higher (cephalad) position relative to the mandible with suture or fascia. The overall effect is to advance the anterior pharyngeal wall from the level of the base of the tongue to the lower part of the hypopharynx (just above the epiglottis). A more anterior tongue position also decreases its opportunity to obstruct the airway while the patient is sleeping supine (Fig. 71.11). This procedure appears to affect multiple segments of the pharyngeal airway.

Another surgical option for treatment of OSA is maxillomandibular advancement. In this procedure the maxilla and mandible are both advanced through an intentional facial fracture and then plated into a new position (Fig. 71.12). This procedure has been used in cases in which other surgical procedures have not been successful in alleviating sleep apnea.

Medical Therapy

A variety of medical therapies other than PAP have been described. Body position therapy (e.g., having the patient sleep on his or her side) is useful when OSA is documented to occur only when the patient sleeps supine. Weight loss has been shown to be effective as a primary therapy for sleep apnea as well as a useful adjunct to CPAP therapy.

Medications that have been tried in the treatment of OSA include protriptyline, fluoxetine, and progesterone. Each has a pharmacologic rationale behind its consideration for therapy. Unfortunately, none has demonstrated much efficacy in the treatment of OSA.

CLINICAL COURSE

The clinical course of OSA is highly variable. If treatment is started, clinical symptoms are diminished, and, presumably, deleterious effects of the disease are eliminated. Untreated, OSA has an uncertain clinical course, because the natural history of the disorder is not well understood. One would expect clinical symptoms to continue relatively unabated. However, few studies have investigated the outcome of patients with untreated OSA. One study found that mortality over a 7-year follow-up period was significantly greater if the apnea index (average number of apneas per hour of sleep) was higher than 20 than if it was lower than 20 (Fig. 71.13). This was a retrospective study and was subject to considerable bias.

A more recent study from Sweden found an increased incidence of cardiovascular disease in middle-age men with OSA over a 7-year period compared with men without OSA. Furthermore, they found that those men effectively treated with CPAP were less likely to have cardiovascular disease compared with men who had not used CPAP during this period. One study looking at mortality in patients with sleep-disordered breathing found that the combination of snoring and daytime sleepiness resulted in increased cardiovascular mortality compared with self-reported snoring without sleepiness, but that the findings were significant for individuals aged less than 60 years. Therefore, SDB with sleepiness appears to have an effect on mortality in large population studies, but the effect seems to be strongest in individuals younger than age 60.

PITFALLS AND CONTROVERSIES

OSA is a common disorder associated with health risks, but it has been difficult to quantify these risks because of confounding factors. It has generally been accepted that OSA impairs automobile driving. Patients with OSA should be counseled about drowsy driving.

Cardiovascular risks have been postulated for untreated OSA but evidence of an increase in cardiovascular morbidity and mortality in patients with OSA has been controversial. The strongest association between OSA and cardiovascular disease is for hypertension. Prospective population-based epidemiologic studies have shown that hypertension developed in more subjects with known OSA over a period of years than it did in subjects without OSA. Studies have shown that treatment with effective CPAP compared with ineffective (placebo) CPAP resulted in a significant lowering of BP in hypertensive patients with OSA. The evidence for a cause-and-effect relationship between OSA and other forms of cardiovascular disease is less clear, although several large cross-sectional population-based studies show a moderate association.

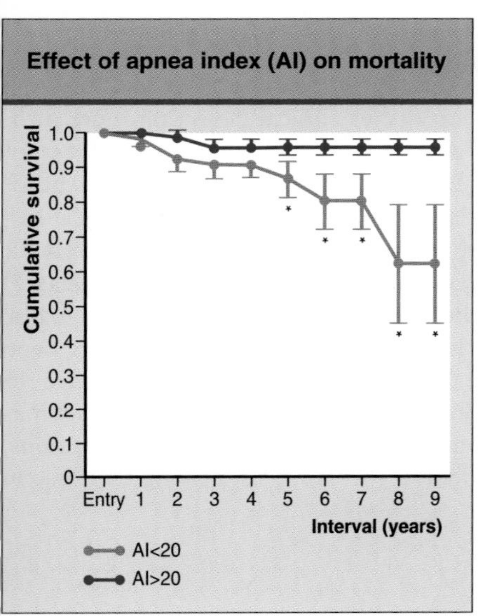

Figure 71.13 Effect of apnea index (AI) on mortality. Cumulative survival of untreated obstructive sleep apnea (OSA) patients based on initial AI. The study was retrospective and subject to bias, but it does suggest that untreated OSA with an AI greater than 20 may be associated with earlier mortality. Asterisks denote $p < 0.05$ for the comparison between the two survival curves at each point. The error bars represent standard error. (Adapted with permission from He J, Kryger MH, Zorick FJ, et al: Mortality and apnea index in obstructive sleep apnea. Chest 88:9-14, 1988.)

Another controversy is the effect of gender on the risk of sleep-disordered breathing. Women appear in large epidemiologic studies to have about one half the prevalence of men for OSA. Despite a lower prevalence, there is preliminary evidence that affected women may have a higher mortality rate. The mechanisms underlying this are unclear, and more work is needed to clarify this potentially important finding.

Adherence to PAP therapy is a problem for many patients. Regardless of the degree of OSA, many patients will not use PAP therapy as much as physicians feel they should. In general, adherence to therapy is better when a patient experiences improvement in symptoms. Nonetheless, the therapy is cumbersome and unattractive to many patients—even ones who admit that they feel better when they use it. For patients with milder disease, CPAP may not be an acceptable therapy for long-term use.

The lack of clinical awareness about sleep disorders, including OSA, is perhaps the largest pitfall to overcome in evaluating and treating patients with a variety of conditions. Information about sleep is needed to highlight the importance of this area for both physicians and the public.

UPPER AIRWAY RESISTANCE SYNDROME

Upper airway resistance syndrome (UARS) is a form of SDB characterized by daytime hypersomnia, increased upper airway resistance during sleep, and the absence of apneas and hypopneas on a polysomnogram (Fig. 71.14).

Epidemiology

The prevalence of UARS is not clear because the definition of the disorder is imprecise compared with that of OSA. It is also more difficult to identify UARS on a polysomnogram than it is to identify relatively unambiguous apneas and hypopneas on a polysomnogram. Furthermore, studies less sensitive than polysomnography would not reliably detect UARS. Measuring excessive sleepiness as a surrogate marker for UARS will not suffice because many other conditions can cause excessive sleepiness, and the measurement of sleepiness itself is imprecise.

Risk Factors

The risk factors have not been as well worked out as they have for OSA. Patients tend to be younger and less obese. Snoring is variable in UARS but is frequently present. Craniofacial abnormalities that may predispose to SDB may affect a higher percentage of patients with UARS than those with OSA.

Pathophysiology

Increased upper airway resistance is the chief pathophysiologic event in UARS. Patients may experience more brief arousals from sleep with lower degrees of upper airway resistance compared with OSA patients. Negative intrathoracic pressure swings

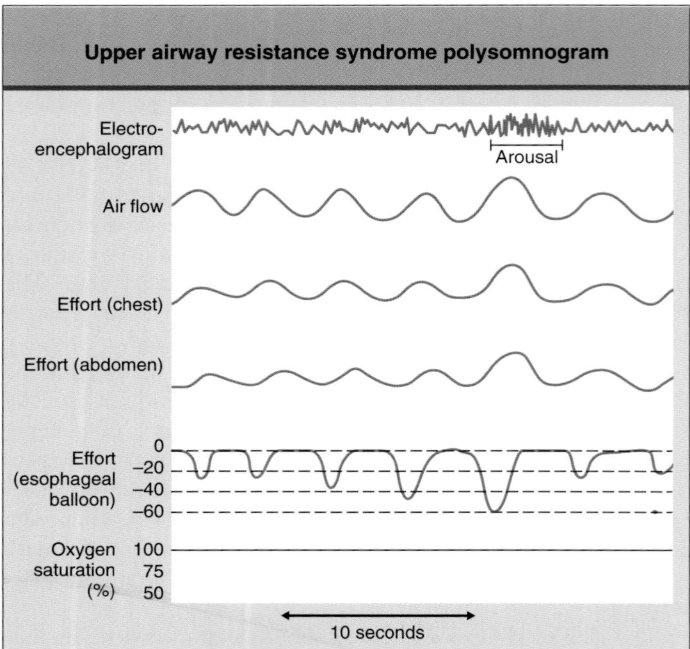

Figure 7.14 Example of polysomnography for upper airway resistance syndrome (UARS). Note that air flow is only minimally perturbed by an increase in upper airway resistance. Respiratory effort recorded in chest and abdomen belts is similarly minimally affected. Respiratory effort as recorded by esophageal pressure shows increasingly negative pleural pressure deflections, which indicate increased respiratory effort because of elevated upper airway resistance. The progression of increasing respiratory effort culminates in an arousal, shown in the electrocardiogram channel.

during obstructed upper airway events is the pathophysiologic process underlying this disorder.

In this respect, the disorder is closely related to OSA. It is likely that UARS and OSA exist together on a continuum of sleep-disordered breathing that begins with mild snoring, progresses through UARS, and ends with OSA.

Clinical Features

Hypersomnia is the chief clinical feature of UARS. This is manifested clinically and can be measured objectively with the Multiple Sleep Latency Test (MSLT). This test measures how long a subject takes to fall asleep in a quiet darkened room when he or she is reclining in a bed; it is repeated four or five times throughout a single day and results in a mean sleep latency value. A mean sleep latency below 10 minutes is abnormal; a value less than 5 minutes is considered pathologic. Snoring is sometimes present but is not necessary for the diagnosis.

Diagnosis

UARS should be considered in patients with excessive daytime sleepiness. Although the diagnosis may be suspected on the basis of clinical features, polysomnography is necessary to confirm the suspicion (see Fig. 71.14). The polysomnogram will exclude OSA from the possible diagnoses, and it should show frequent arousals from sleep associated with increased upper airway resistance. This is most accurately measured by using an esophageal balloon-tipped catheter to measure intraesophageal pressure, a surrogate for intrapleural pressure. Increasingly negative pleural pressure with arousals but without obstructive apneas and hypopneas defines UARS. Because esophageal balloon-tipped catheters are sometimes difficult to work with and are uncomfortable for many patients, a popular alternative approach to diagnosing UARS is to measure nasal airflow with a sensitive airflow monitor based on a pneumotachograph. As upper airway resistance increases, the nasal pneumotachograph monitor shows flattening on the inspiratory limb of the respiratory cycle. Although this method is qualitative, it may be an acceptable clinical alternative to the more invasive approach under the correct clinical circumstances.

Finally, another diagnostic strategy sometimes used in diagnosing UARS is to use a therapeutic trial of CPAP. PAP will decrease upper airway resistance; if clinical improvements are seen after CPAP, then UARS is likely. If no improvement is seen, then UARS is less likely, and other causes of daytime hypersomnia should be considered.

Treatment

Treatment options for UARS include positive airway pressure therapy, oral appliances, and upper airway surgery. The choice of therapy depends chiefly on patient preference. Few clinical trials have examined therapy options for UARS specifically.

Clinical Course and Prevention

Daytime sleepiness associated with UARS is likely to continue unless it is treated, although no studies looking at long-term consequences of patients affected by UARS have been performed. Whether UARS can be prevented is unclear. Avoidance of weight gain would be expected to help prevent UARS, although many patients affected by UARS have a normal body weight. Craniofacial factors associated with UARS are largely genetic in origin and thus are not easily controlled. Surgical therapy may be useful in treatment of these patients.

Pitfalls and Controversies

Lack of a clinical definition makes clinical detection more difficult. Some authorities have even argued that UARS does not exist—that it is a normal variant. Others have proposed that it is a disorder of excessive arousability to normally subclinical respiratory stimuli. At present, the laboratory diagnosis is difficult for some sleep laboratories to manage, as it requires esophageal balloon monitoring for the most accurate diagnosis to be made.

Treatment of UARS is controversial. Nasal CPAP has been shown to be effective therapy, but long-term adherence to therapy is questionable in many cases. Other therapies, such as surgery or dental appliances, should be considered as options, although there is little medical literature supporting their use in this disorder.

SUGGESTED READINGS

Flemons WW: Obstructive sleep apnea. N Engl J Med 347:498-504, 2002.

Jenkinson C, Davies RJO, Mullins R, et al: Comparison of therapeutic and subtherapeutic nasal continuous positive airway pressure for obstructive sleep apnoea: A randomized prospective parallel trial. Lancet 353:2100-2105, 1999.

Peppard P, Young T, Palta M, et al: Longitudinal study of moderate weight change and sleep disordered breathing. JAMA 284:3015-3021, 2000.

Peppard P, Young T, Palta M, et al: Prospective study of the association between sleep-disordered breathing and hypertension. N Engl J Med 342:1378-1384, 2000.

Pepperell J, Ramdassingh-Dow S, Crosthwaite N, et al: Ambulatory blood pressure after therapeutic and subtherapeutic continuous positive airway pressure for obstructive sleep apnoea: a randomised parallel trial. Lancet 359:204-210, 2002.

Riley R, Powell NB, Guilleminault C: Obstructive sleep apnea syndrome: A review of 306 consecutively treated patients. Otolaryngol Head Neck Surg 108:117-125, 1993.

Shahar E, Whitney CW, Redline S, et al: Sleep-disordered breathing and cardiovascular disease. Cross-sectional results of the Sleep Heart Health Study. Am J Respir Crit Care Med 163:19-25, 2001.

Strollo P, Rogers R: Obstructive sleep apnea. N Engl J Med 334:99-104, 1996.

White D: Pathophysiology of obstructive sleep apnea. Thorax 50:797-804, 1995.

Young T, Palta M, Dempsey J, et al: The occurrence of sleep-disordered breathing among middle-aged adults. N Engl J Med 328:1230-1235, 1993.

CHAPTER 72 Central Sleep Apnea and Other Forms of Sleep-Disordered Breathing

Patrick J. Strollo, Jr., and Charles W. Atwood, Jr.

CENTRAL SLEEP APNEA

Epidemiology

Central sleep apnea occurs in between 5% and 10% of all patients who have sleep disordered breathing (SDB). The primary or idiopathic form of central sleep apnea is less common than secondary causes such as congestive heart failure or neurologic conditions such as cerebrovascular disease. Central sleep apnea has been reported to occur in approximately 40% to 50% of patients with advanced heart failure.

Risk Factors

Risk factors include congestive heart failure, neurologic disease, and ascent to high altitude (particularly in individuals who have spent little previous time at altitudes higher than 2500 m). In patients with congestive heart failure, male gender, atrial fibrillation, hypocapnia, and advancing age all increase the risk of central sleep apnea.

Pathophysiology

Transient withdrawal of central respiratory drive to respiratory muscles results in central sleep apnea; this mechanism occurs in a number of ways (Table 72.1). In considering the pathophysiology of central sleep apnea, three subtypes can be described: hypercapnic central sleep apnea, hypocapnic central sleep apnea, and sleep onset apnea.

HYPERCAPNIC CENTRAL SLEEP APNEA

Hypercapnic central sleep apnea results from central hypoventilation in which breathing during wakefulness is usually normal, although daytime hypercapnia can occur. Neuromuscular diseases such as postpolio syndrome, muscular and myotonic dystrophies, and amyotrophic lateral sclerosis are included in this category.

HYPOCAPNIC CENTRAL SLEEP APNEA

Hypocapnic central sleep apnea can be idiopathic as well as associated with congestive heart failure and neurologic disease. As for other forms of central sleep apnea, pathophysiologic mechanisms are not clearly understood, but it is highly dependent on a decreased arterial partial pressure of carbon dioxide (Pa_{CO_2}). Intrinsic properties of the respiratory control system are the most important factors in predisposition to central sleep apnea. Central sleep apnea associated with congestive heart failure is characterized by a crescendo-decrescendo pattern of breathing referred to as Cheyne-Stokes respiration (see Fig. 72.1).

SLEEP ONSET APNEA

A third form of central sleep apnea is that seen at the time of sleep onset in normal humans. Central apneas may arise during the transition between wakefulness and sleep because of transient instabilities in respiratory drive in normal subjects. The mechanism of this form of central sleep apnea is similar to that of the hypocapnic form associated with congestive heart failure. The level of Pa_{CO_2} is the main determinant for respiratory drive in the sleeping human.

Finally, the sensitivity of the arousal mechanism in central sleep apnea is important. In all forms of central sleep apnea, if an arousal does not occur, the cycle of apneas and arousals is broken. In sleep onset central sleep apnea associated with insomnia, sedative medications may be useful in increasing the arousal threshold and decreasing sleep onset arousal. The role of such medications in practice is unclear because of the potential for dependence, concern about precipitating falls in a frail population, and the potential for worsening any underlying obstructive sleep apnea (OSA).

Clinical Features

Hypercapnia associated with central sleep apnea is usually the result of a central hypoventilation disorder or neuromuscular respiratory disease. Affected patients may have a diminished sensation of dyspnea associated with respiratory insufficiency and hypercapnia, although patients who have neuromuscular respiratory disease may complain of dyspnea as the condition progresses. Restless sleep, daytime somnolence, and morning headache may be seen in all forms of hypercapnic central sleep apnea. Right-sided heart failure and secondary polycythemia may develop at an advanced stage. Overt respiratory failure that requires mechanical ventilation is occasionally the presenting complaint and usually occurs after another medical problem, such as bronchitis or pneumonia, has disrupted the existing physiologic homeostasis. The symptoms of central sleep apnea and OSA may differ (Table 72.2).

Patients who have eucapnic or hypocapnic forms of central sleep apnea are typically older, have a more normal body weight, and have coexistent cardiac or neurologic diseases. This holds true for the idiopathic form as well as secondary forms associated with congestive heart failure. Affected patients tend to hyperventilate during wakefulness, and therefore the Pa_{CO_2} is

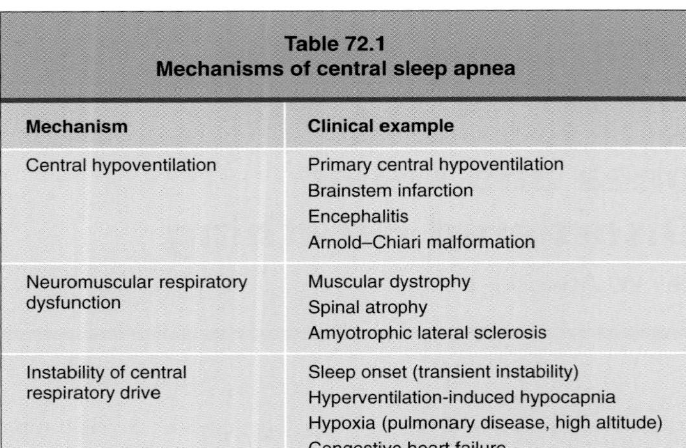

Table 72.1
Mechanisms of central sleep apnea

Mechanism	Clinical example
Central hypoventilation	Primary central hypoventilation Brainstem infarction Encephalitis Arnold–Chiari malformation
Neuromuscular respiratory dysfunction	Muscular dystrophy Spinal atrophy Amyotrophic lateral sclerosis
Instability of central respiratory drive	Sleep onset (transient instability) Hyperventilation-induced hypocapnia Hypoxia (pulmonary disease, high altitude) Congestive heart failure Disorders of the central nervous system

Table 72.2
Signs and symptoms of central sleep apnea versus obstructive sleep apnea

Sign or symptom	Central sleep apnea	Obstructive sleep apnea
Daytime sleepiness	Variable	Yes
Restless sleep	Yes	Yes
Snoring	No	Yes
Nocturnal choking	No	Yes
Nocturnal dyspnea	Variable	Variable
Morning headache	Variable	Variable
Insomnia	Yes	Variable
Nocturnal desaturation	Yes	Yes
Hypercapnia	Variable	Variable

lower than that in patients who have congestive heart failure without central sleep apnea. Symptoms of insomnia, nocturnal dyspnea, and daytime sleepiness (because of sleep fragmentation and frequent arousals) are common, although daytime hypersomnia is less frequent in this group of patients.

Diagnosis

Regardless of the type of central sleep apnea, a high clinical suspicion is essential for its diagnosis. Objective assessment of the breathing pattern during sleep with polysomnography can confirm the diagnosis (Fig. 72.1). Central apneas are distinguished from obstructive apneas by the lack of respiratory effort during the apnea. Examples of central sleep apnea associated with sleep onset and Cheyne-Stokes respiration are shown in Figure 72.1. The potential for underlying cardiovascular and cerebrovascular disease must be assessed. An approach to the diagnostic evaluation and management is outlined in Figure 72.2.

Treatment

Treatment options for central sleep apnea include supplemental oxygen, nasal continuous positive airway pressure (CPAP), bilevel positive airway pressure (BPAP), respiratory stimulant medications, and a combination of these.

If the hypercapnic central sleep apnea results from central hypoventilation or neuromuscular respiratory conditions, the patient benefits most from nocturnal ventilatory assistance, which may be carried out through a tracheostomy or noninvasively by mask ventilation. Patients should avoid benzodiazepines, narcotics, and other sedatives that may suppress respiratory drive.

Supplemental oxygen is useful for alleviating nocturnal hypoxemia, provided it does not induce hypercapnia. This may be of particular concern in central sleep apnea associated with neuromuscular disease. The optimal treatment for nonhypercapnic central sleep apnea has not been defined. Treatment of the underlying cause (e.g., congestive heart failure) is the first step. Therapy can also include supplemental oxygen, respiratory stimulants, and positive-pressure therapy. At present, supplemental oxygen therapy is the mainstay of therapy, as it "stabilizes" the respiratory control centers, although the mechanisms by which this is accomplished are not clear. Acetazolamide has been used successfully to alleviate abnormal respiratory patterns in altitude sickness. Its mechanism of action is to induce a mild degree of metabolic acidosis and increase respiratory drive by inducing a bicarbonate diuresis.

Clinically important improvements in left ventricular function have resulted from CPAP in patients with congestive heart failure, but the number of such patients treated successfully with CPAP is small. In one study, the benefit of CPAP therapy was limited to the group of patients who had higher (>1.6 kPa [>12 mm Hg]) pulmonary capillary wedge pressures (PCWPs). By contrast, the lower PCWP group (<1.6 kPa [<12 mm Hg]) showed a reduction in cardiac index. The mechanism by which CPAP improves central sleep apnea appears related to its improvement in oxygen saturation and a slight elevation in Pa_{CO_2}, which moves arterial Pa_{CO_2} away from the apnea threshold.

Clinical Course

When central sleep apnea is secondary to another condition, such as congestive heart failure, the clinical outcome is in part related to the severity of the underlying disorder. It is currently unclear whether central sleep apnea–Cheyne-Stokes respiration is merely a marker of inadequately treated congestive heart failure or is an independent risk factor for mortality. Regardless, the finding of central sleep apnea–Cheyne-Stokes respiration has been associated with an increased mortality risk.

In most cases, treatment of central sleep apnea, whether with positive-pressure ventilation, respiratory stimulants, supplemental oxygen, or a combination of these therapies, improves clinical symptoms. If severely fragmented sleep can be consolidated and nocturnal dyspnea prevented, the patient almost certainly benefits from the therapy.

Pitfalls and Controversies

Compared with OSA, primary (idiopathic) central sleep apnea is uncommon. Central sleep apnea–Cheyne-Stokes respiration is frequently encountered in patients with advanced congestive

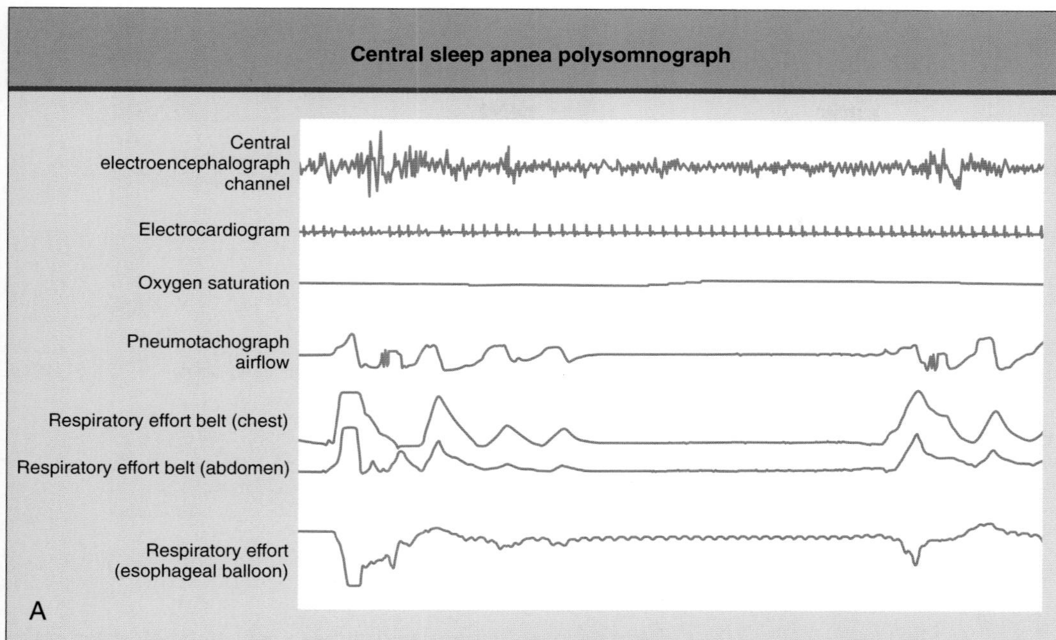

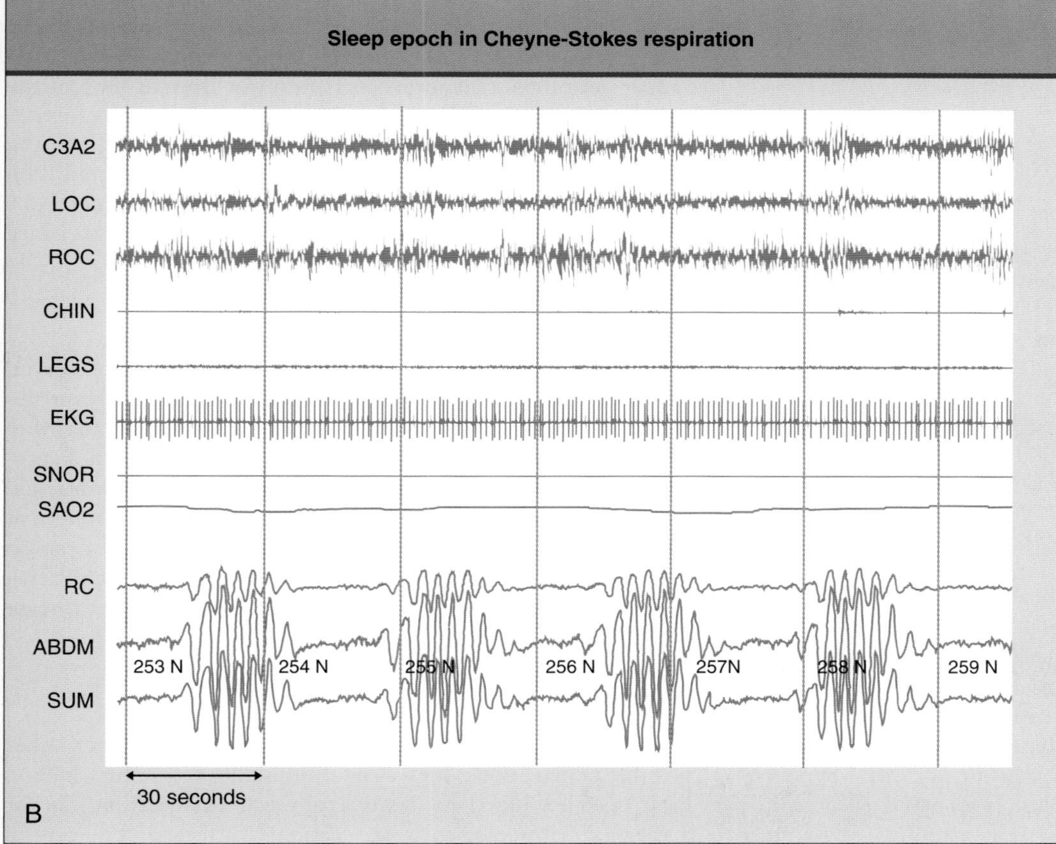

Figure 72.1 A, Example of central sleep apnea polysomnography. The sleep epoch shown is 30 seconds. The patient is awake at the beginning of the tracing. A sleep-onset central apnea, characterized by absence of airflow and respiratory effort, occurs as stage I sleep is entered. An arousal at the end of the epoch ends the apnea. **B,** The sleep epoch shown is Cheyne-Stokes respiration. Note the crescendo-decrescendo pattern of breathing in the effort channels (rib cage, abdomen, and sum). Periods of central apnea are seen following these characteristic periodic breathing events.

heart failure. In advanced congestive heart failure, both OSA and central sleep apnea are frequently not considered. Preliminary data suggest that patients may benefit from treatment, particularly with CPAP. The long-term clinical benefit of treatment for central sleep apnea–Cheyne-Stokes respiration in congestive heart failure is currently uncertain.

DISORDERS OF CENTRAL HYPOVENTILATION

Disorders of central hypoventilation constitute a heterogeneous and uncommon group of disorders characterized by the inability of the central respiratory centers to provide adequate output to the respiratory pump. The hallmark of this disorder is hyper-

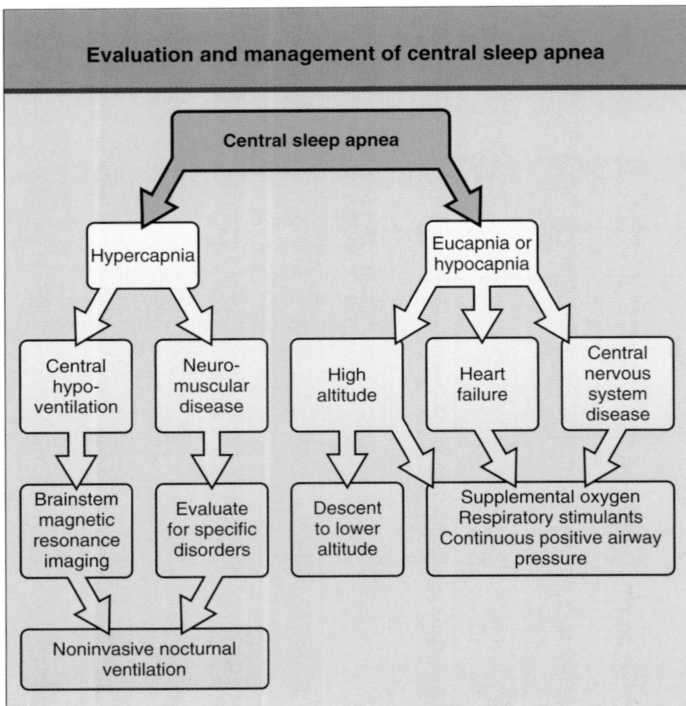

Figure 72.2 Evaluation and management of central sleep apnea.

capnia. Effective treatment involves ventilatory support to optimize gas exchange and improve quality of life.

Epidemiology and Risk Factors

Table 72.3 lists the conditions associated with central hypoventilation.

Trauma accounts for most spinal cord injuries and is the leading cause of central hypoventilation, with approximately 10,000 new cervical spinal injuries occurring each year in the United States. In addition, the prevalence of this disorder is approximately 1 in 400,000.

Although no longer a public health or important clinical problem in the developed world, poliomyelitis continues to be a significant public health problem in developing nations. Patients who have chronic ventilatory failure from the polio epidemics in the 1950s still require treatment. Syringomyelia with or without Chiari malformations (types I and II) is an example of a congenital brain lesion that may result in central hypoventilation. Brain injury and neuronal loss from acute encephalitis, multiple sclerosis, and multiple system atrophy (Shy-Drager syndrome) are examples of rare acquired disorders that may lead to central hypoventilation. Structural lesions caused by brainstem infarctions or neoplasms or following encephalitis are rare but are the most common nontraumatic causes. These conditions result in severe clinical sequelae, and the outcomes tend to be poor. Neurologic conditions, such as multiple sclerosis, multiple system atrophy, or demyelinating disorders, can result in clinically significant hypoventilation, but respiratory failure is rare.

Table 72.3 Classification of disorders of central hypoventilation

Type of neuron	Disorder
Brainstem motoneurons	Primary central hypoventilation
	Congenital malformations (Chiari malformations; syringomyelia)
	Trauma
	Infarction
	Encephalitis
	Tumors
	Chronic metabolic alkalosis
	Multiple sclerosis
	Sarcoidosis
Spinal neurons	Poliomyelitis
	High cervical cord trauma

Pathophysiology

Central hypoventilation can occur as a congenital disorder in the first several hours of life or as an acquired disorder in adulthood, usually as the result of significant brainstem injury. The basic defect is the inability to transduce afferent input from central and/or peripheral chemoreceptors into the efferent limb of the respiratory system. Flat or very decreased respiratory responses to respiratory chemostimuli, such as hypercapnia and hypoxia, may occur. The sleeping state, characterized by the transition from the behavioral control of ventilation to the metabolic control of ventilation, results in more profound gas exchange abnormalities.

Clinical Features

Hypercapnia and hypoxemia are the hallmark signs of central hypoventilation syndromes, regardless of the cause. Hypercapnia can range from mild ($P_{CO_2} < 6.6$ kPa [<50 mm Hg]) to severe ($P_{CO_2} > 8.5$ kPa [>65 mm Hg]). Symptoms may also include progressive lethargy and easy fatigability, daytime hypersomnia, and headache. Dyspnea is variable but is generally not a prominent complaint in central hypoventilation. The symptom of dyspnea may help differentiate patients with central hypoventilation from those with hypoventilation due to neuromuscular disease (Table 72.4).

Diagnosis

The diagnosis of central hypoventilation is made after other possible explanations, such as neuromuscular respiratory failure, have been excluded by history, physical examination, and/or additional physiologic tests. Patients affected by central hypoventilation have impaired ventilatory responses to hypoxia and hypercapnia.

PHYSIOLOGIC TESTS

By measuring ventilatory sensitivity to hypercapnia and hypoxic ventilatory sensitivity, respiratory rate, tidal volume, minute ventilation, inspiratory flow rates, and mouth occlusion pressures in the first 0.1 second of inspiratory activity (P0.1) can be plotted against progressively higher levels of carbon dioxide

Table 72.4
Comparison of clinical features of central hypoventilation and neuromuscular disease

Clinical feature	Central hypoventilation	Neuromuscular respiratory disease
Frequency	Uncommon	Common
Ages affected	Infants through adults	Primarily adults
Hypercapnia	Yes	Yes
Hypoxia	Yes	Yes
Dyspnea	No	Yes
Respiratory mechanics	Normal	Impaired
Ability to hyperventilate	Normal	Impaired
Therapy	Oxygen Chronic ventilator support Diaphragm pacing	Oxygen Chronic ventilator support Disease modifying drugs

or progressively lower oxygen saturation over time. Increases in respiratory rate and minute ventilation occur in response to the ventilatory stimulus given, but the variability in these measurements in normal subjects is considerable. If a response curve with a markedly shallow slope is found, insensitivity to ventilatory stimulants is determined, and central hypoventilation must be considered.

VOLUNTARY HYPERVENTILATION

To distinguish between central and peripheral causes of hypoventilation, the ability to hyperventilate voluntarily and decrease carbon dioxide by 1.3 kPa (10 mm Hg) or more can be measured. In central hypoventilation, maximal voluntary hyperventilation is accomplished easily for short periods of time, as the respiratory pump is not affected. If the cause of hypoventilation is peripheral (e.g., respiratory muscle weakness), the patient may be unable to lower the carbon dioxide by voluntary hyperpnea.

IMAGING STUDIES

Magnetic resonance imaging (MRI) is the procedure of choice for imaging the brainstem and upper spinal cord. Contrast enhancement may be necessary to detect arteriovenous malformations or other small, critically placed lesions. Congenital malformations, such as Chiari malformations or a syrinx, are shown very well by MRI (Fig. 72.3).

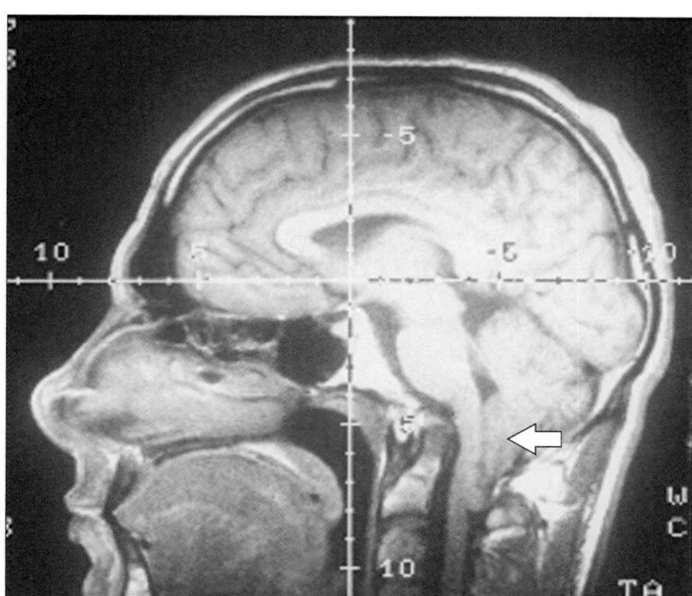

Figure 72.3 Contrast-enhanced magnetic resonance image of an Arnold-Chiari deformity. This 21-year-old man has progressive, nocturnal central hypoventilation as a result of the Chiari type I malformation demonstrated. Note the cerebellar tonsil descent into the spinal canal with impingement of brainstem structures *(arrow)*.

Treatment

Treatment of central hypoventilation depends on its severity, degree of impairment of other systems (e.g., level of mental status, degree of muscle paralysis), and the patient's willingness to use what may be lifelong supportive therapy, such as home ventilation or diaphragmatic pacing.

Treatment for milder cases includes ventilatory stimulants, such as progesterone and methylxanthines, which may successfully delay progression of ventilatory insufficiency. Supplemental oxygen therapy is important for all patients who have documented hypoxemia and may reduce the severity of complications such as secondary polycythemia, pulmonary hypertension, and heart failure and retard progression in respiratory insufficiency.

DIAPHRAGMATIC PACING

The rationale for diaphragmatic pacing is that electric stimulation of the muscle, either directly or via the phrenic nerve, substitutes for the intrinsic respiratory-center output. Newer approaches involve laparoscopic implantation of the pacemaker. Considerable commitment from the patient and medical team is required for this approach to work optimally.

NOCTURNAL VENTILATION

Nocturnal ventilation augments gas exchange during sleep, a time of increased vulnerability of the respiratory system because of the normal hypoventilation associated with sleep. Nocturnal ventilation can be invasive or noninvasive, and the aims are to rest ventilatory muscles and to improve gas exchange.

Invasive Ventilation

Invasive nocturnal ventilation requires a tracheostomy. Prior to the development of noninvasive ventilation techniques that use face masks, invasive ventilation was standard treatment. Because effective noninvasive techniques are now available, the need for a permanent tracheostomy in the management of chronic ventilatory insufficiency has decreased.

Noninvasive Ventilation

Ventilation of patients without the need for a surgical airway can be accomplished using either a negative- or positive-pressure system. Negative-pressure systems, such as an iron lung or a cuirass, were the first type of noninvasive ventilators, and their main advantage over positive-pressure ventilators is that a nasal or oronasal mask, which some patients find uncomfortable, is

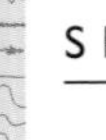

not needed. Many disadvantages exist, however. Negative-pressure ventilators are usually uncomfortable, bulky, and cumbersome, and assistance climbing in and out of them is also sometimes required. The most important problem is that such ventilators tend to induce upper airway collapse and thus cause OSA.

Positive-pressure, noninvasive ventilators are now the mainstay of nocturnal ventilation. They are small, easily portable, and relatively inexpensive. Both pressure-cycled and volume-cycled versions are available. Which type of positive-pressure ventilator to choose is less important than the ability of the patient to learn to use it successfully.

Noninvasive nocturnal positive-pressure ventilation may improve daytime hypersomnia, daytime gas exchange, and secondary polycythemia. It may delay the need for a tracheostomy in patients who have progressive hypoventilation disorders, and it eliminates the need for tracheostomy in patients who have stable forms of hypoventilation, depending on other factors such as secretion control. Swallowing and speech are preserved, which enhances quality of life.

LONG-TERM VENTILATORY SUPPORT

In patients with severely compromised ventilatory function and in those who have difficulty clearing secretions, supplemental ventilatory support may be required long term if the patient desires to live with his or her disease. In cases of encephalitis, brainstem infarction, or arteriovenous malformations that affect the brainstem respiratory centers, nocturnal ventilation alone may not be a viable option; permanent, continuous ventilatory support may be needed. Permanent tracheostomy with mechanical ventilatory support is indicated here. Patients who receive continuous ventilator therapy at home require extensive support from family and outside caregivers. Nonetheless, reasonable quality of life can be achieved for motivated patients and their families.

Clinical Course

The clinical course is variable and depends on the cause and severity of the hypoventilation, its complications, and other comorbidities. The age of onset of primary central hypoventilation ranges from infancy in congenital cases to the seventh decade of life. The average age of onset is about the third to fourth decade. In one case series, half of the 30 cases were acquired. Causes include encephalitis, meningitis, parkinsonism, syringomyelia, vascular malformation, and mental retardation.

Congenital brainstem abnormalities, such as Chiari malformations (see Fig. 72.3), have a prognosis that depends on the degree of neurologic damage associated with the descent of cerebellar tissue into the upper spinal canal, the degree of medullary and spinal cord compression, and associated neurologic conditions such as hydrocephalus or meningocele. These may be detected in infancy or adulthood. Central apnea occurs as a result of impingement of the brainstem respiratory centers at the foramen magnum.

SECONDARY CAUSES OF CENTRAL HYPOVENTILATION

Only a minority of patients who have poliomyelitis develop the paralytic form. Survivors of the outbreaks in the 1950s are still alive, and some require permanent home-ventilator support. The postpolio syndrome is a late complication that is manifested by progressive muscle weakness, fatigue, and joint pain after 20 to 40 years of stability. How often this leads to respiratory muscle dysfunction is not known, but a heightened index of suspicion for this late complication must be maintained.

In a population-based sample of 358 patients with spinal cord injuries, the case-fatality rate was less than 4%. Of patients with cervical cord injuries, 36% experienced neurologic improvement compared with the initial severity of injury, and more than 95% of all patients who had spinal cord injury were discharged home. Unfortunately, respiratory dysfunction remains a significant problem for most patients with cervical cord injury, despite improvement in other areas of function.

The outcome after other central nervous system (CNS) injuries, such as severe encephalitis, infarctions that involve the brainstem respiratory centers, and CNS neoplasms, is usually poor. Involvement of the reticular activating system may result in permanent coma, and patients with such disorders and their family members must be involved in discussions about therapy, as often the only therapy is support using chronic mechanical ventilation.

COMPLICATIONS OF CENTRAL HYPOVENTILATION

Complications of central hypoventilation include pulmonary hypertension, secondary polycythemia, right- and left-sided heart failure, and respiratory failure. Complications related to treatment of this disorder, such as ventilator-associated lung and bronchial infections, must be considered as well.

Pitfalls and Controversies

Disorders of central hypoventilation are rare and easily missed, and their pathophysiology is poorly understood. Central hypoventilation may be primary and/or congenital, or secondary and/or acquired. Development of these disorders typically occurs after a serious brain injury—a severe encephalitis, a neoplasm, or an infarction of the area of the respiratory centers of the medulla. Congenital cases of pure central hypoventilation may also occur, albeit rarely. The prognosis associated with these conditions is poor. Nonetheless, successful clinical management with either noninvasive ventilation or ventilation through a permanent tracheostomy is possible.

SLEEP-DISORDERED BREATHING IN CHRONIC LUNG DISEASE

Epidemiology

Poor sleep is a common complaint with chronic obstructive pulmonary disease (COPD). Most patients do not have OSA, but a fraction have oxygen desaturations less than 85%. The size of the subpopulation of these patients who have nocturnal desaturation is unknown, because measurements of nocturnal oxygen saturation are not routinely carried out.

Risk Factors

Risk factors for nocturnal hypoxemia include severity and type of pulmonary disease, amount of rapid eye movement sleep over the course of a night, and body weight. Patients who have obstructive airway disease appear to be at greater risk of noc-

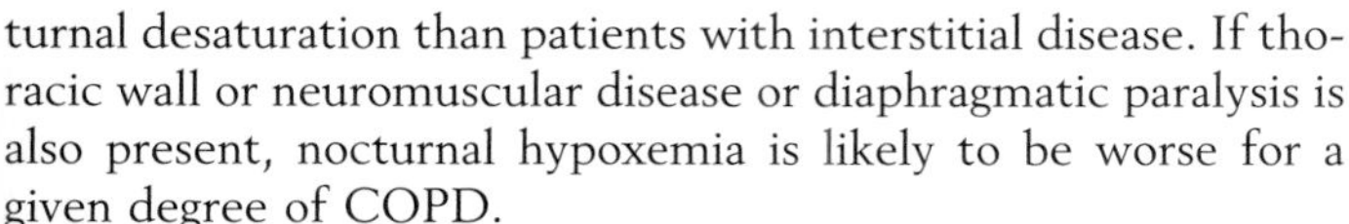

turnal desaturation than patients with interstitial disease. If thoracic wall or neuromuscular disease or diaphragmatic paralysis is also present, nocturnal hypoxemia is likely to be worse for a given degree of COPD.

Diagnosis

Detection of SDB in patients who have COPD and other forms of lung disease is important, and sleep studies must be carried out for those who show symptoms of SDB. Patients in whom cor pulmonale or polycythemia develops despite optimal medical management should undergo sleep studies to detect occult sleep apnea or severe desaturations.

Treatment

All patients with lung disease and who qualify must have continuous oxygen therapy. Some centers empirically increase liter flow by 1 or 2 L/min during sleep. If OSA or other forms of SDB are detected, these patients should be treated with CPAP or BPAP. These patients may not be able to tolerate CPAP therapy, especially if the OSA is mild. If difficulty exhaling against the expiratory pressures of CPAP is identified, a bilevel pressure device may be an option. Occasionally, dramatic improvements in dyspnea and quality of life are seen with nocturnal ventilatory assistance; however, predicting who is likely to benefit is difficult. Clinical trials that examined various methods of nocturnal ventilatory support using positive-pressure breathing delivered by mask frequently showed positive results in the short term but were not able to demonstrate sustained positive results after approximately 3 months of use.

Clinical Course

Nocturnal desaturation in patients who have lung disease complicates the medical care of these patients because it necessitates oxygen therapy and may decrease quality of life. Continuous home oxygen therapy for patients with severe hypoxemic lung disease was shown to prolong life in two large randomized clinical trials conducted in the early 1980s. When patients have only nocturnal desaturation, the benefit of oxygen therapy is less clear. One study compared survival over an average of 70 months between two groups of COPD patients, one of which had less than the expected amount of nocturnal desaturation while the other had greater than the expected amount of nocturnal desaturation. No major differences in survival were detected.

The combination of OSA and COPD can be debilitating and has been termed the *overlap syndrome*. Cor pulmonale, chronic respiratory insufficiency, and secondary polycythemia characterize this syndrome. Treatment is directed at both disorders, with the chief aim being to maintain normal oxygen saturation. Noninvasive ventilation is considered not only for treatment of OSA, but also for treatment of respiratory insufficiency and hypercapnia. Without therapy, affected patients are expected to have a high degree of morbidity and early mortality.

SUGGESTED READINGS

Bonnet MH, Dexter JR, Arand DL: The effect of triazolam on arousal and respiration in central sleep apnea patients. Sleep 13:31-41, 1990.

Connaughton JJ, Catterall JR, Elton RA, et al: Do sleep studies contribute to the management of patients with severe chronic obstructive pulmonary disease? Am Rev Respir Dis 138:341-344, 1988.

DiMarco AF, Onders RP, Kowalski KE, et al: Phrenic nerve pacing in a tetraplegic patient via intramuscular diaphragm electrodes. Am J Respir Crit Care Med 166:1604-1606, 2002.

Gay PC, Edmonds LC: Severe hypercapnia after low-flow oxygen therapy in patients with neuromuscular disease and diaphragmatic dysfunction [comment]. Mayo Clin Proc 70:327-330, 1995.

Gerhart KA: Spinal cord injury outcomes in a population-based sample. J Trauma 31:1529-1535, 1991.

Hillberg R, Johnson DC: Noninvasive ventilation. N Engl J Med 337:1746-1752, 1997.

Lanini B, Misuri G, Gigliotti F, et al: Perception of dyspnea in patients with neuromuscular disease. Chest 120:402-408, 2001.

Leung RS, Bradley TD: Sleep apnea and cardiovascular disease. Am J Respir Crit Care Med 164:2147-2165, 2001.

Martin TJ, Sanders MH: Chronic alveolar hypoventilation: A review for the clinician. Sleep 18:617-634, 1995.

McNicholas WT, Carter JL, Rutherford R, et al: Beneficial effect of oxygen in primary alveolar hypoventilation with central sleep apnea. Am Rev Respir Dis 125:773-775, 1982.

Medical Research Council Working Party: Long term domiciliary oxygen therapy in chronic hypoxic cor pulmonale complicating chronic bronchitis and emphysema. Report of the Medical Research Council Working Party. Lancet 1:681-686, 1981.

Nocturnal Oxygen Therapy Trial Group: Continuous or nocturnal oxygen therapy in hypoxemic chronic obstructive lung disease: A clinical trial. Nocturnal Oxygen Therapy Trial Group. Ann Intern Med 93:391-398, 1980.

Weinberger SE, Schwartzstein RM, Weiss JW: Hypercapnia. N Engl J Med 321:1223-1231, 1989.

Xie A, Skatrud JB, Dempsey JA: Effect of hypoxia on the hypopnoeic and apnoeic threshold for CO(2) in sleeping humans. J Physiol 535:269-278, 2001.

Xie A, Skatrud JB, Puleo DS, et al: Apnea-hypopnea threshold for CO_2 in patients with congestive heart failure. Am J Respir Crit Care Med 165:1245-1250, 2002.

CHAPTER 73 Drugs and the Lungs

Dorothy A. White

Many drugs can cause pulmonary reactions. The list of such drugs grows longer as new complications are linked to drugs and as new drugs appear. Recognition that a pulmonary problem has been caused by administration of a drug is important for several reasons. First, further damage can usually be prevented if use of the offending agent is stopped and, in some cases, if treatment is offered. Second, unnecessary evaluation and treatment for other conditions can be avoided.

Because the list of drugs that cause reactions is long, discussion of each of them is beyond the scope of this book. In this chapter the focus is on general patterns of drug-induced lung injury; several drugs for which pulmonary toxicity is well recognized and described are discussed in more detail.

PATTERNS OF PRESENTATION

Several clinical pulmonary syndromes are related to drug therapy. Parenchymal pulmonary reactions include interstitial pneumonitis and fibrosis, hypersensitivity pneumonitis, noncardiogenic pulmonary edema, acute pneumonia, and the rare entities of pulmonary renal syndrome and pulmonary veno-occlusive disease (Table 73.1). Airway diseases can also occur secondary to drug administration and include bronchospasm, cough, and bronchiolitis obliterans (Table 73.2). Finally, systemic reactions that have pulmonary consequences are noted; these include drug-induced systemic lupus erythematosus and neuromuscular disorders.

Parenchymal Patterns

INTERSTITIAL PNEUMONITIS AND PULMONARY FIBROSIS

The development of interstitial pneumonitis and pulmonary fibrosis is characterized by the subacute to chronic (over weeks to months) development of dyspnea and a dry cough. Fever and systemic symptoms are only rarely present. On physical examination, bibasilar crackles are usually an early finding. With more advanced disease, crackles may be heard throughout the lung fields. Chest radiographs show reticular infiltrates; in advanced cases, restriction of the lung fields and honeycombing are also seen. Pulmonary function tests show a low diffusing capacity for carbon monoxide and varying degrees of restriction.

Pathologically, interstitial pneumonitis or pulmonary fibrosis is characterized by the presence of atypical type II pneumocytes. Type I pneumocytes, which line the alveolar space, are very susceptible to injury induced by drugs. Type II pneumocytes, which are their precursors, proliferate to correct the injury. In the setting of drug-induced injury, the reparative process results in the appearance of abnormal type II cells, which are large and cuboidal and have large and hyperchromatic nuclei, unusual nuclear chromatic patterns, and prominent nucleoli (Fig. 73.1). These cells are often seen with injury from cytotoxic therapy and are suggestive, but not diagnostic, of drug-related injury. With noncytotoxic, drug-induced, interstitial injury, fewer type II cells may be present, or they may be absent. Also present are various degrees of fibrosis and mononuclear cell infiltration; occasionally, mononuclear cell infiltration predominates. The prognosis with interstitial pneumonitis or fibrosis is variable. In some cases resolution or improvement occurs, but progressive fibrosis and respiratory failure can also occur. This type of pattern is most commonly associated with the cytotoxic drugs but can also occur with cardiovascular agents and antimicrobial drugs.

HYPERSENSITIVITY PNEUMONITIS

Drug-induced hypersensitivity pneumonitis is characterized by an acute-to-subacute presentation. Systemic symptoms, with fever, fatigue, myalgias, and arthralgias, are often present. Pulmonary symptoms are cough and dyspnea, but these appear after the systemic symptoms. Eosinophilia is present in 20% to 40% of cases. Chest radiographs typically show airspace disease, which may be focal, lobar, or diffuse in distribution; a peripheral predominance of infiltrates may be present. In some cases Löffler's syndrome (pulmonary infiltrates with eosinophilia) is seen.

Pathologically, acute inflammation with neutrophils and eosinophils and a prominent mononuclear cell infiltration are seen. Two patterns occur. In one pattern, eosinophils are confluent in alveoli and heavily involve the interstitium, a pattern usually associated with a Löffler-like syndrome. The second pattern shows fibrosis and a mixed mononuclear cell infiltrate with interstitial, but not alveolar, eosinophils. Prognosis is generally good with a Löffler-like syndrome but is more variable with the more chronic picture of fibrosis. This pattern of hypersensitivity pneumonitis is associated with a variety of drugs, but most commonly with gold and nitrofurantoin.

NONCARDIOGENIC PULMONARY EDEMA

Noncardiogenic pulmonary edema manifests with acute respiratory distress and may develop over several hours. Chest radiographs show diffuse alveolar filling infiltrates with no cardiomegaly or pleural effusions. Prognosis is generally good if administration of the offending agent is stopped and supportive care is given. This type of injury is commonly associated with aspirin and the opiates.

ACUTE PNEUMONIA

Patients with acute pneumonia have acute distress similar to that seen in noncardiogenic edema. Pathologic studies, however, also

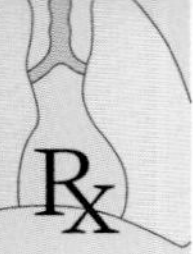

Table 73.1
Major parenchymal pulmonary reactions

Type of reaction	Drugs				
	Cytotoxic	Cardiovascular	Antimicrobial	Anti-inflammatory	Other
Interstitial pneumonitis/ fibrosis	Bleomycin Mitomycin Cyclophosphamide Nitrosoureas Busulfan Gefitinib	Amiodarone Flecainide Mexiletine Tocainide	Nitrofurantoin	Gold	–
Hypersensitivity pneumonitis	Methotrexate Azathioprine	–	Minocycline Nitrofurantoin Pyrimethamine–chloroquine Pyrimethamine–dapsone Sulfasalazine	Gold Penicillamine Nonsteroidal anti-inflammatory drugs	Carbamazepine Phenytoin
Noncardiogenic pulmonary edema	Cytosine arabinoside Gemcitabine	Amiodarone Hydrochlorothiazide Lidocaine (lignocaine) Tocainide	–	Aspirin Nonsteroidal anti-inflammatory drugs	Naloxone Opiates Tocolytic agents
Acute pneumonia	Mitomycin–Vinca alkaloids Paclitaxel Docetaxel	Amiodarone	–	–	–

Table 73.2
Drug-induced bronchospasm

- Aspirin sensitivity
  - Aspirin
  - Nonsteroidal anti-inflammatory drugs
- β-Adrenergic blockers
- Contrast media
- Neuromuscular blocking agents
- Inhaled pentamidine
- Adenosine
- Sotalol
- Dipyridamole (i.v.)
- Taxanes

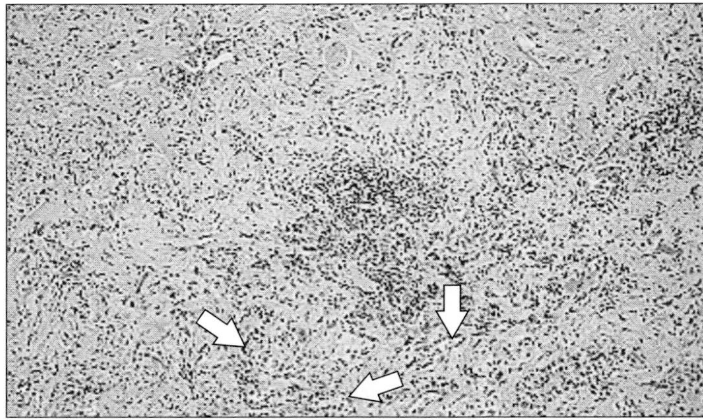

Figure 73.1 Atypical type II pneumocytes. This lung biopsy specimen from a patient with bleomycin toxicity shows extensive fibrosis and inflammatory cell infiltrates. The alveoli are lined by hyperplastic cuboidal cells that protrude into the lumen. These bizarre cells suggest drug-induced injury.

show the presence of interstitial and alveolar inflammation with some degree of fibrosis. Prognosis is variable and less favorable than that with noncardiogenic pulmonary edema. Although improvement often occurs, persistent respiratory impairment may remain and cause significant problems. This effect is most commonly seen with the combination of mitomycin and vinca alkaloids.

PULMONARY VENO-OCCLUSIVE DISEASE

Pulmonary veno-occlusive disease is characterized by occlusion of the pulmonary veins, which leads to pulmonary hypertension. The usual presenting sign is dyspnea of insidious development. Chest radiographs may show Kerley's B lines in the absence of cardiomegaly. Pulmonary veno-occlusive disease has been reported to occur with several cytotoxic drugs, and prognosis is poor.

PULMONARY RENAL SYNDROME

Pulmonary renal syndrome is a rare disorder similar to Goodpasture's syndrome. Patients have dyspnea, hemoptysis, and hematuria. Pathologically, pulmonary hemorrhage is seen, but linear deposits of immunoglobulin are not seen. Pulmonary renal syndrome occurs with penicillamine administration.

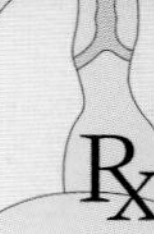

Airway Patterns

BRONCHOSPASM

Bronchospasm can be induced by several drugs, most commonly aspirin, nonsteroidal anti-inflammatory drugs (NSAIDs), β-antagonists, and β-blockers. This reaction usually occurs in patients who have underlying asthma or chronic obstructive airway disease. Bronchospasm occurs minutes to hours after ingestion of the offending drug; it may be severe and difficult to treat. A hypersensitivity reaction with bronchospasm occurs in a high percentage of patients receiving the taxanes, a new class of cancer drugs, but this reaction can be blocked or ameliorated in most cases by premedication with antihistamines and steroids.

COUGH

Angiotensin-converting enzyme (ACE) inhibitors can cause chronic cough in 5% to 15% of patients. It occurs in women more frequently than in men and usually after 1 to 2 months of treatment, but occasionally later. All ACE inhibitors can induce chronic cough, but the direct angiotensin receptor antagonists do not appear to do so. Patients with asthma are not at increased risk. Although airway irritation and bronchoconstriction are possible mechanisms, the mechanism of toxicity is unclear. ACE inhibitors block the metabolism of bradykinins and substance P, leading to an increase of these neuropeptides, which have irritant and bronchoconstrictor effects. Activation of the arachidonic acid pathway by ACE inhibition may also lead to elevated levels of thromboxane, which can potentiate bronchoconstriction. Drug withdrawal results in improvement within a few weeks. Occasionally, a response to inhaled cromolyn occurs.

OBLITERATIVE BRONCHIOLITIS

Obliterative bronchiolitis (OB) is a rare complication of drug therapy and has been described almost exclusively in conjunction with penicillamine use. Patients experience increasing dyspnea and cough. Physical examination may be normal, or squeaks and crackles may be present. Chest radiographs show hyperinflation. Expiratory chest computed tomography (CT) shows air trapping and a mosaic pattern. Pathologically, obliteration of the small conducting airways by concentric luminal narrowing occurs because of an intense lymphocytic infiltration. The occluding plugs of granular tissue common in bronchiolitis obliterans that is not related to drug therapy are not usually found.

DRUG-INDUCED SYSTEMIC LUPUS ERYTHEMATOSUS

Some drugs cause a lupus-like syndrome. The incidence of renal and of neurologic complications is low with drug-induced lupus, but that of pleuropulmonary complications is high. The drugs that most commonly cause this syndrome are hydralazine, procainamide, quinidine, isoniazid, and diphenylhydantoin. Isolated reports suggest that many other drugs cause this problem.

NEUROLOGIC DISORDERS

Many drugs can inhibit neural drive, cause peripheral neuropathy, block neuromuscular functions, or produce myopathy (see Aldrich and Prezant for a review of this subject).

MECHANISMS OF TOXICITY

Several mechanisms are proposed for drug-induced injury to the lungs, and more than one may be operative with any drug. The first is the creation of an imbalance in the oxidant-antioxidant system. Reactive oxygen metabolites, which are formed within phagocytic cells, help in host defense but can produce multiple toxic effects. Antioxidants (such as superoxide dismutase, catalase, and glutathione) can detoxify these reactive molecules and maintain an acceptable balance. Some cytotoxic drugs (e.g., bleomycin, cyclophosphamide, carmustine) are believed to alter the normal balance. Interference with the oxidant-antioxidant system is an unusual mechanism for noncytotoxic drugs but may play a role in toxicity caused by nitrofurantoin.

A second mechanism is an alteration in the fine immunologic balance that exists in the lung, which is open to the atmosphere, and that is designed to protect against invading pathogens but also has mechanisms to prevent excessive reactions and self-destruction. This is an important mechanism of toxicity for many antimicrobial and anti-inflammatory agents. In some cases of drug toxicity, a marked influx of eosinophils occurs, which suggests an acute reaction to antigen and alteration of the immune balance. In many other cases in which eosinophils are not found, experimental evidence also favors immune alteration, as occurs with noncytotoxic drugs such as gold, amiodarone, and nitrofurantoin and the cytotoxic agent methotrexate. Bronchoalveolar lavage in these cases shows an increase in lymphocytes, usually of the suppressor subtype. Enhanced lymphocyte blastogenesis and lymphokine release after exposure of cells to some drugs, notably gold and nitrofurantoin, have also been shown. With some drugs, such as bleomycin, lavage has shown an excess of neutrophils. Complement activation has been noted with the opiates and may also play a role in inducing toxicity. Finally, drugs can also alter pathways with effects on the lung, such as aspirin's inhibition of the cyclooxygenase pathway that leads to the bronchospasm.

Another possible mechanism of drug-induced injury is change in matrix repair by alteration in the balance between collagenosis and collagenolysis. Bleomycin, gold, and penicillamine may effect injury partially through this system. Finally, a neural effect of some drugs that causes increased permeability and leads to pulmonary edema has been suggested as a factor with opiates, major tranquilizers, and salicylates.

SPECIFIC DRUGS

Noncytotoxic Drugs

AMIODARONE

Amiodarone is used for serious ventricular arrhythmias and refractory supraventricular arrhythmias. Its use is often limited by toxicity, which can be ophthalmic, cutaneous, hepatic, thyroid related, or pulmonary. The incidence of pulmonary toxicity is 5% to 15% and is increased in those patients who receive more than 400 mg/day. Three forms of pulmonary toxicity are found, of which interstitial pneumonitis is the most common. Presenting signs and symptoms develop over weeks to months and include cough, dyspnea, and weight loss. The second pattern is that of acute pneumonia, in which patients have the acute-to-subacute onset of fever, cough, and chest pain. In both types, the erythrocyte sedimentation rate (ESR) is elevated and a peripheral leuko-

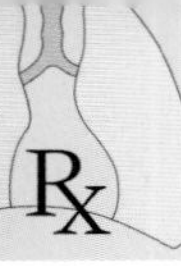

cytosis occurs. Episodes of acute, noncardiogenic pulmonary edema have been described as a serious third type of toxicity, which usually occurs after cardiac and noncardiac surgery, particularly pneumonectomy. A connection with use of high, inspired concentrations of oxygen during surgery is possible.

Chest radiographs show interstitial infiltrates in the chronic pneumonitis pattern, a mixture of interstitial and alveolar infiltrates with acute pneumonia, and diffuse infiltrates with noncardiogenic pulmonary edema. Although less common, focal or lobar infiltrates, pulmonary masses, and pleural effusions have been described. Areas of high density in amiodarone-associated infiltrates are shown on CT scans because large accumulations of macrophages contain amiodarone, which is high in iodine content. These areas of high attenuation are not, however, pathognomonic of amiodarone toxicity, but rather of use of the drug. Gallium scans are positive with amiodarone toxicity.

Pathologically, interstitial and alveolar inflammation and a variable amount of fibrosis are seen. Macrophages of foamy appearance are present in tissue (Fig. 73.2); the foaminess results from phospholipid accumulation, because amiodarone inhibits phospholipase. With acute pneumonia, intra-alveolar hemorrhage and hyaline membrane formation can also be seen. The diagnosis is suspected in any patient who develops respiratory distress while receiving the drug, although congestive heart failure and infection usually must be excluded. Pulmonary function tests show a low diffusing capacity but are nonspecific; a normal diffusing capacity, however, eliminates the diagnosis. A positive gallium scan and elevated ESR are suggestive findings. Treatment consists of discontinuation of the drug. Corticosteroids are often given at a dose of 40 to 60 mg/day, but resolution can take some time, because the half-life of the drug is long (up to 60 days). In cases in which the drug cannot be stopped, a lower dose and concomitant corticosteroids may be useful. High doses of oxygen must be avoided in patients on amiodarone who undergo major surgery, and a substitute drug used if possible.

NITROFURANTOIN

The potential for pulmonary toxicity from nitrofurantoin used for urinary suppression has been recognized for many years. The incidence is less than 1%, but the drug is widely used. Nitrofurantoin causes both a hypersensitivity pneumonitis or, less commonly, a chronic pneumonitis. The hypersensitivity pneumonitis is characterized by systemic symptoms of fever, arthralgias, chest pain, and a maculopapular rash that occurs with pulmonary symptoms of cough and dyspnea. The syndrome usually occurs within the first month of administration of the drug. Eosinophilia is present in most cases. Alveolar filling and interstitial infiltrates are seen, and pleural effusions can occur. In some cases radiographs are normal.

Pathologically, vasculitis and interstitial inflammation, particularly by eosinophils, are seen. Chronic toxicity may occur after months to years of therapy and is not an acute sequela. Dyspnea and cough are seen, and systemic symptoms are less common, although fatigue and weight loss may occur. Chest radiographs show interstitial infiltrates. Peripheral eosinophilia can occur but is less common than with acute toxicity. Positive antinuclear antibodies and rheumatoid factors and elevated immunoglobulins are often found. Biopsies show interstitial inflammation and fibrosis. A toxic reaction to drug metabolites is considered a probable cause.

In most cases a diagnosis is made clinically. The prognosis is good for the hypersensitivity pneumonitis if administration of the drug is discontinued. With chronic toxicity the outcome is less favorable; in approximately 70% of cases, no improvement occurs or some abnormalities persist. Corticosteroids are used, but a beneficial effect has not been proved.

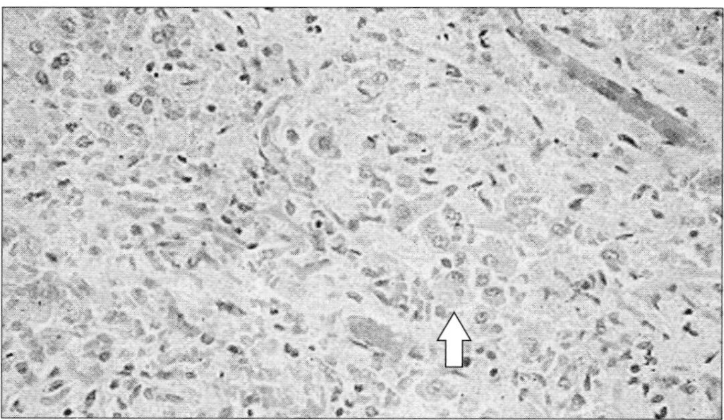

Figure 73.2 Lung histology associated with amiodarone pulmonary toxicity. An interstitial inflammatory infiltrate is seen with vacuolated macrophages. These "foamy" macrophages contain a large amount of abundant, pale cytoplasm of foamy appearance. Although such macrophages are characteristically seen with amiodarone use, they do not mean toxicity has occurred.

GOLD

Gold is used to treat rheumatoid arthritis and other rheumatic diseases, and both parenchymal gold sodium thiomalate and oral gold (auranofin) can cause pulmonary toxicity. The most common manifestation is a hypersensitivity pneumonitis, but occasionally bronchiolitis obliterans with organizing pneumonia (BOOP) and possibly OB may be seen.

The incidence of gold toxicity is less than 1%, and a genetic predisposition to its development is possible. It typically occurs after several months of therapy. Patients experience cough, dyspnea, and a rash, and approximately 40% have eosinophilia. Radiographs show diffuse reticular infiltrates. Pathologically, interstitial inflammation is seen. Gold deposits can be detected in the lung, but their role in toxicity is unknown. Bronchoalveolar lavage studies show increased lymphocytes with a predominance of suppressor or cytotoxic cells. Prognosis is good with discontinuation of the agent and treatment with corticosteroids, which need to be tapered slowly over months. Patients with BOOP that occurs in association with gold therapy have a good response to treatment with corticosteroids, although the prognosis is variable for idiopathic BOOP.

D-PENICILLAMINE

D-Penicillamine, which is used in the treatment of rheumatic disorders and Wilson's disease, has been associated with OB (only in patients who have rheumatoid arthritis), hypersensitivity pneumonitis, and (rarely) a pulmonary renal syndrome. Patients who have OB develop severe dyspnea as well as cough associated with obstructive and restrictive lung function abnormalities. Lung biopsies show infiltration of bronchiolar walls with inflammation and concentric luminal narrowing. The prognosis of patients with OB is poor; little response occurs with use

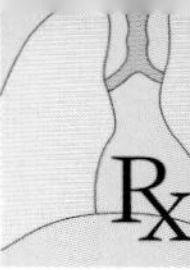

of bronchodilators and corticosteroids, but anecdotal reports indicate success with cyclophosphamide and azathioprine. The mechanism of this unusual airway toxicity is unclear; rheumatoid arthritis has been postulated to induce the injury, but penicillamine interferes with matrix repair and so prolongs the injury and increases the frequency of this entity over that seen with rheumatoid arthritis alone.

Hypersensitivity pneumonitis secondary to D-penicillamine appears to carry a good prognosis and manifests in a pattern that is similar to that seen with other drugs. Patients with the pulmonary renal syndrome have acute respiratory distress and hemoptysis, similar to Goodpasture's syndrome. Prognosis is poor. Patients are treated with immunosuppression, including cyclophosphamide and azathioprine in addition to corticosteroids. The role of plasmapheresis is unknown.

ASPIRIN

Salicylates are associated with acute noncardiogenic edema and exacerbation of bronchospasm. Pulmonary edema usually occurs when salicylate levels are greater than 40 mg/dL. Two groups of patients with this complication have been noted. The first consists of younger patients who have attempted suicide by means of planned overdoses. The second group consists of older individuals with multiple medical problems in whom the overdose is accidental. The clinical presentation includes confusion, focal neurologic findings, tachypnea, inspiratory crackles, proteinuria, primary respiratory alkalosis, and metabolic acidosis. The neurologic findings may lead to a delay in obtaining a history of aspirin ingestion. Treatment is with forced alkaline diuresis and supportive care. Prognosis is good if the diagnosis is made promptly.

Use of aspirin and other NSAIDs may precipitate bronchospasm in some patients with asthma and is often associated with conjunctivitis and rhinitis. The triad of nasal polyps, aspirin sensitivity, and asthma is known as *Samter's syndrome*. The frequency of aspirin-induced bronchospasm is between 5% and 10% of patients with asthma and is more common in those who have perennial rhinitis or nasal polyps. It occurs most frequently in young adults or adolescents. Occasionally, it appears after aspirin has been taken for some time. Bronchospasm usually happens within several hours of taking the drug, but it can occur within minutes. Overproduction of leukotrienes secondary to interference with the cyclooxygenase pathway is probably the mechanism of salicylate-induced bronchospasm. The beneficial effect of the 5-lipoxygenase inhibitor zileuton on the syndrome supports this theory. Avoidance of aspirin and NSAIDs is recommended if possible. Desensitization has been successful in some cases, and leukotriene modifiers are the treatment of choice.

Cytotoxic Drugs

BLEOMYCIN

Bleomycin is known to induce pulmonary fibrosis both in animal models and in patients who receive the drug for a variety of malignancies. The incidence of clinically significant toxicity is 4%; subclinical toxicity detected through pulmonary function tests has been found in 25% of cases. In most cases interstitial pneumonitis or fibrosis is present, but acute pneumonia and hypersensitivity pneumonitis are also occasionally seen. Several risk factors have been identified for toxicity: age greater than 70 years, total dose received, previous radiation to the chest, use of supplemental oxygen, presence of renal insufficiency, and use of multidrug regimens. Studies suggest that although toxicity can occur even at low doses of bleomycin, the incidence increases significantly at doses greater than 400 units (Fig. 73.3). Cases that occur at higher doses are also associated with increased mortality. The synergistic effect of both radiation and high inspired concentrations of oxygen has been documented in both animal models and clinical studies. No safe threshold dose of supplemental oxygen exists, and its use must be avoided in all patients who receive bleomycin or have signs of toxicity.

Patients typically have dyspnea and dry cough of subacute to insidious onset. The physical examination characteristically shows bibasilar crackles, and chest radiographs initially show infiltrates at the bases peripherally (Fig. 73.4). With more

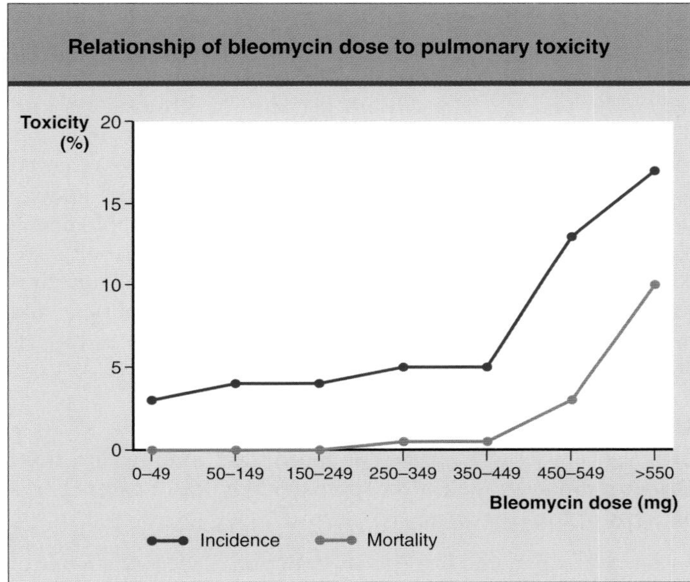

Figure 73.3 Relationship of bleomycin dose to pulmonary toxicity. Bleomycin toxicity occurs even at low doses, but the incidence and mortality increase as the dose exceeds 400 units. (Adapted with permission from Blum RH, Carter SK, Agre K: A clinical review of bleomycin—a new antineoplastic agent. Cancer 31:903-914, 1973. American Cancer Society, by permission of Wiley-Liss, a subsidiary of John Wiley & Sons.)

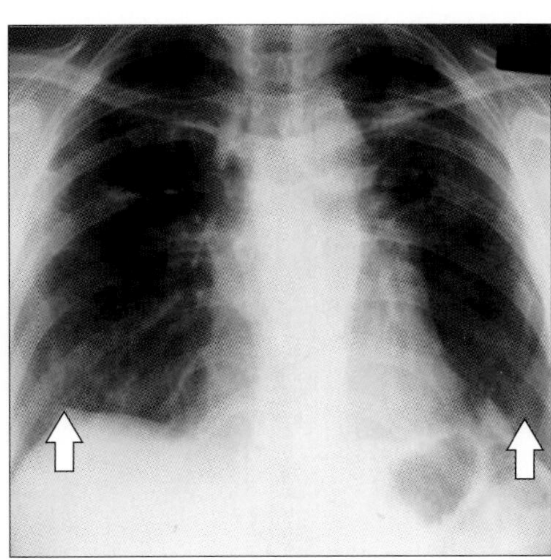

Figure 73.4 Chest radiograph in bleomycin toxicity. Fine bibasilar infiltrates are shown *(arrows)*, suggestive of drug toxicity.

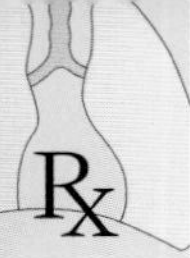

advanced disease, diffuse interstitial infiltrates and small lung fields are seen. Chest CT may reveal subpleural septal thickening and interstitial changes earlier than radiography (Fig. 73.5). Acinar infiltrates can be seen and are more common when hypersensitivity pneumonitis or acute pneumonia is present. Focal infiltrates and nodular densities have also been described.

Pathologically, atypical type II pneumocytes, alveolar and interstitial infiltration, and varying degrees of fibrosis are seen (see Fig. 73.1). Bronchoalveolar lavage studies in animal models and some human cases have shown increased polymorphonuclear cells. Concerns have been raised that use of granulocyte colony-stimulating factor in those receiving the drug might increase the risk of toxicity, but this has not been found to be the case.

Pulmonary function tests in patients who have bleomycin pulmonary toxicity show a decreased diffusing capacity and, in more advanced cases, a restrictive defect. Attempts have been made to use pulmonary function tests for screening, but no clear documentation of efficacy has been established. Such tests continue to be used clinically because of the serious nature of bleomycin toxicity. A significant decrease in diffusing capacity during treatment does not indicate definite toxicity but is a cause of concern, and further investigation may be required to exclude that possibility. Treatment of bleomycin toxicity involves withdrawal of the drug, avoidance of supplemental oxygen, avoidance of chest radiation therapy, and use of corticosteroid therapy in severe cases. Although clinical improvement occurs, residual lung function abnormalities and respiratory symptoms often occur. Mortality can be as high as 50% in those who have severe pneumonitis.

MITOMYCIN

Although not as well studied as bleomycin, mitomycin causes serious pulmonary toxicity in approximately 4% of cases. Three patterns of toxicity occur:

- An acute pneumonitis (most common), seen when mitomycin is used with vinca alkaloids
- Interstitial pneumonitis or fibrosis, similar to that seen with bleomycin use
- Pulmonary infiltrates (rare), associated with microangiopathic hemolytic anemia and uremia

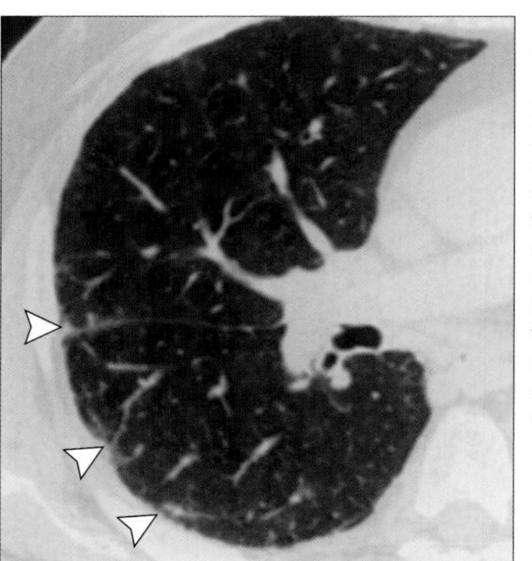

Figure 73.5 Bleomycin toxicity. In a patient receiving bleomycin who had a large decrease in the diffusing capacity, the chest computed tomography (CT) scan showed early changes of septal thickening and increased markings in the subpleural area ***(arrowheads)***. These changes are suggestive of drug toxicity.

In the mitomycin–vinca alkaloid reaction, patients develop severe episodes of respiratory distress usually several hours after they receive a dose of the vinca alkaloid. In some cases the respiratory failure requires intubation. Radiographs show new bilateral interstitial infiltrates. With supportive care and, in most cases, corticosteroids, improvement occurs over several days. Unfortunately, approximately 50% of cases have residual pulmonary impairment similar to that seen with mitomycin-induced pulmonary fibrosis. Lung histology shows fibrosis and a mononuclear cell infiltration. No clear risk factors are identified, and the mechanism of toxicity is unknown.

The interstitial pneumonitis or fibrosis syndrome manifests similar to bleomycin toxicity, with the insidious onset of dyspnea. Chest radiographs show interstitial disease. In many cases the response to corticosteroids is good. The rare entity of mitomycin-induced, microangiopathic hemolytic anemia occurs with pulmonary hemorrhage, which manifests with diffuse pulmonary infiltrates and, sometimes, respiratory failure. Prognosis is poor. Treatment with corticosteroids and possibly plasmapheresis must be attempted.

NITROSOUREAS

The nitrosoureas—carmustine (BCNU) and lomustine—are frequently used for treatment of brain tumors because of their penetration into the central nervous system. They have also been used in high doses as part of regimens before autologous marrow or peripheral stem-cell transplantation. Two patterns of injury have been noted, namely interstitial pneumonitis or fibrosis and acute pneumonia. The first pattern has been described after treatment of brain tumors, and toxicity may not appear for months to years after treatment. In children, respiratory failure may develop up to 10 years later. Several risk factors have been identified: high dose (a relationship exists between increasing dose and risk of toxicity, particularly at doses above 1500 mg/ m^2), pre-existing pulmonary disease, and use in multidrug regimens.

Patients have dyspnea and dry cough of insidious onset. Physical examination reveals bibasilar crackles and occasionally rhonchi. Signs of consolidation have also been reported. Chest radiography can show a variety of findings, which include either upper-lobe infiltration or cystic changes, lower lobe infiltrates, bilateral alveolar filling infiltrates, patchy infiltrates, and nodular densities (Fig. 73.6). Pneumothorax has also been reported. Lung function tests show restriction and occasionally obstruction. Pathologic findings are similar to those found with other cytotoxic agents. Often, however, fibrosis is patchy and little inflammation is present. Treatment with corticosteroids is usually not effective, and discontinuation of the drug is the mainstay of treatment. Prognosis is poor, with a reported mortality of up to 90% in severe cases.

An acute pneumonia-like pattern with the development of diffuse interstitial or alveolar infiltrates can occur several weeks after the use of high-dose carmustine. This form of toxicity is usually responsive to corticosteroids. In some cases in which lung function was monitored after high-dose chemotherapy, marked decreases in the diffusing capacity were noted, presumably because of carmustine toxicity; this improved with cor-

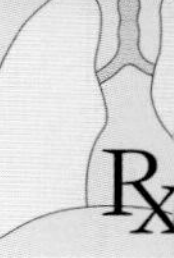

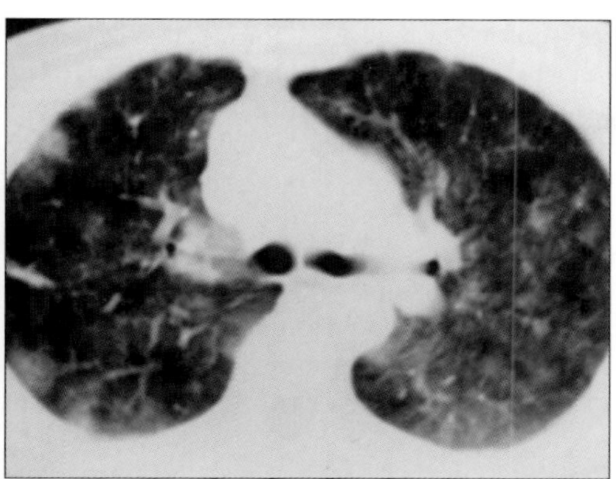

Figure 73.6 Carmustine toxicity. This computed tomography (CT) scan shows the patchy nature of fibrosis after use of carmustine. Respiratory failure developed over several years.

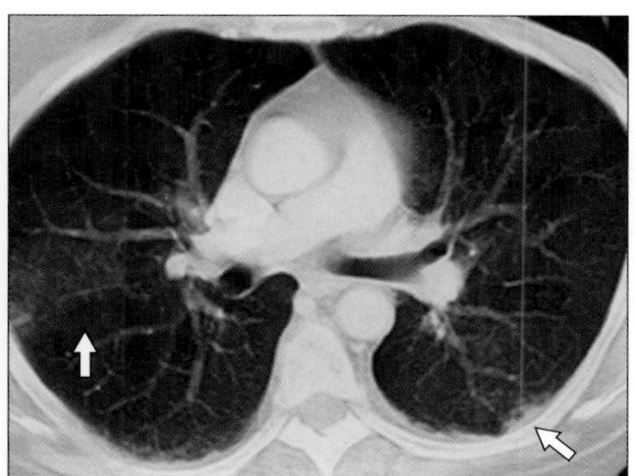

Figure 73.7 Computed tomography (CT) scan in methotrexate toxicity. Patchy acinar infiltrates are seen, consistent with this type of drug toxicity.

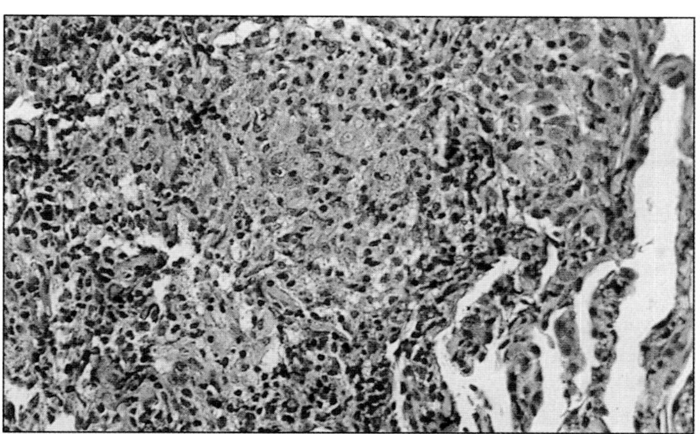

Figure 73.8 Methotrexate toxicity. This biopsy from a patient who had methotrexate pneumonitis shows extensive infiltration with lymphocytes and also loosely formed granulomas. Atypical type II pneumocytes are not seen.

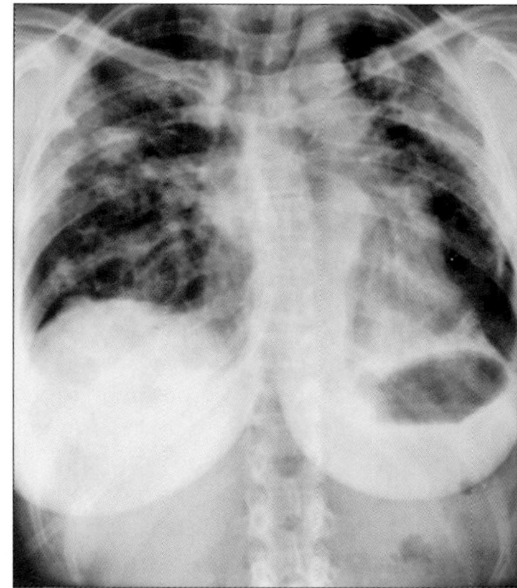

Figure 73.9 Cyclophosphamide toxicity. This patient received high-dose cyclophosphamide for lymphoma and a progressive restrictive disease associated with volume loss on chest radiography and patchy areas of fibrosis developed over several years. She ultimately required a lung transplant. Pathology of the native lung was consistent with a cytotoxically induced injury.

ticosteroid treatment. Some limited evidence exists that use of inhaled steroids during high-dose BCNU treatment may decrease the frequency of pulmonary toxicity.

METHOTREXATE

The antimetabolite methotrexate is used in treatment of leukemia, lymphoma, osteogenic sarcoma, breast cancer, and a variety of inflammatory diseases. Methotrexate has caused a variety of pulmonary complications. The most common is hypersensitivity pneumonitis, but pulmonary fibrosis, noncardiogenic pulmonary edema, and pleuritis have also been described. The frequency of toxicity depends in part on how the drug is used in multidrug regimens, with some combinations reported to have rates of toxicity of up to 40%. Other risk factors are adrenalectomy, corticosteroid tapering, and more frequent administration of methotrexate.

Typically, methotrexate toxicity manifests as a subacute illness over several weeks, with malaise, myalgias, fever, chills, dyspnea, and cough. A skin rash has been noted in some cases. The chest radiograph shows diffuse, bilateral, reticular, reticulonodular, nodular, or patchy alveolar filling infiltrates (Fig. 73.7). Eosinophilia is present in up to 40% of cases. Occasionally, interstitial fibrosis or noncardiogenic edema develops.

Pathologically, lung biopsies show prominent mononuclear cell infiltration with lymphocytes as the predominating cells. A loosely formed granulomatous reaction may also be seen (Fig. 73.8). Overall prognosis is good, and often the response to corticosteroid therapy is dramatic. Occasionally the syndrome resolves spontaneously, but some patients develop pulmonary fibrosis, although mortality is rare.

The presence of systemic symptoms and eosinophilia and the response to corticosteroids suggest that the disorder is immunologically mediated; this theory is also supported by lavage findings that show a lymphocytic predominance with helper cells in some cases and suppressor cells in others. Occasionally, however, a lack of recurrence on rechallenge is reported.

CYCLOPHOSPHAMIDE

The alkylating agent cyclophosphamide is widely used to treat a variety of malignancies. Toxicity is rare, and the usual pattern of pulmonary toxicity is interstitial pneumonitis or fibrosis. The presentation of toxicity is usually insidious and may develop slowly after years of use. A more acute-to-subacute form of toxicity can occur after high-dose therapy. Risk factors have not been identified, partly because cyclophosphamide is almost always used in multidrug regimens with other known pulmonary toxins. Patients have progressive dyspnea. Chest radiographs show patchy areas of fibrosis (Fig. 73.9).

Pathologically, findings are similar to those seen with other cytotoxic drugs. The prognosis is generally poor, although some

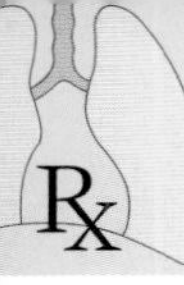

improvement of symptoms can be found with corticosteroids; the fibrosis tends to be progressive.

TAXANES

The taxanes are important new antineoplastic drugs widely used for carcinomas of the lung, breast, ovary, and head and neck and melanoma. They include paclitaxel (Taxol) and docetaxel (Taxotere). A hypersensitivity reaction with dyspnea, bronchospasm, urticaria, erythematous rash, and hypotension occurred initially in up to a third of the patients. Premedication with corticosteroids, antihistamines, and H2-blocker has reduced the incidence to approximately 1%, and the reactions are milder. Transient infiltrates occurring while the patient is on therapy and a syndrome of acute pneumonia have also been noted. Response to corticosteroids has been reported, and the prognosis has been generally good. However, more serious toxicity has occurred when the drugs are combined with radiation therapy. Radiation-recall phenomenon has also been described.

GEMCITABINE

Gemcitabine is a purine-analog antimetabolite with activity in non–small-cell lung cancer, pancreatic cancer, and cancers of the bladder, ovary, and breast. It is increasingly being given because of its broad activity and very favorable toxicity profile, which allows its use in elderly or impaired patients. Myelosuppression is the major dose-limiting toxicity. Pulmonary toxicity ranges from less than 1% to 13% of patients in various studies. Patients typically have dyspnea of insidious development. Radiographs show interstitial infiltrates, which may be reticulonodular, or a diffuse ground-glass appearance consistent with noncardiac pulmonary edema. At times the findings are subtle on radiography and can be seen only on chest CT. Peripheral edema is present in some patients and is believed to be the result of increased vascular permeability. This may be the mechanism that leads to the pulmonary toxicity. Most cases respond to treatment with corticosteroids and discontinuation of the drug. Some cases of pulmonary toxicity have been severe and sudden, with acute respiratory distress syndrome, and fatalities have been reported.

GEFITINIB

Gefitinib (Iressa) is a selective inhibitor of the epidermal growth factor–receptor tyrosine kinase. It has activity in patients with non–small-cell lung cancer, particularly adenocarcinomas. The drug, which is given orally, is well tolerated. The major side effects are diarrhea and skin rash, usually mild. Gefitinib has been in use in Japan, where cases of interstitial pneumonitis have been reported in 1% to 2% of patients. In some patients, concomitant radiotherapy had been given, so the exact frequency of this toxicity is uncertain. Cases manifested as either acute lung injury with patchy diffuse infiltrates or as interstitial pneumonitis. Improvement has occurred in some patients with corticosteroid treatment, but deaths have been attributed to pulmonary toxicity.

DIAGNOSIS

The diagnosis of drug toxicity is often difficult to confirm and must be made clinically. Rechallenge with recurrence is the gold standard but is not practical in most cases, because serious toxicity might be produced. Additionally, with cytotoxic and anti-inflammatory agents, multidrug regimens are often used and it can be difficult to ascribe the reaction to any specific drug. The underlying disease, particularly some autoimmune diseases, may themselves cause pulmonary effects, which makes the diagnosis of a drug effect more difficult. Compounding factors, such as intercurrent infection or progression of tumor, may also affect the lung, which may complicate the diagnosis of drug toxicity. Indeed, the effect of some drugs on the immune system may be directly associated with the development of pulmonary infections. This is the case with tumor necrosis factor-α antagonists, which may induce reactivation of tuberculosis and histoplasmosis.

Unfortunately, radiographic findings are usually nonspecific for drug toxicity, and pathology can be supportive but not pathognomonic of drug-induced injury. Whether to obtain tissue and, if so, whether a transbronchial biopsy will suffice or an open biopsy is needed depend on the individual situation. In cases in which the differential diagnosis is broad, invasive procedures help eliminate other entities and indicate pulmonary toxicity. In cases in which an invasive procedure may carry a high risk (e.g., in cardiac patients) and in which other means are available for diagnosis and treatment of other suspected problems (e.g., bacterial infection or congestive heart failure), a conservative approach is often taken.

The mainstay of diagnosis of drug-induced injury remains a strong clinical suspicion of drug toxicity and knowledge of the types of reactions seen.

PREVENTION

Although risk factors have been described for some drugs, in most cases it is not possible to prevent drug-induced toxicity. Use of antioxidants and antifibrotic agents is being studied in animal models and may have some relevance for prophylactic use with some cytotoxic agents, such as bleomycin and mitomycin. The low incidence of toxicity and the potential side effects of these agents may hinder their use.

Lung function tests have been used to detect the earliest stages of toxicity of some drugs, and diffusing capacity is the most sensitive indicator of drug-induced injury. Such tests have not been found useful with methotrexate, which is understandable given the proposed immunologic mechanism and lack of dose relationship. The tests have also not been shown to be predictive in mitomycin toxicity and, although widely used, have not been proved to help prevent bleomycin pulmonary toxicity.

Use of supplemental oxygen increases the risk of toxicity with bleomycin. Toxicity caused by mitomycin, carmustine, and amiodarone has been proposed to be exacerbated by use of supplemental oxygen. In anyone suspected of toxic reactions to these drugs, prudence dictates that any supplemental oxygen be avoided unless absolutely necessary. If a patient needs surgery, in which high concentrations of oxygen are routinely used during induction of anesthesia, these potential complications must be kept in mind.

PITFALLS AND CONTROVERSIES

Whether screening pulmonary function tests should continue to be carried out in cases of drug-induced toxicity is unclear. These tests are now performed almost exclusively for injury related to

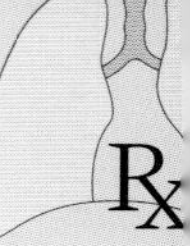

use of cytotoxic drugs, usually bleomycin and occasionally mitomycin and carmustine. They are carried out regularly during therapy; a significant decrease in gas transfer or vital capacity is taken as an indication of subclinical toxicity, and the drug is stopped. Studies have not been undertaken to show the efficacy of this practice, but many oncologists believe that stopping the drug in some patients has prevented toxicity. The use of diffusing capacity as a marker is also complicated, because these cytotoxic drugs are known to affect epithelial or vascular cells that line the alveolar vascular interface and can cause a decrease in the diffusing capacity without indicating the onset of interstitial inflammation or fibrosis. More sophisticated tests separate the vascular and membrane components of the diffusing capacity, but routine use of these is not practical. Better screening tests for toxicity are needed, and if serum or bronchoalveolar biologic markers of fibrosis can be found and validated, they may prove a better method than lung function tests.

One of the most difficult decisions for a clinician in some cases is whether a given drug can be continued or restarted when the diagnosis of drug-induced toxicity is suspected but not clear. In some cases no effective substitute agent is available. Each case must be considered individually, but as a general principle, with drugs that have a high propensity for fibrosis, such as bleomycin and mitomycin, or in cases in which the initial reaction itself was severe and life threatening, the drugs should not be given again, even if toxicity is not proved. In cases of less severe toxicity or in which irreversible fibrosis is unlikely, reinstitution can be considered, if essential. In some cases, as documented with methotrexate and amiodarone, a lower dose or corticosteroid cover may ameliorate or eliminate the reaction.

The greatest pitfall with drug-induced injury is the failure to consider the diagnosis. Except for some cytotoxic agents that have a well-recognized potential for fibrosis, drug-induced lung disease is uncommon, and often less common than many other possible pulmonary complications. A clinician may be personally familiar with only a limited number of reactions and cannot be expected to have detailed knowledge of reactions to all drugs. Once the diagnosis is considered, computerized medical searches, particularly of World Wide Web sites developed to catalogue cases of drug toxicity, can be informative.

SUGGESTED READINGS

Aldrich TK, Prezant DJ: Adverse effects of drugs on the respiratory muscles. Clin Chest Med 11:177-189, 1990.

Camus P, Rosenow E: Iatrogenic respiratory disease. Clin Chest Med (in press).

Cooper JAD, White DA, Matthay RA: Drug induced pulmonary disease. Part 1: Cytotoxic drugs. Am Rev Respir Dis 133:321-340, 1986.

Cooper JAD, White DA, Matthay RA: Drug induced pulmonary disease. Part 2: Noncytotoxic drugs. Am Rev Respir Dis 133:488-505, 1986.

Libby D, White DA: Pulmonary toxicity of drugs used to treat systemic autoimmune disease. Clin Chest Med 19:809-821, 1998.

Ravid D, Leshner M, Lang R, et al: Angiotensin-converting enzyme inhibitors and cough: A prospective evaluation in hypertension and in congestive heart failure. J Clin Pharmacol 34:1116-1120, 1994.

Rosenow EC II, Myers JL, Swensen SJ, Pisoni RJ: Drug induced pulmonary disease: An update. Chest 102:239-250, 1992.

Sunderji R, Kanji Z, Gin K: Pulmonary effects of low dose amiodarone: A review of the risk and recommendations for surveillance. Can J Cardiol 16:1435-1440, 2000.

Drug- Induced Pulmonary Toxicity web site: www.pneumotox.com

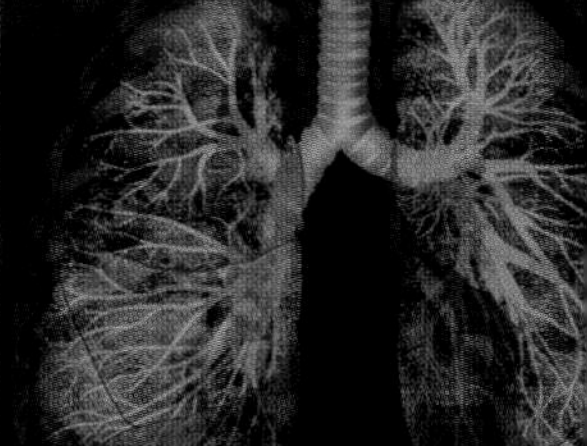

CHAPTER 74 Lung Transplantation

Trevor J. Williams and Gregory I. Snell

HISTORY

In 1946, after returning from the Second World War, surgeon/physiologist Vladimir Demikhov began a program of thoracic organ transplantation in animals and demonstrated that heart, heart-lung, and isolated lung transplantation were technically feasible in a canine model (Table 74.1). Hardy, in 1963, attempted the first human lung transplantation (a single-lung transplant) and found that the transplanted lung was capable of contributing to gas exchange. Unfortunately, this recipient died early of renal failure. In the nearly two decades that followed, none of the more than 40 attempts at lung transplantation was successful.

After a long period of animal experimentation, and with the development of a potent suppressor of T-cell expansion (cyclosporin A), the Stanford University group led by Reitz achieved the first long-term survival in any form of lung replacement, a recipient of heart-lung transplantation (HLTx). Two years later, in 1983, the Toronto Lung Transplantation Group led by Cooper achieved long-term survival in a single lung transplant (SLTx) recipient with idiopathic pulmonary fibrosis (IPF). The Toronto group subsequently performed successful en bloc double-lung (without the heart) transplantation in 1985. This procedure was associated with excessive mortality owing to tracheal anastomotic dehiscence. In 1989, the procedure was modified to the now widely performed bilateral sequential (single) lung transplantation (BLTx) procedure simultaneously in Toronto and San Antonio. More recently, attempts to re-anastomose the bronchial circulation, allowing return to a single tracheal anastomosis, have been reported by a few groups.

Starnes and colleagues at the University of Southern California reported live donor lobe transplantation (LDLTx) in 1991. Initially this was done with two close relatives (typically parents) donating a lower lobe each, although unrelated donors increasingly are being used.

Until 1990, only small numbers of lung transplantations were performed and HLTx was extensively used. Since 1990, there has been a rapid rise in the number of lung transplantations reported worldwide (Fig. 74.1). SLTx and BLTx procedures are performed in almost equal portions, with over 1500 single or bilateral transplantations being performed annually. HLTx is now performed infrequently, usually only for patients with combined end-stage pulmonary and cardiac disease. Very infrequently, retransplantation has been performed. Reports of combined procedures, such as lung-liver and lung-kidney, are still very rare.

The last 10 years have seen the publication of an extensive literature describing the survival, outcome, and complications after lung transplantation, with reliable data now being available up to 10 years post-transplantation. Randomized, controlled trials of lung transplantation for any indication versus best therapy have not been conducted, and even randomized, controlled trials of therapeutic intervention during the transplantation operation, or in postoperative management, are still exceedingly rare.

PROCEDURES

The choice of transplantation procedure (Fig. 74.2) needs to take into account the advantages and disadvantages of the procedure in that individual, surgeon preference and expertise, as well as more global factors such as the extreme shortage of suitable donor organs for lung transplantation and the logistics of organ allocation. Although intuitively BLTx results in more pulmonary reserve, a clear survival advantage is seen in BLTx over SLTx only for chronic obstructive pulmonary disease (COPD) in recipients younger than 60 years of age. Thus, the only almost universally accepted view is that septic lung disease requires BLTx or HLTx, and patients with severe pulmonary or pulmonary vascular disease with combined irreversible cardiac disease require HLTx. The current trend is for BLTx (Fig. 74.3A) to be largely used in bronchiectasis (particularly cystic fibrosis) and COPD. Most programs now would perform BLTx for severe pulmonary hypertension, although this is by no means universal. Rare indications for BLTx include interstitial lung diseases (especially the usual interstitial pneumonia form of IPF), sarcoidosis, lymphangioleiomyomatosis, bronchiolitis obliterans (idiopathic or rheumatoid arthritis associated), lung retransplantation, and other rare indications.

SLTx is most widely applied to COPD (see Fig. 74.3B), although initially it was thought this would lead to hemodynamically significant dynamic hyperinflation of the native lung (Fig. 74.4) in most cases. This has not been borne out, and COPD is the most common indication for SLTx. Idiopathic pulmonary fibrosis is the next most common indication for SLTx. Live donor lobe transplantation can be used for most indications, but in practice this procedure is most commonly used for cystic fibrosis.

Lung transplantation has been used widely in many rare diseases, some of which have been shown to recur in the transplanted lung (Table 74.2). Often, however, the recurrence is of minor functional significance (e.g., sarcoidosis), perhaps because of the transplant-related immunosuppression modifying the primary disease process. Bronchoalveolar cell carcinoma was previously considered to be the only pulmonary malignancy that was amenable to treatment by BLTx, but recently a high rate of recurrence and mortality has been reported.

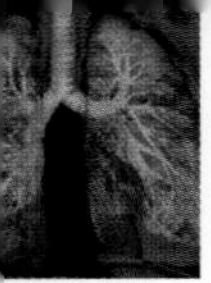

OUTCOME

Survival

In the 1980s, survival often was measured as survival to hospital discharge. From 1990 to 2000, the international registry now run in collaboration between the International Society for Heart and Lung Transplantation (ISHLT) and the United Network for Organ Sharing (UNOS) in the United States (the ISHLT/UNOS Registry) reported a median survival for SLTx of 3.7 years and for BLTx, 4.9 years (Fig. 74.5A). Since 2000, however, survival continues to improve (see Fig. 74.5B). The improved survival is entirely due to improved early (<90-day) survival, without any apparent improvement in the 6% to 8% per year mortality rate in those surviving the first 90 days. Important factors affecting survival are pretransplantation diagnosis (patients with IPF and pulmonary hypertension do worse than those with COPD and cystic fibrosis; see Fig. 74.5C), ventilator dependency, extremes of age (patients <18 or >65 years of age do worse), as well as program activity (programs doing fewer than 10 lung transplantations per year have worse results). More experienced centers seem to achieve better results despite having a more complex patient mix. It is difficult to provide a "benchmark" because of the different case mix of individual centers, but an experienced center would expect an otherwise uncomplicated BLTx recipient to have an 85% 1-year and a 60% to 70% 5-year survival rate.

Table 74.1
Milestones in lung transplantation

1947	Demikhov—canine heart-lung and single lung transplantation
1963	Hardy—first attempt human single lung transplantation
1981	Reitz—first long-term survivor heart-lung transplantation (Stanford)
1983	Cooper—first long-term survivor single-lung transplantation (Toronto)
1983	Cooper—first long-term survivor bilateral lung transplantation (en bloc) (Toronto)
1987	Calhoon and Patterson—first bilateral sequential lung transplantation (San Antonio and Toronto)
1991	Starnes—first live donor lobar transplantation
2001	Steen—successful use of nonbeating heart-lung donor for lung transplantation (Sweden)

Cause of Death

The ISHLT/UNOS Registry now reports the cause of death in four time periods post-lung transplantation (Fig. 74.6). In patients dying within 30 days post-transplantation, graft failure, infection, and cardiac death are the most common causes. Acute rejection is infrequent. These data should be interpreted with great caution, however, because early deaths are often multifactorial and a "convenient" attribution of cause of death may belie an extremely complex sequence of events.

In long-term survivors, two lung allograft complications (see Fig. 74.6) are dominant: infection and chronic rejection in the guise of the bronchiolitis obliterans syndrome (BOS). The two often coexist and are likely to be interrelated in terms of etiology. In patients surviving more than 5 years, the incidence of death due to BOS does not seem to diminish, and deaths due to malignancy or renal failure increase in prevalence.

Physiologic and Functional Outcomes

After successful lung transplantation of any type (but particularly BLTx, HLTx, and LDLTx; Table 74.3), done for any

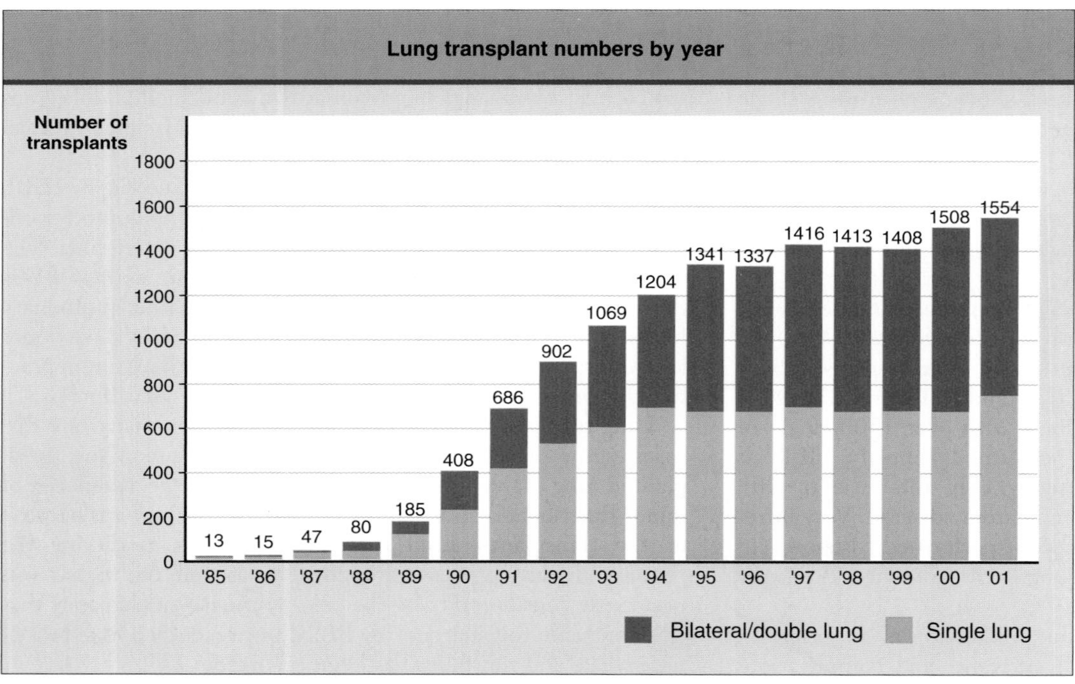

Figure 74.1 Lung transplantation numbers worldwide reported to the International Society for Heart and Lung Transplantation and the United Network for Organ Sharing Registry. Note that lung transplantation numbers have reached a plateau at approximately 1500 to 1600 per year worldwide, with almost equal numbers of bilateral and single-lung transplantations. Not included in this figure is the small number of heart-lung transplantations performed.

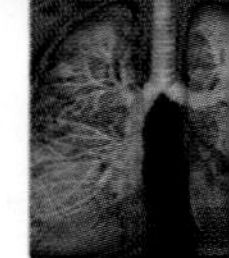

Types of lung transplant				
	Heart-lung	**Bilateral sequential**	**Single lung**	**Live donor lobar**
Incision	Midline sternotomy	Horizontal "clam shell"	Lateral thoracotomy	Horizontal "clam shell"
Anastomoses	Tracheal Right atrial Aortic	Left and right bronchial "Double" left atrial Right and left pulmonary artery	Bronchial Left atrial Pulmonary artery	Lobar bronchus to bronchus Lobar vein to superior pulmonary vein Lobar artery to main pulmonary artery
Advantages	Airway vascularity All indications	Access to pleural space No cardiac allograft Less cardiopulmonary bypass	Easiest procedure Increases recipients	Increases donors Can be done "electively"
Disadvantages	Cardiac allograft Organ 'consumption'	Airway complications Postoperative pain	Airway complications Poor reserve	Complex undertaking Donor morbidity
Common indications	Congenital heart disease with pulmonary hypertension Heart and lung disease Primary pulmonary hypertension	Cystic fibrosis (CF) Bullous emphysema Primary pulmonary hypertension Bronchiectasis	Emphysema Pulmonary fibrosis Primary pulmonary hypertension	Cystic fibrosis (CF) Pulmonary fibrosis Primary pulmonary hypertension

Figure 74.2 Comparison of the four standard lung replacement techniques, including their common indications.

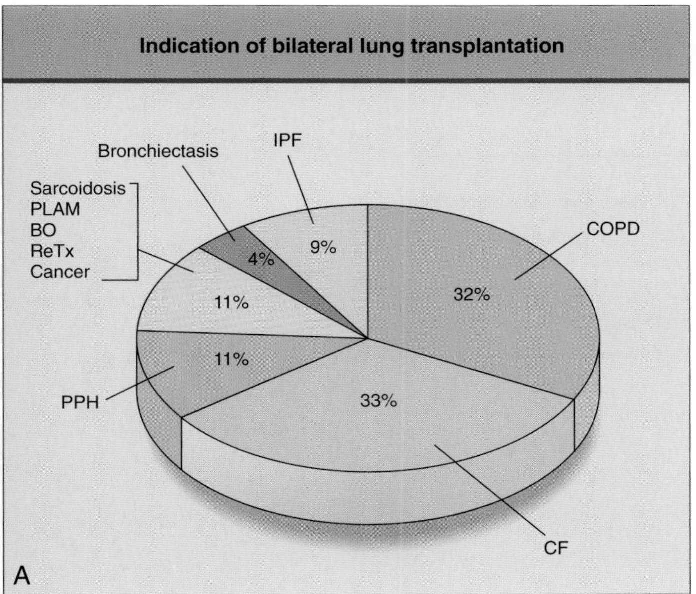

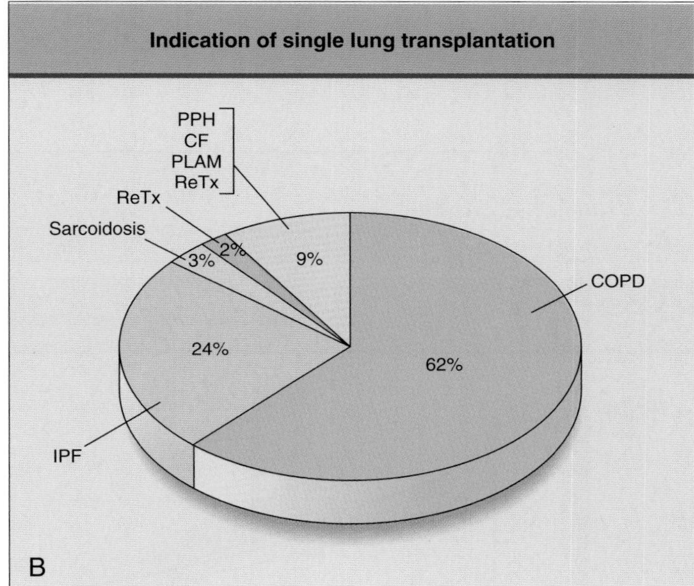

Figure 74.3 Indications for lung transplantation. **A,** The common indications for bilateral lung transplantation. **B,** The common indications for single-lung transplantation. BO, bronchiolitis obliterans; CF, cystic fibrosis; COPD, chronic obstructive pulmonary disease; IPF, idiopathic pulmonary fibrosis; PLAM, pulmonary lymphangioleiomyomatosis; PPH, primary pulmonary hypertension; ReTx, retransplantation. (Data adapted from the International Society for Heart and Lung Transplantation and the United Network for Organ Sharing [ISHLT/UNOS] Registry report, 2002, available at www.ishlt.org.)

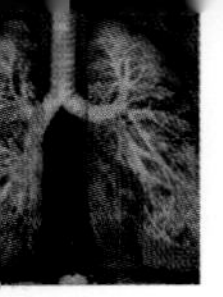

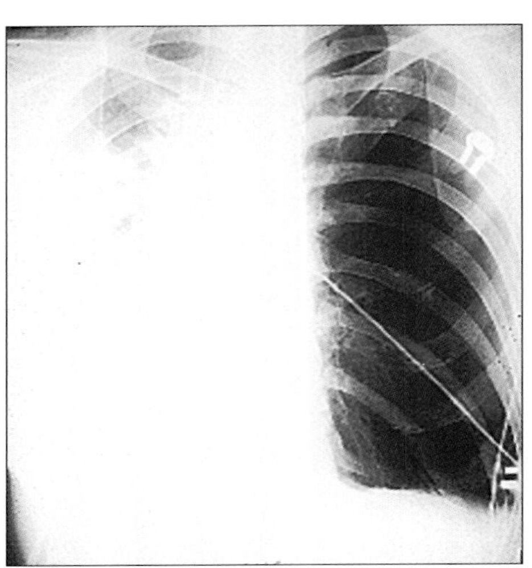

Figure 74.4 Chest radiograph showing right single-lung transplant for emphysema. Severe hyperinflation with mediastinal shift due to overinflation of the native lung and compression of the transplanted right lung is shown.

Table 74.2 Diseases that can recur in pulmonary allograft	
Yes	• Sarcoidosis • Pulmonary lymphangioleiomyomatosis • Bronchoalveolar cell carcinoma • Histiocytosis X (of Langerhans)
Maybe	• Idiopathic pulmonary hemosiderosis • α-antitrypsin deficiency

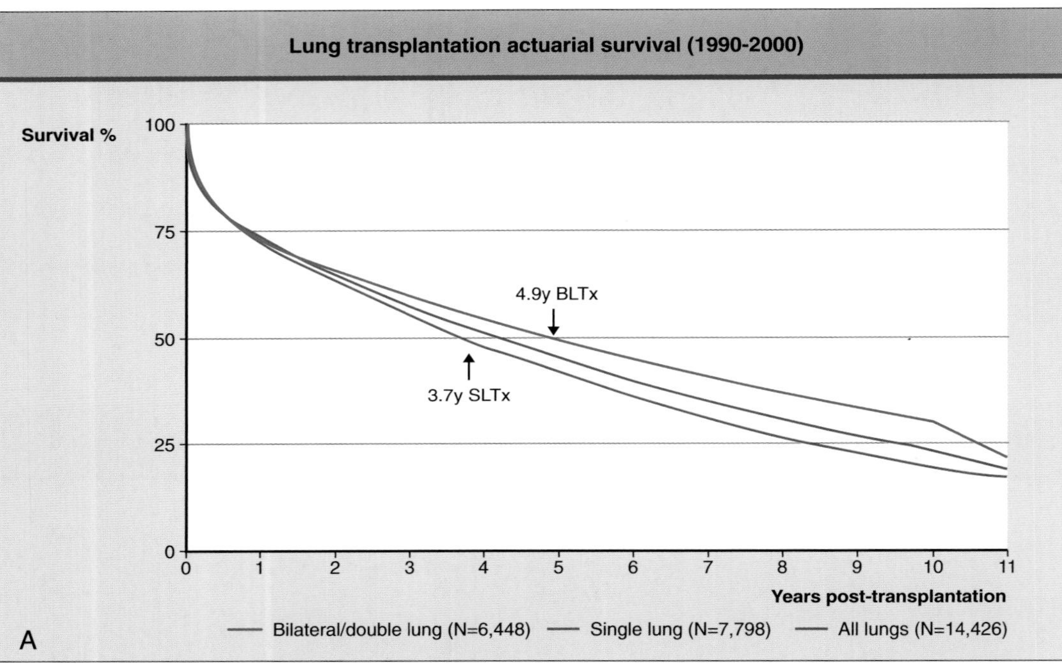

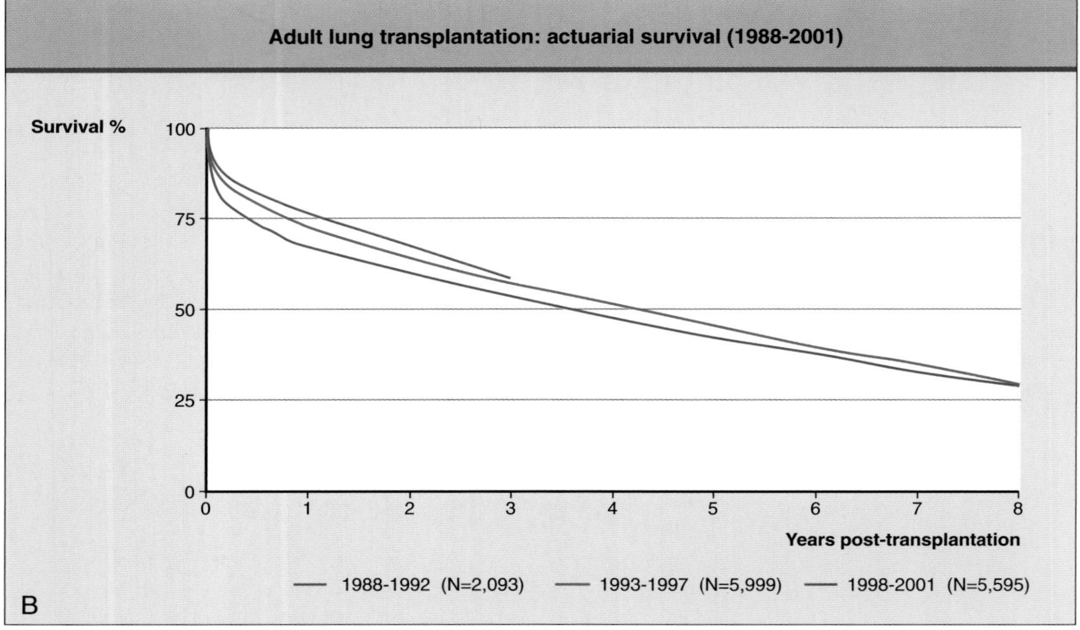

Figure 74.5 Actuarial survival curves for lung transplantation. **A,** Actuarial survival curves from 1990 to 2000, highlighting the superior survival of bilateral lung transplantation. Median survivals for single-lung transplantation and bilateral lung transplantation are shown. **B,** Actuarial survival for adult lung transplantation, 1988 to 2001, by cohorts. The improved survival in the latest cohort compared with the earliest cohort is evident.

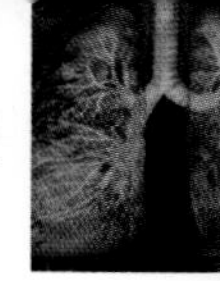

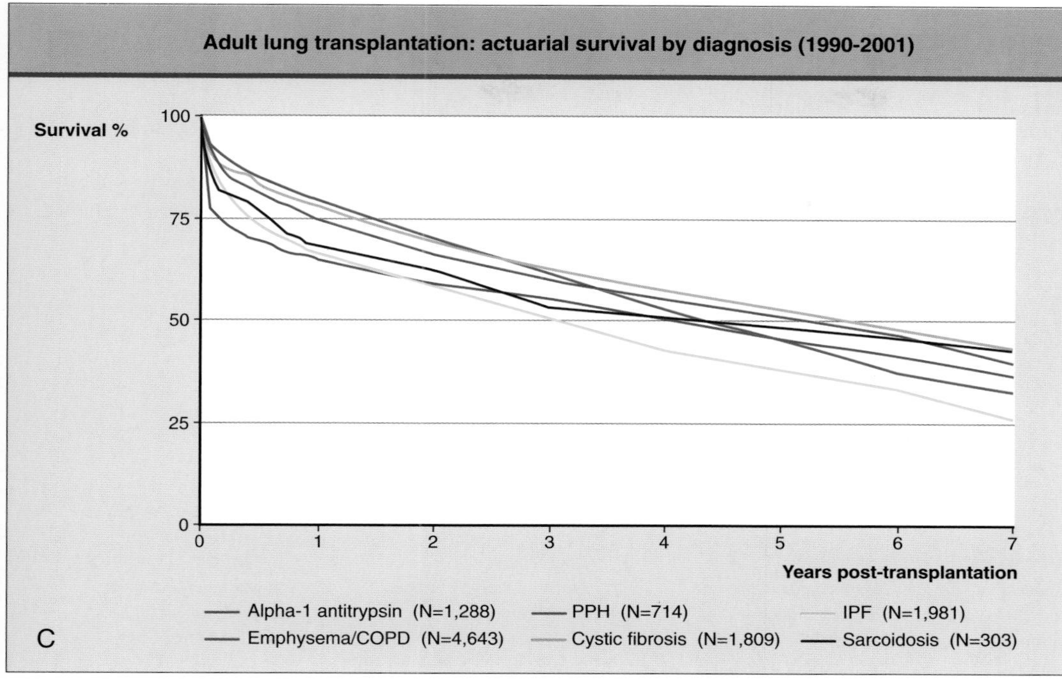

Figure 74.5 (*continued*). **C,** Adult lung transplantation actuarial survival curves from 1990 to 2001 showing distinct differences in survival depending on pretransplantation diagnosis. COPD, chronic obstructive lung disease; IPF, idiopathic pulmonary fibrosis; PPH, primary pulmonary hypertension. (All figures adapted from the International Society for Heart and Lung Transplantation and the United Network for Organ Sharing [ISHLT/UNOS] Registry report, 2002, available at www.ishlt.org.)

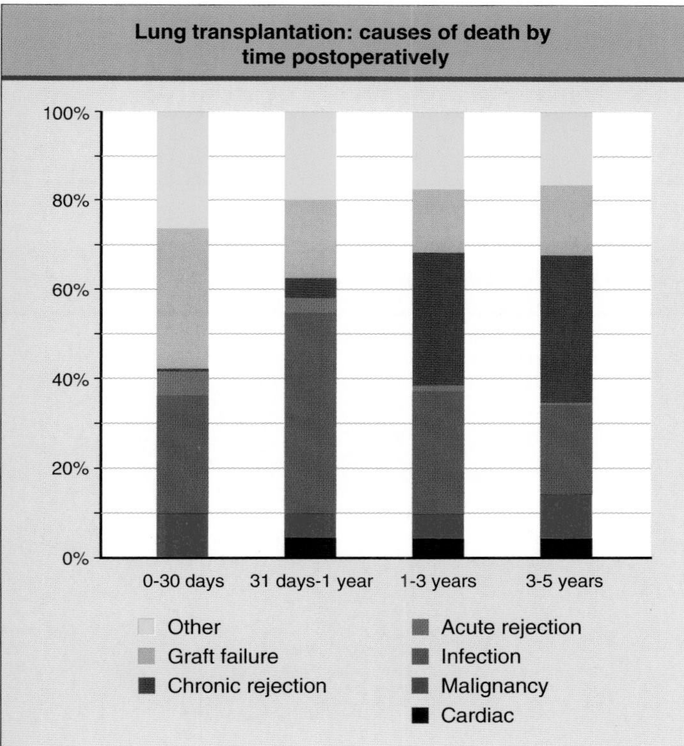

Figure 74.6 Cause of death in time periods after transplantation. Most strikingly, chronic rejection becomes the most common cause of death from 1 year post-transplantation. (Data from the International Society for Heart and Lung Transplantation and the United Network for Organ Sharing [ISHLT/UNOS] Registry report, 2002, available at www.ishlt.org.)

indication, leg tiredness is most commonly reported as the predominant symptom at exercise termination. Cardiac or ventilatory limitation is uncommon.

Lung function (spirometry and diffusing capacity) approaches normal in BLTx and HLTx. Live donor lobe transplant recipients have a persistent, mild, restrictive ventilatory defect with reduced diffusing capacity. SLTx recipients usually have abnormal spirometry results, reflecting the pathologic process in the residual (native) lung (e.g., patients with SLTx for COPD have a persistent mild to moderate obstructive ventilatory defect, and patients with IPF a persistent mild to moderate restriction). On exercise, SLTx recipients with an apparently normally functioning lung allograft may desaturate modestly and even reach ventilatory limitation.

Almost universally, patients with any type of transplant appear limited by peripheral factors on formal cardiopulmonary exercise testing. An early lactic acid threshold and the predominance of symptomatic leg tiredness at exercise termination point to a defect in exercising skeletal muscle oxidative capacity. The muscle injury is most likely due to a combination of severe pretransplantation deconditioning and the toxic effects of post-transplantation medications. When fully recovered, peak oxygen consumption is typically only 45% to 60% predicted regardless of transplant type or indication. Despite this, almost 90% of recipients at 1 year report they are not limited by their health status and have substantially improved quality of life.

RECIPIENT SELECTION

The international transplantation societies have recently attempted to develop uniform recipient selection criteria. This has led to quite wide-ranging discussions and, in part, has focused attention on what specific selection criteria they were actually aiming to achieve. Because the donor lung is such a rare

Table 74.3
Physiologic outcomes by lung transplant type

	Single-lung transplantation	Bilateral lung transplantation	Heart-lung transplantation	Live donar lobar transplantation
Spirometry	Ventilatory defect:	Ventilatory defect:	Ventilatory defect:	Ventilatory defect:
Tx for RLD	Mild to moderate restriction	Mild restriction	Mild restriction	Mild restriction
Tx for OLD	Moderate obstruction	Mild restriction	Mild restriction	Mild restriction
Tx for PVD	Mild restriction	Mild restriction	Mild restriction	Mild restriction
Lung diffusing capacity	Moderately reduced	Mildly reduced	Mildly reduced	Mildly reduced
Alveolar-arterial gradient	Mildly increased	Normal	Normal	Normal
Ventilation ($\dot{V}$)/ perfusion ($\dot{Q}$) scan	In allograft:			
Tx for RLD	$\dot{V}=\dot{Q}$			
Tx for OLD	$\dot{V}>\dot{Q}$			
Tx for PVD	$\dot{V}<\dot{Q}$			
Exercise test features	Low peak work (Wpeak) At ventilatory limitation Mild desaturation Normal heart rate (HR) response Early lactate threshold Peripheral limitation "Deconditioning"	Low Wpeak No ventilatory limitation No desaturation Normal HR response Early lactate threshold Peripheral limitation "Deconditioning"	Low Wpeak No ventilatory limitation No desaturation High resting HR with blunted rise and slow HR recovery rate Early lactate threshold Peripheral limitation "Deconditioning"	Low Wpeak No ventilatory limitation No desaturation Normal HR response Early lactate threshold Peripheral limitation "Deconditioning"
Peak O_2 consumption	45-60% predicted	50-60% predicted	50-60% predicted	50-60% predicted

Tx for RLD = lung transplantation for restrictive lung disease
Tx for OLD = lung transplantation for obstructive lung disease
Tx for PVD = lung transplantation for pulmonary vascular disease

Table 74.4
Indications for lung transplantation

End-stage pulmonary or pulmonary vascular disease with:	
Poor prognosis	Poor quality of life
<50% 2-year survival	New York Heart Association class III/IV At home struggling with all activities of daily living

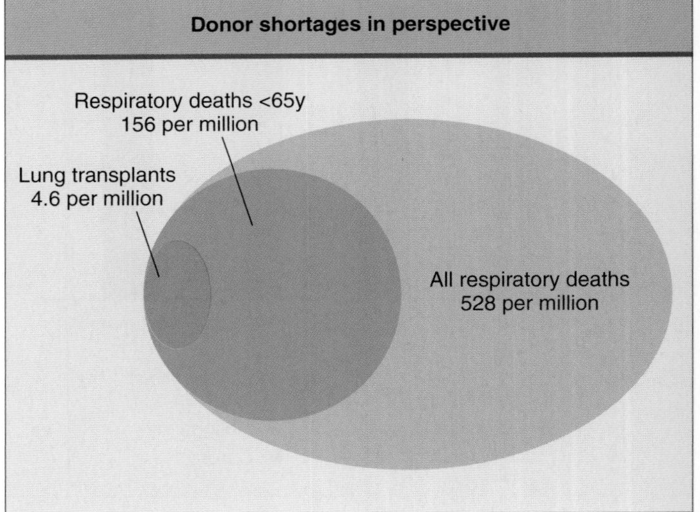

Figure 74.7 Donor shortages in perspective. Lung transplantation is performed in a small fraction of those who may benefit from the procedure. (Death rates from the Australian Bureau of Statistics. Australian Social Trends 2002. Health-Health related Actions: Organ Donation 2002.)

"commodity" (Fig. 74.7), the criteria adopted by any particular organ allocation system need to do more than just identify all who might benefit. The criteria should also identify those with a reasonable chance of prolonged survival with improved quality of life, while reflecting regional and national views on the allocation of scarce resources and complying with the relevant laws.

Generally Accepted Criteria

With programs now achieving a 5-year survival rate of 60% to 70%, patients with chronic lung disease and a predicted survival less than this might be deemed suitable for lung transplantation. Typically patients are assessed and actively listed when their expected survival is 2 years or less (Table 74.4). Waiting times are often long (frequently exceeding 12 to 18 months), however, such that patients with very poor prognoses (<6 months) have a high likelihood of dying while they are on the waiting list. Accordingly, the precise timing of assessment and listing need to take into account patient factors, waiting list factors, and the nature of the organ allocation system being used (e.g., time priority only or clinical priority).

Quality of life is also an important factor in determining when to list. For example, many patients with COPD have a very poor quality of life and, despite no demonstrable survival advantage, are prepared to take the substantial risks associated with transplantation. Assessment at times of recent acute, severe deterioration, or without proper rehabilitation, may cloud the patient's view as to his or her present achievable quality of life. Therapy (including medications, oxygen, psychological assessment and treatment, and rehabilitation) should be maximized before a final decision is made to proceed with lung transplantation on the basis of poor quality of life.

Contraindications

The current contraindications to transplantation (Table 74.5) are the result of expert opinion rather than evidence-based data. They attempt to identify patients who have comorbid factors that predict a poor outcome, may complicate transplantation, or may be exacerbated by the transplantation procedure or the use of immunosuppressive drugs. Lung transplantation programs often have to make two distinct judgments:

1. Is a decision to list for transplantation in the best interest of the specific patient being evaluated?
2. Is transplantation sufficiently likely to have a good outcome to justify the use of a scarce donor organ?

Some contraindications are relative (see Table 74.5), but in combination may lead to an unacceptably high risk. Such decisions require detailed assessment and diligent review and discussion by a multidisciplinary transplantation assessment team (e.g., nutritionists, social workers, psychologists, and physical therapists in addition to physicians).

Table 74.5
Lung transplantation: contraindications

Absolute	Relative
Current cigarette or drug abuse	Unstable clinical status
Malignancy within 5 years (except SCC or BCC)	Severe osteoporosis
Renal impairment creatine clearance < 50mL/min (<0.8mL/sec)	Poor compliance with medication regimens
Cirrhosis or active hepatitis	Inadequate social and financial support
Panresistant organisms	
Hep BsAg, HIV or Hep C PCR positive	
Multisystem diseases	

SCC = squamous cell carcinoma of skin
BCC = basal cell carcinoma of skin
Hep BsAg = Hepatitis B surface antigen
HIV = human immunodeficiency virus antibody
Hep C = Hepatitis C
PCR = polymerase chain reaction

Assessment Process

There is considerable variation in how individual programs approach the assessment process. One proposed generic scheme is shown in Figure 74.8. A number of principles should guide this process, however. First, transplantation should be the last option—all other treatment needs to be properly and exhaustively explored. Second, sufficient investigation is needed by an appropriately skilled multidisciplinary team. A detailed explanation of the decision must then be conveyed empathically to the patient and family in a timely fashion. Third, ample opportunities should be available for the patient and family to obtain information (written and verbal), ask questions, and discuss the procedure so they can make a well-informed decision.

In general, the assessment scheme tries to identify patients with absolute contraindications at the beginning. Early discussion with the transplantation team can often prevent unrealistic expectations in those who will not be offered lung transplantation. In those who have no absolute contraindications, and who make an informed choice, detailed evaluation should then begin. Based on the detailed findings, the assessment team determines transplant type, technical issues, specific risks, and outstanding issues to resolve before listing.

WAITING LIST MANAGEMENT

The potential availability of lung transplantation may confuse the therapeutic objectives in patients with end-stage lung disease. Often patients previously treated with purely palliative

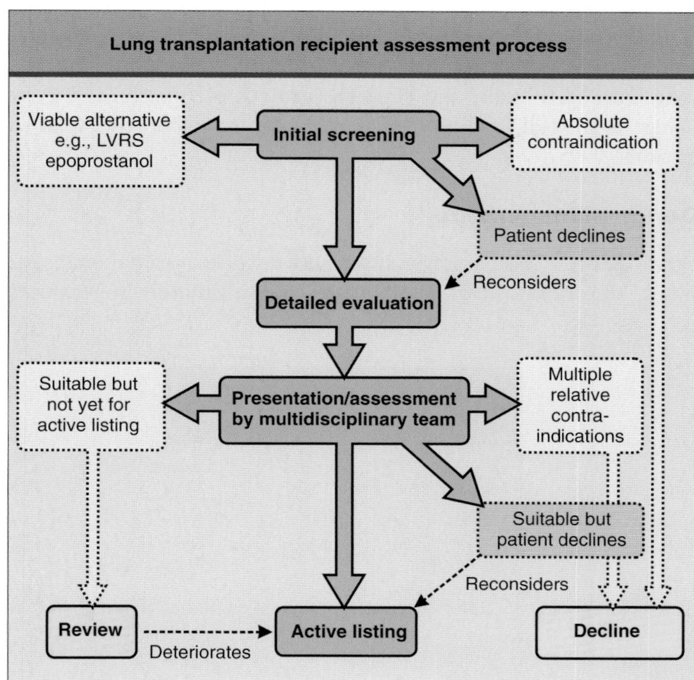

Figure 74.8 An illustrative schema for the lung transplant recipient assessment process. The approach is generally designed to screen out patients who have an absolute contraindication to transplantation or those for whom there may be other viable therapies. Detailed evaluation and assessment by an appropriately qualified multidisciplinary team are essential parts of the process. LVRS, lung volume reduction surgery.

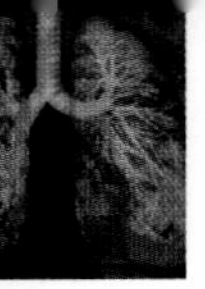

intent are managed actively to try to "bridge" them to transplantation. The new objective on the transplant waiting list is to keep a patient alive in the best possible physical and psychological state until the time of transplantation. Regular review, structured pulmonary rehabilitation, appropriate oxygen therapy, and perhaps the use of noninvasive ventilatory support may be required. Availability of a support group and counseling for patients and caregivers is often crucial. This often falls to the transplantation center. Regular review of waiting list patients is usually practiced, particularly where clinical factors are used in prioritization of organ allocation.

DONOR

Criteria

Conventionally, donors for lung transplantation are brain dead as a result of a catastrophic neurologic event but have a beating heart. They should have no history of respiratory disease, have normal gas exchange and a negative chest radiograph, and be clear of clinically important airway infection. They should also comply with the more generic requirements of multiorgan donors (e.g., be human immunodeficiency virus negative, have no malignancy; Table 74.6).

The extreme shortage of donor lungs (see Fig. 74.7) has led to steady movement toward the use of "extended indication" or marginal donors. This does not appear to have resulted in any worsening of outcomes, although the evolutionary nature of the change makes it difficult to detect all but major effects. Programs or regions using extended indication donors may find an increase in their lung transplantation rates of up to 50%.

A recent Swedish report showed the feasibility of removing lungs as long as 3 hours after the heart had stopped beating. This is likely to be an increasing donor source over the next few years. In the coming decades, xenotransplantation, repopulation of the lung with stem cells, and even the growth of functional organs using stem cell technology may become viable therapeutic options.

Donor Management

Brain death is not a static state and despite optimal management, deterioration of vital organs and ultimately permanent cardiac arrest usually occur within 24 to 48 hours. This process is thought to be exacerbated by the neurohormonal changes associated with brain death. Hormonal manipulation is increasingly being used to stabilize the brain-dead donor. Recipient teams have differing views as to how they wish the multiorgan donor to be managed, particularly with regard to the use of inotropes or fluid resuscitation. The lung is prone to neurogenic pulmonary edema, so avoidance of large fluid volumes is desirable. Bronchoscopic removal of secretions, administration of antibiotics, and the use of positive end-expiratory pressure can often convert marginal donors into acceptable donors with good outcomes.

Donor-Recipient Matching

Matching of donor to recipient in lung transplantation is done primarily on the basis of blood group compatibility and size match (Table 74.7). Whenever possible, recipients who have not been exposed to cytomegalovirus (CMV) and Epstein-Barr virus (EBV) should receive organs from CMV- and EBV-negative donors, although this is often not practical. Lymphocyte crossmatching is desirable although not uniformly practiced.

POSTOPERATIVE CARE

Intensive Care

In the present era, it is most unusual for lung transplant recipients to die on the operating table. Almost all patients are sent to the intensive care unit (ICU) for early management. Key early problems (Fig. 74.9) include early severe graft dysfunction with a differential diagnosis that includes hyperacute rejection (which becomes manifest on reperfusion of the allograft), left atrial/pulmonary venous anastomosis obstruction, or reperfusion pulmonary edema (Fig. 74.10). Patients with these problems continue to deteriorate for 24 to 48 hours after surgery.

Patients may be well enough to extubate rapidly on stabilization in the ICU. Usually, however, a period of a few days of mechanical ventilation, followed by weaning, is required.

Although early allograft function may not be problematic, poor diaphragm function (even paralysis), pain, and a requirement for heavy sedation may prevent weaning, and the situation is often confounded by the development of allograft-related

Table 74.6
Donor selection criteria

	Conventional	Extended
Age	<60 yr	<65 yr (60-65 yr if donor ischemic time <7 hr)
Smoking	<20 pack-years	<30 pack-years
Other respiratory	No history	Asthma acceptable if well controlled
Chest radiograph	Normal	Minor changes OK
Airway secretions	Nil	Acceptable if easily cleared bronchoscopically
Arterial blood gases (ABGs) on positive end-expiratory pressure 10 cm H_2O + FIO_2 100%	PaO_2 > 300 mm Hg	Donor management and repeat ABGs. Use if PaO_2 > 300 mm Hg

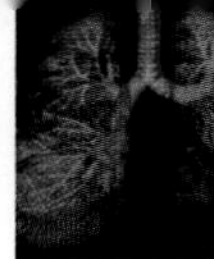

Table 74.7 Donor-recipient matching	
Blood group	Compatible
Size	Matching based on: • Donor predicted total lung capacity (TLC) and recipient measured TLC typically ± 10% • Chest circumference and chest radiographic dimensions also used
Viral exposure	Avoid if feasible: • Cytomegalovirus IgG donor positive into recipient negative • Epstein-Barr virus IgG donor positive into recipient negative
Lymphocyte cross-match	T-cell negative (mandatory) and B-cell negative (desirable)

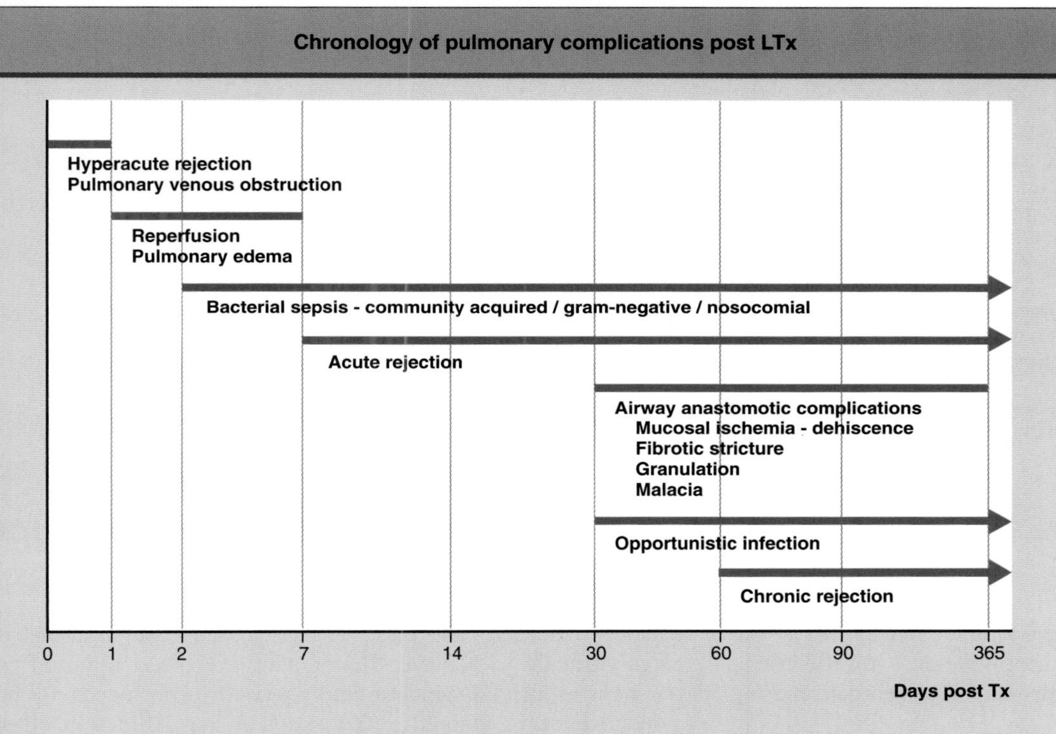

Figure 74.9 The chronology of pulmonary complications in the lung transplant recipient. Some complications occur during a defined time span in the early post-transplantation period, but others occur throughout the follow-up period.

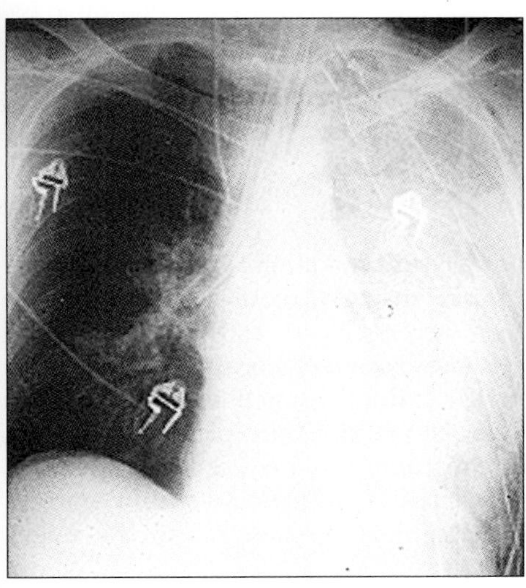

Figure 74.10 Chest radiograph showing typical features of an acute lung injury in the immediate postoperative period after left single-lung transplantation.

sepsis with consolidation or atelectasis. Key objectives at this time include careful fluid monitoring; attempts to keep filling pressures low to limit pulmonary edema due to alveolar-capillary leak, often accepting modest inotropic support; providing excellent pain relief, which is often aided by placement of a thoracic epidural catheter; and meticulous monitoring of renal function. Induction immunosuppression (Table 74.8) usually consists of antilymphocyte globulin (ATGAM, ATG, OKT3) or interleukin-2 receptor antagonists (basiliximab, daclizumab) and high doses of parenteral corticosteroids (methylprednisolone). This is usually followed by a regimen that includes a calcineurin antagonist (cyclosporine or tacrolimus), a cytotoxic agent (azathioprine or mycophenolate mofetil), and a tapering dose of corticosteroid (prednisolone or prednisone).

Severe early graft dysfunction may require prolonged mechanical ventilation or even extracorporeal membrane oxygenation support. In patients with an SLTx for emphysema,

Table 74.8
Immunosuppressive drugs in lung transplantation

	Typical dose	Important side effects
Calcineurin antagonists Cyclosporine Tacrolimus	Maintenance: 5-10 mg/kg/day (target blood levels) 0.2-0.5 mg/kg/day (target blood levels)	Renal impairment Hypertension Hypercholesterolemia Abnormal liver function Headaches Gingival hypertrophy (cyclosporine only) Hirsutism (cyclosporine only) Diabetes (tacrolimus only)
Prednisone/prednisolone Methylprednisolone	Maintenance: 0.2-0.5 mg/kg/day Augmentation for rejection: "Pulse" of 2 g over 3 days for acute rejection	Mood change Weight gain Glucose intolerance Osteopenia Muscle weakness
Azathioprine Mycophenolate mofetil	Maintenance: 1-2 mg/kg/day 2-3 g/day (adult)	Bone marrow suppression Gastrointestinal tract irritation (especially mycophenolate mofetil)
Rapamycin Everolimus	Maintenance: Starting 0.03 mg/kg/day (target blood levels) Not available	Bone marrow suppression Hypercholesterolemia
Interleukin-2 receptor antagonist Basiliximab Daclizumab	Induction of immunosuppression: 20 mg/kg preoperatively and day 4 1 mg/kg preoperatively and days 14, 28, 42, 56	Few and infrequent
Antilymphocyte preparations ATGAM/OKT3	Induction or augmentation for rejection: Various, may target T-lymphocyte levels	Anaphylaxis Sterile meningitis Pulmonary edema Serum sickness

dynamic hyperinflation of the native lung (see Fig. 74.4) or the need to apply positive end-expiratory pressure to the transplanted lung may necessitate independent lung ventilation using two separate ventilators.

Intravenous antibiotics and prophylaxis for viruses such as CMV, EBV, and varicella zoster virus, as well as fungi and protozoa, may need to be instituted. Special attention to gastrointestinal function (especially in patients with cystic fibrosis), neurologic function (especially the awareness of calcineurin inhibitor–induced seizures or leukoencephalopathy), and nutritional state also is necessary. The postoperative period carries a significant mortality and consistent, frequent, and sympathetic communication with the patient and next of kin may help facilitate subsequent difficult discussions.

Postoperative Recovery

Once the patient is out of the ICU, the focus switches to optimizing the immunosuppression regimen and aiding postoperative recovery. Pain management remains a difficult issue, especially after epidural analgesia has been discontinued (around postoperative days 5 to 7). Encouragement in deep breathing, coughing (aided by a physiotherapist), and early ambulation assists in the recovery. With the epidural catheter removed, the balance between adequate analgesia and oversedation is often difficult to achieve. Junior staff are often tempted to try nonsteroidal anti-inflammatory agents. This needs to be avoided because marked deterioration in renal function often results.

Further recovery allows more active rehabilitation, education, and a gradual assumption by the patient of responsibility for complying with a complex medication regimen. With early and detailed discharge planning, the patient can be efficiently and safely discharged to home or to an inpatient rehabilitation facility.

Rehabilitation

Patients are often in poor physical condition at the time of transplantation, with a low muscle mass and reduced skeletal muscle oxidative capacity. Major surgery, sepsis, and the medications (especially calcineurin antagonists and corticosteroids) often exacerbate this muscle injury. Ideally, supervised rehabilitation should start as soon as is practical. In patients requiring prolonged mechanical ventilation, this may occur in the ICU while they are still ventilated. In others, it should start in the hospital before discharge, and continue for several weeks thereafter.

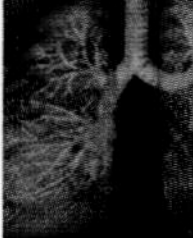

LONG-TERM MANAGEMENT

The main objectives for the treatment team in the long-term management of the lung transplant recipient are obtaining and maintaining optimum immunosuppression (see Table 74.8); early detection and treatment of complications in the allograft (including infection and rejection); monitoring and treatment of nonpulmonary complications of immunosuppression; and serving as a source of support for the recipients and their families.

Most programs use regular chest radiographs, pulmonary function tests, and bronchoscopy (with transbronchial biopsy [TBB] and bronchoalveolar lavage [BAL]) to follow graft function. The management is initially entirely undertaken at the transplantation center, but with time, much of the responsibility can be transferred to the referring physician. Follow-up protocols are highly variable between programs. Routine bronchoscopy with BAL and TBB is usually done at regular intervals in the first 6 months. After that time, practices vary because the yield in an asymptomatic patient is low. The BAL fluid is examined for bacteria, fungi, respiratory viruses, and protozoa. The TBB may reveal features of infection and is graded according to a standard system to quantify acute rejection, airway inflammation, chronic airway rejection, and chronic vascular rejection (Table 74.9). In general, the frequency of these investigations diminishes with time, but may reintensify if allograft problems occur.

Nonpulmonary complications may be detected by symptoms, but typically monitoring of blood pressure, blood tests (including liver function, renal function, and cholesterol), as well as regular physical examination are required. Patients and staff need to be encouraged and supported to report symptoms early because delay often compounds problems.

COMPLICATIONS

Pulmonary

Several features make the pulmonary allograft particularly susceptible to complications: (1) It has impaired mucociliary clearance (in part owing to the airway anastomosis); (2) it is particularly prone to alveolar–capillary leak; (3) it has impaired lymphatic drainage; and (4) there is usually no re-anastomoses of the bronchial artery leading to large airway ischemia. The most common problems are reperfusion pulmonary edema, pneumonia due to gram-negative or hospital-acquired organisms, acute rejection, and chronic rejection in the form of BOS (see Fig. 74.9).

Pulmonary Infections

Patients with pulmonary infections are a major diagnostic and therapeutic challenge after lung transplantation. The cardinal features are fever, cough, increasing dyspnea, sputum production, and an infiltrate on the chest radiograph. Fever may not be universal in the setting of significant immunosuppression. The differential diagnosis (Fig. 74.11) includes nonmicrobial and microbial causes. For microbial causes, the environment that both the donor and recipient have been exposed to will relate to the likely pathogen. The chest radiographic appearance may give some important clues (e.g., a diffuse versus a nodular infiltrate, an infiltrate in the native lung versus the allograft). Bronchoscopy with BAL and TBB is usually the next step. Pathogens may be cultured and identified from BAL fluid, and the TBB may provide evidence indicating that the infection is clinically relevant (e.g., the presence of cytopathic effects resulting from CMV pneumonitis; Fig. 74.12). Rarely, thoracoscopic or open lung biopsy is required to delineate the cause of the pulmonary

Table 74.9
Histologic classification and grading of pulmonary allograft rejection

Acute rejection	
Grade 0 - none	No significant abnormality
Grade 1 - minimal	Infrequent perivascular mononuclear cell infiltrates mainly surrounding venules that are 2-3 cells deep
Grade 2 - mild	More frequent infiltrates, 5 cells or more deep, involving venules and arterioles
Grade 3 - moderate	More exuberant mononuclear cell infiltrate that extends from the perivascular space into the alveolar interstitium
Grade 4 - severe	Infiltrate extending into the alveolar space with pneumocyte damage and at times necrosis of vessels and lung parenchyma
Airway inflammation	Lymphocytic bronchitis/bronchiolitis; pathologist may grade
Chronic airway rejection	
Active	
Inactive	
Chronic vascular rejection - accelerated graft vascular sclerosis	

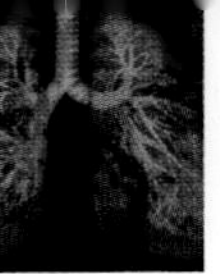

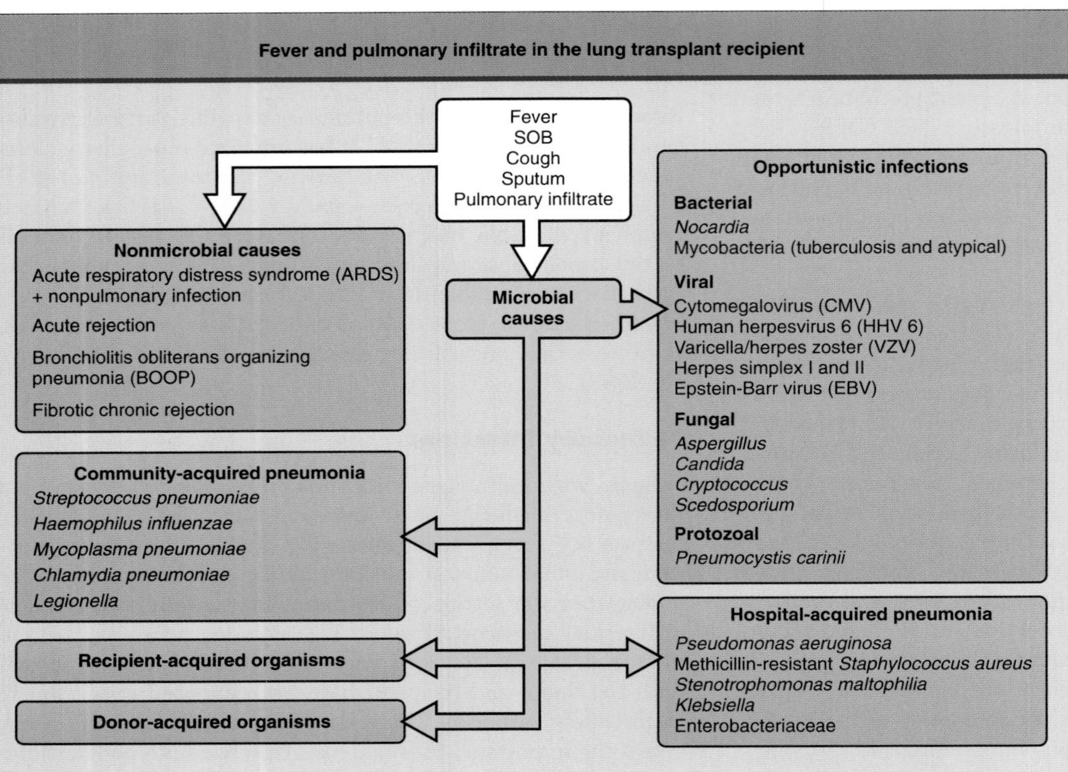

Figure 74.11 A schema for evaluating patients with fever and pulmonary infiltrate after lung transplantation. Nonmicrobial causes need to be considered, as do community-acquired, recipient-acquired, donor-acquired, hospital-acquired, and opportunistic pathogens. SOB, shortness of breath.

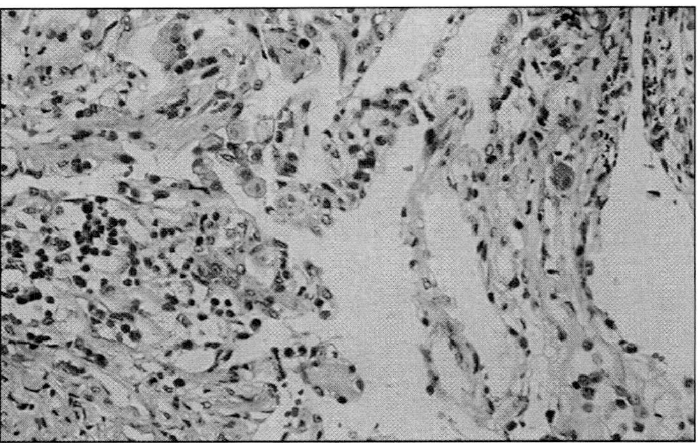

Figure 74.12 Transbronchial lung biopsy showing cytomegalovirus pneumonia with typical owl's eye inclusions.

infiltrate. Unfortunately, none of the investigations is 100% sensitive or 100% specific. Integration of all the available information is required before a decision can be made regarding treatment.

Most infections are due to community-acquired, hospital-acquired, or recipient-colonized persistent pathogens. True opportunistic pathogens are also still important, but the use of antimicrobial prophylaxis has significantly reduced the prevalence of infection and deaths due to CMV and *Pneumocystis carinii*. *Aspergillus fumigatus* and other fungi remain problematic, but it is hoped that the availability of new antifungal agents (liposomal amphotericin, voriconazole, caspofungin) will help. Despite all these approaches, many recipients die of pneumonia both perioperatively and well after the transplantation.

Acute Rejection

The current immunosuppression strategies make acute rejection a rare cause of early death post-transplantation. Many episodes of acute rejection are now detected on surveillance TBB and treated even when patients are asymptomatic. Acute rejection (Table 74.10) can have an abrupt onset of increasing dyspnea, cough, and chest tightness. Oxygen desaturation on exercise may indicate early graft dysfunction. The forced expiratory volume in 1 second (FEV_1), vital capacity, and diffusion capacity may all fall 10% or more. The presence of diffuse pulmonary infiltrates on chest radiography usually reflects a higher grade of acute rejection (A3 or A4; see Table 74.9) or the coexistence of bronchiolitis obliterans organizing pneumonia (BOOP). Unfortunately, none of the features is specific, and histologic confirmation at bronchoscopy using TBB is normally warranted (Fig. 74.13).

Chronic Rejection

BRONCHIOLITIS OBLITERANS SYNDROME

In the last two decades, there has been a substantial improvement in survival after lung transplantation. Almost all the improvement has been due to a reduction in immediate postoperative mortality, with more than 90% of lung transplant recipients now surviving at least to hospital discharge (see Fig. 74.5B). Chronic rejection, most commonly presenting as a clinical syndrome of progressive airflow obstruction with a clear chest radiograph and no other cause, is known as BOS, and this is now the most common cause of death in long-term survivors (see Fig. 74.6).

The pathologic finding seen in BOS (Fig. 74.14) is a proliferative lesion of bronchioles involving fibrin, myofibroblasts, and

Table 74.10
Comparison of acute rejection and bronchiolitis obliterans syndrome

Feature	Acute rejection	Bronchiolitis obliterans syndrome
Peak frequency	First 6 mo	Years > 3 mo
Onset	Abrupt to subacute	Usually subtle
Symptoms	Tightness in chest (immediate postoperative period) Cough (usually not productive) Dyspnea	Dyspnea with heavy exertion Cough (often productive)
Physiologic	Restrictive impairment Desaturation of arterial blood	Obstructive impairment Normoxia until late
Radiologic	Diffuse interstitial infiltrates Pleural effusions	No abnormality until disorder is far advanced Computed tomographic evidence of bronchiectasis and mosaic pattern
Hematologic	Leukocytosis	Normal white blood cell count
Histologic	Perivascular mononuclear cell infiltrates Airway inflammation is variable	Obliterative bronchiolitis Atherosclerosis of pulmonary and bronchial arteries Pleural scarring
Response to treatment	Majority of cases improve rapidly with intravenous corticosteroid	Forced expiratory volume in 1 second at best stabalized Majority of recipients have progressive decline in allograft function

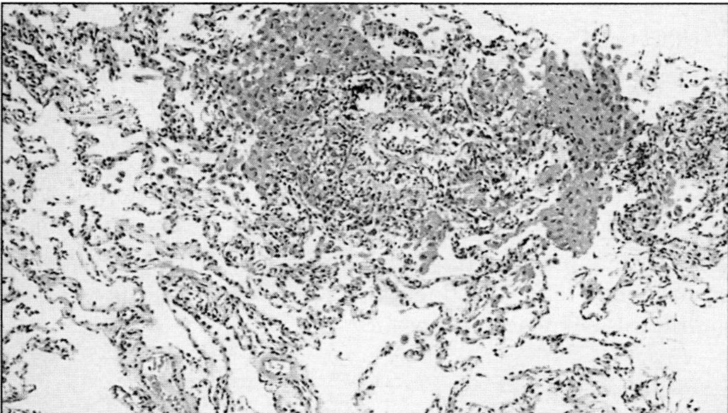

Figure 74.13 Transbronchial lung biopsy specimen showing acute rejection. The lymphocytes surround an arteriole and the infiltrate spreads into surrounding alveolar walls (grade A3).

lymphocytes that may lead to complete occlusion and obliteration of the small airways. Pathologically, the lesion is classified as bronchiolitis obliterans. This pathologic process has many known causes in non–transplant recipients, or may be idiopathic. In the lung transplantation setting, however, this same lesion is called obliterative bronchiolitis (OB). Considerable confusion has arisen because of the poor correlation between the pathologic entity of OB and the clinical syndrome of BOS. For example, OB may be found in lung transplant recipients with

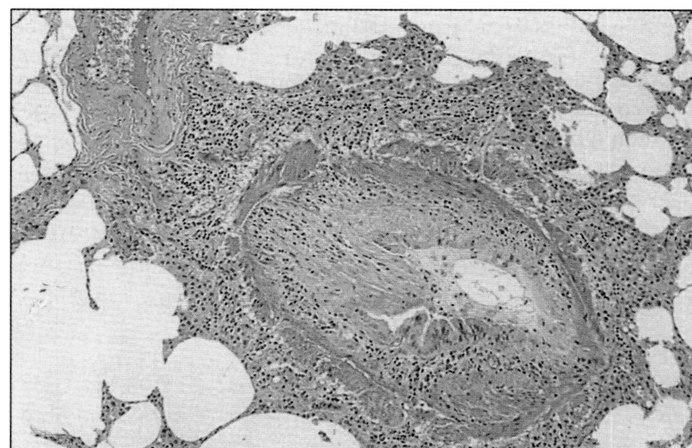

Figure 74.14 Open lung biopsy specimen showing obliterative bronchiolitis. The bronchiolar lumen is obliterated by organizing fibrin, myofibroblasts, and lymphocytes.

normal lung function. Alternatively, OB may not be seen on TBB specimens and may even be difficult to find on open lung biopsy, even in patients with advanced grades of BOS. An expert panel under the auspices of the ISHLT has recommended a standardized approach to the description of chronic rejection focusing on the clinical syndrome of BOS (Table 74.11). The severity of

Table 74.11 Bronchiolitis obliterans syndrome (BOS) grading in lung transplantation	
BOS 0	FEV_1 >90% best post-transplantation
BOS 0p (potential)	FEV_1 81-90% or $FEF_{25-75\%}$ <75% best post-transplantation
BOS 1	FEV_1 66-80% best post-transplantation
BOS 2	FEV_1 51-65% best post-transplantation
BOS 3	FEV_1 >50% best post-transplantation

1. Best post-transplantation defined as the average of the two best measurements at least 3 weeks apart.
2. BOS can be diagnosed only when all other causes of deteriorating lung function have been excluded.
3. The presence or absence of histologic obliterative bronchiolitis should be noted but is not essential to diagnosis.

$FEF_{25-75\%}$, forced expiratory flow at mid-expiratory phase; FEV_1, forced expiratory volume in 1 second.

BOS is based on the percentage fall in FEV_1 below the best achieved post-transplantation FEV_1 value (i.e., BOS 1 = 20% to 34% fall, BOS 2 = 35% to 51% fall, BOS 3 = ≥50% fall).

It is assumed that BOS is due to a late manifestation of the alloimmune response. Persistent acute rejection and lymphocytic bronchitis and bronchiolitis are established risk factors. CMV pneumonitis is also an established risk factor because it may promote alloresponsiveness directly or indirectly as a result of a decision to reduce immunosuppression by the treating physician in response to the infection. High levels of neutrophils and interleukin-8 in the BAL fluid of lung transplant recipients with established BOS have led to speculation that more primitive (innate) immune responses may have an important role. The results of ongoing longitudinal studies will be critical in determining cause and effect regarding these putative mechanisms.

BOS occurs in up to 50% of lung transplant recipients at 3 years, often after a mild viral upper respiratory tract infection. Patients may present with progressive breathlessness or may have recurrent bacterial infections and persistent purulent sputum production (often with computed tomographic [CT] evidence of bronchiectasis). Thus, the cause of death is often attributed to infection when BOS is the underlying cause.

OTHER FORMS OF CHRONIC REJECTION

BOS is the most frequent form of chronic allograft rejection. Rarely, chronic vascular rejection or progressive interstitial fibrosis is seen. BOOP, a subacute form of rejection presenting as increasing breathlessness and a pulmonary infiltrate, sometimes is seen. Although BOOP is often responsive to increased corticosteroids given for a period of several weeks to a few months, in some patients it seems to be a prelude to the development of BOS.

Nonpulmonary Complications

The medications included in the standard immunosuppression regimens have numerous side effects (see Table 74.8). Many may require retargeting of drug levels, different dosing regimens, changing one drug, or treating the specific drug side effects.

Table 74.12 Drugs that can substantially alter the concentration of cyclosporine and tacrolimus in the blood	
Raise blood levels	**Lower blood levels**
Calcium channel blockers: diltiazem, verapamil	Anticonvulsants: phenytoin, carbamazepine, phenobarbitone
Antifungal agents: ketaconazole, itraconazole, fluconazole	Antibiotics: rifampicin, isoniazid, sulfonamide-sulfamethoxazole (high dose)
Macrolide antibiotics: erythromycin, clarithromycin	
Quinalone antibiotics: ciprofloxacin	
Whole grapefruit and grapefruit juice	
Other drugs: metoclopramide, cimetidine	

Cyclosporine and tacrolimus also have a large number of drug interactions, with the levels of these two drugs being substantially altered by other commonly used medications (Table 74.12).

RENAL IMPAIRMENT

Renal impairment is a major problem, with 50% of lung transplant recipients doubling their serum creatinine and 5% to 10% experiencing end-stage renal failure within 5 years after transplantation. Newer, effective immunosuppressives, including mycophenolate mofetil and rapamycin/everolimus, may allow a substantial reduction in the levels of calcineurin antagonists that are currently targeted. Improved targeting of the cyclosporine dose by using 2-hour postdose cyclosporine blood levels (C_2 monitoring) may also help.

NEUROLOGIC

From 5% to 8% of patients on cyclosporine have at least one seizure. The use of anticonvulsant drugs (particularly phenytoin and barbiturates) can substantially lower cyclosporine and tacrolimus levels, and appropriate dose adjustment and monitoring are required. Repeated seizures or progressive deterioration in neurologic state should lead to rapid evaluation, including CT scan and magnetic resonance imaging, to detect the rare, but often rapidly lethal, calcineurin antagonist–induced progressive multifocal leukoencephalopathy.

DIABETES

Pretransplantation disease (e.g., cystic fibrosis) or treatment may already have led to the development of diabetes mellitus. The continued use of oral corticosteroids, particularly in combination with tacrolimus, may lead to continued or newly diagnosed diabetes. Careful blood sugar monitoring during high-dose pulse corticosteroid treatment for acute rejection is required.

OSTEOPOROSIS

Osteoporosis is often found as part of the pretransplantation assessment, but the combination of corticosteroids and a calcineurin antagonist can lead to accelerated osteoporosis. It is hoped that regular monitoring of bone density both before and after transplantation will detect those patients requiring more detailed evaluation and therapy.

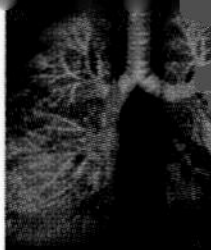

Psychosocial Issues

Lung transplantation can be a deeply emotional situation for patients and their families. Corticosteroids, sedating medications, sleep deprivation, and unremitting pain are a potent mix of contributors, with many patients experiencing an acute organic brain syndrome in the days and weeks after transplantation. Higher doses of corticosteroids can result in profound depression, but also mania and even psychosis. More commonly, however, higher doses of corticosteroids result in sleeplessness and irritability. Forewarning the patient and family can avert a significant domestic crisis.

A close bond is often established among waiting-list patients, and survivor guilt is sometimes seen in those successfully negotiating the transplantation process. Deterioration in graft function (often after a period of good health post-transplantation) can be particularly psychologically devastating. Some family dynamics are based on dependency, and complete recovery of physical health after lung transplantation may result in major change in the dynamics of relationships, sometimes resulting in the breakup of marriages and long-term relationships. A strong psychosocial support team is an essential part of any transplantation program.

CONCLUSION

Lung transplantation offers the possibility of extended life or a period of improved quality of life, but the operation and follow-up period may be accompanied by numerous problems. Obsessional care by an experienced, multidisciplinary team with early intervention for detected problems may improve long-term results. For those with poor quality of life who are otherwise awaiting death, the decision to undergo the procedure may be clear.

SUGGESTED READINGS

Estenne M, Hertz MI: Bronchiolitis obliterans after human lung transplantation. Am J Respir Crit Care Med 166:440-444, 2002.

Hertz MI, Taylor DO, Trulock EP, et al: The registry of the International Society for Heart and Lung Transplantation: Nineteenth official report—2002. J Heart Lung Transplant 21:950-970, 2002.

Ishani A, Erturk S, Hertz MI, et al: Predictors of renal function following lung or heart-lung transplantation. Kidney Int 61:2228-2234, 2002.

Slebos DJ, Scholma J, Marike BH, et al: Longitudinal profile of bronchoalveolar lavage cell characteristics in patients with a good outcome after lung transplantation. Am J Respir Crit Care Med 165:501-507, 2002.

Steen S, Sjoberg T, Pierre L, et al: Transplantation of lungs from a non–heart-beating donor. Lancet 357:825-829, 2001.

Index

Note: Page numbers followed by f indicate figures; those followed by t indicate tables.

B

D

E

F

G

I

J

K

L

M

N

O

P

Q

R

T

U

V

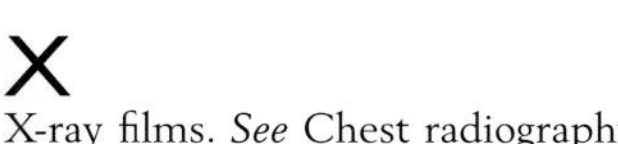

X

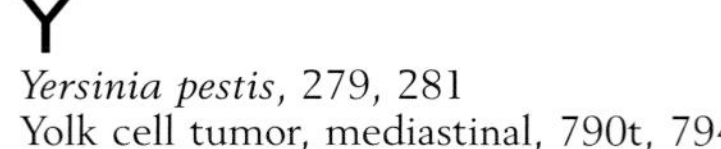

Y

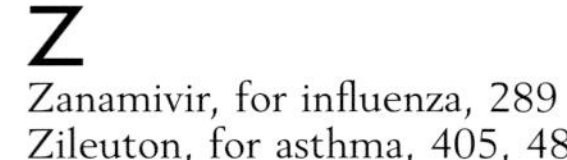

Z